2006
COMPENDIUM
OF SELECTED PUBLICATIONS

THE AMERICAN COLLEGE OF
OBSTETRICIANS AND GYNECOLOGISTS
Women's Health Care Physicians

The *2006 Compendium of Selected Publications* contains current clinical practice documents published by the American College of Obstetricians and Gynecologists (ACOG) as of December 31, 2005. The information in these documents should not be viewed as establishing standards or dictating rigid rules. The guidelines are general and intended to be adapted to many different situations, taking into account the needs and resources particular to the locality, the institution, or the type of practice. Variations and innovations that improve the quality of patient care are to be encouraged rather than restricted. The purpose of these guidelines will be well served if they provide a firm basis on which local norms may be built.

The American College of Obstetricians and Gynecologists
409 12th Street, SW
PO Box 96920
Washington, DC 20090-6920

ISBN: 1-932328-20-3   12345/09876

Publications may be ordered through the ACOG Distribution Center by calling toll free 800-762-2264. To receive order forms via facsimile, call (732) 885-6364 and follow the audio instructions. Publications also may be ordered from the ACOG web site at www.acog.org.

Contents

FOREWORD   V

THE SCOPE OF PRACTICE OF OBSTETRICS AND GYNECOLOGY   VI

CODE OF PROFESSIONAL ETHICS   VII

LISTS OF TITLES BY CATEGORY
    COMMITTEE OPINIONS   XIII
    EDUCATIONAL AND PRACTICE BULLETINS   XVII

Committee Opinions   1

Educational Bulletins   265

Practice Bulletins   325

Technology Assessments   1025

Policy Statements   1055

TITLE INDEX   1071

SUBJECT INDEX   1075

Foreword

The *2006 Compendium of Selected Publications* is a compilation of selected ACOG clinical practice guidelines in effect as of December 31, 2005.

- ■ Committee Opinions: Brief focused documents that address clinical issues of an urgent or emergent nature or nonclinical topics such as policy, economics, and social issues that relate to obstetrics and gynecology. They are consensus statements that may or may not be based on scientific evidence.

- ■ Educational Bulletins: Treatises on specific topics designed to update practicing obstetrician–gynecologists with concise, clinically oriented reviews. Information in these bulletins is supported by satisfactory documentation.

- ■ Practice Bulletins: Evidence-based guidelines developed to indicate a preferred method of diagnosis and management of a condition. The evidence is graded, and peer-reviewed research determines the recommendations in the document.

- ■ Policy Statements: Position papers on key issues approved by the Executive Board.

- ■ Technology Assessments in Obstetrics and Gynecology: Documents that describe specific technologies and their application.

These series are developed by committees of experts and reviewed by leaders in the specialty and the College. Each document is reviewed periodically and either reaffirmed, replaced, or withdrawn to ensure its continued appropriateness to practice. The contribution of the many groups and individuals who participated in the process is gratefully acknowledged.

Each section of the Compendium is devoted to a particular series, and includes those documents considered current at the time of publication. Preceding each section is a complete alphabetic listing of current documents in the series. Those published within the year are indicated with an asterisk. Also provided are lists of titles of all series, grouped by committee or category in order of publication. These lists also include withdrawn titles. An alphabetic listing of all titles is included to complement the subject index.

As the practice of medicine evolves, so too do ACOG documents. As a part of the continuing process of review and revision, many documents initially published as a separate installment of a series evolve to become a part of a broader effort to educate and inform our Fellows. Books such as *Guidelines for Perinatal Care* or *Guidelines for Women's Health Care* carry equal weight as practice guidelines and should be considered adjuncts to the documents in the series. To help make the information more accessible, many individual documents have been consolidated in separate volumes. *Genetics in Obstetrics and Gynecology*, however, is no longer available as a separate volume. All genetics titles are now included in the Compendium.

In another effort to promote access and ease of reference to ACOG information, the Compendium is now provided in CD-ROM format as well as print. Copies are available for sale ($59 for members, $99 for nonmembers) and can be obtained by calling 800-762-2264.

As new documents are released throughout the year, which may replace existing documents in the Compendium, they will be included in ACOG's official journal *Obstetrics & Gynecology*. Single copies can be obtained from the Resource Center (202-863-2518), and the series are available for sale as complete sets or subscriptions (call 800-762-2264 to order). These documents also are available to members on our web site: www.acog.org. To verify the status of documents, contact the Resource Center or check our web site.

We are making every effort to provide health professionals with current, quality information on the practice of obstetrics and gynecology. The *2006 Compendium of Selected Publications* represents still another way to disseminate material designed to promote women's health.

—Ralph W. Hale, MD, Executive Vice President

The Scope of Practice of
Obstetrics and Gynecology

Obstetrics and gynecology is a discipline dedicated to the broad, integrated medical and surgical care of women's health throughout their lifespan. The combined discipline of obstetrics and gynecology requires extensive study and understanding of reproductive physiology, including the physiologic, social, cultural, environmental and genetic factors that influence disease in women. This study and understanding of the reproductive physiology of women gives obstetricians and gynecologists a unique perspective in addressing gender-specific health care issues.

Preventive counseling and health education are essential and integral parts of the practice of obstetricians and gynecologists as they advance the individual and community-based health of women of all ages.

Obstetricians and gynecologists may choose a scope of practice ranging from primary ambulatory health care to concentration in a focused area of specialization.

Approved by the Executive Board
February 6, 2005

Code *of* Professional Ethics

of the American College of Obstetricians and Gynecologists

Obstetrician–gynecologists, as members of the medical profession, have ethical responsibilities not only to patients, but also to society, to other health professionals, and to themselves. The following ethical foundations for professional activities in the field of obstetrics and gynecology are the supporting structures for the Code of Conduct. The Code implements many of these foundations in the form of rules of ethical conduct. Certain documents of the American College of Obstetricians and Gynecologists, including Committee Opinions and *Ethics in Obstetrics and Gynecology*, also provide additional ethical rules. Selections relevant to specific points are set forth in the Code of Conduct, and those particular documents are incorporated into the Code by reference. Noncompliance with the Code, including referenced documents, may affect an individual's initial or continuing Fellowship in the American College of Obstetricians and Gynecologists. These documents may be revised or replaced periodically, and Fellows should be knowledgeable about current information.

Ethical Foundations

I.   The patient–physician relationship: The welfare of the patient *(beneficence)* is central to all considerations in the patient–physician relationship. Included in this relationship is the obligation of physicians to respect the rights of patients, colleagues, and other health professionals. The respect for the right of individual patients to make their own choices about their health care *(autonomy)* is fundamental. The principle of justice requires strict avoidance of discrimination on the basis of race, color, religion, national origin, or any other basis that would constitute illegal discrimination *(justice)*.

II. Physician conduct and practice: The obstetrician–gynecologist must deal honestly with patients and colleagues *(veracity)*. This includes not misrepresenting himself or herself through any form of communication in an untruthful, misleading, or deceptive manner. Furthermore, maintenance of medical competence through study, application, and enhancement of medical knowledge and skills is an obligation of practicing physicians. Any behavior that diminishes a physician's capability to practice, such as substance abuse, must be immediately addressed and rehabilitative services instituted. The physician should modify his or her practice until the diminished capacity has been restored to an acceptable standard to avoid harm to patients *(nonmaleficence)*. All physicians are obligated to respond to evidence of questionable conduct or unethical behavior by other physicians through appropriate procedures established by the relevant organization.

409 12th Street, SW
PO Box 96920
Washington, DC 20090-6920

III. Avoiding conflicts of interest: Potential conflicts of interest are inherent in the practice of medicine. Physicians are expected to recognize such situations and deal with them through public disclosure. Conflicts of interest should be resolved in accordance with the best interest of the patient, respecting a woman's autonomy to make health care decisions. The physician should be an advocate for the patient through public disclosure of conflicts of interest raised by health payer policies or hospital policies.

IV. Professional relations: The obstetrician–gynecologist should respect and cooperate with other physicians, nurses, and health care professionals.

V. Societal responsibilities: The obstetrician–gynecologist has a continuing responsibility to society as a whole and should support and participate in activities that enhance the community. As a member of society, the obstetrician–gynecologist should respect the laws of that society. As professionals and members of medical societies, physicians are required to uphold the dignity and honor of the profession.

Code of Conduct

I. Patient–Physician Relationship

1. The patient–physician relationship is the central focus of all ethical concerns, and the welfare of the patient must form the basis of all medical judgments.

2. The obstetrician–gynecologist should serve as the patient's advocate and exercise all reasonable means to ensure that the most appropriate care is provided to the patient.

3. The patient–physician relationship has an ethical basis and is built on confidentiality, trust, and honesty. If no patient–physician relationship exists, a physician may refuse to provide care, except in emergencies (1). Once the patient–physician relationship exists, the obstetrician–gynecologist must adhere to all applicable legal or contractual constraints in dissolving the patient–physician relationship.

4. Sexual misconduct on the part of the obstetrician–gynecologist is an abuse of professional power and a violation of patient trust. Sexual contact or a romantic relationship between a physician and a current patient is always unethical (2).

5. The obstetrician–gynecologist has an obligation to obtain the informed consent of each patient (3). In obtaining informed consent for any course of medical or surgical treatment, the obstetrician–gynecologist must present to the patient, or to the person legally responsible for the patient, pertinent medical facts and recommendations consistent with good medical practice. Such information should be presented in reasonably understandable terms and include alternative modes of treatment and the objectives, risks, benefits, possible complications, and anticipated results of such treatment.

6. It is unethical to prescribe, provide, or seek compensation for therapies that are of no benefit to the patient.

7. The obstetrician–gynecologist must respect the rights and privacy of patients, colleagues, and others and safeguard patient information and confidences within the limits of the law. If during the process of providing information for consent it is known that results of a particular test or other information must be given to governmental authorities or other third parties, that must be explained to the patient (4).

8. The obstetrician–gynecologist must not discriminate against patients based on race, color, national origin, religion, or any other basis that would constitute illegal discrimination.

II. Physician Conduct and Practice

1. The obstetrician–gynecologist should recognize the boundaries of his or her particular competencies and expertise and must provide only those services and use only those techniques for which he or she is qualified by education, training, and experience.

2. The obstetrician–gynecologist should participate in continuing medical education activities to maintain current scientific and professional knowledge relevant to the medical services he or she renders. The obstetrician–gynecologist should provide medical care involving new therapies or techniques only after undertaking appropriate training and study.

3. In emerging areas of medical treatment where recognized medical guidelines do not exist, the obstetrician–gynecologist should exercise careful judgment and take appropriate precautions to protect patient welfare.

4. The obstetrician–gynecologist must not publicize or represent himself or herself in any untruthful, misleading, or deceptive manner to patients, colleagues, other health care professionals, or the public.

5. The obstetrician–gynecologist who has reason to believe that he or she is infected with the human immunodeficiency virus (HIV) or other serious infectious agents that might be communicated to patients should voluntarily be tested for the protection of his or her patients. In making decisions about patient-care activities, a physician infected with such an agent should adhere to the fundamental professional obligation to avoid harm to patients (5).

6. The obstetrician–gynecologist should not practice medicine while impaired by alcohol, drugs, or physical or mental disability. The obstetrician–gynecologist who experiences substance abuse problems or who is physically or emotionally impaired should seek appropriate assistance to address these problems and must limit his or her practice until the impairment no longer affects the quality of patient care.

III. Conflicts of Interest

1. Potential conflicts of interest are inherent in the practice of medicine. Conflicts of interest should be resolved in accordance with the best interest of the patient, respecting a woman's autonomy to make health care decisions. If there is an actual or potential conflict of interest that could be reasonably construed to affect significantly the patient's care, the physician must disclose the conflict to the patient. The physician should seek consultation with colleagues or an institutional ethics committee to determine whether there is an actual or potential conflict of interest and how to address it.

2. Commercial promotions of medical products and services may generate bias unrelated to product merit, creating or appearing to create inappropriate undue influence. The obstetrician–gynecologist should be aware of this potential conflict of interest and offer medical advice that is as accurate, balanced, complete, and devoid of bias as possible (6, 7).

3. The obstetrician–gynecologist should prescribe drugs, devices, and other treatments solely on the basis of medical considerations and patient needs, regardless of any direct or indirect interests in or benefit from a pharmaceutical firm or other supplier.

4. When the obstetrician–gynecologist receives anything of substantial value, including royalties, from companies in the health care industry, such as a manufacturer of pharmaceuticals and medical devices, this fact should be disclosed to patients and colleagues when material.

5. Financial and administrative constraints may create disincentives to treatment otherwise recommended by the obstetrician–gynecologist. Any pertinent constraints should be disclosed to the patient.

IV. Professional Relations

1. The obstetrician–gynecologist's relationships with other physicians, nurses, and health care professionals should reflect fairness, honesty, and integrity, sharing a mutual respect and concern for the patient.

2. The obstetrician–gynecologist should consult, refer, or cooperate with other physicians, health care professionals, and institutions to the extent necessary to serve the best interests of their patients.

V.   Societal Responsibilities

1.   The obstetrician–gynecologist should support and participate in those health care programs, practices, and activities that contribute positively, in a meaningful and cost-effective way, to the welfare of individual patients, the health care system, or the public good.

2.   The obstetrician–gynecologist should respect all laws, uphold the dignity and honor of the profession, and accept the profession's self-imposed discipline. The professional competence and conduct of obstetrician–gynecologists are best examined by professional associations, hospital peer-review committees, and state medical and licensing boards. These groups deserve the full participation and cooperation of the obstetrician–gynecologist.

3.   The obstetrician–gynecologist should strive to address through the appropriate procedures the status of those physicians who demonstrate questionable competence, impairment, or unethical or illegal behavior. In addition, the obstetrician–gynecologist should cooperate with appropriate authorities to prevent the continuation of such behavior.

4.   The obstetrician–gynecologist must not knowingly offer testimony that is false. The obstetrician–gynecologist must testify only on matters about which he or she has knowledge and experience. The obstetrician–gynecologist must not knowingly misrepresent his or her credentials.

5.   The obstetrician–gynecologist testifying as an expert witness must have knowledge and experience about the range of the standard of care and the available scientific evidence for the condition in question during the relevant time and must respond accurately to questions about the range of the standard of care and the available scientific evidence.

6.   Before offering testimony, the obstetrician–gynecologist must thoroughly review the medical facts of the case and all available relevant information.

7.   The obstetrician–gynecologist serving as an expert witness must accept neither disproportionate compensation nor compensation that is contingent upon the outcome of the litigation (8).

References

1.   American College of Obstetricians and Gynecologists. Seeking and giving consultation. In: Ethics in obstetrics and gynecology. 2nd ed. Washington, DC: ACOG; 2004. p. 77–81.

2.   American College of Obstetricians and Gynecologists. Sexual misconduct. In: Ethics in obstetrics and gynecology. 2nd ed. Washington, DC: ACOG; 2004. p. 101–3.

3.   American College of Obstetricians and Gynecologists. Informed consent. In: Ethics in obstetrics and gynecology. 2nd ed. Washington, DC: ACOG; 2004. p. 9–17.

4.   American College of Obstetricians and Gynecologists. Patient testing. In: Ethics in obstetrics and gynecology. 2nd ed. Washington, DC: ACOG; 2004. p. 26–8.

5.   American College of Obstetricians and Gynecologists. Human immunodeficiency virus. In: Ethics in obstetrics and gynecology. 2nd ed. Washington, DC: ACOG; 2004. p. 29–33.

6.   American College of Obstetricians and Gynecologists. Relationships with industry. In: Ethics in obstetrics and gynecology. 2nd ed. Washington, DC: ACOG; 2004. p. 107–10.

7.   American College of Obstetricians and Gynecologists. Commercial enterprises in medical practice. In: Ethics in obstetrics and gynecology. 2nd ed. Washington, DC: ACOG; 2004. p. 83–5.

8.   American College of Obstetricians and Gynecologists. Expert testimony. In: Ethics in obstetrics and gynecology. 2nd ed. Washington, DC: ACOG; 2004. p. 116–7.

Lists of Titles

Lists of Titles

List of Titles

December 2005

Committee Opinions are intended to provide timely information on controversial issues, ethical concerns, and emerging approaches to clinical management. They represent the considered views of the sponsoring committee based on interpretation of published data in peer-reviewed journals. Committee Opinions are reviewed periodically for continued relevance or needed update. *Note:* Because individual Committee Opinions are withdrawn from and added to the series on a continuing basis, the titles listed in this index may not be identical to those contained in complete sets. Also listed are Technology Assessments, which provide an overview of technology in obstetrics and gynecology.

> The following titles have been withdrawn from circulation:
>
> Committee Opinions
>
> 162 Screening for Tay–Sachs Disease (Replaced by Committee Opinion No. 318)
>
> 164 Incidental Appendectomy (Replaced by Committee Opinion No. 323)

Number	Title	Publication Date	Reaffirmed Date	Page
Committee on Adolescent Health Care				
274	Nonsurgical Diagnosis and Management of Vaginal Agenesis (Obstet Gynecol 2002;100:213–216)	July 2002		**138**
300	Cervical Cancer Screening in Adolescents (Obstet Gynecol 2004;104:885–9)	October 2004		**29**
301	Sexually Transmitted Diseases in Adolescents (Obstet Gynecol 2004;104:891–8)	October 2004		**220**
302	Guidelines for Adolescent Health Research (Obstet Gynecol 2004;104:899–902)	October 2004		**67**
310	Endometriosis in Adolescents (Obstet Gynecol 2005;105:921–7)	April 2005		**46**
*314	Meningococcal Vaccination for Adolescents (Obstet Gynecol 2005;106:667–9)	September 2005		**124**
Committee on Coding and Nomenclature				
205	Tubal Ligation with Cesarean Delivery (Obstet Gynecol Vol. 92, No. 2)	August 1998		**252**
249	Coding Responsibility (Obstet Gynecol Vol. 97, No. 1)	January 2001	2005	**36**
250	Inappropriate Reimbursement Practices by Third-Party Payers (Obstet Gynecol Vol. 97, No. 1)	January 2001		**90**
Committee on Ethics				
†294	At-Risk Drinking and Illicit Drug Use: Ethical Issues in Obstetric and Gynecologic Practice (Obstet Gynecol 2004;103:1021–31)	May 2004		**15**
†297	Nonmedical Use of Obstetric Ultrasonography (Obstet Gynecol 2004;104:423–4)	August 2004		**135**
*321	Maternal Decision Making, Ethics, and the Law (Obstet Gynecol 2005;106:1127–37)	November 2005		**111**
Committee on Genetics				
161	Fragile X Syndrome	October 1995	2000	**62**
183	Routine Storage of Umbilical Cord Blood for Potential Future Transplantation (*Joint with Committee on Obstetric Practice*)	April 1997	2004	**207**

Number	Title	Publication Date	Reaffirmed Date	Page
Committee on Genetics (continued)				
189	Advanced Paternal Age: Risks to the Fetus	October 1997	2003	5
212	Screening for Canavan Disease (Obstet Gynecol Vol. 92, No. 5)	November 1998	2004	216
230	Maternal Phenylketonuria (Obstet Gynecol Vol. 95, No. 1)	January 2000	2004	122
257	Genetic Evaluation of Stillbirths and Neonatal Deaths (Obstet Gynecol Vol. 97, No. 5)	May 2001		64
287	Newborn Screening (Obstet Gynecol 2003;102:887–9)	October 2003		131
296	First-Trimester Screening for Fetal Aneuploidy (*Joint with Committee on Obstetric Practice*) (Obstet Gynecol 2004;104:215–7)	July 2004		58
298	Prenatal and Preconceptional Carrier Screening for Genetic Diseases in Individuals of Eastern European Jewish Descent (Obstet Gynecol 2004;104:425–8)	August 2004		178
*318	Screening for Tay–Sachs Disease (Obstet Gynecol 2005;106:893–4)	October 2005		218
*324	Perinatal Risks Associated With Assisted Reproductive Technology (*Joint with Committees on Obstetric Practice and Gynecologic Practice*) (Obstet Gynecol 2005;106:1143–6)	November 2005		165
*325	Update on Carrier Screening for Cystic Fibrosis (Obstet Gynecol 2005;106:1465–8)	December 2005		253
■ 1	Genetics and Molecular Diagnostic Testing (Obstet Gynecol 2002;100:193–211)	July 2002		1027
Committee on Gynecologic Practice				
186	Role of the Obstetrician–Gynecologist in the Diagnosis and Treatment of Breast Disease	September 1997	2003	205
191	Length of Hospital Stay for Gynecologic Procedures	October 1997	2004	107
203	Hepatitis Virus Infections in Obstetrician–Gynecologists (Obstet Gynecol Vol. 92, No. 1)	July 1998	2001	82
232	Tamoxifen and Endometrial Cancer (Obstet Gynecol Vol. 95, No. 4)	April 2000	2001	235
240	Statement on Surgical Assistants (Obstet Gynecol Vol. 96, No. 2) (*Joint with Committee on Obstetric Practice*)	August 2000	2003	234
243	Performance and Interpretation of Imaging Studies by Obstetrician–Gynecologists (Obstet Gynecol Vol. 96, No. 5)	November 2000	2003	163
253	Nongynecologic Procedures (Obstet Gynecol Vol. 97, No. 3)	March 2001	2004	134
272	Follow-up of Abnormal Screening Mammography (Obstet Gynecol 2002;99:869)	May 2002	2005	61
278	Avoiding Inappropriate Clinical Decisions Based on False-Positive Human Chorionic Gonadotropin Test Results (Obstet Gynecol 2002;100:1057–9)	November 2002		26
280	The Role of the Generalist Obstetrician–Gynecologist in the Early Detection of Ovarian Cancer (*Joint with Society of Gynecologic Oncologists*) (Obstet Gynecol 2002;100:1413–6)	December 2002		240
285	Induced Abortion and Breast Cancer Risk (Obstet Gynecol 2003;102:433–5)	August 2003		96
288	Professional Liability and Gynecology-Only Practice (*Joint with Committees on Obstetric Practice and Professional Liability*) (Obstet Gynecol 2003;102:891)	October 2003		198
292	Primary and Preventive Care: Periodic Assessments (Obstet Gynecol 2003;102:1117–24)	November 2003		190
293	Uterine Artery Embolization (Obstet Gynecol 2004;103:403–4)	February 2004	2004	262
311	Appropriate Use of Laparoscopically Assisted Vaginal Hysterectomy (Obstet Gynecol 2005;105:929–30)	April 2005		13
*313	The Importance of Preconception Care in the Continuum of Women's Health Care (Obstet Gynecol 2005;106:665–6)	September 2005		238
*319	The Role of the Obstetrician–Gynecologist in the Assessment and Management of Obesity (Obstet Gynecol 2005;106:895–9)	October 2005		243
*322	Compounded Bioidentical Hormones (Obstet Gynecol 2005;106:1139–40)	November 2005		40
*323	Elective Coincidental Appendectomy (Obstet Gynecol 2005;106:1141–2)	November 2005		44
*324	Perinatal Risks Associated With Assisted Reproductive Technology (*Joint with Committees on Obstetric Practice and Genetics*) (Obstet Gynecol 2005;106:1143–6)	November 2005		165
■ 3	Saline Infusion Sonohysterography (Obstet Gynecol 2003;102:659–62)	September 2003		1050
■ 4	Hysteroscopy (Obstet Gynecol 2005;106:439–42)	August 2005		1046

Number	Title	Publication Date	Reaffirmed Date	Page

Committee on Health Care for Underserved Women

Number	Title	Publication Date	Reaffirmed Date	Page
307	Partner Consent for Participation in Women's Reproductive Health Research (Obstet Gynecol 2004;104:1467–9)	December 2004		154
308	The Uninsured (Obstet Gynecol 2004;104:1471–4)	December 2004		248
312	Health Care for Homeless Women (Obstet Gynecol 2005;106:429–34)	August 2005		76
*317	Racial and Ethnic Disparities in Women's Health (Obstet Gynecol 2005;106:889–92)	October 2005		199
*316	Smoking Cessation During Pregnancy *(Joint with Committee on Obstetric Practice)* (Obstet Gynecol 2005;106:883–8)	October 2005		228

Committee on Obstetric Practice

Number	Title	Publication Date	Reaffirmed Date	Page
125	Placental Pathology	July 1993	2003	171
174	Use and Abuse of the Apgar Score *(Joint with AAP Committee on Fetus and Newborn)*	July 1996	1999	257
183	Routine Storage of Umbilical Cord Blood for Potential Future Transplantation *(Joint with Committee on Genetics)*	April 1997	2004	207
228	Induction of Labor with Misoprostol (Obstet Gynecol Vol. 94, No. 5)	November 1999	2004	101
234	Scheduled Cesarean Delivery and the Prevention of Vertical Transmission of HIV Infection (Obstet Gynecol Vol. 95, No. 5)	May 2000	2003	213
240	Statement on Surgical Assistants *(Joint with Committee on Gynecologic Practice)* (Obstet Gynecol Vol. 96, No. 2)	August 2000	2003	234
248	Response to Searle's Drug Warning on Misoprostol (Obstet Gynecol Vol. 96, No. 6)	December 2000	2003	203
256	Optimal Goals for Anesthesia Care in Obstetrics *(Joint with American Society of Anesthesiologists)* (Obstet Gynecol Vol. 97, No. 5)	May 2001	2004	150
258	Fetal Pulse Oximetry (Obstet Gynecol 2001;98:523–524)	September 2001	2004	56
260	Circumcision (Obstet Gynecol 2001;98:707–708)	October 2001	2004	34
264	Air Travel During Pregnancy (Obstet Gynecol 2001;98:1187–1188)	December 2001	2004	7
265	Mode of Term Singleton Breech Delivery (Obstet Gynecol 2001;98:1189–1190)	December 2001	2004	127
266	Placenta Accreta (Obstet Gynecol 2002;99:169–170)	January 2002	2005	169
267	Exercise During Pregnancy and the Postpartum Period (Obstet Gynecol 2002;99:171–173)	January 2002	2005	53
268	Management of Asymptomatic Pregnant or Lactating Women Exposed to Anthrax (Obstet Gynecol 2002;99:366–368)	February 2002	2005	108
269	Analgesia and Cesarean Delivery Rates (Obstet Gynecol 2002;99:369–370)	February 2002		9
271	Induction of Labor for Vaginal Birth After Cesarean Delivery (Obstet Gynecol 2002;99:679–680)	April 2002		99
273	Antenatal Corticosteroid Therapy for Fetal Maturation (Obstet Gynecol 2002;99:871–873)	May 2002		11
275	Obstetric Management of Patients with Spinal Cord Injuries (Obstet Gynecol 2002;100:625–7)	September 2002		147
276	Safety of Lovenox in Pregnancy (Obstet Gynecol 2002;100:845–6)	October 2002		211
279	Prevention of Early-Onset Group B Streptococcal Disease in Newborns (Obstet Gynecol 2002;100:1405–12)	December 2002		182
281	Rubella Vaccination (Obstet Gynecol 2002;100:1417)	December 2002		210
282	Immunization During Pregnancy (Obstet Gynecol 2003;101:207–12)	January 2003		84
283	New U.S. Food and Drug Administration Labeling on Cytotec (Misoprostol) Use and Pregnancy (Obstet Gynecol 2003;101:1049–50)	May 2003		129
284	Nonobstetric Surgery in Pregnancy (Obstet Gynecol 2003;102:431)	August 2003		137
288	Professional Liability and Gynecology-Only Practice *(Joint with Committees on Gynecologic Practice and Professional Liability)* (Obstet Gynecol 2003;102:891)	October 2003		198
291	Use of Progesterone to Reduce Preterm Birth (Obstet Gynecol 2003;102:1115–6)	November 2003		260
295	Pain Relief During Labor *(Joint with American Society of Anesthesiologists)* (Obstet Gynecol 2004;104:213)	July 2004		153
296	First-Trimester Screening for Fetal Aneuploidy *(Joint with Committee on Genetics)* (Obstet Gynecol 2004;104:215–7)	July 2004		58

Number	Title	Publication Date	Reaffirmed Date	Page
	Committee on Obstetric Practice (continued)			
299	Guidelines for Diagnostic Imaging During Pregnancy (Obstet Gynecol 2004;104:647–51)	September 2004		**71**
304	Prenatal and Perinatal Human Immunodeficiency Virus Testing: Expanded Recommendations (Obstet Gynecol 2004;104:1119–24)	November 2004		**172**
305	Influenza Vaccination and Treatment During Pregnancy (Obstet Gynecol 2004;104:1125–6)	November 2004		**103**
*315	Obesity in Pregnancy (Obstet Gynecol 2005;106:671–5)	September 2005		**142**
*316	Smoking Cessation During Pregnancy *(Joint with Committee on Health Care for Underserved Women)* (Obstet Gynecol 2005;106:883–8)	October 2005		**228**
*324	Perinatal Risks Associated With Assisted Reproductive Technology *(Joint with Committees on Genetics and Gynecologic Practice)* (Obstet Gynecol 2005;106:1143–6)	November 2005		**165**
*326	Inappropriate Use of the Terms Fetal Distress and Birth Asphyxia (Obstet Gynecol 2005;106:1469–70)	December 2005		**94**
	Committee on Primary Care			
227	Complementary and Alternative Medicine (Obstet Gynecol Vol. 94, No. 5)	November 1999	2004	**37**
	Committee on Professional Liability			
288	Professional Liability and Gynecology-Only Practice *(Joint with Committees on Obstetric Practice and Gynecologic Practice)* (Obstet Gynecol 2003;102:891)	October 2003		**198**
306	Informed Refusal (Obstet Gynecol 2004;104:1465–6)	December 2004		**105**
309	Coping With the Stress of Medical Professional Liability Litigation (Obstet Gynecol 2005;105:453–4)	February 2005		**42**
	Committee on Quality Improvement and Patient Safety			
286	Patient Safety in Obstetrics and Gynecology (Obstet Gynecol 2003;102:883–5)	October 2003		**160**
*320	Partnering With Patients to Improve Safety (Obstet Gynecol 2005;106:1123–5)	November 2005		**157**

Current Committee Opinions and Technology Assessments

■1 ■3 ■4 125 161 174 183 186 189 191 203 205 212 227 228 230 232 234 240 243 248 249 250 253 256 257 258 260 264 265 266 267 268 269 271 272 273 274 275 276 278 279 280 281 282 283 284 285 286 287 288 291 292 293 294 295 296 297 298 299 300 301 302 304 305 306 307 308 309 310 311 312 313 314 315 316 317 318 319 320 321 322 323 324 325 326

Committee Opinions are available on a subscription basis, and complete sets may be purchased. For ordering information, contact the ACOG Distribution Center at 800-762-2264, or order online at sales.acog.org.

*Title issued since publication of last index
†Title issued since publication of *Ethics in Obstetrics and Gynecology*, Second Edition
■ Technology Assessment

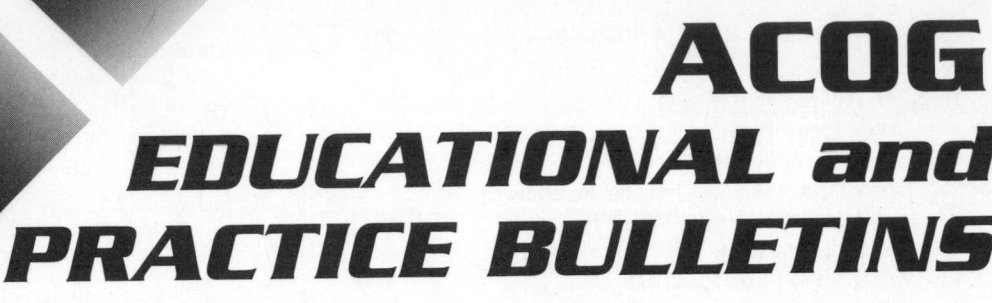

ACOG EDUCATIONAL and PRACTICE BULLETINS

LIST OF TITLES — DECEMBER 2005

Educational and Practice Bulletins provide obstetricians and gynecologists with current information on established techniques and clinical management guidelines. ACOG continuously surveys the field for advances to be incorporated in these series and monitors existing bulletins to ensure they are current. Individual bulletins are withdrawn from and added to the series on a continuing basis.

The following titles have been withdrawn from circulation:

Practice Bulletins

25 Emergency Contraception (Replaced by Practice Bulletin No. 69)
26 Medical Management of Abortion (Replaced by Practice Bulletin No. 67)
62 Intrapartum Fetal Heart Rate Monitoring (Replaced by Practice Bulletin No. 70)

Educational Bulletins

244 Antiphospholipid Syndrome (Replaced by Practice Bulletin No. 68)
260 Smoking Cessation During Pregnancy (Replaced by Committee Opinion No. 316)

Current Bulletins

▶1   ▶3   ▶4   ▶6   ▶7   ▶8   ▶9
▶10 ▶11 ▶12 ▶13 ▶14 ▶15 ▶16
▶17 ▶18 ▶19 ▶20 ▶21 ▶22 ▶23
▶24 ▶27 ▶28 ▶29 ▶30 ▶31 ▶33
▶34 ▶35 ▶36 ▶37 ▶38 ▶39 ▶40
▶41 ▶42 ▶43 ▶44 ▶45 ▶46 ▶47
▶48 ▶49 ▶50 ▶51 ▶52 ▶53 ▶54
▶55 ▶56 ▶57 ▶58 ▶59 ▶60 ▶61
▶63 ▶64 ▶65 ▶66 ▶67 ▶68 ▶69
▶70 227 230 236 248 251 255
258

Number		Page
General		
255	Psychosocial Risk Factors: Perinatal Screening and Intervention (November 1999, Obstet Gynecol Vol. 94, No. 5)	304
258	Breastfeeding: Maternal and Infant Aspects (July 2000, Obstet Gynecol Vol. 96, No. 1)	274
Obstetrics		
▶ 1	Premature Rupture of Membranes (June 1998, Obstet Gynecol Vol. 91, No. 6)	848
▶ 4	Prevention of Rh D Alloimmunization (May 1999, Obstet Gynecol Vol. 93, No. 5)	889
▶ 6	Thrombocytopenia in Pregnancy (September 1999, Obstet Gynecol Vol. 94, No. 3)	950
▶ 8	Management of Herpes in Pregnancy (October 1999, Obstet Gynecol Vol. 94, No. 4)	644
▶ 9	Antepartum Fetal Surveillance (October 1999, Obstet Gynecol Vol. 94, No. 4)	337
▶ 10	Induction of Labor (November 1999, Obstet Gynecol Vol. 94, No. 5)	562
▶ 12	Intrauterine Growth Restriction (January 2000, Obstet Gynecol Vol. 95, No. 1)	591
▶ 13	External Cephalic Version (February 2000, Obstet Gynecol Vol. 95, No. 2)	500
▶ 17	Operative Vaginal Delivery (June 2000, Obstet Gynecol Vol. 95, No. 6)	780
▶ 19	Thromboembolism in Pregnancy (August 2000, Obstet Gynecol Vol. 96, No. 2)	961
▶ 20	Perinatal Viral and Parasitic Infections (September 2000, Obstet Gynecol Vol. 96, No. 3)	810
▶ 22	Fetal Macrosomia (November 2000, Obstet Gynecol Vol. 96, No. 5)	507
▶ 24	Management of Recurrent Early Pregnancy Loss (February 2001, Obstet Gynecol Vol. 97, No. 2)	682
▶ 27	Prenatal Diagnosis of Fetal Chromosomal Abnormalities (May 2001, Obstet Gynecol Vol. 97, No. 5)	867
▶ 29	Chronic Hypertension in Pregnancy (Obstet Gynecol 2001;98:177–185)	418
▶ 30	Gestational Diabetes (Obstet Gynecol 2001;98:525–538)	518
▶ 31	Assessment of Risk Factors for Preterm Birth (Obstet Gynecol 2001;98:709–716)	366
▶ 33	Diagnosis and Management of Preeclampsia and Eclampsia (Obstet Gynecol 2002;99:159–167)	444
▶ 36	Obstetric Analgesia and Anesthesia (Obstet Gynecol 2002;100:177–191)	765
▶ 37	Thyroid Disease in Pregnancy (Obstet Gynecol 2002;100:387–396)	971
▶ 38	Perinatal Care at the Threshold of Viability (Obstet Gynecol 2002;100:617–24)	802

Number		Page

Obstetrics (continued)

▶ 40 Shoulder Dystocia
(Obstet Gynecol 2002;100:1045–50)   **921**

▶ 43 Management of Preterm Labor (Obstet Gynecol
2003;101:1039–47)   **673**

▶ 44 Neural Tube Defects
(Obstet Gynecol 2003;102:203–13)   **754**

▶ 47 Prophylactic Antibiotics in Labor and Delivery
(Obstet Gynecol 2003;102:875–82)   **897**

▶ 48 Cervical Insufficiency
(Obstet Gynecol 2003;102:1091–9)   **409**

▶ 49 Dystocia and Augmentation of Labor
(Obstet Gynecol 2003;102:1445–54)   **479**

▶ 52 Nausea and Vomiting of Pregnancy (Obstet Gynecol
2004;103:803–15)   **741**

▶ 54 Vaginal Birth After Previous Cesarean Delivery
(Obstet Gynecol 2004;104:203–12)   **1015**

▶ 55 Management of Postterm Pregnancy
(Obstet Gynecol 2004;104:639–46)   **665**

▶ 56 Multiple Gestation: Complicated Twin,
Triplet, and High-Order Multifetal Pregnancy
(Obstet Gynecol 2004;104:869–83)   **726**

▶ 58 Ultrasonography in Pregnancy (Obstet Gynecol
2004;104:1449–58)   **981**

▶ 60 Pregestational Diabetes Mellitus (Obstet Gynecol
2005;105:675–85)   **837**

▶ 64 Hemoglobinopathies in Pregnancy (Obstet Gynecol
2005;106:203–11)   **539**

▶*68 Antiphospholipid Syndrome (Obstet Gynecol
2005;106:1113–21)   **357**

▶*70 Intrapartum Fetal Heart Rate Monitoring (Obstet
Gynecol 2005;106:1453–61)   **572**

227 Management of Isoimmunization in Pregnancy
(August 1996)   **290**

230 Assessment of Fetal Lung Maturity
(November 1996)   **267**

236 Teratology (April 1997)   **311**

248 Viral Hepatitis in Pregnancy
(July 1998, Obstet Gynecol Vol. 92, No. 1)   **318**

251 Obstetric Aspects of Trauma Management
(September 1998, Obstet Gynecol Vol. 92, No. 3)   **297**

Gynecology

▶ 3 Medical Management of Tubal Pregnancy
(December 1998, Obstet Gynecol Vol. 92, No. 6)   **719**

▶ 7 Prophylactic Oophorectomy
(September 1999, Obstet Gynecol Vol. 94, No. 3)   **905**

▶ 11 Medical Management of Endometriosis
(December 1999, Obstet Gynecol Vol. 94, No. 6)   **706**

▶ 14 Management of Anovulatory Bleeding
(March 2000, Obstet Gynecol Vol. 95, No. 3)   **623**

Number		Page

▶ 15 Premenstrual Syndrome
(April 2000, Obstet Gynecol Vol. 95, No. 4)   **858**

▶ 16 Surgical Alternatives to Hysterectomy in the
Management of Leiomyomas
(May 2000, Obstet Gynecol Vol. 95, No. 5)   **927**

▶ 18 The Use of Hormonal Contraception
in Women with Coexisting Medical Conditions
(July 2000, Obstet Gynecol Vol. 96, No. 1)   **936**

▶ 21 Prevention of Deep Vein Thrombosis
and Pulmonary Embolism
(October 2000, Obstet Gynecol Vol. 96, No. 4)   **879**

▶ 23 Antibiotic Prophylaxis for Gynecologic Procedures
(January 2001, Obstet Gynecol Vol. 97, No. 1)   **348**

▶ 28 Use of Botanicals for Management
of Menopausal Symptoms
(June 2001, Obstet Gynecol Vol. 97, No. 6)   **1004**

▶ 34 Management of Infertility Caused by Ovulatory
Dysfunction (Obstet Gynecol 2002;99:347–358)   **653**

▶ 35 Diagnosis and Treatment of Cervical Carcinomas
(Obstet Gynecol 2002;99:855–867)   **453**

▶ 39 Selective Estrogen Receptor Modulators
(Obstet Gynecol 2002;100:835–44)   **911**

▶ 41 Polycystic Ovary Syndrome (Obstet Gynecol
2002;100:1389–402)   **823**

▶ 42 Breast Cancer Screening (Obstet Gynecol
2003;101:821–32)   **386**

▶ 45 Cervical Cytology Screening (Obstet Gynecol
2003;102:417–27)   **398**

▶ 46 Benefits and Risks of Sterilization
(Obstet Gynecol 2003;102:647–58)   **374**

▶ 50 Osteoporosis (Obstet Gynecol 2004;103:203–16)   **788**

▶ 51 Chronic Pelvic Pain
(Obstet Gynecol 2004;103:589–605)   **427**

▶ 53 Diagnosis and Treatment of Gestational
Trophoblastic Disease (Obstet Gynecol
2004;103:1365–77)   **466**

▶ 57 Gynecologic Herpes Simplex Virus Infections
(Obstet Gynecol 2004;104:1111–7)   **532**

▶ 59 Intrauterine Device
(Obstet Gynecol 2005;105:223–32)   **581**

▶ 61 Human Papillomavirus (Obstet Gynecol
2005;105:905–18)   **548**

▶ 63 Urinary Incontinence in Women
(Obstet Gynecol 2005:105:1533–45)   **991**

▶ 65 Management of Endometrial Cancer
(Obstet Gynecol 2005;106:413–25)   **631**

▶*66 Management of Abnormal Cervical Cytology and
Histology (Obstet Gynecol 2005;106:645–64)   **603**

▶*67 Medical Management of Abortion
(Obstet Gynecol 2005;106:871–82)   **694**

▶*69 Emergency Contraception (Obstet Gynecol
2005;106:1443–52)   **489**

Practice and Educational Bulletins are available on a subscription basis, and complete sets may be purchased. For ordering information, contact the ACOG Distribution Center at 800-762-2264, or order online at sales.acog.org.

*Title issued since publication of last listing
▶ Practice Bulletin

Committee Opinions

Advanced Paternal Age: Risks to the Fetus (No. 189)   5
Air Travel During Pregnancy (No. 264)   7
Analgesia and Cesarean Delivery Rates (No. 269)   9
Antenatal Corticosteroid Therapy for Fetal Maturation (No. 273)   11
*Appropriate Use of Laparoscopically Assisted Vaginal Hysterectomy (No. 311)   13
At-Risk Drinking and Illicit Drug Use: Ethical Issues in Obstetric
    and Gynecologic Practice (No. 294)   15
Avoiding Inappropriate Clinical Decisions Based
    on False-Positive Human Chorionic Gonadotropin Test Results (No. 278)   26
Cervical Cancer Screening in Adolescents (No. 300)   29
Circumcision (No. 260)   34
Coding Responsibility (No. 249)   36
Complementary and Alternative Medicine (No. 227)   37
*Compounded Bioidentical Hormones (No. 322)   40
*Coping with the Stress of Medical Professional Liability Litigation (No. 309)   42
*Elective Coincidental Appendectomy (No. 323)   44
*Endometriosis in Adolescents (No. 310)   46
Exercise During Pregnancy and the Postpartum Period (No. 267)   53
Fetal Pulse Oximetry (No. 258)   56
First-Trimester Screening for Fetal Aneuploidy (No. 296)   58
Follow-up of Abnormal Screening Mammography (No. 272)   61
Fragile X Syndrome (No. 161)   62
Genetic Evaluation of Stillbirths and Neonatal Deaths (No. 257)   64
Guidelines for Adolescent Health Research (No. 302)   67
Guidelines for Diagnostic Imaging During Pregnancy (No. 299)   71
*Health Care for Homeless Women (No. 312)   76
Hepatitis Virus Infections in Obstetrician–Gynecologists (No. 203)   82
Immunization During Pregnancy (No. 282)   84
Inappropriate Reimbursement Practices by Third Party Payers (No. 250)   90
*Inappropriate Use of the Terms Fetal Distress and Birth Asphyxia (No. 326)   94
Induced Abortion and Breast Cancer Risk (No. 285)   96
Induction of Labor for Vaginal Birth After Cesarean Delivery (No. 271)   99
Induction of Labor with Misoprostol (No. 228)   101
Influenza Vaccination and Treatment During Pregnancy (No. 305)   103
Informed Refusal (No. 306)   105
Length of Hospital Stay for Gynecologic Procedures (No. 191)   107

*Published in 2005

Committee Opinions

Management of Asymptomatic Pregnant
  or Lactating Women Exposed to Anthrax (No. 268)   108
*Maternal Decision Making, Ethics, and the Law (No. 321)   111
Maternal Phenylketonuria (No. 230)   122
*Meningococcal Vaccination for Adolescents (No. 314)   124
Mode of Term Singleton Breech Delivery (No. 265)   127
New U.S. Food and Drug Administration Labeling
  on Cytotec (Misoprostol) Use and Pregnancy (No. 283)   129
Newborn Screening (No. 287)   131
Nongynecologic Procedures (No. 253)   134
Nonmedical Use of Obstetric Ultrasonography (No. 297)   135
Nonobstetric Surgery in Pregnancy (No. 284)   137
Nonsurgical Diagnosis and Management of Vaginal Agenesis (No. 274)   138
*Obesity in Pregnancy (No. 315)   142
Obstetric Management of Patients with Spinal Cord Injuries (No. 275)   147
Optimal Goals for Anesthesia Care in Obstetrics (No. 256)   150
Pain Relief During Labor (No. 295)   153
Partner Consent for Participation in Women's Reproductive Health Research (No. 307)   154
*Partnering with Patients to Improve Safety (No. 320)   157
Patient Safety in Obstetrics and Gynecology (No. 286)   160
Performance and Interpretation of Imaging Studies
  by Obstetrician–Gynecologists (No. 243)   163
*Perinatal Risks Associated with Assisted Reproductive Technology (No. 324)   165
Placenta Accreta (No. 266)   169
Placental Pathology (No. 125)   171
Prenatal and Perinatal Human Immunodeficiency Virus Testing:
  Expanded Recommendations (No. 304)   172
Prenatal and Preconceptional Carrier Screening for Genetic Diseases
  in Individuals of Eastern European Jewish Descent (No. 298)   178
Prevention of Early-Onset Group B Streptococcal Disease in Newborns (No. 279)   182
Primary and Preventive Care: Periodic Assessments (No. 292)   190
Professional Liability and Gynecology-Only Practice (No. 288)   198
*Racial and Ethnic Disparities in Women's Health (No. 317)   199
Response to Searle's Drug Warning on Misoprostol (No. 248)   203
Role of the Obstetrician–Gynecologist in the Diagnosis
  and Treatment of Breast Disease (No. 186)   205
Routine Storage of Umbilical Cord Blood
  for Potential Future Transplantation (No. 183)   207
Rubella Vaccination (No. 281)   210

*Published in 2005

Committee Opinions

Safety of Lovenox in Pregnancy (No. 276)   211

Scheduled Cesarean Delivery and the Prevention of Vertical Transmission
    of HIV Infection (No. 234)   213

Screening for Canavan Disease (No. 212)   216

*Screening for Tay–Sachs Disease (No. 318)   218

Sexually Transmitted Diseases in Adolescents (No. 301)   220

*Smoking Cessation During Pregnancy (No. 316)   228

Statement on Surgical Assistants (No. 240)   234

Tamoxifen and Endometrial Cancer (No. 232)   235

*The Importance of Preconception Care
    in the Continuum of Women's Health Care (No. 313)   238

The Role of the Generalist Obstetrician–Gynecologist
    in the Early Detection of Ovarian Cancer (No. 280)   240

*The Role of the Obstetrician–Gynecologist
    in the Assessment and Management of Obesity (No. 319)   243

The Uninsured (No. 308)   248

Tubal Ligation with Cesarean Delivery (No. 205)   252

*Update on Carrier Screening for Cystic Fibrosis (No. 325)   253

Use and Abuse of the Apgar Score (No. 174)   257

Use of Progesterone to Reduce Preterm Birth (No. 291)   260

Uterine Artery Embolization (No. 293)   262

*Published in 2005

ACOG

Committee on
Genetics

Committee Opinion

Number 189, October 1997

Advanced Paternal Age:
Risks to the Fetus

Advanced maternal age increases the risk of having a liveborn infant with autosomal trisomies 21, 18, or 13, or with the sex chromosome aneuploidies 47,XXY or 47,XXX. Genetic counseling traditionally has been offered when a woman will be 35 years of age or older as of her estimated delivery date. With increased paternal age, however, there does not appear to be an increased risk of chromosomal anomalies in offspring. Insufficient evidence exists to provide a specific cutoff level for assessing risk in association with paternal age.

Although advancing paternal age does affect pregnancy outcome, effects on genetic disease are less completely understood. There is general agreement that advancing paternal age predisposes the fetus to mutations in autosomal dominant diseases such as neurofibromatosis, achondroplasia, Apert syndrome, and Marfan syndrome. The increased risk rises exponentially, rather than linearly, with increasing paternal age. Increasing paternal age may be associated with spontaneous germline mutations in X-linked genes that are transmitted through carrier daughters to affected grandsons. This phenomenon has been called the "grandfather effect" and may occur with several X-linked disorders, including hemophilia A and Duchenne muscular dystrophy.

Although paternal age affects autosomal dominant diseases, the exact risk for any specific disorder is small. Most of the autosomal dominant diseases affect only 1 in 5,000–10,000 individuals, so even a doubling of risk constitutes a very low overall risk. It is the collective risk of autosomal dominant diseases that constitutes the increased risk, not the risk of a particular disorder.

Currently, it is not possible to screen prenatally for all autosomal dominant and X-linked diseases in the presence of advanced paternal age. Fetal ultrasonography may detect some autosomal dominant disorders, but this technique cannot be relied upon as a screening modality. Chromosomal analysis cannot be used to detect these disorders. Only genetic counseling on an individual basis is recommended for couples to address their specific concerns if advancing paternal age is an issue.

Copyright © October 1997
ISSN 1074-861X

The American College of Obstetricians and Gynecologists

409 12th Street, SW
PO Box 96920
Washington, DC 20090-6920

12345/43210

6   COMPENDIUM OF SELECTED PUBLICATIONS

Bibliography

American College of Medical Genetics. Statement on guidance for genetic counseling in advanced paternal age. Bethesda, Maryland: ACMG, 1996

Ashton GC. Mismatches in genetic markers in a large family study. Am J Hum Genet 1980;32:601–613

de Michelena MI, Burstein E, Lama JR, Vasquez JC. Paternal age as a risk factor for Down syndrome. Am J Med Genet 1993;45:679–682

Friedman JM. Genetic disease in the offspring of older fathers. Obstet Gynecol 1981;57:745–749

Hook EB. A search for a paternal-age effect upon cases of 47, +21 in which the extra chromosome is of paternal origin. Am J Hum Genet 1984;36:413–421

McIntosh GC, Olshan AF, Baird PA. Paternal age and the risk of birth defects in offspring. Epidemiology 1995;6:282–288

Olshan AF, Anath CV, Savitz DA. Intrauterine growth retardation as an endpoint in mutation epidemiology: an evaluation based on paternal age. Mutat Res 1995;344:89–94

Olshan AF, Schnitzer PG, Baird PA. Paternal age and the risk of congenital heart defects. Teratology 1994;50:80–84

Risch N, Reich EW, Wishnick MM, McCarthy JG. Spontaneous mutation and parental age in humans. Am J Hum Genet 1987;41:218–248

ACOG

Committee on
Obstetric Practice

Committee Opinion

Number 264, December 2001

Air Travel During Pregnancy

ABSTRACT: In the absence of obstetric or medical complications, pregnant women can observe the same general precautions for air travel as the general population and can fly safely up to 36 weeks of gestation. In-craft environmental conditions such as low cabin humidity and changes in cabin pressure, coupled with the physiologic changes of pregnancy, do result in maternal adaptations, which could have transient effects on the fetus. Pregnant air travelers with medical problems that may be exacerbated by a hypoxic environment, but who must travel by air, should be prescribed supplemental oxygen during air travel. Pregnant women at significant risk for premature labor or with placental abnormalities should avoid air travel. Because air turbulence cannot be predicted and the risk for trauma is significant, pregnant women should be instructed to continuously use their seat belts while seated, as should all air travelers. Pregnant air travelers may take precautions to ease in-flight discomfort, and although no hard evidence exists, preventive measures can be employed to minimize risks.

Air travel during pregnancy is safe for most women and most U.S. airlines allow pregnant women to fly up to 36 weeks of gestation. For specific airline requirements, the patient should check with the specific carrier because documentation of gestational age may be required. For international airlines the cutoff is 35 weeks of gestation.

In the absence of complications, pregnant women can observe the same general precautions while traveling as the general population. Travel is not recommended at any time during pregnancy for women who have either medical or obstetric complications for which likely emergencies cannot be predicted. Such complications may include increased risks for, or evidence of, preterm delivery, pregnancy induced hypertension, poorly controlled type 1 or type 2 diabetes, or sickle cell disease or trait, which may be exacerbated by high altitude. Pregnant women should be informed that the most common obstetric emergencies occur in the first and third trimesters.

Some unconfirmed reports indicate that flight attendants experience twice the incidence (relative risk=1.9) of first trimester spontaneous abortions as other women, but not other employed women. There is no evidence of an increased risk of spontaneous abortion among other air travelers (1). Most airlines restrict the working air travel of flight attendants after 20 weeks of gestation. Airlines also restrict commercial airline pilots from flying once pregnancy is diagnosed.

ISSN 1074-861X

The American College of Obstetricians and Gynecologists
409 12th Street, SW
PO Box 96920
Washington, DC 20090-6920

12345/54321

Air travel during pregnancy. ACOG Committee Opinion No. 264. American College of Obstetricians and Gynecologists. Obstet Gynecol 2001;98:1187–1188

In-craft environmental conditions such as changes in cabin pressure and low humidity, coupled with the physiologic changes of pregnancy, do result in maternal adaptations, which could have transient effects on the fetus. A significant environmental change is the reduction of cabin humidity to less than 25%, which causes hemoconcentration and increases the risk for venous thrombosis and potentially the risk for premature labor.

On long commercial flights traveling at 39,000–41,000 feet, cabin pressure is maintained at the equivalent of an altitude pressure of 8,000 feet. While at 32,000 feet the cabin pressure is set at the equivalent of 6,000 feet. The conditions at a cabin pressure of 8000 feet will create a more hypoxic environment than those at 6000 feet. Acute ascent to 6,000 feet does not elicit ominous fetal responses, but it does produce transient maternal cardiopulmonary adaptations. Among these adaptations are increased heart rate, increased blood pressure, and a significant decrease in aerobic capacity (2, 3). In pregnancy there is limited aerobic capacity. At 6,000 feet the oxygen consumption in pregnant women is 13% (L/min) lower than at sea level (3), in comparison with non-pregnant women for whom the decrease is only 3% lower (4). These changes are associated with a reduction in partial oxygen pressure, which should not affect normal pregnant women, but it could affect those with a compromised cardiovascular system. Therefore, pregnant air travelers with medical problems that may be exacerbated by a hypoxic environment, but who must travel by air, should be prescribed supplemental oxygen during air travel. Pregnant women at significant risk for premature labor or with placental abnormalities should avoid air travel.

Several precautions may ease discomfort for pregnant air travelers. For example, gas-producing foods or drinks should be avoided before scheduled flights since entrapped gases expand at altitude (5). Preventive antiemetic medication should be considered for women with increased nausea.

The risks associated with long hours of air travel immobilization and low cabin humidity, such as lower extremity edema and venous thrombotic events, have recently been the focus of attention for all air travelers. There are no published reports of such events in pregnancy; however, concerns regarding the relationship of venous stasis to in-flight thromboembolism have been raised. Despite the lack of tangible evidence, certain preventive measures can be employed to minimize these risks, ie, support stockings and periodic movement of the lower extremities. Because air turbulence cannot be predicted and the risk for trauma is significant, pregnant women should be instructed to continuously use their seatbelts while seated, as should all air travelers. The seatbelt should be belted low on the hipbones, between the protuberant abdomen and pelvis.

Available information suggests that noise vibration and cosmic radiation present a negligible risk for the pregnant air traveler (6, 7). In the absence of a reasonable expectation for obstetric or medical complications, air travel is safe for pregnant women up to 36 weeks of gestation.

References

1. Daniell WE, Vaughan TL, Millies BA. Pregnancy outcomes among female flight attendants. Aviat Space Environ Med;1990;61:840–884
2. Huch R, Baumann H, Fallenstein F, Schneider KT, Holdener F, Huch A. Physiologic changes in pregnant women and their fetuses during jet air travel. Am J Obstet Gynecol 1986;154:996–1000
3. Artal R, Fortunato V, Welton A, Constantino N, Khodiguian N, Villalobos L, et al. A comparison of cardiopulmonary adaptations to exercise in pregnancy at sea level and altitude. Am J Obstet Gynecol 1995;172:1170–1178; discussion 1178–1180
4. Brooks GA, Fahey TD, White TP, Baldwin KM. Exercise, atmospheric pressure, air pollution, and travel. In: Exercise physiology: human bioenergetics and its applications. 3rd ed. Mountain View, California: Mayfield Publishing Company, 2000:504–436
5. Bia FJ. Medical considerations for the pregnant traveler. Infect Dis Clin N Am 1992;6:371–388
6. Morrell S, Taylor R, Lyle D. A review of health effects of aircraft noise. Aust N Z J Public Health 1997;21:221–236
7. Friedberg W, Faulkner DN, Snyder L, Darden EB Jr, O'Brien K. Galactic cosmic radiation exposure and associated health risks for air carrier crewmembers. Aviat Space Environ Med 1989;60:1104–1108

ACOG Committee Opinion

Committee on Obstetric Practice

Number 269, February 2002

Analgesia and Cesarean Delivery Rates

ABSTRACT: Various studies report conflicting data with regard to the level of risk of cesarean delivery for nulliparous women who receive epidural analgesia before 5 cm of cervical dilatation. As a result, some institutions are requiring that laboring women reach 4–5 cm of dilatation before receiving epidural analgesia. The American College of Obstetricians and Gynecologists wishes to reaffirm the opinion published jointly with the American Society of Anesthesiologists that while under a physician's care, in the absence of a medical contraindication, maternal request is a sufficient medical indication for pain relief during labor. Decisions regarding analgesia should be coordinated among the obstetrician, the anesthesiologist, the patient, and support personnel.

Although neuraxial techniques (epidural, spinal, combined spinal–epidural) provide the most effective and least depressant analgesia for labor, the question of whether their use is associated with an increased risk of cesarean delivery remains controversial. Several randomized prospective studies have shown an increased risk of cesarean delivery with epidural analgesia (1, 2) while others have shown no increased risk with epidural analgesia (3) or combined spinal–epidural analgesia (4). The American College of Obstetricians and Gynecologists (ACOG) Task Force on Cesarean Delivery report, *Evaluation of Cesarean Delivery*, evaluated the potential of several obstetric and nonobstetric factors to affect cesarean delivery rates (5). One of the factors evaluated was the potential contribution of epidural analgesia to the increasing cesarean delivery rate in the United States. The task force noted that the relevant studies varied in size, design, and analysis. Some studies have demonstrated an increased risk of cesarean delivery for nulliparous women who received epidural analgesia before 5 cm of dilatation (1, 6). Conversely, several randomized trials comparing "early" versus "late" epidural analgesia administration reported no difference in cesarean delivery rates and advocated individualized decisions regarding the timing of regional analgesia (7, 8).

After weighing this conflicting data, the task force recommended that when feasible, obstetric practitioners should delay the administration of epidural analgesia in nulliparous women until the cervical dilatation reaches 4–5 cm and that other forms of analgesia be used until that time (5). The task

ISSN 1074-861X

The American College of Obstetricians and Gynecologists
409 12th Street, SW
PO Box 96920
Washington, DC 20090-6920

12345/65432

Analgesia and cesarean delivery rates. ACOG Committee Opinion No. 269. American College of Obstetricians and Gynecologists. Obstet Gynecol 2002;99:369–370 force specifically stated that there is no desire to limit the use of epidural analgesia by women in labor (5). Despite this, it has come to the attention of ACOG that some institutions are now requiring that laboring women reach 4–5 cm of cervical dilatation before receiving epidural analgesia. It is unclear whether these institutions have developed local protocols that are sensitive to patients' needs. Therefore, ACOG reaffirms the opinion it published jointly with the American Society of Anesthesiologists, in which the following statement was articulated: "Labor results in severe pain for many women. There is no other circumstance where it is considered acceptable for a person to experience untreated severe pain, amenable to safe intervention, while under a physician's care. In the absence of a medical contraindication, maternal request is a sufficient medical indication for pain relief during labor (9)."

The American College of Obstetricians and Gynecologists recognizes that many techniques are available for analgesia in laboring patients. The choice of technique, agent, and dosage is based on many factors, including patient preference, medical status, and contraindications. Decisions regarding analgesia should be closely coordinated among the obstetrician, the anesthesiologist, the patient, and skilled support personnel (9).

References

1. Thorp JA, Hu DH, Albin RM, McNitt J, Meyer BA, Cohen GR, et al. The effect of intrapartum epidural analgesia on nulliparous labor: a randomized, controlled, prospective trial. Am J Obstet Gynecol 1993;169:851–858
2. Ramin SM, Gambling DR, Lucas MJ, Sharma SK, Sidawi JE, Leveno KJ. Randomized trial of epidural versus intravenous analgesia during labor. Obstet Gynecol 1995;86: 783–789
3. Sharma SK, Sidawi JE, Ramin SM, Lucas MJ, Leveno KJ, Cunningham FG. Cesarean delivery: a randomized trial of epidural versus patient-controlled meperidine analgesia during labor. Anesthesiology 1997;87:487–494
4. Gambling DR, Sharma SK, Ramin SM, Lucas MJ, Leveno KJ, Wiley J, et al. A randomized study of combined spinal-epidural analgesia versus intravenous meperidine during labor: impact on cesarean delivery rate. Anesthesiology 1998;89:1336–1344
5. American College of Obstetricians and Gynecologists. Task Force on Cesarean Delivery Rates. Evaluation of cesarean delivery. Washington, DC: ACOG, 2000
6. Lieberman E, Lang JM, Cohen A, D'Agostino R Jr, Datta S, Frigoletto FD Jr. Association of epidural analgesia with cesarean delivery in nulliparas. Obstet Gynecol 1996;88: 993–1000
7. Chestnut DH, Vincent RD Jr, McGrath JM, Choi WW, Bates JN. Does early administration of epidural analgesia affect obstetric outcome in nulliparous women who are receiving intravenous oxytocin? Anesthesiology 1994; 80: 1193–1200
8. Chestnut DH, McGrath JM, Vincent RD Jr, Penning DH, Choi WW, Bates JN, et al. Does early administration of epidural analgesia affect obstetric outcome in nulliparous women who are in spontaneous labor? Anesthesiology 1994;80:1201–1208
9. American College of Obstetricians and Gynecologists. Pain relief during labor. ACOG Committee Opinion 231. Washington, DC: ACOG, 2000

ACOG

Committee on Obstetric Practice

Requests for authorization to make photocopies should be directed to:

Copyright Clearance Center
222 Rosewood Drive
Danvers, MA 01923
(978) 750-8400

ISSN 1074-861X

The American College of Obstetricians and Gynecologists
409 12th Street, SW
PO Box 96920
Washington, DC 20090-6920

12345/65432

Antenatal corticosteroid therapy for fetal maturation. ACOG Committee Opinion No. 273. American College of Obstetricians and Gynecologists. Obstet Gynecol 2002;99:871–873

Committee Opinion

Number 273, May 2002   *(Replaces No. 210, October 1998)*

Antenatal Corticosteroid Therapy for Fetal Maturation

ABSTRACT: The National Institute of Child Health and Human Development and the Office of Medical Applications of Research of the National Institutes of Health convened consensus conferences in 1994 and 2000 that recommended giving a single course of corticosteroids to all pregnant women between 24 and 34 weeks of gestation who are at risk of preterm delivery within 7 days. Because of insufficient scientific evidence, the consensus panel also recommended that repeat corticosteroid courses, including so-called "rescue therapy," should not be routinely used but should be reserved for women enrolled in clinical trials. Betamethasone and dexamethasone have been most widely studied and have generally been the preferred corticosteroids for antenatal treatment to accelerate fetal organ maturation. The American College of Obstetricians and Gynecologists' Committee on Obstetric Practice supports the conclusions of the consensus conferences.

In August 2000, the National Institute of Child Health and Human Development and the Office of Medical Applications of Research of the National Institutes of Health reconvened a consensus conference on antenatal steroids, entitled "Consensus Development Conference on Antenatal Corticosteroids Revisited: Repeat Courses," to address the issue of repeated courses of corticosteroids for fetal maturation. The consensus panel from this conference reaffirmed the 1994 consensus panel's recommendation of giving a single course of corticosteroids to all pregnant women between 24 and 34 weeks of gestation who are at risk of preterm delivery within 7 days (1). Because of insufficient scientific evidence, the panel also recommended that repeat corticosteroid courses, including so-called "rescue therapy," should not be routinely used but should be reserved for women enrolled in clinical trials. Several of these randomized trials are in progress. The American College of Obstetricians and Gynecologists' Committee on Obstetric Practice supports the conclusions of the consensus conferences.

There is no convincing scientific evidence that antenatal corticosteroid therapy increases the risk of neonatal infection, although multiple courses have been associated with fetal adrenal suppression (2). Follow-up studies of children aged 12 years and younger exposed to at least one course of corticosteroid treatment indicate there is no apparent risk of adverse neurodevelopmental outcome associated with antenatal corticosteroids. There are inconclusive data that repeated courses of antenatal corticosteroids have been associated with a decrease in birth weight and neonatal head circumference (3, 4). The 2000 consensus panel concluded that studies regarding the possible benefits and risks of repeat courses of corticosteroids are limited because of their study design and "methodologic inconsistencies." The 2000 consensus panel noted that, although there is a suggestion of possible benefit from repeated doses (especially in the reduction and severity of respiratory distress), there also are animal and human data that suggest deleterious effects on the fetus regarding cerebral myelination, lung growth, and function of the hypothalamic–pituitary–adrenal axis. Maternal effects include increased infection and suppression of the hypothalamic–pituitary–adrenal axis (5, 6).

Betamethasone and dexamethasone are the most widely studied and have generally been the preferred corticosteroids used for antenatal treatment to accelerate fetal organ maturation. Both cross the placenta in their active form and have nearly identical biologic activity. Both lack mineralocorticoid activity and have relatively weak immunosuppressive activity with short-term use. Although betamethasone and dexamethasone differ only by a single methyl group, their pharmacokinetics differ. Betamethasone has a longer half-life because of its decreased clearance and larger volume of distribution (7). Meta-analyses of randomized trials have shown that, although both agents decrease the frequency of respiratory distress syndrome, only betamethasone decreases neonatal mortality (8). A recent large, uncontrolled retrospective study suggested that betamethasone also may have significant benefit in decreasing the rate of newborn cystic periventricular leukomalacia by approximately 50% compared with untreated and dexamethasone-treated women (9). The offspring of pregnant mice who were given betamethasone performed neurobehavioral developmental tasks better than the offspring of pregnant mice given dexamethasone (10). Furthermore, betamethasone requires fewer intramuscular injections. Betamethasone use, however, has been associated with a significant transient decrease in fetal movements and heart rate variability (11, 12).

The 2000 consensus panel reviewed all available reports on the safety and efficacy of betamethasone and dexamethasone. It did not find significant scientific evidence to support a recommendation that betamethasone should be used preferentially instead of dexamethasone. Thus, based on this information, the Committee on Obstetric Practice recommends either of the following corticosteroid regimens:

- Betamethasone (12 mg) given intramuscularly every 24 hours for two doses
- Dexamethasone (6 mg) given intramuscularly every 12 hours for four doses in patients at risk for preterm delivery between 24 and 34 weeks of gestation with intact membranes or between 24 and 32 weeks of gestation for patients with ruptured membranes

The use of corticosteroids after 34 weeks of gestation is not recommended unless there is evidence of fetal pulmonary immaturity.

References

1. Antenatal corticosteroids revisited: repeat courses. NIH Consens Statement 2000;17(2):1–10
2. Kairalla AB. Hypothalamic-pituitary-adrenal axis function in premature neonates after extensive prenatal treatment with betamethasone: a case history. Am J Perinatol 1992;9:428–430
3. French NP, Hagan R, Evans SF, Godfrey RN, Newnham JP. Repeated antenatal corticosteroids: size at birth and subsequent development. Am J Obstet Gynecol 1999; 180:114–121
4. Guinn DA, Atkinson MW, Sullivan L, Lee M, MacGregor S, Parilla BV et al. Single vs weekly courses of antenatal corticosteroids for women at risk of preterm delivery: a randomized controlled trial. JAMA 2001;286:1581–1587
5. McKenna DS, Wittber GM, Nagaraja HN, Samuels P. The effects of repeat doses of antenatal corticosteroids on maternal adrenal function. Am J Obstet Gynecol 2000; 183:669–673
6. Abbasi S, Hirsch D, Davis J, Tolosa J, Stouffer N, Debbs R, et al. Effect of single versus multiple courses of antenatal corticosteroids on maternal and neonatal outcome. Am J Obstet Gynecol 2000;182:1243–1249
7. Fanaroff AA, Hack M. Periventricular leukomalacia—prospects for prevention [letter]. N Engl J Med 1999;341:1229–1231
8. Ballard PL, Ballard RA. Scientific basis and therapeutic regimens for use of antenatal glucocorticoids. Am J Obstet Gynecol 1995;173:254–262
9. Baud O, Foix-L'Helias L, Kaminski M, Audiberet F, Jarreau PH, Papiernik E, et al. Antenatal glucocorticoid treatment and cystic periventricular leukomalacia in very premature infants. N Engl J Med 1999;341:1190–1196
10. Rayburn WF, Christensen HD, Gonzalez CL. A placebo-controlled comparison between betamethasone and dexamethasone for fetal maturation: differences in neurobehavioral development of mice offspring. Am J Obstet Gynecol 1997;176:842–850; discussion 850–851
11. Mulder EJ, Derks JB, Visser GH. Antenatal corticosteroid therapy and fetal behavior: a randomised study of the effects of betamethasone and dexamethasone. Br J Obstet Gynaecol 1997;104:1239–1247
12. Senat MV, Minoui S, Multon O, Fernandez H, Frydman R, Ville Y. Effect of dexamethasone and betamethasone on fetal heart rate variability in preterm labour: a randomised study. Br J Obstet Gynaecol 1998;105:749–755

ACOG

ACOG Committee on
Gynecologic Practice

ISSN 1074-861X

The American College of Obstetricians and Gynecologists
409 12th Street, SW
PO Box 96920
Washington, DC 20090-6920

12345/98765

Appropriate use of laparoscopically assisted vaginal hysterectomy. ACOG Committee Opinion No. 311. American College of Obstetricians and Gynecologists. Obstet Gynecol 2005;105:929–30.

Committee Opinion

Number 311, April 2005

Appropriate Use of Laparoscopically Assisted Vaginal Hysterectomy

ABSTRACT: The technique used for hysterectomy should be dictated by the indication for the surgery, patient characteristics, and patient preference. Most patients requiring hysterectomy should be offered the vaginal approach when technically feasible and medically appropriate. If specific additional procedures that can be completed laparoscopically are anticipated before surgery, laparoscopically assisted vaginal hysterectomy may be an appropriate alternative to abdominal hysterectomy. The benefits of laparoscopically assisted vaginal hysterectomy must be weighed against the potentially increased risk and expense of two distinct operative procedures, laparoscopy and vaginal hysterectomy.

The technique used for hysterectomy should be dictated by the indication for the surgery, patient characteristics, and patient preference. Most patients requiring hysterectomy should be offered the vaginal approach when technically feasible and medically appropriate because morbidity appears to be lower with the vaginal approach than with any other method (1–4). Laparoscopically assisted vaginal hysterectomy (LAVH), with or without bilateral salpingo-oophorectomy, usually offers no advantage when a conventional vaginal hysterectomy and bilateral salpingo-oophorectomy can otherwise be performed.

Prospective randomized trials demonstrate that LAVH is associated with faster recovery, less postoperative pain, and similar complication rates when compared with abdominal hysterectomy (1, 5–7). Specific additional procedures that can be completed laparoscopically to facilitate the performance of vaginal hysterectomy include:

- Lysis of adhesions
- Treatment of endometriosis
- Management of uterine leiomyomata that complicate the performance of vaginal hysterectomy
- Ligation of infundibulopelvic ligaments to facilitate difficult ovary removal
- Evaluation of the pelvic and abdominal cavity before hysterectomy

If these procedures are anticipated before surgery, LAVH may be an appropriate alternative to abdominal hysterectomy (8). The laparoscopic approach introduces the potential for additional complications when compared with vaginal hysterectomy. These complications include trocar injuries to vessels and viscera, bowel and omental herniation through large trocar sites, and urinary and bowel injuries (7, 9). The benefits of LAVH must be weighed against the potentially increased risk and expense of two distinct operative procedures, laparoscopy and vaginal hysterectomy, each with its own risks.

References

1. Garry R, Fountain J, Mason S, Hawe J, Napp V, Abbott J, et al. The eVALuate study: two parallel randomised trials, one comparing laparoscopic with abdominal hysterectomy, the other comparing laparoscopic with vaginal hysterectomy [published erratum appears in BMJ 2004; 328:494]. BMJ 2004;328:129.
2. Harkki P, Kurki T, Sjoberg J, Titinen A. Safety aspects of laparoscopic hysterectomy. Acta Obstet Gynecol Scand 2001;80:383–91.
3. Schwartz RO. Complications of laparoscopic hysterectomy. Obstet Gynecol 1993;81:1022–4.
4. Summitt RL Jr, Stovall TG, Lipscomb GH, Ling FW. Randomized comparison of laparoscopy-assisted vaginal hysterectomy with standard vaginal hysterectomy in an outpatient setting. Obstet Gynecol 1992;80:895–901.
5. Summitt RL Jr, Stovall TG, Steege JF, Lipscomb GH. A multicenter randomized comparison of laparoscopically-assisted vaginal hysterectomy and abdominal hysterectomy in abdominal hysterectomy candidates. Obstet Gynecol 1998;92:321–6.
6. Olsson JH, Ellstrom M, Hahlin A. A randomised prospective trial comparing laparoscopic and abdominal hysterectomy. Br J Obstet Gynaecol 1996;103:345–50.
7. Falcone T, Paraiso MF, Mascha E. Prospective randomized clinical trial of laparoscopically assisted vaginal hysterectomy versus total abdominal hysterectomy. Am J Obstet Gynecol 1999;180:955–62.
8. Society of Pelvic Reconstructive Surgeons. Guideline for determining the route and method of hysterectomy for benign conditions. Atlanta (GA): SPRS;2004.
9. Meikle SF, Nugent EW, Orleans M. Complications and recovery from laparoscopy-assisted vaginal hysterectomy compared with abdominal and vaginal hysterectomy. Obstet Gynecol 1997;89:304–11.

ACOG Committee Opinion

Committee on
Ethics

Number 294, May 2004

At-Risk Drinking and Illicit Drug Use: Ethical Issues in Obstetric and Gynecologic Practice

ABSTRACT: *Abuse of alcohol and drugs is a major health problem for American women across differences in socioeconomic status, race, ethnicity, and age, and it is costly to individuals and to society. Obstetrician–gynecologists have an ethical obligation to learn and use a protocol for universal screening questions, brief intervention, and referral to treatment in order to provide patients and their families with medical care that is state-of-the-art, comprehensive, and effective. In this Committee Opinion, the American College of Obstetricians and Gynecologists' Committee on Ethics proposes an ethical rationale for this protocol in both obstetric and gynecologic practice and provides guidelines for resolving common ethical dilemmas related to drug and alcohol use that arise in the clinical setting.*

ISSN 1074-861X

The American College of Obstetricians and Gynecologists
409 12th Street, SW
PO Box 96920
Washington, DC 20090-6920

12345/87654

At-risk drinking and illicit drug use: ethical issues in obstetric and gynecologic practice. ACOG Committee Opinion No. 294. American College of Obstetricians and Gynecologists. Obstet Gynecol 2004;103:1021–31.

Abuse of alcohol and drugs is a major health problem for American women across differences in socioeconomic status, race, ethnicity, and age, and it is costly to individuals and to society. Women who are heavy drinkers (5 or more drinks on 1 occasion on 5 or more days in the past 30 days) represent 5.3% of 18–24 year olds and 3.4% of women aged 25 years or older. Among them, more than 2.5 million U.S. women are estimated to be alcohol dependent (1). Heavy drinking carries a higher risk of cardiac and hepatic complications for women than men. The alcohol-associated mortality rate is 50–100 times higher, and there is an increased burden of mental and physical disability (2). Among pregnant women, 12% admit to drinking some alcohol during the previous month (1), which puts the fetus at risk for fetal alcohol syndrome (FAS), the leading cause of mental retardation in the United States (3). Maternal alcoholism is one of the leading preventable causes of fetal neurodevelopmental disorders (4). The total costs of alcohol misuse and abuse are estimated at more than $667 billion yearly, including $2.8 billion attributable to FAS alone (5). Illicit drug use has major physical and mental health consequences and is associated with increased rates of sexually transmitted infections in women, including hepatitis and human immunodeficiency virus (HIV), as well as depression, domestic violence, poverty, and significant prenatal and neonatal complications (6, 7). In 2001, 8.3% of nonpregnant women and 3.7% of pregnant women reported illicit drug use, but among pregnant women aged 15–17 years, the rate of use increased to 15% (1). Drug abuse costs are estimated at more than $144 billion yearly, including $503 million associated with health care costs for drug-exposed newborns (5).

As a result of intensive research in addiction over the past decade, evidence-based recommendations have been consolidated into a protocol for universal screening questions, brief intervention, and referral to treatment (8). The rate of abstinence from drugs of abuse after treatment (the treatment success rate) is now comparable to the level of medication compliance achieved in diabetes, hypertension, or other chronic illnesses (9). Brief physician advice has been shown unequivocally to be both powerful and feasible in a clinical office setting (8, 10, 11). The American Medical Association has endorsed universal screening (12), and health services researchers have determined that treatment saves $7 for every dollar spent (13). For these reasons, the American College of Obstetricians and Gynecologists (ACOG) recently collaborated with the Physician Leadership on National Drug Policy at Brown University to produce a slide–lecture presentation that addresses the identification and treatment of drug abuse (14). The presentation was distributed to obstetric–gynecologic clerkship and residency program directors and is available at www.acog.org.

Physicians have been slow to implement universal screening, and rates of detection and referral to treatment among nonpregnant women remain very low (15). Studies using simulated patients have demonstrated that women are less likely than men to be screened or referred (16, 17). Physicians lack accurate knowledge about physiology (ie, the equivalency of 1.5 oz of distilled spirits, 12 oz of beer or wine cooler, and 5 oz of wine), risk factors, and sex differences in problem presentation and treatment response (18). These knowledge gaps are compounded by state laws designed to criminalize drug use during pregnancy, by women's fears that they might lose custody of their children, and by the social stigma experienced by women who abuse alcohol or use illicit drugs (19, 20). In one study, for example, the physicians surveyed defined "light drinking" as an average of 1.2 drinks per day, an amount that exceeds the National Institute on Alcohol Abuse and Alcoholism (NIAAA) guidelines

for at-risk drinking for women (21). Furthermore, communicating about difficult issues takes time, requires skills, and is poorly reimbursed by procedure-oriented insurance coverage. Physicians are concerned about the consequences of legally mandated reporting, they lack familiarity with treatment resources, and they do not have the extensive time required to make an appropriate referral (9). These are all problems that must be solved in order to provide medically appropriate and ethically necessary care to women who engage in at-risk drinking or use illicit drugs.

Substance abuse presents complex ethical issues and challenges. This Committee Opinion proposes an ethical rationale for universal screening questions, brief intervention, and referral to treatment in both obstetric and gynecologic practice and provides guidelines for resolving common ethical dilemmas that arise in the clinical setting.

The Ethical Rationale for Universal Screening Questions, Brief Intervention, and Referral to Treatment

Support for universal screening questions, brief intervention, and referral to treatment is derived from 4 basic principles of ethics. These principles are 1) beneficence, 2) nonmaleficence, 3) justice, and 4) respect for autonomy.

Beneficence

Therapeutic intent, or beneficence, is the foundation of medical knowledge, training, and practice. Experts at the NIAAA and the National Institute on Drug Abuse (NIDA) confirm that addiction is not primarily a moral weakness, as it has been viewed in the past, but a "brain disease" that should be included in a review of systems just like any other biologic disease process (22). A medical diagnosis of addiction requires medical intervention in the same manner that a diagnosis of diabetes requires nutritional counseling or therapeutic agents or both. Positive behavior change arises from the trust implicit in the physician–patient relationship, the respect that patients have for physicians' knowledge, and the ability of physicians to help patients see the links between substance use behaviors and real physical consequences. Brief physician advice has been shown to be as effective as conventional treatment for substance abuse and can produce dramatic reductions in drinking and drug use, improved health status, and decreased costs to society (8, 11, 13, 15, 23–25). The Center for Substance Abuse Prevention has now implemented more than 147 projects for pregnant and postpartum women and their children (26), and there are several different successful models for prevention and treatment for women and their families: AR-Cares (27), Choices (28), SafePort (29), Early Start (30), and the Mom/Kid Trial (31).

Given this capacity for dramatic improvement in health status, physicians have an obligation to be therapeutic—in this case to learn the techniques of screening and brief intervention—and to inform themselves as they would if a new test or therapy were developed for any other recognized disease entity. The practice of universal screening questions, brief intervention, and referral to treatment falls well within the purview of the obstetrician–gynecologist's role as a provider of primary care to women and has potential for major impact on recognized obstetric and gynecologic outcomes. Furthermore, if the topic is raised respectfully, the physician–patient relationship may be substantially enhanced, even if no substantive changes in lifestyle are achieved immediately. Therapy is called "patient care" because both physicians and patients recognize and value the commitment of the medical profession to engage in a nurturing relationship in the course of providing carefully selected therapeutic modalities. Nurturance of healthy behaviors through universal screening questions, brief intervention, and referral to treatment is, thus, part of the traditional healing role and an appropriate focus for the obstetrician–gynecologist's role as a primary care provider.

Nonmaleficence

The obligation to do no harm, or nonmaleficence, also applies to universal screening questions, brief intervention, and referral to treatment. Medical care can be compromised if physicians are unaware of a patient's alcohol or drug abuse and, thus, miss related diagnoses or medication interactions with alcohol or illegal substances. If the problem is not identified, major health risks, such as HIV exposure and depression, also may be missed. These are examples of harms that may occur as a result of omission (nondetection of a serious problem). Furthermore, patients may be harmed when substance abuse is treated by a physician as a moral rather than medical

issue (32). Women who abuse alcohol or use illicit drugs are more likely than men to be stigmatized and labeled as hopeless (33). In particular, physicians should avoid using humiliation as a tool to force change because such behavior is ethically inappropriate, engenders resistance, and may act as a barrier to successful treatment and recovery.

Justice

The ethical principle of justice governs access to care and fair distribution of resources. Elimination of health disparities and promotion of quality care for all are at the top of the list of goals for *Healthy People 2010*, the nation's health agenda. Injustice may result from a variety of sources.

Physicians may fail to apply principles of universal screening. When women are less likely to be screened or referred for treatment, their burden of disability is increased and health status decreased. The principle of justice requires that screening questions related to alcohol and drug use should be asked equally of men and women and regardless of race or economic status. It also requires that women be screened with tests such as TWEAK, T-ACE, or the NIAAA quantity and frequency questions that are more accurate in detecting women's patterns of substance abuse, which differ from those of men (34) (see box on next page). Women, for example, are more likely to be hidden drinkers and frequently underreport alcohol use, especially during pregnancy. Tests to detect the problem in women must include questions about tolerance, which are not included in the most commonly employed screen, CAGE, which has a sensitivity of only 75% compared with 87% for TWEAK (35).

Pregnant women are more likely to be screened than nonpregnant women. Although the vulnerability of the fetus is an important concern, the lives of nonpregnant women also have compelling value, and there is much evidence to suggest that women who abuse alcohol or use illicit drugs have coexisting or preexisting conditions (ie, mental health disorders, domestic violence, stress, childhood sexual abuse, poverty, and lack of resources) that put them in a vulnerable status (6, 36, 37). Universal application of screening questions, brief intervention, and referral to treatment eliminates these disparities related to justice.

Additionally, failure to diagnose and treat substance abuse with the same evidence-based approach applied to other chronic illnesses reduces patients'

Substance Abuse Screening

T-ACE

T   **T**olerance: How many drinks does it take to make you feel high? *More than 2 drinks is a positive response—score 2 points.*

A   Have people **A**nnoyed you by criticizing your drinking? *If "Yes"—score 1 point.*

C   Have you ever felt you ought to **C**ut down on your drinking? *If "Yes"—score 1 point.*

E   **E**ye opener: Have you ever had a drink first thing in the morning to steady your nerves or get rid of a hangover? *If "Yes"—score 1 point.*

A total score of 2 or more points indicates a positive screen for pregnancy risk drinking.

Reprinted from The American Journal of Obstetrics & Gynecology, Vol 160, Sokol RJ, Martier SS, Ager JW, The T-ACE questions: practical prenatal detection of risk drinking, 863–8; discussion 868–70, Copyright 1989, with permission from Elsevier.

TWEAK

T   **T**olerance: How many drinks can you hold? *If 5 or more drinks, score 2 points.*

W   Have close friends or relatives **W**orried or complained about your drinking in the past year? *If "Yes" 2 points.*

E   **E**ye Opener: Do you sometimes take a drink in the morning when you get up? *If "Yes" 1 point.*

A   **A**mnesia: Has a friend or family member ever told you about things you said or did while you were drinking that you could not remember? *If "Yes" 1 point.*

K(C) Do you sometimes feel the need to **C**ut down on your drinking? *If "Yes" 1 point.*

The TWEAK is used to screen for pregnant at-risk drinking, defined here as the consumption of 1 oz or more of alcohol per day while pregnant. A total score of 2 points or more indicates a positive screen for pregnancy risk drinking.

Adapted from Chan AW, Pristach EA, Welte JW, Russell M. Use of the TWEAK test in screening for alcoholism/heavy drinking in three populations. Alcohol Clin Exp Res 1993;17:1188–92.

NIAAA Questionnaire

Do you drink? Do you use drugs?

On average, how many days per week do you drink alcohol (beer, wine, liquor)?

On a typical day when you drink, how many drinks do you have?

Positive score: >14 drinks per week for men and >7 drinks per week for women

What is the maximum number of drinks you had on any given occasion during the past month?

Positive score: >4 for men and >3 for women

National Institute on Alcohol Abuse and Alcoholism. Helping patients with alcohol problems: a health practitioner's guide. Bethesda (MD): NIAAA; 2003. Available at: http://www.niaaa.nih.gov/publications/Practitioner/PractitionersGuideFINAL.pdf. Retrieved January 7, 2004.

---

access to health services and resources. Justice requires that physicians counsel patients presenting with drug or alcohol problems and refer them to an appropriate treatment resource when available. No physician would withhold hypertension therapy because the medication compliance rate is only 60%. Physicians who detect the serious medical condition of addiction are equally obligated to intervene.

Respect for Autonomy

On the one hand, no person has a right to use illegal drugs, and a pregnant woman has a moral obligation to avoid use of both illicit drugs and alcohol in order to safeguard the welfare of her fetus. On the other hand, effective intervention with respect to substance abuse by a pregnant or a nonpregnant woman requires that a climate of respect and trust exist within the physician–patient relationship. Patients who

begin to disclose behaviors that are stigmatized by society may be harmed if they feel that their trust is met with disrespect. Criticism and shaming statements actually increase resistance and impede change. Effective interventions, as summarized in the NIAAA Treatment Improvement Protocol (TIP) number 35, are designed to increase motivation to change by respecting autonomy, supporting self-efficacy, and offering hope and resources (8).

Effective intervention also requires that universal screening questions, brief intervention, and referral to treatment be conducted with full protection of confidentiality. Patients who fear that acknowledging substance abuse may lead to disclosure to others will be inhibited from honest reporting to their physicians (38). A difficult dilemma is created by state laws that require physicians to report the nonmedical use of controlled substances by a pregnant woman or that require toxicology tests after delivery when there is evidence of possible use of a controlled substance (eg, Minnesota statutes 626.5561 and 626.5562). Although such laws have the goals of referring the pregnant woman for assessment and chemical dependency treatment if indicated and of protecting fetuses and newborns from harm, these laws may unwittingly result in pregnant women not seeking prenatal care or concealing drug use from their obstetricians. Although it is always appropriate for a physician to negotiate with a patient about her willingness to accept a medical recommendation, respect for autonomy includes respect for refusal to be screened.

Special Responsibilities to Pregnant Patients

Federal warnings about the need to abstain from alcohol use in pregnancy were first issued in 1984. The American College of Obstetricians and Gynecologists recommended screening early in pregnancy in its 1977 *Standards for Ambulatory Obstetric Care*, and a pamphlet was issued in 1982 entitled "Alcohol and Your Unborn Baby." Screening during pregnancy was subsequently supported in a variety of documents and is recommended in a joint publication issued by ACOG and the American Academy of Pediatrics (39). Although obstetricians report screening 97% of pregnant women for alcohol use, only 25% used any of the standard screening tools, and only 20% of those surveyed knew that abstinence is the only known way to avoid all 4 adverse pregnancy outcomes (spontaneous abortion, nervous system impairment, birth defects, and FAS). This is a particularly significant gap in knowledge because there is no level of alcohol use, even the most minimal drinking, that has been determined to be absolutely safe. More than one half of the respondents (63%) reported that they lacked adequate information about referral resources (40). Screening rates for illicit drugs are lower than for alcohol (89%, according to unpublished ACOG survey data).

Ethical issues related to beneficence and nonmaleficence and the ethics of care (41) are similar for pregnant and nonpregnant women and for women who do and do not have children. In each of these cases, universal screening questions, brief intervention, and referral to treatment enables physicians to collaborate with patients to improve their own health, reduce the likelihood of preterm birth and neonatal complications in both current and future pregnancies, and improve the parenting capacity of the family unit.

As noted previously, autonomy issues are particularly challenging in pregnancy. In a survey of obstetricians, pediatricians, and family practice physicians, more than one half of the respondents believed that pregnant women have a legal as well as moral responsibility to ensure that they have healthy newborns (42). Although 61% were concerned that fear of criminal charges would be a barrier to receiving prenatal care, more than one half supported a statute that would permit removal of children from any woman who abused alcohol or drugs (42). This position is particularly troubling because these physicians did not state that there needed to be evidence of physical or emotional neglect (adverse effects on basic needs and safety) for children to be so removed. Both ethical and legal perspectives require that the best interests of the child be served, which requires both protecting children and assisting their mothers to be healthy so as to provide an optimal situation for growth and development.

Physicians' concerns about mothers who abuse alcohol or drugs undoubtedly reflect a desire to protect children. However, recommended screening and referral protocols may be perceived as punitive measures when they are connected with legally mandated testing, or reporting, or both. Such measures endanger the relationship of trust between physician and patient, place the obstetrician in an adversarial relationship with the patient, and possibly conflict with the therapeutic obligation. If pregnant women become reluctant to seek medical care because they fear being reported for alcohol or illegal drug use, these strategies will actually increase the risks to the woman and the fetus rather than reduce the consequences of substance abuse. Furthermore, threats and incarceration have been proved to be ineffective in reducing the incidence of alcohol or drug abuse, and removing children from the home may only subject them to worse risks in the foster care system (43). Treatment is both more effective and less expensive than restrictive policies (44), and it results in a mean net saving of $4,644 in medical expenses per mother/infant pair (45). Moreover, women who have custody of their children complete treatment at a higher rate than those who do not. Putting women in jail, where drugs may be available but treatment is not, jeopardizes the health of pregnant women and that of their existing and future children (46).

Referral to treatment, especially if combined with training in parenting skills, is the clinically appropriate professional action, both medically and ethically (31). Criminal charges against pregnant women on grounds of child abuse have been struck down in almost all cases because courts have upheld the right to privacy, which includes the right to decide whether to have a child, the right to bodily integrity, and the right to "be let alone" (47), and have found that states could better protect fetal health through "education and making available medical care and drug treatment centers for women" (48). The United States Supreme Court recognized the importance of privacy to the physician–patient relationship when it ruled in 2001 to prohibit a public hospital from performing nonconsensual drug tests on pregnant women without a warrant and providing police with positive results (49). Despite a decade of efforts and the 1992 passage of a federal Alcohol Drug Abuse and Mental Health Administration Reorganization Act explicitly prohibiting pregnancy discrimination, few treatment programs focus on the needs of pregnant women. In the absence of appropriate and adequate drug treatment services for pregnant women, criminal charges on grounds of child abuse are unjust in that they indict the woman for failing to seek treatment that actually may not be available to her.

Justice issues also are problematic in that punitive measures are not applied evenly across sex, race, and socioeconomic status. Although several types of legal sanctions against pregnant women who abuse alcohol or drugs are being tested in the courts, there has been no attempt to impose similar sanctions for paternal drug use (50), despite the significant involvement of male partners in pregnant women's substance abuse (51). In a landmark study among pregnant women anonymously tested for drug use, drug prevalence was similar between African-American women and white women, but African-American women were 10 times more likely than white women to be reported as a result of positive screens (52). Similar patterns of injustice have been noted for the types of drugs sanctioned by the legal system. For example, mandatory incarceration and more severe penalties are applied to crack cocaine, which is primarily used by African Americans, than to powder cocaine or heroin, which is primarily used by whites. In the case of *Ferguson v. City of Charleston*, 40 of 41 pregnant women arrested in the immediate postpartum period as a result of cocaine-positive drug screens were

African American. When similarly drawn drug screens were positive for methamphetamine or heroin, which were more commonly used by white patients, physicians were more likely to refer to social services rather than to the courts (49).

Some physicians are reluctant to record information related to alcohol or drug abuse in medical records because of competing obligations. On the one hand, the physician may be concerned about nonmaleficence. Because medical records may not be safe from inappropriate disclosure despite federal and state privacy protections, the patient may experience real harms—such as job loss unrelated to workplace performance issues, eviction from public housing, or termination of insurance—if a diagnosis of dependency is recorded in the medical record. Although legal redress for harms that result from inappropriate transfer of information may be possible, it may not be feasible for a woman in straitened circumstances. On the other hand, the principle of beneficence often requires disclosure of information needed by the medical team to provide appropriate medical care. Without this disclosure, a physician treating the patient for a problem unrelated to pregnancy or an emergency room physician seeing the patient for the first time may miss a major complication related to substance abuse. Concerns about protection of confidentiality and nonmaleficence can be addressed most appropriately by including only medically necessary, accurate information in the medical record and informing the patient about the purpose of any disclosure.

Responsibilities to Neonates

The use of illicit drugs and alcohol during pregnancy has demonstrated adverse effects on the neonate, and these children are subsequently at risk for altered neurodevelopmental outcome and poor health status (53). Detection and treatment are essential precursors of appropriate therapeutic intervention in the immediate setting. Early recognition of parental substance abuse also may lead to interventions designed to decrease associated risks to a child's physical and psychologic health and safety (26–31). Doing so may obviate the necessity for placement in an already overburdened foster care system (54). Underrecognition of prenatal alcohol and drug effects is common, however (55). A toxicology screen and scoring for craniofacial features suggestive of FAS should be performed by the neonate's physician whenever clinically indicated. According to the American Academy of Pediatrics' statement on neonatal drug withdrawal (56), maternal characteristics that suggest a need for biochemical screening of the neonate include no prenatal care, previous unexplained fetal demise, precipitous labor, abruptio placentae, hypertensive episodes, severe mood swings, cerebrovascular accidents, myocardial infarction, and repeated spontaneous abortions. Infant characteristics that may be associated with maternal drug use include preterm birth, unexplained intrauterinc growth restriction, neurobehavioral abnormalities, congenital abnormalities, atypical vascular incidents, myocardial infarction, and necrotizing enterocolitis in otherwise healthy term infants. The legal implications of testing and the need for maternal consent vary from state to state; therefore, physicians should be aware of local laws that may influence regional practice.

Biophysical testing, however, has major limitations (57–59). Both urine and meconium screens have a high rate of false-negative results because of factors related to the timing and amount of the last maternal drug use (for urine) and the failure to detect drug metabolites (for meconium). Hair is associated with a substantial false-positive rate because of passive exposure to minute quantities of illicit substances in the environment. Physicians and nurses often fail to recognize the physical manifestations of FAS (60). Maternal self-report of use or consent to testing, elicited using nonjudgmental, supportive interview techniques within a physician–patient relationship of trust, can thus provide the best information for guiding neonatal treatment and the best prognosis for family intervention. Maternal substance abuse does not by itself guarantee child neglect or prove inadequate parenting capacity (61, 62). Parenting skills programs, assistance with employment and housing issues, and access to substance abuse treatment have been shown to be successful support mechanisms for families of affected neonates, and these elements should be part of a comprehensive approach to substance abuse problems. If there is evidence to suggest the likelihood of neglect or abuse, referral to children's protective services may be indicated (63). A children's protective services referral should never be undertaken as a punitive measure, but with the aim of evaluating circumstances, protecting the child, and providing services to maintain or reunify the family unit if at all possible.

Special Issues for Girls and Adolescent Women

Use of alcohol and illicit drugs among youth is prevalent, and studies that included both male and female youth indicate that age of first use is decreasing. Youth who begin drinking at age 14 years are at least 3 times more likely to experience dependence (using criteria from the *Diagnostic and Statistical Manual of Mental Disorders*, 4th Edition) than those who delay drinking to age 21 years (64). Early onset of drinking increases the likelihood of alcohol-related unintentional injuries (65), motor vehicle crash involvement after drinking (66), unprotected intercourse (67), and getting into fights after drinking, even after controlling for frequency of heavy drinking, alcohol dependence, and other factors related to age of onset (68). A study among a large community sample of lifetime drinkers showed that those who reported first drinking at the ages of 11–14 years experienced a rapid progression to alcohol-related harm, and 16% developed dependence by age 24 years (69). Among youth aged 18–25 years surveyed in 2001, 22.8% drove under the influence of alcohol (1). The use of alcohol and illicit substances by youth and the impact of parental alcohol and substance use on children have adverse health outcomes (70, 71). Prevention (universal screening questions, brief intervention, and referral to treatment) has thus been described by leaders in obstetrics and gynecology and by pediatricians as a moral obligation (72). In 1993, the American Academy of Pediatrics developed substance abuse guidelines for clinical practice. These guidelines have now been refined and developed into competencies that provide practical direction for clinicians engaged in educating, supporting, and treating patients and families affected by substance abuse (73).

Confidentiality is as essential to the physician–patient relationship with children as it is with adults. Many state laws protect the confidentiality of minors with regard to substance abuse detection and treatment (73). Autonomy issues are of particular importance in the detection and treatment of substance abuse for adolescents, who are at a developmental stage in which it is a normative task to test new identities and engage in risk-taking in the process (74). The ACOG Committee on Adolescent Health Care lists the following key points concerning informed consent, parental permission, and assent (75):

- Concern about confidentiality is a major obstacle to the delivery of health care to adolescents. Physicians should address confidentiality issues with the adolescent patient to build a trusting relationship with her and to facilitate a candid discussion regarding her health and health behaviors.

- Physicians also should discuss confidentiality issues with the parent(s) or guardian(s) of the adolescent patient. Physicians should encourage their involvement in the patient's health and health care decisions and, when appropriate, facilitate communication between the two.

- The right of a "mature minor" to obtain selected medical care has been established in most states.

In a document about testing for drugs of abuse in children and adolescents, the American Academy of Pediatrics states that the goal of care is a therapeutic, rather than adversarial relationship with the child and, therefore, makes the following recommendations (76):

- Screening or testing under any circumstances is improper if clinicians cannot be reasonably certain that the laboratory results are valid and that patient confidentiality is ensured.

- Diagnostic testing for the purpose of drug abuse treatment is within the ethical tradition of health care, and in the competent patient, it should be conducted noncovertly, confidentially, and with informed consent in the same context as for other medical conditions.

- Parental permission is not sufficient for involuntary testing of the adolescent with decisional capacity.

- Suspicion that an adolescent is using a psychoactive drug does not justify involuntary testing, and testing adolescents requires their consent unless 1) the patient lacks decision-making capacity or 2) there are strong medical indications or legal requirements to do so.

- Minors should not be immune from the criminal justice system, but physicians should not initiate or participate in a criminal investigation, except when required by law, as in the case of court-ordered drug testing or child abuse reporting.

Guidance for Physicians

The health care system as it is currently constituted creates barriers to the practice of universal screening questions, brief intervention, and referral to treatment for alcohol and drug abuse. Because of a lack of medical school curricular content about addiction, physicians often are unfamiliar with screening procedures. Many institutions do not have appropriate protocols in place for intervention and referral. Time constraints, mandatory reporting laws, and lack of treatment resources may impede both screening and referral, and some of these problems may be beyond the ability of the individual physician to modify. Nevertheless, in fulfillment of the therapeutic obligation, physicians must make a substantial effort to:

- Learn established techniques for rapid, effective screening, intervention, and referral, and practice universal screening questions, brief intervention, and referral to treatment in order to provide benefit and do no harm. Where possible, create a team approach to deal with barriers of time limitations, using the skills of social workers, nurses, and peer educators for universal screening questions, brief intervention, and referral to treatment. Use external resources (ie, hospital social worker, health department, addiction specialist) to develop a list of treatment resources.

- Treat the patient with a substance abuse problem with dignity and respect in order to form a therapeutic alliance.

- Protect confidentiality and the integrity of the physician–patient relationship wherever possible within the requirements of legal obligations, and communicate honestly and directly with patients about what information can and cannot be protected. In states where there are laws requiring disclosure, inform patients in advance about specific items for which disclosure is mandated.

- Recognize that the most effective safeguard for children is treatment for family members who have a substance abuse problem.

- Balance competing obligations carefully, consulting with other physicians or an ethicist if troubling situations arise.

- Participate, whenever possible, in the policy process at institutional, state, and national levels as an advocate for the health care needs of patients.

- Consider whether elements of personal beliefs and values may be resulting in biases in medical practice. Be aware that some physicians minimize the universality and impact of alcohol or prescription drug abuse to protect against evaluating their own alcohol or substance abuse problems. A physician who has questions about his or her own use should seek help.

Conclusion

Substance abuse is a common medical condition that can have devastating physical and emotional consequences for women and their children. The traditional role of healer, the contemporary role of medical expert, and the newer role of primary care physician all require obstetrician–gynecologists to develop an evidence-supported knowledge base about methods for detection and treatment of substance abuse. The close working relationship between the physician and the patient that is both a goal of care and a means to improved health outcomes offers tremendous potential to influence patients' lifestyles positively. Despite this relationship, physicians seldom practice universal screening because of a lack of appreciation of prevalence, misunderstandings about treatment success rates, unfamiliarity with treatment resources, and inadequate knowledge about sex differences in presentation and the course of the disease. However, common barriers to universal screening questions, brief intervention, and referral to treatment can and should be addressed. Physicians have an ethical obligation to learn and use techniques for universal screening questions, brief intervention, and referral to treatment in order to provide patients and their families with medical care that is state-of-the-art, comprehensive, and effective.

References

1. Substance Abuse and Mental Health Services Administration. Results from the 2001 National Household Survey on Drug Abuse: volume I. Summary of national findings. Rockville (MD): SAMHSA; 2002.
2. Smith WB, Weisner C. Women and alcohol problems: a critical analysis of the literature and unanswered questions. Alcohol Clin Exp Res 2000;24:1320–1.
3. National Institute on Alcohol Abuse and Alcoholism. Fetal alcohol exposure and the brain. Alcohol Alert 2000; 50:1–6.
4. American Academy of Pediatrics. Committee on Substance Abuse and Committee on Children with Disabilities. Fetal alcohol syndrome and alcohol-related neurodevelopmental disorders. Pediatrics 2000;106:358–61.
5. Office of National Drug Control Policy. The economic costs of drug abuse in the United States, 1992–1998. Washington, DC: Executive Office of the President; 2001. Publication No. NCJ-190636.
6. Amaro H, Fried LE, Cabral H, Zuckerman B. Violence during pregnancy and substance abuse. Am J Public Health 1990;80:575–9.
7. Hutchins E, DiPietro J. Psychosocial risk factors associated with cocaine use during pregnancy: a case-control study. Obstet Gynecol 1997;90:142–7.
8. Substance Abuse and Mental Health Services Administration. Enhancing motivation for change in substance abuse. Treatment Improvement Protocol (TIP) series; 35. Rockville (MD): SAMHSA; 1999.
9. McLellan AT, Lewis DC, O'Brien CP, Kleber HD. Drug dependence, a chronic medical illness: implications for treatment, insurance, and outcomes evaluation. JAMA 2000;284:1689–95.
10. Bien TH, Miller WR, Tonigan JS. Brief interventions for alcohol problems: a review. Addiction 1993;88:315–35.
11. Fleming MF, Mundt MP, French MT, Manwell LB, Stauffacher EA, Barry KL. Benefit-cost analysis of brief physician advice with problem drinkers in primary care settings. Med Care 2000;38:7–18.
12. Blum LN, Nielsen NH, Riggs JA. Alcoholism and alcohol abuse among women: report of the Council on Scientific Affairs. American Medical Association. J Womens Health 1998;7:861–71.
13. Hubbard RL, French MT. New perspectives on the benefit-cost and cost-effectiveness of drug abuse treatment. NIDA Res Monogr 1991;113:94–113.
14. Chez RA, Andres RL, Chazotte C, Ling FW. Illicit drug use and dependence in women: a slide lecture presentation. Washington, DC: American College of Obstetricians and Gynecologists; 2002. Available at: http://www.acog.org/from_home/departments/underserved/DependenceinWomen.ppt. Retrieved October 27, 2003.
15. Fleming MF, Barry KL. The effectiveness of alcoholism screening in an ambulatory care setting. J Stud Alcohol 1991;52:33–6.
16. Wilson L, Kahan M, Liu E, Brewster JM, Sobell MB, Sobell LC. Physician behavior towards male and female problem drinkers: a controlled study using simulated patients. J Addict Dis 2002;21:87–99.
17. Volk RJ, Steinbauer JR, Cantor SB. Patient factors influencing variation in the use of preventive interventions for alcohol abuse by primary care physicians. J Stud Alcohol 1996;57:203–9.
18. Gearhart JG, Beebe DK, Milhorn HT, Meeks GR. Alcoholism in women. Am Fam Physician 1991;44:907–13.
19. Gomberg ES. Women and alcohol: use and abuse. J Nerv Ment Dis 1993;181:211–9.
20. Marcenko MO, Spense M. Social and psychological correlates of substance abuse among pregnant women. Soc Work Res 1995;19:103–9.
21. Abel EL, Kruger ML, Friedl J. How do physicians define "light," "moderate" and "heavy" drinking? Alcohol Clin Exp Res 1998;22:979–84.
22. National Institute on Drug Abuse. Mind over matter: the brain's response to drugs. Rockville (MD): NIDA; 1997. Available at: http://www.drugabuse.gov/MOM/MOMindex.html. Retrieved October 27, 2003.

23. Chang G, Goetz MA, Wilkins-Haug L, Berman S. A brief intervention for prenatal alcohol use: an in-depth look. J Subst Abuse Treat 2000;18:365–9.

24. Bernstein E, Bernstein J, Levenson S. Project ASSERT: an ED-based intervention to increase access to primary care, preventive services, and the substance abuse treatment system. Ann Emerg Med 1997;30:181–9.

25. Manwell LB, Fleming MF, Mundt MP, Stauffacher EA, Barry KL. Treatment of problem alcohol use in women of childbearing age: results of a brief intervention trial. Alcohol Clin Exp Res 2000;24:1517–24.

26. Rosensweig MA. Reflections on the Center for Substance Abuse Prevention's pregnant and postpartum women and their infants program. Womens Health Issues 1998; 8:206–7.

27. Whiteside-Mansell L, Crone CC, Conners NA. The development and evaluation of an alcohol and drug prevention and treatment program for women and children: The AR-CARES program. J Subst Abuse Treat 1999;16:265–75.

28. Ingersoll K, Floyd L, Sobell M, Velasquez MM. Reducing the risk of alcohol-exposed pregnancies: a study of a motivational intervention in community settings. Project CHOICES Intervention Research Group. Pediatrics 2003;111:1131–5.

29. Metsch LR, Wolfe HP, Fewell R, McCoy CB, Elwood WN, Wohler-Torres B, et al. Treating substance-using women and their children in public housing: preliminary evaluation findings. Child Welfare 2001;80:199–200.

30. Armstrong MA, Gonzales Osejo V, Lieberman L, Carpenter DM, Pantoja PM, Escobar GJ. Perinatal substance abuse intervention in obstetric clinics decreases adverse neonatal outcomes. J Perinatol 2003;23:3–9.

31. Peterson L, Gable S, Saldana L. Treatment of maternal addiction to prevent child abuse and neglect. Addict Behav 1996;21:789–801.

32. Boyd CJ, Guthrie B. Women, their significant others, and crack cocaine. Am J Addict 1996;5:156–66.

33. Ehrmin JT. Unresolved feelings of guilt and shame in the maternal role with substance-dependent African American women. J Nurs Scholarsh 2001;33:47–52.

34. Chang G, Wilkins-Haug L, Berman S, Goetz MA, Behr H, Hiley A. Alcohol use and pregnancy: improving identification. Obstet Gynecol 1998;91:892–8.

35. Cherpitel CJ. Screening in alcohol problems in the emergency department. Ann Emerg Med 1995;26:158–66.

36. Berenson AB, Weimann CM, Wilkinson GS, Jones WA, Anderson GD. Perinatal morbidity associated with violence experienced by pregnant women. Am J Obstet Gynecol 1994;170:1760–6; discussion 1766–9.

37. Sheehan TJ. Stress and low birth weight: a structural modeling approach using real life stressors. Soc Sci Med 1998;47:1503–12.

38. Poland ML, Dombrowski MP, Ager JW, Sokol RJ. Punishing pregnant drug users: enhancing the flight from care. Drug Alcohol Depend 1993;31:199–203.

39. American Academy of Pediatrics, American College of Obstetricians and Gynecologists. Guidelines for perinatal care. 5th ed. Elk Grove Village (IL): AAP; Washington, DC: ACOG; 2003.

40. Diekman ST, Floyd RL, Decoufle P, Schulkin J, Ebrahim SH, Sokol R. A survey of obstetrician–gynecologists on their patients' alcohol use during pregnancy. Obstet Gynecol 2000;95:756–63.

41. American College of Obstetricians and Gynecologists. Ethical decision making in obstetrics and gynecology. In: Ethics in obstetrics and gynecology. 2nd ed. Washington, DC: ACOG; 2004. p. 3–8.

42. Abel EL, Kruger M. Physician attitudes concerning legal coercion of pregnant alcohol and drug abusers. Am J Obstet Gynecol 2002;186:768–72.

43. Drug exposed infants: recommendations. Center for the Future of Children. Future Child 1991;1:8–9.

44. Rydell CP, Everingham SS. Controlling cocaine: supply versus demand programs. Santa Monica (CA): RAND; 1994.

45. Svikis DS, Golden AS, Huggins GR, Pickens RW, McCaul ME, Velez ML, et al. Cost-effectiveness of treatment for drug-abusing pregnant women. Drug Alcohol Depend 1997;45:105–13.

46. Paltrow LM. Punishing women for their behavior during pregnancy: an approach that undermines the health of women and children. In: Wetherington CL, Roman AB, editors. Drug addiction research and the health of women. Bethesda (MD): National Institute on Drug Abuse; 1998. p. 467–501. Available at: http://www.nida.nih.gov/PDF/DARHW/467-502_Paltrow.pdf. Retrieved January 22, 2004.

47. OLMSTEAD v U.S., 277 U.S. 438 (1928).

48. Gostin LO. The rights of pregnant women: the Supreme Court and drug testing. Hastings Cent Rep 2001;31:8–9.

49. Ferguson v. City of Charleston, 532 U.S. 67 (2001).

50. Nelson LJ, Marshall MF. Ethical and legal analyses of three coercive policies aimed at substance abuse by pregnant women (#030790). Robert Wood Johnson Foundation, 1998.

51. Frank DA, Brown J, Johnson S, Cabral H. Forgotten fathers: an exploratory study of mothers' report of drug and alcohol problems among fathers of urban newborns. Neurotoxicol Teratol 2002;24:339–47.

52. Chasnoff IJ, Landress HJ, Barrett ME. The prevalence of illicit-drug or alcohol use during pregnancy and discrepancies in mandatory reporting in Pinellas County, Florida. N Engl J Med 1990;322:1202–6.

53. Wagner CL, Katikaneni LD, Cox TH, Ryan RM. The impact of prenatal drug exposure on the neonate. Obstet Gynecol Clin North Am 1998;25:169–94.

54. United States General Accounting Office. Foster care: health needs of many young children are unknown and unmet. Washington, DC: General Accounting Office; 1995.

55. Stoler JM, Holmes LB. Under-recognition of prenatal alcohol effects in infants of known alcohol abusing women. J Pediatr 1999;135:430–6.

56. Neonatal drug withdrawal. American Academy of Pediatrics Committee on Drugs [published erratum appears in Pediatrics 1998;102:660]. Pediatrics 1998; 101:1079–88.

57. Lester BM, ElSohly M, Wright LL, Smeriglio VL, Verter J, Bauer CR, et al. The Maternal Lifestyle Study: drug use by meconium toxicology and maternal self-report. Pediatrics 2001;107:309–17.

58. Millard DD. Toxicology testing in neonates. Is it ethical and what does it mean? Clin Perinatol 1996;23:491–507.

59. Ostrea EM Jr, Knapp DK, Tannenbaum L, Ostrea AR, Romero A, Salari V, et al. Estimates of illicit drug use during pregnancy by maternal interview, hair analysis and meconium analysis. J Pediatr 2001;138:344–8.
60. Lyons Jones K. Early recognition of prenatal alcohol effects: a pediatrician's responsibility. J Pediatr 1999;135:405–6.
61. Davis SK. Comprehensive interventions for affecting the parenting effectiveness of chemically dependent women. J Obstet Gynecol Neonatal Nurs 1997;26:604–10.
62. Smith BD, Test MF. The risk of subsequent maltreatment allegations in families with substance-exposed infants. Child Abuse Negl 2002;26:97–114.
63. MacMahon JR. Perinatal substance abuse: the impact of reporting infants to child protective services. Pediatrics 1997;100:E1.
64. Grant BF. The impact of a family history of alcoholism on the relationship between the age of onset of alcohol use and DSM-IV alcohol dependence. Results from the National Longitudinal Alcohol Epidemiologic Survey. Alcohol Health Res World 1998;22:144–8.
65. Hingson RW, Heeren T, Jamanka A, Howland J. Age of drinking onset and unintentional injury involvement after drinking. JAMA 2000;284:1527–33.
66. Hingson R, Heeren T, Zakocs R, Winter M, Wechsler H. Age of first intoxication, heavy drinking, driving after drinking and risk of unintentional injury among U.S. college students. J Stud Alcohol 2003;64:23–31.
67. Hingson R, Heeren T, Winter MR, Wechsler H. Early age of first drunkenness as a factor in college students' unplanned and unprotected sex attributable to drinking. Pediatrics 2003;111:34–41.
68. Substance Abuse and Mental Health Services Administration. The relationship between mental health and substance abuse among adolescents. Rockville (MD): SAMHSA; 1999. Available at http://www.samhsa.gov/oas/NHSDA/A-9/TOC.htm. Retrieved January 22, 2004.
69. DeWit DJ, Adlaf EM, Offord DR, Ogborne AC. Age at first alcohol use: a risk factor for the development of alcohol disorders. Am J Psychiatry 2000;157:745–50.
70. American Academy of Pediatrics: Committee on Substance Abuse. Alcohol use and abuse: a pediatric concern. Pediatrics 2001;108:185–9.
71. Fishman M, Bruner A, Adger H Jr. Substance abuse among children and adolescents. Pediatr Rev 1997;18:394–403.
72. Chasnoff IJ. Silent violence: is prevention a moral obligation? Pediatrics 1999;102:145–8.
73. Adger H Jr, MacDonald DI, Wenger S. Core competencies for involvement of health care providers in the care of children and adolescents in families affected by substance abuse. Pediatrics 1999;103:1083–4.
74. Donovan JE, Jessor R, Costa FM. Adolescent problem drinking: stability of psychosocial and behavioral correlates across a generation. J Stud Alcohol 1999;60:352–61.
75. American College of Obstetricians and Gynecologists. Health care for adolescents. Washington, DC: ACOG; 2003.
76. Testing for drugs of abuse in children and adolescents. American Academy of Pediatrics Committee on Substance Abuse. Pediatrics 1996;98:305–7.

ACOG

Committee on
Gynecologic Practice

Committee Opinion

Number 278, November 2002

Avoiding Inappropriate Clinical Decisions Based on False-Positive Human Chorionic Gonadotropin Test Results

ABSTRACT: Clinically significant false-positive human chorionic gonadotropin (hCG) test results are rare. However, some individuals have circulating factors in their serum (eg, heterophilic antibodies or nonactive forms of hCG) that interact with the hCG antibody and cause unusual or unexpected test results. False-positive and false-negative test results can occur with any specimen, and caution should be exercised when clinical findings and laboratory results are discordant. Methods to rule out the presence of interfering substances include using a urine test, rerunning the assay with serial dilutions of serum, preabsorbing serum, and using another assay. Physicians must decide whether the risks of waiting for confirmation of results outweigh the risks of failing to take immediate medical action. Patients should be notified if they are at risk for recurrent false-positive hCG test results, and this information should be included in the patient's medical record.

Clinical management of many gynecologic conditions has improved dramatically over recent decades through the development of very sensitive and highly specific assays for hormones, particularly human chorionic gonadotropin (hCG). These assays have revolutionized the management of ectopic pregnancy and gestational trophoblastic disease, which now have a substantially lower mortality rate as a result of the ability to quantitate circulating (serum) and urinary hCG.

With the technologic improvements, hCG assays are now capable of detecting the presence of a pregnancy before a missed menstrual period. It is vital to remember that, despite technical advances, the ability of laboratory measurements to guide the clinician appropriately in every circumstance is limited (1–3). The purpose of this Committee Opinion is to offer recommendations to better manage situations in which hCG assays may provide false-positive results.

Some individuals have circulating factors in their serum that interact with the hCG antibody. The most common are heterophilic antibodies. These are human antibodies directed against animal-derived antigens used

The American College of Obstetricians and Gynecologists
409 12th Street, SW
PO Box 96920
Washington, DC 20090-6920

12345/65432

Avoiding inappropriate clinical decisions based on false-positive human chorionic gonadotropin test results. ACOG Committee Opinion No. 278. American College of Obstetricians and Gynecologists. Obstet Gynecol 2002;100:1057-9.

in immunoassays (1, 4–9). Individuals who have worked as animal laboratory technicians or in veterinary facilities or who were reared on farms are more likely to develop heterophilic antibodies. Immunoassays of all kinds use animal antibodies. People with heterophilic antibodies might have unusual results in a number of different kinds of assays. However, because the animal antibodies are used in different amounts and with other reagents in each assay system, a person with heterophilic antibodies will not always have an unusual or unexpected result. Results can differ depending on the particular assay used.

Clinically significant false-positive results are rare. One report noted that 5 of 162 women studied had evidence of assay interference sufficient to provide misleading results (10). If results are misleading, they usually are seen with values below 1,000 mIU/mL. To rule out the presence of heterophilic antibodies or other interfering substances, several methods can be used:

- A urine test (either quantitative or qualitative) for hCG can be performed. Because heterophilic antibodies are not present in urine, if the urine test result is negative and the serum test result is persistently positive, interference in the serum immunoassay is confirmed if the serum value is ≥ 50 mIU/mL (3).

- The assay can be rerun with serial dilutions of the serum. Because heterophilic antibodies are directed to reagents in the immunoassay and not hCG, their interaction with the hCG curve will not be linear. Lack of linearity confirms assay interference.

- Some laboratories can preabsorb serum to remove heterophilic antibodies before performing the assay. If the result becomes negative after removal of the heterophilic antibody, interference can be confirmed (11).

There are other ways in which the amount of "true" hCG can be measured differently or even incorrectly by immunoassays. The size of the hCG molecule circulating in the blood of individuals may vary as a result of differences in the protein and carbohydrate structure of hCG. This type of variation is called *microheterogeneity* of hCG, and it sometimes can account for differences in measurements reported by different assays. Additionally, some individuals may produce aberrant forms of hCG that are not biologically active — or are other hormones entirely—that will cross-react with the hCG assays. Still others may partly break down circulating hCG into nonbiologically active forms that react differently with the various assay systems. In these circumstances, substances other than native, biologically active hCG may be recognized by the assay system. Repeating the hCG measurement in a different assay system can best detect this problem.

Wide variations between repeat runs of the same assay could result from serum factors interfering with the assay. Serial dilution of the specimen will be helpful in documenting nonlinearity and confirming the presence of interference.

Finally, inherent assay factors can result in false-positive hCG results. Repeat testing using a different assay system may confirm that the result was falsely positive if the result is now negative.

Patients with evidence of hCG assay interference should be notified that they are at risk for recurrent false-positive hCG assay results. These patients should be instructed to inform all future health care practitioners of this problem, and the information should be included in the patient's medical record.

In summary, modern assay methods have almost eliminated laboratory error. However, false-positive and false-negative test results can occur with any specimen. Caution should be exercised whenever clinical findings and laboratory results are discordant. Although false-positive serum hCG results are rare, if unrecognized, they may lead to unwarranted clinical interventions for conditions such as persistent trophoblastic disease. The physician must judge whether the risks of waiting for confirmation of results outweigh the risks of failing to take immediate action.

References

1. Cole LA, Kardana A. Discordant results in human chorionic gonadotropin assays. Clin Chem 1992;38:263–70.
2. Cole LA, Rinne KM, Shahabi S, Omrani A. False-positive hCG assay results leading to unnecessary surgery and chemotherapy and needless occurrences of diabetes and coma. Clin Chem 1999;45:313–4.
3. Rotmensch S, Cole LA. False diagnosis and needless therapy of presumed malignant disease in women with false-positive human chorionic gonadotropin concentrations. Lancet 2000;355:712–5.
4. Boscato LM, Stuart MC. Incidence and specificity of interference in two-site immunoassays. Clin Chem 1986; 32:1491–5.
5. Boscato LM, Stuart MC. Heterophilic antibodies: a problem for all immunoassays. Clin Chem 1988;34:27–33.

6. Check JH, Nowroozi K, Chase JS, Lauer C, Elkins B, Wu CH. False-positive human chorionic gonadotropin levels caused by a heterophile antibody with the immunoradiometric assay. Am J Obstet Gynecol 1988;158:99–100.

7. Weber TH, Kapyaho KI, Tanner P. Endogenous interference in immunoassays in clinical chemistry. A review. Scand J Clin Lab Invest Suppl 1990;201:77–82.

8. Berglund L, Holmberg NG. Heterophilic antibodies against rabbit serum causing falsely elevated gonadotropin levels. Acta Obstet Gynecol Scand 1989;68:377–8.

9. King IR, Doody MC. False-positive hCG by enzyme immunoassay resulting in repeated chemotherapy. Obstet Gynecol 1995;86:682–3.

10. Rzasa PJ, Caride VJ, Prokop EK. Discordant inter-kit results in the radioimmunoassay for choriogonadotropin in serum. Clin Chem 1984;30:1240–3.

11. Cole LA. Phantom hCG and phantom choriocarcinoma. Gynecol Oncol 1998;71:325–9.

ACOG

Committee on
Adolescent Health Care

Committee Opinion

Number 300, October 2004

The Committee wishes to thank S. Paige Hertweck, MD, for her assistance in the development of this opinion. This document reflects emerging clinical and scientific advances as of the date issued and is subject to change. The information should not be construed as dictating an exclusive course of treatment or procedure to be followed.

ISSN 1074-861X

The American College of Obstetricians and Gynecologists
409 12th Street, SW
PO Box 96920
Washington, DC 20090-6920

12345/87654

Cervical cancer screening in adolescents. ACOG Committee Opinion No. 300. American College of Obstetricians and Gynecologists. Obstet Gynecol 2004;104:885–9.

Cervical Cancer Screening in Adolescents

ABSTRACT: The American Cancer Society recently published a recommendation that cervical cancer screening should begin approximately 3 years after the onset of vaginal intercourse or no later than age 21 years. Once initiated, screening should occur annually for young women. The decision about the initiation of cervical cytology screening in an adolescent patient should be based on the clinician's assessment of risks, including 1) age of first sexual intercourse, 2) behaviors that may place the adolescent patient at greater risk for human papillomavirus infection, and 3) risk of noncompliance with follow-up visits. Patients and parents need to be provided with information about this new recommendation so they understand that there is still a need for preventive health care other than Pap testing. Additional research is needed to facilitate the provision of the best care for adolescent patients and avoid overtreatment of abnormal cervical cytology.

Background

The American Cancer Society (ACS) recommends that cervical cancer screening should begin approximately 3 years after the onset of vaginal intercourse or no later than age 21 years (1). Once initiated, screening should occur annually for adolescents (2). This recommendation is based on the consensus of a national panel of experts who reviewed evidence and concluded that there is little risk of missing an important cervical lesion within 3–5 years after initial exposure to human papillomavirus (HPV). Specific types of HPV (most notably HPV 16, 18, 31, and 45) are associated with nearly all cases of squamous cell cervical cancer (3, 4). The National Cancer Institute's Surveillance, Epidemiology, and End Results program indicates that there were no cases of cervical cancer in females younger than 20 years (5). The ACS further supports this recommendation by stating that screening less than 3 years after the onset of vaginal intercourse may result in overdiagnosis of cervical lesions, which often regress spontaneously, and that inappropriate intervention may cause more harm than good. The ACS recommendation states that it is critical for adolescents who may not need cervical cytology testing to receive gynecologic health care, including preventive measures such as sexually transmitted disease (STD) testing in sexually active patients.

Initiation of Cervical Cancer Screening in Adolescents

Adolescent females have a higher prevalence of abnormal Pap test results (atypical squamous cells of undetermined significance or ASCUS* and above) when compared with adult females (6, 7). However, the severity of lesions tends to be lower in adolescents (7). High-grade squamous intraepithelial lesions (HSIL) still do occur in adolescents. The highest reported prevalence of abnormal Pap test results with evidence of HSIL in adolescents is 18% (6). The decision about the initiation of cervical cytology screening should be based on the clinician's assessment of risks, including 1) age of first sexual intercourse, 2) behaviors that may place the adolescent patient at greater risk for HPV infection, and 3) risk of noncompliance with follow-up visits. Obtaining a complete and accurate sexual history is, therefore, critical.

Assessing Age at First Sexual Intercourse

According to the 2003 Youth Risk Behavior Surveillance Survey, 45% of female high-school students have had sexual intercourse; 62% of female 12th graders have had sexual intercourse (8). Age-specific data show the percentage of female adolescents who have had sexual intercourse increases steadily with age. Specifically, 24% of 15-year-old females, 38% of 16-year-old females, 51% of 17-year-old females, and 62% of 18-year-old females have had sexual intercourse (9). Therefore, most females are sexually active before reaching age 18 years. Non-Hispanic black females and Hispanic females begin sexual activity at younger ages than non-Hispanic white females (8, 9). One study found that only 51% of mothers of sexually active teenagers were aware of such activity (10).

One of the difficulties in caring for the adolescent gynecologic patient is that many adolescents, particularly those who begin sexual activity at a young age or experience abuse, are unlikely to acknowledge sex-

*According to the Bethesda 2001 System for the description of cytologic abnormalities, the epithelial abnormality ASCUS has been replaced by "atypical squamous cells" (ASC) with the subcategories "atypical squamous cells of undetermined significance" (ASC-US) and "atypical squamous cells cannot exclude HSIL" (ASC-H).

ual activity without sensitive and direct questioning (see box "Sexual History Taking"). Therefore, they may not be screened appropriately. The sexual history should include questions about all types of sexual behavior, age at first vaginal intercourse, history of sexual abuse, number of sexual partners, and recent change in sexual partners because these factors have been linked to HPV infection (1, 11–13). An up-to-date history should be completed at each gynecologic visit with an adolescent.

Risk Factors for Human Papillomavirus Infection

Some adolescents may be at increased risk of HPV infection (see box "Risk Factors for Human Papillomavirus"). Prevalence of HPV infection in sexually active young women ranges from 17% to 84%, with most studies reporting prevalence greater than 30% (14). Adolescent females may be more susceptible to HPV infection than adult females because of biologic or physical factors (ie, cervical biologic immaturity) (15–17). Those women who had first intercourse (voluntary or involuntary) at a young age, have a history of other STDs, or have had multiple sexual partners are also at higher risk of HPV infection or cervical intraepithelial neoplasia or both (1, 11–13). According to the 1995 National Survey of Family Growth, 46% of women aged 15–19 years who had sex in the past year had 2 or more partners during the year (18). Immune suppression is another risk factor for HPV infection (see box "Causes of Immunocompromised States"). Studies in women with HIV infection, who undergo dialysis, or who have had a kidney transplant, demonstrate that HPV detection is particularly common with immune suppression (19–22).

Difficulties in Follow-up for High-risk Adolescents

High-risk adolescents often have difficulty obtaining affordable health care. They are, therefore, more likely to receive episodic care and have difficulty in returning for routine follow-up care. In the adolescent, noncompliance with follow-up appointments for abnormal Pap test results ranges from 25% to 66% (23–27).

Abnormal Cervical Cytology and Its Overtreatment in Adolescents

The Pap test is a screening tool, not a diagnostic tool. Those patients with abnormal cytology should be counseled and monitored closely. It is important

---

Sexual History Taking

- Discuss confidentiality
  - —Inform the patient that they have a private and privileged relationship with you and identify any restrictions on the confidential nature of that relationship. For Instance, the physician should explain that if the patient discusses any risk of bodily harm to herself or others, confidentiality will be breached. The physician also should discuss any state or federal privacy laws that affect the confidential nature of the relationship. In addition, state laws may mandate the reporting of physical or sexual abuse of minors.
  - —Inform the patient that if you feel you need to talk to the parent about something that the patient has said, you will discuss that fact and what you plan to say with the patient first.
- Start with nonthreatening topics first and gradually move to more sensitive issues. Have all discussions about sexuality while the adolescent is dressed.
- Introduce the subject of sexual activity by explaining that you ask all of your patients these questions and why this information is important. Discussions should be appropriate for the adolescents' developmental level and should identify risky behaviors.
- Consider using 1 of the following questions to initiate the discussion of the patient's sexual history:
  - —Are you dating anyone?
  - —Are you intimate with anyone?
  - —Are you physically close with anyone?
- Move on to additional questions for clarification. The age of first vaginal intercourse, whether voluntary or involuntary, is critical for proper determination of Pap test recommendations.
- Questions need to leave room for coerced or nonconsensual sexual contact, including sexual violence, abuse, and incest.
  - —Did you choose to have sex?
  - —Has anyone forced you to have sex?

- Questions need to leave room for casual sex partners (who, for example, may not be perceived as "boyfriends").
- Don't assume heterosexual behavior. Establish the sex of partner or partners first. If the patient is heterosexual, consider the following questions:
  - —Many girls are concerned about sex. Some girls have vaginal sex…that is, the boyfriend puts his penis in her vagina… is this something that your friends have done? Have you ever done this or thought about doing it?
  - —Many girls your age have sex. They also have sex in many different ways. Some girls have vaginal sex, that is, the boyfriend puts his penis in their vagina. Has this ever happened for you?
- As you progress with the patient's sexual history, make sure you ask about oral and anal sex, and describe what you mean by this. Anal intercourse can occur among heterosexual adolescents. It may be used by some teenagers specifically to preserve virginity and protect against pregnancy, therefore deterring the use of barrier methods and increasing the risk for human immunodeficiency virus infection and other STDs.
- Questions need to be asked about the number of partners and STD and pregnancy prevention methods used to assess the patient's risks.
- While assuring confidentiality, the provider should encourage adolescents to discuss these issues with their parents. The provider can assist the adolescent in determining how and what to tell her parents about her sexual activity.
- Congratulate the patient for sharing the information with you as a demonstration of her ability to think about her sexual health and be responsible.

Modified from: Asking the Right Questions. STD/HIV Prevention Training Center of New England. Available at http://www.state.ma.us/dph/cdc/stdtcmai/section1.pdf. Retrieved June 14, 2004.

to avoid aggressive management of benign lesions because most cervical intraepithelial neoplasia lesions of grades 1 and 2 regress. There are no data pertaining to the overtreatment of abnormal cervical cytology. It is a concern because the surgical excision or destruction of cervical tissue in a nulliparous adolescent may be detrimental to future fertility and cervical competency. Therapy should not be a part of management in adolescents who have cervical intraepithelial neoplasia 1 (28). An acceptable option

is follow-up without initial colposcopy using a protocol of repeat cytologic testing at 6- and 12-month intervals with a threshold of atypical squamous cells for referral for colposcopy, or of HPV DNA testing at 12 months with a referral for colposcopy if test results are positive for high-risk HPV DNA (29). Cervical intraepithelial neoplasia 2 represents a significant abnormality that typically requires therapy. It can be managed in adolescents with either ablative or excisional therapy or observation (28).

Risk Factors for Human Papillomavirus

- Multiple sexual partners
- Male partner with multiple sexual partners
- History of other sexually transmitted diseases
- Early age of first intercourse (including cases of sexual abuse)

Causes of Immunocompromised States

- Human immunodeficiency virus infection
- Organ transplant
- Cancer chemotherapy
- Chronic steroid use for chronic renal or bowel disease
- Conditions such as lupus

Patient and Parent Education

The new ACS recommendation may be confusing to both adolescents and their parents. Many adolescent girls and their mothers are unaware of the difference between a Pap test and a pelvic examination for any other reason (30). Therefore, they could misinterpret this recommendation as stating that a gynecologic examination or other STD testing is not needed until 3 years after first vaginal intercourse or by age 21 years. In addition, there is concern that adolescents in need of counseling or screening regarding sexual activity may have used the previous recommendation for a Pap test at age 18 as a way to justify a visit to a gynecologist to their parents. Without this justification, it is possible that adolescents will receive less care. Patient and parent education is, therefore, critical. Education should include information about the need for preventive care exclusive of the need for cervical cancer screening and recommended timing for this care. It should be stressed that adolescents should visit an obstetrician–gynecologist before becoming sexually active. Data indicate that currently this is not the case. Most (79%) young women wait 1 month or more after their first intercourse to see a health care provider, with the median wait being 22 months after first intercourse (31). The American College of Obstetricians and Gynecologists recommends that the first visit to an obstetrician–gynecologist for health guidance, screening, and provision of preventive services should take place around ages 13–15 years. This visit is even more important in light of the new cervical cancer screening recommendations and is an ideal time to

begin to provide education about preventive care needs, including the need for STD testing in sexually active adolescents. This visit often does not include a pelvic examination, especially with the onset of urine-based STD screening options. Thereafter, annual preventive health care visits to a gynecologist are strongly recommended (32).

Need for Additional Research

There are limited data on the following issues pertaining to HPV infection in adolescents, and additional research in these areas is needed:

- There are limited data on the incidence of HSIL within 0–3 years after the first exposure to HPV. Based on currently available data, the average time between initial Pap test and HSIL detection is 20 months (7).

- There are limited data on the regression of low-grade squamous intraepithelial lesions and HSIL in adolescents (33). Confirmatory data are needed.

- Data on the progression of low-grade squamous intraepithelial lesions and HSIL in adolescents are lacking. Although not seen in the Surveillance, Epidemiology, and End Results program, international data show invasive carcinoma of the cervix occurs very rarely in adolescents (11).

- There are no data pertaining to the overtreatment of abnormal cervical cytology. Additional research is needed to determine the extent of this problem and appropriate ways to address it.

- Additional research is needed for better understanding of appropriate management of adolescents with cervical cytological abnormalities.

Obtaining additional data in these research areas will facilitate the provision of the best possible care for adolescent patients.

References

1. Saslow D, Runowicz CD, Solomon D, Moscicki AB, Smith RA, Eyre HJ, Cohen C. American Cancer Society guidelines for the early detection of cervical neoplasia and cancer. American Cancer Society. CA Cancer J Clin 2002;52:342–62.
2. Cervical cytology screening. ACOG Practice Bulletin No. 45. American College of Obstetricians and Gynecologists. Obstet Gynecol 2003;102:417–27.
3. Bosch FX, Manos MM, Munoz N, Sherman M, Jansen AM, Peto J, et al. Prevalence of human papillomavirus in cervical cancer: a worldwide perspective. International

biological study on cervical cancer (IBSCC) Study Group. J Natl Cancer Inst 1995;87:796–802.

4. Walboomers JM, Jacobs MV, Manos MM, Bosch FX, Kummer JA, Shah KV, et al. Human papillomavirus is a necessary cause of invasive cervical cancer worldwide. J Pathol 1999;189:12–9.

5. Reis LA, Eisner MP, Kosary CL, Hankey BF, Miller BA, Clegg L, et al, editors. SEER cancer statistics review, 1975-2001. 2002. Available at: http://seer.cancer.gov/csr/1975_2001. Retrieved May 19, 2004.

6. Mount SL, Papillo JL. A study of 10,296 pediatric and adolescent Papanicolaou smear diagnoses in northern New England. Pediatrics 1999;103:539–45.

7. Simsir A, Brooks S, Cochran L, Bourquin P, Ioffe OB. Cervicovaginal smear abnormalities in sexually active adolescents. Implications for management. Acta Cytol 2002;46:271–6.

8. Grunbaum JA, Kann L, Kinchen S, Ross J, Hawkins J, Lowry R, et al. Youth risk behavior surveillance - United States, 2003. MMWR Surveill Summ 2004;53(2):1–96.

9. Abma JC, Sonenstein FL. Sexual activity and contraceptive practices among teenagers in the United States, 1988 and 1995. Vital Health Stat 23. 2001;(21):1–79.

10. Blum RW. Mothers' influence on teen sex: connections that promote postponing sexual intercourse. Center for Adolescent Health and Development, University of Minnesota. Minneapolis (MN): 2002. Available at: http://www.allaboutkids.unm.edu/presskit/MonographMS.pdf. Retrieved July 19, 2004.

11. La Vecchia C, Fransechi S, Decarli A, Fasoli M, Gentile A, Parazzini F, et al. Sexual factors, venereal disease, and the risk of intraepithelial and invasive cervical neoplasia. Cancer 1986;58:935–41.

12. Moscicki AB, Palefsky J, Gonzales J, Schoolnik GK. Human papillomavirus infection in sexually active adolescent females: prevalence and risk factors. Pediatr Res 1990;28:507–13.

13. Moscicki AB, Hills N, Shiboski S, Powell K, Jay N, Hanson E. Risks for incident human papillomavirus infection and low-grade intraepithelial lesion development in young females. JAMA 2001;285:2995–3002.

14. Prevention of genital human papillomavirus infection. Centers for Disease Control and Prevention. 2004. Available at: http://www.cdc.gov/std/HPV/2004HPV%20Report.pdf. Retrieved April 14, 2004.

15. Moscicki AB, Winkler B, Irwin CE Jr, Schachter J. Differences in biologic maturation, sexual behavior, and sexually transmitted disease between adolescents with and without cervical intraepithelial neoplasia. J Pediatr 1989;115:487–93.

16. Shew ML, Fortenberry JD, Miles P, Amortegui AJ. Interval between menarche and first sexual intercourse, related to the risk of human papillomavirus infection. J Pediatr 1994;125:661–6.

17. Moscicki AB, Burt VG, Kanowitz S, Darragh T, Shiboski S. The significance of squamous metaplasia in the development of low grade squamous intraepithelial lesions in young women. Cancer 1999;85:1139–44.

18. Finer LB, Darroch JE, Singh S. Sexual partnership patterns as a behavioral risk factor for sexually transmitted diseases. Fam Plann Perspect 1999;31;228–36.

19. Fairley CK, Chen S, Tabrizi SN, McNeil J, Becker G, Walker R, et al. Prevalence of HPV DNA in cervical specimens in women with renal transplants: a comparison with dialysis-dependent patients and patients with renal impairment. Nephrol Dial Transplant 1994;9:416–20.

20. Moscicki AB, Ellenberg JH, Vermund SH, Holland CA, Darragh T, Crowley-Nowick PA, et al. Prevalence of and risks for cervical human papillomavirus infection and squamous intraepithelial lesions in adolescent girls: impact of infection with human immunodeficiency virus. Arch Pediatr Adolesc Med 2000;154:127–34.

21. Jamieson DJ, Duerr A, Burk R, Klein RS, Paramsothy P, Schuman P, et al. Characterization of genital human papillomavirus infection in women who have or who are at risk of having HIV infection. Am J Obstet Gynecol 2002;186:21–7.

22. Sun XW, Kuhn L, Ellerbrock TV, Chiasson MA, Bush TJ, Wright TC Jr. Human papillomavirus infection in women infected with the human immunodeficiency virus. N Eng J Med 1997;337:1343–9.

23. Cartwright PS, Reed G. No-show behavior in a county hospital colposcopy clinic. Am J Gynecol Health 1990;4:181–7.

24. Michielutte R, Diseker RA, Young LD, May WJ. Noncompliance in screening follow-up among family planning clinic patients with cervical dysplasia. Prev Med 1985;14:248–58.

25. Lavin C, Goodman E, Perlman S, Kelly LS, Emans SJ. Follow-up of abnormal Papanicolaou smears in a hospital-based adolescent clinic. J Pediatr Adolesc Gynecol 1997;10:141–5.

26. Massad LS, Anoina D. Colposcopic and cytologic findings among adolescents referred to two urban teaching hospitals. J Pediatr Adolesc Gynecol 1996;9:190–4.

27. Arora CD, Schmidt DS, Rader AE, Abdul-Karim F, Lazebnik R. Adolescents with ASCUS: are they a high risk group? Clin Pediatr (Phila) 2001;40:133–8.

28. Wright TC Jr, Cox JT, Massad LS, Carlson J, Twiggs LB, Wilkinson EJ. 2001 consensus guidelines for the management of women with cervical intraepithelial neoplasia. American Society for Colposcopy and Cervical Pathology. Am J Obstet Gynecol 2003;189:295–304.

29. Wright TC Jr, Cox JT, Massad LS, Twiggs LB, Wilkinson EJ. 2001 Consensus Guidelines for the management of women with cervical cytological abnormalities. ASCCP-Sponsored Consensus Conference. JAMA 2002;287:2120–9.

30. Blake DR, Weber B, Fletcher KE. Adolescent and young adult women's misunderstanding of the term 'pap smear' [abstract]. J Adolesc Med 2003;32:145.

31. Finer LB, Zabin LS. Does the timing of the first family planning visit still matter? Fam Plann Perspect 1998;30:30–3, 42.

32. American College of Obstetricians and Gynecologists. Health care for adolescents. Washington, DC: ACOG; 2003.

33. Moscicki AB, Hills N, Shiboski S. High rate of regression of low-grade squamous intra-epithelial lesions in adolescents [abstract]. Baltimore (MD): Pediatric Academic Society Annual Meeting; 2002.

ACOG

Committee on Obstetric Practice

Committee Opinion

Number 260, October 2001

Circumcision

ABSTRACT: The American College of Obstetricians and Gynecologists supports the current position of the American Academy of Pediatrics that finds the existing evidence insufficient to recommend routine neonatal circumcision. Given this circumstance, parents should be given accurate and impartial information to help them make an informed decision. There is ample evidence that newborns circumcised without analgesia experience pain and stress. If circumcision is performed, analgesia should be provided.

Some studies have shown potential medical benefits to newborn male circumcision; however, these benefits are modest. The exact incidence of complications after circumcision is not known, but data indicate that the rate is low, and the most common complications are local infection and bleeding. The current position of the American Academy of Pediatrics is that the existing evidence is insufficient to recommend routine neonatal circumcision. The American College of Obstetricians and Gynecologists Committee on Obstetric Practice supports this position. Given this circumstance, parents should be given accurate and impartial information to help them make an informed decision. It is reasonable for parents to take cultural, religious, and ethnic traditions, as well as medical factors, into consideration when making this decision. Circumcision of newborns should be performed only on healthy and stable infants.

There is ample evidence that newborns circumcised without analgesia experience pain and stress. Analgesia has been found to be safe and effective in reducing the pain associated with circumcision. Therefore, if circumcision is performed, analgesia should be provided. Swaddling, sucrose by mouth, and acetaminophen administration may reduce the stress response but are not sufficient for the operative pain and cannot be recommended as the sole method of analgesia. EMLA cream, dorsal penile nerve block, and subcutaneous ring block are all reasonable options, although the subcutaneous ring block may provide the most effective analgesia.

ISSN 1074-861X

The American College of Obstetricians and Gynecologists
409 12th Street, SW
PO Box 96920
Washington, DC 20090-6920

12345/54321

Circumcision. ACOG Committee Opinion No. 260. American College of Obstetricians and Gynecologists. Obstet Gynecol 2001;98:707-708

References

1. Circumcision policy statement. Task Force on Circumcision. American Academy of Pediatrics. Pediatrics 1999;103:686–693
2. Prevention and management of pain and stress in the neonate. American Academy of Pediatrics. Committee on Fetus and Newborn. Committee on Drugs. Section on Anesthesiology. Section on Surgery. Canadian Paediatric Society. Fetus and Newborn Committee. Pediatrics 2000;105:454–461

ACOG Committee Opinion

Committee on
Coding and
Nomenclature

Number 249, January 2001

Coding Responsibility

Physicians are responsible for accurately coding the services they provide to their patients. Likewise, insurers are obligated to process all legitimate insurance claims for covered services accurately and in a timely manner. It is inappropriate for physicians to code or for insurers to process claims incorrectly in order to enhance or reduce reimbursement. When either party engages in such a practice intentionally and repetitively, it should be considered dishonest and may be subject to civil and criminal penalties.

ISSN 1074-861X

The American College of Obstetricians and Gynecologists
409 12th Street, SW
PO Box 96920
Washington, DC 20090-6920

12345/54321

ACOG Committee Opinion

Committee on
Primary Care

The Committee wishes to thank
Ronald A. Chez, MD, for his
assistance in the development of
this opinion. This document
reflects emerging clinical and
scientific advances as of the date
issued and is subject to change.
The information should not be
construed as dictating an exclusive course of treatment or procedure to be followed.

**The American College of
Obstetricians and Gynecologists**
409 12th Street, SW
PO Box 96920
Washington, DC 20090-6920

12345/32109

Number 227, November 1999

Complementary and Alternative Medicine

In 1990, 34% of adults in the United States used complementary and alternative medicine (CAM). In 1997, 42% of adults in the United States and Canada
used CAM, and the use by women was 49%. This trend of increased CAM
use will continue as it is reinforced and supported by continuing media attention; intense commercial efforts by providers of CAM products and services,
including proprietary pharmaceutical companies; third-party reimbursement
for some CAM practices and products; and the increasing over-the-counter
access to CAM products in drugstores and supermarkets. The purpose of this
Committee Opinion is to provide an overview of CAM, to recommend that
physicians ask patients about their use of CAM, and to provide sources of
additional information about the subject.

The physician, in the role of patient advocate, has an ethical responsibility to promote and protect the patient's well-being. This function includes the
ability to engage in a dialogue that honors the patient's values and promotes
shared decision making. Inquiring about the patient's motivation for and use
of CAM and providing information on safety and effectiveness can be integral to this role.

Complementary and alternative medicine can be defined as those
systems, practices, interventions, modalities, professions, therapies, applications, theories, or claims that are currently not an integral part of the dominant or conventional medical system (known as allopathy in North America).
Importantly, over time some of the individual modalities do overlap with or
become integrated into Western medicine. The spectrum of CAM encompasses over 350 different techniques and treatments. These can be classified into
at least seven major categories:

1. *Mind–body interventions* include yoga, relaxation response techniques,
   meditation, t'ai chi, hypnotherapy, spirituality, support groups, and
   biofeedback.
2. *Alternative systems of medical practice* are exemplified by Traditional
   Chinese Medicine. Other systems in this category include homeopathy,
   ayurveda, naturopathy, chiropractic, Native-American medicine, and the
   various forms of acupuncture.

3. *Pharmacologic and biologic* treatments, a diverse and large category, includes folk medicine, medicinal plants, processed blood products, and autogenous vaccines.

4. *Herbal medicine,* another large category, is the use of botanicals with pharmacologic activity. A number of these substances have formed the basis of the Western pharmacopeia. Currently, the public's attention is focused on St. John's wort for depressive disorders, echinacea for upper respiratory infections, valerian for sleep disorders, garlic for hypercholesterolemia, and ginkgo biloba for circulatory disorders.

5. *Diet and nutrition* encompass the use of vitamins, minerals, and nutritional supplements in general, and cancer and cardiovascular disease diets in particular. Treatments include megadosing, elimination of or excessive intake of certain foods, vegetarian and macrobiotic diets, and diets associated with various physicians.

6. *Manual healing methods* include massage, chiropractic and osteopathic manipulation, and biofield therapeutics (eg, Reiki, polarity, reflexology, and therapeutic touch).

7. *Bioelectromagnetic applications* include the use of magnets for musculoskeletal and neurologic pain; low-frequency thermal waves in diathermy; nonionizing, nonthermal applications such as pulsed electromagnetic waves as now used in the treatment of bone fractures; and transcutaneous electrical nerve stimulation for pain relief.

Most patients who use CAM are self-referred and do not tell their physicians they are doing so. Thus, their medical record is incomplete, and the possibility of medical risk cannot be addressed. Patients can be asked questions similar to "Have you used or have you been considering other kinds of treatment or medications for relief of your symptoms or to maintain wellness?" Follow-up questions to a positive answer can include asking when she decided to use CAM, what results she was expecting, how she chose the method, and how it has worked for her. This information can then be documented in the patient's medical record.

Safety is the critical issue when a patient asks about the merit of using a CAM product or intervention. The potential can exist for both direct and indirect risks. These risks can include patient delay in or avoidance of seeking appropriate conventional treatment, a misdiagnosis, toxic reactions from ingested substances, and interference with the mechanism of action of a prescribed drug or treatment.

Over-the-counter herbal preparations and dietary supplements, such as those marketed to relieve menopausal symptoms, may be of particular concern to the obstetrician–gynecologist. As defined in the 1994 Dietary Supplement and Health Education Act passed by Congress and as opposed to prescription items, these products are not subject to standardized manufacture, supporting clinical data, or approval or supervision by the U.S. Food and Drug Administration. Thus, there can be uncertainty as to the identity of the active ingredient and the amount of its dose. Also, the chemical composition may vary from manufacturer to manufacturer and by lot number, and there may be adulteration without this being identified on the label. Some of these problems will be addressed with the new federal regulation requiring that dietary supplement ingredients are labeled in a manner analogous to food labels, increased legislated U.S. Food and Drug Administration authority for these products, and increased attention by the Federal Trade Commission to advertised claims.

Concerns about safety can be tempered for some CAM modalities. For instance, it is unlikely that homeopathic preparations, acupuncture, biofeedback, or prayer will be associated with direct adverse side effects. In contrast, intravenous hydrogen peroxide, chelation therapy, and megadosing of supplements can be toxic and dangerous. Accordingly, when informed that the patient is using CAM, her clinician can advise if there is supporting published research, warn about real or potential dangers, ascertain if it can be continued in conjunction with conventional treatment, and monitor for positive and negative effects over time.

Some patients will request a referral to a local alternative care provider. Any such referral should be made only to a state-licensed provider and at an arm's length relationship. All states license chiropractors, but not all license other CAM providers, such as naturopaths, acupuncturists, or massage therapists. Physicians should be aware of possible liability consequences of such referrals. If the referral itself is negligent because it is inconsistent with reasonable practice, the referring physician may be exposed to liability if the patient is injured by the subsequent treatment. Also, liability may arise if the referring physician supervises the CAM care, jointly treats the patient, or knows or should have known that the CAM provider is incompetent.

It can be anticipated that patients will continue to use CAM with or without physician referral. Accompanying this use is the public's expectation that health insurance plans will reimburse for CAM treatment. A growing number of third-party payers have responded by doing so under a variety of clinical guidelines. This willingness can result in conflict between physicians and CAM providers if important operational issues are not addressed. These issues include the creation of protocols and plans of care for specific diagnoses, procedures for monitoring and follow-up with finite clinical endpoints, evidence for safety and effectiveness, and identified criteria for referral to conventional care.

Each physician can determine to what extent he or she wishes to learn more about various aspects of CAM. There are a number of ways to obtain information. Clinical studies in peer-reviewed, conventional medical journals now appear on a regular basis. In addition to continuing medical education courses, there are peer-reviewed medical journals, textbooks, and newsletters devoted to the subject. Computer databases and webpages specifically oriented to CAM now are accessible by both physicians and patients.

In the coming years, it is probable that there will be a blending of conventional medicine with various CAM therapies as evidence-based research data support clinical decision making in patient care. This comprehensive approach may become known as integrated medical care.

Bibliography

Blumenthal M, ed. The complete German Commission E Monographs. Therapeutic guide to herbal medicines. Austin, TX: American Botanical Council, 1998

Chez RA, Jonas WB, Eisenberg D. The physician and complementary and alternative medicine. In: Jonas WB, Levin JS, eds. Essentials of Complementary and Alternative Medicine. Philadelphia: Lippincott Williams & Wilkins, 1999:31–45

Jonas WB, Levin JS, eds. Essentials of complementary and alternative medicine. Philadelphia: Lippincott Williams and Wilkins, 1999

National Institutes of Health. Alternative medicine: expanding medical horizons: a report to the National Institutes of Health on alternative medical systems and practices in the United States. National Institutes of Health, Workshop on Alternative Medicine, 1995; NIH publication no. 94-066

Newall CA, Anderson LA, Phillipson JD. Herbal medicines, a guide for health-care professionals. London: Pharmaceutical Press, 1996

PDR for Herbal Medicines. Montvale, NJ: Medical Economics Co., 1998

Segen JC. Dictionary of alternative medicine. Stamford, Connecticut: Appleton & Lange, 1998

Resources

Newsletters

Complementary Medicine for the Physician, W.B. Saunders Periodicals Customer Service, 6277 Sea Harbor Drive, Orlando, FL 32887-4800, (800) 654-2452

Alternative Therapies in Women's Health, American Health Consultants, PO Box 740056, Atlanta, GA 30374, (800) 688-2421

Alternative Medicine Alert, American Health Consultants, PO Box 740056, Atlanta, GA 30374, (800) 688-2421

HerbalGram, American Botanical Council, PO Box 144345, Austin, TX 78714-4345, (800) 373-7105

Web Sites

The National Library of Medicine (http://www.ncbi.nlm.nih.gov/PubMed/)

The National Center for Complementary and Alternative Medicine (http://nccam.nih.gov/)

The NIH Office of Dietary Supplements (http://odp.od.nih.gov/ods/)

The Richard and Hinda Rosenthal Center for Complementary & Alternative Medicine (http://cpmcnet.columbia.edu/dept/rosenthal/)

The American Botanical Council (http://www.herbalgram.org/)

HealthWorld Online (http://www.healthy.net/)

Quackwatch (www.quackwatch.com)

ACOG

Committee on
Gynecologic Practice

Committee Opinion

Number 322, November 2005

Compounded Bioidentical Hormones

ABSTRACT: *Compounded bioidentical hormones are plant-derived hormones that are prepared, mixed, assembled, packaged, or labeled as a drug by a pharmacist and can be custom made for a patient according to a physician's specifications. Most compounded products have not undergone rigorous clinical testing for safety or efficacy, and issues regarding purity, potency, and quality are a concern. Compounded hormone products have the same safety issues as those associated with hormone therapy agents that are approved by the U.S. Food and Drug Administration and may have additional risks intrinsic to compounding. There is no scientific evidence to support claims of increased efficacy or safety for individualized estrogen or progesterone regimens.*

Compounded drugs are agents that are prepared, mixed, assembled, packaged, or labeled as a drug by a pharmacist. Unlike drugs that are approved by the U.S. Food and Drug Administration (FDA) to be manufactured and sold in standardized dosages, compounded medications often are custom made for a patient according to a physician's specifications. One category of compounded products is referred to as "bioidentical hormones"; however, there is confusion over what this term implies. *Bioidentical hormones* are plant-derived hormones that are biochemically similar or identical to those produced by the ovary or body.

The steroid hormones most commonly compounded include dehydroepiandrosterone, pregnenolone, testosterone, progesterone, estrone, estradiol, and estriol (1). Bioidentical hormones made by a compounding pharmacist from a health care provider's prescription are available in various routes of administration, including oral, sublingual, and percutaneous or as implants, injectables, and suppositories. Examples of compounded hormones include Biest and Triest preparations. The name Biest (biestrogen) commonly refers to an estrogen preparation based on a ratio of 20% estradiol and 80% estriol on a milligram-per-milligram basis. A similar preparation, Triest (triestrogen), usually contains a ratio of 10% estradiol, 10% estrone, and 80% estriol. It is important to note that these ratios are not based on each agent's estrogenic potency but on the milligram quantity of the different agents added together (2). Purchases of compounded hormones are not typically reimbursed by insurance companies.

The American College of Obstetricians and Gynecologists
409 12th Street, SW
PO Box 96920
Washington, DC 20090-6920

12345/98765

Compounded bioidentical hormones. ACOG Committee Opinion No. 322. American College of Obstetricians and Gynecologists. Obstet Gynecol 2005; 106:1139–40.

Most compounded products have not undergone any rigorous clinical testing for either safety or efficacy, and issues of quality assurance regarding the purity, potency, and quality of compounded products are a concern. From June 2001 to December 2001, the FDA analyzed 29 product samples from 12 compounding pharmacies (3). The types of products varied, but examples include oral, injectable, pellet implants, and inhalation compounds such as hormonal products, steroids, and antibiotics. Although none of the compounded products failed identity testing, 10 of the 29 products (34%) failed one or more standard quality tests performed. Nine of the 10 failing products failed assay or potency tests, with all products failing potency testing demonstrating subpotent results; that is, the products analyzed contained less of the active ingredient than expected. In comparison with these results, the analytical testing failure rate for drug therapies approved by the FDA is less than 2%.

Although many advocates and compounders of bioidentical hormones recommend the use of salivary hormone level testing as a means of offering individualized therapy, hormone therapy does not belong to a class of drugs with an indication for individualized dosing. Individualized dosing is indicated when a narrow therapeutic window exists for a drug or a drug class. Such drugs include those with nonlinear pharmacokinetics, those that are renally eliminated as the active drug, some that are not metabolized during first pass through the liver, and those with clearly defined therapeutic and toxic concentrations based on large population pharmacokinetic studies of serum concentrations. Steroid hormones such as estrogen and progesterone do not meet these criteria and, thus, do not require individualized dosing.

There is no evidence that hormonal levels in saliva are biologically meaningful. Whereas saliva is an ultrafiltrate of the blood and in theory should be amenable to testing for "free" (unbound) concentrations of hormones, this has not proved to be the case (4). The problem with salivary testing and monitoring of free hormone levels is twofold: 1) there is no biologically meaningful relationship between salivary sex steroidal hormone concentrations and free serum hormone concentrations and 2) there is large within-patient variability in salivary hormone concentrations (5–9). Salivary hormone levels vary depending on diet, time of day of testing, the specific hormone being tested, and other variables (6, 7, 10–12).

Currently, the FDA requires manufacturers of products approved by the FDA that contain estrogen and progestogen to use class labeling (the black box warning) reflective of the findings of the Women's

Health Initiative. However, because compounded products are not approved by the FDA and have no official labeling (ie, a package insert), they are exempt from including the contraindications and warnings required by the FDA in class labeling for hormone therapy. Given the lack of well-designed and well-conducted clinical trials of these alternative therapies, compounded hormone products should be considered to have the same safety issues as those associated with hormone therapy agents that are approved by the FDA. They also may have additional risks intrinsic to compounding. There is no scientific evidence to support claims of increased efficacy or safety for individualized estrogen or progesterone regimens.

References

1. Drisko JA. Natural isomolecular hormone replacement: an evidence-based medicine approach. Int J Pharmaceut Compounding 2000;4:414–20.
2. Boothby LA, Doering PL, Kipersztok S. Bioidentical hormone therapy: a review. Menopause 2004;11:356–67.
3. Food and Drug Administration, Center for Drug Evaluation and Research. Report: limited FDA survey of compounded drug products. Available at: http://www.fda.gov/cder/pharmcomp/survey.htm. Retrieved June 15, 2005.
4. Marder MZ, Joshi U, Mandel ID. Estrogen concentration in human parotid and submaxillary saliva. J Dent Res 1979;58:2370.
5. Hardiman P, Thomas M, Osgood V, Vlassopoulou V, Ginsburg J. Are estrogen assays essential for monitoring gonadotropin stimulant therapy? Gynecol Endocrinol 1990;4;261–9.
6. Klee GG, Heser DW. Techniques to measure testosterone in the elderly. Mayo Clin Proc 2000;75 Suppl:S19–25.
7. Lewis JG, McGill H, Patton VM, Elder PA. Caution on the use of saliva measurements to monitor absorption of progesterone form transdermal creams in postmenopausal women. Maturitas 2002;41:1–6.
8. Meulenberg PM, Ross HA, Swinkels LM, Benraad TJ. The effect of oral contraceptives on plasma-free and salivary cortisol and cortisone. Clin Chim Acta 1987;165:379–85.
9. Wren BG, McFarland K, Edwards L, O'Shea P, Sufi S, Gross B, et al. Effect of sequential transdermal progesterone cream on endometrium, bleeding pattern, and plasma progesterone and salivary progesterone levels in postmenopausal women. Climacteric 2000;3:155–60.
10. Bolaji II, Tallon DF, O'Dwyer E, Fottrell PF. Assessment of bioavailability of oral micronized progesterone using a salivary progesterone enzymeimmunoassay. Gynecol Endocrinol 1993;7:101–10.
11. Raff H, Raff JL, Duthie EH, Wilson CR, Sasse EA, Rudman I, et al. Elevated salivary cortisol in the evening in healthy elderly men and women: correlation with bone mineral density. J Gerentol A Biol Sci Med Sci 1999;54:M479–83.
12. Zava DT, Dollbaum CM, Blen M. Estrogen and progestin bioactivity of foods, herbs, and spices. Proc Soc Exp Biol Med 1998;217:369–78.

ACOG

Committee on
Professional Liability

Committee Opinion

Number 309, February 2005   *(Replaces No. 236, June 2000)*

ISSN 1074-861X

The American College of Obstetricians and Gynecologists
409 12th Street, SW
PO Box 96920
Washington, DC 20090-6920

12345/98765

Coping with the stress of medical professional liability litigation. ACOG Committee Opinion No. 309. American College of Obstetricians and Gynecologists. Obstet Gynecol 2005;105:453–4.

Coping With the Stress of Medical Professional Liability Litigation

ABSTRACT: Obstetrician–gynecologists should recognize that being a defendant in a medical professional liability lawsuit can be one of life's most stressful experiences. Coping with the stress of medical professional liability litigation is an ongoing, complex process in which physicians often must struggle to regain a sense of professional mastery and control of their practices. Open communication with family members will assist in reducing emotional isolation and self-blame; however, legal and clinical aspects of a case must be kept confidential. Peer support and individual professional counseling can be of great benefit. Rapid intervention facilitates healthier coping strategies and can restore a sense of equilibrium and self-esteem during an unpredictable time.

The American College of Obstetricians and Gynecologists (ACOG) has long been concerned about the psychologic and emotional impact of medical professional liability litigation on physicians, especially because 76.3% of ACOG Fellows have been sued at least once in their careers (1). Defendant physicians may experience a wide range of distressing emotions and increased stress, which can disrupt their personal lives and the lives of their families, their relationships with patients, and their medical practices. Because a medical professional liability case in obstetrics and gynecology takes an average of 4 years to resolve (1), this stressful period can seem interminable for all involved.

Common responses to medical liability litigation include feelings of shock, outrage, denial, anxiety, guilt, shame, and despair. Coping with medical professional liability litigation is an ongoing, complex process in which physicians often must struggle to regain a sense of professional mastery and control of their practices.

Claims managers and defense attorneys often advise physicians not to speak to anyone regarding any aspect of the medical liability case. Nevertheless, physicians often need to express emotional responses to being sued. Literal adherence to the advice to "speak to no one" can result in isolation, increased stress, and dysfunctional behavior. Guidance on interventions for impaired or dysfunctional physician behavior is addressed elsewhere (2).

Such behavior may jeopardize family relationships and also may affect the physician's ability to function professionally and to represent himself or herself appropriately and effectively during a trial. Therefore, the physician is encouraged to inform family members of the lawsuit, the allegations, the potential for publicity, and any expected testimony while maintaining confidentiality. Children should be told about the lawsuit and their questions honestly answered, commensurate with their age and ability to process the information. Open communication with family members will assist in reducing emotional isolation and self-blame.

Certainly, legal and clinical aspects of a case must be kept confidential. An exception to this rule, however, might be made in the context of professional counseling. Any clinical aspects of a medical professional liability case that are discussed in counseling should be disclosed within the confines of a formal counselor–patient relationship to ensure the confidentiality privilege. Confidentiality may be lost if third parties are present.

Obstetrician–gynecologists should recognize that being a defendant in a medical professional liability lawsuit can be one of life's most stressful experiences. Although negative emotions in response to a lawsuit are normal, physicians may need help from professionals or peers to cope with this stress. Residents, as young physicians in training, may be particularly vulnerable to the psychologic and emotional upheaval that often occurs when named in a medical liability claim. State or local medical societies and medical liability insurance carriers often sponsor support groups for defendant physicians and their families. Support mechanisms for residents also may be available through residency program directors, departmental chairs, departments of risk management, or mentors. In the absence of such services, individual professional counseling can be of great benefit. Rapid intervention facilitates healthier coping strategies and can restore a sense of equilibrium and self-esteem during an unpredictable time.

References

1. American College of Obstetricians and Gynecologists. Overview of the 2003 ACOG Survey on Professional Liability. ACOG Clin Rev 2004;9(6):1, 13–6.
2. American College of Obstetricians and Gynecologists. Guidelines for women's health care. 2nd ed. Washington, DC: ACOG; 2002. p. 21–24.

Bibliography

American Academy of Pediatrics. Coping with malpractice litigation stress. In: Medical liability for pediatricians. 6th ed. Elk Grove Village (IL): AAP; 2004. p. 187–92.

Brazeau CM. Coping with the stress of being sued. Fam Pract Manag 2001;8(5):41–4.

Charles SC. The stress of litigation: do we still have something to fear? Prim Care Update Ob/Gyns 2003;10:60–5.

Charles SC. Coping with a medical malpractice suit. West J Med 2001;174:55–8.

Charles SC. How to handle the stress of litigation. Clin Plast Surg 1999;26:69–77, vii.

Hutchison JR, Hutchison S. The toughest part of being sued. Med Econ 1995;72(23):36–7, 41–4, 48, passim.

Sett KM. The impact of malpractice litigation on physicians. Forum 1998;19(4):13–5.

ACOG

Committee on
Gynecologic Practice

Committee Opinion

Number 323, November 2005   *(Replaces No. 164, December 1995)*

The American College of Obstetricians and Gynecologists
409 12th Street, SW
PO Box 96920
Washington, DC 20090-6920

12345/98765

Elective coincidental appendectomy. ACOG Committee Opinion No. 323. American College of Obstetricians and Gynecologists. Obstet Gynecol 2005;106:1141–2.

Elective Coincidental Appendectomy

ABSTRACT: Because of a lack of evidence from randomized trials, it remains unclear whether the benefits of routine elective coincidental appendectomy outweigh the cost and risk of morbidity associated with this prophylactic procedure. Because the risk–benefit analysis varies according to patient age and history, the decision to perform an elective coincidental appendectomy at the time of an unrelated gynecologic surgical procedure should be based on individual clinical scenarios and patient characteristics and preferences.

Elective coincidental appendectomy is defined as the removal of the appendix at the time of another surgical procedure unrelated to appreciable appendiceal pathology. Cases in which appendectomy may be indicated on the basis of appendiceal pathology are not addressed in this document.

The possible benefits of performing elective coincidental appendectomy include preventing a future emergency appendectomy and excluding appendicitis in patients with complicated differential diagnoses, such as those who have chronic pelvic pain or endometriosis. Other groups that may benefit from elective coincidental appendectomy include women in whom pelvic or abdominal radiation or chemotherapy is anticipated, women undergoing extensive pelvic or abdominal surgery in which major adhesions are anticipated postoperatively, and patients in whom making the diagnosis of appendicitis may be difficult because of diminished ability to perceive or communicate symptoms (eg, the developmentally disabled).

Most studies suggest that there is little, if any, increased morbidity associated with elective coincidental appendectomy at the time of gynecologic surgery, whether performed during an open surgical procedure (1–3) or during laparoscopy (4, 5). However, most of these studies are affected by methodological limitations such as retrospective design, small sample size, and lack of an appropriate control group. One large retrospective study using discharge data from all general hospitals in Ontario during a 10-year period highlights some of the challenges of addressing this issue with data from nonrandomized studies (6). This study compared in-hospital fatality rates, complication rates, and lengths of hospital stay between patients undergoing open primary cholecystectomy with and without incidental appendectomy. Initial results indicated a paradoxical reduction in morbidity and mortality after cholecystectomy when incidental appendectomy was performed. This most likely was because healthier, lower-risk patients are more likely to undergo an elective coincidental appendectomy. However, once multivariate adjustments were made to address these differences in patient characteristics, differences in complication rates were reduced or eliminated. Furthermore, when the study excluded high-risk subgroups, a consistently significant increase in complication rates among low-risk patients who underwent incidental appendectomy was found. These findings suggest that unmeasured or uncontrolled confounding or both make the interpretation of most nonrandomized studies of this topic difficult, but there is probably a small increased risk of nonfatal complications associated with elective coincidental appendectomy.

Given this presumed small but increased risk of complications, the primary debate surrounding elective coincidental appendectomy is whether the additional cost and morbidity incurred at the time of this prophylactic procedure outweigh the cost and risk of morbidity from developing appendicitis in the future. Because the estimated lifetime risk of appendicitis among women is less than 7% (7), a number of elective appendectomies will be required to prevent one case of acute appendicitis. Depending on hospital costs and physician reimbursement rates, the cost-effectiveness of this procedure will vary according to the clinical setting.

Although the incidence of acute appendicitis is greatest between the ages of 10 and 19 years and decreases with age (7), the risks associated with acute appendicitis increase with age. Therefore, the risk–benefit analysis changes according to patient age. A study involving open coincidental appendectomies in otherwise healthy women undergoing gynecologic procedures concluded that the greatest benefit was in patients younger than 35 years (8). The study also concluded that patients between 35 years and 50 years of age might benefit from elective coincidental appendectomy based on specific clinical circumstances. The data, however, did not support elective coincidental appendectomy for patients older than 50 years.

The benefit of elective coincidental appendectomy remains controversial and is still open to debate. It appears, from limited data, that women 35 years of age and younger benefit most from elective coincidental appendectomy. The decision to perform elective coincidental appendectomy at the time of gynecologic procedures should be based on individual clinical scenarios after a discussion of risks and benefits with the patient. In light of the low risk of morbidity based on current limited data, a patient's concern about developing future appendicitis may be considered. If there is a reasonable probability that the benefits outweigh the risks, based on age or history, elective coincidental appendectomy during a primary gynecologic procedure may be appropriate. Because there are clinical situations in which the benefits of an elective coincidental appendectomy may outweigh the risks, insurance companies should be encouraged to pay for this procedure in select cases.

Reference

1. Salom EM, Schey D, Penalver M, Gomez-Marin O, Lambrou N, Almeida Z, et al. The safety of incidental appendectomy at the time of abdominal hysterectomy. Am J Obstet Gynecol 2003;189:1563–7; discussion 1567–8.
2. Tranmer BI, Graham AM, Sterns EE. Incidental appendectomy?—Yes. Can J Surg 1981;24:191–2.
3. Voitk AJ, Lowry JB. Is incidental appendectomy a safe practice? Can J Surg 1988;31:448–51.
4. Chiarugi M, Buccianti P, Decanini L, Balestri R, Lorenzetti L, Franceschi M, et al. "What you see is not what you get." A plea to remove a 'normal' appendix during diagnostic laparoscopy. Acta Chir Belg 2001;101: 243–5.
5. Nezhat C, Nezhat F. Incidental appendectomy during videolaseroscopy. Am J Obstet Gynecol 1991;165: 559–64.
6. Wen SW, Hernandez R, Naylor CD. Pitfalls in nonrandomized outcomes studies. The case of incidental appendectomy with open cholecystectomy. JAMA 1995;274: 1687–91.
7. Addiss DG, Shaffer N, Fowler BS, Tauxe RV. The epidemiology of appendicitis and appendectomy in the United States. Am J Epidemiol 1990;132:910–25.
8. Snyder TE, Selanders JR. Incidental appendectomy—yes or no? A retrospective case study and review of the literature. Infect Dis Obstet Gynecol 1998;6:30–7.

ACOG Committee on Adolescent Health Care

Committee Opinion

The Committee wishes to thank Marc R. Laufer, MD; Joseph Sanfilippo, MD; and Jonathon Solnik, MD; for their assistance in the development of this document.

The American College of Obstetricians and Gynecologists
409 12th Street, SW
PO Box 96920
Washington, DC 20090-6920

12345/98765

Endometriosis in adolescents. ACOG Committee Opinion No. 310. American College of Obstetricians and Gynecologists. Obstet Gynecol 2005;105:921–7.

Number 310, April 2005

Endometriosis in Adolescents

ABSTRACT: Historically thought of as a disease that affects adult women, endometriosis increasingly is being diagnosed in the adolescent population. This disorder, which was originally described more than a century ago, still represents a vague and perplexing entity that frequently results in chronic pelvic pain, adhesive disease, and infertility. The purpose of this Committee Opinion is to highlight the differences in adolescent and adult types of endometriosis. Early diagnosis and treatment during adolescence may decrease disease progression and prevent subsequent infertility.

Incidence

It has been difficult to establish accurate prevalence rates of endometriosis in adult and adolescent women. Documented rates in adolescent patients undergoing laparoscopy for chronic pelvic pain range from 19% to 73%. Goldstein et al (1) reported a 47% prevalence of endometriosis found at laparoscopy in a prospective study of adolescent females with pelvic pain. Other studies have shown that 25–38% of adolescents with chronic pelvic pain have endometriosis (2, 3). In addition, it has been shown that 50–70% of adolescents with pelvic pain not responding to combination hormone therapy (such as oral contraceptive pills [OCPs]) and nonsteroidal antiinflammatory drugs (NSAIDs) have endometriosis at the time of laparoscopy (4, 5).

Endometriosis also has been identified in premenarcheal girls who have started puberty and have some breast development (6, 7). The occurrence of endometriosis before menarche contributes to the argument that one etiology for endometriosis lies in the theory of embryonic müllerian rests or coelomic metaplasia as opposed to retrograde menses. Based on the occurrence of early endometriosis, some authors have argued that "thelarche be recognized as a developmental benchmark, after which endometriosis is included in the differential diagnosis of chronic pelvic pain" (6).

It is common for adult women who have endometriosis to bring in their adolescent daughters for evaluation and early diagnosis. Data from the Endometriosis Association indicate that 66% of adult women reported the onset of pelvic symptoms before age 20 years. Forty-seven percent of these women reported they had to see a doctor five times or more before receiving the diagnosis of endometriosis or referral. As the age of the onset of symptoms decreases, the number of doctors having to be seen to reach a diagnosis increases. Specifically, an average of 4.2 doctors were seen for patients whose symptoms began before age 15 years compared with an average of 2.64 doctors for patients whose symptoms began between the ages of 30 years and 34 years. There are, on average, 9.28 years from the onset of symptoms to the diagnosis (8). Endometriosis is believed to be a progressive disease because the prevalence and severity of the stage of the disease significantly increase with age (9, 10). With early diagnosis and treatment, it is hoped that disease progression and infertility can be limited, but this remains to be proved with prospective research.

Presentation and Characteristics

The typical presentation of an adolescent with endometriosis may be different from that of an adult. One significant difference is that adolescents primarily seek medical attention because of pain rather than a concern for infertility. The most common symptom noted among published reviews is acquired or progressive dysmenorrhea, which was encountered in 64–94% of patients (4, 11). Other common symptoms included acyclic pain (36–91%), dyspareunia (14–25%), and gastrointestinal complaints (2–46%) (11). Adolescents found to have endometriosis most commonly present with both cyclic and acyclic pain (62.6%), as opposed to acyclic pain alone (28.1%), or cyclic pain alone (9.4%) (11).

In young women, pelvic pain associated with endometriosis often interferes with school attendance as well as physical and social activities. Prompt diagnosis and adequate therapy, therefore, may return normal psychosocial development and self-esteem, improve scholastic performance, and lead to a return to normal daily activities.

Diagnosis

History and Physical Examination

A thorough review of history and physical examination are necessary to assess a variety of differential diagnoses of pelvic pain such as appendicitis, pelvic inflammatory disease, müllerian anomalies or outflow obstruction, bowel disease, hernias, musculoskeletal disorders, and psychosocial complaints. Pelvic examination may be difficult, especially in patients who have not had vaginal intercourse.

When evaluating an adolescent for suspected endometriosis or dysmenorrhea, the clinician should aim to rule out a pelvic mass or a congenital anomaly of the reproductive tract. A bimanual examination may not be necessary to evaluate pelvic pain, especially in adolescents who are virgins. If a bimanual examination cannot be performed or is declined, a rectal–abdominal examination in the dorsal lithotomy position may be helpful to determine if a pelvic mass is present, and a cotton-tipped swab can be inserted into the vagina to evaluate for the presence of a transverse vaginal septum, vaginal agenesis, or agenesis of the lower vagina. If a bimanual examination is performed, the clinician should check for the existence of both diffuse and focal pelvic tenderness, and evaluate the pelvis for a displaced uterus or an adnexal mass. An ultrasound examination may be helpful in evaluating the pelvis of a young adolescent who declines a bimanual or rectal–abdominal examination.

Imaging Studies and Serum Markers

Ultrasonography and magnetic resonance imaging are helpful in evaluating anatomical structures, but are not specific for diagnosing endometriosis. An adolescent will rarely have a pelvic mass from an endometrioma or uterosacral nodularity. CA 125, although very sensitive, is not specific and, thus, is not helpful in the diagnosis of adolescent endometriosis. No data exist regarding the use of CA 125 to monitor the clinical progression or regression of disease in adolescents with endometriosis.

Empiric Therapy

If an adolescent younger than 18 years has persistent pain while taking combination hormone therapy and NSAIDs, endometriosis should be suspected and she should be offered a laparoscopic evaluation (discussion follows in section on "Surgical Diagnosis"). If, however, she is older than 18 years and had a negative assessment for an ovarian mass or tumor, she can be offered an empiric trial of gonadotropin-releasing hormone (GnRH) agonist therapy (12, 13). If the pain subsides with the use of GnRH agonist, then a diagnosis of endometriosis can be made. An empiric trial of GnRH agonist is not routinely offered to patients younger than 18 years because the effects of these medications on bone formation and long-term bone density have not been adequately studied. For patients younger than 18 years or who decline empiric therapy, diagnostic and therapeutic laparoscopy can be initiated. An algorithm for therapy is provided in Figure 1 (14).

Surgical Diagnosis

After a comprehensive preoperative evaluation and trial of combination hormone therapy and NSAIDs to treat dysmenorrhea, laparoscopy should be rec-ommended for diagnosing and treating presumed endometriosis in an adolescent. Laparoscopy can be safely performed in adolescents. At the time of surgical diagnosis, most adolescents have Stage I disease as classified by the American Society for Reproductive Medicine classification system (15). Goldstein et al commented that almost 60% of the

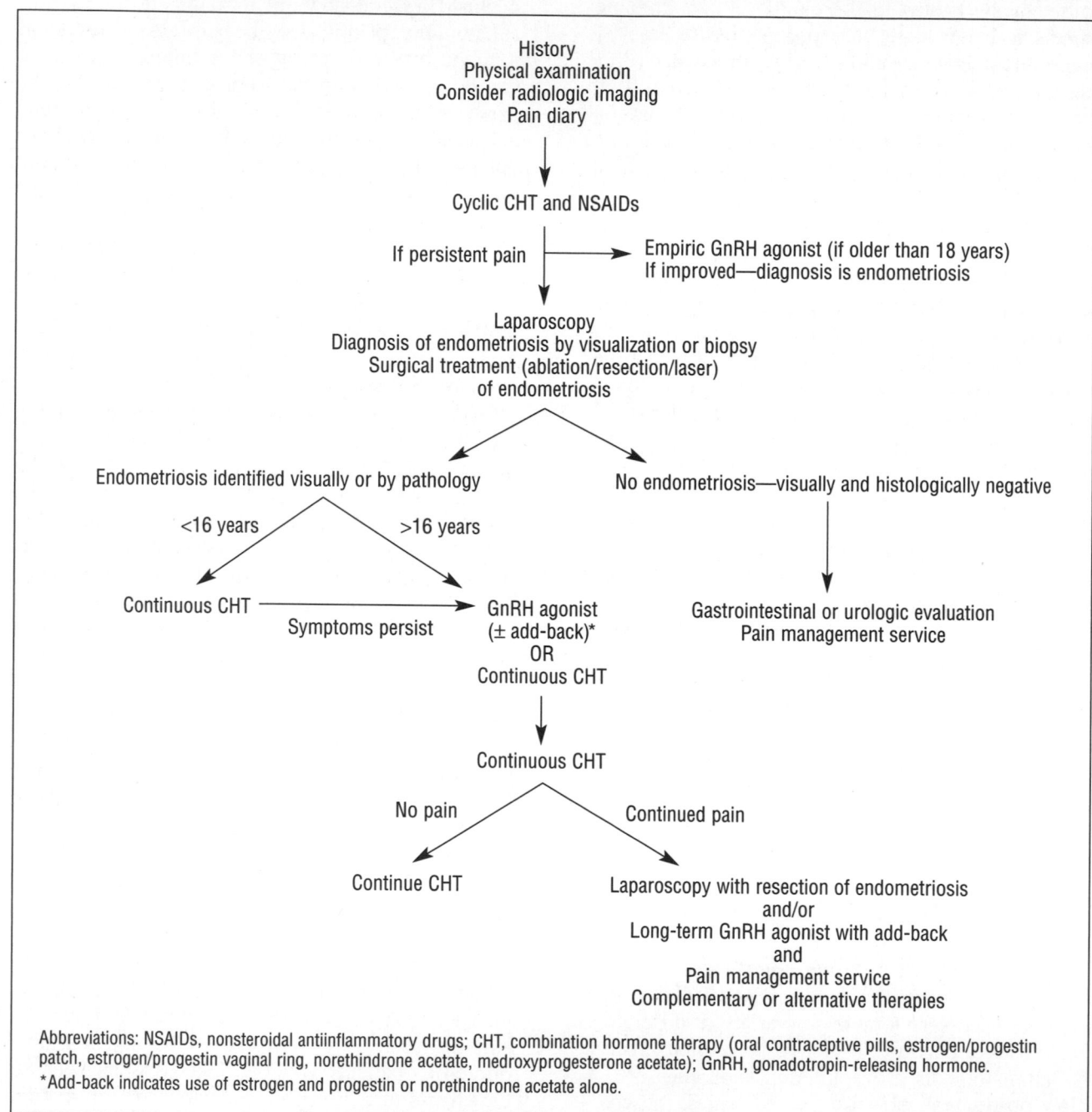

Fig. 1. Protocol for evaluation and treatment of adolescent pelvic pain and endometriosis. (Modified with permission from Bandera CA, Brown LR, Laufer MR. Adolescents and endometriosis. Clin Consult Obstet Gynecol 1995;7:206.)

patients in their cohort had Stage I disease (1), whereas 80% of the cases reported by other researchers had minimal to mild disease (4). Gynecologic surgeons who perform laparoscopy in adolescents with pelvic pain should be familiar with the typical lesions of endometriosis in adolescents, which tend to be red, clear, or white (15) as opposed to the powder-burn lesions seen commonly in adults who have endometriosis. The use of a liquid medium in the pelvis may facilitate the identification of clear lesions, which are very common in adolescents (11).

Müllerian Anomalies and Endometriosis

The development of endometriosis in adolescent patients has been associated with müllerian anomalies with outflow tract obstruction. The published incidence of anomalies of the reproductive system and associated endometriosis has been reported to be as high as 40%, but most studies quote a rate of 5–6%. The clinical outcome in patients with outflow tract obstructions has been reported to differ from those without such obstruction because regression of disease usually has been observed once surgical correction of the anomaly has been accomplished (16).

Treatment

The premise for treating the symptomatic adolescent is based on the concept that endometriosis has been shown to be a progressive disease without a known cure. A physician treating an adolescent with endometriosis should adopt a multidimensional approach and consider the use of the following components: surgery, hormonal manipulation, pain medications, mental health support, complementary and alternative therapies, and education.

Patients younger than 18 years with persistent pelvic pain while taking combination hormone therapy should routinely be offered a laparoscopic procedure for diagnosis and surgical management of endometriosis. The gynecologic surgeon must be familiar with the appearance of endometriosis in adolescents and should remove or destroy all visible lesions of endometriosis. Only procedures that preserve fertility options should be applied; oophorectomy or hysterectomy should not be offered to adolescents.

Long-term follow-up studies of treatments for adolescent endometriosis have not been performed. Current treatments for adolescents have been extrapolated and adapted from the literature of adult cases of endometriosis. The goal of therapy for adolescent endometriosis should be suppression of pain, suppression of disease progression, and preservation of fertility. Consequently, after surgery, all adolescents who have endometriosis should be treated with medical therapy until they have completed child bearing to suppress pain, progression of disease, and resulting potential infertility.

First-line treatment modalities should involve the use of NSAIDs and hormone therapy. Because red lesions have been shown to be active producers of prostaglandins, and adolescents with endometriosis typically report severe dysmenorrhea, NSAIDs may be used in conjunction with hormonal menstrual suppressive therapy to provide sufficient relief. Most pharmacologic agents bring about relief by inducing an anovulatory or a hypoestrogenic state or both. Continuous combination hormone therapy (OCPs, combination hormonal contraceptive patch, or vaginal ring) for menstrual suppression can be used to create a "pseudopregnancy" state, which was described more than 40 years ago (17). This method routinely has been promoted for adolescents who have endometriosis. Although this method may provide effective relief, the Cochrane Database Review 2003 provided data suggesting that further studies are needed to prove long-term benefits (18). Most clinicians advocate continuous use of combination hormone therapy to induce amenorrhea, but this modality can result in significant breakthrough bleeding. One randomized controlled trial compared a 28-day regimen with continuous combination oral contraceptives and found no increase in spotting days after 9 months of therapy, with fewer total bleeding days in the group taking continuous combination oral contraceptives (19). Thus, continuous use of combination hormone therapy is believed to be both safe and effective for adolescents with endometriosis-related pain and, thus, is the first-line hormone therapy for adolescents younger than 16 years with endometriosis. Gonadotropin-releasing hormone agonists are not offered as first-line therapy for adolescents in this age range.

Progestin-only protocols have been used for the treatment of adult endometriosis with mixed results. In a recent critical review, progestins were shown to be as effective as danazol or GnRH agonists (20). Common side effects include irregular bleeding and weight gain. Some studies suggest that these side effects are well tolerated (20), however in a data set of 3,751 women who have endometriosis, treatment with medroxyprogesterone acetate or depot medroxyprogesterone acetate was the least well tolerated and was the least effective in treating pain compared with combination OCPs, GnRH agonists, and pain medications (8). Furthermore, depot medroxyprogesterone acetate used for longer than 2 years has been shown to decrease bone density in adolescents (21, 22, 23). The U.S. Food and Drug Administration has warned against the long-term use of depot medroxyprogesterone acetate because of adverse affects on bone density (24).

Danazol, an androgenic and antiestrogenic agent, is extremely effective in treating symptomatic endometriosis in adults. Doses of 400–800 mg daily have been advocated for 6 months followed by continuous OCP use for maintenance suppression of the hypothalamic–pituitary ovarian axis. This choice of pharmacotherapy was more common in the 1980s, but the androgenic side effects have made this a poor option for adolescents.

Gonadotropin-releasing hormone agonists create a hypoestrogenic state by downregulating the hypothalamic–pituitary axis. Whereas these agents are greatly effective in the treatment of endometriosis-related pain in adolescents, their use alone (without add-back therapy described in the following paragraph) usually is limited to 6 months because of the resultant profound hypoestrogenic state and its subsequent effect on bone mineralization. This is a major issue for an adolescent who is accruing peak bone mineral density. Therefore, it has been suggested that this therapy not be offered as a first-line treatment for adolescents younger than 16 years (14). At 6 months, GnRH agonist induces a 5% loss in trabecular bone mineral density and a 2% loss in femoral neck bone mineral density in adult women. In a cross-sectional study, researchers collected bone mineral density test results of 265 females, aged 8–50 years (25). They determined that the majority of bone mass growth is achieved by age 20 years and that after the age 18 years, no significant differences in bone mass or bone mineral density were noted at most skeletal sites. This emphasizes that a drug-induced hypoestrogenic state could significantly affect peak bone mineralization that occurs during adolescence, particularly in females younger than 16 years.

Investigators have determined that to reduce the symptoms and bone loss related to a hypoestrogenic state, add-back therapy with norethindrone acetate (5 mg per day) or conjugated estrogens/medroxy-progesterone acetate (0.625/2.5 mg per day) can help preserve bone density (26, 27). Add-back therapy has been shown not to influence the primary therapeutic effect and resulted in less bone loss 12 months after cessation of therapy in adult women. There is some evidence in adults to suggest that immediate add-back therapy may result in even less bone loss (28). No data exist on the long-term effects of GnRH agonist use with add-back therapy in the adolescent population and, thus, it should be reserved for adolescents refractory to continuous combination hormone therapy (14, 29). Lifestyle modifications, such as adequate physical exercise and calcium and vitamin D intake, also are essential to maintaining proper bone health when taking GnRH agonists (with or without add-back therapy).

Aside from medical management, surgery also has proved to be an effective form of treatment for adult patients with pain (30). Surgery for the management of endometriosis-related pain is an important option for adolescents, but clearly, radical procedures (oophorectomy, bilateral oophorectomy, or hysterectomy) should be avoided in this age group, even in rare cases of severe endometriosis. A double-blinded randomized controlled trial compared laser vaporization of endometriosis and laser uterosacral nerve ablation with controls in 63 adult patients with proven endometriosis. At 6 months of follow-up, 63% of patients reported significant relief compared with 23% of controls (31). Patients with more advanced disease had better outcomes in pain management compared with those with minimal disease. At 1-year follow-up, 90% of those in the treatment arm who initially responded had continued pain relief (32). Among the symptomatic controls, an even distribution of patients was noted to have progression, regression, and maintenance of disease. Both new and recurrent disease was noted at second look. In a Cochrane review of these data, adult patients were almost 5 times more likely to benefit from surgical management of endometriosis compared with controls (33). One study demonstrated, in a prospective review of 643 patients with pain, or infertility, or both, that there was a significant relationship between pain and the depth of infiltration of the endometriosis implants (9). This study also confirmed that red implants were more common in younger patients and that the depth of invasion increased with age, suggesting that endometriosis is a progressive disease. The concept that endometriosis is a progressive disease supports the recommendation for long-term medical treatment for pain management of adolescent endometriosis and until a woman has completed childbearing. Long-term studies are needed to determine if medical treatment can inhibit the progression of endometriosis diagnosed in adolescents and preserve future fertility.

In addition to surgery and hormonal manipulation, complementary and alternative medicine has been used for the treatment of endometriosis. A multidisciplinary pain management service, including support groups and age-appropriate educational information, may be beneficial for an adolescent with chronic pelvic pain caused by endometriosis.

Summary

Endometriosis can be a debilitating disease that affects adolescent girls and young women. Pediatricians, adolescent health care providers, and gynecologists should recognize that thelarche and the presence of endogenous estrogen can be considered a developmental milestone and benchmark for inclusion of adolescent endometriosis in the differential diagnosis of postpubertal girls and young women with chronic pelvic pain. Adolescent patients typically present with progressive and severe dysmenorrhea, but also may present with acylic pelvic pain. Standard therapy (combination hormone therapy and NSAIDs) for dysmenorrhea should be initiated, and if symptoms do not resolve after 3 months, further evaluation for endometriosis is indicated. Prompt evaluation and consideration of the adverse effects of endometriosis is, therefore, essential in this age group.

Findings of the physical examination of adolescents may vary from the adult population because uterosacral nodularity and endometriomas are found in more advanced disease and, thus, are uncommon in adolescents. A bimanual pelvic examination may not be necessary for further evaluation of pelvic pain and should not be a requirement before the diagnosis of endometriosis and initiation of therapy for adolescents. It is important to evaluate the vagina for a possible obstructive anomaly and the ovaries for a possible ovarian mass. This can be accomplished with an evaluation of the vagina with a cotton-tipped swab and an ultrasound examination of the pelvis.

Endometriosis in adolescents typically presents as early disease (Stage I) and clear, red, and white lesions are the most common. Treatment should focus on conservative measures with surgical and medical interventions. Only procedures that preserve fertility options should be applied. Long-term endometriosis treatment may be required for chronic pain relief. Because there is no cure for endometriosis, long-term treatment should continue until desired family size is reached or fertility no longer needs to be preserved. A multidisciplinary team approach to the adolescent who has endometriosis may be the most rewarding for the adolescent, her family, and the clinician.

Resources

Endometriosis Association
(www.endometriosisassn.org)

The Center for Young Women's Health
(www.youngwomenshealth.org)

References

1. Goldstein DP, De Cholnoky C, Emans SJ. Adolescent endometriosis. J Adolesc Health Care 1980;1:37–41.
2. Vercellini P, Fedele L, Arcaini L, Bianchi S, Rognoni MT, Candiani GB. Laparoscopy in the diagnosis of chronic pelvic pain in adolescent women. J Reprod Med 1989;34:827–30.
3. Kontoravdis A, Hassan E, Hassiakos D, Botsis D, Kontoravdis N, Creatsas G. Laparoscopic evaluation and management of chronic pelvic pain during adolescence. Clin Exp Obstet Gynecol 1999;26:76–7.
4. Reese KA, Reddy S, Rock JA. Endometriosis in an adolescent population: the Emory experience. J Pediatr Adolesc Gynecol 1996;9:125–8.
5. Laufer MR, Goitein L, Bush M, Cramer DW, Emans SJ. Prevalence of endometriosis in adolescent girls with chronic pelvic pain not responding to conventional therapy. J Pediatr Adolesc Gynecol 1997;10:199–202.
6. Batt RE, Mitwally MF. Endometriosis from thelarche to midteens: pathogenesis and prognosis, prevention and pedagogy. J Pediatr Adolesc Gynecol 2003;16:337–47.
7. Marsh EE, Laufer MR. Endometriosis in premenarcheal girls without an associated obstructive anomaly. Fertil Steril 2005;83:758–60.
8. Ballweg ML. Big picture of endometriosis helps provide guidance on approach to teens: comparative historical data show endo starting younger, is more severe. J Pediatr Adolesc Gynecol 2003;16(suppl):S21–6.
9. Koninckx PR, Meuleman C, Demeyere S, Lesaffre E, Comillie FJ. Suggestive evidence that pelvic endometriosis is a progressive disease, whereas deeply infiltrating endometriosis is associated with pelvic pain. Fertil Steril 1991;55:759–65.
10. D'Hooghe TM, Bambra CS, Raeymaekers BM, Koninckx PR. Serial laparoscopies over 30 months show that endometriosis in captive baboons (Papio anubis, Papio cynocephalus) is a progressive disease. Fertil Steril 1996;65:645–9.

11. Laufer MR. Identification of clear vesicular lesions of atypical endometriosis: a new technique. Fertil Steril 1997; 68:739–40.

12. Ling FW. Randomized controlled trial of depot leuprolide in patients with chronic pelvic pain and clinically suspected endometriosis. Pelvic Pain Study Group. Obstet Gynecol 1999;93:51–8.

13. American College of Obstetricians and Gynecologists. Medical management of endometriosis. ACOG Practice Bulletin 11. Washington, DC: ACOG; 1999.

14. Laufer MR, Sanfilippo J, Rose G. Adolescent endometriosis: diagnosis and treatment approaches. J Pediatr Adolesc Gynecol 2003;16(suppl):S3–11.

15. Revised American Society for Reproductive Medicine classification of endometriosis: 1996. Fertil Steril 1997; 67:817–21.

16. Sanfilippo JS, Wakim NG, Schikler KN, Yussman MA. Endometriosis in association with uterine anomaly. Am J Obstet Gynecol 1986;154:39–43.

17. Kistner RW. The treatment of endometriosis by inducing pseudopregnancy with ovarian hormones. Fertil Steril 1959;10:539–56.

18. Moore J, Kennedy S, Prentice A. Modern combined oral contraceptives for pain associated with endometriosis. *The Cochrane Database of Systematic Reviews* 1997, Issue 4. Art. No.: CD001019. DOI: 10.1002/14651858. CD001019.

19. Miller L, Hughes JP. Continuous combination oral contraceptive pills to eliminate withdrawal bleeding: a randomized trial. Obstet Gynecol 2003;101:653–61.

20. Vercellini P, Cortesi I, Crosignani PG. Progestins for symptomatic endometriosis: a critical analysis of the evidence. Fertil Steril 1997;68:393–401.

21. Cromer BA, Blair JM, Mahan JD, Zibners L, Naumovski Z. A prospective comparison of bone density in adolescent girls receiving depot-medroxyprogesterone acetate (Depo-Provera), levonorgestrel (Norplant), or oral contraceptives. J Pediatr 1996;129:671–6.

22. Berenson AB, Radecki CM, Grady JJ, Rickert VI, Thomas A. A prospective, controlled study of the effects of hormonal contraception on bone mineral density. Obstet Gynecol 2001;98:576–82.

23. Lara-Torre E, Edwards CP, Perlman S, Hertweck SP. Bone mineral density in adolescent females using depot medroxyprogesterone acetate. J Pediatr Adolesc Gynecol 2004;17:17–21.

24. Black box warning added concerning long-term use of depo-provera contraceptive injection. FDA talk paper. Rockville (MD): U.S. Food and Drug Administration; 2004. Available at: http://www.fda.gov/bbs/topics/ANSWERS /2004/ANS01325.html. Retrieved December 8, 2004.

25. Matkovic V, Jelic T, Wardlaw GM, Ilich JZ, Goel PK, Wright JK, et al. Timing of peak bone mass in Caucasian females and its implication for the prevention of osteoporosis: inference from a cross-sectional model. J Clin Invest 1994;93:799–808.

26. Barbieri RL. Hormone treatment of endometriosis: the estrogen threshold hypothesis. Am J Obstet Gynecol 1992;166:740–5.

27. Surrey ES, Hornstein MD. Prolonged GnRH agonist and add-back therapy for symptomatic endometriosis: long-term follow-up. Obstet Gynecol 2002;99:709–19.

28. Kiesel L, Schweppe KW, Sillem M, Siebzehnrubl E. Should add-back therapy for endometriosis be deferred for optimal results? Br J Obstet Gynaecol 1996;103(suppl 14):15–7.

29. Lubianca JN, Gordon CM, Laufer MR. "Add-back" therapy for endometriosis in adolescents. J Reprod Med 1998; 43:164–72.

30. Abbott J, Hawe J, Hunter D, Holmes M, Finn P, Garry R. Laparoscopic excision of endometriosis: a randomized, placebo-controlled trial. Fertil Steril 2004;82:878–84.

31. Sutton CJ, Ewen SP, Whitelaw N, Haines P. Prospective, randomized, double-blind, controlled trial of laser laparoscopy in the treatment of pelvic pain associated with minimal, mild and moderate endometriosis. Fertil Steril 1994;62:696–700.

32. Sutton CJ, Pooley AS, Ewen SP, Haines P. Follow-up report on a randomized controlled trial of laser laparoscopy in the treatment of pelvic pain associated with minimal to moderate endometriosis. Fertil Steril 1997;68: 1070–4.

33. Jacobson TZ, Barlow DH, Garry R, Koninckx PR. Laparoscopic surgery for pelvic pain associated with endometriosis. *The Cochrane Database of Systematic Reviews* 2001, Issue 4. Art. No.: CD001300. DOI: 10.1002/ 14651858.CD001300.

ACOG

Committee on Obstetric Practice

Committee Opinion

Number 267, January 2002

Requests for authorization to make photocopies should be directed to:

Copyright Clearance Center
222 Rosewood Drive
Danvers, MA 01923
(978) 750-8400

ISSN 1074-861X

The American College of Obstetricians and Gynecologists
409 12th Street, SW
PO Box 96920
Washington, DC 20090-6920

12345/65432

Exercise during pregnancy and the postpartum period. ACOG Committee Opinion No. 267. American College of Obstetricians and Gynecologists. Obstet Gynecol 2002;99:171–173

Exercise During Pregnancy and the Postpartum Period

ABSTRACT: The physiologic and morphologic changes of pregnancy may interfere with the ability to engage safely in some forms of physical activity. A woman's overall health, including obstetric and medical risks, should be evaluated before prescribing an exercise program. Generally, participation in a wide range of recreational activities appears to be safe during pregnancy; however, each sport should be reviewed individually for its potential risk, and activities with a high risk of falling or those with a high risk of abdominal trauma should be avoided during pregnancy. Scuba diving also should be avoided throughout pregnancy because the fetus is at an increased risk for decompression sickness during this activity. In the absence of either medical or obstetric complications, 30 minutes or more of moderate exercise a day on most, if not all, days of the week is recommended for pregnant women.

The current Centers for Disease Control and Prevention and American College of Sports Medicine recommendation for exercise, aimed at improving the health and well-being of nonpregnant individuals, suggests that an accumulation of 30 minutes or more of moderate exercise a day should occur on most, if not all, days of the week (1). In the absence of either medical or obstetric complications, pregnant women also can adopt this recommendation.

Given the potential risks, albeit rare, thorough clinical evaluation of each pregnant woman should be conducted before recommending an exercise program. In the absence of contraindications (see boxes), pregnant women should be encouraged to engage in regular, moderate intensity physical activity to continue to derive the same associated health benefits during their pregnancies as they did prior to pregnancy.

Epidemiologic data suggest that exercise may be beneficial in the primary prevention of gestational diabetes, particularly in morbidly obese women (BMI >33) (2). The American Diabetes Association has endorsed exercise as "a helpful adjunctive therapy" for gestational diabetes mellitus when euglycemia is not achieved by diet alone (3, 4).

The cardiovascular changes associated with pregnancy are an important consideration for pregnant women both at rest and during exercise. After the

---

Absolute Contraindications to Aerobic Exercise During Pregnancy

- Hemodynamically significant heart disease
- Restrictive lung disease
- Incompetent cervix/cerclage
- Multiple gestation at risk for premature labor
- Persistent second- or third-trimester bleeding
- Placenta previa after 26 weeks of gestation
- Premature labor during the current pregnancy
- Ruptured membranes
- Preeclampsia/pregnancy-induced hypertension

Relative Contraindications to Aerobic Exercise During Pregnancy

- Severe anemia
- Unevaluated maternal cardiac arrhythmia
- Chronic bronchitis
- Poorly controlled type 1 diabetes
- Extreme morbid obesity
- Extreme underweight (BMI <12)
- History of extremely sedentary lifestyle
- Intrauterine growth restriction in current pregnancy
- Poorly controlled hypertension
- Orthopedic limitations
- Poorly controlled seizure disorder
- Poorly controlled hyperthyroidism
- Heavy smoker

---

and have small-for-gestational-age infants (6). However, other reports have failed to confirm these associations suggesting that several factors or conditions have to be present for strenuous activities to affect fetal growth or outcome (7, 8).

In general, participation in a wide range of recreational activities appears to be safe. The safety of each sport is determined largely by the specific movements required by that sport. Participation in recreational sports with a high potential for contact, such as ice hockey, soccer, and basketball, could result in trauma to both the woman and fetus. Similarly, recreational activities with an increased risk of falling, such as gymnastics, horseback riding, downhill skiing, and vigorous racquet sports, have an inherently high risk for trauma in pregnant and nonpregnant women. Those activities with a high risk of falling or for abdominal trauma should be avoided during pregnancy (9). Scuba diving should be avoided throughout pregnancy because during this activity the fetus is at increased risk for decompression sickness secondary to the inability of the fetal pulmonary circulation to filter bubble formation (10).

Exertion at altitudes of up to 6,000 feet appears to be safe; however, engaging in physical activities at higher altitudes carries various risks (11). All women who are recreationally active should be made aware of signs of altitude sickness for which they should stop the exercise, descend from the altitude, and seek medical attention.

Data regarding the effects of exercise on core temperature during pregnancy are limited (12, 13, 14). There have been no reports that hyperthermia associated with exercise is teratogenic.

first trimester, the supine position results in relative obstruction of venous return and, therefore, decreased cardiac output and orthostatic hypotension. For this reason, pregnant women should avoid supine positions during exercise as much as possible. Motionless standing also is associated with a significant decrease in cardiac output so this position should be avoided as much as possible (5).

Epidemiologic studies have long suggested that a link exists between strenuous physical activities, deficient diets, and the development of intrauterine growth restriction. This is particularly true for pregnant women engaged in physical work. It has been reported that pregnant women whose occupations require standing or repetitive, strenuous, physical work (eg, lifting) have a tendency to deliver earlier

---

Warning Signs to Terminate Exercise While Pregnant

- Vaginal bleeding
- Dyspnea prior to exertion
- Dizziness
- Headache
- Chest pain
- Muscle weakness
- Calf pain or swelling (need to rule out thrombophlebitis)
- Preterm labor
- Decreased fetal movement
- Amniotic fluid leakage

Competitive athletes are likely to encounter the same physiologic limitations during pregnancy faced by recreational athletes during pregnancy. The competitors tend to maintain a more strenuous training schedule throughout pregnancy and resume high intensity postpartum training sooner. The concerns of the pregnant, competitive athlete fall into two general categories: 1) the effects of pregnancy on competitive ability, and 2) the effects of strenuous training and competition on pregnancy and the fetus. Such athletes may require close obstetric supervision.

Many of the physiologic and morphologic changes of pregnancy persist 4–6 weeks postpartum. Thus, prepregnancy exercise routines may be resumed gradually as soon as it is physically and medically safe. This will vary from one individual to another with some women able to resume an exercise routine within days of delivery. There are no published studies to indicate that, in the absence of medical complications, rapid resumption of activities will result in adverse effects. Having undergone detraining, resumption of activities should be gradual. No known maternal complications are associated with resumption of training (15). Moderate weight reduction while nursing is safe and does not compromise neonatal weight gain (16). Finally, a return to physical activity after pregnancy has been associated with decreased incidence of postpartum depression, but only if the exercise is stress relieving and not stress provoking (17).

Conclusions and Recommendations

- Recreational and competitive athletes with uncomplicated pregnancies can remain active during pregnancy and should modify their usual exercise routines as medically indicated. The information on strenuous exercise is scarce; however, women who engage in such activities require close medical supervision.

- Previously inactive women and those with medical or obstetric complications should be evaluated before recommendations for physical activity during pregnancy are made. Exercise during pregnancy may provide additional health benefits to women with gestational diabetes.

- A physically active woman with a history of or risk for preterm labor or fetal growth restriction should be advised to reduce her activity in the second and third trimesters.

References

1. American College of Sports Medicine. ACSM's guidelines for exercise testing and prescription. 6th ed. Philadelphia: Lippincott, Williams and Wilkins, 2000
2. Dye TD, Knox KL, Artal R, Aubry RH, Wojtowycz MA. Physical activity, obesity, and diabetes in pregnancy. Am J Epidemiol 1997;146:961–965
3. Jovanovic-Peterson L, Peterson CM. Exercise and the nutritional management of diabetes during pregnancy. Obstet Gynecol Clin North Am 1996;23:75–86
4. Bung P, Artal R. Gestational diabetes and exercise: a survey. Semin Perinatol 1996;20:328–333
5. Clark SL, Cotton DB, Pivarnik JM, Lee W, Hankins GD, Benedetti TJ, et al. Position change and central hemodynamic profile during normal third-trimester pregnancy and post partum. Am J Obstet Gynecol 1991;164:883–887 [erratum in Am J Obstet Gynecol 1991;165:241]
6. Launer LJ, Villar J, Kestler E, deOnis M. The effect of maternal work on fetal growth and duration of pregnancy: a prospective study. Br J Obstet Gynaecol 1990;97;62–70
7. Saurel-Cubizolles MJ, Kaminski M. Pregnant women's working conditions and their changes during pregnancy: a national study in France. Br J Ind Med 1987;44:236–243
8. Ahlborg G Jr, Bodin L, Hogstedt C. Heavy lifting during pregnancy—a hazard to the fetus? A prospective study. Int J Epidemiol 1990;19:90–97
9. Artal R, Sherman C. Exercise during pregnancy: safe and beneficial for most. Phys Sports Med 1999;27:51–52, 54, 57–58
10. Camporesi EM. Diving and pregnancy. Semin Perinatol 1996;20:292–302
11. Artal R, Fortunato V, Welton A, Constantino N, Khodiguian N, Villalobos L, et al. A comparison of cardiopulmonary adaptations to exercise in pregnancy at sea level and altitude. Am J Obstet Gynecol 1995;172:1170–1180
12. Clapp JF 3rd, Capeless EL. Neonatal morphometrics after endurance exercise during pregnancy. Am J Obstet Gynecol 1990;163:1805–1811
13. Artal R, Wiswell RA, Drinkwater BL, eds. Exercise in Pregnancy. 2nd ed. Baltimore: Williams and Wilkins, 1991
14. Soultanakis HN, Artal R, Wiswell RA. Prolonged exercise in pregnancy: glucose homeostasis, ventilatory and cardiovascular responses. Semin Perinatol 1996;20:315–327
15. Hale RW, Milne L. The elite athlete and exercise in pregnancy. Semin Perinatol 1996;20:277–284
16. McCrory MA, Nommsen-Rivers LA, Mole PA, Lonnerdal B, Dewey KG. Randomized trial of the short-term effects of dieting compared with dieting plus aerobic exercise on lactation performance. Am J Clin Nutr 1999;69:959–967
17. Koltyn KF, Schultes SS. Psychological effects of an aerobic exercise session and a rest session following pregnancy. J Sports Med Phys Fitness 1997;37:287–291

ACOG Committee Opinion

Committee on
Obstetric Practice

Number 258, September 2001

The American College of Obstetricians and Gynecologists
409 12th Street, SW
PO Box 96920
Washington, DC 20090-6920

12345/54321

Fetal pulse oximetry. ACOG Committee Opinion No. 258. American College of Obstetricians and Gynecologists. Obstet Gynecol 2001;98:523–524.

Fetal Pulse Oximetry

ABSTRACT: The U.S. Food and Drug Administration recently approved the marketing of the Nellcor N-400 Fetal Oxygen Saturation Monitoring System, a fetal pulse oximeter. The American College of Obstetricians and Gynecologists Committee on Obstetric Practice cannot endorse the adoption of this device in clinical practice at this time because of concerns that its introduction could further escalate the cost of medical care without necessarily improving clinical outcome. The committee recommends that prospective randomized clinical trials be conducted to evaluate the clinical use of this new technology in conjunction with fetal well-being assessment.

Electronic fetal heart rate (FHR) monitoring is used routinely in labor to screen for fetal well-being. The diagnostic value of FHR monitoring is limited. When the FHR tracing is reassuring, it has a predictive value of 99% for fetal well-being, while an abnormal FHR tracing has a positive predictive value of only 50% for fetal compromise. Over the past three decades, the national cesarean delivery rate has increased significantly, in part, as a result of this technology intended to reduce perinatal morbidity and mortality and to prevent long-term neurologic damage. To further refine assessment of fetal well-being in labor, several diagnostic and intervention techniques have been introduced (eg, fetal scalp pH sampling, fetal scalp stimulation, and fetal acoustic stimulation). None of these methods have been universally or routinely adopted by clinicians.

The U.S. Food and Drug Administration (FDA) recently approved the marketing of the Nellcor N-400 Fetal Oxygen Saturation Monitoring System, a fetal pulse oximeter. The device's primary proposed use is as an adjunct to FHR monitoring to continuously monitor fetal intrapartum oxygen saturation in a singleton vertex fetus with a gestational age equal to or greater than 36 weeks in the presence of a nonreassuring heart rate pattern after fetal membranes have ruptured.

It is essential to recognize that the FDA primarily evaluates a device's safety and ability to accurately measure or quantify a certain physiologic function. It appears from the data supplied to the FDA by the company that this device, under certain conditions, can assess fetal oxygenation safely and effectively. The FDA had no additional outcome data available.

In a company-sponsored study, it has been reported that when the Nellcor N-400 Fetal Oxygen Saturation Monitoring System is used in conjunction with FHR monitoring (under specific conditions), there was a reduction in cesarean delivery rates for nonreassuring FHR tracings, but there was no difference in the overall cesarean delivery rates as a result of an increase in cesarean delivery for dystocia (1). Several environmental factors and physiologic events (eg, fetal scalp congestion, color and thickness of fetal hair, skin thickness, vernix caseosa, site of application, fetal presentation, uterine activity, movement artifacts) can affect the accuracy of the fetal pulse oximetry readings. Reliable readings can be obtained approximately 60–70% of the time.

The American College of Obstetricians and Gynecologists Committee on Obstetric Practice currently cannot endorse the adoption of this device in clinical practice. The committee is particularly concerned that the introduction of this technology to clinical practice could further escalate the cost of medical care without necessarily improving clinical outcome. The committee recommends that prospective randomized clinical trials be conducted to evaluate the clinical use of this new technology in conjunction with fetal well-being assessment. Given that this technology is new, attention should be paid to any adverse outcomes, including falsely reassuring fetal pulse oximetry data. Moreover, such untoward events should be reported to FDA MedWatch, the FDA Medical Products Reporting Program.

Reference

1. Garite TJ, Dildy GA, McNamara H, Nageotte MP, Boehm FH, Dellinger EH. A multicenter controlled trial of fetal pulse oximetry in the intrapartum management of nonreassuring fetal heart rate patterns. Am J Obstet Gynecol 2000;183:1049–1058

ACOG

Committee on
Obstetric Practice

Committee on
Genetics

ISSN 1074-861X

The American College of Obstetricians and Gynecologists

409 12th Street, SW
PO Box 96920
Washington, DC 20090-6920

12345/87654

First-trimester screening for fetal aneuploidy. ACOG Committee Opinion No. 296. American College of Obstetricians and Gynecologists. Obstet Gynecol 2004;104:215–17.

Committee Opinion

Number 296, July 2004   *(Replaces No. 223, October 1999)*

First-Trimester Screening for Fetal Aneuploidy

ABSTRACT: First-trimester screening for chromosomal abnormalities offers potential advantages over second-trimester screening. Studies in the 1990s demonstrated an association between chromosomal abnormalities and the ultrasonographic finding of abnormally increased nuchal translucency (an echo-free area at the back of the fetal neck) between 10 and 14 weeks of gestation. First-trimester screening using nuchal translucency, free β-hCG, and pregnancy-associated plasma protein-A has comparable detection rates and positive screening rates for Down syndrome as second-trimester screening using 4 serum markers (alpha-fetoprotein, β-hCG, unconjugated estriol, and inhibin-A). Although first-trimester screening for Down syndrome and trisomy 18 is an option, it should be offered only if certain criteria can be met.

Maternal serum testing in the second trimester of pregnancy (15–20 weeks of gestation) is commonly offered to screen for Down syndrome (trisomy 21), trisomy 18, neural tube defects, and other fetal malformations. This approach detects approximately 60–75% of fetuses with Down syndrome at a screen positive rate of 5% in women younger than 35 years at the time of delivery and detects 85–95% of cases with a screen positive rate of 25% in women older than 35 years at the time of delivery (1). The detection rate for trisomy 18 is approximately 70% when a patient-specific risk of more than 1 in 100 is employed based on maternal age and serum analyte levels (2). First-trimester screening for chromosomal abnormalities offers potential advantages over second-trimester screening. When the results are negative, first-trimester screening may reduce maternal anxiety at an earlier gestational age. When the results are positive, such screening allows the patient to take advantage of first-trimester prenatal diagnosis by chorionic villus sampling or second-trimester amniocentesis (at 15 weeks of gestation or later). If the fetus is found to be affected earlier in the pregnancy, it provides women greater privacy if they elect to terminate the pregnancy. Earlier pregnancy termination is associated with reduced maternal morbidity.

Nuchal Translucency

Studies in the 1990s demonstrated an association between chromosomal abnormalities and the ultrasonographic finding of abnormally increased nuchal translucency (an echo-free area at the back of the fetal neck) between 10 and 14 weeks of gestation (3–5). Early data on nuchal translucency screening showed widely discordant efficacy caused by differences in the study populations, gestational age at screening, the ways in which nuchal translucency measurements were used with serum analytes, ultrasonographic techniques, and the level of training. When measuring nuchal translucency, the fetus should be in the sagittal view as for a crown–rump measurement and care should be taken to distinguish nuchal skin from the amnionic membrane. Interobserver and intraobserver variation in nuchal translucency measurements have been noted. The ability to measure nuchal translucency reliably is dependent on the operator, ultrasound equipment, proper magnification and contrast, fetal position, correct placement of the calipers, and maternal body habitus (6). Ultrasonographer training and ongoing quality assurance are essential if nuchal translucency is used as a screening method (6, 7).

Nuchal translucency increases with gestational age and, hence, a single cutoff value should not be defined as abnormal (3, 4, 8, 9). Like serum screening, nuchal translucency measurements may be reported in multiples of the median, which will be used to modify the patient's age-related risk for Down syndrome. Because small differences in nuchal translucency measurement can have a large impact on the Down syndrome risk prediction, proper quality assurance requires that either center- or ultrasonographer-specific medians need to be monitored closely (10). Nuchal translucency measurement, in the absence of serum screening has a low specificity; therefore, it is not recommended as a screening test for aneuploidy in singleton pregnancies (10).

Increased nuchal translucency also has been associated with other chromosomal abnormalities (eg, trisomy 13; 45,X; and triploidy) and congenital anomalies, in particular, cardiac defects, and some genetic disorders (3, 5, 11). The prevalence of major cardiac defects increases with increasing nuchal translucency thickness (11). Regardless of gestational age, in fetuses with increased nuchal translucency measurement and normal chromosomes, specialized ultrasound examination with detailed assessment of the heart or fetal echocardiography or both are recommended.

Nuchal Translucency With Maternal Serum Screening Markers

Studies have shown that measurement of 2 serum analytes, pregnancy-associated plasma protein-A and free β-hCG, can be used to screen for Down syndrome in the first trimester (7, 12, 13). Pregnancy-associated plasma protein-A tends to be decreased and free β-hCG tends to be increased in Down syndrome. The detection rate with first-trimester biochemical screening is similar to second-trimester screening, approximately 60% with a positive screening rate of 5% (7, 12, 13). A multicenter study of 8,514 patients with singleton pregnancies in the United States demonstrates that combining first-trimester maternal serum screening markers with nuchal translucency measurement is a good alternative to second-trimester serum screening (14). The detection rate for Down syndrome was 78.7% (95% confidence interval [CI], 66.3–88.1) at a cutoff rate of 1:270 with a positive screening rate of 5%. The detection rate for trisomy 18 in women younger than 35 years at the time of delivery was 90.9% (95% CI, 58.7–99.8) at a positive screening rate of 2%.

First-trimester screening using nuchal translucency, free β-hCG, and pregnancy-associated plasma protein-A has comparable detection rates and positive screening rates for Down syndrome as second-trimester screening using 4 serum markers (alpha-fetoprotein, β-HCG, unconjugated estriol, and inhibin-A). The recently completed Serum Urine and Ultrasound Screening Study trial in the United Kingdom suggests that integrated screening (eg, combined first- and second-trimester screening) is the most sensitive and cost-effective test (15). Results from a large multicenter trial in the United States designed to compare the sensitivity of first-trimester screening using nuchal translucency and serum markers with second-trimester serum screening in the same population should be available in the near future. This study also will evaluate the utility of sequential and integrated screening of patients in the first and second trimesters (16).

Although first-trimester screening for Down syndrome and trisomy 18 is an option, it should be offered only if the following criteria can be met:

1. Appropriate ultrasound training and ongoing quality monitoring programs are in place.

2. Sufficient information and resources are available to provide comprehensive counseling to women regarding the different screening options and limitations of these tests.

3. Access to an appropriate diagnostic test is available when screening test results are positive.

References

1. Haddow JE, Palomaki GE, Knight GJ, Williams J, Pulkkinen A, Canick JA, et al. Prenatal screening for Down's syndrome with use of maternal serum markers. N Engl J Med 1992;327:588–93.

2. Benn PA, Leo MV, Rodis JF, Beazoglou T, Collins R, Horne D. Maternal serum screening for fetal trisomy 18: a comparison of fixed cutoff and patient-specific risk protocols. Obstet Gynecol 1999;93:707–11.

3. Nicolaides KH, Azar G, Byrne D, Mansur C, Marks K. Fetal nuchal translucency: ultrasound screening for chromosomal defects in first trimester of pregnancy. BMJ 1992;304:867–9.

4. Nicolaides KH, Brizot ML, Snijders RJ. Fetal nuchal translucency: ultrasound screening for fetal trisomy in the first trimester of pregnancy. Br J Obstet Gynaecol 1994;101:782–6.

5. Taipale P, Hiilesmaa V, Salonen R, Ylostalo P. Increased nuchal translucency as a marker for fetal chromosomal defects. N Engl J Med 1997;337:1654–8.

6. Snijders RJ, Thom EA, Zachary JM, Platt LD, Greene N, Jackson LG, et al. First trimester trisomy screening: nuchal translucency measurement training and quality assurance to correct and unify technique. Ultrasound Obstet Gynecol 2002;19:353–9.

7. Haddow JE, Palomaki GE, Knight GJ, Williams J, Miller WA, Johnson A. Screening of maternal serum for fetal Down's syndrome in the first trimester. N Engl J Med 1998;338:955–61.

8. Pajkrt E, de Graaf IM, Mol BW, van Lith JM, Bleker OP, Bilardo CM. Weekly nuchal translucency measurements in normal fetuses. Obstet Gynecol 1998;91:208–11.

9. Schuchter K, Wald N, Hackshaw AK, Hafner E, Liebhart E. The distribution of nuchal translucency at 10-13 weeks of pregnancy. Prenat Diagn 1998;18:281–6.

10. Malone FD, D'Alton ME. First-trimester sonographic screening for Down syndrome. Society for Maternal-Fetal Medicine. Obstet Gynecol 2003;102:1066–79.

11. Hyett J, Perdu M, Sharland G, Snijders R, Nicolaides KH. Using fetal nuchal translucency to screen for major congenital cardiac defects at 10-14 weeks of gestation: population based cohort study. BMJ 1999;318: 81–5.

12. Wald NJ, Kennard A, Hackshaw AK. First trimester serum screening for Down's syndrome [published erratum appears in Prenat Diagn 1996;16:387]. Prenat Diagn 1995;15:1227–40.

13. Krantz DA, Larsen JW, Buchanan PD, Macri JN. First-trimester Down syndrome screening: free beta-human chorionic gonadotropin and pregnancy-associated plasma protein A. Am J Obstet Gynecol 1996;174:612–6.

14. Wapner R, Thom E, Simpson JL, Pergament E, Silver R, Filkins K, et al. First-trimester screening for trisomies 21 and 18. Trimester Maternal Serum Biochemistry and Fetal Nuchal Translucency Screening (BUN) Study Group. N Eng J Med 2003;349:1405–13.

15. Wald NJ, Rodeck C, Hackshaw AK, Walters J, Chitty L, Mackinson AM. First and second trimester antenatal screening for Down's syndrome: the results of the Serum, Urine, and Ultrasound Screening Study (SURUSS). Health Technol Assess 2003;7(11):1–77.

16. Malone FD, Berkowitz RL, Canick JA, D'Alton ME. First-trimester screening for aneuploidy: research or standard of care? Am J Obstet Gynecol 2000;182:490–6.

ACOG Committee Opinion

Committee on Gynecologic Practice

Number 272, May 2002

Follow-up of Abnormal Screening Mammography

ABSTRACT: Screening mammography facilitates the early diagnosis of breast carcinoma in women. Timely follow-up can optimize the diagnosis and treatment of women with abnormal screening test results. When test results reveal that additional studies are needed, no barriers should prohibit testing during the screening mammography visit.

Screening mammography facilitates the early diagnosis of breast carcinoma in women. Timely follow-up of an abnormal screening mammogram can optimize the diagnosis and treatment of women with abnormal screening test results and may decrease patient anxiety, travel costs, and time off work. Timely follow-up is ethically encouraged and is consistent with the role of physicians as patient advocates.

When interpretation of a screening mammogram indicates that additional diagnostic studies are needed, there should be no barriers imposed by the patient's health insurance policy or other regulations that would prevent the performance of further diagnostic tests during the visit for screening mammography.

ISSN 1074-861X

The American College of Obstetricians and Gynecologists
409 12th Street, SW
PO Box 96920
Washington, DC 20090-6920

12345/65432

Follow-up of abnormal screening mammography. ACOG Committee Opinion No. 272. American College of Obstetricians and Gynecologists. Obstet Gynecol 2002;99:869

Committee on Genetics

Committee Opinion

Number 161, October 1995

Fragile X Syndrome

Fragile X syndrome is the most common inherited form of mental retardation, affecting about 1 in 1,500 males and 1 in 2,500 females from a variety of ethnic backgrounds. Mental retardation ranges from borderline to severe, although most patients have moderate degrees of mental retardation. Other associated phenotypic abnormalities include autistic behaviors, macro-orchidism in adult males, characteristic narrow face with a large jaw, and speech and language problems. The abnormal facial features are subtle and become more noticeable with age, making phenotypic diagnosis difficult, especially in the newborn.

Standard metaphase chromosomal analysis does not consistently demonstrate the cytogenetic abnormality in patients with fragile X syndrome. Using specific culture conditions (folate deprivation), the demonstration of a fragile site on the long (q) arm of the human X chromosome (Xq27-28) was identified in males and some females with fragile X syndrome. The syndrome was originally thought to be transmitted in a classic X-linked recessive fashion; however, the inheritance of fragile X syndrome has proven to be much more complex. Females may be affected. Nearly all males with fragile X and most carrier females who have mental retardation show the fragile site. However, about 20% of males with the mutant gene do not have mental retardation and do not demonstrate cytogenetic evidence of the fragile site. These men are referred to as transmitting males. Two thirds of carrier females are mentally normal, and only one third of these demonstrate cytogenetic findings. These variations in the expression of the fragile site complicate cytogenetic diagnosis, particularly prenatal diagnosis. Molecular diagnostic techniques have now replaced cytogenetic analysis as the diagnostic procedure of choice for the fragile X syndrome.

The molecular cloning of the fragile X mental retardation-1 gene (*FMR*-1) has helped to clarify the molecular basis of the fragile X syndrome. Nearly all of the mutations in the gene involve expansion of a triplet repeat consisting of the bases cytosine–guanine–guanine. This pattern appears to correlate with the fragile site detected by cytogenetic techniques. The number of repeats varies in unaffected individuals (Table 1). A patient with 50–200 repeats is phenotypically normal and is said to have a premutation. When greater than 200 repeats are present, the patient has a full mutation that results in phenotypic fragile X syndrome. The *FMR-1* gene nearly always becomes methylated and inactivated in these patients. The number of repeats and the status of gene

The American College of Obstetricians and Gynecologists
409 12th Street, SW
Washington, DC 20024-2188

Table 1. Mutation in the Fragile X Mental Retardation-1 Gene

Status of Individual	Number of Triplet Repeats (Cytosine–Guanine–Guanine)
Unaffected	6–49
Premutation	50–200
Full mutation	>200

methylation are determined by using DNA-based molecular tests (ie, Southern blot analysis and polymerase chain reaction). Chorionic villus sampling may not be reliable for diagnosis because of different methylation patterns in the trophoblast as compared with the fetus. Although reliable for determining the number of triplet repeats, chorionic villus sampling may not adequately determine the methylation status of the *FMR-1* gene.

Transmission of a disease-producing mutation to a fetus depends upon the sex of the parent and the number of cytosine–guanine–guanine repeats present in the parental gene. Parents at risk for transmission of the disease are those who have either the premutation or the full DNA mutation. When a female carries the premutation and the length of the repeat exceeds 90, premutation genes are much more likely to expand and to result in the birth of an affected child. Males may transmit the premutation gene to their children, but expansion to a full mutation has not been described in the offspring of a male having the premutation gene. Empirically determined risks are available for the purposes of genetic counseling. An antibody-based test using peripheral blood is currently under investigation as a rapid approach to the screening of mentally retarded individuals and neonates for fragile X syndrome (1).

The Committee recommends the following regarding testing for fragile X syndrome:

1. DNA-based molecular analysis is the preferred method of diagnosis for fragile X syndrome and its premutations. Cytogenetic analysis should not be used for the definitive diagnosis of fragile X syndrome.

2. Testing for fragile X syndrome should be considered in any child with developmental delay of uncertain etiology or any individual with mental retardation of uncertain etiology. If there is no DNA evidence for the fragile X syndrome in an individual with mental retardation, standard chromosome analysis may also be considered in order to exclude chromosomal causes of mental retardation such as autosomal trisomies, deletions, duplications, or unbalanced translocations.

3. Patients with a family history of mental retardation or a history of fragile X mental retardation should undergo genetic evaluation to assess their risk for having an affected child.

4. Prenatal testing for fragile X syndrome by amniocentesis should be offered to known carriers of the fragile X premutation or mutation.

References

1. Willemsen R, Mohkamsing S, De Vries B, Devys D, van den Ouweland A, Mandel JL, et al. Rapid antibody test for fragile X syndrome. Lancet 1995;345:1147–1148

2. Warren ST, Nelson DL. Advances in molecular analysis of fragile X syndrome. JAMA 1994;271:536–542

3. Nussbaum RL, Ledbetter DH. The fragile X syndrome. In: Scriver CR, Beaudet AL, Sly WS, Valle D, eds. The metabolic basis of inherited disease. 6th ed. Vol I. New York: McGraw-Hill Inc, 1989:327–341

4. The American College of Medical Genetics policy statement. Fragile X syndrome: diagnostic and carrier testing. Bethesda, Maryland: Working Group of the Genetic Screening Subcommittee of the Clinical Practice Committee, ACMG, July 22, 1994, pages 1–4

ACOG

Committee on Genetics

Committee Opinion

Number 257, May 2001   *(Replaces No. 178, November 1996)*

Genetic Evaluation of Stillbirths and Neonatal Deaths

In the burgeoning field of genetics, a complete evaluation of stillbirths and neonatal deaths yields more information than in the past. Autopsy findings supplemented by genetic studies may provide important information (1). This information may explain the cause of death, direct further investigation of the family, and be particularly valuable in counseling parents about recurrence risks in future pregnancies.

Parental Consent

It is important to obtain parental consent; however, grief stricken parents may be reticent to consent to autopsy examination. They may view it as a violation of the sanctity of the dead body or as serving the physician's interests or curiosity. Even though bereaved parents may not want the information initially, care providers should strongly emphasize that results of the evaluation may be useful to the patient and her family in planning future pregnancies. If still reluctant to consent to a full autopsy, the family should be informed of the value of less invasive methods of evaluation, including photographs, X-rays, and sampling of tissues, such as blood or skin. These methods may help to identify a syndrome or chromosomal abnormality even without full autopsy data. Congenital anomalies are a significant cause of fetal death; 15–20% of stillbirths have a major malformation. Approximately 8% of stillbirths have chromosomal abnormalities and about 20% have dysmorphic features or skeletal abnormalities (2, 3). Malformations often are present in patterns that permit classification into a particular syndrome. Syndrome identification may delineate etiologic and pathogenetic factors that could have predictive significance for recurrence risk and the risk of other associated anomalies (4). Also, it is important to note that in addition to genetic causes, some fetal and neonatal deaths are caused by obstetric or medical complications for which preventive measures may be available.

Management

After a stillbirth or neonatal death, proper management includes a careful perinatal and family history, a physical examination of the fetus or infant (with documentation by description and photography, if possible), and indicated laboratory studies (see box). To ascertain the etiology and provide appropriate counseling to the family, clinical–pathologic correlation is best accomplished by a team comprising obstetricians, pediatricians, neonatologists, pathologists, and geneticists.

History

When stillbirth or neonatal death occurs, the obstetric history including exposures (eg, medications, viral infections), and family history, including a three-generation pedigree if possible, should be reviewed. Any pertinent information in the maternal or paternal pedigree should be documented and investigated further. Relevant original medical records and documentation should be obtained whenever possible. The gestational age by last menstrual period, maternal examinations, laboratory data, and ultrasonograms should be recorded for correlation with the physical examination of the neonate. Possible nongenetic causes also should be considered.

Examination of the Stillbirth

The general examination of the stillborn infant should be done promptly, noting any dysmorphic features and obtaining body measurements, including crown–rump, crown–heel, and foot lengths, as well as weight

---

Management of Stillbirth or Fetal Death*

- Obtain informed consent from parents for autopsy
- Obtain perinatal and family history
- Perform physical examination of fetus and describe findings
- Photograph fetus
- Perform whole body X-rays of fetus
- Perform autopsy of fetus
- Perform gross and microscopic examination of placenta
- Perform cytogenetic studies
- Perform biochemical, molecular genetic, or infectious disease studies as indicated

*If these services are not available at your hospital, consider sending to a regional hospital center or contact your state board of pathology.

(5–8). Foot length is especially useful before 23 weeks of gestation. These measurements help estimate gestational age and evaluate intrauterine growth. Further documentation by frontal and profile photographs, with close-ups of specific abnormalities, is valuable for subsequent review and consultations. Even if parents have declined an autopsy, a description of any obvious abnormalities of the stillbirth should be included in the medical record.

X-rays, examination of the placenta, and autopsy should be considered. This is especially true when dysmorphic features, inconsistent growth measurements, anomalies, hydrops, or growth restriction is present. Whole body X-ray with anterior–posterior and lateral views may reveal an unrecognized skeletal abnormality or further define a grossly apparent deformity. If possible, the infant should be positioned with extremities extended and the epiphyses viewed.

When a full autopsy is performed, it should follow the guidelines for perinatal autopsy published by the College of American Pathologists (www.cap.org) or other standard references (9, 10). The pathologist should be aware of the clinical history and suspected genetic diagnoses so that samples for cytogenetic, metabolic, and molecular studies may be taken.

Examination of the Placenta

Gross and microscopic examination of the placenta, membranes, and umbilical cord may corroborate autopsy findings or explain apparent fetal deformity. Gross evaluation of the umbilical cord and blood vessels, membranes for amniotic bands and other anomalies, and placenta for size and condition should be performed. Histologic study of placental samples also should be performed (11, 12).

Laboratory Studies

Samples of amniotic fluid, umbilical cord blood, or amnion may be obtained for chromosomal and any other relevant studies. Analysis of bile, vitreous humor, urine, and fetal tissue may be helpful if umbilical cord blood is unobtainable (13, 14). Guidelines for the procurement of samples for chromosomal and genetic studies are outlined in the box on the following page.

Chromosomal analysis of amniotic fluid or chorionic villi ideally should be offered as soon as a fetal death is recognized. Although this information can be obtained at the time of delivery, the likelihood of obtaining a karyotype is decreased if there is a long interval between fetal death and delivery. This is

---

Guidelines for the Procurement of Samples for Chromosomal and Genetic Studies

- Obtain consent to take skin, eye, body fluids, and other tissue samples (separate from autopsy consent).
- For cytogenetic and molecular genetic studies, the following samples are acceptable:
  —Umbilical cord blood (3 mL)
  —Skin with attached dermis (1 cm²)
  —Fascia from thigh, inguinal region, or Achilles tendon (1 cm) especially when maceration of the skin is present; and
  —Kidney, skeletal, muscle, liver, lung, and gonads, if indicated.
- Samples should be obtained using sterile techniques as soon as possible.
- Umbilical cord blood should be placed into sterile tube with heparin.
- Tissue samples should be placed in appropriate sterile medium obtained from cytogenetic laboratory or in normal saline if medium is not available. Do not use fixative solutions (eg, formaldehyde).
- Samples should be kept at room temperature.
- Freeze a 1 cm tissue sample.

---

especially true when dysmorphic features, inconsistent growth measurements, anomalies, hydrops, or growth restriction are present, or when a parent carries a balanced chromosomal rearrangement (eg, translocation or inversion) or has a mosaic karyotype. Based on the history, examination of the fetus, radiographic studies, and autopsy findings, specific molecular or biochemical tests may be indicated. For example, fluorescence in situ hybridization studies used to identify a deletion of chromosome 22q11.2 should be considered when a conotruncal cardiac defect (eg, interrupted aortic arch, truncus arteriosus) is detected (15).

Counseling

The results of the autopsy, placental examination, laboratory tests, and cytogenetic studies should be communicated to the involved clinicians and to the family of the deceased infant in a timely manner. Further, the family should be counseled promptly after a consensus is reached. Counseling before the evaluation is complete or before different opinions of the various caregivers have been resolved may increase feelings of guilt or anger in parents who have experienced a perinatal death. When there is an abnormal child or a genetic defect, these feelings often are magnified. Specific testing of the parents may be offered. The results of the tests are important even when no specific diagnosis is identified (16). A list of diagnoses excluded may be useful in counseling the parents. Whether or not there is a specific diagnosis, compassionate counseling of the parents and sensitivity to their needs are required.

References

1. Saller DN Jr, Lesser KB, Harrel U, Rogers BB, Oyer CE. The clinical utility of the perinatal autopsy. JAMA 1995; 273:663–665
2. Pauli RM, Reiser CA. Wisconsin Stillbirth Service Program: II. Analysis of diagnoses and diagnostic categories in the first 1,000 referrals. Am J Med Genet 1994; 50:135–153
3. Pauli RM, Reiser CA, Lebovitz RM, Kirkpatrick SJ. Wisconsin Stillbirth Service Program: I. Establishment and assessment of a community-based program for etiologic investigation of intrauterine deaths. Am J Med Genet 1994;50:116–134
4. Leppig KA, Werler MM, Cann CI, Cook CA, Holmes LB. Predictive value of minor anomalies. I. Association with major malformations. J Pediatr 1987;110:531–537
5. Reed GB, Claireaux AE, Cockburn F, eds. Diseases of the fetus and newborn: pathology, imaging, genetics, and management. 2nd ed. London: Chapman and Hall Medical, 1995
6. Stocker JT, Dehner LP. Pediatric pathology. Philadelphia: Lippincott, 1992
7. Naeye RL. Disorders of the placenta, fetus, and neonate: diagnosis and clinical significance. St Louis: Mosby-Year Book, Inc, 1992
8. Shepard TH, Shi M, Fellingham GW, Fujinaga M, FitzSimmons JM, Fantel AG, et al. Organ weight standards for human fetuses. Pediatr Pathol 1988;8:513–524
9. Valdes-Dapena MA, Huff DS. Perinatal autopsy manual. Collingdale, Pennsylvania: Diane Publishing, 1993
10. Bove KE. Practice guidelines for autopsy pathology: the perinatal and pediatric autopsy. Autopsy Committee of the College of American Pathologists. Arch Pathol Lab Med 1997;121:368–376
11. Benirschke K, Kaufman P. Pathology of the human placenta. 4th ed. New York: Springer-Verlag, 2000
12. Genest DR. Estimating the time of death in stillborn fetuses: II. Histologic evaluation of the placenta; a study of 71 stillborns. Obstet Gynecol 1992;80:585–592
13. Emery JL, Howat AJ, Variend S, Vawter GF. Investigation of inborn errors of metabolism in unexpected infant deaths. Lancet 1988;2:29–31
14. Rashed MS, Ozand PT, Bennett MJ, Barnard JJ, Govindaraju DR, Rinaldo P. Inborn errors of metabolism diagnosed in sudden death cases by acylcarnitine analysis of postmortem bile. Clin Chem 1995;41:1109–1114
15. Goldmuntz E, Clark BJ, Mitchell LE, Jawad AF, Reed L, McDonald-McGinn D, et al. Frequency of 22q11 deletions in patients with conotruncal defects. J Am Coll Cardiol 1998;32:492–498
16. Rushton DI. Prognostic role of the perinatal postmortem. Br J Hosp Med 1994;52:450–454

ACOG

Committee on Adolescent Health Care

The Committee wishes to thank Abigail English, JD; S. Paige Hertweck, MD; Susan Kornetsky, MPH; Audrey Rogers, PhD, MPH; and John Santelli, MD, MPH for their assistance in the development of this opinion. This document reflects emerging clinical and scientific advances as of the date issued and is subject to change. The information should not be construed as dictating an exclusive course of treatment or procedure to be followed.

ISSN 1074-861X

The American College of Obstetricians and Gynecologists
409 12th Street, SW
PO Box 96920
Washington, DC 20090-6920

12345/87654

Guidelines for adolescent health research. ACOG Committee Opinion No. 302. American College of Obstetricians and Gynecologists. Obstet Gynecol 2004;104:899–902.

Committee Opinion

Number 302, October 2004

Guidelines for Adolescent Health Research

ABSTRACT: The risks of exposure to violence, human immunodeficiency virus, and other sexually transmitted diseases; alcohol, tobacco, and prescribed and illicit drug use; and unintended pregnancy, among others, threaten the health and well-being of adolescents in the United States. Research is needed in these and other areas to improve adolescent health care and to aid in health policy decisions. Adolescents often are prevented from participating in such research because of inadequate understanding of their legal status and the ethical considerations regarding their participation in research. There is confusion about what constitutes appropriate levels of protection for studies involving adolescents as research subjects and uncertainty about the need for parental permission. This document is designed to clarify the informed consent and parental permission issues as they pertain to adolescent health research.

Background

A basic criterion for ethical research is the protection of the rights and welfare of people participating in research. The U.S. federal government has promulgated regulations that govern research involving human subjects when the research is supported, conducted, or otherwise subject to regulation by the federal government (1). These federal regulations on protection of human subjects in research, known as the Code of Federal Regulations: Title 45-Public Welfare; Part 46: Protection of Human Subjects (45 CFR Part 46), provide for a nationwide system of local Institutional Review Boards (IRBs). These IRBs must review and approve all federally funded research involving human subjects and are regulated by the Office for Human Research Protections in the Department of Health and Human Services. Most universities and research institutions apply these regulations to privately funded research as well. These regulations serve as guidelines for IRB review and approval. They require that risks to research participants are minimized and that they are reasonable relative to the anticipated benefits and the importance of the knowledge that may be expected to result from the research. The regulations also require that the selection of research participants is equitable and that informed consent is provided from each prospective research participant or the participant's legally authorized representative. Informed consent is the ability to understand the risks and benefits of one's participation in a research activity and to authorize one's participation in this activity freely (2). General requirements for informed consent are described in 45 CFR Part 46, Section 116 (1). Finally, the regulations require that the research plan makes adequate provisions for ensuring the safety of research participants and that adequate provisions are made to protect the privacy of research participants and to maintain the confidentiality of data. Subpart D of 45 CFR Part 46 contains special protections for children who participate as subjects in research.

Research involving adolescents, especially regarding behaviors related to sexuality, often raises questions about how to obtain adequate informed consent and protection of the research participants' confidential receipt of health care services. The Society for Adolescent Medicine provided early leadership to address these concerns. In 1995, they led the development of consensus guidelines to promote the ethical conduct of health research involving adolescents as research participants (3). The society recently issued a revised position statement to support the guidelines (4); the Society for Adolescent medicine also established a code of research ethics to encourage, enhance, and promote ethical standards for the conduct of research in adolescent health (5).

When considering the legal complexities of adolescent health research, it is important to recognize that the age of majority in almost every state is 18 years, and all states recognize the concept of emancipated minors, who generally are allowed to consent for their own health care. In addition, every state has enacted some minor consent laws that allow minors to consent for their own health care, whether or not they are legally emancipated. Such laws may be based on the status of the minor or the services they are seeking. Minors who may consent for their own health care based on their status include those who are married, are members of the armed forces, live apart from their parents, and are parents of a child. In addition, all states allow adolescents who are minors to consent for some categories of health care such as sexually transmitted disease (STD) services (all states), drug and alcohol care (almost all states), contraceptive services and pregnancy related care (a majority of states), outpatient mental health counseling (about one half of states), or sexual assault care (a few states). Some states specify the age at which a minor can begin to consent (6). Researchers in adolescent health should be familiar with current state statutes regarding age of majority and emancipation, as well as with minor consent statutes. An up-to-date listing of these statutes can be found online at http://www.guttmacher.org/pubs/spib.html.

Regulations

In the federal regulations governing research, children are defined in 45 CFR 46 Section 102(a) as "persons who have not attained the legal age for consent to treatments or procedures involved in the research, under the applicable law of the jurisdiction in which the research will be conducted"(1). This definition refers to laws, primarily state laws related to consent for treatment of minors, age of majority, and emancipation status.

Federal regulations governing human subject research require parental permission and child assent for subjects who meet the regulatory definition of "children," ie, those who are younger than the state-mandated age at which people may give legally effective informed consent for treatments or procedures involved in the research. Assent means a child has given affirmative agreement to participate in research. Mere failure to object should not, absent affirmative agreement, be construed as assent. Assent is required when, in the judgment of the IRB, the children are capable of providing it (1).The federal regulations deliberately use the terms "permission" and "assent" to differentiate this process from the usual informed consent process. An individual can provide consent only for himself or herself. Therefore, parents give only permission for their child to be involved in research, not consent. Assent recognizes the importance of the emerging capacity of children to give informed consent for themselves, as well as the ethical importance of obtaining their agreement to participate even if they are not legally authorized to give informed consent.

In 1977, the National Commission for the Protection of Human Subjects of Biomedical and Behavioral Research recommended that individual IRBs be allowed to determine that parental permission is not appropriate in certain research studies, including research involving assessment for or care related to contraception and drug abuse (7). According to the federal regulations (1), informed consent may be waived under 45 CFR Part 46 Section 116(d) and parental permission may be waived under 45 CFR Part 46 Section 408(c).

Four criteria set forth by 45 CFR Part 46 116(d) allow an IRB to waive the requirement to obtain the informed consent for adult research subjects or permission of a parent or guardian for research subjects who are children if: 1) the research involves no more than "minimal risk" (which means that the probability and magnitude of harm or discomfort anticipated in the research are not greater in and of themselves than those ordinarily encountered in daily life or during the performance of routine physical or psychologic examinations or tests [1]), 2) the waiver will not adversely affect the rights and welfare of the subjects, 3) the research could not practically be carried out without a waiver, and 4) whenever appropriate, the subjects will be provided with additional pertinent information after participation (1). This section is commonly used when waiving informed consent for research involving existing data such as medical records.

In addition, 45 CFR Part 46 Section 408(c) specifically allows for a waiver of parental permission under Subpart D, which addresses research with children. Section 408(c) of 45 CFR Part 46 states: "...if an IRB determines that a research protocol is designed for conditions or a subject population for which parental permission is not a reasonable requirement to protect subjects (eg, neglected or abused children), it may waive consent requirements provided an appropriate mechanism for protecting the children who will participate as research subjects is substituted and provided the waiver is not inconsistent with federal, state, or local law.... The choice of an appropriate mechanism would depend on the nature and purpose of the activities described in the protocol, the risk and anticipated benefit to the research subjects, and their age, maturity, status, and condition" (1). In discussing the waiver of parental permission, the National Commission cited as examples of when the requirement might not be a reasonable one: "...[r]esearch designed to identify factors related to the incidence or treatment of certain conditions in adolescents for which, in certain jurisdictions, they legally may receive treatment without parental consent; [and] research in which the subjects are 'mature minors' and the procedures involved entail essentially no more than minimal risk that such individuals might reasonably assume on their own..." (7).

Based on these criteria, either 45 CFR Part 46 Section 408(c) or 45 CFR Part 46 Section 116(d) may be used to waive parental permission in a variety of studies, including, for example, surveys of adolescents. It is important to note that if these surveys are conducted in a school setting, federal educational law governing certain research conducted in schools may apply. Health researchers working in schools are, therefore, advised to become knowledgeable about these laws.

Section 408(c) of 45 CFR Part 46 also may be used to waive parental permission for research areas including STDs, birth control usage, high-risk behaviors, HIV prevention, and situations in which obtaining parental consent may be dangerous to the child (abuse situations). Finally, in certain research studies, adolescent minors would not be considered children and parental permission would not be required. Such research includes certain clinical studies involving pregnancy, family planning, and treatment of STDs where the adolescent minor can legally consent to such services. Again, familiarity with current state statutes on the rights of minors to consent to health care services is essential.

Researchers conducting and IRBs reviewing research involving adolescents should be knowledgeable of the federal regulations and the ethical principles that underlie these regulations. They should understand when parental permission is required and when it may be waived. Personal beliefs and attitudes should not enter into this decision. The Society for Adolescent Medicine's *Guidelines for Adolescent Health Research* (4) provide a comprehensive approach to understanding these issues. Parental permission should not be a barrier to the inclusion of adolescents in studies that meet federal regulations and are designed to improve their health.

Conclusions

1. Researchers developing study protocols and materials for submission for IRB review and approval and the IRBs themselves should be familiar with, and adhere to, current federal regulations, 45 CFR Part 46 (1), and federal and state laws that affect research (including laws regarding age of majority and emancipation, minor consent statutes, and federal educational law governing certain research conducted in schools).

2. Investigators will communicate better with IRB panels regarding the involvement of adolescent participants in research if they understand the purpose of human subject protection regulations

with respect to minors and review the guidelines provided by the Society for Adolescent Medicine (3–5).

3. Under the following circumstances it is reasonable to waive parental permission when adolescents are involved in studies: a) the waiver would not adversely affect the rights and welfare of the adolescent, b) the study poses no more than a minimal risk to adolescents, c) the study could not be practically carried out without a waiver, and d) requiring permission may not be reasonable to protect subjects. Parental permission is not a requirement for research involving the provision of health care for which adolescents do not legally need parental consent. It is important to review 45 CFR Part 46 for the necessary details.

References

1. Protection of human subjects. 45 C.F.R §46 (2003). Available at http://www.access.gpo.gov/nara/cfr/cfr-tablesearch.html#page1. Retrieved July 8, 2004.

2. American College of Obstetricians and Gynecologists. Ethics in obstetrics and gynecology. 2nd ed. ACOG: Washington, DC; 2004.

3. Guidelines for adolescent health research. 1995. Society for Adolescent Medicine. J Adolesc Health 2003;33: 410–5.

4. Santelli JS, Smith Rogers A, Rosenfeld WD, DuRant RH, Dubler N, Morreale M, et al. Guidelines for adolescent health research: A position paper of the Society for Adolescent Medicine. J Adolesc Health 2003;33: 396–409.

5. Code of Research Ethics: position paper of the Society for Adolescent Medicine. J Adolesc Health 1999;24:277–82; discussion 283.

6. English A, Kenney KE. State minor consent laws: a summary. 2nd Ed. Chapel Hill (NC): Center for Adolescent Health & the Law; 2003.

7. The National Commission for the Protection of Human Subjects of Biomedical and Behavioral Research. Research involving children: report and recommendations. Bethesda (MD): U.S. Department of Health Education and Welfare; 1977.

ACOG Committee Opinion

Committee on Obstetric Practice

Number 299, September 2004   *(Replaces No. 158, September 1995)*

Guidelines for Diagnostic Imaging During Pregnancy

ABSTRACT: Undergoing a single diagnostic X-ray procedure does not result in radiation exposure adequate to threaten the well-being of the developing preembryo, embryo, or fetus and is not an indication for therapeutic abortion. When multiple diagnostic X-rays are anticipated during pregnancy, imaging procedures not associated with ionizing radiation, such as ultrasonography and magnetic resonance imaging, should be considered. Additionally, it may be helpful to consult an expert in dosimetry calculation to determine estimated fetal dose. The use of radioactive isotopes of iodine is contraindicated for therapeutic use during pregnancy. Other radiopaque and paramagnetic contrast agents have not been studied in humans, but animal studies suggest that these agents are unlikely to cause harm to the developing human fetus. Although imaging techniques requiring these agents may be diagnostically beneficial, these techniques should be used during pregnancy only if potential benefits justify potential risks to the fetus.

Various imaging modalities are available for diagnostic use during pregnancy. These include X-ray, ultrasonography, magnetic resonance imaging (MRI), and nuclear medicine studies. Of these, diagnostic X-ray is the most frequent cause of anxiety for obstetricians and patients. Much of this anxiety is secondary to a general belief that any radiation exposure is harmful and will result in an anomalous fetus. This anxiety could lead to inappropriate therapeutic abortion and litigation. Actually, most diagnostic radiologic procedures are associated with little, if any, known significant fetal risks. Moreover, according to the American College of Radiology, no single diagnostic X-ray procedure results in radiation exposure to a degree that would threaten the well-being of the developing preembryo, embryo, or fetus (1). Thus, exposure to a single X-ray during pregnancy is not an indication for therapeutic abortion (2, 3).

Some women are exposed to X-rays before the diagnosis of pregnancy. Occasionally, X-ray procedures will be indicated during pregnancy for significant medical problems or trauma. To enable physicians to counsel patients appropriately, the following information is provided about the potential risks and measures that can reduce diagnostic X-ray exposure.

ISSN 1074-861X

The American College of Obstetricians and Gynecologists
409 12th Street, SW
PO Box 96920
Washington, DC 20090-6920

12345/87654

Guidelines for diagnostic imaging during pregnancy. ACOG Committee Opinion No. 299. American College of Obstetricians and Gynecologists. Obstet Gynecol 2004;104:647–51.

X-Ray Exposure

Ionizing radiation can result in the following 3 harmful effects: 1) cell death and teratogenic effects, 2) carcinogenesis, and 3) genetic effects or mutations in germ cells (2, 3). There is little or no information to estimate either the frequency or magnitude of adverse genetic effects on future generations.

Units traditionally used to measure the effects of X-ray include the rad and roentgen equivalents man (rem). Modern units include the gray (Gy) and sievert (Sv). The definitions of these units of measure are summarized in Table 1.

The estimated fetal exposure from some common radiologic procedures is summarized in Table 2. A plain X-ray generally exposes the fetus to very small amounts of radiation. Commonly during pregnancy, the uterus is shielded for nonpelvic procedures. With the exception of barium enema or small bowel series, most fluoroscopic examinations result in fetal exposure of millirads. Radiation exposure from computed tomography (CT) varies depending on the number and spacing of adjacent image sections. Although CT pelvimetry can result in fetal exposures as high as 1.5 rad, exposure can be reduced to approximately 250 mrad (including fetal gonad exposure) by using a low-exposure technique (4).

Spiral (or helical) CT allows continuous scanning of the patient as the couch is moved through the scanner, providing superior speed and image quality. Radiation exposure is affected by slice thickness, the number of cuts obtained, and the "pitch," a ratio defined as the distance the couch travels during one 360-degree rotation divided by the section thickness. The patient dose is proportional to 1 per pitch. Under typical use with a pitch of 1 or greater, the radiation exposure to the fetus from spiral CT is comparable to conventional CT (5).

Cell Death and Teratogenic Effects

Data from an animal study suggest that exposure to high-dose ionizing radiation (ie, much greater than that used in diagnostic procedures) before implantation will most likely be lethal to the embryo (2). In other words, cell death is most likely an "all or none" phenomenon in early embryonic development.

Myriad teratogenic effects have developed in animals exposed to large doses of radiation (ie, 100–200 rad). However, in humans, growth restriction, microcephaly, and mental retardation are the most common adverse effects from high-dose radiation (3, 6, 7). Based on data from atomic bomb survivors, it appears that the risk of central nervous system effects is greatest with exposure at 8–15 weeks of gestation, with no proven risk at less than 8 weeks of gestation or at greater than 25 weeks of gestation (3, 8). Thus, at 8–15 weeks of gestation, the fetus is at greatest risk for radiation-induced mental retardation, and the risk appears to be a "nonthreshold linear function of dose" at doses of at least 20 rad (3, 6, 8, 9). For example, the risk of severe mental retardation in fetuses exposed to ionizing radiation is approximately 40% at 100 rad of exposure and as high as 60% at 150 rad of exposure (3, 8). It has been suggested that a threshold for this adverse effect may exist in the range of 20–40 rad (7, 8). Even multiple diagnostic X-ray procedures rarely result in ionizing radiation exposure to this degree. Fetal risks of anomalies, growth restriction, or abortions are not increased with radiation exposure of less than 5 rad, a level above the range of exposure for diagnostic procedures (2).

Carcinogenesis

The risk of carcinogenesis as a result of in utero exposure to ionizing radiation is unclear but is prob-

Table 1. Some Measures of Ionizing Radiation

Measure	Definition	Unit	Unit
Exposure	Number of ions produced by X-rays per kilogram of air	Roentgen (R)	Roentgen (R)
Dose	Amount of energy deposited per kilogram of tissue	Rad (rad)*	Gray (Gy) 1 Gy = 100 rad
Relative effective dose	Amount of energy deposited per kilogram of tissue normalized for biological effectiveness	Roentgen equivalents man (rem)*	Sievert (Sv) 1 Sv = 100 rem

*For diagnostic X-rays, 1 rad = 1 rem

Cunningham FG, Gant NF, Leveno KJ, Gilstrap LC 3rd, Hauth JC, Wenstrom KD. General considerations and maternal evaluation. In: Williams obstetrics. 21st ed. New York (NY): McGraw-Hill; 2001. p. 1143–58. Reproduced with permission of The McGraw-Hill Companies.

Table 2. Estimated Fetal Exposure From Some Common Radiologic Procedures

Procedure	Fetal Exposure
Chest X-ray (2 views)	0.02–0.07 mrad
Abdominal film (single view)	100 mrad
Intravenous pyelography	≥1 rad*
Hip film (single view)	200 mrad
Mammography	7–20 mrad
Barium enema or small bowel series	2–4 rad
CT† scan of head or chest	<1 rad
CT scan of abdomen and lumbar spine	3.5 rad
CT pelvimetry	250 mrad

*Exposure depends on the number of films
†Abbreviation: CT, computed tomography
Data from Cunningham FG, Gant NF, Leveno KJ, Gilstrap LC 3rd, Hauth JC, Wenstrom KD. General considerations and maternal evaluation. In: Williams obstetrics. 21st ed. New York (NY): McGraw-Hill; 2001. p. 1143–58.

ably very small. It is estimated that a 1–2 rad fetal exposure may increase the risk of leukemia by a factor of 1.5–2.0 over natural incidence and that an estimated 1 in 2,000 children exposed to ionizing radiation in utero will develop childhood leukemia. This is increased from a background rate of approximately 1 in 3,000 (2, 10). If elective abortion were chosen in every instance of fetal exposure to radiation, 1,999 exposed, normal fetuses would be aborted for each case of leukemia prevented (2, 11). It has been estimated that the risk of radiation-induced carcinogenesis may indeed be higher in children compared with adults, but such risks are not likely to exceed 1 in 1,000 children per rad (12). Thus, abortion should not be recommended solely on the basis of exposure to diagnostic radiation.

Ultrasonography

Ultrasonography involves the use of sound waves and is not a form of ionizing radiation. There have been no reports of documented adverse fetal effects for diagnostic ultrasound procedures, including duplex Doppler imaging. Energy exposure from ultrasonography has been arbitrarily limited to 94 mW/cm² by the U.S. Food and Drug Administration. There are no contraindications to ultrasound procedures during pregnancy, and this modality has largely replaced X-ray as the primary method of fetal imaging during pregnancy.

Magnetic Resonance Imaging

With MRI, magnets that alter the energy state of hydrogen protons are used instead of ionizing radiation (13). This technique could prove especially useful for diagnosis and evaluation of fetal central nervous system anomalies and placental abnormalities (eg, accreta, previa).

Nuclear Medicine

Nuclear studies such as pulmonary ventilation–perfusion, thyroid, bone, and renal scans are performed by "tagging" a chemical agent with a radioisotope. The fetal exposure depends on the physical and biochemical properties of the radioisotope (6).

Technetium Tc 99m is one of the most commonly used isotopes and is used for brain, bone, renal, and cardiovascular scans. In general, these latter procedures result in a uterus, embryo, or fetal exposure of less than 0.5 rad (6, 12).

One of the more common nuclear medicine studies performed during pregnancy is the ventilation–perfusion scan for suspected pulmonary embolism. Macroaggregated albumin labeled with Technetium Tc 99m is used for the perfusion portion, and inhaled xenon gas (^{127}Xe or ^{133}Xe) is used for the ventilation portion. The amount of radiation to which the fetus is exposed is extremely small (approximately 50 mrad) (14).

In a 2002 study, investigators calculated the mean fetal radiation exposure resulting from helical (spiral) CT in healthy pregnant women and compared it with reported fetal radiation doses for ventilation–perfusion lung scanning (approximately 100–370 µGy) (15). Although the exposure from ventilation–perfusion is relatively low, the study found that the mean fetal doses associated with helical CT were lower. Although exposure varied with gestational age (3.3–20.2 µGy for the first trimester, 7.9–76.7 µGy for the second trimester, and 51.3–130.8 µGy for the third trimester), 20 of 23 study patients exhibited a mean fetal dose of less than 60 µGy for all 3 trimesters.

Radioactive iodine readily crosses the placenta and can adversely affect the fetal thyroid, especially if used after 10–12 weeks of gestation. Radioactive isotopes of iodine used for treatment of hyperthyroidism are contraindicated during pregnancy, and such therapy should be delayed until after delivery. If a diagnostic scan of the thyroid is essential,

^{123}I or Technetium Tc 99m should be used in place of ^{131}I (14).

Contrast Agents

A variety of oral and intravascular contrast agents are used with X-ray and magnetic imaging procedures. Most radiopaque agents used with CT and conventional radiography contain derivatives of iodine and have not been studied in humans; however iohexol, iopamidol, iothalamate, ioversol, ioxaglate, and metrizamide have been studied in animals and do not appear to be teratogenic (16). Neonatal hypothyroidism has been associated with some iodinated agents taken during pregnancy (17). For this reason, these compounds generally are avoided unless essential for correct diagnosis. Studies requiring views before and after the administration of contrast agents will necessarily have greater radiation exposure. Although some radiopaque agents pass into the breast milk, they have not been associated with problems in nursing babies (16).

Paramagnetic contrast agents used during MRI have not been studied in pregnant women. Animal studies have demonstrated increased rates of spontaneous abortion, skeletal abnormalities, and visceral abnormalities when given at 2–7 times the recommended human dose (18, 19). It is not known if these compounds are excreted into human milk. Generally, these agents should be used during pregnancy only if the potential benefit justifies the potential risk to the fetus as demonstrated in animal studies.

Guidelines

The following guidelines for X-ray examination or exposure during pregnancy are suggested:

1. Women should be counseled that X-ray exposure from a single diagnostic procedure does not result in harmful fetal effects. Specifically, exposure to less than 5 rad has not been associated with an increase in fetal anomalies or pregnancy loss.

2. Concern about possible effects of high-dose ionizing radiation exposure should not prevent medically indicated diagnostic X-ray procedures from being performed on a pregnant woman. During pregnancy, other imaging procedures not associated with ionizing radiation

(eg, ultrasonography, MRI) should be considered instead of X-rays when appropriate.

3. Ultrasonography and MRI are not associated with known adverse fetal effects.

4. Consultation with an expert in dosimetry calculation may be helpful in calculating estimated fetal dose when multiple diagnostic X-rays are performed on a pregnant patient.

5. The use of radioactive isotopes of iodine is contraindicated for therapeutic use during pregnancy.

6. Radiopaque and paramagnetic contrast agents are unlikely to cause harm and may be of diagnostic benefit, but these agents should be used during pregnancy only if the potential benefit justifies the potential risk to the fetus.

References

1. Gray JE. Safety (risk) of diagnostic radiology exposures. In: American College of Radiology. Radiation risk: a primer. Reston (VA): ACR; 1996. p. 15–7.

2. Brent RL. The effect of embryonic and fetal exposure to x-ray, microwaves, and ultrasound: counseling the pregnant and nonpregnant patient about these risks. Semin Oncol 1989;16:347–68.

3. Hall EJ. Scientific view of low-level radiation risks. Radiographics 1991;11:509–18.

4. Moore MM, Shearer DR. Fetal dose estimates for CT pelvimetry. Radiology 1989;171:265–7.

5. Parry RA, Glaze SA, Archer BR. The AAPM/RSNA physics tutorial for residents. Typical patient radiation doses in diagnostic radiology. Radiographics 1999;19: 1289–302.

6. Cunningham FG, Gant NF, Leveno KJ, Gilstrap LC 3rd, Hauth JC, Wenstrom KD. General considerations and maternal evaluation. In: Williams obstetrics. 21st ed. New York (NY): McGraw-Hill; 2001. p. 1143–58.

7. Otake M, Yoshimaru H, Schull WJ. Severe mental retardation among prenatally exposed survivors of the atomic bombing of Hiroshima and Nagasaki: a comparison of the T65DR and DS86 dosimetry systems. Technical report; RERF TR 87-16. Hiroshima: Radiation Effects Research Foundation; 1988.

8. National Research Council. Other somatic and fetal effects. In: Health effects of exposure to low levels of ionizing radiation: BEIR V. Washington, DC: National Academy Press; 1990:352–70.

9. Schull WJ, Otake M. Neurological deficit among survivors exposed to the atomic bombing of Hiroshima and Nagasaki: a reassessment and new directions. In: Kriegel H, Schmahl W, Gerber GB, Stieve FE, editors. Radiation risks to the developing nervous system. Neuherberg, June 18-29, 1985, Munich. Stuttgart: G Fischer Verlag; 1986. p. 399–419.

10. Miller RW. Epidemiological conclusions from radiation toxicity studies. In: Fry RJ, Grahn D, Griem ML, Rust JH, editors. Late effects of radiation: proceedings of the colloquium held at the Center for Continuing Education, the University of Chicago, Illinois, May 1969. New York (NY): Van Nostrand Reinhold; 1970. p. 245–56.

11. Early diagnosis of pregnancy: a symposium. J Reprod Med 1981;26(suppl 4):149–78.

12. Mettler FA Jr, Guiberteau MJ. Essentials of nuclear medicine imaging. 4th ed. Philadelphia (PA): WB Saunders; 1998.

13. Curry TS 3rd, Dowdey JE, Murry RC Jr, editors. Christensen's physics of diagnostic radiology. 4th ed. Philadelphia (PA): Lea & Febiger; 1990.

14. Ginsberg JS, Hirsh J, Rainbow AJ, Coates G. Risks to the fetus of radiologic procedures used in the diagnosis of maternal venous thromboembolic disease. Thromb Haemost 1989;61:189–96.

15. Winer-Muram HT, Boone JM, Brown HL, Jennings SG, Mabie WC, Lombardo GT. Pulmonary embolism in pregnant patients: fetal radiation dose with helical CT. Radiology 2002;224:487–92.

16. Radiopaque agents (diagnostic). MedlinePlus drug information. Available at: http://www.nlm.nih.gov/medlineplus/druginfo/uspdi/202997.html. Retrieved June 17, 2004.

17. Mehta PS, Metha SJ, Vorherr H. Congenital iodide goiter and hypothyroidism: a review. Obstet Gynecol Surv 1983;38:237–47.

18. Gadodiamide (systemic). In: USP DI: drug information for the health care professional. 24th ed. Greenwood Village (CO): Microdemex; 2004. Available at http://uspdi.micromedex.com/v1/excluded/Gadodiamide(Systemic).pdf. Retrieved June 17, 2004.

19. Gadoteridol (systemic). In: USP DI: drug information for the health care professional. 24th ed. Greenwood Village (CO): Microdemex; 2004. Available at: http://uspdi.micromedex.com/v1/excluded/Gadoteridol(Systemic).pdf. Retrieved June 17, 2004.

ACOG

ACOG Committee on
Health Care for
Underserved Women

The Committee wishes to thank Gene Burkett, MD; Ronald Chez, MD; and Eve Espey, MD, for their assistance in the development of this document.

ISSN 1074-861X

The American College of Obstetricians and Gynecologists
409 12th Street, SW
PO Box 96920
Washington, DC 20090-6920

12345/98765

Health Care for Homeless Women. ACOG Committee Opinion No. 312. American College of Obstetricians and Gynecologists. Obstet Gynecol 2005;106:429–34.

Committee Opinion

Number 312, August 2005

Health Care for Homeless Women

Abstract: Homelessness is a considerable social and health problem in the United States with far-reaching effects on the health of homeless women. Homeless women are at higher risk for injury and illness and are less likely to obtain needed health care than women who are not homeless. It is critical to undertake efforts to prevent homelessness. Until this can be accomplished, community-based services targeted specifically to this population that provide both health care and support services are essential. Health care providers can help address the needs of the homeless by identifying their own patients who may be homeless, treating their health problems, offering preventive care, and working with the community to improve the full range of resources available to these individuals.

Approximately 3.5 million Americans are currently homeless (1), and as many as 14% of the U.S. population have been homeless at some time (2) (see box "Definition of Homelessness"). Women make up nearly one third of the homeless population and are one of the fastest growing groups (3). In the population of homeless individuals in families, 84% are women (4). Sixty percent of homeless women have children younger than 18 years, but many do not have custody of their children. There also are children who are homeless in their own right. This group includes runaways (5). Many homeless adolescents left home because of conflicts with parents over their sexual orientation (6). Most homeless adolescents are white and come from suburban and rural areas. They are more likely than other populations to experience depression and substance abuse, to have previously attempted suicide, and to have a history of sexual and physical abuse (7).

Extreme poverty is a universal characteristic of homeless individuals, but not all impoverished individuals become homeless. The shortage of low-income housing is a major precipitating factor to homelessness. It can render homeless even individuals who are not extremely poor. Unemployment or job loss, personal or family crisis, an increase in rent disproportionate to income, or reduction in public health benefits increase the likelihood of loss of a home among those at risk (4). For women, an additional risk factor is early motherhood (8).

Many homeless individuals lack education and money. Thirty-eight percent of homeless individuals did not graduate from high school and another 34% finished only high school. Slightly more than one quarter of homeless individuals have any education beyond high school. The average monthly

Definition of Homelessness

An individual is considered homeless if he or she lacks a fixed, regular, and adequate nighttime residence, or an individual who has a primary nighttime residence that is:

a) a supervised publicly or privately operated shelter designed to provide temporary living accommodations (including welfare hotels, congregate shelters, and transitional housing for the mentally ill);

b) a public or private place that provides a temporary residence for individuals intended to be institutionalized; or

c) a public or private place not designed for, or ordinarily used as, regular sleeping accommodations for human beings.

Interagency Council on the Homeless. Homelessness: programs and the people they serve. Findings of the National Survey of Homeless Assistance Providers and Clients. Washington, DC: U.S. Department of Housing and Urban Development, Office of Policy Development and Research; 1999.

income for a homeless family is $475 (46% of the federal poverty level for a family of three at the time of the study), and for a single homeless individual is $348 (51% of the federal poverty level for one person) (4). Other risk factors include lack of job skills, inadequate social support, problems with alcohol or illicit drugs, mental illness, experiences of violence and victimization, and previous incarceration.

Impact of Homelessness on Women

Homelessness may be difficult to recognize. However, certain circumstances, many of which affect the individual's health, are seen more frequently in this population (see box "Common Characteristics of Homelessness"). Being homeless creates an increased risk for illness and injury resulting in high levels of morbidity and mortality (9). Homeless adolescent and adult women often participate in survival sex, which refers to the selling of sex to meet subsistence needs (10, 11). Approximately 26% of young homeless females reported having participated in survival sex (10). More than two thirds of homeless mothers have a diagnosis of mental illness. Cases of posttraumatic stress disorder, substance abuse disorders, and major depression are disproportionately higher among homeless women compared with other populations (12).

Violence

Violence is common among homeless populations. Homeless individuals are at risk because they lack personal security when living outdoors or in a shelter. Twenty-two percent report having been physically assaulted or beaten up at least once while homeless (4). One study reported that 13% of homeless women, particularly those with mental illness, were sexually assaulted or raped in the past year, compared with 2.7% of the general population (13). Twenty-two percent of homeless adolescents report prior child abuse and 13% report sexual abuse (1, 4).

Gynecologic Health

Among homeless women interviewed in Los Angeles, 66% used no method of contraception even though most had intercourse at least once per week. Fewer than 10% of homeless women report regular condom use although they are at high risk for sexually transmitted diseases (STDs) and human immunodeficiency virus (HIV) infection (14, 15), which are especially problematic in the homeless adolescent population (11). Pelvic inflammatory disease occurred in approximately 28% of homeless women, and 60% had a history of a least one STD (1).

Obstetric Health

Pregnancy and recent birth are highly correlated with becoming homeless in the newly homeless population. At the time they requested emergency shelter, 35% of homeless women were pregnant and 26%

Common Characteristics of Homelessness

- Appearance: unkempt, disheveled, dirty, aggressive, hostile
- Chronic recurrent diseases, including respiratory infections, hepatitis, asthma, arthritis, or tuberculosis
- Multiple STDs or HIV
- Substance abuse (alcohol and other substances)
- Chronic mental illness with or without comorbidity, suicide attempts, posttraumatic stress disorders, stresses associated with sexual identity and orientation
- Repetitive, nonspecific complaints for which a diagnosis cannot be found
- Underweight with history of subnutrition or poor nutritional state
- Domestic violence, including sexual abuse and victimization
- No fixed address or multiple addresses in a short period
- Lack of adherence with physician directives and orders

had given birth in the past year. Only 6% of women in the study who were not homeless were pregnant and only 11% had given birth in the past year (8). Homeless women often have little choice in the timing, the place, the partner, and the circumstances surrounding conception. Factors associated with unintended pregnancy were victimization, survival sex, lack of contraception, uncertain fertility status, desire for intimacy, and lack of hope for the future (16). Women younger than 21 years living on the streets are at much greater risk of having ever been pregnant than are young women living in households (5).

Adverse birth outcomes are substantially higher in homeless women than in the general population (17). In a study conducted in 1997, 17% of babies born to homeless women were low birth weight compared with 11% among those residing in low-income housing (17). The rate of low birth weight at the time of that study was 7.5% for all women (18). Similarly, 19% of births in the homeless population were preterm compared with 11% nationally (17, 18). Homeless women are less likely to receive prenatal care (19, 20). The more severe the homelessness (defined by whether or not the woman was homeless during the first trimester of her pregnancy, the number of times she had been homeless, and the percentage of her life during which she had been homeless), the less likely a woman is to receive prenatal care and the more likely an adverse pregnancy outcome will occur. Older homeless women and those who abuse drugs also are less likely to receive prenatal care. Other predictors of adverse pregnancy outcomes among homeless women include history of preterm birth, antenatal complications, and birth complications; STDs; low income; nulliparity; and being African American (17).

Adverse birth outcomes are higher in African-American homeless women than in homeless women of other races. In the homeless population, 22% of infants born to African-American women were low birth weight, whereas only 16% of Hispanic infants and 5% of non-Hispanic white infants were low birth weight. African-American homeless women are more likely to experience preterm birth. Homeless Native American women also appear to have a large proportion of preterm births and babies with low birth weight (17).

Homeless women may forgo meals in favor of alcohol and other drugs (20). Day-to-day survival stresses are superimposed on emotional distress, which may lead to new or increased substance abuse (20). Homeless pregnant women are prone to urinary tract infections and vaginal infections (20).

Children of homeless women are more likely to be separated from their mothers by social service providers. Forty-four percent of homeless mothers, compared with 8% of mothers receiving public assistance who are not homeless, were separated from their children. Homelessness was the major risk factor in such separation, although substance abuse, domestic violence, and maternal institutionalization also were risk factors. A substantial minority of these children are placed in foster care. (21). This separation from children may lead to emotional strain, anxiety, loss of control, instability, guilt, and insecurity among homeless mothers.

Preventive Health

Homeless women receive breast examinations, mammograms, and Pap tests at lower rates than the general population (22–24). Although no studies have specifically examined cervical dysplasia and cancer in this population, homeless women have many risk factors for inadequate diagnosis, incomplete follow-up, and incomplete treatment because of the competing survival needs.

Use of Health Care

Most homeless people seek care in hospital emergency rooms; only 27% go to an established ambulatory care provider. The younger homeless population is even more likely to receive care in the emergency room. Nearly three quarters of homeless individuals who are hospitalized have conditions that were preventable and could have been treated before admission compared with 41% of low-income individuals who are not homeless (25). Recurrent admission for the same diagnosis is common and occurs in approximately 40% of homeless adults, which imposes a financial burden on hospitals (1).

Barriers to Health Care

Approximately 57% of homeless individuals lack a regular source of care compared with 24% of the poor and 19% of the general population (26). Nearly 25% of homeless individuals who reported a need for medical attention in the previous year were unable to obtain care. The following factors contribute to this situation (1, 4, 27, 28):

- Cost and lack of health insurance (55% of homeless individuals report that they have no medical insurance) and inability to purchase or acquire medications

- Lack of transportation to and from medical facilities
- Competing needs for survival (food, clothing, shelter)
- Mental illness and substance abuse
- Unstable lifestyle interfering with continuity of care and adherence with treatment
- Because an exhibition of toughness is necessary to survive on the streets, homeless individuals may at times deny that they have health problems. They also may have a fear of authority figures, including medical providers.
- Lack of availability of shelters and treatment facilities for the homeless
- Medical providers, including physicians, may prefer not to care for homeless individuals in their offices
- Inadequate inpatient discharge planning and follow-up care because of failure to recognize homelessness
- Lack of health care professionals' knowledge and information on services available within the community for homeless individuals

Recommendations to Improve the Health of Homeless Women

Health care services for a homeless woman should be a part of a multifaceted approach tailored to her needs, perspectives, and values. Acceptance of the individual is critical to the provision of services. Accomplishing these goals is a major challenge to the obstetrician–gynecologist or any other health care provider. Often the resources required, including the necessary professionals and support services, are either not available in the community or difficult for the private provider to obtain. Even though individual obstetrician–gynecologists can and do provide services to homeless patients in their practices, it may be more beneficial for communities to develop organized services targeted specifically to this population that can better provide both health care and support services. Organized services can better implement both the preventive care and the obstetric and gynecologic care recommended in the guidelines of the American College of Obstetricians and Gynecologists (30). Prenatal care that coordinates with social services, rehabilitation programs, and housing programs to shelter homeless women during pregnancy should be the goal.

Health care professionals also can contribute to improved health care for homeless women by participating in the following activities:

- Care for homeless women in individual practices without bias.
- Volunteer or form volunteer groups to provide health care services at homeless shelters and soup kitchens. Adherence to treatment is enhanced when medical care is coupled with services to meet the survival needs of patients. Care should not be withheld because of concerns about lack of adherence.
- Seek donations of medications from pharmaceutical companies for use in homeless clinics and shelters.
- Implement health care programs for the homeless with local hospitals and clinics (see box "J.C. Lewis Health Center: An Example of Success").

J.C. Lewis Health Center: An Example of Success

An example of a successful health care program for homeless women is the J.C. Lewis Health Center. This center is a 32-bed primary and respite care clinic in Savannah, Georgia, that has saved area hospitals $10.3 million in uncompensated care for the homeless. The center allows homeless individuals to gain access to primary care providers who manage acute and episodic health needs and diagnose, control, and monitor chronic health problems such as HIV, hypertension, and diabetes. The operation includes the staffing of four shelter-based primary care clinics across the city where health promotion and primary care divert homeless people from emergency rooms. Wellness care for the homeless includes physical examinations, screening for disease, and patient education. Respite care allows the hospital to release patients too sick to stay in shelters, but not sick enough to stay in the hospital. These individuals would otherwise have remained hospitalized. The health center also coordinates its services with housing and social services to help the individuals obtain permanent housing. Ninety-five percent of the respite care patients ended their homelessness after leaving the program.

Program funding is provided by hospitals (each contribute $250,000 to the program), public support through government grants ($244,000), philanthropic organizations ($164,000), and private citizens ($19,000). In addition, volunteers from the community, including doctors, nurses, and educators, donate their time to the health center, and the center receives in-kind contributions of pharmaceuticals and supplies.

The J.C. Lewis Health Center. Available at: http://www.unionmission.org. Retrieved June 6, 2005.

- Work with medical schools and residency programs to encourage modification of the educational curriculum to increase awareness of the problems associated with homelessness and to involve medical students and residents in care for homeless individuals as part of their training.

- Assess current community programs for homeless individuals and advocate for improved coordination of services between these programs and other special programs such as prenatal care, immunization, tuberculosis treatment, STD clinics, mental health care, and housing and legal aid.

- Advocate for professional liability protections for physicians who volunteer their services to the homeless.

- Encourage federal, state, and local governments to provide adequate funding for the provision of comprehensive health care services, including mental health treatment for all homeless individuals. (See box "Health Care for the Homeless Federal Program.")

Health Care for the Homeless Federal Program

The Health Care for the Homeless program is the only federal program with the sole responsibility of addressing the primary health care needs of homeless individuals. The Health Care for the Homeless program provides primary health care and substance abuse services at locations accessible to individuals who are homeless, emergency care with referrals to hospitals for inpatient care services or other needed services, outreach services to assist difficult-to-reach homeless individuals in gaining access to care, and assistance in establishing eligibility for entitlement programs and housing.

To increase access to services and resources for people who are homeless, the grantees of the Health Care for the Homeless program are encouraged to develop, or actively participate in, local coalitions of health care providers and social service agencies. These collaborations help ensure the adequate and appropriate delivery of services to the clients of the Health Care for the Homeless program. Each individual program determines which service delivery system or combination of systems is appropriate for the people it serves. Programs provide services in a variety of different settings, including traditional clinic sites, shelter-based clinics, and mobile units. In addition, they take health care services to locations where homeless individuals are found, such as streets, parks, and soup kitchens.

Bureau of Primary Health Care. Health Care for the Homeless Information Resource Center. 2004-2005 Health Care for the Homeless Grantee profiles. Available at: http://www.bphc.hrsa.gov/hchirc/directory/text_directory.htm. Retrieved June 6, 2005.

The Prevention of Homelessness

Although it is critical to undertake efforts to improve the health of homeless women, it is even more important to undertake efforts to prevent homelessness. Increased federal, state, and local government support and provision of adequate funding for comprehensive programs for the prevention of homelessness, including increased availability of affordable, usually subsidized, housing are essential to this goal. Numerous studies indicate that affordable housing prevents homelessness more effectively than anything else. This applies to all groups of poor people, including those with persistent and severe mental illness or those with substance abuse problems (29). Additional research is needed to determine other efforts that would be effective at reducing this problem and thereby improve women's health and the overall health of society.

References

1. Gelberg L, Arangua L. Homeless persons. In: Anderson RM, Rice TH, Kominski GF, editors. Changing the U.S. health care system: key issues in health services, policy, and management. San Francisco (CA): Jossey-Bass; 2001. p.332–86.
2. Link BG, Susser E, Stueve A, Phelan J, Moore RE, Struening E. Lifetime and five-year prevalence of homelessness in the United States. Am J Public Health 1994; 84:1907–12.
3. Hodnicki DR, Horner SD, Boyle JS. Women's perspectives on homelessness. Public Health Nurs 1992;9:257–62.
4. Interagency Council on the Homeless. Homelessness: programs and the people they serve. Findings of the National Survey of Homeless Assistance Providers and Clients. Washington, DC: U.S. Department of Housing and Urban Development, Office of Policy Development and Research; 1999.
5. Greene JM, Ringwalt CL. Pregnancy among three national samples of runaway and homeless youth. J Adolesc Health 1998;23:370–7.
6. Farrow JA, Deisher RW, Brown R, Kulig JW, Kipke MD. Health and health needs of homeless and runaway youth. A position paper of the Society for Adolescent Medicine. J Adolesc Health 1992;13:717–26.
7. Pennbridge J, Mackenzie RG, Swofford A. Risk profile of homeless pregnant adolescents and youth. J Adolesc Health 1991;12:534–8.
8. Weitzman BC. Pregnancy and childbirth: risk factors for homelessness? Fam Plann Perspect 1989;21:175–8.
9. Hwang SW. Is homelessness hazardous to your health? Obstacles to the demonstration of a causal relationship. Can J Public Health 2002;93:407–10.
10. Greene JM, Ennett ST, Ringwalt CL. Prevalence and correlates of survival sex among runaway and homeless youth. Am J Public Health 1999;89:1406–9.
11. Bailey SL, Camlin CS, Ennett ST. Substance use and risky sexual behavior among homeless and runaway youth. J Adolesc Health 1998;23:378–88.

12. Bassuk EL, Buckner JC, Perloff JN, Bassuk SS. Prevalence of mental health and substance use disorders among homeless and low-income housed mothers. Am J Psychiatry 1998;155:1561–4.

13. Wenzel SL, Leake BD, Gelberg L. Health of homeless women with recent experience of rape. J Gen Intern Med 2000;15:265–8.

14. Shuler PA, Gelberg L, Davis JE. Characteristics associated with the risk of unintended pregnancy among urban homeless women: use of the Shuler Nurse Practitioner Practice Model in research. J Am Acad Nurse Pract 1995;7:13–22.

15. Gelberg L, Leake BD, Lu MC, Andersen RM, Wenzel SL, Morgenstern H, et al. Use of contraceptive methods among homeless women for protection against unwanted pregnancies and sexually transmitted diseases: prior use and willingness to use in the future. Contraception 2001; 63:277–81.

16. Killion CM. Poverty and procreation among women. An anthropologic study with implications for health care providers. J Nurse Midwifery 1998;43:273–9.

17. Stein JA, Lu MC, Gelberg L. Severity of homelessness and adverse birth outcomes. Health Psychol 2000;19: 524–34.

18. Ventura SJ, Martin JA, Curtin SC, Mathews TJ. Births: final data for 1997. Natl Vital Stat Rep 1999;47(18):1–96.

19. Chavkin W, Kristal A, Seabron C, Guigli PE. The reproductive experience of women living in hotels for the homeless in New York City. NY State J Med 1987; 87: 10–3.

20. Killion CM. Special health care needs of homeless pregnant women. ANS Adv Nurs Sci 1995;18:44–56.

21. Cowal K, Shinn M, Weitzman BC, Stojanovic D, Labay L. Mother-child separations among homeless and housed families receiving public assistance in New York City. Am J Community Psychol 2002;30:711–30.

22. Chau S, Chin M, Chang J, Luecha A, Cheng E, Schlesinger J, et al. Cancer risk behaviors and screening rates among homeless adults in Los Angeles County. Cancer Epidemiol Biomarkers Prev 2002;11:431–8.

23. Long HL, Tulsky JP, Chambers DB, Alpers LS, Robertson MJ, Moss AR, et al. Cancer screening in homeless women: attitudes and behaviors. J Health Care Poor Underserved 1998;9:276–92.

24. Weinreb L, Goldberg R, Perloff J. Health characteristics and medical service use patterns of sheltered homeless and low-income housed mothers. J Gen Intern Med 1998; 13:389–97.

25. Salit SA, Kuhn EM, Hartz AJ, Vu JM, Mosso AL. Hospitalization costs associated with homelessness in New York City. N Engl J Med 1998;338:1734–40.

26. Gallagher TC, Andersen RM, Koegel P, Gelberg L. Determinants of regular source of care among homeless adults in Los Angeles. Med Care 1997;35:814–30.

27. Lim YW, Andersen R, Leake B, Cunningham W, Gelberg L. How accessible is medical care for homeless women? Med Care 2002;40:510–20.

28. Kushel MB, Vittinghoff E, Haas JS. Factors associated with the health care utilization of homeless persons. JAMA 2001;285:200–6.

29. U.S. Department of Housing and Urban Development, U.S. Department of Health and Human Services. Practical lessons: the 1998 National Symposium on Homelessness Research. Available at: http://aspe.hhs.gov/progsys/home less/symposium/toc.htm. Retrieved April 12, 2005.

30. Primary and preventive care: periodic assessments. ACOG Committee Opinion No. 292. American College of Obstetricians and Gynecologists. Obstet Gynecol 2003; 102:1117–24.

ACOG

Committee on
Gynecologic Practice

Committee Opinion

Number 203, July 1998   *(Replaces #199, February 1998)*

Hepatitis Virus Infections in Obstetrician–Gynecologists

The current epidemic of human immunodeficiency virus (HIV) infection has escalated concerns about transmission from infected patients to health care workers. The concerns about HIV have increased attention to hepatitis B virus (HBV). It appears that surgeons who follow recommended infection-control procedures are at little risk of acquiring HIV while caring for HIV-infected patients (1, 2). In contrast, surgeons can readily acquire HBV from infected patients (1, 3).

The College routinely has recommended hepatitis B vaccination for obstetrician–gynecologists who are exposed to blood or blood products. Postvaccination testing for antibodies, which is recommended by the Centers for Disease Control and Prevention, can validate immunization (4). Individuals who are antibody negative after immunization should be tested for hepatitis B surface antigen to identify carriers as a result of previous HBV infection (5). The Committee on Gynecologic Practice supports the recommendation that surgeons who perform invasive procedures and who do not have evidence of immunity to HBV should know their hepatitis B surface antigen status and, if it is positive, also should know their hepatitis B e antigen status (6, 7).

The risk of acquiring hepatitis C virus (HCV) infection appears to be lower than the risk of acquiring HBV and higher than the risk of acquiring HIV (2, 3). Nonetheless, HCV is the most common cause of chronic viral hepatitis, and even chronic HCV infection symptoms typically are silent or minimal (8). Thus, surgeons who perform exposure-prone procedures should consider being tested for anti-HCV antibody and, if positive, should confirm seropositive status by documenting HCV RNA in the serum with reverse transcription polymerase chain reaction testing (8–10). Institutional and local health department rules usually are available to guide health care workers who test positive for bloodborne viruses.

References

1. Henderson DK. Human immunodeficiency virus infection in patients and providers. In: Wenzel RP, ed. Prevention and control of nosocomial infections. 2nd ed. Baltimore: Williams and Wilkins, 1993:42–47
2. Gerberding JL. Management of occupational exposures to blood-borne viruses. N Engl J Med 1995;332:444–451

The American College of Obstetricians and Gynecologists
409 12th Street, SW
PO Box 96920
Washington, DC 20090-6920

12345/21098

3. Shapiro CN. Occupational risk of infection with hepatitis B and hepatitis C virus. Surg Clin N Am 1995;75:1047–1056

4. Centers for Disease Control and Prevention. Protection against viral hepatitis: recommendations of the Immunization Practices Advisory Committee. MMWR 1990;39 (RR-2):13

5. Rhodes RS. Hepatitis B virus, surgeons, and surgery. Bull Am Coll Surg 1995;80(6):32–42

6. Centers for Disease Control and Prevention. Recommendations for preventing transmission of human immunodeficiency virus and hepatitis B virus to patients du82 ring exposure-prone invasive procedures. MMWR 1991;40 (RR-8):1–9

7. American College of Surgeons. Statement on the surgeon and hepatitis B infection. Bull Am Coll Surg 1995;80(5):33–35

8. Sharara AI, Hunt CM, Hamilton JD. Update: hepatitis C. Ann Intern Med 1996;125:658–668

9. Centers for Disease Control and Prevention. Recommendations for follow-up of health-care workers after occupational exposure to hepatitis C virus. MMWR 1997;46:603–606

10. Dore GJ, Kaldor JM, McCaughan GW. Systematic review of role of polymerase chain reaction in defining infectiousness among people infected with hepatitis C virus. BMJ 1997;315:333–337

ACOG Committee Opinion

Committee on
Obstetric Practice

Number 282, January 2003

Immunization During Pregnancy

ABSTRACT: Preconceptional immunization of pregnant women to prevent disease in the offspring, when practical, is preferred to vaccination of pregnant women. The benefits of immunization to the pregnant woman and her neonate usually outweigh the theoretic risks of adverse effects. Current information on the safety of vaccines given during pregnancy is subject to change and can be verified from the Centers for Disease Control and Prevention web site at www.cdc.gov/nip.

The benefits of immunization to the pregnant woman and her neonate usually outweigh the theoretic risks of adverse effects. The theoretic risks of the vaccination of pregnant women with killed virus vaccines have not been identified.

Current recommendations for immunization of pregnant women are presented in Table 1. Although new information continues to confirm the safety of vaccines intentionally or inadvertently given during pregnancy, current information is subject to change because the effects of many diseases and vaccines on the pregnant woman or the fetus may be rare and infrequently reported. (For further information and updates refer to www.cdc.gov/nip.)

In the decision of whether to immunize a pregnant woman with other vaccines not listed in Table 1, the risk for exposure to disease and its deleterious effects on the pregnant woman and the fetus must be balanced against the efficacy of the vaccine and any beneficial effects resulting from it. Preconceptional immunization of women to prevent disease in the offspring, when practical, is preferred to vaccination of pregnant women with certain vaccines. Vaccination of women during the postpartum period, especially for rubella and varicella, should be encouraged. Women susceptible to rubella should be vaccinated with measles–mumps–rubella on postpartum discharge from the hospital.

The American College of Obstetricians and Gynecologists
409 12th Street, SW
PO Box 96920
Washington, DC 20090-6920

12345/76543

Immunization during pregnancy. ACOG Committee Opinion No. 282. American College of Obstetricians and Gynecologists. Obstet Gynecol 2003; 101:207–12.

Table 1. Immunization During Pregnancy

Immunobiologic Agent	Risk from Disease to Pregnant Woman	Risk from Disease to Fetus or Neonate	Type of Immunizing Agent	Risk from Immunizing Agent to Fetus	Indications for Immunization During Pregnancy	Dose Schedule*	Comments
LIVE VIRUS VACCINES							
Measles	Significant morbidity, low mortality; not altered by pregnancy	Significant increase in abortion rate; may cause malformations	Live attenuated virus vaccine	None confirmed	Contraindicated (see immune globulins)	Single dose SC, preferably as measles–mumps–rubella†	Vaccination of susceptible women should be part of postpartum care. Breastfeeding is not a contraindication.
Mumps	Low morbidity and mortality; not altered by pregnancy	Possible increased rate of abortion in first trimester	Live attenuated virus vaccine	None confirmed	Contraindicated	Single dose SC, preferably as measles–mumps–rubella	Vaccination of susceptible women should be part of postpartum care
Poliomyelitis	No increased incidence in pregnancy, but may be more severe if it does occur	Anoxic fetal damage reported; 50% mortality in neonatal disease	Live attenuated virus (oral polio vaccine) and enhanced-potency inactivated virus vaccine‡	None confirmed	Not routinely recommended for women in the United States, except women at increased risk of exposure	*Primary:* Two doses of enhanced-potency inactivated virus SC at 4–8 week intervals and a third dose 6–12 months after the second dose *Immediate protection:* One dose oral polio vaccine (in outbreak setting)	Vaccine indicated for susceptible pregnant women traveling in endemic areas or in other high-risk situations
Rubella	Low morbidity and mortality; not altered by pregnancy	High rate of abortion and congenital rubella syndrome	Live attenuated virus vaccine	None confirmed	Contraindicated, but congenital rubella syndrome has never been described after vaccine	Single dose SC, preferably as measles–mumps–rubella	Teratogenicity of vaccine is theoretic, not confirmed to date; vaccination of susceptible women should be part of postpartum care
Yellow fever	Significant morbidity and mortality; not altered by pregnancy	Unknown	Live attenuated virus vaccine	Unknown	Contraindicated except if exposure is unavoidable	Single dose SC	Postponement of travel preferable to vaccination, if possible

Disease	Effect on maternal health	Effect on fetus/newborn	Vaccine type	Adverse effects	Indications	Dose/schedule	Comments
Varicella	Possible increase in severe pneumonia	Can cause congenital varicella in 2% of fetuses infected during the second trimester	Live attenuated virus vaccine	None confirmed	Contraindicated, but no adverse outcomes reported if given in pregnancy	Two doses needed with second dose given 4–8 weeks after first dose. Should be strongly encouraged	Teratogenicity of vaccine is theoretic, outcomes reported weeks 4–8 not confirmed to date. Vaccination of susceptible women should be considered postpartum

OTHER

Disease	Effect on maternal health	Effect on fetus/newborn	Vaccine type	Adverse effects	Indications	Dose/schedule	Comments
Influenza	Increase in morbidity and mortality during epidemic of new antigenic strain	Possible increased abortion rate; no malformations confirmed	Inactivated virus vaccine	None confirmed	All women who are pregnant in the second and third trimester during the flu season (October–March); women at high risk for pulmonary complications regardless of trimester	One dose IM every year	—
Rabies	Near 100% fatality; not altered by pregnancy	Determined by maternal disease	Killed virus vaccine	Unknown	Indications for prophylaxis not altered by pregnancy; each case considered individually	Public health authorities to be consulted for indications, dosage, and route of administration	—
Hepatitis B	Possible increased severity during third trimester	Possible increase in abortion rate and preterm birth; neonatal hepatitis can occur; high risk of newborn carrier state	Purified surface antigen produced by recombinant technology	None reported	Pre-exposure and postexposure for women at risk of infection	Three-dose series IM at 0, 1, and 6 months	Used with hepatitis B immune globulin for some exposures; exposed newborn needs birth dose vaccination and immune globulin as soon as possible. All infants should receive birth dose of vaccine.
Hepatitis A	No increased risk during pregnancy	—	Inactivated virus	None reported	Pre-exposure and postexposure for women at risk of infection; international travelers	Two-dose schedule 6 months apart	—

(continued)

INACTIVATED BACTERIAL VACCINES

Pneumococcus	No increased risk during pregnancy; no increase in severity of disease	Unknown, but depends on maternal illness	Polyvalent polysaccharide vaccine	None reported	Recommended for women with asplenia; metabolic, renal, cardiac, pulmonary diseases; smokers; immunosuppressed. Indications not altered by pregnancy.	In adults, one SC or IM dose only; consider repeat dose in 6 years for high-risk women	—
Meningococcus	Significant morbidity and mortality; not altered by pregnancy	Unknown, but depends on maternal illness	Quadrivalent polysaccharide vaccine	None reported	Indications not altered by pregnancy; vaccination recommended in unusual outbreak situations	One SC dose; public health authorities consulted	—
Typhoid	Significant morbidity and mortality; not altered by pregnancy	Unknown	Killed or live attenuated oral bacterial vaccine	None confirmed	Not recommended routinely except for close, continued exposure or travel to endemic areas	Killed *Primary:* Two injections SC at least 4 weeks apart. *Booster:* Single dose SC or ID (depending on type of product) *Booster:* Schedule not yet determined	Oral vaccine preferred
Anthrax	Significant morbidity and mortality; not altered by pregnancy	Unknown, but depends on maternal illness	Preparation from cell-free filtrate of *B anthracis*; no dead or live bacteria	None confirmed	Not routinely recommended unless pregnant women work directly with *B anthracis*, imported animal hides, potentially infected animals in high incidence areas (not United States) or military personnel deployed to high-risk exposure areas	Six-dose primary vaccination SC, then annual booster vaccination	Teratogenicity of vaccine theoretical

Table 1. Immunization During Pregnancy *(continued)*

Immunobiologic Agent	Risk from Disease to Pregnant Woman	Risk from Disease to Fetus or Neonate	Type of Immunizing Agent	Risk from Immunizing Agent to Fetus	Indications for Immunization During Pregnancy	Dose Schedule*	Comments
TOXOIDS							
Tetanus–diphtheria	Severe morbidity; tetanus mortality 30%; diphtheria mortality 10%; unaltered by pregnancy	Neonatal tetanus mortality 60%	Combined tetanus–diphtheria toxoids preferred: adult tetanus–diphtheria formulation	None confirmed	Lack of primary series, or no booster within past 10 years	*Primary:* Two doses IM at 1–2-month interval with a third dose 6–12 months after the second. *Booster:* Single dose IM every 10 years after completion of primary series	Updating of immune status should be part of antepartum care
SPECIFIC IMMUNE GLOBULINS							
Hepatitis B	Possible increased severity during third trimester	Possible increase in abortion rate and preterm birth; neonatal hepatitis can occur; high risk of carriage in newborn	Hepatitis B immune globulin	None reported	Postexposure prophylaxis	Depends on exposure; consult Immunization Practices Advisory committee recommendations (IM)	Usually given with hepatitis B virus vaccine; exposed newborn needs immediate postexposure prophylaxis
Rabies	Near 100% fatality; not altered by pregnancy	Determined by maternal disease	Rabies immune globulin	None reported	Postexposure prophylaxis	Half dose at injury site, half dose in deltoid	Used in conjunction with rabies killed virus vaccine
Tetanus	Severe morbidity; mortality 60%	Neonatal tetanus mortality 60%	Tetanus immune globulin	None reported	Postexposure prophylaxis	One dose IM	Used in conjunction with tetanus toxoid

	Possible increase in severe varicella pneumonia	Can cause congenital varicella with increased mortality in neonatal period; very rarely causes congenital defects	Varicella–zoster immune globulin (obtained from the American Red Cross)	None reported	Should be considered for healthy pregnant women exposed to varicella to protect against maternal, not congenital, infection	One dose IM within 96 hours of exposure	Indicated also for newborns of women who developed varicella within 4 days before delivery or 2 days following delivery; approximately 90–95% of adults are immune to varicella; not indicated for prevention of congenital varicella
Varicella							

STANDARD IMMUNE GLOBULINS

	Possible increased severity during third trimester	Probable increase in abortion rate and preterm birth; possible transmission to neonate at delivery if woman is incubating the virus or is acutely ill at that time	Standard immune globulin	None reported	Postexposure prophylaxis, but hepatitis A virus vaccine should be used with hepatitis A immune globulin	0.02 mL/kg IM in one dose of immune globulin	Immune globulin should be given as soon as possible and within 2 weeks of exposure; infants born to women who are incubating the virus or are acutely ill at delivery should receive one dose of 0.5 mL as soon as possible after birth
Hepatitis A							

*Abbreviations: ID, intradermally; IM, intramuscularly; PO, orally; and SC, subcutaneously.

†Two doses necessary for adequate vaccination of students entering institutions of higher education, newly hired medical personnel, and international travelers.

‡Inactivated polio vaccine recommended for nonimmunized adults at increased risk.

Data from General recommendations on immunization. Recommendations of the Advisory Committee on Immunization Practices (ACIP) and the American Academy of Family Physicians (AAFP). Centers for Disease Control. MMWR Recomm Rep;51(RR-2):1–35. Available at http://www.cdc.gov/mmwr/preview/mmwrhtml/rr5102a1.htm. Retrieved October 11, 2002.

ACOG

Committee on
Coding and
Nomenclature

Committee Opinion

Number 250, January 2001

Inappropriate Reimbursement Practices by Third-Party Payers

The American College of Obstetricians and Gynecologists (ACOG) Committee on Coding and Nomenclature believes that physicians must code accurately the services they provide and the diagnoses that justify those services for purposes of appropriate payment. This requirement is consistent with the rules established by the American Medical Association (AMA) Current Procedural Terminology Editorial Panel and published as the *Current Procedural Terminology* (CPT) and with those established by the International Classification of Diseases, Ninth Revision, Clinical Modification (ICD-9-CM), which are published in the American Hospital Association's *ICD-9-CM Coding Clinic*. In fairness, payers should be equally obligated to pay physicians based on the CPT standards and accept for processing all ICD-9-CM codes recorded on the claim. Currently, no such obligation for payers exists.

Inappropriate Billing Denials

Five frequently encountered billing situations account for most payers' inappropriate first-time total or partial denials of correctly coded services. Each of these situations can inappropriately deny payment to physicians for medically indicated and correctly coded services because of payers' payment policies.

1. Inappropriately bundling correctly coded multiple surgical procedures—Current Procedural Terminology clearly describes surgical procedures that may be performed to treat various conditions. Each CPT code describes a specific procedure that was valued under the Resource Based Relative Value Scale (RBRVS) on the basis of a description of the work it entails. Many patients, especially those with complex clinical situations, need more than one surgical procedure to be performed at an operative session. For instance, a patient may require a vaginal hysterectomy because of severe irregular bleeding, but also might require repair of a symptomatic cystocele and rectocele. Because no single CPT code describes this combination of procedures, the physician should apply multiple CPT codes with appropriate modifiers to the secondary procedures as mandated by

ISSN 1074-861X

The American College of Obstetricians and Gynecologists
409 12th Street, SW
PO Box 96920
Washington, DC 20090-6920

12345/54321

CPT rules. Furthermore, the physician should expect reimbursement for all of the provided services defined by the CPT codes.

Despite the accuracy of the above statement regarding reimbursement for multiple procedures, payers often cite the efforts of Medicare to reduce payments for inappropriately unbundled CPT codes by physicians as justification for denial of physician claims for appropriately coded services. Indeed, the Health Care Financing Administration has established the Correct Coding Initiative (CCI), a process for bundling together many services that should not be paid separately. The process continues to undergo refinement with input from the AMA and medical specialty societies.

Unfortunately, some commercial software products that do not adhere to either CPT or CCI guidelines are being used by third-party payers to identify CPT codes for services that will not be reimbursed when coded together. For example, some of these products incorrectly bundle anterior and posterior colporrhaphy with enterocele repair into the code for vaginal hysterectomy, presumably because all of these procedures are performed through a vaginal approach. The AMA Correct Coding and Policy Committee, with input from ACOG staff, has identified many instances of inappropriate denial of reimbursement with some of these commercial bundling products. Physicians should appeal such denials (see the box) and cite the content of this document in requesting appropriate payment for these services.

2. *Ignoring modifiers that explain qualifying circumstances*—Current Procedural Terminology modifiers provide a coding shorthand that helps explain situations for which either increased or reduced payment is justified. There is, at present, no insurance industry standard for recognizing modifiers.

The American College of Obstetricians and Gynecologists believes that third-party payers should follow existing CPT guidelines and coding options, including recognition of all CPT modifiers, to ensure that all circumstances concerning the service performed are recognized. Payers who ignore correctly applied CPT modifiers inappropriately underreimburse physicians for the services provided.

3. *Denying payment for diagnostic and therapeutic procedures performed on the same day of service*—In certain clinical situations, a diagnostic surgical procedure is performed to determine

Seven Steps for Appealing Denied Claims

Take these steps when appealing inappropriate reimbursement practices by third-party payers:

1. Keep in mind that this is a negotiation process that will succeed only if the insurer is convinced that a charge is fair for the patient and the physician. It is important to use accepted coding standards when attempting to show that an insurer's policy is wrong. Polite but direct communication is more likely to achieve desired results than confrontation.

2. Have your staff contact the claims department of the insurer and discuss the reason for denial with the claims processor. These discussions should be based on clinical facts that rely on the Current Procedural Terminology (CPT) code definition of the service and the standard of care implied by the CPT code as it was valued under the Medicare Resource Based Relative Value Scale (RBRVS) system. Document all communication with the insurer (date, person from office making the call, person spoken with, results).

3. If staff is unsuccessful, contact the medical director of the payer yourself. Maintain open lines of communication with the medical director to discuss inappropriate payment policies and accepted coding standards.

4. Involve the state medical society in disputes with insurers. Many state societies will become very involved when patterns of abuse emerge.

5. Contact the American College of Obstetricians and Gynecologists (ACOG) for assistance in dealing with inappropriately denied medically indicated services that are covered by the patient's insurance policy and clearly were correctly reported. Contact ACOG's Department of Health Economics by fax or mail after downloading a complaint form from ACOG's web site (www.acog.org), or call (202) 863-2447 for assistance.

6. Send a copy of any correspondence between the practice and the payer dealing with unresolved problems to the insurance commissioner or equivalent regulatory authority in your state.

7. Involve your patient when inappropriate billing problems cannot be resolved in other ways. Physicians are not responsible for the insurance plan selected by the patient. Many third-party payers will revise their payment policies when they receive a complaint from the patient or patient's employer or union.

whether a therapeutic surgical procedure is required. When this occurs, it often is appropriate for the two procedures to be done at one time rather than at two distinct times. For example, if a diagnostic laparoscopy for a suspected benign condition reveals cancer, the physician may decide to perform a laparotomy to remove the cancer at the same operative session. In such a situation, many payers deny payment for the diagnostic laparoscopy even though performance of both the diagnostic and therapeutic procedures at the same time is medically indicated and requires additional physician work above that of the therapeutic procedure alone. In accordance with CPT guidelines, both procedures should be coded and the physician should be paid for both when the procedures have been documented appropriately and coded correctly. In the example, proper coding for the diagnostic service in addition to a therapeutic procedure would at the present time require the use of modifier –59 to identify the diagnostic procedure as distinct. In addition, however, the diagnostic procedure must be justified with a specific ICD-9-CM diagnostic code, which may or may not be the same as the ICD-9-CM code for the therapeutic procedure.

The practice by payers of bundling diagnostic and therapeutic procedures to reduce physicians' payment is inappropriate. Physicians have a legal obligation to code correctly. Insurers are equally obligated not to alter coding by physicians that is in accordance with approved CPT guidelines.

4. *Precertifying consultations at a predetermined level*—Some payers require precertification of a consultation and typically authorize a predetermined level of service based on the diagnostic information provided by the physician who requested the consultation. By contrast, the CPT guidelines state that the correct level of consultation is determined by the extent of the history, physical examination, and complexity of the medical decision-making process for each patient. This definition of services was used by Medicare under RBRVS to assign the relative value for physician consultation. Each patient who requires a consultation does so with a medical history typically including co-morbidities that can dramatically alter the physician work required to provide this service. Often such co-morbidities will necessitate a more thorough history and physical examination and involve more complex medical decision making than required in their absence. For example, a

request for a consultation to assess fetal well-being in an otherwise healthy patient who has had an uneventful pregnancy will not resemble a consultation for this same problem when the patient has preexisting complications of pregnancy, such as cardiac disease, uncontrolled diabetes mellitus, or a history of poor obstetric outcomes.

Because it is not possible to determine prospectively the level of service that will be required to evaluate and recommend treatment based on the uniqueness of each patient's problems, payers should precertify for an unspecified level of consultation that is paid at the appropriate level once the service has been provided.

5. *Denying diagnostic tests or studies performed at the same encounter as a distinct evaluation and management service*—The CPT manual states:

The actual performance and/or interpretation of diagnostic tests/studies ordered during a patient encounter are not included in the levels of [evaluation and management (E/M)] services. Physician performance of diagnostic tests/studies for which specific CPT codes are available may be reported separately, in addition to the appropriate E/M code.

With this statement, CPT has clarified that diagnostic tests and studies, including colposcopies, biopsies, diagnostic ultrasound examinations, and cystometrics, are ordered on the basis of clinical criteria for each patient and not as a routine service. This definition means that tests performed at the time of an outpatient or other E/M encounter are not to be paid as part of the E/M service, but rather are to be paid separately. The E/M codes in CPT were valued under the Medicare RBRVS fee schedule on the basis of the CPT guidelines; these values do not include any diagnostic tests or studies.

The payer may deny reimbursement of diagnostic tests or studies at the time of an E/M encounter because the payer's payment policies might have been formulated with a lack of understanding of CPT coding standards that separate physician work included with the E/M service from the diagnostic test or study. This lack of understanding may lead the payer to inappropriately include all services provided to the patient at the E/M encounter as part of that service. The payer also may deny payment because the physician failed to add a modifier –25 to the billed E/M code to bypass the payer's established coding edits to ensure appropriate payment for both services.

Possible Remedies

The physician should ensure that his or her billing staff are knowledgeable about:

- What is normally included and what is excluded from the service being billed (This information is provided in the most current edition of ACOG's *OB-GYN Coding Manual: Components of Correct Procedural Coding.**)
- How to link each service billed with one or more specific ICD-9-CM diagnostic codes that specifically justifies the reason for the service (This information is available in the most current edition of ACOG's *ICD-9-CM: Diagnostic Coding in Obstetrics and Gynecology.**)

---

* These resources are available from the American College of Obstetricians and Gynecologists.

- The correct application of CPT modifiers, when indicated (This information may be found in the appendixes of the current AMA CPT manual and in the current edition of ACOG's *CPT Coding in Obstetrics and Gynecology.**)
- Billing rules established by individual payers

The billing office should communicate clearly the indication for performing all coded services on the same date of service by reporting the most specific ICD-9-CM diagnostic codes. In some encounters, the justification for all services rendered may be documented by a single ICD-9-CM code. When a patient has multiple complaints or problems, multiple ICD-9-CM codes should be used.

ACOG

Committee on
Obstetric Practice

Committee Opinion

Number 326, December 2005

Inappropriate Use of the Terms Fetal Distress and Birth Asphyxia

ABSTRACT: The Committee on Obstetric Practice is concerned about the continued use of the term "fetal distress" as an antepartum or intrapartum diagnosis and the term "birth asphyxia" as a neonatal diagnosis. The Committee reaffirms that the term fetal distress is imprecise and nonspecific. The communication between clinicians caring for the woman and those caring for her neonate is best served by replacing the term fetal distress with "nonreassuring fetal status," followed by a further description of findings (eg, repetitive variable decelerations, fetal tachycardia or bradycardia, late decelerations, or low biophysical profile). Also, the term birth asphyxia is a nonspecific diagnosis and should not be used.

The Committee on Obstetric Practice is concerned about the continued use of the term "fetal distress" as an antepartum or intrapartum diagnosis and the term "birth asphyxia" as a neonatal diagnosis. The Committee reaffirms that the term fetal distress is imprecise and nonspecific. The term has a low positive predictive value even in high-risk populations and often is associated with an infant who is in good condition at birth as determined by the Apgar score or umbilical cord blood gas analysis or both. The communication between clinicians caring for the woman and those caring for her neonate is best served by replacing the term fetal distress with "nonreassuring fetal status," followed by a further description of findings (eg, repetitive variable decelerations, fetal tachycardia or bradycardia, late decelerations, or low biophysical profile). Whereas in the past, the term fetal distress generally referred to an ill fetus, nonreassuring fetal status describes the clinician's interpretation of data regarding fetal status (ie, the clinician is not reassured by the findings). This term acknowledges the imprecision inherent in the interpretation of the data. Therefore, the diagnosis of nonreassuring fetal status can be consistent with the delivery of a vigorous neonate.

Because of the implications of the term fetal distress, its use may result in inappropriate actions, such as an unnecessarily urgent delivery under general anesthesia. Fetal heart rate patterns or auscultatory findings should be considered when the degree of urgency, mode of delivery, and type of anesthesia to be given are determined. Performing a cesarean delivery for a non-

The American College of Obstetricians and Gynecologists
409 12th Street, SW
PO Box 96920
Washington, DC 20090-6920

12345/98765

Inappropriate use of the terms fetal distress and birth asphyxia. ACOG Committee Opinion No. 326. American College of Obstetricians and Gynecologists. Obstet Gynecol 2005;106: 1469–70.

reassuring fetal heart rate pattern does not necessarily preclude the use of regional anesthesia.

Since October 1, 1998, all inclusion terms except "metabolic acidemia" have been removed from the International Classification of Diseases code for fetal distress. The Committee believes that there should be uniformity in wording. *The International Classification of Diseases, Ninth Revision, Clinical Modification* code for fetal distress is based on fetal metabolic acidemia and excludes abnormal fetal acid–base balance, abnormality in fetal heart rate or rhythm, fetal bradycardia, fetal tachycardia, and meconium in liquor.

The term birth asphyxia is a nonspecific diagnosis and should not be used. The Committee strongly supports the criteria required to define an acute intrapartum hypoxic event sufficient to cause cerebral palsy, as modified by the ACOG Task Force on Neonatal Encephalopathy and Cerebral Palsy from the template provided by the International Cerebral Palsy Task Force (1) (Box 1).

Criteria to Define an Acute Intrapartum Hypoxic Event as Sufficient to Cause Cerebral Palsy

1.1: Essential criteria (must meet all four)

1. Evidence of a metabolic acidosis in fetal umbilical cord arterial blood obtained at delivery (pH <7 and base deficit ≥12 mmol/L)
2. Early onset of severe or moderate neonatal encephalopathy in infants born at 34 or more weeks of gestation
3. Cerebral palsy of the spastic quadriplegic or dyskinetic type*
4. Exclusion of other identifiable etiologies, such as trauma, coagulation disorders, infectious conditions, or genetic disorders

1.2: Criteria that collectively suggest an intrapartum timing (within close proximity to labor and delivery, eg, 0–48 hours) but are nonspecific to asphyxial insults

1. A sentinel (signal) hypoxic event occurring immediately before or during labor
2. A sudden and sustained fetal bradycardia or the absence of fetal heart rate variability in the presence of persistent, late, or variable decelerations, usually after a hypoxic sentinel event when the pattern was previously normal
3. Apgar scores of 0–3 beyond 5 minutes
4. Onset of multisystem involvement within 72 hours of birth
5. Early imaging study showing evidence of acute nonfocal cerebral abnormality

*Spastic quadriplegia and, less commonly, dyskinetic cerebral palsy are the only types of cerebral palsy associated with acute hypoxic intrapartum events. Spastic quadriplegia is not specific to intrapartum hypoxia. Hemiparetic cerebral palsy, hemiplegic cerebral palsy, spastic diplegia, and ataxia are unlikely to result from acute intrapartum hypoxia (Nelson KB, Grether JK. Potentially asphyxiating conditions and spastic cerebral palsy in infants of normal birth weight. Am J Obstet Gynecol 1998;179:507–13.).

Modified from MacLennan A. A template for defining a causal relation between acute intrapartum events and cerebral palsy: international consensus statement. BMJ 1999;319:1054–9.

References

1. American College of Obstetricians and Gynecologists and American Academy of Pediatrics. Neonatal encephalopathy and cerebral palsy: defining the pathogenesis and pathophysiology. Washington, DC: American College of Obstetricians and Gynecologists; 2003.

ACOG

Committee on Gynecologic Practice

Committee Opinion

Number 285, August 2003

Induced Abortion and Breast Cancer Risk

ABSTRACT: The purpose of this Committee Opinion is to provide a review of recent studies regarding the potential relationship between induced abortion and subsequent breast cancer and to discuss methodologic challenges in this field of study. The American College of Obstetricians and Gynecologists' Committee on Gynecologic Practice concludes that early studies of the relationship between prior induced abortion and breast cancer risk have been inconsistent and are difficult to interpret because of methodologic considerations. More rigorous recent studies argue against a causal relationship between induced abortion and a subsequent increase in breast cancer risk.

In 1995, the American College of Obstetricians and Gynecologists' Committee on Gynecologic Practice concluded that the available evidence was insufficient to support claims that induced abortion has an effect on the later development of breast cancer. It further noted that the available studies were inconsistent and that many of the available case–control studies had methodologic problems. The purpose of this Committee Opinion is to provide a review of more recent studies regarding the potential relationship between induced abortion and subsequent breast cancer and to discuss methodologic challenges in this field of study.

Three systematic reviews of the available studies on the relationship between prior induced abortion and breast cancer risk were performed in 1996 and 1997 (1–3). In the first review, one cohort and 18 case–control studies were identified, and it was concluded that any relationship between induced abortion and breast cancer risk is likely to be small or nonexistent (1). In the second review, 21 studies were reviewed, and it was concluded that induced abortion was associated with an increased risk of breast cancer (odds ratio [OR], 1.3; 95% confidence interval [CI], 1.2–1.4) (2). In the third review, 28 studies of induced abortion and breast cancer risk were examined, and the authors concluded that findings across studies were inconsistent and that definitive conclusions regarding the relationship of induced abortion and breast cancer risk were not possible at that point (3). The authors also concluded that breast cancer risk did not appear to be associated with an increasing number of induced abortions.

ISSN 1074-861X

The American College of Obstetricians and Gynecologists
409 12th Street, SW
PO Box 96920
Washington, DC 20090-6920

12345/76543

Induced abortion and breast cancer risk. ACOG Committee Opinion No. 285. American College of Obstetricians and Gynecologists. Obstet Gynecol 2003;102:433–5.

Two of the three systematic reviews noted two key methodologic considerations in studying any potential relationship between induced abortion and breast cancer (1, 3). The first consideration is that pregnancy may well have a dual effect on breast cancer risk, increasing the short-term risk of breast cancer while providing long-term protection against breast cancer (4–6). This dual effect of parity on breast cancer risk creates a complexity in interpreting available data. For any independent effect of induced abortion on breast cancer risk to be confirmed, investigators would have to demonstrate that terminating a pregnancy creates a larger increase in short-term breast cancer risk than continuing pregnancy to term or that terminating a pregnancy reduced the long-term protection against breast cancer seen with pregnancies continued to term. A second key methodologic consideration in interpreting the evidence for any relationship between abortion and breast cancer risk is the sensitive nature of abortion, which could affect the accuracy in retrospective studies of self-reports of having had an abortion; nearly all studies on this issue have been retrospective.

Cohort studies are less susceptible to bias in data collection than case–control (retrospective) studies. Two cohort studies have been conducted to assess the relationship between induced abortion and breast cancer risk. The first study, from Sweden, found a significantly reduced breast cancer risk after induced abortion (relative risk [RR], 0.8; 95% CI, 0.58–0.99) (7). The second study, from Denmark, found no effect on breast cancer risk (RR, 1; 95% CI, 0.94–1.06) (8). The Swedish study addressed the RR of parous women separate from that of nulliparous women and found that the risk was significantly reduced in the parous group (RR, 0.58; 95% CI, 0.38–0.84) but not in the nulliparous group (RR, 1.09; 95% CI, 0.71–1.56). The Danish study is particularly noteworthy because it used a population-based cohort that linked data from the National Registry of Induced Abortions, which included information on the number and dates of induced abortions, with all new cases of breast cancer identified through the Danish Cancer Registry.

A Dutch case–control study has indicated the potential importance of reporting bias in many of the available case–control studies and the importance of reporting risks of induced abortion separately among parous women and nulliparous women (9).

Among parous women in that study, a history of induced abortion was associated with an increased risk of breast cancer (RR, 1.9; 95% CI, 1.1–3.2). By contrast, among nulliparous women, there was no association between induced abortion and breast cancer risk (RR, 0.9; 95% CI, 0.4–2.3). The authors of the Dutch study concluded that the increased risk among parous women was attributable to reporting bias caused by large differences in the willingness to report having had an abortion in two regions of the country. The population of the one region with an increased risk (RR, 14.6; 95% CI, 1.8–120) was largely composed of members of a religion that officially discourages abortion. The other region had no significant increase in risk (RR, 1.3; 95% CI, 0.7–2.6). Women without breast cancer in the former region may have been less likely than those with breast cancer to acknowledge having had a prior abortion. The authors also documented an underreporting of duration of oral contraceptive use among women in the former region.

The most recent studies, including those completed in China (10), the United Kingdom (11), and the United States (12, 13), argue against a causal link between induced abortion and breast cancer risk. The first of the two U.S. studies evaluated women in western Washington State and concluded that there was no association between prior induced abortion and breast cancer risk (RR, 0.9; 95% CI, 0.7–1.2) (12). The second study used a record linkage methodology in Iowa and likewise found no effect of induced abortion on breast cancer risk (RR, 1.1; 95% CI, 0.8–1.6) (13).

The National Cancer Institute recently convened the Early Reproductive Events and Breast Cancer Workshop to evaluate the current strength of evidence of epidemiologic, clinical, and animal studies addressing the association between reproductive events and the risk of breast cancer (14). The workshop participants concluded that induced abortion is not associated with an increase in breast cancer risk.

The Committee on Gynecologic Practice concludes that early studies of the relationship between prior induced abortion and breast cancer risk have been inconsistent and are difficult to interpret because of methodologic considerations. More rigorous recent studies argue against a causal relationship between induced abortion and a subsequent increase in breast cancer risk.

References

1. Michels KB, Willett WC. Does induced or spontaneous abortion affect the risk of breast cancer? Epidemiology 1996;7:521–8.
2. Brind J, Chinchilli VM, Severs WB, Summy-Long J. Induced abortion as an independent risk factor for breast cancer: a comprehensive review and meta-analysis. J Epidemiol Community Health 1996;50:481–96.
3. Wingo PA, Newsome K, Marks JS, Calle EE, Parker SL. The risk of breast cancer following spontaneous or induced abortion. Cancer Causes Control 1997;8:93–108.
4. Lambe M, Hsieh C, Trichopoulos D, Ekbom A, Pavia M, Adami HO. Transient increase in the risk of breast cancer after giving birth. N Engl J Med 1994;331:5–9.
5. Bruzzi R, Negri E, La Vecchia C, Decarli A, Palli D, Parazzine F, et al. Short term increase in risk of breast cancer after full term pregnancy. BMJ 1988;297:1096–8.
6. Cummings P, Stanford JL, Daling JR, Weiss NS, McKnight B. Risk of breast cancer in relation to the interval since last full term pregnancy. BMJ 1994;308:1672–4.
7. Harris BM, Eklund G, Meirik O, Rutqvist LE, Wiklund K. Risk of cancer of the breast after legal abortion during first trimester: a Swedish register study. BMJ 1989;299:1430–2.
8. Melbye M, Wohlfahrt J, Olsen JH, Frisch M, Westergaard T, Helweg-Larsen K, et al. Induced abortion and the risk of breast cancer. N Engl J Med 1997;336:81–5.
9. Rookus MA, van Leeuwen FE. Induced abortion and risk for breast cancer: reporting (recall) bias in a Dutch case-control study. J Natl Cancer Inst 1996;88:1759–64.
10. Sanderson M, Shu XO, Jin F, Dai Q, Wen W, Hua Y, et al. Abortion history and breast cancer risk: results from the Shanghai Breast Cancer Study. Int J Cancer 2001;92:899–905.
11. Goldacre MJ, Kurina LM, Seagroatt V, Yeates D. Abortion and breast cancer: a case-control record linkage study. J Epidemiol Community Health 2001;55:336–7.
12. Tang MT, Weiss NS, Malone KE. Induced abortion in relation to breast cancer among parous women: a birth certificate registry study. Epidemiology 2000;11:177–80.
13. Lazovich D, Thompson JA, Mink PJ, Sellers TA, Anderson KE. Induced abortion and breast cancer risk. Epidemiology 2000;11:76–80.
14. Summary report: Early Reproductive Events and Breast Cancer Workshop. Bethesda (MD): National Cancer Institute; 2003. Available at http://www.nci.nih.gov/cancerinfo/ere-workshop-report. Retrieved March 28, 2003.

ACOG

**Committee on
Obstetric Practice**

Committee Opinion

Number 271, April 2002

The American College of Obstetricians and Gynecologists
409 12th Street, SW
PO Box 96920
Washington, DC 20090-6920

12345/65432

Induction of labor for vaginal birth after cesarean delivery. ACOG Committee Opinion No. 271. American College of Obstetricians and Gynecologists. Obstet Gynecol 2002;99:679–680

Induction of Labor for Vaginal Birth After Cesarean Delivery

ABSTRACT: A recent population-based study of vaginal birth after cesarean delivery (VBAC) attempts observed uterine rupture rates of 24.5 per 1,000 with prostaglandin-induced labor, while the uterine rupture rates with spontaneous labor and labor induced without prostaglandins were lower (5.2/1,000 and 7.7/1,000 respectively). The authors did not confirm the diagnoses by examining individual medical records, so the actual incidence of uterine rupture may have been overstated. Despite this limitation, the Committee on Obstetric Practice concludes that the risk of uterine rupture during VBAC attempts is substantially increased with the use of various prostaglandin cervical ripening agents for the induction of labor, and their use for this purpose is discouraged.

In an attempt to lower cesarean delivery rates in the United States, attention has been focused on increasing the percentage of vaginal births after cesarean delivery (VBACs). However, reports have suggested a significant risk of uterine rupture with poor outcomes for both the woman and her infant attendant to VBAC attempts (1–3). Although it is clear that the bulk of maternal and perinatal morbidity and mortality are caused by unsuccessful VBAC attempts, there are no reliable ways to predict whether a trial of labor will be successful in an individual patient (3–5). For these reasons, the safety of VBAC has been the subject of intense scrutiny.

In 1996, McMahon and colleagues reported the results of a longitudinal study of 6,138 women with one prior cesarean delivery who subsequently gave birth to singleton infants (6). They observed that major complications (eg, need for hysterectomy, uterine rupture, and operative injury of uterine arteries, ureters, and bladder) were nearly twice as common among women undergoing VBAC attempts compared with those undergoing a repeat cesarean delivery (odds ratio, 1.8; 95% confidence interval [CI], 1.1–3.0). A subsequent study reported an increased risk of major complications with VBAC attempts following the induction of labor (7).

Recently, Lydon-Rochelle and associates reported a population-based, retrospective cohort analysis of the relationship of uterine rupture to VBAC using vital records and abstracted hospital discharge (ICD-9) diagnoses (8). A total of 20,095 women were identified with a history of cesarean delivery for their first delivery and who gave birth to a second child from 1987 through

1996 in Washington state. The risk of uterine rupture was compared among patients with repeat cesarean delivery, deliveries following the spontaneous onset of labor, and labor induced with or without the use of prostaglandins. The authors observed 91 uterine ruptures with rates of 1.6 per 1,000 for repeat cesarean delivery, 5.2 per 1,000 with spontaneous labor, 7.7 per 1,000 when labor was induced without prostaglandins, and 24.5 per 1,000 with prostaglandin-induced labor. Compared with women who gave birth by elective repeat cesarean delivery, the relative risk [RR] of uterine rupture was significantly higher among women with spontaneous labor (RR, 3.3; 95% CI, 1.8–6.0), induction of labor without prostaglandins (RR, 4.9; 95% CI, 2.4–9.7), and induction of labor with prostaglandins (RR, 15.6; 95% CI, 8.1–30.0). There was no significant statistical difference in the risks of uterine rupture between spontaneous labor and labor induced without prostaglandins. In addition, the incidence of infant death was increased 10-fold in the presence of uterine rupture.

The authors acknowledged that they did not confirm the diagnoses of uterine rupture by examining medical records. Furthermore, their use of ICD-9 codes may have caused an overstatement of the actual incidence of uterine ruptures, because of the use of a single code for both uterine incision extension and uterine rupture (8). To the extent that the risk for uterine rupture may have been overstated, the probability of fetal death given uterine rupture may have been underestimated. As reported in the Morbidity and Mortality Weekly Report, only 40% of such ICD-9 coded events are actually caused by uterine rupture (9). Despite this limitation, the Committee on Obstetric Practice concludes that the risk of uterine rupture during VBAC attempts is substantially increased with the use of various prostaglandin cervical ripening agents for the induction of labor. Thus, if induction of labor is necessary for a clear and compelling clinical indication, the potential increased risk of uterine rupture with the use of prostaglandins should be discussed with the patient and documented in the medical record. However, the available data do not appear to preclude the use of oxytocin alone for labor induction or augmentation.

The purpose of this document is to discourage the use of prostaglandins for cervical ripening or the induction of labor in women attempting VBAC. This document should not be interpreted as discouraging the practice of VBAC under the proper circumstances and with the appropriate safeguards (10). The Committee on Obstetric Practice also wishes to reiterate the American College of Obstetricians and Gynecologists' position that misoprostol should not be used in patients with a previous cesarean delivery or major uterine surgery (11–13).

References

1. Farmer RM, Kirschbaum T, Potter D, Strong TH, Medearis AL. Uterine rupture during trial of labor after previous cesarean section. Am J Obstet Gynecol 1991; 165:966–1001
2. Jones RO, Nagashima AW, Hartnett-Goodman MM, Goodlin RC. Rupture of low transverse cesarean scars during trial of labor. Obstet Gynecol 1991;77:815–817
3. Leung AS, Farmer RM, Leung EK, Medearis AL, Paul RH. Risk factors associated with uterine rupture during trial of labor after cesarean delivery: a case-control study. Am J Obstet Gynecol 1993;168:1358–1363
4. Scott JR. Mandatory trial of labor after cesarean delivery: an alternative viewpoint. Obstet Gynecol 1991;77: 811–814
5. Pickhardt MG, Martin JN Jr, Meydrech EF, Blake PG, Martin RW, Perry KG Jr, et al. Vaginal birth after cesarean delivery: are there useful and valid predictors of success or failure? Am J Obstet Gynecol 1992;166:1811–1815; discussion 1815–1819
6. McMahon MJ, Luther ER, Bowes WA Jr, Olshan AF. Comparison of a trial of labor with an elective second cesarean section. N Engl J Med 1996;335:689–695
7. Zelop CM, Shipp TD, Repke JT, Cohen A, Caughey AB, Lieberman E. Uterine rupture during induced or augmented labor in gravid women with one prior cesarean delivery. Am J Obstet Gynecol 1999;181:882–886
8. Lydon-Rochelle M, Holt VL, Easterling TR, Martin DP. Risk of uterine rupture during labor among women with a prior cesarean delivery. N Engl J Med 2001;345:3–8
9. Use of hospital discharge data to monitor uterine rupture—Massachusetts, 1990–1997. MMWR Morb Mortal Wkly Rep 2000;49:245–248
10. American College of Obstetricians and Gynecologists. Vaginal birth after previous cesarean delivery. ACOG Practice Bulletin 5. Washington, DC: ACOG, 1999
11. American College of Obstetricians and Gynecologists. Response to Searle's drug warning on misoprostol. ACOG Committee Opinion 248. Washington, DC: ACOG, 2000
12. American College of Obstetricians and Gynecologists. Induction of labor with misoprostol. ACOG Committee Opinion 228. Washington, DC: ACOG, 1999
13. American College of Obstetricians and Gynecologists. Induction of labor. ACOG Practice Bulletin 10. Washington, DC: ACOG, 1999

ACOG

Committee on
Obstetric Practice

Committee Opinion

Number 228, November 1999

Induction of Labor with Misoprostol

ISSN 1074-861X

The American College of Obstetricians and Gynecologists
409 12th Street, SW
PO Box 96920
Washington, DC 20090-6920

12345/32109

Induction of labor is a common obstetric intervention in the United States, occurring in up to 15% of all pregnancies. The American College of Obstetricians and Gynecologists supports induction of labor as a worthwhile therapeutic option when the benefits of expeditious delivery outweigh the risks of continuing the pregnancy (1). Prostaglandin E_2 (PGE_2), applied locally to the cervix or vagina, has been widely studied as an induction agent, and has been found to be safe and effective (2, 3). Two such agents have been approved by the U.S. Food and Drug Administration for this purpose and are commercially available as dinoprostone preparations. Recent studies have explored the effectiveness and safety of misoprostol for induction of labor. This prostaglandin E_1 analogue is less expensive, more stable, and easier to store than dinoprostone preparations. However, misoprostol currently is approved by the U.S. Food and Drug Administration for the treatment of peptic ulcer disease and not for induction of labor. Moreover, the manufacturer does not plan to pursue approval for this indication (4).

At least 19 prospective, randomized clinical trials involving more than 1,900 patients receiving doses of misoprostol ranging from 25 mcg to 200 mcg in a variety of dosage schedules have been performed. Most researchers have administered misoprostol in tablet form into the posterior fornix of the vagina, but it also has been mixed into a hydroxymethylcellulose gel or applied intracervically.

In general, misoprostol has been found to be an effective agent for the induction of labor. When compared with placebo, misoprostol use decreased oxytocin requirements and achieved higher rates of vaginal delivery within 24 hours of induction. Misoprostol also compared favorably with intracervical and intravaginal PGE_2 preparations; many studies demonstrated shorter times to delivery and reduced oxytocin requirements after misoprostol administration (5). Some studies suggest that misoprostol may reduce the rate of cesarean delivery, but further randomized clinical trials using the 25 mcg dose are required to confirm this observation (5). There have been reports of uterine rupture following misoprostol use for cervical ripening in patients with prior uterine surgery. Thus, until reassuring studies are available, misoprostol is not recommended for cervical ripening in patients who have had prior cesarean delivery or major uterine surgery (6).

When given in doses of 50 mcg or more, misoprostol use has been associated with an increased rate of uterine tachysystole (six or more uterine contractions in 10 minutes in consecutive 10-minute intervals) compared with either placebo or PGE_2 preparations. In two studies in which 50 mcg of misoprostol was administered intravaginally every 4 hours, researchers found increased rates of meconium passage (7) and cesarean delivery due to uterine hyperstimulation syndrome (8) when compared with dinoprostone. However, an increase in neonatal morbidity after misoprostol administration has not been documented. In trials where 25 mcg of misoprostol was administered intravaginally as frequently as every 3 hours, there did not appear to be an increase in uterine tachysystole, hyperstimulation, or meconium passage when compared with PGE_2 (9, 10). Moreover, this dosing regimen appeared to be at least as effective in inducing labor as the PGE_2 preparations.

Currently, misoprostol is available in 100 mcg and 200 mcg tablets, and the 100 mcg tablet is not scored. If misoprostol is used for cervical ripening and induction, one quarter of a 100 mcg tablet (ie, approximately 25 mcg) should be considered for the initial dose.

Given the current evidence, intravaginal misoprostol tablets appear to be effective in inducing labor in pregnant women who have unfavorable cervices. The use of higher doses (50 mcg every 6 hours) may be appropriate in some situations, although increasing the dose appears to be associated most closely with uterine tachysystole and possibly with uterine hyperstimulation and meconium staining of amniotic fluid. Further prospective trials are required to define an optimal dosing regimen for misoprostol. However, misoprostol is not recommended for patients with prior uterine surgery (11). Patients undergoing such therapy should receive fetal heart rate and uterine activity monitoring in a hospital setting until further studies evaluate and confirm the safety of outpatient therapy.

References

1. American College of Obstetricians and Gynecologists. Induction of labor. ACOG Practice Bulletin. Washington, DC: ACOG, 1999
2. Brindley BA, Sokol RJ. Induction and augmentation of labor: basis and methods for current practice. Obstet Gynecol Surv 1988;43:730–743
3. Rayburn WF. Prostaglandin E_2 gel for cervical ripening and induction of labor: a critical analysis. Am J Obstet Gynecol 1989;160:529–534
4. Bauer TA, Brown D, Chai LK. Vaginal misoprostol for term labor induction. Ann Pharmacother 1997;31: 1391–1393
5. Sanchez-Ramos L, Kaunitz AM, Wears RL, Delke I, Gaudier FL. Misoprostol for cervical ripening and labor induction: a meta-analysis. Obstet Gynecol 1997;89: 633–642
6. Hofmeyr GJ. Vaginal misoprostol for cervical ripening and labour induction in late pregnancy. The Cochrane Library 1999; Issue 2:1–18 (Meta-analysis)
7. Wing DA, Jones MM, Rahall A, Goodwin TM, Paul RH. A comparison of misoprostol and prostaglandin E_2 gel for preinduction cervical ripening and labor induction. Am J Obstet Gynecol 1995;172:1804–1810
8. Buser D, Mora G, Arias F. A randomized comparison between misoprostol and dinoprostone for cervical ripening and labor induction in patients with unfavorable cervices. Obstet Gynecol 1997;89:581–585
9. Wing DA, Paul RH. A comparison of different dosing regimens of vaginally administered misoprostol for preinduction cervical ripening and labor induction. Am J Obstet Gynecol 1996;175:158–164
10. Wing DA, Ortiz-Omphroy G, Paul RH. A comparison of intermittent vaginal administration of misoprostol with continuous dinoprostone for cervical ripening and labor induction. Am J Obstet Gynecol 1997;177:612–618
11. Wing DA, Lovett K, Paul RH. Disruption of prior uterine incision following misoprostol for labor induction in women with previous cesarean section. Obstet Gynecol 1998;91:828–830

ACOG Committee Opinion

Committee on Obstetric Practice

Number 305, November 2004

Influenza Vaccination and Treatment During Pregnancy

ABSTRACT: Influenza vaccination is an essential element of prenatal care. The American College of Obstetricians and Gynecologists' Committee on Obstetric Practice supports the Centers for Disease Control and Prevention's expanded recommendation that women who will be pregnant during the influenza season (October through mid May) should be vaccinated. The ideal time to administer the vaccine is October and November; however, it is appropriate to vaccinate patients throughout the influenza season as long as the vaccine supply lasts. This intramuscular, inactivated vaccine may be used in all 3 trimesters. Because of the unknown effects of influenza antiviral drugs on pregnant women and their fetuses, the Committee on Obstetric Practice recommends that these antiviral agents should be used during pregnancy only if the potential benefits justify the potential risks.

Influenza vaccination is an essential element of prenatal care. The risks of serious illness associated with influenza are increased in young children and pregnant women. The influenza epidemic in 2003 resulted in numerous hospitalizations for cardiopulmonary complications among pregnant women and some deaths among young children (1).

The American College of Obstetricians and Gynecologists' Committee on Obstetric Practice supports the Centers for Disease Control and Prevention's expanded recommendation that women who will be pregnant during the influenza season (October through mid May) should be vaccinated (1). The ideal time to administer the vaccine is October and November; however, it is appropriate to vaccinate patients throughout the influenza season as long as the vaccine supply lasts. This intramuscular, inactivated vaccine may be used in all 3 trimesters. One study of influenza vaccination of more than 2,000 pregnant women demonstrated no adverse fetal effects associated with influenza vaccination (2). Any theoretical risk of the vaccination is outweighed by its benefits. Likewise, the benefits of the vaccine outweigh any unproven potential concerns about traces of thimerosal preservative, which exist only in the multidose vials (see http://www.cdc.gov/mmwr/preview/mmwrhtml/rr53e430a1.htm). It should be noted that the intranasal vaccine spray contains a live, attenuated virus and should not be used during pregnancy.

ISSN 1074-861X

The American College of Obstetricians and Gynecologists
409 12th Street, SW
PO Box 96920
Washington, DC 20090-6920

12345/87654

Influenza vaccination and treatment during pregnancy. ACOG Committee Opinion No. 305. American College of Obstetricians and Gynecologists. Obstet Gynecol 2004;104:1125–6.

Immunizing pregnant women also confers protection to their infants; this is an important consideration because infants' aged 0–6 months do not respond to the influenza vaccine. Breastfeeding is not a contraindication for vaccination.

If influenza A develops, amantadine and rimantadine may reduce the duration of illness when given within 2 days of illness onset whereas zanamivir and oseltamivir may reduce the duration of uncomplicated influenza A and B (1). However, no clinical studies have been conducted regarding their safety or efficacy during pregnancy. Therefore, because of the unknown effects of influenza antiviral drugs on pregnant women and their fetuses, the Committee on Obstetric Practice recommends that these antiviral agents should be used during pregnancy only if the potential benefits justify the potential risks. Antiviral agents should not be used as a substitute for influenza vaccination.

References

1. Harper SA, Fukuda K, Uyeki TM, Cox NJ, Bridges CB. Prevention and control of influenza: recommendations of the Advisory Committee on Immunization Practices (ACIP). Centers for Disease Control and Prevention (CDC) Advisory Committee on Immunization Practices (ACIP). MMWR Recomm Rep 2004;53(RR-6):1–40. Available at: http://www.cdc.gov/mmwr/PDF/rr/rr5306.pdf. Retrieved August 6, 2004.
2. Heinonen OP, Shapiro S, Monson RR, Hartz SC, Rosenberg L, Slone D. Immunization during pregnancy against poliomyelitis and influenza in relation to childhood malignancy. Int J Epidemiol 1973;2:229–35.

ACOG

Committee on
Professional Liability

Committee Opinion

Number 306, December 2004   *(Replaces No. 237, June 2000)*

Informed Refusal

ABSTRACT: Informed refusal is a fundamental component of the informed consent process. Informed consent laws have evolved to the "materiality or patient viewpoint" standard. A physician must disclose to the patient the risks, benefits, and alternatives that a reasonable person in the patient's position would want to know to make an informed decision. Throughout this process, the patient's autonomy, level of health literacy, and cultural background should be respected. The subsequent election by the patient to forgo an intervention that has been recommended by the physician constitutes informed refusal. Documentation of the informed refusal process is essential. It should include a notation that the need for the intervention, as well as risks, benefits, and alternatives to the intervention, and possible consequences of refusal, have been explained. The patient's reason for refusal also should be documented.

Informed refusal is inextricably intertwined with the process of informed consent. After addressing the risks, benefits, and alternatives of a proposed medical treatment, surgical procedure, or diagnostic test, an explanation of the risks of refusing or declining the proposed intervention also must be given; this should be considered a fourth element of the consent process. Just as a patient has the right to consent to treatment, she may choose to refuse treatment. Patients are entitled to participate with their physicians in a process of shared decision making (1).

Informed consent laws have evolved from the relatively paternalistic "professional or reasonable physician" standard to the "materiality or patient viewpoint" standard. In the professional or reasonable physician standard, a physician must disclose to a patient the risks and benefits that are customarily disclosed by the medical community for that medical treatment, surgical procedure, or diagnostic test. In the materiality or patient viewpoint standard, a physician must disclose to the patient the risks, benefits, and alternatives that a reasonable person in the patient's position would want to know to make an informed decision. In making such disclosure, a physician also must make allowance for the patient's level of health literacy and cultural background. It often is helpful, for example, to ask the patient to explain in her own words her understanding of the essential elements of this patient–physician exchange of information. As is frequently emphasized, informed consent is a process and not a mere document.

ISSN 1074-861X

The American College of Obstetricians and Gynecologists
409 12th Street, SW
PO Box 96920
Washington, DC 20090-6920

12345/87654

Informed refusal. ACOG Committee Opinion No. 306. American College of Obstetricians and Gynecologists. Obstet Gynecol 2004;104:1465–6.

Once a patient has been informed of the material risks, benefits, and alternatives, as well as the option to refuse, the patient has the right to exercise complete autonomy in deciding whether to undergo the recommended medical treatment, surgical procedure, or diagnostic test; to choose among a variety of treatments, procedures, or tests; or to refuse to undergo these treatments, procedures, or tests. The election by the patient to forgo an intervention that has been recommended by the physician constitutes informed refusal.

In the past, documentation of informed refusal has not been an important element; however, it has become important in the present health care environment. Managed care and increased patient autonomy are 2 factors that warrant a reexamination of the need for documentation of informed refusal. The widespread implementation of managed care and utilization review sometimes has created a conflict between cost containment, sometimes camouflaged as "medical necessity," and best medical practices or even standard medical practices. It is not uncommon for a physician to recommend a medical treatment, surgical procedure, or diagnostic test that will not be paid for by a third-party insurance carrier. Legal precedents have established that an attending physician should act as a patient advocate in such coverage disputes and attempt to convince the managed care organization that coverage is medically indicated. Despite such advocacy, however, there will be situations in which physicians will not prevail on behalf of their patients. In such circumstances, a physician should discuss with the patient whether she wishes to accept personal financial responsibility for the medical treatment, surgical procedure, or diagnostic test, or whether to seek alternative funding. If the patient refuses to undergo the medical treatment, surgical procedure, or diagnostic test for economic or other reasons, the physician should document the informed refusal in the patient's medical record. In some situations the physician might want to obtain a written statement from the patient, acknowledging that the risk of refusal was fully explained.

The increased emphasis on patient autonomy in medical decision making has given rise to other circumstances in which documentation of an informed refusal is appropriate. Despite a physician's medical advice or recommendation, a patient who is informed of the material risks, benefits, and alternatives of particular interventions may elect to forgo them because of cultural or religious beliefs, personal preference, or comfort. This decision should be respected. (Patient choice in the maternal–fetal relationship may require special considerations. Guidance for these issues can be found in another ACOG publication [2].) Alternatively, the patient may weigh the risks and benefits differently than the physician or, simply, the patient may not understand the risk of refusal.

Whenever a patient refuses a medical treatment, surgical procedure, or diagnostic test, the physician should document the informed refusal in the patient's medical record and include the following information:

- The patient's refusal to consent to a medical treatment, surgical procedure, or diagnostic test
- Documentation that the need for the treatment, procedure, or test has been explained
- The reasons stated by the patient for such refusal
- A statement that the consequences of the refusal, including possible jeopardy to health or life, have been described to the patient

References

1. American College of Obstetricians and Gynecologists. Informed consent. In: Ethics in obstetrics and gynecology. 2nd ed. Washington, DC: ACOG; 2004. p. 9–17.
2. American College of Obstetricians and Gynecologists. Patient choice in the maternal–fetal relationship. In: Ethics in obstetrics and gynecology. 2nd ed. Washington, DC: ACOG; 2004. p. 34–6.

ACOG

Committee on
Gynecologic Practice

Committee Opinion

Number 191, October 1997   *(Replaces #134, March 1994)*

Length of Hospital Stay for Gynecologic Procedures

The American College of Obstetricians and Gynecologists is concerned about the compromise in quality of care that can occur as a result of the "cost-saving" measure of reducing length of hospital stay. Length-of-stay normative data record the average stay in hospital days for a given gynecologic procedure and reflect generally recognized practice across geographic areas. These data have changed radically in the past several years and are continuing to change.

Length-of-stay determinants are based upon a range of individual factors, such as concurrent disease process, severity of illness, intensity of care required, and therapeutic approach. Although standard protocols or predetermined number of days for length of stay can offer general guidance, individual patient characteristics, physician judgment, and physician–patient consultation always should determine length of stay in individual cases.

After gynecologic surgery, a patient's readiness for release from the hospital should be based on positive discharge criteria. These criteria generally include (but are not limited to)

- Stable vital signs
- No evidence of untreated infections
- Adequate oral intake
- Satisfactory bowel and urinary tract function

Before discharge, instructions regarding diet, medications, wound and drainage device care, activity, and follow-up should be communicated to the patient or her caregivers. The patient or her caregivers should understand the instructions and be able to provide ongoing care and monitor recovery as needed.

The American College of Obstetricians and Gynecologists

409 12th Street, SW
PO Box 96920
Washington, DC 20090-6920

12345/10987

ACOG

Committee on
Obstetric Practice

Committee Opinion

Number 268, February 2002

The American College of Obstetricians and Gynecologists
409 12th Street, SW
PO Box 96920
Washington, DC 20090-6920

12345/65432

Management of asymptomatic pregnant or lactating women exposed to anthrax. ACOG Committee Opinion No. 268. American College of Obstetricians and Gynecologists. Obstet Gynecol 2002;99:366–368

Management of Asymptomatic Pregnant or Lactating Women Exposed to Anthrax

ABSTRACT: Anthrax infections are diagnosed by isolating Bacillus anthracis *from body fluids or by measuring specific antibodies in the blood of persons suspected to have the disease. It is recommended that asymptomatic pregnant and lactating women who have been exposed to a confirmed environmental contamination or a high-risk source as determined by the local Department of Health (not the women's health care provider) receive prophylactic treatment. A variety of antimicrobial regimens are available. Although some of these drugs may present risks to the developing fetus, these risks are clearly outweighed by the potential morbidity and mortality from anthrax. Guidelines for prophylactic treatment of anthrax and treatment of suspected active cases of anthrax are changing continually, and the Centers for Disease Control and Prevention web site should be consulted for the latest recommendations.*

Anthrax is an infection caused by *Bacillus anthracis*, an aerobic, gram-positive, spore-forming, nonmotile bacillus species. There are three primary clinical manifestations of the disease: 1) cutaneous, 2) inhalational, and 3) gastrointestinal.

Cutaneous: This is the most common presentation, accounting for 95% of naturally occurring infections. The organism's portal of entry is a cut or abrasion on the skin. The areas of greatest exposure are the hands, arms, face or neck. Potential sources of the organism include wool, hides, and leather and hair products of infected animals, particularly goats. Exposure also may result from a bioterrorist act (eg, a contaminated letter). Incubation periods may be as long as 12 days. Skin infection begins as a raised pruritic papule, resembling an insect bite. Within 1–2 days a vesicle develops, followed by a painless ulcer 1–3 cm in diameter with a characteristic black necrotic eschar in the center. Localized lymphangitis and painful lymphadenopathy may occur. Although antibiotic therapy does not appear to change the course of eschar formation and healing, it does decrease the risk of systemic disease. Mortality rates are 20% if untreated, but less than 1% with antibiotic therapy.

Inhalational: This is the most serious presentation, resulting from deposition of spore-bearing particles of 1–5 μm into the alveolar spaces. Macrophages ingest the spores that are then transported to the pulmonary lymphatics where they germinate. The asymptomatic incubation period usually is 1–7 days after exposure, but spores may germinate in the mediastinal lymphatics for up to 60 days. Once germination occurs, replicating bacteria release toxins leading to hemorrhage, edema, and necrosis. Initial symptoms resemble a flulike illness with fever, cough, and headache, but without rhinitis, followed by progressive dyspnea that rapidly progresses to respiratory failure and death within hours. Case-fatality estimates are extremely high, even with supportive care and appropriate antibiotics.

Gastrointestinal: The relatively rare intestinal form of anthrax follows ingestion, deposition, and subsequent germination of spores in the upper or lower gastrointestinal tract. The former leads to the oral-pharyngeal form of the disease marked by oral-esophageal ulcers and regional lymphadenopathy. The latter results in acute inflammation of the intestinal tract with symptoms that include anorexia, malaise, nausea, vomiting, and fever. Subsequently patients infected with gastrointestinal anthrax develop abdominal pain; hematemesis; severe, bloody diarrhea; and sepsis. Intestinal anthrax may be fatal in 25–60% of cases; the effect of early antibiotic therapy is unknown.

Evaluation and Management of Possible Anthrax Exposure Caused by Bioterrorist Acts

The risk of anthrax exposure is remote for people not in direct contact with the contaminated object or site and is greatest for those present in the immediate vicinity of contamination. The disease is not spread by casual contact or by coughing and sneezing.

Active Infection

Anthrax infections are diagnosed by isolating *B anthracis* from the blood, cerebrospinal fluid, skin lesions, or respiratory secretions or by measuring specific antibodies in the blood of persons suspected to have the disease. Rapid diagnostic immunoassays and polymerase chain reaction are available at national reference laboratories. Strategies of antimicrobial treatment of active anthrax infection are

evolving. For the latest recommendations consult the Centers for Disease Control and Prevention (CDC) web site at www.cdc.gov/mmwr and www.bt.cdc.gov.

Exposure

For asymptomatic individuals with low-risk exposure, antimicrobials are not warranted until there is an evident risk of actual exposure based on microbiologically documented anthrax as determined by law enforcement and public health authorities. The woman's health care provider is not the party to validate a threat.

In the current crisis, when screening for exposure is deemed necessary, it is conducted by nasal swab. The resultant secretions can be examined by Gram stain and culture. However, given the lack of reliability of nasal swab screening, postexposure prophylaxis is indicated only after confirmed or high-risk suspected exposure. In the latter cases, treatment can be stopped if anthrax is not documented.

For adult postexposure prophylaxis against anthrax infections, the CDC currently recommends 500 mg of ciprofloxacin orally every 12 hours for 60 days or 100 mg of doxycycline orally every 12 hours for 60 days.

Management of Exposed Asymptomatic Pregnant or Lactating Women

At this time, the Committee on Obstetric Practice recommends that prophylaxis of asymptomatic pregnant and lactating women be limited to those women who have had exposure to a confirmed environmental contamination or who are exposed to a high-risk source as determined by the local Department of Health. Prophylaxis for asymptomatic pregnant or lactating women is 500 mg of ciprofloxacin orally every 12 hours for 60 days (6).

Ciprofloxacin and other fluoroquinolones generally are not used during pregnancy and lactation because of suggested irreversible drug-induced arthropathy associated with such treatment in a variety of species of adolescent animals (1–5). However, no clear evidence of teratogenicity has been demonstrated in humans (1–5). Despite these concerns, the potential morbidity and mortality from anthrax clearly outweighs these risks. Thus, if the bacteria are shown to be sensitive to penicillin, the treatment should be switched to 500 mg of amoxicillin orally three times a day for 60 days (6).

If a woman has been prescribed ciprofloxacin and is found to be pregnant, she should continue her course of antibiotics for the full 60 days (6) unless the bacteria are shown to be penicillin-sensitive. She should then be switched to amoxicillin. A 1999 expert review of published data on experiences with ciprofloxacin concluded that therapeutic doses during pregnancy are unlikely to pose substantial teratogenic risk, but the data are insufficient to state that there is no risk (1). In the case of penicillin- and ciprofloxacin-allergic patients, treatment should consist of doxycycline or penicillin desensitization should be considered if the organism is proved sensitive (6). In this situation, the risks of anthrax would far outweigh the risks of doxycycline to the fetus (ie, dental staining of the primary teeth and possible depressed bone growth and defective dental enamel).

The guidelines for prophylactic treatment of anthrax and treatment of suspected active cases of anthrax are continually evolving. Please refer to www.bt.cdc.gov and www.cdc.gov/mmwr for any updates in CDC treatment guidelines.

References

1. Friedman JM, Polifka JE. Ciprofloxacin. In: Teratogenic effects of drugs: a resource for clinicians (TERIS). 2nd ed. Baltimore: The Johns Hopkins University Press, 2000: 149–150

2. Friedman JM, Polifka JE. Doxycyclicne. In: Teratogenic effects of drugs: a resource for clinicians (TERIS). 2nd ed. Baltimore: The Johns Hopkins University Press, 2000: 238–239

3. Center for Drug Evaluation and Research. U.S. Food and Drug Administration. CIPRO (Ciprofloxacin) use by pregnant and lactating women. Available at http://www.fda.gov/cder/drug/infopage/cipro/cipropreg.htm. Retrieved November 2, 2001

4. Center for Drug Evaluation and Research. U.S. Food and Drug Administration. Drug preparedness and response to bioterrorism. Available at http://www.fda.gov/cder/drug prepare/default.htm. Retrieved November 2, 2001

5. Center for Drug Evaluation and Research. U.S. Food and Drug Administration. Doxycycline (Vibramycin, Monodox, Doryx, Doxy, Atridox, Periodox, Vibra-Tabs) use by pregnant and lactating women. Available at http://www.fda.gov/cder/drug/infopage/penG_doxy/doxy preg.htm. Retrieved November 2, 2001

6. Updated recommendations for antimicrobial prophylaxis among asymptomatic pregnant women after exposure to bacillus anthracis. MMWR Morb Mortal Wkly Rep 2001; 50:960

Resources

Inglesby TV, Henderson DA, Bartlett JG, Ascher MS, Eitzen E, Friedlander AM, et al. Anthrax as a biological weapon: medical and public health management. Working Group on Civilian Biodefense. JAMA 1999;281:1735–1745[erratum JAMA 2000;283:1963]

Update: investigation of anthrax associated with intentional exposure and interim public health guidelines, October 2001. MMWR Morb Mortal Wkly Rep 2001;50:889–893

Use of anthrax vaccine in the United States. MMWR Morb Mortal Wkly Rep 2000;49(RR-15):1–20

ACOG

Committee on
Ethics

Committee Opinion

Number 321, November 2005

Maternal Decision Making, Ethics, and the Law

ABSTRACT: Recent legal actions and policies aimed at protecting the fetus as an entity separate from the woman have challenged the rights of pregnant women to make decisions about medical interventions and have criminalized maternal behavior that is believed to be associated with fetal harm or adverse perinatal outcomes. This opinion summarizes recent, notable legal cases; reviews the underlying, established ethical principles relevant to the highlighted issues; and considers six objections to punitive and coercive legal approaches to maternal decision making. These approaches 1) fail to recognize that pregnant women are entitled to informed consent and bodily integrity, 2) fail to recognize that medical knowledge and predictions of outcomes in obstetrics have limitations, 3) treat addiction and psychiatric illness as if they were moral failings, 4) threaten to dissuade women from prenatal care, 5) unjustly single out the most vulnerable women, and 6) create the potential for criminalization of otherwise legal maternal behavior. Efforts to use the legal system to protect the fetus by constraining pregnant women's decision making or punishing them erode a woman's basic rights to privacy and bodily integrity and are not justified. Physicians and policy makers should promote the health of women and their fetuses through advocacy of healthy behavior; referral for substance abuse treatment and mental health services when indicated; and development of safe, available, and efficacious services for women and families.

Ethical issues that arise in the care of pregnant women are challenging to physicians, politicians, lawyers, and ethicists alike. One of the fundamental goals of medicine and society is to optimize the outcome of pregnancy. Recently, some apparent attempts to foster this goal have been characterized by legal action and policies aimed at specifically protecting the fetus as an entity separate from the woman. These actions and policies have challenged the rights of pregnant women to make decisions about medical interventions and have criminalized maternal behavior that is believed to be associated with fetal harm or adverse perinatal outcomes.

Practitioners who care for pregnant women face particularly difficult dilemmas when their patients reject medical recommendations, use illegal

Requests for authorization to make photocopies should be directed to:

Copyright Clearance Center
222 Rosewood Drive
Danvers, MA 01923
(978) 750-8400

ISSN 1074-861X

The American College of Obstetricians and Gynecologists
409 12th Street, SW
PO Box 96920
Washington, DC 20090-6920

12345/98765

Maternal decision making, ethics, and the law. ACOG Committee Opinion No. 321. American College of Obstetricians and Gynecologists. Obstet Gynecol 2005;106:1127–37.

drugs, or engage in a range of other behaviors that have the potential to cause fetal harm. In such situations, physicians, hospital representatives, and others have at times resorted to legal actions to impose their views about what these pregnant patients ought to do or to effect particular interventions or outcomes. Appellate courts have held, however, that a pregnant woman's decisions regarding medical treatment should take precedence regardless of the presumed fetal consequences of those decisions. In one notable 1990 decision, a District of Columbia appellate court vacated a lower court's decision to compel cesarean delivery in a critically ill woman at 26 weeks of gestation against her wishes, stating in its opinion that "in virtually all cases the question of what is to be done is to be decided by the patient—the pregnant woman—on behalf of herself and the fetus" (1). Furthermore, the court stated that it could think of no "extremely rare and truly exceptional" case in which the state might have an interest sufficiently compelling to override a pregnant patient's wishes (2). Amid often vigorous debate, most ethicists also agree that a pregnant woman's informed refusal of medical intervention ought to prevail as long as she has the ability to make medical decisions (3, 4).

Recent legislation, criminal prosecutions, and legal cases much discussed in both courtrooms and newsrooms have challenged these precedents, raising the question of whether there are circumstances in which a woman who has become pregnant may have her rights to bodily integrity and informed consent overridden to protect her fetus. In Utah, a woman who had used cocaine was charged with homicide for refusing cesarean delivery of a fetus that was ultimately stillborn. In Pennsylvania, physicians obtained a court order for cesarean delivery in a patient with suspected fetal macrosomia. Across the country, pregnant women have been arrested and prosecuted for being pregnant and using drugs or alcohol. These cases and the publicity they have engendered suggest that it is time to revisit the ethical issues involved.

The ethics of caring for pregnant women and an approach to decision making in the context of the maternal–fetal relationship have been discussed in previous statements by the American College of Obstetricians and Gynecologists (ACOG) Committee on Ethics. After briefly reiterating those discussions, this opinion will summarize recent, notable cases; review the underlying, established ethical

principles relevant to the highlighted issues; consider objections to punitive and coercive legal approaches to maternal decision making; and summarize recommendations for attending to future ethical matters that may arise.

Recent Cases

In March 2004, a 28-year-old woman was charged with first-degree murder for refusing to undergo an immediate cesarean delivery because of concerns about fetal well-being and later giving birth to a girl who tested positive for cocaine and a stillborn boy. According to press reports, the woman was mentally ill and intermittently homeless and had been brought to Utah by a Florida adoption agency to give birth to the infants and give them up. She ultimately pled guilty to two counts of child endangerment.

In January 2004, a woman who previously had given birth vaginally to six infants, some of whom weighed close to 12 pounds, refused a cesarean delivery that was recommended because of presumed macrosomia. A Pennsylvania hospital obtained a court order to perform the cesarean delivery and gain custody of the fetus before and after delivery, but the woman and her husband fled to another hospital, where she reportedly had an uncomplicated vaginal delivery of a healthy 11-pound infant.

In September 2003, a 22-year-old woman was prosecuted after her son tested positive for alcohol when he was born in Glens Falls, New York. A few days after the birth, the woman was arrested and charged with two counts of child endangerment for "knowingly feeding her blood," containing alcohol, to her fetus via the umbilical cord. Several months later, her lawyers successfully appealed her conviction.

In May 1999, a 22-year-old woman who was homeless regularly used cocaine while pregnant and gave birth to a stillborn infant in South Carolina. She became the first woman in the United States to be tried and convicted of homicide by child abuse based on her behavior during pregnancy and was given a 12-year prison sentence. The conviction was upheld in the South Carolina Supreme Court, and the U.S. Supreme Court recently refused to hear her appeal. At a postconviction relief hearing, expert testimony supported arguments that the woman had had inadequate representation, but the court held that there was no ineffective assistance of counsel and that she is not entitled to a new trial. This decision is being appealed.

Ethical Considerations

Framing Ethics in Perinatal Medicine

It is likely that the interventions described in the preceding cases were motivated by a shared concept—that a fetus can and should be treated as separable and legally, philosophically, and practically independent from the pregnant woman within whom it resides. This common method of framing ethical issues in perinatal medicine is not surprising given a number of developments in the past several decades. First, since the 1970s, the development of techniques for imaging, testing, and treating fetuses has led to the widespread endorsement of the notion that fetuses are independent patients, treatable apart from the pregnant women upon whom their existence depends (5). Similarly, some bioethical models now assert that physicians have moral obligations to fetal "patients" that are separate from their obligations to pregnant women (6). Finally, a number of civil laws, discussed later in this section, aim to create fetal rights separate from a pregnant woman's rights.

Although frameworks that treat the woman and fetus as separable and independent are meant to simplify and clarify complex issues that arise in obstetrics, many writers have noted that such frameworks tend to distort, rather than illuminate, ethical and policy debates (7). In particular, these approaches have been criticized for their tendency to emphasize the divergent rather than shared interests of the pregnant woman and fetus. This emphasis results in a view of the maternal–fetal relationship as paradigmatically adversarial, when in fact in the vast majority of cases, the interests of the pregnant woman and fetus actually converge.

In addition, these approaches tend to ignore the moral relevance of relationships, including the physically and emotionally intimate relationship between the woman and her fetus, as well as the relationships of the pregnant woman within her broader social and cultural networks. The cultural and policy context, for example, suggests a predominantly child-centered approach to maternal and child health, which has influenced current perspectives on the fetus. The prototype for the federal Maternal and Child Health Bureau dates back to 1912, when the first organization was called into existence by reformers such as Florence Kelley, who stated that "the U.S. should have a bureau to look after the child crop," and Julia Lathrop, who said that "the final

purpose of the Bureau is to serve all children, to try to work out standards of care and protection which shall give to every child his fair chance in the world." The current home page of the Maternal and Child Health Bureau web site cites as its "vision" an equally child-centered goal (8).

At times, in the current clinical and policy contexts, when the woman and fetus are treated as separate individuals, the woman and her medical interests, health needs, and rights as moral agent, patient, and research subject fade from view. Consider, first, women's medical interests as patients. Researchers performing "fetal surgery"—novel interventions to correct fetal anatomic abnormalities—have been criticized recently not only for their tendency to exaggerate claims of success with regard to fetal and neonatal health, but also for their failure to assess the impact of surgery on pregnant women, who also undertake the risks of the major surgical procedures (9). As a result, several centers performing these techniques now use the term "maternal–fetal surgery" to explicitly recognize the fact that a woman's bodily integrity and health are at stake whenever interventions directed at her fetus are performed. Furthermore, a study sponsored by the National Institute of Child Health and Human Development comparing maternal–fetal surgery with postnatal repair of myelomeningocele (the Management of Myelomeningocele Study) is now assessing maternal as well as fetal outcomes, including measurement of reproductive and health outcomes, depression testing, and economic and family health outcomes in women who participate in the clinical trial.

Similarly, new civil laws that aim to treat the fetus as separate and independent have been criticized for their failure both to address the health needs of the woman within whose body the fetus resides and to recognize the converging interests of the woman and fetus. In November 2002, a revision of the state child health insurance program (sCHIP) that expanded coverage to "individual(s) under the age of 19 including the period from conception until birth" was signed into law. The program does not cover pregnant women older than 18 years except when medical interventions could directly affect the well-being of their fetuses. For example, under sCHIP, intrapartum anesthesia is covered, according to the U.S. Department of Health and Human Services, only because "if a woman's pain during a labor and delivery is not reduced or properly relieved, adverse and sometimes disastrous effects can occur for the unborn child" (10).

Furthermore, for beneficiaries of sCHIP, many significant women's health issues, even those that are precipitated by pregnancy (eg, molar gestation, postpartum depression, or traumatic injury from intimate partner violence not impacting the fetus), are not covered as a part of routine antenatal care (11). This approach has been criticized not only for its failure to address the health needs of women, but also for its failure to achieve the narrow goal of improving child health because it ignores the fact that maternal and neonatal interests converge. For instance, postpartum depression is associated with adverse effects in infants, including impaired maternal–infant interaction, delayed cognitive and emotional development, increased anxiety, and decreased self-esteem (12, 13). Thus, the law ignores the fact that a critical component of ensuring the health of newborns is the provision of comprehensive care for their mothers.

Likewise, in April 2004, the Unborn Victims of Violence Act was signed into law, creating a separate federal offense if, during the commission of certain federal crimes, an individual causes the death of, or bodily injury to, a fetus at any stage of pregnancy. The law, however, does not categorize the death of or injury to a pregnant woman as a separate federal offense, or create sentence enhancement for those who assault or murder a woman while pregnant. The statute's sponsors explicitly rejected proposals that had virtually identical criminal penalties but recognized the pregnant woman as the victim, despite the fact that murder is responsible for more pregnancy-associated deaths in the United States than any other cause, including hemorrhage and thromboembolic events (14, 15).

Beyond its impact on maternal and child health, a failure to recognize the interconnectedness of the pregnant woman and fetus has important ethical and legal implications. Because an intervention on a fetus must be performed through the body of a pregnant woman, an assertion of fetal rights must be reconciled with the ethical and legal obligations toward pregnant women *as women*, persons in their own right. Discussions about rights of the unborn often have failed to address these obligations. Regardless of what is believed about fetal personhood, claims about fetal rights require an assessment of the rights of pregnant women, whose personhood within the legal and moral community is indisputable.

Furthermore, many writers have noted a moral injury that arises from abstracting the fetus from the pregnant woman, in its failing to recognize the pregnant woman herself as a patient, person, and rights-bearer. This approach disregards a fundamental moral principle that persons never be treated solely as means to an end, but as ends in themselves. Within the rhetoric of conflict and fetal rights, the pregnant woman has at times been reduced to a vessel—even a "fortress" holding the fetus "prisoner" (16). As George Annas aptly described, "Before birth, we can obtain access to the fetus only through its mother, and in the absence of her informed consent, can do so only by treating her as a fetal container, a nonperson without rights to bodily integrity" (3).

Some writers have argued that at the heart of the distorting influence of the "two-patient" model of the maternal–fetal dyad is the fact that, according to traditional theories that undergird medical ethics, the very notion of a person or a patient is someone who is physically separate from others. Pregnancy, however, is marked by a "particular and particularly thoroughgoing kind of intertwinement" (17). Thus, the pregnant woman and fetus fit awkwardly at best into what the term "patient" is understood to mean. They are neither physically separate, as persons are understood to be, nor indistinguishably fused. A framework that instead defines the professional ethical obligations with a deep sensitivity to relationships of interdependency may help to avoid the distorting influence of the two-patient model as traditionally understood (18). Although this opinion does not specifically articulate a novel comprehensive conceptual model for perinatal ethics, in the discussion that follows, the Committee on Ethics takes as morally central the essential connection between the pregnant woman and fetus.

Ethics Committee Opinions and the Maternal–Fetal Relationship

In the context of a framework that recognizes the interconnectedness of the pregnant woman and fetus and emphasizes their shared interests, certain opinions previously published by the ACOG Committee on Ethics are particularly relevant. These include:

- "Informed Consent" (19)
- "Patient Choice in the Maternal–Fetal Relationship" (20)
- "At-Risk Drinking and Illicit Drug Use: Ethical Issues in Obstetric and Gynecologic Practice" (21)

One fundamental ethical obligation of health care professionals is to respect patients' autonomous decision making and to adhere to the requirement for informed consent for medical intervention. In January 2004, the Committee on Ethics published a revised edition of "Informed Consent" in which the following points are defended:

- "Requiring informed consent is an expression of respect for the patient as a person; it particularly respects a patient's moral right to bodily integrity, to self-determination regarding sexuality and reproductive capacities, and to the support of the patient's freedom within caring relationships."

- "The ethical requirement for informed consent need not conflict with physicians' overall ethical obligation to a principle of beneficence; that is, every effort should be made to incorporate a commitment to informed consent within a commitment to provide medical benefit to patients and thus respect them as whole and embodied persons."

Pregnancy does not obviate or limit the requirement to obtain informed consent. Intervention on behalf of the fetus must be undertaken through the body and within the context of the life of the pregnant woman, and therefore her consent for medical treatment is required, regardless of the treatment indication. However, pregnancy presents a special set of issues. The issues associated with informed refusal of care by pregnant women are addressed in the January 2004 opinion "Patient Choice in the Maternal–Fetal Relationship" (20). This opinion states that in cases of maternal refusal of treatment for the sake of the fetus, "court-ordered intervention against the wishes of a pregnant woman is rarely if ever acceptable." The document presents a review of general ethical considerations applicable to pregnant women who do not follow the advice of their physicians or do not seem to make decisions in the best interest of their fetuses. Although the possibility of a justifiable court-ordered intervention is not completely ruled out, the document presents several recommendations that strongly discourage coercive measures:

- "The obstetrician's response to a patient's unwillingness to cooperate with medical advice . . . should be to convey clearly the reasons for the recommendations to the pregnant woman,

examine the barriers to change along with her, and encourage the development of health-promoting behavior."

- "[Even if] a woman's autonomous decision [seems] not to promote beneficence-based obligations (of the woman or the physician) to the fetus, . . . the obstetrician must respect the patient's autonomy, continue to care for the pregnant woman, and not intervene against the patient's wishes, regardless of the consequences."

- "The obstetrician must keep in mind that medical knowledge has limitations and medical judgment is fallible" and should therefore take great care "to present a balanced evaluation of expected outcomes for both [the woman and the fetus]."

- "Obstetricians should consider the social and cultural context in which these decisions are made and question whether their ethical judgments reinforce gender, class, or racial inequality."

In addition to revisiting questions of how practitioners should address refusal of treatment in the clinic and delivery room, the four cases outlined previously illustrate punitive and coercive policies aimed at pregnant women who engage in behaviors that may adversely affect fetal well-being. The 2004 opinion "At-Risk Drinking and Illicit Drug Use: Ethical Issues in Obstetric and Gynecologic Practice" (21) specifically addresses addiction and the prosecution of women who use drugs and alcohol during pregnancy and recommends strongly against punitive policies:

- "Addiction is not primarily a moral weakness, as it has been viewed in the past, but a 'brain disease' that should be included in a review of systems just like any other biologic disease process."

- "Recommended screening . . . connected with legally mandated testing or reporting . . . endanger[s] the relationship of trust between physician and patient, place[s] the obstetrician in an adversarial relationship with the patient, and possibly conflict[s] with the therapeutic obligation."

- Punitive policies "are unjust in that they indict the woman for failing to seek treatment that actually may not be available to her" and in that they "are not applied evenly across sex, race, and socioeconomic status."

- Physicians must make a substantial effort to "treat the patient with a substance abuse problem with dignity and respect in order to form a therapeutic alliance."

Finally, recent legal decisions affirm that physicians have neither an obligation nor a right to perform prenatal testing for alcohol or drug use without a pregnant woman's consent (22, 23). This includes consent to testing of the woman that could lead to any form of reporting, both to legal authorities for purposes of criminal prosecution and to civil child welfare authorities.

Against Coercive and Punitive Legal Approaches to the Maternal–Fetal Relationship

This section addresses specifically the ethical issues associated with the cases outlined previously and delineates six reasons why restricting patients' liberty and punishing pregnant women for their actions during pregnancy that may affect their fetuses is neither wise nor justifiable. Each raises important objections to punishing pregnant women for actions during pregnancy; together they provide an overwhelming rationale for avoiding such approaches.

1. Coercive and punitive legal approaches to pregnant women who refuse medical advice fail to recognize that all competent adults are entitled to informed consent and bodily integrity.

A fundamental tenet of contemporary medical ethics is the requirement for informed consent, including the right of competent adults to refuse medical intervention. The Committee on Ethics affirms that informed consent for medical treatment is an ethical requirement and is an expression of respect for the patient as a person with a moral right to bodily integrity (19).

The crucial difference between pregnant and nonpregnant individuals, though, is that a fetus is involved whose health interests could arguably be served by overriding the pregnant woman's wishes. However, in the United States, even in the case of two completely separate individuals, constitutional law and common law have historically recognized the rights of all adults, pregnant or not, to informed consent and bodily integrity, *regardless of the impact of that person's decision on others.* For instance, in 1978, a man suffering from aplastic anemia sought a court order to force his cousin, who was the only compatible donor available, to submit

to bone marrow harvest. The court declined, explaining in its opinion:

> For our law to compel the Defendant to submit to an intrusion of his body would change every concept and principle upon which our society is founded. To do so would defeat the sanctity of the individual and would impose a rule which would know no limits. . . . For a society that respects the rights of one individual, to sink its teeth into the jugular vein or neck of its members and suck from it sustenance for another member, is revolting to our hard-wrought concepts of jurisprudence. Forcible extraction of living body tissues causes revulsion to the judicial mind. Such would raise the specter of the swastika and the Inquisition, reminiscent of the horrors this portends. (24)

Justice requires that a pregnant woman, like any other individual, retain the basic right to refuse medical intervention, even if the intervention is in the best interest of her fetus. This principle was challenged unsuccessfully in June 1987 with the case of a 27-year-old woman who was at 25 weeks of gestation when she became critically ill with cancer. Against the wishes of the woman, her family, and her physicians, the hospital obtained a court order for a cesarean delivery, claiming independent rights of the fetus. Both mother and infant died shortly after the cesarean delivery was performed. Three years later, the District of Columbia Court of Appeals vacated the court-ordered cesarean delivery and held that the woman had the right to make health care decisions for herself and her fetus, arguing that the lower court had "erred in subordinating her right to bodily integrity in favor of the state's interest in potential life" (1).

2. Court-ordered interventions in cases of informed refusal, as well as punishment of pregnant women for their behavior that may put a fetus at risk, neglect the fact that medical knowledge and predictions of outcomes in obstetrics have limitations.

Beyond its importance as a means to protect the right of individuals to bodily integrity, the doctrine of informed consent recognizes the right of individuals to weigh risks and benefits for themselves. Women almost always are best situated to understand the importance of risks and benefits in the context of their own values, circumstances, and concerns. Furthermore, medical judgment in obstetrics itself has limitations in its ability to predict outcomes. In this document, the Committee on Ethics has argued that overriding a woman's autonomous choice, whatever its potential consequences, is neither ethically nor legally justified, given her fundamental rights to bodily integrity. Even those who challenge these fundamental rights in favor of protecting the fetus, however, must recognize and communicate that medical judgments in obstetrics are fallible (25). And fallibility—present to various degrees in all medical encounters—is sufficiently high in obstetric decision making to warrant wariness in imposing legal coercion. Levels of certainty underlying medical recommendations to pregnant women are unlikely to be adequate to justify legal coercion and the tremendous impact on the lives and civil liberties of pregnant women that such intervention would entail (26). Some have argued that court-ordered intervention might plausibly be justified only when certainty is especially robust and the stakes are especially high. However, in many cases of court-ordered obstetric intervention, the latter criterion has been met but not the former. Furthermore, evidence-based medicine has revealed limitations in the ability to concretely describe the relationship of maternal behavior to perinatal outcome. Criminalizing women in the face of such scientific and clinical uncertainty is morally dubious. Not only do these approaches fail to take into account the standards of evidence-based medical practice, but they are also unjust, and their application is likely to be informed by bias and opinion rather than objective assessment of risk.

Consider, first, the limitations of medical judgment in predicting birth outcomes based on mode of childbirth. A study of court-ordered obstetric interventions suggested that in almost one third of cases in which court orders were sought, the medical judgment was incorrect in retrospect (27). One clear example of the challenges of predicting outcome is in the management of risk associated with shoulder dystocia in the setting of fetal macrosomia—which is, and should be, of great concern for all practitioners. When making recommendations to patients, however, practitioners have an ethical obligation to recognize and communicate that accurate diagnosis of macrosomia is imprecise (20). Furthermore, although macrosomia increases the risk of shoulder dystocia, it is certainly not absolutely predictive; in fact, most cases of shoulder dystocia occur unpredictably among infants of normal birthweight. Given this uncertainty, ACOG makes recommendations about when cesarean delivery may be considered, not about when it is absolutely indicated. Because of the inability to determine with certainty when a situation is harmful to the fetus or pregnant woman and the inability to guarantee that the pregnant woman will not be harmed by the medical intervention, great care should be exercised to present a balanced evaluation of expected outcomes for both parties (20). The decision about weighing risks and benefits in the setting of uncertainty should remain the pregnant woman's to make in the setting of supportive, informative medical care.

Medical judgment also has limitations in that the relationship of maternal behavior to pregnancy outcome is poorly understood and may be exaggerated in realms often mistaken to be of moral rather than medical concern, such as drug use. For instance, recent child development research has not found the effects of prenatal cocaine exposure that earlier uncontrolled studies reported (28). It is now understood that poverty and its concomitants—poor nutrition and inadequate health care—can account for many of the effects popularly attributed to cocaine. Before these data emerged, the criminal justice approach to drug addiction during pregnancy was fueled to a great degree by what is now understood to be the distorting image of the "crack baby." Such an image served as a "convenient symbol for an aggressive war on drug users [that] makes it easier to advocate a simplistic punitive response than to address the complex causes of drug use" (29). The findings questioning the impact of cocaine on perinatal outcome are among many considerations that bring sharply into question any possible justification for a criminal justice approach, rather than a public health approach, to drug use during pregnancy. Given the incomplete understanding of factors underlying perinatal outcomes in general and the contribution of individual behavioral and socioeconomic factors in particular, to identify homeless and addicted women as personally, morally, and legally culpable for perinatal outcomes is inaccurate, misleading, and unjust.

3. Coercive and punitive policies treat medical problems such as addiction and psychiatric illness as if they were moral failings.

Regardless of the strength of the link between an individual's behaviors and pregnancy outcome, punitive policies directed at women who use drugs are not justified, because these policies are, in effect, punishing women for having a medical problem. Although once considered a sign of moral weakness, addiction is now, according to evidence-based medicine, considered a disease—a compulsive disorder requiring medical attention (30). Pregnancy should not change how clinicians understand the medical nature of addictive behavior. In fact, studies overwhelmingly show that pregnant drug users are very concerned about the consequences of their drug use for their fetuses and are particularly eager to obtain treatment once they find out they are pregnant (31, 32). Despite evidence-based medical recommendations that support treatment approaches to drug use and addiction (21), appropriate treatment is particularly difficult to obtain for pregnant and parenting women and the incarcerated (29). Thus, a disease process exacerbated by social circumstance—not personal, legal, or moral culpability—is at the heart of substance abuse and pregnancy. Punitive policies unfairly make pregnant women scapegoats for medical problems whose cause is often beyond their control.

In most states, governmental responses to pregnant women who use drugs have upheld medical characterizations of addiction. Consistent with long-standing U.S. Supreme Court decisions recognizing that addiction is an illness and that criminalizing it violates the Constitution's Eighth Amendment prohibitions against cruel and unusual punishment, no state has adopted a law that specifically creates unique criminal penalties for pregnant women who use drugs (33). However, in South Carolina, using drugs or being addicted to drugs was *effectively* criminalized when the state supreme court interpreted the word "child" in the state's criminal child endangerment statute to include viable fetuses, making the child endangerment statute applicable to pregnant women whose actions risk harm to a viable fetus (23). In all states, women retain their Fourth Amendment freedom from unreasonable searches, so that pregnant women may not be subject to nonconsensual drug testing for the purpose of criminal prosecution.

Partly on the basis of the understanding of addiction as a compulsive disorder requiring medical attention, medical professionals, U.S. state laws, and the vast majority of courts do not support unique criminal penalties for pregnant women who use drugs.

4. Coercive and punitive policies are potentially counterproductive in that they are likely to discourage prenatal care and successful treatment, adversely affect infant mortality rates, and undermine the physician–patient relationship.

Even if the aforementioned ethical concerns could be addressed, punitive policies would not be justifi-

able on utilitarian grounds, because they would likely result in more harm than good for maternal and child health, broadly construed. Various studies have suggested that attempts to criminalize pregnant women's behavior discourage women from seeking prenatal care (34, 35). Furthermore, an increased infant mortality rate was observed in South Carolina in the years following the *Whitner v State* decision (36), in which the state supreme court concluded that *anything* a pregnant woman does that might endanger a viable fetus (including, but not limited to, drug use) could result in either charges of child abuse and a jail sentence of up to 10 years or homicide and a 20-year sentence if a stillbirth coincides with a positive drug test (23). As documented previously (21), threats and incarceration have been ineffective in reducing the incidence of alcohol and drug abuse among pregnant women, and removing children from the home of an addicted mother may subject them to worse risks in the foster care system. In fact, women who have custody of their children complete substance abuse treatment at a higher rate (37–39).

These data suggest that punishment of pregnant women might not result in women receiving the desired message about the dangers of prenatal substance abuse; such measures might instead send an unintended message about the dangers of prenatal care. Ultimately, fear surrounding prenatal care would likely undermine, rather than enhance, maternal and child health. Likewise, court-ordered interventions and other coercive measures may result in fear about whether one's wishes in the delivery room will be respected and ultimately could discourage pregnant patients from seeking care. Encouraging prenatal care and treatment in a supportive environment will advance maternal and child health most effectively.

5. Coercive and punitive policies directed toward pregnant women unjustly single out the most vulnerable women.

Evidence suggests that punitive and coercive policies not only are ethically problematic in and of themselves, but also unfairly burden the most vulnerable women. In cases of court-ordered cesarean deliveries, for instance, the vast majority of court orders have been obtained against poor women of color (27, 40).

Similarly, decisions about detection and management of substance abuse in pregnancy are fraught with bias, unfairly burdening the most vulnerable despite the fact that addiction occurs consistently across race and socioeconomic status (41). In the landmark case of *Ferguson v City of Charleston*, which involved selective screening and arrest of pregnant women who tested positive for drugs, 29 of 30 women arrested were African American. Studies suggest that affluent women are less likely to be tested for use of illicit drugs than poor women of color, perhaps because of stereotyped but demonstrably inaccurate assumptions about drug use. One study found that despite similar rates of substance abuse across racial and socioeconomic status, African–American women were 10 times more likely than white women to be reported to public health authorities for substance abuse during pregnancy (42). These data suggest that, as implemented, many punitive policies centered on maternal behaviors, including substance use, are deeply unjust in that they reinforce social and racial inequality.

6. Coercive and punitive policies create the potential for criminalization of many types of otherwise legal maternal behavior.

In addition to raising concerns about race and socioeconomic status, punitive and coercive policies may have even broader implications for justice for women. Because many maternal behaviors are associated with adverse pregnancy outcome, these policies could result in a society in which simply being a woman of reproductive potential could put an individual at risk for criminal prosecution. For instance, poorly controlled diabetes is associated with numerous congenital malformations and an excessive rate of fetal death. Periconceptional folic acid deficiency is associated with an increased risk of neural tube defects. Obesity has been associated in recent studies with adverse pregnancy outcomes, including preeclampsia, shoulder dystocia, and antepartum stillbirth (43, 44). Prenatal exposure to certain medications that may be essential to maintaining a pregnant woman's health status is associated with congenital abnormalities. If states were to consistently adopt policies of punishing women whose behavior (ranging from substance abuse to poor nutrition to informed decisions about prescription drugs) has the potential to lead to adverse perinatal outcomes, at what point would they draw the line? Punitive policies, therefore, threaten the privacy and autonomy not only of all pregnant women, but also of all women of reproductive potential.

Recommendations

In light of these six considerations, the Committee on Ethics strongly opposes the criminal prosecution of pregnant women whose activities may appear to cause harm to their fetuses. Efforts to use the legal system specifically to protect the fetus by constraining women's decision making or punishing them for their behavior erode a woman's basic rights to privacy and bodily integrity and are neither legally nor morally justified. The ACOG Committee on Ethics therefore makes the following recommendations:

- In caring for pregnant women, practitioners should recognize that in the majority of cases, the interests of the pregnant woman and her fetus converge rather than diverge. Promoting pregnant women's health through advocacy of healthy behavior, referral for substance abuse treatment and mental health services when necessary, and maintenance of a good physician–patient relationship is always in the best interest of both the woman and her fetus.

- Pregnant women's autonomous decisions should be respected. Concerns about the impact of maternal decisions on fetal well-being should be discussed in the context of medical evidence and understood within the context of each woman's broad social network, cultural beliefs, and values. In the absence of extraordinary circumstances, circumstances that, in fact, the Committee on Ethics cannot currently imagine, judicial authority should not be used to implement treatment regimens aimed at protecting the fetus, for such actions violate the pregnant woman's autonomy.

- Pregnant women should not be punished for adverse perinatal outcomes. The relationship between maternal behavior and perinatal outcome is not fully understood, and punitive approaches threaten to dissuade pregnant women from seeking health care and ultimately undermine the health of pregnant women and their fetuses.

- Policy makers, legislators, and physicians should work together to find constructive and evidence-based ways to address the needs of women with alcohol and other substance abuse problems. This should include the development of safe, available, and efficacious services for women and families.

References

1. In re A.C., 573 A.2d 1235 (D.C. 1990).
2. Annas GJ. Foreclosing the use of force: A.C. reversed. Hastings Cent Rep 1990;20(4):27–9.
3. Annas GJ. Protecting the liberty of pregnant patients [editorial]. N Engl J Med 1987;316:1213–4.
4. Rhoden NK. The judge in the delivery room: the emergence of court-ordered cesareans. Calif Law Rev 1986; 74:1951–2030.
5. Bianchi DW, Crombleholme TM, D'Alton ME. Fetology: diagnosis and management of the fetal patient. New York (NY): McGraw-Hill; 2000.
6. McCullough LB, Chervenak FA. Ethics in obstetrics and gynecology. New York (NY): Oxford University Press; 1994.
7. Harris LH. Rethinking maternal-fetal conflict: gender and equality in perinatal ethics. Obstet Gynecol 2000;96: 786–91.
8. Maternal and Child Health Bureau. Mission statement. Rockville (MD): MCHB; 2005. Available at: http://www.mchb.hrsa.gov/about/default.htm. Retrieved June 17, 2005.
9. Lyerly AD, Gates EA, Cefalo RC, Sugarman J. Toward the ethical evaluation and use of maternal-fetal surgery. Obstet Gynecol 2001;98:689–97.
10. State Children's Health Insurance Program; eligibility for prenatal care and other health services for unborn children. Final rule. Centers for Medicare & Medicaid Services (CMS), HHS. Fed Regist 2002;67:61955–74.
11. Steinbock B. Health care coverage for not-yet-born children. Hastings Cent Rep 2003;33(1):49.
12. Murray L, Cooper P. Effects of postnatal depression on infant development. Arch Dis Child 1997;77:99–101.
13. Murray L, Fiori-Cowley A, Hooper R, Cooper P. The impact of postnatal depression and associated adversity on early mother-infant interactions and later infant outcome. Child Dev 1996;67:2512–26.
14. Horon IL, Cheng D. Enhanced surveillance for pregnancy-associated mortality—Maryland, 1993–1998. JAMA 2001;285:1455–9.
15. Frye V. Examining homicide's contribution to pregnancy-associated deaths [editorial]. JAMA 2001;285:1510–1.
16. Phelan JP. The maternal abdominal wall: a fortress against fetal health care? South Calif Law Rev 1991;65:461–90.
17. Little MO. Abortion, intimacy, and the duty to gestate. Ethical Theory Moral Pract 1999;2:295–312.
18. Mattingly SS. The maternal-fetal dyad. Exploring the two-patient obstetric model. Hastings Cent Rep 1992;22: 13–8.
19. Informed consent. In: American College of Obstetricians and Gynecologists. Ethics in obstetrics and gynecology. 2nd ed. Washington, DC: ACOG; 2004. p. 9–17.
20. Patient choice in the maternal–fetal relationship. In: American College of Obstetricians and Gynecologists. Ethics in obstetrics and gynecology. 2nd ed. Washington, DC: ACOG; 2004. p. 34–6.
21. At-risk drinking and illicit drug use: ethical issues in obstetric and gynecologic practice. ACOG Committee Opinion No. 294. American College of Obstetricians and Gynecologists. Obstet Gynecol 2004;103:1021–31.
22. Ferguson v. City of Charleston, 532 U.S. 67 (2001).
23. Whitner v. State, 328 S.C. 1, 492 S.E.2n 777 (1997).
24. McFall v. Shimp, 10 Pa. D. & C.3d (C.P. 1978).
25. Rhoden NK. Informed consent in obstetrics: some special problems. West N Engl Law Rev 1987;9:67–88.
26. Nelson LJ, Milliken N. Compelled medical treatment of pregnant women. Life, liberty, and law in conflict. JAMA 1988;259:1060–6.
27. Kolder VE, Gallagher J, Parsons MT. Court-ordered obstetrical interventions. N Engl J Med 1987;316:1192–6.
28. Frank DA, Augustyn M, Knight WG, Pell T, Zuckerman B. Growth, development, and behavior in early childhood following prenatal cocaine exposure: a systematic review. JAMA 2001;285:1613–25.
29. Chavkin W. Cocaine and pregnancy—time to look at the evidence [editorial]. JAMA 2001;285:1626–8.
30. Marwick C. Physician leadership on National Drug Policy finds that addiction treatment works. JAMA 1998;279: 1149–50.
31. Murphy S, Rosenbaum M. Pregnant women on drugs: combating stereotypes and stigma. New Brunswick (NJ): Rutgers University Press; 1999.
32. Kearney MH, Murphy S, Rosenbaum M. Mothering on crack cocaine: a grounded theory analysis. Soc Sci Med 1994;38:351–61.
33. Harris LH, Paltrow L. MSJAMA. The status of pregnant women and fetuses in US criminal law. JAMA 2003; 289:1697–9.
34. Poland ML, Dombrowski MP, Ager JW, Sokol RJ. Punishing pregnant drug users: enhancing the flight from care. Drug Alcohol Depend 1993;31:199–203.
35. United States. General Accounting Office. Drug exposed infants: a generation at risk: report to the chairman, Committee on Finance, U.S. Senate. Washington, DC: U.S. General Accounting Office; 1990.
36. The Annie E. Casey Foundation. 2004 kids count data book: moving youth from risk to opportunity. Baltimore (MD): AECF; 2004. Available at: http://www.aecf.org/publications/data/kc2004_e.pdf. Retrieved June 17, 2005.
37. Haller DL, Knisely JS, Elswick RK Jr, Dawson KS, Schnoll SH. Perinatal substance abusers: factors influencing treatment retention. J Subst Abuse Treat 1997;14: 513–9.
38. Hohman MM, Shillington AM, Baxter HG. A comparison of pregnant women presenting for alcohol and other drug treatment by CPS status. Child Abuse Negl 2003;27: 303–17.
39. Kissin WB, Svikis DS, Morgan GD, Haug NA. Characterizing pregnant drug-dependent women in treatment and their children. J Subst Abuse Treat 2001;21: 27–34.
40. Nelson LJ, Marshall MF. Ethical and legal analyses of three coercive policies aimed at substance abuse by pregnant women. Charleston (SC): Medical University of South Carolina, Program in Bioethics; 1998.
41. Mathias R. NIDA survey provides first national data on drug use during pregnancy. NIDA Notes 1995;10(1). Available

at: http://www.nida.nih.gov/NIDA_Notes/NNVol10N1/ NIDASurvey.html. Retrieved June 17, 2005.

42. Chasnoff IJ, Landress HJ, Barrett ME. The prevalence of illicit-drug or alcohol use during pregnancy and discrepancies in mandatory reporting in Pinellas County, Florida. N Engl J Med 1990;322:1202–6.

43. Cedergren MI. Maternal morbid obesity and the risk of adverse pregnancy outcome. Obstet Gynecol 2004;103: 219–24.

44. Cnattingius S, Bergstrom R, Lipworth L, Kramer MS. Prepregnancy weight and the risk of adverse pregnancy outcomes. N Engl J Med 1998;338:147–52.

ACOG Committee Opinion

Committee on
Genetics

Number 230, January 2000

Maternal Phenylketonuria

Phenylketonuria (PKU) is an autosomal recessive disorder of phenylalanine metabolism that, if untreated, can cause severe mental retardation. Phenylketonuria is caused by a deficiency of the enzyme phenylalanine hydroxylase. Children of women with PKU will carry at least one abnormal gene, which is inherited from their homozygous affected mother. Even though the fetus is unlikely to be affected, approximately 1 in 120 children will inherit an abnormal phenylalanine hydroxylase gene from both parents and also have PKU. The remainder of children are carriers and should receive genetic counseling in the future. Phenylalanine crosses the placenta by an active transport process that results in a fetal-to-maternal plasma phenylalanine ratio of 1.5. This results in higher levels of phenylalanine in fetal blood than would be expected based on maternal blood levels.

Routine screening for PKU in newborns and early dietary therapy with a phenylalanine-restricted diet have markedly reduced mental retardation in affected individuals. As a result of these advances in the detection and treatment of PKU, there are large numbers of young adults with PKU who received early dietary treatment for this disorder and have IQs in the normal or near-normal range. The failure of young women with PKU to adhere to dietary restrictions has led to a new public health challenge. The heterozygous fetus is metabolically normal. However, these metabolically normal fetuses of women with PKU who are on an unrestricted diet may develop microcephaly, low birth weight, heart defects, and mental retardation due to maternal hyperphenylalaninemia. Children of women with PKU on unrestricted diets are at a 92% risk for mental retardation, a 73% risk for microcephaly, and a 12% risk for congenital heart defects (1).

In the United States, approximately 3,000 women of reproductive age are affected with PKU. Evidence indicates that women with PKU will benefit from remaining on a phenylalanine-free diet throughout their lives. Many of these women are not currently on phenylalanine-restricted diets, which require the consumption of phenylalanine-free products and supplements that many women find unpalatable. Unless these women are identified and placed on an appropriate diet before and during pregnancy, they are at risk for having children affected with PKU. It has been suggested that dietary control should be implemented at least 3 months prior to conception to help prevent fetal structural defects, including cardiac defects (2). If phenylalanine levels are normalized by 8 weeks of gestation, there is evidence to suggest a reduction in intrauterine growth restriction (3).

The American College of Obstetricians and Gynecologists
409 12th Street, SW
PO Box 96920
Washington, DC 20090-6920

12345/43210

Conclusions and Recommendations

1. All women with PKU should be strongly encouraged to receive family planning and preconceptional counseling.

2. Women with PKU should begin dietary phenylalanine restriction prior to conception (4).

3. Ideally, pregnant women with PKU should be managed in consultation with practitioners from experienced PKU centers.

References

1. Lenke RR, Levy HL. Maternal phenylketonuria and hyperphenylalaninemia. An international survey of the outcome of untreated and treated pregnancies. N Engl J Med 1980; 303:1202–1208

2. Waisbren SE, Hamilton BD, St. James PJ, Shiloh S, Levy HL. Psychosocial factors in maternal phenylketonuria: women's adherence to medical recommendations. Am J Public Health 1995;85:1636–1641

3. Koch R, Friedman E, Azen C, Hanley W, Levy H, Matalon R, et al. The international collaborative study of maternal phenylketonuria status report 1998. MRDD Res Rev 1999;5:117–121

4. Levy HL, Waisbren SE, Lobbregt D, Allred E, Schuler A, Trefz FK, et al. Maternal mild hyperphenylalaninaemia: an international survey of offspring outcome. Lancet 1994; 344: 1589–1594

Bibliography

Koch R, Levy HL, Matalon R, Rouse B, Haney WB, Trefz F, et al. The international collaborative study of maternal phenylketonuria: status report 1994. Acta Paediatr Suppl 1994;407: 111–119

Levy HL, Waisbren SE. Effects of untreated maternal phenylketonuria and hyperphenylalaninemia on the fetus. N Engl J Med 1983;309:1269–1274

Lipson A, Beuhler B, Bartley J, Walsh D, Yu J, O'Halloran M, et al. Maternal hyperphenylalaninemia fetal effects. J Pediatr 1984;104:216–220

Luke B, Keith LG. The challenge of maternal phenylketonuria screening and treatment. J Reprod Med 1990;35:667–673

MacCready RA. Admissions of phenylketonuric patients to residential institutions before and after screening programs of the newborn infant. J Pediatr 1974;85:383–385

Platt LD, Koch R, Azen C, Hanley WB, Levy HL, Matalon R, et al. Maternal phenylketonuria collaborative study, obstetric aspects and outcome: the first 6 years. Am J Obstet Gynecol 1992;166:1150–1162

ACOG Committee Opinion

Committee on
Adolescent Health Care

Number 314, September 2005

Meningococcal Vaccination for Adolescents

The American College of Obstetricians and Gynecologists
409 12th Street, SW
PO Box 96920
Washington, DC 20090-6920

12345/98765

Meningococcal vaccination for adolescents. ACOG Committee Opinion No. 314. American College of Obstetricians and Gynecologists. Obstet Gynecol 2005;106:667–9.

ABSTRACT: *Every year in the United States, approximately 1,400–2,800 individuals are infected with meningococcal disease. The Advisory Committee on Immunization Practices (ACIP) to the Centers for Disease Control and Prevention (CDC) released recommendations in early 2005 to reduce the incidence of meningococcal disease during adolescence and young adulthood. To achieve this goal, routine vaccination of preadolescents with meningococcal conjugate vaccine (MCV4) is now recommended. For adolescents who have not received MCV4, the CDC now recommends vaccination before entry into high school, at approximately 15 years of age. The American College of Obstetricians and Gynecologists supports these recommendations and encourages all health care providers caring for adolescent and young adult patients to provide meningococcal vaccination with MCV4 when appropriate. This includes vaccination of college freshmen who live in dormitories. Pregnant women may be vaccinated with meningococcal polysaccharide vaccine (MPSV4) as indicated. Health care providers also are encouraged to discuss meningococcal vaccination with patients whose children have reached preadolescence, adolescence, or young adulthood and to increase awareness of the signs and symptoms of meningococcal disease.*

Background

Meningococcal disease is caused by bacteria (*Neisseria meningitidis*) that infect the bloodstream and the meninges, resulting in serious illness. Every year in the United States, approximately 1,400–2,800 individuals are infected with meningococcal disease. *Neisseria meningitidis* has become a leading cause of bacterial meningitis in the United States. Ten percent to 14% of individuals with meningococcal disease die, and 11–19% percent of those who survive have permanent disabilities, such as mental retardation, hearing loss, and loss of limbs (1). The disease often begins with generalized symptoms that can be mistaken for a common illness, such as the flu. Meningococcal disease is particularly dangerous because it progresses rapidly and can be fatal within hours (2). Therefore, it is important to prevent the disease, through use of meningococcal vaccination, for individuals at highest risk.

Two meningococcal vaccines are available in the United States, meningococcal polysaccharide vaccine (MPSV4) and meningococcal conjugate vaccine (MCV4). Studies indicate that both vaccines can prevent four types of meningococcal disease (serogroups A, C, Y, W-135). Of all cases of meningococcal disease among individuals 11 years and older, 75% are caused by serogroups C, Y, or W-135. Both vaccines protect approximately 90% of individuals vaccinated.

Meningococcal polysaccharide vaccine is a tetravalent meningococcal polysaccharide vaccine that has been available in the United States since the 1970s. Each dose consists of purified bacterial capsular polysaccharides (50 µg each) from serogroups A, C, Y, and W-135. Meningococcal polysaccharide vaccine is available in single-dose (0.5 mL) and 10-dose (5 mL) vials (1).

Meningococcal conjugate vaccine is a tetravalent meningococcal conjugate vaccine that was licensed for use in the United States in January 2005. A 0.5-mL single dose of vaccine contains 4 µg each of capsular polysaccharide from serogroups A, C, Y, and W-135 conjugated to 48 µg of diphtheria toxoid. Meningococcal conjugate vaccine is available only in single-dose vials and is expected to be more effective, longer lasting, and more capable of preventing transmission of the disease from person to person (1).

These vaccines have been shown to be highly effective at reducing meningococcal disease. However, they do not protect individuals against meningococcal disease caused by serogroup B of *N meningitidis*. This type of bacteria causes one third of all meningococcal cases. More than half of the cases among infants younger than 1 year are caused by serogroup B, for which no vaccine is available in the United States (1).

Studies of vaccination with MPSV4 during pregnancy have not documented adverse effects among either pregnant women or newborns. On the basis of these data, the Centers for Disease Control and Prevention (CDC) states that pregnancy should not preclude vaccination with MPSV4, if indicated. No data are available on the safety of MCV4 during pregnancy (1).

Recommendations of the Advisory Committee on Immunization Practices to the Centers for Disease Control and Prevention

The Advisory Committee on Immunization Practices (ACIP) to the CDC released recommendations in early 2005 to reduce meningococcal disease during adolescence and young adulthood. Routine vaccination of preadolescents 11–12 years of age with MCV4 is now recommended. For adolescents who have not received MCV4, the CDC now recommends vaccination before entry into high school, at approximately 15 years of age. The goal is to implement, within 3 years, routine vaccination with MCV4 of all preadolescents beginning at 11 years of age. Other adolescents and young adults who want to decrease their risk for meningococcal disease also can be given the immunization. The recommendations state that MCV4 is preferred, but MPSV4 is acceptable (1).

Meningococcal vaccination also is recommended for other high-risk groups including (1):

- Anyone traveling to or living in a part of the world where meningococcal disease is endemic
- Anyone who is asplenic or has a damaged spleen
- Anyone who has terminal complement component deficiency (an immune system disorder)
- Anyone possibly exposed to meningitis during an outbreak
- Young men and women entering the military
- College freshmen living in dormitories

College freshmen who live in dormitories are at higher risk for meningococcal disease than other individuals of the same age because lifestyle factors common among freshman college students appear to be linked to the disease. These factors include: living in crowded housing, going to bars, smoking, and having irregular sleeping habits. Because of the feasibility constraints in targeting freshmen in dormitories, the CDC indicates that colleges may elect to target their vaccination campaigns to all matriculating freshmen. The risk for meningococcal disease among nonfreshmen college students is similar to that for the general population of similar age (18–24 years). However, the vaccines are safe and immunogenic and can be provided to nonfreshmen college students who want to reduce their risk for meningococcal disease (1).

ACOG Recommendations

The American College of Obstetricians and Gynecologists supports the recommendations of the ACIP for routine vaccination of preadolescents against meningococcal disease. Several medical professional organizations, including the American Academy of Pediatrics, the Society for Adolescent Medicine, and the American Academy of Family Physicians also support the recommendations of the ACIP (3–5). The American College of Obstetricians and Gynecologists encourages all health care providers caring for adolescent and young adult patients to provide meningococcal vaccination with MCV4 when appropriate. Because of the lack of data regarding the safety of MCV4 during pregnancy, MPSV4 can be considered for adolescents and young adults who are pregnant and those having unprotected sex who may be at risk for unintended pregnancy. Health care providers are encouraged to discuss meningococcal vaccination with patients whose children have reached preadolescence, adolescence, or young adulthood. It is important to increase parents', adolescents', and young adults' awareness of the signs and symptoms of meningococcal disease even though they are frequently nonspecific. This can result in earlier medical care and improved clinical outcomes.

References

1. Bilukha OO, Rosenstein N. Prevention and control of meningococcal disease. Recommendations of the Advisory Committee on Immunization Practices (ACIP). National Center for Infectious Diseases, Centers for Disease Control and Prevention (CDC). MMWR Recomm Rep 2005;54(RR-7):1-21. Available at: http://www.cdc.gov/mmwr/preview/mmwrhtml/rr5407a1.htm. Retrieved June 6, 2005.
2. Centers for Disease Control and Prevention. Meningococcal vaccines: what you need to know. Available at http://www.cdc.gov/nip/publications/vis/vis-mening.rtf. Retrieved May 18, 2005.
3. American Academy of Family Physicians. Meningococcal immunization. Available at: http://www.aafp.org/x34406.xml. Retrieved June 8, 2005.
4. Middleman AB, Rickert VI, Rosenthal SL. Meningococcal vaccine: position statement of the Society for Adolescent Medicine. J Adolesc Health 2005;37:262.
5. Prevention and control of meningococcal disease: recommendations for use of meningococcal vaccines in pediatric patients. Pediatrics 2005;116:496–505.

ACOG

Committee on
Obstetric Practice

Committee Opinion

Number 265, December 2001

Mode of Term Singleton Breech Delivery

ABSTRACT: Recently, researchers conducted a large, international multicenter randomized clinical trial comparing a policy of planned cesarean birth to planned vaginal birth. Given the results of this exceptionally large and well-controlled clinical trial, the American College of Obstetricians and Gynecologists Committee on Obstetric Practice recommends that obstetricians continue their efforts to reduce breech presentations in singleton gestations through the application of external cephalic version whenever possible. As a result of the findings of the study, planned vaginal delivery of a singleton term breech may no longer be appropriate. In those instances in which breech vaginal deliveries are pursued, great caution should be exercised. Patients with persistent breech presentation at term in a singleton gestation should undergo a planned cesarean delivery. A planned cesarean delivery does not apply to patients presenting with advanced labor and likely to have an imminent delivery of a fetus in a breech presentation or to patients whose second twin is in a nonvertex presentation.

During the past decade there has been an increasing trend in the United States to deliver term singleton fetuses in a breech presentation by cesarean delivery. In 1999, the rate of cesarean delivery for mothers in labor with breech presentation was 84.5 (1). The number of practitioners with the skills and experience to perform vaginal breech delivery has decreased. In academic medical centers where faculty support for teaching vaginal breech delivery to residents remains high, there may be insufficient numbers of vaginal breech deliveries to adequately teach this procedure (2).

Recently, researchers conducted a large, international multicenter randomized clinical trial comparing a policy of planned cesarean birth with planned vaginal birth (3). These investigators noted that perinatal mortality, neonatal mortality, and serious neonatal morbidity were significantly lower among the planned cesarean group compared with planned vaginal birth group (17/1039 [1.6%] versus 52/1039 [5.0%]) while there was no difference in maternal morbidity or mortality observed between the groups (3). The benefits of planned cesarean delivery remained after correcting for numerous potential confounding factors, including birth weight, gestational age at delivery, and maternal parity, as well as the potential effect modifier of the experience of the physician. Most concerning was their finding that the reduction

Requests for authorization to make photocopies should be directed to:

Copyright Clearance Center
222 Rosewood Drive
Danvers, MA 01923
(978) 750-8400

ISSN 1074-861X

The American College of Obstetricians and Gynecologists
409 12th Street, SW
PO Box 96920
Washington, DC 20090-6920

12345/54321

Mode of term singleton breech delivery. Committee Opinion No. 265. American College of Obstetricians and Gynecologists. Obstet Gynecol 2001;98:1189–1190 in risk attributable to planned cesarean delivery was greatest among centers in industrialized nations with low overall perinatal mortality rates (0.4% versus 5.7%). Among such settings, typical of current practice in the United States, a policy of planned cesarean birth for breech presentation would result in seven cesarean births to avoid one infant death or serious morbidity. These data are consistent with previously reported increases in poor obstetric outcomes in vaginal breech deliveries (4).

Given the results of this exceptionally large and well-controlled clinical trial, the American College of Obstetricians and Gynecologists Committee on Obstetric Practice recommends that obstetricians continue their efforts to reduce breech presentations in singleton gestations through the application of external cephalic version whenever possible. The success rate for versions ranges from 35% to 86% in the literature with an average of 58% (5,6). As a result of the findings of the study, planned vaginal delivery of a singleton term breech may no longer be appropriate. In those instances in which breech vaginal deliveries are pursued, great caution should be exercised. Patients with a persistent breech presentation at term in a singleton gestation should undergo a planned cesarean delivery. If the patient refuses a planned cesarean delivery, informed consent should be obtained and should be documented. A planned cesarean delivery does not apply to patients presenting with advanced labor and likely to have an imminent delivery of a fetus in a breech presentation or to patients whose second twin is in a nonvertex presentation.

References

1. Ventura SJ, Martin JA, Curtin SC, Menacker F, Hamilton BE. Births: final data for 1999. Natl Vital Stat Rep 2001;49(1):1–100
2. Lavin JP Jr, Eaton J, Hopkins M. Teaching vaginal breech delivery and external cephalic version. A survey of faculty attitudes. J Reprod Med 2000;45:808–812
3. Hannah ME, Hannah WJ, Hewson SA, Hodnett ED, Saigal S, Willan AR. Planned caesarean section versus planned vaginal birth for breech presentation at term: a randomised multicentre trial. Term Breech Trial Collaborative Group. Lancet 2000;356:1375–1383
4. Gifford DS, Morton SC, Fiske M, Kahn K. A meta-analysis of infant outcomes after breech delivery. Obstet Gynecol 1995;85:1047–1054
5. Van Veelen AJ, Van Cappellen AW, Flu PK, Straub MJ, Wallenburg HC. Effect of external cephalic version in late pregnancy on presentation at delivery: a randomized controlled trial. Br J Obstet Gynaecol 1989;96:916–921
6. Mahomed K, Seeras R, Coulson R. External cephalic version at term. A randomized controlled trial using tocolysis. Br J Obstet Gynaecol 1991;98:8–13

Recommended Reading

Cheng M, Hannah M. Breech delivery at term: a critical review of the literature. Obstet Gynecol 1993;82:605–618

The Canadian consensus on breech management at term. SOGC Policy Statement. Society of Obstetricians and Gynaecologists of Canada. J SOGC 1994;16:1839–1848

ACOG

Committee on
Obstetric Practice

Committee Opinion

Number 283, May 2003

The American College of Obstetricians and Gynecologists
409 12th Street, SW
PO Box 96920
Washington, DC 20090-6920

12345/76543

New U.S. Food and Drug Administration labeling on Cytotec (misoprostol) use and pregnancy. ACOG Committee Opinion No. 283. American College of Obstetricians and Gynecologists. Obstet Gynecol 2003;101:1049–50.

New U.S. Food and Drug Administration Labeling on Cytotec (Misoprostol) Use and Pregnancy

ABSTRACT: On April 17, 2002, the U.S. Food and Drug Administration approved a new label for the use of Cytotec (misoprostol) during pregnancy. The new labeling does not contain claims regarding the efficacy and/or safety of Cytotec when it is used for cervical ripening for the induction of labor nor does it stipulate doses or dosing intervals. Therefore, the Committee on Obstetric Practice reminds Fellows that this agent should be used as previously recommended.

On April 17, 2002, the U.S. Food and Drug Administration (FDA) approved a new label for the use of Cytotec (misoprostol) during pregnancy. The FDA describes the major labeling changes and their rationale as follows (see also the FDA's web site at www.fda.gov/medwatch/safety/2002/safety02.htm#cytote). The new labeling:

- Revises the contraindication and precaution that Cytotec should not be used in women who are pregnant by stating that the contraindication is for pregnant women who are using Cytotec to reduce the risk of nonsteroidal antiinflammatory drug (NSAID)-induced stomach ulcers.
  - *Rationale* — The drug has a recognized use by ob-gyns to induce labor, delivery, and is part of the FDA-approved regimen for use with mifepristone to induce abortion in pregnancies of 49 days or less. The contraindication now refers to the drug's approved indication, for reducing the risk of NSAID-induced gastric ulcers.

- Creates a new labor and delivery section of the labeling and provides safety information related to those uses.
  - *Rationale* — 21 CFR 201.57(f)(7) requires labeling to include drug-effect information if a drug has a recognized use during labor or delivery, whether or not the use is stated in the indications section of the labeling.

- Provides new information that uterine rupture, an adverse event reported with Cytotec, is associated with risk factors such as later trimester pregnancies, higher doses of the drug, including the manufactured 100-mcg tablets, prior cesarean delivery or uterine surgery, and having had five or more previous pregnancies.

— *Rationale* —Risk factors allow physicians to identify patients who may be at greater risk for these adverse events. This information may guide safer use of the drug.

The new labeling does not contain claims regarding the efficacy and/or safety of Cytotec when it is used for cervical ripening for the induction of labor nor does it stipulate doses or dosing intervals. Therefore, the Committee on Obstetric Practice reminds Fellows that this agent should be used as previously recommended (see box) (1–3).

Recommended Uses of Cytotec

- If misoprostol is to be used for cervical ripening or labor induction in the third trimester, one quarter of a 100-µg tablet (ie, approximately 25 µg) should be considered for the initial dose. The use of higher doses (50 µg every 6 hours) may be appropriate in some situations, although increasing the dose appears to be associated with uterine tachysystole and possibly with uterine hyperstimulation and meconium staining of amniotic fluid.

- Doses should not be administered more frequently than every 3–6 hours.

- Oxytocin should not be administered less than 4 hours after the last misoprostol dose.

- Patients undergoing cervical ripening or labor induction with misoprostol for labor induction should undergo fetal heart rate and uterine activity monitoring in a hospital setting.

- Misoprostol should not be used for cervical ripening for the induction of labor in patients with a previous cesarean delivery or prior major uterine surgery.

References

1. American College of Obstetricians and Gynecologists. Induction of labor with misoprostol. ACOG Committee Opinion 228. Washington, DC: ACOG; 1999.
2. American College of Obstetricians and Gynecologists. Response to Searle's drug warning on misoprostol. ACOG Committee Opinion 248. Washington, DC: ACOG; 2000.
3. American College of Obstetricians and Gynecologists. Induction of labor. ACOG Practice Bulletin 10. Washington, DC: ACOG; 1999.

ACOG

Committee on
Genetics

Committee Opinion

Number 287, October 2003

Newborn Screening

ABSTRACT: Newborn screening programs have enormous public health benefits and have been effective in identifying newborns who can benefit from early treatment. Because of advances in genetics and technology, newborn screening programs are capable of testing for more than 30 disorders, including infections, genetic diseases, and inherited and metabolic disorders. Many important issues surround the debate on universal screening, including financial resources, level of screening, continuity of care, and informed consent. To date, policy on newborn screening has been fragmented; however, efforts are underway to ensure uniformity and equity for all newborns. Obstetrician–gynecologists can continue to work to improve the health of their patients by informing expectant families of the newborn screening process.

ISSN 1074-861X

The American College of Obstetricians and Gynecologists
409 12th Street, SW
PO Box 96920
Washington, DC 20090-6920

12345/76543

Newborn screening. ACOG Committee Opinion No. 287. American College of Obstetricians and Gynecologists. Obstet Gynecol 2003;102:887–9.

Newborn screening is a public health issue that has moved into the spotlight because of advances in genetic medicine. Although newborn screening tests are designed to detect infants with specific metabolic disorders who would benefit from early diagnosis and treatment, they also may identify couples who are carriers of disorders. Because of advances in genetics and technology, newborn screening programs are capable of testing for more than 30 disorders, including infections, genetic diseases, and inherited and metabolic disorders. Yet, many program and policy issues that surround state-based newborn screening programs remain controversial. Because newborn screening programs vary by state, obstetricians need to be aware of the status of newborn screening in their states and should be prepared to address questions or refer their patients to appropriate sources for additional information.

Dr. Robert Guthrie pioneered newborn screening in the early 1960s. His efforts were aimed at preventing mental retardation by screening for phenylketonuria (PKU) and instituting dietary changes for affected newborns. The blood specimen for the Guthrie test is collected on a piece of filter paper that soaks up a few drops of blood from a newborn's heel after it has been stuck with a lancet. The ideal period for specimen collection is 2–5 days after birth. However, most infants are tested at 24–48 hours of life just before they are discharged from the hospital. For many conditions, the test should be performed after the newborn has been fed but before blood transfusions are given. Specimens are sent to a laboratory to be analyzed by a bacterial inhibition assay, electrophoresis, high-pressure liquid chromatography, or newer technologies, such as tandem mass spectrometry. The hospital of birth, the pediatrician, or both are notified of any positive test results.

Newborn screening programs are designed for maximal sensitivity and specificity; the false-negative rate must be kept at an absolute minimum so that no cases will be missed. However, this results in significant false-positive rates. Therefore, confirmatory testing is essential. A false-positive test result can cause parental anxiety. Counseling by the obstetric provider can be of great value. Prenatal education about newborn screening not only provides parents with an understanding of the reasons for obtaining their newborn's blood specimen, but also informs them that an initial positive test result does not necessarily mean that their child will be affected.

Newborn screening is mandated by state statute or regulation and does not require written parental consent in most states; Maryland and Wyoming require written consent. Many states allow parents to refuse testing based on religious or personal grounds. Hospitals and newborn nurseries usually provide written materials to parents immediately postpartum to inform them of the newborn screening their children will undergo. Many patients will turn to their obstetricians for additional information regarding newborn testing and may ask why their newborns have a bandage on their heels.

Newborn screening programs have expanded in some states to include testing for congenital hypothyroidism, hemoglobinopathies, galactosemia, biotinidase deficiency, congenital adrenal hyperplasia, maple syrup urine disease, medium chain acyl-CoA dehydrogenase deficiency, human immunodeficiency virus (HIV), and toxoplasmosis. Currently, debate continues about which tests should be part of the newborn screening panel. There is no constitutional or federal mandate for newborn screening. Therefore, laws and policies regarding newborn screening are individually determined by each state. Each state program must have a system in place to notify the pediatrician, the parents, or both of the need for follow-up and treatment at a center equipped to care for an infant who receives a positive test result for a metabolic, hematologic, endocrine, infectious, or other congenital disorder.

Phenylketonuria and congenital hypothyroidism are the only tests that are performed in all 50 states and the District of Columbia. Forty-nine states screen for galactosemia, and all states screen at least selected populations for hemoglobinopathies, such as sickle cell disease. Some states screen for infec-

tious diseases, such as HIV and toxoplasmosis, and inherited disorders, such as cystic fibrosis. All states have started to perform newborn hearing screening to identify infants with congenital moderate to profound hearing loss using noninvasive techniques called evoked otoacoustic emissions and auditory brainstem response. The current panel of tests in each state can be viewed at http://genes-r-us.uthscsa.edu/resources/newborn/screenstatus.htm.

The fee charged by state programs for each infant screened is variable and in 2002 ranged from $10 to $60. Some states use public funds for their newborn screening programs and do not bill individuals for newborn screening tests. Commercial laboratories have started to offer additional newborn screening tests to the public. Patients who are considering the expanded newborn screen should discuss the testing with their pediatrician and obtain a kit from the laboratories offering this service before delivery. It is important for parents to recognize that most of these additional disorders are relatively infrequent and many cannot be treated. However, they can occur in families without a positive family history, and early diagnosis and treatment for some of these disorders may prevent serious complications.

A state's financial resources often determine the level of newborn screening (eg, how many conditions for which they can test). The state must consider not only the cost of the test itself but also their financial capacity to provide subspecialty follow-up, services, and treatment. Many state public health agencies report inadequate financial resources to expand programs. This has led to inequity in access to care for newborns across state lines. In response to calls for a universal newborn screening program, the American Academy of Pediatrics (AAP) convened a national Task Force on Newborn Screening in May 1999, cosponsored by the Maternal and Child Health Bureau of the Health Resources and Services Administration. The American Academy of Pediatrics called for participation by both federal and state governments. It recommends that the federal government, acting through its established health care agencies, such as the Health Resources and Services Administration, the National Institutes of Health, and the Centers for Disease Control and Prevention, develop guidelines, standards, and policies for newborn screening and take a leadership role in bringing this information to states. The AAP report *Serving the Family from Birth to the Medical Home* "highlights the need for a more uniform national policy for the selection of newborn screening tests." According to *The Importance of Newborn Screening*, the March of Dimes also has advocated for newborn screening that is "universally available and… uniform quality." The March of Dimes has issued guidelines for a minimum core panel of 10 screening tests that should be included on each state's newborn screening panel. The core panel includes tests for PKU, congenital hypothyroidism, congenital adrenal hyperplasia, biotinidase deficiency, maple syrup urine disease, galactosemia, medium chain acyl-CoA dehydrogenase deficiency, homocystinuria, sickle cell anemia, and hearing loss.

Emerging Technology

Tandem mass spectrometry recently has been added to the methods of newborn screening. This technology enables the testing of a single blood spot for many metabolites, including amino acids, organic acids, and fatty acids. Tandem mass spectrometry allows rapid testing for multiple diseases with high sensitivity and specificity without adding much to the cost of newborn screening. However, for some of these diseases, there are no effective treatments at this time. In addition, adding more diseases to screening panels will increase the need for follow-up services.

It is now feasible to store the blood spots obtained for newborn screening. However, this raises many ethical issues about personal privacy. The medical, ethics, and legal communities as well as the public and legislative representatives continue to grapple with this issue of privacy, including employment and insurance eligibility based on genetic information.

Conclusion

Newborn screening programs have enormous public health benefits and have been effective in identifying newborns who can benefit from early treatment. In addition, many couples have been made aware of their carrier status because of diagnoses in their newborns. There are many important issues surrounding the debate on universal screening, including financial resources, level of screening, continuity of care, and informed consent. To date, policy on newborn screening has been fragmented, but efforts are underway to ensure uniformity and equity for all newborns. Obstetrician–gynecologists can continue to work to improve the health of their patients by informing expectant families of the newborn screening process.

Bibliography

Hiller EH, Landenburger G, Natowicz MR. Public participation in medical policy-making and the status of consumer autonomy: the example of newborn-screening programs in the United States. Am J Public Health 1997;87:1280–8.

Howse JL, Katz M. The importance of newborn screening. Pediatrics 2000;106:595.

Kwon C, Farrell PM. The magnitude and challenge of false-positive newborn screening test results. Arch Pediatr Adolesc Med 2000;154:714–8.

Larsson A, Therrell B. Newborn screening: the role of the obstetrician. Clin Obstet Gynecol 2002;45:697–710; discussion 730–2.

National Newborn Screening and Genetics Resource Center. National Newborn Screening Report—2000. Austin (TX): NNSGRC; 2003.

Piper MA, Lindenmayer JM, Lengerich EJ, Pass KA, Brown WG, Crowder WB, et al. The role of state public health agencies in genetics and disease prevention: results of a national survey. Public Health Rep 2001;116:22–31.

Serving the family from birth to the medical home. Newborn screening: a blueprint for the future—a call for a national agenda on state newborn screening programs. Pediatrics 2000;106: 389–422.

Tandem mass spectrometry in newborn screening. American College of Medical Genetics/American Society of Human Genetics Test and Technology Transfer Committee Working Group. Genet Med 2000;2:267–9.

ACOG

Committee on Gynecologic Practice

Committee Opinion

Number 253, March 2001

(Replaces Statement of Policy on Liposuction, January 1988)

Nongynecologic Procedures

Cosmetic procedures (such as laser hair removal, body piercing, tattoo removal, and liposuction) are not considered gynecologic procedures and, therefore, generally are not taught in approved obstetric and gynecologic residencies. Because these are not considered gynecologic procedures, it is inappropriate for the College to establish guidelines for training. As with other surgical procedures, credentialing for cosmetic procedures should be based on education, training, experience, and demonstrated competence.

This document reflects emerging clinical and scientific advances as of the date issued and is subject to change. The information should not be construed as dictating an exclusive course of treatment or procedure to be followed.

ISSN 1074-861X

The American College of Obstetricians and Gynecologists
409 12th Street, SW
PO Box 96920
Washington, DC 20090-6920

12345/54321

ACOG

Committee on
Ethics

Committee Opinion

Number 297, August 2004

Nonmedical Use of Obstetric Ultrasonography

ABSTRACT: The American College of Obstetricians and Gynecologists (ACOG) has endorsed the "Prudent Use" statement from the American Institute of Ultrasound in Medicine (AIUM) discouraging the use of obstetric ultrasonography for nonmedical purposes (eg, solely to create keepsake photographs or videos). The ACOG Committee on Ethics provides reasons in addition to those offered by AIUM for discouraging this practice.

The American College of Obstetricians and Gynecologists (ACOG) has endorsed the following statement from the American Institute of Ultrasound in Medicine (AIUM) discouraging the use of obstetric ultrasonography for nonmedical purposes (eg, solely to create keepsake photographs or videos) (1):

> The AIUM advocates the responsible use of diagnostic ultrasound. The AIUM strongly discourages the non-medical use of ultrasound for psychosocial or entertainment purposes. The use of either two-dimensional (2D) or three-dimensional (3D) ultrasound to only view the fetus, obtain a picture of the fetus or determine the fetal gender without a medical indication is inappropriate and contrary to responsible medical practice. Although there are no confirmed biological effects on patients caused by exposures from present diagnostic ultrasound instruments, the possibility exists that such biological effects may be identified in the future. Thus ultrasound should be used in a prudent manner to provide medical benefit to the patient.

In addition to the concerns noted by AIUM, the ACOG Committee on Ethics believes that nonmedical use of ultrasonography should be discouraged for the following reasons:

- Nonmedical ultrasonography may falsely reassure women. Even though centers that perform nonmedical ultrasonography and create keepsake photographs and videos of the fetus may offer disclaimers about the limitations of their product, customers may interpret an aesthetically pleasing image or entertaining video as evidence of fetal health and appropriate development. Ultrasonography performed for psychosocial or entertainment purposes may be limited by the extent and duration of the examination, the training of those acquiring the images, and the quality control in place at the ultrasound facility. Women may incorrectly believe that the limited scan is, in fact, diagnostic.

Requests for authorization to make photocopies should be directed to:

Copyright Clearance Center
222 Rosewood Drive
Danvers, MA 01923
(978) 750-8400

ISSN 1074-861X

The American College of Obstetricians and Gynecologists
409 12th Street, SW
PO Box 96920
Washington, DC 20090-6920

12345/87654

Nonmedical use of obstetric ultrasonography. ACOG Committee Opinion No. 297. American College of Obstetricians and Gynecologists. Obstet Gynecol 2004;104:423–4.

- Abnormalities may be detected in settings that are not prepared to discuss and provide follow-up for concerning findings. Without the ready availability of appropriate prenatal health care professionals, customers at sites for nonmedical ultrasonography may be left without necessary support, information, and follow-up for concerning findings. For example, customers may interpret a minor finding (eg, an echogenic intracardiac focus) as a major abnormality, resulting in unnecessary anxiety and concern. Conversely, in the event of concerning findings (eg, oligohydramnios), women may not receive appropriate follow-up. Obstetric ultrasonography is most appropriately obtained as part of an integrated system for delivering prenatal care.

Reference

1. American Institute of Ultrasound in Medicine. Prudent use. AIUM Official Statements. Laurel (MD): AIUM; 1999. Available at http://www.aium.org/provider/statements/_statementSelected.asp?statement=2. Retrieved May 19, 2004.

ACOG

Committee on
Obstetric Practice

Committee Opinion

Number 284, August 2003

Nonobstetric Surgery in Pregnancy

ABSTRACT: Although there are no data to support specific recommendations regarding nonobstetric surgery and anesthesia in pregnancy, it is important for nonobstetric physicians to obtain obstetric consultation before performing nonobstetric surgery. The decision to use fetal monitoring should be individualized, and each case warrants a team approach for optimal safety of the woman and her baby.

The American College of Obstetricians and Gynecologists' Committee on Obstetric Practice acknowledges that the issue of nonobstetric surgery and anesthesia in pregnancy is an important concern for physicians who care for women; however, there are no data to allow us to make specific recommendations. It is important for physicians to obtain obstetric consultation before performing nonobstetric surgery because obstetricians are uniquely qualified to discuss aspects of maternal physiology and anatomy that may affect intraoperative maternal–fetal well-being. The decision to use fetal monitoring should be individualized, and, if used, may be based on gestational age, type of surgery, and facilities available. Ultimately, each case warrants a team approach (anesthesia, obstetrics, surgery) for optimal safety of the woman and her baby.

ISSN 1074-861X

The American College of Obstetricians and Gynecologists
409 12th Street, SW
PO Box 96920
Washington, DC 20090-6920

12345/76543

Nonobstetric surgery in pregnancy. ACOG Committee Opinion No. 284. American College of Obstetricians and Gynecologists. Obstet Gynecol 2003;102:431.

ACOG

Committee on
Adolescent Health Care

Committee Opinion

Number 274, July 2002

Nonsurgical Diagnosis and Management of Vaginal Agenesis

ABSTRACT: Vaginal agenesis occurs once in every 4,000–10,000 females. The most common cause of vaginal agenesis is congenital absence of the uterus and vagina, which is also referred to as müllerian aplasia, müllerian agenesis, or Mayer–Rokitansky–Küster–Hauser syndrome. The condition usually can be managed nonsurgically with the use of successive dilators if it is correctly diagnosed and the patient is sufficiently motivated. Besides correct diagnosis, effective management also includes evaluation for associated congenital, renal, or other anomalies and careful psychologic preparation of the patient before any treatment or intervention. If surgery is preferred, a number of approaches are available; the most common is the Abbe-McIndoe operation.

Vaginal agenesis is an uncommon, but not rare, condition. Given an incidence ranging from 1 per 4,000 to 1 per 10,000 females (1), vaginal agenesis is a condition that general gynecologists will encounter once or twice during their professional careers. The most common etiology of vaginal agenesis is congenital absence of the uterus and vagina, which also is referred to as müllerian aplasia, müllerian agenesis, or Mayer–Rokitansky–Küster–Hauser syndrome. The term *müllerian aplasia* will be used to describe this congenital reproductive anomaly throughout this document. Müllerian aplasia is caused by embryologic failure of the müllerian duct with resultant anomalies in the müllerian structures. The ovaries, given their separate embryologic source, are normal in structure and function.

To manage vaginal agenesis effectively in young women, correct diagnosis of the underlying condition is important. Evaluation for associated congenital, renal, or other anomalies also is essential. Both diagnosis and evaluation usually can be completed without surgery. Careful patient counseling should be provided before any treatment or intervention. Nonsurgical creation of the neovagina should be the first-line approach. These recommendations, as well as surgical approaches for use in the rare situations when nonsurgical approaches are unsuccessful, are discussed.

The American College of Obstetricians and Gynecologists
409 12th Street, SW
PO Box 96920
Washington, DC 20090-6920

12345/65432

Nonsurgical diagnosis and management of vaginal agenesis. Committee Opinion No. 274. American College of Obstetricians and Gynecologists. Obstet Gynecol 2002;100:213–216

Differential Diagnosis

Patients with müllerian aplasia have a normal 46,XX karyotype, normal female phenotype, and normal ovarian hormonal and oocyte function. Puberty and development of secondary sexual characteristics progress normally except that menarche does not occur. Therefore, patients with müllerian aplasia typically present in adolescence with primary amenorrhea. Müllerian aplasia is the second most common etiology of primary amenorrhea, next to gonadal dysgenesis (2).

On physical examination, patients with müllerian aplasia have normal breast development, normal secondary sexual body proportions, body hair, and hymenal tissue. A vagina is absent unless it has been created by sexual encounters. Differential diagnosis of vaginal agenesis includes congenital absence of the uterus and vagina, androgen insensitivity (absence or alteration of androgen-receptor function), a low-lying transverse vaginal septum, and imperforate hymen.

In androgen insensitivity, the gonads are testes producing normal androgens in karyotypic 46,XY individuals. The lack of androgen tissue receptor results in sparse or no pubic and axillary hair. Patients with androgen insensitivity typically have normal breast development at puberty due to peripheral conversion of circulating androgens to estrogen; however, no internal female organs exist. In pubertal females, the differential diagnosis between androgen insensitivity and müllerian aplasia is easily made by assessing serum testosterone levels. A testosterone level in the pubertal male range confirms the diagnosis of androgen insensitivity.

In postpubertal patients, the presence of functioning ovarian tissue seen on pelvic ultrasound examination may serve as a secondary confirmation of the diagnosis of müllerian aplasia, excluding the diagnosis of androgen insensitivity. Chromosomal studies, which are significantly more costly than ultrasonography, are required only in prepubertal children who do not yet produce gonadal steroids.

The differential diagnosis of vaginal agenesis also includes the diagnosis of imperforate hymen and transverse vaginal septum. Patients with these latter conditions will have a normal cervix and fundus, both of which are palpable on rectal examination. In contrast to most patients with müllerian aplasia, the patient with an imperforate hymen will not have the typical fringe of hymenal tissue. The patient with a low transverse vaginal septum will have a normal hymen, like the patient with müllerian aplasia. Ultrasonography can be used to define the müllerian structures in cases where palpation is unrevealing.

Correct diagnosis of the underlying condition affecting the genital anatomy is crucial before any surgical intervention. If the patient is operated on for an incorrect diagnosis, it can be extremely difficult to create a vagina without surgery because of scar tissue.

Evaluation of the Patient with Müllerian Aplasia

Most patients with müllerian aplasia have small rudimentary müllerian bulbs without any endometrial activity. In 2–7% of patients with müllerian aplasia, active endometrium is found in these uterine structures (1). These patients will present with cyclic abdominal pain. Magnetic resonance imaging has been suggested to assess the internal genitalia, although it is rarely needed in the initial evaluation unless ultrasound evaluation for the presence of functional endometrium in a müllerian structure is equivocal (3). Although laparoscopy is not necessary to diagnose müllerian aplasia, it may be useful in the evaluation of patients with cyclic abdominal pain to exclude the possibility of endometrial activity in müllerian structures (4).

Patients with müllerian aplasia often have concomitant congenital malformations, especially of the urinary tract and skeleton, and should be evaluated for these anomalies. Ultrasonography can be used to screen for the more common findings of renal agenesis or a pelvic kidney. This evaluation can be performed during the study of ovarian and müllerian structures. The implications of ureteral duplication in the case of later abdominal or pelvic surgery can be discussed or intravenous pyelography can be used to exclude this possibility.

After the diagnosis of müllerian aplasia, the adolescent should be offered psychologic support to help her adjust. Counseling should emphasize that a normal sex life will be possible after a neovagina has been created. Ultimately, however, infertility will be the most difficult aspect of this disorder for the patient to accept. Discussion of assisted reproductive techniques and use of surrogacy is appropriate. Specifically, it is important to explain that eggs can be harvested from patients with müllerian aplasia. This allows young teens to understand their reproductive potential for becoming a biologic parent and may help them accept the diagnosis and its implications. Referral to a mental health professional may be necessary for some patients.

The best predictor of good emotional outcome after diagnosis and vaginoplasty is a good relationship between the patient and her parents and the ability to show feelings with family and friends (5). Contact with a support group or young women with the same diagnosis may be helpful (4). (More information is available at http://www.mrkh.org.)

Patients should be given a brief, written medical summary of their condition, including a summary of concomitant malformations. This information may be useful if the patient requires urgent medical care or emergency surgery from a provider unfamiliar with müllerian aplasia.

Nonsurgical Creation of a Neovagina

Timing for nonsurgical or surgical creation of a neovagina is elective; however, it is best planned when the patient is emotionally mature. Nonsurgical creation of the vagina is the appropriate first-line approach in the majority of patients because it is the least morbid procedure. In a recently reported series of patients with müllerian aplasia, more than 90% were able to achieve anatomic and functional success by vaginal dilation (6).

Patients are asked to place successive dilators on the perineal dimple for 30 minutes–2 hours a day. Sitting on a race bicycle seat stool provides the perineal pressure and allows the patient to participate in simultaneous productive activities, such as doing homework or practicing a musical instrument (7). If sitting on the bicycle seat stool is too uncomfortable, the patient may have better success using dilators while reclining on a bed after a bath while still wet from bathing. Use of dilators in the management of vaginal agenesis is appropriate and successful in the majority of patients. Mature, highly motivated patients who wish to avoid surgery and are aware that it will take several months to achieve their goal are likely to be successful (7, 8). Because the nonoperative approach is noninvasive and often successful, it is strongly recommended as first-line therapy.

Clinicians often use "buddies," other patients with vaginal agenesis who have successfully dilated, as support to the young woman attempting dilation. Young married patients make excellent buddies. If fertility issues are a major concern to the patient or her family, it may be helpful to find a buddy who has used assisted reproductive techniques to become a mother.

Surgical Creation of a Neovagina

Surgery becomes an option in patients unsuccessful with dilators or if the patient prefers surgery after a thorough discussion of the risks and benefits of the procedure and the available nonsurgical alternatives. The aim of surgery is the creation of a vaginal canal in the correct axis of adequate size and secretory capacity to allow intercourse to occur without the need for continued postoperative dilation. The timing of the surgery depends on the patient and the type or procedure planned. Surgeries often are performed in late adolescence when the patient is more mature and better able to comply with postoperative dilation or instructions. Surgery usually is scheduled during summer vacation to allow for an adequate recovery time without missing school while limiting questions from peers (4, 9).

A number of operations are appropriate for the correction of vaginal agenesis. The approach usually is based on the experience of the operating surgeon. Pediatric surgeons are more likely to use bowel segments for the creation of a neovagina; gynecologists are more likely to use a perineal approach. Whatever technique is chosen, the surgeon must be experienced with the procedure, because the initial surgery is more likely to succeed than are follow-up procedures. Reoperation in these cases increases the chance of operative injury to surrounding tissues and the possibility of a poor functional outcome. At present, there is no consensus in the literature regarding the best option for surgical correction (10).

The most commonly used surgical procedure employed by U.S. gynecologists to create a neovagina is the Abbe-McIndoe operation. This involves the dissection of a space between the rectum and bladder, placement of a mold covered with a split thickness skin graft into the space, and the diligent use of vaginal dilation postoperatively. Postoperative dilation must be continued to prevent significant skin graft contracture. This surgery is inappropriate if the patient rejects the nonsurgical technique because she has concerns about or objections to dilation. If postoperative dilation is not done, the patient will have a nonfunctional vagina.

Newer procedures for the creation of the neovagina are the Vecchietti procedure and laparoscopic modifications of operations previously performed by laparotomy. The Vecchietti procedure involves the creation of a neovagina via dilation with a traction device attached to the abdomen, sutures placed subperitoneally via laparotomy, and a plastic "olive" placed on the vaginal dimple. In the laparoscopic modification, traction sutures are placed laparoscopically. The two techniques are comparable in terms of producing a functional neovagina (11).

Davydov developed a three-stage operation involving dissection of the rectovesical space with abdominal mobilization of the peritoneum with creation of the vaginal fornices and attachment of the peritoneum to the introitus. The newer adaptation involves dissection of the rectovaginal space, with mobilization of the peritoneum from below and laparoscopic assistance from above. This is followed by closure of the abdominal end of the neovagina with a laparoscopically placed pursestring suture (12–14).

Summary

The most important steps in the effective management of vaginal agenesis are correct diagnosis of the underlying condition; evaluation for associated congenital, renal, or other anomalies; and careful psychologic preparation of the patient before any treatment or intervention. If any of these are neglected, the success of the intervention will be compromised.

Laparoscopy is seldom required to make the diagnosis, but may be appropriate in the rare patient presenting with cyclic pelvic pain. Nonsurgical creation of the neovagina should be the first-line approach. In cases where surgical intervention is required, referrals to centers with expertise in this area should be considered. Few surgeons have extensive experience in construction of the neovagina, and the initial surgery has the greatest chance for success. In addition, experts at these centers may be more successful in promoting the nonsurgical approach, given their experience.

References

1. Evans TN, Poland ML, Boving RL. Vaginal malformations. Am J Obstet Gynecol 1981;141:910–920
2. Reindollar RH, Byrd JR, McDonough PG. Delayed sexual development: a study of 252 patients. Am J Obstet Gynecol 1981;140:371–380
3. Fedele L, Dorta M, Brioschi D, Giudici MN, Candiani GB. Magnetic resonance imaging in Mayer-Rokitansky-Kuster-Hauser syndrome. Obstet Gynecol 1990;76:593–596
4. Laufer MR, Goldstein DP. Structural abnormalities of the female reproductive tract. In: Emans SJ, Laufer MR, Goldstein DP, eds. Pediatric and adolescent gynecology. 4th ed. Philadelphia: Lippincott–Raven, 1998:303–362
5. Poland ML, Evans TN. Psychological aspects of vaginal agenesis. J Reprod Med 1985;30:340–344
6. Roberts CP, Haber MJ, Rock JA. Vaginal creation for mullerian agenesis. Am J Obstet Gynecol 2001;185:1349–1352; discussion 1352–1353
7. Williams JK, Lake M, Ingram JM. The bicycle seat stool in the treatment of vaginal agenesis and stenosis. J Obstet Gynecol Neonatal Nurs 1985;14:147–150
8. Rock JA, Reeves LA, Retto H, Baramki TA, Zacur HA, Jones HW Jr. Success following vaginal creation for Mullerian agenesis. Fertil Steril 1983;39:809–813
9. Templeman CL, Lam AM, Hertweck SP. Surgical management of vaginal agenesis. Obstet Gynecol Surv 1999;54:583–591
10. Templeman C, Hertweck SP. Vaginal agenesis: an opinion on the surgical management. J Pediatr Adolesc Gynecol 2000;13:143–144
11. Borruto F, Chasen ST, Chervenak FA, Fedele L. The Vecchietti procedure for surgical treatment of vaginal agenesis: comparison of laparoscopy and laparotomy. Int J Gynaecol Obstet 1999;64:153–158
12. Davydov SN. Colpopoiesis from the peritoneum of the uretorectal space. Obstet Gynecol (Moscow) 1969;12:55–57
13. Adamyan LV. Laparoscopic management of vaginal aplasia with or without functional noncommunicating rudimentary uterus. In: Arregui ME, Fitzgibbons RJ, Katkhouda N, McKernan JB, Reich H, eds. Principles of laparoscopic surgery: basic and advanced techniques. New York: Springer–Verlag, 1995:646–651
14. Adamyan LV. Therapeutic and endoscopic perspectives. In: Nichols DH, Clarke-Pearson DL, eds. Gynecologic, obstetric, and related surgery. 2nd ed. St. Louis: Mosby, 2000:1209–1217

ACOG

Committee on
Obstetric Practice

Committee Opinion

Number 315, September 2005

Obesity in Pregnancy

ABSTRACT: *One third of adult women in the United States are obese. During pregnancy, obese women are at increased risk for several adverse perinatal outcomes, including anesthetic, perioperative, and other maternal and fetal complications. Obstetricians should provide preconception counseling and education about the possible complications and should encourage obese patients to undertake a weight reduction program before attempting pregnancy. Obstetricians also should address prenatal and peripartum care considerations that may be especially relevant for obese patients, including those who have undergone bariatric surgery.*

The prevalence of obesity in the United States has increased dramatically over the past 20 years. The World Health Organization and the National Institutes of Health define *normal weight* as a body mass index (BMI) of 18.5–24.9, *overweight* as a BMI of 25–29.9, and *obesity* as a BMI of 30 or greater. Obesity is further categorized by BMI into Class I (30–34.9), Class II (35–39.9), and Class III or extreme obesity ($\geq$40) (1, 2). (For online BMI calculator, see www.nhlbisupport.com/bmi.) The most recent National Health and Nutrition Examination Survey (NHANES) for 1999–2002 found that approximately one third of adult women are obese (3). This problem is greatest among non-Hispanic black women (49%) compared with Mexican-American women (38%) and non-Hispanic white women (31%) (3).

Obese women are at increased risk for several pregnancy complications; therefore, preconception assessment and counseling are strongly encouraged. Obstetricians should provide education about the possible complications and should encourage obese patients to undertake a weight reduction program, including diet, exercise, and behavior modification, before attempting pregnancy. Specific medical clearance may be indicated for some patients.

At least three cohort studies suggest that obesity is an independent risk factor for spontaneous abortion among women who undergo infertility treatment (4–6). Given this association, obese women should be encouraged to lose weight before beginning infertility therapy. Data also link obesity with spontaneous abortion among women after natural conception (7).

In a prospective multicenter study of more than 16,000 patients, Class I (BMI 30–34.9) and Class II (BMI 35–39.9) obesity was associated with an increased risk of gestational hypertension (odds ratio [OR] = 2.5 and 3.2, respectively), preeclampsia (OR = 1.6 and 3.3), gestational diabetes (OR = 2.6 and 4.0), and fetal macrosomia (OR = 1.7 and 1.9), when compared with

The American College of Obstetricians and Gynecologists
409 12th Street, SW
PO Box 96920
Washington, DC 20090-6920

12345/98765

Obesity in pregnancy. ACOG Committee Opinion No. 315. American College of Obstetricians and Gynecologists. Obstet Gynecol 2005;106:671–5.

a BMI of less than 30 (8). In this same study, the cesarean delivery rate was 20.7% for women with a BMI of 29.9 or less, 33.8% for women with a BMI of 30–34.9, and 47.4% for women with a BMI of 35–39.9. Several other studies consistently report higher rates of preeclampsia, gestational diabetes, and cesarean delivery, particularly for failure to progress, in obese women than in nonobese women (9–12). Operative and postoperative complications include increased rates of excessive blood loss, operative time greater than 2 hours, wound infection, and endometritis (13–15). Surgery in obese women poses anesthetic challenges, such as difficult epidural and spinal placement requiring multiple attempts and intraoperative respiratory events from failed or difficult intubation (16). Sleep apnea occurring in this group of women may further complicate anesthetic management and postoperative care (17).

Height and weight should be recorded for all women at the initial prenatal visit to allow calculation of the BMI. Recommendations for prenatal weight gain should be made based on the Institute of Medicine (IOM) guidelines, which suggest a gain of 25–35 lb for women of normal weight, 15–25 lb for overweight women, and 15 lb for obese women (18). Nutrition consultation should be offered to all obese women, and they should be encouraged to follow an exercise program. This consultation should continue postpartum and before attempting another pregnancy. Consideration should be given to screening for gestational diabetes upon presentation or during the first trimester and repeating it later in pregnancy if the initial screening result is negative. Because these patients are at increased risk for emergent cesarean delivery and anesthetic complications, anesthesiology consultation before delivery is encouraged (19).

It is important to discuss potential intrapartum complications, such as difficulty estimating fetal weight (even with ultrasonography), inability to obtain interpretable external fetal heart rate and uterine contraction patterns, and difficulty performing an emergent cesarean delivery. If an anesthesiology consultation was not obtained antepartum, it should be conducted early in labor to allow adequate time for development of an anesthetic plan.

If obese patients require cesarean delivery, they should receive antibiotic prophylaxis even if surgery is elective (14). Obese women who require cesarean delivery are more likely to have an increased incidence of wound breakdowns and infections (20). Attempts to decrease these postoperative complications have included closure of the subcutaneous layers and the placement of subcutaneous drains.

Investigators have demonstrated that suture closure of the subcutaneous layer after cesarean delivery in obese patients may lead to a significant reduction in the incidence of postoperative wound disruption (21, 22). Postoperative placement of subcutaneous draining systems, however, have not consistently been shown to be of value in reducing postcesarean delivery morbidity (23, 24).

It has been recommended that graduated compression stockings, hydration, and early mobilization be used during and after cesarean delivery in obese patients. Postpartum heparin therapy has been recommended for patients thought to be at high risk for venous thromboembolism (25, 26); however, data are insufficient to determine whether the benefits of heparin prophylaxis in this group of patients outweigh the risks (27, 28).

Women with a BMI of 35 or greater who have preexisting medical conditions, such as hypertension or diabetes, may benefit from a cardiac evaluation (29). Because of the increased likelihood of complicated and emergent cesarean delivery, extremely obese women may require specific resources such as additional blood products, a large operating table, and extra personnel in the delivery room. Particular attention to the type and placement of the surgical incision is needed (ie, placing the incision above the panniculus adiposus) (20, 30). The success rate of attempted vaginal birth after cesarean delivery is very low in extremely obese women (31). There are additional logistical challenges to monitoring labor and performing an emergent cesarean delivery in the extremely obese patient. Therefore, these patients should be counseled about these possible complications of an emergent cesarean delivery.

The number of obese women of childbearing age considering bariatric surgery is increasing, resulting in questions about pregnancy after these types of surgeries. Early case reports and series described various pregnancy complications after bariatric surgery such as gastrointestinal bleeding (32), anemia (33), intrauterine growth restriction (34), and neural tube defects (35, 36). However, recent studies suggest that previous bariatric surgery is not associated with adverse perinatal outcomes (37, 38). Researchers have determined that pregnancies after bariatric surgery are less likely to be complicated by gestational diabetes, hypertension, macrosomia, and cesarean delivery than are pregnancies of obese women who have not had the surgery (38–40).

Bariatric surgical procedures are categorized into two main types: malabsorptive procedures (jejunoileal bypass and biliopancreatic diversion) and restrictive procedures (gastric banding and vertical banded gastroplasty). Both types of procedures can result in deficiencies in iron, vitamin B_{12}, folate, and calcium. Women who have undergone bariatric surgery require the following counseling before and during pregnancy:

- Patients with adjustable gastric banding should be advised that they are at risk of becoming pregnant unexpectedly after weight loss following surgery (39).

- All patients are advised to delay pregnancy for 12–18 months after surgery to avoid pregnancy during the rapid weight loss phase (39).

- Women with a gastric band should be monitored by their general surgeons during pregnancy because adjustment of the band may be necessary (41).

- Patients should be evaluated for nutritional deficiencies and vitamin supplementation where indicated.

In counseling all obese women about potential pregnancy complications, it is important to inform them of the fetal risks (eg, prematurity, stillbirth, neural tube defect, and macrosomia). Some studies have reported a greater rate of premature delivery for obese women than for women of normal weight (9, 42). However, in a study of more than 2,900 obese women, prepregnancy obesity was associated with a lower rate of spontaneous preterm birth (43). A large Swedish cohort study reported a greater risk of antepartum stillbirth among obese patients than among women who had a BMI of less than 20 (42). Data establish that the risk of neural tube defects among obese women is double that among women of normal weight, after correcting for diabetes as a potential confounding factor (44–46). The benefit of folic acid doses higher than 400 µg has not been studied in nondiabetic obese women. Multiple studies have shown that maternal obesity and excessive weight gain during pregnancy are associated with macrosomic and large-for-gestational-age infants (10, 19, 47, 48). Furthermore, these large-for-gestational-age infants are at increased risk for childhood obesity (11, 49). The decision to perform a primary cesarean delivery for these obese women is based on the previously recommended maternal and fetal indications. A cesarean delivery should be considered for those patients who have a fetus with a fetal weight estimated to be greater than 5,000 g if the patient does not have diabetes (50) or greater than 4,500 g if the patient has diabetes (51).

Recommendations for obese women who are pregnant or planning a pregnancy include the following:

- Preconception counseling
- Provision of specific information concerning the maternal and fetal risks of obesity in pregnancy
- Consideration of screening for gestational diabetes upon presentation or in the first trimester, and repeated screening later in pregnancy if results are initially negative
- Assessment and possible supplementation of vitamin B_{12}, folate, iron, and calcium for women who have undergone bariatric surgery
- Possible use of graduated compression stockings, hydration, and early mobilization during and after cesarean delivery
- Anesthesiology consultation
- Continuation of nutrition counseling and exercise program after delivery, and consultation with weight loss specialists before attempting another pregnancy

References

1. World Health Organization. Obesity: preventing and managing the global epidemic. Geneva, Switzerland: World Health Organization; 2000. WHO technical report series 894.
2. National Heart, Lung, and Blood Institute (NHLBI) and National Institute for Diabetes and Digestive and Kidney Diseases (NIDDK). Clinical guidelines on the identification, evaluation and treatment of overweight and obesity in adults. The evidence report. Obes Res 1998;6(suppl 2):51S–210S.
3. Hedley AA, Ogden CL, Johnson CL, Carroll MD, Curtin LR, Flegal KM. Prevalence of overweight and obesity among US children, adolescents, and adults, 1999-2002. JAMA 2004;291:2847–50.
4. Bellver J, Rossal LP, Bosch E, Zuniga A, Corona JT, Melendez F, et al. Obesity and the risk of spontaneous abortion after oocyte donation. Fertil Steril 2003;79:1136–40.
5. Fedorcsak P, Storeng R, Dale PO, Tanbo T, Abyholm T. Obesity is a risk factor for early pregnancy loss after IVF or ICSI. Acta Obstet Gynecol Scand 2000;79:43–8.
6. Wang JX, Davies MJ, Norman RJ. Obesity increases the risk of spontaneous abortion during infertility treatment. Obes Res 2002;10:551–4.
7. Lashen H, Fear K, Sturdee DW. Obesity is associated with increased risk of first trimester and recurrent miscarriage: matched case-control study. Hum Reprod 2004;19:1644–6.
8. Weiss JL, Malone FD, Emig D, Ball RH, Nyberg DA, Comstock CH, et al. Obesity, obstetric complications and cesarean delivery rate—a population-based screening

study. FASTER Research Consortium. Am J Obstet Gynecol 2004;190:1091–7.

9. Baeten JM, Bukusi EA, Lambe M. Pregnancy complications and outcomes among overweight and obese nulliparous women. Am J Public Health 2001:91:436–40.

10. Cedergren MI. Maternal morbid obesity and the risk of adverse pregnancy outcome. Obstet Gynecol 2004;103: 219–24.

11. Sebire NJ, Jolly M, Harris JP, Wadsworth J, Joffe M, Beard RW, et al. Maternal obesity and pregnancy outcome: a study of 287,213 pregnancies in London. Int J Obes Relat Metab Disord 2001;25:1175–82.

12. Young TK, Woodmansee B. Factors that are associated with cesarean delivery in a large private practice: the importance of prepregnancy body mass index and weight gain. Am J Obstet Gynecol 2002;187:312–8; discussion 318–20.

13. Kabiru W, Raynor BD. Obstetric outcomes associated with increase in BMI category during pregnancy. Am J Obstet Gynecol 2004:191:928–32.

14. Myles TD, Gooch J, Santolaya J. Obesity as an independent risk factor for infectious morbidity in patients who undergo cesarean delivery. Obstet Gynecol 2002;100: 959–64.

15. Perlow JH, Morgan MA. Massive maternal obesity and perioperative cesarean morbidity. Am J Obstet Gynecol 1994;170:560–5.

16. Hood DD, Dewan DM. Anesthetic and obstetric outcome in morbidly obese parturients. Anesthesiology 1993;79: 1210–8.

17. Maasilta P, Bachour A, Teramo K, Polo O, Laitinen LA. Sleep-related disordered breathing during pregnancy in obese women. Chest 2001;120:1448–54.

18. Institute of Medicine (US). Nutritional status and weight gain. In: Nutrition during pregnancy. Washington, DC: National Academy Press; 1990. p. 27–233.

19. Rode L, Nilas L, Wojdemann K, Tabor A. Obesity-related complications in Danish single cephalic term pregnancies. Obstet Gynecol 2005;105:537–42.

20. Wall PD, Deucy EE, Glantz JC, Pressman EK. Vertical skin incisions and wound complications in the obese parturient. Obstet Gynecol 2003;102(5 pt):952–6.

21. Cetin A, Cetin M. Superficial wound disruption after cesarean section: effect of the depth and closure of subcutaneous tissue. Int J Gynaecol Obstet 1997;57:17–21.

22. Chelmow D, Rodriguez EJ, Sabatini MM. Suture closure of subcutaneous fat and wound disruption after cesarean section: a meta-analysis. Obstet Gynecol 2004;103: 974–80.

23. Al-Inany H, Youssef G, Abd ElMaguid A, Abdel Hamid M, Naguib A. Value of subcutaneous drainage system in obese females undergoing cesarean section using Pfannenstiel incision. Gynecol Obstet Invest 2002;53: 75–8.

24. Magann EF, Chauhan SP, Rodts-Palenik S, Bufkin L, Martin JN Jr, Morrison JC. Subcutaneous stitch closure versus subcutaneous drain to prevent wound disruption after cesarean delivery: a randomized clinical trial. Am J Obstet Gynecol 2002;186:1119–23.

25. Bates SM, Greer IA, Hirsh J, Ginsberg JS. Use of antithrombotic agents during pregnancy: the Seventh ACCP Conference on Antithrombotic and Thrombolytic Therapy. Chest 2004;126:627S–44S.

26. Royal College of Obstetricians and Gynaecologists. Report of the RCOG working party on prophylaxis against thromboembolism in gynaecology and obstetrics. London: RCOG; 1995.

27. Gates S, Brocklehurst P, Davis LJ. Prophylaxis for venous thromboembolic disease in pregnancy and the early postnatal period. The Cochrane Database of Systematic Reviews 2002, Issue 2. Art. No.: CD001689. DOI: 10. 1002/14651858.CD001689.

28. Hague WM, North RA, Gallus AS, Walters BN, Orlikowski C, Burrows RF, et al. Anticoagulation in pregnancy and the puerperium. Working Group on behalf of the Obstetric Medicine Group of Australasia. Med J Aust 2001;175:258–63.

29. Tomoda S, Tamura T, Sudo Y, Ogita S. Effects of obesity on pregnant women: maternal hemodynamic change. Am J Perinatol 1996;13:73–8.

30. Houston MC, Raynor BD. Postoperative morbidity in the morbidly obese parturient woman: supraumbilical and low transverse abdominal approaches. Am J Obstet Gynecol 2000;182:1033–5.

31. Chauhan SP, Magann EF, Carroll CS, Barrilleaux PS, Scardo JA, Martin JN Jr. Mode of delivery for the morbidly obese with prior cesarean delivery: vaginal versus repeat cesarean section. Am J Obstet Gynecol 2001; 185:349–54.

32. Ramirez MM, Turrentine MA. Gastrointestinal hemorrhage during pregnancy in a patient with a history of vertical-banded gastroplasty. Am J Obstet Gynecol 1995; 173:1630–1.

33. Gurewitsch ED, Smith-Levitin M, Mack J. Pregnancy following gastric bypass surgery for morbid obesity. Obstet Gynecol 1996;88:658–61.

34. Granstrom L, Granstrom L, Backman L. Fetal growth retardation after gastric banding. Acta Obstet Gynecol Scand 1990;69:533–6.

35. Haddow JE, Hill LE, Kloza EM, Thanhauser D. Neural tube defects after gastric bypass. Lancet 1986;1:1330.

36. Martin L, Chavez GF, Adams MJ Jr, Mason EE, Hanson JW, Haddow JE, et al. Gastric bypass surgery as maternal risk factor for neural tube defects. Lancet 1988;1:640–1.

37. Marceau P, Kaufman D, Biron S, Hould FS, Lebel S, Marceau S, et al. Outcome of pregnancies after biliopancreatic diversion. Obes Surg 2004;14:318–24.

38. Sheiner E, Levy A, Silverberg D, Menes TS, Levy I, Katz M, et al. Pregnancy after bariatric surgery is not associated with adverse perinatal outcome. Am J Obstet Gynecol 2004;190:1335–40.

39. Martin LF, Finigan KM, Nolan TE. Pregnancy after adjustable gastric banding. Obstet Gynecol 2000;95: 927–30.

40. Wittgrove AC, Jester L, Wittgrove P, Clark GW. Pregnancy following gastric bypass for morbid obesity. Obes Surg 1998;8:461–4; discussion 465–6.

41. Weiss HG, Nehoda H, Labeck B, Hourmont K, Marth C, Aigner F. Pregnancies after adjustable gastric banding. Obes Surg 2001;11:303–6.

42. Cnattingius S, Bergstrom R, Lipworth L, Kramer MS. Prepregnancy weight and the risk of adverse pregnancy outcomes. N Engl J Med 1998;338:147–52.

43. Hendler I, Blackwell SC, Treadwell MC, Bujold E, Sokol RJ, Sorokin Y. Does advanced ultrasound equipment improve the adequacy of ultrasound visualization of fetal

cardiac structures in the obese gravid woman? Am J Obstet Gynecol 2004;190;1616–9; discussion 1619–20.

44. Shaw GM, Velie EM, Schaffer D. Risk of neural tube defect-affected pregnancies among obese women. JAMA 1996;275:1093–6.

45. Waller DK, Mills JL, Simpson JL, Cunningham GC, Conley MR, Lassman MR, et al. Are obese women at higher risk for producing malformed offspring? Am J Obstet Gynecol 1994;170:541–8.

46. Werler MM, Louick C, Shapiro S, Mitchell AA. Prepregnancy weight in relation to risk of neural tube defects. JAMA 1996;275:1089–92.

47. Stephansson O, Dickman PW, Johansson A, Cnattingius S. Maternal weight, pregnancy weight gain, and the risk of antepartum stillbirth. Am J Obstet Gynecol 2001; 184:463–9.

48. Watkins ML, Rasmussen SA, Honein MA, Botto LD, Moore CA. Maternal obesity and risk for birth defects. Pediatrics 2003;111:1152–8.

49. Hediger ML, Overpeck MD, McGlynn A, Kuczmarski RJ, Maurer KR, Davis WW. Growth and fatness at three to six years of age of children born small- or large-for-gestational age. Pediatrics 1999;104:e33.

50. Spellacy WN, Miller S, Winegar A, Peterson PQ. Macrosomia—maternal characteristics and infant complications. Obstet Gynecol 1985;66:158–61.

51. Lipscomb KR, Gregory K, Shaw K. The outcome of macrosomic infants weighing at least 4500 grams: Los Angeles County + University of Southern California experience. Obstet Gynecol 1995;85:558–64.

ACOG

Committee on
Obstetric Practice

Committee Opinion

Number 275, September 2002   *(Replaces No. 121, April 1993)*

ISSN 1074-861X

The American College of Obstetricians and Gynecologists
409 12th Street, SW
PO Box 96920
Washington, DC 20090-6920

12345/65432

Obstetric management of patients with spinal cord injuries. ACOG Committee Opinion No. 275. American College of Obstetricians and Gynecologists. Obstet Gynecol 2002;100:625–7.

Obstetric Management of Patients with Spinal Cord Injuries

ABSTRACT: *Effective rehabilitation and modern reproductive technology may increase the number of women considering pregnancy who have spinal cord injuries (SCIs). It is important that obstetricians caring for these patients are aware of the specific problems related to SCIs. Autonomic dysreflexia is the most significant medical complication seen in women with SCIs, and precautions should be taken to avoid stimuli that can lead to this potentially fatal syndrome. Women with SCIs may give birth vaginally, but when cesarean delivery is indicated, adequate anesthesia (spinal or epidural if possible) is needed.*

Approximately 11,000 new spinal cord injuries (SCIs) are reported per year in the United States. More than 50% occur in persons between the ages of 16 and 30 years, with women constituting approximately 18% of these cases. Effective rehabilitation and modern reproductive technology may increase the number of these patients considering pregnancy.

Ideally, women with SCIs who are considering pregnancy should have a preconceptional evaluation. Chronic medical conditions and the woman's adaptation to her disability must be evaluated. Baseline pulmonary function and renal studies may be appropriate. Also, it should be recognized that fertility in these patients usually is not affected, and family planning should be discussed.

It is important that obstetricians caring for such patients acquaint themselves with the problems related to SCIs that may occur throughout pregnancy. Common complications affecting women with SCIs include urinary tract infections, decubital ulcers, impaired pulmonary function, and autonomic dysreflexia. Additional potential complications include anemia, deep vein thrombosis, pulmonary emboli, and unattended delivery.

Common Complications

Urinary Tract Infections

Asymptomatic bacteriuria occurs in a majority of patients with SCIs during pregnancy. The incidence of lower urinary tract infections and pyelonephritis also is increased. Incomplete bladder emptying, neurogenic bladder, urinary diversions, and indwelling catheters contribute to this risk. Frequent urine cultures or antibiotic suppression are indicated.

Decubital Ulcers

Decubital ulcers are a frequently preventable complication in women with SCIs. During pregnancy, women with SCIs should have routine skin examinations, frequent position changes, adequate padding, and appropriately sized medical equipment (eg, wheelchairs). Weight gain and edema also may contribute to decubital ulceration.

Pulmonary Function

Impaired pulmonary function may be present in women with high thoracic or cervical spine lesions. For patients with borderline function, ventilatory support and meticulous attention to pulmonary care is necessary during pregnancy and delivery. Supine positioning may further impair pulmonary function. Serial assessments of vital capacity will help assess the need for ventilatory assistance.

Autonomic Dysreflexia

Autonomic dysreflexia is the most significant medical complication occurring in women with SCIs (85% of patients with lesions above T5 through T6 level). This condition is attributed to a loss of hypothalamic control of sympathetic spinal reflexes and occurs in patients with viable spinal cord segments distal to the level of injury. It can occur in patients with incomplete transections. In susceptible patients, afferent stimuli from a hollow viscus (eg, the bladder, bowel, or uterus) and from the skin below the level of the lesion or of the genital areas ascend in the spinothalamic tracts and posterior columns, which causes reflex sympathetic activation unmodified by the supraspinal centers. The resultant catecholamine release and vasoconstriction lead to hypertension associated with headache, bradycardia, tachycardia, cardiac arrhythmia, sweating, flushing, tingling, nasal congestion, piloerection, and, occasionally, respiratory distress. Uteroplacental vasoconstriction may result in fetal hypoxemia.

It is important to avoid stimuli that can lead to autonomic dysreflexia, such as distension or manipulation of the vagina, bladder, urethra, or bowel. During labor, the symptoms of autonomic dysreflexia are commonly synchronous with uterine contractions. The severity of the syndrome during labor

ranges from unpleasant symptoms to hypertensive encephalopathy, cerebrovascular accidents, intraventricular and retinal hemorrhages, and death. Therefore, continual hemodynamic monitoring during labor is mandatory in all at-risk patients.

Although patients with SCIs may perceive no pain during labor, anesthesia should be used to prevent autonomic dysreflexia. Spinal or epidural anesthesia extending to the T10 level is the most reliable method of preventing autonomic dysreflexia by blocking stimuli that arise from pelvic organs. Therefore, antepartum consultation with an anesthesiologist and the establishment of a plan for induction of epidural or spinal anesthesia at the onset of labor is imperative. If autonomic dysreflexia occurs before a regional anesthetic is available or occurs despite regional anesthesia, hypertension may be treated with antihypertensive agents that have a rapid onset and short duration of action (eg, sodium nitroprusside or nitroglycerin), ganglionic blocking agents (eg, trimethaphan), adrenergic blocking agents (eg, guanethidine), or a direct vasodilator (eg, hydralazine).

If there is evidence of autonomic dysreflexia during the second stage of labor, delivery can be expedited by forceps or vacuum assisted delivery with adequate anesthesia. If autonomic dysreflexia during labor cannot be controlled by any means, cesarean delivery may be necessary. Adequate anesthesia, spinal or epidural if possible, is needed for cesarean deliveries in all patients with SCIs.

Ascertainment of Labor

Women with SCIs may give birth vaginally. Women with spinal cord transection above the T10 segment may have painless labor. In a patient with total transection at a lower thoracic level, labor pain may be so reduced that the patient is unaware of uterine contractions, especially during sleep. However, symptoms under the control of the sympathetic nervous system (eg, abdominal or leg spasms, shortness of breath, increased spasticity) concurrent with uterine contractions may make patients aware of labor. Patients should be instructed in uterine palpation techniques to detect contractions at home.

General Support

Excess weight gain may increase the difficulty of moving and transporting pregnant women with SCIs. Muscle-strengthening exercises may be recommended for the upper extremities of nonquadriplegic patients. For all patients, elevation of the legs and range-of-motion exercises may be implemented as pregnancy advances. The possibility of an increased need for social support services also should be addressed.

Bibliography

American Society of Anesthesiologists. Standards for basic anesthetic monitoring. In: ASA standards, guidelines and statements. Park Ridge (IL): ASA; 2000. p. 5–6.

Atterbury JL, Groome LJ. Pregnancy in women with spinal cord injuries. Nurs Clin North Am 1998;33:603–13.

Baker EB, Cardenas DD. Pregnancy in spinal cord injured women. Arch Phys Med Rehabil 1996;77:501–7.

Baker EB, Cardena DD, Benedetti TJ. Risks associated with pregnancy in spinal cord-injured women. Obstet Gynecol 1992;80:425–8.

Hambly PR, Martin B. Anaesthesia for chronic spinal cord lesions. Anaesthesia 1998;53:273–89.

Nobunaga AI, Go BK, Karunas RB. Recent demographic and injury trends in people served by the Model Spinal Cord Injury Care Systems. Arch Phys Med Rehabil 1999;80:1372–82.

Paonessa K, Fernand R. Spinal cord injury and pregnancy. Spine 1991;16:596–8.

Verduyn WH. Spinal cord injured women, pregnancy and delivery. Paraplegia 1986;24:231–40.

ACOG
Committee on
Obstetric Practice

American Society of
Anesthesiologists
Committee on
Obstetric Anesthesia

The American College of Obstetricians and Gynecologists
409 12th Street, SW
PO Box 96920
Washington, DC 20090-6920

12345/54321

Committee Opinion

Number 256, May 2001

Optimal Goals for Anesthesia Care in Obstetrics

This joint statement from the American Society of Anesthesiologists (ASA) and the American College of Obstetricians and Gynecologists (ACOG) has been designed to address issues of concern to both specialties. Good obstetric care requires the availability of qualified personnel and equipment to administer general or regional anesthesia both electively and emergently. The extent and degree to which anesthesia services are available varies widely among hospitals. However, for any hospital providing obstetric care, certain optimal anesthesia goals should be sought. These include:

I. Availability of a licensed practitioner who is credentialed to administer an appropriate anesthetic whenever necessary

    For many women, regional anesthesia (epidural, spinal, or combined spinal epidural) will be the most appropriate anesthetic.

II. Availability of a licensed practitioner who is credentialed to maintain support of vital functions in any obstetric emergency

III. Availability of anesthesia and surgical personnel to permit the start of a cesarean delivery within 30 minutes of the decision to perform the procedure; in cases of vaginal birth after cesarean delivery (VBAC), appropriate facilities and personnel, including obstetric anesthesia, nursing personnel, and a physician capable of monitoring labor and performing cesarean delivery, immediately available during active labor to perform an emergency cesarean delivery (1)

    The definition of immediately available personnel and facilities remains a local decision based on each institution's available resources and geographic location.

IV. Appointment of a qualified anesthesiologist to be responsible for all anesthetics administered

    There are many obstetric units where obstetricians or obstetrician-supervised nurse anesthetists administer anesthetics. The administration of general or regional anesthesia requires both medical judgment and technical skills. Thus, a physician with privileges in anesthesiology should be readily available.

Persons administering or supervising obstetric anesthesia should be qualified to manage the infrequent but occasionally life-threatening complications of major regional anesthesia such as respiratory and cardiovascular failure, toxic local anesthetic convulsions, or vomiting and aspiration. Mastering and retaining the skills and knowledge necessary to manage these complications require adequate training and frequent application.

To ensure the safest and most effective anesthesia for obstetric patients, the director of anesthesia services, with the approval of the medical staff, should develop and enforce written policies regarding provision of obstetric anesthesia. These include:

I. Availability of a qualified physician with obstetric privileges to perform operative vaginal or cesarean delivery during administration of anesthesia

Regional and/or general anesthesia should not be administered until the patient has been examined and the fetal status and progress of labor evaluated by a qualified individual. A physician with obstetric privileges who has knowledge of the maternal and fetal status and the progress of labor, and who approves the initiation of labor anesthesia should be readily available to deal with any obstetric complications that may arise.

II. Availability of equipment, facilities, and support personnel equal to that provided in the surgical suite

This should include the availability of a properly equipped and staffed recovery room capable of receiving and caring for all patients recovering from major regional or general anesthesia. Birthing facilities, when used for analgesia or anesthesia, must be appropriately equipped to provide safe anesthetic care during labor and delivery or postanesthesia recovery care.

III. Personnel other than the surgical team should be immediately available to assume responsibility for resuscitation of the depressed newborn

The surgeon and anesthesiologist are responsible for the mother and may not be able to leave her to care for the newborn even when a regional anesthetic is functioning adequately. Individuals qualified to perform neonatal resuscitation should demonstrate:

A. Proficiency in rapid and accurate evaluation of the newborn condition, including Apgar scoring

B. Knowledge of the pathogenesis of a depressed newborn (acidosis, drugs, hypovolemia, trauma, anomalies, and infection), as well as specific indications for resuscitation

C. Proficiency in newborn airway management, laryngoscopy, endotracheal intubations, suctioning of airways, artificial ventilation, cardiac massage, and maintenance of thermal stability

In larger maternity units and those functioning as high-risk centers, 24-hour in-house anesthesia, obstetric and neonatal specialists are usually necessary. Preferably, the obstetric anesthesia services should be directed by an anesthesiologist with special training or experience in obstetric anesthesia. These units will also frequently require the availability of more sophisticated monitoring equipment and specially trained nursing personnel.

A survey jointly sponsored by the ASA and ACOG found that many hospitals in the United States have not yet achieved the goals mentioned previously. Deficiencies were most evident in smaller delivery units. Some small delivery units are necessary because of geographic considerations. Currently, approximately 50% of hospitals providing obstetric care have fewer than 500 deliveries per year. Providing comprehensive care for obstetric patients in these small units is extremely inefficient, not cost-effective and frequently impossible. Thus, the following recommendations are made:

1. Whenever possible, small units should consolidate.

2. When geographic factors require the existence of smaller units, these units should be part of a well-established regional perinatal system.

The availability of the appropriate personnel to assist in the management of a variety of obstetric problems is a necessary feature of good obstetric care. The presence of a pediatrician or other trained physician at a high-risk cesarean delivery to care for the newborn or the availability of an anesthesiologist during active labor and delivery when VBAC is attempted and at a breech or twin delivery are examples. Frequently, these professionals spend a considerable amount of time standing by for the possibility that their services may be needed emergently but may ultimately not be required to perform the tasks for which they are present. Reasonable compensation for these standby services is justifiable and necessary.

A variety of other mechanisms have been suggested to increase the availability and quality of anesthesia services in obstetrics. Improved hospital design, to place labor and delivery suites closer to the operating rooms, would allow for more efficient supervision of nurse anesthetists. Anesthesia equipment in the labor and delivery area must be comparable to that in the operating room.

Finally, good interpersonal relations between obstetricians and anesthesiologists are important. Joint meetings between the two departments should be encouraged. Anesthesiologists should recognize the special needs and concerns of the obstetrician and obstetricians should recognize the anesthesiologist as a consultant in the management of pain and life-support measures. Both should recognize the need to provide high quality care for all patients.

Reference

1. American College of Obstetricians and Gynecologists. Vaginal birth after previous cesarean delivery. ACOG Practice Bulletin 5. Washington, DC: ACOG, 1999

Bibliography

Committee on Perinatal Health. Toward improving the outcome of pregnancy: the 90s and beyond. White Plains, New York: March of Dimes Birth Defects Foundation, 1993

ACOG

Committee on
Obstetric Practice

American Society of
Anesthesiologists

This document reflects emerging clinical and scientific advances as of the date issued and is subject to change. The information should not be construed as dictating an exclusive course of treatment or procedure to be followed.

ISSN 1074-861X

The American College of Obstetricians and Gynecologists
409 12th Street, SW
PO Box 96920
Washington, DC 20090-6920

12345/87654

Pain relief during labor. ACOG Committee Opinion No. 295. American College of Obstetricians and Gynecologists. Obstet Gynecol 2004;104:213.

Committee Opinion

Number 295, July 2004   *(Replaces No. 231, February 2000)*

Pain Relief During Labor

ABSTRACT: Pain management should be provided whenever medically indicated. The American Society of Anesthesiologists (ASA) and the American College of Obstetricians and Gynecologists (ACOG) believe that women requesting epidural analgesia during labor should not be deprived of this service based on their insurance or inadequate nursing participation in the management of regional analgesic modalities. Furthermore, in an effort to allow the maximum number of patients to benefit from neuraxial analgesia, ASA and ACOG believe that labor nurses should not be restricted from participating in the management of pain relief during labor.

Labor causes severe pain for many women. There is no other circumstance where it is considered acceptable for an individual to experience untreated severe pain, amenable to safe intervention, while under a physician's care. In the absence of a medical contraindication, maternal request is a sufficient medical indication for pain relief during labor. Pain management should be provided whenever medically indicated.

Of the various pharmacologic methods used for pain relief during labor and delivery, neuraxial analgesia techniques (epidural, spinal, and combined spinal–epidural) are the most flexible, effective, and least depressing to the central nervous system, allowing for an alert participating woman and an alert neonate. The American Society of Anesthesiologists (ASA) and the American College of Obstetricians and Gynecologists (ACOG) believe that women requesting epidural analgesia during labor should not be deprived of this service based on their insurance or inadequate nursing participation in the management of regional analgesic modalities. In addition, third-party payers who provide reimbursement for obstetric services should not deny reimbursement for labor analgesia because of an absence of "other medical indications." Although the availability of various methods of labor analgesia will vary from hospital to hospital, within an institution the methods available should not be based on a patient's ability to pay. Furthermore, in an effort to allow the maximum number of patients to benefit from neuraxial analgesia, ASA and ACOG believe that labor nurses should not be restricted from participating in the management of pain relief during labor. Under appropriate physician supervision, labor and delivery nursing personnel who have been properly educated and have demonstrated current competence should be able to participate in the management of epidural infusions, including adjusting dosage and discontinuing infusions.

ACOG

Committee on Health Care for Underserved Women

Committee Opinion

Number 307, December 2004

Partner Consent for Participation in Women's Reproductive Health Research

ABSTRACT: *Recent advances in reproductive medicine include treatment of subfertility as well as investigation of agents that may serve as both contraceptives and potential prophylaxis against sexually transmitted diseases, including potential protection from human immunodeficiency virus (HIV). Although there is no doubt regarding the need for informed consent by women participating in trials evaluating the safety and effectiveness of these novel agents and treatments, there has been some debate regarding the necessity and propriety of requiring consent from the partners of women involved in certain types of clinical trials involving reproductive health. Issues of partner consent are unique to research surrounding women's reproductive health as opposed to research pertaining to women's health, in general. This is due, in part, to a valid concern about a potential effect of the research on the partner. There are, therefore, legitimate reasons to obtain partner consent for a woman's participation in a clinical trial. In the absence of such reason, partner consent should not be mandated.*

Background

A large number of clinical trials are currently being conducted in nearly every therapeutic area, including women's health. Women may be motivated to participate in clinical trials by altruism to further the care of women, by the ability to receive novel and state-of-the-art medical care, or by the benefits of highly supervised medical monitoring of treatment. Often women without health insurance choose to participate in these trials because such trials may provide enhanced access to care, the care provided is often rendered without cost, and there is reimbursement for time and travel. The American College of Obstetricians and Gynecologists supports the development of new devices and medications to advance women's health and reproductive options. The American College of Obstetricians and Gynecologists also endorses the highest ethical and moral conduct of clinical research. All women, regardless of socioeconomic status and race, should have access to enrollment in clinical trials. The decision to enter a clinical trial should be autonomous, without

The information should not be construed as dictating an exclusive course of treatment or procedure to be followed.

The Committee wishes to thank Kurt Barnhart, MD, MSCE; Jeffrey Ecker, MD; and Carol Tauer, PhD; for their assistance in the development of this document.

ISSN 1074-861X

The American College of Obstetricians and Gynecologists
409 12th Street, SW
PO Box 96920
Washington, DC 20090-6920

12345/87654

Partner consent for participation in women's reproductive health research. ACOG Committee Opinion No. 307. American College of Obstetricians and Gynecologists. Obstet Gynecol 2004; 104:1467–9.

coercion, and after informed consent. Informed consent is the ability to understand the risks and benefits of one's participation in a research activity and to authorize one's participation in this activity freely (1).

A research subject is defined as "An individual who participates in a clinical trial, either as a recipient of the investigational product(s) or as a control." (2). In research on women's reproductive health, sometimes both the woman and her partner will be the subjects. For example, in a study designed to identify any risk or harm to a partner of a new contraceptive method, both the woman and her partner may be research subjects. If a partner is a subject in the research, informed consent for both participants is required. This Committee Opinion primarily addresses the need for partner consent in research for which the woman, and not a partner, is the research subject. The respect for the autonomy of research subjects to consent to participation is one of the pillars of The Belmont Report, promulgated by The National Commission for the Protection of Human Subjects of Biomedical and Behavioral Research in 1979 (3). The decision to reproduce or use contraceptives should remain autonomous for a woman even when enrolled in a clinical trial.

It also is important to note that the discussion and recommendations that follow do not pertain to research involving pregnant women. There are specific regulations that apply to federally funded research involving this population (4).

Partner Consent Requirement Inconsistencies

Recent advances in reproductive medicine include treatment of subfertility as well as investigation of agents that may serve as both contraceptives and potential prophylaxis against sexually transmitted diseases, including potential protection from human immunodeficiency virus (HIV). Although there is no doubt regarding the need for informed consent by women participating in trials evaluating the safety and effectiveness of these novel agents and treatments, there has been some debate regarding the necessity and propriety of requiring consent from the partners of women involved in certain types of clinical trials involving reproductive health. Some local institutional review boards (IRB) have requested consent of a woman's partner and at other times a trial sponsor or an individual investigator has made the decision unilaterally. Because of the lack of guidance on this issue, there is great inconsistency regarding requirements for partner consent and the manner in which partner consent is obtained (see box "Methods of Obtaining Partner Consent").

When Is Partner Consent Needed?

Issues of partner consent are unique to research surrounding women's reproductive health as opposed to research pertaining to women's health, in general. This is partly due to a valid concern about a potential impact of the research on the partner. Therefore, there are legitimate reasons to obtain partner consent for a woman's participation in a clinical trial. In the absence of such reason, partner consent should not be mandated. Partner consent should be obtained if:

- A sexual partner is a subject in the same clinical trial as the woman.
- A partner will be exposed to a novel agent and there is a potential for more than minimal risks* of exposure to the investigational agent.
- Data will be collected regarding a partner's acceptance of the investigational agent, or the impact of partner's acceptance of the agent on the female participant.
- Inclusion or exclusion criteria directly relate to a partner, for example, if testing of a partner is required for a woman to enroll in the trial (eg, semen analysis or testing for a sexually transmitted disease).

If, after careful consideration, it is determined that none of the previous conditions apply, partner consent is not warranted because it should not needlessly:

- Impose a barrier to participation for a woman
- Interfere with a woman's choice of reproductive options
- Interfere with a woman's right to make independent decisions about her reproductive health care due to an IRB's or regulatory agency's paternalistic reasons for partner consent

---

*According to applicable federal regulations, "*Minimal risk* means that the probability and magnitude of harm or discomfort anticipated in the research are not greater in and of themselves than those ordinarily encountered in daily life or during the performance of routine physical or psychological examinations or tests." (45 C.F.R §46.102[I]).

Methods of Obtaining Partner Consent

Several methods exist that may be used to obtain partner consent regarding a woman's participation in a clinical trial. The suitability of these methods depends on the particular research study. Some ways of obtaining partner consent include:

- Having a partner attend the screening visit and sign the consent at that time
- Giving a copy of the consent to the participant and having a partner come in for a separate visit to consent
- Mailing the consent and having it mailed back
- Performing the informed consent process over the telephone
- Obtaining a single informed consent that is signed by the woman and partner

Recommendations

Recognizing the complexities of the conduct and consent requirements for trials in women's reproductive health, the following recommendations are made:

- The partner consent requirements of each clinical trial need to be individually evaluated and based on the best available scientific and medical evidence and ethical principles.

- When partner consent is required, efforts should be undertaken to decrease the likelihood that receipt of such consent will be a barrier for participation of a woman interested in enrolling in such a trial. The addition of consent adds complexity to all trials, often resulting in additional visits for the participant and partner. This can result in fewer women enrolling and a decrease in compliance.

- Whenever possible, the choice of a woman to enroll in a clinical trial regarding her reproductive function and health should be hers alone when it does not also include a partner as a research subject. In these instances, the woman, not the IRB or the researcher(s), considering the research study should determine the extent to which a partner is to be involved in the process of informed consent and the decision to participate. For example:

  —In the case of the study of a microbicide or barrier contraception efficacy, the risk to a partner is likely negligible (compared with the female partner) because of minimal contact time. If potential irritation to a male partner is suspected, it should be ruled out in the early stages of clinical investigation.

  —In contraceptive research where the participant may face an unintended pregnancy, a partner may be a potential father with the resultant legal and moral responsibilities for the child. However, the principle of autonomy, allowing a woman to make a choice to enter a trial regarding her reproductive rights, should take precedence (5). The American College of Obstetricians and Gynecologists does not support recognition of distinct paternal rights before the birth of a child (6).

- Regardless of the requirement for partner consent, communication with a partner about reproductive health and contraception use should be encouraged.

References

1. American College of Obstetricians and Gynecologists. Informed consent. In: Ethics in obstetrics and gynecology. 2nd ed. Washington (DC): ACOG; 2004. p. 9–17.
2. International Conference On Harmonisation. Guideline for good clinical practice. ICH Harmonised Tripartite Guideline E6. London: ICH; 1997. Available at: http://www.proclinica.fr/GCPICH.pdf. Retrieved August 26, 2004.
3. The National Commission for the Protection of Human Subjects of Biomedical and Behavioral Research. The Belmont report: ethical principles and guidelines for the protection of human subjects of research. Washington, DC: U.S Department of Health and Human Services; 1979. Available at: http://www.hhs.gov/ohrp/humansubjects/guidance/belmont.htm. Retrieved August 26, 2004.
4. Protection of human subjects. 45 C.F.R §46 (2003). Available at: http://www.access.gpo.gov/nara/cfr/waisidx_03/45cfr46_03.html. Retrieved August 27, 2004.
5. Holder AR. Contraceptive research: do sex partners have rights? IRB 1982;4(2):6–7.
6. American College of Obstetricians and Gynecologists. Research involving women. In: Ethics in obstetrics and gynecology. 2nd ed. Washington (DC): ACOG; 2004. p. 86–91.

ACOG

Committee on
Quality Improvement
and Patient Safety

Committee Opinion

Number 320, November 2005

The American College of Obstetricians and Gynecologists
409 12th Street, SW
PO Box 96920
Washington, DC 20090-6920

12345/98765

Partnering with patients to improve safety. ACOG Committee Opinion No. 320. American College of Obstetricians and Gynecologists. Obstet Gynecol 2005;106:1123–5.

Partnering With Patients to Improve Safety

ABSTRACT: Actively involving patients in their care will lead to increased patient satisfaction, increased diagnostic accuracy, enhanced adherence to therapeutic recommendations, and ultimately, improved health quality. Partnering with patients in the office setting by sharing information and enhancing communication can lead to improved patient health care and satisfaction.

The foundation for a positive physician–patient interaction is formed by establishing a partnership and creating a meaningful dialogue. Accomplishing this in a brief office visit may be challenging, but with adequate planning these encounters can be structured in a positive way. Improving communication with patients, listening to their concerns, and facilitating active partnerships should be central to any patient safety strategy (1). Involving patients in planning and delivering health services also is recommended as a means of improving the quality of services (2). Additionally, several studies indicate that physician–patient communication problems may account for an increase in medical professional liability actions (3, 4).

Information Sharing

Patients are responsible for providing their physicians with the information that is necessary to reach an accurate diagnosis or treatment plan. To facilitate this process, patients should be encouraged to discuss the reasons for their visits and ask questions such as, "What is my primary problem?" "What do I need to do?" and "Why is it important for me to do this?" (5). In response, physicians should actively listen to engage their patients. Physicians also can solicit the patient's concerns and opinions by asking open-ended questions and asking patients to share key information such as their medical history (including illnesses, immunizations, and hospitalizations), medication history (including over-the-counter [OTC] medications, and dietary supplements), and any allergies, reactions, or sensitivities experienced after taking medication.

Health Literacy

According to an Institute of Medicine report, "nearly half of all American adults—90 million people—have difficulty understanding and acting upon health information" (6). The Institute of Medicine defines health literacy as "the degree to which individuals have the capacity to obtain, process, and understand basic health information and services needed to make appropriate health decisions" (6). Cultural barriers also can impede physician–patient communication. Consequently, it is important for clinicians to use proven strategies to facilitate communication with patients. Listed as follows are examples of useful methods:

- Speaking slowly and using plain, nonmedical language
- Limiting the amount of information provided and repeating the information
- Using teach-back or show-me techniques (asking the patient to repeat any instructions given) to confirm that the patient understands
- Making patients feel comfortable to ask questions (7)
- Providing written materials to reinforce oral explanations

Informed Consent

Informed consent is a process, not a form. At the end of this process, the patient should understand her diagnosis, recommended treatment, potential complications, and treatment options. This discussion should be documented in the medical record. It often is helpful to invite the patient to bring a relative or a close friend to this discussion. There are many commercially available videotapes and printed materials, including those produced by ACOG, that can reinforce—but not replace—this process.

Medications

Medication errors are the largest source of preventable adverse events. It is important for patients to provide their physicians with a list of the prescription and nonprescription medications they take. Whenever new prescriptions are given, patients should be told why the medication is being prescribed and given instructions for taking the medication. For example, if a medication is to be taken three times per day, the patient should be told what time of day the medication should be taken, whether it should be taken with food or without food, how much should be taken at one time, how long the medication should be continued, possible interactions with other medications the patient is taking, and whether any medications (including OTC medications), foods, or alcohol are contraindicated while taking this medication. Physicians should encourage their patients to maintain a list of all the medications, including herbal supplements and OTC medications, they are taking and share the list with any other physicians they may be seeing. Medication forms to facilitate this process have been developed by some groups (see Resources).

Follow-up

Physicians should develop a system to track test results and communicate those results to patients. Tracking strategies in the office may include log books or computer prompts. Clinicians should inform their patients that no news is not necessarily good news. Patients should be given a reasonable time frame within which they should expect to hear about their test results, and they should be encouraged to call if they have not heard from the office at the end of that period.

Conclusion

Partnering with patients to improve communication results in increased patient satisfaction, increased diagnostic accuracy, enhanced adherence to therapeutic recommendations, and improved health quality. In addition to the physician, other staff, such as nurses and physician assistants, may play an important role in ensuring appropriate communication. More time may be required during the patient encounter, but overall, these measures will save time, improve patient safety and satisfaction, and will be worth the additional effort.

References

1. Vincent CA, Coulter A. Patient safety: what about the patient? Qual Saf Health Care 2002;11:76–80.
2. Crawford MJ, Rutter D, Manley C, Weaver T, Bhui K, Fulop N, et al. Systematic review of involving patients in the planning and development of health care. BMJ 2002; 325:1263.

3. Hickson GB, Clayton EW, Githens PB, Sloan FA. Factors that prompted families to file medical malpractice claims following perinatal injuries. JAMA 1992;267:1359–63.
4. Hickson GB, Clayton EW, Entman SS, Miller CS, Githens PB, Whetten-Goldstein K, et al. Obstetricians' prior malpractice experience and patients' satisfaction with care. JAMA 1994;272:1583–7.
5. Partnership for Clear Health Communication. Ask me 3: good questions for your good health. Available at: http://www.askme3.org/pdfs/Patient_Eng.pdf. Retrieved July 29, 2005.
6. Institute of Medicine (US). Health literacy. A prescription to end confusion. Washington, DC: National Academies Press; 2004.
7. Weiss BD. Health literacy: a manual for clinicians. Chicago (IL): American Medical Association; 2003.

Resources

National Patient Safety Foundation
www.npsf.org

Institute for Safe Medical Practice
www.ismp.org

ACOG

Committee on
Quality Improvement
and Patient Safety

Committee Opinion

Number 286, October 2003

The American College of Obstetricians and Gynecologists
409 12th Street, SW
PO Box 96920
Washington, DC 20090-6920

12345/76543

Patient safety in obstetrics and gynecology. ACOG Committee Opinion No. 286. American College of Obstetricians and Gynecologists. Obstet Gynecol 2003;102:883–5.

Patient Safety in Obstetrics and Gynecology

ABSTRACT: *Emphasis on patient safety has increased in the past few years mostly in response to the Institute of Medicine report* To Err Is Human: Building a Safer Health System. *Obstetrician–gynecologists should incorporate elements of patient safety into their practices and also encourage others to use these practices.*

The American College of Obstetricians and Gynecologists (ACOG) is committed to improving quality and safety in women's health care. The Institute of Medicine report, *To Err Is Human: Building a Safer Health System*, notes that errors in health care are a significant cause of death and injury (1). Despite disagreements over the actual numbers cited, all health care professionals agree that patient safety is extremely important and should be addressed by the overall health care system. The American College of Obstetricians and Gynecologists continues to emphasize its long-standing commitment to quality and patient safety by codifying a set of objectives that should be adopted by obstetrician–gynecologists in their practices. Obstetrician–gynecologists are encouraged to promulgate these principles in the hospitals and other settings where they practice.

Objectives

I.   Develop a commitment to encourage a culture of patient safety

Safety should be viewed as an essential component of a broader commitment to the provision of optimal health care for women. Promoting safety requires that all those in the health care environment recognize that the potential for errors exists and that teamwork and communication are the basis for fostering change and preventing errors. A culture of safety should be the framework for any effort to reduce medical errors. Women's health care should be delivered in a learning environment that encourages disclosure and exchange of information in the event of errors, near misses, and adverse outcomes.

A systems view of clinical processes also is a key element in supporting this culture. Consequently, all health care systems should be designed with the objective to minimize errors.

The first step in the delivery of safe health care should be to identify and study the patterns and causes of error occurrence within delivery systems. Obstetrician–gynecologists should adopt and develop those safe practices that reduce the likelihood of system failures that can cause adverse outcomes.

The role of leadership, whether in the inpatient or outpatient setting, is essential in facilitating an effective patient safety program. Strong leadership within obstetrics and gynecology is necessary to advocate for the provision of both financial and human resources to achieve patient safety goals. Efforts devoted to optimizing communication and collaboration among the various members of the health care team are equally important in promoting these principles of patient safety.

II. Implement recommended safe medication practices

Most medical errors are caused by problems associated with the use of medications; therefore, efforts to reduce the occurrence of these errors should be ongoing. Although computerized physician order entry systems can be effective in reducing prescribing errors, they are costly and their use is not widespread. In the absence of computerized physician order entry systems, the following steps should be adopted to reduce errors in prescribing and administering medications (2):

- Improve legibility of handwriting

- Avoid use of nonstandard abbreviations

- Check for drug allergies and sensitivities

- Always use a leading 0 for doses of less than 1 unit (eg, 0.1 mg, not .1 mg), and never use a trailing 0 after a decimal (eg, 1 mg, not 1.0 mg): "always lead, never follow"

- All verbal orders should be written down by the individual receiving the order and read back to the prescriber verbatim to ensure accuracy

III. Reduce the likelihood of surgical errors

Surgical errors may involve the performance of the incorrect operation or a procedure on the wrong site or wrong patient. Although these errors occur much less frequently than medication errors, the consequences of these errors are always significant. The attending obstetrician–gynecologist who is ultimately responsible for the patient's care should work with other operating room personnel, such as nurses and anesthesiologists, to be certain that systems are in place to ensure proper patient and procedure identification. The obstetrician–gynecologist also should use a preoperative verification process to confirm, with the patient, the intended procedure to be performed.

IV. Improve communication

According to the *Code of Professional Ethics of the American College of Obstetricians and Gynecologists*, "the patient–physician relationship has an ethical basis and is built on confidentiality, trust, and honesty" (3). It also states "the obstetrician–gynecologist should deal honestly with patients and colleagues.... This includes not misrepresenting himself or herself through any form of communication in an untruthful, misleading, or deceptive manner." The American College of Obstetricians and Gynecologists encourages the development and use of a disclosure policy to communicate an unexpected outcome, as defined by the institution, when it occurs; to take immediate necessary steps to neutralize or limit any harm to the patient; to engage in the critical analysis of the incident; and to learn from the error and, by system redesign, to decrease the likelihood of recurrence. The American College of Obstetricians and Gynecologists believes that it is the moral obligation of every physician to communicate honestly with patients, particularly those who experience an adverse outcome. Open communication and transparency in health care will increase trust, improve patient satisfaction, and may decrease liability exposure (4).

V. Identify and resolve system problems

Generally, most medical errors should be handled in a nonpunitive environment to improve reporting and to gain an understanding of the breadth of problems in health care systems. However, willful violation of rules, repetitive errors despite attempts at corrective action, and criminal or egregious activity in the health care environment may require punitive actions or other interventions to protect patients or staff from harm. To improve patient safety, physicians should openly disclose errors and near misses and encourage their colleagues to do the same. This will promote and increase error reporting and identify potentially hidden problems, as well as motivate providers to find system problems and collaborate to resolve system failures.

VI. Establish a partnership with patients to improve safety

Patients who are involved in making their health care decisions have better outcomes than those who are not (5). According to ACOG's *Ethics in Obstetrics and Gynecology*, the "involvement of patients in [decisions about their own medical care] is good for their health—not only because it is a protection against treatment that patients might consider harmful, but because it contributes positively to their well-being" (6). Patients should be encouraged to ask questions about medical procedures, the medications they are taking, and any other aspect of their care. Patient education materials developed by ACOG and other organizations are available.

VII. Make safety a priority in every aspect of practice

The discipline of obstetrics and gynecology has a long tradition of leadership in quality assessment activities, which have been associated with an increase in patient safety. The quest for patient safety is an ongoing, continuously refined process incorporating information shar-

ing and collaboration into daily practice. Emphasizing compassion, communication, and patient-focused care will aid in creating a culture of excellence. Opportunities to improve patient safety should be used whenever identified.

References

1. Institute of Medicine. To err is human: building a safer health system. Washington, DC: National Academy Press; 2000.
2. Pearlman MD, Erickson TB. Patient safety series: safe medication prescribing. ACOG Clin Rev 2002;7(7):1–2, 11–4.
3. American College of Obstetricians and Gynecologists. Code of professional ethics of the American College of Obstetricians and Gynecologists. Ethics in obstetrics and gynecology. Washington, DC: ACOG; 2002. p. 97–101.
4. Kraman SS, Hamm G. Risk management: extreme honesty may be the best policy. Ann Intern Med 1999;131: 963–7.
5. Kaplan SH, Gandek B, Greenfield S, Rogers W, Ware JE. Patient and visit characteristics related to physicians' participatory decision-making style. Results from the Medical Outcomes Study. Med Care 1995;33:1176–87.
6. American College of Obstetricians and Gynecologists. Ethics in obstetrics and gynecology. Washington, DC: ACOG; 2002.

Resources

Agency for Healthcare Research and Quality
www.ahrq.gov/qual/errorsix.htm

Department of Veterans Affairs (VA) National Center for Patient Safety
www.patientsafety.gov

Joint Commission on Accreditation of Healthcare Organizations
www.jcaho.org/accredited+organizations/patient+safety

National Patient Safety Foundation
www.npsf.org

ACOG

Committee on
Gynecologic Practice

Requests for authorization to make photocopies should be directed to:

Copyright Clearance Center
222 Rosewood Drive
Danvers, MA 01923
(978) 750-8400

ISSN 1074-861X

The American College of Obstetricians and Gynecologists
409 12th Street, SW
PO Box 96920
Washington, DC 20090-6920

12345/43210

Committee Opinion

Number 243, November 2000

Performance and Interpretation of Imaging Studies by Obstetrician–Gynecologists

Obstetrician–gynecologists are experienced in diagnostic imaging methods and receive privileges to perform and interpret imaging studies on the basis of their training, experience, and demonstrated current competence. Obstetrician–gynecologists can perform the immediate and timely interpretation of imaging studies, correlate these studies with clinical findings, counsel the patient, and assume the responsibility for determining the treatment of the patient.

Education and Training

By virtue of their education and experience, obstetrician–gynecologists are qualified to perform the imaging studies that are a necessary and integral part of obstetric–gynecologic care. Training in diagnostic imaging is a part of obstetric–gynecologic residencies, and questions related to this field are a part of the certifying examinations of the American Board of Obstetrics and Gynecology. For example, the performance and interpretation of ultrasound images are required components of obstetric and gynecologic residency training and are monitored by the Residency Review Committee for Obstetrics and Gynecology. In addition to interpreting images in descriptive terms, obstetrician–gynecologists add functional, anatomical, and clinical assessments, resulting in patient-specific information. It is the obstetric–gynecologic interpretation of the images, in concert with the history and physical examination, that determines the course of treatment and carries with it the responsibility for patient care. A written report, signed by the interpreting physician, should be considered an integral part of the performance and interpretation of an imaging study.

Timeliness

For optimal patient care, imaging studies should be performed and interpreted in a timely manner. Many obstetric–gynecologic imaging procedures are performed when the patient is in the obstetrician–gynecologist's office or in

ACOG

Committee on
Obstetric Practice

Committee on
Gynecologic Practice

Committee on
Genetics

ISSN 1074-861X

The American College of Obstetricians and Gynecologists
409 12th Street, SW
PO Box 96920
Washington, DC 20090-6920

12345/98765

Perinatal risks associated with assisted reproductive technology. ACOG Committee Opinion No. 324. American College of Obstetricians and Gynecologists. Obstet Gynecol 2005; 106:1143–6.

Committee Opinion

Number 324, November 2005

Perinatal Risks Associated With Assisted Reproductive Technology

ABSTRACT: Over the past two decades, the use of assisted reproductive technology (ART) has increased dramatically worldwide and has made pregnancy possible for many infertile couples. A growing body of evidence suggests an association between pregnancies resulting from ART and perinatal morbidity (possibly independent of multiple births), although the absolute risk to children conceived through ART is low. Prospective studies are needed to further define the risk of ART to offspring. The single most important health effect of ART for the offspring remains iatrogenic multiple fetal pregnancy. The American College of Obstetricians and Gynecologists supports the effort toward lowering the risk of multiple gestation with ART.

Over the past two decades, the use of assisted reproductive technology (ART) has increased dramatically worldwide and has made pregnancy possible for many infertile couples. The American Society for Reproductive Medicine defines ART as treatments and procedures involving the handling of human oocytes and sperm, or embryos, with the intent of establishing a pregnancy (1). By this definition, ART includes in vitro fertilization (IVF) with or without intracytoplasmic sperm injection (ICSI), but it excludes techniques such as artificial insemination and superovulation drug therapy.

Several studies have been conducted to describe and compare the obstetric outcome of pregnancies resulting from ART with those of pregnancies conceived without treatment. Some retrospective and prospective follow-up studies suggest that pregnancies achieved by ART are associated with an increased risk of prematurity, low birth weight, and neonatal encephalopathy and a higher perinatal mortality rate, even after adjusting for age, parity, and multiple gestation (2, 3). Even in studies limited to singleton ART pregnancies, the prematurity rate is twice as high, and the proportion of infants with low birth weight is three times as high as that of the general population (4, 5). A meta-analysis of 15 studies comprising 12,283 singleton infants conceived by IVF and 1.9 million spontaneously conceived singleton infants showed significantly higher odds of perinatal mortality (odds ratio [OR], 2.2), preterm delivery (OR, 2.0), low birth weight (OR, 1.8), very low birth weight (OR, 2.7), and small for gestational age status (OR, 1.6) in IVF pregnancies, after adjusting for maternal age and parity (6).

It is difficult to determine the degree to which these associations are specifically related to the ART procedures versus any underlying factors within the couple, such as coexisting maternal disease, the cause of infertility, or differences in behavioral risk (eg, smoking). Many of the adverse obstetric outcomes associated with ART may actually be linked to infertility rather than the treatment for this disorder. Continued research is needed to examine possible confounding variables for these observations. Patients undergoing superovulation drug therapy alone, IVF alone, and IVF with ICSI should be examined as three distinct risk populations, and control populations should ideally consist of two separate groups—normal fertile couples and infertile couples who conceive without treatment.

Assisted reproductive technology has been associated with a 30-fold increase in multiple pregnancies compared with the rate of spontaneous twin pregnancies (1% in the general white population). The obstetric and neonatal risks associated with multiple gestation include preeclampsia, gestational diabetes, preterm delivery, and operative delivery. Multifetal births account for 17% of all preterm births (before 37 weeks of gestation), 23% of early preterm births (before 32 weeks of gestation), 24% of low-birth-weight infants (< 2,500 g), and 26% of very-low-birth-weight infants (< 1,500 g) (7–10). In a large population-based cohort study in the United States from 1996 to 1999, the proportion of multiple births attributable to ovulation induction or ART was 33% (11), although the rate of high-order multiple gestations from ART decreased significantly between 1998 and 2001 (12). Methods to limit high-order multiple pregnancies include monitoring hormone levels and follicle number during superovulation and limiting transfer to fewer embryos in IVF cycles (12–14). Transferring two embryos can limit the occurrence of triplets in younger candidates who have a good prognosis without significantly decreasing the overall pregnancy rate (15, 16). The American Society for Reproductive Medicine and the Society for Assisted Reproductive Technology have developed updated recommendations on the number of embryos per transfer to reduce the risk of multiple gestation (1). The multiple gestation risk of ART, unlike that of superovulation, can be effectively managed by limiting the number of embryos transferred. When considering how to minimize multiple gestation, ART can be viewed as the safer and more favorable approach compared with superovulation.

Informing couples of the obstetric risks as well as the socioeconomic consequences of multiple gestations may modify their decisions regarding the number of embryos to be transferred (17). Patients undergoing ART procedures should be counseled in advance regarding the option of multifetal pregnancy reduction to decrease perinatal risks if a high-order multiple pregnancy occurs. Because the intense motivation for a successful outcome and the substantial out-of-pocket cost of ART may increase patients' desire for the transfer of an excessive number of embryos, it is critical that couples be aware of the risk and associated morbidity of high-order multiple gestation.

Most retrospective and prospective follow-up studies of children born as a result of ART have provided evidence for congenital malformation rates similar to those reported in the general population (18–20). In contrast, an Australian study of 4,916 women found that the risk of one or more major birth defects in infants conceived with ART was twice the expected rate (8.6% for ICSI and 9.0% for IVF, compared with 4.2% in the general population) (21). As with other studies, the control group was not ideal because it did not include couples with infertility who conceived without ART. Prospective studies are needed to further define the risk of ART to offspring.

Male factor infertility is now recognized as an inherited disorder for some infertile couples. In vitro fertilization offers the opportunity to achieve pregnancy while increasing the couple's awareness of possible inherited disorders in their offspring. Genetic conditions can predispose to abnormal sperm characteristics that may be passed to male children. In addition, azoospermia is associated with congenital bilateral absence or atrophy of the vas deferens in men with gene mutations associated with cystic fibrosis. Congenital bilateral absence or atrophy of the vas deferens accounts for approximately 2% of all cases of male infertility (22, 23). Therefore, all patients with congenital bilateral absence or atrophy of the vas deferens and their partners considering IVF by sperm extraction procedure with ICSI should be offered genetic counseling to discuss testing for cystic fibrosis.

Approximately 10–15% of azoospermic and severely oligospermic (< 5 million/mL) males have microdeletions of their Y chromosome that can be passed on to their male offspring (24, 25). There is speculation that a deletion could potentially expand in successive generations; however, the reproductive and nonreproductive health implications of this possibility are unknown (26). Some studies have suggested a 1% increased risk for fetal sex chromosome abnormalities following ICSI conception (27–29), but others have yielded conflicting results (30). Subfertile men, with a higher proportion of aneuploid sperm, may have an increased risk of transmitting chromosomal abnormalities to their children (31). These men should be aware of the possible reproductive consequences in their male offspring and the options for prenatal diagnosis.

There is some concern that the micromanipulation of the early embryonic environment in IVF may result in imprinting errors. Genomic imprinting is an epigenetic phenomenon in which one of the two alleles of a subset of genes is expressed differentially according to its parental origin. Imprinting is established early in gametogenesis and maintained in embryogenesis. Recent case series have reported an overrepresentation of two syndromes associated with abnormal imprinting in IVF offspring—Beckwith–Wiedemann syndrome and Angelman's syndrome (32, 33). Both of these conditions may be associated with severe learning disabilities, mental retardation, and congenital malformations. Because these conditions are so rare (1 in 100,000–1 in 300,000), large prospective studies of offspring conceived with ART would be necessary to confirm an increased risk (34). Currently, the risk of imprinting disorders with offspring conceived with ART is largely theoretical but warrants further investigation.

A growing body of evidence suggests an association between ART pregnancies and perinatal morbidity (possibly independent of multiple births), although the absolute risk to children conceived with IVF is low. There is observational evidence linking ART and chromosomal abnormalities following ICSI in severe male factor cases, and concerns have been raised about a possible relationship to genomic imprinting modifications. Given the large sample sizes required to firmly answer these questions, particularly for rare genetic disorders, no causal relationship can be established at this time. It is still unclear to what extent these associations are related to the underlying cause(s) of infertility versus the treatment. It would be prudent to acknowledge these possibilities and to counsel patients accordingly. The single most important health effect of ART for the offspring remains iatrogenic multiple fetal pregnancy. The American College of Obstetricians and Gynecologists supports the effort toward lowering the risk of multiple gestation with ART.

References

1. Guidelines on the number of embryos transferred. Practice Committee of the Society for Assisted Reproductive Technology and the American Society for Reproductive Medicine. Fertil Steril 2004;82 Suppl 1:S1–2.
2. Badawi N, Kurinczuk JJ, Keogh JM, Alessandri LM, O'Sullivan F, Burton PR, et al. Antepartum risk factors for newborn encephalopathy: the Western Australian case-control study. BMJ 1998;317:1549–53.
3. Ozturk O, Bhattacharya S, Templeton A. Avoiding multiple pregnancies in ART: evaluation and implementation of new strategies. Hum Reprod 2001;16:1319–21.
4. Cetin I, Cozzi V, Antonazzo P. Fetal development after assisted reproduction—a review. Placenta 2003;24 Suppl B:S104–13.
5. Schieve LA, Ferre C, Peterson HB, Macaluso M, Reynolds MA, Wright VC. Perinatal outcome among singleton infants conceived through assisted reproductive technology in the United States. Obstet Gynecol 2004; 103:1144–53.
6. Jackson RA, Gibson KA, Wu YW, Croughan MS. Perinatal outcomes in singletons following in vitro fertilization: a meta-analysis. Obstet Gynecol 2004;103: 551–63.
7. Donovan EF, Ehrenkranz RA, Shankaran S, Stevenson DK, Wright LL, Younes N, et al. Outcomes of very low birth weight twins cared for in the National Institute of Child Health and Human Development Neonatal Research Network's intensive care units. Am J Obstet Gynecol 1998;179:742–9.
8. Martin JA, Hamilton BE, Sutton PD, Ventura SJ, Menacker F, Munson ML. Births: final data for 2002. Natl Vital Stat Rep 2003;52:1–113.
9. Powers WF, Kiely JL. The risks confronting twins: a national perspective. Am J Obstet Gynecol 1994;170: 456–61.
10. Stevenson DK, Wright LL, Lemons JA, Oh W, Korones SB, Papile LA, et al. Very low birth weight outcomes of the National Institute of Child Health and Human Development Neonatal Research Network, January 1993 through December 1994. Am J Obstet Gynecol 1998; 179:1632–9.
11. Lynch A, McDuffie R, Murphy J, Faber K, Leff M, Orleans M. Assisted reproductive interventions and multiple birth. Obstet Gynecol 2001;97:195–200.
12. Jain T, Missmer SA, Hornstein MD. Trends in embryo-transfer practice and in outcomes of the use of assisted reproductive technology in the United States. N Engl J Med 2004;350:1639–45.
13. Gleicher N, Oleske DM, Tur-Kaspa I, Vidali A, Karande V. Reducing the risk of high-order multiple pregnancy after ovarian stimulation with gonadotropins. N Engl J Med 2000;343:2–7.
14. Licciardi F, Berkeley AS, Krey L, Grifo J, Noyes N. A two- versus three-embryo transfer: the oocyte donation model. Fertil Steril 2001;75:510–3.

15. Staessen C, Janssenswillen C, Van den Abbeel E, Devroey P, Van Steirteghem AC. Avoidance of triplet pregnancies by elective transfer of two good quality embryos. Hum Reprod 1993;8:1650–3.

16. Templeton A, Morris JK. Reducing the risk of multiple births by transfer of two embryos after in vitro fertilization. N Engl J Med 1998;339:573–7.

17. Grobman WA, Milad MP, Stout J, Klock SC. Patient perceptions of multiple gestations: an assessment of knowledge and risk aversion. Am J Obstet Gynecol 2001;185:920–4.

18. Bergh T, Ericson A, Hillensjo T, Nygren KG, Wennerholm UB. Deliveries and children born after in-vitro fertilisation in Sweden 1982–95: a retrospective cohort study. Lancet 1999;354:1579–85.

19. Ericson A, Kallen B. Congenital malformations in infants born after IVF: a population-based study. Hum Reprod 2001;16:504–9.

20. Wennerholm UB, Bergh C, Hamberger L, Lundin K, Nilsson L, Wikland M. Incidence of congenital malformations in children born after ICSI. Hum Reprod 2000;15:944–8.

21. Hansen M, Kurinczuk JJ, Bower C, Webb S. The risk of major birth defects after intracytoplasmic sperm injection and in vitro fertilization. N Engl J Med 2002;346:725–30.

22. Chillon M, Casals T, Mercier B, Bassas L, Lissens W, Silber S, et al. Mutations in the cystic fibrosis gene in patients with congenital absence of the vas deferens. N Engl J Med 1995;332:1475–80.

23. Dork T, Dworniczak B, Aulehla-Scholz C, Wieczorek D, Bohm I, Mayerova A, et al. Distinct spectrum of CFTR gene mutations in congenital absence of vas deferens. Hum Genet 1997;100:365–77.

24. Dohle GR, Halley DJ, Van Hemel JO, van den Ouwel AM, Pieters MH, Weber RF, et al. Genetic risk factors in infertile men with severe oligozoospermia and azoospermia. Hum Reprod 2002;17:13–6.

25. Feng HL. Molecular biology of male infertility. Arch Androl 2003;49:19–27.

26. Tournaye H. ICSI: a technique too far? Int J Androl 2003;26:63–9.

27. Bonduelle M, Aytoz A, Van Assche E, Devroey P, Liebaers I, Van Steirteghem A. Incidence of chromosomal aberrations in children born after assisted reproduction through intracytoplasmic sperm injection. Hum Reprod 1998;13:781–2.

28. Bonduelle M, Ponjaert I, Van Steirteghem A, Derde MP, Devroey P, Liebaers I. Developmental outcome at 2 years of age for children born after ICSI compared with children born after IVF. Hum Reprod 2003;18:342–50.

29. In't Veld P, Brandenburg H, Verhoeff A, Dhont M, Los F. Sex chromosomal abnormalities and intracytoplasmic sperm injection. Lancet 1995;346:773.

30. Loft A, Petersen K, Erb K, Mikkelsen AL, Grinsted J, Hald F, et al. A Danish national cohort of 730 infants born after intracytoplasmic sperm injection (ICSI) 1994–1997. Hum Reprod 1999;14:2143–8.

31. Calogero AE, Burrello N, De Palma A, Barone N, D'Agata R, Vicari E. Sperm aneuploidy in infertile men. Reprod Biomed Online 2003;6:310–7.

32. Cox GF, Burger J, Lip V, Mau UA, Sperling K, Wu BL, et al. Intracytoplasmic sperm injection may increase the risk of imprinting defects. Am J Hum Genet 2002;71:162–4.

33. DeBaun MR, Niemitz EL, Feinberg AP. Association of in vitro fertilization with Beckwith–Wiedemann syndrome and epigenetic alterations of L1T1 and H19. Am J Hum Genet 2003;72:156–60.

34. Niemitz EL, Feinberg AP. Epigenetics and assisted reproductive technology: a call for investigation. Am J Hum Genet 2004;74:599–609.

ACOG

Committee on
Obstetric Practice

Committee Opinion

Number 266, January 2002

Placenta Accreta

ABSTRACT: The incidence of placenta accreta has increased 10-fold in the past 50 years and now occurs with a frequency of 1 per 2,500 deliveries. Women who have had two or more cesarean deliveries with anterior or central placenta previa have nearly a 40% risk of developing placenta accreta. If the diagnosis or strong suspicion of placenta accreta is formed before delivery, the patient should be counseled about the likelihood of hysterectomy and blood transfusion. Blood products and clotting factors should be available. Cell saver technology should be considered if available as well as the appropriate location and timing for delivery to allow access to adequate surgical personnel and equipment. A preoperative anesthesia assessment should be obtained.

The American College of Obstetricians and Gynecologists
409 12th Street, SW
PO Box 96920
Washington, DC 20090-6920

12345/65432

Placenta accreta. ACOG Committee Opinion No. 266. American College of Obstetricians and Gynecologists. Obstet Gynecol 2002;99:169–170

Placenta accreta occurs when there is a defect of the decidua basalis resulting in abnormally invasive implantation of the placenta. The resultant incomplete separation of the placenta may lead to massive hemorrhage. Furthermore, placenta accreta has been reported to result in a 7% mortality rate as well as intraoperative and postoperative morbidity associated with massive blood transfusions, infection, ureteral damage, and fistula formation (1). Most likely driven by the increasing cesarean delivery rate, the incidence of placenta accreta has increased 10-fold in the past 50 years and now occurs with a frequency of 1 per 2,500 deliveries (2). Risk factors for placenta accreta include placenta previa with or without previous uterine surgery, prior myomectomy, prior cesarean delivery, Asherman's syndrome, submucous leiomyomata, and maternal age older than 35 years (3). Women who have had two or more cesarean deliveries with anterior or central placenta previa have nearly a 40% risk of developing placenta accreta. In the presence of any of these conditions, the obstetric care provider must have a high clinical suspicion for placenta accreta and take appropriate precautions.

Ultrasonography may be helpful to make the diagnosis in the antepartum period. Mounting evidence suggests that magnetic resonance imaging and color Doppler studies also may be useful to define an abnormally implanted placenta (4), although, at this time no diagnostic technique affords the clinician 100% assurance of either ruling in or ruling out the presence of placenta accreta.

If the diagnosis or a strong suspicion is formed before delivery:

- The patient should be counseled about the likelihood of hysterectomy and blood transfusion.
- Blood products and clotting factors should be available.
- Cell saver technology should be considered if available.
- The appropriate location and timing for delivery should be considered to allow access to adequate surgical personnel and equipment.
- A preoperative anesthesia assessment should be obtained.

Profuse hemorrhage can occur when attempting to separate the placenta. If the clinician is extremely confident in the diagnosis, it may be prudent to complete the delivery of the infant and proceed with hysterectomy while the placenta remains attached (3, 5). Profuse hemorrhage after vaginal delivery also may be due to placenta accreta. In this instance, selective pelvic vessel embolization may be an alternative to hysterectomy, or this procedure may decrease blood loss before or after hysterectomy (6).

References

1. O'Brien JM, Barton JR, Donaldson ES. The management of placenta percreta: conservative and operative strategies. Am J Obstet Gynecol 1996;175:1632–1638
2. Miller DA, Chollet JA, Goodwin TM. Clinical risk factors for placenta previa-placenta accreta. Am J Obstet Gynecol 1997;177:210–214
3. Clark SL, Koonings PP, Phelan JP. Placenta previa/accreta and prior cesarean section. Obstet Gynecol 1985;66:89–92
4. Kirkinen P, Helin-Martikainen HL, Vanninen R, Partanen K. Placental accreta: imaging by gray-scale and contrast-enhanced color Doppler sonography and magnetic resonance imaging. J Clin Ultrasound 1998;26:90–94
5. Resnik R. Diagnosis and management of placenta accreta. ACOG Clin Rev 1999;4(2):8–9
6. Clark SL, Phelan JP, Yeh SY, Bruce SR, Paul RH. Hypogastric artery ligation for obstetric hemorrhage. Obstet Gynecol 1985;66:353–356

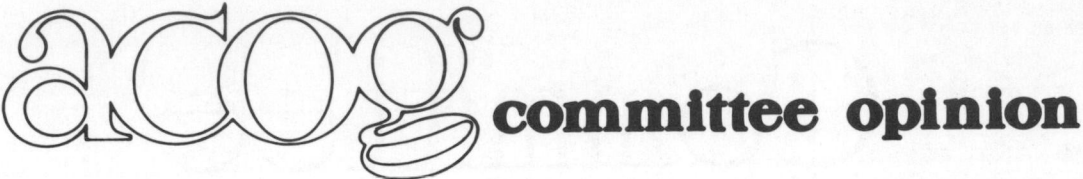

committee opinion

Committee on Obstetrics: Maternal and Fetal Medicine

Number 125—July 1993
(Replaces #102, December 1991)

Placental Pathology

Recently, there has been heightened interest in clinical–pathologic correlation between placental abnormalities and adverse pregnancy outcome. When a skilled and systematic examination of the umbilical cord, membranes, and placenta is performed on properly prepared specimens, insight into antepartum pathophysiology may be gained under certain circumstances.

In most of these instances, such as chorioamnionitis, the diagnosis already will have been made on clinical grounds, with the placental examination providing confirmation. In other cases of poor outcome, a disorder that was not suspected clinically may be revealed by placental pathology. Examples of pathologic findings and the disorders they suggest include the microabscesses of listeriosis and amnion nodosum suggesting long-standing oligohydramnios. The underlying pathophysiology of these lesions has been confirmed by laboratory testing or consistent and specific clinical associations.

The significance of other findings, such as villous edema, hemorrhagic endovasculitis, and chronic villitis, has not been as well delineated. These lesions, among others, have been variously reported to correlate with poor short-term and long-term neonatal outcome. The paucity of properly designed studies of adequate size with appropriate outcome parameters has prevented universal agreement as to positive predictive values, underlying pathophysiology, or even the consistency of clinical correlations with these findings. Furthermore, the distribution of pathologists with the expertise to interpret more subtle placental findings is uneven from region to region. Although a protocol for obtaining routine placental pathologic examination under certain obstetric and neonatal conditions has been recommended (1), there are few data to support the clinical utility of this approach.

In addition to the issue of positive and negative predictive values of the spectrum of placental findings, there are practical concerns regarding examination of the placenta. In some instances, a neonatal problem may not be ascertained until days or weeks after birth, when the placenta is no longer available. Different approaches have been recommended to address this problem, including routinely examining all placentas, securing a small section from each placenta in a fixed state for an indefinite period, and saving all placentas unfixed at 4°C for 1 week before discarding. However, routine determinations of placental pathology are not feasible on either a cost or manpower basis, and a small portion of placenta obtained at random would be unlikely to provide useful information. The practice of saving all placentas for 1 week after delivery would permit ascertaining most neonatal problems in which pathologic examination of the placenta may be appropriate, but the effectiveness of this approach has not been proven.

In conclusion, an examination of the umbilical cord, membranes, and placenta may assist the obstetric care provider in clinical–pathologic correlation when there is an adverse perinatal outcome. However, the scientific basis for clinical correlation with placental pathology is still evolving, and the benefit of securing specimens on a routine basis is as yet unproven. Continued research and education in this field should be encouraged. Research should be designed with the goal of defining clinical indications for placental examination. In contrast, pathologic examination of the stillborn fetus and placenta is always potentially informative. Obstetric providers should be persistent in seeking consent from parents for autopsy examinations.

REFERENCE

1. College of American Pathologists Conference XIX. The examination of the placenta: patient care and risk management. Arch Pathol Lab Med 1991;115: 641–732

The American College of Obstetricians and Gynecologists
409 12th Street, SW • Washington, DC 20024-2188

12345/76543

ACOG

Committee on
Obstetric Practice

Committee Opinion

Number 304, November 2004

The American College of Obstetricians and Gynecologists
409 12th Street, SW
PO Box 96920
Washington, DC 20090-6920

12345/87654

Prenatal and perinatal human immunodeficiency virus testing: expanded recommendations. ACOG Committee Opinion No. 304. American College of Obstetricians and Gynecologists. Obstet Gynecol 2004;104:1119–24.

Prenatal and Perinatal Human Immunodeficiency Virus Testing: Expanded Recommendations

ABSTRACT: Early identification and treatment of all pregnant women with human immunodeficiency virus (HIV) is the best way to prevent neonatal disease. Pregnant women universally should be tested for HIV infection with patient notification as part of the routine battery of prenatal blood tests unless they decline the test (ie, opt-out approach). Repeat testing in the third trimester and rapid HIV testing at labor and delivery are additional strategies to further reduce the rate of perinatal HIV transmission. The Committee on Obstetric Practice makes the following recommendations: follow an opt-out prenatal HIV testing approach where legally possible; repeat offer of HIV testing in the third trimester to women in areas with high HIV prevalence, women known to be at high risk for HIV infection, and women who declined testing earlier in pregnancy, as allowed by state laws and regulations; use conventional HIV testing for women who are candidates for third-trimester testing; use rapid HIV testing in labor for women with undocumented HIV status; and if a rapid HIV test result is positive, initiate antiretroviral prophylaxis (with consent) without waiting for the results of the confirmatory test.

The Centers for Disease Control and Prevention (CDC) estimates that 40,000 new human immunodeficiency virus (HIV) infections still occur in the United States each year (1). This figure includes approximately 300 infants infected via mother to child (vertical) transmission (2). Antiretroviral medications given to women with HIV perinatally and to their newborns in the first weeks of life reduce the vertical transmission rate from 25% to 2% or less (3–6). Even instituting maternal prophylaxis during labor and delivery or neonatal prophylaxis within 24–48 hours of delivery can substantially decrease rates of infection in infants (4). A retrospective review of HIV-exposed infants in New York State showed a transmission rate of approximately 10% when zidovudine prophylaxis was begun intrapartum and for newborns up to 48 hours of life (4). However, when neonatal prophylaxis was begun on day 3 of life or later, the transmission rate was 18.4% compared with 26.6% in the absence of any prophylaxis. Early identification and treatment of pregnant women and treatment of newborns in the first hours of life are essential to prevent neonatal disease.

Prenatal Approaches to Offering Human Immunodeficiency Virus Testing: Opt-In Versus Opt-Out

Variations of 2 prenatal HIV testing strategies are being practiced by obstetric providers in the United States. The opt-in approach is the strategy that requires specific informed consent, usually in writing, and is the foundation for most state laws and regulations in effect today.

The opt-out approach is the strategy in which universal HIV testing with patient notification is a routine component of prenatal care. A pregnant woman is notified that she will be tested for HIV as part of the routine battery of prenatal blood tests unless she declines. If a patient declines HIV testing, this should be noted in the medical record. The use of patient notification provides women the opportunity to decline testing but eliminates the requirement to obtain specific informed consent. Although no states currently have adopted an opt-out approach as defined previously, some states have adopted variations of this approach and others are reviewing the opt-out approach.

The opt-out approach is associated with greater testing rates than the opt-in approach. Medical record surveys, laboratory data, and population-based surveys (1998–2001) report 85% to 98% HIV testing rates in surveyed areas using the opt-out approach, compared with testing rates ranging from 25% to 83% in surveyed areas using the opt-in approach (7). Based on these data, in 2003 the CDC revised its guidelines to recommend the opt-out approach (8). Additionally, the CDC recommends that jurisdictions with statutory barriers to such routine prenatal screening consider revising them.* The American College of Obstetricians and Gynecologists, the American Academy of Pediatrics (9), and the CDC recommend the opt-out approach (8, 9).

Physicians should be aware of and follow their states' prenatal HIV screening requirements. Specific prenatal HIV screening requirements may be verified by contacting state or local public health departments.

---

*Gerberding JL, Jaffe HW. Dear colleague letter from CDC and NCHSTP directors on HIV testing. Atlanta (GA): Centers for Disease Control and Prevention; 2003. Available at: http://www.cdc.gov/hiv/rapid_testing/rt-appendix_a.htm. Retrieved June 30, 2004.

Conventional Prenatal Human Immunodeficiency Virus Testing

The conventional HIV testing algorithm, which generally takes up to 2 weeks to process, begins with a screening test, the enzyme-linked immunosorbent assay (ELISA), that detects antibodies to HIV; if the results are positive, it is followed by a confirmatory test, either a Western blot or an immunofluorescence assay (IFA). A positive ELISA test result is not diagnostic of HIV infection unless confirmed by the Western blot or IFA. The sensitivity and specificity of ELISA with a confirmatory Western blot test are greater than 99%. The false-positive rate for ELISA with a confirmatory Western blot test is 1 in 59,000 tests. If the ELISA test result is positive and the Western blot or IFA test result is negative, the patient is not infected and repeat testing is not indicated.

If the ELISA test result is repeatedly positive and the Western blot result contains some but not all of the viral bands required to make a definitive diagnosis, the test result is labeled indeterminate. Most patients with indeterminate test results are not infected with HIV. However, consultation with a provider well versed in HIV infection is recommended. This specialist may suggest viral load testing or repeat testing later in pregnancy to rule out the possibility of recent infection.

If the screening (eg, ELISA) and confirmatory (eg, Western blot or IFA) test results are both positive, the patient should be given her results in person. The implications of HIV infection and vertical transmission should be discussed with the patient. Additional laboratory evaluation, including CD4 count, HIV viral load, hepatitis C virus antibody, complete blood count with platelet count, and baseline chemistries with liver function tests, will be useful before prescribing antiretroviral prophylaxis. Consultation with a provider well versed in HIV infection is recommended.

Repeat Human Immunodeficiency Virus Testing in the Third Trimester

Routine universal repeat testing in the third trimester may be considered in health care facilities in areas with high HIV prevalence among women of childbearing age (ie, 5 per 1,000 or 0.5% or greater). Additionally, although physicians need to be aware of and follow their states' perinatal HIV screening guidelines, repeat testing in the third trimester, preferably before 36 weeks of gestation, is recommended for pregnant women at high risk for acquiring HIV (10). Criteria for repeat testing can include:

- A history of a sexually transmitted disease
- Illicit drug use or the exchange of sex for money or drugs
- Multiple sex partners during pregnancy or a sex partner(s) known to be HIV-positive or at high risk
- Signs or symptoms suggestive of acute HIV infection at any time during pregnancy

Women who are candidates for third-trimester testing, including those who previously declined testing earlier in pregnancy, should be given a conventional HIV test rather than waiting to receive a rapid test at labor and delivery as allowed by state laws and regulations.

Rapid Human Immunodeficiency Virus Testing

Rapid HIV testing can be used to identify HIV infection in women who arrive at labor and delivery with undocumented HIV status and to provide an opportunity to begin prophylaxis of previously undiagnosed infection before delivery. A negative rapid HIV test result is definitive. A positive HIV test result is not definitive and must be confirmed with a supplemental test, such as a Western blot or IFA (11); however, antiretroviral prophylaxis should be initiated (with consent) without waiting for the results of the confirmatory test to further reduce possible transmission to the infant.

A rapid HIV test is an HIV screening test with results available within hours. Data from several studies indicate that 40–85% (11–14) of infants infected with HIV are born to women whose HIV infection is unknown to their obstetric provider before delivery. Some of these women have had no opportunity to learn their HIV status before labor, and recent data suggest that knowledge of HIV status, even if only obtained in labor, will allow the use of therapies that may reduce rates of vertical transmission. If a rapid test is used in labor and HIV antibodies are detected, the pregnant woman should be encouraged to start antiretroviral prophylaxis. Recommendations for the use of antiretroviral med-

ications in pregnant women infected with HIV-1 are available at http://www.aidsinfo.nih.gov/guidelines/perinatal/PER_062304.html and are updated frequently (15). In some cases, cesarean delivery may provide additional protection against vertical HIV transmission; however, once labor has begun or rupture of membranes has occurred, the utility of cesarean delivery is unknown.

When selecting a rapid HIV test for use during labor and delivery, it is important to consider the accuracy of the test and the site where testing will be performed. Tests that require serum or plasma (eg, Reveal) are more suitable for use in the laboratory, whereas tests that can be performed with whole blood (eg, OraQuick, Uni-Gold) without specimen processing can be performed more easily in the labor and delivery unit (11). Performance evaluations on 3 U.S. Food and Drug Administration (FDA)-approved rapid HIV tests (OraQuick, Reveal, and Uni-Gold) indicate a sensitivity of 100%, 99.8%, and 100% (95% confidence interval), respectively, and a specificity of 99.9%, 99.1% (serum), and 99.7% (95% confidence interval), respectively (11, 16) (Table 1).

The CDC-sponsored Mother-Infant Rapid Intervention at Delivery (MIRIAD) Study Group examined the use of rapid testing using OraQuick or enzyme immunoassay (EIA) in 4,849 prenatal patients with unknown HIV status in a multistate hospital study (16). Human immunodeficiency virus-1 test results were positive for 34 women (HIV prevalence 7/1,000). Data from that study showed a sensitivity for OraQuick of 100% and a specificity of 99.9% with a positive predictive value of 90% compared with 76% for EIA. Offering rapid HIV testing during labor is feasible in obstetric settings, and the OraQuick Rapid HIV-1 Antibody Test, used on whole blood specimens, delivers accurate and timely (20–40 minutes) test results (11).

As with all screening tests before confirmation, the likelihood of a false-positive result is higher in populations with low HIV prevalence when compared with populations with high HIV prevalence. Additionally, at present it is not known how the false-positive rate for rapid testing will compare with the false-positive rate for conventional testing. Available calculated comparisons of the positive predictive values of 3 FDA-approved rapid HIV-1 antibody tests (OraQuick, Reveal, and Uni-Gold) and for the HIV-1 EIA in populations with differing HIV prevalence rates are shown in Table 1.

If the rapid HIV test result is positive, the obstetric provider should take the following steps:

1. Tell the woman she may have HIV infection and that her neonate also may be exposed

2. Explain that the rapid test result is preliminary and that false-positive results are possible

3. Assure the woman that a second test is being done right away to confirm the positive rapid test result

4. Initiate (with consent) antiretroviral prophylaxis without waiting for the results of the confirmatory test to reduce the risk of transmission to the infant

5. Tell the woman that she should postpone breastfeeding until the confirmatory result is available because she should not breastfeed if she is infected with HIV

6. Inform pediatric colleagues of positive maternal test results, as allowed by federal and state privacy laws, so that they may institute the appropriate neonatal prophylaxis

If the results of the rapid test and the confirmatory test are discrepant, both tests should be repeated and consultation with an infectious disease specialist is recommended. Additionally, all antiretroviral prophylaxis should be stopped if the confirmatory test result is negative (11).

Oral fluid based rapid HIV testing (OraQuick Rapid HIV-1/2 Antibody Test) is now available. This may be another option for perinatal testing in the future (see http://www.cdc.gov/hiv and http://www.fda.gov/cber/pma/p01004710.htm).

Recommendations

Given the enormous advances in HIV prophylaxis for pregnant women and newborns, it is clear that early identification and treatment of all pregnant women with HIV is the best way to prevent neona-

Table 1. Estimated Positive Predictive Value of a Single Screening Test for Human Immunodeficiency Virus in Populations With Differing Human Immunodeficiency Virus Prevalence*

Human Immunodeficiency Virus Prevalence (%)	Estimated Positive Predictive Value (%)			
	OraQuick† (blood) (CLIA-waived)	Reveal† (serum) (CLIA-moderate complexity)	Uni-Gold† (blood) (CLIA-moderate complexity)	Single Enzyme Immunoassay (EIA) (CLIA-high complexity)
10	99	92	97	98
5	98	85	95	96
2	95	69	87	91
1	91	53	77	83
0.5	83	36	63	71
0.3	75	25	50	60
0.1	50	10	25	33
Test sensitivity (95% CI)	100	99.8	100	—
Test specificity (95% CI)	99.9	99.1	99.7	99.8

Abbreviation: CI, confidence interval; CLIA, Clinical Laboratory Improvement Act.

*Based on point estimate for specificity from the Mother-Infant Rapid Intervention at Delivery study for OraQuick and enzyme immunoassay (Bulterys M, Jamieson DJ, O'Sullivan MJ, Cohen MH, Maupin R, Nesheim S, et al. Rapid HIV-1 testing during labor: a multicenter study. Mother-Infant Rapid Intervention at Delivery (MIRIAD) Study Group. JAMA 2004;292:219–23.) and from the U.S. Food and Drug Administration summary basis of approval for the other tests (Rapid HIV antibody testing during labor and delivery for women of unknown HIV status: a practical guide and model protocol. Centers for Disease Control and Prevention. Atlanta (GA): CDC; 2004. Available at: http://www.cdc.gov/hiv/rapid/testing/materials/Labor&DeliveryRapidTesting.pdf.). In practice, the specificity and actual positive predictive value may differ from these estimates.

†Trade names are for identification purposes only and do not imply endorsement by the U.S. Department of Health and Human Services, the Centers for Disease Control and Prevention, or the American College of Obstetricians and Gynecologists.

Modified from Rapid HIV antibody testing during labor and delivery for women of unknown HIV status: a practical guide and model protocol. Centers for Disease Control and Prevention. Atlanta (GA): CDC; 2004.

tal disease. Pregnant women universally should be tested for HIV infection with patient notification as part of the routine battery of prenatal blood tests unless they decline the test (opt-out approach). The American College of Obstetricians and Gynecologists, the American Academy of Pediatrics, and the CDC[†] recommend the opt-out approach (8, 9). There are encouraging results from the MIRIAD Study Group (16) and other evidence (3–6, 11) to suggest that antiretroviral prophylaxis started in labor and delivery and for the infant in the first hours of life also can substantially reduce vertical transmission of the HIV virus. Therefore, the Committee on Obstetric Practice makes the following recommendations:

- Follow an opt-out prenatal HIV testing approach where legally possible

- Repeat offer of HIV testing in the third trimester to women in areas with high HIV prevalence, women known to be at high risk for HIV infection, and women who declined testing earlier in pregnancy, as allowed by state laws and regulations

- Use conventional HIV testing for women who are candidates for third-trimester testing

- Use rapid HIV testing in labor for women with undocumented HIV status

- If a rapid HIV test result is positive, initiate antiretroviral prophylaxis (with consent) without waiting for the results of the confirmatory test

References

1. HIV/AIDS update: a glance at the HIV epidemic. Atlanta (GA): Centers for Disease Control and Prevention. Available at: http://www.cdc.gov/nchstp/od/news/At-a-Glance.pdf. Retrieved June 22, 2004.
2. Centers for Disease Control and Prevention. HIV/AIDS Surveillance Report 2002;14:1–40. Available at: http://www.cdc.gov/hiv/stats/hasr1402/2002surveillance Report.pdf. Retrieved June 24, 2004.
3. Recommendations of the U.S. Public Health Service Task Force on the use of zidovudine to reduce perinatal transmission of human immunodeficiency virus. MMWR Recomm Rep 1994;43(RR-11):1–20.

[†]Gerberding JL, Jaffe HW. Dear colleague letter from CDC and NCHSTP directors on HIV testing. Atlanta (GA): Centers for Disease Control and Prevention; 2003. Available at: http://www.cdc.gov/hiv/rapid_testing/rt-appendix_a.htm. Retrieved June 30, 2004.

4. Wade NA, Birkhead GS, Warren BL, Charbonneau TT, French PT, Wang L, et al. Abbreviated regimens of zidovudine prophylaxis and perinatal transmission of human immunodeficiency virus. N Engl J Med 1998;339:1409–14.
5. Mofenson LM, Lambert JS, Stiehm ER, Bethel J, Meyer WA 3rd, Whitehouse J, et al. Risk factors for perinatal transmission of human immunodeficiency virus type 1 in women treated with zidovudine. Pediatric AIDS Clinical Trials Group Study 185 Team. N Engl J Med 1999;341:385–93.
6. Garcia PM, Kalish LA, Pitt J, Minkoff H, Quinn TC, Burchett SK, et al. Maternal levels of plasma human immunodeficiency virus type 1 RNA and the risk of perinatal transmission. Women and Infants Transmission Study Group. N Engl J Med 1999;341:394–402.
7. HIV testing among pregnant women—United States and Canada, 1998–2001. MMWR Morb Mortal Wkly Rep 2002;51:1013–6.
8. Advancing HIV prevention: new strategies for a changing epidemic—United States, 2003. MMWR Morb Mortal Wkly Rep 2003;52:329–32.
9. American Academy of Pediatrics, American College of Obstetricians and Gynecologists. Joint statement on human immunodeficiency virus screening. ACOG Policy Statement 75. Elk Grove Village (IL): AAP; Washington, DC: ACOG; 1999.
10. Revised recommendations for HIV screening of pregnant women. Centers for Disease Control and Prevention. MMWR Recomm Rep 2001;50(RR-19):63–85; quiz CE1-19a2–CE6-19a2.
11. Rapid HIV antibody testing during labor and delivery for women of unknown HIV status: a practical guide and model protocol. Centers for Disease Control and Prevention. Atlanta (GA): CDC; 2004. Available at: http://www.cdc.gov/hiv/rapid/testing/materials/Labor&DeliveryRapidTesting.pdf.
12. Peters V, Liu KL, Dominguez K, Frederick T, Melville S, Hsu H, et al. Missed opportunities for perinatal HIV prevention among HIV-exposed infants born 1996–2000, pediatric spectrum of HIV disease cohort. Pediatrics 2003;111:1186–91.
13. Gross E, Burr CK. HIV counseling and testing in pregnancy. N J Med 2003;100 (suppl):21–6; quiz 67–8.
14. Paul SM, Grimes-Dennis J, Burr CK, DiFerdinando GT. Rapid diagnostic testing for HIV. Clinical indications. N J Med 2002;99:20–4; quiz 24–6.
15. Recommendations for use of antiretroviral drugs in pregnant HIV-infected women for maternal health and interventions to reduce perinatal HIV-1 transmission in the United States. Public Health Service Task Force. Rockville (MD): U.S. Department of Health and Human Services. Available at: http://www.aidsinfo.nih.gov/guidelines/perinatal/PER_062304.html. Retrieved July 16, 2004.
16. Bulterys M, Jamieson DJ, O'Sullivan MJ, Cohen MH, Maupin R, Nesheim S, et al. Rapid HIV-1 testing during labor: a multicenter study. Mother-Infant Rapid Intervention at Delivery (MIRIAD) Study Group. JAMA 2004;292:219–23.

Resources

Publications

American College of Obstetricians and Gynecologists. Scheduled cesarean delivery and the prevention of vertical transmission of HIV infection. ACOG Committee Opinion 234. Washington, DC: ACOG; 2000.

Institute of Medicine (US). Reducing the odds: preventing perinatal transmission of HIV in the United States. Washington, DC: The Institute; 1999.

Organizations

American College of Obstetricians and Gynecologists (http://www.acog.org; http://sales.acog.org)

CDC Division of HIV/AIDS Prevention: (404) 639-0900

Centers for Disease Control and Prevention (http://www.cdc.gov/hiv)

National AIDS Hotline: 800-342-AIDS (2437) (English); 800-344-7432 (Spanish); 800-243-7889 (TTY)

National HIV Telephone Consultation Service (for physician consultation only): 800-933-3413

State public health departments

ACOG

Committee on
Genetics

Committee Opinion

Number 298, August 2004

The American College of Obstetricians and Gynecologists
409 12th Street, SW
PO Box 96920
Washington, DC 20090-6920

12345/87654

Prenatal and preconceptional carrier screening for genetic diseases in individuals of Eastern European Jewish descent. ACOG Committee Opinion No. 298. American College of Obstetricians and Gynecologists. Obstet Gynecol 2004;104:425–8.

Prenatal and Preconceptional Carrier Screening for Genetic Diseases in Individuals of Eastern European Jewish Descent

ABSTRACT: Certain autosomal recessive disease conditions are more prevalent in individuals of Eastern European Jewish (Ashkenazi) descent. Previously, the American College of Obstetricians and Gynecologists recommended that individuals of Eastern European Jewish ancestry be offered carrier screening for Tay–Sachs disease, Canavan disease, and cystic fibrosis as part of routine obstetric care. Based on the criteria used to justify offering carrier screening for Tay–Sachs disease, Canavan disease, and cystic fibrosis, the American College of Obstetricians and Gynecologists' Committee on Genetics recommends that couples of Ashkenazi Jewish ancestry also should be offered carrier screening for familial dysautonomia. Individuals of Ashkenazi Jewish descent may inquire about the availability of carrier screening for other disorders. Carrier screening is available for mucolipidosis IV, Niemann-Pick disease type A, Fanconi anemia group C, Bloom syndrome, and Gaucher's disease.

Carrier screening for specific genetic conditions often is determined by an individual's ancestry. Certain autosomal recessive disease conditions are more prevalent in individuals of Eastern European Jewish (Ashkenazi) descent. Most individuals of Jewish ancestry in North America are descended from Ashkenazi Jewish communities and, thus, are at increased risk for having offspring with one of these conditions. Many of these disorders are lethal in childhood or associated with significant morbidity.

Tay–Sachs disease (TSD) was one of the first disorders amenable to carrier screening. As a result of carrier screening programs established in the 1970s, the incidence of TSD in the North American Ashkenazi Jewish population has decreased by more than 90%. Carrier screening also is recommended for individuals of French Canadian and Cajun descent. Initially, carrier screening was based on the measurement of hexosaminidase A levels (the enzyme deficient in TSD) in serum or leukocytes. As the genes for TSD and other diseases more prevalent in Ashkenazi Jews were identified, DNA carrier tests have been developed. Because each of these disorders is caused by a small number of common mutations, the carrier tests are very sensitive (94–99% detection rates). Previously, the American College of Obstetricians and Gynecologists (ACOG) recommended that individuals of Eastern European Jewish ancestry be offered carrier screening for TSD, Canavan disease, and cystic fibrosis as part of routine obstetric care. Because of recent advances in genetics, additional carrier tests are now available (Table 1).

In 2001, the gene for familial dysautonomia was identified. At least 2 mutations in the familial dysautonomia gene, *IKBKAP*, have been identified in patients with familial dysautonomia of Ashkenazi Jewish descent. One of the mutations (IVS20$^{+6T \rightarrow C}$) is found in more than 99% of patients with familial dysautonomia. It occurs almost exclusively in individuals of Ashkenazi Jewish descent; the carrier rate (1 in 32) is similar to TSD and cystic fibrosis. Familial dysautonomia, a disorder of the sensory and autonomic nervous system, is associated with significant morbidity. Clinical features include abnormal suck and feeding difficulties, episodic vomiting, abnormal sweating, pain and temperature insensitivity, labile blood pressure levels, absent tearing, and scoliosis. Treatment is available, which can improve the length and quality of life, but there currently is no cure. Based on the criteria used to justify offering carrier screening for TSD, Canavan disease, and cystic fibrosis, the ACOG Committee on Genetics recommends that couples of Ashkenazi Jewish ancestry also should be offered carrier screening for familial dysautonomia.

Carrier screening tests are available for several diseases that are less common (carrier rates 1 in 89 to 1 in 127), including Fanconi anemia group C, Niemann-Pick disease type A, Bloom syndrome, and mucolipidosis IV. These conditions are associated with significant neurologic or medical problems and very limited treatment options (see box). Carrier screening also is available for Gaucher's disease, the most common disorder in Eastern European Jews. Although Gaucher's disease affects 1 in 900 individuals, the age of onset (from a few months to 90 years) and severity are variable (see box). Gaucher's disease can be very mild, and treatment is available.

All of these tests have a high sensitivity in the Jewish population. The prevalence of these disorders in non-Jewish populations, except for TSD and cystic fibrosis, is unknown. The sensitivity of these carrier tests in non-Jewish populations has not been established. The mutations may be different and more diverse. Consequently, when only 1 partner is Jewish, it is difficult to assess the risk of having an affected offspring. Therefore, carrier screening of the non-Jewish partner is of limited value.

Based on these recent developments, the ACOG Committee on Genetics makes the following 7 recommendations:

1. The family history of individuals considering pregnancy, or who are already pregnant, should determine whether either member of the couple is of Eastern European (Ashkenazi) Jewish ancestry or has a relative with 1 or more of the genetic conditions listed in Table 1.

Table 1. Recessive Genetic Diseases Frequent Among Individuals of Eastern European Jewish Descent Amenable to Carrier Screening

Disorder	Disease Incidence	Carrier Frequency*	Detection rate*
Tay–Sachs disease	1/3,000	1/30	98% by Hex-A test, 94% by DNA-based test
Canavan disease	1/6,400	1/40	98%
Cystic fibrosis	1/2,500–3,000	1/29	97%
Familial dysautonomia	1/3,600	1/32	99%
Fanconi anemia group C	1/32,000	1/89	99%
Niemann-Pick disease type A	1/32,000	1/90	95%
Mucolipidosis IV	1/62,500	1/127	95%
Bloom syndrome	1/40,000	1/100	95–97%
Gaucher's disease	1/900	1/15	95%

*Non-Jewish carrier frequency and detection rates are unknown except for Tay–Sachs disease. Carrier frequency for Tay–Sachs disease is 1 in 30 if French Canadian or Cajun ancestry and 1 in 300 for others with a 98% carrier detection rate by Hex-A test.

Modified from March of Dimes. Genetic screening pocket facts. White Plains (NY): MOD; 2001.

2. Carrier screening for TSD, Canavan disease, cystic fibrosis, and familial dysautonomia should be offered to Ashkenazi Jewish individuals before conception or during early pregnancy so that a couple has an opportunity to consider prenatal diagnostic testing options. If the woman is already pregnant, it may be necessary to screen both partners simultaneously so that the results are obtained in a timely fashion to ensure that prenatal diagnostic testing is an option.

3. Individuals of Ashkenazi Jewish descent may inquire about the availability of carrier screening for other disorders. Carrier screening is available for mucolipidosis IV, Niemann-Pick disease type A, Fanconi anemia group C, Bloom syndrome, and Gaucher's disease. Patient edu-

cation materials can be made available so that interested patients can make an informed decision about having additional screening tests (see box). Some patients may benefit from genetic counseling.

4. When only 1 partner is of Ashkenazi Jewish descent, that individual should be screened first. If it is determined that this individual is a carrier, the other partner should be offered screening. However, the couple should be informed that the carrier frequency and the detection rate in non-Jewish individuals is unknown for all of these disorders, except for TSD and cystic fibrosis. Therefore, it is difficult to accurately predict the couple's risk of having a child with the disorder.

5. Individuals with a positive family history of 1 of these disorders should be offered carrier screen-

---

Clinical Features of Autosomal Recessive Genetic Diseases Frequent Among Individuals of Eastern European Jewish Descent

Bloom syndrome is a genetic condition associated with increased chromosome breakage, a predisposition to infections and malignancies, prenatal and postnatal growth deficiency, skin findings (such as facial telangiectasias, abnormal pigmentation), and in some cases learning difficulties and mental retardation. The mean age of death is 27 years and usually is related to cancer. No effective treatment currently is available.

Canavan disease is a disorder of the central nervous system characterized by developmental delay, hypotonia, large head, seizures, blindness, and gastrointestinal reflux. Most children die within the first several years of life. Canavan disease is caused by a deficiency of the aspartoacylase enzyme. No treatment currently is available.

Familial dysautonomia is a neurologic disorder characterized by abnormal suck and feeding difficulties, episodic vomiting, abnormal sweating, pain and temperature insensitivity, labile blood pressure levels, absent tearing, and scoliosis. There currently is no cure for familial dysautonomia, but some treatments are available that can improve the length and quality of a patient's life.

Fanconi anemia group C usually presents with severe anemia that progresses to pancytopenia, developmental delay, and failure to thrive. Congenital anomalies are not uncommon, including limb, cardiac, and genital–urinary defects. Microcephaly and mental retardation may be present. Children are at increased risk for leukemia. Some children have been successfully treated with bone marrow transplantation. Life expectancy is 8–12 years.

Gaucher's disease is a genetic disorder that mainly affects the spleen, liver, and bones; it occasionally affects the lungs, kidneys, and brain. It may develop at any age. Some individuals are chronically ill, some are moderately affected, and

others are so mildly affected that they may not know that they have Gaucher's disease. The most common symptom is chronic fatigue caused by anemia. Patients may experience easy bruising, nosebleeds, bleeding gums, and prolonged and heavy bleeding with their menses and after childbirth. Other symptoms include an enlarged liver and spleen, osteoporosis, and bone and joint pain. Gaucher's disease is caused by the deficiency of the β-glucosidase enzyme. Treatment is available through enzyme therapy, which results in a vastly improved quality of life.

Mucolipidosis IV is a neurodegenerative lysosomal storage disorder characterized by growth and psychomotor retardation, corneal clouding, progressive retinal degeneration, and strabismus. Most affected infants never speak, walk, or develop beyond the level of a 1–2 year old. Life expectancy may be normal, and there currently is no effective treatment.

Niemann-Pick disease type A is a lysosomal storage disorder typically diagnosed in infancy and marked by a rapid neurodegenerative course similar to Tay–Sachs disease. Affected children die by age 3–5 years. Niemann-Pick disease type A is caused by a deficiency of the sphingomyelinase enzyme. There currently is no treatment.

Tay–Sachs disease (TSD) is a severe, progressive disorder of the central nervous system leading to death within the first few years of life. Infants with TSD appear normal at birth but by age 5–6 months develop poor muscle tone, delayed development, loss of developmental milestones, and mental retardation. Children with TSD lose their eyesight at age 12–18 months. This condition usually is fatal by age 6 years. Tay–Sachs disease is caused by a deficiency of the hexosaminidase A enzyme. No effective treatment currently is available.

ing for the specific disorder and may benefit from genetic counseling.

6. When both partners are carriers of 1 of these disorders, they should be referred for genetic counseling and offered prenatal diagnosis. Carrier couples should be informed of the disease manifestations, range of severity, and available treatment options. Prenatal diagnosis by DNA-based testing can be performed on cells obtained by chorionic villus sampling or amniocentesis.

7. When an individual is found to be a carrier, his or her relatives are at risk for carrying the same mutation. The patient should be encouraged to inform his or her relatives of the risk and the availability of carrier screening. The provider does not need to contact these relatives because there is no provider–patient relationship with the relatives, and confidentiality must be maintained.

Carrier screening is voluntary. Informed consent and assurance of confidentiality are required. For all of these disorders, a negative screening test result for 1 or both partners significantly reduces the possibility of an affected offspring. However, it does not exclude it because the test sensitivity is less than 100% so not all carriers can be identified.

The number and choice of genetic tests available to patients is likely to increase as a result of the Human Genome Project and advances in technology. For some patients, it can be difficult to decide whether to have a specific test. There are many factors patients may consider, including the prevalence of the disease, the carrier risk, the disease severity and treatment options, cost, and reproductive choices. Counseling by a genetic counselor, geneticist, or physician with expertise in these diseases may assist patients in making an informed decision about carrier testing.

Bibliography

American College of Obstetricians and Gynecologists. Screening for Canavan disease. ACOG Committee Opinion 212. Washington, DC: ACOG, 1998.

American College of Obstetricians and Gynecologists. Screening for Tay–Sachs disease. ACOG Committee Opinion 162. Washington, DC: ACOG, 1995.

Dong J, Edelmann L, Bajwa AM, Kornreich R, Desnick RJ. Familial dysautonomia: detection of the IKBKAP IVS20 (+6T→C) and R696P mutations and frequencies among Ashkenazi Jews. Am J Med Genet 2002;110:253–7.

Eng CM, Desnick RJ. Experiences in molecular-based prenatal screening for Ashkenazi Jewish genetic diseases. Adv Genet 2001;44:275–96.

Zlotogora J, Bach G, Munnich A. Molecular basis of mendelian disorders among Jews. Mol Genet Metab 2000; 69:169–80.

ACOG

Committee on
Obstetric Practice

Committee Opinion

Number 279, December 2002   *(Replaces No. 173, June 1996)*

The American College of Obstetricians and Gynecologists
409 12th Street, SW
PO Box 96920
Washington, DC 20090-6920

12345/65432

Prevention of early-onset group B streptococcal disease in newborns. ACOG Committee Opinion No. 279. American College of Obstetricians and Gynecologists. Obstet Gynecol 2002;100:1405–12.

Prevention of Early-Onset Group B Streptococcal Disease in Newborns

ABSTRACT: During the past two decades, group B streptococci (GBS), or Streptococcus agalactiae, *has emerged as an important cause of perinatal morbidity and mortality. Intrapartum administration of antibiotics to the woman (during labor or after rupture of membranes, but before delivery) has been demonstrated to reduce early-onset neonatal GBS disease. In 1996, the federal Centers for Disease Control and Prevention (CDC), the American College of Obstetricians and Gynecologists, and the American Academy of Pediatrics recommended that obstetric providers adopt either a culture-based or a risk-based approach for the prevention of early-onset GBS. A recent multistate retrospective cohort study of live births in 1998 and 1999 of residents from eight areas of the Active Bacterial Core Surveillance/Emerging Infections Program network suggests that the culture-based approach is superior to the risk-based approach. The Committee on Obstetric Practice supports the new CDC recommendations that obstetric providers adopt a culture-based strategy for the prevention of early-onset GBS disease in the newborn. It is important to acknowledge that complete implementation of this complex strategy will not eliminate all cases of early-onset GBS.*

During the past two decades, group B streptococci (GBS), or *Streptococcus agalactiae*, has emerged as an important cause of perinatal morbidity and mortality (1, 2). The gram-positive organism can colonize the lower gastrointestinal tract, and secondary spread to the genitourinary tract is common. Between 10% and 30% of pregnant women are colonized with GBS in the vagina or rectum (3–6). The organism may cause urinary tract infection, amnionitis, endometritis, sepsis, or, rarely, meningitis (7–12).

Vertical transmission of GBS during labor or delivery may result in invasive infection in the newborn during the first week of life. This is known as early-onset GBS infection, resulting in approximately 1,600 cases and 80 deaths annually (13). Late-onset GBS disease in the newborn may be the result of vertical transmission or of nosocomial or community-acquired infection. Invasive GBS disease in the newborn is characterized primarily by sepsis, pneumonia, or meningitis. The incidence of invasive GBS infections among pregnant women in the United States decreased by 21% from 1993 to 1998 to an incidence of 0.23 per 1,000 live births (1). Morbidity caused by overwhelming sepsis and neurologic sequelae of meningitis also is clinically important but more difficult to estimate.

Factors Associated with Early-Onset Disease

A number of obstetric factors have been associated with an increased likelihood of early-onset GBS disease in the newborn (14). These include maternal colonization of the vagina and rectum with GBS, premature births, prolonged rupture of membranes, or intrapartum fever. The incidence of GBS disease also is higher among infants born to African-American women (15, 16), to Hispanic women, and to women younger than 20 years (16, 17). Neonates born to women with a prior GBS-infected infant (18–20) or women with heavy colonization such as that seen with GBS bacteriuria equal to or greater than 10^4 colony-forming units (CFU) (21–25) or low levels of anti-GBS capsular antibody, also are more likely to be infected (26).

Intrapartum administration of antibiotics to the women (during labor or after rupture of membranes, but before delivery) has been demonstrated to reduce early-onset neonatal GBS disease. Coinciding with active prevention efforts in the 1990s, the incidence of early-onset disease decreased by 70% to 0.5 cases per 1,000 live births in 1999. Projections derived from 1999 active surveillance data from the Active Bacterial Core Surveillance/Emerging Infections Program Network (27) estimate that intrapartum antibiotics prevented nearly 4,500 early-onset cases and 225 deaths that year (1, 2). Other countries that have adopted perinatal GBS prevention guidelines similar to the United States' guidelines have seen comparable decreases in early-onset disease incidence (28–30). Recent estimates of early-onset disease incidence in the United States suggest a slight increase in incidence from 1999 to 2000, consistent with a plateau in the impact of prevention efforts.

Strategies for Intrapartum Antibiotic Prophylaxis

In 1996, the federal Centers for Disease Control and Prevention (CDC) (31), the American College of Obstetricians and Gynecologists (ACOG), and the American Academy of Pediatrics (AAP) recommended that obstetric providers adopt either a culture-based or a risk-based approach for the prevention of early-onset GBS. Using the risk-based approach, women with preterm labor (<37 weeks of gestation), preterm premature rupture of membranes (preterm PROM) (<37 weeks of gestation), rupture of membranes greater than or equal to 18 hours, or maternal fever during labor (≥38°C or 100.4°F) receive intrapartum antibiotic prophylaxis. With both culture-based and risk-based approaches, women with GBS bacteriuria during their current pregnancy or women who previously gave birth to an infant with early-onset GBS disease were candidates for intrapartum antibiotic prophylaxis. The culture-based approach requires obtaining a single swab from the lower vagina (introitus) and perianal area, placing the swab in transport media, and using selective broth media. Use of prenatal cultures remote from term to identify women who are colonized with GBS at delivery may not be accurate, and since 1996, the CDC, ACOG, and AAP have recommended obtaining rectovaginal cultures at 35–37 weeks of gestation with the culture-based approach. All women who are GBS culture positive should be treated with intrapartum antibiotic prophylaxis in labor. Still, intrapartum antibiotic prophylaxis should be administered to women with preterm labor or preterm PROM who are in labor.

A recent multistate retrospective cohort study of live births in 1998 and 1999 of residents from eight areas of the Active Bacterial Core Surveillance/ Emerging Infections Program network suggests that the culture-based approach is superior to the risk-based approach (32). All cases of early-onset GBS identified by population-based surveillance in these areas were identified. The provider's intended strategy was unknown; thus, women without documented prenatal GBS screening were considered to have been managed by the risk-based approach. The study used data abstracted from records of 5,144 births, including 312 early-onset GBS cases. Univariate analysis showed that intrapartum fever equal to or greater than 38°C or a previous infant with GBS disease was associated with the highest risks of early-onset GBS disease with a relative risk (RR) of 5.99 (95% confidence interval [CI], 4.28–8.38) and RR of 3.79 (95% CI, 1.3–11.11), respectively. In addition, all risk factors (ie, preterm delivery, prolonged rupture of membranes ≤18 hours, inadequate prenatal care, black race, Hispanic ethnicity, and maternal age <20 years) except GBS bacteriuria were significantly associated with early-onset GBS. The risk of having an infant with early-onset GBS was significantly lower in the culture cohort relative to the risk cohort with an adjusted RR of 0.46 (95% CI, 0.37–0.60). Moreover, of the 312 infants with early-onset GBS, 63% of the mothers had no risk factors. Even when the women who had no strategy applied were excluded (n=207, including 30 early-onset GBS cases), the culture approach remained protective with an adjusted RR of 0.48 (95% CI, 0.37–0.63).

In addition, a number of small studies have evaluated compliance of hospitals with GBS guideline recommendations and found that a greater proportion of GBS-positive women receive intrapartum prophylaxis under the culture-based approach than with the risk-based approach (28, 32–39). Data from a large cohort of term infants with early-onset GBS infections found that more than one half of the term infants with culture-proven infection were born to women with no obstetric risk factors (40). Based on CDC surveillance data, the risk-based approach fails to identify approximately 50% of infants with GBS sepsis (41).

Commentary

The Committee on Obstetric Practice recognizes that some of these recent studies have methodologic flaws. Still, they represent the best available comparison of the risk-based and culture-based strategies to date. Larger studies or randomized studies are not likely to be conducted; therefore, the Committee supports the new CDC recommendation that obstetric providers adopt a culture-based strategy for the prevention of early-onset GBS disease in the newborn (see Fig. 1). The Committee agrees with the CDC that the risk-based approach is no longer an acceptable alternative except for circumstances where culture results are not available before delivery. Laboratories must process GBS cultures correctly using the recommended selective broth media for results to be accurate. Culture specimens should be collected by swabbing the lower vagina and rectum (ie, through the anal sphincter), not by speculum examination, to maximize the likelihood of GBS recovery (see box). Laboratories also must

Fig. 1. Indications for intrapartum antibiotic prophylaxis to prevent perinatal group B streptococcal disease under a universal prenatal screening strategy based on combined vaginal and rectal cultures collected at 35–37 weeks of gestation from all pregnant women.

Procedures for collecting and processing clinical specimens for group B streptococcal culture and performing susceptibility testing to clindamycin and erythromycin

Procedure for collecting clinical specimens for culture of group B streptococcus at 35–37 weeks of gestation

- Swab the lower vagina (vaginal introitus), followed by the rectum (ie, insert swab through the anal sphincter) using the same swab or two different swabs. Cultures should be collected in the outpatient setting by the health care provider or the patient herself, with appropriate instruction. Cervical cultures are not recommended and a speculum should not be used for culture collection.

- Place the swab(s) into a nonnutritive transport medium. Appropriate transport systems (eg, Amies or Stuart without charcoal) are commercially available. If vaginal and rectal swabs were collected separately, both swabs can be placed into the same container of medium. Transport media will maintain GBS viability for up to 4 days at room temperature or under refrigeration.

- Specimen labels should clearly identify that specimens are for group B streptococcal culture. If susceptibility testing is ordered for penicillin-allergic women, specimen labels should also identify the patient as penicillin allergic and should specify that susceptibility testing for clindamycin and erythromycin should be performed if GBS is isolated.

Procedure for processing clinical specimens for culture of group B streptococcus

- Remove swab(s) from transport medium.* Inoculate swab(s) into a recommended selective broth medium, such as Todd-Hewitt broth supplemented with either gentamicin (8 μg/mL) and nalidixic acid (15 μg/mL), or with colistin (10 μg/mL) and nalidixic acid (15 μg/mL). Examples of appropriate commercially available options include Trans-Vag broth supplemented with 5% defibrinated sheep blood or LIM broth.[†]

- Incubate inoculated selective broth for 18–24 hours at 35°–37°C in ambient air of 5% CO_2. Subculture the broth to a sheep blood agar plate (eg, tryptic soy agar with 5% defibrinated sheep blood).

- Inspect and identify organisms suggestive of GBS (ie, narrow zone of beta hemolysis, gram-positive cocci, catalase negative). Note that hemolysis may be difficult to observe, so typical colonies without hemolysis should also be further tested. If GBS is not identified after incubation for 18–24 hours, reincubate and inspect at 48 hours to identify suspected organisms.

- Various streptococcus grouping latex agglutination tests or other tests for GBS antigen detection (eg, genetic probe) may be used for specific identification, or the cAMP test may be employed for presumptive identification.

Procedure for clindamycin and erythromycin disk susceptibility testing of isolates, when ordered for penicillin-allergic patients[‡]

- Use a cotton swab to make a suspension from an 18–24-hour growth of the organism in saline or Mueller-Hinton broth to match a 0.5 McFarland turbidity standard.

- Within 15 minutes of adjusting the turbidity, dip a sterile cotton swab into the adjusted suspension. The swab should be rotated several times and pressed firmly on the inside wall of the tube above the fluid level. Use the swab to inoculate the entire surface of a Mueller-Hinton sheep blood agar plate. After the plate is dry, use sterile forceps to place a clindamycin (2-μg) disk onto half of the plate and an erythromycin (15-μg) disk onto the other half.

- Incubate at 35°C in 5% CO_2 for 20–24 hours.

- Measure the diameter of the zone of inhibition using a ruler or calipers. Interpret according to NCCLS guidelines for *Streptococcus* species other than *S pneumoniae* (2002 breakpoints:[‡] clindamycin: ≥19 mm = susceptible, 16–18 = intermediate, ≤15 = resistant; erythromycin: ≥21 mm = susceptible, 16–20 = intermediate, ≤ 15 = resistant).

---

cAMP, cyclic adenosine monophosphate; CNA, Columbia colistin–nalidixic acid; LIM broth, Todd-Hewitt with CNA.

*Before inoculation step, some laboratories may choose to roll swab(s) on a single sheep blood agar plate or CNA sheep blood agar plate. This should be done only in addition to, and not instead of, inoculation into selective broth. The plate should be streaked for isolation, incubated at 35–37°C in ambient air or 5% CO_2 for 18–24 hours and inspected for organisms suggestive of GBS as described above. If suspected colonies are confirmed as GBS, the broth can be discarded, thus shortening the time to obtain culture results.

† Source: Fenton, LJ, Harper MH. Evaluation of colistin and nalidixic acid in Todd-Hewitt broth for selective isolation of group B streptococci. J Clin Microbiol 1979;9:167–9. Although Trans-Vag medium is often available without sheep blood, direct comparison of medium with and without sheep blood has shown higher yield when blood is added. LIM broth also may benefit from the addition of sheep blood, although the improvement in yield is smaller and sufficient data are not yet available to support a recommendation.

‡ Source: NCCLS. Performance standard for antimicrobial susceptibility testing. M100-S12, Table 2H, Wayne Pa.: NCCLS, 2002. NCCLS recommends disk diffusion (M-2) or broth microdilution testing (M-7) for susceptibility testing of GBS. Commercial systems that have been cleared or approved for testing of streptococci other than *S pneumoniae* may also be used. Penicillin susceptibility testing is not routinely recommended for GBS because penicillin-resistant isolates have not been confirmed to date.

Schrag S, Gorwitz R, Fultz-Butts K, Schuchat A. Prevention of perinatal group B streptococcal disease. Revised guidelines from CDC. MMWR Recomm Rep 2002;51(RR-11):1–22.

communicate culture results to the obstetric provider, the anticipated site of delivery if possible, and the patient so that intrapartum antibiotic prophylaxis can be given to all GBS-positive women. For women who have GBS bacteriuria in any concentration during the current pregnancy or who have previously given birth to an infant with early-onset GBS disease, GBS cultures are not required. Those women should automatically receive intrapartum prophylaxis. Urine specimens should be labeled to indicate they were obtained from a pregnant woman so laboratories can report any presence of GBS bacteriuria in specimens obtained from pregnant women. If, at anytime during pregnancy, GBS is present in urine in concentrations equal to or greater than 10^5, antibiotics for asymptomatic bacteriuria or a symptomatic urinary tract infection should be administered, as it would be for any other organism in significant concentration (42, 43). Women who had GBS colonization during a previous pregnancy may no longer be colonized during subsequent pregnancies and require GBS culture evaluation with each pregnancy.

Penicillin remains the agent of choice for intrapartum prophylaxis. Ampicillin is an acceptable alternative, but penicillin is preferred. However, data also show that GBS isolates are increasingly resistant to second-line therapies. Up to 15% of GBS isolates are resistant to clindamycin and 7–25% of isolates are resistant to erythromycin (44). This pattern of resistance has led to a change in the recommendations for second-line therapies (see Table 1). Intravenous administration is the only route recommended for intrapartum GBS prophylaxis because of the higher intraamniotic concentrations achieved with this route. Of note, erythromycin does not cross the placenta.

The benefit of GBS prevention must be weighed against the risk to the woman and her fetus of maternal allergic reactions to antibiotics during labor. Although the risk of fatal anaphylaxis has been estimated at 1 per 100,000 (45, 46), the risk of less severe anaphylactic or allergic reactions is important. In the recent CDC surveillance project of more than 5,000 live births, there was a single, nonfatal anaphylactic reaction (13, 47). The Committee agrees with the CDC that local health agencies should establish surveillance systems to monitor the incidence of early-onset neonatal GBS disease, the emergence of infection in women and their newborns that is caused by resistant organisms, and other complications of widespread maternal antibiotic administration such as severe allergic reactions.

The Committee believes that when culture results are not available, intrapartum prophylaxis should be offered only on the basis of the presence

Table 1. Recommended Regimens for Intrapartum Antimicrobial Prophylaxis for Perinatal Group B Streptococcal Disease Prevention*

Regimens	Antimicrobial
Recommended	Penicillin G, 5 million units IV initial dose, then 2.5 million units IV every 4 hours until delivery
Alternative	Ampicillin, 2 g IV initial dose, then 1 g IV every 4 hours until delivery
If penicillin allergic†	
• Patients not at high risk for anaphylaxis	Cefazolin, 2 g IV initial dose, then 1 g IV every 8 hours until delivery
• Patients at high risk for anaphylaxis‡	
—GBS susceptible to clindamycin and erythromycin§	Clindamycin, 900 mg IV every 8 hours until delivery OR Erythromycin, 500 mg IV every 6 hours until delivery
—GBS resistant to clindamycin or erythromycin or susceptibility unknown	Vancomycin,‖ 1 g IV every 12 hours until delivery

GBS, group B streptococci; IV, intravenously.

*Broader-spectrum agents, including an agent active against GBS, may be necessary for treatment of chorioamnionitis.

† History of penicillin allergy should be assessed to determine whether a high risk for anaphylaxis is present. Penicillin-allergic patients at high risk for anaphylaxis are those who have experienced immediate hypersensitivity to penicillin including a history of penicillin-related anaphylaxis; other high-risk patients are those with asthma or other diseases that would make anaphylaxis more dangerous or difficult to treat, such as persons being treated with beta-adrenergic–blocking agents.

‡ If laboratory facilities are adequate, clindamycin and erythromycin susceptibility testing should be performed on prenatal GBS isolates from penicillin-allergic women at high risk for anaphylaxis.

§ Resistance to erythromycin often but not always is associated with clindamycin resistance. If a strain is resistant to erythromycin but appears susceptible to clindamycin, it may still have inducible resistance to clindamycin.

‖ Cefazolin is preferred over vancomycin for women with a history of penicillin allergy other than immediate hypersensitivity reactions, and pharmacologic data suggest it achieves effective intraamniotic concentrations. Vancomycin should be reserved for penicillin-allergic women at high risk for anaphylaxis.

Schrag S, Gorwitz R, Fultz-Butts K, Schuchat A. Prevention of perinatal group B streptococcal disease. Revised guidelines from CDC. MMWR Recomm Rep 2002;51(RR-11):1–22.

of intrapartum risk factors for early-onset GBS disease (see previous description and Fig. 1). The Committee strongly discourages using a hybrid of both strategies (eg, administering intrapartum antibiotics to a woman with rupture of membranes ≥18 hours despite a negative GBS culture at 35–37 weeks of gestation).

The Committee has insufficient data to suggest a specific course of management for women with threatened preterm labor or preterm PROM when delivery is postponed successfully. Determining the timing of intrapartum prophylaxis in these women is challenging. Management of preterm PROM and threatened preterm labor should be guided by clinical considerations. The Committee supports CDC's potential management scheme (see Fig. 2).

The Committee concurs with the CDC that intrapartum prophylaxis is not recommended for women undergoing a planned cesarean delivery in the absence of labor or rupture of membranes, regardless of the GBS colonization status. A retrospective study at a single institution (48) and a review of CDC surveillance data showed that the risk of transmission of GBS from a colonized woman to her infant during a prelabor cesarean delivery with intact membranes is low. Patients expected to undergo planned cesarean deliveries should nonetheless undergo culture screening at 35–37 weeks of gestation because onset of labor or rupture of membranes may occur before the planned cesarean delivery. If intrapartum prophylaxis is administered before a planned cesarean delivery,

*If a hospital chooses to give antibiotics to prolong the latent period, a GBS culture should be obtained before initiating therapy and the results used to guide intrapartum management.

† Penicillin should be continued for a total of at least 48 hours, unless delivery occurs sooner. At the physician's discretion, antibiotic prophylaxis may be continued beyond 48 hours in a GBS culture-positive woman if delivery has not yet occurred. For women who are GBS culture positive, antibiotic prophylaxis should be reinitiated when labor likely to proceed to delivery occurs or recurs.

‡ If antibiotics are used to prolong the latent period, GBS cultures should be obtained prior to initiating therapy and the results used to guide intrapartum management.

§ If delivery has not occurred within 4 weeks, a vaginal and rectal GBS screening culture should be repeated and the patient should be managed as described, based on the result of the repeat culture.

 || Intrapartum antibiotic prophylaxis.

Adapted from Schrag S, Gorwitz R, Fultz-Butts K, Schuchat A. Prevention of perinatal group B streptococcal disease. Revised guidelines from CDC. MMWR Recomm Rep 2002;51(RR-11):1–22.

Fig. 2. Sample algorithm for group B streptococci (GBS) prophylaxis for women with threatened preterm delivery. This algorithm is not an exclusive course of management. Variations that incorporate individual circumstances or institutional preferences may be appropriate.

the timing of administration of antibiotics and the timing of incision should be individualized (49).

The Committee has insufficient data to support or discourage the use of scalp electrodes or fetal scalp/blood pH determinations in women known to be GBS colonized. Furthermore, the risks of membrane stripping in GBS-colonized women have not been investigated in well-designed prospective studies. Therefore, data are insufficient to encourage or discourage this practice in women known to be GBS colonized.

Current rapid tests for the detection of GBS colonization at the time of labor or rupture of membranes do not have sufficient sensitivity and specificity to eliminate the need for culture-based prenatal screening (50, 51).

The Committee on Obstetric Practice recognizes that compliance with the culture-based approach will require the implementation of several steps. Patient and professional materials are available from ACOG (sales.acog.org and www.acog.org) and the CDC (www.cdc.gov.nci-dod/dbmd/gbs). Success of the culture-based approach will require the following:

- Obtaining accurate culture data
- Appropriate processing of the culture by laboratories
- Timely reporting of results to obstetric providers
- Administering intrapartum prophylaxis to culture-positive women

It is important to acknowledge that complete implementation of this complex strategy still will not eliminate all cases of early-onset GBS.

References

1. Schrag SJ, Zywicki S, Farley MM, Reingold AL, Harrison LH, Lefkowitz LB, et al. Group B streptococcal disease in the era of intrapartum antibiotic prophylaxis. N Engl J Med 2000;342:15–20.
2. Early-onset group B streptococcal disease—United States, 1998-1999. Centers for Disease Control and Prevention. MMWR Morb Mortal Wkly Rep 2000;49:793–6.
3. Anthony BF, Okada DM, Hobel CJ. Epidemiology of group B Streptococcus: longitudinal observations during pregnancy. J Infect Dis 1978;137:524–30.
4. Regan JA, Klebanoff MA, Nugent RP. The epidemiology of group B streptococcal colonization in pregnancy. Vaginal Infections and Prematurity Study Group. Obstet Gynecol 1991;77:604–10.
5. Dillon HC Jr, Gray E, Pass MA, Gray BM. Anorectal and vaginal carriage of group B streptococci during pregnancy. J Infect Dis 1982;145:794–9.
6. Boyer KM, Gadzala CA, Kelly PD, Burd LI, Gotoff SP. Selective intrapartum chemoprophylaxis of neonatal group B streptococcal early-onset disease. II. Predictive value of prenatal cultures. J Infect Dis 1983;148:802–9.
7. Pass MA, Gray BM, Dillon HC Jr. Puerperal and perinatal infections with group B streptococci. Am J Obstet Gynecol 1982;143:147–52.
8. Bobitt JR, Ledger WJ. Amniotic fluid analysis. Its role in maternal neonatal infection. Obstet Gynecol 1978;51:56–62.
9. Braun TI, Pinover W, Sih P. Group B streptococcal meningitis in a pregnant woman before the onset of labor. Clin Infect Dis 1995;21:1042–3.
10. Yancey MK, Duff P, Clark P, Kurtzer T, Frentzen BH, Kubilis P. Peripartum infection associated with vaginal group B streptococcal colonization. Obstet Gynecol 1994;84:816–9.
11. Fox BC. Delayed-onset postpartum meningitis due to group B streptococcus. Clin Infect Dis 1994;19:350.
12. Aharoni A, Potasman I, Levitan Z, Golan D, Sharf M. Postpartum maternal group B streptococcal meningitis. Rev Infect Dis 1990;12:273–6.
13. Schrag S, Gorwitz R, Fultz-Butts K, Schuchat A. Prevention of perinatal group B streptococcal disease. Revised guidelines from CDC. MMWR Recomm Rep 2002;51(RR-11):1–22.
14. Boyer KM, Gotoff SP. Strategies for chemoprophylaxis of GBS early-onset infections. Antibiot Chemother 1985;35:267–80.
15. Zangwill KM, Schuchat A, Wenger JD. Group B streptococcal disease in the United States, 1990: report from a multistate active surveillance system. Mor Mortal Wkly Rep CDC Surveill Summ 1992;41(6):25–32.
16. Schuchat A, Oxtoby M, Cochi S, Sikes RK, Hightower A, Plikaytis B, et al. Population-based risk factors for neonatal group B streptococcal disease: results of a cohort study in metropolitan Atlanta. J Infect Dis 1990;162:672–7.
17. Schuchat A, Deaver-Robinson K, Plikaytis BD, Zangwill KM, Mohle-Boetani J, Wenger JD. Multistate case-control study of maternal risk factors for neonatal group B streptococcal disease. The Active Surveillance Study Group. Pediatr Infect Dis J 1994;13:623–9.
18. Carstensen H, Christensen KK, Grennert L, Persson K, Polberger S. Early-onset neonatal group B streptococcal septicaemia in siblings. J Infect 1988;17:201–4.
19. Faxelius G, Bremme K, Kvist-Christensen K, Christensen P, Ringertz S. Neonatal septicemia due to group B streptococci-perinatal risk factors and outcome of subsequent pregnancies. J Perinat Med 1988;16:423–30.
20. Christensen KK, Dahlander K, Linden V, Svenningsen N, Christensen P. Obstetrical care in future pregnancies after fetal loss in group B streptococcal septicemia. A prevention program based on bacteriological and immunological follow-up. Eur J Obstet Gynecol Reprod Biol 1981;12:143–50.
21. Pass MA, Gray BM, Khare S, Dillon HC Jr. Prospective studies of group B streptococcal infections in infants. J Pediatr 1979;95:437–43.
22. Wood EG, Dillon HC Jr. A prospective study of group B streptococcal bacteriuria in pregnancy. Am J Obstet Gynecol 1981;140:515–20.
23. Moller M, Thomsen AC, Borch K, Dinesen K, Zdravkovic M. Rupture of fetal membranes and premature delivery

associated with group B streptococci in urine of pregnant women. Lancet 1984;2(8394):69–70.

24. Liston TE, Harris RE, Foshee S, Null DM Jr. Relationship of neonatal pneumonia to maternal urinary and neonatal isolates of group B streptococci. South Med J 1979;72:1410–2.

25. Persson K, Christensen KK, Christensen P, Forsgren A, Jorgensen C, Persson PH. Asymptomatic bacteriuria during pregnancy with special reference to group B streptococci. Scand J Infect Dis 1985;17:195–9.

26. Baker CJ, Kasper DL. Correlation of maternal antibody deficiency with susceptibility to neonatal group B streptococcal infection. N Engl J Med 1976;294:753–6.

27. Schuchat A, Hilger T, Zell E, Farley M, Reingold A, Harrison L, et al. Active bacterial core surveillance of the emerging infections program network. Emerging Infect Dis 2001;7:92–9.

28. Jeffery HE, Moses Lahra M. Eight-year outcome of universal screening and intrapartum antibiotics for maternal group B streptococcal carriers. Pediatrics 1998;101:E2.

29. Isaacs D, Royle JA. Intrapartum antibiotics and early onset neonatal sepsis caused by group B streptococcus and by other organisms in Australia. Australasian Study Group for Neonatal Infections. Pediatr Infect Dis J 1999;18:524–8.

30. Davies HD, Adair CE, Schuchat A, Low DE, Sauve RS, McGeer A. Physicians' prevention practices and incidence of neonatal group B streptococcal disease in 2 Canadian regions. CMAJ 2001;164:479–85.

31. Prevention of perinatal group B streptococcal disease: a public health perspective. Centers for Disease Control and Prevention. MMWR Recomm Rep1996;45:1–24.

32. Schrag SJ, Zell ER, Lynfield R, Roome A, Arnold KE, Craig AS, et al. A population-based comparison of strategies to prevent early-onset group B streptococcal disease in neonates. N Engl J Med 2002;347:233–9.

33. Hafner E, Sterniste W, Rosen A, Schuchter K, Plattner M, Asboth F, et al. Group B streptococci during pregnancy: a comparison of two screening and treatment protocols. Am J Obstet Gynecol 1998;179:677–81.

34. Lieu TA, Mohle-Boetani JC, Ray GT, Ackerson LM, Walton DL. Neonatal group B streptococcal infection in a managed care population. Perinatal Group B Streptococcal Infection Study Group. Obstet Gynecol 1998;92:21–7.

35. Factor SH, Levine OS, Nasser A, Potter J, Fajardo A, O'Sullivan MJ, et al. Impact of a risk-based prevention policy on neonatal group B streptococcal disease. Am J Obstet Gynecol 1998;179:1568–71.

36. Cheon-Lee E, Amstey MS. Compliance with the Centers for Disease Control and Prevention antenatal culture protocol for preventing group B streptococcal neonatal sepsis. Am J Obstet Gynecol 1998;179:77–9.

37. Katz VL, Moos MK, Cefalo RC, Thorp JM Jr, Bowes WA Jr, Wells SD. Group B streptococci: results of a protocol of antepartum screening and intrapartum treatment. Am J Obstet Gynecol 1994;170:521–6.

38. Gilson GJ, Christensen F, Romero H, Bekes K, Silva L, Qualls CR. Prevention of group B streptococcus early-onset neonatal sepsis: comparison of the Center for Disease Control and Prevention screening-based protocol to a risk-based protocol in infants at greater than 37 weeks' gestation. J Perinatol 2000;20:491–5.

39. Brozanski BS, Jones JG, Krohn MA, Sweet RL. Effect of a screening-based prevention policy on prevalence of early-onset group B streptococcal sepsis. Obstet Gynecol 2000;95:496–501.

40. Bromberger P, Lawrence JM, Braun D, Saunders B, Contreras R, Petitti DB. The influence of intrapartum antibiotics on the clinical spectrum of early-onset group B streptococcal infection in term infants. Pediatrics 2000;106:244–50.

41. Rosenstein NE, Schuchat A. Opportunities for prevention of perinatal group B streptococcal disease: a multistate surveillance analysis. The Neonatal Group B Streptococcal Disease Study Group. Obstet Gynecol 1997;90:901–6.

42. Persson K, Bjerre B, Elfstrom L, Polberger S, Forsgren A. Group B streptococci at delivery: high count in urine increases risk for neonatal colonization. Scand J Infect Dis 1986;18:525–31.

43. Persson K, Bjerre B, Elfstrom L, Forsgren A. Longitudinal study of group B streptococcal carriage during late pregnancy. Scand J Infect Dis 1987;19:325–9.

44. Pearlman MD, Pierson CL, Faix RG. Frequent resistance of clinical group B streptococci isolates to clindamycin and erythromycin. Obstet Gynecol 1998;92:258–61.

45. Schwartz B, Schuchat A, Oxtoby MJ, Cochi SL, Hightower A, Broome CV. Invasive group B streptococcal disease in adults. A population-based study in metropolitan Atlanta. JAMA 1991;266:1112–4.

46. Hardman JG, Limbird LE, Molinoff PB, Ruddon RW, Gilman AG, editors. Goodman and Gilman's the pharmacological basis of therapeutics. 9th ed. New York: McGraw-Hill; 1996.

47. Dunn AB, Blomquist J, Khouzami V. Anaphylaxis in labor secondary to prophylaxis against group B Streptococcus: a case report. J Reprod Med 1999;44:381–4.

48. Ramus RM, McIntire DD, Wendel GD Jr. Antibiotic chemoprophylaxis for group B strep is not necessary with elective cesarean section at term [abstract]. Am J Obstet Gynecol 1999;180:S85.

49. Hager WD, Schuchat A, Gibbs R, Sweet R, Mead P, Larsen JW. Prevention of perinatal group B streptococcal infection: current controversies. Obstet Gynecol 2000;96:141–5.

50. Yancey MK, Armer T, Clark P, Duff P. Assessment of rapid identification tests for genital carriage of group B streptococci. Obstet Gynecol 1992;80:1038–47.

51. Walker CK, Crombleholme WR, Ohm-Smith MJ, Sweet RL. Comparison of rapid tests for detection of group B streptococcal colonization. Am J Perinatol 1992;9:304–8.

ACOG

Committee on
Gynecologic Practice

Committee Opinion

Number 292, November 2003   *(Replaces No. 246, December 2000)*

The American College of Obstetricians and Gynecologists
409 12th Street, SW
PO Box 96920
Washington, DC 20090-6920

12345/76543

Primary and preventive care: periodic assessments. ACOG Committee Opinion No. 292. American College of Obstetricians and Gynecologists. Obstet Gynecol 2003;102:1117–24.

Primary and Preventive Care: Periodic Assessments

ABSTRACT: Periodic assessments provide an excellent opportunity for obstetricians and gynecologists to provide preventive screening, evaluation, and counseling. This Committee Opinion provides the recommendations of the American College of Obstetricians and Gynecologists' Committee on Gynecologic Practice for routine assessments in primary and preventive care for women based on age and risk factors.

The following charts are updated versions of those previously published by the American College of Obstetricians and Gynecologists (ACOG) in *Guidelines for Women's Health Care* (2002) and Committee Opinion No. 246. This version replaces those previous versions. The policies and recommendations of ACOG committees regarding specific aspects of the health care of women have been incorporated; they may differ from the recommendations of other groups. These recommendations are for nonpregnant women.

Periodic assessments provide an excellent opportunity to counsel patients about preventive care. These assessments, yearly or as appropriate, should include screening, evaluation, and counseling based on age and risk factors. Personal behavioral characteristics are important aspects of a woman's health. Positive behaviors, such as exercise, should be reinforced, and negative ones, such as smoking, should be discouraged. The following guidelines indicate routine assessments for women based on age groups and risk factors (Table 1) and list leading causes of death and morbidity for each age group identified by various sources (see box). It is recognized that variations may be required to adjust to the needs of a specific individual. For example, certain risk factors may influence additional assessments and interventions. Physicians should be alert to high-risk factors (indicated by an asterisk and further elucidated in Table 1). During evaluation, the patient should be made aware of high-risk conditions that require targeted screening or treatment.

The material in these charts is based heavily on evidence of effectiveness and cost-effectiveness. It should be recognized, however, that making these determinations is both complex and inexact in the present environment. Nonetheless, the progress that has been made is encouraging, and the goal is desirable and of great importance. Although there will be differences of opinion regarding some specific recommendations, the major benefit to be derived should not be lost in debating those issues.

Periodic Assessment
Ages 13–18 Years

Screening

History

Reason for visit

Health status: medical, surgical, family

Dietary/nutrition assessment

Physical activity

Use of complementary and alternative medicine

Tobacco, alcohol, other drug use

Abuse/neglect

Sexual practices

Physical Examination

Height

Weight

Blood pressure

Secondary sexual characteristics (Tanner staging)

Pelvic examination (when indicated by the medical history)

Skin*

Laboratory Testing

Periodic

Cervical cytology (annually beginning at approximately 3 years after initiation of sexual intercourse)

High-Risk Groups*

Hemoglobin level assessment

Bacteriuria testing

Sexually transmitted disease testing

Human immunodeficiency virus (HIV) testing

Genetic testing/counseling

Rubella titer assessment

Tuberculosis skin testing

Lipid profile assessment

Fasting glucose testing

Hepatitis C virus testing

Colorectal cancer screening†

Evaluation and Counseling

Sexuality

Development

High-risk behaviors

Preventing unwanted/unintended pregnancy

—Postponing sexual involvement

—Contraceptive options, including emergency contraception

Sexually transmitted diseases

—Partner selection

—Barrier protection

Fitness and Nutrition

Dietary/nutrition assessment (including eating disorders)

Exercise: discussion of program

Folic acid supplementation (0.4 mg/d)

Calcium intake

Psychosocial Evaluation

Interpersonal/family relationships

Sexual identity

Personal goal development

Behavioral/learning disorders

Abuse/neglect

Satisfactory school experience

Peer relationships

Cardiovascular Risk Factors

Family history

Hypertension

Dyslipidemia

Obesity

Diabetes mellitus

Health/Risk Behaviors

Hygiene (including dental); fluoride supplementation*

Injury prevention

—Safety belts and helmets

—Recreational hazards

—Firearms

—Hearing

—Occupational hazards

—School hazards

—Exercise and sports involvement

Skin exposure to ultraviolet rays

Suicide: depressive symptoms

Tobacco, alcohol, other drug use

Immunizations

Periodic

Tetanus–diphtheria booster (once between ages 11 years and 16 years)

Hepatitis B virus vaccine (1 series for those not previously immunized)

High-Risk Groups

Influenza vaccine

Hepatitis A virus vaccine

Pneumococcal vaccine

Measles–mumps–rubella vaccine

Varicella vaccine

Leading Causes of Death‡

1. Accidents
2. Malignant neoplasms
3. Homicide
4. Suicide
5. Diseases of the heart
6. Congenital anomalies

Leading Causes of Morbidity‡

Acne

Asthma

Chlamydia

Diabetes mellitus

Headache

Infective, viral, and parasitic diseases

Mental disorders, including affective and neurotic disorders

Nose, throat, ear, and upper respiratory infections

Sexual assault

Sexually transmitted diseases

Urinary tract infections

Vaginitis

*See Table 1.

†Only for those with a family history of familial adenomatous polyposis or 8 years after the start of pancolitis. For a more detailed discussion of colorectal cancer screening, see Smith RA, von Eschenbach AC, Wender R, Levin B, Byers T, Rothenberger D, et al. American Cancer Society guidelines for the early detection of cancer: update of early detection guidelines for prostate, colorectal, and endometrial cancers. Also: update 2001–testing for early lung cancer detection [published erratum appears in CA Cancer J Clin 2001;51:150]. CA Cancer J Clin 2001;51:38–75; quiz 77–80.

‡See box.

Periodic Assessment
Ages 19–39 Years

Screening

History

Reason for visit

Health status: medical, surgical, family

Dietary/nutrition assessment

Physical activity

Use of complementary and alternative medicine

Tobacco, alcohol, other drug use

Abuse/neglect

Sexual practices

Urinary and fecal incontinence

Physical Examination

Height

Weight

Blood pressure

Neck: adenopathy, thyroid

Breasts

Abdomen

Pelvic examination

Skin*

Laboratory Testing

Periodic

Cervical cytology (annually beginning no later than age 21 years; every 2–3 years after 3 consecutive negative test results if age 30 years or older with no history of cervical intraepithelial neoplasia 2 or 3, immunosuppression, human immunodeficiency virus [HIV] infection, or diethylstilbestrol exposure in utero)†

High-Risk Groups*

Hemoglobin level assessment

Bacteriuria testing

Mammography

Fasting glucose testing

Sexually transmitted disease testing

Human immunodeficiency virus testing

Genetic testing/counseling

Rubella titer assessment

Tuberculosis skin testing

Lipid profile assessment

Thyroid-stimulating hormone screening

Hepatitis C virus testing

Colorectal cancer screening

Bone density screening

Evaluation and Counseling

Sexuality

High-risk behaviors

Contraceptive options for prevention of unwanted pregnancy, including emergency contraception

Preconceptional and genetic counseling for desired pregnancy

Sexually transmitted diseases

—Partner selection

—Barrier protection

Sexual function

Fitness and Nutrition

Dietary/nutrition assessment

Exercise: discussion of program

Folic acid supplementation (0.4 mg/d)

Calcium intake

Psychosocial Evaluation

Interpersonal/family relationships

Domestic violence

Work satisfaction

Lifestyle/stress

Sleep disorders

Cardiovascular Risk Factors

Family history

Hypertension

Dyslipidemia

Obesity

Diabetes mellitus

Lifestyle

Health/Risk Behaviors

Hygiene (including dental)

Injury prevention

—Safety belts and helmets

—Occupational hazards

—Recreational hazards

—Firearms

—Hearing

—Exercise and sports involvement

Breast self-examination‡

Chemoprophylaxis for breast cancer (for high-risk women aged 35 years or older)§

Skin exposure to ultraviolet rays

Suicide: depressive symptoms

Tobacco, alcohol, other drug use

Immunizations

Periodic

Tetanus–diphtheria booster (every 10 years)

High-Risk Groups*

Measles–mumps–rubella vaccine

Hepatitis A virus vaccine

Hepatitis B virus vaccine

Influenza vaccine

Pneumococcal vaccine

Varicella vaccine

Leading Causes of Death‖

1. Malignant neoplasms
2. Accidents
3. Diseases of the heart
4. Suicide
5. Human immunodeficiency virus (HIV) disease
6. Homicide

Leading Causes of Morbidity‖

Acne

Appendicitis

Arthritis

Asthma

Back symptoms

Cancer

Chlamydia

Depression

Diabetes mellitus

Gynecologic disorders

Headache/migraine

Hypertension

Infective, viral, and parasitic diseases

Joint disorders

Menstrual disorders

Mental disorders, including affective and neurotic disorders

Nose, throat, ear, and upper respiratory infections

Obesity

Sexual assault/domestic violence

Sexually transmitted diseases

Skin rash/dermatitis

Substance abuse

Urinary tract infections

---

*See Table 1.

†For a more detailed discussion of cervical cytology screening, including the use of human papillomavirus DNA testing and screening after hysterectomy, see Cervical cytology screening. ACOG Practice Bulletin No. 45. American College of Obstetricians and Gynecologists. Obstet Gynecol 2003;102:417–27.

‡Despite a lack of definitive data for or against breast self-examination, breast self-examination has the potential to detect palpable breast cancer and can be recommended.

§For a more detailed discussion of risk assessment and chemoprevention therapy, see Selective estrogen receptor modulators. ACOG Practice Bulletin No. 39. American College of Obstetricians and Gynecologists. Obstet Gynecol 2002;100:835–43.

‖See box.

Periodic Assessment
Ages 40–64 Years

Screening

History

Reason for visit

Health status: medical, surgical, family

Dietary/nutrition assessment

Physical activity

Use of complementary and alternative medicine

Tobacco, alcohol, other drug use

Abuse/neglect

Sexual practices

Urinary and fecal incontinence

Physical Examination

Height

Weight

Blood pressure

Oral cavity

Neck: adenopathy, thyroid

Breasts, axillae

Abdomen

Pelvic examination

Skin*

Laboratory Testing

Periodic

Cervical cytology (every 2–3 years after 3 consecutive negative test results if no history of cervical intraepithelial neoplasia 2 or 3, immunosuppression, human immunodeficiency virus [HIV] infection, or diethylstilbestrol exposure in utero)†

Mammography (every 1–2 years beginning at age 40 years; yearly beginning at age 50 years)

Lipid profile assessment (every 5 years beginning at age 45 years)

Yearly fecal occult blood testing *or* flexible sigmoidoscopy every 5 years *or* yearly fecal occult blood testing plus flexible sigmoidoscopy every 5 years *or* double contrast barium enema every 5 years *or* colonoscopy every 10 years (beginning at age 50 years)

Fasting glucose testing (every 3 years after age 45 years)

Thyroid-stimulating hormone screening (every 5 years beginning at age 50 years)

High-Risk Groups*

Hemoglobin level assessment

Bacteriuria testing

Fasting glucose testing

Sexually transmitted disease testing

Bone density screening

Human immunodeficiency virus testing

Tuberculosis skin testing

Lipid profile assessment

Thyroid-stimulating hormone screening

Hepatitis C virus testing

Colorectal cancer screening

Evaluation and Counseling

Sexuality‡

High-risk behaviors

Contraceptive options for prevention of unwanted pregnancy, including emergency contraception

Sexually transmitted diseases

—Partner selection

—Barrier protection

Sexual functioning

Fitness and Nutrition

Dietary/nutrition assessment

Exercise: discussion of program

Folic acid supplementation (0.4 mg/d until age 50 years)

Calcium intake

Psychosocial Evaluation

Family relationships

Domestic violence

Work satisfaction

Retirement planning

Lifestyle/stress

Sleep disorders

Cardiovascular Risk Factors

Family history

Hypertension

Dyslipidemia

Obesity

Diabetes mellitus

Lifestyle

Health/Risk Behaviors

Hygiene (including dental)

Hormone therapy

Injury prevention

—Safety belts and helmets

—Occupational hazards

—Recreational hazards

—Exercise and sports involvement

—Firearms

—Hearing

Breast self-examination§

Chemoprophylaxis for breast cancer (for high-risk women)‖

Skin exposure to ultraviolet rays

Suicide: depressive symptoms

Tobacco, alcohol, other drug use

Immunizations

Periodic

Influenza vaccine (annually beginning at age 50 years)

Tetanus–diphtheria booster (every 10 years)

High-Risk Groups

Measles–mumps–rubella vaccine

Hepatitis A virus vaccine

Hepatitis B virus vaccine

Influenza vaccine

Pneumococcal vaccine

Varicella vaccine

Leading Causes of Death¶

1. Malignant neoplasms
2. Diseases of the heart
3. Cerebrovascular diseases
4. Chronic lower respiratory disease
5. Diabetes mellitus
6. Accidents
7. Chronic liver disease and cirrhosis
8. Suicide
9. Human immunodeficiency virus (HIV) disease

Leading Causes of Morbidity¶

Arthritis/osteoarthritis

Asthma

Back symptoms

Cancer

Cardiovascular disease

Depression

Diabetes mellitus

Headache/migraine

Hypertension

Menopause

Mental disorders, including affective and neurotic disorders

Mononeuritis of upper limb and mononeuritis multiplex

Nose, throat, ear, and upper respiratory infections

Obesity

Pneumonia

Sexually transmitted diseases

Skin conditions/dermatitis

Ulcers

Urinary tract infections

Vision impairment

---

*See Table 1.

†For a more detailed discussion of cervical cytology screening, including the use of human papillomavirus DNA testing and screening after hysterectomy, see Cervical cytology screening. ACOG Practice Bulletin No. 45. American College of Obstetricians and Gynecologists. Obstet Gynecol 2003;102:417–27.

‡Preconceptional and genetic counseling is appropriate for certain women in this age group.

§Despite a lack of definitive data for or against breast self-examination, breast self-examination has the potential to detect palpable breast cancer and can be recommended.

‖For a more detailed discussion of risk assessment and chemoprevention therapy, see Selective estrogen receptor modulators. ACOG Practice Bulletin No. 39. American College of Obstetricians and Gynecologists. Obstet Gynecol 2002;100:835–43.

¶See box.

Periodic Assessment
Ages 65 and Older

Screening

History

Reason for visit

Health status: medical, surgical, family

Dietary/nutrition assessment

Physical activity

Use of complementary and alternative medicine

Tobacco, alcohol, other drug use, and concurrent medication use

Abuse/neglect

Sexual practices

Urinary and fecal incontinence

Physical Examination

Height

Weight

Blood pressure

Oral cavity

Neck: adenopathy, thyroid

Breasts, axillae

Abdomen

Pelvic examination

Skin*

Laboratory Testing

Periodic

Cervical cytology (every 2–3 years after 3 consecutive negative test results if no history of cervical intraepithelial neoplasia 2 or 3, immunosuppression, human immunodeficiency virus [HIV] infection, or diethylstilbestrol exposure in utero)†

Urinalysis

Mammography

Lipid profile assessment (every 5 years)

Yearly fecal occult blood testing *or* flexible sigmoidoscopy every 5 years *or* yearly fecal occult blood testing plus flexible sigmoidoscopy every 5 years *or* double contrast barium enema every 5 years *or* colonoscopy every 10 years

Fasting glucose testing (every 3 years)

Bone density screening‡

Thyroid-stimulating hormone screening (every 5 years)

*High-Risk Groups**

Hemoglobin level assessment

Sexually transmitted disease testing

Human immunodeficiency virus testing

Tuberculosis skin testing

Thyroid-stimulating hormone screening

Hepatitis C virus testing

Colorectal cancer screening

Evaluation and Counseling

Sexuality

Sexual functioning

Sexual behaviors

Sexually transmitted diseases

—Partner selection

—Barrier protection

Fitness and Nutrition

Dietary/nutrition assessment

Exercise: discussion of program

Calcium intake

Psychosocial Evaluation

Neglect/abuse

Lifestyle/stress

Depression/sleep disorders

Family relationships

Work/retirement satisfaction

Cardiovascular Risk Factors

Hypertension

Dyslipidemia

Obesity

Diabetes mellitus

Sedentary lifestyle

Health/Risk Behaviors

Hygiene (including dental)

Hormone therapy

Injury prevention

—Safety belts and helmets

—Prevention of falls

—Occupational hazards

—Recreational hazards

—Exercise and sports involvement

—Firearms

Visual acuity/glaucoma

Hearing

Breast self-examination§

Chemoprophylaxis for breast cancer (for high-risk women)ǁ

Skin exposure to ultraviolet rays

Suicide: depressive symptoms

Tobacco, alcohol, other drug use

Immunizations

Periodic

Tetanus–diphtheria booster (every 10 years)

Influenza vaccine (annually)

Pneumococcal vaccine (once)

*High-Risk Groups**

Hepatitis A virus vaccine

Hepatitis B virus vaccine

Varicella vaccine

Leading Causes of Death¶

1. Diseases of the heart
2. Malignant neoplasms
3. Cerebrovascular diseases
4. Chronic lower respiratory diseases
5. Alzheimer's disease
6. Influenza and pneumonia
7. Diabetes mellitus

Leading Causes of Morbidity¶

Arthritis/osteoarthritis

Asthma

Back symptoms

Cancer

Cardiovascular disease

Chronic obstructive pulmonary diseases

Diabetes mellitus

Hearing and vision impairment

Hypertension

Mental disorders, including affective and neurotic disorders

Nose, throat, ear, and upper respiratory infections

Obesity

Osteoporosis

Pneumonia

Septicemia

Skin lesions/dermatoses/dermatitis

Ulcers

Urinary tract infections

Urinary tract (other conditions, including urinary incontinence)

Vertigo

---

*See Table 1.

†For a more detailed discussion of cervical cytology screening, including the use of human papillomavirus DNA testing and screening after hysterectomy, see Cervical cytology screening. ACOG Practice Bulletin No. 45. American College of Obstetricians and Gynecologists. Obstet Gynecol 2003;102:417–27.

‡In the absence of new risk factors, subsequent bone density screening should not be performed more frequently than every 2 years.

§Despite a lack of definitive data for or against breast self-examination, breast self-examination has the potential to detect palpable breast cancer and can be recommended.

ǁFor a more detailed discussion of risk assessment and chemoprevention therapy, see Selective estrogen receptor modulators. ACOG Practice Bulletin No. 39. American College of Obstetricians and Gynecologists. Obstet Gynecol 2002;100:835–43.

¶See box.

Table 1. High-Risk Factors

Intervention	High-Risk Factor
Bacteriuria testing	Diabetes mellitus
Bone density screening*	Postmenopausal women younger than 65 years: personal history of fracture as an adult; history of fracture in a first-degree relative; Caucasian; dementia; poor health or frailty; current cigarette smoking; low body weight (<127 lb); estrogen deficiency caused by early (age <45 years) menopause, bilateral ovariectomy, or prolonged (>1 year) premenopausal amenorrhea; low lifelong calcium intake; alcoholism; impaired eyesight despite adequate correction; recurrent falls; inadequate physical activity. All women: certain diseases or medical conditions and those who take certain drugs associated with an increased risk of osteoporosis
Colorectal cancer screening†	Colorectal cancer or adenomatous polyps in first-degree relative younger than 60 years or in 2 or more first-degree relatives of any ages; family history of familial adenomatous polyposis or hereditary nonpolyposis colon cancer; history of colorectal cancer, adenomatous polyps, inflammatory bowel disease, chronic ulcerative colitis, or Crohn's disease
Fasting glucose testing	Overweight (body mass index ≥25 kg/m^2); family history of diabetes mellitus; habitual physical inactivity; high-risk race/ethnicity (eg, African American, Hispanic, Native American, Asian, Pacific Islander); have given birth to a newborn weighing more than 9 lb or history of gestational diabetes mellitus; hypertension; high-density lipoprotein cholesterol level ≤35 mg/dL; triglyceride level ≥250 mg/dL; history of impaired glucose tolerance or impaired fasting glucose; polycystic ovary syndrome; history of vascular disease
Fluoride supplementation	Live in an area with inadequate water fluoridation (<0.7 ppm)
Genetic testing/counseling	Considering pregnancy and: will be 35 years or older at time of delivery; patient, partner, or family member with history of genetic disorder or birth defect; exposure to teratogens; or African, Acadian, European Caucasian, Eastern European (Ashkenazi) Jewish, Mediterranean, or Southeast Asian ancestry
Hemoglobin level assessment	Caribbean, Latin American, Asian, Mediterranean, or African ancestry; history of excessive menstrual flow
HAV vaccination	Chronic liver disease; clotting factor disorders; illegal drug users; individuals who work with HAV-infected nonhuman primates or with HAV in a research laboratory setting; individuals traveling to or working in countries that have high or intermediate endemicity of hepatitis A
HBV vaccination	Hemodialysis patients; patients who receive clotting factor concentrates; health care workers and public safety workers who have exposure to blood in the workplace; individuals in training in schools of medicine, dentistry, nursing, laboratory technology, and other allied health professions; injecting drug users; individuals with more than 1 sexual partner in the previous 6 months; individuals with a recently acquired STD; all clients in STD clinics; household contacts and sexual partners of individuals with chronic HBV infection; clients and staff of institutions for the developmentally disabled; international travelers who will be in countries with high or intermediate prevalence of chronic HBV infection for more than 6 months; inmates of correctional facilities
HCV testing	History of injecting illegal drugs; recipients of clotting factor concentrates before 1987; chronic (long-term) hemodialysis; persistently abnormal alanine aminotransferase levels; recipient of blood from a donor who later tested positive for HCV infection; recipient of blood or blood-component transfusion or organ transplant before July 1992; occupational percutaneous or mucosal exposure to HCV-positive blood
HIV testing	Seeking treatment for STDs; drug use by injection; history of prostitution; past or present sexual partner who is HIV positive or bisexual or injects drugs; long-term residence or birth in an area with high prevalence of HIV infection; history of transfusion from 1978 to 1985; invasive cervical cancer. Offer to women seeking preconceptional evaluation.

(continued)

Table 1. High-Risk Factors *(continued)*

Intervention	High-Risk Factor
Influenza vaccination	Anyone who wishes to reduce the chance of becoming ill with influenza; chronic cardiovascular or pulmonary disorders including asthma; chronic metabolic diseases, including diabetes mellitus, renal dysfunction, hemoglobinopathies, and immunosuppression (including immunosuppression caused by medications or by HIV); residents of nursing homes and other long-term care facilities; individuals likely to transmit influenza to high-risk individuals (eg, household members and care-givers of elderly, those with medical indications, and adults with high-risk conditions); health care workers; day care workers
Lipid profile assessment	Family history suggestive of familial hyperlipidemia; family history of premature (age <50 years for men, age <60 years for women) cardiovascular disease; diabetes mellitus; multiple coronary heart disease risk factors (eg, tobacco use, hypertension)
Mammography	Women who have had breast cancer or who have a first-degree relative (ie, mother, sister, or daughter) or multiple other relatives who have a history of premenopausal breast or breast and ovarian cancer
MMR vaccination	Adults born in 1957 or later should be offered vaccination (1 dose of MMR) if there is no proof of immunity or documentation of a dose given after first birthday; individuals vaccinated in 1963–1967 should be offered revaccination (2 doses); health care workers, students entering college, international travelers, and rubella-negative postpartum patients should be offered a second dose.
Pneumococcal vaccination	Chronic illness, such as cardiovascular disease, pulmonary disease, diabetes mellitus, alcoholism, chronic liver disease, cerebrospinal fluid leaks, functional asplenia (eg, sickle cell disease) or splenectomy; exposure to an environment where pneumococcal outbreaks have occurred; immuno-compromised patients (eg, HIV infection, hematologic or solid malignancies, chemotherapy, steroid therapy). Revaccination after 5 years may be appropriate for certain high-risk groups.
Rubella titer assessment	Childbearing age and no evidence of immunity
STD testing	History of multiple sexual partners or a sexual partner with multiple contacts, sexual contact with individuals with culture-proven STD, history of repeated episodes of STDs, attendance at clinics for STDs; routine screening for chlamydial infection for all sexually active women aged 25 years or younger and other asymptomatic women at high risk for infection; routine screening for gonorrheal infection for all sexually active adolescents and other asymptomatic women at high risk for infection
Skin examination	Increased recreational or occupational exposure to sunlight; family or personal history of skin cancer; clinical evidence of precursor lesions
Thyroid-stimulating hormone screening	Strong family history of thyroid disease; autoimmune disease (evidence of subclinical hypothy-roidism may be related to unfavorable lipid profiles)
Tuberculosis skin testing	Human immunodeficiency virus infection; close contact with individuals known or suspected to have tuberculosis; medical risk factors known to increase risk of disease if infected; born in country with high tuberculosis prevalence; medically underserved; low income; alcoholism; intravenous drug use; resident of long-term care facility (eg, correctional institutions, mental institutions, nursing homes and facilities); health professional working in high-risk health care facilities
Varicella vaccination	All susceptible adults and adolescents, including health care workers; household contacts of immunocompromised individuals; teachers; day-care workers; residents and staff of institutional settings, colleges, prisons, or military installations; adolescents and adults living in households with children; international travelers; nonpregnant women of childbearing age

Abbreviations: HAV, hepatitis A virus; HBV, hepatitis B virus; HCV, hepatitis C virus; HIV, human immunodeficiency virus; MMR, measles–mumps–rubella; STD, sexually transmitted disease.

*For a more detailed discussion of bone density screening, see Bone density screening for osteoporosis. ACOG Committee Opinion No. 270. American College of Obstetricians and Gynecologists. Obstet Gynecol 2002;99:523–5.

†For a more detailed discussion of colorectal cancer screening, see Smith RA, von Eschenbach AC, Wender R, Levin B, Byers T, Rothenberger D, et al. American Cancer Society guidelines for the early detection of cancer: update of early detection guidelines for prostate, colorectal, and endometrial cancers. Also: update 2001—testing for early lung cancer detection [published erratum appears in CA Cancer J Clin 2001;51:150]. CA Cancer J Clin 2001;51:38–75; quiz 77–80.

Sources of Leading Causes of Mortality and Morbidity

Leading causes of mortality are provided by the Mortality Statistics Branch at the National Center for Health Statistics. Data are from 2000, the most recent year for which final data are available. The causes are ranked.

Leading causes of morbidity are unranked estimates based on information from the following sources:

- National Health Interview Survey, 1998
- National Ambulatory Medical Care Survey, 2001
- National Health and Nutrition Examination Survey III, 1998
- National Hospital Discharge Survey, 2001
- National Nursing Home Survey, 1997
- U.S. Department of Justice National Crime Victimization Survey
- U.S. Centers for Disease Control and Prevention Sexually Transmitted Disease Surveillance, 2001
- U.S. Centers for Disease Control and Prevention HIV/AIDS Surveillance Report, 2001

ACOG Committee Opinion

Committee on
Gynecologic Practice

Committee on
Obstetric Practice

Committee on
Professional Liability

Number 288, October 2003

Professional Liability and Gynecology-Only Practice

ABSTRACT: Some Fellows of the American College of Obstetricians and Gynecologists limit the scope of their practices solely to gynecology. The College considers early pregnancy complications (often up to 12–14 weeks of gestation) to be within the definition of gynecology. Liability insurance should cover the role of gynecologists in the management of early pregnancy-related conditions.

Some Fellows of the American College of Obstetricians and Gynecologists limit the scope of their practices to gynecology and do not request professional liability coverage for obstetrics. The College considers early pregnancy complications (often up to 12–14 weeks of gestation) to be within the definition of gynecology. Management of conditions such as ectopic pregnancy and spontaneous and elective abortion, including early and mid-trimester abortion, often are included in such a practice. Liability insurance should cover this role of gynecologists in the management of such early pregnancy-related conditions.

ISSN 1074-861X

The American College of
Obstetricians and Gynecologists
409 12th Street, SW
PO Box 96920
Washington, DC 20090-6920

12345/76543

Professional liability and gynecology-only practice. ACOG Committee Opinion No. 288. American College of Obstetricians and Gynecologists. Obstet Gynecol 2003;102:891.

ACOG

Committee on Health Care for Underserved Women

Committee Opinion

Number 317, October 2005

Racial and Ethnic Disparities in Women's Health

The Committee on Health Care for Underserved Women wishes to thank Raymond L. Cox, MD, MBA, for his invaluable assistance in the development of this document.

The American College of Obstetricians and Gynecologists
409 12th Street, SW
PO Box 96920
Washington, DC 20090-6920

12345/98765

Racial and ethnic disparities in women's health. ACOG Committee Opinion No. 317. American College of Obstetricians and Gynecologists. Obstet Gynecol 2005;106:889–92

ABSTRACT: Significant racial and ethnic disparities exist in women's health. These health disparities largely result from differences in socioeconomic status and insurance status. Although many disparities diminish after taking these factors into account, some remain because of health care system-level, patient-level, and provider-level factors. The American College of Obstetricians and Gynecologists strongly supports the elimination of racial and ethnic disparities in the health and the health care of women. Health professionals are encouraged to engage in activities to help achieve this goal.

Health disparities can be defined as "differences in the incidence, prevalence, mortality, and burden of diseases and other adverse health conditions that exist among specific population groups in the United States" (1). These differences can be assessed according to a variety of factors including gender, race or ethnicity, education, income, disability, geographic location, or sexual orientation (2). Although significant health disparities occur between men and women and among certain groups of women based on the factors mentioned previously, disparities are most likely to be experienced by women who are members of racial and ethnic minority groups. For example, disease and premature death occur disproportionately in minority women compared with non-Hispanic white women (3).

Approximately 44 million women in the United States, nearly one third of all women in this country, are members of racial and ethnic minority groups. African-American women and women of Hispanic origin together comprise roughly one quarter of the total population of U.S. women (4). The Hispanic population accounted for 22% of the 4 million births in the United States in 2003 (5). The largest segment of the immigrant population in the United States is from Latin America (6).

It is important to note that race and ethnicity are primarily social characteristics much more than they are biologic categories. However, race and ethnicity can provide useful information to women's health care providers about environmental, cultural, behavioral, and medical factors that may affect their patients' health. Also, the frequency of certain genetic variations may differ between racial or ethnic groups. For instance, there is an increased frequency of mutations for certain genetic diseases, such as Tay-Sachs disease, in individuals of Ashkenzic Jewish descent. These differences in the frequency of genetic variations generally are related to a common ancestral lineage (founder effect).

Genetic polymorphisms associated with increased susceptibility to disease also may vary in frequency in different racial and ethnic groups (7). Another consideration is the issue of gene-environment interaction. Genetic variations, even those that do not vary in frequency among racial or ethnic groups, may enhance susceptibility to an environmental exposure that occurs more frequently in a particular racial or ethnic group. Thus, although race and ethnicity are primarily social constructs, the impact of common ancestral lineage on the segregation and frequency of genetic variations in combination with the influence of cultural factors on environmental exposures cannot be ignored. All of these factors should be considered when trying to elucidate the multifactorial causes of health disparities.

Examples of Racial and Ethnic Health Disparities Among Women

- During 1991–1995, heart disease death rates remained the highest for African-American women, followed by white, American Indian/Alaskan Native, and Asian/Pacific Islander women, with more than a twofold difference between the lowest and highest rates (8).

- Asian/Pacific Islander women, especially those who are Vietnamese; black women; and Hispanic white women have higher incidence rates of invasive cervical cancer than non-Hispanic white women (9, 10). Cervical cancer mortality rates are higher among American Indian/Alaskan Natives than among all racial and ethnic populations (3.7 per 100,000 population and 2.6 per 100,000 population, respectively) despite lower incidence (11).

- When compared with white women, black women have a higher mortality rate (34.7 per 100,000 compared with 25.9 per 100,000) for breast cancer despite a lower breast cancer incidence rate (10).

- Seventy-eight percent of the female population with acquired immunodeficiency syndrome (AIDS) is African American or Hispanic. Although American Indian/Alaskan Native

women have a lower annual rate of new AIDS cases (4.8 per 100,000) than non-Hispanic black (50.2 per 100,000) and Hispanic (12.4 per 100,000) women, the rate is still more than twice the rate for non-Hispanic white women (2.0 per 100,000) (12).

- Non-Hispanic black and some Hispanic populations have preterm births at rates 60% and 27% higher, respectively, than the rate for non-Hispanic white women (13).

- African-American women have higher infant, fetal, and perinatal mortality rates than white women (14) (see Table 1).

- Although maternal mortality ratios for all ethnic groups have declined over the past half century, racial and ethnic disparities in maternal mortality have actually increased (15, 16). African-American women are three to six times more likely to have a pregnancy-related death than white women (16).

Understanding the Causes of Health Disparities

Many health disparities are directly related to inequities in income, housing, safety, education, and job opportunities; they largely result from differences in socioeconomic status and insurance status. Although many disparities diminish after taking these factors into account, some remain because of health care system-level, patient-level, and provider-level factors (17).

The current U.S. health care financing paradigm inadvertently may contribute to disparities in health outcomes. The United States is the only developed country that does not extend health care as a right of citizenship. In the United States, health care is

Table 1. Infant, Fetal, and Perinatal Mortality by Race of Mother

Race of Mother	Infant Mortality Rate	Fetal Mortality Rate	Perinatal Mortality Rate
White	5.8	5.5	5.9
Black or African American	14.4	11.9	12.8

National Center for Health Statistics. Health, United States, 2004: with chartbook on trends in the health of Americans. Hyattsville (MD): NCHS; 2004. Available at: http://www.cdc.gov/nchs/data/hus/hus04.pdf. Retrieved June 23, 2005.

driven by market forces; the ultimate goal of the health care business is to maximize profit. For these reasons, this health care system contributes to a lack of access for citizens who are either uninsured or underinsured. The varying geographic availability of health care institutions also may contribute to racial and ethnic disparities in health care.

Access to health insurance coverage and care and utilization of care is significantly different for minority women. The following examples illustrate this point:

- Hispanic and African-American women are more likely to be uninsured than white women. In 2001, 16% of white women, 20% of African-American women, and 37% of Hispanic women 18–64 years of age were uninsured (18).

- Asian-American and Hispanic women are most likely to have not received preventive care in the past year. In 1998, 29% of Asian-American women and 21% of Hispanic women received no preventive services in the previous year compared with 16% of white women and 7% of African-American women. (19).

- The proportion of Asian-American women obtaining Pap tests was considerably lower than that for white women. Only approximately one half (49%) of Asian-American women reported receiving a Pap test in the previous year compared with 64% of white women (19).

- Non-Hispanic black, Hispanic, and American Indian women are more than twice as likely as non-Hispanic white women to begin prenatal care in the third trimester or not at all (5).

Evidence suggests that factors such as stereotyping and prejudice on the part of health care providers may contribute to racial and ethnic disparities in health (17). Additionally, cultural differences between the health care provider and patient can cause communication problems between the patient and the provider and can lead to an inaccurate understanding of the patient's symptoms. Ambiguities between health care providers' and patients' understanding and interpretation of information may contribute to disparities in care (17). For example, language and literacy barriers interfere with physician–patient communication and can contribute to culturally derived mistrust of the health care system and to reduced adherence to health care provider recommendations. Use of traditional or folk remedies can interfere with science-based treatments. There also are lifestyle risk factors, such as unhealthy diets, low levels of physical activity, and alcohol and tobacco use, which contribute to morbidity and mortality and are more prevalent among certain populations (3).

ACOG Recommendations

The American College of Obstetricians and Gynecologists strongly supports the elimination of racial and ethnic disparities in women's health and health care as well as gender disparities in health and health care. The elimination of disparities in women's health and health care requires a comprehensive, multilevel strategy that involves all members of society. Our goal as health care providers and leaders must be to optimize individuals' health status and the quality of health care. We encourage health professionals to engage in the following activities:

1. Advocate for universal access to basic affordable health care (20).

2. Improve cultural competency in the physician–patient relationship and engage in cross-cultural educational activities to improve communication and language skills (21).

3. Use national best practice guidelines to reduce unintended variation in health care outcomes by gender, race, and ethnicity.

4. Provide high quality, compassionate, and ethically sound health care services to all. Engage in dialogue with patients to determine their care expectations, and counsel patients regarding the benefits of preventive health care and early screening, intervention, and treatment.

5. Advocate for increased public awareness of the benefits of preventive health care and early screening and intervention.

6. Encourage and become active in recruiting minorities to the health professions.

7. Advocate for improved access to programs that develop fluency in English among non-English speaking populations.

8. Acquire team-building skills to help attract and retain qualified nurses and other health professionals for provision of quality services to underserved women.

9. Conduct research to determine causes of health disparities and develop and evaluate interventions to address these causes.

10. Advocate for the continued collection of race-based data which is important in understanding disparities. Advocate for increased funding for this research.

11. Increase training of health care providers about racial, ethnic, and gender disparities in health and health care.

12. Support safety net providers, including public health systems, urban academic centers, and other health care delivery systems that are more likely to provide health care to minority populations.

References

1. Fauci AS. Slideshow: The NIH Strategic Plan to Address Health Disparities. Bethesda (MD): National Institutes of Allergy and Infectious Diseases; 2000. Available at: http://www.niaid.nih.gov/director/healthdis.htm. Retrieved June 23, 2005.

2. U.S. Department of Health and Human Services. Healthy people 2010: understanding and improving health. 2nd ed. Washington, DC: U.S. Government Printing Office; 2000. Available at: http://www.healthypeople.gov/Document/pdf/uih/2010uih.pdf. Retrieved June 23, 2005.

3. Clark A, Fong C, Romans M. Health disparities among U.S. women of color: an overview. Washington, DC: The Jacobs Institute of Women's Health; 2002.

4. U.S. Bureau of the Census. Population by age, sex, race, and Hispanic or Latino origin for the United States: 2000(PHC-T-9). Washington, DC: The Bureau; 2001. Available at: http://www.census.gov/population/www/cen2000/phc-t9.html. Retrieved June 23, 2005.

5. Hamilton BE, Martin JA, Sutton PD. Births: preliminary data for 2003. Natl Vital Stat Rep 2004;53(9):1–17.

6. Larsen LJ. The foreign-born population in the United States: 2003: population characteristics. Current Population Reports, P20-539. Washington, DC: US Census Bureau; 2004. Available at: http://www.census.gov/prod/2004pubs/p20–551.pdf. Retrieved June 23, 2005.

7. Romero R, Kuivaniemi H, Tromp G, Olson J. The design, execution, and interpretation of genetic association studies to decipher complex diseases. Am J Obstet Gynecol 2002;187:1299–312.

8. Casper ML, Barnett E, Halverson JA, Elmes GA, Braham VE, Majeed ZA, et al. Racial and ethnic disparities in heart disease among women. In: Women and heart disease: an atlas of racial and ethnic disparities in mortality.

2nd ed. Atlanta (GA): Centers for Disease Control and Prevention; Morgantown (WV): West Virginia University, Office for Social Environment and Health Research; 2000. Available at: ftp://ftp.cdc.gov/pub/Publications/womens_atlas/00-atlas-all.pdf. Retrieved June 22, 2005. p. 19–24.

9. Satcher D. American women and health disparities [editorial]. J Am Med Womens Assoc 2001;56:131–2, 160.

10. Ries LA, Eisner MP, Kosary CL, Hankey BF, Miller BA, Clegg L, et al., editors. SEER cancer statistics review, 1975–2002. Bethesda (MD): National Cancer Institute; 2005. Available at: http://seer.cancer.gov/csr/1975_2002. Retrieved June 23, 2005.

11. Cancer mortality among American Indians and Alaska Natives—United States, 1994–1998. Centers for Disease Control and Prevention. MMWR Morb Mortal Wkly Rep 2003;52:704–7.

12. Centers for Disease Control and Prevention. HIV/AIDS Surveillance Report, 2003;15:1–46. Available at: http://www.cdc.gov/hiv/stats/2003SurveillanceReport.pdf. Retrieved June 22, 2005.

13. Martin JA, Hamilton BE, Sutton PD, Ventura SJ, Menacker F, Munson ML. Births: final data for 2002. Natl Vital Stat Rep 2003;52(10):1–113.

14. National Center for Health Statistics. Health, United States, 2004: with chartbook on trends in the health of Americans. Hyattsville (MD): NCHS; 2004. Available at: http://www.cdc.gov/nchs/data/hus/hus04.pdf. Retrieved June 23, 2005.

15. Differences in maternal mortality among black and white women—United States, 1990. MMWR Morb Mortal Wkly Rep 1995;44:6–7, 13–4.

16. State-specific maternal mortality among black and white women—United States, 1987–1996. MMWR Morb Mortal Wkly Rep 1999;48:492–6.

17. Institute of Medicine (US). Unequal treatment: confronting racial and ethnic disparities in healthcare. Washington, DC: The Institutes 2002.

18. Kaiser Family Foundation. Racial and ethnic disparities in women's health coverage and access to care: findings from the 2001 Kaiser Women's Health Survey. Menlo Park (CA): KFF; 2004. Available at: http://www.kff.org/womenshealth/loader.cfm?url=/commonspot/security/getfile.cfm&PageID=33087. Retrieved June 23, 2005.

19. Collins KS, Schoen C, Joseph S, Duchon L, Simantov E, Yellowitz M. Health concerns across a woman's lifespan: The Commonwealth Fund 1998 Survey of Women's Health. New York (NY): The Commonwealth Fund; 1999.

20. The uninsured. ACOG Committee Opinion No. 308. American College of Obstetricians and Gynecologists. Obstet Gynecol 2004;104:1471–4.

21. American College of Obstetricians and Gynecologists. Cultural competency, sensitivity and awareness in the delivery of health care. In: Special issues in women's health. Washington, DC: ACOG; 2005. p. 11–20.

ACOG

Committee on
Obstetric Practice

Committee Opinion

Number 248, December 2000

Response to Searle's Drug Warning on Misoprostol

On August 23, 2000, G.D. Searle & Co. issued a letter entitled "Important Drug Warning Concerning Unapproved Use of Intravaginal or Oral Misoprostol in Pregnant Women for Induction of Labor or Abortion." This letter cautions that Cytotec (misoprostol) is indicated for prevention of nonsteroidal-antiinflammatory-drug-induced gastric ulcers and states, *"…Cytotec administration by any route is contraindicated in women who are pregnant because it can cause abortion."* The letter further states that Searle has become aware of the drug's use for induction of labor or as a cervical ripening agent prior to termination of pregnancy. Moreover, the letter notes serious adverse events, including uterine hyperstimulation and uterine rupture, which have resulted in fetal and maternal death. Finally, the company cautions, *"In addition to the known and unknown acute risks to the mother and fetus, the effect of Cytotec on the later growth, development, and functional maturation of the child when Cytotec is used for induction of labor or cervical ripening has not been established."*

The American College of Obstetricians and Gynecologists (ACOG) is concerned about the content, timing, and tone of this letter. Given that misoprostol is commonly employed in conjunction with mifepristone (RU 486) to achieve nonsurgical early pregnancy terminations, the arrival of the Searle letter within weeks of the U.S. Food and Drug Administration's (FDA) approval of mifepristone could limit the use of this new option for reproductive choice. Also, although the letter correctly points out the potentially serious, but relatively rare, risks of misoprostol when employed for cervical ripening and labor induction, it fails to comment on the extensive clinical experience with this agent and the large body of published reports supporting its safety and efficacy when used appropriately. A recent review of the Cochrane Pregnancy and Childbirth group trials registry identified 26 clinical trials of misoprostol for cervical ripening or induction of labor or both (1). These studies indicate misoprostol is more effective than prostaglandin E_2 in achieving vaginal deliveries within 24 hours and reduces the need for and total amount of oxytocin augmentation. Although these studies do suggest misoprostol is associated with a higher incidence of uterine hyperstimulation and meconium-stained amniotic fluid, these complications were more common with higher doses (>25 µg) of misoprostol. Other recent reviews and

The American College of Obstetricians and Gynecologists
409 12th Street, SW
PO Box 96920
Washington, DC 20090-6920

12345/43210

clinical trials support these conclusions (2–4). No studies indicate that intrapartum exposure to misoprostol (or other prostaglandin cervical ripening agents) has any long-term adverse health consequences to the fetus in the absence of fetal distress, nor is there a plausible biologic basis for such a concern.

A review of published reports and of MedWatch, the FDA medical products reporting program, indicates the vast majority of adverse maternal and fetal outcomes associated with misoprostol therapy resulted from the use of doses greater than 25 µg, dosing intervals more frequent than 3–6 hours, addition of oxytocin less than 4 hours after the last misoprostol dose, or use of the drug in women with prior cesarean delivery or major uterine surgery. Grand multiparity also appears to be a relative risk factor for uterine rupture.

Thus, based on recently published series and a detailed review of adverse outcomes reported to the FDA, the ACOG Committee on Obstetric Practice strongly endorses its previous conclusion, published in Committee Opinion Number 228 (November 1999), *Induction of Labor with Misoprostol*, which states, *"Given the current evidence, intravaginal misoprostol tablets appear effective in inducing labor in pregnant women who have unfavorable cervices"* (5). Nonetheless, the committee would like to emphasize that the following clinical practices appear to minimize the risk of uterine hyperstimulation and rupture in patients undergoing cervical ripening or induction in the third trimester:

1. If misoprostol is to be used for cervical ripening or labor induction in the third trimester, one quarter of a 100-µg tablet (ie, approximately 25 µg) should be considered for the initial dose.

2. Doses should not be administered more frequently than every 3–6 hours.

3. Oxytocin should not be administered less than 4 hours after the last misoprostol dose.

4. Misoprostol should not be used in patients with a previous cesarean delivery or prior major uterine surgery.

The use of higher doses of misoprostol (eg, 50 µg every 6 hours) to induce labor may be appropriate in some situations, although there are reports that such doses increase the risk of complications, including uterine hyperstimulation and uterine rupture (6). There is insufficient clinical evidence to address the safety or efficacy of misoprostol in patients with multifetal gestations or suspected fetal macrosomia.

In conclusion, the ACOG Committee on Obstetric Practice reaffirms that misoprostol is a safe and effective agent for cervical ripening and labor induction when used appropriately. Moreover, misoprostol also contributes to the obstetrician–gynecologist's resources as an effective treatment for serious postpartum hemorrhage in the presence of uterine atony (7–12).

References

1. Hofmeyr GJ, Gulmezoglu AM. Vaginal misoprostol for cervical ripening and labour induction in late pregnancy (Cochrane Review). In: The Cochrane Library, Issue 3, 2000. Oxford: Update Software
2. Wing DA. Labor induction with misoprostol. Am J Obstet Gynecol 1999;181:339–345
3. Nunes F, Rodrigues R, Meirinho M. Randomized comparison between intravaginal misoprostol and dinoprostone for cervical ripening and induction of labor. Am J Obstet Gynecol 1999;181:626–629
4. Blanchette HA, Nayak S, Erasmus S. Comparison of the safety and efficacy of intravaginal misoprostol (prostaglandin E1) with those of dinoprostone (prostaglandin E2) for cervical ripening and induction of labor in a community hospital. Am J Obstet Gynecol 1999;180:1551–1559
5. American College of Obstetricians and Gynecologists. Induction of labor with misoprostol. ACOG Committee Opinion 228. Washington, DC: ACOG, 1999
6. American College of Obstetricians and Gynecologists. Induction of labor. ACOG Practice Bulletin 10. Washington, DC: ACOG, 1999
7. El-Refaey H, O'Brien P, Morafa W, Walder J, Rodeck C. Use of oral misoprostol in the prevention of postpartum haemorrhage. Br J Obstet Gynaecol 1997;104:336–339
8. O'Brien P, El-Refaey H, Gordon A, Geary M, Rodeck CH. Rectally administered misoprostol for the treatment of postpartum hemorrhage unresponsive to oxytocin and ergometrine: a descriptive study. Obstet Gynecol 1998;92:212–214
9. Bamigboye AA, Hofmeyr GJ, Merrell DA. Rectal misoprostol in the prevention of postpartum hemorrhage: a placebo-controlled trial. Am J Obstet Gynecol 1998;179:1043–1046
10. Surbek DV, Fehr PM, Hosli I, Holzgreve W. Oral misoprostol for third stage of labor: a randomized placebo-controlled trial. Obstet Gynecol 1999;94:255–258
11. Hofmeyr GJ, Nikodem VC, de Jager M, Gelbart BR. A randomised placebo controlled trial of oral misoprostol in the third stage of labour. Br J Obstet Gynaecol 1998;105:971–975
12. Bamigboye AA, Merrell DA, Hofmeyr GJ, Mitchell R. Randomized comparison of rectal misoprostol with Syntometrine for management of third stage of labor. Acta Obstet Gynecol Scand 1998;77:178–181

ACOG

Committee on
Gynecologic Practice

Committee Opinion

Number 186, September 1997   *(Replaces #140, June 1994)*

Role of the Obstetrician–Gynecologist in the Diagnosis and Treatment of Breast Disease

Obstetrician–gynecologists are in a favorable position to diagnose breast disease in their patients. The American College of Obstetricians and Gynecologists (ACOG) has adopted the goals of assisting in educating obstetrician–gynecologists in the diagnosis and treatment of benign breast disease and in reducing mortality from breast cancer. As an initial step toward these goals, ACOG has developed the following guidelines for the early diagnosis of breast disease:

1. Breast examination by visual inspection and palpation should be an integral part of initial obstetric and all complete gynecologic examinations.

2. Patients should be instructed in the technique of life-long periodic self-examination of the breast and informed of the importance of self-examination.

3. Patients should be encouraged to undergo screening by mammography in accordance with ACOG guidelines. Earlier or more frequent screening is recommended for women who have had breast cancer or who have a first-degree relative (ie, mother, sister, or daughter) or multiple other relatives who have a history of premenopausal breast or breast and ovarian cancer.

4. Obstetrician–gynecologists should perform diagnostic procedures when indicated.

5. When indicated, referrals should be made to physicians who specialize in the diagnosis and treatment of the type of breast disease that is suspected.

6. Institutions that credential physicians to perform breast surgery should apply the same criteria for clinical competence to obstetrician–gynecologists as to other physicians requesting to obtain or maintain such privileges.

7. A persistent palpable breast mass requires evaluation. Mammography alone is not sufficient to rule out malignant pathology in a patient with a palpable breast mass. Ultrasonography or magnified mammographic imaging of the breast containing the mass may provide additional information and may identify cystic structures or variations in normal breast architecture that account for the palpable abnormality.

The American College of Obstetricians and Gynecologists

409 12th Street, SW
PO Box 96920
Washington, DC 20090-6920

12345/10987

When cyst aspiration is performed, the fluid may be discarded if it is clear (transparent and not bloody) and the mass disappears. Otherwise, the patient should be considered a candidate for a breast biopsy.

Solid masses usually require histologic diagnosis. Fine-needle aspiration or stereotactic needle biopsy may be an alternative to open breast biopsy in some cases. If breast cancer or a specific benign condition is not detected by fine-needle aspiration or needle core biopsy, open biopsy is necessary. Because the incidence of breast cancer is extremely low in patients younger than 20 years of age, patients in this age group who have solid masses that appear to be benign when examined by ultrasonography can be monitored without biopsy at the discretion of the physician. These guidelines apply both to pregnant and to nonpregnant women.

8. When a patient is referred to another physician for management of a breast disorder, following are the responsibilities of the obstetrician–gynecologist:

- Explain to the patient that she needs further care
- Provide names of qualified physicians from whom the patient can receive care
- Answer the patient's questions
- Document these steps and include a detailed description of the clinical findings in the medical record

The American College of Obstetricians and Gynecologists encourages both basic and clinical research into the etiology, early diagnosis, and treatment of all breast disease. Postgraduate education, including residency training programs in obstetrics and gynecology and continuing medical education, should include education in the early diagnosis and management of all forms of breast disease. Obstetrician–gynecologists also should take advantage of opportunities to educate other physicians involved in the health care of women about the diagnosis and treatment of breast disease.

Bibliography

American College of Obstetricians and Gynecologists. Nonmalignant conditions of the breast. ACOG Technical Bulletin 156. Washington, DC: ACOG, 1991

American College of Obstetricians and Gynecologists. Carcinoma of the breast. ACOG Technical Bulletin 158. Washington, DC: ACOG, 1991

American College of Obstetricians and Gynecologists. Guidelines for women's health care. Washington, DC: ACOG, 1996

American College of Obstetricians and Gynecologists. Routine cancer screening. ACOG Committee Opinion 185. Washington, DC: ACOG, 1997

Brenner RJ, Fajardo L, Fisher PR, Dershaw DD, Evans WP, Bassett L, et al. Percutaneous core biopsy of the breast: effect of operator experience and number of samples on diagnostic accuracy. AJR Am J Roentgenol 1996;166:341–346

Mainiero MB, Philpotts LE, Lee CH, Lange RC, Carter D, Tocino I. Stereotaxic core needle biopsy of breast microcalcifications: correlation of target accuracy and diagnosis with lesion size. Radiology 1996;198:665–669

Mitnick JS, Vazquez MF, Feiner HD, Pressman P, Roses DF. Mammographically detected breast lesions: clinical importance of cytologic atypia in stereotaxic fine-needle aspiration biopsy samples. Radiology 1996;198:319–322

ACOG

Committee on
Obstetric Practice

Committee
on Genetics

Committee Opinion

Number 183, April 1997

Routine Storage of Umbilical Cord Blood for Potential Future Transplantation

Reconstitution of the bone marrow can be a life-saving procedure in the treatment of hematologic disease (eg, Fanconi anemia) or advanced malignancy. The necessary hematopoietic stem and progenitor cells are usually obtained from allogeneic or autologous bone marrow. If autologous marrow is not an option, then a human leukocyte antigen (HLA)-identical sibling is the donor most likely to result in successful engraftment and minimization of the risk of graft-versus-host (GVH) disease. Most people do not have an HLA-identical sibling available, and they must look outside of their families. There is a national registry of potential bone marrow donors, but finding an identical match and convincing that individual to undergo the unpleasant donation procedure is not always easy. Many individuals who could potentially benefit from transplantation die while awaiting donors.

A recently recognized potential source for hematopoietic stem and progenitor cells is human fetal cord blood. Early results from more than 200 transplants of human cord stem cells, primarily to treat childhood malignancies, seem very encouraging for several reasons. There appears to be a relatively high success rate for the procedure even in the face of HLA mismatches at one or more loci. There also appears to be a somewhat lower risk for GVH disease than that which is true for traditional bone marrow transplantation. These encouraging preliminary reports have generated considerable enthusiasm because the 4 million births per year in the United States would appear to provide a large reservoir of genetically diverse, potentially transplantable specimens. Large volumes of cord blood are now being "wasted" as "discarded human material" that could theoretically be easily collected, typed, screened for infections, and banked cryogenically for transplantation.

The use of this technology raises a number of scientific, legal, and ethical issues that need to be addressed:

- Should cord blood specimens be collected and banked centrally for allogeneic transplantation in a system analogous to the way that we now handle blood, or would parents be well-advised to bank their own child's cord blood at birth for potential future autologous use should it ever be necessary?

The American College of Obstetricians and Gynecologists
409 12th Street, SW
PO Box 96920
Washington, DC 20090-6920

12345/10987

- What is the probability that any individual will ever need his or her own cord blood for transplantation? If that need does arise 18 years later, what is the probability that a specimen stored for 18 years will still be viable?

- Most transplants to date have been done in babies and young children. More cells are needed to reconstitute the bone marrow of persons of larger size. What percentage of cord blood specimens will have adequate numbers of cells to reconstitute the bone marrow of adults?

- Are cord blood stem and progenitor cells more efficient at reconstituting marrow than are cells obtained from adult marrow? Would fewer cells on a per-kilogram body weight basis be as effective?

- Could the number of stem and progenitor cells in a specimen of cord blood be expanded in vitro to provide enough cells for a reliable reconstitution of the bone marrow of persons of adult size?

- If the apparently lower incidence of GVH disease compared with adult marrow sources is real, it may represent reduced immunocompetence of cord stem and progenitor cells. This may be disadvantageous in treating patients with cancer. It may also permit a higher incidence of second primary cancers in transplant survivors.

- As many as 38% of cord blood specimens may be contaminated with maternal cells. What effect will this contamination with adult cells that are (presumably) immunocompetent have upon graft success rate?

- In the future, there may be other medical approaches to manage these diseases.

- Should this technology continue to show promise, and the decision is made to establish cord blood banks, should cord blood continue to be regarded as "discarded human material?"

- Could cord blood be collected routinely at deliveries without consent?

- All specimens would need to be tested for infectious and selected genetic diseases before use. Should parents be informed if their child's specimen tests positive for an infection (eg, human immunodeficiency virus) or genetic disease?

- If nonpaternity is discovered in the course of testing, should that be disclosed to the mother, father, or child?

- Physicians should resist the pressures of marketing, and they should evaluate thoroughly the potential benefits and risks—emotional as well as physical—of all new medical interventions.

Privately owned for-profit companies have been established to bank cord blood samples for potential future use by those individuals or their family members. There is a significant cost associated with the initial specimen processing (approximately $1,500) and an annual storage fee (approximately $100). Given the low probability of needing a stem cell transplant (which has been estimated at between 1 in 1,000 and 1 in 200,000 by age 18) and the other uncertainties regarding success rates with increasing body mass and time in storage, is this a "good" investment? In view of the apparent success rate, despite HLA mismatch, will there be an advantage to receiving one's own banked cells, or could one do just as well with someone else's cord blood? Once banked, to whom do the cells there belong? Do they belong to the parents who paid the fees or the child from whom they came? Do the parents have the right to give them away or sell them, or should they be held for the person from whom they came until he or she reaches the age of majority? If the cells are to be used for someone other than the person from whom they came, must both parents agree or is consent from one adequate? What happens if the parents disagree?

There are clearly many questions about this technology that remain to be answered. Some are relatively simple, such as the success rate of the procedure for various diseases and at various body weights. These simply await a larger number of cases. Some will be more difficult, such as the viability of cells in long-term storage; these questions will take time to answer. The most difficult will be the moral, ethical, and social questions, which need extensive public discussion and may never all be resolved to everyone's satisfaction. Until there is a fuller understanding of all of these issues, we must proceed with considerable circumspection. Parents should not be sold this service without a realistic assessment of their likely return on their investment. Commercial cord blood banks should not represent the service they sell as "doing everything possible" to ensure the health of children. Parents and grandparents should not be made to feel guilty if they are not eager or able to invest these considerable sums in such a highly speculative venture.

Bibliography

Broxmeyer HE. Questions to be answered regarding umbilical cord blood hematopoietic stem and progenitor cells and their use in transplantation. Transfusion 1995;35:694-702

Kurtzberg J, Laughlin M, Graham ML, Smith C, Olson JF, Halperin EC, et al. Placental blood as a source of hematopoietic stem cells for transplantation into unrelated recipients. N Engl J Med 1996;335:157-166

Laporte JP, Gorin NC, Rubinstein P, Lesage S, Portnoi MF, Barbu V, et al. Cord-blood transplantation from an unrelated donor in an adult with chronic myelogenous leukemia. N Engl J Med 1996;335:167-170

Marshall E. Clinical promise, ethical quandary. Science 1996;271:586-588

Rubinstein P, Rosenfield RE, Adamson JW, Stevens CE. Stored placental blood for unrelated bone marrow reconstitution. Blood 1993;81:1679-1690

Scaradavou A, Carrier C, Mollen N, Stevens C, Rubenstein P. Detection of maternal DNA in placental/umbilical cord blood by locus-specific amplification of the noninherited maternal HLA gene. Blood 1996;88:1494-1500

Silberstein LE, Jefferies LC. Placental-blood banking—a new frontier in transfusion medicine. N Engl J Med 1996;335:199-201

Wagner JE, Rosenthal J, Sweetman R, Shu XO, Davies SM, Ramsay NK, et al. Successful transplantation of HLA-matched and HLA-mismatched umbilical cord blood from unrelated donors: analysis of engraftment and acute graft-versus-host disease. Blood 1996:88:795-802

ACOG

Committee on Obstetric Practice

Committee Opinion

Number 281, December 2002

Rubella Vaccination

ABSTRACT: The incidence of rubella decreased from 0.45 per 100,000 in 1990 to 0.1 per 100,000 in 1999. Although there is a nationwide shortage of rubella vaccine, women who are rubella susceptible during pregnancy should receive MMR (measles–mumps–rubella) vaccination postpartum. In October 2001, the federal Centers for Disease Control and Prevention changed the recommendations concerning the pregnancy interval after receiving rubella vaccine. This interval has been reduced from 3 months to 1 month.

The incidence of rubella decreased from 0.45 per 100,000 in 1990 to 0.1 per 100,000 in 1999 (1). There have been cluster outbreaks, especially among persons born outside of the United States. Although there is a nationwide shortage of rubella vaccine, women who are rubella susceptible during pregnancy should receive MMR (measles–mumps–rubella) vaccination postpartum. The appropriate test for assessing rubella immunity is the immunoglobulin G serology. There is no contraindication to giving MMR vaccination while breastfeeding. Receipt of rubella vaccination in a new mother does not pose a risk of transmission of the virus to the newborn or to other children in her household. Receipt of rubella vaccination during pregnancy is not an indication for interruption of that pregnancy.

In October 2001, the federal Centers for Disease Control and Prevention changed the recommendations concerning the pregnancy interval after receiving rubella vaccine. This interval has been reduced from 3 months to 1 month (2). The safe interval for measles and mumps vaccination was already 1 month.

References

1. Reef SE, Frey TK, Theall K, Abernathy E, Burnett CL, Icenogle J, et al. The changing epidemiology of rubella in the 1990s: on the verge of elimination and new challenges for control and prevention. JAMA 2002;287:464-72.
2. Revised ACIP recommendation for avoiding pregnancy after receiving a rubella-containing vaccine. MMWR Morb Mortal Wkly Rep 2001;50:1117.

The American College of Obstetricians and Gynecologists
409 12th Street, SW
PO Box 96920
Washington, DC 20090-6920

12345/65432

Rubella vaccination. ACOG Committee Opinion No. 281. American College of Obstetricians and Gynecologists. Obstet Gynecol 2002;100:1417.

ACOG Committee Opinion

Committee on Obstetric Practice

Number 276, October 2002

ISSN 1074-861X

The American College of Obstetricians and Gynecologists
409 12th Street, SW
PO Box 96920
Washington, DC 20090-6920

12345/65432

Safety of Lovenox in pregnancy. Committee Opinion No. 276. American College of Obstetricians and Gynecologists. Obstet Gynecol 2002;100:845–6.

Safety of Lovenox in Pregnancy

ABSTRACT: *Lovenox (enoxaparin sodium) therapy appears to be safe and efficacious for pregnant women who are candidates for either prophylactic or therapeutic heparin. However, the use of enoxaparin and other low-molecular-weight heparins for therapeutic anticoagulation is not recommended for pregnant women with prosthetic heart valves. Additionally, enoxaparin should be used with caution or discontinued before administration of epidural for pain relief during labor.*

Aventis Pharmaceuticals has issued a letter to health professionals describing the addition of warnings and precautions to their Lovenox Injection (enoxaparin sodium) prescribing information. The "Warnings" section notes that Lovenox Injection is not recommended for thromboprophylaxis in patients with prosthetic heart valves because of reports of valvular thrombosis in patients who were apparently adequately anticoagulated. The cases reported by the manufacturer and in the literature suggest a relatively frequent occurrence of valvular thromboses in pregnant women treated with low-molecular-weight heparin, possibly caused by the hypercoagulability of pregnancy (1, 2). The American College of Obstetricians and Gynecologists' (ACOG) Committee on Obstetric Practice concurs that low-molecular-weight heparins should not be used for anticoagulation in pregnant women with prosthetic heart valves.

The "Precautions" section now includes a paragraph in the "Pregnancy" subsection that reports the occurrence of congenital anomalies in infants of women treated with Lovenox Injection during pregnancy, but it notes that a "cause and effect relationship has not been established nor has the incidence been shown to be higher than in the general population." The Committee on Obstetric Practice does not believe that Lovenox Injection presents a teratogenic risk for the following three reasons: 1) the agent does not cross the placenta, providing no biologic plausibility for such a risk (3); 2) a large study by Lepercq and associates described pregnancy outcomes in 604 women treated with enoxaparin during 624 pregnancies and observed a congenital anomaly rate of 2.5%, which is consistent with the rate in the general population (4); and 3) the variety of anomalies reported by Aventis Pharmaceuticals, and their rare occurrence, suggests no specific pathogenic pattern or increased frequency.

Aventis Pharmaceuticals also states that there "have been post-marketing reports of fetal death when pregnant women received Lovenox® Injection" and warns of the risk of hemorrhage in women receiving enoxaparin during pregnancy. However, a review by the Committee on Obstetric Practice of the reported events actually suggests the occurrence of both fetal deaths and hemorrhage is rare despite the high-risk nature of this population. This is borne out in the survey of enoxaparin users by Lepercq and associates who observed a 1.1% fetal death rate and noted that none of the fetal or neonatal adverse events was related to enoxaparin (4). This study noted enoxaparin-related hemorrhage occurred in 1 of 624 pregnancies, and the occurrence of recurrent maternal venous thrombotic events in this high-risk population was 1.3%.

Enoxaparin therapy appears to be safe and efficacious when used in pregnant women. The Committee on Obstetric Practice reiterates the recommendations made by ACOG that "Patients who are candidates for either prophylactic or therapeutic heparin may be given enoxaparin or dalteparin during pregnancy" (5). In addition, the Committee on Obstetric Practice recommends against the use of enoxaparin and other low-molecular-weight heparins for therapeutic anticoagulation in pregnant women with prosthetic heart valves. Enoxaparin should not be used 18–24 hours before administration of epidural for pain relief during labor (6).

References

1. Rowan JA, McCowan LM, Raudkivi PJ, North RA. Enoxaparin treatment in women with mechanical heart valves during pregnancy. Am J Obstet Gynecol 2001; 185:633–7.
2. Lev-Ran O, Kramer A, Gurevitch J, Shapira I, Mohr R. Low-molecular-weight heparin for prosthetic heart valves: treatment failure. Ann Thorac Surg 2000;69:264–5; discussion 265–6.
3. Dimitrakakis C, Papageorgiou P, Papageorgiou I, Antzaklis A, Sakarelou N, Michalas S. Absence of transplacental passage of the low molecular weight heparin enoxaparin. Haemostasis 2000;30:243–8.
4. Lepercq J, Conard J, Borel-Derlon A, Damon JY, Boudignat O, Francoual C, et al. Venous thromboembolism during pregnancy: a retrospective study of enoxaparin safety in 624 pregnancies. BJOG 2001;108:1134–40.
5. American College of Obstetricians and Gynecologists. Thromboembolism in pregnancy. ACOG Practice Bulletin 19. Washington DC: ACOG; 2000.
6. Horlocker TT, Wedel DJ. Neuraxial block and low-molecular-weight heparin: balancing perioperative analgesia and thromboprophylaxis. Reg Anesth Pain Med 1998;23(suppl 2):164–77.

ACOG

Committee on
Obstetric Practice

Committee Opinion

Number 234, May 2000   *(Replaces No. 219, August 1999)*

Scheduled Cesarean Delivery and the Prevention of Vertical Transmission of HIV Infection

Prevention of transmission of the human immunodeficiency virus (HIV) from mother to fetus or newborn (vertical transmission) is a major goal in the care of pregnant women infected with HIV. An important advance in this regard was the demonstration that treatment of the mother with zidovudine (ZDV) during pregnancy and labor and of the neonate for the first 6 weeks after birth could reduce the transmission rate from 25% to 8% (1).

Continuing research into vertical transmission of HIV suggests that a substantial number of cases occur as the result of fetal exposure to the virus during labor and delivery; the precise mechanisms are not known. Transmission could occur by transplacental maternal–fetal microtransfusion of blood contaminated with the virus during uterine contractions or by exposure to the virus in maternal cervicovaginal secretions and blood at delivery. Data also indicate that the risk of vertical transmission is proportional to the concentration of virus in maternal plasma (viral load). At very low concentrations of virus in maternal plasma (viral load less than 1,000 copies per milliliter), the observed incidence of vertical transmission among 141 mother–infant pairs was 0 with a 95% upper confidence bound of about 2% (2, 3).

In theory, the risk of vertical transmission in mothers with high viral loads could be reduced by performing cesarean deliveries before the onset of labor and before rupture of membranes (termed *scheduled cesarean delivery* in this document). Early studies of the relationship between the mode of delivery and the risk of vertical transmission yielded inconsistent results. Data from two prospective cohort studies (4, 5), an international randomized trial (6), and a meta-analysis of individual patient data from 15 prospective cohort studies, including more than 7,800 mother–child pairs (7), indicate that there is a significant relationship between the mode of delivery and vertical transmission of HIV. This body of evidence, accumulated mostly before the use of highly active antiretroviral therapy (HAART) and without any data regarding maternal viral load, indicates that scheduled cesarean delivery reduces the likelihood of vertical transmission of HIV compared with either unscheduled cesarean delivery or vaginal delivery. This finding holds true whether or not the patient is receiving ZDV therapy. Whether cesarean deliv-

The American College of Obstetricians and Gynecologists
409 12th Street, SW
PO Box 96920
Washington, DC 20090-6920

12345/43210

ery offers any benefit to women on HAART or to women with low or undetectable maternal viral loads is unknown. Data are insufficient to address the question of how long after the onset of labor or rupture of membranes the benefit is lost. It is clear that maternal morbidity is greater with cesarean delivery than with vaginal delivery, as is true for women not infected with HIV (8–10). Increases in postpartum morbidity seem to be greatest among women infected with HIV who have low CD4 cell counts (9).

Although many issues remain unresolved because of insufficient data, there is consensus that the following should be recommended:

- Patients should be counseled that in the absence of antiretroviral therapy, the risk of vertical transmission is approximately 25%. With ZDV therapy, the risk is reduced to 5–8%. When care includes both ZDV therapy and scheduled cesarean delivery, the risk is approximately 2%. A similar risk of 2% or less is seen among women with viral loads of less than 1,000 copies per milliliter, even without the systematic use of scheduled cesarean delivery. No combination of therapies can guarantee that a newborn will not become infected (a 0% transmission rate).

- Women infected with HIV, whose viral loads are greater than 1,000 copies per milliliter, should be counseled regarding the potential benefit of scheduled cesarean delivery to further reduce the risk of vertical transmission of HIV beyond that achievable with antiretroviral therapy alone.

- Neonates of women at highest risk for vertical transmission, with relatively high plasma viral loads, are most likely to benefit from scheduled cesarean delivery. Data are insufficient to demonstrate a benefit for neonates of women with plasma viral loads of less than 1,000 copies per milliliter. The available data indicate no reduction in the transmission rate if cesarean delivery is performed after the onset of labor or rupture of membranes. The decision regarding the route of delivery must be individualized in these circumstances.

- The patient's autonomy in making the decision regarding route of delivery must be respected. A patient's informed decision to undergo vaginal delivery must be honored, with cesarean delivery performed only for other accepted indications and with patient consent.

- Patients should receive antiretroviral chemotherapy during pregnancy according to currently accepted guidelines for adults (11). This should not be interrupted around the time of cesarean delivery. For those patients receiving ZDV, adequate levels of the drug in the blood should be achieved if the infusion is begun 3 hours preoperatively (1), according to the dosing schedule recommended by the Centers for Disease Control and Prevention (www.cdc.gov/hiv/treatment).

- Because morbidity is increased in HIV-infected women undergoing cesarean delivery, physicians should consider using prophylactic antibiotics during all such cesarean deliveries.

- The American College of Obstetricians and Gynecologists generally recommends that scheduled cesarean deliveries not be performed before 39 completed weeks of gestation. In women with HIV infection, however, delivery at 38 completed weeks of gestation is recommended to reduce the likelihood of onset of labor or rupture of membranes before delivery.

- Best clinical estimates of gestational age should be used for planning cesarean delivery. Amniocentesis to determine fetal lung maturity in pregnant women infected with HIV should be avoided whenever possible.

- Current recommendations for adults indicate that plasma viral load should be determined at baseline and then every 3 months or following changes in therapy (11). Plasma viral load should be monitored, according to these guidelines, during pregnancy as well. The patient's most recently determined viral load should be used to direct counseling regarding mode of delivery.

- Preoperative maternal health status affects the degree of risk of maternal morbidity associated with cesarean delivery. All women should be clearly informed of the risks associated with cesarean delivery. Ultimately, the decision to perform a cesarean delivery must be individualized in each case according to circumstances.

A skin-penetrating injury (eg, needlestick or scalpel laceration) is a risk to care providers during all deliveries, vaginal or cesarean. This risk is not greater during cesarean delivery, although there generally are more health care personnel present and, thus, at risk during a cesarean delivery than during a vaginal delivery (12). Appropriate care and precautions against such injuries always should be taken, but these concerns should not affect decisions regarding route of delivery (13).

In summary, cesarean delivery performed before the onset of labor and before rupture of membranes effectively reduces the risk of vertical transmission of HIV infection. Scheduled cesarean delivery should be discussed and recommended for women with viral loads greater than 1,000 copies per milliliter whether or not they are taking antiretroviral therapy. As with all complex clinical decisions, the choice of delivery must be individualized. Discussion of the option of scheduled cesarean delivery should begin as early as possible in pregnancy with every pregnant woman with HIV infection to give her an adequate opportunity to consider the choice and plan for the procedure. The risks, which are greater for the mother, must be balanced with the benefits expected for the neonate. The patient's autonomy must be respected when making the decision to perform a cesarean delivery, because the potential for maternal morbidity is significant.

References

1. Connor EM, Sperling RS, Gelber R, Kiselev P, Scott G, O'Sullivan MJ, et al. Reduction of maternal-infant transmission of human immunodeficiency virus type 1 with zidovudine treatment. Pediatric AIDS Clinical Trials Group Protocol 076 Study Group. N Engl J Med 1994;331:1173–1180

2. Mofenson LM, Lambert JS, Stiehm ER, Bethel J, Meyer WA 3rd, Whitehouse J, et al. Risk factors for perinatal transmission of human immunodeficiency virus type 1 in women treated with zidovudine. Pediatric AIDS Clinical Trials Group Study 185 Team. N Engl J Med 1999;341:385–393

3. Garcia PM, Kalish LA, Pitt J, Minkoff H, Quinn T, Burchett SK, et al. Maternal levels of plasma human immunodeficiency virus type 1 RNA and the risk of perinatal transmission. Women and Infants Transmission Study Group. N Engl J Med 1999;341:394–402

4. Kind C, Rudin C, Siegrist CA, Wyler CA, Biedermann K, Lauper U, et al. Prevention of vertical HIV transmission: additive protective effect of elective cesarean section and zidovudine prophylaxis. AIDS 1998;12:205–210

5. Mandelbrot L, Le Chenadec J, Berrebi A, Bongain A, Benifla JL, Delfraissy JF, et al. Perinatal HIV-1 transmission: interaction between zidovudine prophylaxis and mode of delivery in the French Perinatal Cohort. JAMA 1998;280:55–60

6. The European Mode of Delivery Collaboration. Elective caesarean-section versus vaginal delivery in prevention of vertical HIV-1 transmission: a randomized clinical trial. Lancet 1999;353:1035–1039

7. The International Perinatal HIV Group. The mode of delivery and the risk of vertical transmission of human immunodeficiency virus type 1: a meta-analysis of 15 prospective cohort studies. N Engl J Med 1999;340:977–987

8. Nielsen TF, Hakegaard KH. Postoperative cesarean section morbidity: a prospective study. Am J Obstet Gynecol 1983; 146:911–915

9. Semprini AE, Castagna C, Ravizza M, Fiore S, Savasi V, Muggiasca ML, et al. The incidence of complications after cesarean section in 156 HIV-positive women. AIDS 1996; 9:913–917

10. Bulterys M, Chao A, Dushimimana A, Saah A. Fatal complications after cesarean section in HIV-infected women. AIDS 1996;10:923–924

11. Centers for Disease Control and Prevention. Report of the NIH Panel to define principles of therapy of HIV infection and guidelines for the use of antiretroviral agents in HIV-infected adults and adolescents. MMWR Morb Mortal Wkly Rep 1998;47(RR-5):1–82

12. Duff P, Robertson AW, Read JA. Single-dose cefazolin versus cefonicid for antibiotic prophylaxis in cesarean delivery. Obstet Gynecol 1987;70:718–721

13. Centers for Disease Control. Update: universal precautions for prevention of transmission of human immunodeficiency virus, hepatitis B virus, and other bloodborne pathogens in health-care settings. MMWR Morb Mortal Wkly Rep 1988;37:377–382;387–388

Bibliography

Rodman JH, Robbins BL, Flynn PM, Fridland A. A systematic and cellular model for zidovudine plasma concentrations and intracellular phosphorylation in patients. J Infect Dis 1996;174: 490–499

ACOG Committee Opinion

Committee on Genetics

Number 212, November 1998

Screening for Canavan Disease

Canavan disease is a severe progressive genetic disorder of the central nervous system. The clinical features of Canavan disease usually appear after the first few months of life and include developmental delay, macrocephaly, hypotonia, and poor head control. As the disease progresses, seizures, optic atrophy, gastrointestinal reflux, and deterioration of swallowing develop. Most children with Canavan disease die in the first decade of life. Presently, there is no cure or effective therapy for Canavan disease.

Canavan disease is caused by a deficiency of the enzyme aspartoacylase, which leads to increased excretion of its substrate, N-acetylaspartic acid (NAA). A diagnosis of Canavan disease is established by determining an increased level of urinary NAA by organic acid analysis. These abnormally high levels of NAA lead to demyelination and spongy degeneration of the brain, which cause the neurologic features of Canavan disease.

As in Tay–Sachs disease, Canavan disease is inherited as an autosomal recessive condition and is more prevalent among individuals of Eastern European Jewish (Ashkenazi) background. It is estimated that the carrier frequency in the Ashkenazi Jewish population is approximately 1 per 40. Thus, the risk for an affected offspring in this population approximates 1 in 6,400 births. Unlike Tay–Sachs disease, however, there do not appear to be other high-risk ethnic populations, although Canavan disease has been reported in individuals of non-Ashkenazi Jewish background.

Molecular studies have revealed two specific mutations in the aspartoacylase gene on chromosome 17. These account for approximately 97% of the mutations causing Canavan disease in the Ashkenazi Jewish population. One is a mutation in codon 285 of the aspartoacylase gene, and the other is a mutation in codon 231. Screening of Ashkenazi Jewish individuals can be performed by analyzing for these two mutations. In non-Jewish persons, the mutations may be different and more diverse. The most common mutation is in codon 305, which has been noted in approximately 36% of the 70 identified alleles from unrelated non-Jewish individuals.

Carrier screening for Canavan disease requires molecular diagnostic methods. Simple enzymatic assays, as commonly used in Tay–Sachs screening, cannot be used for Canavan disease because the activity of the deficient enzyme, aspartoacylase, is not detectable in blood. Testing for the three most common Canavan disease mutations will identify about 97% of Ashkenazi Jewish carriers and 40–50% of non-Jewish carriers.

When both parents are carriers of identifiable Canavan disease mutations, prenatal diagnosis by chorionic villus sampling (CVS) or amniocentesis can be accomplished using DNA analysis. In couples where one or both members have unknown mutations, biochemical analysis of NAA levels in the amniotic fluid can be used reliably. Elevated NAA levels can be used to detect an affected fetus. The analysis should be done in a laboratory that has personnel who have expertise in performing this test. Enzyme analysis of aspartoacylase in cultured fetal cells from CVS or amniocentesis is not reliable.

Based on the preceding information, the Committee on Genetics makes the following recommendations:

1. Ideally, molecular carrier screening for Canavan disease should be offered preconceptionally if both members of the couple are of Ashkenazi Jewish genetic background. This screening could be combined with screening for Tay–Sachs disease because both disorders are more common in this group. Many specialized laboratories already offer screening for both diseases. Those with a family history consistent with Canavan disease also should be offered screening, which should be voluntary; informed consent and assurance of confidentiality are required. If potential carriers have not been screened preconceptionally, screening may be offered during early pregnancy.

2. If only one partner is of high risk (of Ashkenazi Jewish descent or with a family history consistent with Canavan disease), this partner should be screened first. Ideally, this should be performed preconceptionally. If it is determined that the high-risk partner is a carrier, the other partner should be offered screening. The couple, however, must be informed of the limitations of testing. If the woman is already pregnant, it may be necessary to screen both partners simultaneously so that results are obtained in a timely fashion and to ensure that all options are available for the couple.

3. If it is determined by DNA-based analysis that both partners are carriers of Canavan disease, prenatal diagnosis should be offered either by CVS or amniocentesis, using DNA-based testing of the fetal cells.

Bibliography

American College of Medical Genetics Board of Directors. Position statement on carrier testing for Canavan disease. Bethesda, Maryland: January 10, 1998

American College of Obstetricians and Gynecologists. Screening for Tay–Sachs disease. ACOG Committee Opinion 162. Washington, DC: ACOG, 1995

Bennett MJ, Gibson KM, Sherwood WG, Divry P, Rolland MO, Elpeleg ON, et al. Reliable prenatal diagnosis of Canavan disease (aspartoacylase deficiency): comparison of enzymatic and metabolite analysis. J Inherit Metab Dis 1993;16:831–836

Kaul R, Gao GP, Matalon M, Aloya M, Su Q, Jin M, et al. Identification and expression of eight novel mutations among non-Jewish patients with Canavan disease. Am J Hum Genet 1996;59:95–102

Kronn D, Oddoux C, Philips J, Ostrer H. Prevalence of Canavan disease heterozygotes in the New York metropolitan Ashkenazi Jewish population. Am J Hum Genet 1995;57:1250–1252

Matalon R. Canavan disease: diagnosis and molecular analysis. Genetic Testing 1997;1:21–25

Matalon R, Michals K, Kaul R. Canavan disease: from spongy degeneration to molecular analysis. J Pediatr 1995;127:511–517

ACOG Committee Opinion

Committee on Genetics

Number 318, October 2005 *(Replaces No. 162, November 1995)*

Screening for Tay–Sachs Disease

ABSTRACT: *Tay–Sachs disease (TSD) is a severe progressive neurologic disease that causes death in early childhood. Carrier screening should be offered before pregnancy to individuals and couples at high risk, including those of Ashkenazi Jewish, French–Canadian, or Cajun descent and those with a family history consistent with TSD. If both partners are determined to be carriers of TSD, genetic counseling and prenatal diagnosis should be offered.*

Tay–Sachs disease (TSD) is a lysosomal storage disease in which GM_2 gangliosides accumulate throughout the body. The accumulation of these gangliosides in the central nervous system results in a severe progressive neurologic disease that causes death in early childhood.

The TSD carrier rate in Jewish individuals of Eastern European descent (Ashkenazi) is approximately 1 in 30; the carrier rate for non-Jewish individuals is estimated to be 1 in 300. It has been determined that individuals of French–Canadian and Cajun descent also have a greater carrier frequency than the general population.

The enzyme hexosaminidase occurs in two principal forms, Hexosaminidase A and Hexosaminidase B. Hexosaminidase A is composed of one α subunit and one β subunit, whereas Hexosaminidase B is composed of two β subunits. Tay–Sachs disease is caused by a deficiency of Hexosaminidase A, whereas Sandhoff disease is caused by a deficiency of both Hexosaminidase A and Hexosaminidase B. Both of these diseases are transmitted in an autosomal recessive fashion. Laboratories report Hexosaminidase A levels as a percentage of total hexosaminidase activity. Hexosaminidase A is almost completely absent in patients with classical TSD. The percentage of Hexosaminidase A activity in carriers usually is less than 55% of total activity, whereas Hexosaminidase A activity in noncarriers generally is more than 60% of total activity. Tay–Sachs disease can be diagnosed prenatally by measuring hexosaminidase activity in samples obtained by amniocentesis or by chorionic villus sampling.

Carrier screening can be performed by molecular analysis, biochemical analysis, or both. Molecular analyses of the α subunit gene for TSD have been reported in both Jewish and non-Jewish populations. Molecular analysis of three mutations will detect 94% of carriers in the Ashkenazi Jewish population, compared with biochemical analysis, which will detect 98% of carriers.

The American College of Obstetricians and Gynecologists
409 12th Street, SW
PO Box 96920
Washington, DC 20090-6920

12345/98765

Screening for Tay–Sachs disease. ACOG Committee Opinion No. 318. American College of Obstetricians and Gynecologists. Obstet Gynecol 2005;106:893–4.

Different mutations have been found in other ethnic groups. Biochemical analysis should be used in low-risk populations because molecular analysis detects less than 50% of carriers in these populations.

Test results of biochemical carrier screening using serum are inaccurate when performed in women who are pregnant or taking oral contraceptives. If the serum test is used for pregnant women, many of them will be misclassified as carriers. If biochemical testing is to be done in women who are pregnant or taking oral contraceptives, leukocyte testing must be used. If both partners are determined to be carriers of TSD, genetic counseling and prenatal diagnosis should be offered.

When the serum test result is inconclusive, biochemical analysis should be performed on leukocytes from peripheral blood. DNA analysis may be helpful for those individuals whose leukocyte test results are inconclusive and those individuals whose test results are positive to rule out a rare pseudodeficiency condition.

Pseudodeficiency refers to a state in which asymptomatic individuals have a low amount of Hexosaminidase A activity when tested with conventional artificial substrate. However, these normal individuals without Hexosaminidase A are able to catalyze the breakdown of natural substrate GM_2 ganglioside. Pseudodeficiency mutations comprise approximately one third of the mutations identified in non-Jewish individuals. Because some of these individuals are compound heterozygotes for a Tay–Sachs mutation and a pseudodeficiency allele, the delineation of their precise genotype for reproductive purposes usually requires further biochemical assessment complemented with DNA analysis.

Based on the preceding information, the Committee on Genetics makes the following recommendations:

1. Screening for TSD should be offered before pregnancy if both members of a couple are of Ashkenazi Jewish, French–Canadian, or Cajun descent. Those with a family history consistent with TSD also should be offered screening.

2. When one member of a couple is at high risk (ie, of Ashkenazi Jewish, French–Canadian, or Cajun descent or has a family history consistent with TSD) but the other partner is not, the high-risk partner should be offered screening. This is particularly important if there is uncertainty about ancestry or if there is a family history consistent with TSD. If the high-risk partner is determined to be a carrier, the other partner also should be offered screening. If the woman is already pregnant, it may be necessary to offer screening to both partners simultaneously to ensure that results are obtained promptly and that all options are available to the couple.

3. Biochemical analysis should be used for individuals in low-risk populations.

4. If TSD biochemical screening is performed in women who are pregnant or taking oral contraceptives, leukocyte testing must be used.

5. Ambiguous screening test results or positive screening test results in individuals should be confirmed by biochemical and DNA analysis for the most common mutations. This will detect patients who carry genes associated with mild disease or pseudodeficiency states. Referral to a specialist in genetics may be helpful in these cases.

6. If both partners are determined to be carriers of TSD, genetic counseling and prenatal diagnosis should be offered.

Bibliography

Prenatal and preconceptional carrier screening for genetic diseases in individuals of Eastern European Jewish descent. ACOG Committee Opinion 298. American College of Obstetricians and Gynecologists. Obstet Gynecol 2004;104: 425–8.

Kaback M, Lim-Steele J, Dabholkar D, Brown D, Levy N, Zeiger K. Tay-Sachs disease—carrier screening, prenatal diagnosis, and the molecular era. An international perspective, 1970 to 1993. The International TSD Data Collection Network. JAMA 1993;270:2307–15.

Mules EH, Hayflick S, Dowling CE, Kelly TE, Akerman BR, Gravel RA, et al. Molecular basis of hexosaminidase A deficiency and pseudodeficiency in the Berks County Pennsylvania Dutch. Hum Mutat 1992;1:298–302.

Prence EM, Natowicz MR, Zalewski I. Unusual thermolability properties of leukocyte beta-hexosaminidase: implications in screening for carriers of Tay-Sachs disease. Clin Chem 1993;39:1811–4.

Triggs-Raine BL, Feigenbaum AS, Natowicz M, Skomorowski MA, Schuster SM, Clarke JT, et al. Screening for carriers of Tay-Sachs disease among Ashkenazi Jews. A comparison of DNA-based and enzyme-based tests. N Engl J Med 1990; 323:6–12.

ACOG

Committee on Adolescent Health Care

The Committee wishes to thank Melisa Holmes, MD, Stephen Vermillion, MD, and David Soper, MD, for their assistance in the development of this opinion. This document reflects emerging clinical and scientific advances as of the date issued and is subject to change. The information should not be construed as dictating an exclusive course of treatment or procedure to be followed.

ISSN 1074-861X

The American College of Obstetricians and Gynecologists
409 12th Street, SW
PO Box 96920
Washington, DC 20090-6920

12345/87654

Sexually transmitted diseases in adolescents. ACOG Committee Opinion No. 301. American College of Obstetricians and Gynecologists. Obstet Gynecol 2004;104:891–8.

Committee Opinion

Number 301, October 2004

Sexually Transmitted Diseases in Adolescents

ABSTRACT: *Sexually transmitted diseases are common among adolescents in the United States. Female adolescents face numerous obstacles to care and experience a disproportionate burden related to the sequelae of sexually transmitted diseases. These diseases are a primary cause of short and long-term morbidity in adolescents that can result in infertility, chronic pelvic pain, ectopic pregnancy, vertical transmission to newborns, malignancy, chronic illness, and even death. Clinicians treating female adolescents should be prepared to offer confidential and comprehensive counseling, screening, and treatment according to established guidelines. They should also work within their communities and at the state and national levels to assure access to medical care for all adolescents. Adolescence is a period during which life-long health behaviors are established. It is, therefore, a critical time for promoting responsible behaviors and reducing risks through health promotion and prevention strategies.*

Epidemiology

Approximately 18.9 million new cases of sexually transmitted diseases (STDs) occurred in 2000, of which 9.1 million (48%) were among persons aged 15–24 years (1). Many STDs are found at disproportionately high rates in the female adolescent population, especially among high-risk populations such as homeless and runaway adolescents and adolescents in detention facilities (2–4). The Centers for Disease Control and Prevention (CDC) estimates that more than 1 in 10 sexually active female adolescents have chlamydial infection (5). In 2002, as in previous years, females aged 15–24 years had the highest rates of gonorrhea compared with females in all other age categories (2). Prevalence of human papillomavirus infection in sexually active young women ranges from 17% to 84%, with most studies reporting prevalence greater than 30% (6). The incidence of hepatitis B virus (HBV) per year has decreased from an average of 260,000 cases in the 1980s to approximately 78,000 cases in 2001. The greatest decrease has occurred among children and adolescents as a result of routine HBV vaccination. It is estimated that there are 1.25 million chronically infected Americans, of whom 20–30% acquired the HBV infection in childhood (7). It is estimated that at least one half of all new human immunodeficiency virus (HIV) infections in the United States are among individuals younger than 25 years (8). In 2000, the estimated direct medical costs of STDs acquired by individuals aged 15–24 years in the United States were $6.5 billion (in year 2000 dollars). Many of these costs are borne inordinately by female adolescents. For example, the average lifetime cost per case of chlamydial infection to female adolescents is $244 compared with a per-case cost of $20 to male adolescents (8).

Risk Factors

Although many of the issues pertaining to high-risk sexual behavior and STDs are common to both adolescents and adults, they often are intensified among adolescents and contribute to their high prevalence rates of STDs. This is caused by developmental changes that affect adolescents physically, behaviorally, and emotionally, as well as access-related and financial barriers to health care.

Adolescents often engage in high-risk sexual behaviors as they respond to their physical and emotional changes and strive for peer approval. Depending on their developmental status, some adolescents may not possess the foresight to recognize and understand the potential consequences of their risky behaviors, such as the potential fatality related to the acquisition of HIV. This lack of foresight often is compounded by the use of alcohol or drugs or both.

The likelihood of adolescents engaging in sexual intercourse increases steadily with age. In 2003, 28% of girls in the ninth grade and 62% of girls in the 12th grade reported having sexual intercourse (9). Adolescents who have sexual intercourse at an early age are more likely to have multiple partners, more likely to have had nonvoluntary or unwanted sex, and less likely to use barrier protection (10). Although approximately two thirds of adolescents report having used condoms, only 45% report using condoms consistently (11). In addition, condom use among adolescents is greater in the early stages of the relationship and decreases significantly as the relationship progresses, leaving adolescents vulnerable to STDs (12). Although many adolescents may say that they have only 1 sexual partner, they change partners frequently. Specifically, 14.4% of high-school students already have had 4 or more sexual partners during their lifetime (9). Within 1 year, the majority of sexually active female adolescents will have sex with more than 1 sexual partner or with a partner who also has other sexual partners (13).

Use of alcohol and other substances that impair judgment can increase the likelihood of engaging in sexual intercourse without a condom, with multiple partners, or with high-risk partners. Adolescents with tattoos or body piercings may be at an increased risk for STDs, particularly HBV infection because of the nature of the piercing process and the vulnerability of open sores to infection.

Biologic factors also contribute to the female adolescent's greater risk for acquiring an STD compared with adult women. During puberty and the early postpubertal years, the cervix develops a prominent ectropion with a large area of exposed columnar epithelium undergoing active metaplasia. The columnar epithelium is the primary site of invasion by both chlamydial and gonococcal agents (14). Adolescents also may have "immature" local immunity and low levels of existing antibodies against certain infections (15).

Barriers to Care

Confidentiality concerns limit the use of medical care by adolescents. Adolescents are more willing to communicate with and seek health care from physicians who assure confidentiality (16). A recent study of girls younger than 18 years attending family planning clinics found that 47% of girls would no longer attend if their parents had to be notified that they were seeking prescription birth control pills or devices, and another 10% would delay or discontinue STD testing and treatment (17). A study of pediatric patients in North Carolina found that whereas 92% of sexually active adolescent patients (primarily female) would consent to STD testing if their parents would not find out, the proportion decreased to 38% if their parents might find out and to 35% if their parents definitely would find out that they were tested (18). Physicians are encouraged to establish office policies regarding confidential care for adolescents and clearly communicate these policies to adolescents and their parents. Although providing confidentiality to adult patients is relatively easy, parental consent and billing issues for the treatment of adolescents can make confidentiality for adolescents a much more complex task. All states have statutes allowing minors to receive services related to STD testing and treatment without parental consent or involvement. The laws may specify the age at which minors can begin to consent to such care (19, 20). Physicians providing care for an adolescent population should be familiar with current state statutes on the rights of minors to consent to health care services, as well as those laws that affect confidentiality. Providers should encourage and, when appropriate, facilitate communication between a minor and her parent(s) (21).

The subtle and asymptomatic nature of many STDs further inhibits adolescents from seeking medical attention or adhering to prescribed treatment regimens. Adolescents may not be able to distinguish whether aspects of their health are physically normal or abnormal. They may fear a physical examination, which they perceive as painful; may be embarrassed about a pelvic examination; or may be concerned about the discovery of sexual activity or sexual abuse that they are afraid to reveal. In addition, they may be reluctant to face a diagnosis of an STD because it may have implications regarding the fidelity of their partner and the stability of their relationship.

Clinician-related barriers to STD testing also exist and include concern over lack of confidentiality, clinician discomfort with discussion of sexual behavior with adolescents, and clinician belief that their patients are not sexually active or that the prevalence of certain STDs is low in their patient population. These barriers result in lower than recommended STD screening rates (22).

The costs associated with diagnosis and treatment of STDs also may be a significant barrier to care. Adolescents who have insurance coverage for these services through their parents may not want to use this insurance for fear of loss of confidentiality. Others may be uninsured. In both cases, referral to a publicly funded clinic may be appropriate. Transportation difficulties may further impede access to care.

Screening and Prevention Recommendations

Nonpregnant Adolescent Patients

The provision of health guidance, screening, and preventive health care services is an essential component of reproductive health care for adolescents that should begin between the ages 13 years and 15 years. The provision of additional services beyond guidance and screening should be based on the information obtained at the initial visit. If the patient has had sexual intercourse, testing for STDs is appropriate. A pelvic examination also may be appropriate (21). In addition, adolescents who have had sexual intercourse should have their initial Pap test approx-

imately 3 years after first vaginal–penile coitus, but no later than age 21 years (21, 23). Because the potential for risky behaviors is significant during adolescence, the initial consultation visit should be followed by annual preventive health care visits (21).

Oral–genital contact is a common behavior among adolescents and, along with anal–genital contact, contributes to the transmission of STDs. One study indicated that 9% of high-school virgins engaged in heterosexual fellatio with ejaculation, 10% engaged in heterosexual cunnilingus, and 1% engaged in heterosexual anal intercourse. Condom use for fellatio was rare (24). Vulva-to-vulva sex also can transmit STDs. Generally, STDs, including HIV, are less common in lesbians than in heterosexual women, but they can be passed from woman to woman. Also, many women who identify themselves as lesbians may have or may have had sexual intercourse with men. Because all of these activities increase the risk of acquiring an STD, clinicians should not limit their patient interview to questions about heterosexual vaginal–penile intercourse. Clinicians also should ascertain if their adolescent patients are in new relationships because being in a new sexual partnership is an important predictor of incident STDs (25). In addition, sexually active adolescents should receive screening annually for the following conditions:

- Gonorrhea and chlamydia (21, 26)—Urine screening should be considered when adolescents are reluctant to have pelvic examinations or are seen where pelvic examinations are not feasible (21).
- Cervical neoplasia—This screening should start approximately 3 years after first vaginal–penile coitus, but no later than age 21 years (21, 23).

Adolescents who have any of the following characteristics or who have a history of these characteristics should be screened annually for HIV and syphilis:

- STDs
- Multiple sexual partners or high-risk sexual partner
- Exchange of sex for drugs or money
- Intravenous drug use
- Blood transfusion before 1985 (HIV only)
- Admittance to jail or other detention facility
- Live in areas with high prevalence of HIV and syphilis (21, 26)

Counseling of adolescents before HIV testing should include a risk assessment profile, explanation of testing procedures, implications of test results, informed consent for testing, and the development of risk reduction strategies. It also may be helpful for the adolescent to identify an adult who knows she is being tested and will provide support. This is particularly helpful in cases of a positive HIV test result. In addition to informing the patient of the results of the test, posttest counseling should include a review of the meaning of the results and reinforcement of prevention strategies. Adolescents with negative test results who are still considered at risk may benefit from additional counseling services. Adolescent patients with confirmed positive HIV test results should receive additional psychologic and social counseling (27).

Because the risk of STDs increases with exposure to multiple partners, adolescents who are sexually active need to understand this risk and should be encouraged to limit that exposure. Some experts recommend that female adolescent patients be seen every 6 months for STD screening regardless of the number of sexual partners (28). The CDC recommends that all female adolescents and women with chlamydial infections be rescreened 3 or 4 months after treatment is completed. It also strongly encourages providers to rescreen all women treated for chlamydial infection at their next office visit within the following 12 months, regardless of whether the patient believes that her partner(s) was treated (27).

All adolescents should receive annual health guidance regarding sexuality. Such guidance should include counseling about what constitutes responsible, consensual sexual behavior and that abstinence from sexual intercourse is the only definitive way to prevent pregnancy and STDs (21). Abstinence from all risky behaviors also should be encouraged. These risky behaviors should be defined because in a study of college students, 24% defined anal intercourse, 37% defined oral intercourse, and 47% defined oral–anal contact as "abstinent" behavior (29). All sexually active adolescents should be encouraged to use condoms consistently and correctly with all sexual partners no matter what other birth control method is used. Recent studies indicate a potential association between use of hormonal contraception (depotmedroxyprogesterone acetate or oral contraceptives) and increased acquisition of cervical chlamydial and gonoccocal infections (30). Counseling should stress the effectiveness of latex condoms in reducing the risk of pregnancy and the STDs most likely to cause serious morbidity and mortality (21). When used consistently and correctly, male latex condoms are effective in preventing the sexual transmission of HIV infection and can reduce the risk for other STDs (eg, gonorrhea, chlamydia, and trichomonas). However, because condoms do not cover all exposed areas, they are likely to be more effective in preventing infections transmitted by fluids from mucosal surfaces (eg, gonorrhea, chlamydia, trichomoniasis, and HIV) than in preventing those transmitted by skin-to-skin contact (eg, herpes simplex virus, human papillomavirus, syphilis, and chancroid) (27, 31). Polyurethane condoms should be promoted among those allergic to latex although data regarding the effectiveness of this type of condom at preventing STDs are sparse (32).

Pregnant Adolescent Patients

Pregnant adolescents should be counseled about the effects of STDs on themselves and their fetuses. They should receive repetitive reinforcement that condoms should be used during pregnancy for STD prevention (33). They should be screened for syphilis, HBV, and gonorrhea early in pregnancy. It is important to note that pregnancy is not a contraindication to HBV or hepatitis B immune globulin vaccine administration (27, 34). The American College of Obstetricians and Gynecologists (ACOG) recommends HIV testing of all pregnant women, with patient notification, as a routine component of prenatal care. If the patient declines HIV testing, it should be documented in the patient's record. However, physicians need to be aware of and follow their own states' prenatal HIV screening guidelines (35, 36). Repeat testing for HIV in the third trimester can be considered for high-risk patients, including those who use illicit drugs, exchange sex for money or drugs, have a history of STDs, have multiple sexual partners during pregnancy, have HIV-infected or high-risk partners, or have signs or symptoms suggestive of acute HIV infection at any time during the pregnancy (27). Testing for other STDs should be offered on the basis of the patient's history and physical examination or in response to public health guidelines.

Screening for chlamydia is recommended during the third trimester for women younger than 25 years. Screening during the first trimester for chlamydia might enable prevention of its adverse effects during pregnancy; however, evidence for preventing these adverse effects during pregnancy is limited (27). Among high-risk patients, repeat testing for gonorrhea, syphilis, and HBV should occur in the third trimester (27, 34). Health care providers should inquire regularly about changes in sexual partners because diligent rescreening is especially important in the adolescent population.

Adolescent Victims of Sexual Assault

Identification of STDs after a sexual assault is important for the psychologic and medical treatment of the patient. Appropriately sensitive care should be offered because of the trauma the patient has experienced. It is helpful to have a trained counselor available during the examination or to provide a referral for counseling. Although the clinical management of adolescent patients who have experienced sexual assault is the same as that of the adult patients who have experienced sexual assault (37), legal reporting requirements will vary by state depending on the age of the victim and her relationship with the perpetrator. It is important for clinicians to know their local reporting requirements, which can be obtained from their state attorney general's office or medical board. Provision of emergency contraception should be considered if the sexual assault occurred within 72 hours before the examination.

Specific Treatment Guidelines

Current treatment recommendations regarding antimicrobial therapy for specific STDs are available in the CDC 2002 Guidelines for Treatment of Sexually Transmitted Diseases (27). It is especially important when treating an adolescent for an STD to use on-site single-dose antibiotics whenever possible and to give presumptive treatment because of the difficulties in getting adolescents to return for treatment. This also is an opportunity to facilitate STD prevention by providing condoms to adolescents. Current recommendations on immunizations have been developed by ACOG (38, 39).

Reporting and Partner Notification

Success in controlling STDs requires vigorous ongoing prevention efforts, accurate identification, administration of appropriate treatments, and timely reporting of partner notification and treatment. Providers should encourage their patients to make partners aware of potential STD risk and urge them

to seek diagnosis and treatment (27). Many local or state health departments offer assistance in partner notification specifically for patients who have received the diagnosis of HIV, syphilis, gonorrhea, chlamydia, and HBV. Health departments protect the privacy of patients in partner notification services, and in some cases, this is preferable to direct communication between the patient and her partner. Identifying an STD in an adolescent who denies sexual activity or is hesitant to address partner notification may lead to the discovery of forced or coerced sex. In such cases, partner notification becomes secondary and providing appropriate support, evaluation, and legal reporting takes precedence.

In the United States, syphilis, gonorrhea, and acquired immunodeficiency syndrome (AIDS) are reportable diseases in every state. Human immunodeficiency virus infection and chancroid are reportable in many states. The requirements for reporting other STDs vary among states. Reporting may be provider initiated or laboratory based or both. All clinicians should be familiar with their local STD reporting requirements. Sexually transmitted disease and HIV test results are maintained in the strictest of confidence and, in most jurisdictions, are protected by statute from subpoena (27).

Conclusion

The American College of Obstetricians and Gynecologists considers STDs in the adolescent population a significant public health concern in need of attention. As such, ACOG advocates for improved access to health care for this population. Clinicians can work within their communities and at the state and national levels to assure access to medical care for all adolescents, especially homeless and runaway adolescents and those in detention facilities. Most importantly, clinicians can help to address this problem when caring for adolescent patients. Specifically, when providing health care for adolescents who have not yet become sexually active, abstinence from all risky behaviors should be encouraged. For sexually active adolescents, it is crucial to promote safe sexual behaviors, provide contraceptive information, encourage condom use, perform recommended STD screenings, prescribe appropriate antimicrobial therapies for infections, follow requirements for reporting and partner notification, and ensure continued support and follow-up care.

References

1. Weinstock H, Berman S, Cates W Jr. Sexually transmitted diseases among American youth: incidence and prevalence estimates, 2000. Perspect Sex Reprod Health 2004; 36:6–10.
2. Centers for Disease Control and Prevention. Sexually transmitted disease surveillance 2002. Atlanta (GA): CDC; 2003.
3. Widom R, Hammett TM. HIV/AIDS and STDs in juvenile facilities. Research in Brief. 1996. Available at: http://www.ncjrs.org/pdffiles/hivjuve.pdf. Retrieved June 24, 2004.
4. National Coalition for the Homeless. Homeless youth. NCH Fact Sheet II. 1999. Available at: http://www.nationalhomeless.org/youth.html. Retrieved June 24, 2004.
5. Centers for Disease Control and Prevention. Tracking the hidden epidemics: trends in STDs in the United States 2000. 2001. Available at: http://www.cdc.gov/nchstp/od/news/RevBrochure/pdftoc.htm. Retrieved June 24, 2004.
6. Centers for Disease Control and Prevention. Prevention of genital human papillomavirus infection: report to Congress. 2004. Available at: http://www.cdc.gov/std/HPV/2004HPV%20Report.pdf. Retrieved June 24, 2004.
7. Centers for Disease Control and Prevention. Hepatitis B fact sheet. 2003. Available at: http://www.cdc.gov/ncidod/diseases/hepatitis/b/bfact.pdf. Retrieved June 24, 2004.
8. Cates JR, Herndon NL, Schulz SL, Darroch JE. Our voices, our lives, our futures: youth and sexually transmitted diseases. 2004. Available at: http://www.jomc.unc.edu/youthandSTDs/ourvoicesreport.pdf. Retrieved June 24, 2004.
9. Grunbaum JA, Kann L, Kinchen S, Ross J, Hawkins J, Lowry R, et al. Youth risk behavior surveillance - United States, 2003. MMWR Surveill Summ 2004;53(2):1–96.
10. Moore KA, Driscoll A. Partners, predators, peers, protectors: males and teen pregnancy: new data analyses of the 1995 National Survey of Family Growth. In: Moore KA, Driscoll AK, Ooms T, editors. Not just for girls: the roles of boys and men in teen pregnancy prevention. Washington, DC: National Campaign to Prevent Teen Pregnancy; 1997. p. 5–10.
11. Sonenstein FL, Ku L, Lindberg LD, Turner CF, Pleck JH. Changes in sexual behavior and condom use among teenaged males: 1988 to 1995. Am J Public Health 1998; 88:956–9.
12 Ku L, Sonenstein FL, Pleck JH. The dynamics of young men's condom use during and across relationships. Fam Plann Perspect 1994;26:246–51.
13. Finer LB, Darroch JE, Singh S. Sexual partnership patterns as a behavioral risk factor for sexually transmitted diseases. Fam Plann Perspect 1999;31:228–36.
14. Cates W Jr. The epidemiology and control of sexually transmitted diseases in adolescents. Adolesc Med 1990; 1:409–28.
15. Holmes KK, Mardh PA, Sparling PF, Lemon SM, Stamm WE, Piot P, et al, editors. Sexually transmitted diseases. 3rd edition. New York (NY): McGraw-Hill; 1999.
16. Ford CA, Millstein SG, Halpern-Felsher BL, Irwin CE Jr. Influence of physician confidentiality assurances on adolescents' willingness to disclose information and seek future health care. A randomized controlled trial. JAMA 1997;278;1029–34.
17. Reddy DM, Fleming R, Swain C. Effect of mandatory parental notification on adolescent girls' use of sexual health care services. JAMA 2002;288:710–4.
18. Ford CA, Best D, Miller WC. The pediatric forum: confidentiality and adolescents' willingness to consent to sexually transmitted disease testing. Arch Pediatr Adolesc Med 2001;155:1072–3.
19. The Alan Guttmacher Institute. Minors' access to STD services. State Policies in Brief. 2004. Available at: http://www.guttmacher.org/statecenter/spibs/spib_MASS.pdf. Retrieved June 24, 2004.
20. Center for Adolescent Health & the Law. State minor consent laws: a summary. 2nd ed. Chapel Hill (NC): CAHL; 2003.
21. American College of Obstetricians and Gynecologists. Health care for adolescents. Washington DC: ACOG; 2003.
22. Huppert JS, Adams Hillard PJ. Sexually transmitted disease screening in teens. Curr Womens Health Rep 2003; 3:451–8.
23. American College of Obstetricians and Gynecologists. Committee Opinion No. 300. Cervical cancer screening in the adolescent female. Washington, DC: ACOG; 2004.
24. Schuster MA, Bell RM, Kanouse DE. The sexual practices of adolescent virgins: genital sexual activities of high school students who have never had vaginal intercourse. Am J Public Health 1996;86:1570–6.
25. Niccolai LM, Ethier KA, Kershaw TS, Lewis JB, Meade CS, Ickovics JR. New sex partner acquisition and sexually transmitted disease risk among adolescent females. J Adolesc Health 2004;34:216–23.
26. HIV prevention through early detection and treatment of other sexually transmitted diseases—United States. Recommendations of the Advisory Committee for HIV and STD prevention. MMWR Recomm Rep 1998;47(RR-12):1–24.
27. Sexually transmitted diseases treatment guidelines 2002. Centers for Disease Control and Prevention. MMWR Recomm Rep 2002;51(RR-6):1–78. Available at: http://www.cdc.gov/STD/treatment/rr5106.pdf. Retrieved July 7, 2004.
28. Burstein GR, Gaydos CA, Diener-West M, Howell MR, Zenilman JM, Quinn TC. Incident chlamydia trachomatis infections among inner-city adolescent females. JAMA 1998;280:521–6.
29. Horan PF, Phillips J, Hagan NE. The meaning of abstinence for college students. J HIV/AIDS Prev Educ Adolesc Child 1998;2(2):51–66.
30. Morrison CS, Bright P, Wong EL, Kwok C, Yacobson I, Gaydos CA, et al. Hormonal contraceptive use, cervical ectopy, and the acquisition of cervical infections. Sex Transm Dis 2004;31:561–7.
31. National Institute of Allergy and Infectious Diseases, National Institutes of Health. Workshop summary: scientific evidence on condom effectiveness for sexually transmitted disease (STD) prevention. 2001. Available at: http://www.niaid.nih.gov/dmid/stds/condomreport.pdf. Retrieved June 24, 2004.

32. Frezieres RG, Walsh TL, Nelson AL, Clark VA, Coulson AH. Evaluation of the efficacy of a polyurethane condom: results from a randomized, controlled clinical trial. Fam Plann Perspect 1999;31:81–7.

33. Niccolai LM, Ethier KA, Kershaw TS, Lewis JB, Ickovics JR. Pregnant adolescents at risk: sexual behaviors and sexually transmitted disease prevalence. Am J Obstet Gynecol 2003;188:63–70.

34. American Academy of Pediatrics, American College of Obstetricians and Gynecologists. Guidelines for perinatal care. 5th ed. Elk Grove Village (IL): AAP; Washington, DC: ACOG; 2002.

35. American Academy of Pediatrics, American College of Obstetricians and Gynecologists. Joint statement on human immunodeficiency virus screening. ACOG Policy Statement 75. Elk Grove Village (IL): AAP; Washington, DC: ACOG; 1999.

36. Revised guidelines for HIV counseling, testing, and referral and revised recommendations for HIV screening of pregnant women. Centers for Disease Control and Prevention. MMWR Recomm Rep 2001;50(RR-19): 1–86; quiz CE1-19a2-CE6-19a2.

37. American College of Obstetricians and Gynecologists. Sexual assault. ACOG Educational Bulletin 242. Washington, DC: ACOG; 1997.

38. Primary and preventive care: periodic assessments. ACOG Committee Opinion No. 292. American College of Obstetricians and Gynecologists. Obstet Gynecol 2003; 102:1117–24.

39. Immunization during pregnancy. ACOG Committee Opinion No. 282. American College of Obstetricians and Gynecologists. Obstet Gynecol 2003;101:207–12.

Resources

Publications

The American College of Obstetricians and Gynecologists Tool Kit for Teen Care offers a fact sheet on the topic of STDs that may be helpful for patients and providers alike. This fact sheet is available online at http://www.acog.org/goto/teens. For information on the entire kit, go to sales.acog.org or contact the Department of Adolescent Health Care at 202-863-2497. Other ACOG resources are listed as follows:

> American College of Obstetricians and Gynecologists. Health Care for Adolescents. Washington, DC: ACOG; 2003.
>
> Patient Education Pamphlets
>
> > How to Prevent Sexually Transmitted Diseases (1999) (AP009) (SP009—Spanish)
> >
> > Genital Herpes (1999) (AP054)
> >
> > Gonorrhea, Chlamydia, and Syphilis (2000) (AP071)
> >
> > Hepatitis B Virus in Pregnancy (2000) (AP093)
> >
> > HIV Infection in Women (2000) (AP082)
> >
> > Human Papillomavirus Infection (2003) (AP073)
> >
> > Protecting Yourself Against Hepatitis B (1998) (AP125)

Web Sites

We have provided web sites and contact information for the following organizations because they have information that may be of interest to our readers. The American College of Obstetricians and Gynecologists does not necessarily endorse the views expressed or the facts presented by these organizations or on these web sites. Furthermore, ACOG does not endorse any commercial products that may be advertised or available from these organizations or on these web sites.

Advocates for Youth
2000 M St NW, Ste 750
Washington, DC 20036
Telephone: 202-419-3420
Fax: 202-419-1448
www.advocatesforyouth.org
E-mail: questions@advocatesforyouth.org

Alan Guttmacher Institute
120 Wall Street, 21st Fl
New York, NY 10005
Telephone: 212-248-1111
Fax: 212-248-1951
www.guttmacher.org
E-mail: info@guttmacher.org

American Academy of Family Physicians
11400 Tomahawk Creek Parkway
Leawood, KS 66211-2672
Telephone: 800-274-2237 or 913-906-6000
www.aafp.org
E-mail: fp@aafp.org

American Academy of Pediatrics
141 Northwest Point Boulevard
Elk Grove Village, IL 60007-1098
Telephone: 847-434-4000
Fax: 847-434-8000
www.aap.org
E-mail: kidsdocs@aap.org

American Social Health Association
PO Box 13827
Research Triangle Park, NC 27709
Telephone: 919-361-8400
Fax: 919-361-8425
www.ashastd.org
E-mail: std-hivnet@ashastd.org

AWARE Foundation
1015 Chestnut Street, Suite 1225
Philadelphia, PA 19107-4302
Telephone: 215-955-9847
www.awarefoundation.org
E-mail: info@awarefoundation.org

Centers for Disease Control and Prevention
National Center for Chronic Disease Prevention
  and Health Promotion
Division of Adolescent and School Health
www.cdc.gov/HealthyYouth/index.htm
E-mail: healthyyouth@cdc.gov

Centers for Disease Control and Prevention
Office of Women's Health
1600 Clifton Road, MS E-89
Atlanta, GA 30333
Telephone: 404-498-2300
Fax: 404-498-2370
www.cdc.gov/health/od/spotlight/nwhw/default.htm
E-mail: owh@cdc.gov

Johns Hopkins AIDS Service
www.hopkins-aids.edu

National Sexually Transmitted Disease Hotline
Telephone: 800-227-8922

National Women's Health Information Center
Telephone: 800-994-WOMAN
www.4woman.org

Planned Parenthood Federation of America, Inc.
434 W 33rd St.
New York, NY 10001
Telephone: 215-541-7800
Fax: 212-245-1845
www.plannedparenthood.org
E-mail: communications@ppfa.org

Sexuality Information and Education Council
  of the United States
130 West 42nd Street, Suite 350
New York, NY 10036-7802
Telephone: 212-819-9770
Fax: 212-819-9776
www.siecus.org
E-mail: siecus@siecus.org

The Society of Obstetricians and Gynecologists of Canada
Sexuality and U
www.sexualityandu.ca

ACOG

Committee on Health Care for Underserved Women

Committee on Obstetric Practice

The Committees would like to thank Kelli Mudd Miller, MD, and Kirsten Smith, MD, for their assistance in the development of this bulletin.

ISSN 1074-861X

The American College of Obstetricians and Gynecologists
409 12th Street, SW
PO Box 96920
Washington, DC 20090-6920

12345/98765

Smoking cessation during pregnancy. ACOG Committee Opinion No. 316. American College of Obstetricians and Gynecologists. Obstet Gynecol 2005;106:883–8.

Committee Opinion

Number 316, October 2005

(Replaces Educational Bulletin 260, September 2000)

Smoking Cessation During Pregnancy

ABSTRACT: Smoking is one of the most important modifiable causes of poor pregnancy outcomes in the United States. An office-based protocol that systematically identifies pregnant women who smoke and offers treatment has been proved to increase quit rates. For pregnant women who are light to moderate smokers, a short counseling session with pregnancy-specific educational materials often is an effective intervention for smoking cessation. The 5 A's is an office-based intervention developed for use by trained practitioners. Techniques for smoking reduction, pharmacotherapy, and health care support systems can help smokers quit.

Epidemiology

Increased public education measures and public health campaigns in the United States have led to a decline in smoking during pregnancy (1). Pregnancy appears to motivate women to make lifestyle changes; approximately 46% of prepregnancy smokers quit during pregnancy (1). From 1990 to 2003, the rate of smoking reported by pregnant women decreased from 18.4% (2) to 11% (3). The smoking rate during pregnancy in 2002 for women ages 18 and 19 years was 18%, higher than that for pregnant women of any other age (4).

Consequences of Maternal Smoking

The biologic evidence that maternal smoking has a detrimental effect on the fetus includes fetal hypoxia from increased carboxyhemoglobin; reduced blood flow to the uterus, placenta, and fetus; and direct effects of nicotine and other compounds in tobacco smoke on the placenta and fetus (5). Health risks associated with smoking during pregnancy include intrauterine growth restriction, placenta previa, and abruptio placentae (5). Adverse pregnancy outcomes include premature rupture of membranes (6, 7), low birth weight, and perinatal mortality (5). Evidence also suggests that smoking is associated with an increase in ectopic pregnancies (5). It is estimated that eliminating smoking during pregnancy would reduce infant deaths by 5% (8) and reduce the incidence of singleton low-birth-weight infants by 10.4% (9).

There is a strong association between smoking during pregnancy and sudden infant death syndrome (SIDS) (5). Children born to mothers who smoke during pregnancy are at increased risk for asthma (10), infantile colic (11), and childhood obesity (12). Successful smoking cessation before the third trimester eliminates much of the reduced birth weight caused by maternal smoking (5). Women who continue to smoke during pregnancy must achieve very low levels of tobacco use to see improvements in infant birth weight, and they must quit entirely if their infants are to have birth weights similar to those of women who do not smoke (13).

Intervention

Both cessation of tobacco use and prevention of relapse to smoking are key clinical intervention strategies during pregnancy. Techniques for helping patients to stop smoking have included counseling, cognitive and behavioral therapy, hypnosis, acupuncture, and pharmacologic therapy. A 5–15-minute counseling session performed by appropriately trained health care providers is most effective with pregnant women who smoke fewer than 20 cigarettes per day (14). This intervention, known as the 5 A's, is appropriate for use during routine prenatal office visits and includes the following five steps: Ask, Advise, Assess, Assist, and Arrange. The intervention is adapted from the U.S. Public Health Service clinical practice guideline, "Treating Tobacco Use and Dependence" (14). Its effectiveness can be enhanced for those who smoke any amount by referring the patient to a pregnancy-specific smoker's "quitline." The approach described in the box and outlined as follows guides the provider through the interaction and in documentation of the treatment (14).

1. **Ask** about smoking status. Providers should ask the patient at the first prenatal visit to choose a statement that best describes her smoking status from a list of statements on smoking behavior (see the box). Using this multiple-choice method is more likely to elicit an accurate response than asking a question that elicits a simple "yes" or "no" answer. A smoking cessation chart, a tobacco use sticker, or a vital signs stamp that includes smoking status may be useful in the medical record to remind providers to ask patients about smoking status at follow-up visits (see resource box).

2. **Advise** patients who smoke to stop by providing clear, strong advice to quit with personalized messages about the benefits of quitting and the impact of continued smoking on the woman, fetus, and newborn. Congratulate patients who report having stopped smoking and affirm their efforts with a statement about the benefits of quitting.

3. **Assess** the patient's willingness to attempt to quit smoking within the next 30 days. One approach to this assessment is to say, "Quitting smoking is one of the most important things you can do for your health and your baby's health. If we can give you some help, are you willing to try?" If the patient is willing, the provider can move to the next step. If the patient is unwilling to try, providers may consider having a brief discussion with the patient to educate and reassure her about quitting (14). Quitting advice, assessment, and assistance should be offered at subsequent prenatal care visits.

4. **Assist** patients who are interested in quitting by providing pregnancy-specific, self-help smoking cessation materials (see resource box). Enhance the patient's problem-solving skills by asking when and where she typically smokes and suggesting how she might avoid these situations that trigger the desire to smoke. Offer support on the importance of 1) having a smoke-free space at home, 2) seeking out a "quitting buddy" such as a former smoker or nonsmoker both at work and at home, and 3) understanding nicotine withdrawal, such as irritability and cravings. Communicate caring and concern and encourage the patient to talk about the process of quitting.

   The provider also may refer the patient to a smoker's quitline. Telephone quitlines offer information, direct support, and ongoing counseling and have been very successful in helping pregnant smokers quit and remain smoke free (15). Great Start (1-866-66-START) is a national pregnancy-specific smoker's quitline operated by the American Legacy Foundation. Some states also have proactive direct fax referral capability for providers to connect pregnant smokers directly to their state quitline. By dialing the national quitline network (1-800-QUIT NOW), callers are routed immediately to their state smoker's quitline.

5. **Arrange** follow-up visits to track the progress of the patient's attempt to quit smoking. For current and former smokers, smoking status should be monitored throughout pregnancy, providing opportunities to congratulate and support success, reinforce steps taken toward quitting, and advise those still considering a cessation attempt.

Although counseling and pregnancy-specific materials are effective cessation aids for many pregnant women, some women continue to smoke. These women often are heavily addicted to nicotine and should be *Asked* and *Advised* and *Assessed* about smoking at follow-up visits. Women who continue to smoke may benefit from screening for alcohol use and other drug use (16). If the alcohol or drug use screen result is positive, information about the risks associated with alcohol and drug use during pregnancy should be added to the *Advise* step, and specific strategies for abstaining from alcohol and drugs should be discussed in the *Assist* step. Clinicians also may consider referring patients for additional psychosocial treatment (14).

Although quitting smoking early in pregnancy yields the greatest benefits for the pregnant woman and fetus, quitting at any point can be beneficial (14). The benefits of cutting down are difficult to measure or verify. The effort of women who cut down should be reinforced, but these women also should be reminded that quitting entirely brings the best results for their health, the health of the fetus, and that of their babies (17).

Approximately 60–80% of women who quit smoking during pregnancy return to smoking within a year postpartum (1). Former smokers should be counseled in the third trimester and at the postpartum visit and subsequent gynecology visits concerning relapse to smoking (18).

Pharmacotherapy

The use of nicotine replacement products or other pharmaceuticals for smoking cessation aids during pregnancy and lactation have not been sufficiently evaluated to determine their efficacy or safety. Nicotine gum, lozenges, patches, inhalers, and special-dose antidepressants that reduce withdrawal symptoms, such as bupropion, should be considered for use during pregnancy and lactation only when nonpharmacologic treatments (eg, counseling) have failed. If the increased likelihood of

---

Smoking Cessation Intervention for Pregnant Patients

Ask—1 minute

- Ask the patient to choose the statement that best describes her smoking status:

  A. I have NEVER smoked or have smoked FEWER THAN 100 cigarettes in my lifetime.

  B. I stopped smoking BEFORE I found out I was pregnant, and I am not smoking now.

  C. I stopped smoking AFTER I found out I was pregnant, and I am not smoking now.

  D. I smoke some now, but I have cut down on the number of cigarettes I smoke SINCE I found out I was pregnant.

  E. I smoke regularly now, about the same as BEFORE I found out I was pregnant.

If the patient stopped smoking before or after she found out she was pregnant (B or C), reinforce her decision to quit, congratulate her on success in quitting, and encourage her to stay smoke free throughout pregnancy and postpartum.

If the patient is still smoking (D or E), document smoking status in her medical record, and proceed to Advise, Assess, Assist, and Arrange.

Advise—1 minute

- Provide clear, strong advice to quit with personalized messages about the benefits of quitting and the impact of smoking and quitting on the woman, fetus, and newborn.

Assess—1 minute

- Assess the willingness of the patient to attempt to quit within 30 days.

If the patient is ready to quit, proceed to Assist.

If the patient is not ready, provide information to motivate the patient to quit and proceed to Arrange.

Assist—3 minutes

- Suggest and encourage the use of problem-solving methods and skills for smoking cessation (eg, identify situations that trigger the desire to smoke).
- Provide social support as part of the treatment (eg, "We can help you quit").
- Arrange social support in the smoker's environment (eg, identify a "quit buddy" and smoke-free space).
- Provide pregnancy-specific, self-help smoking cessation materials.

Arrange—1 minute or more

- Assess smoking status at subsequent prenatal visits and, if patient continues to smoke, encourage cessation.

Adapted from Melvin CL, Dolan-Mullen P, Windsor RA Jr, Whiteside HP, Goldenberg RL. Recommended cessation counselling for pregnant women who smoke: a review of the evidence. Tob Control 2000;9(suppl 3):III80–4. Reproduced with permission from the BMJ Publishing Group.

Resources for Smoking Cessation

The American College of Obstetricians and Gynecologists Resources for the Clinician

American College of Obstetricians and Gynecologists. Smoking cessation during pregnancy: a clinician's guide to helping pregnant women quit smoking. Washington, DC: ACOG; 2002. Contains guidelines, a tool kit for the clinician, lecture guide, and CD-ROM. Request a copy by e-mail to: smoking@acog.org. Lecture guide is available online. Go to www.acog.org/goto/smoking.

Dartmouth Medical School. Smoking cessation for pregnancy and beyond: learn proven strategies to help your patients quit. Hanover (NH): Dartmouth Medical School; 2004. Available for purchase from the ACOG Distribution Center (800-762-2264, sales.acog.org): Item No. AA423; price: $25.

American College of Obstetricians and Gynecologists. Smoking and women's health. In: Special issues in women's health. Washington, DC: ACOG; 2005. p. 151–67. Available for purchase from the ACOG Distribution Center (800-762-2264, sales.acog.org): Item No. AA451; price: $59; ACOG members: $45. Available online to members. Go to www.acog.org/goto/underserved.

American College of Obstetricians and Gynecologists "Ask about tobacco use" chart stickers. Washington, DC: ACOG. Available for purchase from the ACOG Distribution Center (800-762-2264, sales.acog.org): Item No. AA268; price: $19/260 stickers; ACOG members: $15/260 stickers.

Other Resources for the Clinician

The following resources are for information purposes only. Referral to these sources and web sites does not imply the endorsement of ACOG. This list is not meant to be comprehensive. The exclusion of a source or web site does not reflect the quality of that source or web site. Please note that web sites are subject to change without notice.

Many states offer free or low-cost smoking cessation counseling services consisting of telephone quitlines, group or individual counseling programs, and materials to help the smoker quit and prevent relapse. Check with the state or local public health office or tobacco control program to access these resources.

Helping pregnant women quit smoking: progress and future directions. Nicotine Tob Res 2004; 6(suppl 2): S95–277.

National Partnership to Help Pregnant Smokers Quit: has tools on helping patients quit, assessing smokers' quitlines, and obtaining Medicaid reimbursement for smoking cessation services. Posters are also available.
Web: www.helppregnantsmokersquit.org.
E-mail: info@helppregnantsmokersquit.org.

British Medical Association. Smoking and reproductive life: the impact of smoking on sexual, reproductive and child health. London (UK): BMA; 2004. Available at: www.bma.org.uk/ap.nsf/Content/smokingreproductivelife/$file/smoking.pdf. Retrieved June 22, 2005.

Treating tobacco use and dependence: clinician's packet. A how-to guide for implementing the Public Health Service Clinical Practice Guidelines. Washington, DC: U.S. Public Health Service; 2003. Available at: www.surgeongeneral.gov/tobacco/clincpack.html. Retrieved June 22, 2005.

Web Sites

American Cancer Society
www.cancer.org

The American Heart Association
www.americanheart.org

The Centers for Disease Control and Prevention: Tobacco Information and Prevention Source (TIPS).
www.cdc.gov/tobacco
TIPS contains documents for health providers to implement tobacco control programs

The National Cancer Institute
www.cancer.gov

National Partnership to Help Pregnant Smokers Quit
www.helppregnantsmokersquit.org/quit/toll_free.asp
The partnership has a listing of states with pregnancy-specific quitlines.

Smoke-Free Families
www.smokefreefamilies.org

Smokefree.gov
www.smokefree.gov
Web site has multiple cessation strategies and information for smokers.

Resources for Patients

American College of Obstetricians and Gynecologists, Smoke-Free Families. Need help putting out that cigarette? Washington, DC: ACOG; Chapel Hill (NC): Smoke-Free Families; 2001. Available in English and Spanish for purchase from the ACOG Distribution Center (800-762-2264, sales.acog.org): Item Nos. AA424 and AA4245; price: $10/10 booklets.

You can quit smoking: support and advice from your prenatal care provider. Available at: www.surgeongeneral.gov/tobacco/prenatal.pdf. Retrieved June 22, 2005. Available for multiple orders from AHRQ (PO Box 8547, Silver Spring MD 20907-8547, 800-358-9295): Item No. AHRQ 00-0052.

Recomendaciones y apoyo de su médico de cuidados, Spanish language. Available at: www.surgeongeneral.gov/tobacco/prenatalsp.pdf. Retrieved June 22, 2005. Available for multiple orders from AHRQ (PO Box 8547, Silver Spring MD 20907-8547, 800-358-9295): Item No. AHRQ 00-0065.

American Legacy Foundation. Great start quitline. Available at: www.americanlegacy.org/greatstart/html/quitline.html. Retrieved: June 22, 2005. 866-66-START for toll free help Monday–Friday 8:00 AM–8:00 PM (Eastern Time) and Saturday 9:00 AM–4:00 PM. Counseling in English or Spanish.

smoking cessation, with its potential benefits, outweighs the unknown risk of nicotine replacement and potential concomitant smoking, nicotine replacement products or other pharmaceuticals may be considered (14). Because potential benefits seem to outweigh potential risks, research to determine the safety and efficacy of pharmacotherapy is underway. Some tobacco control experts have reported that if nicotine replacement therapy is used during pregnancy, products with intermittent dosages, such as the gum or inhaler, should be tried first (19). If the nicotine patch is used, it can be removed at night to reduce fetal nicotine exposure (20). Nicotine replacement therapy also may be considered during lactation. Optimally, smokers can be treated with these pharmacotherapies before conception.

Support Systems

The Agency for Healthcare Research and Quality has recommended systems changes to help health care providers identify and treat tobacco users (14). These changes require the partnership of health care administrators and insurers, and include the following strategies: 1) provide education, resources, and feedback to promote provider involvement in smoking cessation; 2) promote hospital policies that support and provide smoking cessation services; 3) include effective smoking cessation treatments as paid or covered services in all health benefits packages; and 4) reimburse clinicians and specialists for delivery of effective tobacco dependence treatments and include these interventions among the defined duties of the clinicians (14).

Coding

Office visits specifically addressing smoking cessation may be coded using International Classification of Diseases, Ninth Revision, Clinical Modification (ICD-9-CM) code 305.1 (tobacco use disorder, tobacco dependence from the Mental Health section) with Current Procedural Terminology* (CPT®) code 99401 or 99211:

---

* Current Procedural Terminology (CPT) is copyright 2004 American Medical Association. All rights reserved. No fee schedules, basic units, relative values or related listings are included in CPT. The AMA assumes no liability for the data contained herein. CPT® is a trademark of the American Medical Association.

- CPT code 99401 (preventive medicine counseling lasting approximately 15 minutes): If counseling is done by the physician at the time of a regular antepartum visit, use modifier 25 on code 99401. If counseling is done by the physician at another encounter, separate from the antepartum visit, no modifier is needed with code 99401.
- CPT code 99211: If a nurse counsels the patient, and if nurses are recognized by the insurance company as qualified providers of the service, code 99211 would be used instead of code 99401. If the nurse is not recognized as a caregiver, the services will not be covered unless provided by the physician.

Note that not all payers reimburse for counseling outside of the global package and some do not cover preventive services at all.

Many private and public insurers are changing policy to provide coverage for smoking cessation counseling for pregnant women. Although coverage for such counseling may have been denied previously, it may be prudent for the clinician to continue to submit for reimbursement for these services.

References

1. Colman GJ, Joyce T. Trends in smoking before, during, and after pregnancy in ten states. Am J Prev Med 2003;24:29–35.
2. Smoking during pregnancy—United States—1990–2002. Centers for Disease Control and Prevention. MMWR Morb Mortal Wkly Rep 2004;53:911–5.
3. Hamilton BE, Martin JA, Sutton PD. Births: preliminary data for 2003. Centers for Disease Control and Prevention, National Center for Health Statistics. Natl Vital Stat Rep 2004;53(a):1–17.
4. National Center for Health Statistics. Health, United States, 2004: with chartbook on trends in the health of Americans. Hyattsville (MD): NCHS; 2004. Available at: http://www.cdc.gov/nchs/data/hus/hus04.pdf. Retrieved June 20, 2005.
5. U.S. Department of Health and Human Services. The health consequences of smoking: a report of the Surgeon General. Washington, DC: HHS; 2004. Available at: www.cdc.gov/tobacco/sgr/sgr_2004/chapters.htm. Retrieved June 20, 2005.
6. Castles A, Adams EK, Melvin CL, Kelsch C, Boulton ML. Effects of smoking during pregnancy. Five meta-analyses. Am J Prev Med 1999;16:208–15.
7. Spinillo A, Nicola S, Piazzi G, Ghazal K, Colonna L, Baltaro F. Epidemiological correlates of preterm premature rupture of membranes. Int J Gynaecol Obstet 1994; 47:7–15.

8. Salihu HM, Aliyu MH, Pierre-Louis BJ, Alexander GR. Levels of excess infant deaths attributable to maternal smoking during pregnancy in the United States. Matern Child Health J 2003;7:219–27.

9. Ventura SJ, Hamilton BE, Mathews TJ, Chandra A. Trends and variations in smoking during pregnancy and low birth weight: evidence from the birth certificate, 1990-2000. Pediatrics 2003;111:1176–80.

10. Li YF, Langholz B, Salam MT, Gilliland FD. Maternal and grandmaternal smoking patterns are associated with early childhood asthma. Chest 2005;127:1232–41.

11. Sondergaard C, Henriksen TB, Obel C, Wisborg K. Smoking during pregnancy and infantile colic. Pediatrics 2001;108:342–6.

12. von Kries R, Toschke AM, Koletzko B, Slikker W Jr. Maternal smoking during pregnancy and childhood obesity. Am J Epidemiol 2002;156:954–61.

13. England LJ, Kendrick JS, Wilson HG, Merritt RK, Gargiullo PM, Zahniser SC. Effects of smoking reduction during pregnancy on the birth weight of term infants. Am J Epidemiol 2001;154:694–701.

14. Fiore MC, Bailey WC, Cohen SJ, Dorfman SF, Goldstein MG, Gritz ER. Treating tobacco use and dependence. Clinical practice guideline. Rockville (MD): U.S. Department of Health and Human Services, Public Health Service; 2000.

15. Tomson T, Helgason AR, Gilljam H. Quitline in smoking cessation: a cost-effectiveness analysis. Int J Technol Assess Health Care 2004;20:469–74.

16. Ockene J, Ma Y, Zapka J, Pbert L, Valentine Goins K, Stoddard A. Spontaneous cessation to smoking and alcohol use among low-income pregnant women. Am J Prev Med 2002;23:150–9.

17. Melvin CL, Dolan-Mullen P, Windsor RA, Whiteside HP Jr, Goldenberg RL. Recommended cessation counselling for pregnant women who smoke: a review of the evidence. Tob Control 2000;9(suppl 3):III80–4.

18. Dolan Mullen P. How can more smoking suspension during pregnancy become lifelong abstinence? Lessons learned about predictors, interventions, and gaps in our accumulated knowledge. Nicotine Tob Res 2004;6(suppl 2):S217–38.

19. Benowitz N, Dempsey D. Pharmacotherapy for smoking cessation during pregnancy. Nicotine Tob Res 2004;6 (suppl 2):S189–202.

20. Windsor R, Oncken C, Henningfield J, Hartmann K, Edwards N. Behavioral and pharmacological treatment methods for pregnant smokers: issues for clinical practice. J Am Med Womens Assoc 2000;55:304–10.

ACOG Committee Opinion

Committee on
Gynecologic Practice

Committee on
Obstetric Practice

Number 240, August 2000   *(Replaces No. 145, November 1994)*

Statement on Surgical Assistants

Competent surgical assistants should be available for all major obstetric and gynecologic operations. In many cases, the complexity of the surgery or the patient's condition will require the assistance of one or more physicians to provide safe, quality care. Often, the complexity of a given surgical procedure cannot be determined prospectively. Procedures including, but not limited to, operative laparoscopy, major abdominal and vaginal surgery, and cesarean delivery may warrant the assistance of another physician to optimize safe surgical care.

The primary surgeon's judgment and prerogative in determining the number and qualifications of surgical assistants should not be overruled by public or private third-party payers. Surgical assistants should be appropriately compensated.

The American College of Obstetricians and Gynecologists
409 12th Street, SW
PO Box 96920
Washington, DC 20090-6920

12345/43210

ACOG

Committee on
Gynecologic Practice

Committee Opinion

Number 232, April 2000   *(Replaces No. 169, February 1996)*

Tamoxifen and Endometrial Cancer

Tamoxifen, a nonsteroidal antiestrogen agent, is used widely as adjunctive therapy for women with breast cancer. Its efficacy has been recognized by the U.S. Food and Drug Administration, which has approved tamoxifen for the following indications:

- Adjuvant treatment of breast cancer
- Metastatic breast cancer
- Reduction in breast cancer incidence in high-risk women

As the use of tamoxifen to treat both patients with breast cancer and women at risk for the disease becomes more widespread, gynecologists will be consulted more frequently for advice on the proper follow-up of these individuals. Unfortunately, data from prospective trials are insufficient to give definitive guidelines. The purpose of this Committee Opinion is to recommend care to prevent and detect endometrial cancer in women taking tamoxifen.

Tamoxifen is one of a class of agents known as selective estrogen receptor modulators (SERMs). Although the primary therapeutic effect of tamoxifen is derived from its antiestrogenic properties, this agent also has modest estrogenic activity. In standard dosages, tamoxifen may be associated with endometrial proliferation, hyperplasia, polyp formation, and invasive carcinoma.

Most studies have found the increased relative risk of developing endometrial cancer while taking tamoxifen to be two to three times higher than that of an age-matched population (1–3). The level of risk of endometrial cancer in women treated with tamoxifen is dose and time dependent. Studies suggest that the stage, grade, histology, or biology of tumors that develop in individuals treated with tamoxifen (20 mg/d) is no different from those that arise in the general population (3, 4). However, some reports have indicated that women treated with a higher dosage of tamoxifen (40 mg/d) are more prone to develop more biologically aggressive tumors (5).

The rate of endometrial cancer occurrence among tamoxifen users who were administered 20 mg/d in the National Surgical Adjuvant Breast and Bowel Project (NSABP) was 1.6 per 1,000 patient years, compared with 0.2 per 1,000 patient years among control patients taking placebo (3). In this study, the 5-year disease-free survival rate from breast cancer was 38% higher in the tamoxifen group than in the placebo group, suggesting that the small risk of developing endometrial cancer is outweighed by the significant survival benefit provided by tamoxifen therapy for women with breast cancer (3).

The American College of Obstetricians and Gynecologists
409 12th Street, SW
PO Box 96920
Washington, DC 20090-6920

12345/43210

The survival advantage with 5 years of tamoxifen therapy continued with long-term follow-up, but extending the duration of tamoxifen use to 10 years failed to improve the survival benefit gained from 5 years of tamoxifen use (6).

The association between tamoxifen treatment and endometrial cancer is being scrutinized because data support a chemopreventive role for tamoxifen in women at high risk for developing breast cancer. The NSABP prevention trial (P-1) data suggest their risk for both invasive and noninvasive breast cancer is reduced markedly with tamoxifen prophylaxis. In this trial, the risk ratio for developing endometrial cancer was 2.53 in women using tamoxifen compared with women receiving a placebo (7). The Pilot Breast Cancer Prevention Trial showed that 39% of healthy postmenopausal women who were administered tamoxifen at a dosage of 20 mg/d had a histologically abnormal endometrium, compared with 10% of the placebo-treated control group (8). However, no case of endometrial cancer was identified in this small cohort of 111 postmenopausal women.

Several approaches are being explored for screening asymptomatic women using tamoxifen for abnormal endometrial proliferation or endometrial cancer. Correlation may be poor between ultrasonographic measurements of endometrial thickness and abnormal pathology in asymptomatic tamoxifen users because of tamoxifen-induced subepithelial stromal hypertrophy (9). In asymptomatic women using tamoxifen, screening for endometrial cancer with routine transvaginal ultrasonography, endometrial biopsy, or both has not been shown to be effective (10–13).

Although the concurrent use of progestin reduces the risk of endometrial hyperplasia and cancer in patients receiving unopposed estrogen, the impact of progestin on the course of breast cancer and on the endometrium of women receiving tamoxifen is not known. Therefore, such use cannot be advocated as a means of lowering risk in women taking tamoxifen.

On the basis of these data, the committee recommends the following:

- Women taking tamoxifen should be monitored closely for symptoms of endometrial hyperplasia or cancer and should have a gynecologic examination at least once every year.
- Women taking tamoxifen should be educated about the risks of endometrial proliferation, endometrial hyperplasia, and endometrial cancer. Women should be encouraged to promptly report any abnormal vaginal symptoms, including bloody discharge, spotting, staining, or leukorrhea.
- Any abnormal vaginal bleeding, bloody vaginal discharge, staining, or spotting should be investigated.
- Because screening tests have not been effective in increasing the early detection of endometrial cancer in women using tamoxifen and may lead to more invasive and costly diagnostic procedures, they are not recommended.
- Tamoxifen use should be limited to 5 years' duration because a benefit beyond this time has not been documented.
- If atypical endometrial hyperplasia develops, appropriate gynecologic management should be instituted, and the use of tamoxifen should be reassessed. If tamoxifen therapy must be continued, hysterectomy should be considered in women with atypical endometrial hyperplasia. Tamoxifen use may be reinstituted following hysterectomy for endometrial carcinoma in consultation with the physician responsible for the woman's breast care.

References

1. Sismondi P, Biglia N, Volpi E, Giai M, de Grandis T. Tamoxifen and endometrial cancer. Ann N Y Acad Sci 1994;734:310–321
2. Bissett D, Davis JA, George WD. Gynaecological monitoring during tamoxifen therapy. Lancet 1994;344:1244
3. Fisher B, Costantino JP, Redmond CK, Fisher ER, Wickerham DL, Cronin WM. Endometrial cancer in tamoxifen-treated breast cancer patients: findings from the National Surgical Adjuvant Breast and Bowel Project (NSABP) B-14. J Natl Cancer Inst 1994;86:527–537
4. Barakat RR, Wong G, Curtin JP, Vlamis V, Hoskins WJ. Tamoxifen use in breast cancer patients who subsequently develop corpus cancer is not associated with a higher incidence of adverse histologic features. Gynecol Oncol 1994;55:164–168
5. Magriples U, Naftolin F, Schwartz PE, Carcangiu ML. High-grade endometrial carcinoma in tamoxifen-treated breast cancer patients. J Clin Oncol 1993;11:485–490
6. Fisher B, Dignam J, Bryant J, DeCillis A, Wickerham DL, Wolmark N, et al. Five versus more than five years of tamoxifen therapy for breast cancer patients with negative lymph nodes and estrogen receptor-positive tumors. J Natl Cancer Inst 1996;88:1529–1542
7. Fisher B, Costantino JP, Wickerham DL, Redmond CK, Kavanah M, Cronin WM, et al. Tamoxifen for prevention of breast cancer: report of the National Surgical Adjuvant Breast and Bowel Project P-1 Study. J Natl Cancer Inst 1998;90:1371–1388
8. Kedar RP, Bourne TH, Powles TJ, Collins WP, Ashley SE, Cosgrove DO, et al. Effects of tamoxifen on uterus and ovaries of postmenopausal women in a randomised breast cancer prevention trial. Lancet 1994;343:1318–1321
9. Achiron R, Lipitz S, Sivan E, Goldenberg M, Horovitz A, Frenkel Y, et al. Changes mimicking endometrial neoplasia in postmenopausal, tamoxifen-treated women with breast cancer: a transvaginal Doppler study. Ultrasound Obstet Gynecol 1995;6:116–120

10. Bertelli G, Venturini M, Del Mastro L, Garrone O, Cosso M, Gustavino C, et al. Tamoxifen and the endometrium: findings of pelvic ultrasound examination and endometrial biopsy in asymptomatic breast cancer patients. Breast Cancer Res Treat 1998;47:41–46

11. Cecchini S, Ciatto S, Bonardi R, Mazzotta A, Grazzini G, Pacini P, et al. Screening by ultrasonography for endometrial carcinoma in postmenopausal breast cancer patients under adjuvant tamoxifen. Gynecol Oncol 1996;60: 409–411

12. Love CD, Muir BB, Scrimgeour JB, Leonard RC, Dillon P, Dixon JM. Investigation of endometrial abnormalities in asymptomatic women treated with tamoxifen and an evaluation of the role of endometrial screening. J Clin Oncol 1999;17:2050–2054

13. Seoud M, Shamseddine A, Khalil A, Salem Z, Saghir N, Bikhazi K, et al. Tamoxifen and endometrial pathologies: a prospective study. Gynecol Oncol 1999;75:15–19

ACOG

Committee on
Gynecologic Practice

Committee Opinion

The Committee wishes to thank the ACOG Preconception Care Work Group co-chairs, Michele G. Curtis, MD, and Paula J. Adams Hillard, MD, and members, Hani K. Atrash, MD, MPH; Alfred Brann Jr, MD; Siobhan M. Dolan, MD, MPH; Ann Lang Dunlop, MD; Ann Weathersby, CNM, MSN; and Gerald Zelinger, MD, for their assistance in the development of this opinion.

The American College of Obstetricians and Gynecologists
409 12th Street, SW
PO Box 96920
Washington, DC 20090-6920

12345/98765

The importance of preconception care in the continuum of women's health care. ACOG Committee Opinion No. 313. American College of Obstetricians and Gynecologists. Obstet Gynecol 2005;106:665–6

Number 313, September 2005

The Importance of Preconception Care in the Continuum of Women's Health Care

ABSTRACT: The goal of preconception care is to reduce the risk of adverse health effects for the woman, fetus, or neonate by optimizing the woman's health and knowledge before planning and conceiving a pregnancy. Because reproductive capacity spans almost four decades for most women, optimizing women's health before and between pregnancies is an ongoing process that requires access to and the full participation of all segments of the health care system.

Although most pregnancies result in good maternal and fetal outcomes, some pregnancies may result in adverse health effects for the woman, fetus, or neonate. Although some of these outcomes cannot be prevented, optimizing a woman's health and knowledge before planning and conceiving a pregnancy—also referred to as preconception care or prepregnancy care—may eliminate or reduce the risk. For example, initiation of folic acid supplementation at least 1 month before pregnancy reduces the incidence of neural tube defects such as spina bifida and anencephaly (1–3). Similarly, adequate glucose control in a woman with diabetes before conception and throughout pregnancy can decrease maternal morbidity, spontaneous abortion, fetal malformation, fetal macrosomia, intrauterine fetal death, and neonatal morbidity (4).

Nearly half of all pregnancies in the United States are unintended (5). Therefore, the challenge of preconception care lies not only in addressing pregnancy planning for women who seek medical care and consultation specifically in anticipation of a planned pregnancy but also in educating and screening all reproductively capable women on an ongoing basis to identify potential maternal and fetal risks and hazards to pregnancy before and between pregnancies.

This Committee Opinion reinforces the importance of preconception care, provides resources for the woman's health care clinician, and proposes that every reproductively capable woman create a reproductive health plan. The specific clinical content of preconception care is outlined elsewhere (6–8).

Several national and international medical organizations and advocacy groups have focused on the optimization of health before conception, resulting in the development of clinical recommendations and educational materials (see Resources). Core preconception care considerations addressed by all include the following factors:

- Undiagnosed, untreated, or poorly controlled medical conditions
- Immunization history
- Medication and radiation exposure in early pregnancy
- Nutritional issues
- Family history and genetic risk
- Tobacco and substance use and other high-risk behaviors
- Occupational and environmental exposures
- Social issues
- Mental health issues

As medical care rapidly advances, the list of issues to consider when planning a pregnancy continues to grow.

Clinicians should encourage women to formulate a reproductive health plan and should discuss it in a nondirective way at each visit. Such a plan would address the individual's or couple's desire for a child or children (or desire not to have children); the optimal number, spacing, and timing of children in the family; and age-related changes in fertility. Because many women's plans change over time, creating a reproductive health plan requires an ongoing conscientious assessment of the desirability of a future pregnancy, determination of steps that need to be taken either to prevent or to plan for and optimize a pregnancy, and evaluation of current health status and other issues relevant to the health of a pregnancy.

A question such as "Are you considering pregnancy, or could you possibly become pregnant?" can initiate several preconception care interventions, including those listed as follows:

- A dialogue regarding the patient's readiness for pregnancy
- An evaluation of her overall health and opportunities for improving her health
- Education about the significant impact that social, environmental, occupational, behavioral, and genetic factors have in pregnancy
- Identification of women at high risk for an adverse pregnancy outcome

If pregnancy is not desired, current contraceptive use and options should be discussed to assist the patient in identifying the most appropriate and effective method for her.

Preconception and interpregnancy care are components of a larger health care goal—optimizing the health of every woman (9). Because reproductive capacity spans almost four decades for most women, optimizing women's health before and between pregnancies is an ongoing process that requires access to and the full participation of all segments of the health care system.

References

1. Czeizel AE, Dudas I. Prevention of the first occurrence of neural-tube defects by periconceptional vitamin supplementation. N Engl J Med 1992;327:1832–5.
2. Prevention of neural tube defects: results of the Medical Research Council Vitamin Study. MRC Vitamin Study Research Group. Lancet 1991;338:131–7.
3. Botto LD, Moore CA, Khoury MJ, Erickson JD. Neural-tube defects. N Engl J Med 1999;341:1509–19.
4. Pregestational diabetes mellitus. ACOG Practice Bulletin No. 60. American College of Obstetricians and Gynecologists. Obstet Gynecol 2005;105:675–85.
5. Henshaw SK. Unintended pregnancy in the United States. Fam Plann Perspect 1998;30:24–9, 46.
6. American Academy of Pediatrics, American College of Obstetricians and Gynecologists. Guidelines for perinatal care. 5th ed. Elk Grove Village (IL): AAP; Washington, DC: ACOG; 2002.
7. American College of Obstetricians and Gynecologists. Guidelines for women's health care. 2nd ed. Washington, DC: ACOG; 2002.
8. American College of Obstetricians and Gynecologists, American College of Medical Genetics. Preconception and prenatal carrier screening for cystic fibrosis. Clinical and laboratory guidelines. Washington, DC: ACOG; 2001.
9. American College of Obstetricians and Gynecologists. Access to women's health care. ACOG Statement of Policy. Washington, DC: ACOG; 2003.

Resources

American College of Obstetricians and Gynecologists
www.acog.org

American Academy of Family Physicians
www.aafp.org

American Academy of Pediatrics
www.aap.org

American College of Nurse-Midwives
www.acnm.org

American Society for Reproductive Medicine
www.asrm.org

Association of Women's Health, Obstetric and Neonatal Nurses
www.awhonn.org

Centers for Disease Control and Prevention National Center on Birth Defects and Developmental Disabilities
www.cdc.gov/ncbddd

March of Dimes
www.marchofdimes.com

ACOG Committee Opinion

Committee on
Gynecologic Practice

Society of
Gynecologic
Oncologists

Number 280, December 2002

The Role of the Generalist Obstetrician–Gynecologist in the Early Detection of Ovarian Cancer

The American College of Obstetricians and Gynecologists
409 12th Street, SW
PO Box 96920
Washington, DC 20090-6920

12345/65432

The role of the generalist obstetrician–gynecologist in the early detection of ovarian cancer. ACOG Committee Opinion No. 280. American College of Obstetricians and Gynecologists. Obstet Gynecol 2002;100:1413–16.

ABSTRACT: The purpose of this Committee Opinion is to define the role of the generalist obstetrician–gynecologist in the early detection of ovarian cancer. Currently, it appears that the best way to detect early ovarian cancer is for both the patient and her clinician to have a high index of suspicion of the diagnosis in the symptomatic woman. In evaluating symptoms, physicians should perform a physical examination, including a pelvic examination. In premenopausal women with symptoms, a CA 125 measurement has not been shown to be useful in most circumstances. In postmenopausal women with a pelvic mass, a CA 125 measurement may be helpful in predicting a higher likelihood of a malignant tumor than a benign tumor, which may be useful in making consultation or referral decisions or both. A woman with a suspicious or persistent complex adnexal mass requires surgical evaluation by a physician trained to appropriately stage and debulk ovarian cancer. Data suggest that currently available screening tests do not appear to be beneficial for screening low-risk, asymptomatic women. An annual gynecologic examination with an annual pelvic examination is recommended for preventive health care.

Although ovarian cancer is the second most common female reproductive cancer, preceded by cancer of the uterine corpus, more women die from ovarian cancer than from cervical and uterine cancer combined. In the United States, it is estimated that ovarian cancer will be diagnosed in 23,300 women, and 13,900 women will die from this malignancy in 2002. The principal reason for these poor outcomes is the advanced stage of disease at diagnosis in 70–75% of cases and an overall 5-year survival of only 20–30%. However, women with a diagnosis of stage I disease achieve a 90–95% probability of cure. The purpose of this Committee Opinion is to define the role of the generalist obstetrician–gynecologist in the early detection of ovarian cancer.

The poor prognosis of ovarian cancer often is attributed to the fact that it is a "silent" cancer, with symptoms appearing only late in the disease process. This is a misconception, in that studies have shown that women with ovarian cancers are symptomatic often several months before the diagnosis, even with early-stage disease. In a survey of 1,725 women with ovarian cancer, 70% recalled having symptoms for 3 months or longer before the diagnosis, and

35% recalled having symptoms for at least 6 months (1). About three fourths of these women had abdominal symptoms and half had pain or constitutional symptoms. Overall, only 5% were asymptomatic, including only 11% of those with stage I and stage II disease. Pelvic examinations and tests to evaluate symptoms in these women were done more frequently by obstetrician–gynecologists than by other primary care physicians, resulting in earlier disease diagnosis.

Currently, it appears that the best way to detect early ovarian cancer is for both the patient and her clinician to have a high index of suspicion of the diagnosis in the symptomatic woman. This requires education of both as to the symptoms commonly associated with ovarian cancer. Persistent symptoms such as an increase in abdominal size, abdominal bloating, fatigue, abdominal pain, indigestion, inability to eat normally, urinary frequency, pelvic pain, constipation, back pain, urinary incontinence of recent onset, or unexplained weight loss should be evaluated with ovarian cancer being included in the differential diagnosis. Because ovarian cancer occurs most frequently in the postmenopausal woman (median age, approximately 60 years), these symptoms should not be ignored in these women. Unfortunately, many women and clinicians are quick to attribute such symptoms to menopause, aging, dietary changes, stress, or functional bowel problems. As a result, delays of weeks or months often occur before medical advice is sought or diagnostic studies are performed.

In evaluating these symptoms, physicians should perform a physical examination, including a pelvic examination. Imaging studies (including vaginal ultrasonography) may be helpful before making the diagnosis of irritable bowel syndrome, depression, stress, or other diagnoses. In premenopausal women with symptoms, a CA 125 measurement has not been shown to be useful in most circumstances because elevated levels of CA 125 are associated with a variety of common benign conditions, including uterine leiomyomata, pelvic inflammatory disease, endometriosis, adenomyosis, pregnancy, and even menstruation. In postmenopausal women with a pelvic mass, a CA 125 measurement may be helpful in predicting a higher likelihood of a malignant tumor than a benign tumor, which may be useful in making consultation or referral decisions or both; however, a normal CA 125 measurement alone does not rule out ovarian cancer because up to 50% of early-stage cancers and 20–25% of advanced cancers are associated with normal values. The longer the delay in evaluating symptoms or suspicious findings by either the patient or the clinician, the more likely advanced disease will be found.

Diagnostic criteria based on physical examination and imaging techniques that should be used to consider referral to or consultation with a gynecologic oncologist are as follows:

- Postmenopausal women who have a pelvic mass that is suspicious for a malignant ovarian neoplasm, as suggested by at least one of the following indicators: elevated CA 125 level; ascites; a nodular or fixed pelvic mass; evidence of abdominal or distant metastasis; a family history of one or more first-degree relatives with ovarian or breast cancer

- Premenopausal women who have a pelvic mass that is suspicious for a malignant ovarian neoplasm, as suggested by at least one of the following indicators: very elevated CA 125 level (eg, >200 U/mL); ascites; evidence of abdominal or distant metastasis; a family history of one or more first-degree relatives with ovarian or breast cancer

A woman with a suspicious or persistent complex adnexal mass requires surgical evaluation. In these circumstances, a physician trained to appropriately stage and debulk ovarian cancer, such as a gynecologic oncologist, should perform the operation. This should be done in a hospital facility that has the necessary support and consultative services (eg, pathology) to optimize the patient's outcome. When a malignant ovarian tumor is discovered and the appropriate operation cannot be properly performed, a gynecologic oncologist should be consulted.

Of particular concern is the observation that many women with early-stage disease do not undergo appropriate surgical staging. Patients whose comprehensive surgical staging confirms early-stage disease have a much better prognosis than those patients who were thought to have early-stage disease but did not undergo comprehensive surgical staging, presumably because occult disease was missed. In the absence of clinically apparent malignant disease, intraoperative pathology consultation should be obtained if cancer remains a concern. If an apparent early-stage malignancy is present, comprehensive surgical staging should be performed, preferably during the same operation. At the time of surgery for a pelvic mass, samples for peritoneal cytology should be obtained when the abdomen is entered. The mass should be removed intact through an incision that permits thorough staging and surgical management of the primary tumor and possible sites of metastasis. After the liver, spleen, and all peritoneal surfaces, including both hemidiaphragms, are inspected and palpated, a bilateral pelvic and paraaortic lymphadenectomy is performed along with an omentectomy, peritoneal biopsies, removal of the uterus and adnexa, and biopsies or removal of any suspicious lesions. When the cancer appears to be confined to one ovary, especially if it is low grade, it may be appropriate to modify the staging procedure by leaving the uterus and the uninvolved ovary in place for younger women who wish to preserve their fertility.

Unfortunately, there is no screening test for ovarian cancer that has proved effective in screening low-risk asymptomatic women. Measurement of CA 125 levels and completion of pelvic ultrasonography (both abdominal and transvaginal) have been the two tests most thoroughly evaluated. One group of researchers evaluated 22,000 women with CA 125 screening, followed by pelvic ultrasonography if an elevated tumor marker was present (2, 3). More than 98% of women had normal CA 125 values. Of the remaining group, 41 (0.1%) had both increased CA 125 values and abnormal ultrasonograms and underwent surgical assessment. Only 11 women (0.05% of women screened) had ovarian cancer, which was stage III in 7 women. The false-positive rate among those undergoing surgery was 73%. Another group of researchers evaluated 14,469 asymptomatic women with transvaginal ultrasonography, performing 57,214 scans over a period of several years (4). During the period of evaluation, only 11 of 180 women who had surgery for abnormal adnexal masses (6% of operations and 0.07% of women screened) had primary epithelial ovarian cancers, 6 of whom had cancers beyond stage I. Unfortunately, 4 additional women developed primary epithelial ovarian cancers (stage II and stage III) within 12 months of a normal scan. In a mass screening study of 51,500 women conducted over several years using transvaginal ultrasonography, 324 women were identified with abnormalities requiring surgery (5). Only 17 of these women (5% of operations and 0.03% of women screened) were found to have primary epithelial ovarian cancers.

Data suggest that currently available tests do not appear to be beneficial for screening low-risk, asymptomatic women because their sensitivity, specificity, positive predictive value, and negative predictive value have all been modest at best. Because of the low incidence of disease, reported to be approximately one case per 2,500 women per year, it has been estimated that a test with even 100% sensitivity and 99% specificity would have a positive predictive value of only 4.8%, meaning 20 of 21 women undergoing surgery would not have primary ovarian cancer. Unfortunately, no test available approaches this level of sensitivity or specificity.

Hereditary ovarian cancer is estimated to represent only 5–10% of all ovarian cancers. Based on current data, a woman with a germline mutation of *BRCA1* or *BRCA2* has a lifetime risk of 15–45% of developing ovarian cancer. There are no data demonstrating that screening improves early detection of ovarian cancer in this population. These women should be offered genetic counseling to address issues that relate to their high risk of breast and ovarian cancer and the potential impact of these genetic mutations on their offspring. Even if this group were screened for ovarian cancer on a regular basis, more than 90% of all potential ovarian cancer patients would remain unscreened.

Despite varying recommendations regarding the frequency of cervical cytology screening, the Committee on Gynecologic Practice and the Society of Gynecologic Oncologists still believe that an annual gynecologic examination with an annual pelvic examination is recommended for preventive health care. Although newer tumor markers and proteomics are undergoing investigation and appear promising for screening, it is unclear whether they will help identify high-risk women or facilitate the early diagnosis of more women with ovarian cancer. Currently, there are no techniques that have proved to be effective in the routine screening of asymptomatic low-risk women for ovarian cancer.

References

1. Goff BA, Mandel L, Muntz HG, Melancon CH. Ovarian carcinoma diagnosis. Cancer 2000;89:2068–75.
2. Jacobs IJ, Skates SJ, MacDonald N, Menon U, Rosenthal AN, Davies AP, et al. Screening for ovarian cancer: a pilot randomized controlled trial. Lancet 1999;353:1207–10.
3. Jacobs I, Davies AP, Bridges J, Stabile I, Fay T, Lower A, et al. Prevalence screening for ovarian cancer in postmenopausal women by CA 125 measurement and ultrasonography. BMJ 1993;306:1030–4.
4. van Nagell JR Jr, DePriest PD, Reedy MB, Gallion HH, Ueland FR, Pavlik EJ, et al. The efficacy of transvaginal sonographic screening in asymptomatic women at risk for ovarian cancer. Gynecol Oncol 2000;77:350–6.
5. Sato S, Yokoyama Y, Sakamoto T, Futagami M, Saito Y. Usefulness of mass screening for ovarian carcinoma using transvaginal ultrasonography. Cancer 2000;89:582–8.

ACOG

Committee on
Gynecologic Practice

ISSN 1074-861X

The American College of Obstetricians and Gynecologists
409 12th Street, SW
PO Box 96920
Washington, DC 20090-6920

12345/98765

The role of the obstetrician–gynecologist in the assessment and management of obesity. ACOG Committee Opinion No. 319. American College of Obstetricians and Gynecologists. Obstet Gynecol 2005;106:895–9.

Committee Opinion

Number 319, October 2005

The Role of the Obstetrician–Gynecologist in the Assessment and Management of Obesity

ABSTRACT: *Approximately one third of all women in the United States are obese. Obstetrician–gynecologists should evaluate all women for obesity by calculating a body mass index (BMI) measurement and should offer appropriate interventions or referrals to promote a healthy weight and lifestyle.*

The purpose of this Committee Opinion is to address the role of the obstetrician–gynecologist in the assessment and management of obesity in nonpregnant adult women. Definitions of overweight and obesity will be reviewed, the importance of calculating the body mass index (BMI) will be outlined, and resources for counseling and referral will be provided. The impact of obesity on pregnancy and the assessment of overweight and obesity in adolescents are addressed elsewhere (1, 2).

Background

Obesity, defined as a BMI of 30 or greater, is the fastest-growing health problem in the United States, and its prevalence has increased sharply over the past 20 years (3). Approximately one third of all U.S. women are obese (3). Obesity is more prevalent in lower-income and minority women; 49% of African–American women and 38% of Mexican–American women are obese, compared with 31% of white women (3). Obesity has been associated with increased morbidity, including type 2 diabetes, hypertension, infertility, heart disease, gallbladder disease, osteoarthritis, and a variety of cancers, including breast, uterine, and colon cancers (4–7). Endometrial cancer is the most common gynecologic malignancy, and obese women are almost five times more likely than nonobese women (BMI 20–22.9) to develop endometrial cancer (8). Obesity and overweight are associated with an increased risk for heart disease, the leading cause of death of American women (4, 5, 9). An estimated 112,000 individuals die annually of obesity-associated causes (10).

Assessment

The patient's medical, social, and family history should be reviewed for weight-related conditions. To determine if the patient is overweight or obese, the BMI should be calculated. If the patient's BMI is 30 or greater, the severity of obesity (Class I, II, or III) should be noted (Table 1).

Central adiposity, defined as a waist circumference greater than 35 inches (>88 cm) in women, may further identify women at risk for obesity-related morbidity (11). Waist circumference is measured at the end of a normal expiration of breath by placing a measuring tape around the abdomen at the level of the iliac crest.

Table 1. Body Mass Index Calculation, Chart, and Categories

The Body Mass Index (BMI) is an indirect measure of body fat and is used to determine obesity. The BMI is calculated as weight in kilograms (kg) divided by the square of height in meters (m²).

$$BMI = \frac{weight\ (kg)}{height\ squared\ (m^2)}$$

Using a BMI chart is an easy and rapid way of identifying the BMI for all adult patients.

Body Mass Index Table

	Normal						Overweight					Obese										Extreme Obesity														
BMI	19	20	21	22	23	24	25	26	27	28	29	30	31	32	33	34	35	36	37	38	39	40	41	42	43	44	45	46	47	48	49	50	51	52	53	54
Height (inches)																Body Weight (pounds)																				
58	91	96	100	105	110	115	119	124	129	134	138	143	148	153	158	162	167	172	177	181	186	191	196	201	205	210	215	220	224	229	234	239	244	248	253	258
59	94	99	104	109	114	119	124	128	133	138	143	148	153	158	163	168	173	178	183	188	193	198	203	208	212	217	222	227	232	237	242	247	252	257	262	267
60	97	102	107	112	118	123	128	133	138	143	148	153	158	163	168	174	179	184	189	194	199	204	209	215	220	225	230	235	240	245	250	255	261	266	271	276
61	100	106	111	116	122	127	132	137	143	148	153	158	164	169	174	180	185	190	195	201	206	211	217	222	227	232	238	243	248	254	259	264	269	275	280	285
62	104	109	115	120	126	131	136	142	147	153	158	164	169	175	180	186	191	196	202	207	213	218	224	229	235	240	246	251	256	262	267	273	278	284	289	295
63	107	113	118	124	130	135	141	146	152	158	163	169	175	180	186	191	197	203	208	214	220	225	231	237	242	248	254	259	265	270	278	282	287	293	299	304
64	110	116	122	128	134	140	145	151	157	163	169	174	180	186	192	197	204	209	215	221	227	232	238	244	250	256	262	267	273	279	285	291	296	302	308	314
65	114	120	126	132	138	144	150	156	162	168	174	180	186	192	198	204	210	216	222	228	234	240	246	252	258	264	270	276	282	288	294	300	306	312	318	324
66	118	124	130	136	142	148	155	161	167	173	179	186	192	198	204	210	216	223	229	235	241	247	253	260	266	272	278	284	291	297	303	309	315	322	328	334
67	121	127	134	140	146	153	159	166	172	178	185	191	198	204	211	217	223	230	236	242	249	255	261	268	274	280	287	293	299	306	312	319	325	331	338	344
68	125	131	138	144	151	158	164	171	177	184	190	197	203	210	216	223	230	236	243	249	256	262	269	276	282	289	295	302	308	315	322	328	335	341	348	354
69	128	135	142	149	155	162	169	176	182	189	196	203	209	216	223	230	236	243	250	257	263	270	277	284	291	297	304	311	318	324	331	338	345	351	358	365
70	132	139	146	153	160	167	174	181	188	195	202	209	216	222	229	236	243	250	257	264	271	278	285	292	299	306	313	320	327	334	341	348	355	362	369	376
71	136	143	150	157	165	172	179	186	193	200	208	215	222	229	236	243	250	257	265	272	279	286	293	301	308	315	322	329	338	343	351	358	365	372	379	386
72	140	147	154	162	169	177	184	191	199	206	213	221	228	235	242	250	258	265	272	279	287	294	302	309	316	324	331	338	346	353	361	368	375	383	390	397
73	144	151	159	166	174	182	189	197	204	212	219	227	235	242	250	257	265	272	280	288	295	302	310	318	325	333	340	348	355	363	371	378	386	393	401	408
74	148	155	163	171	179	186	194	202	210	218	225	233	241	249	256	264	272	280	287	295	303	311	319	326	334	342	350	358	365	373	381	389	396	404	412	420
75	152	160	168	176	184	192	200	208	216	224	232	240	248	256	264	272	279	287	295	303	311	319	327	335	343	351	359	367	375	383	391	399	407	415	423	431
76	156	164	172	180	189	197	205	213	221	230	238	246	254	263	271	279	287	295	304	312	320	328	336	344	353	361	369	377	385	394	402	410	418	426	435	443

Weight category	BMI
Underweight	<18.5
Normal weight	18.5–24.9
Overweight	25–29.9
Obesity (Class I)	30–34.9
Obesity (Class II)	35–39.9
Extreme Obesity (Class III)	≥40

The practical guide: identification, evaluation, and treatment of overweight and obesity in adults. National Heart, Lung, and Blood Institute and North American Association for the Study of Obesity. Bethesda (MD): National Institutes of Health; 2000.

Blood pressure measurements, fasting lipid panels, and fasting blood glucose measurements may be appropriate for identifying comorbidities. However, no single laboratory test or diagnostic evaluation is indicated for all patients with obesity, and the tests and evaluations performed should be based on the patient's symptoms and risk factors and the clinician's index of suspicion for specific comorbidities (12).

Management

Weight management is a challenge for patients and their physicians. For many women, achieving and maintaining a healthy weight is a difficult and lifelong process. Improved health through weight loss and appropriate increased physical activity should be the goal. Counseling to support improvements in diet and physical activity are considered first-line interventions, although pharmacotherapy and surgery may be appropriate for some women (Table 2). The U.S. Preventive Services Task Force found the most successful nonsurgical approaches to be intensive, weight-focused counseling (more than one session per month) or multicomponent, intensive interventions that combine nutrition and exercise counseling with supportive, skill-building behavioral interventions (13). If available, referral for further evaluation and treatment should be considered whenever the resources of the clinician are insufficient to meet the patient's current needs, for women with a BMI of 40 or greater, and for women with a BMI of 35 or greater with comorbidities or who have failed appropriate prior intervention(s).

Reinforcing the importance of weight loss and exercise and assessing the patient's readiness to make behavioral changes should be the initial approach. The clinician should inform the patient in a sensitive manner that her weight is a health concern and assist her in developing a weight loss and exercise plan. Asking the patient if she is concerned about her weight and has ever tried to lose weight will help the clinician determine if she is interested in weight management. Applying the stages of change model, as adapted for overweight and obesity, may help determine patient motivation and interest in weight loss (Table 3). Educational handouts for the patient to read at home can be discussed at a follow-up visit. Setting an initial goal of losing 5–10% of total body weight over a 6-month period is realistic and achievable and can decrease the severity of obesity-associated risk factors (14). Contact information for community resources, support groups, and weight loss programs may be provided (see Patient Resources). Evaluation by a nutritionist may be of benefit, in addition to follow-up visits with a clinician to monitor progress and provide support. Patients can be informed that some insurance carriers may provide coverage for weight loss interventions.

Orlistat and sibutramine hydrochloride monohydrate have been approved by the U.S. Food and Drug Administration for patients with a BMI of 30 or greater and for those with a BMI of 27 or greater and other risk factors (eg, hypertension, diabetes, or dyslipidemia) when used in combination with lifestyle changes (see Table 2). These agents are the two most studied pharmacologic treatments for obesity, although efficacy and safety beyond 12 months have not been investigated in randomized, controlled trials (15, 16). Orlistat is a gastrointestinal lipase inhibitor that limits fat absorption. Side

Table 2. Guide to Selecting Treatment

Treatment	Body Mass Index Category				
	25–26.9	27–29.9	30–34.9	35–39.9	≥40
Diet, physical activity, and behavior therapy	With comorbidities	With comorbidities	+	+	+
Pharmacotherapy		With comorbidities	+	+	+
Surgery			With comorbidities	With comorbidities	With comorbidities

The + represents the use of indicated treatment regardless of comorbidities.

The practical guide: identification, evaluation, and treatment of overweight and obesity in adults. National Heart, Lung, and Blood Institute and North American Association for the Study of Obesity. Bethesda (MD): National Institutes of Health; 2000.

Table 3. Stages of Change Model to Assess Readiness for Weight Loss

Stage	Characteristic	Patient Verbal Cue	Appropriate Intervention	Sample Dialogue
Precontemplation	Unaware of problem, no interest in change	"I'm not really interested in weight loss. It's not a problem."	Provide information about health risks and benefits of weight loss	"Would you like to read some information about the health aspects of obesity?"
Contemplation	Aware of problem, beginning to think of changing	"I know I need to lose weight, but with all that's going on in my life right now, I'm not sure I can."	Help resolve ambivalence; discuss barriers	"Let's look at the benefits of weight loss, as well as what you may need to change."
Preparation	Realizes benefits of making changes and thinking about how to change	"I have to lose weight, and I'm planning to do that."	Teach behavior modification; provide education	"Let's take a closer look at how you can reduce some of the calories you eat and how to increase your activity during the day."
Action	Actively taking steps toward change	"I'm doing my best. This is harder than I thought."	Provide support and guidance, with a focus on the long term	"It's terrific that you're working so hard. What problems have you had so far? How have you solved them?"
Maintenance	Initial treatment goals reached	"I've learned a lot through this process."	Relapse control	"What situations continue to tempt you to overeat? What can be helpful for the next time you face such a situation?"

Assessment and management of adult obesity: a primer for physicians, assessing readiness and making treatment decisions. American Medical Association and the Robert Wood Johnson Foundation, Copyright 2003.

effects are common and include fecal urgency, flatulence, and oily rectal discharge. A recent literature review found six trials that demonstrated significant weight loss (2.8–4.5 kg in 6–12.5 months) by patients who took orlistat (120 mg, taken 3 times daily before meals) compared with patients who took a placebo (17). In three trials reporting response rates, 14–38% of patients treated with orlistat lost 10% of their body weight. This degree of weight loss was 9–19% more common in patients who received orlistat than patients who received a placebo (17). Sibutramine is a dopamine, norepinephrine, and serotonin reuptake inhibitor for which the method of action for weight loss is unknown. Side effects include increases in blood pressure and heart rate. Six clinical trials of sibutramine (10–20 mg daily) versus placebo have shown at 6–12 months of treatment that patients taking sibutramine have a weight loss of 2.8–7.8 kg more than patients taking a placebo (17). Loss of 10% of body weight occurred in 6–34% of patients who took sibu-

tramine; this degree of weight loss was 5–27% more common in patients who took sibutramine than in patients who received a placebo (17). Unfortunately, discontinuation of pharmacotherapy may lead to rapid weight regain.

In some patients with severe obesity (BMI > 40) or patients with a BMI of 35 or greater with comorbid conditions, surgical intervention may be an option if nonsurgical methods of weight loss have failed (4). Surgical options can promote substantial, long-term weight loss (17). These patients should be evaluated by a comprehensive bariatric treatment team.

Conclusion

Obstetrician–gynecologists should evaluate all women for obesity by calculating BMI. Clinicians should offer patients appropriate interventions or referrals to promote a healthy weight and lifestyle.

References

1. Obesity in pregnancy. ACOG Committee Opinion 315. American College of Obstetricians and Gynecologists. Obstet Gynecol 2005;106:671–5.
2. American College of Obstetricians and Gynecologists. Health care for adolescents. Washington, DC: ACOG; 2003.
3. Hedley AA, Ogden CL, Johnson CL, Carroll MD, Curtin LR, Flegal KM. Prevalence of overweight and obesity among U.S. children, adolescents, and adults, 1999–2002. JAMA 2004;291:2847–50.
4. Clinical guidelines on the identification, evaluation, and treatment of overweight and obesity in adults—the evidence report. National Institutes of Health [published erratum appears in Obes Res 1998;6:464]. Obes Res 1998;6 Suppl 2:51S–209S.
5. Office of the Surgeon General. The Surgeon General's call to action to prevent and decrease overweight and obesity 2001. Rockville (MD): U.S. Department of Health and Human Services, Public Health Service, Office of the Surgeon General; 2001.
6. World Health Organization. Obesity: preventing and managing the global epidemic. WHO Technical Report Series 894. Geneva, Switzerland: World Health Organization; 2000.
7. Azziz R. Reproductive endocrinologic alterations in female asymptomatic obesity. Fertil Steril 1989;52: 703–25.
8. Schouten LJ, Goldbohm RA, van den Brandt PA. Anthropometry, physical activity, and endometrial cancer risk: results from the Netherlands Cohort Study. J Natl Cancer Inst 2004;96:1635–8.
9. Mosca L, Appel LJ, Benjamin EJ, Berra K, Chandra-Strobos N, Fabunmi RP, et al. Evidence-based guidelines for cardiovascular disease prevention in women. American Heart Association. Circulation 2004;109: 672–93.
10. Flegal KM, Graubard BI, Williamson DF, Gail MH. Excess deaths associated with underweight, overweight, and obesity. JAMA 2005;293:1861–7.
11. Janssen I, Katzmarzyk PT, Ross R. Body mass index, waist circumference, and health risk: evidence in support of current National Institutes of Health guidelines. Arch Intern Med 2002;162:2074–9.
12. Kushner RF, Weinsier RL. Evaluation of the obese patient. Practical considerations. Med Clin North Am 2000;84:387–99, vi.
13. Screening for obesity in adults: recommendations and rationale. U.S. Preventive Services Task Force. Ann Intern Med 2003;139:930–2.
14. Goldstein DJ. Beneficial health effects of modest weight loss. Int J Obes Relat Metab Disord 1992;16:397–415.
15. Li Z, Maglione M, Tu W, Mojica W, Arterburn D, Shugarman LR, et al. Meta-analysis: pharmacologic treatment of obesity. Ann Intern Med 2005;142:532–46.
16. Snow V, Barry P, Fitterman N, Qaseem A, Weiss K. Pharmacologic and surgical management of obesity in primary care: a clinical practice guideline from the American College of Physicians. Clinical Efficacy Assessment Subcommittee of the American College of Physicians. Ann Intern Med 2005;142:525–31.
17. McTigue KM, Harris R, Hemphill B, Lux L, Sutton S, Bunton AJ, et al. Screening and interventions for obesity in adults: summary of the evidence for the U.S. Preventive Services Task Force. Ann Intern Med 2003;139:933–49.

Physician Resources

American Medical Association—Roadmaps for Clinical Practice series: Assessment and management of adult obesity
www.ama-assn.org/ama/pub/category/10931.html

American Society for Bariatric Surgery
www.asbs.org

ACOG Clinical Updates in Women's Health Care—Weight control: assessment and management
www.clinicalupdates.org

National Heart, Lung, and Blood Institute—Clinical guidelines on the identification, evaluation, and treatment of overweight and obesity in adults
www.nhlbi.nih.gov/guidelines/obesity/ob_home.htm

The Surgeon General's call to action to prevent and decrease overweight and obesity
www.surgeongeneral.gov/topics/obesity

U.S. Preventive Services Task Force—Screening for obesity in adults
www.ahrq.gov/clinic/uspstf/uspsobes.htm

Patient Resources

American Obesity Association
www.obesity.org

American Society of Bariatric Physicians
www.asbp.org

MedlinePlus: Weight Loss and Dieting
www.nlm.nih.gov/medlineplus/weightlossanddieting.html

National Heart, Lung, and Blood Institute Obesity Education Initiative
www.nhlbi.nih.gov/about/oei/index.htm

Overeaters Anonymous
www.overeatersanonymous.org

TOPS—Take Off Pounds Sensibly
www.tops.org

Weight-control Information Network
www.win.niddk.nih.gov

ACOG

Committee on Health Care for Underserved Women

The Committee wishes to thank Kurt Barnhart, MD, MSCE, for his assistance in the development of this document.

ISSN 1074-861X

The American College of Obstetricians and Gynecologists
409 12th Street, SW
PO Box 96920
Washington, DC 20090-6920

12345/87654

The uninsured. ACOG Committee Opinion No. 308. American College of Obstetricians and Gynecologists. Obstet Gynecol 2004;104:1471–4.

Committee Opinion

Number 308, December 2004

The Uninsured

ABSTRACT: The United States is one of the few industrialized nations in the world that does not guarantee access to health care for its population. Access to health care for all women is a paramount concern of obstetrician–gynecologists and the American College of Obstetricians and Gynecologists. Lack of health care coverage creates access issues that affect women, practitioners, and the health care system as a whole. The number of women in the United States without health care coverage grew 3 times faster than the number of men without such coverage during the late 1990s and early 2000s. A change in our currently fragmented health care system is warranted because the lack of coverage clearly matters to the millions of uninsured Americans. Pregnant women and infants are among the most vulnerable populations in the country and the American College of Obstetricians and Gynecologists believes that providing them with full insurance coverage must be a primary step in the process of providing coverage for all Americans. However, it is only the first step; it is critical to expand coverage for all Americans. Health professionals can play a pivotal role in improving access to needed health care by helping society understand the importance of broadening health insurance coverage.

The United States is one of the few industrialized nations in the world that does not guarantee access to health care for its population. Of the 30 countries in the Organization of Economic Cooperation and Development, only Mexico and Turkey have a higher uninsured rate than the United States (1). Millions of women are caught in the gaps in the current health care system, leaving them in a vulnerable position regarding their health status. The number of women in the United States who are uninsured grew 3 times faster than the number of men without health insurance during the late 1990s and early 2000s (2). In 2003, it was estimated that of the 45 million Americans (15.6% of the total population) without health insurance for the entire year, 21.2 million were women (14.4% of all women) (3, 4). This represents an increase from 2002 when it was estimated that of the 43.6 million Americans (15.2% of the total population) without health insurance for the entire year, 20.2 million were women (13.9% of all women) (5). Approximately 13% of all pregnant women are uninsured (6).

Access to health care for all women is a paramount concern of obstetrician–gynecologists and the American College of Obstetricians and Gynecologists (ACOG). Lack of health care coverage creates access issues that affect women, practitioners, and the health care system as a whole. These issues have an effect on ACOG's core missions of education and service and are exacerbated by the ailing professional liability system.

Effect on Women's Reproductive Health and Health Care

Having health insurance does not guarantee good health, but not having insurance is guaranteed to put Americans at higher risk for poorer health outcomes and economic disaster. The uninsured receive less preventive care, receive diagnoses at more advanced disease stages, and, once diseases are diagnosed, tend to receive less therapeutic care (drugs and surgical interventions) (7). Acquisition of health insurance reduces mortality rates for the uninsured by 10–15% (8). In terms of women's reproductive health and health care, the lack of health insurance may affect women in the following ways:

- Lack of insurance limits women's options for contraception (9).

- Uninsured women receive fewer prenatal care services than their insured counterparts (1).

- Eighteen percent of uninsured pregnant women reported that they did not receive some "needed" medical care versus 7.6% of privately insured and 8.1% of Medicaid-enrolled pregnant women (10).

- Uninsured pregnant women are more likely to experience an adverse maternal outcome (1).

- Uninsured newborns are more likely to experience adverse health outcomes than insured newborns. Infants of uninsured women are more likely to die than are those of insured women (1).

- Uninsured women with breast cancer have a 30–50% higher risk of dying than insured women (1). This is not surprising given that uninsured women aged 50–64 years are 3 times less likely to have had a mammogram or clinical breast examination in the past 2 years compared with insured women (11).

- Uninsured women aged 18–64 years are 3 times less likely to have had a needed Pap test in the past 3 years (11), contributing to a 60% greater risk of late-stage diagnosis of cervical cancer among uninsured women compared with insured women (12).

The Capacity of the Health Care System to Serve the Uninsured

Uninsured patients receive health care via 3 primary sources—hospitals (including academic medical centers), office-based physicians, and clinics and direct care programs. The cost of uncompensated care is staggering; in 2004, it was estimated to be $40.7 billion. Despite the disincentives for providing such care, all of the aforementioned sources have taken on part of the burden. Most uncompensated care expenses are incurred by hospitals, where services are most costly. In 2001, hospitals accounted for $25.6 billion (63%) in uncompensated care. Office-based physicians and direct care programs or clinics accounted for $7.3 billion (18%) and $7.7 billion (19%) respectively, in uncompensated care (13). A 2001 Commonwealth Fund study found that the level of care provided by academic health centers to those who were unable to pay for their services increased as a percentage of gross patient revenues by more than 40% in the past decade (14). The number of patients treated at hospitals who are unable to pay is increasing as the number of uninsured grows. This is especially true for academic medical centers. All of the efforts to provide care to those unable to pay create adverse effects on profit margins, which in turn imperil the mission of institutions and facilities to provide health care for all patients, not just the uninsured.

The proportion of private physicians providing care to the uninsured is decreasing and those who provide such care are spending less time doing so (15). Specifically, the number of physicians providing any care to individuals unable to pay decreased from 76.3% in 1997 to 71.5% in 2001. In addition, the proportion of providers who spend more than 5% of their practice time treating patients who are unable to pay decreased between 1997 and 2001, while the proportion of providers who spend less than 5% of their practice time treating a low volume of such patients increased. In addition, the professional liability insurance crisis is threatening the availability of physicians and their capacity to provide care to the uninsured.

Conclusions

Allowing health care to be driven by market forces has led to a lack of access for many of our citizens.

Provision of care to patients who are unable to pay by private physicians and the safety net of community clinics, public hospitals, and academic medical centers does not substitute for health insurance. A change in our currently fragmented health care system is, therefore, warranted because the lack of coverage clearly matters to the millions of uninsured Americans. This lack of coverage affects job decisions, financial security, access to care, and health status.

Health professionals can play a pivotal role in improving access to needed health care by helping society understand the importance of broadening health insurance coverage. Health care providers need to be advocates for the goal of securing quality, affordable coverage for every American with active support of proposed local, state, and national legislation. There are formidable obstacles to major progress in increasing the number of people who are insured. Among them are fiscal limitations, the political climate, and philosophical differences in approaches to resolving this problem.

In 1993, ACOG developed U.S. MaternaCare, which is a proposal designed to ensure that all women in the United States have access to a full range of pregnancy related services, including family planning and infant care. Pregnant women and infants are among the most vulnerable populations in the country, and ACOG believes that providing them with full insurance coverage must be a primary step in the process of providing coverage for all Americans. However, it is only the first step; it is critical to expand the basic benefits and coverage for all Americans. As a proposal for universal insurance coverage, U.S. MaternaCare was designed around a set of principles that ACOG continues to support. It uses and builds upon the existing strengths of the U.S. health care system, including multiple financing and delivery systems. It calls for coverage for all women regardless of their citizenship status, and includes a basic set of benefits that must be offered to all women. It asserts that any health care reform proposal must address issues of quality assurance, cost containment, and professional liability reform (16). Until these goals are achieved, continued support of the safety net system and provision of care in the community and office setting for the uninsured is essential. For a listing of resources on the topic of the uninsured, go to http://www.acog.org/goto/underserved.

References

1. Institute of Medicine. Insuring America's health: principles and recommendations. Washington, DC: The Institute; 2004.
2. Labrew JM. Diagnosing disparities in health insurance for women: a prescription for change. New York (NY): The Commonwealth Fund; 2001. Available at: http://www.cmwf.org/programs/insurance/lambrew_disparities_493.pdf. Retrieved August 5, 2004.
3. DeNavas-Walt C, Proctor BD, Mills RJ. Income, poverty, and health insurance coverage in the United States: 2003. Current Population Reports. Washington, DC: U.S. Census Bureau; 2004. Available at: http://www.census.gov/prod/2004pubs/p60-226.pdf. Retrieved August 31, 2004.
4. U.S. Census Bureau. 2004 annual social and economic supplement. Current Population Survey. Washington, DC: Census Bureau; 2004. Available at: http://ferret.bls.census.gov/macro/032004/health/h01_001.htm. Retrieved August 31, 2004.
5. Mills RJ, Bhandari S. Health insurance coverage in the United States: 2002. Consumer income. Current Population Reports. Washington, DC: U.S. Census Bureau; 2003. Available at: http://www.census.gov/prod/2003pubs/p60223.pdf. Retrieved August 5, 2004.
6. Thorpe KE, Flome J, Joski P. The distribution of health insurance coverage among pregnant women, 1999. New York (NY): March of Dimes; 2001. Available at: http://www.modimes.com/files/2001FinalThorpeReport.pdf. Retrieved August 5, 2004.
7. American College of Physicians - American Society of Internal Medicine. No health insurance? It's enough to make you sick. Philadelphia (PA): ACP-ASIM; 1999. Available at: http://www.acponline.org/uninsured/lack-consents.htm. Retrieved August 5, 2004.
8. Hadley J. Sicker and poorer: the consequences of being uninsured. A review of the research on the relationship between health insurance, health, work, income, and education. The Kaiser Commission on Medicaid and the Uninsured. Menlo Park (CA): The Henry J Kaiser Family Foundation; 2002. Available at: http://www.kff.org/uninsured/upload/13970_1.pdf. Retrieved September 2, 2004.
9. Sonfield A, Gold RB. New study documents major strides in drive for contraceptive coverage. Guttmacher Rep Pub Pol 2004;7(2):4–5, 14.
10. Bernstein AB. Insurance status and use of health services by pregnant women. Washington, DC: Alpha Center; 1999. Available at: http://www.marchofdimes.com/files/bernstein_paper.pdf. Retrieved September 2, 2004.
11. Ayanian JZ, Weissman JS, Schneider EC, Ginsburg JA, Zaslavsky AM. Unmet health needs of uninsured adults in the United States. JAMA 2000;284:2061–9.
12. Ferrante JM, Gonzalez EC, Roetzheim RG, Pal N, Woodard L. Clinical and demographic predictors of late-stage cervical cancer. Arch Fam Med 2000;9:439–45.
13. Hadley J, Holahan J. The cost of care for the uninsured: what do we spend, who pays, and what would full coverage add to medical spending? Issue update. The Kaiser Commission on Medicaid and the Uninsured. Menlo Park

(CA): The Henry J Kaiser Family Foundation; 2004. Available at: http://www.kff.org/uninsured/7084.cfm. Retrieved August 5, 2004.

14. The Commonwealth Fund. A shared responsibility: academic health centers and the provision of care to the poor and uninsured. A report of The Commonwealth Fund Task Force on Academic Health Centers. New York (NY): Commonwealth Fund; 2001. Available at: http://www.cmwf.org/programs/taskforc/AHC_indigent care_443.pdf. Retrieved August 5, 2004.

15. Cunningham PJ. Mounting pressures: physicians serving Medicaid patients and the uninsured, 1997-2001. Track Rep 2002;(6):1–4.

16. American College of Obstetricians and Gynecologists. U.S. MaternaCare. A proposal for universal access to maternity care. Washington, DC: ACOG; 1993. Available at: http://www.acog.org/departments/dept_notice.cfm?recno =18&bulletin=2650. Retrieved August 5, 2004.

ACOG Committee Opinion

Committee
on Coding and
Nomenclature

Number 205, August 1998

Tubal Ligation with Cesarean Delivery

Tubal ligation at the time of cesarean delivery requires significant additional physician work even though the technical work of the procedure is brief. Informed consent by the patient requires considerably more counseling by the physician regarding potential risks and benefits of this procedure than is necessary with alternative means of sterilization and contraception. Also, many states require completion of special informed consent documents in addition to the customary consent forms required by hospitals. These forms must be completed before scheduling the procedure.

Patients have the right to change their minds. Thus, it is important to reconfirm the patient's decision shortly before the operation.

Tubal ligation with cesarean delivery involves removal of a segment of fallopian tube, which is sent for histologic confirmation. With most cesarean deliveries, tissue is not evaluated by a pathologist. Accordingly, it is important for the surgeon to verify the pathology report, which adds an additional component to post-service work.

The risk of professional liability for operative complications is increased with this procedure. This risk is low, but real. Furthermore, sterilization failure occurs in about 1 in 100 cases even though the operation was performed properly. This failure also carries a liability risk.

Because tubal ligation is a discrete extra service, it should be coded accordingly: 59510 or 59618—routine obstetric care including antepartum care, cesarean delivery, and postpartum care—and 58611—ligation or transection of fallopian tube(s) done at the time of cesarean delivery or intra-abdominal surgery.

ACOG
Committee
on Genetics

Committee Opinion

Number 325, December 2005

Update on Carrier Screening for Cystic Fibrosis

ABSTRACT: In 2001, the American College of Obstetricians and Gynecologists and the American College of Medical Genetics introduced guidelines for prenatal and preconception carrier screening for cystic fibrosis. The American College of Obstetricians and Gynecologists has updated current guidelines for cystic fibrosis screening practices among obstetrician–gynecologists.

Prenatal and preconception carrier screening for cystic fibrosis was introduced into routine obstetric practice in 2001. *Preconception and Prenatal Carrier Screening for Cystic Fibrosis: Clinical and Laboratory Guidelines* (1), developed by the American College of Obstetricians and Gynecologists (ACOG) and the American College of Medical Genetics (ACMG), was sent to all ACOG members in practice. According to a survey of ACOG members 2 years later, most obstetricians are offering cystic fibrosis carrier screening to their pregnant patients (2). As recommended in the guidelines, most obstetricians ask their patients if there is a family history of cystic fibrosis and provide the pregnant patients with information on cystic fibrosis. In contrast, significantly fewer obstetrician–gynecologists offer nonpregnant patients cystic fibrosis carrier screening unless a patient requests the information or has a family history. After cystic fibrosis carrier screening was implemented, the ACMG convened a work group to review the prevalence of mutations in the general population and to evaluate the cystic fibrosis carrier screening program in the United States. The purpose of this document is to provide an update on cystic fibrosis carrier screening.

The goal of cystic fibrosis carrier screening is to identify couples at risk for having a child with classic cystic fibrosis. The ACOG/ACMG guidelines recommended that cystic fibrosis carrier screening be offered to Caucasian couples (including Ashkenazi Jews) who are planning a pregnancy or seeking prenatal care and be made available to all patients. This recommendation took into account differences in cystic fibrosis prevalence and test sensitivity. Cystic fibrosis is more common (ie, has higher carrier rate) in Caucasians (including Ashkenazi Jews) than in other populations, and the screening test detects a higher percentage of carriers in this population than in other popu-

The American College of Obstetricians and Gynecologists
409 12th Street, SW
PO Box 96920
Washington, DC 20090-6920

12345/98765

Update on carrier screening for cystic fibrosis. ACOG Committee Opinion No. 325. American College of Obstetricians and Gynecologists. Obstet Gynecol 2005;106:1465–8.

lations (Table 1). In practice, two thirds of obstetricians offer cystic fibrosis carrier screening to all pregnant patients rather than using the selective criteria. Because it is becoming increasingly difficult to assign a single ethnicity, it is reasonable to offer cystic fibrosis carrier screening to all pregnant patients, provided that women are aware of their carrier risk and of the test limitations. The sensitivity of the screening test and the carrier risk vary among different ethnic groups. The results often are reported with a table of the residual carrier risk for each ethnic group, and it is the physician's responsibility to interpret the results based on the patient's ethnicity. A negative carrier screening test result can reduce but not eliminate the risk of being a cystic fibrosis carrier.

Generally, it is more cost-effective and practical to perform initial carrier screening for the patient. If the patient is a cystic fibrosis carrier then her partner should be tested. Concurrent screening of the patient and her partner is preferred if there are time constraints for decisions regarding prenatal diagnostic testing or termination of the affected pregnancy. If a woman is a carrier of a cystic fibrosis mutation and her partner is unavailable for testing, genetic counseling to review the risk of having an affected child and prenatal testing options and limitations in this situation may be helpful.

Preconception carrier screening allows carrier couples to consider the fullest range of reproductive options. A significant proportion of obstetrician–gynecologists are not offering screening to their nonpregnant patients unless there is a family history or the patient specifically requests screening. Knowledge of the risk for having an affected child may influence a carrier couple's decision to conceive, to use donor gametes, and to consider preimplantation or prenatal genetic testing.

The initial guidelines recommended that laboratories screen a panel of 25 pan-ethnic mutations that were present in at least 0.1% of patients with cystic fibrosis. Based on a review of the first 2 years of laboratory data from screening the general population, the ACMG Cystic Fibrosis Carrier Screening Work Group recommended that two mutations (I148T and 1078delT) be removed from the panel because they do not cause classic cystic fibrosis or occur less frequently than 0.1%. The work group did not recommend additions to the panel at this time because they would not substantially increase the test sensitivity but acknowledged that some laboratories may choose to add mutations to the standard panel to increase the sensitivity of testing for specific ethnic groups.

Cystic fibrosis screening may identify a 5T/7T/9T variant, located in a noncoding region of the gene for cystic fibrosis, the cystic fibrosis transmembrane regulator (CFTR) gene. During the first 2 years of carrier testing, some laboratories reported this variant indiscriminately, resulting in some confusion in the interpretation of test results. Testing for the variant as a reflex test is appropriate only when the R117H mutation is detected. Classic cystic fibrosis occurs when 5T is on the same chromosome with R117H and there is a CFTR mutation of the other chromosome. Other combinations of the 5T variant with a CFTR mutation on the opposite chromosome are not known to have a clinical significance in females. Males with this genotype are at increased risk for congenital bilateral absence of the vas deferens and atypical cystic fibrosis. Couples with the R117H mutation will benefit from genetic counseling.

Complete analysis of the CFTR gene by DNA sequencing is not appropriate for routine carrier screening. This type of testing generally is reserved for patients with cystic fibrosis, a family history of

Table 1. Cystic Fibrosis Detection and Carrier Rates Before and After Testing

Racial or Ethnic Group	Detection Rate	Carrier Rate Before Testing	Carrier Risk After Negative Test Result
Ashkenazi Jewish	94%	1/24	Approximately 1/400
Non-Hispanic Caucasian	88%	1/25	Approximately 1/208
Hispanic American	72%	1/46	Approximately 1/164
African American	65%	1/65	Approximately 1/186
Asian American	49%	1/94	Approximately 1/184

cystic fibrosis, infertile males with congenital bilateral absence of the vas deferens, or a positive newborn screening test result when mutation testing using an expanded panel of mutations has a negative result.

The decision to have cystic fibrosis carrier screening should be by informed choice. Patients should receive information about cystic fibrosis and its inheritance pattern. Educational brochures are available from ACOG (sales.acog.org) and a brief description is included in this document. It is important for patients and their partners to recognize the sensitivity and limitations of testing as well as their reproductive options. Molecular testing does not identify all carriers. The ability to identify carriers differs based on ethnic origin, ranging from less than 50% in Asian Americans to up to 94% in the Ashkenazi Jewish population (Table 1). Therefore, a negative carrier screening test result will reduce but not eliminate the risk of being a cystic fibrosis carrier. When both parents are carriers of CFTR mutations that cause the disease, prenatal diagnosis by chorionic villus sampling or amniocentesis can be accomplished using DNA analysis.

Based on the preceding information, the Committee on Genetics provides the following recommendations:

1. Information about cystic fibrosis screening should be made available to all couples. It is reasonable to offer cystic fibrosis carrier screening to all couples regardless of race or ethnicity as an alternative to selective screening.

2. Cystic fibrosis carrier screening should be offered before conception or early in pregnancy when both partners are of Caucasian, European, or Ashkenazi Jewish ethnicity. Patients may elect to use either sequential or concurrent carrier screening; the latter option may be preferred if there are time constraints for decisions regarding prenatal diagnostic testing or termination of the affected pregnancy.

3. For individuals with a family history of cystic fibrosis, medical records indicating the CFTR mutation in the affected family member should be obtained whenever possible. If the mutation has not been identified, screening with an expanded panel of mutations or, in some cases, complete analysis of the CFTR gene by sequencing may be indicated. Genetic counseling in this situation usually is beneficial.

4. Individuals who have a reproductive partner with cystic fibrosis or congenital bilateral absence of the vas deferens may benefit from screening with an expanded panel of mutations or, in some cases, a complete analysis of the CFTR gene by sequencing.

5. When both partners are cystic fibrosis carriers, genetic counseling is recommended to review prenatal testing and reproductive options. Prenatal diagnosis by chorionic villus sampling or amniocentesis, using DNA-based testing of the fetal cells, should be offered. If the partner is unavailable for testing, genetic counseling may be helpful.

6. Cystic fibrosis carrier screening may identify individuals with two cystic fibrosis mutations who have not previously received a diagnosis of cystic fibrosis. These individuals may have a milder form of cystic fibrosis and should be referred to a specialist in cystic fibrosis for further evaluation. Genetic counseling also is beneficial.

Information on Cystic Fibrosis to Share With Your Patients

Cystic fibrosis is a progressive, multisystem disease that primarily affects the pulmonary, pancreatic, gastrointestinal, biliary, and reproductive systems. Individuals with cystic fibrosis typically present with cough, wheezing, failure to thrive, loose stools, abdominal pain, and, in males, infertility secondary to congenital bilateral absence of the vas deferens. Treatment involves pancreatic enzymes, proper nutrition, and respiratory therapy with aggressive treatment of infection. The current median survival is approximately 30 years, and the cause of death usually is respiratory failure. Approximately 15% of individuals with cystic fibrosis are pancreatic sufficient and have a milder disease course and a median survival of 56 years.

Cystic fibrosis is an autosomal recessive genetic condition. Therefore, when a patient and her partner are both carriers of a mutation in the cystic fibrosis gene, they have a one-in-four chance of having a child with cystic fibrosis. More than 1,300 mutations have been identified in the gene for cystic fibrosis, but screening for 23 common mutations is available and can reduce a couple's risk for having a child with cystic fibrosis. The risk of being a carrier depends on an individual's ethnicity and family history.

References

1. American College of Obstetricians and Gynecologists, American College of Medical Genetics. Preconception and prenatal carrier screening for cystic fibrosis: clinical and laboratory guidelines. Washington, DC: ACOG; Bethesda (MD): ACMG; 2001.
2. Morgan MA, Driscoll DA, Mennuti MT, Schulkin J. Practice patterns of obstetrician–gynecologists regarding preconception and prenatal screening for cystic fibrosis. Genet Med 2004;6:450–5.

Bibliography

Cystic fibrosis mutation database. Available at: http://www. genet. sickkids.on.ca/cftr/. Retrieved March 18, 2005.

Grosse SD, Boyle CA, Botkin JR, Comeau AM, Kharrazi M, Rosenfeld M, et al. Newborn screening for cystic fibrosis: evaluation of benefits and risks and recommendations for state newborn screening programs. MMWR Recomm Rep 2004; 53(RR-13):1–36.

Morgan MA, Driscoll DA, Zinberg S, Schulkin J, Mennuti MT. Impact of self-reported familiarity with guidelines for cystic fibrosis carrier screening. Obstet Gynecol 2005;105:1355–61.

Muller F, Simon-Bouy B, Girodon E, Monnier N, Malinge MC, Serre JL. Predicting the risk of cystic fibrosis with abnormal ultrasound signs of fetal bowel: results of a French molecular collaborative study based on 641 prospective cases. French Collaborative Group. Am J Med Genet 2002;110:109–15.

Watson MS, Cutting GR, Desnick RJ, Driscoll DA, Klinger K, Mennuti M, et al. Cystic fibrosis population carrier screening: 2004 revision of American College of Medical Genetics mutation panel [published errata appear in Genet Med 2004;6:548; Genet Med 2005;7:286]. Genet Med 2004;6:387–91.

ACOG
Committee on
Obstetric Practice

American Academy
of Pediatrics
Committee on
Fetus and Newborn

Committee Opinion

Number 174, July 1996   *(Replaces #49, November 1986)*

The American College of Obstetricians and Gynecologists
409 12th Street, SW
PO Box 96920
Washington, DC 20090-6920

12345/09876

Use and Abuse of the Apgar Score

The Apgar score, devised in 1952 by Dr. Virginia Apgar, is a quick method of assessing the clinical status of the newborn infant (1, 2). Ease of scoring has led to its use in many studies of outcome. However, its misuse has led to an erroneous definition of asphyxia. Intrapartum asphyxia implies fetal hypercarbia and hypoxemia, which if prolonged will result in eventual metabolic acidemia. Because the intrapartum disruption of uterine or fetal blood flow is rarely, if ever, absolute, *asphyxia* is an imprecise, general term. Terms such as *hypercarbia, hypoxia,* and *metabolic, respiratory,* or *lactic acidemia* are more precise, both for immediate assessment of the newborn and for retrospective assessment of intrapartum management. Although the Apgar score continues to provide a convenient "shorthand" for reporting the status of the newborn and the effectiveness of resuscitation, the purpose of this statement is to place the Apgar score in its proper perspective.

The Apgar score comprises five components: heart rate, respiratory effort, muscle tone, reflex irritability, and color, each of which is given a score of 0, 1, or 2 (Table 1). Reliable Apgar scores require assessment of individual components of the score by trained personnel.

Factors That May Affect the Apgar Score

Although rarely stated, it is important to recognize that elements of the Apgar score such as tone, color, and reflex irritability are partially dependent on the physiologic maturity of the infant. The healthy premature infant with no evidence of anoxic insult, acidemia, or cerebral depression may thus receive a low score only because of immaturity (3, 4).

A number of maternal medications and infant conditions may influence Apgar scores, including, but not limited to, neuromuscular or cerebral malformations that may decrease tone and respiratory effort. Cardiorespiratory conditions may also decrease the infant's heart rate, respiration, and tone. Infection may interfere with tone, color, and response to resuscitative efforts. Additional information is required to interpret Apgar scores properly in infants receiving resuscitation. Thus, to equate the presence of a low Apgar score solely with asphyxia or hypoxia represents a misuse of the score.

Table 1. Apgar Score: Five Components and Score Definitions

	Score		
Component	0	1	2
Heart rate	Absent	Slow (<100 beats/min)	>100 beats/min
Respirations	Absent	Weak cry, hypoventilation	Good, strong cry
Muscle tone	Limp	Some flexion	Active motion
Reflex irritability	No response	Grimace	Cry or active withdrawal
Color	Blue or pale	Body pink, extremities blue	Completely pink

Adapted from Apgar V, Holaday DA, James LS, Weisbrot IM, Berrien C. Evaluation of the newborn infant: second report. JAMA 1958;168:1985–1988

Apgar Score and Subsequent Disability

A low 1-minute Apgar score does not correlate with the infant's future outcome. The 5-minute Apgar score, and particularly the change in the score between 1 and 5 minutes, is a useful index of the effectiveness of resuscitation efforts. However, even a 5-minute score of 0–3, although possibly a result of hypoxia, is limited as an indicator of the severity of the problem and correlates poorly with future neurologic outcome (5, 6). An Apgar score of 0–3 at 5 minutes is associated with an increased risk of cerebral palsy in term infants, but this increase is only from 0.3% to 1% (5, 6). A 5-minute Apgar score of 7–10 is considered "normal." Scores of 4, 5, and 6 are intermediate and are not markers of high levels of risk of later neurologic dysfunction. As previously mentioned, such scores are affected by physiologic immaturity, medication, the presence of congenital malformations, and other factors.

Because Apgar scores at 1 and 5 minutes correlate poorly with either cause or outcome, the scores alone should not be considered evidence of or a consequence of substantial asphyxia. Therefore, a low 5-minute Apgar score alone does not demonstrate that later development of cerebral palsy was caused by perinatal asphyxia.

Correlation of the Apgar score with future neurologic outcome increases when the score remains 0–3 at 10, 15, and 20 minutes but still does not indicate the cause of future disability (5, 7). The term *asphyxia* in a clinical context should be reserved to describe a combination of damaging acidemia, hypoxia, and metabolic acidosis. A neonate who has had "asphyxia" proximate to delivery that is severe enough to result in acute neurologic injury should demonstrate all of the following:

- Profound metabolic or mixed acidemia (pH <7.00) on an umbilical cord arterial blood sample, if obtained
- An Apgar score of 0–3 for longer than 5 minutes
- Neonatal neurologic manifestations (eg, seizures, coma, or hypotonia)

- Multisystem organ dysfunction (eg, cardiovascular, gastrointestinal, hematologic, pulmonary, or renal system)

The Apgar score alone cannot establish hypoxia as the cause of cerebral palsy. A term infant with an Apgar score of 0–3 at 5 minutes whose 10-minute score improved to 4 or higher has a 99% chance of not having cerebral palsy at 7 years of age (5). Conversely, 75% of children with cerebral palsy had normal Apgar scores at birth (5).

Cerebral palsy is the only neurologic deficit clearly linked to perinatal asphyxia. Although mental retardation and epilepsy may accompany cerebral palsy, there is no evidence that they are caused by perinatal asphyxia unless cerebral palsy is also present, and even then a relationship is in doubt (8, 9).

Conclusion

Apgar scores are useful in assessing the condition of the infant at birth. Their use in other settings, such as collection of a child's Apgar score upon entry to school, is inappropriate. Low Apgar scores may be indicative of a number of maternal and infant factors. Apgar scores alone should not be used as evidence that neurologic damage was caused by hypoxia that results in neurologic damage or by inappropriate intrapartum management. In the infant who later is found to have cerebral palsy, low 1-minute or 5-minute Apgar scores are not sufficient evidence that the damage was due to hypoxia or inappropriate intrapartum management. Hypoxia as a cause of acute neurologic injury and adverse neurologic outcome occurs in infants who demonstrate the four perinatal findings listed in this Committee Opinion and in whom other possible causes of neurologic damage have been excluded. In the absence of such evidence, subsequent neurologic deficiencies cannot be ascribed to perinatal asphyxia or hypoxia (10, 11).

References

1. Apgar V. A proposal for a new method of evaluation of the newborn infant. Curr Res Anesth Analg 1953;32:260–267

2. Apgar V, Holaday DA, James LS, Weisbrot IM, Berrien C. Evaluation of the newborn infant: second report. JAMA 1958;168:1985–1988

3. Catlin EA, Carpenter MW, Brann BS IV, Mayfield SR, Shaul PW, Goldstein M, et al. The Apgar score revisited: influence of gestational age. J Pediatr 1986;109:865–868

4. Amon E, Sibai BM, Anderson GD, Mabie WC. Obstetric variables predicting survival of the immature newborn (less than or equal to 1000 gm): a five-year experience in a single perinatal center. Am J Obstet Gynecol 1987;156: 1380–1389

5. Nelson KB, Ellenberg JH. Apgar scores as predictors of chronic neurologic disability. Pediatrics 1981;68:36–44

6. Stanley FJ. Cerebral palsy trends: implications for perinatal care. Acta Obstet Gynecol Scand 1994;73:5–9

7. Freeman JM, Nelson KB. Intrapartum asphyxia and cerebral palsy. Pediatrics 1988;82:240–249

8. Levene MI, Sands C, Grindulis H, Moore JR. Comparison of two methods of predicting outcome in perinatal asphyxia. Lancet 1986;1:67–69

9. Paneth N. The causes of cerebral palsy: recent evidence. Clin Invest Med 1993;16:95–102

10. Brann AW Jr, Dykes FD. The effects of intrauterine asphyxia on the full-term neonate. Clin Perinatol 1977;4: 149–161

11. Nelson KB, Leviton A. How much of neonatal encephalopathy is due to birth asphyxia? Am J Dis Child 1991;145: 1325–1331

ACOG Committee Opinion

Committee on
Obstetric Practice

Number 291, November 2003

Use of Progesterone to Reduce Preterm Birth

ABSTRACT: Preterm birth affects 12% of all births in the United States. Recent studies support the hypothesis that progesterone supplementation reduces preterm birth in a select group of women (ie, those with a prior spontaneous birth at <37 weeks of gestation). Despite the apparent benefits of progesterone in this high-risk population, the ideal progesterone formulation is unknown. The American College of Obstetricians and Gynecologists Committee on Obstetric Practice believes that further studies are needed to evaluate the use of progesterone in patients with other high-risk obstetric factors, such as multiple gestations, short cervical length, or positive test results for cervicovaginal fetal fibronectin. When progesterone is used, it is important to restrict its use to only women with a documented history of a previous spontaneous birth at less than 37 weeks of gestation because unresolved issues remain, such as optimal route of drug delivery and long-term safety of the drug.

Preterm birth affects 12% of all births in the United States. This statistic has led multiple investigators to identify those women at greatest risk (eg, those with prior preterm delivery, maternal weight <50 kg, African-American race, bleeding, and concurrent sexually transmitted diseases). Despite identification of these risk factors, no interventions to date have been associated with a decrease in preterm delivery rates.

A recent large randomized placebo-controlled trial comparing 17α hydroxyprogesterone caproate "17P" therapy to prevent preterm birth in a select, high-risk group of women (documented history of a previous spontaneous preterm birth <37 weeks of gestation) was conducted for the National Institute of Child Health and Human Development (NICHD) Maternal-Fetal Medicine Units Network (1). A total of 459 women with a history of previous spontaneous births at less than 37 weeks of gestation were enrolled between 16 weeks and 20 weeks of gestation. Of note, the mean gestational age of their previous preterm deliveries was 30.7 weeks. They were randomly assigned to receive weekly intramuscular injections of 17P (n = 306) or placebo (n = 153). The study was stopped early when results showed a significant protection against recurrent preterm birth for all races of women who received 17P (Table 1).

A recent small randomized placebo-controlled trial of supplemental vaginal progesterone (100 mg daily) in 142 women at high risk for preterm birth

The American College of Obstetricians and Gynecologists
409 12th Street, SW
PO Box 96920
Washington, DC 20090-6920

12345/76543

Use of progesterone to reduce preterm birth. ACOG Committee Opinion No. 291. American College of Obstetricians and Gynecologists. Obstet Gynecol 2003;102:1115–6.

Table 1. Rates of Preterm Labor with Progesterone Therapy or Placebo

Gestation	Placebo Group (n = 153)	Progesterone Group (n = 306)	Relative Risk	Confidence Interval	P
<37 wk	54.9%	36.3%	0.66	0.54–0.81	.0001
<35 wk	30.7%	20.6%	0.67	0.48–0.93	.0165
<32 wk	19.6%	11.4%	0.58	0.37–0.91	.0180

Data from Meis PJ, Klebanoff M, Thom E, Dombrowski MP, Sibai B, Moawad AH, et al. Prevention of recurrent preterm delivery by 17 alpha-hydroxy-progesterone caproate. N Engl J Med 2003;348:2379–85.

(women with at least 1 previous spontaneous preterm birth, prophylactic cervical cerclage, and uterine malformation) revealed that for delivery at less than 34 weeks of gestation, the preterm birth rate was significantly lower among women receiving progesterone than among those receiving placebo (2.7% versus 18.6%) (2). The results of this study and the NICHD trial support the hypothesis that progesterone supplementation reduces preterm birth in a select very high-risk group of women.

Despite the apparent benefits of progesterone in a high-risk population, the ideal progesterone formulation is unknown. The 17P used in the NICHD trial was specially formulated for research and is not currently commercially available on a wide scale. Progesterone has been studied only as a prophylactic measure in asymptomatic women, not as a tocolytic agent. Whether vaginal progesterone is equally efficacious remains to be proved in a larger population. The American College of Obstetricians and Gynecologists Committee on Obstetric Practice believes that further studies are needed to evaluate the use of progesterone in patients with other high-risk obstetric factors, such as multiple gestations, short cervical length, or positive test results for cervicovaginal fetal fibronectin. When progesterone is used, it is important to restrict its use to only women with a documented history of a previous spontaneous birth at less than 37 weeks of gestation because unresolved issues remain, such as optimal route of drug delivery and long-term safety of the drug.

References

1. Meis PJ, Klebanoff M, Thom E, Dombrowski MP, Sibai B, Moawad AH, et al. Prevention of recurrent preterm delivery by 17 alpha-hydroxyprogesterone caproate. N Engl J Med 2003;348:2379–85.
2. da Fonseca EB, Bittar RE, Carvalho MH, Zugaib M. Prophylactic administration of progesterone by vaginal suppository to reduce the incidence of spontaneous preterm birth in women at increased risk: a randomized placebo-controlled double-blind study. Am J Obstet Gynecol 2003;188:419–24.

ACOG Committee Opinion

Committee on Gynecologic Practice

Number 293, February 2004

Uterine Artery Embolization

ABSTRACT: Uterine artery embolization for the treatment of symptomatic uterine leiomyomata has become increasingly popular. Based on current evidence, it appears that uterine artery embolization, when performed by experienced physicians, provides good short-term relief of bulk-related symptoms and a reduction in menstrual flow. Complication rates associated with the procedure are low, but in rare cases can include hysterectomy and death. There is insufficient evidence to ensure its safety in women desiring to retain their fertility, and pregnancy-related outcomes remain understudied. The American College of Obstetricians and Gynecologists' Committee on Gynecologic Practice considers the procedure investigational or relatively contraindicated in women wishing to retain fertility. The use of uterine artery embolization in postmenopausal women is rarely, if ever, indicated. The Committee strongly recommends that women who wish to undergo uterine artery embolization have a thorough evaluation with an obstetrician–gynecologist to help facilitate optimal collaboration with interventional radiologists and to ensure the appropriateness of this therapy, taking into account the reproductive wishes of the patient. It is also recommended that all patients considering uterine artery embolization be adequately informed about potential complications.

Uterine artery embolization for the treatment of symptomatic uterine leiomyomata has become increasingly popular. The concept of selective arterial embolization was originally used in obstetrics and gynecology in 1979 to treat postpartum hemorrhage (1). It subsequently was used as an alternative to surgical removal of uterine leiomyomata in 1995 (2). This procedure typically is performed by inserting a catheter into the common femoral artery to access the uterine arteries. The uterine arteries are then embolized using polyvinyl alcohol particles or tris-acryl gelatin microspheres. Supplemental metal coils also may be used to assist with vascular occlusion.

To date, most data regarding patient satisfaction, leiomyomata and uterine size reduction, fertility, and complications are derived from case reports and case series. In general, these reports have shown a short-term reduction in leiomyomata and uterine size, as well as a short-term clinical improvement in bulk-related symptoms and reduction in menstrual bleeding. Recently, a large multicenter series reporting on 538 women and a nonrandomized controlled study have been published, which confirm these short-term findings (3, 4). In the latter study, though limited in sample size (n=51), patient satis-

The American College of Obstetricians and Gynecologists

409 12th Street, SW
PO Box 96920
Washington, DC 20090-6920

12345/87654

Uterine artery embolization. ACOG Committee Opinion No. 293. American College of Obstetricians and Gynecologists. Obstet Gynecol 2004;103:403–4 faction was followed for up to 5 years and was found to be comparable to myomectomy.

Complications from uterine artery embolization have likewise become more apparent as case reports have been published and as results from larger case series have become available. Reported complications include infection, abscess, sepsis, hysterectomy, permanent amenorrhea, labial necrosis, focal bladder necrosis, vesicouterine fistula, uterine wall defects, groin hematoma, pulmonary emboli, and, rarely, death. In addition, embolization of an undiagnosed leiomyosarcoma has been reported. In a large series of 400 patients undergoing uterine artery embolization, the following complication rates were reported: febrile morbidity, 2%; hemorrhage, 0.75%; performance of unintended procedure, 2.5%; life-threatening events, 0.5%; and readmission within 14 days of procedure, 3.5%. Overall, the complication rate, using these clinical indicators for perioperative morbidity, was 5% (5). The loss of ovarian function has been reported to be as high as 14% with uterine artery embolization (6). Embolic microspheres have been documented histologically in the ovarian arterial vasculature in patients undergoing the procedure (7). Although transient postoperative pain occurs in most cases, persistent postoperative pain leads to hysterectomy in less than 1% of cases (8).

Approximately 50 cases of pregnancy have been reported in patients who have undergone elective uterine artery embolization. Of the resulting births, 58% were delivered by cesarean birth, 28% were preterm births, and 13% of patients experienced postpartum hemorrhage (9). Further data are needed to draw conclusions regarding the safety of uterine artery embolization in patients desiring to become pregnant.

Based on current evidence, it appears that uterine artery embolization, when performed by experienced physicians, provides good short-term relief of bulk-related symptoms as well as a reduction of menstrual flow. Complication rates associated with the procedure are low, but in rare cases can include hysterectomy and death. There is insufficient evidence in the current literature to ensure safety in women desiring to retain their fertility. Furthermore, pregnancy-related outcomes remain understudied. Therefore, the procedure should be considered investigational or relatively contraindicated in women wishing to retain fertility. The use of uterine artery embolization in postmenopausal women is rarely, if ever, indicated.

It is strongly recommended that women who wish to undergo uterine artery embolization have a thorough evaluation with an obstetrician–gynecologist to help facilitate optimal collaboration with interventional radiologists and to ensure the appropriateness of this therapy, taking into account the reproductive wishes of the patient. It also is recommended that all patients considering uterine artery embolization be adequately informed about potential complications.

References

1. Heaston DK, Mineau DE, Brown BJ, Miller FJ Jr. Transcatheter arterial embolization for control of persistent massive puerperal hemorrhage after bilateral surgical hypogastric artery ligation. AJR Am J Roentgenol 1979;133:152–4.
2. Ravina JH, Herbreteau D, Ciraru-Vigneron N, Bouret JM, Houdart E, Aymard A, et al. Arterial embolisation to treat uterine myomata. Lancet 1995;346:671–2.
3. Pron G, Bennett J, Common A, Wall J, Asch M, Sniderman K, et al. The Ontario Uterine Fibroid Embolization Trial. Part 2. Uterine fibroid reduction and symptom relief after uterine artery embolization for fibroids. Fertil Steril 2003;79:120–7.
4. Broder MS, Goodwin S, Chen G, Tang LJ, Costantino MM, Nguyen MH, et al. Comparison of long-term outcomes of myomectomy and uterine artery embolization. Obstet Gynecol 2002;100:864–8.
5. Spies JB, Spector A, Roth AR, Baker CM, Mauro L, Murphy-Skrynarz K. Complications after uterine artery embolization of leiomyomas. Obstet Gynecol 2002;100: 873–80.
6. Chrisman HB, Saker MB, Ryu RK, Nemcek AA Jr, Gerbie MV, Milad MP, et al. The impact of uterine fibroid embolization on resumption of menses and ovarian function. J Vasc Interv Radiol 2000;11:699–703.
7. Payne JF, Robboy SJ, Haney AF. Embolic microspheres within ovarian arterial vasculature after uterine artery embolization. Obstet Gynecol 2002;100:883–6.
8. Pron G, Mocarski E, Cohen M, Colgan T, Bennett J, Common A, et al. Hysterectomy for complications after uterine artery embolization for leiomyoma: results from a Canadian multicenter clinical trial. J Am Assoc Gynecol Laparosc 2003;10:99–106.
9. Goldberg J, Pereira L, Berghella V. Pregnancy after uterine artery embolization. Obstet Gynecol 2002;100: 869–72.

Educational Bulletins

Assessment of Fetal Lung Maturity (No. 230)   267

Breastfeeding: Maternal and Infant Aspects (No. 258)   274

Management of Isoimmunization in Pregnancy (No. 227)   290

Obstetric Aspects of Trauma Management (No. 251)   297

Psychosocial Risk Factors: Perinatal Screening and Intervention (No. 255)   304

Teratology (No. 236)   311

Viral Hepatitis in Pregnancy (No. 248)   318

Educational Bulletins

ACOG EDUCATIONAL BULLETIN

Number 230, November 1996

Assessment of Fetal Lung Maturity

Approximately 300,000–500,000 of the deliveries in the United States each year are preterm. Preterm birth causes significant neonatal morbidity and mortality, which are often due to difficulty in providing oxygen transfer to an immature neonatal pulmonary system (1).

The pulmonary system is among the last of the fetal organ systems to become functionally mature. Thus, pulmonary maturity has been assumed to connote adequate maturation in other fetal systems. This assumption may not be true in fetuses relatively remote from term (2). Documentation of fetal pulmonary maturity should not be used as the sole indication for delivery of a preterm infant. Although preterm delivery may be indicated in many situations, delivery of fetuses with immature pulmonary systems should be avoided when possible.

Direct methods of assessing fetal pulmonary maturity have been available for more than 20 years, and a number of new tests have been introduced (3, 4). Proper use of these tests can aid the clinician in determining the optimal time for delivery.

Indications for Assessing Maturity

Fetal pulmonary maturity should be confirmed before elective delivery at less than 39 weeks of gestation unless fetal maturity can be inferred from any of the following criteria:

- Fetal heart tones have been documented for 20 weeks by nonelectronic fetoscope or for 30 weeks by Doppler.
- It has been 36 weeks since a serum or urine human chorionic gonadotropin pregnancy test was found to be positive by a reliable laboratory.
- Ultrasound measurement of the crown–rump length at 6–11 weeks of gestation supports a gestational age equal to or greater than 39 weeks.
- Ultrasound measurement at 12–20 weeks of gestation supports a clinically determined gestational age of 39 weeks or greater.

If any of the aforementioned criteria confirms a gestational age of 39 weeks or more in a patient with normal menstrual cycles (no oral contraceptive use immediately prior to conception), it is appropriate to schedule delivery at 39 weeks

This Educational Bulletin was developed under the direction of the Committee on Educational Bulletins of the American College of Obstetricians and Gynecologists as an aid to obstetricians and gynecologists. The College wishes to thank William N. P. Herbert, MD, for his assistance in the development of this bulletin. This document is not to be construed as establishing a standard of practice or dictating an exclusive course of treatment. Rather, it is intended as an educational tool that presents current information on obstetric–gynecologic issues.

of gestation or beyond in accordance with menstrual dates. Ultrasonography may be considered confirmatory of menstrual dates if there is a gestational age agreement within 1 week by crown–rump measurements obtained at 6–11 weeks of gestation or within 10 days by an average of multiple measurements obtained between 12–20 weeks of gestation. Unless circumstances preclude continued expectant management, awaiting the onset of spontaneous labor is another option for some patients (5).

Amniocentesis for fetal pulmonary assessment is rarely warranted before 33 weeks of gestation because test results confirming lung maturity are unlikely. Confirmation of a mature fetal pulmonary system does not preclude consideration of the fetal risk of intraventricular hemorrhage and necrotizing enterocolitis.

Physiology and Pathophysiology

Fetal Lung Development

Knowledge of the development of the fetal pulmonary system and the evolution of surfactant production is helpful in understanding the tests performed for fetal lung maturity. The development of the fetal pulmonary system begins about 3 weeks after conception and continues for about 8 years after birth. The pulmonary tree development begins in the glandular period, which ends at about 16 weeks of gestation. During the canalicular period (16–24 weeks of gestation), early bronchioles develop and the epithelium vascularizes and differentiates. The alveolar (or terminal sac) period is the last stage of pulmonary development, which extends from about 24 weeks of gestation well into childhood. Bronchiolar division during this period leads to the development of thin spherical saccules, known as alveoli, that are lined by type II pneumocytes. The concomitant proliferation of capillaries around these alveoli makes effective gas exchange possible after delivery.

The type II pneumocytes produce intracellular stores, or "packages," of phospholipids called lamellar bodies, which can be released into the alveolar spaces. Surfactant is the name given to this group of "surface-active" phospholipid compounds that can reduce the surface tension within the alveolar spaces following delivery. Low surface tension within the alveoli allows these sacs to remain expanded during respiratory activity permitting continuous and maximally effective gas exchange. As a result of in utero "respiratory" activity, these substances enter the amniotic fluid cavity, where they can be measured.

The most prominent of these surfactant compounds is lecithin (phosphotidylcholine). The phospholipid compound phosphatidylglycerol (PG) appears later, and documentation of its presence is the basis of several of the commonly used tests for fetal lung maturity. Other phospholipids (phosphatidylinositol, phosphatidylethanola-

mine), a variety of proteins, and cholesterol contribute to this group of surface-active substances within the lung as well.

Respiratory Distress Syndrome

A deficiency in the quantity of surfactant in premature infants leads to higher surface tension within the alveoli, which can cause alveolar collapse and make gas exchange more difficult. Impaired gas exchange can result in neonatal hypoxia, with further worsening of pulmonary status manifested by acidosis and increased shunting within the lungs. Signs of respiratory distress syndrome (RDS) include neonatal tachypnea, grunting, retractions, and cyanosis, often occuring within several hours of birth. Radiography of the infant's chest revealing atelectasis, air bronchograms, and a diffuse reticulogranular infiltrate is suggestive of RDS.

Other complications associated with RDS include necrotizing enterocolitis, patent ductus arteriosus, intraventricular hemorrhage, and infection, which can result in long-term disability or death. Some survivors of RDS will suffer long-term pulmonary sequelae in the form of bronchopulmonary dysplasia (6). The Centers for Disease Control and Prevention reports that 2,000 of the 20,000–30,000 infants who develop RDS each year will die (7). Despite the positive impact of antepartum corticosteroid therapy and neonatal administration of surfactant compounds, RDS continues to be a significant cause of neonatal morbidity and mortality.

Classification of Fetal Maturity Tests

Fetal pulmonary testing can be categorized as either indirect or direct measures of fetal lung maturation. Indirect tests do not measure pulmonary function per se but rather evaluate the age or size of the fetus. From these parameters, maturity can be inferred and neonatal respiratory function predicted. Such methods include obstetric estimation of gestational age (menstrual history, first appearance of fetal heart tones, and physical examination), ultrasound examination (identification or evaluation of gestational sac, crown–rump length, biparietal diameter, etc), and the rarely used amniotic fluid analysis for fetal fat cells or creatinine.

Direct tests of fetal maturity measure either the concentration of particular components of pulmonary surfactant (biochemical tests) or the surface-active effects of these phospholipids (biophysical tests). Biochemical tests include determining the lecithin–sphingomyelin ratio (L/S) and identifying PG. Biophysical tests include the foam stability index (FSI) and fluorescence polarization. Although these tests differ in their techniques, all predict pulmonary maturity (the absence of RDS) with much greater certainty than they predict pulmonary immaturity (the presence of RDS) (3) (Table 1).

Tests of Fetal Maturity

Lecithin–Sphingomyelin Ratio

The first widely accepted direct test for assessment of fetal pulmonary status was the L/S ratio (8). This test evaluates a change in the relative amounts of lecithin (phosphatidylcholine) and sphingomyelin (a sphingolipid of unknown origin) in amniotic fluid samples as gestational age increases. Until about 32–33 weeks of gestation, the concentrations of these two substances are quite similar; thereafter, the concentration of lecithin increases significantly compared with the relatively constant concentration of sphingomyelin. In the absence of complications, the densitometric ratio of these two components reaches 2.0 at about 35 weeks of gestation. Infants delivered after attaining an L/S ratio of 2.0 or higher rarely develop RDS. This value of 2.0 has become the commonly accepted standard value indicating maturity in the fetus of a nondiabetic woman. However, correlation with clinical outcome in individual centers should precede acceptance of this threshold for pulmonary maturity, as variations within and between laboratories can be considerable. The predictive value of a negative result (value less than 2.0) is quite low.

Determination of the L/S ratio involves thin-layer chromatography after organic solvent extraction. Commercial versions of this test are available. Identification of lecithin and sphingomyelin is accomplished by using any one of a number of different staining procedures, with planimetry or densitometry used to compare the relative amounts of lecithin and sphingomyelin. This methodology is quite cumbersome and labor intensive despite numerous modifications to the original technique.

As with many tests of fetal maturity, blood and meconium can interfere with test interpretation (4). Plasma is rich in lipids that can be difficult to distinguish from phospholipids in surfactant. A bloody amniotic fluid sample may be difficult to interpret. The L/S ratio in plasma is similar to the maturity threshold (2.0) found in amniotic fluid. Theoretically, L/S values significantly lower or higher than 2.0 should be reliable, but caution is advised in relying on results from bloody amniotic fluid samples. Likewise, the mucoid nature of meconium may obscure the thin-layer chromatography pattern and interfere with the accuracy of the L/S values. Moreover, with some L/S procedures, a heme derivative in meconium may resemble PG on the thin-layer chromatography plate.

Since amniotic fluid contains enzymes, improper storage conditions can affect the L/S ratio (9). An amniotic fluid sample should be centrifuged shortly after it is obtained. If the determination is not performed immediately or if the sample is transported to an outside laboratory, the specimen should be frozen, preferably at –20°C (9). The L/S ratio decreases if an uncentrifuged sample either remains at room temperature for at least 1 hour or is cooled but not frozen for more than 12 hours. Failure to properly handle the amniotic fluid specimen can result in invalid conclusions and difficulty in interpretation of the results.

Phosphatidylglycerol

Phosphatidylglycerol is a minor constituent of surfactant that generally appears in sufficient quantity to be measured several weeks after the increase in lecithin concentration (10). Because PG enhances the spread of phospholipids on the alveolar surface, its presence indicates a more advanced state of fetal pulmonary maturity.

Phosphatidylglycerol determination can be accomplished by thin-layer chromatography, either alone or as an extension of L/S ratio testing. In addition, a slide-agglutination test has been developed using antisera specific for PG.

An advantage of PG determination in assessing fetal maturity is the fact that it is not generally affected by blood, meconium, or other contaminants. This characteristic allows PG determination by using vaginal pool samples from patients who have experienced spontaneous rupture of membranes. A disadvantage of using PG for assessing fetal maturity is its relatively late appearance in pregnancy. Compared with results of other tests, an "immature" result (negative PG) is associated with a greater proportion of patients who will deliver infants who do not develop RDS (11).

"Shake" Test and Foam Stability Index

Prediction of pulmonary maturity based on the ability of pulmonary surfactant to generate and maintain a stable foam in the presence of ethanol was first reported in 1972 (12). In this biophysical test, the addition of ethanol to amniotic fluid eliminates foam formation caused by "nonsurfactant" substances in the amniotic fluid. The generation of a stable ring of foam by shaking amniotic fluid and ethanol in a test tube demonstrates the presence of surface-active material in the amniotic fluid. Serial dilutions with ethanol allow determination of the concentration of surfactant.

This procedure has been modified and named the FSI, which uses a series of test tubes containing successively greater amounts of 95% ethanol in an attempt to quantitate surface-active properties over a wider range of concentrations (13). In effect, a single cut-off point of 47 or 48 or greater is used to indicate fetal maturity. A commercial version of this test is available. Amniotic fluid should not be placed in a siliconized collection tube if the "shake" test or FSI is used, as stable foam will result from this contamination. The presence of blood or meconium in samples interferes with the results of these tests as well.

Table 1. Commonly Used Direct Tests of Fetal Maturity

Test*	Technique	Time/Ease of Testing†	Threshold	Typical Predictive Value (%)		Relative Cost	Notes
				Mature	Immature		
Lecithin/sphingomyelin ratio	Thin-layer chromatography	4+	2.0–3.5	95–100	33–50	High	Many variations in technique; laboratory variation significant
Phosphatidylglycerol	Thin-layer chromatography	4+	"Present" (usually means >3% of total phospholipid)	95–100	23–53	High	Not affected by blood, meconium; vaginal pool samples satisfactory
	Antisera	1+	0.5 = low positive 2.0 = high positive	95–100	23–53	Commercial version—moderate	Not affected by blood, meconium; vaginal pool samples satisfactory
Foam stability index	Ethanol added to amniotic fluid, solution shaken, presence of stable bubbles at meniscus noted	2+	≥47 or 48	95	51	Laboratory—low Commercial version—moderate	Affected by blood, meconium, vaginal pool debris, silicone-coated test tubes
Fluorescence polarization	Fluorescence polarization	1+	≥55 mg/g of albumin‡	96–100	47–61	Moderate	Minimal intraassay and interassay variability; simple testing procedure
Optical density (OD) at 650 nm	Spectrophotometric reading	1+	OD ≥0.15	98	13	Low	Simple technique
Lamellar body counts	Counts using commercial hematology counter	2+	30,000–40,000 (still investigational)	97–98	29–35	Low	Promising technique

*Commercial versions are available for all tests except optical density and lamellar body counts.

†Range in complexity: 1+ indicates procedure is simple, is available all the time, requires only short procedure time, and personnel effort is not intensive; 4+ indicates procedure is complex or difficult, time consuming, and therefore, frequently not available at all times.

‡The manufacturer has reformulated the product and revised the testing procedure. Currently, the threshold for maturity is 55; with the original assay it was 70.

Fluorescence Polarization

Fetal maturity testing using fluorescence polarization is based on competitive binding of a fluorescent probe to albumin and surfactant. When the probe is bound to albumin, net polarization values are high; when bound to surfactant, polarization values are low. In amniotic fluid samples, the fluorescence polarization measured by an automated analyzer reflects the ratio of surfactant to albumin, a value that correlates with lung maturity. Recent modifications of this concept provide a simple, automated, rapid test that is widely available and varies minimally between laboratories. In the recently modified commercial version of this assay, the ratio indicating maturity is at or above 55 mg of surfactant per gram of albumin in the nondiabetic patient. Preliminary use of this test in patients with diabetes is promising (14).

This assay compares favorably with other direct tests (15, 16), but blood and meconium contamination interfere with its interpretation. Sufficient testing on amniotic fluid samples obtained vaginally has not been done.

Optical Density at 650 nm

Measuring optical absorbance of amniotic fluid at a wavelength of 650 nm is a rapid indirect biophysical test for fetal maturity. It is based on the concept that the opalescence of mature amniotic fluid is due to an increasing number of lamellar bodies, which scatter light. After centrifugation, amniotic fluid samples are analyzed on a spectrophotometer, an instrument commonly available in hospital laboratories. An optical density reading of absorbancy of 0.15 or greater is used as the indicator of pulmonary maturity. It is a simple procedure that compares favorably with other methods of fetal maturity assessment (3, 17). The degree of centrifugation and presence of blood and meconium can alter the validity of this method.

Lamellar Body Counts

Lamellar bodies represent packages of surfactant that are extruded into the alveoli from within type II pneumocytes. The similarity of lamellar body size to platelet size permits the use of a standard hematologic counter to determine lamellar body concentrations. Values of approximately 30,000–50,000/μL appear to indicate pulmonary maturity; however, alterations in technique and determinations on different commercial hematology counters yield varying results for maturity assessment (3, 17, 18). Neither bilirubin nor meconium interferes with this test, but erythrocytes lower the lamellar body number density.

Other Amniotic Fluid Tests of Maturity

Other direct and indirect tests of fetal pulmonary status have been introduced. Direct enzymatic assays have been developed for lecithin, sphingomyelin, and PG, but their use in predicting respiratory outcome has not been evaluated adequately. The lack of commercial kits and preparation costs limit use of these assays. Surfactant proteins (apoproteins) are nonphospholipid markers of fetal maturity that have been investigated for use in maturity assessment. Immunoassay for the presence of the surfactant apoproteins SP-A and SP-B in amniotic fluid has permitted such evaluation, but further investigations are necessary to clarify the usefulness of this approach.

Imaging

Ultrasonography has replaced radiographic techniques for assessing fetal age. A biparietal diameter of 9.2 cm or more, a femur length of 7.3 cm or more, the presence and size of epiphyseal ossification centers, placental grading (classification based on chorionic convolutions and calcifications), and other imaging determinations have been evaluated as means to assess maturity (19–21). Some fetuses at term, however mature, may lack these findings, and some fetuses with these characteristics may be immature (eg, maternal diabetes complicated by macrosomia). In general, ultrasound assessment of gestational age (indirectly evaluating for maturity) in the third trimester is inferior to the other methods available.

Effect of Associated Conditions on Fetal Lung Maturity

Accelerated fetal lung maturity has been reported to occur with a number of obstetric conditions, including hypertensive disorders, hemoglobinopathies, narcotics addiction, intrauterine growth restriction, classes of diabetes that are long-standing or associated with complications, premature rupture of membranes, multiple gestation, and smoking. Conversely, a delay in fetal lung maturation has been reported in patients with certain other classes of diabetes, nonhypertensive renal disease, and isoimmunization. For virtually all of these conditions, however, conflicting results concerning their effect on pulmonary maturation and testing have been reported.

Fetal lung maturity in patients with diabetes is the condition that has been studied most extensively, yet consensus is still lacking. While some have reported altered maturity test results and an increased rate of RDS in newborns of diabetic patients, others have reported no difference in either test results or clinical outcome. Causes other than deficient surfactant may be responsible for some cases of respiratory distress (22).

Other Considerations

Administration of corticosteroids to pregnant women at risk for preterm delivery has been shown to be effective in decreasing the prevalence, severity, and complications of RDS (23). Corticosteroids accelerate pulmonary maturity by stimulation of both the synthesis and release of surfactant from the type II pneumocytes into the alveolar spaces. In general, fetal maturity test results measured soon after steroid administration are affected minimally. This is probably due in part to the time interval required between steroid administration and the synthesis and release of the surface-active materials into the alveolar spaces and subsequently into the amniotic fluid.

Amniotic fluid present in the vagina following spontaneous rupture of membranes can be used for fetal maturity assessment. As noted, PG is not present in other tissue fluids and, for this reason, has particular importance in assessing maturity in patients from whom vaginal pool specimens can be obtained. Unfortunately, PG is often absent in preterm patients with fetal pulmonary maturity and may be present in others who are not mature because of bacterial contamination. There is no consensus on the utility of other tests using vaginal samples.

Comparison Among Tests

Various characteristics of commonly used tests to assess fetal maturity are compared in Table 1. Although the L/S ratio was the first direct test used to assess fetal maturity, other tests perform equally well and, because of technical aspects of the testing procedure for L/S ratio determination, have become more widely used. Regardless of the test used, the predictive value of all mature results is over 95%. That is, if the result of any test indicates maturity, the likelihood that RDS will be diagnosed in a delivered infant is less than 5%. Conversely, all available tests share a relatively poor predictive value in assessing the likelihood of the presence of RDS. The predictive values for RDS of immature test results range from approximately 30% to 60%. Other test characteristics, including cost, ease of test performance, availability, and reproducibility, are important factors in selecting maturity tests.

Testing Strategies

With the introduction of newer tests for fetal maturity assessment, it has become a common practice to order multiple tests routinely for the assessment of fetal maturity. Results are often reported as a "lung profile" or "pulmonary profile." Since a mature result on any one of the commonly used tests of fetal lung maturity is strongly predictive of the absence of RDS, the practice of multiple testing on a routine basis should be questioned. Little additional information will be gained by the performance of multiple assays. When multiple tests are performed, discordant results are sometimes found, which is not surprising because these tests measure various components or

aspects of maturity by different means. Obviously, costs are increased when multiple tests are obtained.

Because of the strong predictive value of a single mature result, the strategy of ordering tests individually, but within a defined protocol, is logical. This so-called "cascade" (24) or "sequential" (25) testing involves the performance of a rapid, inexpensive test initially, with a subsequent test ordered only if the result of the initial test is immature. Such a practice can provide clinicians with around-the-clock availability of a test for fetal maturity and yet maximizes laboratory efficiency by decreasing the overall number of tests performed. The testing sequence should be determined jointly between clinicians and laboratory personnel.

Women with diabetes are thought by some to have altered fetal lung maturation or fetal maturity test results or both; thus, some practitioners approach the assessment of these women differently from that of women who do not have diabetes. In the woman whose diabetes is well controlled, awaiting the appearance of PG may be justified, as its presence seems to provide the strongest evidence of pulmonary maturity. However, it must be remembered that PG may be absent in approximately 20% of women with gestational or overt diabetes at a gestational age as late as 38–39 weeks (26). In a recent multicenter study, only 2 of 13 patients with a mature fluorescence polarization test and absent PG delivered infants who developed RDS. Neither required intubation or prolonged oxygen therapy (14). Other strategies for managing patients with diabetes include delaying delivery until two separate tests (eg, FSI, L/S) indicate fetal lung maturity or using a higher threshold for maturity on which to proceed with delivery.

Regardless of which method of fetal lung maturity assessment is chosen, it should be emphasized that no mature result from one test or a group of tests can completely eliminate the risk of RDS or other neonatal complications (2). The risk of adverse outcome with delivery on the basis of lung maturity assessment must be weighed against the potential risk of untoward outcome by permitting the pregnancy to continue in utero.

References

1. Parilla BV, Dooley SL, Jansen RD, Socol ML. Iatrogenic respiratory distress syndrome following elective repeat cesarean delivery. Obstet Gynecol 1993;81:392–395 (Level III)

2. Wigton TR, Tamura RK, Wickstrom E, Atkins V, Deddish R, Socol ML. Neonatal morbidity after preterm delivery in the presence of documented lung maturity. Am J Obstet Gynecol 1993;169:951–955 (Level II-3)

3. Dubin SB. The laboratory assessment of fetal lung maturity. Am J Clin Pathol 1992;97:836–849 (Level III)

4. Spillman T, Cotton DB. Current perspectives in assessment of fetal pulmonary surfactant status with amniotic fluid. Crit Rev Clin Lab Sci 1989;27:341–389 (Level III)

5. American College of Obstetricians and Gynecologists. Fetal maturity assessment prior to elective repeat cesarean delivery. ACOG Committee Opinion 98. Washington, DC: ACOG, 1991 (Level III)

6. Whitsett JA, Pryhuber GS, Rice WR, Warner BB, Wert SE. Acute respiratory disorders. In: Avery GB, Fletcher MA, MacDonald MG, eds. Neonatology pathophysiology and management of the newborn. Philadelphia: JB Lippincott Company 1994;429–452 (Level III)

7. National Center for Health Statistics. Births, marriages, divorces, and deaths for 1993. Monthly vital statistics report; vol 42, no. 12. Hyattsville, Maryland: Public Health Service, 1994 (Level III)

8. Gluck L, Kulovich MV, Borer RC Jr, Brenner PH, Anderson GG, Spellacy WN. Diagnosis of respiratory distress by amniocentesis. Am J Obstet Gynecol 1971;109: 440–445 (Level II-3)

9. Blumenfeld TA. Clinical laboratory tests for fetal lung maturity. Pathol Annu 1975;10:21–36 (Level III)

10. Hallman M, Kulovich M, Kirkpatrick E, Sugarman RG, Gluck L. Phosphatidylinositol and phosphatidylglycerol in amniotic fluid: indices of lung maturity. Am J Obstet Gynecol 1976;125:613–617 (Level II-3)

11. Lewis DF, Towers CV, Major CA, Asrat T, Nageotte MP, Freeman RK, et al. Use of amniostat-FLM in detecting the presence of phosphatidylglycerol in vaginal pool samples in preterm premature rupture of membranes. Am J Obstet Gynecol 1993;169:573–576 (Level II-3)

12. Clements JA, Platzker ACG, Tierney DF, Hobel CJ, Creasy RK, Margolis AJ, et al. Assessment of the risk of the respiratory-distress syndrome by a rapid test for surfactant in amniotic fluid. N Engl J Med 1972;286:1077–1081 (Level II-3)

13. Sher G, Statland BE, Freer DE, Kraybill EN. Assessing fetal lung maturation by the foam stability index test. Obstet Gynecol 1978;52:673–677 (Level II-3)

14. Livingston EG, Herbert WNP, Hage ML, Chapman JF, Stubbs TM. Use of the TDx-FLM assay in evaluating fetal lung maturity in an insulin-dependent diabetic population. Obstet Gynecol 1995;86:826–829 (Level III)

15. Herbert WNP, Chapman JF, Schnoor MM. Role of the TDx FLM assay in fetal lung maturity. Am J Obstet Gynecol 1993;168:808–812 (Level II-3)

16. Hagen E, Link JC, Arias F. A comparison of the accuracy of the TDx-FLM assay, lecithin–sphingomyelin ratio, and phosphatidylglycerol in the prediction of neonatal respiratory distress syndrome. Obstet Gynecol 1993;82:1004–1008 (Level II-3)

17. Ashwood ER, Palmer SE, Taylor JS, Pingree SS. Lamellar body counts for rapid fetal lung maturity testing. Obstet Gynecol 1993;81:619–624 (Level II-3)

18. Delance CR, Bowie LJ, Dohnal JC, Farrell EE, Neerhof MG. Amniotic fluid lamellar body count: a rapid and reliable fetal lung maturity test. Obstet Gynecol 1995;86:235–239 (Level II-2)

19. Mahony BS, Bowie JD, Killam AP, Kay HH, Cooper C. Epiphyseal ossification centers in the assessment of fetal maturity: sonographic correlation with the amniocentesis lung profile. Radiology 1986;159:521–524 (Level II-3)

20. Goldstein I, Lockwood C, Belanger K, Hobbins J. Ultrasonographic assessment of gestational age with the distal, femoral and proximal tibial ossification centers in the third

trimester. Am J Obstet Gynecol 1988;158:127–130 (Level II-3)

21. Tahilramaney MP, Platt LD, Golde SH. Use of femur length measured by ultrasonography to predict fetal maturity. J Perinatol 1991;11:157–160 (Level II-3)

22. Kjos SL, Walther FJ, Montoro M, Paul RH, Diaz F, Stabler M. Prevalence and etiology of respiratory distress in infants of diabetic mothers: predictive value of fetal lung maturation tests. Am J Obstet Gynecol 1990;163:898–903 (Level II-3)

23. Effect of corticosteroids for fetal maturation on perinatal outcomes. NIH Consens Statement 1994 Feb 28–Mar 2; 12(2):1–24 (Level III)

24. Garite TJ, Freeman RK, Nageotte MP. Fetal maturity cascade: a rapid and cost-effective method for fetal lung maturity testing. Obstet Gynecol 1986;67:619–622 (Level II-3)

25. Herbert WNP, Chapman JF. Clinical and economic considerations associated with testing for fetal lung maturity. Am J Obstet Gynecol 1986;155:820–823 (Level II-3)

26. Ojomo EO, Coustan DR. Absence of evidence of pulmonary maturity at amniocentesis in term infants of diabetic mothers. Am J Obstet Gynecol 1990;163:954–957 (Level II-3)

The references in this bulletin are graded according to the method outlined by the U.S. Preventive Services Task Force:

I   Evidence obtained from at least one properly designed randomized controlled trial

II-1   Evidence obtained from well-designed controlled trials without randomization

II-2   Evidence obtained from well-designed cohort or case–control analytic studies, preferably from more than one center or research group

II-3   Evidence obtained from multiple time series, with or without intervention, or dramatic results in uncontrolled experiments

III   Opinions of respected authorities, based on clinical experience, descriptive studies, or reports of expert committees

Other publications from ACOG:

- **Committee Opinions**, focused updates on emerging areas
- **Practice Patterns**, evidence-based guidelines
- **Criteria Sets**, baseline guidelines for review of diagnostic and management procedures

**The American College of Obstetricians and Gynecologists
409 12th Street, SW
PO Box 96920
Washington, DC 20090-6920**

12345/09876

ACOG EDUCATIONAL BULLETIN

Number 258, July 2000

Breastfeeding: Maternal and Infant Aspects

Breastfeeding rates decreased significantly in the past half century as formula feeding gained popularity. In 1971, only 24.7% of mothers left the hospital breastfeeding. Recently, breastfeeding initiation rates have been increasing, reaching 64.3% in 1998, according to the Mothers' Survey (Ross Products Division, Abbott Laboratories, Inc., Columbus, Ohio). These increases reflect a growing awareness of the advantages of breast milk over formula. Improvement in breastfeeding initiation rates, however, has been uneven, as women attempt to overcome practical obstacles.

Evidence continues to mount regarding the value of breastfeeding for both women and their infants. Human milk provides developmental, nutritional, and immunologic benefits to the infant that cannot be duplicated by formula feeding. Breastfeeding also provides significant benefits to women. It is critical that women be prepared to make an informed choice in deciding what is best for them, their families, and their babies. Obstetrician–gynecologists and other health professionals caring for pregnant women should regularly impart accurate information about breastfeeding to expectant mothers and be prepared to support them should any problems arise while breastfeeding.

This document will focus primarily on breastfeeding by healthy mothers with healthy infants born at term. Human milk and breastfeeding are recommended for premature newborns and mother–infant pairs with other special needs; however, specific information in this regard is beyond the scope of this document.

This Educational Bulletin was developed under the direction of the Committees on Health Care for Underserved Women and Obstetric Practice of the American College of Obstetricians and Gynecologists. The college wishes to thank John T. Queenan, MD, for his assistance in the development of this bulletin. This document is not to be construed as establishing a standard of practice or dictating an exclusive course of treatment. Rather, it is intended as an educational tool that presents current information on obstetric–gynecologic issues.

Benefits of Breastfeeding

Research in the United States and throughout the world indicates that breastfeeding and human milk provide benefits to infants, women, families, and society. These studies have been done in a variety of settings, resulting in information derived from culturally and economically diverse populations.

Infants

The benefits of breastfeeding for the infant have been established in the following areas. Human milk provides species-specific and age-specific nutrients for the infant (1). Colostrum, the fluid secreted immediately following the infant's birth, conveys a high level of immune protection, particularly secretory immunoglobulin A (IgA). During the first 4–7 days following delivery, protein and mineral concentrations decrease and water, fat, and lactose increase. Milk composition continues to change to match infant nutritional needs. In addition to the right balance of nutrients and immunologic factors, human milk contains factors that act as biologic signals for promoting cellular growth and differentiation. It also contains multiple substances with antimicrobial properties, which protect against infection (1, 2). Human milk alone, however, may not provide adequate iron for premature newborns, infants whose mothers have low iron stores, and infants older than 6 months.

In 1997, the American Academy of Pediatrics (AAP) published a policy statement, "Breastfeeeding and the Use of Human Milk" (3). The statement was developed by the AAP Work Group on Breastfeeding, which evaluated the research literature on relationships between breastfeeding and infant health and development. The statement's summary paragraph (see the box below) on established infant protective effects, as well as positive associations (which require further study), is well referenced. Obstetrician–gynecologists who review these sources of evidence for infant benefit will be better prepared to care for the women in their practices.

Women

The benefits of breastfeeding for women are well documented. During the immediate postpartum period, the oxytocin released during milk let-down causes increased uterine contractions and lessens maternal blood loss (4). Evidence exists that the hormones of lactation (oxytocin and prolactin) contribute to feelings of relaxation and attachment (5). Breastfeeding is associated with a decreased risk of developing ovarian and premenopausal breast cancer (6, 7). Breastfeeding also delays postpartum ovulation, supporting birth spacing (8–10). Although breastfeeding causes some bone demineralization, studies indicate that "catch-up" remineralization occurs following weaning; some studies also show a lower incidence of osteoporosis and hip fracture after menopause (11, 12). The incidence of pregnancy-induced long-term obesity also is reduced (13).

There are psychologic benefits as well. A woman who breastfeeds her baby is able to take advantage of the natural dynamics of nurturing and bonding.

Families and Society

Studies indicate that the breastfed child has fewer illnesses and, therefore, fewer visits to the doctor and hospital (14). This translates into less absenteeism from work for the mother and lower medical expenses. The improvement in work productivity may be significant for society as well, because women now constitute a large portion of the workforce. More than 60% of all women return to outside employment during the first year following birth of a child.

Breastfeeding, while demanding maternal time and attention, can save individual families and society considerable money compared with formula feeding (15). On a national scale, disposal of formula cans, bottles, and bottle liners may be an ecologic consideration.

Obstacles to Breastfeeding

Women need to know that breastfeeding, like other aspects of having a new baby, may be demanding as well as rewarding. They should be assured that they will have support and that there are options for problem solving and for addressing the practical obstacles they may face. Some women will decide the challenges outweigh the benefits for themselves and their babies, given the overall circumstances of their lives. However, physicians and other health professionals should recognize the potential effectiveness of applying their knowledge and skills to encourage and support women in initiating and continuing breastfeeding.

Modern society creates some of the obstacles to breastfeeding. Short hospital stays make the teaching of breastfeeding a challenge. Lack of spousal or partner support and family custom may discourage breastfeeding. Having to return to work is an obstacle, which is being diminished for some women as more employers learn that

---

Research on Established and Potential Protective Effects of Human Milk and Breastfeeding on Infants

Research in the United States, Canada, Europe and other developed countries, among predominantly middle-class populations, provides strong evidence that human milk feeding decreases the incidence and/or severity of diarrhea, lower respiratory infection, otitis media, bacteremia, bacterial meningitis, botulism, urinary tract infection, and necrotizing enterocolitis. There are a number of studies that show a possible protective effect of human milk feeding against sudden infant death syndrome, insulin-dependent diabetes mellitus, Crohn's disease, ulcerative colitis, lymphoma, allergic diseases, and other chronic digestive diseases. Breastfeeding has also been related to possible enhancement of cognitive development.

American Academy of Pediatrics, Work Group on Breastfeeding. Breastfeeding and the use of human milk. Pediatrics 100;1997: 1035–1039 (Paragraph includes 39 citations.)

encouraging breastfeeding as a policy improves employee morale and decreases absenteeism (16, 17). An unfriendly social environment may make it difficult to breastfeed in public. The effect of these obstacles can be mitigated by educating the families, employers, and society. All share in the benefits and, through positive attitudes and workplace and public policies, also can support women who are willing to breastfeed.

Who Can Breastfeed

Breastfeeding is a natural function; nearly every woman can breastfeed her child. Mother and newborn can more easily learn the basics and how to deal with the challenges if they have skilled and experienced support. Mothers who have cesarean deliveries should be reassured that they can breastfeed their newborns as well as those women having vaginal deliveries. Specific infections such as endometritis or mastitis are not contraindications to breastfeeding.

Women with structural problems such as hypoplastic or tubular breasts may have difficulty producing sufficient milk. True inverted nipples are rare but generally preclude nursing; most women with nipples that appear flat or inverted can breastfeed, given appropriate assistance in the early days of lactation. Pumping for a minute or two before offering the breast to the newborn has been shown to facilitate latch-on (1). Lactation is not possible for women who have had breast surgery involving the complete severing of the lactiferous ducts. However, some women may breastfeed after reduction mammoplasty or augmentation mammoplasty with implants, and most women can breastfeed after breast biopsies.

Mothers with premature infants also can breastfeed. A mother's milk has specific properties that match the needs of her premature newborn. However, nutrition requirements for the premature newborn are different and require special attention. Some babies with cleft lips or palate may be able to breastfeed. The soft breast tissue may fill the defect and enable the infant to develop a seal. Sometimes a palatal obturator allows the infant to breastfeed and not aspirate milk. A newborn that is premature or has other special needs may benefit from breastfeeding but requires individual evaluation by appropriate experts.

Who Should Not Breastfeed

Although it is true that most women can breastfeed, there are exceptions. These exceptions should be understood by all clinicians so that a patient's frustration and disappointment can be minimized. The number of contraindi-cations is small (18). Women who should not breastfeed are those who:

- Take street drugs or do not control alcohol use
- Have an infant with galactosemia
- Are infected with the human immunodeficiency virus (HIV)
- Have active, untreated tuberculosis
- Take certain medications
- Are undergoing treatment for breast cancer (1)

Women who use illegal drugs should not breastfeed because it is unknown which agent or how much of the agent the infant will be exposed to. Alcohol is a toxin, so a breastfeeding woman should minimize or avoid it, and a mother who drinks significant amounts of alcohol should not breastfeed (2).

Infants with galactosemia should neither breastfeed, because this will exacerbate the condition, nor consume any formula containing lactose (eg, cows' milk). They need special lactose-free formula.

Some infections contraindicate breastfeeding; others require precautions. Approaches to breastfeeding vary according to the infection and the environment. Comprehensive information about breastfeeding in relation to the following common maternal infections and others is available for further reference (1). Women in the United States who have HIV infections should not breastfeed because breast milk can carry HIV and pass the infection to the infant. In some countries with high infant mortality rates, however, the benefits of breastfeeding in providing nutrition and preventing infections may still outweigh the risks of transmitting HIV.

If a woman has active pulmonary tuberculosis, the repeated and prolonged close contact involved in feeding exposes the infant to risk of airborne infection. Therefore the woman should neither breastfeed nor bottle feed her newborn until she has been appropriately treated for at least 2 weeks and is otherwise considered to be noncontagious. The infant can be given the mother's expressed breast milk because it does not contain *Mycobacterium tuberculosis* (1).

Similarly, if a woman has varicella, she should be isolated from the infant and neither breastfeed nor bottle feed while she is clinically infectious. Once the infant has received varicella-zoster immune globulin (1), the woman can provide expressed breast milk for the infant if there are no skin lesions on the breasts. An immunocompetent woman who develops herpes zoster infection (shingles) can continue breastfeeding if lesions are covered and are not on the breast. Maternal antibodies delivered through the placenta and breast milk will prevent the disease or diminish its severity. An infant may be given varicella-zoster immune globulin in these circumstances as an added precaution (1).

Breastfeeding also is contraindicated in women who have active herpes simplex infections on the breast until the lesion is cleared. In women with cytomegalovirus infection, both the virus and maternal antibodies are present in breast milk. Because of the antibodies, otherwise healthy infants born at term with congenital or acquired cytomegalovirus infections usually do better if they are breastfed. A study of infants who developed infections during breastfeeding found the infants also developed an immune response, did not develop the disease, and rarely manifested symptoms (18).

Hepatitis infections do not preclude breastfeeding. With appropriate immunoprophylaxis, including hepatitis B immune globulin (HBIG) and hepatitis vaccine, breastfeeding of babies born to women positive for hepatitis B surface antigen poses no additional risk for the transmission of hepatitis B virus (19). If a woman has acute hepatitis A infection, her infant can breastfeed after receiving immune serum globulin and vaccine (1). The average rate of hepatitis C virus (HCV) infection reported in infants born to HCV-positive women is 4% for both breastfed and bottle-fed infants. Therefore maternal HCV is not considered a contraindication to breastfeeding (20).

Many medications are compatible with breastfeeding. The AAP Committee on Drugs reviewed the current data on the transfer of drugs and other chemicals in human milk. The committee classified drugs for safety in breastfeeding on a scale of 1 (contraindicated) to 6 (compatible) (21). Generally, breastfeeding is contraindicated for women taking antineoplastic, thyrotoxic, and immunosuppressive agents (Table 1) (19). Medications with relative contraindications may sometimes be used cautiously by timing doses to immediately follow a feeding.

Education on Breastfeeding

Teaching the pregnant woman and her partner about childbirth and breastfeeding is an integral part of good prenatal care. Other family members who could support breastfeeding may be included. Education can occur in the physician's office or clinic. Alternatively, hospitals and other organizations provide education for pregnant women and their partners. The advice and encouragement of the obstetrician–gynecologist are critical in making the decision to breastfeed. Other health professionals such as pediatricians, nurses, and certified lactation specialists play an important role, as do mother-to-mother groups and other lay organizations. The health benefits of breastfeeding warrant efforts in professional cooperation and

Table 1. Medications Contraindicated During Breastfeeding

Medication	Reason
Bromocriptine	Suppresses lactation; may be hazardous to the mother
Cocaine	Cocaine intoxication
Cyclophosphamide	Possible immune suppression; unknown effect on growth or association with carcinogenesis; neutropenia
Cyclosporine	Possible immune suppression; unknown effect on growth or association with carcinogenesis
Doxorubicin*	Possible immune suppression; unknown effect on growth or association with carcinogenesis
Ergotamine	Vomiting, diarrhea, convulsions (at doses used in migraine medications)
Lithium	One third to one half of therapeutic blood concentration in infants
Methotrexate	Possible immune suppression; unknown effect on growth or association with carcinogenesis; neutropenia
Phencyclidine	Potent hallucinogen
Phenindione	Anticoagulant; increased prothrombin and partial thromboplastin time in one infant; not used in United States
Radioactive iodine and other radiolabeled elements	Contraindications to breastfeeding for various periods

*Medication is concentrated in human milk.

American Academy of Pediatrics, American College of Obstetricians and Gynecologists. Guidelines for perinatal care. 4th ed. Elk Grove Village, Illinois: AAP; Washington, DC: ACOG, 1997

coordination among all health care workers to educate and encourage women and their families to choose breastfeeding. Patient education materials can reinforce the message (see the boxes, "Patient Education Materials" and "References for Health Care Workers and Patients Seeking In-depth Information").

Some women who choose to breastfeed were breastfed themselves or had a sibling who was breastfed, which established it as normal behavior in their household. These women would probably benefit from some education and reinforcement concerning breastfeeding. Women whose family and friends have not shared breastfeeding experiences also approach pregnancy with a desire to do what is healthiest for their babies. Guidance and consideration of life situations are important in helping these women and their families make a decision about feeding their infants. Information about the benefits and challenges of breastfeeding compared with the use of formula will help them make good decisions. The obstetrician–gynecologist often

---

Patient Education Materials

Breast-feeding your baby. Patient Education Pamphlet AP029. Washington, DC: American College of Obstetricians and Gynecologists, 1997

Breastfeeding: loving support for a bright future. Q & A. Physicians' breastfeeding support kit. Tampa, Florida: Best Start Social Marketing, 1998

Working & breastfeeding. Can you do it? Yes, you can! Alexandria, Virginia: National Healthy Mothers, Healthy Babies Coalition, 1997

Ten steps to support parents' choice to breastfeed their baby. American Academy of Pediatrics Task Force on Breastfeeding. Elk Grove Village, Illinois: AAP, 1999

References for Health Care Workers and Patients Seeking In-depth Information

American Academy of Pediatrics and the American College of Obstetricians and Gynecologists. Guidelines for perinatal care. 4th ed. Elk Grove Village, Illinois: AAP, and Washington, DC: ACOG, 1997

American Academy of Pediatrics Committee on Drugs. The transfer of drugs and other chemicals into human milk. Pediatrics 1994;93:137–150.

American Academy of Pediatrics, Work Group on Breastfeeding. Breastfeeding and the use of human milk. Pediatrics 1997;100:1035–1039

ABM News and Views. The Newsletter of The Academy of Breastfeeding Medicine. Lenexa, Kansas: ABM

Lawrence RA. A review of the medical benefits and contraindications to breastfeeding in the United States. Maternal and Child Health Technical Information Bulletin. Arlington, Virginia: National Center for Education in Maternal and Child Health, 1997

Lawrence RA, Lawrence RM. Breastfeeding: a guide for the medical profession. 5th ed. St. Louis, Missouri: Mosby, 1999

U.S. Department of Health and Human Services, Health Resources & Services Administration, Maternal and Child Health Bureau, U.S. Department of Agriculture, Food and Nutrition Service. Physicians' breastfeeding support kit. Tampa, Florida: Best Start Social Marketing, 1998

---

can allay a woman's anxieties and suggest solutions or resources to make breastfeeding a practical choice for her and her family.

Periodic Gynecologic Examinations

Obstetrician–gynecologists can begin to educate women who have their reproductive lives ahead of them by mentioning breastfeeding during the breast examination portion of routine gynecologic visits, if appropriate. Women whose anatomy appears to be normal can be told that if they decide to have a baby, there are no structural impediments to breastfeeding.

First Obstetric Visit

The initial prenatal visit is the optimal time to encourage or reinforce the decision to breastfeed. It is also an ideal time to let the patient know the advantages of breastfeeding over formula feeding. Most patients seek information and guidance from their doctors. The importance of the physician's recommendation should never be underestimated. If a woman has not yet made a decision to breastfeed, this and subsequent visits may provide an opportunity for her to do so. During the breast examination, the physician can perform a breastfeeding-specific examination and answer any questions about the usual pattern of changes in the breasts during pregnancy and breastfeeding. If there are no structural problems, the woman can be reassured about her ability to breastfeed. If her nipples appear to be inverted, she should know that appearance is not necessarily prognostic and she may be able to breastfeed, but that techniques to assist in nipple eversion are not recommended during pregnancy because of the potential for stimulating contractions.

Antenatal Breastfeeding Instruction

In the past, when hospital stays were longer, women could receive fairly adequate education about breastfeeding before discharge. Today, with shorter hospital stays, it is imperative that pregnant women come to the hospital for delivery with a good foundation of knowledge gained during the antepartum period. Prenatal education groups have been shown to be particularly effective in increasing duration of breastfeeding (22). Education in the hospital can then focus on operational aspects of breastfeeding such as latch-on and feeding techniques.

The woman who is appropriately counseled on breastfeeding options and chooses not to breastfeed should be reassured that her milk production will abate during the first few days after delivery. Hormone treatment to stop milk production is no longer recommended. She should be treated with a well-fitted support bra, analgesics, and ice packs to relieve the pain. She also can be assured that if she changes her mind, she may still be able to initiate breastfeeding within the first few days.

Hospital Stay

Shortened hospital stays for childbirth have made the teaching of breastfeeding difficult. Certain protocols and practices, however, will increase rates of successful breastfeeding (see the box, "Ten Hospital Practices to Encourage and Support Breastfeeding") (23).

Delivery

The immediate postpartum period should allow the woman and her newborn to experience optimal bonding with immediate physical contact, preferably skin to skin. The initial feeding should occur as soon after birth as possible, preferably in the first hour when the baby is awake, alert, and ready to suck. Newborn eye prophylaxis, weighing, measuring, and other such examinations can be done after the feeding. Such procedures usually can be performed later in the woman's room.

Rooming-In

Today, all hospitals should make trained personnel available to provide breastfeeding support and should offer 24-hour rooming-in to maximize the interaction between the woman and her newborn. Separation of a breastfeeding woman and newborn should be avoided whenever possible. Most newborn care and procedures, including bathing, blood drawing, physical examinations, and administration of medication and phototherapy, can be performed in the mother's room. In this way, mother and baby can benefit together from the nursing care available (3).

The rooming-in experience allows a woman and her newborn to start the adjustment to a breastfeeding routine. Normally a newborn will show signs of hunger, such as increased alertness or activity, mouthing, or rooting. Crying is a late sign of hunger. Newborns should be nursed approximately 8–12 times every 24 hours until satiety; time at breast varies but may be 10 to 15 minutes on each breast (3).

Instruction

Hospital personnel should have adequate time allotted to each patient, no matter when the delivery occurs, and provide a specific program on practical aspects of breastfeeding that women master before discharge. Trained staff should assess breastfeeding behavior of the woman and newborn during the first 24–48 hours after birth for correct nursing positions, latch-on, and adequacy of newborn swallowing. They also should ensure that the woman is skilled in the technique of manual expression of milk (3).

Before discharge the woman should be educated about age-appropriate elimination patterns of her newborn during the first week after birth. At least six urinations per day and three to four stools per day are to be expected by 5–7 days of age. She can be shown how to keep simple records for the first few weeks, noting the frequency and length of feedings and the number of stools and wet diapers, for discussion with her care providers. She should understand expected patterns of newborn weight loss and gain (3). Before gaining, the breastfeeding newborn may lose 5–7% of birth weight in the first week. When the loss is greater than 5–7% or reaches that level in the first 3 days, a clinician should evaluate the breastfeeding process to address any problems before they become serious. A loss of up to 10% is the maximum acceptable. Follow-up should confirm that the newborn is beginning to regain weight after the first week (1).

Ten Hospital Practices to Encourage and Support Breastfeeding*

- Maintain a written breastfeeding policy that is communicated to all health care staff.

- Train all pertinent health care staff in skills necessary to implement this policy.

- Inform all pregnant women about the benefits of breastfeeding.

- Offer all mothers the opportunity to initiate breastfeeding within 1 hour of birth.

- Show breastfeeding mothers how to breastfeed and how to maintain lactation even if they are separated from their infants.

- Give breastfeeding infants only breast milk unless medically indicated.

- Facilitate rooming-in; encourage all mothers and infants to remain together during their hospital stay.

- Encourage unrestricted breastfeeding when baby exhibits hunger cues or signals or on request of mother.

- Encourage exclusive suckling at the breast by providing no pacifiers or artificial nipples.

- Refer mothers to established breastfeeding and mother's support groups and services, and foster the establishment of those services when they are not available.

*The 1994 report of the Healthy Mothers, Healthy Babies National Coalition Expert Work Group recommended that the UNICEF-WHO Baby Friendly Hospital Initiative be adapted for use in the United States as the United States Breastfeeding Health Initiative, using the adapted 10 steps above.

Randolph L, Cooper L, Fonseca-Becker F, York M, McIntosh M. Baby Friendly Hospital Initiative feasibility study: final report. Healthy Mothers, Healthy Babies National Coalition Expert Work Group. Alexandria, Virginia: HMHB, 1994

Latch-On

Breastfeeding should not be painful, but minor discomfort is common during the first 2 weeks. Painful breastfeeding almost always results from poor positioning or latch-on, which should be immediately corrected. ACOG's "Breast-feeding Your Baby" pamphlet is an example of a resource that can be used to help women with positioning and latch-on (24). Discomfort may occur temporarily as the woman's milk supply is beginning to be established. Any significant pain or tenderness should be assessed promptly by a physician.

Latch-on is one of the most important steps to successful breastfeeding. There are several helpful approaches, including gently stroking the newborn's lower lip with the nipple to get the baby to open his or her mouth wide, or gently pulling the newborn's chin down. The newborn should take a large amount of breast into his or her mouth, generally an inch or more of the areola with the nipple pointing toward the soft palate. The mother may hold her breast to facilitate this position, using a hand position comfortable for her. The nipple and the areola elongate into a teat, and the baby's tongue should be slightly cupped beneath it. The mother should adopt a comfortable position and draw the baby to the breast. The newborn should be held close, facing the mother, with his chin and the tip of his nose touching but not completely occluded by the breast. Usually, it is wise to alternate the breast used to initiate the feeding and to equalize the time spent at each breast over the day. The mother can break the suction by gently inserting her finger in the newborn's mouth before taking him off the breast.

Home

All breastfeeding women and their babies who are discharged from the hospital in less than 48 hours after delivery should be seen by a pediatrician or other knowledgeable health care practitioner when the baby is 2–4 days old. This is important in order to evaluate health status of the newborn (eg, weight, hydration, and hyperbilirubinemia) at this critical age, as well as to observe the woman and newborn during breastfeeding (3).

Women can be reassured that eating a well-balanced diet generally will provide the nutrients their infants need. On average, it is estimated that women will need approximately 500 kcal per day more than nonpregnant and nonlactating recommended levels, and the additional maternal food intake generally will provide additional needed vitamins and minerals (with the possible exceptions of calcium and zinc). Women of childbearing age need to maintain a calcium intake of 1,000 mg per day at all times, including during pregnancy and lactation

(1,300 for adolescents through 18 years of age). Dietary intake is the preferred source of all needed nutrients. However, many women breastfeed on a lower calorie intake level than suggested, consuming bodily stores instead. This will result in gradual weight loss and is not likely to affect breastfeeding, but further questions may need to be asked about sources of magnesium, vitamin B_6, folate, calcium, and zinc (2, 25, 26). Corrective measures can be suggested for improving nutrient intakes of women with restrictive eating patterns (2). Women should be encouraged to drink plenty of fluids to satisfy their thirst and maintain adequate hydration. They need not avoid certain foods (spicy or strong flavored) because of breastfeeding unless the infant seems to react negatively to specific foods.

The spouse or partner can play a vital support role for the breastfeeding woman by encouraging her, bringing the newborn to her for feeding, changing the newborn, and holding the newborn. Couples may find that caring for a baby can complicate their own relationship, including a desired resumption of sexual intercourse. They may be encouraged to discuss emotional adjustments to their new family status as well as physical problems of soreness, fatigue, and vaginal dryness secondary to lactation. When a woman is ready to resume sexual intercourse, prelubricated latex condoms can be recommended to prevent infection and ease vaginal dryness.

Phone-In Resource

The departure of a woman and her newborn from the hospital can be a joyous but daunting experience. The family is now responsible for the care and feeding of the newborn. Whether or not they have a support system at home, a phone-in resource is needed for ongoing instruction and advice. The obstetrician–gynecologist's office, the place where the woman has received most of her care, should be that resource or at least provide links to other resources in the community, such as lactation specialists and support groups.

Contraception

Women should be encouraged to consider their future plans for additional childbearing during prenatal care and be given information and services that will help them meet their goals. This is especially important for a woman who breastfeeds, because there are fewer variables in her nutrition status if the next pregnancy is delayed until she has completed breastfeeding.

In nonbreastfeeding women, the average time to first ovulation is 45 days (range, 25–72 days) (27). Many women resume intercourse well before they return for their postpartum checkup, thus some women are at risk of becoming pregnant.

For breastfeeding women, however, the situation is different. Exclusive breastfeeding helps prevent pregnancy for the first 6 months after delivery, but should be relied on only temporarily and when it meets carefully observed criteria of the lactational amenorrhea method (LAM) (see "Lactational Amenorrhea Method").

Nonhormonal Methods

If a breastfeeding woman needs or wants more protection from pregnancy, options are available that do not affect breastfeeding or pose even a theoretical risk to the infant. *She should first consider the nonhormonal methods such as copper intrauterine contraceptive devices, condoms, or other barrier methods* (see the box, "ACOG Recommendations for Nonhormonal Contraception for Breastfeeding Women"). Condoms have additional, noncontraceptive advantages. Female sterilization or vasectomy may be considered by couples desiring permanent methods of birth control (27).

Hormonal Methods

Hormonal contraception offers effective protection from becoming pregnant. Several factors should be considered before prescribing hormonal contraception for the lactating woman. Contradictory lines of thought have resulted in conflicting recommendations that have been put forward by generally authoritative sources. The ACOG recommendations represent a more practical approach to the woman's needs, based on relevant research.

Progestin-Only Contraceptives

Progestin-only contraceptives, including progestin-only tablets (minipills), depot medroxyprogesterone acetate

---

ACOG Recommendations for Nonhormonal Contraception for Breastfeeding Women

Exclusive breastfeeding up to 6 months meeting lactational amenorrhea method criteria (see "Lactational Amenorrhea Method")

Additional protection if desired

- Prelubricated latex condoms
- Other barrier methods
- Copper intrauterine contraceptive devices
- Male or female sterilization if permanent contraception is desired

---

(DMPA), and levonorgestrel implants, do not affect the quality of breast milk and may slightly increase the volume of milk and duration of breastfeeding compared with nonhormonal methods (28–32). Accordingly, progestin-only methods are the hormonal contraceptives of choice for breastfeeding women. Nonetheless, some authorities have recommended delays of various lengths before introduction of progestin-only contraceptives on the basis of two sets of theoretical concerns:

- The normal 2–3-day postdelivery decrease of progesterone is part of the process that initiates lactation. There is theoretical concern that giving progestins in the first few days before lactation is established could interfere with optimal lactation. Note that DMPA enters the milk at approximately the same level found in the woman's blood; by contrast norgestrel and norethindrone enter the milk at only one tenth the level in the woman's blood. The injectable route of administration also may result in a comparatively high initial dose (27).

- Progestin methods carry a theoretical risk to the newborn because of exposure to exogenous steroids at a time when the newborn's system is very immature in its ability to metabolize drugs. Because of this concern, research studies presented to the FDA for drug approval investigated only the effects of these methods administered several weeks after birth. Because documentation of experience with earlier initiation was not presented to the FDA, package inserts recommend initiation of progestin-only oral contraceptives at 6 weeks for women who are exclusively breastfeeding and at 3 weeks for those who are breastfeeding with supplementation. Most authorities recommend introduction of long-acting progestin-only injectables or implants 6 weeks after delivery for breastfeeding women (27, 33, 34).

To balance these conservative recommendations, it is important to understand that the few studies that included early administration of progestin-only methods—oral contraceptives at 1 week postpartum (35, 36) and injectable medroxyprogesterone acetate at 2 days (37) and 7 days (38)—found no adverse effects on the newborn or on breastfeeding. In the absence of evidence that earlier introduction of progestin-only contraceptives has adverse effects on the newborn and on breastfeeding, the labeling for progestin-only oral contraceptives focuses instead on what is known about fertility after childbirth. Taking only biologic factors into account, contraception is not needed in the first 3 weeks postpartum because of a delay in return of ovulation in all women. And this delay is extended for women who breastfeed exclusively. An implied prohibition on earlier administration is more in the nature of a pragmatic rather than a scientific resolution of the question. From the perspective of routine clinical practice, it would appear reasonable to apply the same rationale, even though conservative, to the initiation of DMPA and implants in postpartum breastfeeding women. However, the package labeling for these methods has the effect of being even more conservative as noted, outlining a 6-week start for all breastfeeding women, with no flexibility. Sometimes, however, there are practical reasons a breastfeeding woman may consider initiating hormonal contraception while in the hospital or shortly after. For example, there may be uncertainty about opportunities for follow-up visits. The breastfeeding woman and her physician can then weigh the reasons for early use of these contraceptives against potential disadvantages, make an appropriate decision, and continue to evaluate the woman's individual breastfeeding experience if hormonal contraceptives are chosen.

Combination Estrogen–Progestin Contraceptives

The postpartum patient has a hypercoagulable state that predisposes her to venous thrombosis (39). The use of estrogen-containing contraceptives during this phase of approximately 3 weeks after childbirth could contribute to this state. Furthermore, estrogen–progestin contraceptives have been shown to reduce the quantity and quality of breast milk. The World Health Organization recommends that the breastfeeding woman wait at least 6 months after childbirth to start using them (33). Labeling required by the FDA for combined oral contraceptives states, "If possible, the nursing mother should be advised not to use oral contraceptives but to use other forms of contraception until she has completely weaned her child" (34). These conservative approaches emanate for the most part from earlier combination oral contraceptive studies using higher doses of estrogens. Low-dose tablets (35 µg or lower) probably have a lesser effect on quality and quantity of breast milk. Effects are variable and if there are strong reasons the woman wishes to start combined estrogen–progestin contraceptive use earlier, she should understand and weigh the potential disadvantages. If estrogen–progestin contraceptives are prescribed, they should not be started before 6 weeks postpartum, and the physician should continue to evaluate the woman's individual breastfeeding experience.

The summary recommendations given in the box, "ACOG Recommendations for Hormonal Contraception If Used by Breastfeeding Women," with regard to progestin-only methods are based on the conservative timing outlined in labeling. Exceptions may be considered for earlier use on an individual basis. With combined estrogen–progestin contraceptives, a minimum 6-week delay is prudent

because practical obstacles in developing successful breastfeeding techniques are likely to be resolved by 6 weeks. Most women experience reduced milk volume as a result of estrogen ingestion; this may be dealt with more easily after breastfeeding skills and patterns are established, should combined contraceptives be chosen despite this disadvantage. FDA labeling, however, is more conservative than the summary recommendation offered for combined estrogen–progestin contraceptives here. As noted earlier, prelubricated condoms are a good interim contraceptive choice and will address vaginal dryness associated with breastfeeding as well as help prevent infection.

Lactational Amenorrhea Method

Women who breastfeed can make use of the natural contraceptive effect of lactation. The LAM is most appropriate for women who plan to fully breastfeed 6 months or longer. If the baby is fed only mother's milk or is given supplemental nonbreast-milk feedings only to a minor extent and the woman has not experienced her first postpartum menses, then breastfeeding provides more than 98% protection from pregnancy in the first 6 months following delivery (27, 40, 41). Four prospective clinical trials of the contraceptive effect of LAM demonstrated cumulative 6-month life-table, perfect-use pregnancy rates of 0.5%, 0.6%, 1.0%, and 1.5% among women who relied solely on it. Women should be advised that for significant fertility impact, intervals between feedings should not exceed 4 hours during the day or 6 hours at night (Fig. 1). Supplemental feedings should not exceed 5–10% of the total (42–46). For example, more than one supplemental feeding out of every 10 might increase the

---

ACOG Recommendations for Hormonal Contraception If Used by Breastfeeding Women

- Progestin-only oral contraceptives prescribed or dispensed at discharge from the hospital to be started 2–3 weeks postpartum (eg, the first Sunday after the newborn is 2 weeks old)

- Depot medroxyprogesterone acetate initiated at 6 weeks postpartum*

- Hormonal implants inserted at 6 weeks postpartum*

- Combined estrogen–progestin contraceptives, if prescribed, should not be started before 6 weeks postpartum, and only when lactation is well established and the infant's nutritional status well-monitored

*There are certain clinical situations in which earlier initiation might be considered.

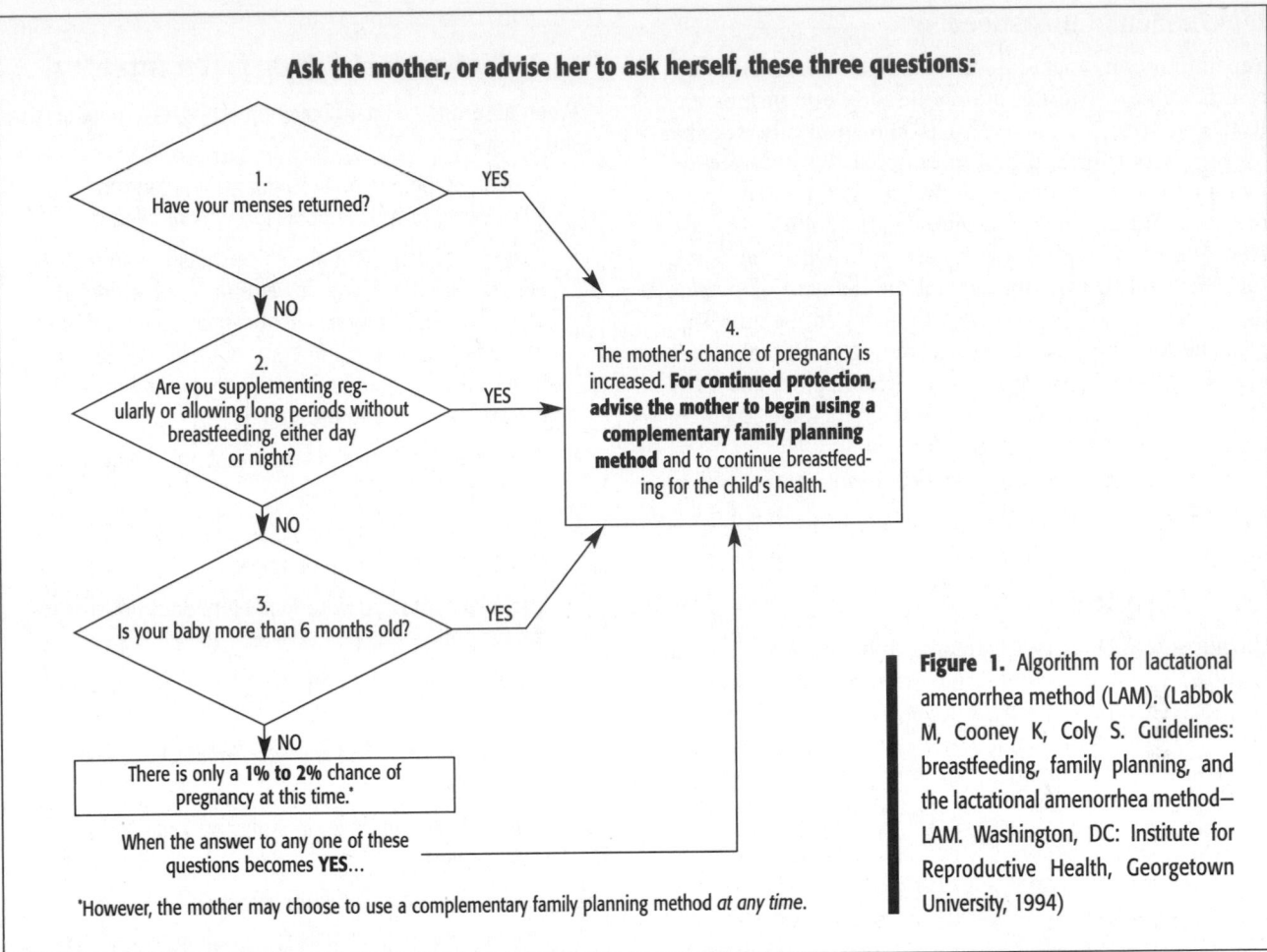

Ask the mother, or advise her to ask herself, these three questions:

1. Have your menses returned? — YES →

NO ↓

2. Are you supplementing regularly or allowing long periods without breastfeeding, either day or night? — YES →

NO ↓

3. Is your baby more than 6 months old? — YES →

NO ↓

There is only a **1% to 2%** chance of pregnancy at this time.*

When the answer to any one of these questions becomes **YES**...

4. The mother's chance of pregnancy is increased. **For continued protection, advise the mother to begin using a complementary family planning method** and to continue breastfeeding for the child's health.

*However, the mother may choose to use a complementary family planning method *at any time*.

Figure 1. Algorithm for lactational amenorrhea method (LAM). (Labbok M, Cooney K, Coly S. Guidelines: breastfeeding, family planning, and the lactational amenorrhea method—LAM. Washington, DC: Institute for Reproductive Health, Georgetown University, 1994)

likelihood of returning fertility. Feeding practices other than direct breastfeeding, insofar as they may reduce the vigor and frequency of suckling and the maternal neuro-endocrine response, increase the probability of returning ovulation (47). If there is uncertainty regarding the extent to which a given woman is breastfeeding, it would be prudent to recommend additional contraception.

Maintaining Milk Supply

Regular breastfeeding generally ensures adequate milk supply. As the baby grows and requires more milk, the woman's supply, which is demand driven, increases to accommodate the baby's needs.

Bottle Supplements and Pacifiers

The use of pacifiers and supplemental bottle feeding have been considered deterrents to sustained breastfeeding. Studies do not provide clear evidence that bottle feeding and pacifiers directly interfere with breastfeeding. A recent prospective cohort study indicated that pacifier use in the first 6 weeks was independently associated with declines in the duration of full and overall breastfeeding in the long term, but not short term (during the first 3 months of life). Women who introduced pacifiers early tended to breastfeed fewer times per day. The authors suggested that maternal behavior, such as extending intervals between feedings and decisions to begin weaning, may lead to introduction of pacifiers. They suggested that pacifier use, through an association with infrequent breastfeeding, may mediate (rather than cause) the declines observed in breastfeeding duration (48). It is important to help mothers understand that substituting for or delaying breastfeedings may ultimately reduce milk supply because of the reduction in stimulation of milk production that depends on infant suckling. Another study found that fluid supplements offered by bottle with or without the use of pacifiers during the first 5 days of life were not associated with a lower frequency or shorter duration of breastfeeding during the first 6 months of life (49).

Interruption of Breastfeeding

Separation of mother and infant should be avoided whenever possible, especially during the early establishment of lactation (first 3 weeks). If it is known in advance that hospitalization or a trip, for example, will require the mother to be separated from the infant for more than a day, careful planning can ensure that the ability to breastfeed will be preserved and breast milk will be available for the infant. During the separation, regular pumping of the breasts should be sufficient to maintain the milk supply. The milk may be saved for feeding the infant. When the separation is because of hospitalization, the milk should be discarded if it is judged to contain anesthetic or contraindicated medications. When the mother and infant are reunited, the reestablishment of normal breastfeeding generally progresses well.

Sore Nipples

Having sore nipples is a common problem for the breastfeeding woman. It usually results from poor positioning or latch-on (see box, "Positioning and Latch-On for Breastfeeding"). The first-line treatment should be counseling about these basic techniques (24). Purified lanolin cream and breast shells (to protect the nipples from friction between feedings) may be initiated to facilitate healing (50).

Mastitis

Mastitis occurs in 1–2% of breastfeeding women (51). It most commonly occurs between the first and fifth weeks postpartum but may be seen any time throughout the first year (52). Mastitis is manifested by a sore, reddened area on one breast and often is accompanied by chills, fever, and malaise. A segment of the breast becomes hard and erythematous, the fever can be as high as 40°C, and the mother feels ill.

The differential diagnosis includes clogged milk duct, marked engorgement, and a rare condition, inflammatory breast carcinoma. Clogged milk ducts present as localized tender masses. They respond to warm wet compresses and manually massaging the loculated milk towards the nipple. Breast engorgement is always bilateral with generalized involvement. It occurs most commonly in the first 2 weeks postpartum. The major feature that differentiates it from inflammatory breast cancer is the knowledge of previous negative breast examination results during the pregnancy. If examination results have been normal, breast engorgement is the more likely diagnosis (51). Inflammatory breast cancer is a lethal form of breast cancer. It presents as unilateral erythema, heat, and induration that is more diffuse and recurrent (53).

Positioning and Latch-On for Breastfeeding

When observing an infant being breastfed, take note of the following:

- Position of mother, body language, and tension. Pillows may provide support for arms or infant.

- Position of infant. Ventral surface should be to mother's ventral surface, with lower arm, if not swaddled, around mother's thorax. Infant cannot swallow if head has to turn to breast, and grasp of areola will be poor. Infant's head should be in crook of arm and moved toward breast by arm movement.

- Position of mother's hand on breast not in way of proper grasp by infant

- Position of infant's lips on areola about 1–1½ inches (2.5–3.7 cm) from base of nipple

- Lower lip not folded in so that infant does not suck it; lips flanged

- Actual events around presenting breast and assisting infant to latch on

- Response of infant to lower lip stimulus by opening mouth wide

- Motion of masseter muscle during suckling and sounds of swallowing

- Mother comfortable with no breast pain

Lawrence RA, Lawrence RM. Breastfeeding: a guide for the medical profession. 5th ed. St. Louis, Missouri: Mosby, 1999

The most common causative agent in mastitis is *Staphylococcus aureus*, occurring in 40% of cases (54). It is also the most common cause of abscess. Other common organisms in mastitis are *Hemophilus influenzae* and *H parainfluenzae*, *Escherichia coli*, *Enterococcus faecalis*, *Klebsiella pneumoniae*, *Enterobacter cloacae*, *Serratia marcescens*, and *Pseudomonas pickettii* (53).

The condition usually can be treated successfully with narrow-spectrum antibiotic therapy (first choice for women who are not allergic is dicloxacillin, 500 mg four times daily), hydration, bedrest, and acetaminophen. The mother should continue to breastfeed or express the milk from both breasts because it is important to empty the affected breast. In some cases, the woman may be advised to discard the milk until she has been treated for 24 hours.

If mastitis is not treated aggressively, an abscess may develop. Treatment is successful in curing mastitis if started early; the most common cause of recurrent mastitis is inadequate treatment. Delayed administration of antibiotics is associated with an increased incidence of breast abscess. Many staphylococcal infections are caused by organisms sensitive to penicillin or a cephalosporin. Dicloxacillin may be started empirically (55). Women who are allergic to penicillin may be given erythromycin. If the infection is caused by resistant, penicillinase-producing staphylococci, an antibiotic such as vancomycin or cefotetan should be given and continued until 2 days after the infection subsides, a minimum of 10–14 days.

Abscess

Abscess is diagnosed by a palpable mass or failure to defervesce within 48–72 hours of antibiotic therapy. Generally, abscesses are treated with incision and drainage. Multiple abscesses may require multiple incisions, with a finger inserted to break down the locules. Breast milk should be discarded for the first 24 hours after surgery, with breastfeeding resuming thereafter if there is no drainage into the breast milk (1). Recently, ultrasonographically guided needle aspiration was shown to be successful in treating abscesses in 18 of 19 women (56).

Working Mothers and Time Away

Over half of mothers are employed outside the home. In some situations, the mother is able to feed her infant at work, but this is not common. Health professionals can help the mother consider the method by which she plans to feed her infant when she returns to work. Employers are increasingly supportive of accommodating the needs of their breastfeeding employees (16). If a woman wants to continue to breastfeed or breast-milk feed, she should plan to pump her breasts to maintain her milk supply and to provide stored milk for the caregiver to feed the infant in her absence. A mother can be reassured that continuing breastfeeding and use of breast milk to whatever degree she finds possible will benefit her infant.

Expressing Milk

Several methods are available to collect milk. Health professionals should ensure that breastfeeding women can successfully express milk by hand. Because use of a breast pump is more efficient, rental or purchase of a pump can be considered. In general, electric pumps are more efficient than hand pumps. Pumping both breasts simultaneously is more effective and saves time.

On occasion, women have to educate employers about the necessity of time and location to pump breasts during the workday. The influence of the physician in creating a better environment should not be underestimated. A physician's letter or phone call to the employer explaining how simple but vital the breastfeeding employee's needs are can be effective.

Storage of Milk

Breast milk can be stored in the refrigerator or on ice in glass or plastic containers. The use of refrigerated milk within 2 days is recommended, which is well before appreciable bacterial growth usually occurs. Breast milk intended for longer storage should be frozen as soon as possible and kept at the lowest and most constant temperatures available; for example, a deep freezer is preferable to a refrigerator freezer with a self-defrost cycle. Milk should be dated and used in date order to avoid loss of beneficial properties over time. Frozen milk can be thawed quickly under running water or gradually in the refrigerator. It should not be left out at room temperature for more than 4–8 hours, exposed to very hot water, or put in the microwave. Once the milk has thawed, it can be kept in the refrigerator for 24 hours (1, 57).

Breastfeeding Expectations in Daily Life

Despite sporadic instances of authorities forbidding breastfeeding in public, there is an increased level of acceptance of breastfeeding nationally. Supportive laws and policies are becoming the trend. Recently, breastfeeding mothers have had increasing success in leading active lives. Couples commonly take their babies with them to meetings, outings, restaurants, and while traveling. Women can be skillful at unobtrusively feeding their babies in public. There are many baby-friendly restaurants that welcome families and have a positive approach to breastfeeding.

Physicians' offices and other health facilities should welcome and encourage breastfeeding by providing educational material and an atmosphere receptive to breastfeeding women. All staff members should be aware of the value and importance of breastfeeding and understand that their contacts with patients can help them decide to breastfeed and encourage them to continue (see the box, "Office Tips").

Formula companies try to attract the interest of pregnant women with gift packs. Care providers should be aware that the giving of gift packs with formula to breastfeeding women is commonly a deterrent to continuation of breastfeeding (58, 59). A professional recommendation of the care and feeding products in the gift pack is implied. Physicians may conclude that noncommercial educational alternatives or gift packs without health-related items are preferable.

Office Tips

- Make ACOG Patient Education Pamphlets and other patient education materials available in waiting and examination rooms.

- Offer a call-in telephone number for advice—yours or another health care resource available in the community or hospital of birth.

- Provide information about and phone numbers of lactation consultants, such as La Leche League, in your community.

- Show videos on breastfeeding; if women's health videos normally play in waiting room, include those on breastfeeding so all patients see them, not just pregnant or breastfeeding patients.

- Provide seating, such as pillows and a rocking chair for women with infants, that keeps breastfeeding in mind.

- Have pumps and an appropriate room for employees and patients. If in a medical office complex with other practices, make its availability known to other employees (they may be your patients) or collaborate in setting up a room elsewhere in the building.

- Identify a staff member interested in being a special resource on breastfeeding in the office and facilitate further training for the individual in order to assist you, other staff, and patients.

- Develop breastfeeding statistics for your practice and encourage staff by showing changes over time on displays in staff areas.

- Ask about hospital policies and practices and offer to help with staff training and patient orientation materials.

- Find out about breastfeeding skills, interests, and services of family physician and pediatric colleagues in the community. Encourage women and parents to choose a supportive caregiver for the infant and meet with him or her during pregnancy.

How Long to Breastfeed

During the first 6 months of life, exclusive breastfeeding is the preferred feeding approach for the healthy infant born at term. It provides optimal nutrients for growth and development of the infant. The ACOG recommends that exclusive breastfeeding be continued until the infant is about 6 months old. A longer breastfeeding experience is, of course, beneficial. The professional objectives are to encourage and enable as many women as possible to breastfeed and to help them continue as long as possible.

Gradual introduction of iron-enriched solid foods in the second half of the first year should complement the breast milk diet (3). The AAP recommends that breastfeeding continue for at least 12 months, and thereafter for as long as is mutually desired (3). "Vitamin D and iron may need to be given before 6 months of age in selected groups of infants (vitamin D for infants whose mothers are vitamin D-deficient or those infants not exposed to adequate sunlight, iron for those who have low iron stores or anemia)" (3).

Weaning

The weaning process should be gradual. Eliminating a feeding every 2–3 days will achieve a comfortable transition for the infant and prevent engorgement in the mother. An infant weaned before 12 months should receive iron-fortified infant formula rather than cows' milk (3). If an infant is less than 9 months, weaning can be accomplished by substituting a bottle or cup for a breastfeeding. If an infant is 9 months or older, he or she may use a cup and substitute other foods for breastfeeding.

Abrupt weaning can be difficult for the mother and the baby. When this is necessary, certain measures can be helpful. The mother should wear a support bra. She does not need to restrict fluids. She may manually express sufficient milk to relieve the engorgement, but not so much that more milk production is stimulated. Cool compresses will reduce engorgement. Hormonal therapy is not recommended.

Weaning creates a hormonal milieu conducive to remineralization of bone and maternal replenishment. This may be a consideration favoring delay of the next pregnancy until the mother has completed breastfeeding.

Breast Cancer Detection

Because of normal changes in the breasts during pregnancy and lactation, cancer detection by palpation becomes more difficult. Breast self-examination is recommended, as it is for all women; however, in general, significant changes are difficult to distinguish from the normal changes in the breast during breastfeeding. Any suspicious lesion should be investigated. Studies indicate there are delays in diagnosis of breast cancer during pregnancy and lactation, including greater intervals between palpation of a lesion and diagnosis. These delays result in an increased risk of metastatic disease at diagnosis and a reduced chance of diagnosis at stage I (60). If a mass or other abnormality is detected during lactation, it should be fully evaluated, including biopsy, if indicated. Breastfeeding can continue during the evaluation. During lactation, mammograms are less reliable because of the associated increase in breast tissue density, which may make the test more difficult to interpret (53).

With these difficulties in detection during pregnancy and lactation as a backdrop, clinical breast examinations of women who may become pregnant are especially important. In addition, increasing age is one of many risk factors for breast cancer. Women are having babies in their late 30s and early 40s, and screening may be difficult during a 1- or 2-year period of pregnancy and lactation. This may influence some women who would not otherwise be candidates for mammography to consider it with their physicians as part of the total clinical evaluation before pregnancy.

Healthy People 2010

The goal set by the U.S. Public Health Service for *Healthy People 2010* is to "increase the proportion of mothers who breastfeed their babies" with specific targets for breastfeeding of 75% in the early postpartum period, 50% at 6 months, and 25% at 12 months (61). These are basically the same levels that were called for in *Healthy People 2000* except that the 12-month target has been added. Significant progress has been made from the rates of the early 90s. By 1998, the most recent year for which data are available, the proportion of mothers choosing to breastfeed reached a high of 64.3% after a concerted effort on the part of health professionals and support people. The highest breastfeeding rates are among college-educated women, those older than the age of 30, those living in the Mountain or Pacific census regions, and those not enrolled in WIC (Special Supplemental Nutrition Program for Women, Infants, and Children). Breastfeeding initiation rates are lowest among black women, women younger than 20 years old, women enrolled in WIC, those who did not complete high school, and those living in the East South Central census region (Mothers' Survey, Ross Products Division, Abbott Laboratories, Inc., Columbus, Ohio).

Some concentrated educational efforts also have had a statistical impact in specific populations (62). Women enrolled in WIC, because of increased breastfeeding support, are among those with the most rapid increases in rates of breastfeeding, although their rates remain well below national averages. Between 1990 and 1998, the most rapidly increasing initiation rate was among black women, the demographic group with the lowest breastfeeding rate (44.9% in-hospital compared with 64.3% nationally) in 1998 despite this increase (Mothers' Survey).

In 1998, the breastfeeding rate at 6 months reached 28.6%, the highest rate in the nearly 30 years such data have been collected. The highest 6-month rates are among mothers with the same demographic and socioeconomic characteristics as those who have the highest in-hospital breastfeeding rates. Younger women, black women, WIC participants, women in the East South Central census region, and women who are employed full time outside the home have the lowest 6-month breastfeeding rates (Mothers' Survey).

With the cooperation of many dedicated caregivers, it appears that the 2010 goals may be achievable. However, even if 75% of women initiate breastfeeding, two thirds of them will need to continue breastfeeding, to reach the proposed 6-month target of 50% of all women breastfeeding. Obstetrician–gynecologists should ensure that women have the correct information to make an informed decision and, together with pediatricians, they should ensure that each woman has the help and support necessary to continue to breastfeed successfully (63). The combined efforts of all health care providers will be necessary to meet this goal.

References

1. Lawrence RA, Lawrence RM. Breastfeeding: a guide for the medical profession. 5th ed. St. Louis, Missouri: Mosby, 1999

2. Institute of Medicine. Subcommittee on Nutrition During Lactation, Committee on Nutritional Status During Pregnancy and Lactation, Food and Nutrition Board. Nutrition during lactation. Washington, DC: National Academy Press, 1991

3. American Academy of Pediatrics, Work Group on Breastfeeding. Breastfeeding and the use of human milk. Pediatrics 1997;100:1035–1039

4. Chua S, Arulkumaran S, Lim I, Selamat N, Ratham SS. Influence of breastfeeding and nipple stimulation on postpartum uterine activity. Br J Obstet Gynaecol 1994;101: 804–805

5. Carter CS, Altemus M. Integrative functions of lactational hormones in social behavior and stress management. Ann N Y Acad Sci 1997;807:164–174

6. Rosenblatt KA, Thomas DB. Lactation and the risk of epithelial ovarian cancer. The WHO Collaborative Study of Neoplasia and Steroid Contraceptives. Int J Epidemiol 1993;22:192–197

7. Newcomb PA, Storer BE, Longnecker MP, Mittendorf R, Greenberg ER, Clapp RW, et al. Lactation and a reduced risk of premenopausal breast cancer. N Engl J Med 1994; 330:81–87

8. Kennedy KI, Visness CM. Contraceptive efficacy of lactational amenorrhoea. Lancet 1992;339:227–230

9. Gray RH, Campbell OM, Apelo R, Eslami SS, Zacur H, Ramos RM, et al. Risk of ovulation during lactation. Lancet 1990;335:25–29

10. Labbok MH, Colie C. Puerperium and breast-feeding. Curr Opin Obstet Gynecol 1992;4:818–825

11. Melton LJ 3d, Bryant SC, Wahner HW, O'Fallon WM, Malkasian GD, Judd HL, et al. Influence of breastfeeding and other reproductive factors on bone mass later in life. Osteoporos Int 1993;3:76–83

12. Cumming RG, Klineberg RJ. Breastfeeding and other reproductive factors and the risk of hip fractures in elderly women. Int J Epidemiol 1993;22:684–691

13. Dewey KG, Heinig MJ, Nommsen LA. Maternal weight-loss patterns during prolonged lactation. Am J Clin Nutr 1993;58:162–166

14. Ball TM, Wright AL. Health care costs of formula-feeding in the first year of life. Pediatrics 1999;103:870–876

15. Montgomery DL, Splett PL. Economic benefit of breast-feeding infants enrolled in WIC. J Am Diet Assoc 1997; 97:379–385

16. Jacobson M, Kolarek MH, Newton B. Business, babies and the bottom line: corporate innovations and best practices in maternal and child health. Washington, DC: Washington Business Group on Health, 1996

17. Cohen R, Mrtek MB, Mrtek RG. Comparison of maternal absenteeism and infant illness rates among breast-feeding and formula-feeding women in two corporations. Am J Health Promot 1995;10:148–153

18. Lawrence RA. A review of the medical benefits and contraindications to breastfeeding in the United States. Maternal and Child Health Technical Information Bulletin. Arlington, Virginia: National Center for Education in Maternal and Child Health, 1997

19. American Academy of Pediatrics, American College of Obstetricians and Gynecologists. Guidelines for perinatal care. 4th ed. Elk Grove Village, Illinois: AAP; Washington, DC: ACOG, 1997

20. Recommendations for prevention and control of hepatitis C virus (HCV) infection and HCV-related chronic disease. Centers for Disease Control and Prevention. MMWR Morb Mortal Wkly Rep 1998;47(RR-19):1–39

21. American Academy of Pediatrics Committee on Drugs. The transfer of drugs and other chemicals into human milk. Pediatrics 1994;93:137–150

22. Pugin E, Valdes V, Labbok MH, Perez A, Aravena R. Does prenatal breastfeeding skills group education increase the effectiveness of a comprehensive breastfeeding promotion program? J Hum Lact 1996;12(1):15–19

23. Randolph L, Cooper L, Fonseca-Becker F, York M, McIntosh M. Baby friendly hospital initiative feasibility study: final report. Healthy Mothers Healthy Babies National Coalition Expert Work Group. Alexandria, Virginia: HMHB, 1994

24. American College of Obstetricians and Gynecologists. Breast-feeding your baby. ACOG Patient Education Pamphlet AP029. Washington, DC: ACOG, 1997

25. Institute of Medicine. Standing Committee on the Scientific Evaluation of Dietary Reference Intakes, Food and Nutrition Board. Dietary reference intakes for calcium, phosphorus, magnesium, vitamin D, and fluoride. Washington, DC: National Academy Press, 1997

26. Institute of Medicine. Committee on Nutritional Status During Pregnancy and Lactation, Food and Nutrition Board. Nutrition services in perinatal care. 2nd ed. Washington, DC: National Academy Press, 1992

27. Hatcher RA, Trussell J, Stewart F, Cates W Jr, Stewart GK, Guest F, et al. Contraceptive technology. 17th rev. ed. New York: Ardent Media, Inc, 1998

28. Tankeyoon M, Dusitsin N, Chalapati S, Koetsawang S, Saibiang S, Sas M, et al. Effects of hormonal contraceptives on milk volume and infant growth. WHO Special Programme of Research, Development, and Research Training in Human Reproduction, Task Force on Oral Contraceptives. Contraception 1984;30:505–522

29. World Health Organization (WHO) Task Force on Oral Contraceptives. Effects of hormonal contraceptives on milk composition and infant growth. Stud Fam Plann 1988;19:361–369

30. Speroff L, Darney P. A clinical guide for contraception. 2nd ed. Baltimore, Maryland: Williams & Wilkins, 1996

31. Abdulla KA, Elwan SI, Salem HS, Shaaban MM. Effect of early postpartum use of the contraceptive implants, NOR-PLANT, on the serum levels of immunoglobulins of the mothers and their breastfed infants. Contraception 1985; 32:261–266

32. Shaaban MM, Salem HT, Abdullah KA. Influence of levonorgestrel contraceptive implants, NORPLANT, initiated early postpartum upon lactation and infant growth. Contraception 1985;32:623–635

33. World Health Organization. Division of Family and Reproductive Health. Improving access to quality care in family planning: medical eligibility criteria for contraceptive use. Geneva: WHO, 1996

34. Physicians' Desk Reference. 53rd ed. Montvale, New Jersey: Medical Economics, Inc, 1999

35. McCann MF, Moggia AV, Higgins JE, Potts M, Becker C. The effects of a progestin-only oral contraceptive (levonorgestrel 0.03 mg) on breast-feeding. Contraception 1989;40:635–648

36. Moggia AV, Harris GS, Dunson TR, Diaz R, Moggia MS, Ferrer MA, et al. A comparative study of a progestin-only oral contraceptive versus non-hormonal methods in lactating women in Buenos Aires, Argentina. Contraception 1991;44:31–43

37. Guiloff E, Ibarra-Polo A, Zañartu J, Toscanini C, Mischler TW, Gómez-Rogers C. Effect of contraception on lactation. Am J Obstet Gynecol 1974;118:42–45

38. Karim M, Ammar R, el Mahgoub S, el Ganzoury B, Fikri F, Abdou I. Injected progestogen and lactation. BMJ 1971; 1:200–203

39. WHO Task Force on Oral Contraceptives. Contraception during the postpartum period and during lactation: the effects on women's health. Int J Gynaecol Obstet 1987;25 (suppl):13–26

40. Kennedy KI, Rivera R, McNeilly AS. Consensus statement on the use of breastfeeding as a family planning method. Contraception 1989;39:477–496

41. World Health Organization. Task Force on Methods for the Natural Regulation of Fertility. The WHO multinational study of breast-feeding and lactational amenorrhea. III. Pregnancy during breast-feeding. Fertil Steril 1999;72;431–440

42. Perez A, Labbok MH, Queenan JT. Clinical study of the lactational amenorrhoea method for family planning. Lancet 1992;339:968–970

43. Ramos R, Kennedy KI, Visness CM. Effectiveness of lactational amenorrhea in prevention of pregnancy in Manila, the Philippines: non-comparative prospective trial. BMJ 1996;313:909–912

44. Labbok MH, Hight-Laukaran V, Peterson AE, Fletcher V, von Hertzen H, Van Look PF. Multicenter study of the Lactational Amenorrhea Method (LAM): I. Efficacy, duration and implications for clinical application. Contraception 1997;55:327–336

45. Kazi A, Kennedy KI, Visness CM, Khan T. Effectiveness of the lactational amenorrhea method in Pakistan. Fertil Steril 1995;64:717–723

46. Labbok M, Cooney K, Coly S. Guidelines: breastfeeding, family planning, and the lactational amenorrhea method— LAM. Washington, DC: Institute for Reproductive Health, Georgetown University, 1994

47. Campbell OM, Gray RH. Characteristics and determinants of postpartum ovarian function in women in the United States. Am J Obstet Gynecol 1993;169:55–60

48. Howard CR, Howard FM, Lanphear B, deBlieck EA, Eberly S, Lawrence RA. The effects of early pacifier use on breastfeeding duration. Pediatrics 1999;103:E33

49. Schubiger G, Schwarz U, Tonz O. UNICEF/WHO baby-friendly hospital initiative: does the use of bottles and pacifiers in the neonatal nursery prevent successful breastfeeding? Neonatal Study Group. Eur J Pediatr 1997;156:874–877

50. Brent N, Rudy SJ, Redd B, Rudy TE, Roth LA. Sore nipples in breast-feeding women: a clinical trial of wound dressings vs conventional care. Arch Pediatr Adolesc Med 1998;152:1077–1082

51. Stehman FB. Infections and inflammations of the breast. In: Hindle WH, ed. Breast disease for gynecologists. Norwalk, Connecticut: Appleton & Lange, 1990:151

52. Niebyl JR, Spence MR, Parmley TH. Sporadic (nonepidemic) puerperal mastitis. J Reprod Med 1978;20: 97–100

53. Hankins GD, Clark SL, Cunningham FG, Gilstrap LC III. Breast disease during pregnancy and lactation. In: Hankins GD, Clark SL, Cunningham FG, Gilstrap LC III, eds. Operative obstetrics. Norwalk, Connecticut: Appleton & Lange, 1995:667–694

54. Matheson I, Aursnes I, Horgen M, Aabo O, Melby K. Bacteriological findings and clinical symptoms in relation to clinical outcome in puerperal mastitis. Acta Obstet Gynecol Scand 1988;67:723–726

55. Hindle WH. Other benign breast problems. Clin Obstet Gynecol 1994;37:916–924

56. Karstrup S, Solvig J, Nolsoe CP, Nilsson P, Khattar S, Loren I, et al. Acute puerperal breast abscesses: US-guided drainage. Radiology 1993;188:807–809

57. Arnold LDW. Recommendations for collection, storage and handling of a mother's milk for her own infant in the hospital setting. 3rd ed. Denver: Human Milk Banking Association of North America, 1999

58. Howard C, Howard F, Lawrence R, Andresen E, DeBlieck E, Weitzman M. Office prenatal formula advertising and its effect on breast-feeding patterns. Obstet Gynecol 2000;95:296–303

59. Pérez-Escamilla R, Pollitt E, Lönnerdal B, Dewey KG. Infant feeding policies in maternity wards and their effect on breast-feeding success: an analytical overview. Am J Public Health 1994;84:89–97

60. Zemlickis D, Lishner M, Degendorfer P, Panzarella T, Burke B, Sutcliffe SB, et al. Maternal and fetal outcome after breast cancer in pregnancy. Am J Obstet Gynecol 1992;166:781–787

61. Healthy people 2010, volume II. Washington, DC: U.S. Department of Health and Human Services, 2000: 16-46–16-48

62. Ryan AS. The resurgence of breastfeeding in the United States. Pediatrics 1997;99:E12

63. Freed GL, Clark SJ, Cefalo RC, Sorenson JR. Breast-feeding education of obstetrics-gynecology residents and practitioners. Am J Obstet Gynecol 1995;173:1607–1613

ACOG EDUCATIONAL BULLETIN

Number 227, August 1996

Management of Isoimmunization in Pregnancy

This Educational Bulletin was developed under the direction of the Committee on Educational Bulletins of the American College of Obstetricians and Gynecologists as an aid to obstetricians and gynecologists. The College wishes to thank Michael L. Socol, MD, for his assistance in the development of this bulletin. This document is not to be construed as establishing a standard of practice or dictating an exclusive course of treatment. Rather, it is intended as an educational tool that presents current information on obstetric–gynecologic issues.

When any fetal blood group factor inherited from the father is not possessed by the mother, antepartum or intrapartum fetal–maternal bleeding may stimulate an immune reaction by the mother. Maternal immune reactions can also occur from blood product transfusion. The formation of maternal antibodies to a foreign antigen may be followed by various degrees of transplacental passage of these antibodies into the fetal circulation. Depending on the degree of antigenicity and the amount and type of antibody involved, this transplacental passage may lead to hemolytic disease of the newborn.

The reproductive history of a woman with isoimmunization is of considerable importance in recognizing and determining the prognosis for a subsequent isoimmunized pregnancy. For example, if a D-negative, isoimmunized woman becomes pregnant with a D-positive fetus, the severity of the hemolytic disease will usually be equal to or greater than that of the previous pregnancy. Occasionally, the disease progression may be such that early-onset fetal hydrops may occur in a patient who experienced only mildly affected prior pregnancies. In rare cases, hemolytic disease in the current pregnancy may be less severe than in a prior pregnancy. Regardless of obstetric history, all pregnant women should undergo laboratory examinations at the first prenatal visit to determine the possibility of isoimmunization. Tests should include determination of ABO and D types as well as a screen for the presence of antibodies by an indirect Coombs test (antibody screen).

Factors that minimize the chance of isoimmunization to the D antigen are detailed elsewhere (1). There are no preventive strategies against sensitization to blood factors other than the D antigen. Although some of these antibodies are not clinically significant, most do gain access to the fetus across the placenta and can potentially cause fetal anemia and hydrops. Fortunately, ABO incompatibility, which is a common cause of subclinical and mild hemolytic disease of the newborn, does not cause clinical or severe erythroblastosis. Therefore, no antenatal testing, either by titer or by amniocentesis, is necessary when there is a history of ABO incompatibility.

Replaces Number 148, October 1990

Clinically Significant Antibodies

CDE System

Anti-D isoimmunization remains the most common cause of erythroblastosis fetalis. Antibodies formed in response to the D antigen are of the immunoglobulin G (IgG) type. Consequently, they can cross the placenta and hemolyze fetal erythrocytes. Whereas most clinically significant blood group sensitizations noted during pregnancy are still secondary to anti-D incompatibility, sensitization to antigens other than D in the CDE system is not uncommon and can cause severe disease.

Other Antibodies

The most frequently encountered antibodies other than D are Lewis antibodies (Le^a and Le^b). Like most cold agglutinins, Lewis antigens do not cause erythroblastosis fetalis because they are predominantly of the IgM type and they are poorly expressed on fetal and newborn erythrocytes. In contrast, Kell antibodies (k, K, Kp^a, Kp^b, Js^a, Js^b) can produce erythroblastosis fetalis. Kell isoimmunization is often caused by prior transfusion, since Kell compatibility is usually not considered when blood is crossmatched. Fortunately, 90% of partners of Kell-immunized women are Kell negative themselves. Less common, but just as likely to cause erythroblastosis fetalis, are some of the Duffy antigens. Additional antibodies known to cause hemolytic disease are listed in Table 1. Care of patients with sensitization to antigens other than D that are known to cause hemolytic disease should be the same as that for patients with D isoimmunization. A possible exception is Kell sensitization, in which amniotic fluid analysis has been reported to correlate poorly with the severity of fetal anemia (2). These patients may benefit from more aggressive fetal assessment; however, optimal management of Kell-sensitized patients is controversial (3).

Clinical Management

Once it has been established that a pregnant woman is sensitized to an antigen that may cause erythroblastosis, the genotype of the fetus's father should be determined. This is most useful for the atypical antigens because isoimmunization is often secondary to a transfusion. If the father of the fetus does not possess the antigen, the fetus is not at risk. If the father is a heterozygote there is only a 50% chance that the fetus has inherited the blood group antigen and the pregnancy is affected. The most likely zygosity for the D antigen can also be predicted as the alleles at the C, D, and E loci are inherited together, and some combinations are more frequent than others. Because it is not possible to test for the presence of D antigens, zygosity can be determined only by looking at the combination. Clinically, however, determining this genotype is of limited value for the couple receiving counseling after a severely affected pregnancy. Unless the D-positive partner has previously fathered a D-negative child, it is impossible to state with certainty that he is a heterozygote.

Antibody Titers

Maternal serum antibody titers can be measured by a variety of techniques (4). Agglutination of erythrocytes in saline measures maternal IgM antibody, and this is too large a molecule to cross the placenta. Albumin is a more viscous medium; therefore, the smaller IgG molecules are capable of agglutinating erythrocytes, but the contribution by IgM is not eliminated. The most sensitive and accurate barometer for clinical practice is the indirect Coombs test.

The usefulness of maternal serum antibody titers is determined by the patient's reproductive history. If a patient has never had a pregnancy complicated by Rh-related neonatal morbidity other than hyperbilirubinemia treated by phototherapy, antibody titers are the initial step of management. An antibody titer should be determined at the first prenatal visit, at 20 weeks of gestation, and approximately every 4 weeks thereafter. When the antibody titer is ≤ 1:8, whether directed to D or another paternal antigen capable of causing severe erythroblastosis, no intervention is necessary; when the titer is ≥ 1:16 in albumin or 1:32 by indirect antiglobulin (indirect Coombs test), amniocentesis or percutaneous umbilical cord blood sampling (cordocentesis) should be considered (5).

TABLE 1. ISOIMMUNIZATION RESULTING FROM IRREGULAR ANTIBODIES*

Blood Group System	Antigen
Rh	C, c, e, E
Kell	K, k, Ko, Kp^a, Kp^b, Js^a, Js^b
Duffy	Fy^a, Fy^b, Fy^3
Kidd	Jk^a, Jk^b, Jk^3
MNSs	M, N, S, s, U, Mi^a, Mt^a, Vw, Mur, Hil, Hut
Lutheran	Lu^a, Lu^b
Diego	Di^a, Di^b
Xg	Xg^a
P	PP$_1$p^k(Tj^a)
Public antigens	Yt^a, Yt^b, Lan, En^a, Ge, Jr^a, Co^a, Co^{a-b-}
Private antigens	Batty, Becker, Berrens, Biles, Evans, Gonzales, Good, Heibel, Hunt, Jobbins, Radin, Rm, Ven, Wright^a, Wright^b, Zd

* Lewis (Le^a, Le^b) and I antigens are not causes of hemolytic disease of the newborn.

Modified from Socol ML. Management of blood group isoimmunization. In: Gleicher N. Principles and practice of medical therapy in pregnancy. 2nd ed. Norwalk, Connecticut: Appleton and Lange, 1992:1051

If a patient has had a prior affected pregnancy (neonatal exchange transfusion, early delivery, or intrauterine transfusion), antibody titers are not necessary because amniocentesis or percutaneous umbilical cord blood sampling will be required. The timing of the initial procedure is determined by past clinical history. It is usually performed at least 4–8 weeks earlier than the prior gestational age at which significant morbidity occurred, with some clinicians beginning at 20 weeks or even earlier.

Amniocentesis and Percutaneous Umbilical Cord Blood Sampling

Since the mid-1960s, amniocentesis with spectrophotometric examination of the amniotic fluid has been the accepted method for assessing the severity of erythroblastosis in utero. Amniotic fluid bilirubin is most likely derived from fetal tracheal and pulmonary secretions. It can be quantitated by spectrophotometrically measuring absorbance at the 450-nm wavelength in a specimen of amniotic fluid that has been shielded from light. The deviation from linearity (change in optical density at 450 nm [ΔOD_{450}]) is determined by measuring the difference between this absorbance and a straight line drawn from points 365 nm to 535 nm on the spectrophotometric curve. Contamination of amniotic fluid by meconium and by erythrocytes and their porphyrin breakdown products can significantly alter spectrophotometric analysis at 450 nm, but these problems can be largely overcome by chloroform extraction of the amniotic fluid (6). Heme pigment will also generate a peak at the 405-nm wavelength, and in the absence of blood contamination this may be indicative of severe hemolysis (4).

Fetal status is determined by plotting the ΔOD_{450} measurement on a Liley graph (Fig. 1) (7). Readings in zone III (uppermost zone) suggest severe hemolytic disease with a high probability of fetal death within 7–10 days. Readings in zone I (lowest zone) are reassuring although neonatal exchange transfusion may be necessary occasionally. There are no reliable data concerning the optimal frequency for repeated sampling. In general, amniocentesis is repeated every 1–4 weeks if the ΔOD_{450} measurement is in zone II (middle zone) and every 3–4 weeks if it has dropped into zone I. The frequency depends on where in zone II the value falls and the pattern established in previous procedures. Declining values are encouraging although they do not preclude mild hemolytic disease. Stable or rising ΔOD_{450} measurements are causes of concern.

Patients with results in zone I or low zone II can be allowed to proceed to term, at which point labor should be induced. In most cases, patients in the middle of zone II can progress to 36–38 weeks of gestation, at which time delivery should be accomplished, by induction of labor if possible. Depending on gestational age, patients in zone III should either be delivered or should receive intrauterine fetal transfusion. Similar considerations may apply to a rising titer in upper zone II. Delivery is often by cesarean birth because of an unfavorable cervix, but a trial of labor is not contraindicated.

Percutaneous umbilical cord blood sampling has improved the obstetric care of isoimmunized patients because of the ability to evaluate fetal status precisely. This is particularly true in the middle trimester, when amniotic fluid from unaffected fetuses will also contain bilirubin. Peak values of bilirubin are present between 20 and 24 weeks of gestation. The Liley curve was generated from pregnancies of at least 28 weeks of gestation. In the past, obstetricians have derived values for pregnancies of 20–27 weeks of gestation by extrapolating backwards from the Liley curve; however, such extrapolations may be inappropriate (8). In either the second or the third trimester, knowledge of the specific fetal hematocrit enables the physician to take a more rational approach to the need for, volume of, and timing of fetal transfusions. Hematologic values for normal fetuses from 15 to 30 weeks of gestation are shown in Table 2 (9, 10). In some instances, findings may even indicate that the fetus does not possess the blood group antigen in question and therefore requires no further evaluation. Perhaps most importantly, the use of amniocentesis in conjunction with percutaneous umbilical cord blood sampling allows a more aggressive approach at an earlier gestational age.

In spite of the enthusiasm that percutaneous umbilical cord blood sampling has generated for fetal diagnosis and therapy, some caution should be exercised. First, a chart of spectrophotometric measurements from sensitized pregnancies in the middle trimester has been constructed that may minimize the benefit of fetal blood sampling as the primary assessment of fetal status (11). Second, determination of fetal blood type, particularly for the D antigen, can be accomplished by polymerase chain reaction on fetal amniocytes and therefore does not always require a fetal blood sample (12). It should be emphasized, however, that these tests should be done in specialized laboratories with considerable experience in polymerase chain reaction testing. Third, liberal use of percutaneous umbilical cord blood sampling may induce an anamnestic immune response in the mother secondary to fetal–maternal hemorrhage, thereby accelerating the disease process (13, 14). Fourth, the loss rate with percutaneous umbilical cord blood sampling is generally agreed to be greater than that with amniocentesis. Consequently, whereas fetal blood sampling as the principal means of fetal assessment in isoimmunized pregnancies appears safe and effective in experienced hands (15, 16), most clinicians continue to rely primarily on amniocentesis.

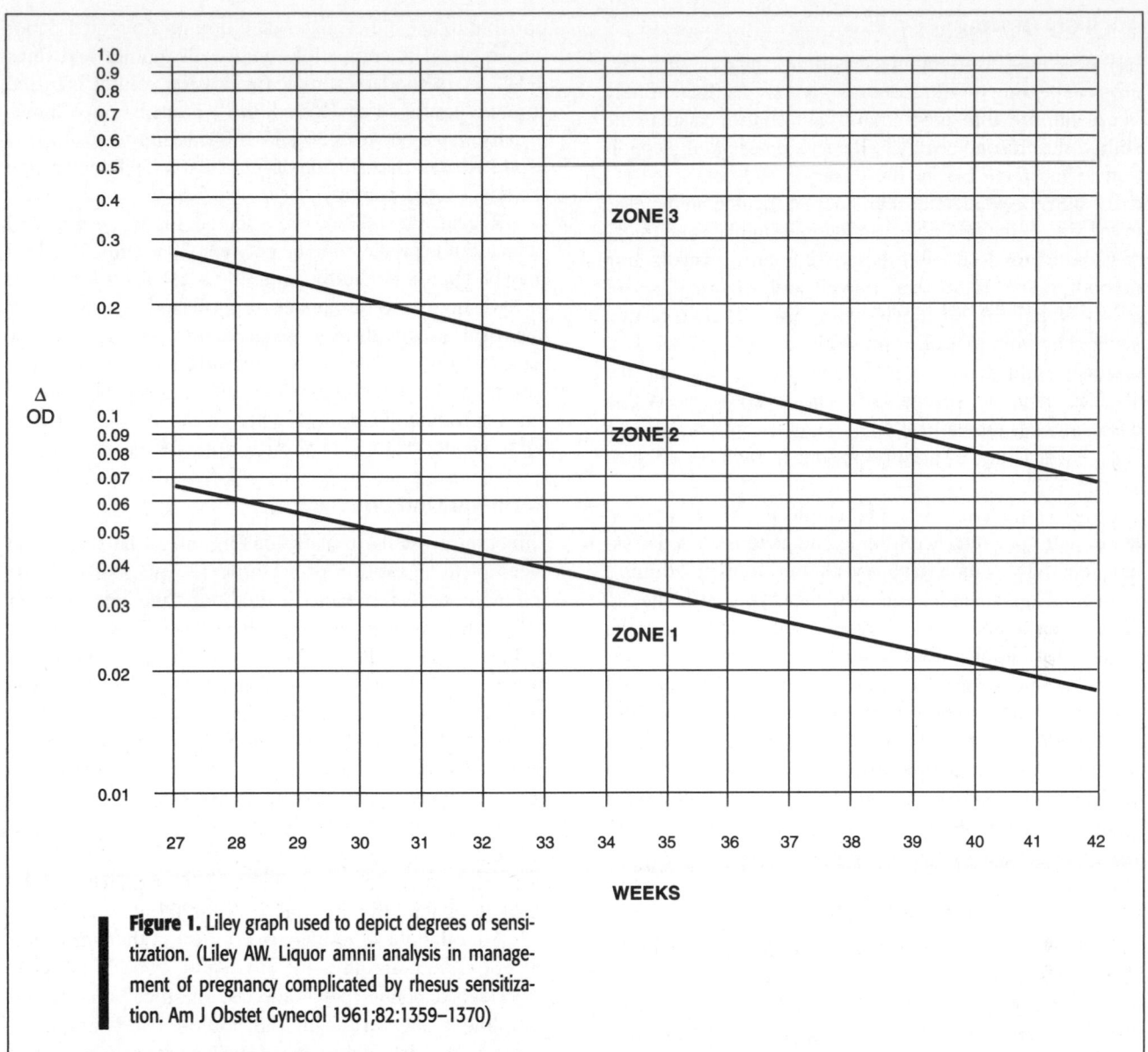

Figure 1. Liley graph used to depict degrees of sensitization. (Liley AW. Liquor amnii analysis in management of pregnancy complicated by rhesus sensitization. Am J Obstet Gynecol 1961;82:1359–1370)

TABLE 2. HEMATOLOGIC VALUES FOR NORMAL FETUSES*

Hematologic Value†	Gestational Age (Weeks)					
	15	16–17	18–20	21–22	23–25	26–30
Hgb (g/100 ml)	10.9 ± 0.7	12.5 ± 0.8	11.48 ± 0.78	12.29 ± 0.89	12.4 ± 0.77	13.36 ± 1.18
RBC (×10⁹/L)	2.43 ± 0.26	2.68 ± 0.21	2.66 ± 0.29	2.97 ± 0.27	3.06 ± 0.27	3.52 ± 0.32
MCV (±1)	143 ± 8	143 ± 12	133.9 ± 8.83	130 ± 6.17	126.2 ± 6.23	118.2 ± 5.7

*Values are for normal fetuses from 15 to 30 weeks of estimated gestational age.

†Hgb indicates hemoglobin; RBC, red blood cells; MCV, mean corpuscular volume.

Ancillary Testing

In the severely isoimmunized patient, signs of early hydrops appearing on ultrasonography may facilitate timely intervention. More problematic and controversial is the ability of ultrasonography to detect a deteriorating condition in the fetus before the onset of hydrops. Reported early signs of worsening fetal anemia include an increase in the size of the fetal liver, an increase in placental thickness, pericardial effusion, polyhydramnios, visualization of both sides of the fetal bowel, and abnormalities of pulsed Doppler flow-velocity waveforms. There is no evidence, however, that ultrasound markers can reliably distinguish mild from severe hemolytic disease in the absence of fetal hydrops (17). One study suggests that hydramnios is the earliest sign of significant fetal anemia (18), but it is not invariably present in severely affected cases.

Electronic fetal heart rate monitoring allows dynamic evaluation of fetal well-being and central nervous system reactivity. Some severely anemic fetuses exhibit a sinusoidal heart rate pattern, which has been attributed to the absence of autonomic nervous system control over the heart, high-output cardiac failure, or tissue hypoxia of the fetal heart and central nervous system. Nonreactive, suboptimal, or pathologic fetal heart rate patterns have also been reported more commonly in sensitized fetuses who were hypoxic and anemic than in those who had normal oxygen levels and were not anemic. Characteristics of the fetal heart rate pattern, however, did not accurately predict the degree of anemia or oxygenation (19).

Intrauterine Fetal Transfusion

Before physicians were able to gain direct access to the fetal circulation, intraperitoneal fetal transfusion was indicated if serial spectrophotometric measurements rose into upper zone II before 30 weeks of gestation or into zone III before 32–34 weeks of pregnancy. The infused blood was absorbed into the fetal circulation via the subdiaphragmatic lymphatic system. In the nonhydropic fetus, the rate of absorption was estimated to be 10–15% per 24 hours. Absorption was slower if hydrops was already evident (4).

Because of erratic absorption, especially in hydropic fetuses, intravascular fetal transfusion (20, 21) has largely replaced the intraperitoneal technique, although some investigators advocate a combined intravascular and intraperitoneal approach in select circumstances (22, 23). The fetal hematocrit level at which to initiate transfusion is somewhat arbitrary, but the value of 25% seems reasonable (24). Transfusions are performed using type O, Rh-negative, cytomegalovirus-negative, washed, irradiated packed cells cross-matched against maternal blood. After the fetal blood type is determined, it may occasionally be possible to use either maternal blood or a targeted donor whose blood is compatible with both mother and fetus (25). One method to estimate transfusion volume is by the formula described by Rodeck (26). Transfusion volumes usually range between 30 and 100 ml, and fetal blood is aspirated at the conclusion of the transfusion to determine the adequacy of therapy.

Repeat transfusions are planned for when the fetal hematocrit is predicted to be between 20% and 25%. This may be approximated by assuming a 1% decline per day or by using one of a number of published equations (27, 28). In fetuses with more severe hemolytic anemia, few fetal erythrocytes survive the initial transfusion interval. Therefore, the interval between first and second transfusions is usually 7–14 days, whereas the interval between subsequent transfusions or birth is 21–28 days.

Perinatal Outcome

Direct intravascular transfusion eliminates the erratic and incomplete absorption of erythrocytes inherent with the intraperitoneal approach. In addition, the intravascular technique allows more precise evaluation of the need for and adequacy of therapy by measurements of the initial and final fetal hematocrits. Consequently, it is not surprising that perinatal survival rates for severely isoimmunized fetuses following intravascular transfusion are now reported in excess of 80% (16, 21, 29–32). The improved survival rate is especially noteworthy when the early gestational ages at which therapy is being attempted are considered. Also encouraging is the improved outcome for hydropic fetuses. In one series, 16 of 20 pregnancies complicated by fetal hydrops had successful outcomes (33).

Although these results are promising, there are complications with any invasive procedure. Even in the most experienced hands, percutaneous umbilical cord blood sampling alone results in procedure-related pregnancy loss of approximately 1% (34). The procedure-related mortality for intravascular transfusion has been reported to be between 4% and 9% (29–31, 33). Additional significant morbidity has included nonremediable prolonged fetal heart rate decelerations that required emergent cesarean delivery (35) and increases in maternal antibody titer, presumably secondary to fetal–maternal hemorrhage (13, 14). When weighing the procedure-related risks against those for the neonate in the nursery, one should seriously consider delivery rather than performing an intravascular transfusion after 34 completed weeks of pregnancy.

Summary

Isoimmunization is diagnosed by a positive antibody screen and requires identification of the specific antigen responsible, classification of the antigen into either a clinically significant or a benign group, and titration of the level of antibody response. The paternal antigen status and zygosity should be determined whenever possible. Repetitive amniocentesis or fetal blood sampling may be required to monitor the fetal condition adequately. Early and continued consultation with experts in the management of this condition is key to developing an appropriate therapeutic plan that includes proper management at delivery and optimal neonatal support. New technologies and expertise now allow better outcome for severely affected fetuses.

References

1. American College of Obstetricians and Gynecologists. Prevention of D isoimmunization. ACOG Technical Bulletin 147. Washington, DC: ACOG, 1990 (Level III)

2. Caime ME, Mueller-Heubach E. Kell sensitization in pregnancy. Am J Obstet Gynecol 1986;154:85–90 (Level III)

3. Weiner CP, Widness JA. Decreased fetal erythropoiesis and hemolysis in Kell hemolytic anemia. Am J Obstet Gynecol 1996;174:547–551 (Level II-3)

4. Bowman JM. Maternal blood group isoimmunization. In: Creasy RK, Resnik R, eds. Maternal–fetal medicine: principles and practice. 3rd ed. Philadelphia: WB Saunders, 1994:711–743 (Level III)

5. Bowman JM, Pollock JM. Transplacental fetal hemorrhage after amniocentesis. Obstet Gynecol 1985;66:749–754 (Level II-3)

6. Brazie JV, Bowes WA Jr, Ibbott FA. An improved, rapid procedure for the determination of amniotic fluid bilirubin and its use in the prediction of the course of Rh-sensitized pregnancies. Am J Obstet Gynecol 1969;104:80–86 (Level III)

7. Liley AW. Liquor amnii analysis in the management of pregnancy complicated by rhesus sensitization. Am J Obstet Gynecol 1961;82:1359–1370 (Level III)

8. Nicolaides KH, Rodeck CH, Mibashan RS, Kemp JR. Have Liley charts outlived their usefulness? Am J Obstet Gynecol 1986;155:90–94 (Level III)

9. Forestier F, Daffos F, Galacteros F, Bardakjian J, Rainaut M, Beuzard Y. Hematological values of 163 normal fetuses between 18 and 30 weeks of gestation. Pediatr Res 1986; 20:342–346 (Level II-3)

10. Millar DS, Davis LR, Rodeck CH, Nicolaides KH, Mibashan RS. Normal blood cell values in the early midtrimester fetus. Prenat Diagn 1985;5:367–373 (Level III)

11. Queenan JT, Tomai TP, Ural SH, King JC. Deviation in amniotic fluid optical density at a wavelength of 450 nm in Rh-immunized pregnancies from 14 to 40 weeks' gestation: a proposal for clinical management. Am J Obstet Gynecol 1993;168:1370–1376 (Level III)

12. Fisk NM, Bennett P, Warwick RM, Letsky EA, Welch R, Vaughan JI, et al. Clinical utility of fetal RhD typing in alloimmunized pregnancies by means of polymerase chain reaction on amniocytes or chorionic villi. Am J Obstet Gynecol 1994;171:50–54 (Level III)

13. Nicolini U, Kochenour NK, Greco P, Letsky EA, Johnson RD, Contreras M, et al. Consequences of fetomaternal haemorrhage after intrauterine transfusion. BMJ 1988;297: 1379–1381 (Level III)

14. MacGregor SN, Silver RK, Sholl JS. Enhanced sensitization after cordocentesis in a rhesus-isoimmunized pregnancy. Am J Obstet Gynecol 1991;165:382–383 (Level III)

15. Weiner CP, Williamson RA, Wenstrom KD, Sipes SL, Grant SS, Widness JA. Management of fetal hemolytic disease by cordocentesis. I. Prediction of fetal anemia. Am J Obstet Gynecol 1991;165:546–553 (Level II-3)

16. Weiner CP, Williamson RA, Wenstrom KD, Sipes SL, Widness JA, Grant SS, et al. Management of fetal hemolytic disease by cordocentesis. II. Outcome of treatment. Am J Obstet Gynecol 1991;165:1302–1307 (Level II-3)

17. Nicolaides KH, Fontanarosa M, Gabbe SG, Rodeck CH. Failure of ultrasonographic parameters to predict the severity of fetal anemia in Rhesus isoimmunization. Am J Obstet Gynecol 1988;158:920–926 (Level II-2)

18. Chitkara U, Wilkins I, Lynch L, Mehalek K, Berkowitz RL. The role of sonography in assessing severity of fetal anemia in Rh- and Kell-isoimmunized pregnancies. Obstet Gynecol 1988;71:393–398 (Level III)

19. Nicolaides KH. Studies on fetal physiology and pathophysiology in Rhesus disease. Semin Perinatol 1989;13:328–337 (Level III)

20. Socol ML, MacGregor SN, Pielet BW, Tamura RK, Sabbagha RE. Percutaneous umbilical transfusion in severe rhesus isoimmunization: resolution of fetal hydrops. Am J Obstet Gynecol 1987;157:1369–1375 (Level III)

21. Harman CR, Bowman JM, Manning FA, Menticoglou SM. Intrauterine transfusion—intraperitoneal versus intravascular approach: a case–control comparison. Am J Obstet Gynecol 1990;162:1053–1059 (Level II-2)

22. Pattison N, Roberts A. The management of severe erythroblastosis fetalis by fetal transfusion: survival of transfused adult erythrocytes in the fetus. Obstet Gynecol 1989; 74:901–904 (Level II-3)

23. Moise KJ, Giancarlo M, Fisher DJ, Huhta JC, Cano LE, Carpenter RJ Jr. Acute fetal hemodynamic alterations after intrauterine transfusion for treatment of severe red blood cell alloimmunization. Am J Obstet Gynecol 1990;163: 776–784 (Level II-3)

24. Reece EA, Copel JA, Scioscia AL, Grannum PAT, DeGennaro N, Hobbins JC. Diagnostic fetal umbilical blood sampling in the management of isoimmunization. Am J Obstet Gynecol 1988;159:1057–1062 (Level III)

25. Gonsoulin WJ, Moise KJ Jr, Milam JD, Sala JD, Weber VW, Carpenter RJ Jr. Serial maternal blood donations for intrauterine transfusion. Obstet Gynecol 1990;75:158–162 (Level II-3)

26. Rodeck CH, Nicolaides KH, Warsof SL, Fysh WJ, Gamsu HR, Kemp JR. The management of severe rhesus iso-immunization by fetoscopic intravascular transfusions. Am J Obstet Gynecol 1984;150:769–774 (Level III)

27. Plecas DV, Chitkara U, Berkowitz GS, Lapinski RH, Alvarez M, Berkowitz RL. Intrauterine intravascular transfusion for severe erythroblastosis fetalis: how much to transfuse? Obstet Gynecol 1990;75:965–969 (Level II-3)

28. MacGregor SN, Socol ML, Pielet BW, Sholl JS, Silver RK. Prediction of hematocrit decline after intravascular fetal transfusion. Am J Obstet Gynecol 1989;161:1491–1493 (Level II-3)

29. Ney JA, Socol ML, Dooley SL, MacGregor SN, Silver RK, Millard DD. Perinatal outcome following intravascular transfusion in severely isoimmunized fetuses. Int J Gynaecol Obstet 1991;35:41–46 (Level II-3)

30. Berkowitz RL, Chitkara U, Wilkins IA, Lynch L, Plosker H, Bernstein HH. Intravascular monitoring and management of erythroblastosis fetalis. Am J Obstet Gynecol 1988;158: 783–795 (Level III)

31. Barss VA, Benacerraf BR, Frigoletto FD, Greene MF, Penso C, Saltzman DH, et al. Management of isoimmunized pregnancy by use of intravascular techniques. Am J Obstet Gynecol 1988;159:932–937 (Level III)

32. Parer JT. Severe Rh isoimmunization—current methods of in utero diagnosis and treatment. Am J Obstet Gynecol 1988;158:1323–1329 (Level III)

33. Grannum PAT, Copel JA, Moya FR, Scioscia AL, Robert JA, Winn HN, et al. The reversal of hydrops fetalis by intravascular intrauterine transfusion in severe isoimmune fetal anemia. Am J Obstet Gynecol 1988;158:914–919 (Level III)

34. Daffos F, Capella-Pavlovsky M, Forestier F. Fetal blood sampling during pregnancy with use of a needle guided by ultrasound: a study of 606 consecutive cases. Am J Obstet Gynecol 1985;153:655–660 (Level III)

35. Pielet BW, Socol ML, MacGregor SN, Ney JA, Dooley SL. Cordocentesis: an appraisal of risks. Am J Obstet Gynecol 1988;159:1497–1500 (Level III)

The references in this bulletin are graded according to the method outlined by the U.S. Preventive Services Task Force:

I   Evidence obtained from at least one properly designed randomized controlled trial

II-1 Evidence obtained from well-designed controlled trials without randomization

II-2 Evidence obtained from well-designed cohort or case–control analytic studies, preferably from more than one center or research group

II-3 Evidence obtained from multiple time series, with or without intervention, or dramatic results in uncontrolled experiments

III   Opinions of respected authorities, based on clinical experience, descriptive studies, or reports of expert committees

ACOG EDUCATIONAL BULLETIN

Number 251, September 1998

Obstetric Aspects of Trauma Management

This Educational Bulletin was developed under the direction of the Committee on Educational Bulletins of the American College of Obstetricians and Gynecologists as an aid to obstetricians and gynecologists. The College wishes to thank Mark Pearlman, MD, and Cosmas van de Ven, MD, for their assistance in the development of this bulletin. This document is not to be construed as establishing a standard of practice or dictating an exclusive course of treatment. Rather, it is intended as an educational tool that presents current information on obstetric–gynecologic issues.

Trauma has become one of the leading causes of morbidity and mortality of women in the world, resulting in nearly one million deaths each year. It also has become one of the leading causes of morbidity and mortality during pregnancy (1, 2). It is estimated that physical trauma complicates approximately 1 in every 12 pregnancies, with motor vehicle crashes being the most significant contributor to fetal death due to trauma (3). Nearly 50,000 of the estimated 250 million people in the United States die each year from motor vehicle crashes. This rate is equivalent to approximately 20 deaths due to motor vehicle crashes for every 100,000 persons in the United States.

The incidence and severity of injuries can be lessened by the appropriate use of automobile safety restraints. Physicians should counsel patients about such use and reassure them of the safety of these devices during pregnancy. Despite these precautions, injuries will occur during pregnancy and obstetrician–gynecologists should be equipped to handle them.

Optimum management of the seriously injured pregnant woman requires an integrated effort of multiple specialties, starting with emergency medical technicians, emergency medicine physicians, trauma surgeons, and other specialists, depending on the type of injury. Obstetricians play a central role in the management of injured pregnant women. Their knowledge and expertise are vital to management decisions regarding both the woman and the fetus. The effects of various drugs on uterine blood flow, potential teratogenic and mutagenic effects of diagnostic radiation and medications, the effect of surgery on pregnancy, and the assessment of gestational age are critical management issues. In addition, complications of pregnancy unrelated to the trauma may be superimposed in the injured gravida (eg, pregnancy-induced hypertension, placenta previa) and are best managed by the obstetrician. The obstetrician may be consulted regarding the condition of a pregnant trauma patient or, more commonly, may be the primary physician caring for the patient following trauma. In either case, the approach must be systematic, ensuring that the woman is medically stable prior to evaluation of the fetus.

Obstetricians who are involved with the care of pregnant trauma patients should seek consultation with experienced trauma surgeons. It also is helpful for all physicians to be knowledgeable about advanced trauma life-support measures.

Replaces Number 151, January 1991, and Number 161, November 1991

Incidence

In industrialized nations, approximately two thirds of all trauma during pregnancy results from motor vehicle crashes. Other frequent causes of trauma during pregnancy are falls and direct assaults to the abdomen (3, 4). According to the National Safety Council, female drivers are more likely to be involved in automobile accidents than male drivers (84 female drivers versus 73 male drivers per 10 million miles driven) (5).

Domestic violence has reached epidemic proportion in the United States. It is estimated that approximately 2 million women per year are reported to have been assaulted by their male partners (6). Researchers have found a prevalence of violence against pregnant women ranging from 1% to 20% (7). Domestic violence and battery were found to occur in 1 of every 12 pregnant women in an inner-city setting (8). Among victims of physical abuse, moderate or severe violence during pregnancy was reported by 20% of women in the Baltimore area, 17% in Houston, 7% in Galveston, and 7% in Toronto (9, 10). Sixty percent of victims report two or more episodes of physical assault during pregnancy (11). This latter statistic emphasizes the importance of early identification of physical abuse during pregnancy and implementation of effective intervention methods, which are discussed elsewhere (6).

Maternal Mortality

Trauma, either accidental (as in traffic accidents) or intentional (as in homicide or domestic violence), is a leading cause of death in women of reproductive age (1). Trauma also is the leading cause of nonobstetric maternal death (12); for example, it accounted for an average of 22% of all maternal deaths in Iowa and caused nearly one half of 95 maternal deaths from 1986 to 1989 in Cook County, Illinois (2).

Fetal Mortality

Accurate statistics on the number of fetal losses due to trauma each year are not available. Estimates extrapolated from published case series suggest that between 1,300 and 3,900 pregnancies are lost each year in the United States as a result of trauma (13).

Life-threatening maternal trauma (eg, maternal shock, head injury resulting in coma, emergency laparotomy for maternal indications) is associated with a 40–50% fetal loss rate, whereas minor or non–life-threatening injuries resulted in a 1–5% pregnancy loss (14). Because minor injuries are more common, most fetal losses result from minor maternal injuries (4, 15, 16). It is estimated that abruptio placentae is a complication in 40–50% of pregnant women who sustain severe trauma, compared with the 1–5% incidence in pregnant women

who experience non–life-threatening trauma (4, 16–19). Several series of fetal losses resulting from trauma indicate that more than 50% of fetal losses occur in association with seemingly minor or insignificant maternal trauma (4, 15, 16, 18, 20).

Numerous retrospective studies have attempted to predict fetal or neonatal outcome based on an injury severity score. However, one study suggests that injury severity scoring is not a good predictor of adverse fetal outcome (21).

Types of Trauma

Blunt Abdominal Trauma

The evaluation and management of blunt abdominal trauma during pregnancy involves several key issues. Gestational age at the time of injury, extent and severity of maternal injury, and mechanism of injury should be considered.

The gestational age at the time of injury is valuable in determining the need for fetal assessment as well as in managing the mother's condition. The possibility of fetal viability in an extrauterine environment (ie, beyond 24–26 weeks of gestation) can significantly change management decisions if there is evidence of fetal compromise. Furthermore, enlargement of the uterus beyond 18–20 weeks of gestation compresses both the inferior vena cava and aorta in the supine position, increasing the likelihood of hypotension and decreased uterine perfusion. Finally, the type of maternal and fetal injury patterns may depend to a great extent on gestational age at the time of injury. For example, direct injury to the uterus and fetus prior to 13 weeks of gestation is extremely unlikely because they are protected by the bony pelvis. Generally, trauma in the first trimester does not cause pregnancy loss, with the exception of profound hypotension and associated hypoperfusion of the uterus and its contents. Although it is not the highest priority in managing the injured gravida, gestational age should be assessed as soon as feasible.

Fetal loss resulting from blunt abdominal trauma may result from abruptio placentae or other placental injury, direct fetal injury, uterine rupture, maternal shock, or death or some combination thereof. Several studies of trauma and fetal loss show that at least 50% of fetal losses with known etiology were the result of abruptio placenta (4, 15, 16, 18). In one report of severe car crashes involving pregnant women, maternal loss of life was the most frequent cause of fetal death (17).

There are several potential mechanisms of abruptio placentae due to trauma. Differences in tissue properties between the elastic myometrium and the relatively inelastic placenta can result in a shearing at the tissue interface. Because fluid is noncompressible, intrusion of the elastic uterine wall will result in displacement of amniotic fluid and distention of the other parts of the uterus. Therefore, a shear force can occur regardless of placental location. The risk of abruptio placentae appears to be independent of the placental location (3).

Direct fetal injury (eg, skull fracture) complicates less than 1% of all pregnancies in which trauma occurs. Although case reports of fetal skull fractures have been described following relatively minor trauma, most cases result from significant maternal injury later in gestation (22, 23).

Uterine rupture is an infrequent but life-threatening complication of trauma. It occurs in only 0.6% of all injuries during pregnancy and tends to complicate trauma resulting from direct abdominal impact associated with substantial force (24, 25). The extent of uterine injury can be variable, and it may result in serosal hemorrhage or abrasions; avulsion of the uterine vasculature with hemorrhage; complete disruption of the myometrial wall with extrusion of the fetus, placenta, or umbilical cord into the abdominal cavity; or complete uterine avulsion. Approximately 75% of reported cases of uterine rupture involve the fundus. The presentation of uterine rupture can range from subtle findings (eg, uterine tenderness, nonreassuring fetal heart rate patterns) without changes in maternal vital signs, to rapid onset of maternal hypovolemic shock. Signs of peritoneal irritation, such as distention, rebound tenderness, guarding, and rigidity are frequently detected upon examination but may be less pronounced during pregnancy.

Pelvic Fractures

Pelvic fractures may result in significant retroperitoneal bleeding, which is associated with substantial morbidity and mortality. When combined with the possibility of intraperitoneal bleeding, pelvic fractures are frequently associated with hypovolemic shock. Associated injuries of the bladder or urethral disruption can result in hematuria and also may pose difficulty in placing a urinary catheter.

Pelvic fracture is not a definite contraindication for vaginal delivery. Even in the presence of a slightly displaced pelvic fracture, safe vaginal delivery can be accomplished. However, a severe, dislocated, or unstable fracture or a large healing callus may preclude an attempt at vaginal delivery.

Penetrating Trauma

Most penetrating abdominal trauma results from gunshot wounds or stab wounds. Penetrating abdominal trauma during pregnancy has a remarkably disparate prognosis for the fetus and the woman (26, 27). Fetal loss due to penetrating trauma usually occurs through direct injury or by injury to the cord or placenta. Maternal outcome generally is more favorable because the maternal viscera are shielded by the uterus and its contents, which absorbs much of the projectile energy.

The extent and severity of maternal and fetal injury due to gunshot wounds depends on a number of factors including the size and velocity of the bullet; the anatomic region penetrated; the angle of entry; deflection of the bullet's trajectory by muscle, bone, or viscera; the gestational age of the fetus; and the distance from which the bullet was fired. Frequently, more internal damage occurs than that suggested by the appearance of the entrance wound.

The enlarged uterus tends to protect the bowel from injury when stab wounds penetrate the lower abdomen because the bowel is displaced into the upper abdomen. However, as a result of cephalad displacement of the bowel by the enlarging uterus, stab wounds to the upper abdomen can frequently result in more complex bowel injury than in the nonpregnant woman.

Management

The primary goal and initial efforts in managing the injured pregnant woman should be evaluation and stabilization of maternal vital signs. If attention is drawn to the fetus before the woman is stabilized, serious or life-threatening maternal injuries may be overlooked, or circumstances that can compromise fetal oxygenation (eg, maternal hypoxemia, hypovolemia, or supine hypotension) may be ignored, lessening the likelihood of both maternal and fetal survival.

A systematic approach begins with a primary survey of the woman by securing and maintaining an airway, ensuring adequate breathing, and maintaining adequate circulatory volume. The placement of two large-bore (14–16 gauge) intravenous lines is necessary in most seriously injured trauma patients. Supplemental oxygen should be administered by nasal cannula, mask, or endotracheal intubation as required to maintain a hemoglobin saturation of 90% or greater. Crystalloid in the form of lactated Ringer's solution or normal saline should be given over the first 30–60 minutes of acute resuscitation as a 3:1 replacement based on blood loss. The use of vasopressors to restore maternal blood pressure should be avoided until appropriate volume replacement has been administered. Although these agents may reduce uterine blood flow in normovolemic patients, they should not be withheld if needed in the resuscitation of the mother. Displacement of the uterus off the inferior vena cava and abdominal aorta with the patient in a supine position is helpful in trauma patients beyond midpregnancy. This can be effected by having the patient lie in the lateral decubitus position. If the patient must remain supine (eg, if a spinal injury is suspected or if cardiopulmonary resuscitation is being administered), manual displacement of the uterus laterally with a hand or placement of a wedge under a backboard will accomplish this goal.

Following stabilization, a more detailed secondary survey of the patient, including fetal evaluation, should be performed. All body regions must be thoroughly examined. Pregnancy should not alter necessary treatment and evaluation of the trauma patient. The abdomen is of particular importance, because a substantial percentage of serious injuries involve the uterus, intraperitoneal structures, and retroperitoneum. The uterus should be examined for evidence of gross deformity, tenderness, or contractions.

Computed tomography can be used to evaluate patients who have suffered significant trauma. Computed tomographic scanning of the abdomen exposes the fetus to approximately 3.5 rad, depending on the number and thickness of the images and the equipment used. As with any procedure involving ionizing radiation, scanning closer to the uterus increases fetal exposure. Fetal exposure exceeding 20 rad may be sufficient to induce adverse effects in early pregnancy (28).

Open peritoneal lavage can be effective in the diagnosis of intraperitoneal hemorrhage during pregnancy (29). Open lavage with sharp dissection and opening of the anterior abdominal peritoneum under direct vision, usually periumbilically, is advocated over a blind needle insertion to lessen the likelihood of injury to the uterus or to other displaced intraabdominal organs. Peritoneal lavage is unnecessary if clinically obvious intraperitoneal bleeding is present. Following are some indications for peritoneal lavage after trauma during pregnancy:

- Abdominal signs or symptoms suggestive of intraperitoneal bleeding
- Altered sensorium
- Unexplained shock
- Major thoracic injuries
- Multiple major orthopedic injuries

Penetrating trauma requires the complete undressing of the patient for careful inspection of all entrance and exit wounds because occasionally victims are shot or stabbed multiple times, and entrance and exit wounds of high-velocity projectiles are unpredictable. Radiographs of the area in multiple projections often are helpful to localize a bullet if an exit wound is not seen. The uterus and its contents can often stop the progression of a projectile, limiting the extent of maternal injury to the abdominal wall and the uterus. Signs of peritoneal irritation are less reliable during pregnancy, however, and changes in vital signs due to blood loss may occur rela-

tively late because of the increase in blood volume related to pregnancy. The general approach to management of abdominal gunshot wounds involves exploratory laparotomy, although laparotomy can be used selectively (26). Although stab wounds that do not appear to penetrate beyond the abdominal wall have been managed nonoperatively, evidence of peritoneal penetration usually requires exploratory laparotomy, particularly if there are signs of intraperitoneal hemorrhage or bowel perforation (30). The indications for tetanus prophylaxis do not change in pregnancy, and appropriate candidates should be vaccinated.

If adequate oxygenation and uterine perfusion are maintained, the fetus usually tolerates surgery and anesthesia well. Intraoperative fetal heart rate monitoring should be considered if the fetus is viable. A Doppler device or ultrasound transducer wrapped in a sterile plastic bag may be used for this purpose. When the uterus has been penetrated by an object or projectile, the fetus probably has been injured. If the fetus is alive, the decision to perform cesarean delivery should be weighed against the likelihood of fetal survival. Factors involved in this decision include gestational age, the condition of the fetus based on any antenatal testing that may have been performed, the extent of injury to the uterus (ie, a cesarean hysterectomy may be necessary with extensive injuries), and whether the gravid uterus allows adequate exploration of the peritoneal cavity. These decisions often are made jointly with the trauma surgeon. The need to perform a laparotomy, by itself, is not an indication to proceed with cesarean delivery. If the uterus has been penetrated and delivery must proceed, a pediatric surgeon and a neonatologist should be available if possible.

Fetal Assessment

The use of electronic fetal cardiac and uterine activity monitoring in pregnant trauma victims beyond 20 weeks of gestation may be predictive of abruptio placentae. Placental abruption did not occur in trauma patients in whom uterine contractions occurred at a frequency of less than one every 10 minutes during 4 hours of monitoring (16, 18). Of those women who had uterine contractions of greater frequency, however, almost 20% had placental abruption (16). Abnormal fetal heart tracings, including tachycardia and late deceleration, were seen frequently in cases of abruptio placentae.

Because abruption usually becomes apparent shortly after injury, monitoring should be initiated as soon as the woman is stabilized. Recommended minimum time of posttrauma monitoring includes 4 hours (3, 18) and 2–6 hours (31). However, none of these times have been validated by large, prospective studies. Monitoring should be continued and further evaluation carried out if uterine contractions, a nonreassuring fetal heart rate pattern, vaginal bleeding, significant uterine tenderness or irritability, serious maternal injury, or rupture of the amniotic membranes is present. If these findings are not present, the patient may be discharged or transferred (20). Upon discharge, the patient should be instructed to return if she develops vaginal bleeding, leakage of fluid, decreased fetal movement, or severe abdominal pain.

The use of ultrasonography following trauma during pregnancy does not appear to be as sensitive as cardiotocographic monitoring for diagnosing abruptio placentae (4, 16, 18, 20). However, ultrasonography is useful in the setting of trauma during pregnancy for establishing gestational age, locating the placenta, determining fetal wellbeing and extent of fetal injury or demise, and estimating amniotic fluid volume. In the woman, ultrasonography also may reveal the presence of intraabdominal fluid and increase the index of suspicion for intraperitoneal hemorrhage.

Fetal–Maternal Hemorrhage

Complications of fetal–maternal hemorrhage in trauma patients include fetal and neonatal anemia, fetal cardiac arrhythmias, and fetal death. There is no evidence that laboratory testing for fetal–maternal hemorrhage (eg, Kleihauer–Betke test) can predict adverse immediate sequelae due to hemorrhage (32). Among women who exhibit signs of fetal–maternal hemorrhage due to trauma, the mean estimated blood volume of injected fetal blood usually is less than 15 mL, and more than 90% of the hemorrhages are less than 30 mL (4, 16). Therefore, administration of 300 µg (one ampule) of D immune globulin would protect nearly all D-negative trauma victims from D alloimmunization. The routine use of the Kleihauer–Betke assay or other similar quantitative assays of fetal–maternal hemorrhage may be useful in identifying those few unsensitized, D-negative trauma patients who are found to have more than 30 mL transfusion. Additional D immune globulin (300 µg for every 30 mL of whole blood transfused) may be administered to these patients. Administration of D immune globulin at any time within the first 72 hours following fetal–maternal hemorrhage appears to provide protection from alloimmunization. Consideration should be given to administering D immune globulin to all unsensitized D-negative pregnant patients who have experienced abdominal trauma.

Special Considerations

Perimortem Cesarean Delivery

Although there are no clear guidelines regarding perimortem cesarean delivery, fetal survival is unlikely if more than 15–20 minutes have transpired since the loss of maternal vital signs. There are insufficient data on which to base conclusions regarding the appropriateness of abdominal delivery when efforts at resuscitation have failed. Based on isolated case reports, cesarean delivery should be considered for both maternal and fetal benefit 4 minutes after a woman has experienced cardiopulmonary arrest in the third trimester (33).

Safety Restraint Use During Pregnancy

There is substantial evidence that seat belt use during pregnancy protects both the mother and the fetus (17, 34, 35). Nonetheless, many pregnant women do not wear seat belts properly (13). Prenatal education on the use of seat belts improves compliance of seat belt use as well as improves knowledge of proper use (13). Current recommendations indicate that throughout pregnancy, safety belts should be used with both the lap belt and shoulder harness in place. The lap belt portion should be placed under the pregnant woman's abdomen, over both anterior superior iliac spines and the pubic symphysis. The shoulder harness should be positioned between the breasts. There should not be excessive slack in either belt, and both the lap and shoulder restraints should be applied as snugly as comfort will allow. Placement of the lap belt over the dome of the uterus significantly increases pressure transmission to the uterus and has been associated with significant uterine and fetal injury (36, 37). Based on preliminary data using a crash dummy that simulates a pregnant woman, there does not appear to be extraordinary force transmission to the pregnant uterus when seat belts are properly placed (37).

Airbag deployment during pregnancy does not appear to be associated with an increased risk for either maternal or fetal injury. Based on limited existing information, it does not appear reasonable to recommend disabling airbags during pregnancy.

Summary

Trauma is one of the leading causes of death of young people in this country; in many cases, it is preventable. The appropriate use of safety restraint systems in automobiles, compliance with traffic laws, and early identification and intervention in suspected cases of domestic violence are all preventive measures that may reduce the likelihood of both maternal and fetal morbidity and mortality. The obstetrician–gynecologist plays a central role both in the education of pregnant women and in the early identification of suspected abuse.

When trauma has occurred, an organized approach to management is critically important to optimize outcome. The first priority is treatment and stabilization of the woman; only then should attention be directed to the fetus. Electronic fetal and uterine monitoring is an important component of management beyond midtrimester trauma.

References

1. Dannenberg AL, Carter DM, Lawson HW, Ashton DM, Dorfman SF, Graham EH. Homicide and other injuries as causes of maternal death in New York City, 1987 through 1991. Am J Obstet Gynecol 1995;172:1557–1564

2. Fildes J, Reed L, Jones N, Martin M, Barrett J. Trauma: the leading cause of maternal death. J Trauma 1992;32:643–645

3. Pearlman MD, Tintinalli JE, Lorenz RP. A prospective controlled study of outcome after trauma during pregnancy. Am J Obstet Gynecol 1990;162:1502–1510

4. Goodwin TM, Breen MT. Pregnancy outcome and fetomaternal hemorrhage after noncatastrophic trauma. Am J Obstet Gynecol 1990;162:665–671

5. National Safety Council. Accident facts. Chicago: National Safety Council, 1997

6. American College of Obstetricians and Gynecologists. Domestic violence. ACOG Technical Bulletin 209. Washington, DC: ACOG, 1995

7. Gazamararian JA, Lazorick S, Spitz AM, Ballard TJ, Saltzman LE, Marks JS. Prevalence of violence against pregnant women. JAMA 1996;275:1915–1920

8. Helton AS, McFarlane J, Anderson ET. Battered and pregnant: a prevalence study. Am J Public Health 1987;77:1337–1339

9. Berenson AB, Stiglich NJ, Wilkinson GS, Anderson GD. Drug abuse and other risk factors for physical abuse in pregnancy among white non-Hispanic, black, and Hispanic women. Am J Obstet Gynecol 1991;164:1491–1499

10. McFarlane J, Parker B, Soeken K, Bullock L. Assessing for abuse during pregnancy. Severity and frequency of injuries and associated entry into prenatal care. JAMA 1992;267:3176–3178

11. Stewart DE, Cecutti A. Physical abuse in pregnancy. Can Med Assoc J 1993;149:1257–1263

12. Varner MW. Maternal mortality in Iowa from 1952 to 1986. Surg Gynecol Obstet 1989;168:555–562

13. Pearlman MD, Phillips ME. Safety belt use during pregnancy. Obstet Gynecol 1996;88:1026–1029

14. Pearlman MD, Tintinalli JE. Evaluation and treatment of the gravida and fetus following trauma during pregnancy. Obstet Gynecol Clin North Am 1991;18:371–381

15. Fries MH, Hankins GDV. Motor vehicle accident associated with minimal maternal trauma but subsequent fetal demise. Ann Emerg Med 1989;18:301–304

16. Pearlman MD, Tintinalli JE, Lorenz RP. Blunt trauma during pregnancy. N Engl J Med 1990;323:1609–1613

17. Crosby WM, Costiloe JP. Safety of lap-belt restraint for pregnant victims of automobile collisions. N Engl J Med 1971;284:632–636

18. Dahmus MA, Sibai BM. Blunt abdominal trauma: are there predictive factors for abruptio placentae or maternal–fetal distress? Am J Obstet Gynecol 1993;169:1054–1059

19. Rothenberger D, Quattlebaum FW, Perry JF Jr, Zabel J, Fischer RP. Blunt maternal trauma: a review of 103 cases. J Trauma 1978;18:173–179

20. Williams JK, McClain L, Rosemurgy AS, Colorado NM. Evaluation of blunt abdominal trauma in the third trimester of pregnancy: maternal and fetal considerations. Obstet Gynecol 1990;75:33–37

21. Biester EM, Tomich PG, Esposito TJ, Weber L. Trauma in pregnancy: normal revised trauma score in relation to other markers of maternofetal status—a preliminary study. Am J Obstet Gynecol 1997;176:1206–1212

22. Evrard JR, Sturner WQ, Murray EJ. Fetal skull fracture from an automobile accident. Am J Forensic Med Pathol 1989;10:232–234

23. Hartl R, Ko K. In utero skull fracture: case report. J Trauma 1996;41:549–552

24. Astarita DC, Feldman B. Seat belt placement resulting in uterine rupture. J Trauma 1997;42:738–740

25. Buchsbaum HJ. Accidental injury complicating pregnancy. Am J Obstet Gynecol 1968;102:752–769

26. Awwad JT, Azar GB, Seoud MA, Mroueh AM, Karam KS. High-velocity penetrating wounds of the gravid uterus: review of 16 years of civil war. Obstet Gynecol 1994;83:259–264

27. Kissinger DP, Rozycki GS, Morris JA Jr, Knudson M, Copes WS, Bass SM, et al. Trauma in pregnancy: predicting pregnancy outcome. Arch Surg 1991;126:1079–1086

28. American College of Obstetricians and Gynecologists. Guidelines for diagnostic imaging during pregnancy. ACOG Committee Opinion 158. Washington, DC: ACOG, 1995

29. Esposito TJ, Gens DR, Smith LG, Scorpio R. Evaluation of blunt abdominal trauma occurring during pregnancy. J Trauma 1989;29:1628–1632

30. Grubb DK. Nonsurgical management of penetrating uterine trauma in pregnancy: a case report. Am J Obstet Gynecol 1992;166:583–584

31. American Academy of Pediatrics, American College of Obstetricians and Gynecologists. Guidelines for perinatal care. 4th ed. Elk Grove Village, Illinois: AAP; Washington, DC: ACOG, 1997

32. Boyle J, Kim J, Walerius H, Samuels P. The clinical use of the Kleihauer–Betke test in Rh positive patients. Am J Obstet Gynecol 1996;174:343

33. Katz VL, Dotters DJ, Droegemueller W. Perimortem cesarean delivery. Obstet Gynecol 1986;68:571–576

34. Crosby WM, King AI, Stout LC. Fetal survival following impact: improvement with shoulder harness restraint. Am J Obstet Gynecol 1972;112:1101–1106

35. Wolf ME, Alexander BH, Rivara FP, Hickok DE, Maier RV, Starzyk PM. A retrospective cohort study of seatbelt use and pregnancy outcome after a motor vehicle crash. J Trauma 1993;34:116–119

36. McCormick RD. Seat belt injury: case of complete transection of pregnant uterus. J Am Osteopath Assoc 1968;67:1139–1141

37. Pearlman MD, Viano D. Automobile crash simulation with the first pregnant crash test dummy. Am J Obstet Gynecol 1996;175:977–981

ACOG EDUCATIONAL BULLETIN

Number 255, November 1999

Psychosocial Risk Factors: Perinatal Screening and Intervention

The American College of Obstetricians and Gynecologists has long been concerned about the psychosocial issues faced by women and their families during the childbearing years that affect their mental and physical well being. Many of these issues are more prevalent in the adolescent population. Screening for psychosocial risk factors may help predict a woman's attentiveness to personal health matters, her use of prenatal services, and the health status of her offspring (1).

Many physicians who care for women have had little training in managing the psychosocial issues that women encounter (2). An emerging body of evidence indicates that patients place high value on attention to these issues and report greater satisfaction with physician visits when there is more "psychosocial talk" and less "biomedical talk" (3). Health care providers, therefore, need to be encouraged to screen for psychosocial risk factors and to provide or refer patients for essential services to manage psychosocial problems. This can be accomplished through training to increase provider awareness of and interest in these issues as well as ways to respond to them. Adequate reimbursement by third-party payers for the necessary services also is essential.

Background

Although it is acknowledged that addressing psychosocial issues during pregnancy is important and has the potential to reduce costs to the individual and society (4), there are no screening tools widely available that have been shown to have high degrees of sensitivity and specificity. The Healthy Start Program of the Florida Department of Health, however, has designed one particularly well-regarded screening system, which has been used and refined by this program since 1992. Other tools exist, but none have been identified that have been evaluated as extensively as the Healthy Start tool. In addition, the Healthy Start tool provides a more concise and simple

Psychosocial Screening Tool

1. Do you have any problems that prevent you from keeping your health care appointments?

2. How many times have you moved in the past 12 months? 0 1 2 3 >3

3. Do you feel unsafe where you live?

4. Do you or any members of your household go to bed hungry?

5. In the past 2 months, have you used any form of tobacco?

6. In the past 2 months, have you used drugs or alcohol (including beer, wine, or mixed drinks)?

7. In the past year, has anyone hit you or tried to hurt you?

8. How do you rate your current stress level—low or high?

9. If you could change the timing of this pregnancy, would you want it earlier, later, not at all, or no change?

Modified and reprinted with permission from Florida's Healthy Start Prenatal Risk Screening Instrument. Florida Department of Health. DH 3134. September 1997

Given the sensitive nature of psychosocial assessment, every effort should be made to screen in private, especially when inquiring about domestic or intimate partner violence. Even then, patients may not be comfortable discussing problems with physicians until a trusting relationship has been formed. Because problems may arise during the pregnancy that were not present at the initial visit, it is best to perform psychosocial screening once each trimester to increase the likelihood of identifying important issues and reducing poor birth outcomes. A recent study indicates that women who were screened for psychosocial issues once each trimester were half as likely as women who were not screened to have a low-birth-weight or preterm baby (5). Documentation should include the nature of any problems identified, the chosen intervention(s), and plans for follow-up. A suggested format for this documentation can be found at the end of this document.

Psychosocial risk factors also should be considered in discharge planning after delivery. Many of the psychosocial issues that increase the risk for poor pregnancy outcome also can affect the health and welfare of the newborn. It is essential that women with significant psychosocial problems stay in the hospital after delivery as long as necessary to assess adequately the health of the mother and the newborn; education of the woman about postpartum and infant care also occurs during this time. In the absence of complications, a 48-hour hospital stay after a normal vaginal delivery and a 96-hour stay after a cesarean delivery is recommended (6).

Barriers to Care

Inadequate insurance coverage, inability to pay for health care services, and not knowing where to go to receive care are a few of the most common barriers to health care. Others include lack of transportation and day care and language difficulties (7). These barriers are especially problematic for adolescents. For individuals faced with these barriers, referral to an appropriate social service agency may be useful. These agencies can sometimes help women navigate the health care system. In particular, they can help her enroll in Medicaid, which covers the costs of medical care and transportation to and from medical and social service appointments and also subsidizes or provides free day care. Through flexible scheduling of appointments, inquiring about difficulties a patient may have with keeping appointments, and assisting with solutions, the provider increases the likelihood of compliance with prenatal care recommendations. Following are brief interventions for several of the most common barriers to care.

means of collecting psychosocial data that can be used for self-reporting or interview style information retrieval (see the box for a modified version of this screening tool). Each topic identified in this tool will be discussed in this Educational Bulletin. Many of the topics are discussed more fully in various ACOG documents (see ACOG Resources).

Even though at first glance some of the questions appear to be relevant only for low-income populations, psychosocial screening of all patients presenting for pregnancy evaluation or prenatal care is an important step toward improving women's health and birth outcomes. When screening is done, every effort should be made to provide the brief interventions that are described in the following discussion. Through a brief intervention, the provider can identify areas of concern, validate major issues with the patient, provide information and, if indicated, make suggestions for possible changes. If necessary, the provider can refer the patient for further evaluation or intervention. For screening to be effective, a well-developed process for referrals is necessary. If assistance is needed with locating appropriate referral sites, local or state health officials can be contacted.

Transportation

Transportation difficulties are commonly cited as a barrier to prenatal visits (8), particularly for women residing in rural areas (9). Many women lack transportation to and from health care appointments and rely on either public transportation or the willingness of friends and family to transport them. If a patient is not certain how she will get to appointments, the health care provider should discuss options available to her.

Day Care

For a patient who already has children, finding and paying for appropriate child care while attending appointments can be another barrier to care (10). Caring for elderly or disabled family members may pose a similar challenge. For patients who cannot arrange day care, establishing an office setting that can accommodate children and relatives is helpful.

Interference by Others

Sometimes a patient's spouse, partner, or parent may not want her to keep medical appointments. Although patients often are not directly forthcoming with this information, providers can obtain important details about the patient by asking about interference from family members, domestic or family violence, and safety issues when patients miss appointments. Flexible scheduling, assistance with transportation, or social service assistance may improve compliance with ongoing perinatal care.

Language

Because barriers to care are magnified when the patient does not speak English, it is important to use translators when possible. If this is not possible, providers can ask the patient to identify a family member or friend who can act as a translator. This may be a less desirable choice, however, because information may be intentionally or unintentionally translated incorrectly. For example, in cases of domestic violence, if the abusive spouse is translating, he might omit a question about safety in the home, misrepresent the patient's response, or retaliate. Another partial solution is to provide written materials in appropriate languages for patients who do not speak English. If communication is not adequate, it must be decided whether the patient should remain in the practice or be referred to a facility with better access to translators.

Frequent Moves

Frequent moves can indicate a variety of problems. For example, the patient may be having difficulty finding acceptable housing that is affordable. If this is the case, the patient can be referred to the appropriate social service agency for assistance. These local agencies also can provide information about other resources in the area, including health services, social support groups, and child care resources. Inquiring about the patient's feelings of isolation also is important. If this is a problem, referral to any available neighborhood support groups or a counselor can be helpful. In addition, frequent moves may reflect violence in the home or may indicate problems with the law that can cause stress.

Safety

Safety concerns can pertain to either safety in the house or safety in the neighborhood. In either case, if there is immediate danger to the patient, alternative housing should be discussed. If there are children who are not safe in the household, a referral to the state's child protection agency may be required. The state agency can be contacted for specific reporting requirements. If the safety concern relates specifically to the house, such as structural defects, rat or insect infestation, or sanitation issues, further inquiry can determine the necessary referral or intervention.

If the danger is a result of intimate partner violence, referrals, including one to a battered women's shelter, should be made. If there are no shelters or safe houses available, hospital beds may be provided on an emergency basis in some cases. It is important to assess the potential for life-threatening situations and develop safety plans with the patient, understanding that the likelihood of serious injury often is highest when the woman attempts to leave her abuser. Physicians need to be aware that the patient is the best judge of her own safety. She, therefore, may choose to return home despite receiving advice to the contrary, and the physician must honor her decision.

Nutrition

Nutritional problems can be found in women of every socioeconomic status and range from an inability to acquire and prepare food to eating disorders. If the woman cannot afford a sufficient supply of food, she should be referred to food pantries and soup kitchens in her area. All low-income women should receive information about the Special Supplemental Food Program for Women, Infants and Children (WIC) and food stamp programs. Referrals to the appropriate social service agency to apply for these or other available benefits can be helpful.

Women of low socioeconomic status often live in environments that do not allow for the storage, refrigeration, or preparation of food. Many nutritionists are trained in alternative methods of food storage and preparation and would, therefore, be able to assist the patient upon referral. The nutritionist also could assess the patient's diet and suggest healthy foods that are inexpensive.

Additional questions should be asked, especially of adolescents and young women, about eating habits such as fasting or meal skipping, which are indicative of anorexia and bulimia. If it is determined that the patient has an eating disorder, referral to a psychiatrist who specializes in this issue and a nutritionist for counseling about food management is essential. All WIC programs have nutritionists who are required to counsel patients on these matters. Hospitalization also may be required for patients with eating disorders. Poor weight gain also may reflect substance abuse, domestic violence, or depression.

Tobacco Use

Smoking tobacco is associated with increased perinatal mortality; bleeding complications of pregnancy; and a higher incidence of small-for-gestational age babies, low-birth-weight babies, and preterm delivery (11). It is estimated that a 10% reduction in fetal and infant deaths would be achieved if all pregnant women stopped smoking (12). There also is increasing evidence that Attention Deficit Hyperactivity Disorder (ADHD) and other behavioral or learning problems that affect school-aged children may be linked to maternal smoking during pregnancy (13). Therefore, it is essential that patients be screened for tobacco use and provided information on smoking cessation and why it is necessary to stop smoking during pregnancy. Interventions by clinicians that are as brief as 5–15 minutes have been shown to be effective at increasing smoking cessation rates (14).

Substance Use

Women who use substances have increased risks of preterm delivery, fetal growth restriction, fetal alcohol syndrome, fetal death, and possible long-term neurobehavioral effects (15). They also are at increased risk for sexually transmitted diseases, including human immunodeficiency virus (HIV). Women who use substances often obtain prenatal care late in the pregnancy, achieve poor weight gain, and frequently miss appointments, all of which can have negative effects on the health of the woman and the fetus. Substance abuse, by either the woman or her partner, also is associated with domestic violence. Asking patients about substance abuse at the time of the first prenatal visit is essential; questions about her partner's use of substances also may be helpful. If

either inquiry indicates an area of concern, additional assessment is required (15).

Intimate Partner Violence

The incidence of abuse during pregnancy is high, with reports ranging from 1% to 20% of all pregnant women (16). Many studies report that violence often begins in pregnancy; if already present, it may escalate (17). Research also suggests that violence may increase during the postpartum period (18). Given these findings, it would be useful to screen every woman for intimate partner violence at least once in each trimester; whenever bruising, improbable injury, or depressed mood is noted; and at the postpartum visit. It also is important to know the various characteristics that may serve as markers for abuse. Women who are abused are more likely to receive inadequate prenatal care. In particular, abused pregnant women seek prenatal care later in pregnancy (19), miss more appointments, and are more likely to cancel appointments on short notice than nonabused pregnant women (20).

Stress

Stress is defined as any real or perceived trauma—whether it is physical or psychologic—that results in the release of stress hormones. Folklore has always taken it for granted that stress, such as acute anxiety, sorrow, or worry disturbs the fetus and causes physical harm (21). The observation that maternal stress is measurably related to neonatal activity and irritability in both lower animals and in humans has been documented by research during the past 30 years (22). Recent studies support that women who are anxious during pregnancy tend to have smaller babies and that women with high levels of stress hormones are more likely to deliver preterm (23, 24).

Practitioners should identify patients under stress. The stress associated with pregnancy itself, concerns about labor and delivery, and projected fears about parenting can sometimes be reduced by providing counseling and information during the course of prenatal care. Other patients may require evaluation and treatment by mental health practitioners to help identify and resolve distress.

Unintended Pregnancy

Approximately 49% of all pregnancies are unintended at the time of conception (25). This percentage is considerably higher among adolescents. An unintended pregnancy generally is defined as a pregnancy that was mistimed or unwanted at the time of conception. Research has shown that having an unintended pregnancy is a predictor of insufficient prenatal care, which results in an increased risk of a poor birth outcome. Women with unintended pregnancies are more likely to smoke and drink and have a greater likelihood of delivering a low-birth-weight infant. Their infants are more likely to die within the first year of life (26). In addition, the incidence of unintended pregnancy is higher among women who have been battered (27) and battering is more common during an unplanned pregnancy (28).

Unintended pregnancies often become accepted pregnancies that produce much-loved and wanted children. However, women with pregnancies that remain unwanted should be counseled about the full range of reproductive options, which include abortion and adoption. Women must be allowed to make independent decisions about their own pregnancies. This choice remains a woman's right and must be respected.

Summary

Addressing the broad range of psychosocial issues with which pregnant women are confronted is an essential step toward improving women's health and birth outcomes. This may be difficult to do completely in a private physician's office setting, therefore, an effective system of referrals is helpful. To increase the likelihood of successful interventions, psychosocial screening should be performed on a regular basis and documented in the patient's prenatal record.

ACOG Resources

American College of Obstetricians and Gynecologists. Depression in women. ACOG Technical Bulletin 182. Washington, DC: ACOG, 1993

American College of Obstetricians and Gynecologists. Domestic violence: the role of the physician in identification, intervention, and prevention. Slide lecture kit. Washington, DC: ACOG, 1995

American College of Obstetricians and Gynecologists. Domestic violence. ACOG Educational Bulletin 209. Washington, DC: ACOG, 1995

American College of Obstetricians and Gynecologists. Mandatory reporting of domestic violence. ACOG Committee Opinion 200. Washington, DC: ACOG, 1998

American College of Obstetricians and Gynecologists. Nutrition and women. ACOG Educational Bulletin 229. Washington, DC: ACOG, 1996

American College of Obstetricians and Gynecologists. Smoking and women's health. ACOG Educational Bulletin 240. Washington, DC: ACOG, 1997

American College of Obstetricians and Gynecologists. Substance abuse. ACOG Technical Bulletin 194. Washington, DC: ACOG, 1994

American College of Obstetricians and Gynecologists. Substance abuse in pregnancy. ACOG Technical Bulletin 195. Washington, DC: ACOG, 1994

Bibliography

American Academy of Pediatrics Committee on Drugs. The transfer of drugs and other chemicals into human milk. Pediatrics 1994;93:137–150

Briggs GG, Freeman RK, Yaffe SJ. Drugs in pregnancy and lactation. 5th ed. Baltimore: Williams & Wilkins, 1998

Dolan-Mullen P, Ramirez G, Groff JY. A meta-analysis of randomized trials of prenatal smoking cessation interventions. Am J Obstet Gynecol 1994;171:1328–1334

Haller E. Eating disorders. A review and update. West J Med 1992;157:658–662

Henningfield JE. Nicotine medications for smoking cessation. N Engl J Med 1995;333:1196–1203

Hutchins E, DiPietro J. Psychosocial risk factors associated with cocaine use during pregnancy: a case-control study. Obstet Gynecol 1997;90:142–147

Laken MP, Hutchins E. Building and sustaining systems of care for substance-using pregnant women and their infants: Lessons learned. Arlington, Virginia: National Center for Education in Maternal and Child Health, 1995

MacGregor SN, Keith LG, Bachicha JA, Chasnoff IJ. Cocaine abuse during pregnancy: correlation between prenatal care and perinatal outcome. Obstet Gynecol 1989;74:882–885

Morse B, Gehshan S, Hutchins E. Screening for substance abuse during pregnancy: improving care, improving health. Arlington, Virginia: National Center for Education in Maternal and Child Health, 1997

Tofler IR, Stryer BK, Micheli LJ, Herman LR. Physical and emotional problems of elite female gymnasts. N Engl J Med 1996;335:281–283

Working Group on Nicotine Dependence. Practice guideline for the treatment of patients with nicotine dependence. American Psychiatric Association. Am J Psychiatry 1996;153:1–31

References

1. Goldenberg RL, Patterson ET, Freese MP. Maternal demographic, situational and psychosocial factors and their relationship to enrollment in prenatal care: a review of the literature. Women Health 1992;19:133–151

2. Goldberg D. A classification of psychological distress for use in primary care setting. Soc Sci Med 1992;35:189–193

3. Bertakis KD, Roter D, Putnam SM. The relationship of physician medical interview style to patient satisfaction. J Fam Pract 1991;32:175–181

4. Curry MA. Nonfinancial barriers to prenatal care. Women Health 1989;15:85–99

5. Wilkinson DS, Korenbrot CC, Greene J. A performance indicator of psychosocial services in enhanced prenatal care of Medicaid-eligible women. Matern Child Health J 1998;2:131–143

6. American Academy of Pediatrics, American College of Obstetricians and Gynecologists. Guidelines for perinatal care. 4th ed. Elk Grove Village, Illinois: AAP; Washington, DC: ACOG, 1997

7. Brown SS. Drawing women into prenatal care. Fam Plann Perspect 1989;21:73–80

8. Aved BM, Irwin MM, Cummings LS, Findeisen N. Barriers to prenatal care for low-income women. West J Med 1993;158:493–498

9. McDonald TP, Coburn AF. Predictors of prenatal care utilization. Soc Sci Med 1988;27:167–172

10. Kugler JP, Yeash J, Rumbaugh PC. The impact of sociodemographic, health care system, and family function variables on prenatal care utilization in a military setting. J Fam Pract 1993;37:143–147

11. American College of Obstetricians and Gynecologists. Smoking and women's health. ACOG Educational Bulletin 240. Washington, DC: ACOG, 1997

12. Kleinman JC, Pierre MB Jr, Madans JH, Land GH, Schramm WF. The effects of maternal smoking on fetal and infant mortality. Am J Epidemiol 1988;127:274–282

13. Milberger S, Biederman J, Faraone SV, Chen L, Jones J. Is maternal smoking during pregnancy a risk factor for attention deficit hyperactivity disorder in children? Am J Psychiatry 1996;153:1138–1142

14. Dolan Mullen P, Melvin CL, Windsor RA. A Review of the Evidence to Recommend Cessation Counseling for Pregnant Women Who Smoke. Smoke-Free Families Program, Department of Obstetrics and Gynecology, School of Medicine, University of Alabama at Birmingham, Birmingham, Alabama, 1999

15. American College of Obstetricians and Gynecologists. Substance abuse in pregnancy. ACOG Technical Bulletin 195. Washington, DC: ACOG, 1994

16. Gazmararian JA, Lazorick S, Spitz AM, Ballard TJ, Saltzman LE, Marks JS. Prevalence of violence against pregnant women. JAMA 1996:1915–1920

17. Hillard PJ. Physical abuse in pregnancy. Obstet Gynecol 1985;66:185–190

18. Stewart DE. Incidence of postpartum abuse in women with a history of abuse during pregnancy. CMAJ 1994;151:1601–1604

19. McFarlane J, Parker B, Soeken K, Bullock L. Assessing for abuse during pregnancy. Severity and frequency of injuries and associated entry into prenatal care. JAMA 1992;267:3176–3178

20. American Medical Association. Diagnostic and treatment guidelines on domestic violence. Chicago: AMA, 1994

21. Benedek T. The psychobiology of pregnancy. In: Anthony EJ, Benedek T, eds. Parenthood: Its psychology and psychopathology. London: J & A Churchill Ltd., 1970:137–151

22. Herrenkohl LR. The impact of prenatal stress on the developing fetus and child. In: Cohen RL, ed. Psychiatric consultation in childbirth settings. New York: Plenum, 1988:21–35

23. Teixeira JM, Fisk NM, Glover V. Association between maternal anxiety in pregnancy and increased uterine artery resistance index: cohort based study. BMJ 1999;318:153–157

24. Wadhwa PD, Porto M, Garite TJ, Chicz-DeMet A, Sandman CA. Maternal corticotropin-releasing hormone levels in the early trimester predict length of gestation in human pregnancy. Am J Obstet Gynecol 1998;179:1079–1085

25. National Center for Health Statistics. Healthy People 2000 review, 1998-99. Hyattsville, Maryland: Public Health Service, 1999

26. The best intentions: unintended pregnancy and the well-being of children and families. Committee on Unintended Pregnancy, Institute of Medicine, National Academy of Sciences. Washington, DC: National Academy Press, 1995

27. Stewart DE, Cecutti A. Physical abuse in pregnancy. CMAJ 1993;149:1257–1263

28. Fergusson DM, Horwood LJ, Kershaw KL, Shannon FT. Factors associated with reports of wife assault in New Zealand. J Marriage Fam 1986;48:407–412

Psychosocial Risk Assessment

	YES	NO	
	☐	☐	1. Do you have any problems that prevent you from keeping your health care appointments?
	0 1 2 3 >3		2. How many times have you moved in the past 12 months?
	☐	☐	3. Do you feel unsafe where you live?
	☐	☐	4. Do you or any members of your household go to bed hungry?
	☐	☐	5. In the past 2 months, have you used any form of tobacco?
	☐	☐	6. In the past 2 months, have you used drugs or alcohol (including beer, wine, and mixed drinks)?
	☐	☐	7. In the past year, has anyone hit you or tried to hurt you?
	low	high	8. How do you rate your current stress level—low or high?
	a b c d		9. If you could change the timing of this pregnancy, would you want it (a) earlier, (b) later, (c) not at all, (d) no change?

Patient Name: _____

Patient No.: _____

Date	Area of Concern	Intervention	Recommendation/Referral	Follow-up	Initials

Modified and reprinted with permission from Florida's Healthy Start Prenatal Risk Screening Instrument. Florida Department of Health. DH 3134. October 1996

ACOG EDUCATIONAL BULLETIN

Number 236, April 1997

Teratology

Teratology is the study of abnormal fetal development. Major defects are apparent at birth in about 3% of the general population, and in about 4.5% by 5 years of age. An exact cause or mechanism for the defect can be determined in less than 50% of cases. Some substances, organisms, and physical agents are known to be teratogens, capable of causing abnormal fetal development.

Although obstetricians are often asked about potentially teratogenic agents, the present discussion is limited to those agents proved by cumulative information to be harmful to a fetus. Other agents are suspected but not documented teratogens. Expert consensus on the safety of such agents does not exist and may be impossible to achieve.

Practical information for determining the teratogenicity of common environmental, infectious, and pharmacologic agents is outlined in this bulletin. Important factors to consider in determining the risk of teratogenesis include the exact identity and dose of the apparent teratogen, the stage of embryogenesis during which the exposure occurred, and the genetic sensitivity of the mother and fetus.

Factors Influencing Teratogenic Effect

Some agents cause major defects if fetal exposure occurs during a specific critical period but cause no harmful effect at another time. For example, ru-bella can cause multiple anatomic defects when fetal infection occurs during the first trimester of pregnancy but causes only chronic infection in the newborn when exposure occurs during the third trimester. After organogenesis has been completed (13 weeks of gestation), the observable effect of an environmental agent may be limited to fetal growth restriction or a minimal reduction in organ size and to functional rather than gross structural defects.

Individual variation in susceptibility to a constant dose of a given agent also influences teratogenic effect. Each child of a chronic alcoholic may display different manifestations of fetal alcohol syndrome, possibly because of genotypic differences in sensitivity to alcohol. This may also explain why high doses of a known teratogen have no effect on some exposed fetuses. The occurrence of threshold phenomena can explain why low doses of some agents have no teratogenic effect. Furthermore, an effect of a low dose that is statistically insignificant in a small sample might be shown to be biologically significant if a larger population were studied.

This Educational Bulletin was developed under the direction of the Committee on Educational Bulletins of the American College of Obstetricians and Gynecologists as an aid to obstetricians and gynecologists. This document is not to be construed as establishing a standard of practice or dictating an exclusive course of treatment. Rather, it is intended as an educational tool that presents current information on obstetric–gynecologic issues.

Replaces Number 233, February 1997

Study of Teratogenic Drugs

For most drugs, animal studies have been used extensively to determine possible teratogenic effects. Although such studies may be helpful, their results do not always reliably predict human response.

When studies of birth defects in humans are evaluated, the statistics presented should be reviewed with caution. Results of retrospective and uncontrolled studies, as well as individual case reports, may be misleading about the risk of exposure to specific drugs during pregnancy, especially those commonly used during gestation. Some offspring of any large population of women using a drug during pregnancy will be born with birth defects. These events may lead to spurious claims of a causal relationship. Differentiating the effects of a specific pharmacologic agent from the effects of the illness for which it was prescribed can also be difficult as it involves determining the natural prevalence rate—the rate at which the defect occurs in a population—and the increased risk known to be attributable to the drug used to treat that population. Often, studies of large populations are required to determine the risk from teratogenic agents. Large, carefully done, controlled prospective studies can help resolve questions raised by retrospective studies and case reports. Current data from well-designed prospective studies, when available, should be emphasized in counseling.

Counseling

Counseling regarding environmental or teratogenic exposure should be performed in a sympathetic, supportive, and informative manner so that the patient is not unduly alarmed or burdened by guilt. Most patient inquiries are related to low-level risks.

Certain patients, however, have been exposed to agents that are known to be associated with significant increased risk for fetal malformation or mental retardation. The physician may wish to consult with or refer such a patient to a health professional with special education or experience in teratology and birth defects. Prenatal testing also may be indicated. After patients are fully informed of the risks, some request pregnancy termination. Psychologic support of the patient's decision should be provided. In particular, follow-up counseling is advised for patient education and emotional support after abortion or after the birth of an affected baby. Technical multispecialty support for the abnormal infant is essential.

Specific techniques for prenatal diagnosis and management of teratogenic effects are beyond the scope of this bulletin. Amniocentesis for chromosome karyotyping is not appropriate for detecting birth defects caused by environmental teratogens. Detailed targeted ultrasonography may be used to diagnose some structural defects and effects produced by teratogenic agents (1). Serologic testing, ultrasonography, chorionic villus sampling, amniocentesis, and fetal blood sampling may be used in the prenatal diagnosis of congenital cytomegalovirus, rubella, toxoplasmosis, and varicella infections. Open neural tube defects and midline ventral fusion defects may often be detected by ultrasonography or maternal serum screening (2). However, patients should be counseled that ultrasonography can never exclude the presence of teratogenic effects.

Although general statements may be made about the teratogenetic potential of prescription drugs, maternal condition and treatment needs should also be considered, weighing the benefit to the mother with the risk to the fetus. The U.S. Food and Drug Administration has defined five risk categories (A, B, C, D, X) that are used by manufacturers to rate their products for use during pregnancy and are reported in the *Physicans' Desk Reference* (3):

- **Category A**: Controlled studies in women fail to demonstrate a risk to the fetus in the first trimester (and there is no evidence of a risk in later trimesters), and the possibility of fetal harm appears remote. Vitamin C is an example of a category A substance when its use does not exceed the recommended daily allowance.

- **Category B**: Either animal reproduction studies have not demonstrated fetal risk but no controlled studies in pregnant women have been reported, or animal reproduction studies have shown an adverse effect (other than a decrease in fertility) that was not confirmed in controlled studies in women in the first trimester (and there is no evidence of risk in later trimesters). Ampicillin is an example of a category B drug.

- **Category C**: Either studies in animals have revealed adverse effects on the fetus (teratogenic, embryocidal, or other) but no controlled studies in women have been reported, or studies in women and animals are not available. Drugs should be given only if the potential benefit justifies the potential risk to the fetus. Zidovudine used to decrease perinatal transmission of human immunodeficiency virus (HIV) is an example of a category C drug.

- **Category D**: Positive evidence of human fetal risk exists, but the benefits from use in pregnant women may be acceptable despite the risk (eg, if the drug is needed for a life-threatening condition or for a serious disease for which safer drugs cannot be used or are ineffective). Phenytoin is an example of a category D drug.

- **Category X**: Studies in animals or human beings have demonstrated fetal abnormalities, or evidence exists of fetal risk based on human experience, or both, and the risk in pregnant women clearly outweighs any possible benefit. The drug is contraindicated in women who are or may become pregnant. Isotretinoin is an example of a category X drug.

Examples of agents of common concern to pregnant patients but for which there is not adequate evidence to document teratogenicity or adverse effect are listed in the box. Paternal exposure to any agent is not thought to be teratogenic.

Table 1 lists some drugs, chemicals, and infectious agents for which the preponderance of evidence suggests a

---

Agents Not Documented Teratogens*

Following are examples of agents for which there is limited evidence of varying degrees to document teratogenicity:

Drugs and chemicals

    Acetaminophen

    Acyclovir

    Antiemetics (eg, phenothiazines, trimethobenzamide)

    Antihistamines (eg, doxylamine)

    Aspartame

    Aspirin

    Caffeine

    Hair spray

    Marijuana

    Metronidazole

    Minor tranquilizers (eg, meprobamate, chlordiazepoxide, fluoxetine)

    Occupational chemical agents

    Oral contraceptives

    Pesticides

    Trimethoprim–sulfamethoxazole

    Vaginal spermicides

    Zidovudine

Infections

    Herpes simplex type 2 virus

    Parvovirus B19

Electromagnetic fields from video display terminals

Heat

*Paternal exposure to any agent has not been shown to be teratogenic.

---

significant teratogenic risk, as well as the most commonly encountered effects. The organisms that cause cytomegalovirus infections, rubella, syphilis, toxoplasmosis, and varicella infections are classified as fetal pathogens because they damage fully or partially formed tissues by direct infection. However, they are not limited to inducing abnormal development during organogenesis. Causes of neonatal damage (eg, herpes infection passed from mother to child during labor) rather than fetal damage are excluded from the table. Also excluded are agents such as cigarette smoke, which causes fetal hypoxia, ischemia, and growth restriction, but does not cause structural defects. The omission of certain agents is not meant to imply that their safety has been proved.

The use of illicit substances is poorly reported so it is difficult to delineate the precise incidence of use in the general population and in the population of women who have infants with particular birth defects. Thus, it is difficult to know if such drugs are teratogenic.

Sources of Current Teratogen Information

Several sources of useful current information regarding potential teratogens are available. These include computerized databases both on-line and on diskette. Another source is the Organization of Teratogen Information Services, which consolidates teratology information nationwide and reports it by region. Numerous teratogen information services are available throughout the United States to serve specific geographic areas. For information on the teratogen service in a particular area, contact:

Eastern United States
Massachusetts Teratogen Information Service
Boston, Massachusetts
(617) 466-8474
        or
Western United States
Pregnancy Riskline
Salt Lake City, Utah
(801) 328-2229

Computerized teratology and reproductive risk databases provide up-to-date summaries of electronic resource teratology information. Databases commonly available are listed in the box.

References

1. American College of Obstetricians and Gynecologists. Ultrasonography in pregnancy. ACOG Technical Bulletin 187. Washington, DC: ACOG, 1993 (Level III)

```
┌──────────────────────────────────────────────┐
│                                                │
│          Computer Teratology and              │
│   Reproductive Risk Information Databases      │
│                                                │
│  Micromedex, Inc.                              │
│  REPRORISK (REPROTEXT, REPROTOX, Shepard's     │
│  Catalog of                                    │
│  Teratogenic Agents and TERIS)                 │
│  Englewood, CO                                 │
│  (800) 525-9083                                │
│                                                │
│                                                │
│  National Library of Medicine, MEDLARS         │
│  Service Desk                                  │
│  GRATEFUL MED (TOXLINE, TOXNET and MEDLINE)    │
│  Bethesda, MD                                  │
│  (800) 638-8480                                │
│                                                │
│                                                │
│  Reproductive Toxicology Center                │
│  REPROTOX                                      │
│  Columbia Hospital for Women Medical Center    │
│  Washington, DC                                │
│  (202) 293-5137                                │
│                                                │
│                                                │
│  Shepard's Catalog of Teratogenic Agents       │
│  University of Washington                      │
│  Seattle, WA                                   │
│  (206) 543-3373                                │
│                                                │
│                                                │
│  Teratogen Information System                  │
│  TERIS and Shepard's Catalog of Teratogenic    │
│  Agents                                        │
│  Seattle, WA                                   │
│  (206) 543-2465                                │
│                                                │
└──────────────────────────────────────────────┘
```

2. American College of Obstetricians and Gynecologists. Maternal serum screening. ACOG Educational Bulletin 228. Washington, DC: ACOG, 1996 (Level III)

3. U.S. Food and Drug Administration. Pregnancy labeling. FDA Drug Bulletin 1979;9:23–24 (Level III)

Suggested Reading

American College of Obstetricians and Gynecologists. Diagnosis and management of fetal death. ACOG Technical Bulletin 176. Washington, DC: ACOG, 1993

American College of Obstetricians and Gynecologists. Early pregnancy loss. ACOG Technical Bulletin 212. Washington, DC: ACOG, 1995

American College of Obstetricians and Gynecologists. Maternal serum screening. ACOG Educational Bulletin 228. Washington, DC: ACOG, 1996

American College of Obstetricians and Gynecologists. Perinatal viral and parasitic infections. ACOG Technical Bulletin 177. Washington, DC: ACOG 1993

American College of Obstetricians and Gynecologists. Preconceptional care. ACOG Technical Bulletin 205. Washington, DC: ACOG, 1995

American College of Obstetricians and Gynecologists. Seizure disorders in pregnancy. ACOG Educational Bulletin 231. Washington, DC: ACOG, 1996

American College of Obstetricians and Gynecologists. Substance abuse in pregnancy. ACOG Technical Bulletin 195. Washington, DC: ACOG, 1994

American Medical Association Drug Evaluation Annual 1995. Chicago: AMA, 1995

Briggs GG, Freeman RK, Yaffe SJ. Drugs in pregnancy and lactation. 4th ed. Baltimore: Williams and Wilkins, 1994

Cefalo RC, Moos MK. Preconceptional health care: a practical guide. 2nd ed. St Louis: Mosby, 1995

Friedman JM, Polifka JE. Teratogenic effects of drugs: a resource for clinicians (TERIS). Baltimore: Johns Hopkins University Press, 1994

Gilstrap LC, Little BB. Drugs and pregnancy. New York: Elsevier, 1992

Heinonen OP, Slone D, Shapiro S. Birth defects and drugs in pregnancy. Boston: John Wright, PSG Inc, 1982

Paul M. Occupational and environmental reproductive hazards: a guide for clinicians. Baltimore: Williams and Wilkins, 1993

Rayburn WH, Zuspan FP. Drug therapy in obstetrics and gynecology. 3rd ed. St Louis: Mosby Year Book, Inc, 1992

Shepard TH. Catalog of teratogenic agents. 8th ed. Baltimore: Johns Hopkins University Press, 1995

Table 1. Teratogenic Agents

Agent	Effects	Comments
Drugs and chemicals		
Alcohol	Growth restriction before and after birth, mental retardation, microcephaly, midfacial hypoplasia producing atypical facial appearance, renal and cardiac defects, various other major and minor malformations	Nutritional deficiency, smoking, and multiple drug use confound data. Risk due to ingestion of one to two drinks per day is not well defined but may cause a small reduction in average birth weight. Fetuses of women who ingest six drinks per day are at a 40% risk of developing some features of the fetal alcohol syndrome.
Androgens and testosterone derivatives (eg, danazol)	Virilization of female, advanced genital development in males	Effects are dose dependent and related to the stage of embryonic development at the time of exposure. Given before 9 weeks of gestation, labioscrotal fusion can be produced; clitoromegaly can occur with exposure at any gestational age. Risk related to incidental brief androgenic exposure is minimal.
Angiotensin-converting enzyme (ACE) inhibitors (eg, enalapril, captopril)	Fetal renal tubular dysplasia, oligohydramnios, neonatal renal failure, lack of cranial ossification, intrauterine growth restriction	Incidence of fetal morbidity is 30%. The risk increases with second- and third-trimester use, leading to in utero fetal hypotension, decreased renal blood flow, and renal failure.
Coumarin derivatives (eg, warfarin)	Nasal hypoplasia and stippled bone epiphyses are most common; other effects include broad short hands with shortened phalanges, ophthalmologic abnormalities, intrauterine growth restriction, developmental delay, anomalies of neck and central nervous system	Risk for a seriously affected child is considered to be 15–25% when anticoagulants that inhibit vitamin K are used in the first trimester, especially during 6–9 weeks of gestation. Later drug exposure may be associated with spontaneous abortion, stillbirths, central nervous system abnormalities, abruptio placentae, and fetal or neonatal hemorrhage.
Carbamazepine	Neural tube defects, minor craniofacial defects, fingernail hypoplasia, microcephaly, developmental delay, intrauterine growth restriction	Risk of neural tube defect, mostly lumbosacral, is 1–2% when used alone during first trimester and increased when used with other antiepileptic agents.
Folic acid antagonists (methotrexate and aminopterin)	Increased risk for spontaneous abortions, various anomalies	These drugs are contraindicated for the treatment of psoriasis in pregnancy and must be used with extreme caution in the treatment of malignancy. Cytotoxic drugs are potentially teratogenic. Effects of aminopterin are well documented. Folic acid antagonists used during the first trimester produce a malformation rate of up to 30% in fetuses that survive.
Cocaine	Bowel atresias; congenital malformations of the heart, limbs, face and genitourinary tract; microcephaly; intrauterine growth restriction; cerebral infarctions	Risks may be affected by other factors and concurrent abuse of multiple substances. Maternal and pregnancy complications include sudden death and placental abruption.
Diethylstilbestrol	Clear-cell adenocarcinoma of the vagina or cervix, vaginal adenosis, abnormalities of cervix and uterus, abnormalities of the testes, possible infertility in males and females	Vaginal adenosis is detected in more than 50% of women whose mothers took these drugs before 9 weeks of gestation. Risk for vaginal adenocarcinoma is low. Males exposed in utero may have a 25% incidence of epididymal cysts, hypotrophic testes, abnormal spermatozoa, and induration of the testes.
Lead	Increased abortion rate, stillbirths	Fetal central nervous system development may be adversely affected. Determining preconceptional lead levels for those at risk may be useful.
Lithium	Congenital heart disease, in particular, Ebstein anomaly	Risk of heart malformations due to first-trimester exposure is low. The effect is not as significant as reported in earlier studies. Exposure in the last month of gestation may produce toxic effects on the thyroid, kidneys, and neuromuscular systems.

(Continued)

Table 1. Teratogenic Agents (*continued*)

Agent	Effects	Comments
Drugs and Chemicals (*continued*)		
Organic mercury	Cerebral atrophy, microcephaly, mental retardation, spasticity, seizures, blindness	Cerebral palsy can occur even when exposure is in the third trimester. Exposed individuals include consumers of fish and grain contaminated with methyl mercury.
Phenytoin	Intrauterine growth restriction, mental retardation, microcephaly, dysmorphic craniofacial features, cardiac defects, hypoplastic nails and distal phalanges	The full syndrome is seen in less than 10% of children exposed in utero, but up to 30% have some manifestations. Mild to moderate mental retardation is found in some children who have severe physical stigmata. The effect may depend on whether the fetus inherits a mutant gene that decreases production of epoxide hydrolase, an enzyme necessary to decrease the teratogen phenytoin epoxide.
Streptomycin and kanamycin	Hearing loss, eighth-nerve damage	No ototoxicity in the fetus has been reported from use of gentamicin or vancomycin.
Tetracycline	Hypoplasia of tooth enamel, incorporation of tetracycline into bone and teeth, permanent yellow–brown discoloration of deciduous teeth	Drug has no known effect unless exposure occurs in second or third trimester.
Thalidomide	Bilateral limb deficiencies, anotia and microtia, cardiac and gastrointestinal anomalies	Of children whose mothers used thalidomide between 35 and 50 days of gestation, 20% show the effect.
Trimethadione and paramethadione	Cleft lip or cleft palate; cardiac defects; growth deficiency; microcephaly; mental retardation; characteristic facial appearance; ophthalmologic, limb, and genitourinary tract abnormalities	Risk for defects or spontaneous abortion is 60–80% with first-trimester exposure. A syndrome including V-shaped eyebrows, low-set ears, high arched palate, and irregular dentition has been identified. These drugs are no longer used during pregnancy due to the availability of more effective, less toxic agents.
Valproic acid	Neural tube defects, especially spina bifida; minor facial defects	Exposure must occur prior to normal closure of neural tube during first trimester to produce open defect (incidence of approximately 1%).
Vitamin A and its derivatives (eg, isotretinoin, etretinate, and retinoids)	Increased abortion rate, microtia, central nervous system defects, thymic agenesis, cardiovascular effects, craniofacial dysmorphism, microphthalmia, cleft lip and palate, mental retardation	Isotretinoin exposure before pregnancy is not a risk because the drug is not stored in tissue. Etretinate has a long half-life and effects occur long after drug is discontinued. Topical application does not have a known risk.
Infections		
Cytomegalovirus	Hydrocephaly, microcephaly, chorioretinitis, cerebral calcifications, symmetric intrauterine growth restriction, microphthalmos, brain damage, mental retardation, hearing loss	Most common congenital infection. Congenital infection rate is 40% after primary infection and 14% after recurrent infection. Of infected infants, physical effects as listed are present in 20% after primary infection and 8% after secondary infection. No effective therapy exists.
Rubella	Microcephaly, mental retardation, cataracts, deafness, congenital heart disease; all organs may be affected	Malformation rate is 50% if the mother is infected during first trimester. Rate of severe permanent organ damage decreases to 6% by midpregnancy. Immunization of children and nonpregnant adults is necessary for prevention. Immunization is not recommended during pregnancy, but the live attenuated vaccine virus has not been shown to cause the malformations of congenital rubella syndrome.
Syphilis	If severe infection, fetal demise with hydrops; if mild, detectable abnormalities of skin, teeth, and bones	Penicillin treatment is effective for *Treponema pallidum* eradication to prevent progression of damage. Severity of fetal damage depends on duration of fetal infection; damage is worse if infection is greater than 20 weeks. Prevalence is increasing; need to rule out other sexually transmitted diseases.

(*Continued*)

Table 1. Teratogenic Agents (*continued*)

Agent	Effects	Comments
Infections (*continued*)		
Toxoplasmosis	Possible effects on all systems but particularly central nervous system: microcephaly, hydrocephaly, cerebral calcifications. Chorioretinitis is most common. Severity of manifestations depends on duration of disease.	Low prevalence during pregnancy (0.1–0.5%); initial maternal infection must occur during pregnancy to place fetus at risk. *Toxoplasma gondii* is transmitted to humans by raw meat or exposure to infected cat feces. In the first trimester, the incidence of fetal infection is as low as 9% and increases to approximately 59% in the third trimester. The severity of congenital infection is greater in the first trimester than at the end of gestation. Treat with pyrimethamine, sulfadiazine, or spiramycin.
Varicella	Possible effects on all organs, including skin scarring, chorioretinitis, cataracts, microcephaly, hypoplasia of the hands and feet, and muscle atrophy	Risk of congenital varicella is low, approximately 2–3% and occurs between 7 and 21 weeks of gestation. Varicella–zoster immune globulin is available regionally for newborns exposed in utero during last 4–7 days of gestation. No effect from herpes zoster.
Radiation	Microcephaly, mental retardation	Medical diagnostic radiation delivering less than 0.05 Gy* to the fetus has no teratogenic risk. Estimated fetal exposure of common radiologic procedures is 0.01 Gy or less (eg, intravenous pyelography, 0.0041 Gy).

*1 gray = 100 rad.

The references in this bulletin are graded according to the method outlined by the U.S. Preventive Services Task Force:

I   Evidence obtained from at least one properly designed randomized controlled trial

II-1   Evidence obtained from well-designed controlled trials without randomization

II-2   Evidence obtained from well-designed cohort or case–control analytic studies, preferably from more than one center or research group

II-3   Evidence obtained from multiple time series, with or without intervention, or dramatic results in uncontrolled experiments

III   Opinions of respected authorities, based on clinical experience, descriptive studies, or reports of expert committees

Other publications from ACOG:

- **Committee Opinions**, focused updates on emerging areas
- **Practice Patterns**, evidence-based guidelines
- **Criteria Sets**, baseline guidelines for review of diagnostic and management procedures

ACOG EDUCATIONAL BULLETIN

Number 248, July 1998

Viral Hepatitis in Pregnancy

Viral hepatitis is one of the most serious infections that can occur in pregnant women. Six different forms of viral hepatitis have now been defined. This bulletin describes the various types of hepatitis, their implications during pregnancy, the risk of perinatal transmission, and treatment.

Etiology, Epidemiology, and Natural History

Hepatitis A

In the United States, approximately one third of cases of acute hepatitis are caused by hepatitis A virus. The virus usually is transmitted by person-to-person contact through fecal–oral contamination. Poor hygiene, poor sanitation, and intimate personal or sexual contact facilitate transmission. Epidemics frequently result from exposure to contaminated food and water. In obstetric populations in the United States, the patients at greatest risk for hepatitis A infection are those who recently have emigrated from, or traveled to, developing nations where hepatitis A is endemic, particularly in Southeast Asia, Africa, Central America, Greenland, Mexico, and the Middle East. In the United States, the incidence of acute hepatitis A in pregnancy is approximately 1/1,000.

Hepatitis A is caused by an RNA virus. Its incubation period ranges from 15 to 50 days; the mean is 28–30 days. Feces contain the highest concentration of virus particles, and virus excretion reaches its maximum late in the incubation period and early in the prodromal phase of the illness. The duration of viremia is short, and the virus normally is not excreted in urine or other body fluids.

Serious complications of hepatitis A are uncommon. Among all acutely ill patients who require hospitalization, the overall fatality rate does not exceed 2/1,000 cases in the United States. A chronic carrier state of hepatitis A does not exist. In addition, perinatal transmission of the virus has not been demonstrated (1). Hepatitis A immune globulin is recommended for household contacts and contacts in day care centers and custodial institutions. It should be given as soon as possible after exposure; it is ineffective if given more than 2 weeks after exposure. A vaccine is available, which may be taken during pregnancy (2).

This Educational Bulletin was developed under the direction of the Committee on Educational Bulletins of the American College of Obstetricians and Gynecologists as an aid to obstetricians and gynecologists. This document is not to be construed as establishing a standard of practice or dictating an exclusive course of treatment. Rather, it is intended as an educational tool that presents current information on obstetric–gynecologic issues.

Replaces Number 174, November 1992

Hepatitis B

Hepatitis B is caused by a small DNA virus. The intact virus is termed the Dane particle. Hepatitis B virus contains three principal antigens. Hepatitis B surface antigen (HBsAg) is present on the surface of the virus and also circulates freely in the serum in spherical and filamentous forms. The middle portion of the Dane particle contains hepatitis B core antigen (HBcAg). The core antigen is present only in hepatocytes and does not circulate in the serum. Hepatitis B e antigen (HBeAg) is encoded by the same portion of the viral genome that codes for the core antigen. The presence of HBeAg indicates an extremely high viral inoculum and active virus replication (1, 3).

Hepatitis B infection occurs throughout the world. In the United States, it is responsible for 40–45% of all cases of hepatitis. Approximately 300,000 new cases of hepatitis B occur annually, and more than 1 million Americans are chronic carriers. Acute hepatitis B occurs in 1–2/1,000 pregnancies. Chronic infection is present in 5–15/1,000 pregnancies (3, 4), but is more prevalent among certain ethnic groups (ie, Asians, Inuits).

Hepatitis B virus is transmitted by parenteral and sexual contact. Individuals at greatest risk of becoming infected are those who have multiple sexual partners, inject drugs percutaneously, or have sexual partners who engage in these risk-taking behaviors. Other important risk factors are receipt of blood products and household or institutional contact.

All blood donors are screened routinely for HBsAg. Thus, transmission of hepatitis B virus by transfusion of blood or blood products is rare (1). Drug addiction is an important risk factor for horizontal transmission of hepatitis B virus. Sexual contact is an efficient mechanism for spreading the virus. Approximately 25% of the regular sexual contacts of infected individuals will themselves become seropositive.

The mortality associated with acute hepatitis B is approximately 1%. Of patients who become infected, 85–90% experience complete resolution of their physical findings and develop protective levels of the antibody. The other 10–15% of patients become chronically infected; they continue to have detectable serum levels of HBsAg but are asymptomatic and have no biochemical evidence of hepatic dysfunction. In 15–30% of those chronically infected, viral replication continues and is manifested by persistence of the e antigen and active viral DNA synthesis. These individuals are at risk for the subsequent development of chronic or persistent hepatitis and cirrhosis, and approximately 4,000–5,000 die annually of complications of chronic liver disease (5, 6), including hepatocellular carcinoma.

Because hepatitis B virus is highly pathogenic and infectious, perinatal transmission of infection occurs with disturbing regularity. Approximately 10–20% of women who are seropositive for HBsAg transmit the virus to their neonates in the absence of immunoprophylaxis. In women who are seropositive for both HBsAg and HBeAg, the frequency of vertical transmission increases to approximately 90%.

In patients with acute hepatitis B, the frequency of vertical transmission also depends on the time during gestation that maternal infection occurs. When maternal infection occurs in the first trimester, up to 10% of neonates will be seropositive for HBsAg (1, 3). In women acutely infected in the third trimester, 80–90% of offspring will be infected (3).

Between 85% and 95% of cases of perinatal transmission of hepatitis B virus occur as a consequence of intrapartum exposure of the infant to contaminated blood and genital tract secretions. The remaining cases result from hematogenous transplacental dissemination, breastfeeding, and close postnatal contact between the infant and the infected parent. Infants of women who are HBsAg positive at the time of delivery should receive both hepatitis B immune globulin (HBIG) and hepatitis B vaccine within 12 hours of birth, followed by two more injections of hepatitis B vaccine in the first 6 months of life.

Hepatitis C

Hepatitis C virus (previously termed nonA, nonB hepatitis) is a single-stranded RNA virus that appears to infect as much as 0.6% of the pregnant population (7, 8). The principal risk factors for acquiring hepatitis C virus are the same as for hepatitis B.

Approximately 50% of patients with acute hepatitis C develop biochemical evidence of chronic liver disease. Of these individuals, at least 20% subsequently have chronic active hepatitis or cirrhosis. Vertical transmission has been well documented and is proportional in likelihood to the titer of hepatitis C virus RNA present in the mother's blood (7, 9). Approximately 7–8% of hepatitis C virus-positive women transmit hepatitis C virus to their offspring (7, 8). Vertical transmission of hepatitis C may be more likely if the mother also is infected with human immunodeficiency virus (HIV) (8, 10). Currently, no method has been found to prevent prenatal transmission. Many experts believe that hepatitis C virus-positive women should not breastfeed because there is a 2–3% risk of vertical transmission. Unlike hepatitis B, antibodies to hepatitis C are not protective.

Hepatitis D

Hepatitis D requires hepatitis B virus for replication and expression and so occurs only in people already infected with hepatitis B. In acute hepatitis B, once HBsAg clears the bloodstream, so does hepatitis D. Approximately 20–25% of chronic hepatitis B virus carriers ultimately are coinfected with hepatitis D virus (11, 12). In acute hepatitis D, immunoglobulin M (IgM) antibodies against hepatitis D predominate, whereas IgG antibodies may be found in chronic infections.

Chronic hepatitis D produces severe disease more often than other forms of chronic hepatitis. Of patients with chronic hepatitis D, 70–80% ultimately develop cirrhosis and portal hypertension, 15% of whom suffer an unusually rapid progression to cirrhosis within 2 years of the initial onset of acute illness. Mortality due to hepatic failure approaches 25% (11–13). In contrast, only 15–30% of patients with chronic hepatitis B virus infection develop cirrhosis and portal hypertension, and the disease progression typically is much slower.

Vertical transmission of hepatitis D virus has been documented. Transmission is uncommon, however, because the measures used to prevent perinatal infection with hepatitis B virus are almost uniformly effective in preventing infection by hepatitis D.

Hepatitis E

The epidemiologic features of hepatitis E are similar to those of hepatitis A. Although the disease has been reported only rarely in the United States, it is endemic in several developing nations, similar to those mentioned for hepatitis A. In these regions, maternal mortality often has been alarmingly high. In the 1980s, India and Burma reported 10–18% of pregnant women with hepatitis E died as a complication of their infection (14). Most of these women lived under conditions of extreme poverty. Women who have a higher standard of living and greater access to medical care are unlikely to have the same high rate of mortality.

Although acute hepatitis E can be a serious disease, it usually is self-limited and does not result in a chronic carrier state (14, 15). As with hepatitis A, hepatitis E is transmitted via contaminated food or water, though less efficiently. Vertical transmission of hepatitis E has been reported (16).

Hepatitis G

Hepatitis G infection is more likely in people already infected with hepatitis B or C or who have a history of intravenous drug use (17). In a study of 47 women infected with HIV or hepatitis C virus, 9 of whom also were infected with the hepatitis G virus, the risk of vertical transmission was higher for hepatitis G than it was for the other two agents (18). Hepatitis G probably does not cause chronic active hepatitis or cirrhosis.

Clinical Manifestations

The usual subjective symptoms in patients with acute viral hepatitis are malaise, fatigue, anorexia, nausea, and right upper quadrant or epigastric pain. Typical physical findings include jaundice, upper abdominal tenderness, and hepatomegaly, although many cases of hepatitis are anicteric. The patient's urine usually is darkened, and the stool may be acholic. In cases of fulminant hepatitis, signs of coagulopathy and encephalopathy may be evident.

In patients with hepatitis A or E, these clinical manifestations usually are temporally related to recent travel to an endemic area or exposure to an infected person. Similarly, hepatitis B, C, D, or G typically ensues after parenteral exposure to contaminated blood or sexual contact with an infected partner. The evolution of acute clinical illness in patients with hepatitis D often follows a biphasic course. In the initial phase of infection, patients with hepatitis D are indistinguishable from individuals with acute hepatitis B. Two to four weeks after apparent resolution of symptoms, patients have a relapse, which usually is of a milder nature and is associated with a second episode of elevation in serum transaminases. At this time serologic assays for hepatitis D virus usually are positive.

As noted previously, among those patients originally infected with hepatitis B, C, or D virus whose acute symptoms resolve, some become chronic carriers of viral antigens. The same may be true for hepatitis G, although a carrier state has yet to be identified. Although most viral hepatitis carriers initially are asymptomatic, up to one third subsequently develop chronic active or persistent hepatitis or cirrhosis. Once cirrhosis ensues, patients demonstrate the typical signs of end-stage liver disease, such as jaundice, muscle wasting, ascites, spider angioma, palmar erythema, and, ultimately, hepatic encephalopathy. Hepatitis C is probably the leading cause of hepatocellular carcinoma in the United States, whereas hepatitis B virus is the leading cause worldwide.

Diagnosis

Jaundice, a primary symptom of hepatitis infection, also occurs with numerous other disorders. The principal disorders that should be considered in the differential diagnosis of jaundice in pregnancy are shown in Table 1. Testing strategies should be directed toward discriminating among clinically likely diagnoses.

General Tests

Coincident with the onset of symptoms, patients with acute hepatitis usually have a marked increase in the serum concentration of alanine aminotransferase (ALT, previously SGPT) and aspartate aminotransferase (AST, previously SGOT). In addition, the serum bilirubin concentration often is increased. In patients who are mod-

Table 1. Disorders to Consider in the Differential Diagnosis of Jaundice in Pregnancy

Condition	Distinguishing Characteristics
Viral hepatitis	Mild to marked elevation in serum transaminases Positive viral serology Prominent inflammatory infiltrate with hepatocellular disarray
Acute fatty liver of pregnancy	Minimal elevation in transaminases Little if any inflammatory infiltrate with prominent microvesicular fat deposition
Toxic injury	History of drug exposure (eg, tetracycline, isoniazid, erythromycin estolate, alpha methyldopa)
Cholestasis of pregnancy	Pruritus Elevation of bile salts Cholestasis with little inflammation
Severe preeclampsia	Hypertension, edema, proteinuria, oliguria Elevated blood urea nitrogen, creatinine, uric acid, transaminases, and lactate dehydrogenase Thrombocytopenia
Mononucleosis	Flulike illness Positive heterophile antibody Elevated transaminases
Cytomegalovirus (CMV) hepatitis	CMV antibodies Positive viral culture or polymerase chain reaction Elevated transaminases
Autoimmune hepatitis	Antinuclear antibodies, liver–kidney microsomal antibodies Elevated transaminases

erately to severely ill, coagulation abnormalities and hyperammonemia also may be present. Although liver biopsy is rarely indicated in pregnancy, viral hepatitis may be distinguished histologically from other causes of hepatic injury by its characteristic pattern of extensive hepatocellular injury and inflammatory infiltrate. Initial evaluation of the patient with suspected viral hepatitis should include tests for: anti-HA IgM, HBsAg, and HC PCR. In selected patients, additional testing can include anti-HBc IgM, HD PCR, anti-HE, and anti-HG.

Specific Tests

If hepatitis is suspected based on the initial evaluation and general tests, the type of virus is determined through laboratory analysis.

Hepatitis A

The diagnosis of acute hepatitis A is confirmed by detecting IgM antibodies to the virus. A chronic carrier state for this infection does not exist, but IgG antibodies to hepatitis A virus will persist in patients with previous exposure to the virus (1).

Hepatitis B

In the acute stage of hepatitis B virus infection, the diagnosis is confirmed by the identification of the surface antigen and the IgM antibody to the core antigen. The presence of e antigen is indicative of an exceptionally high viral inoculum and active virus replication, and implies a high degree of infectivity. Chronic hepatitis B virus infection is characterized by the persistence of the surface antigen in the liver and serum. The time of infection can be evaluated by measuring IgG and IgM antibodies to HBcAg. Typically, the IgG hepatitis B core antibody (HBcAb) appears 6 months or more after infection, with the IgM moiety being predominant prior to that time.

Occasionally patients with acute hepatitis B will demonstrate HBsAg only briefly and will develop anti-HBc (IgM) as their only marker of acute hepatitis B infection. Anti-HBc (IgM) may be helpful in HBsAg-negative patients in whom hepatitis B is strongly suspected (19).

Hepatitis C

The diagnosis of hepatitis C is confirmed by the identification of the antibody to hepatitis C virus. However, the antibody may not be present until 6–16 weeks after the onset of clinical illness. Hepatitis C viral RNA can be detected by polymerase chain reaction assay of serum soon after infection as well as in chronic disease.

Hepatitis D

Laboratory tests that may be used to confirm the diagnosis of acute hepatitis D are detection of D antigen in hepatic tissue or serum and identification of the IgM antibody to hepatitis D virus. D antigenemia usually persists in patients with chronic hepatitis D despite the appearance of the IgG antibody to the virus. Thus, as in hepatitis C and HIV infection, viremia and end-organ damage can continue despite the presence of the antibody to the virus (11, 12).

Hepatitis E and G

The diagnoses of infection with hepatitis E and hepatitis G are similar. In both cases, the infection is documented by the presence of virus-specific antibodies.

Management

General Supportive Measures

Patients with acute hepatitis should be hospitalized if they have encephalopathy, coagulopathy, or severe debilitation. Nutritional needs should be addressed within the context of the severity of the disease. Fluid and electrolyte abnormalities should be corrected. If a coagulopathy is present, administration of erythrocytes, platelets, and clotting factors such as fresh frozen plasma or cryoprecipitate may be necessary. Activity should be limited, and the patient should be protected from upper abdominal trauma.

Women who are less severely ill may be treated as outpatients. They should reduce their level of activity, avoid upper abdominal trauma, and maintain good nutrition as well. Infected women also should avoid intimate contact with household members and sexual partners until these individuals receive appropriate prophylaxis outlined as follows.

Specific Immunotherapy

Hepatitis A

Currently, no antiviral agent is available for treatment of acute hepatitis A. An inactivated-virus vaccine that is safe in pregnancy is available. Women at risk for infection with hepatitis A, such as those traveling to endemic areas, should be vaccinated (2).

Patients who have close personal or sexual contact with an individual who has hepatitis A should receive immune globulin if they have not been immunized. Immune globulin does not pose a risk to either a pregnant woman or her fetus, and therefore the preparation should be administered during pregnancy if indicated. For postexposure prophylaxis, a single intramuscular dose of 1 mL should be administered as soon as possible after contact with the infected individual. Administration of immune globulin more than 2 weeks after exposure is not effective in preventing or ameliorating the severity of hepatitis A (1).

Hepatitis B

Although interferon alfa has been shown to alter the natural history of acute hepatitis B, C, and D virus infection, it has multiple side effects including myelosuppression, autoantibody formation, thyroid disturbances, and possible cardiotoxicity. Interferon alfa should be avoided during pregnancy because of its possible abortifacient effects. Accordingly, prevention of infection is of paramount importance. Specific immunotherapy with hepatitis B immune globulin (HBIG) has been effective (20).

Vaccination. Individuals who have risk factors should be vaccinated against infection. In general, it is cost-effective to screen for the antibody to hepatitis B virus in women who belong to groups with a high risk of infection. In most other risk groups, antibody screening prior to vaccination is probably not indicated.

Two vaccines for hepatitis B virus, Recombivax HB and Engerix-B, have been developed. The original vaccine (Heptavax-B), licensed in 1982 but not currently available, was prepared by purification of surface antigen extracted from the serum of hepatitis B virus carriers. Because of concerns, later disproven, that this vaccine might transmit HIV infection, many individuals who were appropriate candidates for the vaccine refused to receive it. Currently available vaccines prepared from yeast cultures by using recombinant DNA technology clearly pose no risk of transmission of HIV infection. They are highly immunogenic and result in seroconversion in more than 95% of recipients (1).

The vaccine should be administered into the deltoid muscle. Intragluteal and intradermal injections result in lower rates of seroconversion. Pregnancy is not a contraindication to vaccination. In fact, susceptible pregnant women who are at risk for hepatitis B infection should be specifically targeted for vaccination.

Individuals who have been exposed to hepatitis B virus before they are vaccinated should receive passive immunization with HBIG and undergo the immunization series—preferably in the contralateral arm. Hepatitis B immune globulin is prepared from pooled plasma that has an HBsAg antibody titer of at least 1/100,000, as determined by radioimmunoassay. The preparation is administered intramuscularly in a dose of 0.06 mL/kg. When exposure has occurred as a result of sexual contact, the patient should receive a single dose of HBIG within 14 days of contact. For prophylaxis after percutaneous or mucous membrane injury, treatment should include an initial injection of HBIG, followed by a second dose 1 month later. These regimens are approximately 75% effective in preventing hepatitis B virus infection. If an antibody response is documented, clinical hepatitis B virus infection is rare (1). However, because of the high rate of usually conferred protection, evaluation of immune status at any interval is not deemed necessary (1). Human immunodeficiency virus infection has not been transmitted by HBIG. In addition, pregnancy is not a contraindication to administration of HBIG (1).

Perinatal Management. The combination of passive and active immunization, as outlined here, has been particularly effective in reducing the frequency of perinatal transmission of hepatitis B virus. Several investigations conducted in Asian nations have shown that passive and active immunization of the newborn is 85–95% effective in preventing perinatal transmission of hepatitis B virus.

The Centers for Disease Control and Prevention and the American College of Obstetricians and Gynecologists recommend hepatitis B virus screening for all pregnant women. Pregnant women should be routinely tested for HBsAg during an early prenatal visit. If, at the time of admission to the hospital for delivery, the test has not been performed or the results are not available, the HBsAg test should be done. Women in high-risk groups who initially test negative for hepatitis B virus should be targeted for vaccination if they have not been vaccinated previously. Seropositive women should be encouraged to inform their children and sexual partners of the need for testing and vaccination. Serum transaminases should be measured in seropositive women to detect biochemical evidence of chronic active hepatitis. If the test results are abnormal or if the liver is palpable, the patient should be evaluated further to determine whether the disease is acute or chronic.

The Centers for Disease Control and Prevention recommends universal active immunization of all infants born in the United States (6). The immunization schedule for infants of women who have been screened and are negative should be started preferably before discharge, but by no later than 2 months of age. Infants of women who are known to be HBsAg positive or whose status is unknown should have both passive and active immunization treatment. It should be given simultaneously at different sites intramuscularly and started within 12 hours after birth. Such a strategy will prevent postnatal and neonatal acquisition of hepatitis B virus in most cases. The physician responsible for the care of a newborn delivered to a mother with chronic hepatitis B should be informed of the mother's carrier status so that the appropriate doses of hepatitis B virus vaccine and HBIG can be given as soon as possible following delivery.

Hepatitis C and D
Treatment with interferon alfa produced clinical improvement in 28–46% of patients with chronic hepatitis C. Unfortunately, however, approximately 50% of patients who initially improved suffered a relapse within 6 months of the cessation of therapy. In addition, pregnant women were specifically excluded from the investigation (21). Similar results are seen with hepatitis D.

Precautions for Health Care Workers
Each year, approximately 12,000 health care workers in the United States contract hepatitis B virus infection as a result of an occupational injury. Of these individuals, about 200 experience a fulminant course and die. Another 1,000–1,200 become chronic carriers of the surface antigen (22).

The principal mechanism of transmission of hepatitis B virus from patient to health care worker is through injury from a sharp object, such as a needle or scalpel, that is contaminated with infected blood. Of the individuals exposed in these ways, 10–20% subsequently become seropositive for HBsAg. Although most remain asymptomatic, they are still at increased risk for development of chronic liver disease (1, 22). Another important, but less frequent, mechanism of transmission is a splash injury, resulting in contact between skin or mucosal surfaces and contaminated secretions or blood.

Physicians and other health care workers should use standard precautions to reduce their risk of acquiring hepatitis B virus infection (23). The primary element of universal precautions is the use of appropriate barrier precautions by all health care personnel to prevent the exposure of their skin and mucous membranes to the blood or other body fluids of any patient. Most important, all health care workers who may have direct or indirect exposure to patients should be immunized.

Reports have been published documenting transmission of hepatitis B from infected health care workers, including obstetrician–gynecologists, to patients during invasive procedures (24). In each instance in which complete serologic testing has been performed, the health care workers were seropositive for both surface and e antigens.

Summary
Hepatitis A is an uncommon complication of pregnancy and is not associated with perinatal transmission. In contrast, hepatitis B virus infection is more common and

clearly poses a serious risk to the household contacts and neonates of infected mothers. Accordingly, all pregnant women should be tested for hepatitis B virus. Universal vaccination of all neonates with hepatitis B vaccine is now recommended. Infants delivered to HBsAg seropositive mothers also should receive HBIG and vaccination immediately after birth. Hepatitis E is extremely rare in the United States and is quite similar to hepatitis A, although perinatal transmission does occur with hepatitis E. Hepatitis C and D, which are transmitted parenterally and by sexual contact, have been associated with vertical transmission. No immunoprophylaxis currently is available for neonates of mothers with hepatitis C or E virus. Immunization against hepatitis B is protective against vertical transmission of hepatitis D.

References

1. Centers for Disease Control. Protection against viral hepatitis. Recommendations of the Immunization Practices Advisory Committee (ACIP). MMWR 1990;39(RR-2):1–26

2. Totos G, Gizaris V, Papaevangelou G. Hepatitis A vaccine: persistence of antibodies 5 years after the first vaccination. Vaccine 1997;15:1252–1253

3. Sweet RL. Hepatitis B infection in pregnancy. Obstetrics/Gynecology Report 1990;2:128–139

4. Snydman DR. Hepatitis in pregnancy. N Engl J Med 1985; 313:1398–1401

5. Hoofnagle JH. Chronic hepatitis B. N Engl J Med 1990; 323:337–339

6. Centers for Disease Control. Hepatitis B virus: A comprehensive strategy for eliminating transmission in the United States through universal childhood vaccination: recommendations of the Immunization Practices Advisory Committee (ACIP). MMWR 1991;40(RR-13):1–25

7. Ohto H, Terazawa S, Sasaki N, Sasaki N, Hino K, Ishiwata C, et al. Transmission of hepatitis C virus from mothers to infants. N Engl J Med 1994;330:744–750

8. Silverman NS, Snyder M, Hodinka RL, McGillen P, Knee G. Detection of hepatitis C virus antibodies and specific hepatitis C virus ribonucleic acid sequences in cord bloods from a heterogeneous prenatal population. Am J Obstet Gynecol 1995;173:1396–1400

9. Matsubara T, Sumazaki R, Takita H. Mother-to-infant transmission of hepatitis C virus: a prospective study. Eur J Pediatr 1995;154:973–978

10. Zucotti GV, Ribero ML, Giovannini M, Fasola M, Riva E, Portera G, et al. Effect of hepatitis C genotype on mother-to-infant transmission of virus. J Pediatr 1995;127:278–280

11. Hoofnagle JH. Type D (delta) hepatitis. JAMA 1989;261:1321–1325 [Erratum in JAMA 1989;261:3552]

12. Rizzetto M. The delta agent. Hepatology 1983;3:729–737

13. Shattock AG, Irwin FM, Morgan BM, Hillary IB, Kelly MG, Fielding JF, et al. Increased severity and morbidity of acute hepatitis in drug abusers with simultaneously acquired hepatitis B and hepatitis D virus infections. BMJ 1985;290:1377–1380

14. Bradley DW, Maynard JE. Etiology and natural history of post-transfusion and enterically-transmitted non-A, non-B hepatitis. Semin Liver Dis 1986;6:56–66

15. Velázquez O, Stetler HC, Avila C, Ornelas G, Alvarez C, Hadler SC, et al. Epidemic transmission of enterically transmitted non-A, non-B hepatitis in Mexico, 1986-1987. JAMA 1990;263:3281–3285

16. Khuroo MS, Kamill S, Jameel S. Vertical transmission of hepatitis E virus. Lancet 1995;345:1025–1026

17. Linnen J, Wages J Jr, Zhang-Keck Z-Y, Fry KE, Krawzynski KZ, Alter H, et al. Molecular cloning and disease association of hepatitis G virus: a transfusion-transmissible agent. Science 1996;271:505–508

18. Feucht HH, Zollner B, Polywka S, Laufs R. Vertical transmission of hepatitis G. Lancet 1996;347:615–616

19. Kryger P. Significance of anti-HBc IgM in the differential diagnosis of viral hepatitis. J Virol Methods 1985;10:283–289

20. Vassiliadis S, Athanassakis I. Type II interferon may be a potential hazardous therapeutic agent during pregnancy. Br J Haematol 1992;82:782–783

21. Davis GL, Balart LA, Schiff ER, Lindsay K, Bodenheimer HC Jr, Perillo RP, et al. Treatment of chronic hepatitis C with recombinant interferon alfa. N Engl J Med 1989; 321:1501–1506

22. Jagger J, Hunt EH, Brand-Elnaggar J, Pearson RD. Rates of needle-stick injury caused by various devices in a university hospital. N Engl J Med 1988;319:284–288

23. Occupational Safety and Health Administration. Bloodborne pathogens (29 CFR 1910.1030). Fed Regis. December 6, 1991; 56:64004–64182

24. Welch J, Webster M, Tilzey AJ, Noah ND, Banatvala JE. Hepatitis B infections after gynaecological surgery. Lancet 1989;1:205–206

Practice Bulletins

Reading the Medical Literature:
  Applying Evidence to Practice   **329**

Antepartum Fetal Surveillance (No. 9)   337

Antibiotic Prophylaxis for Gynecologic Procedures (No. 23)   348

*Antiphospholipid Syndrome (No. 68)   357

Assessment of Risk Factors for Preterm Birth (No. 31)   366

Benefits and Risks of Sterilization (No. 46)   374

Breast Cancer Screening (No. 42)   386

Cervical Cytology Screening (No. 45)   398

Cervical Insufficiency (No. 48)   409

Chronic Hypertension in Pregnancy (No. 29)   418

Chronic Pelvic Pain (No. 51)   427

Diagnosis and Management of Preeclampsia and Eclampsia (No. 33)   444

Diagnosis and Treatment of Cervical Carcinomas (No. 35)   453

Diagnosis and Treatment of Gestational Trophoblastic Disease (No. 53)   466

Dystocia and the Augmentation of Labor (No. 49)   479

*Emergency Contraception (No. 69)   489

External Cephalic Version (No. 13)   500

Fetal Macrosomia (No. 22)   507

Gestational Diabetes (No. 30)   518

Gynecologic Herpes Simplex Virus Infections (No. 57)   532

*Hemoglobinopathies in Pregnancy (No. 64)   539

*Human Papillomavirus (No. 61)   548

Induction of Labor (No. 10)   562

*Intrapartum Fetal Heart Rate Monitoring (No. 70)   572

*Intrauterine Device (No. 59)   581

Intrauterine Growth Restriction (No. 12)   591

*Management of Abnormal Cervical Cytology and Histology (No. 66)   603

Management of Anovulatory Bleeding (No. 14)   623

*Management of Endometrial Cancer (No. 65)   631

*Published in 2005

Practice Bulletins

Management of Herpes in Pregnancy (No. 8)   644

Management of Infertility Caused by Ovulatory Dysfunction (No. 34)   653

Management of Postterm Pregnancy (No. 55)   665

Management of Preterm Labor (No. 43)   673

Management of Recurrent Early Pregnancy Loss (No. 24)   682

*Medical Management of Abortion (No. 67)   694

Medical Management of Endometriosis (No. 11)   706

Medical Management of Tubal Pregnancy (No. 3)   719

Multiple Gestation: Complicated Twin, Triplet,
and High-Order Multifetal Pregnancy (No. 56)   726

Nausea and Vomiting of Pregnancy (No. 52)   741

Neural Tube Defects (No. 44)   754

Obstetric Analgesia and Anesthesia (No. 36)   765

Operative Vaginal Delivery (No. 17)   780

Osteoporosis (No. 50)   788

Perinatal Care at the Threshold of Viability (No. 38)   802

Perinatal Viral and Parasitic Infections (No. 20)   810

Polycystic Ovary Syndrome (No. 41)   823

*Pregestational Diabetes Mellitus (No. 60)   837

Premature Rupture of Membranes (No. 1)   848

Premenstrual Syndrome (No. 15)   858

Prenatal Diagnosis of Fetal Chromosomal Abnormalities (No. 27)   867

Prevention of Deep Vein Thrombosis and Pulmonary Embolism (No. 21)   879

Prevention of Rh D Alloimmunization (No. 4)   889

Prophylactic Antibiotics in Labor and Delivery (No. 47)   897

Prophylactic Oophorectomy (No. 7)   905

Selective Estrogen Receptor Modulators (No. 39)   911

Shoulder Dystocia (No. 40)   921

Surgical Alternatives to Hysterectomy in the Management of Leiomyomas (No. 16)   927

*Published in 2005

Practice Bulletins

The Use of Hormonal Contraception in Women
   with Coexisting Medical Conditions (No. 18)   936

Thrombocytopenia in Pregnancy (No. 6)   950

Thromboembolism in Pregnancy (No. 19)   961

Thyroid Disease in Pregnancy (No. 37)   971

Ultrasonography in Pregnancy (No. 58)   981

*Urinary Incontinence in Women (No. 63)   991

Use of Botanicals for Management of Menopausal Symptoms (No. 28)   1004

Vaginal Birth After Previous Cesarean Delivery (No. 54)   1015

*Published in 2005

Practice Bulletins

Reading the Medical Literature

Applying Evidence to Practice

Developed under the direction
of the ACOG Committee on
Practice Patterns:

James R. Scott, MD, Chair

Daniel W. Cramer, MD, ScD

Herbert B. Peterson, MD

Benjamin P. Sachs, MD

Mary L. Segars Dolan, MD, MPH

Stanley Zinberg, MD
　Director of Practice Activities

Nancy E. O'Reilly, MHS
　Manager, Practice Activities

Peter J. Sebeny
　Research Associate

Reading the Medical Literature *is designed as a resource for Fellows of the American College of Obstetricians and Gynecologists (ACOG) and others to offer a better understanding of evidence-based medicine, particularly as it relates to the development of ACOG's clinical practice guidelines. As evidence-based medicine continues to develop and to be integrated into clinical practice, an understanding of its basic elements is critical in translating the medical literature into appropriate clinical practice. The emphasis on evidence-based medicine has taken on new and greater importance as the environment of clinical practice grows more diverse, with increased access to more information by both physicians and patients and the changing allocation of resources. Practice guidelines are a formal synthesis of evidence, developed according to a rigorous research and review process. This document provides an overview of ACOG's guideline development process, including elements of study design that are linked to the strength of the evidence.* Reading the Medical Literature *is not intended to serve as a comprehensive overview of the scientific methods of epidemiology and study design. Rather, it is provided to serve as a readily available introduction to and overview of the topic.*

In 1995, ACOG began developing scientifically based practice guidelines, formerly known as Practice Patterns and subsequently as Practice Bulletins. The guidelines are derived from the best available evidence of clinical efficacy and consideration of costs, with recommendations explicitly linked to the evidence. These evidence-based practice guidelines are intended to be a means of improving the quality of health care, decreasing its cost, and diminishing professional liability. They are proscriptive in nature and, therefore, directive in their approach.

This document describes how ACOG Practice Committees identify, evaluate, and synthesize evidence from the medical literature to produce practice guidelines. In particular, this document briefly describes various study

329

designs evaluated in the production of evidence-based guidelines and the decision-making steps used to construct evidence-based recommendations on clinical issues. Also highlighted are potential major flaws in study design that affect the validity and applicability of study results, as well as the strength of the evidence. This document includes a glossary of commonly encountered epidemiologic and biostatistic terms found in reports of scientific evidence, as well as suggestions for further reading.

Selection of Topics

Topics developed into evidence-based practice guidelines are selected based on clinical issues in obstetrics and gynecology with unexplained variations in practice or because there are differences between what is known scientifically and what is practiced. Once a topic has been identified, objectives of the guideline are developed and research questions are formulated to guide the literature search. The research questions highlight the most important aspects of a particular clinical issue, focusing on areas relevant to practice and useful in patient management.

Searching the Literature

In the ACOG Resource Center, medical librarians with extensive subject expertise perform a literature search based on the clinical questions and objectives. The search includes a review of the MEDLINE database, the Cochrane Library, ACOG's internal resources and documents, and other databases as appropriate. In addition, ACOG librarians review more than 200 journals. This process locates relevant articles from journals not indexed in MEDLINE and those not yet indexed.

The search is limited to documents published in English, and a specific strategy may be used to refine the search further. This filter strategy restricts the search by study design or publication type and is similar to the process used by the Cochrane Library. No further screening or elimination of records is done by the librarians. Updated searches are conducted as the topic is developed or further revised.

Literature Analysis

After results of the literature search are compiled, the study abstracts are reviewed to assess the relevance of each study or report. Those articles appropriate for further critical appraisal are obtained and subdivided according to the research question they address. The bibliographies of these articles are also reviewed to identify additional studies that may not have been identified in the initial literature search.

The data in the literature are evaluated to provide answers to the clinical questions. The articles obtained for review are organized by study design to ascertain the possible strengths and weaknesses inherent in each study, as well as the quality of evidence they may provide. Certain aspects of a clinical issue may not be addressed in research studies, and expert opinion may be used and identified as such.

The levels of evidence used are based on the method used by the U.S. Preventive Services Task Force. The U.S. Preventive Services Task Force was a 20-member panel of scientific and medical experts charged with developing recommendations on appropriate use of clinical interventions. Their recommendations were based on a systematic review of the evidence of clinical effectiveness.

Types of Study Designs

Intervention Studies

Level I Evidence

Commonly referred to as clinical trials, intervention studies are characterized by the investigators' roles in assigning subjects to exposed and nonexposed groups and following the subjects to assess outcome. Intervention studies may involve the use of a comparison group, which may include subjects under another treatment, drug, test, or placebo.

Randomized controlled trials are characterized by the prospective assignment of subjects, through a random method, into an experimental group and a control (placebo) group. The experimental group receives the drug or treatment to be evaluated, while the control group receives a placebo, no treatment, or the standard of care. Both groups are followed for the outcome(s) of interest. Randomization is the most reliable method to ensure that the participants in both groups are as similar as possible with respect to all known or unknown factors that might affect the outcome.

 Example

Postmenopausal women are identified from a population and randomly assigned either to a study group that will be prescribed hormone replacement therapy or to a control group that will be prescribed a placebo. Both groups of women are observed prospectively to determine who in each group subsequently develops endometrial cancer. The rate at which women prescribed hormone replacement therapy develop endometrial cancer is compared to that of women in the control group.

Major Study Flaws

- Randomization was not valid and resulted in a differential assignment of treatment that affected the outcomes.
- The sample size was too small to detect a clinically important difference.
- Poor compliance or loss to follow-up was significant enough to affect the outcomes.

Level II-1 Evidence

Controlled trials without randomization are intervention studies in which allocation to either the experimental or control group is not based on randomization, making assignment subject to biases that may influence study results. Conclusions drawn from these types of studies are considered to be less reliable than those from randomized controlled trials.

 Example

Postmenopausal women are identified from a population and assigned in a nonrandomized manner either to a study group that will be prescribed hormone replacement therapy or to a control group that will be prescribed a placebo. Both groups of women are observed prospectively to determine who subsequently develops endometrial cancer. The rate at which women prescribed hormone replacement therapy develop endometrial cancer is compared to that of women in the control group.

 Major Study Flaws

- Nonrandom group assignment resulted in unequal distribution of known and unknown factors that may influence the outcome.
- Other potential flaws are the same as those for randomized controlled trial (Level I).

Observational Studies

Level II-2 Evidence

There are two types of observational studies in this category: cohort and case-control. In these studies, the investigator has no role in assignment of study exposures but, rather, observes the natural course of events of exposure and outcome.

The starting point for a *cohort study* is exposure status. Subjects are classified on the basis of the presence or absence of exposure to a risk factor, a treatment, or an intervention and then followed for a specified period to determine the presence or absence of disease. Cohort studies can be of two different types determined by the timing

of initiation of the study: retrospective (nonconcurrent) or prospective (concurrent) studies. In a *prospective cohort study*, the groups of exposed and unexposed subjects have been identified and the investigator must conduct follow-up for an adequate period to ascertain the outcome of interest. In a *retrospective cohort study*, both the exposure and outcomes of interest already have occurred by the initiation of the study. The rate of disease in the exposed group is divided by the rate of disease in the unexposed group, yielding a rate ratio or relative risk.

 Example

A group of postmenopausal women who have been prescribed hormone replacement therapy is identified (study group), as is an otherwise similar group of postmenopausal women who have not been prescribed hormone replacement therapy (control group). The study and control groups are observed to determine who subsequently develops endometrial cancer. The rate at which women using hormone replacement therapy develop endometrial cancer is compared with that of women not using hormone replacement therapy who also develop endometrial cancer.

 Major Study Flaws

- Criteria for determining exposure status were inadequately defined.
- The assessments of the outcome for the exposed and nonexposed groups differed in a biased manner.
- The nonexposed comparison group was inappropriate.

A *case-control study* is a retrospective study in which a group of subjects with a specified outcome (cases) and a group without that same outcome (controls) are identified. Thus, the starting point for a case-control study is disease status. Investigators then compare the extent to which each subject was previously exposed to the variable of interest such as a risk factor, a treatment, or an intervention. A disadvantage of this study type is that assessment of exposure may have been influenced by disease status, including the possibility that cases recalled their exposure differently than controls. The odds of exposure in the case group compared with the odds of exposure in the control group provide the measure of association between the disease and exposure (odds ratio).

 Example

Researchers conduct a case-control study to assess the relationship between hormone replacement therapy and endometrial cancer. A group of women who have recently developed endometrial cancer (cases) and a group of women with similar characteristics who did not develop endometrial cancer (controls) are identified. The use of hormone replacement therapy for each woman in the case group and the control group is determined to assess exposure history. The odds that women who developed endometrial cancer had used hormone replacement therapy are compared with the odds that women who did not develop endometrial cancer had used hormone replacement therapy. These odds are calculated to determine any association of hormone replacement therapy to endometrial cancer.

 Major Study Flaws

- The case or control group preferentially included or excluded subjects with a particular exposure history.
- Cases or controls were selectively more likely to recall or admit to a particular exposure.
- The possibility of known or unknown factors that may have been related to both exposure status and outcome were not adequately considered and assessed.

Level II-3 Evidence

Cross-sectional studies are observational studies that assess the status of individuals with respect to the presence or absence of both exposure and outcome at a particular time. In this type of study, one is unlikely to be able to discern the temporal relationship between an exposure and outcome. Results from cross-sectional studies can yield correlations and disease prevalence. Prevalence is defined as the proportion of individuals with a disease at a specific time; in contrast, incidence is the number of new cases occurring over a specified period.

Uncontrolled investigational studies report the results of treatment or interventions in a particular group, but lack a control group for comparison. They may demonstrate impressive results, but in the absence of a control group the results may be attributable to factors other than the intervention or treatment.

Of all observational studies, cross-sectional and uncontrolled investigational studies provide the least evidence of causation.

 Example

Postmenopausal women are identified from a population and surveyed at a particular time about their current intake of calcium. Bone densitometry is evaluated in these women at the same time to identify signs of osteoporosis. In this cross-sectional study, a measure of calcium intake in women with and without signs of osteoporosis is compared.

 Major Study Flaws

- It is usually not possible to determine the temporal relationship between disease and exposure.
- Other factors that may contribute to the disease, particularly past exposure to factors other than the factor under study, are not taken into consideration.

Level III Evidence

These studies provide limited information about the relationship between exposure and the outcome of interest. This category includes *descriptive studies*, such as case reports and case series, and *expert opinion*, which is often based on clinical experience.

A *case study* describes clinical characteristics or other interesting features of a single patient or a series of patients. The latter is referred to as a *case series*.

Expert opinion often is used to make recommendations. This type of evidence includes findings from expert panels and committees and the opinions of respected experts in a particular field.

Other Study Designs

A *meta-analysis* is a systematic structured process, not merely a literature review. It combines results from more than one investigation to obtain a weighted average of the effect of a variable or intervention on a defined outcome. This approach can increase precision of the exposure to the outcome measured, although it is important to add that the validity of the conclusions of the meta-analysis depends largely on the quality of its component studies. Results are usually presented in a graph that illustrates the measure of association by each study type and the overall summary association (Fig. 1).

A *decision analysis* is a type of study that uses mathematical models of the sequences of multiple strategies to determine which are optimal. The basic framework is the decision tree in which branches of the tree represent key probabilities or decisions. Decision analysis is driven by key assumptions. Ideally the assumptions are based on data that may include findings from meta-analyses. Often a decision analysis is undertaken when there are inadequate data to perform a meta-analysis (Fig. 2).

Cost-benefit analysis and *cost-effectiveness analysis* are related analytic methods that compare health care practices or techniques in terms of their relative economic efficiencies

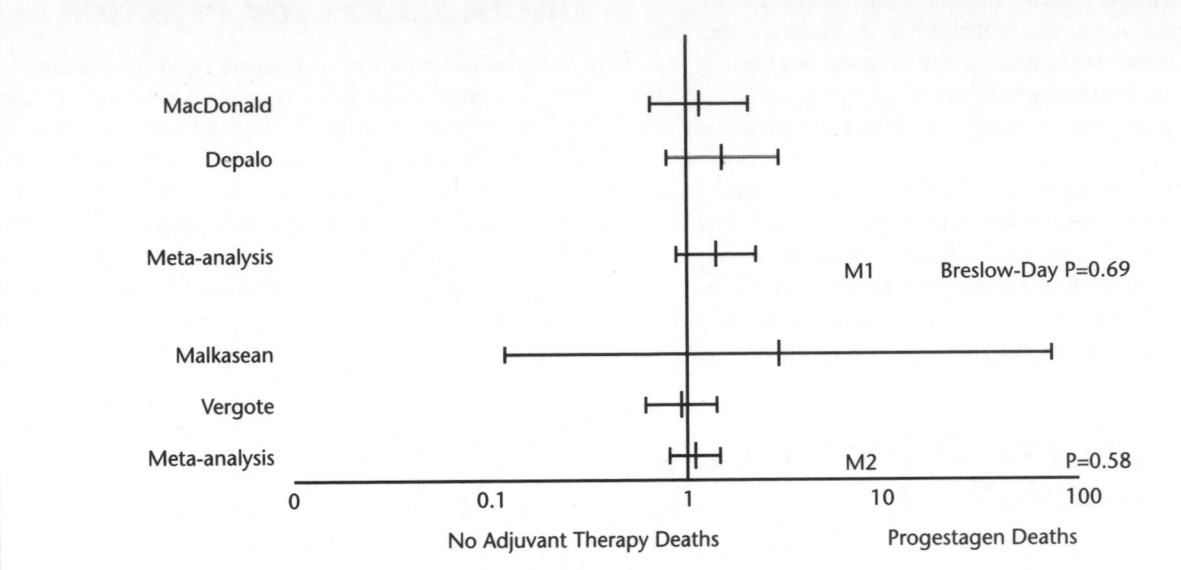

Fig. 1. Effects on endometrial cancer deaths: progestagen versus no adjuvant treatment.

(Reprinted from the European Journal of Obstetrics, Gynecology, and Reproductive Biology, Vol. 65. Martin-Hirsch PL, Lilford RJ, Jarvis GJ. Adjuvant progestagen therapy for the treatment of endometrial cancer: review and meta-analyses of published randomized controlled trials, p. 205, © 1996, with permission from Elsevier Science Ireland Ltd, Bay 15K, Shannon Industrial Estate, Co. Clare, Ireland.)

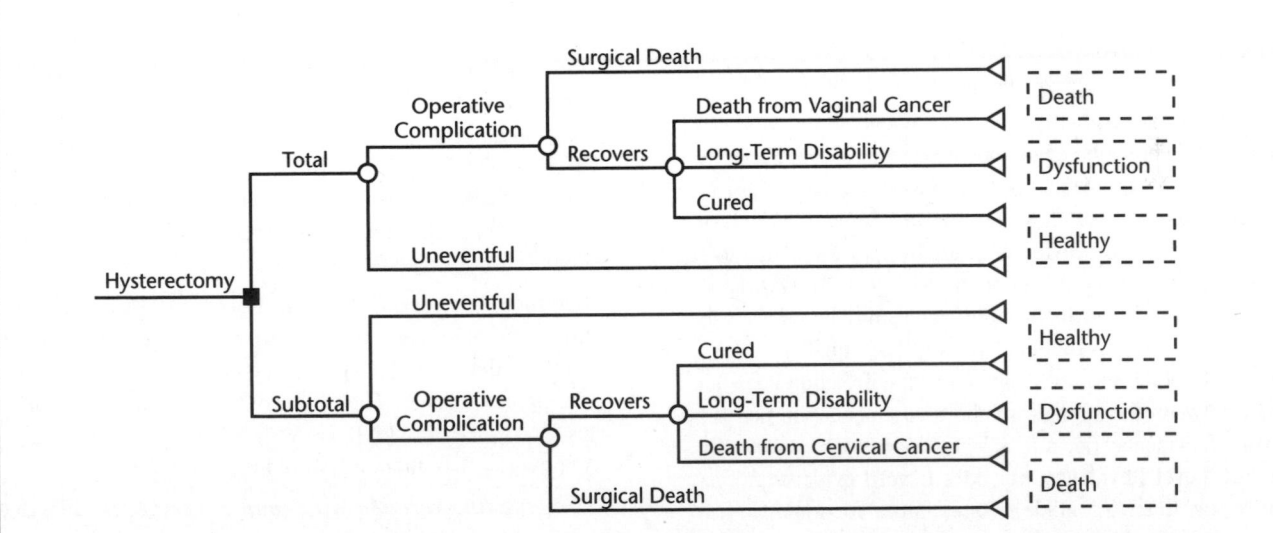

Fig. 2. Decision model. Square at far left, choice between two treatment options: total or subtotal hysterectomy. Round nodes, chance outcomes; end branches, final outcome states.

(Scott JR, Sharp HT, Dodson MK, Norton PA, Warner HR. Subtotal hysterectomy in modern gynecology: a decision analysis. Am J Obstet Gynecol 1997;176:1187. Reprinted with permission.)

in providing health benefits. In a *cost-effectiveness analysis*, the net monetary costs of a health care intervention are compared with some measure of clinical outcome or effectiveness. In a *cost-benefit analysis*, the net monetary costs of a health care intervention typically are compared with the net monetary costs of the clinical outcome or effectiveness. Therefore, a cost-benefit analysis compares costs associated with an intervention with monetary benefits from the use of that intervention. The advantage of a cost-benefit analysis is the ability to use dollars for comparison across interventions. The disadvantage is the difficulty in assigning a monetary value to health status or quality of life.

Developing Evidence-Based Recommendations

Having stated the clinical question and assembled and graded the literature using the levels just outlined, recommendations are formulated according to the quality and quantity of evidence. Based on the highest available level of evidence, recommendations are provided and graded according to the following categories:

A   There is good evidence to support the recommendation.

B   There is fair evidence to support the recommendation.

C   There is insufficient evidence to support the recommendation; however, the recommendation may be made on other grounds.

D   There is fair evidence against the recommendation.

E   There is good evidence against the recommendation.

This method explicitly links recommendations to the evidence. Determination of the quality of the evidence and the strength of recommendations are based on good, fair, or insufficient evidence. These descriptors address the levels of evidence and also provide a qualitative review of the evidence in terms of its methodologic strengths and weaknesses. A prerequisite for inclusion of each study in the analysis is that it provides overall evidence of "good quality."

It is important to note that an exact correlation does not exist between the strength of the recommendation and the level of evidence (ie, an "A" grade does not necessarily require Level I evidence, nor does Level I evidence necessarily lead to an "A" grade). For example, for some clinical issues a randomized trial is not possible for medical or ethical reasons, and recommendations must be based on evidence from other types of studies (Level II-2, II-3). In other cases, high-quality studies have produced conflicting results, or evidence of significant benefit is offset by evidence of important harm from the intervention. Although these studies may be randomized controlled trials (Level I), insufficient or conflicting evidence would result in a "C" recommendation.

Implications for Practice

Medicine will continue to face the rapid introduction of new technologies, rationing of health resources, and increasing attention to the quality and outcomes of medical care. Physicians will have to acquire the skills necessary to review the medical literature critically to identify the best evidence in managing patients. This process for developing practice guidelines identifies available evidence and constructs recommendations based on the best evidence so that obstetrician–gynecologists can continue to provide the highest quality of care.

 # Glossary*

Accuracy: The degree to which a measurement or an estimate based on measurements represents the true value of the attribute that is being measured.

Bias: Deviation of results or inferences from the truth, or processes leading to such deviation; it is any trend in the collection, analysis, interpretation, publication, or review of data that can lead to conclusions that are systematically different from the truth. Three frequently occurring types of bias include selection bias, information bias, and confounding. *Selection bias* is error due to systematic differences in characteristics between those who are selected for study and those who are not. *Information bias*, also called observational bias, is a flaw in measuring exposure or outcome data that results in different quality (accuracy) of information between comparative groups. Recall bias is an example of information bias. The third example of bias, *confounding*, describes a situation in which the effects of two processes are not separated; it is the distortion of the apparent effect of an exposure on risk brought about by the association with other factors that can influence the outcome.

Confidence interval: An indication of the variability of a point estimate, such as an odds ratio or relative risk. In general, the wider the confidence interval, the less precise the point estimate. The 95% confidence interval is often used. As an example, if the 95% confidence interval does not overlap 1.0, then one would reject the null hypothesis.

Confounding variable (syn: confounder): A variable that can cause or prevent the outcome of interest, is not an intermediate variable, and is associated with the factor under investigation. Unless it is possible to adjust for confounding variables, their effects cannot be distinguished from those factor(s) being studied. Bias can occur when adjustment is made for any factor that is caused in part by the exposure and is also correlated with the outcome.

---

* Adapted from *A Dictionary of Epidemiology*, third edition. Last JM, ed. Used by permission of Oxford University Press.

Incidence: The number of instances of illness commencing, or persons falling ill, during a given period in a specified population. More generally, the number of new events (eg, new cases of a disease in a defined population) within a specified period.

Null hypothesis (test hypothesis): The statistical hypothesis that one variable has no association with another variable or set of variables, or that two or more population distributions do not differ from one another. In simplest terms, the null hypothesis states that the results observed in a study, experiment, or test are no different from what might have occurred as a result of the operation of chance alone.

Odds ratio (syn: cross product ratio, relative odds): The ratio of two odds. The exposure odds ratio for a set of case control data is the ratio of the odds in favor of exposure among the cases (*a/b*) to the odds in favor of exposure among noncases (*c/d*). A 2 × 2 table (Table 1) can be used to illustrate this calculation of odds ratios.

Table 1. Odds Ratio Calculations*

	Exposed	Unexposed
Disease	a	b
No disease	c	d

*The odds ratio is *ad/bc.*

P-value: The probability that a test statistic would be as extreme or more extreme than observed if the null hypothesis were true. The letter *P*, followed by the abbreviation n.s. (not significant) or by the symbol < (less than) and a decimal notation such as 0.01 or 0.05, is a statement of the probability that the difference observed could have occurred by chance if the groups were really alike (ie, under the null hypothesis). Investigators may arbitrarily set their own significance levels, but in most biomedical and epidemiologic work, a study result whose probability value is less than 5% (P <0.05) or 1% (P <0.01) is considered sufficiently unlikely to have occurred by chance and would justify the designation "statistically significant." By convention, most investigators choose P <0.05 as statistically significant.

Power (statistical power): The ability of a study to demonstrate an association if one exists. The power of the study is determined by several factors, including the frequency of the condition under study, the magnitude of the effect, the study design, and sample size.

Prevalence: The number of events (eg, instances of a given disease or other condition) in a given population at a des-

ignated time; sometimes used to mean prevalence rate. When used without qualification, the term usually refers to the situation at a specified time (point prevalence).

Relative risk: The ratio of risk of disease or death among the exposed to that of the risk among the unexposed; this usage is synonymous with risk ratio. If the relative risk is above 1.0, then there is a positive association between the exposure and the disease; if it is less than 1.0, then there is a negative association.

Sensitivity and specificity: Sensitivity is the proportion of truly diseased persons in the screened population who are identified as diseased by the screening test. Specificity is the proportion of truly nondiseased persons who are so identified by the screening test. Table 2 illustrates these quantities.

In screening and diagnostic tests, the probability that a person with a positive test is a true positive (ie, does have the condition) is referred to as the *predictive value* of a positive test. The *predictive value* of a negative test is the probability that a person with a negative test does not have the condition. The predictive value of a screening test is determined by the sensitivity and specificity of the test and by the prevalence of the condition for which the test is being used.

$$\text{Positive predictive value} = a/a+b$$

$$\text{Negative predictive value} = d/c+d$$

Table 2. Sensitivity and Specificity Calculations

Screening Test Results	True Status		Total
	Diseased	Not Diseased	
Positive	a	b	a + b
Negative	c	d	c + d
Total	a + c	b + d	a + b + c + d

a = Diseased individuals detected by the test (true positives)
b = Nondiseased individuals positive by the test (false positives)
c = Diseased individuals not detected by the test (false negatives)
d = Nondiseased individuals negative by the test (true negatives)
Sensitivity = *a/a+c*; specificity = *d/b+d*.

Type I error: The error of rejecting a true null hypothesis (ie, declaring that a difference exists when it does not).

Type II error: The error of failing to reject a false null hypothesis (ie, declaring that a difference does not exist when in fact it does).

▶ Suggested Reading

Asilomar Working Group on Recommendations for Reporting of Clinical Trials in the Biomedical Literature. Checklist of information for inclusion in reports of clinical trials. Ann Intern Med 1996;124:741–743

Chalmers TC, Smith H Jr, Blackburn B, Silverman B, Schroeder B, Reitman D, et al. A method for assessing the quality of a randomized control trial. Control Clin Trials 1981; 2:31–49

DuRant RH. Checklist for the evaluation of research articles. J Adolesc Health 1994;15:4–8

Grisso JA. Making comparisons. Lancet 1993;342:157–160

Guyatt GH, Sackett DL, Cook DJ. Users' guides to the medical literature. II. How to use an article about therapy or prevention. A. Are the results of the study valid? Evidence-Based Medicine Working Group. JAMA 1993;270:2598–2601

Guyatt GH, Sackett DL, Cook DJ. Users' guides to the medical literature. II. How to use an article about therapy or prevention. B. What were the results and will they help me in caring for my patients? Evidence-Based Medicine Working Group. JAMA 1994;271:59–63

Guyatt GH, Sackett DL, Sinclair JC, Hayward R, Cook DJ, Cook RJ. Users' guides to the medical literature. IX. A method for grading health care recommendations. Evidence-Based Medicine Working Group. JAMA 1995;274:1800–1804

Hadorn DC, Baker D, Hodges JS, Hicks N. Rating the quality of evidence for clinical practice guidelines. J Clin Epidemiol 1996;49:749–754

Hayward RS, Wilson MC, Tunis SR, Bass EB, Guyatt G. Users' guides to the medical literature. VIII. How to use clinical practice guidelines. A. Are the recommendations valid? The Evidence-Based Medicine Working Group. JAMA 1995; 274:570–574

Jaeschke R, Guyatt GH, Sackett DL. Users' guides to the medical literature. III. How to use an article about a diagnostic test. B. What are the results and will they help me in caring for my patients? The Evidence-Based Medicine Working Group. JAMA 1994;271:703–707

Laupacis A, Wells G, Richardson WS, Tugwell P. Users' guides to the medical literature. V. How to use an article about prognosis. Evidence-Based Medicine Working Group. JAMA 1994;272:234–237

Naylor CD, Guyatt GH. Users' guides to the medical literature. X. How to use an article reporting variations in the outcomes of health services. The Evidence-Based Medicine Working Group. JAMA 1996;275:554–558

Naylor CD, Guyatt GH. Users' guides to the medical literature. XI. How to use an article about a clinical utilization review. Evidence-Based Medicine Working Group. JAMA 1996;275: 1435–1439

Oxman AD. Checklists for review articles. BMJ 1994;309: 648–651

Oxman AD, Cook DJ, Guyatt GH. Users' guides to the medical literature. VI. How to use an overview. Evidence-Based Medicine Working Group. JAMA 1994;272:1367–1371

Oxman AD, Sackett DL, Guyatt GH. Users' guides to the medical literature. I. How to get started. The Evidence-Based Medicine Working Group. JAMA 1993;270:2093–2095

Peipert JF, Gifford DS, Boardman LA. Research design and methods of quantitative synthesis of medical evidence. Obstet Gynecol 1997;90:473–478

Richardson WS, Detsky AS. Users' guides to the medical literature. VII. How to use a clinical decision analysis. A. Are the results of the study valid? Evidence-Based Medicine Working Group. JAMA 1995;273:1292–1295

Wilson MC, Hayward RS, Tunis SR, Bass EB, Guyatt G. Users' guides to the medical literature. VIII. How to use clinical practice guidelines. B. What are the recommendations and will they help you in caring for your patients? The Evidence-Based Medicine Working Group. JAMA 1995;274:1630–1632

ACOG PRACTICE BULLETIN

CLINICAL MANAGEMENT GUIDELINES FOR
OBSTETRICIAN–GYNECOLOGISTS

NUMBER 9, OCTOBER 1999

(Replaces Technical Bulletin Number 188, January 1994)

This Practice Bulletin was developed by the ACOG Committee on Practice Bulletins—Obstetrics with the assistance of Dwight J. Rouse, MD. The information is designed to aid practitioners in making decisions about appropriate obstetric and gynecologic care. These guidelines should not be construed as dictating an exclusive course of treatment or procedure. Variations in practice may be warranted based on the needs of the individual patient, resources, and limitations unique to the institution or type of practice.

Antepartum Fetal Surveillance

The goal of antepartum fetal surveillance is to prevent fetal death. Antepartum fetal surveillance techniques based on assessment of fetal heart rate patterns have been in clinical use for almost three decades. More recently, real-time ultrasonography and Doppler velocimetry have been used to evaluate fetal well-being. Antepartum fetal surveillance techniques are now routinely used to assess the risk of fetal death in pregnancies complicated by preexisting maternal conditions (eg, type 1 diabetes mellitus) as well as those in which complications have developed (eg, intrauterine growth restriction). This document will review the current indications for and techniques of antepartum fetal surveillance and outline management guidelines for antepartum fetal surveillance, consistent with the best contemporary scientific evidence.

Background

Physiology of Fetal Heart Response and Fetal Behavioral State Alteration

In both animals and humans, fetal heart rate pattern, level of activity, and degree of muscular tone are sensitive to hypoxemia and acidemia (1–4). Redistribution of fetal blood flow in response to hypoxemia may result in diminished renal perfusion and oligohydramnios (5). Surveillance techniques such as cardiotocography, real-time ultrasonography, and maternal perception of fetal movement can identify the fetus that is either suboptimally oxygenated or, with increasing degrees of placental dysfunction, acidemic. Identification of suspected fetal compromise provides the opportunity to intervene before progressive metabolic acidosis can lead to fetal death. However, acute, catastrophic changes in fetal status, such as those that can occur with abruptio placentae or an umbilical cord accident, are generally not predicted by tests of fetal well-being. Therefore, fetal deaths from such events are not as amenable to prevention.

In humans, the range of normal umbilical blood gas parameters has been established by cordocentesis performed in pregnancies in which the fetus ultimately proved to be healthy, and ranges vary by gestational age (6). Although the degree of hypoxemia and acidemia at which various indices of fetal well-being become abnormal is not known with precision, it can be estimated, based on data from published studies. In one investigation, the fetal biophysical profile (BPP) was performed immediately before cordocentesis. Fetuses with a nonreactive nonstress test (NST) were found to have a mean (± standard deviation) umbilical vein pH of 7.28 ± 0.11. Cessation of fetal movement appears to occur at lower pH levels; fetuses with abnormal movement were found to have an umbilical vein pH of 7.16 ± 0.08 (7). Thus, a reasonable correlation between certain measurable aspects of fetal heart rate and behavior and evidence of fetal metabolic compromise can be inferred.

However, when abnormal antepartum fetal surveillance results are compared with evidence of hypoxia or acidemia, the degree of acid–base disturbance may range from mild to severe. Furthermore, factors other than acid–base and oxygenation status (eg, prematurity, fetal sleep–wake cycle, maternal medication exposure, and fetal central nervous system abnormalities) can adversely affect biophysical parameters. Finally, neither the degree nor the duration of intrauterine hypoxemia and acidemia necessary to adversely affect short- and long-term neonatal outcome has been established with any precision.

Antepartum Fetal Surveillance Techniques

Several antepartum fetal surveillance techniques (tests) are in use. These include fetal movement assessment, NST, contraction stress test (CST), BPP, modified BPP, and umbilical artery Doppler velocimetry.

Fetal Movement Assessment

A diminution in the maternal perception of fetal movement often but not invariably precedes fetal death, in some cases by several days (8). This observation provides the rationale for fetal movement assessment by the mother ("kick counts") as a means of antepartum fetal surveillance.

Although several counting protocols have been employed, neither the optimal number of movements nor the ideal duration for counting movements has been defined. Thus, numerous protocols have been reported and appear to be acceptable. In one approach, the woman lies on her side and counts distinct fetal movements (9). Perception of 10 distinct movements in a peri-

od of up to 2 hours is considered reassuring. Once 10 movements have been perceived, the count may be discontinued. In another approach, women are instructed to count fetal movements for 1 hour three times per week (10). The count is considered reassuring if it equals or exceeds the woman's previously established baseline count. In the absence of a reassuring count, further fetal assessment is recommended.

Contraction Stress Test

The CST is based on the response of the fetal heart rate to uterine contractions. It relies on the premise that fetal oxygenation will be transiently worsened by uterine contractions. In the suboptimally oxygenated fetus, the resultant intermittent worsening in oxygenation will, in turn, lead to the fetal heart rate pattern of late decelerations. Uterine contractions also may provoke or accentuate a pattern of variable decelerations caused by fetal umbilical cord compression, which in some cases is associated with oligohydramnios.

With the patient in the lateral recumbent position, the fetal heart rate and uterine contractions are simultaneously recorded with an external fetal monitor. If at least three spontaneous contractions of 40 seconds' duration each or longer are present in a 10-minute period, no uterine stimulation is necessary. If fewer than three contractions of at least 40 seconds' duration occur in 10 minutes, contractions are induced with either nipple stimulation or intravenous administration of dilute oxytocin.

Nipple stimulation usually is successful in inducing an adequate contraction pattern and allows completion of testing in approximately half the time required when intravenous oxytocin is given (11). In one nipple stimulation technique, the woman is instructed to rub one nipple through her clothing for 2 minutes or until a contraction begins (11). If by that time the contraction frequency has not become adequate (as defined previously), stimulation is stopped and restarted again after 5 minutes. If nipple stimulation is unsuccessful, or if the use of oxytocin is preferred, an intravenous infusion of dilute oxytocin may be initiated at a rate of 0.5 mU/min and doubled every 20 minutes until an adequate contraction pattern is achieved (12).

The CST is interpreted according to the presence or absence of late fetal heart rate decelerations (13), which are defined as decelerations that reach their nadir after the peak of the contraction and that usually persist beyond the end of the contraction. The results of the CST are categorized as follows:

- Negative: no late or significant variable decelerations

- Positive: late decelerations following 50% or more of contractions (even if the contraction frequency is fewer than three in 10 minutes)

- Equivocal–suspicious: intermittent late decelerations or significant variable decelerations

- Equivocal–hyperstimulatory: fetal heart rate decelerations that occur in the presence of contractions more frequent than every 2 minutes or lasting longer than 90 seconds

- Unsatisfactory: fewer than three contractions in 10 minutes or an uninterpretable tracing

Relative contraindications to the CST generally include conditions associated with an increased risk of preterm labor and delivery, uterine rupture, or uterine bleeding. These include the following (12):

- Preterm labor or certain patients at high risk of preterm labor

- Preterm membrane rupture

- History of extensive uterine surgery or classical cesarean delivery

- Known placenta previa

Nonstress Test

The NST is based on the premise that the heart rate of the fetus that is not acidotic or neurologically depressed will temporarily accelerate with fetal movement. Heart rate reactivity is thought to be a good indicator of normal fetal autonomic function. Loss of reactivity is associated most commonly with a fetal sleep cycle but may result from any cause of central nervous system depression, including fetal acidosis.

With the patient in the lateral tilt position, the fetal heart rate is monitored with an external transducer. Ideally, the patient should not have smoked recently, because this may adversely affect test results (14). The tracing is observed for fetal heart rate accelerations that peak (but do not necessarily remain) at least 15 beats per minute above the baseline and last 15 seconds from baseline to baseline. It may be necessary to continue the tracing for 40 minutes or longer to take into account the variations of the fetal sleep–wake cycle. Acoustic stimulation of the nonacidotic fetus may elicit fetal heart rate accelerations that appear to be valid in the prediction of fetal well-being. Such stimulation offers the advantage of safely reducing overall testing time without compromising detection of the acidotic fetus (15–17). To perform acoustic stimulation, an artificial larynx (ideally one of the commercially available models especially designed for this purpose) is positioned on the maternal abdomen and a stimulus of 1–2 seconds is applied. This may be repeated up to three times for progressively longer durations of up to 3 seconds to elicit fetal heart rate accelerations.

Nonstress test results are categorized as reactive or nonreactive. Various definitions of reactivity have been used. Using the most common definition, the NST is considered reactive (normal) if there are two or more fetal heart rate accelerations (as defined previously) within a 20-minute period, with or without fetal movement discernible by the woman (18). A nonreactive NST is one that lacks sufficient fetal heart rate accelerations over a 40-minute period. The NST of the noncompromised preterm fetus is frequently nonreactive: from 24 to 28 weeks of gestation, up to 50% of NSTs may not be reactive (19), and from 28 to 32 weeks of gestation, 15% of NSTs are not reactive (20, 21).

Variable decelerations may be observed in up to 50% of NSTs (22). If nonrepetitive and brief (<30 seconds), they indicate neither fetal compromise nor the need for obstetric intervention (22). Repetitive variable decelerations (at least 3 in 20 minutes), even if mild, have been associated with an increased risk of cesarean delivery for a nonreassuring intrapartum fetal heart rate pattern (23, 24). Fetal heart rate decelerations during an NST that persist for 1 minute or longer are associated with a markedly increased risk of both cesarean delivery for a nonreassuring fetal heart rate pattern and fetal demise (25–27).

Biophysical Profile

The BPP consists of an NST combined with four observations made by real-time ultrasonography (28). Thus, the BPP comprises five components:

1. Nonstress test (which, if all four ultrasound components are normal, may be omitted without compromising the validity of the test results) (28)

2. Fetal breathing movements (one or more episodes of rhythmic fetal breathing movements of 30 seconds or more within 30 minutes)

3. Fetal movement (three or more discrete body or limb movements within 30 minutes)

4. Fetal tone (one or more episodes of extension of a fetal extremity with return to flexion, or opening or closing of a hand)

5. Determination of the amniotic fluid volume (a single vertical pocket of amniotic fluid exceeding 2 cm is considered evidence of adequate amniotic fluid) (29, 30)

Each of the five components is assigned a score of either 2 (normal or present as defined previously) or 0 (abnormal, absent, or insufficient). A composite score of 8 or 10 is normal, a score of 6 is considered equivocal, and a score of 4 or less is abnormal. Regardless of the composite score, in the presence of oligohydramnios (largest vertical pocket of amniotic fluid volume ≤ 2 cm), further evaluation is warranted (30).

Modified Biophysical Profile

In the late second- or third-trimester fetus, amniotic fluid reflects fetal urine production. Placental dysfunction may result in diminished fetal renal perfusion, leading to oligohydramnios (5). Amniotic fluid volume assessment can therefore be used to evaluate long-term uteroplacental function. This observation fostered the development of what has come to be termed the "modified BPP" as a primary mode of antepartum fetal surveillance. The modified BPP combines the NST (with the option of acoustic stimulation), as a short-term indicator of fetal acid–base status, with the amniotic fluid index (AFI), which is the sum of measurements of the deepest cord-free amniotic fluid pocket in each of the abdominal quadrants, as an indicator of long-term placental function (15). An AFI greater than 5 cm generally is considered to represent an adequate volume of amniotic fluid (31). Thus, the modified BPP is considered normal if the NST is reactive and the AFI is more than 5, and abnormal if either the NST is nonreactive or the AFI is 5 or less.

Umbilical Artery Doppler Velocimetry

Doppler ultrasonography is a noninvasive technique used to assess the hemodynamic components of vascular impedance. Umbilical artery Doppler flow velocimetry has been adapted for use as a technique of fetal surveillance, based on the observation that flow velocity waveforms in the umbilical artery of normally growing fetuses differ from those of growth-restricted fetuses. Specifically, the umbilical flow velocity waveform of normally growing fetuses is characterized by high-velocity diastolic flow, whereas with intrauterine growth restriction, there is diminution of umbilical artery diastolic flow (32–34). In some cases of extreme intrauterine growth restriction, flow is absent or even reversed. The perinatal mortality rate in such pregnancies is quite high (35). Abnormal flow velocity waveforms have been correlated histopathologically with small-artery obliteration in placental tertiary villi (36) and functionally with fetal hypoxia and acidosis (37), as well as with perinatal morbidity and mortality (35). Commonly measured flow indices, based on the characteristics of peak systolic frequency shift (S), end-diastolic frequency shift (D), and mean peak frequency shift over the cardiac cycle (A), include the following:

- Systolic to diastolic ratio (S/D)
- Resistance index (S-D/S)
- Pulsatility index (S-D/A)

Randomized studies (38–44) of the utility of umbilical artery Doppler velocimetry generally have defined abnormal flow as either absent end diastolic flow, or a flow index greater than two standard deviations above the mean for gestational age. To maximize interpretability, multiple waveforms should be assessed, and wall-filter settings should be set low enough (typically <150 Hz) to avoid masking diastolic flow.

Clinical Considerations and Recommendations

▶ *Is there compelling evidence that any form of antepartum fetal surveillance decreases the risk of fetal demise or otherwise improves perinatal outcome?*

There is a dearth of evidence from randomized controlled trials that antepartum fetal surveillance decreases the risk of fetal death (45). Moreover, in one comprehensive review, antepartum fetal surveillance was categorized as a form of care "likely to be ineffective or harmful" (46). In spite of its unproven value, antepartum fetal surveillance is widely integrated into clinical practice in the developed world. Therefore, a definitive evaluation of antepartum fetal surveillance (which would require the random allocation of gravidas to prenatal care that included some form of antepartum fetal surveillance versus prenatal care that did not include any form of antepartum fetal surveillance) is unlikely to be conducted in a setting that can be generalized to current U.S. obstetric practice. In the absence of a definitive, relevant randomized clinical trial, evidence for the value of antepartum fetal surveillance will remain circumstantial and rest principally on the observation that antepartum fetal surveillance has been consistently associated with rates of fetal death that are substantially lower than the rates of fetal death in both untested (and presumably lower-risk) contemporaneous pregnancies from the same institutions (15, 16, 47) and pregnancies with similar complicating factors that were managed before the advent of currently employed techniques of antepartum fetal surveillance (historic controls). However, these perceived benefits of antepartum fetal surveillance may be influenced by the low incidence of adverse fetal outcome in the general population. The lower the incidence of adverse outcomes, the more likely favorable outcomes will be achieved regardless of test performance.

▶ *What are the indications for antepartum fetal surveillance?*

Because antepartum fetal surveillance results have not been definitively demonstrated to improve perinatal outcome, all indications for antepartum testing must be considered somewhat relative. In general, antepartum fetal surveillance has been employed in pregnancies in which the risk of antepartum fetal demise is increased. Accordingly, some of the conditions under which testing may be appropriate include the following:

- Maternal conditions
  - Antiphospholipid syndrome
  - Hyperthyroidism (poorly controlled)
  - Hemoglobinopathies (hemoglobin SS, SC, or S-thalassemia)
  - Cyanotic heart disease
  - Systemic lupus erythematosus
  - Chronic renal disease
  - Type 1 diabetes mellitus
  - Hypertensive disorders
- Pregnancy-related conditions
  - Pregnancy-induced hypertension
  - Decreased fetal movement
  - Oligohydramnios
  - Polyhydramnios
  - Intrauterine growth restriction
  - Postterm pregnancy
  - Isoimmunization (moderate to severe)
  - Previous fetal demise (unexplained or recurrent risk)
  - Multiple gestation (with significant growth discrepancy)

▶ *When during gestation should antepartum fetal surveillance be initiated?*

Choosing the appropriate point in gestation to begin antepartum testing depends on balancing several considerations, including the prognosis for neonatal survival, the severity of maternal disease, the risk of fetal death, and the potential for iatrogenic prematurity complications resulting from false-positive test results. The importance of the last consideration is illustrated by the experience of one large center, in which 60% of infants delivered because of an abnormal antepartum test result had no evidence of short-term or long-term fetal compromise (16). Both theoretic models (48) and large clinical studies (49, 50) confirm that initiating testing at 32–34 weeks of gestation is appropriate for most at-risk patients. However, in pregnancies with multiple or particularly worrisome high-risk conditions (eg, chronic hypertension with suspected intrauterine growth restriction), testing might begin as early as 26–28 weeks of gestation.

▶ *What is the proper frequency of testing?*

How frequently to perform fetal testing depends on several factors, including clinical judgment. If the indication for testing is not persistent (eg, a single episode of decreased fetal movement followed by reassuring testing in an otherwise uncomplicated pregnancy), it need not be repeated. When the clinical condition that prompted testing persists, the test should be repeated periodically until delivery to monitor for continued fetal well-being. If the maternal medical condition is stable and CST results are negative, the CST is typically repeated in 1 week (12). Other tests of fetal well-being (NST, BPP, or modified BPP) are typically repeated at weekly intervals (16), but in the presence of certain high-risk conditions, such as postterm pregnancy, type 1 diabetes, intrauterine growth restriction, or pregnancy-induced hypertension, some investigators have performed twice-weekly NST, BPP, or modified BPP testing. Any significant deterioration in the maternal medical status requires fetal reevaluation, as does any acute diminution in fetal activity, regardless of the amount of time that has elapsed since the last test.

▶ *How reassuring is a normal test result?*

In most cases, a normal test result is highly reassuring, as reflected in the false-negative rate of antepartum fetal surveillance, defined as the incidence of stillbirth occurring within 1 week of a normal test result. The stillbirth rate, corrected for lethal congenital anomalies and unpredictable causes of demise, was 1.9 per 1,000 in the largest series of NSTs (5,861) versus 0.3 per 1,000 in 12,656 CSTs (13), 0.8 per 1,000 in 44,828 BPPs (51), and 0.8 per 1,000 in 54,617 modified BPPs (16). Based on these data, the negative predictive value of the NST is 99.8%, and greater than 99.9% for the CST, BPP, and modified BPP. Although similar data from a large series are not available for umbilical artery Doppler velocimetry, in one randomized clinical trial among women with pregnancies complicated by intrauterine growth restriction (38), no stillbirths occurred in 214 pregnancies in which umbilical artery Doppler velocimetry was the primary means of antepartum fetal surveillance (negative predictive value of 100%). The low false-negative rate of these tests depends on an appropriate response to any significant deterioration in the maternal clinical status, including retesting of the fetal condition. As mentioned previously, these tests generally do not predict stillbirths related to acute changes in maternal–fetal status, such as those that occur with abruptio placentae or an umbilical cord accident. Moreover, recent, normal antepartum fetal test results should not preclude the use of intrapartum fetal monitoring.

▶ How should one respond to an abnormal test result?

An abnormal fetal test result should always be considered in the context of the overall clinical picture, taking into account the substantial possibility that the test result is falsely positive. Certain acute maternal conditions (eg, diabetic ketoacidosis, pneumonia with hypoxemia) can result in abnormal test results, which generally will become normal as the maternal condition improves. In these circumstances, stabilizing the maternal condition and retesting the fetus may be appropriate.

In cases where an abnormal test result is not associated with any clinical evidence of worsening in the maternal status, a sequenced approach to the investigation of the fetal condition should be undertaken. Such an approach takes advantage of the high negative predictive value generally exhibited by all commonly used antepartum tests (see above), and minimizes the potential for unnecessary delivery based on a false-positive (ie, abnormal) test result. False-positive rates, in contrast to false-negative rates, have typically not been calculated using the outcome of stillbirth. This is because most antepartum tests were introduced into clinical practice before an unbiased evaluation of their sensitivity and specificity. In clinical practice, abnormal test results usually are followed by another test or delivery is effected, which obscures the relationship between a positive test result and the subsequent risk of stillbirth. Therefore, in the absence of unbiased evaluations, the positive predictive value of antepartum tests has been estimated using surrogate markers, such as the rate of positive follow-up test results when the primary test result is positive. For example, it has been observed that up to 90% of nonreactive NSTs are followed by a negative CST result (18). Based on this observation, the positive predictive value of an NST is only 10%. Another way that the false-positive rate of fetal testing has been estimated is to calculate the incidence of abnormal test results that prompt delivery but are not associated with evidence of fetal compromise, as manifested by a nonreassuring intrapartum fetal heart rate, meconium-stained amniotic fluid, 5-minute Apgar scores of less than 7, or birth weight greater than the 10th percentile for gestational age. By this latter definition, in one large series, a testing scheme in which abnormal modified BPPs were followed by full BPPs had a false-positive rate of 60% (positive predictive value = 40%) (18). In another study in which the physicians were blinded to test results, a CST was found to have a positive predictive value of less than 35% (52).

Therefore, the response to an abnormal test result should be tailored to the clinical situation. Maternal reports of decreased fetal movement should be evaluated by an NST, CST, BPP, or modified BPP; these results, if normal, usually are sufficient to exclude imminent fetal jeopardy. A nonreactive NST or an abnormal modified BPP generally should be followed by additional testing (either a CST or a full BPP). A positive CST result suggests that NST nonreactivity is a consequence of hypoxia-induced acidosis, whereas a negative result implies that the NST nonreactivity exists for another reason, such as a premature fetus, maternal exposure to certain drugs or medications, a fetal sleep cycle, or preexisting neurologic damage. In many circumstances, a positive CST result generally indicates that delivery is warranted. However, the combination of a nonreactive NST and a positive CST result is associated frequently with serious fetal malformation and justifies ultrasonographic investigation for anomalies whenever possible (53). Indeed, evaluation for grossly abnormal fetal anatomy should precede any intervention for suspected fetal compromise whenever possible.

A BPP score of 6 is considered equivocal; in the term fetus, this score generally should prompt delivery, whereas in the preterm fetus, it should result in a repeat BPP in 24 hours (30). In the interim, maternal corticosteroid administration should be considered for pregnancies of less than 34 weeks of gestation. Repeat equivocal scores should result either in delivery or continued intensive surveillance. A BPP score of 4 usually indicates that delivery is warranted, although in extremely premature pregnancies, management should be individualized. Biophysical profiles less than 4 should result in expeditious delivery. Regardless of the overall score, oligohydramnios always requires further evaluation.

In the absence of obstetric contraindications, delivery of the fetus with an abnormal test result often may be attempted by induction of labor, with continuous monitoring of both the fetal heart rate and contractions.

▶ Are there clinical circumstances in which one test is distinguished by its utility or lack thereof?

A large-scale, definitive randomized trial comparing the relative efficacy of one technique of antepartum fetal testing to another has not yet been performed. Accordingly, in most clinical situations, no single antepartum fetal test can be considered superior to any other.

As mentioned previously, in certain clinical situations, the CST is considered relatively contraindicated (increased risk of preterm labor and delivery, uterine rupture, and uterine bleeding), although even in these situations the value of the information provided by the test may outweigh its potential risks.

▶ *When should oligohydramnios prompt delivery?*

Amniotic fluid volume is estimated using ultrasonography. One widely used definition of oligohydramnios is no measurable vertical pocket of amniotic fluid greater than 2 cm (29), and another is an AFI of 5 cm or less (31). Nevertheless, from a clinical standpoint, an ideal cutoff level for intervention using the AFI has yet to be established. Determining when to intervene for oligohydramnios depends on several factors, including gestational age, the maternal and fetal clinical condition as determined by other indices of fetal well-being, and the actual measured AFI value. Because rupture of the fetal membranes can cause diminished amniotic fluid volume, an evaluation for membrane rupture may be appropriate.

In postterm pregnancy, oligohydramnios is common and is associated with an increased risk of meconium staining of the amniotic fluid and cesarean delivery for nonreassuring fetal heart rate (54, 55). Thus, oligohydramnios has been considered an indication for delivery of the postterm pregnancy (15), although the effectiveness of this approach in improving perinatal outcome has not been established by randomized investigation.

In a term pregnancy complicated by oligohydramnios, delivery often is the most appropriate course of action. However, management should be individualized, and in certain situations, delivery may be safely postponed (eg, an uncomplicated pregnancy with an AFI of 5 cm but otherwise reassuring fetal testing and an unfavorable cervix at 37 weeks of gestation).

In the preterm fetus, depending on the maternal and fetal condition, expectant management may be the most appropriate course of action (eg, with preterm premature rupture of membranes or in the presence of fetal anomalies). Once oligohydramnios is diagnosed, if delivery is not undertaken, follow-up amniotic fluid volume and fetal growth assessments are indicated. If the oligohydramnios is persistent, close monitoring of the maternal condition and ongoing antepartum fetal surveillance should be performed to guide further management. If the oligohydramnios results from fetal membrane rupture, follow-up amniotic fluid volume assessment often may be safely omitted.

▶ *What is the role of Doppler velocimetry?*

At least three randomized trials (38, 56, 57) have evaluated the utility of umbilical artery Doppler velocimetry as a technique of antepartum fetal surveillance in pregnancies complicated by suspected intrauterine growth restriction.

In the first and largest of these trials (38), 214 pregnancies were allocated to Doppler umbilical artery velocimetry as the primary technique of fetal surveillance, and 212 were allocated to cardiotocography (NST). Overall, women in the Doppler group were significantly less likely to undergo obstetric intervention, including antepartum hospital admission, labor induction, and emergency cesarean delivery for nonreassuring fetal status. On average, women in the Doppler group underwent antenatal testing less frequently (4 times) than women in the cardiotocography group (8 times). Other perinatal outcomes, such as gestational age at birth, birthweight, Apgar scores, and cesarean birth rates, did not differ between the groups.

Subsequent trials (56, 57) have supported the findings of less frequent antenatal monitoring (56) and shorter durations of maternal hospitalization (56, 57) in the Doppler group. However, rates of obstetric interventions, such as antepartum admission and labor induction, were not lower in the Doppler groups, and perinatal outcome was not improved. On balance, the available evidence suggests that primary antepartum surveillance of suspected intrauterine growth restriction with umbilical artery Doppler velocimetry can achieve at least equivalent (and possibly better) fetal and neonatal outcomes as primary antepartum surveillance based on results of the NST. Furthermore, frequency of antepartum testing and certain aspects of obstetric intervention are reduced with use of Doppler (58). If umbilical artery Doppler velocimetry is used, decisions regarding timing of delivery should be made using a combination of information from the Doppler ultrasonography and other tests of fetal well-being, such as amniotic fluid volume assessment, NST, CST, and BPP, along with careful monitoring of maternal status.

No benefit has been demonstrated for umbilical artery velocimetry for conditions other than suspected intrauterine growth restriction, such as postterm gestation, diabetes mellitus, systemic lupus erythematosus, or antiphospholipid syndrome. Doppler ultrasonography has not been shown to be of value as a screening test for detecting fetal compromise in the general obstetric population, and its use for this purpose cannot be recommended (59). In addition to the umbilical artery, it is possible to evaluate blood flow in major fetal vessels. Multiple investigators have observed a correlation between increased flow resistance (elevated S/D ratio) in the umbilical artery and decreased resistance to flow (reduced S/D ratio) in the middle cerebral artery. This phenomenon has been attributed to a "brain sparing" adaptive response to fetal hypoxemia, and it has been suggested that the ratio of middle cerebral artery S/D ratio to umbilical artery S/D ratio might serve as a useful predictor of fetal compromise (60). However, the only randomized clinical trial of middle cerebral artery Doppler velocimetry failed to demonstrate any clinical benefit to assessing this parameter (61). Moreover, women in this trial who were allocated to standard fetal evaluation plus assessment of the ratio of middle cerebral artery or umbilical artery Doppler flow, or both, were delivered on average 5.7 days earlier after the institution of fetal testing than women who were allocated to standard fetal evaluation without assessment of middle cerebral artery blood flow. This suggests that incorporation of middle cerebral artery Doppler flow assessment into clinical practice might increase unnecessary intervention. Therefore, at present, middle cerebral artery Doppler flow measurement should be considered investigational.

▶ Should all women perform daily fetal movement assessment?

Whether programs of fetal movement assessment actually can reduce the risk of stillbirth is not clear. Only two randomized trials have addressed this issue. The first was conducted in a mixed high-risk (39%) and low-risk (61%) population of 3,111 Danish women who, after 32 weeks of gestation, were randomly assigned to an experimental (counting) group or a control group (10). Women in the experimental group were asked to count fetal movements for 1 hour three times a week and to contact their hospital immediately if they detected fewer movements than their previously established baseline. The control group of women were given no special fetal movement assessment instructions but were asked about fetal movement at their prenatal visits. Of the 1,583 women in the counting group, three experienced stillbirths of normally formed infants weighing more than 1,500 g, versus 12 stillbirths among the 1,569 women in the control group (P<0.05). Of women allocated to the counting group, 80% complied well with the protocol for counting, and 4% were evaluated for decreased fetal movement. The rates of operative vaginal birth and cesarean delivery did not differ significantly between the groups.

The second randomized study to evaluate fetal movement allocated 68,000 women at 28–32 weeks of gestation to a counting policy (in which normal fetal movement was defined as the perception of 10 movements within 10 hours) or to routine care in which no special counting policies were employed (62). Women in the counting group with fewer than 10 movements in 10 hours for two successive days were instructed to alert their care provider, at whose discretion further evaluation was undertaken. Overall fetal death rates were low in this trial and did not differ significantly between the two groups (2.9/1,000 in the counting group versus 2.7/1,000 in the control group). More women in the counting group

(7% versus 5%) underwent fetal heart rate testing, and more (5% versus 4%) were admitted antenatally to the hospital. However, the rates of labor induction and elective cesarean delivery did not differ significantly between the two groups. It should be noted that in the counting group, only 46% of women with decreased fetal movement alerted their care providers. Compliance for both recording fetal movements and reporting when they were diminished was even lower for women who experienced a stillbirth.

Consistent evidence that a formal program of fetal movement assessment will result in a reduction in fetal deaths is lacking. Moreover, whether fetal movement assessment adds benefit to an established program of regular fetal surveillance has not been evaluated. One of the two randomized studies of fetal movement assessment suggests that its use may reduce stillbirths; the other does not. Formal movement assessment may increase, by a small degree, the number of antepartum visits and fetal evaluations. In the randomized trials, however, this increased surveillance did not result in a higher rate of intervention (10, 62).

Summary

The following recommendations are based on limited or inconsistent scientific evidence (Level B):

- ▶ Women with high-risk factors for stillbirth should undergo antepartum fetal surveillance using the NST, CST, BPP, or modified BPP.

- ▶ Initiating testing at 32–34 weeks of gestation is appropriate for most pregnancies at increased risk of stillbirth, although in pregnancies with multiple or particularly worrisome high-risk conditions, testing may be initiated as early as 26–28 weeks of gestation.

- ▶ When the clinical condition that has prompted testing persists, a reassuring test should be repeated periodically (either weekly or, depending on the test used and the presence of certain high-risk conditions, twice weekly) until delivery. Any significant deterioration in the maternal medical status or any acute diminution in fetal activity requires fetal reevaluation, regardless of the amount of time that has elapsed since the last test.

- ▶ An abnormal NST or modified BPP usually should be further evaluated by either a CST or a full BPP. Subsequent management should then be predicated on the results of the CST or BPP, the gestational age, the degree of oligohydramnios (if assessed), and the maternal condition.

▶ Oligohydramnios, defined as either no ultrasonographically measurable vertical pocket of amniotic fluid greater than 2 cm or an AFI of 5 cm or less, requires (depending on the degree of oligohydramnios, the gestational age, and the maternal clinical condition) either delivery or close maternal or fetal surveillance.

▶ In the absence of obstetric contraindications, delivery of the fetus with an abnormal test result often may be attempted by induction of labor with continuous monitoring of the fetal heart rate and contractions. If repetitive late decelerations are observed, cesarean delivery generally is indicated.

▶ Recent, normal antepartum fetal test results should not preclude the use of intrapartum fetal monitoring.

▶ Umbilical artery Doppler velocimetry has been found to be of benefit only in pregnancies complicated by intrauterine growth restriction. If used in this setting, decisions regarding timing of delivery should be made using a combination of information from the Doppler ultrasonography and other tests of fetal well-being, along with careful monitoring of maternal status.

▶ Middle cerebral artery Doppler velocimetry should be considered an investigational approach to antepartum fetal surveillance.

References

1. Boddy K, Dawes GS, Fisher R, Pinter S, Robinson JS. Foetal respiratory movements, electrocortical and cardiovascular responses to hypoxaemia and hypercapnia in sheep. J Physiol 1974;243:599–618 (Level III)

2. Manning FA, Platt LD. Maternal hypoxemia and fetal breathing movements. Obstet Gynecol 1979;53:758–760 (Level III)

3. Murata Y, Martin CB Jr, Ikenoue T, Hashimoto T, Taira S, Sagawa T, et al. Fetal heart rate accelerations and late decelerations during the course of intrauterine death in chronically catheterized rhesus monkeys. Am J Obstet Gynecol 1982;144:218–223 (Level III)

4. Natale R, Clewlow F, Dawes GS. Measurement of fetal forelimb movements in the lamb in utero. Am J Obstet Gynecol 1981;140:545–551 (Level III)

5. Seeds AE. Current concepts of amniotic fluid dynamics. Am J Obstet Gynecol 1980;138:575–586 (Level III)

6. Weiner CP, Sipes SL, Wenstrom K. The effect of fetal age upon normal fetal laboratory values and venous pressure. Obstet Gynecol 1992;79:713–718 (Level III)

7. Manning FA, Snijders R, Harman CR, Nicolaides K, Menticoglou S, Morrison I. Fetal biophysical profile score. VI. Correlation with antepartum umbilical venous fetal pH. Am J Obstet Gynecol 1993;169:755–763 (Level II-2)

8. Pearson JF, Weaver JB. Fetal activity and fetal wellbeing: an evaluation. BMJ 1976;1(6021):1305–1307 (Level III)

9. Moore TR, Piacquadio K. A prospective evaluation of fetal movement screening to reduce the incidence of antepartum fetal death. Am J Obstet Gynecol 1989;160:1075–1080 (Level II-2)

10. Neldam S. Fetal movements as an indicator of fetal wellbeing. Dan Med Bull 1983;30:274–278 (Level II-1)

11. Huddleston JF, Sutliff G, Robinson D. Contraction stress test by intermittent nipple stimulation. Obstet Gynecol 1984;63:669–673 (Level II-3)

12. Freeman RK. The use of the oxytocin challenge test for antepartum clinical evaluation of uteroplacental respiratory function. Am J Obstet Gynecol 1975;121:481–489 (Level III)

13. Freeman RK, Anderson G, Dorchester W. A prospective multi-institutional study of antepartum fetal heart rate monitoring. I. Risk of perinatal mortality and morbidity according to antepartum fetal heart rate test results. Am J Obstet Gynecol 1982;143:771–777 (Level II-3)

14. Graca LM, Cardoso CG, Clode N, Calhaz-Jorge C. Acute effects of maternal cigarette smoking on fetal heart rate and fetal body movements felt by the mother. J Perinat Med 1991;19:385–390 (Level III)

15. Clark SL, Sabey P, Jolley K. Nonstress testing with acoustic stimulation and amniotic fluid volume assessment: 5973 tests without unexpected fetal death. Am J Obstet Gynecol 1989;160:694–697 (Level II-3)

16. Miller DA, Rabello YA, Paul RH. The modified biophysical profile: antepartum testing in the 1990s. Am J Obstet Gynecol 1996;174:812–817 (Level II-3)

17. Smith CV, Phelan JP, Platt LD, Broussard P, Paul RH. Fetal acoustic stimulation testing. II. A randomized clinical comparison with the nonstress test. Am J Obstet Gynecol 1986;155:131–134 (Level I)

18. Evertson LR, Gauthier RJ, Schifrin BS, Paul RH. Antepartum fetal heart rate testing. I. Evolution of the nonstress test. Am J Obstet Gynecol 1979;133:29–33 (Level II-3)

19. Bishop EH. Fetal acceleration test. Am J Obstet Gynecol 1981;141:905–909 (Level II-2)

20. Lavin JP Jr, Miodovnik M, Barden TP. Relationship of nonstress test reactivity and gestational age. Obstet Gynecol 1984;63:338–344 (Level II-3)

21. Druzin ML, Fox A, Kogut E, Carlson C. The relationship of the nonstress test to gestational age. Am J Obstet Gynecol 1985;153:386–389 (Level III)

22. Meis PJ, Ureda JR, Swain M, Kelly RT, Penry M, Sharp P. Variable decelerations during nonstress tests are not a sign of fetal compromise. Am J Obstet Gynecol 1986;154:586–590 (Level II-3)

23. Anyaegbunam A, Brustman L, Divon M, Langer O. The significance of antepartum variable decelerations. Am J Obstet Gynecol 1986;155:707–710 (Level II-2)

24. O'Leary JA, Andrinopoulos GC, Giordano PC. Variable decelerations and the nonstress test: an indication of cord compromise. Am J Obstet Gynecol 1980;137:704–706 (Level III)

25. Bourgeois FJ, Thiagarajah S, Harbert GM Jr. The significance of fetal heart rate decelerations during nonstress testing. Am J Obstet Gynecol 1984;150:213–216 (Level III)

26. Druzin ML, Gratacos J, Keegan KA, Paul RH. Antepartum fetal heart rate testing. VII. The significance of fetal bradycardia. Am J Obstet Gynecol 1981;139:194–198 (Level III)

27. Pazos R, Vuolo K, Aladjem S, Lueck J, Anderson C. Association of spontaneous fetal heart rate decelerations during antepartum nonstress testing and intrauterine growth retardation. Am J Obstet Gynecol 1982;144:574–577 (Level II-2)

28. Manning FA, Morrison I, Lange IR, Harman CR, Chamberlain PF. Fetal biophysical profile scoring: selective use of the nonstress test. Am J Obstet Gynecol 1987;156:709–712 (Level II-3)

29. Chamberlain PF, Manning FA, Morrison I, Harman CR, Lange IR. Ultrasound evaluation of amniotic fluid volume. I. The relationship of marginal and decreased amniotic fluid volumes to perinatal outcome. Am J Obstet Gynecol 1984;150:245–249 (Level II-3)

30. Manning FA, Harman CR, Morrison I, Menticoglou SM, Lange IR, Johnson JM. Fetal assessment based on fetal biophysical profile scoring. IV. An analysis of perinatal morbidity and mortality. Am J Obstet Gynecol 1990;162:703–709 (Level II-3)

31. Rutherford SE, Phelan JP, Smith CV, Jacobs N. The four-quadrant assessment of amniotic fluid volume: an adjunct to antepartum fetal heart rate testing. Obstet Gynecol 1987;70:353–356 (Level III)

32. Erskine RL, Ritchie JW. Umbilical artery blood flow characteristics in normal and growth-retarded fetuses. Br J Obstet Gynaecol 1985;92:605–610 (Level II-2)

33. Gudmundsson S, Marsal K. Umbilical and uteroplacental blood flow velocity waveforms in pregnancies with fetal growth retardation. Eur J Obstet Gynecol Reprod Biol 1988;27:187–196 (Level III)

34. Reuwer PJ, Bruinse HW, Stoutenbeek P, Haspels AA. Doppler assessment of the fetoplacental circulation in normal and growth-retarded fetuses. Eur J Obstet Gynecol Reprod Biol 1984;18:199–205 (Level II-2)

35. Karsdorp VH, van Vugt JM, van Geijn HP, Kostense PJ, Arduini D, Montenegra N, et al. Clinical significance of absent or reversed end diastolic velocity waveforms in umbilical artery. Lancet 1994;344:1664–1668 (Level II-2)

36. Giles WB, Trudinger BJ, Baird PJ. Fetal umbilical artery flow velocity waveforms and placental resistance: pathological correlation. Br J Obstet Gynaecol 1985;92:31–38 (Level II-2)

37. Nicolaides KH, Bilardo CM, Soothill PW, Campbell S. Absence of end diastolic frequencies in umbilical artery: a sign of fetal hypoxia and acidosis. BMJ 1988;297:1026–1027 (Level III)

38. Almstrom H, Axelsson O, Cnattingius S, Ekman G, Maesel A, Ulmsten U, et al. Comparison of umbilical-artery velocimetry and cardiotocography for surveillance of small-for-gestational-age fetuses. Lancet 1992;340:936–940 (Level I)

39. Johnstone FD, Prescott R, Hoskins P, Greer IA, McGlew T, Compton M. The effect of introduction of umbilical Doppler recordings to obstetric practice. Br J Obstet Gynaecol 1993;100:733–741 (Level I)

40. Newnham JP, O'Dea MR, Reid KP, Diepeveen DA. Doppler flow velocity waveform analysis in high risk pregnancies: a randomized controlled trial. Br J Obstet Gynaecol 1991;98:956–963 (Level I)

41. Omtzigt AM, Reuwer PJ, Bruinse HW. A randomized controlled trial on the clinical value of umbilical Doppler velocimetry in antenatal care. Am J Obstet Gynecol 1994;170:625–634 (Level I)

42. Pattinson RC, Norman K, Odendaal HJ. The role of Doppler velocimetry in the management of high risk pregnancies. Br J Obstet Gynaecol 1994;101:114–120 (Level I)

43. Trudinger BJ, Cook CM, Giles WB, Connelly A, Thompson RS. Umbilical artery flow velocity waveforms in high-risk pregnancy. Randomised controlled trial. Lancet 1987;1(8526):188–190 (Level I)

44. Tyrrell SN, Lilford RJ, Macdonald HN, Nelson EJ, Porter J, Gupta JK. Randomized comparison of routine vs highly selective use of Doppler ultrasound and biophysical scoring to investigate high risk pregnancies. Br J Obstet Gynaecol 1990;97:909–916 (Level I)

45. Thacker SB, Berkelman RL. Assessing the diagnostic accuracy and efficacy of selected antepartum fetal surveillance techniques. Obstet Gynecol Surv 1986;41:121–141 (Level III)

46. Enkin M, Keirse MJNC, Renfrew M, Neilson J. A guide to effective care in pregnancy and childbirth. 2nd ed. Oxford: Oxford University Press, 1995:410 (Level III)

47. Nageotte MP, Towers CV, Asrat T, Freeman RK. Perinatal outcome with the modified biophysical profile. Am J Obstet Gynecol 1994;170:1672–1676 (Level I)

48. Rouse DJ, Owen J, Goldenberg RL, Cliver SP. Determinants of the optimal time in gestation to initiate antenatal fetal testing: a decision-analytic approach. Am J Obstet Gynecol 1995;173:1357–1363 (Decision Analysis)

49. Lagrew DC, Pircon RA, Towers CV, Dorchester W, Freeman RK. Antepartum fetal surveillance in patients with diabetes: when to start? Am J Obstet Gynecol 1993;168:1820–1826 (Level III)

50. Pircon RA, Lagrew DC, Towers CV, Dorchester WL, Gocke SE, Freeman RK. Antepartum testing in the hypertensive patient: when to begin. Am J Obstet Gynecol 1991;164:1563–1570 (Level III)

51. Manning FA, Morrison I, Harman CR, Lange IR, Menticoglou S. Fetal assessment based on fetal biophysical profile scoring: experience in 19,221 referred high-risk pregnancies. II. An analysis of false-negative fetal deaths. Am J Obstet Gynecol 1987;157:880–884 (Level II-3)

52. Staisch KJ, Westlake JR, Bashore RA. Blind oxytocin challenge test and perinatal outcome. Am J Obstet Gynecol 1980;138:399–403 (Level II-2)

53. Garite TJ, Linzey EM, Freeman RK, Dorchester W. Fetal heart rate patterns and fetal distress in fetuses with congenital anomalies. Obstet Gynecol 1979;53:716–720 (Level II-2)

54. Leveno KJ, Quirk JG Jr, Cunningham FG, Nelson SD, Santos-Ramos R, Toofanian A, et al. Prolonged pregnancy. I. Observations concerning the causes of fetal distress. Am J Obstet Gynecol 1984;150:465–473 (Level III)

55. Phelan JP, Platt LD, Yeh SY, Broussard P, Paul RH. The role of ultrasound assessment of amniotic fluid volume in the management of the postdate pregnancy. Am J Obstet Gynecol 1985;151:304–308 (Level II-2)

56. Haley J, Tuffnell DJ, Johnson N. Randomised controlled trial of cardiotocography versus umbilical artery Doppler in the management of small for gestational age fetuses. Br J Obstet Gynaecol 1997;104:431–435 (Level I)

57. Nienhuis SJ, Vles JS, Gerver WJ, Hoogland HJ. Doppler ultrasonography in suspected intrauterine growth retardation: a randomized clinical trial. Ultrasound Obstet Gynecol 1997;9:6–13 (Level I)

58. Neilson JP, Alfirevic Z. Doppler ultrasound for fetal assessment in high risk pregnancies (Cochrane Review). In: The Cochrane Library, Issue 3, 1999. Oxford: Update Software (Meta-analysis)

59. Mason GC, Lilford RJ, Porter J, Nelson E, Tyrell S. Randomised comparison of routine versus highly selective use of Doppler ultrasound in low risk pregnancies. Br J Obstet Gynaecol 1993;100:130–133 (Level I)

60. Mari G, Deter RL. Middle cerebral artery flow velocity waveforms in normal and small-for-gestational-age fetuses. Am J Obstet Gynecol 1992;166:1262–1270 (Level II-2)

61. Ott WJ, Mora G, Arias F, Sunderji S, Sheldon G. Comparison of the modified biophysical profile to a "new" biophysical profile incorporating the middle cerebral artery to umbilical artery velocity flow systolic/diastolic ratio. Am J Obstet Gynecol 1998;178:1346–1353 (Level I)

62. Grant A, Elbourne D, Valentin L, Alexander S. Routine formal fetal movement counting and risk of antepartum late death in normally formed singletons. Lancet 1989;2(8659):345–349 (Level I)

The MEDLINE database, the Cochrane Library, and ACOG's own internal resources and documents were used to conduct a literature search to locate relevant articles published between January 1985 and February 1999. The search was restricted to articles published in the English language. Priority was given to articles reporting results of original research, although review articles and commentaries also were consulted. Abstracts of research presented at symposia and scientific conferences were not considered adequate for inclusion in this document. Guidelines published by organizations or institutions such as the National Institutes of Health and the American College of Obstetricians and Gynecologists were reviewed, and additional studies were located by reviewing bibliographies of identified articles. When reliable research was not available, expert opinions from obstetrician–gynecologists were used.

Studies were reviewed and evaluated for quality according to the method outlined by the U.S. Preventive Services Task Force:

I   Evidence obtained from at least one properly designed randomized controlled trial.

II-1   Evidence obtained from well-designed controlled trials without randomization.

II-2   Evidence obtained from well-designed cohort or case–control analytic studies, preferably from more than one center or research group.

II-3   Evidence obtained from multiple time series with or without the intervention. Dramatic results in uncontrolled experiments also could be regarded as this type of evidence.

III   Opinions of respected authorities, based on clinical experience, descriptive studies, or reports of expert committees.

Based on the highest level of evidence found in the data, recommendations are provided and graded according to the following categories:

Level A—Recommendations are based on good and consistent scientific evidence.

Level B—Recommendations are based on limited or inconsistent scientific evidence.

Level C—Recommendations are based primarily on consensus and expert opinion.

ISSN 1099-3630

The American College of
Obstetricians and Gynecologists
409 12th Street, SW
PO Box 96920
Washington, DC 20090-6920

12345/32109

ACOG PRACTICE BULLETIN

CLINICAL MANAGEMENT GUIDELINES FOR
OBSTETRICIAN–GYNECOLOGISTS

NUMBER 23, JANUARY 2001

(Replaces Educational Bulletin Number 237, June 1997)

This Practice Bulletin was developed by the ACOG Committee on Practice Bulletins— Gynecology with the assistance of David Soper, MD. The information is designed to aid practitioners in making decisions about appropriate obstetric and gynecologic care. These guidelines should not be construed as dictating an exclusive course of treatment or procedure. Variations in practice may be warranted based on the needs of the individual patient, resources, and limitations unique to the institution or type of practice.

Antibiotic Prophylaxis for Gynecologic Procedures

Antibiotic use, especially prophylactic antibiotic use, has been associated with the selection of antibiotic-resistant bacteria. Indiscriminate use of antimicrobial prophylaxis promotes this dangerous side effect. There are acknowledged consequences of prophylactic antibiotics for institutions as well as for individual patients. It is important for clinicians to understand when antibiotic prophylaxis is indicated and when it is inappropriate. The purpose of this document is to review the evidence for appropriate antibiotic prophylaxis for gynecologic surgery and other procedures.

Background

Pathophysiology and Microbiology of Gynecologic Infections

As the number and virulence of contaminating bacteria increase in a surgical site, so does the risk for postoperative infection. Surgery and the use of foreign material, such as sutures, further potentiate the risk of infection. At the same time, systemic and local host immune mechanisms function to contain inoculated bacteria and prevent infection. Antibiotics in the tissues provide a pharmacologic means of defense that augments the natural host immunity. Bacterial resistance mechanisms may contribute to the pathogenesis of operative-site infection by enabling organisms to evade the prophylactically administered antibiotics (1).

Operative-site infections after a hysterectomy result from the ascending spread of microorganisms from the upper vagina and endocervix to the vaginal cuff and paravaginal tissues dissected during the procedure (2). Bacterial vaginosis, a complex alteration of vaginal flora resulting in an increased concentration of potentially pathogenic anaerobic bacteria, is associated with an increased risk of posthysterectomy cuff cellulitis (3). However, there is a lack of data showing that pretreatment for bacterial vaginosis before hysterectomy reduces the rate of postoperative cuff cellulitis. These microorganisms also can be spread to the abdominal incision at the time of surgery; in addition, the skin microorganisms *Staphylococcus epidermidis* and *Staphylococcus aureus* may lead to an abdominal-incision infection. Gynecologic surgical procedures, such as laparotomy or laparoscopy, do not breach surfaces colonized with bacteria from the vagina, and infections following these procedures more commonly result from contaminating skin bacteria only.

Procedures breaching the endocervix, such as hysterosalpingogram, sonohysterography, intrauterine device (IUD) insertion, endometrial biopsy, and dilation and curettage, may seed the endometrium and the fallopian tubes with microorganisms found in the upper vagina and endocervix. Prevention and treatment of these postoperative infections, either endometritis or pelvic inflammatory disease (PID), should take into consideration the polymicrobial nature of these infections.

The risk of developing bacterial endocarditis is related to a patient's risk of bacteremia and the significance of an underlying cardiac lesion. Most cases of infective endocarditis are caused by gram-positive cocci that originate from the mouth or the skin.

Theory of Antimicrobial Prophylaxis

State-of-the-art aseptic technique has been associated with a dramatic decrease in operative-site infections, but bacterial contamination of the operative site is inevitable. The in vivo interaction between the inoculated bacteria and prophylactically administered antibiotic is one of the most important determinants of the state of the surgical site. Systemic antibiotic prophylaxis is based on the belief that antibiotics in the host tissues can augment natural immune-defense mechanisms and help to kill bacteria that are inoculated into the wound. Only a narrow window of antimicrobial efficacy is available, requiring the administration of antibiotics either shortly before or at the time of bacterial inoculation (eg, when the incision is made, viscus entered, or pedicles clamped). A delay of only 3–4 hours can result in ineffective prophylaxis (4). The induction of anesthesia represents a convenient time for initiating antibiotic prophylaxis in major gynecologic procedures. Current data indicate that for lengthy procedures, additional, intraoperative doses of an antibiotic, given at intervals of one or two times the half-life of the drug, maintain adequate levels throughout the operation (5). A second dose of the prophylactic antibiotic also may

be appropriate in surgical cases with an increased blood loss (>1,500 mL). Neither subsequent doses nor treatment for several days before a procedure is indicated for prophylaxis. The use of prophylaxis implies that the patient is presumed to be free of infection at the time of the procedure. During a procedure when a patient is found to be at greater risk for disease, use of therapeutic antibiotics should be considered.

Pharmacology and Spectrum of Activity of Antibiotics Used in Prophylaxis

The cephalosporins have emerged as the drugs of choice for the vast majority of operative procedures because of their broad antimicrobial spectrum and low incidence of allergy and side effects. Cefazolin (1 g) is the most commonly used agent because of its reasonably long half-life (1.8 hours) and low cost. It is the frequent choice for clean procedures, and most clinical studies indicate that it is equivalent to cephalosporins which have improved in vitro activity against anaerobic bacteria in clean-contaminated procedures such as hysterectomy. Table 1 lists antibiotic regimens by procedure.

Table 1. Antimicrobial Prophylactic Regimens by Procedure

Procedure	Antibiotic	Dose
Vaginal/abdominal hysterectomy*	Cefazolin	1 or 2 g single dose IV
	Cefoxitin	2 g single dose IV
	Cefotetan	1 or 2 g single dose IV
	Metronidazole	500 mg single dose IV
Laparoscopy	None	
Laparotomy	None	
Hysteroscopy	None	
Hysterosalpingogram	Doxycycline†	100 mg twice daily for 5 days orally
IUD insertion	None	
Endometrial biopsy	None	
Induced abortion/D&C	Doxycycline	100 mg orally 1 hour before procedure and 200 mg orally after the procedure
	Metronidazole	500 mg twice daily orally for 5 days
Urodynamics	None	

Abbreviations: IV, intravenously; IUD, intrauterine device; D&C, dilation and curettage.

*A convenient time to administer antibiotic prophylaxis is just before induction of anesthesia.

†If hysterosalpingogram demonstrates dilated tubes. No prophylaxis is indicated for a normal study.

Adverse Reactions to Antibiotics

Adverse effects for the patient include allergic reactions ranging in severity from minor skin rashes to anaphylaxis. Pseudomembranous colitis is an uncommon complication of prophylactic antibiotics. Overall, attack rates for antibiotic-associated diarrhea in hospitals range from 3.2% to 29% (6, 7). Nearly 15% of hospitalized patients receiving β-lactam antibiotics develop diarrhea (7), and rates for those receiving clindamycin range from 10% to 25% (8). Predisposing host factors and circumstances affecting the frequency and severity of disease include advanced age, underlying illness, recent surgery, and recent administration of bowel motility-altering drugs (9).

Anaphylaxis, the most immediate and most life-threatening risk of prophylaxis, is rare. Anaphylactic reactions to penicillin reportedly occur in 0.2% of courses of treatment, with a fatality rate of 0.0001% (10). The induction of bacterial resistance may be a consequence of prophylactic antibiotic use. The most common example of this is the selection of *Enterococcus* sp. as a result of cephalosporin use. However, no clinically relevant ill effects have been reported as a result of this particular type of alteration in the flora of the lower genital tract (11).

Patients with a history of an adverse reaction or allergy to an antibiotic recommended for prophylaxis should not be administered that particular drug. However, given the wide range of antibiotics available for prophylaxis, it would be unlikely to have to avoid giving antibiotic prophylaxis because of the inability to find an appropriate agent.

Clinical Considerations and Recommendations

▶ *What constitutes appropriate antibiotic prophylaxis for the following situations?*

When choosing a prophylactic antimicrobial agent, the practitioner should consider the following factors. The agent selected must: 1) be of low toxicity, 2) have an established safety record in patients, 3) not be routinely used for the treatment of serious infections, 4) have a spectrum of activity that includes the microorganisms most likely to cause infection, 5) reach a useful concentration in relevant tissues during the procedure, 6) be administered for a short duration, and 7) be administered in a manner that will ensure it is present in surgical sites at the time of the incision (11).

Hysterectomy—Vaginal, Abdominal, or Laparoscopically Assisted. More than 25 prospective randomized clinical trials and two meta-analyses support the use of prophylactic antibiotics to significantly reduce postoperative infectious morbidity and decrease length of hospitalization in women undergoing abdominal hysterectomy (12, 13). Most studies show no particular antibiotic regimen to be superior to all others. A single study performed in women undergoing abdominal hysterectomy showed that, when compared with cefotetan, cefazolin prophylaxis was associated with a significantly increased risk for major operative-site infection and postoperative pelvic abscess (14). Patients undergoing vaginal or abdominal hysterectomy should receive antibiotic prophylaxis.

Laparoscopy and Laparotomy. No data are available to recommend antibiotic prophylaxis in clean abdominal surgery not involving vaginal or intestinal operations. Studies evaluating the use of antibiotics to prevent wound infections after hernia repair and total or partial mastectomy fail to show a benefit. Antibiotic prophylaxis is not recommended in patients undergoing diagnostic laparoscopy or exploratory laparotomy.

Hysterosalpingography, Sonohysterography, and Hysteroscopy. Hysterosalpingography (HSG) is a commonly performed procedure to evaluate infertile couples for tubal factor infertility. Post-HSG PID is an uncommon (1.4–3.4%) but potentially serious complication in this patient population (15, 16). Patients with dilated tubes at the time of HSG have a higher rate (11%) of post-HSG PID (15). The possibility of lower genital tract infection with chlamydia should be considered before performing this procedure (16). In a retrospective review, investigators observed no cases of post-HSG PID in patients with nondilated tubes (0/398) (15). In 56 women with dilated tubes, doxycycline was effective in preventing infection. In 51 of these 56 cases, after dilated tubes were noted during the HSG, the antibiotic was administered. The other five patients received their doxycycline before the HSG.

In patients with no history of pelvic infection, HSG can be performed without prophylactic antibiotics. If HSG demonstrates dilated tubes, the patient should be given doxycycline, 100 mg twice daily for 5 days, to reduce the incidence of post-HSG PID (17). In patients with a history of pelvic infection, doxycycline can be started before the procedure and continued if dilated tubes are found. Another option in patients with a history of pelvic infection is to begin antibiotics if dilated tubes are discovered. In patients thought to have an active pelvic infection, HSG should not be performed.

No data are available on which to base a recommendation for prophylaxis in patients undergoing sonohysterography, but reported rates of postprocedure infection are negligible (0/300 in one series) (18). Sonohysterography is a relatively new procedure, technically similar to HSG. The risks probably are similar to those of HSG, and the same considerations should be taken into account. Prophylaxis should be based on the individual patient's risk of PID; routine use of antibiotic prophylaxis is not recommended.

Infectious complications following hysteroscopic surgery are uncommon and estimated to occur in 0.18–1.5% of cases (19). A single prospective study has evaluated the utility of amoxicillin/clavulanate antibiotic prophylaxis in preventing bacteremia associated with hysteroscopic endometrial laser ablation or endometrial resection (20). Although the incidence of bacteremia was lower in the antibiotic group than in the placebo group (2% versus 16%), most of the microorganisms isolated were of dubious clinical significance (anaerobic staphylococci) and may have resulted from contamination. Interestingly, postoperative fever was noted twice as often in the patients receiving antimicrobial prophylaxis. Postoperative infection requiring antibiotic therapy was not significantly different between the two groups, with 11.4% and 9% of patients requiring antibiotics in the placebo and antibiotic groups, respectively.

Other retrospective case series evaluating endometrial ablation reported similarly low rates of infection. In a series of 568 patients treated without antimicrobial prophylaxis, one woman (0.18%) developed endometritis (21). A second series reported 2 of 600 women (0.3%) developed mild pelvic infections, of whom one received antimicrobial prophylaxis and one did not (22). However, in a series of 200 women undergoing operative hysteroscopy without prophylactic antibiotics, investigators reported three cases of severe pelvic infection, although all three of these women had a history of PID (23). Given the low risk of infection and lack of evidence of efficacy, antibiotics are not of value for the general patient population undergoing these procedures.

Intrauterine Device Insertion, Endometrial Biopsy. The IUD is a highly effective contraceptive, but concern about the perceived risk of PID limits its use. Most of the risk of IUD-related infection occurs in the first few weeks to months after insertion, suggesting that contamination of the endometrial cavity at the time of insertion is the infecting mechanism rather than the IUD or string itself. Four randomized clinical trials have now been performed using doxycycline or azithromycin as antibiotic prophylaxis (24–27). Pelvic inflammatory disease occurred uncommonly with or without the use of antibiotic prophylaxis. A Cochrane Collaboration review concluded that either doxycycline or azithromycin before IUD insertion confers little benefit (28). When the results of the four studies were combined, a reduction in unscheduled visits to the provider was seen but not in the only trial performed in the United States. In the U.S. trial, however, all patients were screened for gonorrhea and chlamydia, and some with positive results were excluded from the study. The cost-effectiveness of screening for sexually transmitted diseases (STDs) before IUD insertion remains unclear because of limited data. The only randomized controlled trial performed in the United States concluded that in women screened for STDs before IUD insertion, prophylactic antibiotics provide no benefit (27).

No data are available on infectious complications of endometrial biopsy. The incidence is presumed to be negligible. It is recommended that this procedure be performed without the use of antimicrobial prophylaxis.

Induced Abortion and Dilation and Curettage. Eleven of 15 randomized clinical trials support the use of antibiotic prophylaxis at the time of suction curettage abortion. In a meta-analysis of 11 placebo-controlled, blinded clinical trials, the overall summary relative risk (RR) estimate for developing postabortal infection of the upper genital tract in women receiving antibiotic therapy compared with those receiving placebo was 0.58 (95% confidence interval [CI], 0.47–0.71) (29). Of high-risk women, those with a history of PID had a summary RR of 0.56 (CI, 0.37–0.84); women with a positive chlamydia culture at abortion had a summary RR of 0.38 (CI, 0.15–0.92). Of low-risk women, those with no reported history of PID had a summary RR of 0.65 (CI, 0.47–0.90); in women with a negative chlamydia culture, the RR was 0.63 (CI, 0.42–0.97). The overall 42% decreased risk of infection in women given periabortal antibiotics confirms that prophylactic antibiotics are effective for these women, regardless of risk.

The optimal antibiotic and dosing regimens remain unclear. Both tetracyclines and nitro-imidazoles provide significant and comparable protection against postabortal PID. One of the most effective and inexpensive regimens reported in a meta-analysis was doxycycline, 100 mg orally 1 hour before the abortion followed by 200 mg after the procedure. It is estimated that the cost of treating a single case of postabortal PID as an outpatient far exceeds the cost of doxycycline prophylaxis (29). In a prospective, randomized trial, antibiotic prophylaxis showed no benefit before treatment of incomplete abortion (30).

Preoperative Bowel Preparation. Occasionally the gynecologic surgeon runs the risk of both small- and large-bowel injuries because of the presence of pelvic adhesions resulting from either previous surgery or an inflammatory process, such as PID or endometriosis. In these cases, it is reasonable to consider preparing the bowel for surgery with a mechanical bowel preparation and using an antibiotic regimen that is effective in preventing infection among patients undergoing elective bowel surgery. Eight randomized clinical trials confirm the effectiveness of prophylactic parenteral antibiotics administered preoperatively with or without a prior oral antibiotic bowel preparation in decreasing the rate of postoperative infection, such as wound and intraabdominal infections (5). It is unclear whether any one regimen is superior, but broad-spectrum cephalosporins, such as cefotetan or cefoxitin, were commonly used.

Endocarditis Prophylaxis. As many as 75% of patients who develop endocarditis after undergoing a surgical procedure have preexisting cardiac abnormalities. To date, no randomized controlled trials have definitively established the efficacy of endocarditis prophylaxis, but most authorities agree that prophylaxis should be offered to susceptible patients. Patients with high- and moderate-risk structural cardiac defects may benefit from antimicrobial prophylaxis (see the box, right). In addition, bacteremia is associated with certain surgical procedures; therefore, in patients with underlying cardiac structural defects who are undergoing these procedures, antimicrobial prophylaxis is recommended (see the box, next page). Suggested regimens are listed in Table 2.

In the absence of obvious infection, bacteremia is uncommon after cervical biopsy or IUD insertion or removal, and prophylaxis is not indicated. In the presence of infection, removal of an IUD or other genitourinary procedures require endocarditis prophylaxis. Antibiotics administered for prevention of surgical-site infection are not sufficient for endocarditis prophylaxis. However, most experts agree that prophylactic agents for endocarditis provide sufficient coverage against surgical-site infection. For patients with significant heart disease being treated by a specialist, it may be helpful to consult the specialist for additional information if necessary.

Urodynamic Studies or Bladder Catheterization. Several studies suggest that prophylactic antibiotics are not effective in preventing urinary tract infections resulting from urodynamic testing. One study identified 2 of 45 women (4%) not given antibiotics following urodynamic testing whose postprocedure urine cultures were positive, compared with 0 of 51 women given macrodantin, 50 mg three times a day for 3 days after testing (31). A second study identified 10 of 49 women (18.9%) not given antibiotics after urodynamic testing whose urine

cultures were positive, compared with 4 of 49 women (8.9%) who received prophylaxis and had positive urine cultures (32). The differences in both studies were not statistically significant. Because neither study reported on "symptomatic infection" nor the microbiology of the postprocedure bacteriuria, the site could have been contaminated with a nonuropathogen. However, given the prevalence of asymptomatic bacteriuria in women, approximately 8% of women had unsuspected bacteriuria at the time of urodynamic testing. Because bacteriuria and urinary tract infection can be a cause of detrusor instability, pretest screening by urine culture or urinalysis, or both, is recommended.

Cardiac Conditions Associated with Endocarditis

Endocarditis Prophylaxis Recommended

High-Risk Category

Prosthetic cardiac valves, including bioprosthetic and homograft valves
Previous bacterial endocarditis
Complex cyanotic congenital heart disease (eg, single-ventricle states, transposition of the great arteries, tetralogy of Fallot)
Surgically constructed systemic pulmonary shunts or conduits

Moderate-Risk Category

Most other congenital cardiac malformations (other than those listed above and below)
Acquired valvar dysfunction (eg, rheumatic heart disease)
Hypertrophic cardiomyopathy
Mitral valve prolapse with valvar regurgitation, thickened leaflets, or both

Endocarditis Prophylaxis Not Recommended

Negligible-Risk Category (Risk No Greater Than That of the General Population)
Isolated secundum atrial septum defect
Surgical repair of atrial septal defect, ventricular septal defect, or patent ductus arteriosus (without residua beyond 6 months)
Previous coronary artery bypass graft surgery
Mitral valve prolapse without valvar regurgitation
Physiologic, functional, or innocent heart murmurs
Previous Kawasaki syndrome without valvar dysfunction
Previous rheumatic fever without valvar dysfunction
Cardiac pacemakers (intravascular and epicardial) and implanted defibrillators

Dajani AS, Taubert KA, Wilson W, Bolger AF, Bayer A, Ferrieri P, et al. Prevention of bacterial endocarditis: recommendations by the American Heart Association. JAMA 1997;277:1795. Copyrighted 1997, American Medical Association.

Endocarditis Prophylaxis by Surgical Procedure

Endocarditis Prophylaxis Recommended

Gastrointestinal Tract*
  Surgical operations that involve intestinal mucosa
Genitourinary Tract
  Cystoscopy
  Urethral dilation
  Other genitourinary procedures only in presence of
  infection

Endocarditis Prophylaxis Not Recommended

Genitourinary Tract
  Vaginal hysterectomy†
  In uninfected tissue:
    Urethral catheterization
    Uterine dilation and curettage
    Therapeutic abortion
    Sterilization procedures
    Insertion or removal of intrauterine devices

*Prophylaxis is recommended for high-risk patients; optional
for medium-risk patients.

†Prophylaxis is optional for high-risk patients.

Adapted from Dajani AS, Taubert KA, Wilson W, Bolger AF, Bayer A,
Ferrieri P, et al. Prevention of bacterial endocarditis: recommenda-
tions by the American Heart Association. JAMA 1997;277:1797.
Copyrighted 1997, American Medical Association.

Urinary tract infection after one-time bladder catheterization has been reported to be approximately 2%
(33). No randomized trials have compared antibiotic prophylaxis with placebo in trying to further decrease the
incidence of urinary tract infection. Therefore, given the
low risk of infection, antibiotic prophylaxis is not indicated for this procedure.

▶ *Which antibiotics should be used in the
patient with penicillin allergy?*

Allergic reactions occur in 0.7–4% of courses of treatment with penicillin (34). Four types of immunopatho-
logic reactions have been described, all of which have
been seen with β-lactam antibiotics: 1) immediate hypersensitivity reactions, 2) cytotoxic antibodies, 3) immune
complexes, and 4) cell-mediated hypersensitivity (35).
Approximately 5–20% of patients indicate a history of
reactions to β-lactam antibiotics.

Like penicillins, cephalosporins possess a β-lactam
ring; however, the five-membered thiazolidine ring is
replaced by a six-membered dihydrothiazine ring. The
overall incidence of adverse reactions from cephalosporins ranges from 1% to 10%, with rare anaphylaxis
(<0.02%). In patients with histories of penicillin allergy,
the incidence of cephalosporin reactions is increased
minimally. Postmarketing studies of second- and third-
generation cephalosporins showed no increase in allergic
reactions to cephalosporins in patients with histories of
penicillin allergy. One reaction occurred in 98 patients
(1%) with positive penicillin skin test results, and six
reactions occurred in 310 patients (2%) with negative test
results (36). The incidence of clinically relevant cross-
reactivity between the penicillins and cephalosporins is

Table 2. Prophylactic Regimens for Prevention of Endocarditis in Susceptible Patients Undergoing Genitourinary or Gastrointestinal Procedures

Situation	Agents	Regimen*
High-risk patients	Ampicillin plus gentamicin	Ampicillin, 2 g IM or IV, plus gentamicin, 1.5 mg/kg (not to exceed 120 mg) within 30 minutes of starting the procedure; 6 hours later, ampicillin, 1 g IM/IV, or amoxicillin, 1 g orally
High-risk patients allergic to ampicillin/amoxicillin	Vancomycin plus gentamicin	Vancomycin, 1 g IV over 1 to 2 hours, plus gentamicin, 1.5 mg/kg IV/IM (not to exceed 120 mg); complete injection/infusion within 30 minutes of starting the procedure
Moderate-risk patients	Amoxicillin or ampicillin	Amoxicillin, 2 g orally 1 hour before procedure, or ampicillin, 2 g IM/IV within 30 minutes of starting the procedure
Moderate-risk patients allergic to ampicillin/amoxicillin	Vancomycin	Vancomycin, 1 g IV over 1 to 2 hours; complete infusion within 30 minutes of starting the procedure

Abbreviations: IM, intramuscularly; IV, intravenously.

*No second dose of vancomycin or gentamicin is recommended.

Adapted from Dajani AS, Taubert KA, Wilson W, Bolger AF, Bayer A, Ferrieri P, et al. Prevention of bacterial endocarditis: recommendations by the American Heart Association. JAMA 1997;277:1799. Copyrighted 1997, American Medical Association.

small, but rare anaphylactic reactions have occurred (37). Patients with a history of an immediate hypersensitivity reaction to penicillin should not receive cephalosporin antibiotics, given that alternative drugs are available for prophylaxis. Alternative agents include metronidazole, doxycycline, clindamycin, and the quinolones. Cephalosporin prophylaxis is acceptable in those patients with a history of penicillin allergy not felt to be immunoglobulin-E (IgE) mediated (immediate hypersensitivity).

▶ *How cost-effective is antibiotic prophylaxis?*

Prophylactic antibiotics add considerable cost to the routine care of surgical patients. However, the prevention of postoperative infection decreases hospital stay and the use of other resources to assess and treat infections not otherwise prevented by antimicrobial prophylaxis. A 1983 study found an average net savings of $102 per patient in women undergoing hysterectomy who received prophylactic antibiotics (38). This savings would be eroded by use of the more expensive cephalosporins unless they were considerably more effective than cefazolin or cefotetan. Likewise, the inexpensive prophylactic regimens used for the prevention of postabortal PID are cost-effective as noted previously. It is estimated that more than $500,000 would be saved each year in the United States in direct treatment costs alone by providing antibiotic prophylaxis to women at average risk undergoing induced abortion (29).

Summary

The following recommendations are based on good and consistent scientific evidence (Level A):

▶ Patients undergoing hysterectomy should receive antimicrobial prophylaxis.

▶ Pelvic inflammatory disease complicating IUD insertion is uncommon. The cost-effectiveness of screening for gonorrhea and chlamydia before insertion is unclear; in women screened and found to be negative, prophylactic antibiotics appear to provide no benefit.

▶ Women undergoing surgically induced abortion are candidates for antibiotic prophylaxis.

▶ Appropriate prophylaxis for women undergoing surgery that may involve the bowel includes a mechanical bowel preparation with or without oral antibiotics and the use of a broad-spectrum parenteral antibiotic, given preoperatively.

The following recommendations are based on limited or inconsistent scientific evidence (Level B):

▶ In patients with no history of pelvic infection, HSG can be performed without prophylactic antibiotics. If HSG demonstrates dilated tubes, antibiotic prophylaxis should be given to reduce the incidence of postHSG PID.

▶ Routine antibiotic prophylaxis is not recommended in patients undergoing hysteroscopic surgery.

▶ Cephalosporin antibiotics may be used for antimicrobial prophylaxis in women with a history of penicillin allergy not manifested by an immediate hypersensitivity reaction.

The following recommendations are based primarily on consensus and expert opinion (Level C):

▶ Antibiotic prophylaxis is not recommended in patients undergoing exploratory laparotomy or diagnostic laparoscopy.

▶ Use of antibiotic prophylaxis with saline infusion sonography should be based on clinical considerations, including individual risk factors.

▶ Patients with high- and moderate-risk structural cardiac defects undergoing certain surgical procedures may benefit from antimicrobial prophylaxis.

▶ Patients with a history of anaphylactic reaction to penicillin should not receive cephalosporins.

▶ Pretest screening for bacteriuria or urinary tract infection by urine culture or urinalysis, or both, is recommended in women undergoing urodynamic testing. Those with positive results should be given antibiotic treatment.

References

1. Kernodle DS, Kaiser AB. Postoperative infections and antimicrobial prophylaxis. In: Mandell GL, Bennett JE, Dolin R, eds. Mandell, Douglas, and Bennett's principles and practice of infectious diseases. 5th ed. Philadelphia: Churchill Livingstone, 2000:3177–3191 (Level III)

2. Hemsell DL. Gynecologic postoperative infections. In: Pastorek JG II, ed. Obstetric and gynecologic infectious disease. New York: Raven Press, 1994:141–149 (Level III)

3. Soper DE, Bump RC, Hurt WG. Bacterial vaginosis and trichomoniasis vaginitis are risk factors for postoperative cuff cellulitis after abdominal hysterectomy. Am J Obstet Gynecol 1990;163:1016–1021; discussion 1021–1023 (Level II-2)

4. Burke JF. The effective period of preventive antibiotic action in experimental incisions and dermal lesions. Surgery 1961;50:161–168; discussion 184–185 (Level II-2)

5. Dellinger EP, Gross PA, Barrett TL, Krause PJ, Martone WJ, McGowan JE, et al. Quality standard for antimicrobial prophylaxis in surgical procedures. Infectious Disease Society of America. Clin Infect Dis 1994;18:422–427 (Level III)

6. McFarland LV. Diarrhea acquired in the hospital. Gastroenterol Clin North Am 1993;22:563–577 (Level III)

7. McFarland LV, Surawicz CM, Greenberg RN, Elmer GW, Moyer KA, Melcher SA, et al. Prevention of beta-lactam-associated diarrhea by Saccharomyces boulardii compared with placebo. Am J Gastroenterol 1995;90:439–448 (Level I)

8. Bartlett JG. Antibiotic-associated diarrhea. Clin Infect Dis 1992;15:573–581 (Level III)

9. Thielman NM. Antibiotic-associated colitis. In: Mandell GL, Bennett JE, Dolin R, eds. Mandell, Douglas, and Bennett's principles and practice of infectious diseases. 5th ed. Philadelphia: Churchill Livingstone, 2000: 1111–1126 (Level III)

10. Idsoe O, Guthe T, Willcox RR, Weck AL de. Nature and extent of penicillin side-reactions, with particular reference to fatalities from anaphylactic shock. Bull World Health Organ 1968;38:159–188 (Level III)

11. Hemsell DL. Prophylactic antibiotics in gynecologic and obstetric surgery. Rev Infect Dis 1991;13(Suppl 10): S821–S841 (Level III)

12. Tanos V, Rojansky N. Prophylactic antibiotics in abdominal hysterectomy. J Am Coll Surg 1994;179:593–600 (Meta-analysis)

13. Mittendorf R, Aronson MP, Berry RE, Williams MA, Kupelnick B, Klickstein A, et al. Avoiding serious infections associated with abdominal hysterectomy: a meta-analysis of antibiotic prophylaxis. Am J Obstet Gynecol 1993;169:1119–1124 (Meta-analysis)

14. Hemsell DL, Johnson ER, Hemsell PG, Nobles BJ, Little BB, Heard MC. Cefazolin is inferior to cefotetan as single-dose prophylaxis for women undergoing elective total abdominal hysterectomy. Clin Infect Dis 1995;20: 677–684 (Level I)

15. Pittaway DE, Winfeld AC, Maxson W, Daniell J, Herbert C, Wentz AC. Prevention of acute pelvic inflammatory disease after hysterosalpingography: efficacy of doxycycline prophylaxis. Am J Obstet Gynecol 1983;147:623–626 (Level II-2)

16. Moller BR, Allen J, Toft B, Hansen KB, Taylor-Robinson D. Pelvic inflammatory disease after hysterosalpingography associated with Chlamydia trachomatis and Mycoplasma hominis. Br J Obstet Gynaecol 1984;91: 1181–1187 (Level III)

17. Speroff L, Glass RH, Kase NG. Female infertility. In: Clinical gynecologic endocrinology and infertility. 5th ed. Baltimore: Williams & Wilkins, 1994:809–839 (Level III)

18. Goldstein SR. Sonohysterography. In: Goldstein SR, Timor-Tritsch IE. Ultrasound in gynecology. New York: Churchill Livingstone, 1995:203–221 (Level III)

19. Baggish MS. Complications of hysteroscopic surgery. In: Baggish MS, Barbot J, Valle RF, eds. Diagnostic and operative hysteroscopy. 2nd ed. St. Louis: Mosby, 1999: 367–379 (Level III)

20. Bhattacharya S, Parkin DE, Reid TM, Abramovich DR, Mollison J, Kitchener HC. A prospective randomised study of the effects of prophylactic antibiotics on the incidence of bacteraemia following hysteroscopic surgery. Eur J Obstet Gynecol Reprod Biol 1995;63:37–40 (Level I)

21. Baggish MS, Sze EH. Endometrial ablation: a series of 568 patients treated over an 11-year period. Am J Obstet Gynecol 1996;174:908–913 (Level II-3)

22. Garry R, Shelley-Jones D, Mooney P, Phillips G. Six hundred endometrial laser ablations. Obstet Gynecol 1995; 85:24–29 (Level II-2)

23. McCausland VM, Fields GA, McCausland AM, Townsend DE. Tuboovarian abscesses after operative hysteroscopy. J Reprod Med 1993;38:198–200 (Level II-3)

24. Walsh T, Grimes D, Frezieres R, Nelson A, Bernstein L, Coulson A, et al. Randomised controlled trial of prophylactic antibiotics before insertion of intrauterine devices. IUD Study Group. Lancet 1998;351:1005–1008 (Level I)

25. Walsh TL, Bernstein GS, Grimes DA, Frezieres R, Bernstein L, Coulson AH. Effect of prophylactic antibiotics on morbidity associated with IUD insertion: results of a pilot randomized controlled trial. IUD Study Group. Contraception 1994;50:319–327 (Level I)

26. Ladipo OA, Farr G, Otolorin E, Konje JC, Sturgen K, Cox P, et al. Prevention of IUD-related pelvic infection: the efficacy of prophylactic doxycycline at IUD insertion. Adv Contracept 1991;7:43–54 (Level I)

27. Sinei SK, Schulz KF, Lamptey PR, Grimes DA, Mati JK, Rosenthal SM, et al. Preventing IUCD-related pelvic infection: the efficacy of prophylactic doxycycline at insertion. Br J Obstet Gynaecol 1990;97:412–419 (Level I)

28. Grimes DA, Schulz KF. Antibiotic prophylaxis for intrauterine contraceptive device insertion (Cochrane Review). In: The Cochrane Library, Issue 4, 2000. Oxford: Update Software.

29. Sawaya GF, Grady D, Kerlikowske K, Grimes DA. Antibiotics at the time of induced abortion: the case for universal prophylaxis based on a meta-analysis. Obstet Gynecol 1996;87:884–890 (Meta-analysis)

30. Prieto JA, Eriksen NL, Blanco JD. A randomized trial of prophylactic doxycycline for curettage in incomplete abortion. Obstet Gynecol 1995;85:692–696 (Level I)

31. Bergman A, McCarthy TA. Antibiotic prophylaxis after instrumentation for urodynamic testing. Br J Urol 1983; 55:568–569 (Level II-1)

32. Baker KR, Drutz HP, Barnes MD. Effectiveness of antibiotic prophylaxis in preventing bacteriuria after multichan-

nel urodynamic investigations: a blind, randomized study in 124 female patients. Am J Obstet Gynecol 1991;165: 679–681 (Level I)

33. Walter S, Vejlsgaard R. Diagnostic catheterization and bacteriuria in women with urinary incontinence. Br J Urol 1978;50:106–108 (Level II-3)

34. Parker CW. Drug allergy (first of three parts). N Engl J Med 1975;292:511–514 (Level III)

35. Gell PG, Coombs RR. Classification of allergic reactions responsible for clinical hypersensitivity and disease. In: Gell PG, Coombs RR, Hachmann PJ, eds. Clinical aspects of immunology. Oxford: Blackwell Scientific Publications, 1975:761–781 (Level III)

36. Anne S, Reisman RE. Risk of administering cephalosporin antibiotics to patients with histories of penicillin allergy. Ann Allergy Asthma Immunol 1995;74:167–170 (Level III)

37. Weiss ME, Adkinson NF Jr. β-lactam allergy. In: Mandell GL, Bennett JE, Dolin R, eds. Mandell, Douglas, and Bennett's principles and practice of infectious diseases. 5th ed. Philadelphia: Churchill Livingstone, 2000: 299–305 (Level III)

38. Shapiro M, Schoenbaum SC, Tager IB, Munoz A, Polk BF. Benefit-cost analysis of antimicrobial prophylaxis in abdominal and vaginal hysterectomy. JAMA 1983;249: 1290–1294 (Cost-benefit analysis)

The MEDLINE database, the Cochrane Library, and ACOG's own internal resources and documents were used to conduct a literature search to locate relevant articles published between January 1985 and May 2000. The search was restricted to articles published in the English language. Priority was given to articles reporting results of original research, although review articles and commentaries also were consulted. Abstracts of research presented at symposia and scientific conferences were not considered adequate for inclusion in this document. Guidelines published by organizations or institutions such as the National Institutes of Health and the American College of Obstetricians and Gynecologists were reviewed, and additional studies were located by reviewing bibliographies of identified articles. When reliable research was not available, expert opinions from obstetrician–gynecologists were used.

Studies were reviewed and evaluated for quality according to the method outlined by the U.S. Preventive Services Task Force:

I Evidence obtained from at least one properly designed randomized controlled trial.
II-1 Evidence obtained from well-designed controlled trials without randomization.
II-2 Evidence obtained from well-designed cohort or case–control analytic studies, preferably from more than one center or research group.
II-3 Evidence obtained from multiple time series with or without the intervention. Dramatic results in uncontrolled experiments also could be regarded as this type of evidence.
III Opinions of respected authorities, based on clinical experience, descriptive studies, or reports of expert committees.

Based on the highest level of evidence found in the data, recommendations are provided and graded according to the following categories:

Level A—Recommendations are based on good and consistent scientific evidence.

Level B—Recommendations are based on limited or inconsistent scientific evidence.

Level C—Recommendations are based primarily on consensus and expert opinion.

ISSN 1099-3630

The American College of Obstetricians and Gynecologists
409 12th Street, SW, PO Box 96920
Washington, DC 20090-6920

12345/54321

ACOG PRACTICE BULLETIN

CLINICAL MANAGEMENT GUIDELINES FOR
OBSTETRICIAN–GYNECOLOGISTS

NUMBER 68, NOVEMBER 2005

(Replaces Educational Bulletin 244, February 1998)

This Practice Bulletin was developed by the ACOG Committee on Practice Bulletins— Obstetrics with the assistance of M. Sean Esplin, MD. The information is designed to aid practitioners in making decisions about appropriate obstetric and gynecologic care. These guidelines should not be construed as dictating an exclusive course of treatment or procedure. Variations in practice may be warranted based on the needs of the individual patient, resources, and limitations unique to the institution or type of practice.

Antiphospholipid Syndrome

Antiphospholipid syndrome is an autoimmune disorder defined by the presence of characteristic clinical features and specified levels of circulating antiphospholipid antibodies (Table 1). Because approximately 70% of individuals with antiphospholipid syndrome are female (1), it is reasonably common among women of reproductive age. Antiphospholipid antibodies are a diverse group of antibodies with specificity for protein binding negatively charged phospholipids on cell surfaces. Despite the prevalence and clinical significance of antiphospholipid syndrome, there is controversy about the indications for antiphospholipid syndrome testing and the tests that should be ordered to diagnose the condition. Much of the debate results from a lack of well-designed and controlled studies on the diagnosis and management of antiphospholipid syndrome. The purpose of this document is to evaluate the data for diagnosis and treatment of antiphospholipid syndrome.

Background

The lupus anticoagulant and anticardiolipin antibodies, the most widely accepted antibodies of clinical use, have been associated with a variety of medical problems, including arterial and venous thromboses, autoimmune thrombocytopenia, and fetal loss (2–7). In addition to fetal loss, several obstetric complications have been associated with antiphospholipid antibodies, including preeclampsia, intrauterine growth restriction, placental insufficiency, and preterm delivery (8, 9). *Primary antiphospholipid syndrome* refers to patients with antiphospholipid syndrome but no other recognized autoimmune disorders (3, 4, 10). However, other autoimmune conditions such as systemic lupus erythematosus often coexist with the condition. When it occurs in the setting of other autoimmune disease, it is referred to as *secondary antiphospholipid syndrome* (2, 4).

Antiphospholipid Antibodies

The two antiphospholipid antibodies that are best characterized are lupus anticoagulant and anticardiolipin antibodies. Although many women with lupus anticoagulant also have anticardiolipin antibodies, the correlation is imperfect (1, 11). Approximately 80% of patients with lupus anticoagulant have anticardiolipin antibodies, and 20% of patients positive for anticardiolipin antibodies have lupus anticoagulant. Although some investigators suggest that lupus anticoagulant and anticardiolipin antibodies are the same antibody detected by different methods (12), the fact that lupus anticoagulant and anticardiolipin antibodies may be separated in the laboratory (13) would indicate that they may be related but different immunoglobulins. Regardless, lupus anticoagulant and anticardiolipin antibodies are both independently associated with the clinical features of antiphospholipid syndrome, and the presence of only one of these antibodies is adequate for the laboratory diagnosis of antiphospholipid syndrome.

Lupus Anticoagulant

Lupus anticoagulant is present in many individuals without systemic lupus erythematosus and is associated with thrombosis, not anticoagulation. The presence of lupus anticoagulant is assessed indirectly, and a series of tests are needed for the laboratory diagnosis (Table 1). The initial laboratory test for lupus anticoagulant can be one of several phospholipid-dependent clotting assays, such as the activated partial thromboplastin time (APTT), kaolin plasma clotting time, and dilute Russell's viper venom time. Lupus anticoagulants are antibodies directed against plasma proteins (such as β_2-glycoprotein I, prothrombin, or annexin V) that bind to anionic or hexagonal phase phospholipids (14, 15). Lupus anticoagulants paradoxically block phospholipid-dependent clotting assays by interfering with the assembly of the prothrombin complex. The sensitivity and specificity of each test for lupus anticoagulant are greatly affected by the reagents used and vary among laboratories.

Because prolonged clotting times in these assays can result from factors other than lupus anticoagulant, such as improperly processed specimens, anticoagulant medications, clotting factor deficiencies, and factor-specific inhibitors, plasma suspected of containing lupus anticoagulant based on a prolonged clotting time is subjected to additional testing. If the prolonged clotting time is caused by a factor deficiency, the addition of normal plasma (containing the missing factor) results in a normal clotting time on repeat testing. In contrast, if an inhibitor such as lupus anticoagulant is present, the clotting time remains prolonged despite the addition of normal plasma. A second confirmatory test involving the addition or removal of phospholipid from the assay has been recommended. For example, preincubation of plasma with phospholipid binds and removes lupus anticoagulant from the sample being tested and normalizes clotting time. Regardless of the assays used, lupus anticoagulant cannot be quantified and is reported only as present or absent.

Anticardiolipin Antibodies

Like lupus anticoagulants, anticardiolipin antibodies react to the complex of negatively charged phospholipids, such as cardiolipin or phosphatidylserine bound to proteins such as β_2-glycoprotein I, prothrombin, or annexin V. However, these antibodies are detected by conventional immunoassays using purified cardiolipin as the phospholipid matrix. Historically, interlaboratory variation in this assay resulted in inappropriate diagnosis and various treatments and outcomes (16, 17). The development of standard sera, available from the Antiphospholipid Standardization Laboratory in Atlanta, Georgia (18), has greatly improved the reliability of this test among different laboratories. Assays using these standard positive serum calibrators are quite reliable and allow for the semiquantitation of antibody levels. Standard sera have been assigned numeric values termed GPL (immunoglobulin G [IgG] binding), MPL (IgM binding), and APL (IgA binding) units. Test results are reported as negative, low-positive, medium-positive, or high-positive.

Low-positive anticardiolipin antibodies (<20 GPL or MPL units) of any quantity are of questionable clinical significance and should not be considered diagnostic of antiphospholipid syndrome (19). The relevance of positive test results for IgA anticardiolipin antibodies of any level also is uncertain. Low levels of IgG anticardiolipin antibodies and IgM anticardiolipin antibodies are sometimes found in healthy individuals (18) and can result from infection (20) and nonspecific binding. In the general obstetric population, the prevalence of anticardiolipin antibodies has been reported to be between 2.7% and 7.0% (21–23). In contrast, several studies have shown a correlation between increasing titers of anticardiolipin antibodies and disorders related to antiphospholipid antibodies (5, 19, 24). Thus, only medium to high levels of IgG (>20 GPL units) or IgM (>20 MPL units) anticardiolipin antibodies or positive lupus anticoagulant are considered sufficient laboratory criteria for the diagnosis of antiphospholipid syndrome (2, 4). Positive test results for antiphospholipid antibodies can be transient and should be confirmed on two occasions at least several weeks apart (4, 25). The diagnosis of antiphospholipid syndrome is not based on laboratory testing alone. Rather, a diagnosis of antiphospholipid syndrome must be based on an appropriate clinical history and laboratory criteria.

Other Antibodies Associated With Antiphospholipid Syndrome

The antibody responsible for the biologic false-positive serologic test for syphilis (BFP STS) also is an antiphospholipid antibody and often is present in patients with lupus anticoagulant or anticardiolipin antibodies. Compared with lupus anticoagulant and anticardiolipin antibodies, the BFP STS correlates poorly with the development of medical problems associated with antiphospholipid antibodies. Thus, the BFP STS is not recommended in the routine evaluation of antiphospholipid syndrome. Laboratories often report antibodies to other phospholipids (ie, antiphosphatidylserine, antiphosphatidylinositol, antiphosphatidylethanolamine, antiphosphatidylcholine, and antiphosphatidylglycerol). However, these assays have not been subjected to quality control or standardization and are of uncertain clinical value. In contrast, tests for antiphospholipid antibodies other than lupus anticoagulant and anticardiolipin antibodies that appear to correlate with thrombotic risk include antiprothrombin, antiannexin V, and anti-β_2-glycoprotein I antibodies. However, although they may prove useful in the future, they cannot be recommended for clinical use at this time.

Medical Complications of Antiphospholipid Syndrome

The most common and serious complications associated with antiphospholipid syndrome are venous and arterial thromboses (4, 5, 26). Most thrombotic events (65–70%) are venous (27, 28). Approximately 2% of all patients with venous thrombosis will test positive for antiphospholipid antibodies (29). Although the most frequent site of venous thrombosis is a lower extremity, thrombosis can occur in almost any blood vessel in the body, and occlusions in unusual locations should prompt clinicians to consider the diagnosis of antiphospholipid syndrome. It is estimated that between 0.5% and 2% of the asymptomatic people incidentally found to have antiphospholipid antibodies eventually will develop thromboses each year (30). Up to one half of

patients with an antiphospholipid syndrome–associated thrombosis will have at least one pulmonary embolus. One retrospective cohort study of 147 subjects found a thrombosis recurrence rate of 25% per year in untreated patients with antiphospholipid syndrome and prior thrombosis, but that recurrence can be minimized with anticoagulation (27).

The risk of thrombosis is significantly increased during pregnancy in patients with antiphospholipid syndrome. In a large cohort study, up to 25% of thrombotic events in patients with antiphospholipid syndrome occurred during pregnancy or the postpartum period (31). These findings were confirmed in prospective studies indicating a 5–12% risk of thrombosis during pregnancy or the puerperium in women with antiphospholipid syndrome (8, 9).

Arterial thrombosis also is associated with antiphospholipid antibodies and can occur in atypical sites, such as retinal, subclavian, digital, or brachial arteries. Stroke is the most common arterial event, and the most frequently involved vessel is the middle cerebral artery. Transient ischemic attacks (TIAs) and amaurosis fugax also are associated with antiphospholipid antibodies (19, 31). Antiphospholipid antibodies are present in 4–6% of otherwise healthy individuals with stroke who are younger than 50 years (32, 33). Coronary occlusions also are reported (3). Individuals with unexplained arterial thrombosis, stroke, amaurosis fugax, or transient ischemic attacks should undergo testing for antiphospholipid antibodies.

Autoimmune thrombocytopenia occurs in 40–50% of individuals with primary antiphospholipid syndrome (2, 3, 34). Thrombocytopenia associated with antiphospholipid antibodies is extremely difficult to distinguish from idiopathic thrombocytopenic purpura, although the pertinent platelet antigens appear to differ in antiphospholipid syndrome and idiopathic thrombocytopenic purpura. Thrombocytopenia caused by idiopathic thrombocytopenic purpura is treated the same as thrombocytopenia caused by antiphospholipid syndrome.

A variety of other medical conditions have been associated with antiphospholipid antibodies, including autoimmune hemolytic anemia, livedo reticularis, cutaneous ulcers, chorea gravidarum, multiinfarct dementia, and transverse myelitis (2, 3). A recently described condition termed *catastrophic antiphospholipid syndrome* occurs in some individuals who develop progressive thromboses and multiorgan failure (35). Others have a severe illness postpartum primarily consisting of cardiopulmonary failure and fever, as well as renal insufficiency and multiple thromboses (36–38).

Obstetric Complications

A large proportion of pregnancy losses related to antiphospholipid antibodies are second-trimester or third-trimester fetal deaths. Although fetal deaths normally account for only a small proportion of all pregnancy losses in the general population (39), 50% of pregnancy losses in a cohort of 76 women (333 pregnancies) with antiphospholipid syndrome were fetal deaths (40). Of the 76 women in this study, 80% had at least one fetal death.

Antiphospholipid antibodies also are associated with recurrent early pregnancy loss. Observational studies have consistently documented positive test results for antiphospholipid antibodies in a higher proportion of women with recurrent spontaneous abortion than in controls (25, 41–49). Most studies report positive test results for antiphospholipid antibodies in 5–20% of women with recurrent pregnancy loss. However, many positive results are low titer or IgM isotype only. Although low levels of antiphospholipid antibodies may prove relevant to obstetric outcome, as stated earlier, they identify a distinct population at lower risk for disorders related to antiphospholipid antibodies than patients with antiphospholipid syndrome (19). In contrast to recurrent pregnancy loss, antiphospholipid antibodies are not associated with sporadic preembryonic or embryonic pregnancy loss (50).

Preeclampsia is associated with antiphospholipid syndrome (8, 9). In one observational study of 54 women, 50% of those with antiphospholipid syndrome had preeclampsia and 25% had severe preeclampsia (8). Between 11% and 17% of women with preeclampsia will test positive for antiphospholipid antibodies (51–54). The association is strongest in women with severe, early onset (<34 weeks of gestation) preeclampsia. However, term preeclampsia is not associated with increased levels of antiphospholipid antibodies (55).

Intrauterine growth restriction (IUGR) complicates pregnancies in women with antiphospholipid syndrome, occurring in 15–30% in most series (8, 9, 43, 56). There is conflicting evidence of the link between antiphospholipid antibodies and IUGR (57). Although some studies have not found a correlation between antiphospholipid antibodies and IUGR (22, 58), this discrepancy may result from the inclusion of some women with low-positive test results for antiphospholipid antibodies (9, 24, 43).

Uteroplacental insufficiency, preeclampsia, and IUGR all increase the risk of indicated preterm delivery in women with antiphospholipid syndrome. The risk is greatest in women with high titers of antiphospholipid antibodies who meet strict criteria for antiphospholipid syndrome. In one report, approximately one third of pregnancies in women with antiphospholipid syndrome resulted in live births that occurred before 34 weeks of gestation (8).

Clinical Considerations and Recommendations

▶ *Who should be tested for antiphospholipid antibodies?*

The principal manifestations of antiphospholipid syndrome are venous or arterial thromboses, pregnancy loss, and morbidity. Generally accepted indications for antiphospholipid antibody testing are listed in Table 1. Although most are straightforward, the obstetric indications are a matter of some controversy. In part, this results from poorly characterized obstetric details in available studies and the need for additional information. The preliminary criteria for antiphospholipid syndrome (10) developed in 1999 by an international group of experts recognized obstetric complications occurring in both the preembryonic–embryonic period and the fetal–neonatal periods and divided them into three categories, one encompassing early pregnancy loss and the other two relating primarily to complications in second or third trimesters. Thus, the accepted obstetric clinical criteria are 1) one or more unexplained deaths of a morphologically normal fetus at or beyond the 10th week of gestation, 2) one or more premature births of a morphologically normal neonate at or before the 34th week of gestation resulting from preeclampsia, eclampsia, or placental insufficiency, or 3) three or more unexplained consecutive spontaneous abortions before the 10th week of gestation. Unexplained venous or arterial thrombosis, or a small-vessel thrombosis (in the absence of inflammation of the vessel wall), are the nonobstetric clinical criteria for antiphospholipid syndrome.

Other conditions associated with antiphospholipid syndrome include hemolytic anemia, autoimmune thrombocytopenia, amaurosis fugax, livedo reticularis, systemic lupus erythematosus, and a false-positive RPR. These conditions are not considered clinical criteria for antiphospholipid syndrome; therefore, testing individuals with these conditions alone is not warranted.

Antiphospholipid antibodies, especially low-level or IgM anticardiolipin antibodies, are present in a few healthy people (18, 21) and are probably meaningless. Clinicians who test for antiphospholipid antibodies in women without clinical features of antiphospholipid syndrome may be left with an uninterpretable positive test result and a management dilemma. It is best to avoid such

Table 1. Preliminary Classification Criteria for Antiphospholipid Syndrome*

Criteria	Definition
Clinical	
Obstetric	1) Three or more consecutive spontaneous abortions before the 10th week of gestation
	2) One or more unexplained fetal deaths at or beyond the 10th week of gestation
	3) Severe preeclampsia or placental insufficiency necessitating birth before the 34th week of gestation
Vascular thrombosis	1) Unexplained venous thrombosis
	2) Unexplained arterial thrombosis
	3) Small-vessel thrombosis in any tissue or organ, without significant evidence of inflammation of the vessel wall
Laboratory	
Anticardiolipin	Anticardiolipin antibody of IgG or IgM isotype in medium to high titers, on two or more occasions at least 6 weeks apart, measured by standardized enzyme-linked immunosorbent assay
Lupus anticoagulant	Lupus anticoagulant present in plasma, on two or more occasions at least 6 weeks apart, detected according to guidelines of the International Society on Thrombosis and Hemostasis, in the following steps:
	1) Demonstration of a prolonged phospholipid-dependent coagulation screening test (eg, activated partial thromboplastin time, kaolin clotting time, dilute Russell's viper venom time, dilute prothrombin time)
	2) Failure to correct the prolonged screening test by mixing with normal platelet-poor plasma
	3) Shortening or correction of the prolonged screening test by the addition of excess phospholipids
	4) Exclusion of other coagulopathies (eg, factor VIII inhibitor, heparin) as clinically indicated

*Definite antiphospholipid syndrome is considered to be present if at least one of the clinical criteria and one of the laboratory criteria are met.

Adapted from Wilson WA, Gharavi AE, Koike T, Lockshin MD, Branch DW, Piette JC, et al. International consensus statement on preliminary classification criteria for definite antiphospholipid syndrome: report of an international workshop. Arthritis Rheum 1999;42:1309–11. Copyright © Wiley-Liss Inc. Reprinted with permission of Wiley-Liss Inc., a subsidiary of John Wiley & Sons, Inc.

problems by testing only patients with disorders clearly related to antiphospholipid antibodies.

▶ *What laboratory criteria are used for the diagnosis of antiphospholipid syndrome?*

The initial diagnosis of antiphospholipid syndrome requires testing for anticardiolipin antibodies by enzyme-linked immunosorbent assay and lupus anticoagulant with two sensitive phospholipid-dependent clotting assays. A positive screening test result for lupus anticoagulant must be further investigated according to established criteria (Table 1). A prolongation of the phospholipid-based clotting assay must be confirmed by mixing with normal plasma. The subsequent normalization of the clotting time is an indication of other causes and not the presence of antiphospholipid antibodies. Although lupus anticoagulant is interpreted as either present or absent, anticardiolipin must be abnormal in moderate to high (>20 GPL or >20 MPL) titers to be considered clinically significant. Positive results require a repeat test after several weeks to exclude a transient, clinically unimportant antibody. Other antibodies, such as antiphosphatidylserine, antiphosphatidylinositol, antiphosphatidylethanolamine, antiphosphatidylcholine, and antiphosphatidylglycerol, are not used as laboratory criteria for the diagnosis of antiphospholipid syndrome.

▶ *How should antiphospholipid syndrome be managed during pregnancy and the postpartum period?*

The goals of treatment for antiphospholipid syndrome during pregnancy are to improve maternal and fetal–neonatal outcome by reducing the risk of pregnancy loss, preeclampsia, placental insufficiency, and preterm birth and to reduce or eliminate the maternal thrombotic risk of antiphospholipid syndrome during pregnancy. Two recent reviews (59, 60) have emphasized that case series and treatment trials tend to include individuals whose antiphospholipid syndrome diagnosis falls into one of two groups: those with a history of thrombotic events and those without a history.

Treatment of women with antiphospholipid syndrome without a thrombotic event is controversial. A recent meta-analysis suggested that, for women with recurrent miscarriage as the clinical criteria, prophylactic heparin and low-dose aspirin may reduce pregnancy loss by 50% (61). This combined therapy appears superior to low-dose aspirin alone or prednisone. Few data from controlled trials are available on the efficacy of various treatment regimens for women with antiphospholipid syndrome with other obstetric clinical events (severe preeclampsia, uteroplacental insufficiency). Many experts recommend prophylactic heparin and aspirin in these women. For women with antiphospholipid syndrome without a history of a thrombotic event, some physicians recommend initiation of heparin before conception, although no clinical trial supports this recommendation. Most experts recommend 6–8 weeks of postpartum thromboprophylaxis in women with obstetric antiphospholipid syndrome (59).

For women with antiphospholipid syndrome who have had a thrombotic event, most experts recommend full heparin anticoagulation (62). Patients enrolled in most published series also received low-dose aspirin, but the benefit of adding aspirin is unknown. Several approaches to the peripartum management of anticoagulation therapy in these patients are available, thus treatment should be individualized.

Anticoagulation should be continued for a minimum of 6 weeks postpartum to minimize the risk of maternal thromboembolism (59). After delivery, this can be safely accomplished with coumarin. Patients with antiphospholipid syndrome should be referred to an internist or hematologist after delivery to prescribe anticoagulation therapy outside of pregnancy.

Other therapies that have been suggested for treatment of pregnant women with antiphospholipid syndrome include corticosteroids and intravenous immunoglobulin (IVIG). Several case series have reported a 60–70% rate of successful pregnancies in women with antiphospholipid syndrome treated with prednisone and low-dose aspirin (63). However, a meta-analysis of therapeutic trials showed no reduction in pregnancy loss in women treated with prednisone and low-dose aspirin (61). Direct comparison of studies is difficult because subjects had different clinical and laboratory features and dosing regimens, and many trials were nonrandomized and poorly controlled. Thus, the efficacy of prednisone in pregnancies complicated by antiphospholipid syndrome remains uncertain.

Treatment with IVIG has been promising in a small number of cases refractory to heparin or prednisone (64–66). Obstetric complications have been rare in patients treated with IVIG (66). However, most of these women also were treated with heparin or prednisone and low-dose aspirin. A recent small randomized controlled study demonstrated no greater benefit from IVIG (plus heparin and aspirin) than with heparin and aspirin alone (67). Because the efficacy of IVIG has not been proved in appropriately designed studies and the drug is extremely expensive, it is not recommended as primary therapy.

▶ *Should women with antiphospholipid syndrome have antepartum surveillance?*

Pregnant women with antiphospholipid syndrome should be examined frequently and instructed about the signs and symptoms of preeclampsia and thrombosis. The primary goal of prenatal visits after 20 weeks of gestation is the detection of preeclampsia or growth restriction. Because of the risk for growth restriction, consideration should be given to serial ultrasonographic assessment. Antepartum testing should be considered after 32 weeks of gestation, or earlier if there are signs of growth restriction.

▶ *What is appropriate long-term management of antiphospholipid syndrome?*

Long-term risks for women with antiphospholipid syndrome include thrombosis and stroke. In studies of women with antiphospholipid syndrome, including studies of women without prior thrombosis, one half developed thromboses during 3–10 years of follow-up and 10% developed systemic lupus erythematosus (30, 31, 68). The studied populations were highly selected referral populations; thus selection may have been biased toward severe disease. However, no method currently predicts which patients with antiphospholipid syndrome using anticoagulants will develop recurrent thrombosis once treatment is discontinued. In addition, no evidence exists to support long-term treatment when thrombotic events occur in the presence of other risk factors (30). Therefore, for long-term management, patients with antiphospholipid syndrome should be referred to a physician with expertise in treatment of the syndrome, such as an internist or hematologist.

Pregnancy and the use of estrogen-containing oral contraceptives appear to increase the risk for thrombosis in women with antiphospholipid syndrome. In retrospective analyses of women with antiphospholipid syndrome, most thromboses occurred in association with pregnancy or oral contraceptive use (8, 31). Thus, estrogen-containing oral contraceptives in women with well-characterized antiphospholipid syndrome should be avoided.

Summary of Recommendations and Conclusions

The following recommendation is based on limited or inconsistent scientific evidence (Level B):

▶ Testing for antiphospholipid antibodies should be limited to those women with appropriate medical or obstetric histories.

The following recommendations are based primarily on consensus and expert opinion (Level C):

▶ Women with antiphospholipid syndrome and no thrombotic history should receive prophylactic doses of heparin and low-dose aspirin during pregnancy and the postpartum period (6–8 weeks).

▶ Women with antiphospholipid syndrome and previous history of thrombosis should receive full anticoagulation throughout pregnancy and the postpartum period (6–8 weeks).

▶ Women with antiphospholipid syndrome should be referred to an internist or hematologist for long-term follow-up.

▶ Women with antiphospholipid syndrome should avoid estrogen-containing oral contraceptives.

▶ Because of the risk for growth restriction, consideration should be given to serial ultrasonographic assessment. Antepartum testing should be considered after 32 weeks of gestation, or earlier if there are signs of growth restriction.

References

1. Lockshin MD. Antiphospholipid antibody. Babies, blood clots, biology. JAMA 1997;277:1549–51. (Level III)

2. Alarcon-Segovia D, Perez-Vazquez ME, Villa AR, Drenkard C, Cabiedes J. Preliminary classification criteria for the antiphospholipid syndrome within systemic lupus erythematosus. Semin Arthritis Rheum 1992;21:275–86. (Level II-2)

3. Asherson RA, Khamashta MA, Ordi-Ros J, Derksen RH, Machin SJ, Barquinero J, et al. The "primary" antiphospholipid syndrome: major clinical and serological features. Medicine (Baltimore) 1989;68:366–74. (Level III)

4. Harris EN. Syndrome of the black swan. Br J Rheumatol 1987;26:324–6. (Level III)

5. Harris EN, Chan JK, Asherson RA, Aber VR, Gharavi AE, Hughes GR. Thrombosis, recurrent fetal loss, and thrombocytopenia. Predictive value of the anticardiolipin antibody test. Arch Intern Med 1986;146:2153–6. (Level II-3)

6. Levine JS, Branch DW, Rauch J. The antiphospholipid syndrome. N Engl J Med 2002;346:752–63. (Level III)

7. Viard JP, Amoura Z, Bach JF. Association of anti-beta 2 glycoprotein I antibodies with lupus-type circulating anticoagulant and thrombosis in systemic lupus erythematosus. Am J Med 1992;93:181–6. (Level II-3)

8. Branch DW, Silver RM, Blackwell JL, Reading JC, Scott JR. Outcome of treated pregnancies in women with antiphospholipid syndrome: an update of the Utah experience. Obstet Gynecol 1992;80:614–20. (Level II-3)

9. Lima F, Khamashta MA, Buchanan NM, Kerslake S, Hunt BJ, Hughes GR. A study of sixty pregnancies in patients with the antiphospholipid syndrome. Clin Exp Rheumatol 1996;14:131–6. (Level II-3)

10. Wilson WA, Gharavi AE, Koike T, Lockshin MD, Branch DW, Piette JC, et al. International consensus statement on preliminary classification criteria for definite antiphospholipid syndrome: report of an international workshop. Arthritis Rheum 1999;42:1309–11. (Level III)

11. Triplett DA, Brandt JT, Musgrave KA, Orr CA. The relationship between lupus anticoagulants and antibodies to phospholipid. JAMA 1988;259:550–4. (Level II-3)

12. Pierangeli SS, Harris EN, Gharavi AE, Goldsmith G, Branch DW, Dean WL. Are immunoglobulins with lupus anticoagulant activity specific for phospholipids? Br J Haematol 1993;85:124–32. (Level II-3)

13. Chamley LW, Pattison NS, McKay EJ. Separation of lupus anticoagulant from anticardiolipin antibodies by ion-exchange and gel filtration chromatography. Haemostasis 1991;21:25–9. (Level III)

14. Passam F, Krilis S. Laboratory tests for antiphospholipid syndrome: current concepts. Pathology 2004;36:129–38. (Level III)

15. Roubey R. Autoantibodies to phospholipid-binding plasma proteins: a new review of lupus anticoagulants and other "antiphospholipid" autoantibodies. Blood 1994;84:2854–67. (Level III)

16. Coulam CB, McIntyre JA, Wagenknecht D, Rote N. Interlaboratory inconsistencies in detection of anticardiolipin antibodies. Lancet 1990;335:865. (Level II-3)

17. Peaceman AM, Silver RK, MacGregor SN, Socol ML. Interlaboratory variation in antiphospholipid antibody testing. Am J Obstet Gynecol 1992;166:1780–4; discussion 1784–7. (Level III)

18. Harris EN, Spinnato JA. Should anticardiolipin tests be performed in otherwise healthy pregnant women? Am J Obstet Gynecol 1991;165:1272–7. (Level II-2)

19. Silver RM, Porter TF, van Leeuwen I, Jeng G, Scott JR, Branch DW. Anticardiolipin antibodies: clinical consequences of "low titers." Obstet Gynecol 1996;87:494–500. (Level II-3)

20. Vaarala O, Palosuo T, Kleemola M, Aho K. Anticardiolipin response in acute infections. Clin Immunol Immunopathol 1986;41:8–15. (Level II-3)

21. Lockwood CJ, Romero R, Feinberg RF, Clyne LP, Coster B, Hobbins JC. The prevalence and biologic significance of lupus anticoagulant and anticardiolipin antibodies in a general obstetric population. Am J Obstet Gynecol 1989;161:369–73. (Level II-2)

22. Lynch A, Marlar R, Murphy J, Davila G, Santos M, Rutledge J, et al. Antiphospholipid antibodies in predicting adverse pregnancy outcome. A prospective study. Ann Intern Med 1994;120:470–5. (Level II-2)

23. Yasuda M, Takakuwa K, Tokunaga A, Tanaka K. Prospective studies of the association between anticardiolipin antibody and outcome of pregnancy. Obstet Gynecol 1995;86:555–9. (Level II-2)

24. Lockshin MD, Druzin ML, Qamar T. Prednisone does not prevent recurrent fetal death in women with antiphospholipid antibody. Am J Obstet Gynecol 1989;160:439–43. (Level II-3)

25. Rai RS, Regan L, Clifford K, Pickering W, Dave M, Mackie I, et al. Antiphospholipid antibodies and beta 2-glycoprotein-I in 500 women with recurrent miscarriage: results of a comprehensive screening approach. Hum Reprod 1995;10:2001–5. (Level II-3)

26. Hughes GR, Harris NN, Gharavi AE. The anticardiolipin syndrome. J Rheumatol 1986;13:486–9. (Level III)

27. Khamashta MA, Cuadrado MJ, Mujic F, Taub NA, Hunt BJ, Hughes GR. The management of thrombosis in the antiphospholipid-antibody syndrome. N Engl J Med 1995;332:993–7. (Level II-2)

28. Rosove MH, Brewer PM. Antiphospholipid thrombosis: clinical course after the first thrombotic event in 70 patients. Ann Intern Med 1992;117:303–8. (Level II-2)

29. Malm J, Laurell M, Nilsson IM, Dahlback B. Thromboembolic disease—critical evaluation of laboratory investigation. Thromb Haemost 1992;68:7–13. (Level II-2)

30. Erkan D, Merrill JT, Yazici Y, Sammaritano L, Buyon JP, Lockshin MD. High thrombosis rate after fetal loss in antiphospholipid syndrome: effective prophylaxis with aspirin. Arthritis Rheum 2001;44:1466–7. (Level III)

31. Silver RM, Draper ML, Scott JR, Lyon JL, Reading J, Branch DW. Clinical consequences of antiphospholipid antibodies: an historic cohort study. Obstet Gynecol 1994; 83:372–7. (Level II-3)

32. Brey RL, Hart RG, Sherman DG, Tegeler CH. Antiphospholipid antibodies and cerebral ischemia in young people. Neurology 1990;40:1190–6. (Level II-2)

33. Ferro D, Quintarelli C, Rasura M, Antonini G, Violi F. Lupus anticoagulant and the fibrinolytic system in young patients with stroke. Stroke 1993;24:368–70. (Level II-2)

34. Harris EN, Asherson RA, Gharavi AE, Morgan SH, Derue G, Hughes GR. Thrombocytopenia in SLE and related autoimmune disorders: association with anticardiolipin antibody. Br J Haematol 1985;59:227–30. (Level II-3)

35. Asherson RA, Cervera R, Piette JC, Font J, Lie JT, Burcoglu A, et al. Catastrophic antiphospholipid syndrome. Clinical and laboratory features of 50 patients. Medicine (Baltimore) 1998;77:195–207. (Level III)

36. Hochfeld M, Druzin ML, Maia D, Wright J, Lambert RE, McGuire J. Pregnancy complicated by primary antiphospholipid antibody syndrome. Obstet Gynecol 1994; 83:804–5. (Level III)

37. Kochenour NK, Branch DW, Rote NS, Scott JR. A new postpartum syndrome associated with antiphospholipid antibodies. Obstet Gynecol 1987;69:460–8. (Level III)

38. Kupferminc MJ, Lee MJ, Green D, Peaceman AM. Severe postpartum pulmonary, cardiac, and renal syndrome associated with antiphospholipid antibodies. Obstet Gynecol 1994;83:806–7. (Level III)

39. Goldstein SR. Embryonic death in early pregnancy: a new look at the first trimester. Obstet Gynecol 1994;84:294–7. (Level III)

40. Oshiro BT, Silver RM, Scott JR, Yu H, Branch DW. Antiphospholipid antibodies and fetal death. Obstet Gynecol 1996;87:489–93. (Level II-2)

41. Balasch J, Creus M, Fabregues F, Reverter JC, Carmona F, Tassies D, et al. Antiphospholipid antibodies and human reproductive failure. Hum Reprod 1996;11: 2310–5. (Level II-2)

42. Barbui T, Cortelazzo S, Galli M, Parazzini F, Radici E, Rossi E, et al. Antiphospholipid antibodies in early repeated abortions: a case-controlled study. Fertil Steril 1988; 50:589–92. (Level II-2)

43. Kutteh WH. Antiphospholipid antibody-associated recurrent pregnancy loss: treatment with heparin and low-dose aspirin is superior to low-dose aspirin alone. Am J Obstet Gynecol 1996;174:1584–9. (Level II-1)

44. MacLean MA, Cumming GP, McCall F, Walker ID, Walker JJ. The prevalence of lupus anticoagulant and anticardiolipin antibodies in women with a history of first trimester miscarriages. Br J Obstet Gynaecol 1994;101: 103–6. (Level II-3)

45. Out HJ, Kooijman CD, Bruinse HW, Derksen RH. Histopathological findings in placentae from patients with intra-uterine fetal death and anti-phospholipid antibodies. Eur J Obstet Gynecol Reprod Biol 1991;41:179–86. (Level II-3)

46. Parazzini F, Acaia B, Faden D, Lovotti M, Marelli G, Cortelazzo S. Antiphospholipid antibodies and recurrent abortion. Obstet Gynecol 1991;77:854–8. (Level II-2)

47. Parke AL, Wilson D, Maier D. The prevalence of antiphospholipid antibodies in women with recurrent spontaneous abortion, women with successful pregnancies, and women who have never been pregnant. Arthritis Rheum 1991;34:1231–5. (Level II-3)

48. Petri M, Golbus M, Anderson R, Whiting-O'Keefe Q, Corash L, Hellmann D. Antinuclear antibody, lupus anticoagulant, and anticardiolipin antibody in women with idiopathic habitual abortion. A controlled, prospective study of forty-four women. Arthritis Rheum 1987;30: 601–6. (Level II-2)

49. Yetman DL, Kutteh WH. Antiphospholipid antibody panels and recurrent pregnancy loss: prevalence of anticardiolipin antibodies compared with other antiphospholipid antibodies. Fertil Steril 1996;66:540–6. (Level II-2)

50. Infante-Rivard C, David M, Gauthier R, Rivard GE. Lupus anticoagulants, anticardiolipin antibodies, and fetal loss. A case-control study. N Engl J Med 1991;325:1063–6. (Level II-2)

51. Branch DW, Andres R, Digre KB, Rote NS, Scott JR. The association of antiphospholipid antibodies with severe preeclampsia. Obstet Gynecol 1989;73:541–5. (Level II-2)

52. Milliez J, Lelong F, Bayani N, Jannet D, el Medjadji M, Latrous H, et al. The prevalence of autoantibodies during third-trimester pregnancy complicated by hypertension or idiopathic fetal growth retardation. Am J Obstet Gynecol 1991;165:51–6. (Level II-2)

53. Moodley J, Bhoola V, Duursma J, Pudifin D, Byrne S, Kenoyer DG. The association of antiphospholipid antibodies with severe early-onset pre-eclampsia. S Afr Med J 1995;85:105–7. (Level III)

54. Sletnes KE, Wisloff F, Moe N, Dale PO. Antiphospholipid antibodies in pre-eclamptic women: relation to growth retardation and neonatal outcome. Acta Obstet Gynecol Scand 1992;71:112–7. (Level II-2)

55. Scott RA. Anti-cardiolipin antibodies and pre-eclampsia. Br J Obstet Gynaecol 1987;94:604–5. (Level III)

56. Caruso A, De Carolis S, Ferrazzani S, Valesini G, Caforio L, Mancuso S. Pregnancy outcome in relation to uterine artery flow velocity waveforms and clinical characteristics in women with antiphospholipid syndrome. Obstet Gynecol 1993;82:970–7. (Level II-3)

57. Polzin WJ, Kopelman JN, Robinson RD, Read JA, Brady K. The association of antiphospholipid antibodies with

pregnancies complicated by fetal growth restriction. Obstet Gynecol 1991;78:1108–11. (Level II-2)

58. Pattison NS, Chamley LW, McKay EJ, Liggins GC, Butler WS. Antiphospholipid antibodies in pregnancy: prevalence and clinical associations. Br J Obstet Gynaecol 1993;100:909–13. (Level II-3)

59. Branch DW, Khamashta MA. Antiphospholipid syndrome: obstetric diagnosis, management, and controversies. Obstet Gynecol 2003;101:1333–44. (Level III)

60. Derksen RH, Khamashta MA, Branch DW. Management of the obstetric antiphospholipid syndrome. Arthritis Rheum 2004;50:1028–39. (Level III)

61. Empson M, Lassere M, Craig JC, Scott JR. Recurrent pregnancy loss with antiphospholipid antibody: a systematic review of therapeutic trials. Obstet Gynecol 2002;99:135–44. (Level III)

62. Bates SM, Greer IA, Hirsh J, Ginsberg JS. Use of antithrombotic agents during pregnancy: the Seventh ACCP Conference on Antithrombotic and Thrombolytic Therapy. Chest 2004;126(suppl 3):627S–44S. (Level III)

63. Lubbe WF, Walkom P, Alexander CJ. Hepatic and splenic haemorrhage as a complication of toxaemia of pregnancy in a patient with circulating lupus anticoagulant. N Z Med J 1982;95:842–4. (Level III)

64. Carreras LD, Perez GN, Vega HR, Casavilla F. Lupus anticoagulant and recurrent fetal loss: successful treatment with gammaglobulin. Lancet 1988;2:393–4. (Level III)

65. Scott JR, Branch DW, Kochenour NK, Ward K. Intravenous immunoglobulin treatment of pregnant patients with recurrent pregnancy loss caused by antiphospholipid antibodies and Rh immunization. Am J Obstet Gynecol 1988;159:1055–6. (Level III)

66. Spinnato JA, Clark AL, Pierangeli SS, Harris EN. Intravenous immunoglobulin therapy for the antiphospholipid syndrome in pregnancy. Am J Obstet Gynecol 1995;172:690–4. (Level III)

67. Branch DW, Peaceman AM, Druzin M, Silver RK, El-Sayed Y, Silver RM, et al. A multicenter, placebo-controlled pilot study of intravenous immune globulin treatment of antiphospholipid syndrome during pregnancy. The Pregnancy Loss Study Group. Am J Obstet Gynecol 2000;182:122–7. (Level I)

68. Shah NM, Khamashta MA, Atsumi T, Hughes GR. Outcome of patients with anticardiolipin antibodies: a 10 year follow-up of 52 patients. Lupus 1998;7:3–6. (Level II-2)

The MEDLINE database, the Cochrane Library, and the American College of Obstetricians and Gynecologists' own internal resources and documents were used to conduct a literature search to locate relevant articles published between January 1985 and June 2005. The search was restricted to articles published in the English language. Priority was given to articles reporting results of original research, although review articles and commentaries also were consulted. Abstracts of research presented at symposia and scientific conferences were not considered adequate for inclusion in this document. Guidelines published by organizations or institutions such as the National Institutes of Health and ACOG were reviewed, and additional studies were located by reviewing bibliographies of identified articles. When reliable research was not available, expert opinions from obstetrician–gynecologists were used.

Studies were reviewed and evaluated for quality according to the method outlined by the U.S. Preventive Services Task Force:

I   Evidence obtained from at least one properly designed randomized controlled trial.

II-1 Evidence obtained from well-designed controlled trials without randomization.

II-2 Evidence obtained from well-designed cohort or case–control analytic studies, preferably from more than one center or research group.

II-3 Evidence obtained from multiple time series with or without the intervention. Dramatic results in uncontrolled experiments also could be regarded as this type of evidence.

III   Opinions of respected authorities, based on clinical experience, descriptive studies, or reports of expert committees.

Based on the highest level of evidence found in the data, recommendations are provided and graded according to the following categories:

Level A—Recommendations are based on good and consistent scientific evidence.

Level B—Recommendations are based on limited or inconsistent scientific evidence.

Level C—Recommendations are based primarily on consensus and expert opinion.

ISSN 1099-3630

The American College of Obstetricians and Gynecologists
409 12th Street, SW, PO Box 96920, Washington, DC 20090-6920

12345/98765

Antiphospholipid syndrome. ACOG Practice Bulletin No. 68. American College of Obstetricians and Gynecologists. Obstet Gynecol 2005;106:1113–21.

ACOG PRACTICE BULLETIN

CLINICAL MANAGEMENT GUIDELINES FOR
OBSTETRICIAN–GYNECOLOGISTS

NUMBER 31, OCTOBER 2001

(Replaces Technical Bulletin Number 206, June 1995; Committee Opinion Number 172, May 1996; Committee Opinion Number 187, September 1997; Committee Opinion Number 198, February 1998; and Committee Opinion Number 251, January 2001)

This Practice Bulletin was developed by the ACOG Committee on Practice Bulletins— Obstetrics with the assistance of Jodi F. Abbott, MD. The information is designed to aid practitioners in making decisions about appropriate obstetric and gynecologic care. These guidelines should not be construed as dictating an exclusive course of treatment or procedure. Variations in practice may be warranted based on the needs of the individual patient, resources, and limitations unique to the institution or type of practice.

Assessment of Risk Factors for Preterm Birth

Preterm birth is the second leading cause of neonatal mortality in the United States (1) (second only to birth defects), and preterm labor is the cause of most preterm births (2). Neonatal intensive care has improved the survival rate for babies at the cusp of viability, but it also has increased the proportion of survivors with disabilities (3). The incidence of multiple births also has increased along with the associated risk of preterm delivery (4). Interventions to delay preterm delivery in these settings have not shown conclusive effectiveness. Because the morbidity of babies born after 34–35 weeks of gestation has diminished, most efforts to identify preterm deliveries have focused on deliveries before this age. This document describes the various methods proposed for predicting preterm birth and the evidence for their roles in clinical practice.

Background

Preterm labor is defined as regular contractions associated with cervical change before the completion of 37 weeks of gestation. Spontaneous preterm birth includes preterm labor, preterm spontaneous rupture of membranes, and cervical incompetence; it does not include indicated preterm delivery for maternal or fetal conditions (5). Preterm delivery accounted for 11.8% of births in the United States in 1999; this figure has increased steadily from 9.4% in 1981 (6).

The pathophysiologic events that trigger preterm parturition are largely unknown but may include decidual hemorrhage (abruption), mechanical factors (uterine overdistention or cervical incompetence), and hormonal changes (perhaps mediated by fetal or maternal stress) (7–9). In addition, several bacterial infections have been associated with preterm labor. Commonly identified organisms are *Ureaplasma urealyticum, Mycoplasma hominis, Gardnerella* vaginalis, *Peptostreptococcus,* and *Bacteroides* species (10). Because these bacteria usually are of low virulence, it is unclear whether they are truly etiologic or are associated with an acute inflammatory response of another etiology.

Value of Predicting Risk

The ability to predict whether a woman is at risk of preterm delivery has value only if an intervention is available that is likely to improve the outcome. The opportunity to administer maternal corticosteroid ther-apy is an important intervention recommended by the National Institutes of Health because it is strongly associated with decreased morbidity and mortality (11–13). In addition, maternal tocolytic therapy may prolong pregnancy for up to 48 hours in some women, during which time corticosteroids can be administered (14). Because tocolytic and steroid therapy may result in untoward maternal and fetal consequences, use of these therapies should be limited to women with true preterm labor at high risk for spontaneous preterm birth. Finally, in women being managed at hospitals without appropriate neonatal resources, identifying women at risk allows for appropriate maternal transport to a tertiary care center. Conversely, identifying those women at low risk for preterm delivery would avert the use of unnecessary interventions.

Risk Factors

Risk factors for preterm birth include demographic characteristics, behavioral factors, and aspects of obstetric history. Demographic characteristics that carry a high risk for preterm birth include nonwhite race (African American relative risk [RR]=3.3), age younger than 17 years or older than 35 years (RR=1.47–1.95), low socioeconomic status (RR=1.83–2.65), and low prepregnancy weight (odds ratio=2.72) (15, 16). Maternal his-tory of preterm birth, particularly in the second trimester, has a strong statistical association with the risk of preterm delivery (17); this risk appears to be associated with prior spontaneous preterm birth with or without rupture of membranes and increases the relative risk sixfold to eightfold. Risk also increases with vaginal bleeding in more than one trimester (18). Controversy exists as to whether an excessively physically stressful job can lead to early delivery; one study has shown an increase in spontaneous preterm birth associated with long periods of standing (>40 hours per week) (19). Smoking increases the risk of preterm birth (20) and low birth weight, and some evidence suggests it increases the risk for spontaneous abortion (21). Despite the identification of a number of risk factors, attempts to determine the risk of preterm delivery based on historic and epidemiologic risk scoring systems (22–24) have been unable to reliably identify women who will give birth preterm.

Biologic Markers for Predicting Preterm Birth

Home Uterine Activity Monitoring

Tocodynamometry has long been used for hospital-based evaluation of uterine contractions. Home uterine activity monitoring (HUAM) has been proposed as a method for predicting preterm birth in high-risk women. It consists of a combination of telemetric recordings of uterine contractions with the use of a tocodynamometer and daily telephone calls from a health care practitioner to offer patient support and advice. Uterine activity beyond an arbitrary cutoff triggers notification of the patient's health care practitioner. This approach was based on the observation that some women who subsequently give birth before term have an increase in uterine activity earlier in pregnancy than women who give birth at term (25) and that these prodromal uterine contractions otherwise may not be recognized by the patient.

Salivary Estriol

Activation of the fetal hypothalamic pituitary–adrenal axis precedes some spontaneous preterm births. Adrenal production of dehydroepiandrosterone results in increased placental estrogen synthesis. Observational studies have shown that maternal levels of serum estradiol and salivary estriol increase before the onset of spontaneous term and preterm labor (26). These findings prompted the design of a test to predict preterm delivery by measuring salivary estriol; however, maternal estriol levels show diurnal variation, peaking at night (27). Also, estriol levels may be suppressed by betamethasone administration (28).

Bacterial Vaginosis

Bacterial vaginosis (BV) is a common alteration of the normal vaginal flora and has been found in 10–25% of patients in general gynecologic and obstetric clinics and in up to 64% of patients in clinics for sexually transmitted diseases (29). Fifty percent of women with BV are asymptomatic (30). Bacterial vaginosis also has been found more frequently in African-American women (22%) than in white women (8%) (10, 31). The presence of BV has been associated with preterm delivery independent of other known risk factors (32, 33).

Fetal Fibronectin Screening

Fetal fibronectin (fFN) is a basement membrane protein produced by the fetal membranes that functions as an adhesion binder of the placenta and membranes to the decidua (34, 35). It is normally present in cervical secretions until 16–20 weeks of gestation. Numerous trials have shown both an association with the presence of fFN and preterm birth (5, 34, 36) and a decrease in the risk of preterm birth when the test result for the presence of this protein is negative. The basis for the association of fFN and preterm birth is unclear. It has been hypothesized that fFN is a marker for the disruption of the chorioamnion and underlying decidua due to inflammation with or without infection (34). A positive midtrimester fFN test result has been associated with subsequently diagnosed maternal and fetal infection (37).

Cervical Ultrasonography

Transvaginal cervical ultrasonography has been shown to be a reliable and reproducible way to assess the length of the cervix (38). A prospective blinded trial showed an association between cervical length and preterm delivery (39). This study established the normal distribution of cervical length in pregnancy after 22 weeks of gestation. It also looked at various cervical measurements as criteria for the prediction of preterm delivery.

Clinical Considerations and Recommendations

▶ Does the use of HUAM predict preterm birth?

The usefulness of HUAM as a screening test depends on both its ability to detect women at higher risk for preterm birth as well as the effectiveness of any intervention to then prevent preterm birth. At least 13 randomized controlled trials examining the efficacy of HUAM have published results (40–52). The studies vary in design, criteria for inclusion of patients, and measurements of endpoints and outcomes. These differences make comparisons difficult. Furthermore, many of these studies had limitations with their research design, including sample size (power) or numbers of patients, that preclude reaching conclusions about the usefulness of HUAM. Results vary, with some trials reporting no difference and some reporting a difference in outcome in monitored and unmonitored women. The largest study involved 2,422 women at risk and showed no improvement in outcome (41).

Earlier studies that showed a reduction in the incidence of preterm birth with HUAM have been criticized for their flawed design (53, 54); some studies have been identified as having biases and errors sufficient to warrant dismissing the results (55). The U.S. Preventive Services Task Force performed an independent review and concluded the device was not effective (56). Although the U.S. Food and Drug Administration has approved a HUAM device for women with a prior preterm birth, there is no demonstrated role for HUAM in

the prevention of preterm birth. Data are insufficient to support a benefit from HUAM in preventing preterm birth (13, 57, 58); therefore, this system of care is not recommended.

▶ Does salivary estriol determination predict preterm birth?

There have been two prospective trials evaluating whether salivary estriol levels can predict preterm delivery (59, 60); they showed that salivary estriol was more predictive than traditional risk assessment. However, the results of the second trial showed a relatively poor sensitivity of 71%, specificity of 77%, and a false-positive rate of 23% (using delivery before 37 weeks of gestation as the outcome measure) (60). Because the test carries a high percentage of false-positive results, its use could add significantly to the cost of prenatal care, particularly if used in a low-risk population. Although the hormonal pathway etiology for some cases of preterm birth is intriguing, trials with salivary estriol testing to predict preterm birth have failed to establish its usefulness for anything more than investigational purposes at present.

▶ Do screening and treatment for BV affect the likelihood of preterm birth?

Trials of screening and treatment for BV in pregnant women to reduce the incidence of preterm delivery have been conducted in mixed populations with varying results. Some small studies found screening and treatment of women at risk for preterm birth reduced the risk of preterm birth (61, 62), but other studies have not confirmed these findings (63, 64).

A recent meta-analysis reviewed five trials involving 1,504 women (65). The analysis included trials of women without risk factors for preterm birth as well as studies that screened general obstetric populations. Treatments used in these trials included amoxicillin, clindamycin, and metronidazole. Although investigators found antibiotic therapy effective at eradicating BV, the difference in the rate of preterm birth between the two groups was not statistically significant. However, looking at the subgroup of women with a previous preterm birth, the difference was significant, with an odds ratio of 0.37 (95% confidence interval, 0.23–0.60). This meta-analysis did not include results from the most recent and largest double-blind, randomized controlled trial. This trial of 1,953 women found no difference in the rates of preterm birth between the treatment and placebo groups, and no subgroup demonstrated a statistically significant difference in preterm birth rates (64).

Although some trials have shown an association with the presence of BV and preterm birth, most large trials designed to determine whether treatment of BV can prevent preterm birth have failed. Currently, there are insufficient data to suggest screening and treating women at either low or high risk will reduce the overall rate of preterm birth (66). There is speculation that BV could be either a marker or a cause of choriodecidual inflammation without intraamniotic infection (24). However, research testing this hypothesis by serial fFN screening in women with BV was unable to confirm an association (67).

▶ *Does screening for fFN predict preterm birth?*

A meta-analysis of 27 studies showed consistent moderate success using fFN screening to predict preterm birth (68). Using delivery at less than 34 weeks of gestation as the outcome, sensitivity was 61% and specificity was 83% (68). A study that analyzed the relationship between fFN, short cervix, BV, and designated traditional risk factors for spontaneous preterm birth showed the highest association of preterm birth with positive fFN test result, followed by a cervical length less than 25 mm and a history of preterm birth (69). The negative predictive value of the fFN test to identify symptomatic women who are actually at low risk for imminent preterm delivery ranges from 69% to 92% before 37 weeks of gestation, with a greater than 95% likelihood of not delivering within 14 days of a negative test result (13, 70, 71).

Although a negative test result appears to be useful in ruling out preterm delivery that is imminent (ie, within 2 weeks) (13, 72, 73), the clinical implications of a positive test result have not been evaluated fully because no obstetric intervention has been shown to decrease the risk of preterm delivery. The test should not be routinely used to screen low-risk, asymptomatic women, because the incidence of preterm birth in this population is low and the test, therefore, has limited usefulness (68).

If the test is to be used in specific high-risk groups, the following criteria should be met: intact amniotic membranes, minimal cervical dilatation (<3 cm), and sampling performed no earlier than 24 weeks and 0 days of gestation and no later than 34 weeks and 6 days of gestation (74). If the test is to be clinically useful, the results must be available from a laboratory within a time frame that allows for clinical decision making (ideally within 24 hours).

▶ *Does cervical ultrasonography predict preterm birth?*

Numerous studies have confirmed the association of cervical shortening with preterm delivery, but they have varied widely in their predictive value (13, 75–77). A review of 35 studies using cervical length (determined by ultrasonography) to predict preterm delivery found sensitivities ranging from 68% to 100%, with specificities from 44% to 79% (78).

A prospective trial of more than 2,900 women evaluated by serial transvaginal ultrasonography at 24 weeks of gestation and again at 28 weeks of gestation showed the RR of preterm delivery increased as the cervical length decreased. Specifically, at 28 weeks of gestation, when cervical lengths were 40 mm or less, RR was 2.80; at 35 mm or less, RR was 3.52; at 30 mm or less, RR was 5.39; at 26 mm or less, RR was 9.57; at 22 mm or less, RR was 13.88; and at 13 mm or less, RR was 24.94 (39).

Despite the usefulness of cervical length determination by ultrasonography as a predictor of preterm labor, routine use is not recommended because of the lack of proven treatments affecting outcome (79). Until effective treatment options are identified, cervical length measurement has limited clinical application.

▶ *Should fFN and cervical ultrasonography be used together to better identify those at highest risk?*

In a multicenter trial, investigators found a short cervix (defined as <25 mm), particularly if associated with a positive fFN test result, to be a strong predictor of preterm birth (80). A more recent trial by the National Institute of Child Health and Human Development looked at the sequential use of both methods to try to stratify risk groups as well as discern etiologies of preterm birth (69) (see Table 1). The presence of either a cervix less than 25 mm in length at less than 35 weeks of gestation or a positive fFN test result was strongly associated with preterm birth, especially in women with a history of preterm birth. These data were particularly useful in decreasing the assessed risk of preterm birth in women with classic risk factors and negative results of one or both tests. The success of interventions once a short cervix is identified or positive fFN test result is determined remains uncertain (13).

Table 1. Recurrence Risk of Spontaneous Preterm Birth at <35 Weeks of Gestation According to Cervical Length and Fetal Fibronectin in Women with a Prior Preterm Birth

Cervical Length (mm)	Fetal Fibronectin + (%)	Fetal Fibronectin – (%)
25	65	25
26–35	45	14
>35	25	7

Fetal fibronectin and cervical length assessed at 24 weeks of gestation. Cervical length assessed by transvaginal ultrasonography.

Data from: Iams JD, Goldenberg RL, Mercer BM, Moawad A, Thom E, Meis PJ, et al. The Preterm Prediction Study: recurrence risk of spontaneous preterm birth. National Institute of Child Health and Human Development Maternal-Fetal Medicine Units Network. Am J Obstet Gynecol 1998;178:1035–1040

Summary of Recommendations

The following recommendation is based on good and consistent scientific evidence (Level A):

► There are no current data to support the use of salivary estriol, HUAM, or BV screening as strategies to identify or prevent preterm birth.

The following recommendations are based on limited or inconsistent scientific evidence (Level B):

► Screening for risk of preterm labor by means other than historic risk factors is not beneficial in the general obstetric population.

► Ultrasonography to determine cervical length, fFN testing, or a combination of both may be useful in determining women at high risk for preterm labor. However, their clinical usefulness may rest primarily with their negative predictive value given the lack of proven treatment options to prevent preterm birth.

► Fetal fibronectin testing may be useful in women with symptoms of preterm labor to identify those with negative values and a reduced risk of preterm birth, thereby avoiding unnecessary intervention.

References

1. Murphy SL. Deaths: final data for 1998. Natl Vital Stat Rep 2000;48(11):1–108 (Level III)

2. Tucker JM, Goldenberg RL, Davis RO, Copper RL, Winkler CL, Hauth JC. Etiologies of preterm birth in an indigent population: is prevention a logical expectation? Obstet Gynecol 1991;77:343–347 (Level II-3)

3. Wood NS, Marlow N, Costeloe K, Gibson AT, Wilkinson AR. Neurologic and developmental disability after extremely preterm birth. EPICure Study Group. N Engl J Med 2000;343:378–384 (Level II-2)

4. Preterm singleton births—United States, 1989–1996. MMWR Morb Mortal Wkly Rep 1999;48:185–189 (Level III)

5. Iams JD. Preterm birth. In: Gabbe SG, Niebyl JR, Simpson JL, eds. Obstetrics: normal and problem pregnancies. 3rd ed. New York: Churchill Livingstone, 1996:743–820 (Level III)

6. Ventura SJ, Martin JA, Curtin SC, Menacker F, Hamilton BE. Births: final data for 1999. Nat Vital Stat Rep 2001;49(1):1–100 (Level III)

7. Goldenberg RL, Iams JD, Mercer BM, Meis PJ, Moawad AH, Copper RL, et al. The preterm prediction study: the value of new vs. standard risk factors in predicting early and all spontaneous preterm births. NICHD MFMU Network. Am J Public Health 1998;88:233–238 (Level III)

8. Norwitz ER, Robinson JN, Challis JR. The control of labor. N Engl J Med 1999;341:660–666 (Level III)

9. Lockwood CJ. Stress-associated preterm delivery: the role of corticotropin-releasing hormone. Am J Obstet Gynecol 1999;180:S264–S266 (Level III)

10. Goldenberg RL, Hauth JC, Andrews WW. Intrauterine infection and preterm delivery. N Engl J Med 2000; 342:1500–1507 (Level III)

11. Effect of corticosteroids for fetal maturation on perinatal outcomes. NIH Consens Statement 1994;12(2):1–24 (Level III)

12. Antenatal corticosteroids revisited: repeat courses. NIH Consens Statement 2000;17(2):1–10 (Level III)

13. Agency for Healthcare Research and Quality. Management of preterm labor. Evidence Report/Technology Assessment no. 18. Rockville, Maryland: AHRQ, 2000. AHRQ publication no. 00-E021 (Level III)

14. Gyetvai K, Hannah ME, Hodnett ED, Ohlsson A. Any tocolytic drug for preterm labour (Protocol for a Cochrane Review). In: The Cochrane Library, Issue 2, 2001. Oxford: Update Software (Level III)

15. Lumley J. The epidemiology of preterm birth. Baillieres Clin Obstet Gynaecol 1993;7:477–498 (Level III)

16. Wen SW, Goldenberg RL, Cutter GR, Hoffman HJ, Cliver SP. Intrauterine growth retardation and preterm delivery: perinatal risk factors in an indigent population. Am J Obstet Gynecol 1990;162:213–218 (Level II-2)

17. Ekwo EE, Gosselink CA, Moawad A. Unfavorable outcome in penultimate pregnancy and premature rupture of membranes in successive pregnancy. Obstet Gynecol 1992;80:166–172 (Level II-2)

18. Strobino B, Pantel-Silverman J. Gestational vaginal bleeding and pregnancy outcome. Am J Epidemiol 1989;129:806–815 (Level II-2)

19. Luke B, Mamelle N, Keith L, Munoz F, Minogue J, Papiernik E, et al. The association between occupational factors and preterm birth: a United States nurses' study. Research Committee of the Association of Women's Health, Obstetric and Neonatal Nurses. Am J Obstet Gynecol 1995;173:849–862 (Level II-2)

20. Cnattingius S, Granath F, Petersson G, Harlow BL. The influence of gestational age and smoking habits on the risk of subsequent preterm deliveries. N Eng J Med 1999;341:943–948 (Level II-2)

21. Walsh RA. Effects of maternal smoking on adverse pregnancy outcomes: examination of the criteria of causation. Hum Biol 1994;66:1059–1092 (Level II-3)

22. Creasy RK, Gumer BA, Liggins GC. System for predicting spontaneous preterm birth. Obstet Gynecol 1980;55:692–695 (Level II-3)

23. Main DM, Gabbe SG, Richardson D, Strong S. Can preterm deliveries be prevented? Am J Obstet Gynecol 1985;151:892–898 (Level I)

24. Mercer BM, Goldenberg RL, Dao A, Moawad AH, Iams JD, Meis PJ, et al. The preterm prediction study: a clinical

risk assessment system. Am J Obstet Gynecol 1996;174:1885–1893; discussion 1893–1895 (Level II-2)

25. Nageotte MP, Dorchester W, Porto M, Keegan KA Jr, Freeman RK. Quantitation of uterine activity preceding preterm, term and postterm labor. Am J Obstet Gynecol 1988;158:1254–1259 (Level II-2)

26. Goodwin TM. A role for estriol in human labor, term and preterm. Am J Obstet Gynecol 1999;180:S208–S213 (Level III)

27. McGregor JA, Hastings C, Roberts T, Barrett J. Diurnal variation in salivary estriol level during pregnancy: a pilot study. Am J Obstet Gynecol 1999;180:S223–S225 (Level III)

28. Hendershott CM, Dullien V, Goodwin TM. Serial betamethasone administration: effect on maternal salivary estriol levels. Am J Obstet Gynecol 1999;180:S219–S222 (Level II-2)

29. Hallen A, Pahlson C, Forsum U. Bacterial vaginosis in women attending STD clinic: diagnostic criteria and prevalence of mobiluncus spp. Genitourin Med 1987;63:386–389 (Level III)

30. Eschenbach DA. History and review of bacterial vaginosis. Am J Obstet Gynecol 1993;169:441–445 (Level III)

31. Royce RA, Jackson TP, Thorp JM Jr, Hillier SL, Rabe LK, Pastore LM, et al. Race/ethnicity, vaginal flora patterns, and pH during pregnancy. Sex Transm Dis 1999;26: 96–102 (Level II-2)

32. Meis PJ, Goldenberg RL, Mercer B, Moawad A, Das A, McNellis D, et al. The preterm prediction study: significance of vaginal infections. National Institute of Child Health and Human Development Maternal-Fetal Medicine Units Network. Am J Obstet Gynecol 1995;173:1231–1235 (Level II-2)

33. Hillier SL, Nugent RP, Eschenbach DA, Krohn MA, Gibbs RS, Martin DH, et al. Association between bacterial vaginosis and preterm delivery of a low-birth-weight infant. The Vaginal Infections and Prematurity Study Group. N Engl J Med 1995;333:1737–1742 (Level II-2)

34. Lockwood CJ, Senyei AE, Dische MR, Casal D, Shah KD, Thung SN, et al. Fetal fibronectin in cervical and vaginal secretions as a predictor of preterm delivery. N Engl J Med 1991;325:669–674 (Level II-2)

35. Feinberg RF, Kliman HJ, Lockwood CJ. Is oncofetal fibronectin a trophoblast glue for human implantation? Am J Pathol 1991;138:537–543 (Level II-2)

36. Lockwood CJ, Wein R, Lapinski R, Casal D, Berkowitz G, Alvarez M, et al. The presence of cervical and vaginal fetal fibronectin predicts preterm delivery in an inner-city obstetric population. Am J Obstet Gynecol 1993;169:798–804 (Level II-2)

37. Goldenberg RL, Thom E, Moawad AH, Johnson F, Roberts J, Caritis SN. The preterm prediction study: fetal fibronectin, bacterial vaginosis, and peripartum infection. NICHD Maternal Fetal Medicine Units Network. Obstet Gynecol 1996;87:656–660 (Level II-2)

38. Sonek JD, Iams JD, Blumenfeld M, Johnson F, Landon M, Gabbe S. Measurement of cervical length in preg-nancy: comparison between vaginal ultrasonography and digital examination. Obstet Gynecol 1990;76:172–175 (Level II-2)

39. Iams JD, Goldenberg RL, Meis PJ, Mercer BM, Moawad A, Das A, et al. The length of the cervix and the risk of spontaneous premature delivery. National Institute of Child Health and Human Development Maternal Fetal Medicine Unit Network. N Engl J Med 1996;334: 567–572 (Level II-2)

40. Brown HL, Britton KA, Brizendine EJ, Hiett AK, Ingram D, Turnquest MA, et al. A randomized comparison of home uterine activity monitoring in the outpatient management of women treated for preterm labor. Am J Obstet Gynecol 1999;180:798–805 (Level I)

41. Dyson DC, Crites YM, Ray DA, Armstrong MA. Prevention of preterm birth in high-risk patients: the role of education and provider contact versus home uterine monitoring. Am J Obstet Gynecol 1991;164:756–762 (Level I)

42. Dyson DC, Danbe KH, Bamber JA, Crites YM, Rield DR, Maier JA, et al. Monitoring women at risk for preterm labor. N Engl J Med 1998;338;15–19 (Level I)

43. Iams JD, Johnson FF, O'Shaugnessy RW, West LC. A prospective random trial of home uterine monitoring in pregnancies at increased risk of preterm labor. Part II. Am J Obstet Gynecol 1987;157:638–643 (Level I)

44. Iams JD, Johnson FF, O'Shaughnessy RW. A prospective random trial of home uterine activity monitoring in pregnancies at increased risk of preterm labor. Am J Obstet Gynecol 1988;159:595–603 (Level I)

45. Blondel B, Breat G, Berthoux Y, Berland M, Melher B, Rudigoz RC, et al. Home uterine activity monitoring in France: a randomized controlled trial. Am J Obstet Gynecol 1992;167:424–429 (Level I)

46. Hill WC, Fleming AD, Martin RW, Hamer C, Knuppel RA, Lake MF, et al. Home uterine activity monitoring is associated with a reduction in preterm birth. Obstet Gynecol 1990;76:13S–18S (Level I)

47. Knuppel RA, Lake MF, Watson DL, Welch RA, Hill WC, Fleming AD, et al. Preventing preterm birth in twin gestation: home uterine activity monitoring and perinatal nursing support. Obstet Gynecol 1990;76:24S–27S (Level II-1)

48. Morrison JC, Martin JN Jr, Martin RW, Gookin KS, Wiser WL. Prevention of preterm birth by ambulatory assessment of uterine activity: a randomized study. Am J Obstet Gynecol 1987;156:536–543 (Level I)

49. Mou SM, Sunderji SG, Gall S, How H, Patel V, Gray M, et al. Multicenter randomized clinical trial of home uterine activity monitoring for the detection of preterm labor. Am J Obstet Gynecol 1991;165:858–866 (Level I)

50. Nagey DA, Bailey-Jones C, Herman AA. Randomized comparison of home uterine activity monitoring and routine care in patients discharged after treatment for preterm labor. Obstet Gynecol 1993;82:319–323 (Level II-1)

51. Wapner RJ, Cotton DB, Artal R, Librizzi RJ, Ross MG. A randomized multicenter trial assessing a home uterine activity monitoring device used in the absence of daily nursing contact. Am J Obstet Gynecol 1995;172: 1026–1034 (Level I)

52. Watson DL, Welch RA, Mariona FG, Lake MF, Knuppel RA, Martin RW, et al. Management of preterm labor patients at home: does daily uterine activity monitoring

and nursing support make a difference? Obstet Gynecol 1990;76:32S–35S (Level I)

53. Grimes DA, Schulz KF. Randomized controlled trials of home uterine activity monitoring: a review and critique. Obstet Gynecol 1992;79:137–142 (Level III)

54. Sachs BP, Hellerstein S, Freeman R, Frigoletto F, Hauth JC. Home monitoring of uterine activity. Does it prevent prematurity? N Engl J Med 1991;325:1374–1377 (Level III)

55. Keirse MJ, Van Hoven M. Reanalysis of a multireported trial on home uterine activity monitoring. Birth 1993;20:117–122 (Level III)

56. Home uterine activity monitoring for preterm labor. Review article. US Preventive Services Task Force. JAMA 1993;270:371–376 (Level III)

57. A multicenter randomized controlled trial of home uterine monitoring: active versus sham device. The Collaborative Home Uterine Monitoring Study Group (CHUMS). Am J Obstet Gynecol 1995;173:1120–1127 (Level I)

58. Colton T, Kayne HL, Zhang Y, Heeren T. A metaanalysis of home uterine activity monitoring. Am J Obstet Gynecol 1995;173:1499–1505 (Meta-analysis)

59. McGregor JA, Jackson GM, Lachelin GC, Goodwin TM, Artal R, Hastings C, et al. Salivary estriol as risk assessment for preterm labor: a prospective trial. Am J Obstet Gynecol 1995;173:1337–1342 (Level II-2)

60. Heine RP, McGregor JA, Dullien VK. Accuracy of salivary estriol testing compared to traditional risk factor assessment in predicting preterm birth. Am J Obstet Gynecol 1999;180:S214–S218 (Level II-2)

61. Morales WJ, Schorr S, Albritton J. Effect of metronidazole in patients with preterm birth in preceding pregnancy and bacterial vaginosis: a placebo-controlled, double-blind study. Am J Obstet Gynecol 1994;171:345–347; discussion 348–349 (Level I)

62. Hauth JC, Goldenberg RL, Andrews WW, DuBard MB, Copper RL. Reduced incidence of preterm delivery with metronidazole and erythromycin in women with bacterial vaginosis. N Engl J Med 1995;333:1732–1736 (Level I)

63. Joesoef MR, Schmid GP, Hillier SL. Bacterial vaginosis: review of treatment options and potential clinical indications for therapy. Clin Infect Dis 1999;28:S57–S65 (Level III)

64. Carey JC, Klebanoff MA, Hauth JC, Hillier SL, Thom EA, Ernest JM, et al. Metronidazole to prevent preterm delivery in pregnant women with asymptomatic bacterial vaginosis. National Institute of Child Health and Human Development Network of Maternal-Fetal Medicine Units. N Engl J Med 2000;342:534–540 (Level I)

65. Brocklehurst P, Hannah M, McDonald H. Interventions for treating bacterial vaginosis in pregnancy (Cochrane Review). In: The Cochrane Library, Issue 2, 2001. Oxford: Update Software (Meta-analysis)

66. Berg AO. Screening for bacterial vaginosis in pregnancy. Recommendations and rationale. Am J Prev Med 2001;20(3 Suppl):59–61 (Level III)

67. Goldenberg RL, Andrews WW, Guerrant RL, Newman M, Mercer B, Iams J, et al. The preterm prediction study: cer-

vical lactoferin concentration, other markers of lower genital tract infection, and preterm birth. National Institute of Child Health and Human Development Maternal-Fetal Medicine Units Network. Am J Obstet Gynecol 2000;182:631–635 (Level II-2)

68. Leitich H, Egarter C, Kaider A, Hohlagschwandtner M, Berghammer P, Hussein P. Cervicovaginal fetal fibronectin as a marker for preterm delivery: a meta-analysis. Am J Obstet Gynecol 1999;180:1169–1176 (Meta-analysis)

69. Goldenberg RL, Iams JD, Das A, Mercer BM, Meis PJ, Moawad AH, et al. The Preterm Prediction Study: sequential cervical length and fetal fibronectin testing for the prediction of spontaneous preterm birth. National Institute of Child Health and Human Development Maternal-Fetal Medicine Network. Am J Obstet Gynecol 2000;182:636–643 (Level III)

70. Inglis SR, Jeremias J, Kuno K, Lescale K, Peeper Q, Chervenak FA, et al. Detection of tumor necrosis factor-alpha, interleukin-6, and fetal fibronectin in the lower genital tract during pregnancy: relation to outcome. Am J Obstet Gynecol 1994;171:5–10 (Level II-3)

71. Malak TM, Sizmur F, Bell SC, Taylor DJ. Fetal fibronectin in cervicovaginal secretions as a predictor of preterm birth. Br J Obstet Gynaecol 1996;103:648–653 (Level II-3)

72. Revah A, Hannah ME, Sue-A-Quan AK. Fetal fibronectin as a predictor of preterm birth: an overview. Am J Perinatol 1998;15:613–621 (Level III)

73. Benattar C, Taieb J, Fernandez H, Lindendaum A, Frydman R, Ville Y. Rapid fetal fibronectin swab-test in preterm labor patients treated by betamimetics. Eur J Obstet Gynecol Reprod Biol 1997;72:131–135 (Level II-3)

74. Peaceman AM, Andrews WW, Thorp JM, Cliver SP, Lukes A, Iams JD, et al. Fetal fibronectin as a predictor of preterm birth in patients with symptoms: a multicenter trial. Am J Obstet Gynecol 1997;177:13–18 (Level II-2)

75. Crane JM, Van den Hof M, Armson BA, Liston R. Transvaginal ultrasound in the prediction of preterm delivery: singleton and twin gestations. Obstet Gynecol 1997;90:357–363 (Level II-2)

76. Berghella V, Tolosa JE, Kuhlman K, Weiner S, Bolognese RJ, Wapner RJ. Cervical ultrasonography compared with manual examination as a predictor of preterm delivery. Am J Obstet Gynecol 1997;177:723–730 (Level II-2)

77. Watson WJ, Stevens D, Welter S, Day D. Observations on the sonographic measurement of cervical length and the risk of preterm birth. J Matern Fetal Med 1999;8:17–19 (Level II-2)

78. Leitich H, Brunbauer M, Kaider A, Egarter C, Husslein P. Cervical length and dilatation of the internal cervical os detected by vaginal ultrasonography as markers for preterm delivery: a systematic review. Am J Obstet Gynecol 1999;181:1465–1472 (Level III)

79. Ultrasound cervical assessment in predicting preterm birth. SOGC Clinical Practice Guidelines 102. J SOGC 2001;23:418–421 (Level III)

80. Iams JD, Goldenberg RL, Mercer BM, Moawad A, Thom E, Meis PJ, et al. The Preterm Prediction Study: recurrence

risk of spontaneous preterm birth. National Institute of Child Health and Human Development Maternal-Fetal Medicine Units Network. Am J Obstet Gynecol 1998;178:1035–1040 (Level II-2)

The MEDLINE database, the Cochrane Library, and ACOG's own internal resources and documents were used to conduct a literature search to locate relevant articles published between January 1985 and May 2000. The search was restricted to articles published in the English language. Priority was given to articles reporting results of original research, although review articles and commentaries also were consulted. Abstracts of research presented at symposia and scientific conferences were not considered adequate for inclusion in this document. Guidelines published by organizations or institutions such as the National Institutes of Health and the American College of Obstetricians and Gynecologists were reviewed, and additional studies were located by reviewing bibliographies of identified articles. When reliable research was not available, expert opinions from obstetrician–gynecologists were used.

Studies were reviewed and evaluated for quality according to the method outlined by the U.S. Preventive Services Task Force:

I   Evidence obtained from at least one properly designed randomized controlled trial.

II-1   Evidence obtained from well-designed controlled trials without randomization.

II-2   Evidence obtained from well-designed cohort or case–control analytic studies, preferably from more than one center or research group.

II-3   Evidence obtained from multiple time series with or without the intervention. Dramatic results in uncontrolled experiments could also be regarded as this type of evidence.

III   Opinions of respected authorities, based on clinical experience, descriptive studies, or reports of expert committees.

Based on the highest level of evidence found in the data, recommendations are provided and graded according to the following categories:

Level A—Recommendations are based on good and consistent scientific evidence.

Level B—Recommendations are based on limited or inconsistent scientific evidence.

Level C—Recommendations are based primarily on consensus and expert opinion.

ISSN 1099-3630

The American College of Obstetricians and Gynecologists
409 12th Street, SW, PO Box 96920
Washington, DC 20090-6920

12345/54321

Assessment of risk factors for preterm birth. ACOG Practice Bulletin No. 31. American College of Obstetricians and Gynecologists. Obstet Gynecol 2001;98:709–716

ACOG PRACTICE BULLETIN

CLINICAL MANAGEMENT GUIDELINES FOR
OBSTETRICIAN–GYNECOLOGISTS
NUMBER 46, SEPTEMBER 2003

(Replaces Technical Bulletin Number 222, April 1996)

This Practice Bulletin was developed by the ACOG Committee on Practice Bulletins— Gynecology with the assistance of Amy Pollack, MD. The information is designed to aid practitioners in making decisions about appropriate obstetric and gynecologic care. These guidelines should not be construed as dictating an exclusive course of treatment or procedure. Variations in practice may be warranted based on the needs of the individual patient, resources, and limitations unique to the institution or type of practice.

Benefits and Risks of Sterilization

Bilateral tubal sterilization and vasectomy are both safe and effective permanent methods of contraception; more than 220 million couples worldwide use them as their contraceptive method of choice (1). Sterilization continues to be the most commonly used contraceptive method in the United States, with 11 million U.S. women relying on the method. Approximately 700,000 tubal sterilizations (2) and 500,000 vasectomies (3) are performed in the United States annually. The purpose of this document is to review the evidence for the safety and effectiveness of sterilization in comparison with other forms of contraception, as well as evidence of the likelihood that a woman will regret having had a sterilization procedure.

Background

Prevalence of Sterilization Compared With Other Contraceptive Methods

Sterilization accounts for 39% of contraceptive method use by U.S. women of reproductive age (15–44 years) and their partners. Of those, 28% had tubal sterilization, and 11% have partners who had a vasectomy. In comparison, 27% of the same population use oral contraceptives, 21% use male condoms, 3% use injectable contraceptives, 2% use diaphragms, and 1% use intrauterine devices (IUDs) (4). Tubal sterilization is the only permanent female contraceptive method available to U.S. women.

Tubal Sterilization

Timing

Tubal sterilization can be performed postpartum, after spontaneous or therapeutic abortion, or as an interval procedure (unrelated in time to a pregnancy).

Key factors affecting the choice and timing of sterilization are a mix of individual patient preference, medical assessment of acute risk, and access to services. The timing of the procedure influences both the surgical approach and the method of tubal occlusion. In the United States, approximately one half of all tubal sterilizations are performed as interval procedures (2). Postpartum sterilization is performed after 10% of all hospital deliveries (5); approximately 3.5% of all sterilizations are performed after an elective or spontaneous abortion (6).

Postpartum sterilization is performed at the time of cesarean delivery or after a vaginal delivery and should not extend the patient's hospital stay. Ideally, postpartum minilaparotomy is performed before the onset of significant uterine involution but following a full assessment of maternal and neonatal well-being. Postpartum minilaparotomy may be performed using local anesthesia with sedation, regional anesthesia, or general anesthesia. Postpartum sterilization requires counseling and informed consent before labor and delivery (7, 8). Consent should be obtained during prenatal care, when the patient can make a considered decision, review the risks and benefits of the procedure, and consider alternative contraceptive methods. In all cases of intrapartum or postpartum medical or obstetric complications, the physician should consider postponing sterilization to a later date (5). The federal and state regulations that address the timing of consent also are important to consider (9).

Postabortion sterilization can be performed safely after uncomplicated spontaneous or induced abortion without added risk over interval sterilization (10). After a first- or second-trimester abortion, both laparoscopic and minilaparotomy sterilization are acceptable. With either approach, a single anesthetic for the abortion and the sterilization may be used to avoid additional risk.

Tubal sterilization can be performed as an interval procedure at any time during the menstrual cycle. A same-day, highly sensitive, pregnancy test (urine test capable of detecting human chorionic gonadotropin levels as low as 20 mIU/mL) (11) will detect pregnancies as early as 1 week after conception (12). Performing the procedure during the patient's follicular phase and patient use of an effective method of contraception before sterilization further reduces the likelihood of concurrent pregnancy. Dilation and curettage concurrent with all interval sterilizations as a routine practice is not recommended on the basis of effectiveness, cost, and morbidity (13).

Methods of Surgical Sterilization

Laparoscopy. The laparoscopic approach is the one most commonly used for interval sterilization procedures and usually is performed as an outpatient procedure. The advantages of laparoscopy over other surgical approaches include the opportunity to inspect the abdominal and pelvic organs. Furthermore, laparoscopy results in barely visible incision scars and a rapid return to full activity for the patient. The disadvantages of laparoscopy include the cost and fragility of the equipment; the special training required; and the risk of bowel, bladder, or major vessel injury after insertion of the needle or trocar. The use of general anesthesia also increases risk.

Minilaparotomy. In the United States, minilaparotomy is most commonly used for postpartum procedures and in patients considered at high risk for laparoscopic procedures. Minilaparotomy is performed by using a 2–3-cm incision placed in relation to the uterine fundus. In contrast with laparoscopy, minilaparotomy requires only basic surgical instruments and training.

Transcervical Approaches. Transcervical approaches to sterilization involve gaining access to the fallopian tubes through the cervix. A device or occlusive material is then placed hysteroscopically or blindly to block each tube. In November 2002, the U.S. Food and Drug Administration approved the use of Essure, a new transcervical sterilization device that is placed hysteroscopically, which avoids entry into the peritoneal cavity. Backup contraception is needed for 3 months, at which time a hysterosalpingography is performed to confirm occlusion. Short-term efficacy studies suggest a rate equal to or greater than other tubal sterilization methods. However, long-term efficacy rates are not yet available (14).

Transvaginal Approach. Although performed infrequently, sterilization by the vaginal route remains an option. Fimbriectomy, Pomeroy, and other tubal occlusion methods traditionally used with laparoscopic techniques can be performed via posterior colpotomy. The advantages include less patient preparation (eg, bladder catheterization), the absence of abdominal incision, and potentially less pain for the patient with an earlier return to routine activity. Contraindications include suspicion of major pelvic adhesions, enlarged uterus, and inability to place the patient in the lithotomy position. One major disadvantage is the need for adequate vaginal surgical training (15) to minimize potential complications, such as cellulitis, pelvic abscess, hemorrhage, proctotomy, or cystotomy.

Methods of Occlusion

Electrocoagulation. Electrocoagulation for tubal occlusion is used exclusively with laparoscopic sterilization. Bipolar coagulation is now the most commonly used laparoscopic occlusion method in the United States. It results in a more localized injury to the fallopian tube than does the unipolar method, which is associated with thermal bowel injury. To maximize the effectiveness of bipolar coagulation, at least 3 cm of the isthmic portion of the fallopian tube must be completely coagulated by using sufficient energy (25 W) delivered in a cutting waveform (16, 17). Use of a current meter, rather than a visual endpoint or a defined period, more accurately indicates complete coagulation.

Mechanical Methods. Mechanical occlusion devices commonly used in the United States include the silicone rubber band (Falope ring), the spring-loaded clip (Hulka-Clemens clip), and the titanium clip lined with silicone rubber (Filshie clip). Mechanical methods have no associated risk of electrical burn and destroy less of the fallopian tube (approximately 5 mm for clips and 2 cm for rings), making microsurgical reversal more likely to succeed. Special applicators are necessary for each of these mechanical occlusion devices, and each requires skill for proper application. The silicone band can only be applied to a fallopian tube that is sufficiently mobile to allow it to be drawn into the applicator. All of these devices are most likely to be effective when used to occlude a normal fallopian tube; tubal adhesions or thickened or dilated fallopian tubes increase the risk of misapplication and subsequent failure. Spontaneous clip migration or expulsion is rare (18, 19).

Ligation Methods. A variety of techniques for ligating and resecting a portion of both fallopian tubes have been described, including the Pomeroy, modified Pomeroy, and Parkland methods; the Uchida and Irving methods are rarely used in the United States (8). Tubal occlusion at the time of cesarean delivery, laparotomy for other indications, and minilaparotomy usually are performed by using ligation techniques. Care should be taken to excise a sufficient section of the fallopian tube to ensure complete transection of the tubal lumen.

Chemical Methods. Chemical sclerosing agents have been investigated for many years for their potential use as blindly placed transcervical tubal blocking agents. Although some have shown promise, none are currently approved for use in the United States (20, 21).

Vasectomy

Prevalence and Practice

Vasectomy performed as an outpatient procedure has been popular in the United States since 1965. More than 5 million men had undergone vasectomy by 1988 (22). No nationwide surveillance system exists to monitor trends in vasectomies performed; however, surveys in 1991 and 1995 found that almost 500,000 men had a vasectomy in each of those years (3, 23). When compared with tubal sterilization, vasectomy is safer, less expensive, and appears to be at least as effective. In the United States, urologists, general surgeons, and family physicians perform vasectomy procedures in their offices using local anesthesia. Vasectomy failure rates range from 0% to 2%, with most studies reporting pregnancy rates of less than 1% (24).

Complications

Minor complications of vasectomy, such as infection at the site of incision, bleeding and hematoma formation, granuloma formation, and epididymitis, are reported to occur at rates of 5–10% (25). In comparison with the incisional technique, the no-scalpel vasectomy technique has a lower incidence of hematoma formation (0.1–2.1% versus 0.3–10.7%) and infection (0.2–0.9% versus 1.3–4%) (24, 26, 27). Vasectomy-related major morbidity and mortality are extremely rare in the United States (24).

Late Sequelae

Multiple large epidemiologic studies have examined the relationship of both atherosclerosis and immunologic disease with vasectomy and have concluded there is no causal relationship (28–30). In 1994, both a retrospective cohort study of 74,000 men and a case–control study of 794 men provided convincing evidence that vasectomy is not associated with an increased risk of testicular cancer (31, 32).

In 1993, researchers published the first large cohort studies to show a weak but statistically significant increased risk for prostate cancer in a subgroup of men at least 20 years after vasectomy (33). Two subsequent studies failed to confirm these findings (30, 31). Recently, a large, national, population-based, randomized, case–control study from New Zealand concluded that vasectomy does not increase the risk of prostate cancer even when men are examined 25 years postvasectomy (34).

The nerves involved in male erectile function and ejaculation are not affected by vasectomy, and, when studied, measures of impotence were similar in men who had undergone vasectomy and those who had not. "Postvasectomy pain syndrome," or chronic testicular pain, has been described in the literature and is poorly understood.

Clinical Considerations and Recommendations

▶ *How safe is tubal sterilization?*

Tubal sterilization is a safe method of contraception. Death from tubal sterilization is a rare event, and overall complication rates are low. Mortality rates in the United States have been estimated at 1–4 deaths per 100,000 procedures (35–38). Most deaths in the United States have been attributed to hypoventilation and cardiopulmonary arrest during general anesthesia. In an early U.S. study, 11 of 29 sterilization-related deaths occurred in women with underlying medical conditions (39). A more recent study found no mortality among 9,475 women who underwent interval laparoscopic tubal ligation (40).

Major complications from tubal sterilization are uncommon and vary by study definition, occurring at levels that range from 1% to 3.5% (18, 19, 40). Using a standard definition of complications, including intraoperative and postoperative events, overall complication rates for tubal sterilization are estimated to be 0.9–1.6 per 100 procedures (40); unintended major surgery (laparotomy) represented 0.9 per 100 cases. This complication rate did not vary significantly according to the method of occlusion used. Intraoperative complications include unintended, unplanned major surgery needed because of a problem related to the tubal surgery, transfusion, a life-threatening event, or death. Postoperative complications include unintended major surgery, transfusion, febrile morbidity, a life-threatening event, rehospitalization, or death caused by a complication within 42 days of surgery. General anesthesia, previous abdominal or pelvic surgery, obesity, and diabetes were independent predictors of complication (40).

When sterilization is performed concurrent with cesarean delivery, any higher associated morbidity has been attributed to the indications for which the cesarean delivery was performed (41). The risk of complications was similarly low for women undergoing tubal sterilization after abortion when compared with the risks of sterilization alone (10).

▶ *How effective is tubal sterilization compared with other female contraceptive methods?*

Tubal sterilization is far more effective than short-term, user-dependent, reversible contraceptive methods. Data from the 1995 U.S. National Survey of Family Growth indicate that within 1 year of starting any reversible method, 90 per 1,000 typical users experience a contraceptive failure (42). By method, contraceptive failure occurs in the first year of use for 70 per 1,000 women using oral contraceptives, 90 per 1,000 women relying on the male condom, 32 per 1,000 women using injectable methods, 81 per 1,000 women using the diaphragm, and 198 per 1,000 women using periodic abstinence.

Failure rates of tubal sterilization are roughly comparable with those of the IUD. The U.S. Collaborative Review of Sterilization (CREST), a large, prospective, multicenter observational study of 10,685 women conducted by the Centers for Disease Control and Prevention in 1996, concluded that although tubal sterilization is highly effective, the risk of sterilization failure is substantially higher than previously reported (43). Analysis of CREST data found a 5-year cumulative life-table probability of failure of aggregated sterilization methods of 13 per 1,000 procedures (43), compared with a 5-year cumulative failure rate for the copper T 380-A IUD of 14 per 1,000 procedures (44). The 5-year cumulative pregnancy rate for levonorgestrel-releasing IUDs ranges between 5 and 11 per 1,000 procedures (45–47).

The risk of sterilization failure persists for years after the procedure and varies by method, age, and race and ethnicity. The younger a woman was at the time of sterilization, the more likely she was to have had sterilization failure (43).

The CREST data reported that the 10-year cumulative probability for sterilization failure varied by sterilization method and ranged from 7.5 per 1,000 to 36 per 1,000 procedures. Postpartum partial salpingectomy had the lowest 5-year and 10-year cumulative pregnancy rates: 6.3 per 1,000 and 7.5 per 1,000 procedures, respectively. The 5-year and 10-year pregnancy rates, respectively, for other occlusion methods are as follows (43):

- Bipolar coagulation: 16.5 per 1,000 and 24.8 per 1,000 procedures
- Silicone band methods: 10 per 1,000 and 17.7 per 1,000 procedures
- Spring clip: 31.7 per 1,000 and 36.5 per 1,000 procedures

Secondary analysis of 5-year failure rates with bipolar coagulation performed in different decades found that failure was significantly lower in later periods, reflecting improved technique with the method: 19.5 per 1,000 procedures for 1978–1982 versus 6.3 per 1,000 procedures for 1985–1987 (16). The 10-year cumulative risk of pregnancy was highest among women sterilized at a young age with bipolar coagulation (54.3/1,000) and clip application (52.1/1,000). The study cautions that the reported failure rates should not be considered in isolation of other variables that influence overall outcome.

Although pregnancy after sterilization is uncommon, there is substantial risk that any poststerilization pregnancy will be ectopic. Analysis of CREST data found that one third of poststerilization pregnancies (47/143) were ectopic (48). For all methods of sterilization except postpartum partial salpingectomy, women younger than 30 years were more likely to experience ectopic pregnancy than women older than 30 years (a reflection of the greater overall fecundity of younger women). Non-Hispanic blacks had 4 times the relative risk (RR) of ectopic pregnancy than non-Hispanic whites. Women with a history of pelvic inflammatory disease (PID) had 2.7 times the RR of women without a history of PID.

▶ Does the technique used for sterilization affect the risk of ectopic pregnancy?

The risk of ectopic pregnancy varies substantially with the method and timing of sterilization. Based on CREST study data, the 10-year cumulative probability of ectopic pregnancy after tubal sterilization by any method was 7.3 per 1,000 procedures. Bipolar coagulation had the highest cumulative probability of ectopic pregnancy (17.1/1,000), and postpartum partial salpingectomy had the lowest cumulative probability (1.5/1,000).

Bipolar coagulation had a cumulative probability 10 times higher than unipolar coagulation (17.1/1,000 versus 1.8/1,000) and 2–2.5 times higher than the spring clip (8.5/1,000) and the silicone band (7.3/1,000). It should be noted that these figures reflect procedures that took place before the routine use of a current meter, and pregnancy rates have since decreased (16). Also, current data are not available specifically for ectopic pregnancies. Interval partial salpingectomy was 5 times more likely to result in ectopic pregnancy than was postpartum partial salpingectomy, although this finding was felt to be caused by chance or selection bias (48).

For all methods except postpartum partial salpingectomy, the probability of ectopic pregnancy was greater for women sterilized before age 30 years than for women sterilized at age 30 years or older. Women sterilized by bipolar tubal coagulation before age 30 years had a 10-year cumulative probability of ectopic pregnancy of 31.9 per 1,000 procedures, approximately 4 times the cumulative probability of women aged 30 years and older. Postpartum partial salpingectomy was the only method reported by the CREST study that did not have a higher 10-year cumulative probability of ectopic pregnancy in younger women (48). For all methods of occlusion, the risk of ectopic pregnancy did not diminish with the length of time since the tubal sterilization.

▶ How do the safety and effectiveness of tubal sterilization compare with the IUD?

Both tubal sterilization and modern IUDs are safe methods of contraception. Death from tubal sterilization is rare, with case fatality levels reported to be between 1 and 4 deaths per 100,000 procedures (35–38). Because IUDs are not inserted under general anesthesia and IUD insertion is not a surgical procedure, death caused by IUD insertion is a rare event, with only anecdotal reports in the literature in the past (49).

Major complications from tubal sterilization are uncommon and vary by study definition. Most major complications associated with the IUD occur around the time of insertion and include uterine perforation and infection. Perforation rates vary based on the type of IUD and study design, but a rate of less than 1 in 1,000 insertions generally is recognized (50). The risk of PID is highest immediately after and up to 20 days after IUD insertion, varies according to geographic region, and is inversely related to age and parity (51, 52). One large study reported an IUD discontinuation rate from PID or infection of 4 cases in 2,795 insertions (51). The PID rate after insertion of a levonorgestrel IUD may be lower (45, 46).

The copper T 380-A IUD and the levonorgestrel IUD are highly effective methods of contraception, roughly comparable with tubal sterilization, with cumulative 5-year failure rates of 1.4 and 0.5 pregnancies per 100 women, respectively (45, 53). The failure rate of levonorgestrel IUDs remains low and stable across all age groups; however, some copper IUDs have a failure rate that varies inversely with the patient's age (54). Sterilization failure rates also are inversely related to the patient's age (43). One third of all sterilization failures will result in ectopic pregnancy, whereas approximately 20% of all IUD failures will result in an ectopic pregnancy (43, 45).

When intrauterine pregnancy occurs after tubal sterilization, there is no known added risk to the woman or her fetus. In contrast, when an intrauterine pregnancy is diagnosed in an IUD user and the IUD is not removed, there is a 3 times greater risk of spontaneous abortion in the first trimester, a highly increased risk of septic abortion in the second trimester (RR, 26; 95% confidence interval, 6–108), and a 3 times greater risk of preterm birth in the third trimester (55–57).

▶ How do the safety and effectiveness of tubal sterilization compare with vasectomy?

Vasectomy is safer than tubal sterilization because it is a less invasive surgical procedure and because it is performed using local anesthesia. Tubal sterilization involves entry into the peritoneal cavity and usually is performed under general or regional anesthesia.

Although specific data are lacking on mortality related to vasectomy, knowledgeable observers state that such deaths are extremely rare in the United States (24). Mortality from tubal sterilization, although rare, occurs at levels that are measurable, ranging from 1 to 4 deaths per 100,000 procedures (35–38). Major complications from vasectomy also are extremely rare (24). Major complications from tubal sterilization are uncommon and vary by definition.

Short-term effectiveness of vasectomy—with reported failures of less than 1%—is comparable with that of tubal sterilization. Tubal sterilization provides immediate contraceptive protection, whereas men remain fertile for several months after vasectomy and require semen analysis to fully determine the success of the procedure. Neither female nor male sexual function appears to be affected after tubal sterilization or vasectomy (30, 58).

Assuming that vasectomy and tubal sterilization provide similar protection against pregnancy, women who have had tubal sterilization are at increased RR of ectopic pregnancy in the case of failures, with estimated absolute incidence of ectopic pregnancy of 0.32 per 1,000 women-years in women who had tubal sterilization and 0.005 per 1,000 women-years in women whose partners had vasectomy (59). By comparison, the estimated absolute incidence of ectopic pregnancy in women using no contraception is 2.6 per 1,000 women-years (59).

▶ Does tubal sterilization cause menstrual abnormalities?

The long-term health effects of tubal sterilization on menstrual pattern disturbance (posttubal ligation syndrome) appear to be negligible. Early studies of menstrual disturbances after sterilization failed to account for confounding variables, such as presterilization use of hormonal contraceptives, that generally mask underlying menstrual dysfunction and, in particular, heavy bleeding and intermenstrual bleeding (60–62). Most recent prospective studies that account for these factors have found little or no difference in menstrual patterns between women before and after sterilization or between sterilized women and nonsterilized controls in the first 1–2 years of follow-up (61, 63–69).

A recent analysis of the CREST data prospectively examined menstrual patterns of 9,514 women for 5 years after interval tubal sterilization and compared them with those of women whose partners underwent vasectomy (70). The study found that women who underwent sterilization were no more likely than the control group to report persistent changes in their menstrual cycle length or intermenstrual bleeding. However, they were more likely to have beneficial changes in their menstrual cycle, including decreased amount of bleeding, number of days of bleeding, and menstrual pain. Although an increase in "cycle irregularity" was reported in one study subset, this was considered likely to be caused by chance. The method of tubal occlusion did not have a significant impact on the findings.

▶ Are women who undergo tubal sterilization more likely to have a hysterectomy?

Women who undergo tubal sterilization appear to be 4–5 times more likely to undergo hysterectomy than those whose partners underwent vasectomy (71). In one analysis of CREST data, this increased risk was found to persist across all ages and methods for a 14-year follow-up period (71). The reported association between sterilization and hysterectomy tends to be strong (RR, 1.6–4.4) (67, 71–75). Some older studies suggested a significantly greater risk of hysterectomy for women sterilized at a young age (73, 75), but more recent studies found no difference based on age (71). Increased risk was independent of the method of tubal occlusion used (71, 73) but was associated with a presterilization history of menstrual or other benign gynecologic disorders (71). A history of endometriosis or uterine leiomyomata was associated with the highest long-term probability of hysterectomy at 14 years poststerilization (71). These findings are consistent with the results from previous studies (76–78).

There is no known biologic mechanism to support a causal relationship between tubal sterilization and subsequent hysterectomy. Nonbiologic mechanisms are speculative. Women who choose one surgical procedure may be more likely to undergo another for the management of gynecologic conditions. Women who have had tubal sterilization may be more likely to perceive themselves or be perceived as appropriate candidates for hysterectomy, given that fertility preservation is no longer a factor in decision making (71, 75).

▶ Does tubal sterilization have noncontraceptive benefits?

The long-term protective effect of tubal sterilization on ovarian cancer incidence (RR, 0.29–0.69) has been confirmed by multiple observational studies (79–82). This protective effect persists after adjusting for age, use of oral contraceptives, and parity (80). In addition, a case–control study of 4,742 women found no association between tubal sterilization and breast cancer (81). Most prospective studies have shown either no consistent change or no improvement in sexual interest or pleasure after sterilization (83, 84).

Although tubal sterilization does not protect against sexually transmitted diseases (including human immunodeficiency virus [HIV]) (85, 86), it has been shown to reduce the spread of organisms from the lower genital tract to the peritoneal cavity and thus protect against PID. This protection is incomplete, however, as suggested by rare case reports of PID and tuboovarian abscess in women who have undergone sterilization (87–89).

▶ *What is the risk that a patient will regret having had tubal sterilization, and how can the risk be reduced?*

Most women who choose sterilization as a contraceptive method do not regret their decision (90–92); however, information and counseling about sterilization should be provided with the intent to minimize regret among individual women. Although there are certain key indicators for future regret—such as young age at the time of sterilization—many indicators of regret are part of individual social circumstances, which should be explored with the patient before a decision is made.

Poststerilization regret measured by self-report or by request for information on reversal ranges from 0.9% to 26% (90, 93–97). Prospective CREST study data analysis found that the cumulative probability of regret over 14 years of follow-up was 12.7% (90). However, the probability was 20.3% for women aged 30 years or younger at the time of sterilization, compared with 5.9% for women older than 30 years at the time of sterilization.

Regarding the timing of sterilization, previous reports have identified postpartum sterilization as a risk factor for increased regret (83, 98–101). Analysis of CREST data found similar levels of regret for interval sterilization within 1 year of delivery (22.3%) as for postpartum sterilization after vaginal delivery (23.7%) and cesarean delivery (20.7%). The cumulative probability of regret diminished steadily with the interval between delivery and sterilization (90). Postabortion sterilization was not associated with increased regret when compared with interval sterilization (90, 101–103).

The most common reason for regret is the desire for more children. Younger women who choose sterilization have more time to change their minds and life circumstances. Women sterilized before age 25 years were 18 times more likely to request reversal over the course of follow-up than women older than 30 years at the time of sterilization. Other risk factors for increased regret include having received less information about the procedure, having had less access to information or support for other contraceptive method use (104), and having made the decision under pressure from a spouse or because of medical indications (94, 100).

Data from the CREST study have been analyzed to report reversal requests as a different indicator for regret. The 14-year cumulative probability of requesting reversal information was 14.3% but was as high as 40.4% in women who underwent sterilization between ages 18 and 24 years—almost 4 times higher than for women older than 30 years at the time of sterilization (92). The number of living children was not associated with a request for reversal information. Although the overall cumulative probability of obtaining reversal was 1.1%, this number does not include women who selected in vitro fertilization to attempt pregnancy instead of reversal. Data on poststerilization users of in vitro fertilization are not available.

Because tubal sterilization is common and regret is not uncommon, it is important to attempt to reduce regret with thorough and effective counseling that takes into account the risk factors described previously. Both the patient and her partner, when appropriate, should be counseled (see box). Because young age at the time of sterilization, regardless of parity or marital status, is associated with significant levels of regret, individualized counseling of younger women is critical. Full consideration should be given to all temporary contraceptive options. Ambivalence should be addressed directly, taking into account the elective nature of the procedure. In particular, ambivalence displayed in the postpartum period just before sterilization should be seriously weighed against any advantage and considered an indication for interval sterilization.

Components of Presterilization Counseling

- Permanent nature of the procedure
- Alternative methods available, including male sterilization
- Reasons for choosing sterilization
- Screening for risk indicators for regret
- Details of the procedure, including risks and benefits of anesthesia
- The possibility of failure, including ectopic pregnancy
- The need to use condoms for protection against sexually transmitted diseases, including human immunodeficiency virus infection
- Completion of informed consent process
- Local regulations regarding interval from time of consent to procedure

Data from Pollack AE, Soderstrom RM. Female tubal sterilization. In: Corson SL, Derman RJ, Tyrer LB, editors. Fertility control. 2nd ed. London (ON): Goldin Publishers; 1994. p. 295–6.

Summary of Recommendations

The following recommendations are based on good and consistent scientific evidence (Level A):

▶ Tubal sterilization may be recommended as a safe and effective method for women who desire permanent contraception. Women should be counseled that tubal ligation is not intended to be reversible; therefore, those who do not want permanent contraception should be counseled to consider other methods of contraception.

▶ Patients should be advised that neither tubal sterilization nor vasectomy provides any protection against sexually transmitted diseases, including HIV infection.

▶ Patients should be advised that the morbidity and mortality of tubal ligation, although low, is higher than that of vasectomy, and the efficacy rates of the 2 procedures are similar.

▶ Patients should be counseled that tubal sterilization is more effective than short-term, user-dependent reversible methods.

▶ Patients should be counseled that failure rates of tubal sterilization are comparable with those of IUDs.

The following recommendations are based primarily on consensus and expert opinion (Level C):

▶ If a patient has a positive pregnancy test result after a tubal ligation, ectopic pregnancy should be ruled out.

▶ Indications for hysterectomy in women with previous tubal sterilization should be the same as for women who have not had tubal sterilization.

References

1. EngenderHealth. Contraceptive sterilization: global issues and trends. New York: EngenderHealth; 2002. (Level III)

2. MacKay AP, Kieke BA Jr, Koonin LM, Beattie K. Tubal sterilization in the United States, 1994–1996. Fam Plann Perspect 2001;33:161–5. (Level II-3)

3. Magnani RJ, Haws JM, Morgan GT, Gargiullo PM, Pollack AE, Koonin LM. Vasectomy in the United States, 1991 and 1995. Am J Public Health 1999;89:92–4. (Level II-3)

4. Piccinino LJ, Mosher WD. Trends in contraceptive use in the United States:1982–1995. Fam Plann Perspect 1998;30:4–10, 46. (Level II-3)

5. Pollack AE, Soderstrom RM. Female tubal sterilization. In: Corson SL, Derman RJ, Tyrer LB, editors. Fertility control. 2nd ed. London (ON): Goldin Publishers; 1994. p. 293–317. (Level III)

6. Centers for Disease Control. Surgical sterilization surveillance: tubal sterilization 1976–1978. Atlanta (GA): CDC; 1981. (Level II-3)

7. American College of Obstetricians and Gynecologists. Tubal ligation with cesarean delivery. ACOG Committee Opinion 205. Washington, DC: ACOG; 1998. (Level III)

8. Peterson HB, Pollack AE, Warshaw JS. Tubal sterilization. In: Rock JA, Thompson JD, editors. Te Linde's Operative Gynecology. 8th ed. Philadelphia (PA): Lippincott-Raven; 1997. p. 529–47. (Level III)

9. American College of Obstetricians and Gynecologists. Ethics in obstetrics and gynecology. Washington, DC: ACOG; 2002. (Level III)

10. Akhter HH, Flock ML, Rubin GL. Safety of abortion and tubal sterilization performed separately versus concurrently. Am J Obstet Gynecol 1985;152:619–23. (Level II-3)

11. Lipscomb GH, Spellman JR, Ling FW. The effect of same-day pregnancy testing on the incidence of luteal phase pregnancy. Obstet Gynecol 1993;82:411–3. (Level II-3)

12. Kasliwal A, Farquharson RG. Pregnancy testing prior to sterilisation. BJOG 2000;107:1407–9. (Level III)

13. Lichter ED, Laff SP, Friedman EA. Value of routine dilatation and curettage at the time of interval sterilization. Obstet Gynecol 1986;67:763–5. (Level III)

14. Valle RF, Carignan CS, Wright TC. Tissue response to the STOP microcoil transcervical permanent contraceptive device: results from a prehysterectomy study. Fertil Steril 2001;76:974–80. (Level III)

15. Hartfield VJ. Female sterilization by the vaginal route: a positive reassessment and comparison of 4 tubal occlusion methods. Aust N Z J Obstet Gynaecol 1993;33: 408–12. (Level II-1)

16. Peterson HB, Xia Z, Wilcox LS, Tylor LR, Trussell J. Pregnancy after tubal sterilization with bipolar electrocoagulation. U.S. Collaborative Review of Sterilization Working Group. Obstet Gynecol 1999;94:163–7. (Level II-2)

17. Soderstrom RM, Levy BS, Engel T. Reducing bipolar sterilization failures. Obstet Gynecol 1989;74:60–3. (Level III)

18. Sokal D, Gates D, Amatya R, Dominik R. Two randomized controlled trials comparing the tubal ring and filshie clip for tubal sterilization. Fertil Steril 2000;74: 525–33. (Level I)

19. Dominik R, Gates D, Sokal D, Cordero M, Lasso de la Vega J, Remes Ruiz A, et al. Two randomized controlled trials comparing the Hulka and Filshie Clips for tubal sterilization. Contraception 2000;62:169–75. (Level I)

20. Hieu DT, Tan TT, Tan ND, Nguyet PT, Than P, Vinh DQ. 31,781 cases of non-surgical female sterilization with quinacrine pellets in Vietnam. Lancet 1993;342:213–7. (Level II-1)

21. Mumford SD, Kessel E. Sterilization needs in the 1990s: the case for quinacrine nonsurgical female sterilization. Am J Obstet Gynecol 1992;167:1203–7. (Level III)

22. Mosher WD, Pratt WF. Use of contraception and family planning services in the United States, 1988. Am J Public Health 1990;80:1132–3. (Level II-3)

23. Marquette CM, Koonin LM, Antarsh L, Gargiullo PM, Smith JC. Vasectomy in the United States, 1991. Am J Public Health 1995;85:644–9. (Level II-3)

24. Peterson HB, Huber DH, Belker AM. Vasectomy: an appraisal for the obstetrician–gynecologist. Obstet Gynecol 1990;76:568–72. (Level III)

25. Alderman PM. Complications in a series of 1224 vasectomies. J Fam Pract 1991;33:579–84. (Level III)

26. Sokal D, McMullen S, Gates D, Dominik R. A comparative study of the no scalpel and standard incision approaches to vasectomy in 5 countries. The Male Sterilization Investigator Team. J Urol 1999;162:1621–5. (Level I)

27. Arellano Lara S, Gonzales Barrera JL, Hernandez Ono A, Moreno Alcazar O, Espinosa Perez J. No-scalpel vasectomy: review of the first 1,000 cases in a family medicine unit. Arch Med Res 1997;28:517–22. (Level II-3)

28. Giovannucci E, Tosteson TD, Speizer FE, Vessey MP, Colditz GA. A long-term study of mortality in men who have undergone vasectomy. N Engl J Med 1992;326:1392–8. (Level II-2)

29. Nienhuis H, Goldacre M, Seagroatt V, Gill L, Vessey M. Incidence of disease after vasectomy: a record linkage retrospective cohort study. BMJ 1992;304:743–6. (Level III)

30. Schuman LM, Coulson AH, Mandel JS, Massey FJ Jr, O'Fallon WM. Health Status of American Men—a study of post-vasectomy sequelae. J Clin Epidemiol 1993;46:697–958. (Level II-2)

31. Moller H, Knudsen LB, Lynge E. Risk of testicular cancer after vasectomy: cohort study of over 73,000 men. BMJ 1994;309:295–9. (Level II-2)

32. Aetiology of testicular cancer: association with congenital abnormalities, age at puberty, infertility, and exercise. United Kingdom Testicular Cancer Study Group. BMJ 1994;308:1393–9. (Level II-2)

33. Giovannucci E, Ascherio A, Rimm EB, Colditz GA, Stampfer MJ, Willett WC. A prospective cohort study of vasectomy and prostate cancer in US men. JAMA 1993;269:873–7. (Level II-2)

34. Cox B, Sneyd MJ, Paul C, Delahunt B, Skegg DC. Vasectomy and risk of prostate cancer. JAMA 2002;287:3110–5. (Level II-2)

35. Escobedo LG, Peterson HB, Grubb GS, Franks AL. Case-fatality rates for tubal sterilization in U.S. hospitals, 1979 to 1980. Am J Obstet Gynecol 1989;160:147–50. (Level III)

36. Hulka JF, Phillips JM, Peterson HB, Surrey MW. Laparoscopic sterilization: American Association of Gynecologic Laparoscopists' 1993 membership survey. J Am Assoc Gynecol Laparosc 1995;2:137–8. (Level III)

37. Peterson HB, Ory HW, Greenspan JR, Tyler CW Jr. Deaths associated with laparoscopic sterilization by unipolar electrocoagulating devices, 1978 and 1979. Am J Obstet Gynecol 1981;139:141–3. (Level II-3)

38. Peterson HB, Hulka JF, Phillips JM, Surrey MW. Laparoscopic sterilization. American Association of Gynecologic Laparoscopists 1991 membership survey. J Reprod Med 1993;38:574–6. (Level III)

39. Peterson HB, DeStefano F, Rubin GL, Greenspan JR, Lee NC, Ory HW. Deaths attributable to tubal sterilization in the United States, 1977–81. Am J Obstet Gynecol 1983;146:131–6. (Level II-3)

40. Jamieson DJ, Hillis SD, Duerr A, Marchbanks PA, Costello C, Peterson HB. Complications of interval laparoscopic tubal sterilization: findings from the United States Collaborative Review of Sterilization. Obstet Gynecol 2000;96:997–1002. (Level II-2)

41. Chi IC, Petta CA, McPheeters M. A review of safety, efficacy, pros and cons, and issues of puerperal tubal sterilization—an update. Adv Contracept 1995;11:187–206. (Level III)

42. Trussell J, Vaughan B. Contraceptive failure, method-related discontinuation and resumption of use: results from the 1995 National Survey of Family Growth. Fam Plann Perspect 1999;31:64–72, 93. (Level II-3)

43. Peterson HB, Xia Z, Hughes JM, Wilcox LS, Tylor LR, Trussell J. The risk of pregnancy after tubal sterilization: findings from the U.S. Collaborative Review of Sterilization. Am J Obstet Gynecol 1996;174:1161–8; discussion 1168–70. (Level II-2)

44. Fortney JA, Feldblum PJ, Raymond EG. Intrauterine devices. The optimal long-term contraceptive method? J Reprod Med 1999;44:269–74. (Level III)

45. Andersson K, Odlind V, Rybo G. Levonorgestrel-releasing and copper-releasing (Nova T) IUDs during five years of use: a randomized comparative trial. Contraception 1994;49:56–72. (Level I)

46. Sivin I, el Mahgoub S, McCarthy T, Mishell DR Jr, Shoupe D, Alvarez F, et al. Long-term contraception with the levonorgesterel 20 mcg/day (LNg 20) and the copper T 380Ag intrauterine devices: a five-year randomized study. Contraception 1990;42:361–78. (Level I)

47. Luukkainen T, Allonen H, Haukkamaa M, Lahteenmaki P, Nilsson CG, Toivonen J. Five years' experience with levonorgesterel-releasing IUDs. Contraception 1986;33:139–48. (Level I)

48. Peterson HB, Xia Z, Hughes JM, Wilcox LS, Tylor LR, Trussell J. The risk of ectopic pregnancy after tubal sterilization. U.S. Collaborative Review of Sterilization Working Group. N Engl J Med 1997;336:762–7. (Level II-2)

49. Kahn HS, Tyler CW Jr. Mortality associated with use of IUDs. JAMA 1975;234:57–9. (Level III)

50. Long-term reversible contraception. Twelve years of experience with the TCu380A and TCu220C. Contraception 1997;56:341–52. (Level I)

51. Farley TM, Rosenberg MJ, Rowe PJ, Chen JH, Meirik O. Intrauterine devices and pelvic inflammatory disease:

an international perspective. Lancet 1992;339:785–8. (Level III)

52. Lee NC, Rubin GL, Ory HW, Burkman RT. Type of intrauterine device and the risk of pelvic inflammatory disease. Obstet Gynecol 1983;62:1–6. (Level II-2)

53. The TCu380A, TCu220C, multiload 250 and Nova T IUD at 3, 5 and 7 years of use—results from three randomized multicentre trials. World Health Organization. Special Programme of Research, Development and Research Training in Human Reproduction: Task Force on Safety and Efficacy of Fertility Regulating Methods. Contraception 1990;42:141–58. (Level I)

54. Luukkainen T, Toivonen J. Levonorgestrel-releasing IUD as a method of contraception with therapeutic properties. Contraception 1995;52:269–76. (Level III)

55. Chaim W, Mazor M. Pregnancy with an intrauterine device in situ and preterm delivery. Arch Gynecol Obstet 1992;252:21–4. (Level II-2)

56. Foreman H, Stadel BV, Schlesselman S. Intrauterine device usage and fetal loss. Obstet Gynecol 1981;58:669–77. (Level II-2)

57. Tatum HJ, Schmidt FH, Jain AK. Management and outcome of pregnancies associated with the Copper T intrauterine contraceptive device. Am J Obstet Gynecol 1976;126:869–79. (Level II-2)

58. Massey FJ Jr, Bernstein GS, O'Fallon WM, Schuman LM, Coulson AH, Crozier R, et al. Vasectomy and health. Results from a large cohort study. JAMA 1984;252:1023–9. (Level II-2)

59. Franks AL, Beral V, Cates W Jr, Hogue CJ. Contraception and ectopic pregnancy risk. Am J Obstet Gynecol 1990;163:1120–3. (Level III)

60. Alder E, Cook A, Gray J, Tyrer G, Warner P, Bancroft J, et al. The effects of sterilisation: a comparison of sterilized women with wives of vasectomized men. Contraception 1981;23:45–54. (Level III)

61. Gentile GP, Kaufman SC, Helbig DW. Is there any evidence for a post-tubal sterilization syndrome? Fertil Steril 1998;69:179–86. (Level III)

62. Poma PA. Tubal sterilization and later hospitalizations. J Reprod Med 1980;25:272–8. (Level II-2)

63. Bhiwandiwala PP, Mumford SD, Feldblum PJ. Menstrual pattern changes following laparoscopic sterilization with different occlusion techniques: a review of 10,004 cases. Am J Obstet Gynecol 1983;145:684–94. (Level II-3)

64. DeStefano F, Perlman JA, Peterson HB, Diamond EL. Long-term risk of menstrual disturbances after tubal sterilization. Am J Obstet Gynecol 1985;152:835–41. (Level II-2)

65. Foulkes J, Chamberlain G. Effects of sterilization on menstruation. South Med J 1985;78:544–7. (Level II-2)

66. Rivera R, Gaitan JR, Ruiz R, Hurley DP, Arenas M, Flores C, et al. Menstrual patterns and progesterone circulating levels following different procedures of tubal occlusion. Contraception 1989;40:157–69. (Level I)

67. Rulin MC, Davidson AR, Philliber SG, Graves WL, Cushman LF. Long-term effect of tubal sterilization on menstrual indices and pelvic pain. Obstet Gynecol 1993;82:118–21. (Level II-2)

68. Sahwi S, Toppozada M, Kamel M, Anwar MY, Ismail AA. Changes in menstrual blood loss after four methods of female tubal sterilization. Contraception 1989;40:387–98. (Level I)

69. Thranov I, Hertz JB, Kjer JJ, Andresen A, Micic S, Nielsen J, et al. Hormonal and menstrual changes after laparoscopic sterilization by Falope-rings or Filschie-clips. Fertil Steril 1992;57:751–5. (Level II-3)

70. Peterson HB, Jeng G, Folger SG, Hillis SA, Marchbanks PA, Wilcox LS. The risk of menstrual abnormalities after tubal sterilization. U.S. Collaborative Review of Sterilization Working Group. N Engl J Med 2000;343:1681–7. (Level II-2)

71. Hillis SD, Marchbanks PA, Tylor LR, Peterson HB. Higher hysterectomy risk for sterilized than nonsterilized women: findings from the U.S. Collaborative Review of Sterilization. The U.S. Collaborative Review of Sterilization Working Group. Obstet Gynecol 1998;91:241–6. (Level II-2)

72. Cohen MM. Long-term risk of hysterectomy after tubal sterilization. Am J Epidemiol 1987;125:410–9. (Level II-2)

73. Goldhaber MK, Armstrong MA, Golditch IM, Sheehe PR, Petitti DB, Friedman GD. Long-term risk of hysterectomy among 80,007 sterilized and comparison women at Kaiser Permanente, 1971–1987. Am J Epidemiol 1993;138:508–21. (Level II-2)

74. Kendrick JS, Rubin GL, Lee NC, Schulz KF, Peterson HB, Nolan TF. Hysterectomy performed within 1 year after tubal sterilization. Fertil Steril 1985;44:606–10. (Level II-2)

75. Stergachis A, Shy KK, Grothaus LC, Wagner EH, Hecht JA, Anderson G, et al. Tubal sterilization and the long-term risk of hysterectomy. JAMA 1990;264:2893–8. (Level II-2)

76. Carlson KJ, Nichols DH, Schiff I. Indications for hysterectomy. N Engl J Med 1993;328:856–60. (Level III)

77. Pokras R, Hufnagel VG. Hysterectomy in the United States, 1965–84. Am J Public Health 1988;78:852–3. (Level II-3)

78. Wilcox LS, Koonin LM, Pokras R, Strauss LT, Xia Z, Peterson HB. Hysterectomy in the United States, 1988–1990. Obstet Gynecol 1994;83:549–55. (Level III)

79. Green A, Purdie D, Bain C, Siskind V, Russell P, Quinn M, et al. Tubal sterilisation, hysterectomy and decreased risk of ovarian cancer. Survey of Women's Health Study Group. Int J Cancer 1997;71:948–51. (Level II-2)

80. Hankinson SE, Hunter DJ, Colditz GA, Willett WC, Stampfer MJ, Rosner B, et al. Tubal ligation, hysterectomy and risk of ovarian cancer. A prospective study. JAMA 1993;270:2813–8. (Level II-2)

81. Irwin KL, Weiss NS, Lee NC, Peterson HB. Tubal sterilization, hysterectomy, and the subsequent occurrence of epithelial ovarian cancer. Am J Epidemiol 1991;134: 362–9. (Level II-2)

82. Miracle-McMahill HL, Calle EE, Kosinski AS, Rodriguez C, Wingo PA, Thun MJ, et al. Tubal ligation and fatal ovarian cancer in a large prospective cohort study. Am J Epidemiol 1997;145:349–57. (Level II-2)

83. Cooper JE, Bledin KD, Brice B, Mackenzie S. Effects of female sterilization: one year follow-up in a prospective controlled study of psychological and psychiatric outcomes. J Psychosom Res 1985;29:13–22. (Level II-2)

84. Costello C, Hillis SD, Marchbanks PA, Jamieson DJ, Peterson HB. The effect of interval tubal sterilization on sexual interest and pleasure. Obstet Gynecol 2002;100: 511–7. (Level II-2)

85. Surgical sterilization among women and use of condoms—Baltimore, 1989–1990. MMWR Morb Mortal Wkly Rep 1992;41:568–9, 575. (Level II-2)

86. HIV-risk behaviors of sterilized and nonsterilized women in drug-treatment programs—Philadelphia, 1989–1991. MMWR Morb Mortal Wkly Rep 1992;41:149–52. (Level II-2)

87. Green MM, Vicario SJ, Sanfilippo JS, Lochhead SA. Acute pelvic inflammatory disease after surgical sterilization. Ann Emerg Med 1991;20:344–7. (Level III)

88. Reedy MB, Galan HL, Patterson KM. Acute pelvic inflammatory disease after tubal sterilization. A report of three cases. J Reprod Med 1994;39:752–4. (Level III)

89. Weeks AG, Entman SS. Gonococcal peritonitis after tubal ligation. A case report. J Reprod Med 1991;36:683–4. (Level III)

90. Hillis SD, Marchbanks PA, Tylor LR, Peterson HB. Poststerilization regret: findings from the United States Collaborative Review of Sterilization. Obstet Gynecol 1999;93:889–95. (Level II-2)

91. Jamieson DJ, Kaufman SC, Costello C, Hillis SD, Marchbanks PA, Peterson HB. A comparison of women's regret after vasectomy versus tubal sterilization. Obstet Gynecol 2002;1073–9. (Level II-2)

92. Schmidt JE, Hillis SD, Marchbanks PA, Jeng G, Peterson HB. Requesting information about and obtaining reversal after tubal sterilization: findings from the U.S. Collaborative Review of Sterilization. Fertil Steril 2000;74:892–8. (Level II-2)

93. Bartfai G, Kaali SG. Late sequelae following laparoscopic female sterilization. Int J Fertil 1989;34:67–70. (Level II-3)

94. Boring CC, Rochat RW, Becerra J. Sterilization regret among Puerto Rican women. Fertil Steril 1988;49: 973–81. (Level II-2)

95. Kjer JJ. Regret of laparoscopic sterilization. Eur J Obstet Gynecol Reprod Biol 1990;35:205–10. (Level II-2)

96. Rosenfeld JA, Zahorik PM, Saint W, Murphy G. Women's satisfaction with birth control. J Fam Pract 1993;36:169–73. (Level II-2)

97. Tang CS, Chung TK. Psychosexual adjustment following sterilization: a prospective study on Chinese women. J Psychosom Res 1997;42:187–96. (Level II-2)

98. Chick PH, Frances M, Paterson PJ. A comprehensive review of female sterilisation—tubal occlusion methods. Clin Reprod Fertil 1985;3:81–97. (Level III)

99. Miller WB, Shain RN, Pasta DJ. The predictors of post-sterilization regret in married women. J Appl Soc Psychol 1991;21:1083–110. (Level II-2)

100. Neuhaus W, Bolte A. Prognostic factors for preoperative consultation of women desiring sterilization: findings of a retrospective analysis. J Psychosom Obstet Gynecol 1995;16:45–50. (Level III)

101. Wilcox LS, Chu SY, Eaker ED, Zeger SL, Peterson HB. Risk factors for regret after tubal sterilization: 5 years of follow-up in a prospective study. Fertil Steril 1991;55: 927–33. (Level II-2)

102. Cheng MC, Cheong J, Ratnam SS, Belsey MA, Edstrom KE, Pinol A, et al. Psychosocial sequelae of abortion and sterilization: a controlled study of 200 women randomly allocated to either a concurrent or interval abortion and sterilization. Asia Oceania J Obstet Gynecol 1986;12: 193–200. (Level I)

103. Wilcox LS, Chu SY, Peterson HB. Characteristics of women who considered or obtained tubal reanastomosis: results from a prospective study of tubal sterilization. Obstet Gynecol 1990;75:661–5. (Level II-2)

104. Hardy E, Bahamondes L, Osis MJ, Costa RG, Faundes A. Risk factors for tubal sterilization regret, detectable before surgery. Contraception 1996;54:159–62. (Level II-2)

The MEDLINE database, the Cochrane Library, and ACOG's own internal resources and documents were used to conduct a literature search to locate relevant articles published between between January 1985 and January 2003. The search was restricted to articles published in the English language. Priority was given to articles reporting results of original research, although review articles and commentaries also were consulted. Abstracts of research presented at symposia and scientific conferences were not considered adequate for inclusion in this document. Guidelines published by organizations or institutions such as the National Institutes of Health and the American College of Obstetricians and Gynecologists were reviewed, and additional studies were located by reviewing bibliographies of identified articles. When reliable research was not available, expert opinions from obstetrician–gynecologists were used.

Studies were reviewed and evaluated for quality according to the method outlined by the U.S. Preventive Services Task Force:

I   Evidence obtained from at least one properly designed randomized controlled trial.

II-1   Evidence obtained from well-designed controlled trials without randomization.

II-2   Evidence obtained from well-designed cohort or case–control analytic studies, preferably from more than 1 center or research group.

II-3   Evidence obtained from multiple time series with or without the intervention. Dramatic results in uncontrolled experiments also could be regarded as this type of evidence.

III   Opinions of respected authorities, based on clinical experience, descriptive studies, or reports of expert committees.

Based on the highest level of evidence found in the data, recommendations are provided and graded according to the following categories:

Level A—Recommendations are based on good and consistent scientific evidence.

Level B—Recommendations are based on limited or inconsistent scientific evidence.

Level C—Recommendations are based primarily on consensus and expert opinion.

ISSN 1099-3630

**The American College of
Obstetricians and Gynecologists
409 12th Street, SW
PO Box 96920
Washington, DC 20090-6920**

12345/76543

Benefits and risks of sterilization. ACOG Practice Bulletin No. 46. American College of Obstetricians and Gynecologists. Obstet Gynecol 2003;102:647–58.

ACOG PRACTICE BULLETIN

CLINICAL MANAGEMENT GUIDELINES FOR
OBSTETRICIAN–GYNECOLOGISTS
NUMBER 42, APRIL 2003

This Practice Bulletin was developed by the ACOG Committee on Practice Bulletins—Gynecology with the assistance of William H. Hindle, MD. The information is designed to aid practitioners in making decisions about appropriate obstetric and gynecologic care. These guidelines should not be construed as dictating an exclusive course of treatment or procedure. Variations in practice may be warranted based on the needs of the individual patient, resources, and limitations unique to the institution or type of practice.

Breast Cancer Screening

Early detection of breast cancer has been shown to decrease the mortality rate (1). Technology continues to evolve to improve the accuracy of detection. In addition, the process of individual risk assessment is evolving, and new factors that affect risk are being identified. The purpose of this document is to clarify the rationale for current breast cancer screening guidelines and evaluate the evidence regarding screening techniques. It also focuses on mammography and other detection techniques as screening tools to identify nonpalpable lesions; the use of mammography for diagnostic purposes when a lesion is palpated is addressed briefly.

Background

Incidence

Breast cancer is the most common malignancy among U.S. women (excluding skin cancer); it is the second leading cause of death from cancer among American women (lung cancer is first). A woman's lifetime risk (80-year life-span) of developing breast cancer is 12.5%, or 1 in 8 (Table 1) (2). It is estimated that in 2003, 211,300 new cases of invasive breast cancer will be diagnosed (32% of all cancers in women), and 39,800 deaths will be attributable to breast cancer (15% of all cancer deaths in women) (3). In addition, 55,700 new cases of in situ breast cancer are expected to be diagnosed in 2003 (1).

Current Mammography Screening Guidelines

The most recent breast cancer screening guidelines recommend that mammography be performed every 1–2 years for women aged 40–49 years and annually thereafter (4). Most guidelines have dropped the suggestion to obtain routine baseline mammograms in women younger than 40 years. Most have recommended annual screening mammography and clinical breast examination for women aged 50 years and older. However, published and public controversy about the potential benefits and risks of screening mammography continues.

Table 1. Age-Specific Probabilities of Developing Breast Cancer*

If Current Age is	Then the Probability of Developing Breast Cancer in the Next 10 Years is:†	or the Probability of Developing Breast Cancer is 1 in:
20	0.05%	2,044
30	0.40%	249
40	1.49%	67
50	2.77%	36
60	3.45%	29
70	4.16%	24

*Among those free of cancer at beginning of age interval. Based on cases diagnosed 1995–1997. Percentages and "1 in" numbers may not be numerically equivalent because of rounding.

†Probability derived using NCI DEVCAN software. American Cancer Society, Surveillance Research, 2001.

American Cancer Society. Breast Cancer Facts & Figures 2001–2002. American Cancer Society, Inc. Atlanta (GA): ACS; 2002. p. 9.

Of the eight published randomized, controlled trials of screening for breast cancer with mammography, questions have been raised regarding trial design, randomization, exclusions, reallocations, contamination (the number of women in the control group who underwent mammography on their own), compliance (the number of women in the study group who, for whatever reason, did not undergo screening mammography), mammography screening of the control group before they entered the study, verification of a disease-specific cause of death, autopsy rates, and variations in cancer therapy (5–15). The variability of the design, technology, methodology, interpretation, and endpoints of most of the trials does not permit meaningful comparisons. All the screening mammography trials were designed and carried out before the current stringent and exacting format for a population-based randomized trial was established. No consensus exists regarding the optimum details of the design and formatting of a population-based, randomized clinical trial to assess breast cancer screening.

Rationale for Mammography Screening
Mathematical Model

In 1966, Macdonald estimated invasive breast cancer doubling times to range from 23 to 209 days, with an average of 128 days for localized cancer and 85 days for metastatic cancer (16). A graph based on mathematical calculation of 100-day doubling time revealed an 8-year preclinical phase and a 4-year clinical phase of breast cancer growth, which occurs before the usual size when breast cancer is diagnosed. Later, Gullino reported a range of 45–260 days for invasive breast cancer doubling time and modified the 100-day doubling time graph (17), which was subsequently modified by Wertheimer to demonstrate the potential benefit of screening mammography (18).

Thus, by mathematical estimation, a typical ductal adenocarcinoma with a constant mean doubling time of 100 days would have been present for more than 11 years before it grew to a generally palpable size of 2 cm. Mammography screening could potentially identify a nonpalpable mass of approximately 1 mm to 1 cm during its preclinical phase 3 years before it became palpable (16–19).

Validation of the Model

Validation of the calculations of time of metastasis came from a 1992 study that monitored 767 patients with node-negative breast cancer for a median of 18 years (20). It revealed that 89% of the patients with T1 N0 M0 cancers of 1 cm or less were cured by primary surgery (mastectomy and axillary dissection). Numerous other studies have subsequently confirmed similar results, with 90% of patients experiencing 10-year (or longer) disease-free survival periods after cancers of 1 cm or less were detected by mammography, indicating the probability that the cancers had not yet metastasized before they were diagnosed and treated (21–25).

Studies Documenting the Value of Mammography

Most studies of mammography use mortality as the endpoint, so the value of screening often is solely based on mortality rates. Few studies take into account the effects of early detection on quality of life or the fact that treatment at earlier stages carries less morbidity.

In 1966, a preliminary report described the Health Insurance Plan of Greater New York, a randomized, controlled trial initiated in 1963 (15). Women aged 40–64 years were randomly assigned to a study or control group (30,000 women in each group). After an initial screening (two-view mammography and clinical examination), the study group was offered annual rescreening for 3 additional years. Ten-year and 18-year follow-up reports validated the clinical application of mammography for breast cancer screening (26–28). An approximate 25% lower breast cancer mortality rate was demonstrated for the screened group (28).

In 1982, the Breast Cancer Detection Demonstration Project established the applicability of breast cancer screening with mammography to identify nonpalpable lesions. The Breast Cancer Detection Demonstration Project consisted of 29 nationwide centers, which recruited more than 280,000 women between the ages of 35 and 74 years (mean age: 49.5 years) for breast cancer screening by means of physical examination and mammography. The 5-year result demonstrated that 8.7% of breast cancers were detected by physical examination only, 41.6% were detected by mammography only, and 47.3% were detected by both mammography and physical examination (29). Of infiltrating breast cancers smaller than 1 cm, 52.6% were detected only by mammography. Among the 4,240 women in whom breast cancer was detected and treated, the 10-year survival rate was 79% (30).

In 1985, the Swedish Two-County clinical trial demonstrated a 31% decrease in mortality from breast cancer with the use of screening mammography from 1978 to 1984 when 77,080 women who were invited to receive mammography screening were compared with 55,985 controls who were not offered screening (12). Subsequent long-term analysis of the Swedish trial data revealed a 63% decrease in breast cancer mortality in women aged 40–69 years when the women who had mammography screening between 1988 and 1996 were compared with women from 1968 to 1977, when screening mammography was not available (31). When adjusted for selection bias and inclusion of the nonattendees, the overall decrease in mortality was 48% in the screened group (31). Modeling studies of annual screening estimated a 36% decrease in breast cancer mortality among women aged 40–49 years (32). Twenty-year follow-up data for women aged 40–69 years confirmed an overall 32% reduction in breast cancer mortality (relative risk [RR], 0.68; 95% confidence interval [CI], 0.59–0.80) (33).

In the Gothenburg Breast Cancer Screening Trial, women aged 39–49 years had mammography screening every 18 months for five cycles; 11,724 women were enrolled in the screening study group, and 14,217 were in the control group (34). A 44% reduction in mortality (RR, 0.56; $P = 0.042$; 95% CI, 0.32–0.98) was demonstrated in the screened group versus the control group. The Malmo Mammographic Screening Program that updated results for mammography screening of women younger than 50 years had a breast cancer mortality reduction of 36% (RR, 0.64; 95% CI, 0.45–0.89) (35).

Long-term analyses also predict decreases in mortality. Mammography programs in the United Kingdom and the Netherlands project mortality reductions of 24%

and 29%, respectively (36). In the United States between 1990 and 1999, the breast cancer mortality rate decreased by 17% (37), which correlates with the increasing use of mammography (38). However, it has been suggested that the decrease in breast cancer mortality in the United States is approximately 39%, which is an estimate that includes the 36.8% increased incidence of breast cancer between 1980 and 1999 (39).

Meta-analyses

Meta-analyses in 1995 and 2002 of screening mammography randomized clinical trials revealed a 26% (RR, 0.74; 95% CI, 0.66–0.83) and 27% (RR, 0.73; 95% CI, 0.59–0.93) reduction in breast cancer mortality, respectively (5, 40). A meta-analysis of the accuracy of screening mammography reported a true-positive rate ranging from 83% to 95% and a false-positive rate ranging from 0.9% to 6.5% (41). A meta-analysis in 1997 of updated data on women aged 40–49 years in eight randomized controlled trials with an average follow-up time of 12.7 years documented an 18% (RR, 0.82; 95% CI, 0.71–0.95) mortality reduction for women invited to screening (42). In 2002, a subsequent meta-analysis of seven randomized clinical trials with data for women younger than 50 years revealed a similar 18% (RR, 0.82; 95% CI, 0.66–1.02) breast cancer mortality reduction with screening mammography (5). The 2002 updated overview of the Swedish screening mammography randomized trials (129,750 subjects and 117,260 controls) with a median follow-up of 15.8 years confirmed a significant 21% (RR, 0.79; 95% CI, 0.70–0.89) breast cancer mortality reduction (43).

Frequency and Timing of Mammography Screening

Using Health Insurance Plan of Greater New York data, it has been calculated that beginning screening at age 40 years instead of age 50 years reduces breast cancer mortality by 14 per 10,000 women per year (95% CI, 4–32/10,000) (44). Initiating screening at this age, however, increases the number of noncancer biopsies.

On the basis of Health Insurance Plan of Greater New York and Breast Cancer Detection Demonstration Project data, the estimated lead-time (the time between detection on mammography and when the lesion is clinically detectable) for invasive breast cancer is 1.7 years (range: 0.4–3 years), which suggests that the optimal screening interval would be no more than 1.7 years (19). A study of 105 interval breast cancers (ie, those diagnosed between screening rounds) noted that for true interval cancers, one quarter were fast growing (14/57) and were characterized by young age, absence of calcification, and lymph-node-positive cancers (45). The observed 5-year survival rate for women with fast-growing true interval cancers was 54% compared with 80% for women with slower-growing cancers.

The Falun (Sweden) Meeting Committee and collaborators reviewed the Swedish Two-County Trial's 34% mortality rate reduction for women who entered the trial at age 50–69 years and who were screened every 33 months (46). They estimated a 39% mortality reduction with screening every 2 years and a 45% mortality reduction with annual screening.

Review of the available data on mammography screening for women aged 40–49 years indicates that with high-quality mammography and screening intervals of 12–18 months, an equivalent breast cancer mortality reduction can be achieved in women aged 40–49 years as for women aged 50 years and older (47). As a group, younger women (eg, aged 40–49 years) have a shorter detectable preclinical phase of breast cancer than women aged 50 years and older; that is, the duration of time when a cancer can be detected by mammography before the cancer is palpable is shorter in women aged 40–49 years. These findings suggest that a short screening interval may be particularly important in younger women (32, 39, 47, 48).

Other studies have found that women aged 40–49 years who have an observed 13% mortality reduction with screening every 2 years have an estimated 36% mortality reduction with annual screening (39, 46). Several modeling studies of women aged 40–49 years indicate similar greater mortality benefits from annual screening (48–50).

Not all investigators agree that more frequent screening in younger women is beneficial. The Canadian National Breast Screening Study I randomized 50,430 women aged 40–49 years to annual mammography, breast physical examination, and breast self-examination or usual community health care with annual follow-up (51). After 11–16 years of follow-up, no difference in the rate of breast cancer mortality was found between the groups. In addition, the study was sufficiently large enough to demonstrate that at most one death per 10,000 women per year would be prevented or caused by mammography screening. The authors concluded that for women younger than 50 years, the benefits of screening mammography are uncertain with the availability of breast self-examination, clinical breast examination, diagnostic mammography, and effective cancer therapy. They noted that the adverse consequences of false-positive mammography results also should be considered. Two detailed analyses of mammography for women aged 40–49 years concluded that mammography screening was relatively cost-ineffective because of the decreased efficacy of mammography (related to a higher percentage of women with dense breast tissue) and the low incidence of breast cancer in this age group (52, 53).

A historical, prospective cohort study of 971 women who were aged 40–49 years at the time their breast cancer was diagnosed revealed that those with cancer detected by mammography had smaller mean tumor sizes, had tumors that were more often localized, and had better survival rates than patients whose cancers were detected by breast self-examination, patients' incidental findings, or clinical breast examination (54). All the differences were statistically significant even when survival was adjusted for the lead-time bias for cancer detected by mammography (54). Detailed analysis of the Nijmegen population-based breast cancer screening data indicates that some small cancers detected by mammography metastasize early and are clinically diagnosed at an advanced stage (55–57). Furthermore, the women aged 40–49 years had proportionally more lymph-node-positive cancers at the time of diagnosis compared with women older than 50 years (55, 56). Other studies have confirmed more rapid breast cancer growth rates in younger women (eg, those aged 40–49 years) (58, 59). These studies also found that decreased mammogram sensitivity in women younger than 50 years was not a function of breast density (58, 59). This apparently more aggressive biologic behavior of cancers in women aged 40–49 years and analysis of age-related breast cancer screening efficiency in the Swedish Two-County trial led to recommendations for more frequent screening (eg, annual) for women aged 40–49 years (50, 59, 60).

Adverse Consequences of Screening Mammography

Initial concerns about the risk of radiation (eg, induction of breast cancer by radiation) have largely been allayed by improvements in mammography technique, technology, and clinical experience (61–63). False-positive mammograms (ie, those with perceived abnormalities requiring further evaluation to verify that the lesion is not cancer) are a continuing concern (62, 64). False-positive screening mammograms require diagnostic mammography with supplementary views, ultrasonography, and even biopsy in 20–30% of cases in an attempt to reach an accurate diagnosis (62, 64). Psychosocial consequences of screening mammography have been identified and reviewed (65, 66). These psychologic, behavioral, and quality-of-life issues seem to be intrinsic to the fear of breast cancer (67).

Other Screening Techniques

Clinical breast examination and breast self-examination as breast cancer screening methods have been the subject of multiple studies with conflicting conclusions. As primary screening for breast cancer, both methods lack the support of published rigorous clinical trials, particularly when the endpoint is decreased breast cancer mortality. Furthermore, both methods only detect palpable lesions. For breast cancer screening, the American Cancer Society recommends clinical breast examination every 3 years for women aged 20–39 years and annually beginning at age 40 years (60).

Ultrasonography is an established adjunct to mammography in the imaging evaluation. It is useful in evaluating inconclusive mammographic findings, in evaluating young patients and other women with dense breast tissue, in guiding tissue core-needle biopsy and other biopsy techniques, and in differentiating a cyst from a solid mass. Magnetic resonance imaging can be a useful adjunct to diagnostic mammography, but cost, duration of the examination, and injection of contrast material prohibit its use as a routine, population-based screening technique. Color Doppler ultrasonography, computer-aided detection, positron emission tomography, scinti-mammography, step-oblique mammography, and thermography have shown promise in specific, selected situations but remain under clinical investigation and have not been proposed as effective screening techniques. A detailed review of breast imaging and related technologies (as of 2001) is available elsewhere (68).

Clinical Considerations and Recommendations

▶ Is breast self-examination effective in the general population?

A critical review by the U.S. Preventive Services Task Force in 1987 found no controlled prospective trials on the effect of breast self-examination on breast cancer mortality and noted consistently low sensitivity of breast self-examination, estimated at 20–30%, compared with clinical breast examination and mammography (69). In 2002, an updated and more extensive review by the U.S. Preventive Services Task Force found insufficient evidence for or against breast self-examination (70).

A prospective study of 604 patients with breast cancer revealed that only 7.6% of the 448 women who practiced regular breast self-examination had detected their own cancers, and those who did showed no survival advantage (71). The Shanghai breast self-examination trial of 266,000 women aged 39–72 years randomized to receive either breast self-examination instruction plus follow-up or no information on breast cancer screening reported essentially no difference in the number of deaths from breast cancer between the two groups (135 versus 131, respectively) after 10–11 years of follow-up (72). Although

breast cancers were detected at an earlier stage in the women who received instruction, the difference between the two groups was not statistically significant and yielded no clinical differences in terms of mortality. However, women in the instruction group were more likely to undergo breast biopsy for benign lesions (72).

An analysis by the Canadian Task Force on Preventive Health Care revealed fair evidence that breast self-examination had no benefit and good evidence that it was harmful. This group concluded that among women aged 40–69 years, routine teaching of breast self-examination should be excluded from breast cancer screening (73). Increased physician visits and higher rates of benign breast biopsies were documented to be adverse effects of breast self-examination (73, 74). In addition, studies were cited that revealed patients experienced increased worry, anxiety, and depression associated with breast self-examination (73). Despite a lack of definitive data for or against breast self-examination, breast self-examination has the potential to detect palpable breast cancer and can be recommended.

▶ Is clinical breast examination effective for breast cancer screening? If so, how frequently should it be performed?

Pooled data for all controlled trials and case–control studies in which clinical breast examination was used for breast cancer screening revealed a sensitivity of 54% and a specificity of 94%. Although the evidence was indirect, the review supported the use and effectiveness of clinical breast examination (75). The frequency of clinical breast examination was not addressed.

An analysis of 752,081 clinical breast examinations from the National Breast and Cervical Cancer Early Detection Program found that 6.9% were coded as abnormal, and five cancers were palpated per 1,000 clinical breast examinations (76). This study found clinical breast examination to have a sensitivity of 58.8%, specificity of 93.4%, and a positive predictive value of 4.3%. In addition, clinical breast examination detected 7.4 cancers per 1,000 women with normal screening mammograms (95% CI, 6.3–8.4).

Multiple reviews have supported the combination of clinical breast examination and mammography for breast cancer screening for women aged 50–69 years (77–80). Analysis of the Swedish trial revealed that in women aged 50–74 years, the mean size of the invasive cancers detected by physical examination was 23.1 mm, whereas the mean size of the cancers detected by mammography was 13.4 mm (59).

In a retrospective, computer-aided study of breast cancers missed by clinical breast examination or mammography, the threshold of palpability was 6 mm, and the majority of the cancers detected by clinical breast examination were larger than 16 mm (in a consecutive series of 509 breast cancers) (81). In further analysis of 553 consecutive breast cancers, 9% were not detected by the mammograms.

Studies of efficacy have looked only at annual clinical breast examination; no studies have addressed other intervals. Therefore, there are no data on which to base a recommendation on the frequency of clinical breast examination. However, it seems prudent to perform clinical breast examination annually, perhaps with the annual physical examination.

▶ How frequently should mammography be performed?

Various groups have offered recommendations on the frequency of mammography screening. Each group places different values on competing considerations, such as published evidence, cost-effectiveness, efficiency, accuracy, adverse consequences, specificity, sensitivity, false-positive results, false-negative results, positive predictive value, patient compliance, availability of health care resources, conflicting health care needs, and potential benefits.

The U.S. Preventive Services Task Force updated its 1996 guidelines after reviewing the evidence about the efficacy of breast self-examination, clinical breast examination, and mammography in reducing breast cancer mortality (82). It recommends screening mammography every 1–2 years for women aged 40 years and older. The American Cancer Society recommends annual screening mammography beginning at age 40 years (60). Data from the Swedish trial and others suggest that an interval of every 1–2 years may be appropriate for women aged 50–74 years (33, 83, 84).

In light of available data, the optimal screening interval appears to be every 1–2 years for women aged 40–49 years and annually thereafter. Current data do not clearly support a recommendation as to whether mammography annually or every 2 years is superior. The U.S. Preventive Services Task Force notes:

> "The absolute probability of benefits of regular mammography increases along a continuum with age, whereas the likelihood of harms from screening (false-positive results and unnecessary anxiety, biopsies, and cost) diminishes from ages 40 to 70. The balance of benefits and potential harms, therefore, grows more favorable as women age. The precise age at which the potential benefits of mammography justify the possible harms is a subjective choice" (82).

▶ What elements of patient history should be used to determine risk and to guide screening?

Most women in whom invasive breast cancer is diagnosed do not have unique identifiable risk factors (67, 85). The incidence of breast cancer increases with advancing age (86). A personal history of breast cancer, either invasive or in situ, is a clinically meaningful risk factor (67, 85). Although the Agency for Healthcare Research and Quality has not evaluated genetic risk factors, it recommends against modifying the workup on the basis of risk factors other than age (Table 2) (85).

Table 2. Factors That Increase the Relative Risk for Breast Cancer in Women

Relative Risk	Factor
Relative risk >4	Certain inherited genetic mutations for breast cancer
	Two or more first-degree relatives with breast cancer diagnosed at an early age
	Personal history of breast cancer
	Age (≥65 vs <65 years, although risk increases across all ages until age 80 years)
Relative risk 2.1–4	One first-degree relative with breast cancer
	Nodular densities on mammogram (>75% of breast volume)
	Atypical hyperplasia
	High-dose ionizing radiation to the chest
	Ovaries not surgically removed (age <40 years)
Relative risk 1.1–2	High socioeconomic status
	Urban residence
	Northern U.S. residence
Reproductive factors	Early menarche (age <12 years)
	Late menopause (age ≥55 years)
	No term pregnancies (for breast cancer diagnosed at age ≥40 years)
	Late age at first term pregnancy (≥30 years)
	Never breastfed a child
Other factors that affect circulating hormones or genetic susceptibility	Postmenopausal obesity
	Alcohol consumption
	Recent hormone therapy
	Recent oral contraceptive use
	Tall stature
	Personal history of cancer of endometrium, ovary, or colon
	Jewish heritage

Reprinted with permission from Elsevier Science (The Lancet, 1995, Vol 346, 883–7).

▶ *Should anyone be screened before age 40 years?*

Despite an estimated 50–80% lifetime risk of breast cancer for those who carry the *BRCA1* or *BRCA2* mutation, few have advised any changes in the population-based guidelines for screening mammography in this high-risk group (87, 88). Acknowledging that no surveillance data or related clinical trials are available for *BRCA1* or *BRCA2* carriers, the Cancer Genetics Studies Consortium has offered Level-III provisional recommendations of 1) education regarding monthly breast self-examination, 2) annual or semiannual clinical breast examination beginning at age 25–35 years, and 3) annual mammography beginning at age 25–35 years (88).

▶ *Is there an upper age range when the risks of mammography outweigh the benefits?*

Figure 1 illustrates the progressively increasing incidence and mortality rates of invasive breast cancer through age 84 years (2). The majority of the screening mammography clinical trials had an upper age limit criteria ranging from 64 to 74 years. Medical co-morbidity and life expectancy should be considered in a breast cancer screening program for women aged 75 years or older because the benefit-to-risk ratio of screening mammography continues to shift adversely with advancing age. A consensus of recommendations does not exist. However,

a meta-analysis concluded that screening mammography in women aged 70–79 years is moderately cost-effective and yields a small increase in life expectancy (89).

▶ *How should a palpable breast mass be evaluated?*

A palpable breast mass requires a follow-up examination and additional diagnostic testing. It has been suggested that in younger women (defined by some institutions as age younger than 40 years) with dense breast tissue, evaluation of a palpable mass begins with an ultrasound examination performed by an individual experienced in breast imaging, followed by diagnostic mammography, if necessary. For those women aged 40 years and older with a palpable mass, it has been suggested that evaluation begin with diagnostic mammography and include ultrasound breast imaging, if useful, performed by an individual experienced in diagnostic breast imaging. Screening mammography is not sufficient to rule out malignancy (85). A solid, dominant, persistent mass requires tissue diagnosis by fine needle aspiration or biopsy (85).

Ultrasonography may be useful to define a cystic lesion. If a cyst is aspirated and the fluid is clear (transparent and not bloody), there is no need for cytology (85). If the cyst does not disappear after aspiration or recurs within 6 weeks, surgical follow-up should be considered.

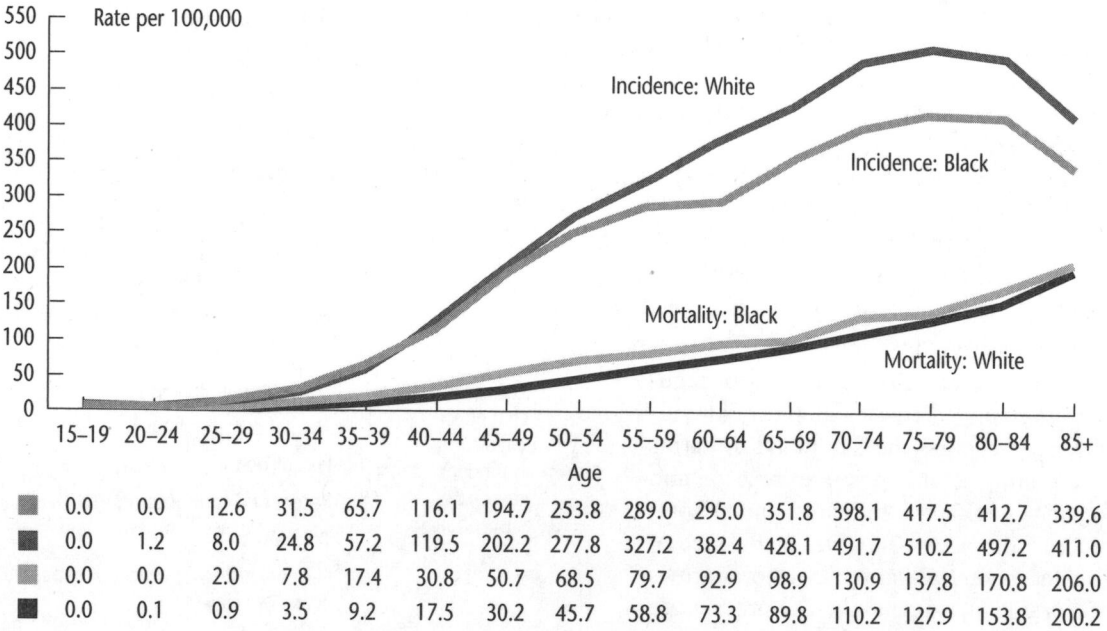

	15–19	20–24	25–29	30–34	35–39	40–44	45–49	50–54	55–59	60–64	65–69	70–74	75–79	80–84	85+
■	0.0	0.0	12.6	31.5	65.7	116.1	194.7	253.8	289.0	295.0	351.8	398.1	417.5	412.7	339.6
■	0.0	1.2	8.0	24.8	57.2	119.5	202.2	277.8	327.2	382.4	428.1	491.7	510.2	497.2	411.0
■	0.0	0.0	2.0	7.8	17.4	30.8	50.7	68.5	79.7	92.9	98.9	130.9	137.8	170.8	206.0
■	0.0	0.1	0.9	3.5	9.2	17.5	30.2	45.7	58.8	73.3	89.8	110.2	127.9	153.8	200.2

Figure 1. Female breast cancer—age-specific incidence and death rates, by race, United States, 1994–1998. (American Cancer Society. Breast Cancer Facts & Figures 2001–2002. American Cancer Society, Inc. Atlanta [GA]: ACS; 2002. p. 2.)

▶ *When a nonpalpable mass is detected by mammography, how should management proceed?*

When a nonpalpable mass is perceived on screening mammography, the patient should be referred to a professional experienced in the diagnosis of breast cancer. This individual can perform a complete imaging workup and make subsequent recommendations.

▶ *If a woman feels a mass that is not palpable to the clinician, how should management proceed?*

Mammography is useful in evaluating women who suspect they have a breast mass that the clinician cannot palpate (90, 91). In such cases, focused ultrasound imaging may be a component of the complete imaging evaluation at any age (92, 93). A nonpalpable mass may require needle localization biopsy or stereotactic biopsy.

▶ *Who should be referred for genetic counseling?*

Women may benefit from genetic counseling and testing if their family history, including age at diagnosis and type of all cancers (in any relatives, female and male), suggests a possible autosomal dominant cancer pattern or if a *BRCA* mutation has been discovered in their family (88, 94). Genetic counseling will address the risks and benefits of the test.

Summary of Recommendations

The following recommendations are based on limited and inconsistent scientific evidence (Level B):

▶ Women aged 40–49 years should have screening mammography every 1–2 years.

▶ Women aged 50 years and older should have annual screening mammography.

The following recommendations are based primarily on consensus and expert opinion (Level C):

▶ Despite a lack of definitive data for or against breast self-examination, breast self-examination has the potential to detect palpable breast cancer and can be recommended.

▶ All women should have clinical breast examinations annually as part of the physical examination.

References

1. American Cancer Society. Cancer facts & figures 2003. Atlanta (GA): ACS; 2003. (Level II-3)
2. American Cancer Society. Breast cancer facts & figures 2001–2002. Atlanta (GA): ACS; 2001. (Level II–3)
3. Jemal A, Thomas A, Murray T, Thun M. Cancer statistics, 2002. CA Cancer J Clin 2002;52:23–47. (Level II–3)
4. American College of Obstetricians and Gynecologists. Routine cancer screening. ACOG Committee Opinion 247. Washington, DC: ACOG; 2000. (Level III)
5. Humphrey LL, Helfand M, Chan BK, Woolf SH. Breast cancer screening: a summary of the evidence for the U.S. Preventive Services Task Force. Ann Intern Med 2002;137:347–60. (Meta-analysis)
6. Miller AB, Baines CJ, To T, Wall C. Canadian National Breast Screening Study: 1. Breast cancer detection and death rates among women aged 40 to 49 years. CMAJ 1992;147:1459–76. (Level I)
7. Miller AB, Baines CJ, To T, Wall C. Canadian National Breast Screening Study: 2. Breast cancer detection and death rates among women aged 50 to 59 years. CMAJ 1992;147:1477–88. (Level I)
8. Alexander FE, Anderson TJ, Brown HK, Forrest AP, Hepburn W, Kirkpatrick AE, et al. The Edinburgh randomised trial of breast cancer screening: results after 10 years of follow-up. Br J Cancer 1994;70:542–8. (Level I)
9. Bjurstam N, Bjorneld L, Duffy SW, Smith TC, Cahlin E, Eriksson O, et al. The Gothenburg breast cancer screening trial: preliminary results on breast cancer mortality for women aged 39–49. J Natl Cancer Inst Monogr 1997;(22):53–5. (Level I)
10. Andersson I, Aspegren K, Janzon L, Landberg T, Lindholm K, Linell F, et al. Mammographic screening and mortality from breast cancer: the Malmo mammographic screening trial. BMJ 1988;297:943–8. (Level I)
11. Frisell J, Glas U, Hellstrom L, Somell A. Randomised mammographic screening for breast cancer in Stockholm. Design, first round results and comparisons. Breast Cancer Res Treat 1986;8:45–54. (Level I)
12. Tabar L, Fagerberg CJ, Gad A, Baldetorp L, Holmberg LH, Grontoft O, et al. Reduction in mortality from breast cancer after mass screening with mammography. Randomised trial from the Breast Cancer Screening Working Group of the Swedish National Board of Health and Welfare. Lancet 1985;1:829–32. (Level I)
13. Olsen O, Gotzsche PC. Cochrane review on screening for breast cancer with mammography. Lancet 2001;358:1340–2. (Meta-analysis)
14. Olsen O, Gotzsche PC. Screening for breast cancer with mammography (Cochrane Review). In: The Cochrane Library, Issue 4, 2002. Oxford: Update Software. (Meta-analysis)
15. Shapiro S, Strax P, Venet L. Evaluation of periodic breast cancer screening with mammography. Methodology and early observations. JAMA 1966;195:731–8. (Level I)

16. Macdonald I. The natural history of mammary carcinoma. Am J Surg 1966;111:435–42. (Level III)

17. Gullino PM. Natural history of breast cancer. Progression from hyperplasia to neoplasia as predicted by angiogenesis. Cancer 1977;39:2697–2703. (Level III)

18. Wertheimer MD, Costanza ME, Dodson TF, D'Orsi C, Pastides H, Zapka JG. Increasing the effort toward breast cancer detection. JAMA 1986;255:1311–5. (Level III)

19. Walter SD, Day NE. Estimation of the duration of a preclinical disease state using screening data. Am J Epidemiol 1983;118:865–86. (Level III)

20. Rosen PP, Groshen S, Kinne DW. Survival and prognostic factors in node-negative breast cancer: results of long-term follow-up studies. J Natl Cancer Inst Monogr 1992;(11):159–62. (Level II-2)

21. Tabar L, Dean PB, Kaufman CS, Duffy SW, Chen HH. A new era in the diagnosis of breast cancer. Surg Oncol Clin N Am 2000;9:233–77. (Level III)

22. Tabar L, Chen HH, Duffy SW, Yen MF, Chiang CF, Dean PB, et al. A novel method for prediction of long-term outcome of women with T1a, T1b, and 10–14 mm invasive breast cancers: a prospective study. Lancet 2000;355: 429–33. (Level II-2)

23. Joensuu H, Pylkkanen L, Toikkanen S. Late mortality from pT1N0M0 breast carcinoma. Cancer 1999;85: 2183–9. (Level II-2)

24. Lopez MJ, Smart CR. Twenty-year follow-up of minimal breast cancer from the Breast Cancer Detection Demonstration Project. Surg Oncol Clin N Am 1997; 6:393–401. (Level II-2)

25. Arnesson LG, Smeds S, Fagerberg G. Recurrence-free survival in patients with small breast cancer. An analysis of cancers 10 mm or less detected clinically and by screening. Eur J Surg 1994;160:271–6. (Level II–2)

26. Shapiro S, Venet W, Strax P, Venet L, Roeser R. Ten- to fourteen-year effect of screening on breast cancer mortality. J Natl Cancer Inst 1982;69:349–55. (Level I)

27. Shapiro S, Venet W, Strax P, Venet L. Mortality and case survival. In: Periodic screening for breast cancer: the health insurance plan project and its sequelae, 1963–1986. Baltimore (MD): Johns Hopkins University Press; 1988. p. 59–83. (Level III)

28. Shapiro S. Periodic screening for breast cancer: the HIP Randomized Controlled Trial. Health Insurance Plan. J Natl Cancer Inst Monogr 1997;(22):27–30. (Level I)

29. Baker LH. Breast Cancer Detection Demonstration Project: five-year summary report. CA Cancer J Clin 1982;32:194–225. (Level II-3)

30. Seidman H, Gelb SK, Silverberg E, LaVerda N, Lubera JA, et al. Survival experience in the Breast Cancer Detection Demonstration Project. CA Cancer J Clin 1987;37:258–90. (Level II-3)

31. Tabar L, Vitak B, Chen HH, Yen MF, Duffy SW, Smith RA. Beyond randomized controlled trials: organized mammographic screening substantially reduces breast carcinoma mortality. Cancer 2001;91:1724–31. (Level II–2)

32. Tabar L, Duffy SW, Vitak B, Chen HH, Prevost TC. The natural history of breast carcinoma: what have we learned from screening? Cancer 1999;86:449–62. (Level I)

33. Tabar L, Vitak B, Chen HH, Duffy SW, Yen MF, Chiang CF, et al. The Swedish Two–County Trial twenty years later. Updated mortality results and new insights from long-term follow-up. Radiol Clin North Am 2000;38: 625–51. (Level I)

34. Bjurstam N, Bjorneld L, Duffy SW, Smith TC, Cahlin E, Eriksson O, et al. The Gothenburg breast cancer screening trial: preliminary results on breast cancer mortality for women aged 39–49. J Natl Cancer Inst Monogr 1997; (22):53–5. (Level I)

35. Andersson I, Janzon L. Reduced breast cancer mortality in women under age 50: updated results from the Malmo Mammographic Screening Program. J Natl Cancer Inst Monogr 1997;(22):63–7. (Level I)

36. van den Akker-van Marle E, de Koning H, Boer R, van der Maas P. Reduction in breast cancer mortality due to the introduction of mass screening in The Netherlands: comparison with the United Kingdom. J Med Screen 1999;6:30–4. (Level II–3)

37. National Cancer Institute. SEER cancer statistics review, 1973–1999. Bethesda (MD): NCI; 2002. Available at http:// seer.cancer.gov/csr/1973_1999/. Retrieved December 13, 2002. (Level II–3)

38. Breen N, Wagener DK, Brown ML, Davis WW, Ballard-Barbash R. Progress in cancer screening over a decade: results of cancer screening from the 1987, 1992, and 1998 National Health Interview Surveys. J Natl Cancer Inst 2001;93:1704–13. (Level II–3)

39. Feig SA. Effect of service screening mammography on population mortality from breast carcinoma. Cancer 2002;95:451–7. (Level III)

40. Kerlikowske K, Grady D, Rubin SM, Sandrock C, Ernster V. Efficacy of screening mammography. A meta-analysis. JAMA 1995;273:149–54. (Meta-analysis)

41. Mushlin AI, Kouides RW, Shapiro DE. Estimating the accuracy of screening mammography: a meta-analysis. Am J Prev Med 1998;14:143–53. (Meta-analysis)

42. Hendrick RE, Smith RA, Rutledge JH 3rd, Smart CR. Benefit of screening mammography in women aged 40–49: a new meta-analysis of randomized controlled trials. J Natl Cancer Inst Monogr 1997;(22):87–92. (Meta-analysis)

43. Nystrom L, Andersson I, Bjurstam N, Frisell J, Nordenskjold B, Rutqvist LE. Long-term effects of mammography screening: updated overview of the Swedish randomised trials. Lancet 2002;359:909–19. (Level III)

44. Baker SG. Evaluating the age to begin periodic breast cancer screening using data from a few regularly scheduled screenings. Biometrics 1998;54:1569–78. (Level III)

45. Brekelmans CT, van Gorp JM, Peeters PH, Collette HJ. Histopathology and growth rate of interval breast carcinoma. Characterization of different subgroups. Cancer 1996;78:1220–8. (Level II-3)

46. Breast–cancer screening with mammography in women aged 40–49 years. Swedish Cancer Society and the Swedish National Board of Health and Welfare. Int J Cancer 1996;68:693–9. (Level III)

47. Smith RA. Breast cancer screening among women younger than age 50: a current assessment of the issues. CA Cancer J Clin 2000;50:312–36. (Meta-analysis)

48. Feig SA. Increased benefit from shorter screening mammography intervals for women ages 40–49 years. Cancer 1997;80:2035–9. (Level III)

49. Michaelson JS, Halpern E, Kopans DB. Breast cancer: computer simulation method for estimating optimal intervals for screening. Radiology 1999;212:551–60. (Level III)

50. Feig SA. Strategies for improving sensitivity of screening mammography for women aged 40 to 49 years [editorial]. JAMA 1996;276:73–4. (Level III)

51. Miller AB, To T, Baines CJ, Wall C. The Canadian National Breast Screening Study-1: breast cancer mortality after 11 to 16 years of follow-up. A randomized screening trial of mammography in women age 40 to 49 years. Ann Intern Med 2002;137:305–12. (Level I)

52. Salzmann P, Kerlikowske K, Phillips K. Cost-effectiveness of extending screening mammography guidelines to include women 40 to 49 years of age. Ann Intern Med 1997;127:955–65. (Level III)

53. Vogel VG. Screening younger women at risk for breast cancer. J Natl Cancer Inst Monogr 1994;(16):55–60. (Level III)

54. McPherson CP, Swenson KK, Jolitz G, Murray CL. Survival of women ages 40–49 years with breast carcinoma according to method of detection. Cancer 1997;79:1923–32. (Level II–2)

55. Peer PG, Verbeek AL, Mravunac M, Hendriks JH, Holland R. Prognosis of younger and older patients with early breast cancer. Br J Cancer 1996;73:382–5. (Level II–3)

56. Peer PG, Holland R, Hendriks JH, Mravunac M, Verbeek AL. Age-specific effectiveness of the Nijmegen population-based breast cancer-screening program: assessment of early indicators of screening effectiveness. J Natl Cancer Inst 1994;86:436–41. (Level II–1)

57. Peer PG, van Dijck JA, Hendriks JH, Holland R, Verbeek AL. Age-dependent growth rate of primary breast cancer. Cancer 1993;71:3547–51. (Level II–2)

58. Kerlikowske K, Grady D, Barclay J, Sickles EA, Ernster V. Effect of age, breast density, and family history on the sensitivity of first screening mammography. JAMA 1996;276:33–8. (Level II–2)

59. Tabar L, Fagerberg G, Chen HH, Duffy SW, Smart CR, Gad A, et al. Efficacy of breast cancer screening by age. New results from the Swedish Two-County Trial. Cancer 1995;75:2507–17. (Level I)

60. Smith RA, Cokkinides V, von Eschenbach AC, Levin B, Cohen C, Runowicz CD, et al. American Cancer Society guidelines for the early detection of cancer. CA Cancer J Clin 2002;52:8–22. (Level III)

61. Feig SA, Hendrick RE. Radiation risk from screening mammography of women aged 40–49 years. J Natl Cancer Inst Monogr 1997;(22):119–24. (Level III)

62. Harris R. Variation of benefits and harms of breast cancer screening with age. J Natl Cancer Inst Monogr 1997;(22):139–43. (Level III)

63. Mattsson A, Ruden BI, Hall P, Wilking N, Rutqvist LE. Radiation-induced breast cancer: long-term follow-up of radiation therapy for benign breast disease. J Natl Cancer Inst 1993;85:1679–85. (Level II)

64. Elmore JG, Barton MB, Moceri VM, Polk S, Arena PJ, Fletcher SW. Ten-year risk of false positive screening mammograms and clinical breast examinations. N Engl J Med 1998;338:1089–96. (Level II–2)

65. Rimer BK, Bluman LG. The psychosocial consequences of mammography. J Natl Cancer Inst Monogr 1997;(22):131–8. (Level III)

66. Lerman C, Trock B, Rimer BK, Boyce A, Jepson C, Engstrom PF. Psychological and behavioral implications of abnormal mammograms. Ann Intern Med 1991;114:657–61. (Level II–3)

67. Overmoyer B. Breast cancer screening. Med Clin North Am 1999;83:1443–66, vi–vii. (Level III)

68. Breast imaging and related technologies. In: Institute of Medicine. Committee on the Early Detection of Breast Cancer. Mammography and beyond: developing technologies for the early detection of breast cancer. Washington, DC: National Academy Press; 2001. p. 55–104. (Level III)

69. O'Malley MS, Fletcher SW. US Preventative Services Task Force. Screening for breast cancer with breast self-examination. A critical review. JAMA 1987;257:2196–203. (Level III)

70. Humphrey LL, Helfand M, Chan BK, Woolf SH. Breast cancer screening: a summary of the evidence for the U.S. Preventive Services Task Force. Ann Intern Med 2002;137:347–60. (Meta-analysis)

71. Auvinen A, Elovainio L, Hakama M. Breast self–examination and survival from breast cancer: a prospective follow-up study. Breast Cancer Res Treat 1996;38:161–8. (Level II–2)

72. Thomas DB, Gao DL, Ray RM, Wang WW, Allison CJ, Chen FL, et al. Randomized trial of breast self-examination in Shanghai: final results. J Natl Cancer Inst 2002;94:1445–57. (Level I)

73. Baxter N. Preventive health care, 2001 update: should women be routinely taught breast self-examination to screen for breast cancer? CMAJ 2001;164:1837–46. (Level III)

74. Ellman R, Moss SM, Coleman D, Chamberlain J. Breast self-examination programmes in the trial of early detection of breast cancer: ten year findings. Br J Cancer 1993;68:208–12. (Level II-2)

75. Barton MB, Harris R, Fletcher SW. The rational clinical examination. Does this patient have breast cancer? The screening clinical breast examination: should it be done? How? JAMA 1999;282:1270–80. (Level III)

76. Bobo JK, Lee NC, Thames SF. Findings from 752,081 clinical breast examinations reported to a national screening program from 1995 through 1998. J Natl Cancer Inst 2000;92:971–6. (Level II–2)

77. Shen Y, Zelen M. Screening sensitivity and sojourn time from breast cancer early detection clinical trials: mammograms and physical examinations. J Clin Oncol 2001;19: 3490–9. (Level II–2)

78. Jatoi I. Breast cancer screening. Am J Surg 1999;177: 518–24. (Level III)

79. Primic-Zakelj M. Screening mammography for early detection of breast cancer. Ann Oncol 1999;10 (suppl 6):121–7. (Level III)

80. Fletcher SW, Black W, Harris R, Rimer BK, Shapiro S. Report of the International Workshop on Screening for Breast Cancer. J Natl Cancer Inst 1993;85:1644–56. (Level III)

81. Reintgen D, Berman C, Cox C, Baekey P, Nicosia S, Greenberg H, et al. The anatomy of missed breast cancers. Surg Oncol 1993;2:65–75. (Level II–2)

82. Screening for breast cancer: recommendation and rationale. Ann Intern Med 2002;137:344–6. (Level III)

83. Benedet JL, Bender H, Jones H 3rd, Ngan HY, Pecorelli S. FIGO staging classifications and clinical practice guidelines in the management of gynecologic cancers. FIGO Committee on Gynecologic Oncology. Int J Gynaecol Obstet 2000;70:209–62. (Level III)

84. Tabar L, Fagerberg G, Day NE, Holmberg L. What is the optimum interval between mammographic screening examinations? An analysis based on the latest results of the Swedish two-county breast cancer screening trial. Br J Cancer 1987;55:547–51. (Level I)

85. Agency for Healthcare Research and Quality. Diagnosis and management of specific breast abnormalities. Evidence Report/Technology Assessment 33. Rockville (MD): AHRQ; 2001. AHRQ publication no. 01–E046. (Level III)

86. National Cancer Institute. SEER cancer statistics review, 1973–1998. Bethesda (MD): NCI; 2001. Available at http://seer.cancer.gov/csr/1973_1998/. Retrieved December 13, 2002. (Level II–3)

87. Hulka BC, Stark AT. Breast cancer: cause and prevention. Lancet 1995;346:883–7. (Level III)

88. Burke W, Daly M, Garber J, Botkin J, Kahn MJ, Lynch P, et al. Recommendations for follow-up care of individuals with an inherited predisposition to cancer. II. BRCA1 and BRCA2. Cancer Genetics Studies Consortium. JAMA 1997;277:997–1003. (Level III)

89. Kerlikowske K, Salzmann P, Phillips KA, Cauley JA, Cummings SR. Continuing screening mammography in women aged 70 to 79 years: impact on life expectancy and cost-effectiveness. JAMA 1999;282:2156–63. (Level III)

90. Hindle WH, Davis L, Wright D. Clinical value of mammography for symptomatic women 35 years of age and younger. Am J Obstet Gynecol 1999;180:1484–90. (Level III)

91. Williams SM, Kaplan PA, Petersen JC, Lieberman RP. Mammography in women under age 30: is there clinical benefit? Radiology 1986;161:49–51. (Level III)

92. Kolb TM, Lichy J, Newhouse JH. Occult cancer in women with dense breasts: detection with screening US— diagnostic yield and tumor characteristics. Radiology 1998;207:191–9. (Level II–3)

93. Lister D, Evans AJ, Burrell HC, Blamey RW, Wilson AR, Pinder SE, et al. The accuracy of breast ultrasound in the evaluation of clinically benign discrete, symptomatic breast lumps. Clin Radiol 1998;53:490–2. (Level II–3)

94. Claus EB, Risch N, Thompson WD. Autosomal dominant inheritance of early-onset breast cancer. Implications for risk reduction. Cancer 1994;73:643–51. (Level III)

The MEDLINE database, the Cochrane Library, and ACOG's own internal resources and documents were used to conduct a literature search to locate relevant articles published between between January 1985 and July 2002. The search was restricted to articles published in the English language. Priority was given to articles reporting results of original research, although review articles and commentaries also were consulted. Abstracts of research presented at symposia and scientific conferences were not considered adequate for inclusion in this document. Guidelines published by organizations or institutions such as the National Institutes of Health and the American College of Obstetricians and Gynecologists were reviewed, and additional studies were located by reviewing bibliographies of identified articles. When reliable research was not available, expert opinions from obstetrician–gynecologists were used.

Studies were reviewed and evaluated for quality according to the method outlined by the U.S. Preventive Services Task Force:

I   Evidence obtained from at least one properly designed randomized controlled trial.

II-1 Evidence obtained from well-designed controlled trials without randomization.

II-2 Evidence obtained from well-designed cohort or case–control analytic studies, preferably from more than one center or research group.

II-3 Evidence obtained from multiple time series with or without the intervention. Dramatic results in uncontrolled experiments also could be regarded as this type of evidence.

III Opinions of respected authorities, based on clinical experience, descriptive studies, or reports of expert committees.

Based on the highest level of evidence found in the data, recommendations are provided and graded according to the following categories:

Level A—Recommendations are based on good and consistent scientific evidence.

Level B—Recommendations are based on limited or inconsistent scientific evidence.

Level C—Recommendations are based primarily on consensus and expert opinion.

ISSN 1099-3630

**The American College of
Obstetricians and Gynecologists
409 12th Street, SW
PO Box 96920
Washington, DC 20090-6920**

12345/76543

Breast cancer screening. ACOG Practice Bulletin No. 42. American College of Obstetricians and Gynecologists. Obstet Gynecol 2003;101:821–32.

ACOG PRACTICE BULLETIN

CLINICAL MANAGEMENT GUIDELINES FOR
OBSTETRICIAN–GYNECOLOGISTS

NUMBER 45, AUGUST 2003

(Replaces Committee Opinion Number 152, March 1995)

This Practice Bulletin was developed by the ACOG Committee on Practice Bulletins— Gynecology with the assistance of Alan G. Waxman, MD, MPH. The information is designed to aid practitioners in making decisions about appropriate obstetric and gynecologic care. These guidelines should not be construed as dictating an exclusive course of treatment or procedure. Variations in practice may be warranted based on the needs of the individual patient, resources, and limitations unique to the institution or type of practice.

Cervical Cytology Screening

Although cervical cancer was the leading cause of cancer death in American women as recently as the 1930s, both the incidence and mortality from cervical cancer have decreased by almost one half since the early 1970s, largely as a result of widespread screening with the Pap test (1–3). However, the annual incidence rate has remained at approximately 8 cases per 100,000 women over the past few years (4). New technology for performing cervical cytology is evolving rapidly, as are recommendations for classifying and interpreting the results. The purpose of this document is to provide a review of the best available evidence on screening for cervical cancer. Specific equipment and techniques for performing cervical cytology and interpretation of the results are discussed elsewhere.

Background

Value of Cervical Cytology

Although the incidence and mortality from cervical cancer have decreased substantially in the past several decades among women in the United States, cervical cancer remains the third most common gynecologic malignancy (2, 5). In countries where cytologic screening is not widely available, cervical cancer remains common. Worldwide, it is the second most common cancer among women, the third most common cause of cancer-related death, and the most common cause of mortality from gynecologic malignancy (3, 6, 7). When cervical cytology screening programs have been introduced into communities, however, marked reductions in cervical cancer incidence have followed (7–9).

Cervical cytology screening is, in many respects, the ideal screening test (8). Cervical cancer has a defined premalignant phase of many years, which allows repeated tests to significantly reduce the impact of individual false-negative test results. Cervical cytology is inexpensive and is readily accepted among American women. In 1998, 79% of women aged 18 years and older had cervical cytology screening in the preceding 3 years (10). Treatment is effective in reducing the chance of progression to invasive disease.

Despite effective screening measures and treatment, it is estimated that 50% of the women who receive cervical cancer diagnoses each year have never had cervical cytology screening. Another 10% had not been screened within the 5 years before diagnosis (11). Thus, one approach to reducing the incidence and mortality of cervical cancer would be to increase screening rates among women who currently are not screened or undergo screening infrequently (5).

Addressing Errors in Cervical Cytology

In some cases, cervical cancer is undetected despite a recent screening test because of errors in sampling, interpretation, or follow-up. Sampling errors occur when dysplastic cells on the cervix are not transferred to the slide; errors of interpretation are attributed to lack of recognition of abnormal cells in the laboratory. These two sources of false-negative test results are associated with 30% of the new cases of cervical cancer each year (12, 13).

The problem of errors in interpretation is compounded by inconsistency among cytologists. When results of monolayer cytology specimens were reviewed by quality control pathologists, only negative and low-grade squamous intraepithelial lesion (LSIL) readings had greater than 50% consistency (14). Most revised results were downgraded to lesser diagnoses. Of those reported as atypical squamous cells of undetermined significance (ASCUS), 39% were downgraded to negative on further review. Of those originally interpreted as high-grade squamous intraepithelial lesions (HSIL), 50% were reinterpreted as LSIL, ASCUS, or negative.

The 1998 Clinical Laboratory Improvement Amendments (CLIA), passed in response to claims of poor or absent quality control practices in U.S. cytology laboratories, limited the number of cervical cytology tests a technician could read each day to a maximum of 100. In addition, CLIA mandated that each laboratory rescreen at least 10% of the cervical cytology tests that have negative results (15).

Techniques of Cervical Cytology

Sampling involves collecting exfoliated cells from the ectocervix and endocervical canal and transferring them to a glass microscope slide or into a liquid transport medium for review. Patient preparation and proper provider technique can help optimize the collection of cells:

- Cells should be collected before the bimanual examination.

- Care should be taken to avoid contaminating the sample with lubricant.
- If testing for sexually transmitted diseases is indicated, cell collection for cervical cytology should be undertaken first.
- Ideally, the entire portio of the cervix should be visible when the sample is obtained.
- Routine swabbing of the discharge from the cervix may result in cytologic samples of scant cellularity (16).
- In an effort to reduce air-drying artifact, the specimen should be transferred and fixed as quickly as possible.

When performing cervical cytology by standard preparation, a single slide, combining both the endocervical and ectocervical samples, or two separate slides can be used. The most important consideration is rapid fixation. If liquid-based preparations are used, rapid immersion in liquid media is equally important.

New Screening and Interpretation Devices

Many methods to refine and improve cervical cytology have been proposed (17). In the 1980s, new devices were developed for enhancing the collection of exfoliated cells from the cervix. These included nylon brushes for sampling the endocervix and "broom" sampling devices, which simultaneously sample both the ectocervix and endocervix. These devices have been shown to increase the amount of cells captured from the transformation zone and to increase the amount of dysplastic cells collected when compared with cotton-tipped applicators and wooden Ayre's spatulas (18, 19). In 1996, the U.S. Food and Drug Administration (FDA) approved the first of two currently available liquid-based thin-layer cytology preparations for cervical screening. In addition, automated, computer-based technologies have been marketed that use digitally scanned images to facilitate primary screening and the CLIA-mandated rescreening of cervical cytology tests that have negative results.

Cytologic Reporting

The nomenclature for reporting cervical cytology results has undergone several changes since the publication of the original Papanicolaou system. The Bethesda System of reporting is the most widely used system in the United States (20). First proposed in 1988, it was revised in 1991 and again in 2001 (21–23). The most important changes in the 2001 revised terminology are listed as follows (23):

- Specimen adequacy—Slides are to be reported as "satisfactory" or "unsatisfactory" for interpretation.

"Satisfactory, but limited by ..." is no longer reported as a separate category under the heading "specimen adequacy." The presence or absence of an endocervical or transformation zone component is described in the narrative portion of the laboratory report, as are other quality indicators, such as partly obscuring inflammation or blood. If a slide is categorized as unsatisfactory, the reason should be specified. If abnormalities are found on an otherwise unsatisfactory slide, it will, by definition, be considered satisfactory for interpretation.

- Negative for intraepithelial lesion or malignancy—This designation should be used for slides with no cytologic evidence of neoplasia. This category includes findings previously designated as "benign cellular changes." When specific organisms are identified (eg, *Trichomonas vaginalis, Candida* species, shift in flora suggestive of bacterial vaginosis, bacteria consistent with *Actinomyces* species, and cellular changes consistent with herpes simplex virus), they are reported and categorized as "negative for intraepithelial lesion or malignancy." Other nonneoplastic findings, including reactive cellular changes associated with inflammation, radiation, or an intrauterine device, as well as glandular cells posthysterectomy or atrophy, also may be included in this category. Endometrial cells found in a woman aged 40 years or older will be listed under this category, but the finding of endometrial cells will not be reported routinely if noted in a woman younger than 40 years.

- Atypical squamous cells—The epithelial abnormality ASCUS has been replaced by "atypical squamous cells" (ASC) with the subcategories "atypical squamous cells of undetermined significance" (ASC-US) and "atypical squamous cells cannot exclude HSIL" (ASC-H). The modifier of "favor reactive" was eliminated. The category ASC-H was introduced to include those cytologic changes suggestive of HSIL but lacking sufficient criteria for definitive interpretation. The literature suggests ASC-H should represent 5–15% of the total pool of ASC but would have a significantly higher predictive value for diagnosing cervical intraepithelial neoplasia (CIN) of grades 2 or 3 than ASC-US (24, 25).

- Atypical glandular cells—This term designates cells exhibiting atypia that are of glandular rather than squamous origin and replaces the term "atypical glandular cells of undetermined significance." The finding of atypical glandular cells on cytology is more likely to be associated with both squamous and glandular abnormalities than is ASC-US, and the workup required of atypical glandular cells is more aggressive (26, 27). The 2001 terminology subdivides atypical glandular cells by cell type, ie, atypical endocervical cells, atypical endometrial cells, or atypical glandular cells not otherwise specified. Although the subdivision of "favor neoplastic" is maintained in the 2001 reporting system, favor reactive is not. In addition, because sufficient cytologic criteria exist to designate endocervical adenocarcinoma and adenocarcinoma in situ, these two findings are reported when identified.

- Low-grade squamous intraepithelial lesions—As in the original terminology, the 2001 nomenclature combines cytologic findings of CIN 1 (mild dysplasia) and those consistent with human papillomavirus (HPV) infections into the category LSIL (22, 28, 29).

- High-grade squamous intraepithelial lesions—The 2001 nomenclature maintains the category of HSIL, which combines CIN 2 and CIN 3 (moderate dysplasia, severe dysplasia, and carcinoma in situ). Although the natural history of CIN 2 lies between CIN 1 and CIN 3, the virology of CIN 2 is more like CIN 3 than CIN 1 in its likelihood of representing aneuploidy and monoclonal proliferation with a single high-risk HPV type (29).

- The absence of endocervical cells or a transformation zone component on the cervical cytology sample may reflect that the transformation zone was not well sampled. This finding is common in pregnant women and in postmenopausal women in whom the transformation zone has receded onto the canal. Data conflict as to whether the lack of these cells is associated with an increase in squamous intraepithelial lesions. Women with this finding whose recent cervical cytology test results have been normal without intervening findings of ASC-US or worse may be monitored by repeat cervical cytology screening in 1 year. Others, including those with incompletely evaluated abnormal test results, incompletely visualized cervix, immunocompromised status, and poor prior screening, should have repeat cervical cytology screening within 6 months. Pregnant women lacking endocervical cells or transformation zone component should have repeat cervical cytology screening postpartum (30).

Natural History of Cervical Neoplasia

Infection with HPV is a necessary factor in the development of cervical neoplasia; however, most HPV-infected women will not develop significant cervical abnormalities (7, 29, 31–33). The infection is easily transmitted during sexual intercourse. Most women, especially younger women, have an effective immune response that clears the infection or reduces the viral load to undetectable levels in an average of 8–24 months (32, 34–36). Factors that determine which HPV infections will develop into squamous intraepithelial lesions have been poorly identified. Cigarette smoking may be a co-factor, and a compromised immune system appears to play a role in some women (7, 29, 32).

Despite decades of study, the natural history of cervical intraepithelial lesions is still not completely understood. The once widely held concept that low-grade lesions are necessary precursors to the high-grade lesions that, in turn, may progress to invasive cancer has been questioned as the sole pathogenesis (32, 33, 37). It has been observed, for example, that many women present with CIN 2 or CIN 3 without prior CIN 1 lesions. Foci of CIN 1 and CIN 3 with different HPV types have been reported in the same cervical lesion, which raises the possibility that concomitant development of different grades of CIN may occur (37). A few cases of invasive cancer of the cervix have been reported despite continuous and appropriate screening.

Multiple longitudinal studies have attempted to document rates of "progression" and "regression" of CIN. A review of the literature since 1950 reported that 57% of patients with CIN 1 and 32% with CIN 3 undergo spontaneous regression (38). However, the same review reported that 1.7% of all patients with CIN of any grade progress to invasive cancer, ranging from 1% for CIN 1 to more than 12% for CIN 3. Progression from CIN 3 to invasive cancer has been reported in up to 36% of cases (29). A review of 30 years of the literature calculated pooled rates of progression from LSIL and HSIL to invasive cancer to be 0.15% and 1.44%, respectively, over 24 months (39). In that analysis, 47% of LSIL and 35% of HSIL regressed to normal during the 2-year observation period. Conclusions from reviews of multiple natural history studies must be interpreted with caution. The studies included in these reviews used varying diagnostic criteria (biopsy or cytology or both), populations, and duration of follow-up. Moreover, they did not account for the poor reproducibility inherent in both cytologic and histologic diagnoses (14).

Clinical Considerations and Recommendations

▶ *When should screening begin?*

Cervical neoplasia develops in susceptible individuals in response to a sexually transmitted infection with a high-risk type of HPV (28, 29, 31, 40). The cervix is especially vulnerable to this infection during adolescence when squamous metaplasia is most active. Human papillomavirus infections are commonly acquired by young women (34, 35), but, in most, they are cleared by the immune system within 1–2 years without producing neoplastic changes. The risk of neoplastic transformation increases in those women whose infections persist (35, 41). Most cervical squamous intraepithelial lesions do not progress to cervical cancer (29, 38, 39). The small proportion of women who do develop invasive squamous cancer generally do so over many years, and the transition from CIN to cancer takes longer in younger women (29). Cervical cancer screening in adolescents within the first 3 years after initiation of sexual intercourse is not likely to result in the identification of HSIL or cancer. In addition, earlier onset of screening may increase anxiety, morbidity, and expense from increased follow-up procedures. Furthermore, squamous cell cervical cancer is exceedingly rare in the first two decades of life (4). Therefore, it seems reasonable to begin cervical cancer screening approximately 3 years after initiation of sexual intercourse, but no later than age 21 years. Recognizing the time course in the progression of CIN and the unpredictable nature of follow-up in younger women, cytologic screening may be initiated earlier at the discretion of the clinician.

▶ *What is the optimal frequency of cervical cytology screening?*

The optimal number of negative cervical cytology test results needed to reduce the false-negative rate to a minimum has not been demonstrated (3, 42). Several studies have shown that in an organized program of cervical cancer screening, annual cytology examinations offer little advantage over screening performed at 2- or 3-year intervals (43–45). These studies showed minimal difference in the acquisition of cervical cancer or HSIL at screening intervals of 1, 2, or 3 years in women who had at least one prior normal screening result and who were enrolled in health care programs that provided and monitored cervical cytology screening.

Several practical considerations must be examined before biennial or triennial screening can be adopted as a national standard. Published studies have assumed a program of cervical cancer screening and follow-up. In the current U.S. practice climate, a woman's care provider may change frequently, as employment and insurance carriers change. Consequently, the physician may be unable to determine a woman's screening history—ie, the date of her last cervical cytology test, frequency and results of her prior tests, or prior abnormal test results and their management. Patients are frequently inaccurate in recalling the timing and results of recent screening, more often underestimating the time elapsed and incorrectly recalling abnormal results as normal (46–49). In addition, the high false-negative rate of cytology screening remains a concern, as does the relatively poor reproducibility inherent in cervical cytology (14). Performing multiple screening tests at regular intervals remains the best way to ensure existing premalignant cervical disease has been ruled out before extending the interval between screenings. This is especially true for young women who have a high likelihood of acquiring a high-risk type of HPV (34, 35).

There is room to individualize screening frequency in a woman who is known to have a negative history and several recent annual cervical cytology tests. The chance such a patient will develop CIN 2 or CIN 3 is extremely low, and screening at intervals of every 2–3 years is a safe, cost-effective approach. It is important to educate patients about the nature of cervical cytology, its limitations, and the rationale for prolonging the screening interval. Physicians also should inform their patients that annual gynecologic examinations are still appropriate even if cervical cytology is not performed at each visit.

Annual cytology screening should be recommended for women younger than 30 years. Women aged 30 years and older who have had three consecutive cervical cytology test results that are negative for intraepithelial lesions and malignancy may be screened every 2–3 years. Certain risk factors have been associated with CIN in observational studies; women with any of the following risk factors may require more frequent cervical cytology screening:

- Women who are infected with human immunodeficiency virus (HIV)

- Women who are immunosuppressed (such as those who have received renal transplants)

- Women who were exposed to diethylstilbestrol in utero

Women infected with HIV should have cervical cytology screening twice in the first year after diagnosis and annually thereafter (22, 50). Women treated in the past for CIN 2 or CIN 3 or cancer remain at risk for persistent or recurrent disease and should continue to be screened annually (51, 52). Women with previously normal cervical cytology results whose most recent cervical cytology sample lacked endocervical cells or transformation zone components and those with partly obscuring red or white blood cells should be rescreened in 1 year (30).

▶ *When is it appropriate to recommend discontinuing screening?*

Although the rate of new-onset cervical cancer plateaus at age 65 years in U.S. women in general, among certain subsets—most notably, African-American women—the incidence increases steadily across the age spectrum (2, 7). Most new cases are seen in unscreened or infrequently screened women. It is difficult to set an upper age limit for cervical cancer screening. Postmenopausal women screened within the prior 2–3 years have been shown to have a very low risk of developing abnormal cytology (53, 54).

The American Cancer Society recommends that screening may be discontinued at age 70 years in low-risk women (5). The U.S. Preventive Services Task Force has set age 65 years as the upper limit of screening (55). An older woman who is sexually active and has had multiple partners may be at lower risk for new-onset CIN than a younger woman because of her decreased rate of metaplasia and less accessible transformation zone; however, she is still at some risk for acquiring HPV and CIN. A woman with a previous history of abnormal cytology also is at risk; women in both of these categories should continue to have routine cervical cytology examinations.

Primary vaginal cancer represents a very small fraction of gynecologic malignancies (5). The vaginal mucosa lacks a transformation zone. Women who have had a hysterectomy and have no history of CIN are at very low risk of developing vaginal cancer. Cytologic screening in this group has a low rate of diagnosing an abnormality and a very low positive predictive value. In a study of 9,610 Pap tests performed among women who had a hysterectomy for benign indications an average of 19 years previously, only 1.1% had cytologic abnormalities. Biopsies of these women showed no vaginal intraepithelial neoplasia grade 3 or cancer (54). Continued routine vaginal cytology examinations in such women are not cost-effective and may cause anxiety and overtreatment. Thus, women who have had a total hysterectomy and have no prior history of high-grade CIN may discontinue screening.

Women who had high-grade cervical intraepithelial lesions before hysterectomy can develop recurrent intraepithelial neoplasia or carcinoma at the vaginal cuff several years postoperatively (56, 57). Women who have had a hysterectomy and have a history of CIN 2 or CIN 3—or in whom a negative history cannot be documented—should continue to be screened annually until three consecutive satisfactory negative cervical cytology results are obtained. Routine screening may then be discontinued. A woman who has had three consecutive satisfactory negative examinations following treatment for

CIN 2 or CIN 3 before she had a hysterectomy also may discontinue screening.

Before considering whether a woman who has had a hysterectomy should continue regular cytology screening, the provider should be sure the woman's cervical cytology history is accurate. The history should confirm that she had benign findings at the time of hysterectomy and that her cervix was removed as part of the hysterectomy. However, when a woman's past cervical cytology and surgical history are not available to the physician, screening recommendations may need to be modified.

▶ How do the various methods of cervical cytology compare in terms of effectiveness?

Cervical cytology is the basis of the most effective and cost-effective cancer screening program ever implemented. Cervical cytology, however, is not a diagnostic test (1). The sensitivity of cervical cytology recently has been reported to be lower than the previously estimated 60–85% (29). A recent comprehensive review of the literature evaluated the accuracy of screening cervical cytology in screened populations with a low prevalence of cervical disease (42). For inclusion in this review, a study was required to have sufficient verification of both negative and positive cervical cytology to calculate sensitivity and specificity. Only three studies met the inclusion criteria to evaluate the standard preparation for cervical cytology at a threshold of ASCUS or worse and estimate its ability to diagnose CIN 1 or more severe lesions. At these thresholds, the standard preparation had a sensitivity of 51% and a specificity of 98%. The authors also calculated performance measures based on nine studies that permitted evaluation at the cytologic threshold of LSIL. The mean sensitivity was 47%, and specificity was 95% (58).

Studies comparing the accuracy of liquid-based thin-layer cervical cytology with the standard preparation have used 1 of 2 study designs. The split sample design prepares the specimen by first placing cells on a glass slide for a standard preparation, then suspending the remaining cells in liquid medium for liquid-based cytology. This design has the potential to falsely decrease the sensitivity of the liquid-based preparation. The direct-to-vial technique, however, prepares the entire specimen for liquid-based cytology but compares a screened population with historic controls. Although most studies have included confirmation of positive test results with colposcopy and biopsy, which allows an estimate of sensitivity, few have used sufficient verification of negative cervical cytology to determine specificity. With both study designs, liquid-based cytology diagnosed from 36% to more than 200% more cases of LSIL and from 26% to 103% more cases of HSIL than the conventional method (59–63). True-positive rates documented with biopsy were improved with the use of liquid-based cytology in some but not all studies (60–64).

Although liquid-based thin-layer cervical cytology appears to have increased sensitivity for detecting cancer precursor lesions over the conventional method, the degree to which sensitivity is increased is unknown. Equally important, the difference in specificity between the liquid-based and conventional tests has not been determined. Although an increase in sensitivity will permit earlier detection of cancer precursor lesions, any decrease in specificity can result in increased cost and morbidity from false-positive diagnoses. The conventional test, although disappointing in its documented sensitivity, has proved effective in reducing cervical cancer rates where screening programs exist. Liquid-based products can be effective in population screening as well. Their reported increase in sensitivity may make them especially useful in women who are screened infrequently. Providers selecting a cervical cytology method should consider the screening history of their patient, the cost of the test, and the possible effects of false-negative or false-positive results.

▶ Is the recommended frequency of screening affected by the method of screening?

The American Cancer Society recommends that women younger than 30 years undergo cervical cancer screening annually if the conventional method is used or every 2 years if a liquid-based method is used (5). However, there are very limited data to support this approach. The recommendation of biennial cytology using the liquid-based method discounts the possibility of false-negative results, a consideration with both liquid-based and conventional methodologies. Moreover, the increased sensitivity of liquid-based methods over conventional methods is small with studies showing overlapping confidence intervals. According to FDA-required labeling, the ThinPrep technique may be marketed as better able to detect LSIL and HSIL than the conventional Pap test, and the SurePath technique may be marketed as equivalent to the conventional Pap test (17).

▶ When is HPV testing appropriate?

Although it is estimated that up to 100% of women with histologic CIN 2 or CIN 3 will test positive for a high-risk type of HPV, many women harbor the virus in their lower genital tracts without showing cytologic or histologic changes (31, 32, 34, 40, 65). Currently, only one product, Hybrid Capture II, is FDA-approved for testing for cervical HPV DNA. It assesses exfoliated cervical cells for the presence of 1 or more of 13 high- and intermediate-risk HPV types. Although the test appears to be very sensitive, rare cross-reactivity with low-risk HPV types and HPV types of undetermined significance has been reported. The clinical implications of this finding are unknown (66).

Its utility has been well demonstrated for the primary triage of cervical cytology tests read as ASC-US (23, 67–70). In this setting, high-risk HPV DNA testing has been shown to have a sensitivity ranging from 78% to 96% for the detection of CIN 2 or CIN 3, with rates of referral for colposcopy ranging from 31% to 56%. The use of "reflex" HPV testing has been recommended as a convenient and cost-effective approach to evaluating ASC-US (68, 71, 72). The technique involves collecting a sample for high-risk HPV DNA testing at the same time as cervical cytology screening and evaluating it only if the cytology is read as ASC-US. Reflex HPV testing may be done by testing from residual preservative if liquid-based cytology is used or by performing a separate HPV DNA test at the same time as cervical cytology and storing it for use if ASC-US is the result.

High-risk HPV DNA test results would be expected to be positive when cervical cytology results indicate HSIL, so the test has little utility in this setting. Likewise, up to 83% of women with LSIL diagnosed by cervical cytology have been shown to be positive for high-risk HPV types, thus limiting the usefulness of the test in this setting as well (73). Because HPV is more prevalent in younger women and the rate of CIN 2 and CIN 3 increases with age, it has been suggested that HPV DNA testing might be a more selective test in older women (68). However, stratifying results by age demonstrated only minimal differences in the sensitivity of HPV DNA testing when used as a triage test for ASCUS results (74). The rate of referral to colposcopy decreased with age, however, from 68% in women younger than 29 years to 31% for women aged 29 years and older (74).

Another clinical setting in which HPV DNA testing may be useful is in the secondary triage of women with a cytologic diagnosis of ASC-US, ASC-H, or LSIL in whom colposcopy is negative or biopsy fails to reveal CIN. A protocol of follow-up in 1 year with HPV DNA testing has been suggested as an alternative to repeat cytology in this group, with repeat colposcopy for those with positive test results (71).

▶ *When cervical cytology and HPV DNA testing are used together, can women be screened less frequently?*

The FDA has recently approved the combination of cervical cytology and HPV DNA testing for primary screening for cervical cancer for women aged 30 years and older. This new indication for the use of HPV DNA testing was based on information from several large studies (71, 75–78). These studies demonstrated that women aged 30 years and older who had both negative cervical cytology test results and negative high-risk type HPV-DNA test results were at extremely low risk of developing CIN 2 or CIN 3 during the next 3–5 years. This risk was much lower than the risk for women who had only cytology and tested negative. Because the FDA approval for the use of HPV DNA as a primary screening modality was based on clinical study data, whether the combination of virus screening and cytology will perform equally well when applied to population-based screening practice is unknown.

Any woman aged 30 years or older who receives negative test results on both cervical cytology screening and HPV DNA testing should be rescreened no more frequently than every 3 years. The combined use of these modalities has been shown to increase sensitivity but also decrease specificity and increase cost. However, it has been estimated that the increase in screening interval will offset the cost of this new screening regimen (79).

It is important to note that the FDA approval for use of this approach is only for the panel of high-risk HPV types. In addition, the combination of cytology and HPV DNA screening should be restricted to women aged 30 years and older because transient HPV infections are common in women younger than 30 years, and a positive test result may lead to unnecessary additional evaluation and treatment. Routine testing using cytology alone remains an acceptable screening plan.

Summary of Recommendations

The following recommendations are based on good and consistent scientific evidence (Level A):

▶ Annual cervical cytology screening should begin approximately 3 years after initiation of sexual intercourse, but no later than age 21 years.

▶ Women younger than 30 years should undergo annual cervical cytology screening.

▶ Women aged 30 years and older who have had three consecutive negative cervical cytology screening test results and who have no history of CIN 2 or CIN 3, are not immunocompromised and are not HIV infected, and were not exposed to diethylstilbestrol in utero may extend the interval between cervical cytology examinations to every 2–3 years.

▶ Evidence-based data indicate both liquid-based and conventional methods of cervical cytology are acceptable for screening.

▶ Women who have undergone hysterectomy with removal of the cervix for benign indications and who have no prior history of CIN 2 or CIN 3 or worse may discontinue routine cytology testing.

The following recommendations are based on limited and inconsistent scientific evidence (Level B):

▶ Women previously treated for CIN 2 or CIN 3 who have completed their posttreatment follow-up should be monitored annually until at least three consecutive negative cytology screening results are documented.

▶ The use of a combination of cervical cytology and HPV DNA screening is appropriate for women aged 30 years and older. If this combination is used, women who receive negative results on both tests should be rescreened no more frequently than every 3 years.

▶ Women who have undergone hysterectomy with removal of the cervix and have a history of CIN 2 or CIN 3 should continue to be screened annually until three consecutive negative vaginal cytology test results are achieved.

The following recommendations are based primarily on consensus and expert opinion (Level C):

▶ Physicians should consider individualization in determining the time to begin screening, the interval between cervical cytology examinations, the age at which cervical cytology testing is no longer needed, and the testing methodology to be used. In addition to considering risk factors for cervical cancer, the provider ideally should be able to determine the patient's past screening history and reliably monitor the patient in the future.

▶ Evidence is inconclusive to establish an upper age limit for cervical cancer screening. If screening is discontinued, risk factors should be assessed during the annual examination to determine if reinitiating screening is appropriate.

▶ Yearly testing using cytology alone remains an acceptable screening plan.

▶ Regardless of the frequency of cervical cytology screening, women should be counseled that annual examinations, including pelvic examination, are still recommended.

References

1. Janicek MF, Averette HE. Cervical cancer: prevention, diagnosis, and therapeutics. CA Cancer J Clin 2001;51: 92–114; quiz 115–8. (Level III)

2. Annual report to the nation on the status of cancer, 1973–1999: supplemental materials. Bethesda (MD): National Cancer Institute. Available at http://seer.cancer.gov/reportcard/supplemental.html. Retrieved January 22, 2003. (Level II-3)

3. Sawaya GF, Brown AD, Washington AE, Garber AM. Clinical Practice. Current approaches to cervical-cancer screening. N Engl J Med 2001;344:1603–7. (Level III)

4. Reis LA, Eisner MP, Kosary CL, Hankey BF, Miller BA, Clegg L, et al, editors. SEER cancer statistics review, 1973–1999. Bethesda (MD): National Cancer Institute; 2002. Available at http://seer.cancer.gov/csr/1973_1999/. Retrieved January 16, 2003. (Level II-3)

5. American Cancer Society. Cancer facts & figures 2003. Atlanta (GA): ACS; 2003. Available at http://www.cancer.org/downloads/STT/CAFF2003PWSecured.pdf. Retrieved January 22, 2003. (Level II-3)

6. World Health Organization. The world health report 2002: reducing risks, promoting healthy life. Geneva: WHO; 2002. Available at http://www.who.int/whr/2002/download/en/. Retrieved January 22, 2003. (Level II-3)

7. Herrero R. Epidemiology of cervical cancer. J Natl Cancer Inst Monogr 1996;(21):1–6. (Level III)

8. Eddy DM. Screening for cervical cancer. Ann Intern Med 1990;113:214–26. (Level III)

9. van der Graaf Y, Klinkhamer PJ, Vooijs GP. Effect of population screening for cancer of the uterine cervix in Nijmegen, The Netherlands. Prev Med 1986;15:582–90. (Level II-3)

10. U.S. Department of Health and Human Services. Healthy people 2010. Vol 1–2. 2nd ed. Washington, DC: U.S. Government Printing Office; 2000. (Level III)

11. Cervical cancer. NIH Consens Statement 1996;14:1–38; quiz 4p. (Level III)

12. Sawaya GF, Grimes DA. New technologies in cervical cytology screening: a word of caution. Obstet Gynecol 1999;94:307–10. (Level III)

13. Shingleton HM, Patrick RL, Johnston WW, Smith RA. The current status of the Papanicolaou smear. Ca Cancer J Clin 1995;45:305–20. (Level III)

14. Stoler MH, Schiffman M. Interobserver reproducibility of cervical cytologic and histologic interpretations: realistic estimates from the ASCUS-LSIL Triage Study. JAMA 2001;285:1500–5. (Level II-3)

15. Centers for Disease Control and Prevention. Regulations for implementing the Clinical Laboratory Improvement Amendments of 1988: a summary. MMWR Recomm Rep 1992;(RR-2):1–17. (Level III)

16. Hild-Mosley KA, Lindblade JA, Julian TM. The management of cervical mucus in obtaining a Papanicolaou smear. J Low Genital Tract Dis 1997;1:1–3. (Level I)

17. Cervical cytology screening. ACOG Technology Assessment No. 2. American College of Obstetricians and Gynecologists. Obstet Gynecol 2002;100:1423–7. (Level III)

18. Hutchinson M, Fertitta L, Goldbaum B, Hamza M, Vanerian S, Isenstein L. Cervex-Brush and Cytobrush. Comparison of their ability to sample abnormal cells for cervical smears. J Reprod Med 1991;36:581–6. (Level II-2)

19. Martin-Hirsch P, Lilford R, Jarvis G, Kitchener HC. Efficacy of cervical-smear collection devices: a systematic review and meta-analysis. Lancet 1999;354:1763–70. (Meta-analysis)

20. The 1988 Bethesda System for reporting cervical/vaginal cytological diagnoses. National Cancer Institute Workshop. JAMA 1989;262:931–4. (Level III)

21. Broder S. From the National Institutes of Health. JAMA 1992;267:1892. (Level III)

22. Kurman RJ, Solomon D. The Bethesda System for reporting cervical/vaginal cytologic diagnoses: definitions, criteria, and explanatory notes for terminology and specimen adequacy. New York: Springer-Verlag; 1994. (Level III)

23. Solomon D, Davey D, Kurman R, Moriarty A, O'Connor D, Prey M, et al. The 2001 Bethesda System: terminology for reporting results of cervical cytology. JAMA 2002; 287:2114–9. (Level III)

24. Sherman ME, Tabbara SO, Scott DR, Kurman RJ, Glass AG, Manos MM, et al. "ASCUS, rule out HSIL": cytologic features, histologic correlates, and human papillomavirus detection. Mod Pathol 1999;12:335–42. (Level II-2)

25. Sherman ME, Solomon D, Schiffman M. Qualification of ASCUS. A comparison of equivocal LSIL and equivocal HSIL cervical cytology in the ASCUS LSIL Triage Study. Am J Clin Pathol 2001;116:386–94. (Level II-2)

26. Veljovich DS, Stoler MH, Andersen WA, Covell JL, Rice LW. Atypical glandular cells of undetermined significance: a five-year retrospective histopathologic study. Am J Obstet Gynecol 1998;179:382–90. (Level III)

27. Kinney WK, Manos MM, Hurley LB, Ransley JE. Where's the high-grade cervical neoplasia? The importance of minimally abnormal Papanicolaou diagnoses. Obstet Gynecol 1998;91:973–6. (Level III)

28. Lorincz AT, Reid R, Jenson AB, Greenberg MD, Lancaster W, Kurman RJ. Human papillomavirus infection of the cervix: relative risk associations of 15 common anogenital types. Obstet Gynecol 1992;79:328–37. (Level II-2)

29. Mitchell MF, Tortolero-Luna G, Wright T, Sarkar A, Richards-Kortum R, Hong WK, et al. Cervical human papillomavirus infection and intraepithelial neoplasia: a review. J Natl Cancer Inst Monogr 1996;(21):17–25. (Level III)

30. Davey DD, Austin RM, Birdsong G, Buck HW, Cox JT, Darragh TM, et al. ASCCP patient management guidelines: pap test specimen adequacy and quality indicators. J Low Genital Tract Dis 2002;6:195–9. (Level III)

31. Walboomers JM, Jacobs MV, Manos MM, Bosch FX, Kummer JA, Shah KV, et al. Human papillomavirus is a necessary cause of invasive cervical cancer worldwide. J Pathol 1999;189:12–9. (Level II-2)

32. Schiffman MH, Brinton LA. The epidemiology of cervical carcinogenesis. Cancer 1995;76:1888–901. (Level III)

33. Kiviat N. Natural history of cervical neoplasia: overview and update. Am J Obstet Gynecol 1996;175:1099–104. (Level III)

34. Ho GY, Bierman R, Beardsley L, Chang CJ, Burk RD. Natural history of cervicovaginal papillomavirus infection in young women. N Engl J Med 1998;338:423–8. (Level II-2)

35. Moscicki AB, Shiboski S, Broering J, Powell K, Clayton L, Jay N, et al. The natural history of human papillomavirus infection as measured by repeated DNA testing in adolescent and young women. J Pediatr 1998;132: 277–84. (Level II-2)

36. Woodman CB, Collins S, Winter H, Bailey A, Ellis J, Prior P, et al. Natural history of cervical human papillomavirus infection in young women: a longitudinal cohort study. Lancet 2001;357:1831–6. (Level II-2)

37. Park J, Sun D, Genest DR, Trivijitsilp P, Suh I, Crum CP. Coexistence of low and high grade squamous intraepithelial lesions of the cervix: morphologic progression or multiple papillomaviruses? Gynecol Oncol 1998;70:386–91. (Level II-3)

38. Ostor AG. Natural history of cervical intraepithelial neoplasia: a critical review. Int J Gynecol Pathol 1993;12: 186–92. (Meta-analysis)

39. Melnikow J, Nuovo J, Willan AR, Chan BK, Howell LP. Natural history of cervical squamous intraepithelial lesions: a meta-analysis. Obstet Gynecol 1998;92: 727–35. (Meta-analysis)

40. Bosch FX, Manos MM, Munoz N, Sherman M, Jansen AM, Peto J, et al. Prevalence of human papillomavirus in cervical cancer: a worldwide perspective. International Biological Study on Cervical Cancer (IBSCC) Study Group. J Natl Cancer Inst 1995;87:796–802. (Level II-2)

41. Ho GY, Burk RD, Klein S, Kadish AS, Chang CJ, Palan P, et al. Persistent genital human papillomavirus infection as a risk factor for persistent cervical dysplasia. J Natl Cancer Inst 1995;87:1365–71. (Level II-2)

42. Agency for Health Care Policy and Research. Evaluation of cervical cytology. Evidence Report/Technology Assessment no 5. Rockville (MD): AHCPR; 1999. AHCPR Publication no. 99-E010. (Meta-analysis)

43. Screening for squamous cervical cancer: duration of low risk after negative results of cervical cytology and its implication for screening policies. IARC Working Group on evaluation of cervical cancer screening programmes. Br Med J (Clin Res Ed) 1986;293:659–64. (Level II-3)

44. Sawaya GF, Kerlikowske K, Lee NC, Gildengorin G, Washington AE. Frequency of cervical smear abnormalities within 3 years of normal cytology. Obstet Gyncol 2000;96:219–23. (Level II-3)

45. Eddy DM. The frequency of cervical cancer screening. Comparison of a mathematical model with empirical data. Cancer 1987;60:1117–22. (Level III)

46. Boyce JG, Fruchter RG, Romanzi L, Sillman FH, Maiman M. The fallacy of the screening interval for cervical smears. Obstet Gynecol 1990;76:627–32. (Level II-2)

47. Mamoon H, Taylor R, Morrell S, Wain G, Moore H. Cervical screening: population-based comparisons between self-reported survey and registry-derived Pap test rates. Aust N Z J Public Health 2001;25:505–10. (Level II-2)

48. Eaker S, Adami HO, Sparen P. Reasons women do not attend screening for cervical cancer: a population-based study in Sweden. Prev Med 2001;32:482–91. (Level II-2)

49. Sawyer JA, Earp JA, Fletcher RH, Daye FF, Wynn TM. Accuracy of women's self-report of their last Pap smear. Am J Public Health 1989;79:1036–7. (Level II-2)

50. 1999 USPHS/IDSA guidelines for the prevention of opportunistic infections in persons infected with human immunodeficiency virus. U.S. Public Health Service (USPHS) and Infectious Diseases Society of America (IDSA). MMWR Recomm Rep 1999;48(RR-10):1–59, 61–6. (Level III)

51. Baldauf JJ, Dreyfus M, Ritter J, Cuenin C, Tissier I, Meyer P. Cytology and colposcopy after loop electrosurgical excision: implications for follow-up. Obstet Gynecol 1998;92:124–30. (Level II-2)

52. Flannelly G, Langhan H, Jandial L, Mana E, Campbell M, Kitchener H. A study of treatment failures following large loop excision of the transformation zone for the treatment of cervical intraepithelial neoplasia. Br J Ostet Gynaecol 1997;104:718–22. (Level II-3)

53. Sawaya GF, Grady D, Kerlikowske K, Valleur JL, Barnabei VM, Bass K, et al. The positive predictive value of cervical smears in previously screened postmenopausal women: the Heart and Estrogen/Progestin Replacement Study (HERS). Ann Intern Med 2000;133:942–50. (Level II-2)

54. Pearce KF, Haefner HK, Sarwar SF, Nolan TE. Cytopathological findings on vaginal Papanicolaou smears after hysterectomy for benign gynecologic disease. N Engl J Med 1996;335:1559–62. (Level II-3)

55. U.S. Preventive Services Task Force. Screening for cervical cancer. Rockville (MD): Agency for Healthcare Research and Quality; 2003. Available at http://www.ahrq.gov/clinic/3rduspstf/cervcan/cervcanwh.pdf. Retrieved January 24, 2003. (Level III)

56. Kalogirou D, Antoniou G, Karakitsos P, Botsis D, Papadimitriou A, Giannikos L. Vaginal intraepithelial neoplasia (VAIN) following hysterectomy in patients treated for carcinoma in situ of the cervix. Eur J Gynaecal Oncol 1997;18:188–91. (Level II-2)

57. Sillman FH, Fruchter RG, Chen YS, Camilien L, Sedlis A, McTigue E. Vaginal intraepithelial neoplasia: risk factors for persistence, recurrence, and invasion and its management. Am J Obstet Gynecol 1997;176:93–9. (Level II-2)

58. Nanda K, McCrory DC, Myers ER, Bastian LA, Hasselblad V, Hickey JD, et al. Accuracy of the Papanicolaou test in screening for and follow-up of cervical cytologic abnormalities: a systematic review. Ann Intern Med 2000;132:810–9. (Level III)

59. Diaz-Rosario LA, Kabawat SE. Performance of a fluid-based, thin-layer Papanicolaou smear method in the clinical setting of an independent laboratory and an outpatient screening population in New England. Arch Pathol Lab Med 1999;123:817–21. (Level II-2)

60. Carpenter AB, Davey DD. ThinPrep Pap Test: performance and biopsy follow-up in a university hospital. Cancer 1999;87:105–12. (Level II-2)

61. Papillo JL, Zarka MA, St John TL. Evaluation of the ThinPrep Pap test in clinical practice. A seven-month, 16,314-case experience in northern Vermont. Acta Cytol 1998;42:203–8. (Level II-2)

62. Hartmann KE, Nanda K, Hall S, Myers E. Technologic advances for evaluation of cervical cytology: is newer better? Obstet Gynecol Surv 2001;56:765–74. (Level III)

63. Hutchinson ML, Zahniser DJ, Sherman ME, Herrero R, Alfaro M, Bratti MC, et al. Utility of liquid-based cytology for cervical carcinoma screening: results of a population-based study conducted in a region of Costa Rica with a high incidence of cervical carcinoma. Cancer 1999;87:48–55. (Level II-2)

64. Vassilakos P, Schwartz D, de Marval F, Yousfi L, Broquet G, Mathez-Loic F, et al. Biopsy-based comparison of liquid-based, thin-layer preparations to conventional Pap smears. J Reprod Med 2000;45:11–6. (Level II-2)

65. Herrero R, Hildesheim A, Bratti C, Sherman ME, Hutchinson M, Morales J, et al. Population-based study of human papillomavirus infection and cervical neoplasia in rural Costa Rica. J Natl Cancer Inst 2000;92:464–74. (Level II-2)

66. Peyton CL, Schiffman M, Lorincz AT, Hunt WC, Mielzynska I, Bratti C, et al. Comparison of PCR- and hybrid capture-based human papillomavirus detection systems using multiple cervical specimen collection strategies. J Clin Microbiol 1998;36:3248–54. (Level II-2)

67. Manos MM, Kinney WK, Hurley LB, Sherman ME, Shieh-Ngai J, Kurman RJ, et al. Identifying women with cervical neoplasia: using human papillomavirus DNA testing for equivocal Papanicolaou results. JAMA 1999;281:1605–10. (Level II-2)

68. Wright TC Jr, Lorincz A, Ferris DG, Richart RM, Ferenczy A, Mielzynska I, et al. Reflex human papillomavirus deoxyribonucleic acid testing in women with abnormal Papanicolaou smears. Am J Obstet Gynecol 1998;178:962–6. (Level II-2)

69. Shlay JC, Dunn T, Byers T, Baron AE, Douglas JM Jr. Prediction of cervical intraepithelial neoplasia grade 2–3 using risk assessment and human papillomavirus testing in women with atypia on Papanicolaou smears. Obstet Gynecol 2000;96:410–6. (Cost-effectiveness analysis)

70. Bergeron C, Jeannel D, Poveda J, Cassonnet P, Orth G. Human papillomavirus testing in women with mild cytologic atypia. Obstet Gynecol 2000;95:821–7. (Level II-1)

71. Wright TC Jr, Cox JT, Massad LS, Twiggs LB, Wilkinson EJ. 2001 Consensus Guidelines for the management of

women with cervical cytological abnormalities. JAMA 2002;287:2120–9. (Level III)

72. Kim JJ, Wright TC, Goldie SJ. Cost-effectiveness of alternative triage strategies for atypical squamous cells of undetermined significance. JAMA 2002;287:2382–90. (Cost-effectiveness analysis)

73. Human papillomavirus testing for triage of women with cytologic evidence of low-grade squamous intraepithelial lesions: baseline data from a randomized trial. The Atypical Squamous Cells of Undetermined Significance/Low-Grade Squamous Intraepithelial Lesion Triage Study (ALTS) Group. J Natl Cancer Inst 2000;92: 397–402. (Level I)

74. Sherman ME, Schiffman M, Cox JT. Effects of age and human papilloma viral load on colposcopy triage: data from the randomized Atypical Squamous Cells of Undetermined Significance/Low-Grade Squamous Intraepithelial Lesion Triage Study (ALTS). J Natl Cancer Inst 2002;94:102–7. (Level I)

75. Petry KU, Menton S, van Loenen-Frosch F, De Carvalho Gomes H, Holz B, Schopp B, et al. Inclusion of HPV-testing in routine cervical cancer screening for women above 29 years in Germany: results for 8466 patients. Br J Cancer 2003;88:1570–7. (Level II-2)

76. Belinson J, Qiao YL, Pretorius R, Zhang WH, Elson P, Li L, et al. Shanxi Province Cervical Cancer Screening Study: a cross-sectional comparative trial of multiple techniques to detect cervical neoplasia. Gynecol Oncol 2001;83:439–44. (Level II-2)

77. Schiffman M, Herrero R, Hildescheim A, Sherman ME, Bratti M, Wacholder S, et al. HPV DNA testing in cervical cancer screening: results from women in a high-risk province of Costa Rica. JAMA 2000;283:87–93. (Level I)

78. Sherman ME, Lorincz AT, Scott DR, Wacholder S, Castle PE, Glass AG, et al. Baseline cytology, human papillomavirus testing, and risk for cervical neoplasia: a 10-year cohort analysis. J Natl Cancer Inst 2003;95:46–52. (Level II-2)

79. Mandelblatt JS, Lawrence WF, Womack SM, Jacobson D, Yi B, Hwang YT, et al. Benefits and costs of using HPV testing to screen for cervical cancer. JAMA 2002;287: 2372–81. (Cost-effectiveness analysis)

The MEDLINE database, the Cochrane Library, and ACOG's own internal resources and documents were used to conduct a literature search to locate relevant articles published between January 1985 and May 2003. The search was restricted to articles published in the English language. Priority was given to articles reporting results of original research, although review articles and commentaries also were consulted. Abstracts of research presented at symposia and scientific conferences were not considered adequate for inclusion in this document. Guidelines published by organizations or institutions such as the National Institutes of Health and the American College of Obstetricians and Gynecologists were reviewed, and additional studies were located by reviewing bibliographies of identified articles. When reliable research was not available, expert opinions from obstetrician–gynecologists were used.

Studies were reviewed and evaluated for quality according to the method outlined by the U.S. Preventive Services Task Force:

I Evidence obtained from at least one properly designed randomized controlled trial.

II-1 Evidence obtained from well-designed controlled trials without randomization.

II-2 Evidence obtained from well-designed cohort or case–control analytic studies, preferably from more than one center or research group.

II-3 Evidence obtained from multiple time series with or without the intervention. Dramatic results in uncontrolled experiments also could be regarded as this type of evidence.

III Opinions of respected authorities, based on clinical experience, descriptive studies, or reports of expert committees.

Based on the highest level of evidence found in the data, recommendations are provided and graded according to the following categories:

Level A—Recommendations are based on good and consistent scientific evidence.

Level B—Recommendations are based on limited or inconsistent scientific evidence.

Level C—Recommendations are based primarily on consensus and expert opinion.

ISSN 1099-3630

The American College of Obstetricians and Gynecologists
409 12th Street, SW, PO Box 96920
Washington, DC 20090-6920

12345/76543

Cervical cytology screening. ACOG Practice Bulletin No. 45. American College of Obstetricians and Gynecologists. Obstet Gynecol 2003;102:417–27.

ACOG PRACTICE BULLETIN

CLINICAL MANAGEMENT GUIDELINES FOR
OBSTETRICIAN–GYNECOLOGISTS

NUMBER 48, NOVEMBER 2003

This Practice Bulletin was developed by the ACOG Committee on Practice Bulletins— Obstetrics with the assistance of James H. Harger, MD. The information is designed to aid practitioners in making decisions about appropriate obstetric and gynecologic care. These guidelines should not be construed as dictating an exclusive course of treatment or procedure. Variations in practice may be warranted based on the needs of the individual patient, resources, and limitations unique to the institution or type of practice.

Cervical Insufficiency

The inability of the uterine cervix to retain a pregnancy to term is referred to as cervical insufficiency. Controversy exists in the medical literature pertaining to issues of pathophysiology, screening, and management of cervical insufficiency. The purpose of this document is to provide a review of current evidence on cervical insufficiency, including screening of asymptomatic at-risk women, and offer management guidelines.

Background

Definition

The terms "cervical insufficiency" and "cervical incompetence" have been used to describe the inability of the uterine cervix to retain a pregnancy in the absence of contractions or labor. Historically, the function of the cervix has been the primary consideration: the cervix was either considered to be fully functional (competent) or nonfunctional (incompetent). The distinction between the 2 states was based on a history of painless cervical dilation after the first trimester with subsequent expulsion of the pregnancy out of the uterus without contractions or labor. More recently, with the advent of ultrasonographic assessment, cervical function has been viewed more as a continuous variable with a range of degrees of competency that may be expressed differently in subsequent pregnancies.

Incidence and Prevalence

The lack of objective findings and clear diagnostic criteria make the incidence of cervical insufficiency difficult to ascertain. According to the National Center for Health Statistics, in 2000, 23,000 discharge records from short-stay hospitals included the diagnosis of cervical incompetence (1). Older studies provided crude estimates by reporting the number of deliveries in a medical facility during the period when a given number of cerclages were performed.

Midrange estimates have suggested that the ratio of cerclage procedures to deliveries ranged from 1 per 222 (2) to 1 per 182 deliveries (3). A Danish study from 1980 to 1990 applied the diagnosis of cervical insufficiency to 2,756 women, resulting in an incidence of 4.6 cerclages per 1,000 births, or 1 per 217 deliveries (4). At the extremes of the frequency range, an American study of 110 cerclages in the 1950s suggested 1 cerclage for every 1,842 deliveries (5), while an Israeli study of 410 cerclages in a 5-year period reported 1 cerclage for every 54 deliveries (6). This wide disparity reflects confusion about the diagnostic criteria for—as well as uncertainty about the proper treatment of—cervical insufficiency.

The success rate of cerclage is equally difficult to estimate. Some studies suggest cerclage is not necessarily an effective treatment. Others report a more than 70% chance of a normal birth without cerclage in the next pregnancy after recurrent pregnancy loss (7, 8). Although these studies lacked any controls, later studies used patients as their own controls. These studies reported infant viability to be only 25% before cerclage was used and 75–90% in the next pregnancy when cerclage was used (9). The lack of properly designed studies allows for speculation regarding the frequency and necessity of cerclage (10).

Causes

Several investigators have postulated that most cases of cervical insufficiency occur as a result of surgical trauma to the cervix from conization, loop electrosurgical excision procedures, overdilation of the cervix during pregnancy termination, or obstetric lacerations, although data confirming this association are limited (11–13). Other proposed etiologies include congenital müllerian anomalies, deficiencies in cervical collagen and elastin, and in utero exposure to diethylstilbestrol (DES).

Emerging Theories

Several investigators have proposed an alternative, multifactorial model for cervical insufficiency. It reflects data generated by serial transvaginal ultrasound measurements of cervical length, dilation, and funneling of the membranes into the cervical canal and comparison of the measurements with pregnancy outcome (11–13). This model takes into account individual observations that the cervix during pregnancy is a dynamic structure responding to different factors, and that cervical compliance and length vary from woman to woman. In this model, cervical length is a marker for cervical competence operating as a continuum, where cervical insufficiency may represent the lowermost end of the continuum (11).

Diagnostic Criteria

The diagnosis of cervical insufficiency remains elusive. Historically, cervical dilation associated with painful uterine contractions or bleeding was believed to represent preterm labor or abruption or both. The diagnosis of cervical insufficiency has been made, historically, based on the presence of painless cervical dilation. A history of prior cervical trauma, pregnancy loss in the second or early third trimester, pelvic pressure, increased mucoid discharge, or cervical dilation without appreciable discomfort or perceived contractions and hourglassing membranes was considered sufficient to make the diagnosis of cervical insufficiency.

Various diagnostic tests have been suggested to confirm the presence of cervical insufficiency. These include hysterosalpingography and radiographic imaging of balloon traction on the cervix (14), assessing the patulous cervix with Hegar or Pratt dilators, the use of a balloon elastance test (15), and calculation of a cervical resistance index using graduated cervical dilators (16). None of these tests have been validated in rigorous scientific studies.

Ultrasonographic assessment of normal cervices during pregnancy demonstrates that cervical length normally has a wide range before 20 weeks of gestation, perhaps because endovaginal ultrasonography cannot easily distinguish between the upper portion of the true cervix and the myometrium of the lower uterine segment during that period of gestation. Studies using transvaginal ultrasonography have demonstrated that in women who gave birth at term, the cervical length is stable in the first 30 weeks of pregnancy, whereas in the last trimester, the cervix shortens progressively. One study demonstrated a mean cervical length of approximately 4 cm (4.16 +/− 1.02 cm) between 14 and 28 weeks of gestation in normal pregnancies, which gradually decreased between 28 and 40 weeks of gestation (3.23 +/− 1.16 cm) (17). These findings were confirmed by other studies (18, 19), one of which demonstrated that cervical length was almost constant during the first 16 weeks of pregnancy and then gradually decreased from 4.3 cm to 2.5 cm at term (19). Gravidity and parity do not seem to influence cervical length.

Ultrasound evidence of cervical effacement—ie, funneling—can be found when the internal cervical os is marked by visible separation of the 2 sidewalls of the upper end of the cervical canal, producing a wedge-shaped space. Noninvasive stress techniques, including transfundal pressure, coughing, and standing, have been used to elicit ultrasonographic cervical changes (20). Lastly, serial ultrasound assessment of cervical length in women between 24 and 28 weeks of gestation has been correlated with preterm delivery, the relative risk of preterm delivery increasing with decreasing cervical length (12).

Treatment Options

Historically, several surgical and nonsurgical modalities have been proposed to treat cervical insufficiency. Nonsurgical approaches, including modified activity, bed rest, pelvic rest, and pessaries, have been used but have not yet been proved to be effective (21). The standard cerclage methods currently used are modifications of the Shirodkar and McDonald techniques. The Shirodkar procedure attempts to place the suture as close to the internal os as possible. The bladder and rectum are dissected from the cervix in a cephalad manner, the suture is placed and tied, and the mucosa is replaced over the knot (5, 22). Currently, polyester fiber or polypropylene sutures are commonly used.

The most commonly used cerclage technique is the McDonald procedure, in which a simple purse-string suture of monofilament suture (such as silk or polypropylene) or polyester fiber tape is inserted at the cervicovaginal junction (23). Retrospective analyses have not demonstrated the superiority of one technique over another (3).

Transabdominal cervicoisthmic cerclage is rarely indicated and generally is reserved for patients with congenital cervical hypoplasia, a cervix badly lacerated or scarred because of prior surgery or obstetric injury, or in the case of failed transvaginal cerclage procedures. If indicated, patients generally are referred to a physician with prior experience in managing such cases. After dissection of the bladder from the lower uterine segment, a polyester fiber suture band is tunneled around the upper cervix. The knot can be left in place between pregnancies with subsequent cesarean delivery or can be tied posteriorly and cut through a posterior colpotomy incision if indicated (24–27).

Clinical Considerations and Recommendations

▶ *Is there a role for routine ultrasound screening of the cervix?*

Serial ultrasound assessments of the cervix in low-risk women have demonstrated both low sensitivity and low positive-predictive values (28), which means numerous false-positive test results would be needed to detect even 1 true positive case of preterm cervical shortening. As a result, ultrasonography lacks enough discriminatory power to recommend its routine use for screening.

▶ *What is the role of ultrasonography in evaluating the cervix of a woman who has had a prior pregnancy loss?*

Ultrasonography may play a role in the woman with a history of 1 or more pregnancy losses in the second or early third trimesters. One prospective observational study of 106 women at high risk for preterm delivery found 12.3% of the women demonstrated an open internal os at rest or cervical shortening and funneling in response to fundal pressure at or before 24 weeks of gestation (29). This study found a specificity for preterm delivery of 0.94 (29). In addition, a prospective, nonrandomized study monitored 168 asymptomatic high-risk women from 14 to 24 weeks of gestation with serial transvaginal ultrasound evaluation of the cervix (30). Among 63 (37.5%) patients identified as having a cervical length less than 25 mm or funneling of more than 25% or both, 23 (37%) had preterm deliveries; whereas among 105 patients with no cervical changes, 8 (8%) had preterm deliveries (relative risk, 4.8; 95% confidence interval 2.3, 10.1). These studies suggest that serial transvaginal ultrasound examination may be considered in women with a history of second- or early third-trimester deliveries. Because the upper portion of the cervix is not easily distinguished from the lower uterine segment in early pregnancy, such assessments should begin no earlier than 16–20 weeks of gestation. There is no role for ultrasonography as a screening tool for cervical insufficiency in women with a history of first-trimester pregnancy losses.

▶ *In whom is a cerclage indicated?*

Historically, patient selection for elective cerclage has been based on congenital or acquired visible defects in the ectocervix or classic historical features of cervical incompetence (see box). Four randomized clinical trials have reported on the efficacy of elective cerclage in women chosen because of various historical features alone. Three of the trials found no significant improvement in outcomes among women treated with cerclage (31–33).

The largest study, the Medical Research Council/ Royal College of Obstetricians and Gynaecologists' international, randomized, intent-to-treat trial of 1,292 women with singleton pregnancies at risk for preterm delivery, divided the study subjects into 6 mutually exclusive cohorts: 1) history of 1 second-trimester abortion or preterm delivery and no history of cone biopsy or

Historical Features of Cervical Insufficiency

- History of 2 or more second-trimester pregnancy losses (excluding those resulting from preterm labor or abruption)
- History of losing each pregnancy at an earlier gestational age
- History of painless cervical dilation of up to 4–6 cm
- Absence of clinical findings consistent with placental abruption
- History of cervical trauma caused by
  - Cone biopsy
  - Intrapartum cervical lacerations
  - Excessive, forced cervical dilation during pregnancy termination

Data from Harger JH. Cerclage and cervical insufficiency: an evidence-based analysis. Obstet Gynecol 2002;100:1313–27.

cervical amputation, 2) history of 2 second-trimester abortions or preterm deliveries and no history of cone biopsy or cervical amputation, 3) history of 3 or more second-trimester abortions or preterm deliveries and no history of cone biopsy or cervical amputation, 4) history of cone biopsy or cervical amputation, 5) previous first-trimester spontaneous abortion, cervical or uterine anomaly on examination, or previous termination of pregnancy, and 6) twin gestation (34). Only in the subgroup of 107 women with at least 3 previous second-trimester pregnancy losses or preterm deliveries was there a significant benefit in reducing the frequency of delivery before 33 weeks of gestation (15% in the cerclage group versus 32% in the control group, $P \leq .05$). In the other 5 subgroups, there was no statistically significant improvement in neonatal outcome or preterm delivery rate.

On the basis of this limited clinical information, elective cerclage for purely historical factors generally should be confined to patients with 3 or more otherwise unexplained second-trimester pregnancy losses or preterm deliveries. In keeping with the protocols used in these randomized trials, the cerclage should be performed at 13–16 weeks gestation after ultrasound evaluation has demonstrated the presence of a live fetus with no apparent anomalies.

Urgent, or therapeutic, cerclage often is recommended for women who have ultrasonographic changes consistent with a short cervix or the presence of funneling. These women usually are undergoing ultrasonography because they have risk factors for early delivery or may have reported nonspecific symptoms, such as backache, uterine contractions, vaginal spotting, pelvic pressure, or mucoid vaginal discharge. Numerous retrospective studies have addressed this group of urgent cerclages, with variable results (35–39). One randomized trial of 61 women with ultrasonographic evidence of dilation of the internal cervical os between 16 and 24 weeks of gestation compared women assigned to receive a McDonald cerclage (n = 31) with women who did not receive a cerclage (n = 30) (40). All patients were evaluated with amniocentesis and urogenital cultures and treated with indomethacin and antibiotics before randomization. There was no significant difference in gestational age at delivery or perinatal outcome between the 2 groups. The final results of the Cervical Incompetence Prevention Randomized Cerclage Trial (CIPRACT) yielded different conclusions (41). In this study of 35 women, preterm delivery before 34 weeks of gestation occurred in 7 of the 16 women (44%) treated with bed rest alone, compared with none (0/19) in those treated with McDonald cerclage plus bed rest ($P = .002$). In addition, neonatal morbidity was significantly higher in the bed rest alone group (8/16) than the cerclage-plus-bed rest group (1/19, $P = .005$). However, small patient numbers limit both of these studies. In addition, given the limited number of well-designed randomized studies on urgent cerclage, the management of women who have ultrasound findings of a short cervix or funneling remains speculative, and the decision to proceed with cerclage should be made with caution.

Women who present with advanced cervical dilation in the absence of labor and abruption have historically been candidates for emergency cerclage. No randomized trials have studied this situation. Although retrospective studies are numerous (39, 42–45), their findings are limited by selection bias, inadequate patient numbers, and inconsistent selection criteria.

▶ How should the finding of a short cervix in the second trimester be treated?

Assessment of cervical length may occur as part of a complete obstetric ultrasonographic survey or in response to patient symptoms or previous obstetric history. If transvaginal ultrasonography before 16–20 weeks of gestation identifies a short cervix, the examination should be repeated because of the inability to adequately distinguish the cervix from the lower uterine segment in early pregnancy (11–13). Identification of a short cervix at or after 20 weeks of gestation should prompt assessment of 1) the fetus for anomalies, 2) uterine activity to rule out preterm labor, and 3) maternal factors to rule out chorioamnionitis. Reduction of other factors affecting preterm labor may be considered, such as modification of activity, cessation of coitus, and cessation of tobacco use. In addition, serial evaluations may be performed (particularly in patients with pelvic pressure, backache, or increased mucoid discharge) every few days to avoid missing rapid changes in cervical dilation or until the trend in cervical length can be characterized.

A patient with a history of 3 or more midtrimester pregnancy losses or preterm deliveries may be candidates for elective cerclage (34). In patients with a history of fewer second-trimester pregnancy losses, urgent cerclage is not supported by evidence-based studies, and further transvaginal ultrasound surveillance may be the more prudent approach.

If cervical shortening or funneling is detected, the appropriate management remains unclear, and the decision to proceed with urgent cerclage should be made with caution. Cervical change documented before fetal viability is a better indication for cerclage than cervical change identified after fetal viability has been achieved.

Lastly, a woman with advanced cervical effacement or dilatation or both should be counseled about the paucity of data to support the efficacy of emergency cerclage, as well as the potential associated maternal and neonatal morbidity. However, emergency cerclage may be considered in such women in the absence of clinical chorioamnionitis or labor.

▶ How should the finding of a short cervix in the third trimester be treated?

The appropriate evaluation of a woman whose cervical length is below the tenth percentile (25 mm) for gestational age at or after fetal viability includes ultrasound assessment of fetal anatomy to exclude anomalies, tocodynamometry to detect the presence of uterine contractions, and assessment of maternal factors to exclude chorioamnionitis. If the woman is in labor, tocolytic therapy may delay delivery long enough to promote fetal lung maturation with maternal glucocorticoid therapy. The presence of chorioamnionitis warrants immediate delivery and the use of broad-spectrum antibiotics. In the absence of labor or chorioamnionitis, modification of activity, pelvic rest, and tobacco cessation, in addition to expectant management, may be considered. The role of cerclage in the treatment of patients with cervical insufficiency after fetal viability has not been adequately assessed.

▶ Is there a role for scheduled early or first-trimester cerclage in patients with a suspicious clinical history (eg, a few contractions or short or dilated cervix at 20 weeks of gestation)?

There are no well-designed studies that compare first-trimester cerclage with the success rate of the standard timing of cerclage at 14–16 weeks of gestation. In spite of the current accuracy and resolution of first-trimester

ultrasound fetal assessment, cerclage in the first trimester might have an adverse impact on the pregnancy and could result in suturing the cervix with an abnormal fetus in the uterus. The evidence-based risk-benefit ratio does not support first-trimester cerclage, even with transabdominal procedures.

▶ Is cerclage placement associated with an increase in morbidity?

Rupture of membranes, chorioamnionitis, and suture displacement are the most common complications associated with cerclage placement, and their incidence varies widely in relation to the timing and indications for the cerclage. Elective cerclage placement is associated with rupture of membranes in 1.1–18% of published reports and chorioamnionitis within 4 weeks of surgery in 0.7–7.7% of cases (Table 1) (3, 38). Postoperative displacement of the cerclage is reported in 3–13% of elective cerclages and is believed to occur as a result of contractile activity from the foreign-body effect of the cerclage suture (3).

Urgent and emergency cerclages are associated with a higher incidence of morbidity as a result of cervical shortening and exposure of the fetal membranes to the vaginal ecosystem. Retrospective studies of emergency cerclage revealed a risk of ruptured membranes within

Table 1. Cerclage Placement: Incidence of Complication

Type of Cerclage	Complication	Percentage (%)
Elective	Rupture of membranes	0.8–18
	Chorioamnionitis	1–6.2
Urgent	Rupture of membranes	3–65.2
	Chorioamnionitis	Approximately 30–35
Emergency	Rupture of membranes	0–51
	Chorioamnionitis	Approximately 9–37

Data from Harger JH. Comparison of success and morbidity in cervical cerclage procedures. Obstet Gynecol 1980;56:543–8; Hassan SS, Romero R, Maymon E, Berry SM, Blackwell SC, Treadwell MC, et al. Does cervical cerclage prevent preterm delivery in patients with a short cervix? Am J Obstet Gynecol 2001;184:1325–9; discussion 1329–31; Kuhn RJ, Pepperell RJ. Cervical ligation: a review of 242 pregnancies. Aust N Z J Obstet Gynaecol 1977;17:79–83; Kurup M, Goldkrand JW. Cervical incompetence: elective, emergent, or urgent cerclage. Am J Obstet Gynecol 1999;181:240–6; Latta RA, McKenna B. Emergent cervical cerclage: predictors of success or failure. J Matern Fetal Med 1996;5:22–7; Lipitz S, Libshitz A, Oelsner G, Kokia E, Goldenberg M, Mashiach S, et al. Outcome of second-trimester, emergency cervical cerclage in patients with no history of cervical incompetence. Am J Perinatol 1996;13:419–22; Novy MJ, Gupta A, Wothe DD, Gupta S, Kennedy KA, Gravett MG. Cervical cerclage in the second trimester of pregnancy: a historical cohort study. Am J Obstet Gynecol 2001;184:1447–54; discussion 1454–6; Olatunbosun OA, al-Nuaim L, Turnell RW. Emergency cerclage compared with bed rest for advanced cervical dilatation in pregnancy. Int Surg 1995;80:170–4; Peters WA 3rd, Thiagarajah S, Harbert GM Jr. Cervical cerclage: twenty years' experience. South Med J 1979;72:933–7; and Rana J, Davis SE, Harrigan JT. Improving the outcome of cervical cerclage by sonographic follow-up. J Ultrasound Med 1990;9:275–8.

2 weeks of the operation of up to 65% of the patients (37). Chorioamnionitis occurred in 9–37% of the patients studied (see Table 1) (38, 45).

Transabdominal cerclage can be complicated by rupture of membranes and chorioamnionitis. It carries the added risk of intraoperative hemorrhage from the uterine veins when the cerclage band is tunneled between the bifurcation of the uterine artery, as well as the known risks associated with laparotomy (24–27, 46, 47). Lastly, life-threatening complications of uterine rupture and maternal septicemia are extremely rare but have been reported with all types of cerclage.

▶ *Should perioperative antibiotics and tocolytics be used in association with cerclage placement?*

Many investigators have used various antibiotic and tocolytic regimens in an attempt to reduce postoperative uterine contractions and infection after cerclage placement (39). Studies using perioperative antibiotics have been small, nonrandomized, and inconclusive. One case–control study comparing cerclage patients with controls noted no difference in pregnancy outcome or the rate of bacterial colonization in cerclage patients who were treated with antibiotics compared with untreated patients (48). The use of unnecessary antibiotics may lead to the development of resistant strains of bacteria and other morbidity for the woman and her fetus. Thus, caution should be used if this unproven practice is considered.

No randomized studies have shown that use of tocolytic therapy after cerclage is efficacious. In most retrospective or observational studies, multivariable regression analysis has not been performed to separate the confounding effects of antibiotics, bed rest, and tocolytics. The lack of clear benefit for these adjunctive treatments suggests that these drugs should be used with caution.

▶ *Does a patient who was exposed to diethylstilbestrol require cerclage?*

Diethylstilbestrol appears to cause some congenital cervical malformations, and there is concern that in utero exposure also may cause functional deficiencies in the cervix, leading to cervical insufficiency (49, 50). To date no definitive epidemiologic studies have proved that cervical insufficiency is more frequent in women exposed to DES than in comparable controls. In addition, there are no randomized trials of cerclage in such patients. One retrospective analysis (51) and one case–control study (52) noted similar pregnancy outcomes between DES-exposed

women treated with cerclage and those managed conservatively without surgery. Therefore, a woman exposed to DES may be evaluated for cervical insufficiency using the same clinical criteria as a nonexposed woman.

▶ *Does a patient who has had a cervical biopsy need cerclage?*

No studies are available on the incidence of cervical insufficiency based on the extent of prior cervical surgery. A simple punch biopsy or limited loop electrosurgical excision procedure is less likely to remove or disrupt much of the functional structure of the cervix. An extensive cervical conization, however, is more likely to produce functional, as well as anatomical, damage to the cervix. Generally, prophylactic cerclage is not warranted unless there is evidence that the biopsy disrupted the functional capacity of the cervix or if severe anatomical damage is apparent. It may be prudent to await the outcome of at least 1 pregnancy before assuming that cervical insufficiency is present. Serial evaluation of the cervix after 16–20 weeks of gestation may help establish the diagnosis of cervical insufficiency. If there is anatomic absence of the portio vaginalis, a transabdominal cerclage might be indicated (24–27, 46, 47).

▶ *When is removal of cerclage indicated in a patient with preterm labor or preterm rupture of membranes?*

Small, retrospective, nonrandomized studies have reported disparate results of delaying cerclage removal after preterm rupture of membranes. One study reported no difference in infection rates and neonatal outcome between patients with premature rupture of membranes who underwent immediate cerclage removal and controls without cerclage (53). A later study reported high neonatal mortality (70%), mainly caused by neonatal sepsis, in 10 preterm infants delivered after delayed cerclage removal, compared with a 20% perinatal mortality rate with immediate cerclage removal (54). Two articles reached differing conclusions on this issue. One comparison of 25 immediate cerclage removals with 37 delayed removals found a prolonged latent period between rupture of membranes and delivery without improvement of neonatal morbidity or mortality and no increase in maternal infectious morbidity (55). Another report comparing 30 immediate cerclage removals with 51 delayed removals found no significant prolongation of latency, again with no improvement in neonatal outcome (56). Because the available studies are small and nonrandomized, the optimal timing of cerclage removal is unclear.

Summary of Recommendations

The following recommendations are based on limited or inconsistent scientific evidence (Level B):

▶ Serial assessments in low-risk women to screen for cervical insufficiency are of low yield and should not be done routinely.

▶ Serial ultrasound examinations should be considered in a patient with historical risk factors for cervical insufficiency and should be initiated between 16 and 20 weeks of gestation or later.

▶ An elective cerclage can be considered in a patient with a history of 3 or more unexplained midtrimester pregnancy losses or preterm deliveries.

▶ Women exposed to DES in utero may be evaluated for cervical insufficiency using the same clinical criteria as nonexposed individuals.

The following recommendations are based primarily on consensus and expert opinion (Level C):

▶ The evaluation of a patient with cervical shortening or funneling should include a comprehensive ultrasonographic assessment of the fetus to rule out anomalies, as well as physical and laboratory assessments to rule out labor and chorioamnionitis.

▶ Given the advances in neonatal care and the potential maternal and fetal morbidity associated with cerclage, surgical correction of cervical insufficiency should be limited to pregnancies before fetal viability has been achieved.

References

1. Kozac LJ, Hall MJ, Owings MF. National Hospital Discharge Survey: 2000 annual summary with detailed diagnosis and procedure data. Vital Health Stat 13 2002;(153):1–94. (Level II-3)

2. Kuhn RJ, Pepperell RJ. Cervical ligation: a review of 242 pregnancies. Aust N Z J Obstet Gynaecol 1977;17:79–83. (Level II-2)

3. Harger JH. Comparison of success and morbidity in cervical cerclage procedures. Obstet Gynecol 1980;56:543–8. (Level II-3)

4. Lidegaard O. Cervical incompetence and cerclage in Denmark 1980–1990. A register based epidemiological survey. Acta Obstet Gynecol Scand 1994;73:35–8. (Level II-3)

5. Barter RH, Dusbabek JA, Riva HL, Parks J. Surgical closure of the incompetent cervix during pregnancy. Am J Obstet Gynecol 1958;75:511–24. (Level III)

6. Toaff R, Toaff ME, Ballas S, Ophir A. Cervical incompetence: diagnostic and therapeutic aspects. Isr J Med Sci 1977;13:39–49. (Level II-2)

7. Phung Thi Tho, Byrd JR, McDonough PG. Etiologies and subsequent reproductive performance of 100 couples with recurrent abortion. Fertil Steril 1979;32:389–95. (Level III)

8. Harger JH, Archer DF, Marchese SG, Muracca-Clemens M, Garver KL. Etiology of recurrent pregnancy losses and outcome of subsequent pregnancies. Obstet Gynecol 1983; 62:574–81. (Level II-2)

9. Harger JH. Cervical cerclage: patient selection, morbidity, and success rates. Clin Perinatol 1983;10:321–41. (Level III)

10. Drakeley AJ, Roberts D, Alfirevic Z. Cervical stitch (cerclage) for preventing pregnancy loss in women (Cochrane Review). In: The Cochrane Library, Issue 3, 2003. Oxford: Update Software. (Meta-analysis)

11. Iams JD, Johnson FF, Sonek J, Sachs L, Gebauer C, Samuels P. Cervical competence as a continuum: a study of ultrasonographic cervical length and obstetric performance. Am J Obstet Gynecol 1995;172:1097–103; discussion 1104–6. (Level II-2)

12. Iams JD, Goldenberg RL, Meis PJ, Mercer BM, Moawad A, Das A, et al. The length of the cervix and the risk of spontaneous premature delivery. National Institute of Child Health and Human Development Maternal Fetal Medicine Unit Network. N Engl J Med 1996;334:567–72. (Level II-2)

13. Shellhaas CS, Iams JD. Ambulatory management of preterm labor. Clin Obstet Gynecol 1998;41:491–502. (Level I)

14. Rubovits FE, Cooperman NR, Lash AF. Habitual abortion: a radiographic technique to demonstrate the incompetent internal os of the cervix. Am J Obstet Gynecol 1953;66: 269–80. (Level III)

15. Kiwi R, Neuman MR, Merkatz IR, Selim MA, Lysikiewicz A. Determination of the elastic properties of the cervix. Obstet Gynecol 1988;71:568–74. (Level III)

16. Anthony GS, Calder AA, MacNaughton MC. Cervical resistance in patients with previous spontaneous midtrimester abortion. Br J Obstet Gynaecol 1982;89:1046–9. (Level II-2)

17. Andersen HF. Transvaginal and transabdominal ultrasonography of the uterine cervix during pregnancy. J Clin Ultrasound 1991;19:77–83. (Level II-3)

18. Kushnir O, Vigil DA, Izquierdo L, Schiff M, Curet LB. Vaginal ultrasonographic assessment of cervical length changes during normal pregnancy. Am J Obstet Gynecol 1990;162:991–3. (Level II-3)

19. Okitsu O, Mimura T, Nakayama T, Aono T. Early prediction of preterm delivery by transvaginal ultrasonography. Ultrasound Obstet Gynecol 1992;2:402–9. (Level II-2)

20. Guzman ER, Pisatowski DM, Vintzileos AM, Benito CW, Hanley ML, Ananth CV. A comparison of ultrasonographically detected cervical changes in response to transfundal pressure, coughing, and standing in predicting cervical incompetence. Am J Obstet Gynecol 1997;177:660–5. (Level II-2)

21. Newcomer J. Pessaries for the treatment of incompetent cervix and premature delivery. Obstet Gynecol Surv 2000; 55:443–8. (Level III)

22. Shirodkar VN. A new method of operative treatment for habitual abortions in the second trimester of pregnancy. Antiseptic 1955;52:299–300. (Level III)

23. McDonald IA. Suture of the cervix for inevitable miscarriage. J Obstet Gynaecol Br Emp 1957;64:346–50. (Level III)

24. Gibb DM, Salaria DA. Transabdominal cervicoisthmic cerclage in the management of recurrent second trimester miscarriage and preterm delivery. Br J Obstet Gynaecol 1995;102:802–6. (Level III)

25. Wallenburg HC, Lotgering FK. Transabdominal cerclage for closure of the incompetent cervix. Eur J Obstet Gynecol Reprod Biol 1987;25:121–9. (Level III)

26. van Dongen PW, Nijhuis JG. Transabdominal cerclage. Eur J Obstet Gynecol Reprod Biol 1991;41:97–104. (Level III)

27. Anthony GS, Walker RG, Cameron AD, Price JL, Walker JJ, Calder AA. Transabdominal cervico-isthmic cerclage in the management of cervical incompetence. Eur J Obstet Gynecol Reprod Biol 1997;72:127–30. (Level III)

28. Andersen HF, Nugent CE, Wanty SD, Hayashi RH. Prediction of risk for preterm delivery by ultrasonographic measurement of cervical length. Am J Obstet Gynecol 1990;163:859–67. (Level II-2)

29. Macdonald R, Smith P, Vyas S. Cervical incompetence: the use of transvaginal sonography to provide an objective diagnosis. Ultrasound Obstet Gynecol 2001;18:211–6. (Level III)

30. Berghella V, Daly SF, Tolosa JE, DiVito MM, Chalmers R, Garg N, et al. Prediction of preterm delivery with transvaginal ultrasonography of the cervix in patients with high-risk pregnancies: does cerclage prevent prematurity? Am J Obstet Gynecol 1999;181:809–15. (Level II-2)

31. Dor J, Shalev J, Mashiach S, Blankstein J, Serr DM. Elective cervical suture of twin pregnancies diagnosed ultrasonically in the first trimester following induced ovulation. Gynecol Obstet Invest 1982;13:55–60. (Level I)

32. Lazar P, Gueguen S, Dreyfus J, Renaud R, Pontonnier G, Papiernik E. Multicentered controlled trial of cervical cerclage in women at moderate risk of preterm delivery. Br J Obstet Gynaecol 1984;91:731–5. (Level I)

33. Rush RW, Isaacs S, McPherson K, Jones L, Chalmers I, Grant A. A randomized controlled trial of cervical cerclage in women at high risk of spontaneous preterm delivery. Br J Obstet Gynaecol 1984;91:724–30. (Level I)

34. Final report of the Medical Research Council/Royal College of Obstetricians and Gynaecologists multicentre randomised trial of cervical cerclage. MRC/RCOG Working Party on Cervical Cerclage. Br J Obstet Gynaecol 1993;100:516–23. (Level I)

35. Dijkstra K, Funai EF, O'Neill L, Rebarber A, Paidas MJ, Young BK. Change in cervical length after cerclage as a predictor of preterm delivery. Obstet Gynecol 2000;96: 346–50. (Level II-2)

36. Guzman ER, Forster JK, Vintzileos AM, Ananth CV, Walters C, Gipson K. Pregnancy outcomes in women treated with elective versus ultrasound-indicated cervical cerclage. Ultrasound Obstet Gynecol 1998;12:323–7. (Level II-3)

37. Hassan SS, Romero R, Maymon E, Berry SM, Blackwell SC, Treadwell MC, et al. Does cervical cerclage prevent preterm delivery in patients with a short cervix? Am J Obstet Gynecol 2001;184:1325–9; discussion 1329–31. (Level II-2)

38. Kurup M, Goldkrand JW. Cervical incompetence: elective, emergent, or urgent cerclage. Am J Obstet Gynecol 1999; 181:240–6. (Level II-3)

39. Novy MJ, Gupta A, Wothe DD, Gupta S, Kennedy KA, Gravett MG. Cervical cerclage in the second trimester of pregnancy: a historical cohort study. Am J Obstet Gynecol 2001;184:1447–54; discussion 1454–6. (Level II-2)

40. Rust OA, Atlas RO, Reed J, van Gaalen J, Balducci J. Revisiting the short cervix detected by transvaginal ultrasound in the second trimester: why cerclage therapy may not help. Am J Obstet Gynecol 2001;185:1098–105. (Level I)

41. Althuisius SM, Dekker GA, Hummel P, Bekedam DJ, van Geijn HP. Final results of the Cervical Incompetence Prevention Randomized Cerclage Trial (CIPRACT): therapeutic cerclage with bed rest versus bed rest alone. Am J Obstet Gynecol 2001;185:1106–12. (Level I)

42. Barth WH Jr, Yeomans ER, Hankins GD. Emergent cerclage. Surg Gynecol Obstet 1990;170:323–6. (Level III)

43. Latta RA, McKenna B. Emergent cervical cerclage: predictors of success or failure. J Matern Fetal Med 1996; 5:22–7. (Level II-2)

44. Lipitz S, Libshitz A, Oelsner G, Kokia E, Goldenberg M, Mashiach S, et al. Outcome of second-trimester, emergency cervical cerclage in patients with no history of cervical incompetence. Am J Perinatol 1996;13:419–22. (Level II-3)

45. Olatunbosun OA, al-Nuaim L, Turnell RW. Emergency cerclage compared with bed rest for advanced cervical dilatation in pregnancy. Int Surg 1995;80:170–4. (Level II-2)

46. Mahran M. Transabdominal cervical cerclage during pregnancy. A modified technique. Obstet Gynecol 1978;52: 502–6. (Level III)

47. Novy MJ. Transabdominal cervicoisthmic cerclage: a reappraisal 25 years after its introduction. Am J Obstet Gynecol 1991;164:1635–41; discussion 1641–2. (Level II-2)

48. Kessler I, Shoham Z, Lancet M, Blickstein I, Yemini M, Miskin A, et al. Complications associated with genital colonization in pregnancies with and without cerclage. Int J Gynaecol Obstet 1988;27:359–63. (Level II-2)

49. Ludmir J, Landon MB, Gabbe SG, Samuels P, Mennuti MT. Management of the diethylstilbestrol-exposed pregnant patient: a prospective study. Am J Obstet Gynecol 1987;157:665–9. (Level II-2)

50. Mangan CE, Borow L, Burtnett-Rubin MM, Egan V, Giuntoli RL, Mikuta JJ. Pregnancy outcome in 98 women exposed to diethylstilbestrol in utero, their mothers, and unexposed siblings. Obstet Gynecol 1982;59:315–9. (Level II-2)

51. Levine RU, Berkowitz KM. Conservative management and pregnancy outcome in diethylstilbestrol-exposed women with and without gross genital tract abnormalities. Am J Obstet Gynecol 1993;169:1125–9. (Level II-2)

52. Michaels WH, Thompson HO, Schreiber FR, Berman JM, Ager J, Olson K. Ultrasound surveillance of the cervix during pregnancy in diethylstilbestrol-exposed offspring. Obstet Gynecol 1989;73:230–9. (Level II-2)

53. Blickstein I, Katz Z, Lancet M, Molgilner BM. The outcome of pregnancies complicated by preterm rupture of the membranes with and without cerclage. Int J Gynaecol Obstet 1989;28:237–42. (Level II-2)

54. Ludmir J, Bader T, Chen L, Lindenbaum C, Wong G. Poor perinatal outcome associated with cerclage in patients with premature rupture of membranes. Obstet Gynecol 1994;84:823–6. (Level II-2)

55. Jenkins TM, Berghella V, Shlossman PA, McIntyre CJ, Maas BD, Pollock MA, et al. Timing of cerclage removal after preterm premature rupture of membranes: maternal and neonatal outcomes. Am J Obstet Gynecol 2000;183:847–52. (Level II-3)

56. McElrath TF, Norwitz ER, Lieberman ES, Heffner LJ. Management of cervical cerclage and preterm premature rupture of the membranes: should the stitch be removed? Am J Obstet Gynecol 2000;183:840–6. (Level II-2)

The MEDLINE database, the Cochrane Library, and ACOG's own internal resources and documents were used to conduct a literature search to locate relevant articles published between January 1985 and July 2003. The search was restricted to articles published in the English language. Priority was given to articles reporting results of original research, although review articles and commentaries also were consulted. Abstracts of research presented at symposia and scientific conferences were not considered adequate for inclusion in this document. Guidelines published by organizations or institutions such as the National Institutes of Health and the American College of Obstetricians and Gynecologists were reviewed, and additional studies were located by reviewing bibliographies of identified articles. When reliable research was not available, expert opinions from obstetrician–gynecologists were used.

Studies were reviewed and evaluated for quality according to the method outlined by the U.S. Preventive Services Task Force:

I Evidence obtained from at least 1 properly designed randomized controlled trial.

II-1 Evidence obtained from well-designed controlled trials without randomization.

II-2 Evidence obtained from well-designed cohort or case–control analytic studies, preferably from more than 1 center or research group.

II-3 Evidence obtained from multiple time series with or without the intervention. Dramatic results in uncontrolled experiments also could be regarded as this type of evidence.

III Opinions of respected authorities, based on clinical experience, descriptive studies, or reports of expert committees.

Based on the highest level of evidence found in the data, recommendations are provided and graded according to the following categories:

Level A—Recommendations are based on good and consistent scientific evidence.

Level B—Recommendations are based on limited or inconsistent scientific evidence.

Level C—Recommendations are based primarily on consensus and expert opinion.

ISSN 1099-3630

The American College of Obstetricians and Gynecologists
409 12th Street, SW, PO Box 96920, Washington, DC 20090-6920

12345/76543

Cervical insufficiency. ACOG Practice Bulletin No. 48. The American College of Obstetricians and Gynecologists. Obstet Gynecol 2003;102:1091–9.

ACOG PRACTICE BULLETIN

CLINICAL MANAGEMENT GUIDELINES FOR
OBSTETRICIAN–GYNECOLOGISTS

NUMBER 29, JULY 2001

(Replaces Technical Bulletin Number 219, January 1996)

This Practice Bulletin was developed by the ACOG Committee on Practice Bulletins—Obstetrics with the assistance of Larry C. Gilstrap III, MD and Susan M. Ramin, MD. The information is designed to aid practitioners in making decisions about appropriate obstetric and gynecologic care. These guidelines should not be construed as dictating an exclusive course of treatment or procedure. Variations in practice may be warranted based on the needs of the individual patient, resources, and limitations unique to the institution or type of practice.

Chronic Hypertension in Pregnancy

Chronic hypertension occurs in up to 5% of pregnant women; rates vary according to the population studied and the criteria used for confirming the diagnosis (1, 2). This complication may result in significant maternal, fetal, and neonatal morbidity and mortality. There has been confusion over the terminology and criteria used to diagnose this complication, as well as the benefit and potential harm of treatment during pregnancy. The purpose of this document is to review the effects of chronic hypertension on pregnancy, to clarify the terminology and criteria used to define and diagnose it during pregnancy, and to review the available evidence for treatment options.

Background

Definition

According to the National High Blood Pressure Education Program Working Group on High Blood Pressure in Pregnancy, chronic hypertension is defined as hypertension present before the 20th week of pregnancy or hypertension present before pregnancy (3). The blood pressure (BP) criteria used to define hypertension are a systolic pressure of ≥140 mmHg, a diastolic pressure of ≥90 mmHg, or both (see the box). Chronic hypertension during pregnancy is most commonly classified as mild (BP >140/90 mmHg) or as severe (BP ≥180/110 mmHg) (4). The diagnosis is relatively easy to make in women taking antihypertensive medications before conception. However, the diagnosis can be difficult to establish or distinguish from preeclampsia when the woman presents with hypertension late in gestation. In this latter scenario, hypertension that persists longer than the postpartum period (12 weeks post delivery) is classified as chronic.

Hypertension should be documented on more than one occasion. According to the National High Blood Pressure Education Program Working

Criteria for Diagnosis of Chronic Hypertension in Pregnancy

- Mild: Systolic blood pressure ≥140 mmHg
          Diastolic blood pressure ≥90 mmHg
- Severe: Systolic blood pressure ≥180 mmHg
          Diastolic blood pressure ≥110 mmHg
- Use of antihypertensive medications before pregnancy
- Onset of hypertension before 20th week of gestation
- Persistence of hypertension beyond the usual postpartum period

Group on High Blood Pressure in Pregnancy, the diastolic blood pressure is that pressure at which the sound disappears (Korotkoff phase V) (3). In order to reduce inaccurate readings, an appropriate size cuff should be used (length 1.5 times upper arm circumference or a cuff with a bladder that encircles 80% or more of the arm). Pressure should be taken with the patient in an upright position, after a 10-minute or longer rest period. For patients in the hospital, the blood pressure can be taken with either the patient sitting up or in the left lateral recumbent position with the patient's arm at the level of the heart (5). The patient should not use tobacco or caffeine for 30 minutes preceding the measurement (6, 7). Although validated electronic devices can be used, a mercury sphygmomanometer is preferred (6, 7).

Chronic hypertension usually can be distinguished from preeclampsia because preeclampsia typically appears after 20 weeks of gestation in a woman who was normotensive before pregnancy. Moreover, preeclampsia resolves during the postpartum period. Additionally, preeclampsia is frequently associated with proteinuria and characteristic symptoms such as headache, scotomata, or epigastric pain. Women with preeclampsia also may have hemolysis, elevated liver enzymes, and low platelet count (HELLP syndrome). However, the development of superimposed preeclampsia in pregnant women with chronic hypertension is relatively common and is often difficult to diagnose. The acute onset of proteinuria and worsening hypertension in women with chronic hypertension is suggestive of superimposed preeclampsia.

An additional diagnostic complication may arise in women with chronic hypertension who begin prenatal care after 20 weeks of gestation. A physiologic decrease in blood pressure normally occurs early in the second trimester, and may be exaggerated in women with chronic hypertension. This decrease may lead to an erroneous assumption that the blood pressure is normal at this stage of gestation (3). By the third trimester, the blood pressure usually returns to its prepregnancy level (5).

Effects of Chronic Hypertension on Pregnancy

Chronic hypertension complicates pregnancy and is associated with several adverse outcomes, including premature birth, intrauterine growth restriction (IUGR), fetal demise, placental abruption, and cesarean delivery (4). The incidence of these potential adverse effects is related to the degree and duration of hypertension and to the association of other organ system involvement or damage. As many as one third of women with severe chronic hypertension may have a small-for-gestational-age (SGA) infant, and two thirds may have a preterm delivery (8). In a study of 211 pregnant women with mild chronic hypertension, the uncorrected perinatal mortality rate was 28 per 1,000 and was highest in the 21 pregnancies complicated by superimposed preeclampsia. The perinatal mortality rate was 5 per 1,000 in the 190 pregnancies not complicated by preeclampsia (9).

In another study, pregnancy outcomes were reviewed in 44 pregnant women with severe chronic hypertension in the first trimester (10). Slightly more than half developed superimposed preeclampsia; in this subgroup of patients, perinatal death and neonatal morbidity were significantly increased. Comparing women who developed superimposed preeclampsia with women who did not, the incidence of prematurity was 100% versus 38%, the incidence of SGA infants was 78% versus 15%, and the perinatal mortality rate was 48% versus 0%.

Other studies also have reported an increase in perinatal mortality of 2–4 times more than the general population (11–13). For example, a study of 337 pregnancies complicated by chronic hypertension reported a perinatal mortality rate of 45 per 1,000 compared with a rate of 12 per 1,000 in the general population (11).

A study of outcomes in 763 pregnant women with chronic hypertension indicated that women with baseline proteinuria (300 mg or greater of urinary protein in 24 hours at initial evaluation at 13–26 weeks of gestation) were at significant risk of preterm delivery (odds ratio [OR], 3.1; 95% confidence interval [CI], 1.8–5.3) and SGA infants (OR, 2.8; 95% CI, 1.6–5.0) independent of superimposed preeclampsia (14). The development of preeclampsia (defined as new-onset proteinuria) was significantly associated with perinatal death (OR, 2.3; 95% CI, 1.1–4.8). Preeclampsia also was associated with an increase in placental abruption (3% versus 1%). In a meta-analysis of seven case–control and six cohort studies, the risk of placental abruption was related to both cigarette smoking and chronic hypertension, as well as preeclampsia (15). A systematic review of the management of chronic hypertension during pregnancy revealed that chronic hypertension doubled the risk for placental abruption (OR, 2.1; 95% CI, 1.1, 3.9) and tripled the risk for perinatal mortality (OR, 3.4; 95% CI, 3.0, 3.7) (4, 16). Several of the studies included in this review also showed an association between chronic hypertension and preeclampsia (variously defined) and preterm, SGA, or low-birth-weight infants when compared with normotensive women or the general obstetric population. The risk of these complications was increased even in the absence of superimposed preeclampsia, although the absolute increased risk from mild hypertension could not be calculated from the available data (4).

Effects of Pregnancy on Hypertension

Several physiologic changes occur in pregnant women that can affect chronic hypertension. One of the most significant changes is the increase in blood volume, which may further burden an already stressed heart and, along with the decrease in colloid oncotic pressure, may lead to cardiac decompensation. Another important change is the physiologic decrease in blood pressure, which begins by the end of the first trimester and reaches its lowest level at 16–18 weeks of gestation (16). This change can mask either the course or the detection of chronic hypertension in early pregnancy (3). Besides superimposed preeclampsia or eclampsia, pregnancy complicated by chronic hypertension (especially if severe) may be associated with worsening or malignant hypertension, central nervous system hemorrhage, cardiac decompensation, and renal deterioration or failure.

Clinical Considerations and Recommendations

▶ *In the initial evaluation of a pregnant woman with hypertension, which clinical tests are useful?*

The age of onset, results of previous evaluation, severity and duration of hypertension, and physical examination are important determinants of which clinical tests may be useful. Ideally, a woman with chronic hypertension should be evaluated before conception to ascertain potentially reversible causes and possible end-organ involvement (eg, heart or kidney). Women who have had hypertension for several years are more likely to have cardiomegaly, ischemic heart disease, renal involvement, and retinopathy (3). Thus, these women are more likely to benefit from various specialized clinical tests at the initial evaluation during pregnancy or preconceptionally. Tests may include electrocardiography, echocardiography, ophthalmologic examination, and renal ultrasonography (7). The information obtained from these tests may prove useful in assessing risks of hypertension during pregnancy, as well as providing information for prenatal counseling. Women with significant left ventricular hypertrophy secondary to

hypertension may experience cardiac decompensation and heart failure as pregnancy progresses.

Women with significant renal disease (serum creatinine >1.4 mg/dL) may experience deterioration of renal function, although it may be difficult to separate the effects of pregnancy from the disease process (3, 17, 18). Many women with the diagnosis of peripartum cardiomyopathy are found to have underlying causes, chronic hypertension being one of the most common (19, 20). However, most pregnant women with mild chronic hypertension have uneventful pregnancies with no end-organ involvement.

▶ *Are other adjunctive tests useful in evaluating a pregnant woman with hypertension?*

Many women with chronic hypertension are under the care of a primary care physician and already have been evaluated for causes of secondary hypertension, such as pheochromocytoma or Cushing's disease. However, young women in whom hypertension has been diagnosed for the first time in early pregnancy, especially those with severe hypertension (systolic pressure ≥180 mmHg or diastolic pressure ≥110 mmHg), are more likely to have secondary hypertension and to benefit from further evaluation for potentially reversible causes (3). Women with paroxysmal hypertension, frequent "hypertensive crisis," seizure disorders, or anxiety attacks should be evaluated for pheochromocytoma with measurements of 24-hour urine vanillylmandelic acid, metanephrines, or unconjugated catecholamines (21). Magnetic resonance imaging after the first trimester or computed tomography also may be useful for adrenal tumor localization (19).

Cushing's syndrome is rare in pregnancy and is difficult to diagnose because of pregnancy-related changes in steroids (22). Fortunately, this condition is diagnosed in most women before pregnancy. Primary aldosteronism also is rare in pregnancy. Women with this disorder may present with severe hypertension and hypokalemia. Imaging studies may be helpful in demonstrating an adrenal adenoma.

A young woman (younger than 30 years) with severe hypertension (especially with no family history) who has not been previously evaluated may benefit from Doppler flow studies or magnetic resonance angiography to detect renal artery stenosis (7). Renal artery stenosis appears to be more prevalent in patients with type-2 diabetes and coexistent hypertension (23, 24). Negative results from renal ultrasonography do not rule out renal artery stenosis.

▶ *Are laboratory tests useful in evaluating a pregnant woman with essential hypertension?*

In pregnant women with known essential hypertension (primary hypertension or hypertension not secondary to underlying renal or adrenal disease), baseline laboratory evaluations that may prove clinically useful include tests of renal function such as serum creatinine, blood urea nitrogen, and 24-hour urine evaluation for total protein and creatinine clearance (1, 7, 25). This initial laboratory assessment is important in identifying women with underlying renal disease because this complication may adversely affect pregnancy outcome (26). The subsequent development of proteinuria in a woman with essential hypertension also may be helpful in identifying the development of superimposed preeclampsia.

As pregnancy progresses, other laboratory tests—in addition to repeating those mentioned previously—may be clinically useful in evaluating worsening renal disease and in diagnosing superimposed preeclampsia. These include liver function tests, hemoglobin/hematocrit evaluation, and platelet count (27). Periodic measurement of urine protein may be useful in detecting worsening renal disease or the development of superimposed preeclampsia (28). It has been reported that the random protein-creatinine ratio may be useful for the quantitation of proteinuria during pregnancy. The correlation coefficient between this ratio and the 24-hour urine total protein was 0.94 (29). Investigators also reported high sensitivity and specificity between the protein/creatinine ratio from a single urine sample and proteinuria of 300 mg or greater in a 24-hour specimen (30).

Although an elevated serum uric acid level represents a useful confirmatory test for the diagnosis of preeclampsia, it has very poor predictive value among patients without preexisting hypertension. However, when the patient has chronic hypertension, the serum uric acid level may be of some value. One investigator has reported that a serum uric acid level of ≥5.5 mg/dL could identify women with an increased likelihood of having superimposed preeclampsia (31).

▶ *Who are candidates for treatment of chronic hypertension in pregnancy?*

Women with mild hypertension (140–179 mmHg systolic or 90–109 mmHg diastolic pressure) generally do well during pregnancy and do not, as a rule, require antihypertensive medication (3). There is, to date, no scientific evidence that antihypertensive therapy will improve perinatal outcome (25, 32–34). In a review of 263 women with mild hypertension randomized to methyldopa, labetalol, or no treatment at 6–13 weeks of gestation, treatment with antihypertensive medications did not decrease the incidence of complications such as IUGR, superimposed preeclampsia, placental abruption, or perinatal mortality (25).

There also is a paucity of scientific data regarding the most appropriate management of women with well-con-

trolled or mild hypertension already taking antihypertensive medications at the time of pregnancy. Although such therapy may offer long-term benefits to the mother, such therapy is of unproven short-term benefit and could interfere with uteroplacental blood flow and fetal growth (3, 35). In one review of 298 pregnant women in whom antihypertensive medications were stopped or whose dosage was reduced, there was no difference in the incidence of preeclampsia, placental abruption, or perinatal death compared with untreated groups (11). In a meta-analysis of 623 women with mild chronic hypertension from 7 trials comparing antihypertensive treatment to no treatment, treatment was associated with a decrease in the incidence of severe hypertension but did not improve perinatal outcomes (36). In a follow-up meta-analysis that included these 7 trials of pregnant women with chronic hypertension and 38 trials of women with late-onset hypertension receiving therapy versus no therapy, there was an increase in the frequency of SGA infants associated with treatment-induced reduction in mean arterial pressure (35).

Thus, the data are inconclusive with regard to both the benefits and potential adverse fetal effects of treatment of mild chronic hypertension during pregnancy. It would seem reasonable not to start antihypertensive therapy in women with mild hypertension who become pregnant unless they have other complicating factors (eg, cardiovascular or renal disease) and to either stop or reduce medication in women who are already taking antihypertensive therapy. As suggested by the National High Blood Pressure Education Program Working Group on High Blood Pressure in Pregnancy, therapy could be increased or reinstituted for women with blood pressures exceeding 150–160 mmHg systolic or 100–110 mmHg diastolic (3). In women with severe chronic hypertension (systolic pressure ≥180 mmHg or diastolic pressure ≥110 mmHg), antihypertensive therapy should be initiated or continued (10).

In addition, a systematic review of management of chronic hypertension during pregnancy concluded that "the evidence base regarding pharmacologic management of chronic hypertension during pregnancy is too small to either prove or disprove moderate to large benefits (>20 percent improvements) of antihypertensive therapy" (16). The report further concluded that the efficacy of antihypertensive therapy for chronic hypertension in pregnant women was still uncertain. In this latter systematic review, the authors also were unable to identify trials that compared nonpharmacologic interventions with antihypertensive agents or with no interventions for chronic hypertension.

▶ *What medications are most often prescribed for the treatment of chronic hypertension in pregnancy?*

Although there are numerous antihypertensive agents that have been used for the treatment of chronic hypertension during pregnancy, methyldopa has been commonly used. It is preferred by most practitioners, and it appears to be relatively safe (3, 16, 37, 38). Methyldopa appears to have limited effects on uteroplacental blood flow (3, 32, 33, 38).

Labetalol, a combined alpha- and beta-blocker, also can be used during pregnancy as an alternative to methyldopa. In one study on the treatment of chronic hypertension with labetalol versus methyldopa, the authors reported no differences in outcomes between the two medications (25).

In a meta-analysis of beta-receptor blockers prescribed for pregnancies complicated by hypertension, there was an increase in SGA infants born to those women who took oral beta-blockers for mild hypertension (OR, 2.46; 95% CI, 1.02, 5.92) (39). Calcium-channel blockers or antagonists also have been used with limited experience (1, 3). In one randomized study that compared nifedipine (n=145) versus expectant management (n=138) for mild hypertension in pregnancy, there was no benefit to pregnancy outcome but also no increase in adverse effects (34).

Diuretics also have been used to treat chronic hypertension, but there has been concern regarding the potential effect of these medications on normal blood volume expansion associated with pregnancy. In one study of 20 women with mild hypertension, diuretics prevented normal expansion of the blood volume but did not adversely affect perinatal outcome (40). Moreover, a meta-analysis of 9 trials involving diuretics during pregnancy reported no increase in adverse perinatal effects (41). The National High Blood Pressure Education Program Working Group on High Blood Pressure in Pregnancy concluded, "If diuretics are indicated, they are safe and efficacious agents that can markedly potentiate the response to other antihypertensive agents and are not contraindicated in pregnancy except in settings in which uteroplacental perfusion is already reduced (preeclampsia and IUGR)" (3).

▶ *Are certain medications used to treat chronic hypertension contraindicated during pregnancy?*

Angiotensin–converting enzyme (ACE) inhibitors are contraindicated during the second and third trimesters of pregnancy. Although the data regarding their use during pregnancy are limited to captopril, enalapril, and lisino-

pril, the teratogenic risk appears to be similar for the entire drug class. These ACE inhibitors have been associated with severely underdeveloped calvarial bone, renal failure, oligohydramnios, anuria, renal dysgenesis, pulmonary hypoplasia, IUGR, fetal death, neonatal renal failure, and neonatal death (42–46). Fetal risks with ACE inhibitors depend on timing and dose. For example, the use of ACE inhibitors during the first trimester (before renal tubular function begins) has not been associated with an increase in birth defects (47, 48).

▶ *Is there a role for fetal surveillance in pregnancies complicated by hypertension?*

There is no consensus as to the most appropriate fetal surveillance test(s) or the interval and timing of testing in women with chronic hypertension. Thus, such testing should be individualized and based on clinical judgment and on severity of disease. A recent systematic review concluded that there are no conclusive data to address either the benefits or the harms of various monitoring strategies for pregnant women with chronic hypertension (16). However, other studies have indicated that most of the increased morbidity associated with this condition is secondary to superimposed preeclampsia or IUGR (3). Thus, these investigators recommend that baseline ultrasonography be obtained at 18–20 weeks of gestation and that ultrasonography should be repeated at 28–32 weeks of gestation and monthly thereafter until delivery to monitor fetal growth. If growth restriction is detected or suspected, fetal status should be monitored frequently with nonstress testing or biophysical profile testing (3). If growth restriction is not present and superimposed preeclampsia is excluded, these tests are not indicated (3).

▶ *Should patients with chronic hypertension be delivered before term?*

Pregnant women with uncomplicated chronic hypertension of a mild degree generally can be delivered vaginally at term (25); most have good maternal and neonatal outcomes (3). Cesarean delivery should be reserved for other obstetric indications. Women with mild hypertension during pregnancy and a prior adverse pregnancy outcome (eg, stillbirth) may be candidates for earlier delivery after documentation of fetal lung maturity (as long as fetal status is reassuring). Women with severe chronic hypertension during pregnancy most often either deliver prematurely or have to be delivered prematurely for fetal or maternal indications (10).

There are no randomized clinical trials that specifically address the timing of delivery in women with chronic hypertension and superimposed preeclampsia. However, the combination of chronic hypertension and superimposed preeclampsia represents a complicated situation, and the clinician should consider consultation with someone who has expertise in such clinical matters. Delivery should be considered in all women with superimposed severe preeclampsia at or beyond 28 weeks of gestation and in women with mild superimposed preeclampsia at or beyond 37 weeks of gestation (49). Women with superimposed severe preeclampsia in whom it is elected to continue the pregnancy should be monitored in a center with maternal and neonatal intensive care capability (49). In women with superimposed severe preeclampsia and the HELLP syndrome (a form of severe preeclampsia) delivery should be considered, even remote from term.

▶ *Are there intrapartum concerns unique to pregnant women with chronic hypertension?*

The majority of pregnant women with chronic hypertension have uncomplicated mild hypertension and can be managed the same as normal, nonhypertensive women during the intrapartum period. In contrast, women with severe hypertension or hypertension that is complicated by cardiovascular or renal disease may present special problems during the intrapartum period. Women with severe hypertension may require antihypertensive medications for acute elevation of blood pressure. Although no well-designed studies specifically address the treatment of severe chronic hypertension during the intrapartum period, it is generally recommended that antihypertensive medications be given to women with preeclampsia for systolic blood pressure of >160 mmHg or diastolic blood pressure of 105–110 mmHg or greater (3).

Women with chronic hypertension complicated by significant cardiovascular or renal disease require special attention to fluid load and urine output because they may be susceptible to fluid overload with resultant pulmonary edema. There are insufficient data to address the benefits and potential harm of central invasive hemodynamic monitoring in women with pregnancy related hypertensive disorders (3, 50).

There are limited data to address the issue of analgesia or anesthesia in pregnant women with chronic hypertension. In one study of 327 women with severe hypertension in labor (158 of whom had chronic hypertension), there was no increase in maternal pulmonary edema, renal failure, or cesarean delivery in women with an epidural (n=209) or without an epidural (n=118). However, there was a higher cesarean delivery rate in the subgroup of women with chronic hypertension who received an epidural (51). There also were no significant differences in neonatal outcomes between the two groups. Mild hypertension was not addressed in this cohort. The authors concluded that the data regarding safety of epidural anesthesia in women with severe hypertension are limited by both the heterogeneity of diagnoses and the uncontrolled nature of the study. It would seem reasonable to conclude that if regional anesthetic techniques are used in women with severe hypertension, clinicians with specialized training in obstetric anesthesia should be available.

General anesthesia may pose a risk in pregnant women with severe hypertension or superimposed preeclampsia. Intubation and extubation may be associated with acute and significant elevations in blood pressure and an agent such as labetalol usually is given acutely to minimize this effect (3). Ketamine, because of its association with hypertension, is not considered first line therapy for the induction of general anesthesia (52).

Magnesium sulfate should be used for women with superimposed severe preeclampsia to prevent seizures. However, its benefit in women with mild preeclampsia is unclear (3).

▶ *How is chronic hypertension distinguished from preeclampsia when the woman presents late in pregnancy?*

It is often difficult, if not impossible, to distinguish worsening chronic hypertension from superimposed severe preeclampsia, especially when the patient presents late in pregnancy. In the woman with chronic hypertension and renal disease, it may not be possible to distinguish between the two entities. If the same woman has only hypertension without proteinuria and no symptoms of preeclampsia, such as headache, epigastric pain, or scotomata, the diagnosis may be more difficult. However, the vast majority of young, nulliparous women presenting with hypertension for the first time during late pregnancy will have preeclampsia. In addition to testing for proteinuria, other tests that may be helpful include hemoglobin and hematocrit evaluation, platelet count, and liver function tests. These latter tests are useful in the diagnosis of the HELLP syndrome. Oliguria and an elevated hemoglobin/hematocrit level usually indicate hemoconcentration—more indicative of preeclampsia. Serum creatinine levels also may be elevated in women with preeclampsia.

Summary of Recommendations

The following recommendation is based on good and consistent scientific evidence (Level A):

▶ Angiotensin-converting enzyme inhibitors are contraindicated during pregnancy and are associated with fetal and neonatal renal failure and death.

The following recommendations are based on limited or inconsistent scientific evidence (Level B):

▶ Antihypertensive therapy should be used for pregnant women with severe hypertension for maternal benefit.

▶ Methyldopa and labetalol are appropriate first-line antihypertensive therapies.

▶ Treatment of women with uncomplicated mild chronic hypertension is not beneficial because it does not improve perinatal outcome.

▶ The beta-blocker atenolol may be associated with growth restriction and is not recommended for use in pregnancy.

The following recommendations are based primarily on consensus and expert opinion (Level C):

▶ Women with chronic hypertension should be evaluated for potentially reversible etiologies, preferably prior to pregnancy.

▶ Women with long-standing hypertension should be evaluated for end-organ disease, including cardiomegaly, renal insufficiency, and retinopathy, preferably prior to pregnancy.

▶ When chronic hypertension is complicated by IUGR or preeclampsia, fetal surveillance is warranted.

References

1. Haddad B, Sibai BM. Chronic hypertension in pregnancy. Ann Med 1999;31:246–252 (Level III)

2. National High Blood Pressure Education Program Working Group Report on High Blood Pressure in Pregnancy. Am J Obstet Gynecol 1990;163:1691–1712 (Level III)

3. Report of the National High Blood Pressure Education Program Working Group on High Blood Pressure in Pregnancy. Am J Obstet Gynecol 2000;183:S1–S22 (Level III)

4. Ferrer RL, Sibai BM, Mulrow CD, Chiquette E, Stevens KR, Cornell J. Management of mild chronic hypertension during pregnancy: a review. Obstet Gynecol 2000;96: 849–860 (Level III)

5. Garovic VD. Hypertension in pregnancy: diagnosis and treatment. Mayo Clin Proc 2000;75:1071–1076 (Level III)

6. Helewa MF, Burrows RF, Smith J, Williams K, Brain P, Rabkin SW. Report of the Canadian Hypertension Society Consensus Conference: 1. Definitions, evaluation and classification of hypertensive disorders in pregnancy. CMAJ 1997;157:715–725 (Level III)

7. The sixth report of the Joint National Committee on prevention, detection, evaluation, and treatment of high blood pressure. Arch Intern Med 1997;157:2413–2446 [erratum in Arch Intern Med 1998;158:573] (Level III)

8. McCowan LM, Buist RG, North RA, Gamble G. Perinatal morbidity in chronic hypertension. Br J Obstet Gynaecol 1996;103:123–129 (Level II-2)

9. Sibai BM, Abdella TN, Anderson GD. Pregnancy outcome in 211 patients with mild chronic hypertension. Obstet Gynecol 1983;61:571–576 (Level II-3)

10. Sibai BM, Anderson GD. Pregnancy outcome of intensive therapy in severe hypertension in first trimester. Obstet Gynecol 1986;67:517–522 (Level II-2)

11. Rey E, Couturier A. The prognosis of pregnancy in women with chronic hypertension. Am J Obstet Gynecol 1994; 171:410–416 (Level II-3)

12. Ananth CV, Savitz DA, Bowes WA Jr. Hypertensive disorders of pregnancy and stillbirth in North Carolina, 1988 to 1991. Acta Obstet Gynecol Scand 1995;74:788–793 (Level II-3)

13. Jain L. Effect of pregnancy-induced and chronic hypertension on pregnancy outcome. J Perinatol 1997; 17:425–427 (Level II-3)

14. Sibai BM, Lindheimer M, Hauth J, Caritis S, VanDorsten P, Klebanoff M, et al. Risk factors for preeclampsia, abruptio placentae, and adverse neonatal outcomes among women with chronic hypertension. National Institute of Child Health and Human Development Network of Maternal-Fetal Medicine Units. N Engl J Med 1998; 339:667–671 (Level I)

15. Ananth CV, Smulian JC, Vintzileos AM. Incidence of placental abruption in relation to cigarette smoking and hypertensive disorders during pregnancy: a meta-analysis of observational studies. Obstet Gynecol 1999;93: 622–628 (Meta-analysis)

16. Agency for Healthcare Research and Quality. Manage-ment of chronic hypertension during pregnancy. Evidence Report/Technology Assessment no. 14. AHRQ Publication No. 00-E011. Rockville, Maryland: AHRQ, 2000 (Level III)

17. Cunningham FG, Cox SM, Harstad TW, Mason RA, Pritchard JA. Chronic renal disease and pregnancy outcome. Am J Obstet Gynecol 1990;163:453–459 (Level II-3)

18. Jones DC. Pregnancy complicated by chronic renal disease. Clin Perinatol 1997;24:483–496 (Level III)

19. Cunningham FG, Pritchard JA, Hankins GD, Anderson PL, Lucas MK, Armstrong KF. Peripartum heart failure: idiopathic cardiomyopathy or compounding cardiovascular events? Obstet Gynecol 1986;67:157–168 (Level III)

20. Mabie WC, Hackman BB, Sibai BM. Pulmonary edema associated with pregnancy: echocardiographic insights and implications for treatment. Obstet Gynecol 1993;81: 227–234 (Level II-3)

21. Botchan A, Hauser R, Kupfermine M, Grisaru D, Peyser MR, Lessing JB. Pheochromocytoma in pregnancy: case report and review of the literature. Obstet Gynecol Surv 1995;50:321–327 (Level III)

22. Buescher MA, McClamrock HD, Adashi EY. Cushing syndrome in pregnancy. Obstet Gynecol 1992;79: 130–137 (Level III)

23. Valabhji J, Robinson S, Poulter C, Robinson AC, Kong C, Henzen C, et al. Prevalence of renal artery stenosis in subjects with type 2 diabetes and coexistent hypertension. Diabetes Care 2000;23:539–543 (Level II-3)

24. Courreges JP, Bacha J, Aboud E, Pradier P. Prevalence of renal artery stenosis in type 2 diabetes. Diabetes Metab 2000;26 Suppl 4:90–96 (Level II-3)

25. Sibai BM, Mabie WC, Shamsa F, Villar MA, Anderson GD. A comparison of no medication versus methyldopa or labetalol in chronic hypertension during pregnancy. Am J Obstet Gynecol 1990;162:960–966; discussion 966–967 (Level I)

26. Katz AL, Davison JM, Hayslett JP, Singson E, Lindheimer MD. Pregnancy in women with kidney disease. Kidney Intl 1980;18:192–206 (Level II-3)

27. Weinstein L. Syndrome of hemolysis, elevated liver enzymes, and low platelet count: a severe consequence of hypertension in pregnancy. Am J Obstet Gynecol 1982: 142:159–167 (Level II-3)

28. Evans W, Lensmeyer JP, Kirby RS, Malnory ME, Broekhuizen FF. Two-hour urine collection for evaluating renal function correlates with 24-hour urine collection in pregnant patients. J Matern Fetal Med 2000;9:233–237 (Level II-3)

29. Robert M, Sepandj F, Liston RM, Dooley KC. Random protein-creatinine ratio for the quantitation of proteinuria in pregnancy. Obstet Gynecol 1997;90:893–895 (Level II-2)

30. Ramos JG, Martins-Costa SH, Mathias MM, Guerin YL, Barros EG. Urinary protein/creatinine ratio in hypertensive pregnant women. Hypertens Pregnancy 1999;18: 209–218 (Level II-3)

31. Lim KH, Friedman SA, Ecker JL, Kao L, Kilpatrick SJ. The clinical utility of serum uric acid measurements in hypertensive diseases of pregnancy. Am J Obstet Gynecol 1998;178:1067–1071 (Level II-2)

32. Cunningham FG, MacDonald PC, Gant NF, Leveno KJ, Gilstrap LC III, Hankins GD, et al. Endocrine disorders. In: Williams obstetrics. 20th ed. Stamford, Connecticut: Appleton & Lange, 1997:1223–1238 (Level III)

33. Sibai BM. Treatment of hypertension in pregnant women. N Engl J Med 1996;335:257–265 (Level III)

34. Nifedipine versus expectant management in mild to moderate hypertension in pregnancy. Gruppo di Studio Ipertensione in Gravidanza. Br J Obstet Gynaecol 1998; 105:718–722 (Level I)

35. von Dadelszen P, Ornstein MP, Bull SB, Logan AG, Koren G, Magee LA. Fall in mean arterial pressure and fetal growth restriction in pregnancy hypertension: a meta-analysis. Lancet 2000;355:87–92 (Meta-analysis)

36. Magee LA, Ornstein MP, von Dadelszen P. Fortnightly review: management of hypertension in pregnancy. BMJ 1999;318:1332–1336 (Meta-analysis)

37. Ounsted M, Cockburn J, Moar VA, Redman CW. Maternal hypertension with superimposed pre-eclampsia: effects on child development at 7 1/2 years. Br J Obstet Gynaecol 1983;90:644–649 (Level II-2)

38. Montan S, Anandakumar C, Arulkumaran S, Ingemarsson I, Ratnam SS. Effects of methyldopa on uteroplacental and fetal hemodynamics in pregnancy-induced hypertension. Am J Obstet Gynecol 1993;168:152–156 (Level III)

39. Magee LA, Elran E, Bull SB, Logan A, Koren G. Risks and benefits of beta-receptor blockers for pregnancy hypertension: overview of the randomized trials. Eur J Obstet Gynecol Reprod Biol 2000;88:15–26 (Meta-analysis)

40. Sibai BM, Grossman RA, Grossman HG. Effects of diuretics on plasma volume in pregnancies with long-term hypertension. Am J Obstet Gynecol 1984;150:831–835 (Level II-1)

41. Collins R, Yusuf S, Peto R. Overview of randomized trials of diuretics in pregnancy. Br Med J (Clin Res Ed) 1985; 290:17–23 (Meta-analysis)

42. Barr M Jr, Cohen MM Jr. ACE inhibitor fetopathy and hypocalvaria: the kidney-skull connection. Teratology 1991;44:485–495 (Level III)

43. Hanssens M, Keirse MJ, Vankelecom F, Van Assche FA. Fetal and neonatal effects of treatment with angiotensin-converting enzyme inhibitors in pregnancy. Obstet Gynecol 1991;78:128–135 (Level III)

44. Briggs GG, Freeman RK, Yaffe SJ. Drugs in pregnancy and lactation: a reference guide to fetal and neonatal risk. 5th ed. Baltimore: Williams & Wilkins, 1998 (Level III)

45. Buttar HS. An overview of the influence of ACE inhibitors on fetal-placental circulation and perinatal development. Mol Cell Biochem 1997;176:61–71 (Level III)

46. Pryde PG, Sedman AB, Nugent CE, Barr M Jr. Angiotensin-converting enzyme inhibitor fetopathy. J Am Soc Nephrol 1993;3:1575–1582 (Level III)

47. Postmarketing surveillance for angiotensin-converting enzyme inhibitor use during the first trimester of pregnancy—United States, Canada, and Israel, 1987–1995. MMWR Morb Mortal Wkly Rep 1997;46:240–242 (Level III)

48. Bar J, Hod M, Merlob P. Angiotensin converting enzyme inhibitors use in the first trimester of pregnancy. Int J Risk Saf Med 1997;10:23–26 (Level III)

49. Sibai BM. Management of pre-eclampsia remote from term. Eur J Obstet Gynecol Reprod Biol 1991;42:S96–S101 (Level III)

50. Practice guidelines for obstetrical anesthesia: a report by the American Society of Anesthesiologists Task Force on Obstetrical Anesthesia. Anesthesiology 1999;90:600–611 (Level III)

51. Hogg B, Hauth JC, Caritis SN, Sibai BM, Lindheimer M, Van Dorsten JP, et al. Safety of labor epidural anesthesia for women with severe hypertensive disease. National Institute of Child Health and Human Development Maternal-Fetal Medicine Units Network. Am J Obstet Gynecol 1999;181:1096–1101 (Level II-3)

52. Cheek TG, Samuels P. Pregnancy-induced hypertension. In: Datta S, ed. Anesthetic and obstetric management of high-risk pregnancy. 2nd ed. St. Louis: Mosby, 1996: 386–411 (Level III)

The MEDLINE database, the Cochrane Library, and ACOG's own internal resources and documents were used to conduct a literature search to locate relevant articles published between January 1985 and August 2000. The search was restricted to articles published in the English language. Priority was given to articles reporting results of original research, although review articles and commentaries also were consulted. Abstracts of research presented at symposia and scientific conferences were not considered adequate for inclusion in this document. Guidelines published by organizations or institutions such as the National Institutes of Health and the American College of Obstetricians and Gynecologists were reviewed, and additional studies were located by reviewing bibliographies of identified articles. When reliable research was not available, expert opinions from obstetrician–gynecologists were used.

Studies were reviewed and evaluated for quality according to the method outlined by the U.S. Preventive Services Task Force:

I   Evidence obtained from at least one properly designed randomized controlled trial.

II-1   Evidence obtained from well-designed controlled trials without randomization.

II-2   Evidence obtained from well-designed cohort or case–control analytic studies, preferably from more than one center or research group.

II-3   Evidence obtained from multiple time series with or without the intervention. Dramatic results in uncontrolled experiments could also be regarded as this type of evidence.

III   Opinions of respected authorities, based on clinical experience, descriptive studies, or reports of expert committees.

Based on the highest level of evidence found in the data, recommendations are provided and graded according to the following categories:

Level A—Recommendations are based on good and consistent scientific evidence.

Level B—Recommendations are based on limited or inconsistent scientific evidence.

Level C—Recommendations are based primarily on consensus and expert opinion.

ISSN 1099-3630

The American College of Obstetricians and Gynecologists
409 12th Street, SW,
PO Box 96920
Washington, DC 20090-6920

12345/54321

Chronic Hypertension in Pregnancy. ACOG Practice Bulletin No. 29. American College of Obstetricians and Gynecologists. Obstet Gynecol 2001;98:177–185

ACOG PRACTICE BULLETIN

CLINICAL MANAGEMENT GUIDELINES FOR
OBSTETRICIAN–GYNECOLOGISTS

NUMBER 51, MARCH 2004

This Practice Bulletin was developed by the ACOG Committee on Practice Bulletins— Gynecology with the assistance of Fred Howard, MD. The information is designed to aid practitioners in making decisions about appropriate obstetric and gynecologic care. These guidelines should not be construed as dictating an exclusive course of treatment or procedure. Variations in practice may be warranted based on the needs of the individual patient, resources, and limitations unique to the institution or type of practice.

Chronic Pelvic Pain

Chronic pelvic pain is a common disorder of women that often presents a diagnostic dilemma. It is frequently difficult to cure or manage adequately. Many gynecologic and nongynecologic disorders appear to cause or be associated with chronic pelvic pain. Treatment usually is directed to specific diseases that cause chronic pelvic pain, but sometimes there is no clear etiology for pain, and treatment must be directed to alleviating the symptoms. The purpose of this document is to provide information on the differential diagnosis of chronic pelvic pain and review the available evidence on treatment options for women with chronic pelvic pain.

Background

Definition and Prevalence

Pain is defined as an unpleasant sensory and emotional experience associated with actual or potential tissue damage or is described in terms of such damage (1). Pain is always subjective. Many patients report pain in the absence of tissue damage or any likely pathophysiologic cause; in such cases, pain may have a psychologic basis. If patients regard their experience as pain and report it in the same ways as pain caused by tissue damage, it should be accepted as pain. The definition of pain avoids tying pain to the stimulus.

There is no generally accepted definition of chronic pelvic pain. In gynecologic publications, most (but not all) authors have used duration of 6 or more months as the major criterion of the definition of chronicity. Specifying only duration allows for significant ambiguity, which has led to marked inconsistency of the patient populations included in published studies of chronic pelvic pain. An acceptable definition of chronic pelvic pain at least needs to specify temporal characteristics and location and possibly severity. Possible temporal characteristics include cyclic (eg, dysmenorrhea), intermittent (eg, dyspareunia), or noncyclic pain. Many have preferred to use only noncyclic pain in the definition of chronic pelvic pain because they think the potential etiologic disorders causing noncyclic pain differ from those associated with dysmenorrhea or dyspareunia. "Pelvic" often is assumed to be an adequate description of location, but visceral pelvic pain often is vaguely sensed at the periumbilical area, whereas somatic pelvic pain usually is well localized, for example, in the sacroiliac joint point at the posterior buttocks area. Additionally, chronic vulvar pain may or may not be included as chronic pelvic pain, depending on the definition of location. In reviewing any research on the causes or treatments of chronic pelvic pain, it is crucial to know which definition was used.

One proposed definition of chronic pelvic pain is noncyclic pain of 6 or more months' duration that localizes to the anatomic pelvis, anterior abdominal wall at or below the umbilicus, the lumbosacral back, or the buttocks and is of sufficient severity to cause functional disability or lead to medical care. A lack of physical findings does not negate the significance of a patient's pain, and normal examination results do not preclude the possibility of finding pelvic pathology.

Although the prevalence of chronic pelvic pain in the general population is not accurately established, available data suggest it is far more common than generally recognized. Approximately 15–20% of women aged 18–50 years have chronic pelvic pain of greater than 1 year's duration (2, 3).

Etiology of Chronic Pelvic Pain

Potential visceral sources of chronic pelvic pain include the reproductive, genitourinary, and gastrointestinal tracts; potential somatic sources include the pelvic bones, ligaments, muscles, and fascia. Chronic pelvic pain may result from psychologic disorders or neurologic diseases, both central and peripheral. It also may be useful to classify etiologies of chronic pelvic pain into gynecologic and nongynecologic causes, but clearly an obstetrician–gynecologist may diagnose and treat many nongynecologic disorders.

Few, if any, of the diseases thought to cause chronic pelvic pain meet traditional epidemiologic criteria of causality. Sufficient evidence strongly suggests that several of the most common disorders in women with chronic pelvic pain are causal, such as endometriosis, interstitial cystitis, and irritable bowel syndrome (see box and Table 1). For many of the diseases often listed as causes of chronic pelvic pain, only limited evidence or expert opinion supports an etiologic relationship. Although the etiologic relationships of many of the proposed disorders are not well established, in clinical practice, most are treated if diagnosed in women with chronic pelvic pain. This ambiguity makes it difficult to interpret cause and effect with regard to treatment in most studies of women with chronic pelvic pain.

Gynecologic Conditions That May Cause or Exacerbate Chronic Pelvic Pain, by Level of Evidence

Level A*
- Endometriosis†
- Gynecologic malignancies (especially late stage)
- Ovarian retention syndrome (residual ovary syndrome)
- Ovarian remnant syndrome
- Pelvic congestion syndrome
- Pelvic inflammatory disease†
- Tuberculous salpingitis

Level B‡
- Adhesions†
- Benign cystic mesothelioma
- Leiomyomata†
- Postoperative peritoneal cysts

Level C§
- Adenomyosis
- Atypical dysmenorrhea or ovulatory pain
- Adnexal cysts (nonendometriotic)
- Cervical stenosis
- Chronic ectopic pregnancy
- Chronic endometritis
- Endometrial or cervical polyps
- Endosalpingiosis
- Intrauterine contraceptive device
- Ovarian ovulatory pain
- Residual accessory ovary
- Symptomatic pelvic relaxation (genital prolapse)

*Level A: good and consistent scientific evidence of causal relationship to chronic pelvic pain
†Diagnosis frequently reported in published series of women with chronic pelvic pain
‡Level B: limited or inconsistent scientific evidence of causal relationship to chronic pelvic pain
§Level C: causal relationship to chronic pelvic pain based on expert opinions
Data from Howard FM. Chronic pelvic pain. Obstet Gynecol 2003; 101:594–611.

The proportion of women with chronic pelvic pain and a specific diagnosis (or diagnoses) is unclear and varies greatly in reported series. A large, primary care

Table 1. Nongynecologic Conditions That May Cause or Exacerbate Chronic Pelvic Pain, by Level of Evidence

Level of Evidence	Urologic	Gastrointestinal	Musculoskeletal	Other
Level A*	Bladder malignancy	Carcinoma of the colon	Abdominal wall myofascial pain (trigger points)	Abdominal cutaneous nerve entrapment in surgical scar
	Interstitial cystitis†	Constipation	Chronic coccygeal or back pain†	Depression†
	Radiation cystitis	Inflammatory bowel disease	Faulty or poor posture	Somatization disorder
	Urethral syndrome	Irritable bowel syndrome†	Fibromyalgia	
			Neuralgia of iliohypogastric, ilioinguinal, and/or genitofemoral nerves	
			Pelvic floor myalgia (levator ani or piriformis syndrome)	
			Peripartum pelvic pain syndrome	
Level B‡	Uninhibited bladder contractions (detrusor dyssynergia)	—	Herniated nucleus pulposus	Celiac disease
	Urethral diverticulum		Low back pain†	Neurologic dysfunction
			Neoplasia of spinal cord or sacral nerve	Porphyria
				Shingles
				Sleep disturbances
Level C§	Chronic urinary tract infection	Colitis	Compression of lumbar vertebrae	Abdominal epilepsy
	Recurrent, acute cystitis	Chronic intermittent bowel obstruction	Degenerative joint disease	Abdominal migraine
	Recurrent, acute urethritis	Diverticular disease	Hernias: ventral, inguinal, femoral, spigelian	Bipolar personality disorders
	Stone/urolithiasis		Muscular strains and sprains	Familial Mediterranean fever
			Rectus tendon strain	
	Urethral caruncle		Spondylosis	

*Level A: good and consistent scientific evidence of causal relationship to chronic pelvic pain

†Diagnosis frequently reported in published series of women with chronic pelvic pain

‡Level B: limited or inconsistent scientific evidence of causal relationship to chronic pelvic pain

§Level C: causal relationship to chronic pelvic pain based on expert opinions

Data from Howard FM. Chronic pelvic pain. Obstet Gynecol 2003;101:594–611.

database from the United Kingdom found diagnoses related to the urinary and gastrointestinal tracts were more common than gynecologic diagnoses (30.8% urinary, 37.7% gastrointestinal, and 20.2% gynecologic) (4). Furthermore, many women with chronic pelvic pain have more than 1 disease that might lead to pain; 25–50% of women who receive medical care in primary care practices have more than 1 diagnosis (4–6). The most common diagnoses are endometriosis, adhesions, irritable bowel syndrome, and interstitial cystitis (2, 7–9).

Women with diagnoses that involve more than 1 organ system have greater pain than women with only 1

system involved. For example, 43% of patients with chronic pelvic pain without gastrointestinal or urologic symptoms had moderate or severe pain (mean visual analog scale score: 3.8), whereas 71% of women with chronic pelvic pain and both gastrointestinal and urologic symptoms had moderate to severe pain (mean visual analog scale score: 5.4) (6). Consistency of pain also is greater in women with multisystem symptoms. Women with chronic pelvic pain are more likely than those in the general population to have dysmenorrhea (81% versus 58%) and dyspareunia (41% versus 14%). The severity of pain with intercourse and with menses is greater in women with chronic pelvic pain who have gastrointestinal and urologic symptoms than in those with no gastrointestinal or urologic symptoms.

Populations at Increased Risk of Chronic Pelvic Pain

Demographic profiles of large surveys suggest that women with chronic pelvic pain are no different from women without chronic pelvic pain in terms of age, race and ethnicity, education, socioeconomic status, or employment status (2, 6). Women with chronic pelvic pain may be slightly more likely to be separated or divorced (2). Women with chronic pelvic pain tend to be of reproductive age; however, age does not appear to be a specific risk factor (6). Women develop chronic pelvic pain at all ages, although the prevalence of different diagnoses seems to vary at different ages.

Physical and Sexual Abuse

Most published evidence suggests a significant association of physical and sexual abuse with various chronic pain disorders (10, 11). Studies have found that 40–50% of women with chronic pelvic pain have a history of abuse (12–16). Whether abuse (physical or sexual) specifically causes chronic pelvic pain is not clear, nor is a mechanism established by which abuse might lead to the development of chronic pelvic pain (17, 18). Women with a history of sexual abuse and high somatization scores have been found to be more likely to have nonsomatic pelvic pain, suggesting the link between abuse and chronic pelvic pain may be psychologic or neurologic (19, 20).

Evidence suggests that abuse may result in biophysical changes. For example, one study found that, after controlling for history of psychiatric disturbance, adult survivors had lower thresholds for pain (21). It also has been suggested that chronic or traumatic stimulation (especially in the pelvic or abdominal region) heightens sensitivity, resulting in persistent pain, such as abdominal and pelvic pain, or other bowel symptoms (22, 23). In women with chronic pelvic pain, as in all women, if a history of abuse is obtained, it is important to ensure that the women are not currently being abused and in danger.

Pelvic Inflammatory Disease

Approximately 18–35% of all women with acute pelvic inflammatory disease (PID) develop chronic pelvic pain (24, 25). The actual mechanisms by which chronic pelvic pain results from PID are not known, and not all women with reproductive organ damage secondary to acute PID develop chronic pelvic pain. Whether acute PID is treated with outpatient or inpatient regimens does not appear to significantly alter the odds of developing subsequent chronic pelvic pain (34% with outpatient therapy versus 30% with inpatient therapy) (24).

Endometriosis

Although endometriosis may be a direct cause of chronic pelvic pain, it also may indirectly place women at increased risk for chronic pelvic pain. For example, evidence suggests that women with endometriosis have increased episodes and pain severity of urinary calculoses than women without endometriosis (26). Similar results have been demonstrated for vaginal pain. Such viscero–visceral interactions may have a significant role in chronic pelvic pain in women and may explain why some women with a history of endometriosis have persistent pelvic pain after their endometriosis is gone.

Endometriosis is diagnosed laparoscopically in approximately 33% of women with chronic pelvic pain (other frequent laparoscopic diagnoses are adhesive disease in 24% of patients and no visible pathology in 35% of patients) (27). Although abnormal examination findings correlate in 70–90% of cases with abnormal laparoscopic findings (28, 29), more than one half of those with abnormal laparoscopic findings have normal findings on preoperative pelvic examinations (30).

Interstitial Cystitis

Women with interstitial cystitis are at significant risk of having chronic pelvic pain. Interstitial cystitis is a chronic inflammatory condition of the bladder. It is clinically characterized by irritative voiding symptoms of urgency and frequency in the absence of objective evidence of another disease that could cause the symptoms (31, 32). Pelvic pain is reported by up to 70% of women with interstitial cystitis, and occasionally it is the presenting symptom or chief complaint (32). It has been suggested that as many as 38–85% of women presenting to gynecologists with chronic pelvic pain may have interstitial cystitis (8, 33).

Irritable Bowel Syndrome

Irritable bowel syndrome is a common functional bowel disorder of uncertain etiology. It is characterized by a chronic, relapsing pattern of abdominopelvic pain and bowel dysfunction with constipation or diarrhea. Irritable bowel syndrome appears to be one of the most common disorders associated with chronic pelvic pain. It seems to occur much more commonly in women with chronic pelvic pain than in the general population; symptoms consistent with irritable bowel syndrome are found in 50–80% of women with chronic pelvic pain (9, 34). The current diagnostic criteria for irritable bowel syndrome are the Rome II criteria (see box).

Obstetric History

Pregnancy and childbirth can cause trauma to the musculoskeletal system, especially the pelvis and back, and may lead to chronic pelvic pain. Although few well-designed trials have assessed the relationship, historical risk factors associated with pregnancy and pain include lumbar lordosis, delivery of a large infant, muscle weakness and poor physical conditioning, a difficult delivery, vacuum or forceps delivery, and use of gynecologic stirrups for delivery (35). Conversely, women who have never been pregnant may have disorders that can cause both infertility and chronic pelvic pain, such as endometriosis, chronic PID, or pelvic adhesive disease.

Past Surgery

A history of abdominopelvic surgery is associated with chronic pelvic pain. In some cases, the relationship is relatively clear, such as unrecognized spillage of gallstones at the time of cholecystectomy (36, 37) or osteitis pubis or osteomyelitis after the Marshall–Marchietti–Kranz procedure (38). Prior cervical surgery for dysplasia may cause cervical stenosis, which has been associated with endometriosis (39). Additionally, among women without preoperative pelvic pain, 3–9% develop pelvic pain or back pain in the 2 years after hysterectomy (40). A recent case–control study suggests that cesarean delivery also may be a risk factor for chronic pelvic pain (odds ratio of 3.7) (41).

Musculoskeletal Disorders

Musculoskeletal disorders as causes of or risk factors for chronic pelvic pain have not been widely discussed in gynecologic publications. They may be more important, however, than generally recognized.

Pain that started with a pregnancy or immediately postpartum may suggest peripartum pelvic pain syndrome. This syndrome is thought to be caused by strain of the ligaments in the pelvis and lower spine from a combination of factors, including specific hormonal changes, damage to pelvic ligaments, muscle weakness, and the weight of the fetus and gravid uterus (35).

Faulty posture, in particular an exaggerated lumbar lordosis and thoracic kyphosis (called "typical pelvic pain posture"), may account for up to 75% of cases of chronic pelvic pain (42). Faulty posture is a contributing cause of weak, deconditioned muscles, which allow for imbalances in the pelvis with formation of trigger points and hypertonicity and, as a result, pelvic pain.

Other musculoskeletal disorders may cause or contribute to pelvic pain. These include trigger points, fibromyalgia, lumbar vertebral disorders, and pelvic floor myalgia.

Diagnostic Studies

A detailed history and physical examination are the basis for differential diagnosis. In a woman with chronic pelvic pain, the history and physical examination should take into account the risk factors noted previously, as well as the various conditions associated with chronic pelvic pain (see box "Gynecologic Conditions That May Cause or Exacerbate Chronic Pelvic Pain, by Level of Evidence" and Table 1). The history and physical examination also should seek to identify the location, severity, quality, and timing of the woman's pain. Because of the many nongynecologic conditions associated with chronic pelvic pain, interdisciplinary evaluation and management may be needed.

Up to two thirds of women with chronic pelvic pain do not undergo diagnostic testing, never receive a diagnosis, and are never referred to a specialist for evaluation

---

Rome II Criteria for Irritable Bowel Syndrome

At least 12 weeks (need not be consecutive) in the preceding 12 months of abdominal discomfort or pain that has 2 of 3 features:

1. Relieved with defecation

2. Onset associated with a change in frequency of stool

3. Onset associated with a change in stool form or appearance

The following symptoms are not essential for the diagnosis, but their presence increases diagnostic confidence and may be used to identify subgroups of irritable bowel syndrome:

- Abnormal stool frequency (more than 3 per day or fewer than 3 per week)

- Abnormal stool form (lumpy, hard or loose, watery) in more than 25% of defecations

- Abnormal stool passage (straining, urgency, or feeling of incomplete evacuation) in more than 25% of defecations

- Passage of mucus in more than 25% of defecations

- Bloating or feeling of abdominal distention in more than 25% of days

Modified from Thompson WG, Longstreth GF, Drossman DA, Heaton KW, Irvine EJ, Muller-Lissner SA. Functional bowel disorders and functional abdominal pain. Gut 1999;45(Suppl 2):II43–7.

or treatment (2, 5). Diagnostic studies should be based on the history and physical examination.

Diagnostic Imaging

Transvaginal ultrasonography is particularly useful for evaluation of the pelvis. In patients with a pelvic mass, ultrasonography may help identify the origin of the mass as uterine, adnexal, gastrointestinal, or from the bladder. Magnetic resonance imaging or computed tomography may be useful in rare cases when ultrasound findings are abnormal.

Laparoscopy

Chronic pelvic pain is the indication for at least 40% of all gynecologic laparoscopies (27). Endometriosis and adhesions account for more than 90% of the diagnoses in women with discernible laparoscopic abnormalities, and laparoscopy is indicated in women thought to have either of these conditions. When endometriosis is suspected on the basis of visual findings during laparoscopy, biopsies and histologic confirmation of suspicious areas are important (43) because the visual diagnosis is incorrect in 10–90% of cases (44). Often, adolescents are excluded from laparoscopic evaluation on the basis of their age, but several series show that endometriosis is as common in adolescents with chronic pelvic pain as in the rest of the population (45, 46).

Conscious laparoscopic pain mapping, a diagnostic laparoscopy performed under local anesthesia, can be performed with the goal of identifying sources of pain in women with chronic pelvic pain. It has been suggested that conscious laparoscopic pain mapping can lead to the treatment of subtle or atypical areas of disease that might have been overlooked if the procedure had been done under general anesthesia or may even help patients avoid surgical treatment when no painful lesions are identified (47). However, no substantial data confirm improved diagnostic accuracy or improved clinical outcomes with conscious laparoscopic pain mapping (48–50).

Evaluation of Symptoms of Urinary Tract Infection

An intravesical potassium sensitivity test evaluates pain and urgency after intravesical instillation of 40 mL of potassium chloride (0.4 mEq/mL) compared with symptoms after instillation of 40 mL of water (51). Among patients with interstitial cystitis, 70–90% have positive results on intravesical potassium sensitivity testing. Up to 85% of women evaluated by obstetrician–gynecologists for chronic pelvic pain may have positive intravesical potassium sensitivity test results (8). Whether these findings represent a high prevalence of interstitial cystitis in women with chronic pelvic pain or viscero–visceral convergence in women with reproductive tract disease has not been determined. Furthermore, the diagnostic validity of the intravesical potassium sensitivity test for interstitial cystitis is still controversial (52, 53).

The interstitial cystitis symptom index is a validated questionnaire that reliably predicts the diagnosis of interstitial cystitis and may be used to help determine whether cystoscopy is indicated (54). For example, 72% of women with a score of 5 or more on the interstitial cystitis symptom index and significant dyspareunia pain levels have intersitial cystitis identified cystoscopically (33). Cystoscopic criteria for interstitial cystitis are the presence of glomerulations (petechiae) or Hunner ulcer with bladder distention to 80–100 cm water pressure under anesthesia and decreased bladder capacity (less than 350 mL) without anesthesia (55). The reliability of bladder glomerulations as a diagnostic criterion for interstitial cystitis has been questioned because similar findings are possible in women without voiding symptoms (56).

Clinical Considerations and Recommendations

▶ *Is there evidence to support the following medical approaches to treatment of chronic pelvic pain?*

Antidepressants

Tricyclic antidepressants and selective serotonin reuptake inhibitors (SSRIs) have been approved for treating depression, but new research has shown they can be effective in treating other conditions in patients who do not have depression. Tricyclic antidepressants, such as imipramine, amitriptyline, desipramine, and doxepin, have been shown in placebo-controlled studies to improve pain levels and pain tolerance in some, but not all, chronic pain syndromes (57). It is not clear how effective other antidepressants, such as SSRIs, are in the treatment of chronic pain syndromes (58–61).

Few studies have evaluated the use of antidepressants for chronic pelvic pain (62). One uncontrolled evaluation of the tricyclic antidepressant nortriptyline showed a decrease of pain intensity and duration, but one half of the patients discontinued nortriptyline before completing the study because of drug side effects at doses of 100 mg or less (63). A placebo-controlled, crossover study of the SSRI sertraline, 50 mg twice daily for 6 weeks, showed no improvement in pelvic pain (64).

At this time, evidence is insufficient to substantiate efficacy of antidepressants for the treatment of chronic pelvic pain, although the efficacy of tricyclic antidepressants for other pain syndromes suggests they also might be efficacious for chronic pelvic pain. Nonetheless, the substantial association of depression with chronic pelvic pain supports the use of antidepressants for the specific treatment of depression.

Local Anesthetic Injection of Trigger Points

Chronic pain syndromes associated with myofascial trigger points have been clinically recognized for quite some time (65). Observational data on the use of local anesthetic injection of trigger points of the abdominal wall, vagina, and sacrum for relief of chronic pelvic pain have demonstrated a response rate of 68% (66).

Analgesics

Extensive evidence demonstrates that nonsteroidal anti-inflammatory drugs, including COX-2 inhibitors, relieve various types of pain, including dysmenorrhea (67, 68). No clinical trials have addressed chronic pelvic pain specifically, but moderate analgesic efficacy, as shown for other types of pain, would be anticipated.

Opioids are increasingly used in the treatment of chronic pain (69). Randomized clinical trials suggest significant analgesic effects but not necessarily improvement in functional or psychologic status (70–72). Risk of addiction has been low in patients with chronic pain. There are no published studies of opioid treatment for chronic pelvic pain.

▶ *Is there evidence to support the use of hormonal therapy for treatment of chronic pelvic pain?*

Combined Oral Contraceptives

Oral contraceptives provide significant relief from primary dysmenorrhea (73). They suppress ovulation, markedly reduce spontaneous uterine activity, stabilize estrogen and progesterone levels, abrogate menstrual increases in prostaglandin levels, and reduce the amount of pain and symptoms associated with menses. These effects also are thought to make oral contraceptives effective in the treatment of other gynecologic pain disorders.

Oral contraceptives often are recommended for endometriosis-associated chronic pelvic pain (74), but there are limited data from clinical trials to support this recommendation. One clinical trial suggested combined oral contraceptives are comparable to the gonadotropin-releasing hormone (GnRH) agonist goserelin in relieving chronic pelvic pain and dyspareunia—but less effective in relieving dysmenorrhea—in women with endometriosis (75). A trial evaluating postoperative administration of monophasic combined oral contraceptives after surgical resection of endometriomas suggested oral contraceptives do not significantly affect the long-term recurrence of endometriosis (76). No data address the use of cyclic versus noncyclic combined oral contraceptives. Other hormonal contraceptive methods, such as the levonorgestrel-releasing intrauterine device, may be effective for treatment of dysmenorrhea associated with endometriosis, but evidence is limited (77).

Gonadotropin-Releasing Hormone Agonists

Gonadotropin-releasing hormone agonists are analogues of naturally occurring gonadotropin-releasing hormones that "down-regulate" hypothalamic–pituitary gland production and the release of luteinizing hormone and follicle-stimulating hormone leading to dramatic reductions in estradiol levels. The GnRH agonists available in the United States are nafarelin, goserelin, and leuprolide. Numerous clinical trials show GnRH agonists are more effective than placebo and as effective as danazol in relieving endometriosis-associated pelvic pain (78–86). However, one clinical trial designed to evaluate empiric treatment of chronic pelvic pain with suspected endometriosis suggested GnRH agonists have the same efficacy in women with symptoms consistent with endometriosis, whether or not they actually have endometriosis (87). Although this finding is based on a relatively small number of cases, it strongly suggests the response to GnRH agonists does not depend on surgical confirmation of endometriosis in women with symptoms suggestive of endometriosis-associated chronic pelvic pain. One possible explanation for this finding may be that although obstetrician–gynecologists generally assume GnRH agonist treatment is specific for endometriosis-associated pelvic pain, in fact, symptoms of pelvic congestion syndrome (88), irritable bowel syndrome (89–92), and interstitial cystitis (93) also vary with the menstrual cycle and respond to GnRH agonist treatment.

Good evidence from studies of prolonged treatment of endometriosis-associated pelvic pain indicates that loss of bone density, one of the major adverse effects of GnRH agonists, can be abrogated by add-back treatment with estrogen and progestogen or progestogen only, without significant loss of efficacy (94–96). Postoperative treatment with GnRH agonists also appears to be efficacious in women with endometriosis (97, 98). In addition, observational data suggest GnRH agonists may be used to treat pelvic pain associated with ovarian retention syndrome (residual ovary syndrome) and ovarian remnant syndrome (98, 99).

Progestins

Clinical trials suggest progestins are effective in the treatment of chronic pelvic pain associated with endometriosis and pelvic congestion syndrome. Medroxyprogesterone acetate, 30–100 mg per day, effectively decreases pain from endometriosis and pelvic congestion syndrome in most studies (100–103). Other progestational agents not available in the United States, such as gestrinone and lynestrenol, also are effective in the treatment of endometriosis-associated pelvic pain (104, 105). Norethindrone is sometimes recommended for treatment of endometriosis-associated pelvic pain but has only been studied in uncontrolled trials (106).

▶ *What is the evidence for efficacy of proposed nonmedical treatments?*

Many modalities of treatment other than medications and surgery have been recommended for chronic pelvic pain, including exercise, physical therapy, and dietary modifications. Very few of these treatments have been studied in clinical trials.

Exercise

Although most studies suggest dysmenorrhea is decreased by exercise, there are no definitive data to support this suggestion (107, 108). Additionally, no data address the efficacy of exercise for relief of chronic pelvic pain.

Physical Therapy

Observational studies suggest various physical therapy modalities are effective for pain relief. Electrotherapy, fast- and slow-twitch exercises of the striated muscles of the pelvic floor, and manual therapy of myofascial trigger points in the pelvic floor have shown improvement of pain in 65–70% of patients (109, 110). For peripartum pelvic pain syndrome, physical therapy showed no efficacy over that of a pelvic belt with no exercise (111).

▶ *Are surgical approaches effective for treatment of chronic pelvic pain?*

Various surgical treatments aimed primarily at treating endometriosis, including excision or destruction of endometriotic tissue and hysterectomy, have been pro-

posed to relieve chronic pelvic pain. Other surgical approaches also have been considered.

Excision or Destruction of Endometriotic Tissue

It is suggested that conservative surgical treatment of endometriosis results in significant pain relief for 1 year in 45–85% of women, but only one clinical trial compared conservative surgical treatment with placebo therapy (112, 113). The design of this trial limits its generalizability (only laparoscopic laser ablation of lesions was performed, only women with endometriosis in stages I through III were included, and only 6 patients had stage III endometriosis), but it confirms the efficacy of conservative surgical treatment. Laparoscopic laser treatment of endometriosis showed pain relief at 6 months in 62% of patients versus 20% in the group that underwent diagnostic laparoscopy only.

The recurrence rate of endometriosis after conservative surgical treatment has been reported to range from 15% to 100% (114). The average time to recurrence after initial surgery by laparotomy is 40–50 months. However, the time to recurrence may reflect the thoroughness of the original surgery or effectiveness of subsequent medical treatment.

Hysterectomy

It is estimated that chronic pelvic pain is the principal preoperative indication for 10–12% of hysterectomies (115). In the Maine Women's Health Study (a prospective cohort study), 18% of women had hysterectomies for a primary indication of chronic pelvic pain (116, 117). In the same study, 45% of the women who had hysterectomies for leiomyomata had more than 8 days of pain per month, and 66% of those with bleeding as the preoperative indication had similar pain, which suggests pain is a secondary indication for hysterectomy in many women. In this study, women with chronic pelvic pain treated with hysterectomy had significantly improved outcomes at 1 year compared with women treated medically. Outcomes were better in mean days of pain per month and severity of pain, as well as in indicators of quality of life. Only one half of these women had specific diagnoses, such as endometriosis, leiomyomata, or adhesions.

The Maryland Women's Health Study, also a prospective cohort study but without a control group, showed that almost 90% of women had relief of pain at 1 and 2 years after hysterectomy (40). Data from the United States Collaborative Review of Sterilization, a prospective cohort study, showed that at 1 year after hysterectomy for chronic pelvic pain, 74% of women had complete resolution of pain, and 21% had decreased pain

(118). A retrospective study of hysterectomy for chronic pelvic pain with no extrauterine pathology found that 78% of women were pain-free at follow-up of at least 1 year (119). In 65% of these women, no uterine pathology was detected. Finally, a small study of women with chronic pelvic pain caused by pelvic congestion (demonstrated by venography and ultrasonography) reported marked improvement or relief of pain in 35 of 36 patients after hysterectomy and bilateral salpingo-oophorectomy (120).

Hysterectomy appears to have a role in the treatment of many women with chronic pelvic pain. Although based only on observational studies, it appears that at least 75% of women who have a hysterectomy for chronic pelvic pain thought to be caused by gynecologic disease experience pain relief at 1 year of follow-up.

Adhesiolysis

Adhesions are commonly thought to be a potential cause of chronic pelvic pain, and evidence from conscious laparoscopic pain mapping suggests some women have painful adhesions (50). Observational studies suggest that up to 85% of women improve after adhesiolysis (121), but the only clinical trial of adhesiolysis suggests that only women with dense adhesions involving bowel show any decrease in pain after surgical adhesiolysis (122).

Nerve Stimulation

Sacral nerve stimulation is beneficial in the treatment of chronic voiding dysfunction. Its use in women with voiding dysfunction and chronic pelvic pain has suggested potential efficacy for treatment of chronic pelvic pain. Uncontrolled studies of sacral nerve stimulation in women with chronic pelvic pain and no voiding disorder suggest that 60% of women show significant improvement in their pain levels (123–125).

Presacral Neurectomy

Innervation from the superior hypogastric plexus (presacral nerve) supplies the cervix, uterus, and proximal fallopian tubes with afferent nociception. Surgical resection of this plexus is sometimes useful for central dysmenorrhea unresponsive to other treatments. Approximately three fourths of patients with this symptom have a greater than 50% decrease in pain after presacral neurectomy (126, 127). Presacral neurectomy is significantly more effective for the treatment of primary dysmenorrhea than uterine nerve ablation (128).

Clinical trials show that as a component of conservative surgery for endometriosis-associated pelvic pain, presacral neurectomy provides additional pain relief mostly of midline pain associated with menses, with little additional effect on dyspareunia and nonmenstrual pain (129, 130). Similar results are obtained in women without endometriosis; that is, only central dysmenorrhea appears to be decreased, with no significant effect on noncentral or nonmenstrual pain (131). Overall, regardless of pathology, pain that is localized in the lateral pelvic area, as opposed to central pelvic pain, has a notably lower response to treatment by presacral neurectomy.

It has been suggested that performing superior hypogastric plexus blocks before deciding to do a presacral neurectomy may improve the outcomes with surgery or avoid the need for surgery altogether (132), but only small case series have been published in support of this concept (133). It also has been suggested that repeated superior hypogastric blocks may reverse central sensitization and sympathetically maintained pelvic pain resulting in prolonged relief of pain (134).

Uterine Nerve Ablation

Uterine nerve ablation involves transecting or resecting the uterosacral ligaments at their insertions into the uterus, which interrupts a significant portion of the cervical sensory nerve fibers. One small clinical trial found uterine nerve ablation significantly decreased the severity of primary dysmenorrhea for at least 3 months ($P < .05$) (135). Uterine nerve ablation is less effective for the treatment of primary dysmenorrhea than presacral neurectomy (128).

Adding uterine nerve ablation to surgical treatment of endometriosis-associated pelvic pain or dysmenorrhea does not improve the outcome of surgical treatment (136, 137). No evidence demonstrates that uterine nerve ablation improves nonmenstrual chronic pelvic pain.

▶ *Is counseling or psychotherapy effective for treatment of chronic pelvic pain?*

Psychosomatic factors appear to have a prominent role in chronic pelvic pain (138), which suggests that psychiatric or psychologic evaluation and treatment should be routine in women with chronic pelvic pain. Various modes of psychotherapy, including cognitive therapy, operant conditioning, and behavioral modification, appear to be helpful in women with chronic pelvic pain, but most of the data are observational (139) or include psychotherapy as part of multidisciplinary treatment (140). One randomized clinical trial of psychotherapy for pelvic congestion syndrome suggested that adding psychotherapy to medical treatment improved the response over that obtained with medical treatment only (102).

Up to 50% of women with chronic pelvic pain have a history of physical or sexual abuse (14, 141). Traumatized patients who experienced abuse as children generally benefit from mental health care. For patients who have not sought such care, obstetrician–gynecologists can be powerful allies in patients' healing by offering support and referral. Efforts should be made to refer patients to mental health professionals with significant experience in abuse-related issues.

When referring a patient to another health care professional, it is especially helpful to indicate to the patient that her past abuse may be contributing to her current health problems and that further evaluation by a therapist would be beneficial. This is likely more effective than telling the patient that her symptoms are all "psychologic" and that she should see a therapist (142). It is important to secure the patient's express authorization before speaking to the therapist when collaborative practice between the obstetrician–gynecologist and therapist is warranted. If appropriate, to reassure the patient, the physician should emphasize his or her ongoing involvement in the patient's case.

▶ *Are complementary or alternative medicine therapies effective for treating chronic pelvic pain?*

Herbal and Nutritional Therapies

Treatment of dysmenorrhea has been studied in clinical trials of magnesium, vitamin B_6, vitamin B_1, omega-3 fatty acids, and a Japanese herbal combination (Japanese angelica root, peony root, hoelen, atractylodes lancea root, alisma root, cnidium root). Vitamin B_1 (100 mg daily) and magnesium (doses varied) were significantly more effective than a placebo in numerous studies, but data were insufficient to recommend the other therapies for dysmenorrhea (143). Published clinical trials of herbal or nutritional therapies for nonmenstrual pain are lacking.

Magnetic Field Therapy

The application of magnets to abdominal trigger points appears to improve disability and reduce pain when compared with placebo magnets (144). However, only one clinical trial evaluated the use of magnet therapy, and it had significant methodologic flaws. Whether magnetic field therapy is helpful for other types of chronic pelvic pain is not known, but limited observational data suggest potential usefulness for endometriosis-associated pain, dyspareunia, and dysmenorrhea (145).

Acupuncture

Clinical trials evaluating the efficacy of acupuncture, acupressure, and transcutaneous nerve stimulation therapies have been performed only for primary dysmenorrhea, not for nonmenstrual pelvic pain. All 3 modalities are better than placebo in the treatment of dysmenorrhea (146–149). Only case reports support acupuncture as a modality to treat nonmenstrual chronic pelvic pain (150).

Summary of Recommendations

The following recommendations are based on good and consistent scientific evidence (Level A):

▶ Combined oral contraceptives should be considered as a treatment option to decrease pain from primary dysmenorrhea.

▶ Gonadotropin-releasing hormone agonists are effective in relieving pelvic pain associated with endometriosis and irritable bowel syndrome, as well as in women with symptoms consistent with endometriosis who do not have endometriosis. Thus, empiric treatment with GnRH agonists without laparoscopy should be considered as an acceptable approach to treatment.

▶ Nonsteroidal antiinflammatory drugs, including COX-2 inhibitors, should be considered for moderate pain and are particularly effective for dysmenorrhea.

▶ Progestins in daily, high doses should be considered as an effective treatment of chronic pelvic pain associated with endometriosis and pelvic congestion syndrome.

▶ Laparoscopic surgical destruction of endometriosis lesions should be considered to decrease pelvic pain associated with stages I–III endometriosis.

▶ Presacral neurectomy may be considered for treatment of centrally located dysmenorrhea but has limited efficacy for chronic pelvic pain or pain that is not central in its location. Uterine nerve ablation or transection of the uterosacral ligament also can be considered for centrally located dysmenorrhea, but it appears to be less effective than presacral neurectomy. Combining uterine nerve ablation or presacral neurectomy with surgical treatment of endometriosis does not further improve overall pain relief.

▶ Adding psychotherapy to medical treatment of chronic pelvic pain appears to improve response over that of medical treatment alone and should be considered.

The following recommendations are based on limited or inconsistent scientific evidence (Level B):

▶ Gonadotropin-releasing hormone agonists should be considered as a treatment option for chronic pelvic pain because they have been shown to relieve endometriosis-associated pelvic pain.

▶ Surgical adhesiolysis should be considered to decrease pain in women with dense adhesions involving the bowel, but it is unclear if lysis of other types of adhesions is effective.

▶ Hysterectomy is an effective treatment for chronic pelvic pain associated with reproductive tract symptoms that results in pain relief in 75–95% of women and should be considered.

▶ Sacral nerve stimulation may decrease pain in up to 60% of women with chronic pelvic pain and should be considered as a treatment option.

▶ Various physical therapy modalities appear to be helpful in the treatment of chronic pelvic pain and should be considered as a treatment option.

▶ Nutritional supplementation with vitamin B_1 or magnesium may be recommended to decrease pain of dysmenorrhea.

▶ Injection of trigger points of the abdominal wall, vagina, and sacrum with local anesthetic may provide temporary or prolonged relief of chronic pelvic pain and should be considered.

▶ Treatment of abdominal trigger points by the application of magnets to the trigger points may be recommended to improve disability and reduce pain.

▶ Acupuncture, acupressure, and transcutaneous nerve stimulation therapies should be considered to decrease pain of primary dysmenorrhea.

The following recommendations are based primarily on consensus and expert opinion (Level C):

▶ A detailed history and physical examination are the basis for differential diagnosis of chronic pelvic pain and should be used to determine appropriate diagnostic studies.

▶ Antidepressants may be helpful in the treatment of chronic pelvic pain.

▶ Opioid analgesics can be used to provide effective relief of severe pain with a low risk of addiction but do not necessarily improve functional or psychologic status and are not well studied in patients with chronic pelvic pain.

References

1. Merskey H, Bogduk N, editors. Classification of chronic pain. IASP Task Force on Taxonomy. 2nd ed. Seattle (WA): IASP Press; 1994. p. 209–14. (Level III)

2. Mathias SD, Kuppermann M, Liberman RF, Lipschutz RC, Steege JF. Chronic pelvic pain: prevalence, health-related quality of life, and economic correlates. Obstet Gynecol 1996;87:321–7. (Level II-2)

3. Jamieson DJ, Steege JF. The prevalence of dysmenorrhea, dyspareunia, pelvic pain, and irritable bowel syndrome in primary care practices. Obstet Gynecol 1996; 87:55–8. (Level II-2)

4. Zondervan KT, Yudkin PL, Vessey MP, Dawes MG, Barlow DH, Kennedy SH. Patterns of diagnosis and referral in women consulting for chronic pelvic pain in UK primary care. Br J Obstet Gynaecol 1999;106: 1156–61. (Level II-2)

5. Zondervan KT, Yudkin PL, Vessey MP, Dawes MG, Barlow DH, Kennedy SH. Prevalence and incidence in primary care of chronic pelvic pain in women: evidence from a national general practice database. Br J Obstet Gynaecol 1999;106:1149–55. (Level II-3)

6. Zondervan KT, Yudkin PL, Vessey MP, Jenkinson CP, Dawes MG, Barlow DH, et al. Chronic pelvic pain in the community—symptoms, investigations, and diagnoses. Am J Obstet Gynecol 2001;184:1149–55. (Level II-2)

7. Prior A, Wilson K, Whorwell PJ, Faragher EB. Irritable bowel syndrome in the gynecological clinic. Survey of 798 new referrals. Dig Dis Sci 1989;34:1820–4. (Level II-2)

8. Parsons CL, Bullen M, Kahn BS, Stanford EJ, Willems JJ. Gynecologic presentation of interstitial cystitis as detected by intravesical potassium sensitivity. Obstet Gynecol 2001;98:127–32. (Level II-2)

9. Longstreth GF, Preskill DB, Youkeles L. Irritable bowel syndrome in women having diagnostic laparoscopy or hysterectomy. Relation to gynecologic features and outcome. Dig Dis Sci 1990;35:1285–90. (Level II-2)

10. Green CR, Flowe-Valencia H, Rosenblum L, Tait AR. The role of childhood and adulthood abuse among women presenting for chronic pain management. Clin J Pain 2001;17:359–64. (Level II-2)

11. Walling MK, Reiter RC, O'Hara MW, Milburn AK, Lilly G, Vincent SD. Abuse history and chronic pain in women: I. Prevalences of sexual abuse and physical abuse. Obstet Gynecol 1994;84:193–9. (Level II-2)

12. Rapkin AJ, Kames LD, Darke LL, Stampler FM, Naliboff BD. History of physical and sexual abuse in

women with chronic pelvic pain. Obstet Gynecol 1990; 76:92–6. (Level II-2)

13. Reiter RC, Gambone JC. Demographic and historic variables in women with idiopathic chronic pelvic pain. Obstet Gynecol 1990;75:428–32. (Level II-2)

14. Jamieson DJ, Steege JF. The association of sexual abuse with pelvic pain complaints in a primary care population. Am J Obstet Gynecol 1997;177:1408–12. (Level II-2)

15. Collett BJ, Cordle CJ, Stewart CR, Jagger C. A comparative study of women with chronic pelvic pain, chronic nonpelvic pain, and those with no history of pain attending general practitioners. Br J Obstet Gynaecol 1998; 105:87–92. (Level II-2)

16. Walker E, Katon W, Harrop-Griffiths J, Holm L, Russo J, Hickok LR. Relationship of chronic pelvic pain to psychiatric diagnoses and childhood sexual abuse. Am J Psychiatry 1988;145:75–80. (Level II-2)

17. Heim C, Ehlert U, Hanker JP, Hellhammer DH. Abuse-related posttraumatic stress disorder and alterations of the hypothalamic-pituitary-adrenal axis in women with chronic pelvic pain. Psychsom Med 1998;60:309–18. (Level II-2)

18. Harrop-Griffiths J, Katon W, Walker E, Holm L, Russo J, Hickok L. The association between chronic pelvic pain, psychiatric diagnoses, and childhood sexual abuse. Obstet Gynecol 1988;71:589–94. (Level II-2)

19. Ehlert U, Heim C, Hellhammer DH. Chronic pelvic pain as a somatoform disorder. Psychother Psychosom 1999; 68:87–94. (Level II-2)

20. Reiter RC, Shakerin LR, Gambone JG, Milburn AK. Correlation between sexual abuse and somatization in women with somatic and nonsomatic chronic pelvic pain. Am J Obstet Gynecol 1991;165:104–9. (Level II-2)

21. Scarinci IC, McDonald-Haile J, Bradley LA, Richter JE. Altered pain perception and psychosocial features among women with gastrointestinal disorders and history of abuse: a preliminary model. Am J Med 1994;97:108–18. (Level II-2)

22. Cervero F, Janig W. Visceral nociceptors: a new world order? Trends Neurosci 1992;15:374–8. (Level III)

23. Drossman DA. Physical and sexual abuse and gastrointestinal illness: what is the link? Am J Med 1994;97: 105–7. (Level III)

24. Ness RB, Soper DE, Holley RL, Peipert J, Randall H, Sweet RL, et al. Effectiveness of inpatient and outpatient treatment strategies for women with pelvic inflammatory disease: results from the Pelvic Inflammatory Disease Evaluation and Clinical Health (PEACH) Randomized Trial. Am J Obstet Gynecol 2002;186:929–37. (Level I)

25. Westrom L. Effect of acute pelvic inflammatory disease on fertility. Am J Obstet Gynecol 1975;121:707–13. (Level II-2)

26. Giamberardino MA, De Laurentis S, Affaitati G, Lerza R, Lapenna D, Vecchiet L. Modulation of pain and hyperalgesia from the urinary tract by algogenic conditions of the reproductive organs in women. Neurosci Lett 2001;304: 61–4. (Level II-2)

27. Howard FM. The role of laparoscopy in chronic pelvic pain: promise and pitfalls. Obstet Gynecol Surv 1993;48: 357–87. (Level III)

28. Kresch AJ, Seifer DB, Sachs LB, Barrese I. Laparoscopy in 100 women with chronic pelvic pain. Obstet Gynecol 1984;64:672–4. (Level II-2)

29. Ripps BA, Martin DC. Focal pelvic tenderness, pelvic pain, and dysmenorrhea in endometriosis. J Reprod Med 1991;36:470–2. (Level III)

30. Cunanan RG Jr, Courey NG, Lippes J. Laparoscopic findings in patients with pelvic pain. Am J Obstet Gynecol 1983;146:589–91. (Level II-3)

31. Summitt RL Jr. Urogynecologic causes of chronic pelvic pain. Obstet Gynecol Clin North Am 1993;20:685–98. (Level III)

32. Ramahi AJ, Richardson DA. A practical approach to the painful bladder syndrome. J Reprod Med 1990;35:805–9. (Level III)

33. Clemons JL, Arya LA, Myers DL. Diagnosing interstitial cystitis in women with chronic pelvic pain. Obstet Gynecol 2002;100:337–41. (Level II-2)

34. Walker EA, Katon WJ, Jemelka R, Alfrey H, Bowers M, Stenchever MA. The prevalence of chronic pelvic pain and irritable bowel syndrome in two university clinics. J Psychosom Obstet Gynecol 1991;12(suppl):65–75. (Level III)

35. Mens JM, Vleeming A, Stoeckart R, Stam HJ, Snijders CJ. Understanding peripartum pelvic pain. Implications of a patient survey. Spine 1996;21:1363–9; discussion 1369–70. (Level III)

36. Pfeifer ME, Hansen KA, Tho SP, Hines RS, Plouffe L Jr. Ovarian cholelithiasis after laparoscopic cholecystectomy associated with chronic pelvic pain. Fertil Steril 1996;66:1031–2. (Level III)

37. Dulemba JF. Spilled gallstones causing pelvic pain. J Am Assoc Gynecol Laparosc 1996;3:309–11. (Level III)

38. Sexton DJ, Heskestad L, Lambeth WR, McCallum R, Levin LS, Corey GR. Postoperative pubic osteomyelitis misdiagnosed as osteitis pubis—report of four cases and review. Clin Infect Dis 1993;17:695–700. (Level III)

39. Barbieri RL. Stenosis of the external cervical os: an association with endometriosis in women with chronic pelvic pain. Fertil Steril 1998;70:571–3. (Level III)

40. Kjerulff KH, Langenberg PW, Rhodes JC, Harvey LA, Guzinski GM, Stolley PD. Effectiveness of hysterectomy. Obstet Gynecol 2000;95:319–26. (Level II-3)

41. Almeida EC, Nogueira AA, Candido dos Reis FJ, Rosa e Silva JC. Cesarean section as a cause of chronic pelvic pain. Int J Gynaecol Obstet 2002;79:101–4. (Level II-2)

42. King PM, Myers CA, Ling FW, Rosenthal RH. Musculoskeletal factors in chronic pelvic pain. J Psychosom Obstet Gynaecol 1991;12(suppl):87–98. (Level II-3)

43. Walter AJ, Hentz JG, Magtibay PM, Cornella JL, Magrina JF. Endometriosis: correlation between his-

tologic and visual findings at laparoscopy. Am J Obstet Gynecol 2001;184:1407–11; discussion 1411–3. (Level II-2)

44. Howard FM. The role of laparoscopy as a diagnostic tool in chronic pelvic pain. Baillieres Best Pract Res Clin Obstet Gynaecol 2000;14:467–94. (Level III)

45. Laufer MR, Goitein L, Bush M, Cramer DW, Emans SJ. Prevalence of endometriosis in adolescent girls with chronic pelvic pain not responding to conventional therapy. J Pediatr Adolesc Gynecol 1997;10:199–202. (Level II-2)

46. Vercellini P, Fedele L, Arcaini L, Bianchi S, Rognoni MT, Candiani GB. Laparoscopy in the diagnosis of chronic pelvic pain in adolescent women. J Reprod Med 1989; 34;827–30. (Level III)

47. Almeida OD Jr, Val-Gallas JM. Conscious pain mapping. J Am Assoc Gynecol Laparosc 1997;4:587–90. (Level III)

48. Demco LA. Effect on negative laparoscopy rate in chronic pelvic pain patients using patient assisted laparoscopy. JSLS 1997;1:319–21. (Level III)

49. Almeida OD Jr. Microlaparoscopic conscious pain mapping in the evaluation of chronic pelvic pain: a case report [published erratum appears in JSLS 2002;6:192]. JSLS 2002;6:81–3. (Level III)

50. Howard FM, El-Minawi AM, Sanchez RA. Conscious pain mapping by laparoscopy in women with chronic pelvic pain. Obstet Gynecol 2000;96:934–9. (Level III)

51. Parsons CL, Stein PC, Bidair M, Lebow D. Abnormal sensitivity to intravesical potassium in intersitial cystitis and radiation cystitis. Neurourol Urodyn 1994;13:515–20. (Level I)

52. Gregoire M, Liandier F, Naud A, Lacombe L, Fradet Y. Does the potassium stimulation test predict cystometric, cystoscopic outcome in interstital cystitis? J Urol 2002; 168:556–7. (Level II-2)

53. Chambers GK, Fenster HN, Cripps S, Jens M, Taylor D. An assessment of the use of intravesical potassium in the diagnosis of interstitial cystitis. J Urol 1999;162: 699–701. (Level II-2)

54. O'Leary MP, Sant GR, Fowler JF Jr, Whitmore KE, Spolarich-Kroll J. The intersitial cystitis symptom index and problem index. Urology 1997;49(5A suppl):58–63. (Level II-2)

55. Messing EM. The diagnosis of intersitial cystitis. Urology 1987;29(suppl):4–7. (Level III)

56. Waxman JA, Sulak PJ, Kuehl TJ. Cystoscopic findings consistent with intersitial cystitis in normal women undergoing tubal ligation. J Urol 1998;160:1663–7. (Level II-2)

57. Onghena P, Van Houdenhove BV. Antidepressant-induced analgesia in chronic non-malignant pain: a meta-analysis of 39 placebo controlled studies. Pain 1992;49:205–19. (Meta-analysis)

58. Rani PU, Naidu MU, Prasad VB, Rao TR, Shobha JC. An evaluation of antidepressants in rheumatic pain conditions. Anesth Analg 1996;83:371–5. (Level I)

59. Saper JR, Silberstein, SD, Lake AE 3rd, Winters ME. Double-blind trial of fluoxetine: chronic daily headache and migraine. Headache 1994;34:497–502. (Level I)

60. Max MB, Lynch SA, Muir J, Shoaf SE, Smoller B, Dubner R. Effects of desipramine, amitriptyline, and fluoxetine on pain in diabetic neuropathy. N Engl J Med 1992;326:1250–6. (Level II-3)

61. Schreiber S, Vinokur S, Shavelzon V, Pick CG, Zahavi E, Shir Y. A randomized trial of fluoxetine versus amitriptyline in musculo-skeletal pain. Isr J Psychiatry Relat Sci 2001;38:88–94. (Level I)

62. Walker EA, Sullivan MD, Stenchever MA. Use of antidepressants in the management of women with chronic pelvic pain. Obstet Gynecol Clin North Am 1993; 20:743–51. (Level III)

63. Walker EA, Roy-Byrne PP, Katon WJ, Jemelka R. An open trial of nortriptyline in women with chronic pelvic pain. Int J Psychiatry Med 1991;21:245–52. (Level III)

64. Engel CC Jr, Walker EA, Engel AL, Bullis J, Armstrong A. A randomized, double-blind crossover trial of sertraline in women with chronic pelvic pain. J Psychosom Res 1998;44:203–7. (Level II-3)

65. Simons DG, Travell JG, Simons LS. Travell & Simons' myofascial pain and dysfunction: the trigger point manual. Vol. I: upper half of body. 2nd ed. Baltimore (MD): Lippincott Williams and Wilkins; 1999. (Level III)

66. Slocumb JC. Neurological factors in chronic pelvic pain: trigger points and the abdominal pelvic pain syndrome. Am J Obstet Gynecol 1984;149:536–43. (Level III)

67. Owen PR. Prostaglandin synthetase inhibitors in the treatment of primary dysmenorrhea: outcome trials reviewed. Am J Obstet Gynecol 1984;148:96–103. (Level III)

68. Marjoribanks J, Proctor ML, Farquhar C. Nonsteroidal anti-inflammatory drugs for primary dysmenorrhoea (Cochrane Review). In: The Cochrane Library, Issue 4, 2003. Chichester, UK: John Wiley & Son, Ltd. (Meta-analysis)

69. Portenoy RK. Current pharmacotherapy of chronic pain. J Pain Symptom Manage 2000;19(suppl):S16–20. (Level III)

70. Moulin DE, Iezzi A, Amireh R, Sharpe WK, Boyd D, Merskey H. Randomised trial of oral morphine for chronic non-cancer pain. Lancet 1996;347:143–7. (Level I)

71. Jamison RN, Raymond SA, Slawsby EA, Nedeljkovic SS, Katz NP. Opioid therapy for chronic noncancer back pain. A randomized prospective study. Spine 1998;23: 2591–600. (Level I)

72. Wilder-Smith CH, Hill L, Spargo K, Kalla A. Treatment of severe pain from osteoarthritis with slow-release tramadol or dihydrocodeine in combination with NSAID's: a randomised study comparing analgesia, antinociception, and gastrointestinal effects. Pain 2001;91:23–31. (Level I)

73. Proctor ML, Roberts H, Farquhar CM. Combined oral contraceptive pill (OCP) as treatment for primary dysmenorrhoea (Cochrane Review). In: The Cochrane

Library, Issue 4, 2003. Chichester, UK: John Wiley & Son, Ltd. (Meta-analysis)

74. Propst AM, Laufer MR. Endometriosis in adolescents. Incidence, diagnosis, and treatment. J Reprod Med 1999; 44:751–8. (Level III)

75. Vercellini P, Trespidi L, Colombo A, Vendola N, Marchini M, Crosignani PG. A gonadotrophin-releasing hormone agonist versus a low-dose oral contraceptive for pelvic pain associated with endometriosis. Fertil Steril 1993;60: 75–9. (Level I)

76. Muzii L, Marana R, Caruana P, Catalano GF, Margutti F, Panici PB. Postoperative administration of monophasic combined oral contraceptives after laparoscopic treatment of ovarian endometriomas: a prospective, randomized trial. Am J Obstet Gynecol 2000;183:588–92. (Level I)

77. Vercellini P, Aimi G, Panazza S, De Giorgi O, Pesole A, Crosignani PG. A levonorgestrel-releasing intrauterine system for the treatment of dysmenorrhea associated with endometriosis: a pilot study. Fertil Steril 1999;72:505–8. (Level II-3)

78. Bergqvist A, Bergh T, Hogstrom L, Mattsson S, Nordenskjold F, Rasmussen C. Effects of triptorelin versus placebo on the symptoms of endometriosis. Fertil Steril 1998;69:702–8. (Level I)

79. Goserelin depot versus danazol in the treatment of endometriosis the Australian/New Zealand experience. Aust N Z J Obstet Gynaecol 1996;36:55–60. (Level I)

80. Henzl MR, Corson SL, Moghissi K, Buttram VC, Berqvist C, Jacobson J. Administration of nasal nafarelin as compared with oral danazol for endometriosis. A multicenter double-blind comparative clinical trial. N Engl J Med 1988;318:485–9. (Level I)

81. Kennedy SH, Williams IA, Brodribb J, Barlow DH, Shaw RW. A comparison of nafarelin acetate and danazol in the treatment of endometriosis. Fertil Steril 1990;53: 998–1003. (Level I)

82. Nafarelin for endometriosis: a large-scale, danazol-controlled trial of efficacy and safety, with 1-year follow-up. Nafarelin European Endometriosis Trial Group. Fertil Steril 1992;57:514–22. (Level I)

83. Prentice A, Deary AJ, Goldbeck-Wood S, Farquhar C, Smith SK. Gonadotrophin-releasing hormone analogues for pain associated with endometriosis (Cochrane Review). In: The Cochrane Library, Issue 4, 2003. Chichester, UK: John Wiley & Son, Ltd. (Meta-analysis)

84. Rock JA, Truglia JA, Caplan RJ. Zoladex (goserelin acetate implant) in the treatment of endometriosis: a randomized comparison with danazol. The Zoladex Endometriosis Study Group. Obstet Gynecol 1993;82: 198–205. (Level I)

85. Wheeler JM, Knittle JD, Miller JD. Depot leuprolide versus danazol in treatment of women with symptomatic endometriosis. I. Efficacy results. Am J Obstet Gynecol 1992;167:1367–71. (Level I)

86. Dlugi AM, Miller JD, Knittle J. Lupron depot (leuprolide acetate for depot suspension) in the treatment of endometriosis: a randomized, placebo-controlled, double-blind study. Lupron Study Group. Fertil Steril 1990;54: 419–27. (Level I)

87. Ling FW. Randomized controlled trial of depot leuprolide in patients with chronic pelvic pain and clinically suspected endometriosis. Pelvic Pain Study Group. Obstet Gynecol 1999;93:51–8. (Level I)

88. Soysal ME, Soysal S, Vicdan, Ozer S. A randomized controlled trial of goserelin and medroxyprogesterone acetate in the treatment of pelvic congestion. Hum Reprod 2001;16:931–9. (Level I)

89. Mathias JR, Clench MH, Reeves-Darby VG, Fox LM, Hsu PH, Roberts PH, et al. Effect of leuprolide acetate in patients with moderate to severe functional bowel disease. Double-blind, placebo-controlled study. Dig Dis Sci 1994;39:1155–62. (Level I)

90. Mathias JR, Clench MH, Roberts PH, Reeves-Darby VG. Effect of leuprolide acetate in patients with functional bowel disease. Long-term follow-up after double-blind, placebo-controlled study. Dig Dis Sci 1994;39:1163–70. (Level I)

91. Mathias JR, Ferguson KL, Clench MH. Debilitating "functional" bowel disease controlled by leuprolide acetate, gonadotropin-releasing hormone (GnRH) analog. Dig Dis Sci 1989;34:761–6. (Level III)

92. Houghton LA, Lea R, Jackson N, Whorwell PJ. The menstrual cycle affects rectal sensitivity in patients with irritable bowel syndrome but not healthy volunteers. Gut 2002;50:471–4. (Level II-2)

93. Lentz GM, Bavendam T, Stenchever MA, Miller JL, Smalldridge J. Hormonal manipulation in women with chronic, cyclic irritable bladder symptoms, and pelvic pain. Am J Obstet Gynecol 2002;186:1268–71; discussion 1271–3. (Level III)

94. Hornstein MD, Surrey ES, Weisberg GW, Casino LA. Leuprolide acetate depot and hormonal add-back in endometriosis: a 12-month study. Lupron Add-Back Study Group. Obstet Gynecol 1998;91:16–24. (Level I)

95. Surrey ES, Hornstein MD. Prolonged GnRH agonist and add-back therapy for symptomatic endometriosis: long-term follow-up. Obstet Gynecol 2002;99:709–19. (Level I)

96. Leather AT, Studd JW, Watson NR, Holland EF. The prevention of bone loss in young women treated with GnRH analogues with "add-back" estrogen therapy. Obstet Gynecol 1993;81:104–7. (Level I)

97. Parazzini F, Fedele L, Busacca M, Falsetti L, Pellegrini S, Venturini PL, et al. Postsurgical medical treatment of advanced endometriosis: results of a randomized clinical trial. Am J Obstet Gynecol 1994;171:1205–7. (Level I)

98. Siddall-Allum J, Rae T, Rogers V, Witherow R, Flanagan A, Beard RW. Chronic pelvic pain caused by residual ovaries and ovarian remnants. Br J Obstet Gynaecol 1994;101:979–85. (Level III)

99. Carey MP, Slack MC. GnRH analogue in assessing chronic pelvic pain in women with residual ovaries. Br J Obstet Gynaecol 1996;103:150–3. (Level III)

100. Telimaa S, Ronnberg L, Kauppila A. Placebo-controlled comparison of danazol and high-dose medroxyprogesterone acetate in the treatment of endometriosis after conservative surgery. Gynecol Endocrinol 1987;1:363–71. (Level I)

101. Telimaa S, Puolakka J, Ronnberg L, Kauppila A. Placebo-controlled comparison of danazol and high-dose medroxyprogesterone acetate in the treatment of endometriosis. Gynecol Endocrinol 1987;1:13–23. (Level I)

102. Farquhar CM, Rogers V, Franks S, Pearce S, Wadsworth J, Beard RW. A randomized controlled trial of medroxyprogesterone acetate and psychotherapy for the treatment of pelvic congestion. Br J Obstet Gynaecol 1989;96:1153–62. (Level I)

103. Harrison RF, Barry-Kinsella C. Efficacy of medroxyprogesterone treatment in infertile women with endometriosis: a prospective, randomized, placebo-controlled study. Fertil Steril 2000;74:24–30. (Level I)

104. Gestrinone versus a gonadotropin-releasing hormone agonist for the treatment of pelvic pain associated with endometriosis: a multicenter, randomized, double-blind study. Gestrinone Italian Study Group. Fertil Steril 1996;66:911–9. (Level I)

105. Regidor PA, Regidor M, Schmidt M, Ruwe B, Lubben G, Fortig P, et al. Prospective randomized study comparing the GnRH-agonist leuprorelin acetate and the gestagen lynestrenol in the treatment of severe endometriosis. Gynecol Endocrinol 2001;15:202–9. (Level I)

106. Muneyyirci-Delale O, Karacan M. Effect of norethindrone acetate in the treatment of symptomatic endometriosis [published erratum appears in Int J Fertil Womens Med 1999;44:215]. Int J Fertil Womens Med 1998;43:24–7. (Level III)

107. Sundell G, Milsom I, Andersch B. Factors influencing the prevalence and severity of dysmenorrhoea in young women. Br J Obstet Gynaecol 1990;97:588–94. (Level II-2)

108. Golomb LM, Solidum AA, Warren MP. Primary dysmenorrhea and physical activity. Med Sci Sports Exerc 1998;30:906–9. (Level III)

109. Weiss JM. Pelvic floor myofascial trigger points: manual therapy for interstitial cystitis and the urgency-frequency syndrome. J Urol 2001;166:2226–31. (Level III)

110. Petros PP, Skilling PM. Pelvic floor rehabilitation in the female according to the integral theory of female urinary incontinence. First report. Eur J Obstet Gynecol Reprod Biol 2001;94:264–9. (Level III)

111. Mens JM, Snijders CJ, Stam HJ. Diagonal trunk muscle exercises in peripartum pelvic pain: a randomized clinical trial. Phys Ther 2000;80:1164–73. (Level I)

112. Sutton CJ, Ewen SP, Whitelaw N, Haines P. Prospective, randomized, double-blind, controlled trial of laser laparoscopy in the treatment of pelvic pain associated with minimal, mild, and moderate endometriosis. Fertil Steril 1994;62:696–700. (Level I)

113. Sutton CJ, Pooley AS, Ewen SP, Haines P. Follow-up report on a randomized controlled trial of laser laparoscopy in the treatment of pelvic pain associated with minimal to moderate endometriosis. Fertil Steril 1997;68:1070–4. (Level III)

114. Candiani GB, Fedele L, Vercellini P, Bianchi S, Di Nola G. Repetitive conservative surgery for recurrence of endometriosis. Obstet Gynecol 1991;77:421–4. (Level III)

115. Lee NC, Dicker RC, Rubin GL, Ory HW. Confirmation of the preoperative diagnoses for hysterectomy. Am J Obstet Gynecol 1984;150:283–7. (Level III)

116. Carlson KJ, Miller BA, Fowler FJ Jr. The Maine Women's Health Study: II. Outcomes of nonsurgical management of leiomyomas, abnormal bleeding, and chronic pelvic pain. Obstet Gynecol 1994;83:566–72. (Level II-3)

117. Carlson KJ, Miller BA, Fowler FJ Jr. The Maine Women's Health Study: I. Outcomes of hysterectomy. Obstet Gynecol 1994;83:556–65. (Level II-3)

118. Hillis SD, Marchbanks PA, Peterson HB. The effectiveness of hysterectomy for chronic pelvic pain. Obstet Gynecol 1995;86:941–5. (Level II-2)

119. Stovall TG, Ling FW, Crawford DA. Hysterectomy for chronic pelvic pain of presumed uterine etiology. Obstet Gynecol 1990;75:676–9. (Level II-2)

120. Beard RW, Kennedy RG, Gangar KF, Stones RW, Rogers V, Reginald PW, et al. Bilateral oophorectomy and hysterectomy in the treatment of intractable pelvic pain associated with pelvic congestion. Br J Obstet Gynaecol 1991;98:988–92. (Level II-3)

121. Steege JF, Stout AL. Resolution of chronic pelvic pain after laparoscopic lysis of adhesions. Am J Obstet Gynecol 1991;165:278–81; discussion 281–3. (Level II-2)

122. Peters AA, Trimbos-Kemper GC, Admiraal C, Trimbos JB, Hermans J. A randomized clinical trial on the benefit of adhesiolysis in patients with intraperitoneal adhesions and chronic pelvic pain. Br J Obstet Gynaecol 1992;99:59–62. (Level I)

123. Aboseif S, Tamaddon K, Chalfin S, Freedman S, Kaptein J. Sacral neuromodulation as an effective treatment for refractory pelvic floor dysfunction. Urology 2002;60:52–6. (Level II-3)

124. Siegel S, Paszkiewicz E, Kirkpatrick C, Hinkel B, Oleson K. Sacral nerve stimulation in patients with chronic intractable pelvic pain. J Urol 2001;166:1742–5. (Level III)

125. Everaert K, Devulder J, De Muynck M, Stockman S, Depaepe H, De Looze D, et al. The pain cycle: implications for the diagnosis and treatment of pelvic pain syndromes. Int Urogynecol J Pelvic Floor Dysfunct 2001;12:9–14. (Level II-2)

126. Black WT Jr. Use of presacral sympathectomy in the treatment of dysmenorrhea: a second look after twenty-five years. Am J Obstet Gynecol 1964;89:16–22. (Level III)

127. Lee RB, Stone K, Magelssen D, Belts RP, Benson WL. Presacral neurectomy for chronic pelvic pain. Obstet Gynecol 1986;68:517–21. (Level II-3)

128. Chen FP, Chang SD, Chu KK, Soong YK. Comparison of laparoscopic presacral neurectomy and laparoscopic uterine nerve ablation for primary dysmenorrhea. J Reprod Med 1996;41:463–6. (Level I)

129. Candiani GB, Fedele L, Vercellini P, Bianchi S, Di Nola G. Presacral neurectomy for the treatment of pelvic pain associated with endometriosis: a controlled study. Am J Obstet Gynecol 1992;167:100–3. (Level I)

130. Tjaden B, Schlaff WD, Kimball A, Rock JA. The efficacy of presacral neurectomy for the relief of midline dysmenorrhea. Obstet Gynecol 1990;76:89–91. (Level III)

131. Chen FP, Soong YK. The efficacy and complications of laparoscopic presacral neurectomy in pelvic pain. Obstet Gynecol 1997;90:974–7. (Level II-3)

132. Sheld HH, Karamitsos CA, Parker EO 3rd, Shapiro BS. The use of superior hypogastric plexus block in the diagnosis of chronic pelvic pain. Am J Gynecol Health 1992;6:96–100. (Level III)

133. Bourke DL, Foster DC, Valley MA, Robinson JC. Superior hypogastric nerve block as predictive of presacral neurectomy success: a preliminary report. Am J Pain Manage 1996;6:9–12. (Level III)

134. Wechsler RJ, Maurer PM, Halpern EJ, Frank ED. Superior hypogastric plexus block for chronic pelvic pain in the presence of endometriosis: CT techniques and results. Radiology 1995;196:103–6. (Level III)

135. Lichten EM, Bombard J. Surgical treatment of primary dysmenorrhea with laparoscopic uterine nerve ablation. J Reprod Med 1987;32:37–41. (Level II-1)

136. Yen YK, Liu WM, Yuan CC, Ng HT. Addition of laparoscopic uterine nerve ablation to laparoscopic bipolar coagulation of uterine vessels for women with uterine myomas and dysmenorrhea. J Am Assoc Gynecol Laparosc 2001;8:573–8. (Level I)

137. Sutton C, Pooley AS, Jones KD, Dover RW, Haines P. A prospective, randomized, double-blind controlled trial of laparoscopic uterine nerve ablation in the treatment of pelvic pain associated with endometriosis. Gynaecol Endosc 2001;10:217–22. (Level I)

138. Renaer M, Vertommen H, Nijs P, Wagemans L, Van Hemelrijck T. Psychological aspects of chronic pelvic pain in women. Am J Obstet Gynecol 1979;134:75–80. (Level II-2)

139. Albert H. Psychosomatic group treatment helps women with chronic pelvic pain. J Psychosom Obstet Gynaecol 1999;20:216–25. (Level II-3)

140. Peters AA, van Dorst E, Jellis B, van Zuuren E, Hermans J, Trimbos JB. A randomized clinical trial to compare two different approaches in women with chronic pelvic pain. Obstet Gynecol 1991;77:740–4. (Level I)

141. Reiter RC. A profile of women with chronic pelvic pain. Clin Obstet Gynecol 1990;33:130–6. (Level II-2)

142. Laws A. Sexual abuse history and women's medical problems. J Gen Intern Med 1993;8:441–3. (Level III)

143. Proctor ML, Murphy PA. Herbal and dietary therapies for primary and secondary dysmenorrhoea (Cochrane Review). In: The Cochrane Library, Issue 4, 2003. Chichester, UK: John Wiley & Son, Ltd. (Meta-analysis)

144. Brown CS, Ling FW, Wan JY, Pilla AA. Efficacy of static magnetic field therapy in chronic pelvic pain: a double-blind pilot study. Am J Obstet Gynecol 2002; 187:1581–7. (Level I)

145. Jorgensen WA, Frome BM, Wallach C. Electrochemical therapy of pelvic pain: effects of pulsed electromagnetic fields (PEMF) on tissue trauma. Eur J Surg Suppl 1994;(574):83–6. (Level III)

146. Proctor ML, Smith CA, Farquhar CM, Stones RW. Transcutaneous electrical nerve stimulation and acupuncture for primary dysmenorrhoea (Cochrane Review). In: The Cochrane Library, Issue 4, 2003. Chichester, UK: John Wiley & Son, Ltd. (Meta-analysis)

147. Taylor D, Miaskowski C, Kohn J. A randomized clinical trial of the effectiveness of an acupressure device (relief brief) for managing symptoms of dysmenorrhea. J Altern Complement Med 2002;8:357–70. (Level I)

148. Helms JM. Acupuncture for the management of primary dysmenorrhea. Obstet Gynecol 1987;69:51–6. (Level I)

149. Milsom I, Hedner N, Mannheimer C. A comparative study of the effect of high-intensity transcutaneous nerve stimulation and oral naproxen on intrauterine pressure and menstrual pain in patients with primary dysmenorrhea. Am J Obstet Gynecol 1994;170:123–9. (Level II-3)

150. Thomas CT, Napolitano PG. Use of acupuncture for managing chronic pelvic pain in pregnancy. A case report. J Reprod Med 2000;45:944–6. (Level III)

The MEDLINE database, the Cochrane Library, and ACOG's own internal resources and documents were used to conduct a literature search to locate relevant articles published between January 1985 and November 2003. The search was restricted to articles published in the English language. Priority was given to articles reporting results of original research, although review articles and commentaries also were consulted. Abstracts of research presented at symposia and scientific conferences were not considered adequate for inclusion in this document. Guidelines published by organizations or institutions such as the National Institutes of Health and the American College of Obstetricians and Gynecologists were reviewed, and additional studies were located by reviewing bibliographies of identified articles. When reliable research was not available, expert opinions from obstetrician–gynecologists were used.

Studies were reviewed and evaluated for quality according to the method outlined by the U.S. Preventive Services Task Force:

I   Evidence obtained from at least 1 properly designed randomized controlled trial.

II-1   Evidence obtained from well-designed controlled trials without randomization.

II-2   Evidence obtained from well-designed cohort or case–control analytic studies, preferably from more than 1 center or research group.

II-3   Evidence obtained from multiple time series with or without the intervention. Dramatic results in uncontrolled experiments also could be regarded as this type of evidence.

III   Opinions of respected authorities, based on clinical experience, descriptive studies, or reports of expert committees.

Based on the highest level of evidence found in the data, recommendations are provided and graded according to the following categories:

Level A—Recommendations are based on good and consistent scientific evidence.

Level B—Recommendations are based on limited or inconsistent scientific evidence.

Level C—Recommendations are based primarily on consensus and expert opinion.

ISSN 1099-3630

**The American College of
Obstetricians and Gynecologists
409 12th Street, SW
PO Box 96920
Washington, DC 20090-6920**

12345/87654

Chronic pelvic pain. ACOG Practice Bulletin No. 51. American College of Obstetricians and Gynecologists. Obstet Gynecol 2004;103: 589–605.

ACOG PRACTICE BULLETIN

CLINICAL MANAGEMENT GUIDELINES FOR
OBSTETRICIAN–GYNECOLOGISTS

NUMBER 33, JANUARY 2002

This Practice Bulletin was developed by the ACOG Committee on Practice Bulletins— Obstetrics with the assistance of Larry C. Gilstrap III, MD, and Susan M. Ramin, MD. The information is designed to aid practitioners in making decisions about appropriate obstetric and gynecologic care. These guidelines should not be construed as dictating an exclusive course of treatment or procedure. Variations in practice may be warranted based on the needs of the individual patient, resources, and limitations unique to the institution or type of practice.

Diagnosis and Management of Preeclampsia and Eclampsia

Hypertensive disease occurs in approximately 12–22% of pregnancies, and it is directly responsible for 17.6% of maternal deaths in the United States (1, 2). However, there is confusion about the terminology and classification of these disorders. This bulletin will provide guidelines for the diagnosis and management of hypertensive disorders unique to pregnancy (ie, preeclampsia and eclampsia), as well as the various associated complications. Chronic hypertension has been discussed elsewhere (3).

Background

Definition

The National High Blood Pressure Education Program Working Group (hereafter referred to as the "Working Group") has recommended that the term "gestational hypertension" replace the term "pregnancy-induced hypertension" to describe cases in which elevated blood pressure without proteinuria develops in a woman after 20 weeks of gestation and blood pressure levels return to normal postpartum (4). According to the criteria established by the Working Group, in pregnant women, hypertension is defined as a systolic blood pressure level of 140 mm Hg or higher or a diastolic blood pressure level of 90 mm Hg or higher that occurs after 20 weeks of gestation in a woman with previously normal blood pressure (4). As many as one quarter of women with gestational hypertension will develop proteinuria, ie, preeclampsia (5).

Preeclampsia is a syndrome defined by hypertension and proteinuria that also may be associated with myriad other signs and symptoms, such as edema, visual disturbances, headache, and epigastric pain. Laboratory abnormalities may include hemolysis, elevated liver enzymes, and low platelet counts (HELLP syndrome). Proteinuria may or may not be present in patients with HELLP syndrome. Proteinuria is defined as the presence of 0.3 g or more of protein in a 24-hour urine specimen. This finding usually correlates with a finding of 1+ or greater but should be confirmed using a random urine dipstick evaluation and a 24-hour or "timed" collection (4). See the box for the criteria for diagnosing preeclampsia. Many practitioners have traditionally used these criteria to diagnose preeclampsia, although they have not been substantiated by research, and other definitions exist. These also are the criteria frequently used in research protocols. Severe preeclampsia is defined in the box.

In the past, hypertension indicative of preeclampsia has been defined as an elevation of more than 30 mm Hg systolic or more than 15 mm Hg diastolic above the patient's baseline blood pressure; however, this definition has not proved to be a good prognostic indicator of outcome (6, 7). The so-called "30–15 rule" is not part of the criteria for preeclampsia established by the Working Group (4). According to the Working Group, however, women who demonstrate an elevation of more than 30 mm Hg systolic or more than 15 mm Hg diastolic above baseline "warrant close observation."

Eclampsia is defined as the presence of new-onset grand mal seizures in a woman with preeclampsia. Other causes of seizures in addition to eclampsia include a bleeding arteriovenous malformation, ruptured aneurysm, or idiopathic seizure disorder. These diagnoses may be more likely in cases in which new-onset seizures occur after 48–72 hours postpartum.

The diagnostic criteria for superimposed preeclampsia include "new-onset proteinuria" in a woman with hypertension before 20 weeks of gestation, a sudden increase in proteinuria if already present in early gestation, a sudden increase in hypertension, or the development of HELLP syndrome (4). Women with chronic hypertension who develop headache, scotomata, or epigastric pain also may have superimposed preeclampsia.

Diagnosis of Severe Preeclampsia

Preeclampsia is considered severe if one or more of the following criteria is present:

- Blood pressure of 160 mm Hg systolic or higher or 110 mm Hg diastolic or higher on two occasions at least 6 hours apart while the patient is on bed rest
- Proteinuria of 5 g or higher in a 24-hour urine specimen or 3+ or greater on two random urine samples collected at least 4 hours apart
- Oliguria of less than 500 mL in 24 hours
- Cerebral or visual disturbances
- Pulmonary edema or cyanosis
- Epigastric or right upper-quadrant pain
- Impaired liver function
- Thrombocytopenia
- Fetal growth restriction

Epidemiology and Risk Factors

The exact incidence of preeclampsia is unknown but it has been reported to be approximately 5–8% (8, 9). Preeclampsia is primarily a disorder of first pregnancies. Other risk factors include multifetal gestations, preeclampsia in a previous pregnancy, chronic hypertension, pregestational diabetes, vascular and connective tissue disease, nephropathy, antiphospholipid antibody syndrome, obesity, age 35 years or older, and African-American race (1, 8, 10–12).

The precise role of genetic and environmental factors on the risk and incidence of preeclampsia is unclear, although emerging data suggest the tendency to develop preeclampsia may have a genetic basis (13–15). Women with thrombophilias also may have a genetic predisposition to preeclampsia.

Pathophysiology

The etiology of preeclampsia is unknown, although much of the literature has focused on the degree of trophoblastic invasion by the placenta (4). In cases of preeclampsia, invasion by the trophoblast appears to be incomplete (16–18). Moreover, the severity of hypertension may be related to the degree of trophoblastic invasion (19). Preeclampsia also may be associated with significant alterations in the immune response (4).

Criteria for Diagnosis of Preeclampsia*

- Blood pressure of 140 mm Hg systolic or higher or 90 mm Hg diastolic or higher that occurs after 20 weeks of gestation in a woman with previously normal blood pressure
- Proteinuria, defined as urinary excretion of 0.3 g protein or higher in a 24-hour urine specimen

*Preeclampsia is a pregnancy-specific syndrome that usually occurs after 20 weeks of gestation.

Data from Report of the National High Blood Pressure Education Program Working Group Report on High Blood Pressure in Pregnancy. Am J Obstet Gynecol 2000;183:S1–S22

Vascular Changes

Hemoconcentration, in addition to hypertension, is a significant vascular change, because women with the preeclampsia–eclampsia syndrome may not develop the normal hypervolemia of pregnancy (20). Changes in vascular reactivity may be mediated by prostaglandins (21, 22). The interaction of various vasoactive agents, such as prostacyclin (vasodilator), thromboxane A_2 (potent vasoconstrictor), nitric oxide (potent vasodilator), and endothelins (potent vasoconstrictors) cause another pathophysiologic change seen in preeclampsia: intense vasospasm. The vasospasm and subsequent hemoconcentration are associated with contraction of the intravascular space. Because of capillary leak and decreased colloid oncotic pressure often associated with this syndrome, attempts to expand the intravascular space in these women with vigorous fluid therapy may result in elevation of the pulmonary capillary wedge pressure and even pulmonary edema. A study using invasive hemodynamic monitoring in women with preeclampsia found that before aggressive intravenous fluid therapy, the women had hyperdynamic ventricular function with low pulmonary capillary wedge pressure (23). However, after aggressive fluid therapy, the pulmonary capillary wedge pressure increased significantly above normal levels (23).

Hematologic Changes

Various hematologic changes also may occur in women with preeclampsia, especially when the preeclampsia is severe. Both thrombocytopenia and hemolysis may occur as part of the HELLP syndrome, although the etiology is unknown. Interpretation of hematocrit levels in the face of severe preeclampsia should take into consideration that hemolysis or hemoconcentration or both may occur. Thus, the hematocrit level may be very low because of hemolysis or very high secondary to hemoconcentration in the absence of hemolysis. Lactate dehydrogenase is present in erythrocytes in high concentration. A disproportionate elevation of levels of lactate dehydrogenase in serum may be a sign of hemolysis.

Hepatic Changes

Hepatic function may be significantly altered in women with severe preeclampsia. Alanine aminotransferase and aspartate aminotransferase may be elevated. Hyperbilirubinemia may occur, especially in the presence of hemolysis. Hepatic hemorrhage, which usually manifests as a subcapsular hematoma, also may occur, especially in women with preeclampsia and upper abdominal pain (24). Rarely, hepatic rupture, which is associated with a high mortality rate, occurs (25).

HELLP Syndrome

Women with severe preeclampsia and hepatic involvement may develop HELLP syndrome. In one study, HELLP syndrome occurred in approximately 20% of women with severe preeclampsia (26). As with severe preeclampsia, HELLP syndrome is associated with an increased risk of adverse outcomes, including placental abruption, renal failure, subcapsular hepatic hematoma, recurrent preeclampsia, preterm delivery, and even fetal or maternal death (26–30).

Neurologic and Cerebral Manifestations

Eclampsia remains a cause of maternal mortality (31, 32), usually in association with intracranial hemorrhage (33). Although uncommon, temporary blindness (lasting a few hours to up to a week) also may accompany severe preeclampsia and eclampsia (34). Other nervous system manifestations include headache, blurred vision, scotomata (4), and hyperreflexia.

Renal Changes

As a result of vasospasm, the normal expected increase in glomerular filtration rate and renal blood flow and the expected decrease in serum creatinine may not occur in women with preeclampsia, especially if the disease is severe. Oliguria, commonly (albeit arbitrarily) defined as less than 500 mL in 24 hours, also may occur secondary to the hemoconcentration and decreased renal blood flow. Rarely, persistent oliguria may reflect acute tubular necrosis, which may lead to acute renal failure (8).

Fetal Changes

As a result of impaired uteroplacental blood flow or placental infarction, manifestations of preeclampsia also may be seen in the fetal placental unit. These include intrauterine growth restriction, oligohydramnios, placental abruption, and nonreassuring fetal status demonstrated on antepartum surveillance.

Clinical Considerations and Recommendations

▶ *Are there effective methods for identifying women at risk for preeclampsia?*

No single screening test for preeclampsia has been found to be reliable and cost-effective (35–37). Uric acid is one of the most commonly used tests but it has a positive predictive value of only 33% and has not proved useful in predicting preeclampsia (38). Doppler velocimetry of the uterine arteries was reported not to be a useful test for screening pregnant women at low risk for preeclampsia (35, 39).

▶ *How should the blood pressure be taken?*

According to the Working Group, the diastolic blood pressure is that pressure at which the sound disappears (Korotkoff phase V) (4). To reduce inaccurate readings, an appropriate size cuff should be used (length 1.5 times upper arm circumference or a cuff with a bladder that encircles 80% or more of the arm). The blood pressure level should be taken with the patient in an upright position, after a 10-minute or longer rest period. For patients in the hospital, the blood pressure can be taken with either the patient sitting up or in the left lateral recumbent position with the patient's arm at the level of the heart (40). The patient should not use tobacco or caffeine for 30 minutes preceding the measurement (37, 41). Although validated electronic devices can be used, a mercury sphygmomanometer is preferred because it is the most accurate device (37, 41).

▶ *What is the optimal treatment for preeclampsia?*

The decision to deliver a patient with preeclampsia must balance both the maternal and fetal risks. Continued observation is appropriate for the woman with a preterm fetus only if she has mild preeclampsia (4). Such therapy consists of fetal and maternal evaluation. No randomized trials have determined the best tests for fetal evaluation. The Working Group recommends weekly nonstress tests, biophysical profiles, or both, which should be repeated as indicated according to maternal condition. Testing is recommended twice weekly for suspected fetal growth restriction or oligohydramnios. Daily fetal movement assessment also may prove useful. The Working Group also recommends ultrasound examination for fetal growth and amniotic fluid assessment every 3 weeks (4).

Maternal evaluation consists primarily of frequent evaluation for worsening preeclampsia. Initial laboratory tests consist of evaluation of platelet count, liver enzymes, and renal function and a 12-hour to 24-hour urine collection for protein (4). With mild disease and no progression, these tests can be repeated weekly. The tests should be repeated sooner if disease progression is questionable.

The management of a woman with severe preeclampsia remote from term is best accomplished in a tertiary care setting or in consultation with an obstetrician–gynecologist with training, experience, and demonstrated competence in the management of high-risk pregnancies, such as a maternal–fetal medicine subspecialist (4, 42–44). Laboratory evaluation and fetal surveillance may be indicated on a daily basis depending on the severity and progression of the disorder (4).

No large randomized clinical trials have compared conservative versus aggressive management of women with HELLP syndrome. Considering the serious nature of this complication, it seems reasonable to conclude that women with HELLP syndrome should be delivered regardless of their gestational age. Expectant management of this syndrome in women before 32 weeks of gestation should be undertaken only in tertiary care centers or as part of randomized clinical trials with appropriate safeguards and consent (4).

▶ *Is there a role for outpatient management in women with preeclampsia?*

According to the Working Group (4):

"Hospitalization is often initially recommended for women with new-onset preeclampsia. After maternal and fetal conditions are serially assessed, subsequent management may be continued in the hospital, at a day-care unit, or at home on the basis of the initial assessment. Prolonged hospitalization for the duration of pregnancy allows rapid intervention in case of fulminant progression to hypertensive crisis, eclampsia, or abruptio placentae. These complications are rare in compliant women who have mild [disease].... Ambulatory management at home or at a day-care unit has been evaluated as an option for monitoring women with mild gestational hypertension or preeclampsia remote from term. A number of observational and randomized studies suggest a place for ambulatory management of selected women. If day care or home management is selected, it should include frequent maternal and fetal evaluation and access to health care providers. If worsening of preeclampsia is diagnosed, as determined by laboratory findings, symptoms, and clinical signs, hospitalization is indicated."

Women who have difficulty with compliance, including logistic barriers, who manifest signs of disease progression or who have severe preeclampsia should be hospitalized.

▶ *Is medical management beneficial during labor and delivery in women with preeclampsia?*

The two main goals of management of women with preeclampsia during labor and delivery are prevention of seizures or eclampsia and control of hypertension. Although there is no unanimity of opinion regarding the prophylactic use of magnesium sulfate for the prevention of seizures in women with mild preeclampsia or gestational hypertension, a significant body of evidence attests to the efficacy of magnesium sulfate in women with severe preeclampsia and eclampsia. A randomized, controlled trial of 822 women with severe preeclampsia (699 evaluated) receiving either intravenous magnesium sulfate or placebo reported one case (0.3%) of eclampsia among the 345 women in the magnesium group versus 11 (3.2%) of 340 in the placebo group (relative risk, 0.09; 95% confidence interval, 0.01–0.69; $P = 0.003$) (45). A review of the literature on magnesium sulfate therapy in women with either preeclampsia or eclampsia identified 19 randomized controlled trials, five retrospective studies, and eight observational studies (46). In the randomized controlled trials of women with eclampsia, recurrent seizures occurred in 23% of 935 women who received either phenytoin or diazepam compared with 9.4% of 932 women who received magnesium sulfate. In the randomized trials of women with severe preeclampsia, seizures occurred in 2.8% of 793 women treated with antihypertensives compared with only 0.9% in women treated with magnesium sulfate. Thus, the data support the use of magnesium sulfate to prevent seizures in women with severe preeclampsia or eclampsia (31, 45–47).

Although no large randomized clinical trials have compared treatment with placebo, antihypertensive therapy is generally recommended for diastolic blood pressure levels of 105–110 mm Hg or higher (4, 8, 48). Hydralazine and labetalol are the two agents most commonly used for this purpose (see box).

▶ What is the optimal mode of delivery for women with preeclampsia?

For mild preeclampsia, vaginal delivery at term is preferred. No randomized clinical trials have evaluated the optimal method of delivery for women with severe preeclampsia or eclampsia. Two retrospective studies comparing induction of labor with cesarean delivery in women with severe preeclampsia remote from term concluded that induction of labor was reasonable and was not "harmful" to low-birth-weight infants (49, 50). The decision to perform cesarean delivery should be individualized.

Antihypertensive Treatment for Preeclampsia

Hydralazine: 5–10-mg doses intravenously every 15–20 minutes until desired response is achieved*

Labetalol: 20-mg intravenous bolus dose followed by 40 mg if not effective within 10 minutes; then, 80 mg every 10 minutes to maximum total dose of 220 mg†

*Cunningham FG, Gant NF, Leveno KJ, Gilstrap LC III, Hauth JC, Wenstrom KD. Hypertensive disorders in pregnancy. In: Williams obstetrics. 21st ed. New York: McGraw-Hill, 2001:567–618

†Report of the National High Blood Pressure Education Program Working Group on High Blood Pressure in Pregnancy. Am J Obstet Gynecol 2000;183:S1–S22

▶ Is anesthesia contraindicated during labor and delivery in women with preeclampsia?

With improved techniques over the past two decades, regional anesthesia has become the preferred technique for women with severe preeclampsia and eclampsia—both for labor and delivery (4). A secondary analysis of women with severe preeclampsia in the National Institute of Child Health and Human Development's Maternal–Fetal Medicine Units Network trial of low-dose aspirin reported that epidural anesthesia was not associated with an increased rate of cesarean delivery, pulmonary edema, or renal failure (51). Moreover, general anesthesia carries more risk to pregnant women than does regional anesthesia (52). However, regional anesthesia is generally contraindicated in the presence of a coagulopathy because of the potential for hemorrhagic complications.

▶ How should women with eclampsia be managed?

Women with eclampsia require prompt intervention. When an eclamptic seizure occurs, the woman should be medically stabilized. First, it is important to control convulsions and prevent their recurrence with intravenous or intramuscular magnesium sulfate (8). One protocol is a 4-g to 6-g loading dose diluted in 100 mL fluid and administered intravenously for 15–20 minutes, followed by 2 g per hour as a continuous intravenous infusion (8). Antihypertensive medications should be used for women with diastolic blood pressure levels of 105–110 mm Hg or higher.

The patient with eclampsia should be delivered in a timely fashion. Fetal bradycardia frequently occurs during an eclamptic seizure; usually, this can be managed by maternal treatment, and cesarean delivery is not necessary. Once the patient is stabilized, the method of delivery should depend, in part, on factors such as gestational age, fetal presentation, and the findings of the cervical examination.

▶ Is there a role for invasive hemodynamic monitoring?

Most women with severe preeclampsia or eclampsia can be managed without invasive hemodynamic monitoring. A review of 17 women with eclampsia reported that use of a pulmonary artery catheter aided in clinical management decisions (53). However, no randomized trials support their routine use in women with severe preeclampsia. Invasive hemodynamic monitoring may prove beneficial in preeclamptic women with severe cardiac disease, severe renal disease, refractory hypertension, oliguria, or pulmonary edema (8, 54–56).

▶ *Can preeclampsia be prevented?*

Much of the obstetric research in the past several decades has been directed at finding ways to prevent preeclampsia and eclampsia. Recent studies have focused on low-dose aspirin, calcium supplementation, and antioxidant therapy. Most evidence suggests that low-dose aspirin therapy is of little, if any, benefit in preventing preeclampsia in low-risk women (4, 57–60).

Although there is some controversy regarding the use of calcium supplementation to prevent preeclampsia, large, randomized, controlled trials have shown no benefit (58, 61, 62). Recently, antioxidant therapy with 1,000 mg per day of vitamin C and 400 mg per day of vitamin E has shown promise in preventing preeclampsia (63). These results need to be confirmed in larger randomized trials.

Summary of Recommendations

The following recommendations are based on good and consistent scientific evidence (Level A):

▶ Magnesium sulfate should be used for the prevention and treatment of seizures in women with severe preeclampsia or eclampsia.

▶ If analgesia/anesthesia is required, regional or neuraxial analgesia/anesthesia should be used because it is efficacious and safe for intrapartum management of women with severe preeclampsia in the absence of coagulopathy.

▶ Low-dose aspirin has not been shown to prevent preeclampsia in women at low risk and, therefore, is not recommended.

▶ Daily calcium supplementation has not been shown to prevent preeclampsia and, therefore, is not recommended.

The following recommendations are based on limited or inconsistent scientific evidence (Level B):

▶ The management of a woman with severe preeclampsia remote from term is best accomplished in a tertiary care setting or in consultation with an obstetrician–gynecologist with training, experience, and demonstrated competence in the management of high-risk pregnancies, such as a maternal–fetal medicine subspecialist.

▶ Practitioners should be aware that although various laboratory tests may be useful in the management of women with preeclampsia, to date there is no reliable predictive test for preeclampsia.

▶ Invasive hemodynamic monitoring should be considered in preeclamptic women with severe cardiac disease, renal disease, refractory hypertension, pulmonary edema, or unexplained oliguria.

The following recommendations are based primarily on consensus and expert opinion (Level C):

▶ Women should be considered as having severe preeclampsia if they have blood pressure levels of 160 mm Hg systolic or higher or 110 mm Hg diastolic or higher on two occasions at least 6 hours apart while the patient is on bed rest, proteinuria of 5 g or higher in a 24-hour urine specimen or 3+ or greater on two random urine samples collected at least 4 hours apart, oliguria of less than 500 mL in 24 hours, cerebral or visual disturbances, pulmonary edema or cyanosis, epigastric or right upper-quadrant pain, elevated liver enzymes, thrombocytopenia, or fetal growth restriction.

▶ Expectant management should be considered for women remote from term who have mild preeclampsia.

▶ Antihypertensive therapy (with either hydralazine or labetalol) should be used for treatment of diastolic blood pressure levels of 105–110 mm Hg or higher.

References

1. Walker JJ. Pre-eclampsia. Lancet 2000;356:1260–1265 (Level III)

2. Koonin LM, MacKay AP, Berg CJ, Atrash HK, Smith JC. Pregnancy-related mortality surveillance—United States, 1987–1990. Mor Mortal Wkly Rep CDC Surveill Summ 1997;46(4):17–36 (Level III)

3. Chronic hypertension in pregnancy. ACOG Practice Bulletin No. 29. American College of Obstetricians and Gynecologists. Obstet Gynecol 2001;98:177–185 (Level III)

4. Report of the National High Blood Pressure Education Program Working Group on High Blood Pressure in Pregnancy. Am J Obstet Gynecol 2000;183:S1–S22 (Level III)

5. Saudan P, Brown MA, Buddle ML, Jones M. Does gestational hypertension become pre-eclampsia? Br J Obstet Gynaecol 1998;105:1177–1184 (Level II-2)

6. North RA, Taylor RS, Schellenberg JC. Evaluation of a definition of pre-eclampsia. Br J Obstet Gynaecol 1999;106:767–773 (Level II-2)

7. Levine RJ, Ewell MG, Hauth JC, Curet LB, Catalano PM, Morris CD, et al. Should the definition of preeclampsia include a rise in diastolic blood pressure >/= 15 mm Hg to a level < 90 mm Hg in association with proteinuria? Am J Obstet Gynecol 2000;183:787–792 (Level II-2)

8. Cunningham FG, Gant NF, Leveno KJ, Gilstrap LC III, Hauth JC, Wenstrom KD. Hypertensive disorders in pregnancy. In: Williams obstetrics. 21st ed. New York: McGraw-Hill, 2001:567–618 (Level III)

9. Hauth JC, Ewell MG, Levine RJ, Esterlitz JR, Sibai B, Curet LB, et al. Pregnancy outcomes in healthy nulliparas who developed hypertension. Calcium for Preeclampsia Prevention Study Group. Obstet Gynecol 2000;95:24–28 (Level II-2)

10. Sibai BM, Ewell M, Levine RJ, Klebanoff MA, Esterlitz J, Catalano PM, et al. Risk factors associated with preeclampsia in healthy nulliparous women. The Calcium for Preeclampsia Prevention (CPEP) Study Group. Am J Obstet Gynecol 1997;177:1003–1010 (Level II-2)

11. Sibai BM, Hauth J, Caritis S, Lindheimer MD, MacPherson C, Klebanoff M, et al. Hypertensive disorders in twin versus singleton gestations. National Institute of Child Health and Human Development Network of Maternal–Fetal Medicine Units. Am J Obstet Gynecol 2000;182:938–942 (Level II-3)

12. Conde-Agudelo A, Belizan JM. Risk factors for preeclampsia in a large cohort of Latin American and Caribbean women. BJOG 2000;107:75–83 (Level II-2)

13. Chesley LC, Cooper DW. Genetics of hypertension in pregnancy: possible single gene control of pre-eclampsia and eclampsia in the descendants of eclamptic women. Br J Obstet Gynaecol 1986;93:898–908 (Level II-2)

14. Ward K, Hata A, Jeunemaitre X, Helin C, Nelson L, Namikawi C, et al. A molecular variant of angiotensinogen associated with preeclampsia. Nat Genet 1993;4:59–61 (Level III)

15. Morgan T, Craven C, Lalouel JM, Ward K. Angiotensinogen Thr^{235} variant is associated with abnormal physiologic change of the uterine spiral arteries in first-trimester decidua. Am J Obstet Gynecol 1999;180:95–102 (Level II-2)

16. Zhou Y, Fisher SJ, Janatpour M, Genbacev O, Dejana E, Wheelock M, et al. Human cytotrophoblasts adopt a vascular phenotype as they differentiate: a strategy for successful endovascular invasion? J Clin Invest 1997;99:2139–2151 (Level II-2)

17. Zhou Y, Damsky CH, Chiu K, Roberts JM, Fisher SJ. Preeclampsia is associated with abnormal expression of adhesion molecules by invasive cytotrophoblasts. J Clin Invest 1993;91:950–960 (Level III)

18. Fox H. The placenta in pregnancy hypertension. In: Rubin PC, ed. Handbook of hypertension, volume 10: hypertension in pregnancy. New York: Elsevier, 1988:16–37 (Level III)

19. Madazli R, Budak E, Calay Z, Aksu MF. Correlation between placental bed biopsy findings, vascular cell adhesion molecule and fibronectin levels in pre-eclampsia. BJOG 2000;107:514–518 (Level II-2)

20. Pritchard JA, Cunningham FG, Pritchard SA. The Parkland Memorial Hospital protocol for treatment of eclampsia: evaluation of 245 cases. Am J Obstet Gynecol 1984;148:951–963 (Level III)

21. Cunningham FG, Cox K, Gant NF. Further observations on the nature of pressor responsivity to angiotensin II in human pregnancy. Obstet Gynecol 1975;46:581–583 (Level III)

22. Gant NF, Chand S, Whalley PJ, MacDonald PC. The nature of pressor responsiveness to angiotensin II in human pregnancy. Obstet Gynecol 1974;43:854–860 (Level III)

23. Hankins GD, Wendel GD Jr, Cunningham FG, Leveno KJ. Longitudinal evaluation of hemodynamic changes in eclampsia. Am J Obstet Gynecol 1984;150:506–512 (Level III)

24. Manas KJ, Welsh JD, Rankin RA, Miller DD. Hepatic hemorrhage without rupture in preeclampsia. N Engl J Med 1985;312:424–426 (Level III)

25. Rinehart BK, Terrone DA, Magann EF, Martin RW, May WL, Martin JN Jr. Preeclampsia-associated hepatic hemorrhage and rupture: mode of management related to maternal and perinatal outcome. Obstet Gynecol Surv 1999;54:196–202 (Level III)

26. Sibai BM, Ramadan MK, Usta I, Salama M, Mercer BM, Friedman SA. Maternal morbidity and mortality in 442 pregnancies with hemolysis, elevated liver enzymes, and low platelets (HELLP syndrome). Am J Obstet Gynecol 1993;169:1000–1006 (Level II-3)

27. Sibai BM, Ramadan MK, Chari RS, Friedman SA. Pregnancies complicated by HELLP syndrome (hemolysis, elevated liver enzymes, and low platelets): subsequent pregnancy outcome and long-term prognosis. Am J Obstet Gynecol 1995;172:125–129 (Level II-3)

28. Barton JR, Sibai BM. Hepatic imaging in HELLP syndrome (hemolysis, elevated liver enzymes, and low platelet count). Am J Obstet Gynecol 1996;174:1820–1825; discussion 1825–1827 (Level II-2)

29. Sullivan CA, Magann EF, Perry KG Jr, Roberts WE, Blake PG, Martin JN Jr. The recurrence risk of the syndrome of hemolysis, elevated liver enzymes, and low platelets (HELLP) in subsequent gestations. Am J Obstet Gynecol 1994;171:940–943 (Level II-3)

30. Isler CM, Rinehart BK, Terrone DA, Martin RW, Magann EF, Martin JN Jr. Maternal mortality associated with HELLP (hemolysis, elevated liver enzymes, and low platelets) syndrome. Am J Obstet Gynecol 1999;181:924–928 (Level III)

31. Which anticonvulsant for women with eclampsia? Evidence from the Collaborative Eclampsia Trial. Lancet 1995;345:1455–1463 [erratum Lancet 1995;346:258] (Level I)

32. Mattar F, Sibai BM. Eclampsia. VIII. Risk factors for maternal morbidity. Am J Obstet Gynecol 2000;182:307–312 (Level II-3)

33. Richards A, Graham D, Bullock R. Clinicopathological study of neurologic complications due to hypertensive disorders of pregnancy. J Neurol Neurosurg Psychiatry 1988;51:416–421 (Level II-3)

34. Cunningham FG, Fernandez CO, Hernandez C. Blindness associated with preeclampsia and eclampsia. Am J Obstet Gynecol 1995;172:1291–1298 (Level III)

35. Friedman SA, Lindheimer MD. Prediction and differential diagnosis. In: Lindheimer MD, Roberts JM, Cunningham FG, eds. Chesley's hypertensive disorders in pregnancy. 2nd ed. Stamford, Connecticut: Appleton & Lange, 1999:201–227 (Level III)

36. Stamilio DM, Sehdev HM, Morgan MA, Propert K, Macones GA. Can antenatal clinical and biochemical markers predict the development of severe preeclampsia? Am J Obstet Gynecol 2000;182:589–594 (Level II-2)

37. Helewa ME, Burrows RF, Smith J, Williams K, Brain P, Rabkin SW. Report of the Canadian Hypertension Society Consensus Conference: 1. Definitions, evaluation and classification of hypertensive disorders in pregnancy. CMAJ 1997;157:715–725 (Level III)

38. Lim KH, Friedman SA, Ecker JL, Kao L, Kilpatrick SJ. The clinical utility of serum uric acid measurements in hypertensive disease of pregnancy. Am J Obstet Gynecol 1998;178:1067–1071 (Level II-2)

39. Irion O, Masse J, Forest JC, Moutquin JM. Prediction of pre-eclampsia, low birthweight for gestation and prematurity by uterine artery blood flow velocity waveform analysis in low risk nulliparous women. Br J Obstet Gynaecol 1998;105:422–429 (Level II-3)

40. Garovic VD. Hypertension in pregnancy: diagnosis and treatment. Mayo Clin Proc 2000;75:1071–1076 (Level III)

41. The sixth report of the Joint National Committee on prevention, detection, evaluation, and treatment of high blood pressure. Arch Intern Med 1997;157:2413–2446 [erratum Arch Intern Med 1998;158:573] (Level III)

42. Sibai BM, Akl S, Fairlie F, Moretti M. A protocol for managing severe preeclampsia in the second trimester. Am J Obstet Gynecol 1990;163:733–738 (Level II-3)

43. Sibai BM, Mercer BM, Schiff E, Friedman SA. Aggressive versus expectant management of severe preeclampsia at 28 to 32 weeks' gestation: a randomized controlled trial. Am J Obstet Gynecol 1994;171:818–822 (Level I)

44. Odendaal HJ, Pattinson RC, Bam R, Grove D, Kotze TJ. Aggressive or expectant management for patients with severe preeclampsia between 28–34 weeks' gestation: a randomized controlled trial. Obstet Gynecol 1990;76:1070–1075 (Level I)

45. Coetzee EJ, Dommisse J, Anthony J. A randomized controlled trial of intravenous magnesium sulphate versus placebo in the management of women with severe preeclampsia. Br J Obstet Gynaecol 1998;105:300–303 (Level I)

46. Witlin AG, Sibai BM. Magnesium sulfate therapy in preeclampsia and eclampsia. Obstet Gynecol 1998;92:883–889 (Level III)

47. Lucas MJ, Leveno KJ, Cunningham FG. A comparison of magnesium sulfate with phenytoin for the prevention of eclampsia. N Engl J Med 1995;333:201–205 (Level I)

48. Sibai BM. Treatment of hypertension in pregnant women. N Engl J Med 1996;335:257–265 (Level III)

49. Nassar AH, Adra AM, Chakhtoura N, Gomez-Marin O, Beydoun S. Severe preeclampsia remote from term: labor induction or elective cesarean delivery? Am J Obstet Gynecol 1998;179:1210–1213 (Level II-3)

50. Alexander JM, Bloom SL, McIntire DD, Leveno KJ. Severe preeclampsia and the very low birth weight infant: is induction of labor harmful? Obstet Gynecol 1999;93:485–488 (Level II-3)

51. Hogg B, Hauth JC, Caritis SN, Sibai BM, Lindheimer M, Van Dorsten JP, et al. Safety of labor epidural anesthesia for women with severe hypertensive disease. National Institute of Child Health and Human Development Maternal-Fetal Medicine Units Network. Am J Obstet Gynecol 1999;181:1096–1101 (Level II-2)

52. Hawkins JL, Koonin LM, Palmer SK, Gibbs CP. Anesthesia-related deaths during obstetric delivery in the United States, 1979–1990. Anesthesiology 1997;86:277–284 (Level II-2)

53. Gilbert WM, Towner DR, Field NT, Anthony J. The safety and utility of pulmonary artery catheterization in severe preeclampsia and eclampsia. Am J Obstet Gynecol 2000;182:1397–1403 (Level II-3)

54. Clark SL, Cotton DB, Hankins GD, Phelan JP. Critical care obstetrics. 3rd ed. Malden, Massachusetts: Blackwell Science, 1997 (Level III)

55. Hallak M. Hypertension in pregnancy. In: James DK, Steer PJ, Weiner C, Gonik B, eds. High risk pregnancy: management options. 2nd ed. London, Saunders, 1999:639–663 (Level III)

56. Easterling TR, Benedetti TJ, Schmucker BC, Carlson KL. Antihypertensive therapy in pregnancy directed by noninvasive hemodynamic monitoring. Am J Perinatol 1989;6:86–89 (Level II-3)

57. Heyborne KD. Preeclampsia prevention: lessons from the low-dose aspirin therapy trials. Am J Obstet Gynecol 2000;183:523–528 (Level III)

58. Sibai BM. Prevention of preeclampsia: a big disappointment. Am J Obstet Gynecol 1998;179:1275–1278 (Level III)

59. Caritis S, Sibai B, Hauth J, Lindheimer MD, Klebanoff M, Thom E, et al. Low-dose aspirin to prevent preeclampsia in women at high risk. National Institute of Child Health and Human Development Network of Maternal-Fetal Medicine Units. N Engl J Med 1998;338:701–705 (Level I)

60. Goffinet F, Aboulker D, Paris-Llado J, Bucourt M, Uzan M, Papiernik E, et al. Screening with a uterine Doppler in low risk pregnant women followed by low dose aspirin in women with abnormal results: a multicenter randomised controlled trial. BJOG 2001;108:510–518 (Level I)

61. Levine RJ, Hauth JC, Curet LB, Sibai BM, Catalano PM, Morris CD, et al. Trial of calcium to prevent preeclampsia. N Engl J Med 1997;337:69–76 (Level I)

62. Crowther CA, Hiller JE, Pridmore B, Bryce R, Duggan P, Hague WM, et al. Calcium supplementation in nulliparous women for the prevention of pregnancy-induced hypertension, preeclampsia and preterm birth: an Australian randomized trial. FRACOG and the ACT Study Group. Aust N Z J Obstet Gynaecol 1999;39:12–18 (Level I)

63. Chappell LC, Seed PT, Briley AL, Kelly FJ, Lee R, Hunt BJ, et al. Effect of antioxidants on the occurrence of preeclampsia in women at increased risk: a randomised trial. Lancet 1999;354:810–816 (Level I)

The MEDLINE database, the Cochrane Library, and ACOG's own internal resources and documents were used to conduct a literature search to locate relevant articles published between January 1985 and January 2001. The search was restricted to articles published in the English language. Priority was given to articles reporting results of original research, although review articles and commentaries also were consulted. Abstracts of research presented at symposia and scientific conferences were not considered adequate for inclusion in this document. Guidelines published by organizations or institutions such as the National Institutes of Health and the American College of Obstetricians and Gynecologists were reviewed, and additional studies were located by reviewing bibliographies of identified articles. When reliable research was not available, expert opinions from obstetrician–gynecologists were used.

Studies were reviewed and evaluated for quality according to the method outlined by the U.S. Preventive Services Task Force:

I   Evidence obtained from at least one properly designed randomized controlled trial.

II-1   Evidence obtained from well-designed controlled trials without randomization.

II-2   Evidence obtained from well-designed cohort or case–control analytic studies, preferably from more than one center or research group.

II-3   Evidence obtained from multiple time series with or without the intervention. Dramatic results in uncontrolled experiments could also be regarded as this type of evidence.

III   Opinions of respected authorities, based on clinical experience, descriptive studies, or reports of expert committees.

Based on the highest level of evidence found in the data, recommendations are provided and graded according to the following categories:

Level A—Recommendations are based on good and consistent scientific evidence.

Level B—Recommendations are based on limited or inconsistent scientific evidence.

Level C—Recommendations are based primarily on consensus and expert opinion.

ISSN 1099-3630

**The American College of
Obstetricians and Gynecologists
409 12th Street, SW
PO Box 96920
Washington, DC 20090-6920**

12345/65432

Diagnosis and management of preeclampsia and eclampsia. ACOG Practice Bulletin No. 33. American College of Obstetricians and Gynecologists. Obstet Gynecol 2002;99:159–167

ACOG PRACTICE BULLETIN

CLINICAL MANAGEMENT GUIDELINES FOR
OBSTETRICIAN–GYNECOLOGISTS

NUMBER 35, MAY 2002

(Replaces Committee Opinion Number 242, October 2000)

This Practice Bulletin was developed by the ACOG Committee on Practice Bulletins— Gynecology with the assistance of Benjamin E. Greer, MD, and Wui-Jin Koh, MD. The information is designed to aid practitioners in making decisions about appropriate obstetric and gynecologic care. These guidelines should not be construed as dictating an exclusive course of treatment or procedure. Variations in practice may be warranted based on the needs of the individual patient, resources, and limitations unique to the institution or type of practice.

Diagnosis and Treatment of Cervical Carcinomas

Invasive cervical carcinoma, once the most common reproductive-tract cancer in the United States, has recently fallen to the rank of third most common. Globally, cervical cancer is a major health problem, with a yearly incidence of 371,000 cases and an annual death rate of 190,000 (1). The International Federation of Gynecology and Obstetrics (FIGO) recently revised its staging criteria. In addition, new evidence has documented conclusively that survival rates for women with cervical cancer improve when radiotherapy is combined with cisplatin-based chemotherapy. This document will describe staging criteria and treatment for cervical carcinoma. For practical purposes, it will focus on the squamous and adenocarcinoma histologies only.

Background

Prevalence

The American Cancer Society estimated that 12,900 new cases of cervical cancer would be diagnosed in the United States in 2001 and that 4,400 deaths from cervical cancer would result (2). Cervical cancer comprises approximately 16% of the estimated 80,300 cases of reproductive-tract cancers among women in the United States. Seventy-eight percent of cases occur in developing countries where cervical cancer is the second most frequent cause of cancer-related death in women. The substantial decrease in incidence and mortality in developed countries is thought to be a result of effective screening.

Risk Factors

Human papillomavirus is considered the most important factor contributing to the development of cervical intraepithelial neoplasia and cervical cancer. Countries with a high incidence of cervical cancer also have a high prevalence of human papillomavirus (1). Other epidemiologic risk factors associated with cervical intraepithelial neoplasia and cervical cancer include history of sexual intercourse at an early age, multiple sexual partners, sexually transmitted diseases (including chlamydia), and smoking (3). Additional risk factors include a male partner or partners who have had multiple sexual partners; previous history of squamous dysplasias of the cervix, vagina, or vulva; and immunosuppression, such as after organ transplantation or patients with acquired immunodeficiency syndrome.

Diagnosis

The signs and symptoms of early cervical carcinoma include watery vaginal discharge, intermittent spotting, and postcoital bleeding. Often the symptoms go unrecognized by the patient. Because of the accessibility of the cervix, accurate diagnosis often can be made with cytologic screening, colposcopically directed biopsy, or biopsy of a gross or palpable lesion (4). In cases of suspected microinvasion and early-stage cervical carcinoma, cone biopsy of the cervix is indicated to evaluate the possibility of invasion or to define the depth and extent of microinvasion. Cold knife cone biopsy provides the most accurate evaluation of the margins.

Histology

The two major histologic types of invasive cervical carcinomas are squamous cell carcinomas and adenocarcinomas. Squamous cell carcinomas comprise 80% of cases, and adenocarcinoma or adenosquamous carcinoma comprise approximately 15%. The remaining cases are made up of various rare histologies, which may have very different biologic behavior.

Management

Early carcinomas of the cervix usually can be managed by surgical techniques or radiation therapy. The more advanced carcinomas require primary treatment with radiation therapy. Many changes in radiation therapy techniques have occurred in the past decade. These include incorporation of higher energy external beam equipment, improved field design to cover anatomic regions at risk, increased use of tomographic imaging, recognition of the adverse impact of prolonged treatment, increased familiarity with high-dose-rate brachytherapy, and, more recently, the use of chemotherapy concurrent with radiation therapy.

Clinical Considerations and Recommendations

▶ *How are patients with cervical carcinoma categorized or staged?*

Staging of gynecologic cancers attempts to define the anatomic extent of a given cancer. This allows for scientific comparison of treatment results from different centers or protocols. The three major staging systems are those of FIGO, the American Joint Committee on Cancer, and the International Union Against Cancer. Cancer registries approved by the American College of Surgeons use the American Joint Committee on Cancer's TNM (tumor, nodes, metastasis) staging system. However, the scientific literature reports gynecologic oncology statistics using the FIGO system. It is recommended that the FIGO system be used to facilitate comparisons of international data.

Staging of invasive cervical cancer with the FIGO system is achieved by clinical evaluation. Other gynecologic cancers are staged surgically. The current FIGO nomenclature for cancer of the cervix was first adopted in 1994 (5) (see box, "Carcinoma of the Cervix Uteri: FIGO Nomenclature").

Careful clinical examination should be performed on all patients. Examinations should be conducted by experienced examiners and may be performed under anesthesia. Pretreatment evaluation of women with cervical carcinoma often can be helpful if provided by an obstetrician–gynecologist with advanced surgical training, experience, and demonstrated competence, such as a gynecologic oncologist. The procedure may be scheduled to occur at the same time the patient is undergoing another procedure requiring anesthesia. Once established, the clinical stage must not be revised because of subsequent findings, even if the cancer recurs. The box, "Guidelines for Clinical Staging of Invasive Cervical Carcinoma," identifies key points in staging disease. These guidelines are made up of examinations generally available throughout the world. Strict adherence to the rules for staging provides the framework for making valid scientific comparison of results.

Various optional examinations, such as ultrasonography, computed tomography (CT), magnetic resonance imaging (MRI), lymphangiography, laparoscopy, and fine-needle aspiration, are valuable for treatment planning. Surgical findings provide extremely accurate information about the extent of disease and will guide treatment plans but will not change the results of clinical staging. The occasional hysterectomy specimen with unsuspected extensive invasive cervical carcinoma cannot change the previously documented clinical stage.

While not required as part of FIGO staging procedures, in the United States, various radiologic tests are frequently undertaken to help define the extent of tumor growth and guide therapy decisions, especially in patients with locally advanced disease (ie, stage IIb or more advanced). Computed tomography of the abdomen and pelvis is the most widely used imaging study. Early evaluation of the efficacy of CT scans in detecting paraaortic adenopathy noted a very high specificity

---

Carcinoma of the Cervix Uteri: FIGO Nomenclature

Stage 0 Carcinoma in situ, cervical intraepithelial neoplasia Grade III

Stage I The carcinoma is strictly confined to the cervix (extension to the corpus would be disregarded).

Ia Invasive carcinoma that can be diagnosed only by microscopy. All macroscopically visible lesions—even with superficial invasion—are allotted to Stage Ib carcinomas. Invasion is limited to a measured stromal invasion with a maximal depth of 5.0 mm and a horizontal extension of not more than 7.0 mm. Depth of invasion should not be more than 5.0 mm taken from the base of the epithelium of the original tissue—superficial or glandular. The involvement of vascular spaces—venous or lymphatic—should not change the stage allotment.

Ia1 Measured stromal invasion of not more than 3.0 mm in depth and extension of not more than 7.0 mm

Ia2 Measured stromal invasion of more than 3.0 mm and not more than 5.0 mm with an extension of not more than 7.0 mm

Ib Clinically visible lesions limited to the cervix uteri or preclinical cancers greater than Stage Ia

Ib1 Clinically visible lesions not more than 4.0 cm

Ib2 Clinically visible lesions more than 4.0 cm

Stage II Cervical carcinoma invades beyond the uterus, but not to the pelvic wall or to the lower third of the vagina

IIa No obvious parametrial involvement

IIb Obvious parametrial involvement

Stage III The carcinoma has extended to the pelvic wall. On rectal examination, there is no cancer-free space between the tumor and the pelvic wall. The tumor involves the lower third of the vagina. All cases with hydronephrosis or nonfunctioning kidney are included, unless they are known to be due to other causes.

IIIa Tumor involves lower third of the vagina, with no extension to the pelvic wall

IIIb Extension to the pelvic wall or hydronephrosis or nonfunctioning kidney

Stage IV The carcinoma has extended beyond the true pelvis, or has involved (biopsy proved) the mucosa of the bladder or rectum. Bullous edema, as such, does not permit a case to be allotted to Stage IV.

IVa Spread of the growth to adjacent organs (bladder or rectum or both)

IVb Spread to distant organs

Benedet JL, Odicino F, Maisonneuve P, Beller U, Creasman WT, Heintz AP, et al. Carcinoma of the cervix uteri. J Epidemiol Biostat 2001;6:7–43

(96%) but low sensitivity (34%) (6). However, with technologic advancements leading to increased imaging resolution, accuracy of CT scanning has improved (7). Recent experience has suggested MRI is as accurate as CT in assessing nodal involvement and provides better definition of the extent of local tumors within the pelvis (7). Some investigators have advocated the use of lymphangiography as the standard for noninvasive assessment of retroperitoneal adenopathy, but a recent review has shown that contemporary CT and MRI results are as accurate as lymphangiography and are preferable given that more information is provided on local tumor infiltration (7). Early experience with a new imaging modality, positron emission tomography (PET), shows considerable promise in further increasing the accuracy of noninvasive radiologic staging. The sensitivity of PET has been reported to be 75%, and the specificity 92% (8).

Guidelines for Clinical Staging of Invasive Cervical Carcinoma

- Examinations should include inspection, palpation, colposcopy, endocervical curettage, hysteroscopy, cystoscopy, proctoscopy, intravenous pyelography, and X-ray examination of lungs and skeleton.

- Conization of the cervix is considered a clinical examination.

- Suspected bladder or rectal involvement should be confirmed histologically.

- If there is a question about the most appropriate stage, the earlier stage should be assigned.

Data from Benedet JL, Odicino F, Maisonneuve P, Beller U, Creasman WT, Heintz AP, et al. Carcinoma of the cervix uteri. J Epidemiol Biostat 2001;6:7–43

▶ How is stage Ib1 carcinoma distinguished from stage Ib2?

In 1994, FIGO revised its staging criteria, subdividing stage Ib carcinoma of the cervix into stage Ib1 (≤4 cm in diameter) and stage Ib2 (>4 cm diameter). When the tumor is confined to the cervix, the size of the primary tumor has been shown to have a significant impact on survival rates in stage Ib cervical cancer, regardless of primary treatment modality (9, 10). A large, prospective Gynecologic Oncology Group surgical–pathologic study demonstrated that in stage Ib carcinoma of the cervix, tumor size of 3 cm or more was an independent adverse prognostic factor for decreased disease-free survival (11). Other independent risk factors in this study were capillary-space involvement and depth of cervical stromal invasion. A large study of patients treated by radiation therapy or radiation therapy followed by hysterectomy demonstrated significantly better survival rates for patients with stage Ib tumors of less than 4 cm in diameter than for those with tumors greater than 4 cm (12). Another study demonstrated the effect of tumor size on outcomes in patients treated with radiation therapy alone (ie, without surgery or chemotherapy). Five-year disease-free survival rates for women with stage Ib cancer were 100% for lesions less than 1 cm in diameter, 93% for those 1–1.9 cm, 98% for those 2–2.9 cm, 83% for those 3–3.9 cm, and 76% for lesions of 4 cm or more (13).

Retrospective analysis has evaluated patients who had radical hysterectomies and lymph node dissections for stage Ib1 and Ib2 cancers of the cervix (14). Patients with stage Ib2 disease had a significantly worse 5-year survival rate (72.8%) when compared with those who had stage Ib1 tumors (90%). Also, in this study, in 38.7% of cases of stage Ib1 disease and 72.9% of cases of stage Ib2 disease patients received postoperative radiation therapy for high-risk indications such as positive lymph nodes, parametrial disease, positive surgical margins, and deep stromal invasion involving the outer third of the cervix. The high percentage of postoperative radiation required in patients with stage Ib2 disease suggests that primary radiation should be considered for these patients and may be supplemented by surgical or radiologic evaluation to assess retroperitoneal nodal status.

▶ Is surgical evaluation of cervical carcinoma appropriate?

As discussed earlier, the results of surgical evaluation should not influence the stage determined by using the FIGO clinical staging system. However, it is well recognized that the presence of lymph node metastasis is the most important adverse predictor of survival. Although surgical evaluation of cervical cancer remains controversial, it is the best method of assessing nodal involvement. Retroperitoneal surgical lymph node dissection of the pelvic and paraaortic lymph nodes provides important information about treatment planning and prognosis. Patients with positive lymph nodes can have radiation fields modified appropriately to cover areas at risk. Resection of positive lymph nodes is thought to provide therapeutic benefit (15, 16). Therefore, surgical evaluation allows individualization of therapy and may result in better clinical outcomes.

▶ How is microinvasive cervical cancer diagnosed and treated?

The concept of microinvasive carcinoma of the cervix as a distinct clinical entity was introduced by Mestwerdt in 1947 (17). The premise for this specific diagnosis was to define a subset of patients with early carcinomas of the cervix who had a favorable prognosis. It is important to remember these lesions are defined microscopically and cannot be visualized on gross inspection. The appropriate definition of this entity has been debated for more than 50 years. The main issues affecting the definition are the maximum depth of stromal invasion, the significance of lymphatic-vascular space invasion, tumor volume, and confluence of the invasion pattern as related to the frequency of pelvic node metastasis, vaginal recurrence, and ultimate survival. These prognostic factors are important determinants of treatment necessary for the best survival with the lowest morbidity and, in certain circumstances, may influence decisions regarding preservation of the uterus for future pregnancy.

The definition of microinvasive carcinoma of the cervix was modified by FIGO seven times between 1961 and 1994, indicating a lack of universal consensus. This section will focus on the rationale for the 1994 definitions and the treatment options based on the best available scientific data.

During the 1970s, the concept of volumetric measurements for early small cancers, rather than just unidimensional consideration of penetration depth, was being developed. Estimation of volume is most accurate by using the three largest diameters of the lesions. The rigorous technique for volumetric assessment requires examining up to 100 sections per cone specimen. This labor-intensive process was not well accepted. Bidimensional planar measurements were recommended without testing. In 1988, FIGO changed the definition of stage Ia2 tumor to include a specified maximal depth of invasion of 5 mm and a maximal horizontal spread of 7 mm. This was based on the presumption that the overall volume of the microcarcinoma should not exceed

350 mm³. One study concluded that a microcarcinoma with a tumor volume of less than 500 mm³ generally was not associated with metastasis (18).

The 1988 FIGO definition of 5 mm of depth for stage Ia2 was in conflict with the Society of Gynecologic Oncologists' definition of 3 mm or less for microinvasive disease, which had been used in the United States since 1974. In 1994, FIGO modified its definition of stage Ia1 to 3 mm or less of invasion. Currently, stage Ia1 is defined as a depth of invasion no greater than 3 mm and no wider than 7 mm, and stage Ia2 is defined as a depth of invasion greater than 3 mm but no greater than 5 mm and no wider than 7 mm. Lymphatic-vascular invasion should not alter the stage.

Despite this background and these definitions, diagnosis of microinvasive squamous carcinoma of the cervix is difficult. The FIGO staging guidelines presume the diagnosis will be made with a cone biopsy. Cold knife cone biopsies may be more accurate than loop electrosurgical excision procedure (LEEP) cones, because the margins are very important. Cautery artifact, loss of tissue, and thermal destruction account for the inaccuracy of information provided by LEEP specimens. In the United States, patients with abnormal Pap test results undergo colposcopy and biopsy for diagnosis. Colposcopic biopsies usually are performed before conization. The biopsy removes part of the lesion and, therefore, alters the apparent depth of invasion as seen on the cone specimen (19). Another potential problem in evaluation involves the accepted techniques of pathologic study. After initial fixation in formalin, cone biopsy specimens are divided into quadrants and step-sectioned. Maximal extent of horizontal spread could be underestimated by this procedure. In addition, there are difficulties in interpretation of the histology by pathologists. In two large studies that employed pathology re-review of cases initially diagnosed as microinvasive cervical carcinomas, 40–50% of the cases were excluded because they did not meet the criteria for microinvasion (20, 21). In 20–40%, no invasion was thought to be present, and in 6–7%, the depth of invasion was greater than 5 mm.

Understanding the concepts behind definition and diagnosis of microinvasive carcinoma of the cervix is important to understanding the biology and behavior of the disease. A comprehensive review of the current literature found that nodal metastasis is the most consistent and strongest predictor of survival for patients with early invasive cervical cancers (22). There is a relationship between depth of invasion and nodal metastasis.

Minimally invasive lesions—those with invasion up to 3 mm—have a lymph node metastatic risk rate of 1.2% and a death rate of less than 1%. However, lesions greater than 3 mm and no greater than 5 mm of invasion have a 7.8% rate of nodal metastasis and a death rate of 2.4%. One study that included only lesions of less than 5 mm depth found nodal metastasis when the lateral spread was greater than 7 mm (23).

According to the FIGO criteria, patients with stage Ia1 carcinoma could be treated with simple hysterectomy without nodal dissection or conization in selected cases. Those patients with invasion greater than 3 mm and no greater than 5 mm (stage Ia2) should undergo radical hysterectomy and pelvic lymphadenectomy (4, 22).

Although lymphatic-vascular invasion should not alter the FIGO stage, it is an important factor in treatment decisions. The risk of recurrence with lymphatic-vascular involvement is 3.1% if the extent of invasion is 3 mm or less and 15.7% if it is greater than 3 mm and no greater than 5 mm (22). Therefore, the presence of lymphatic-vascular invasion would suggest the need for more radical treatment to obtain the optimal outcome. Evaluation in consultation with an obstetrician–gynecologist with advanced surgical training, experience, and demonstrated competence, such as a gynecologic oncologist, often helps to determine the extent of surgery needed and the optimal use of adjunctive therapy.

Preservation of fertility has become increasingly important as more women are delaying having families. A treatment dilemma arises for women with cervical carcinoma who have not started or completed childbearing but desire the option to become pregnant. For both ethical and medical–legal reasons, patients who opt for conservative management should fully understand the risks involved. Recent reports have described the use of radical trachelectomy with or without lymph node dissection (24, 25). This procedure should be considered experimental and may be carried out best in consultation with an obstetrician–gynecologist with advanced surgical training, experience, and demonstrated competence, such as a gynecologic oncologist.

Treatment of microinvasive squamous carcinoma of the cervix deserves careful attention to details and individualization of therapy based on histologic evaluation. The concept of microinvasive adenocarcinoma has not been generally accepted.

▶ *How is early-stage (Ib–IIa) carcinoma treated?*

Both treatment strategies for stage Ib and early-stage IIa invasive carcinoma include 1) a primary surgical approach with radical hysterectomy and pelvic lymphadenectomy or 2) primary radiation therapy with external beam radiation and either high-dose-rate or low-dose-rate brachytherapy. A review of collective observational experiences reported in the literature demonstrates a 5-year survival rate of 87–92% using either approach (26).

Until recently, there have been no prospective randomized studies comparing surgery and radiation therapy. An Italian randomized trial provides information about primary surgery and radiation therapy but does not include the addition of concurrent or neoadjuvant chemotherapy (27). This study compared radical hysterectomy and primary radiotherapy with adjuvant radiation therapy in high-risk surgically treated patients. Stratification for stage Ib and Ib2 was included. Pathologic findings indicated identical 5-year overall and disease-free survival rates in the radiation therapy group and the surgical group with tailored postoperative radiation therapy. Severe morbidity occurred in 28% of patients in the surgery and postoperative radiation therapy group and in 12% of patients in the radiation therapy–only group ($P = 0.0004$). In this study, adjuvant radiation therapy after primary surgery was used in 54% of patients with tumors measuring 4 cm or less and in 84% of patients with tumor diameters greater than 4 cm. Significant prognostic factors included tumor diameter, positive lymphangiography, and adenocarcinoma histology as identified on univariate and multivariate analyses.

Although the two modalities were found to be similarly effective in the randomized trials, the rate and types of complications differ. The preference of treatment depends on the situation, the physician's input, and the patient's age, health, and tumor characteristics.

Those who favor radical surgery point out that it leaves the vagina in more functional condition, while radiation therapy results in a reduction in length, caliber, and lubrication of the vagina. In premenopausal women, ovarian function can be preserved with surgery. The surgical approach also provides the opportunity for pelvic and abdominal exploration and provides better clinical and pathologic information with which to individualize treatment. Surgery may be preferred over radiation therapy in women who have diverticular disease, tuboovarian abscess, or appendiceal abscess; have had prior radiation therapy; have congenital pelvic located kidney; or are psychotic or noncompliant. Proponents of radiation therapy advocate primary radiation to avoid surgical morbidity or mortality, risk of blood loss and transfusion, and excessive anesthesia time.

▶ *What is the role of adjuvant therapy following primary surgery in early-stage carcinoma?*

The identification of various pathologic risk factors, such as lymph node metastases, following primary surgical management of early-stage cervical cancer portends a higher rate of relapse and decreased survival rates (28). Historically, attempts to improve outcome mainly focused on the role of adjuvant pelvic radiation therapy,

with inconsistent results. More careful analysis of patterns of failure following radical hysterectomy has led to better stratification of patients into risk groups and incorporated testing of systemic chemotherapy agents in those considered at high risk of distant failure (28).

Two randomized clinical trials have greatly advanced our understanding of the role of postoperative therapy in cervical cancer (29, 30). Patients with histologically documented extracervical disease—specifically those with pelvic nodal involvement, positive margins, or parametrial extension—are treated with concurrent pelvic radiation therapy and cisplatin-based chemotherapy. The use of combined adjuvant chemotherapy and radiation therapy in these high-risk patients following primary surgery significantly improves relapse-free survival and overall survival rates when compared with radiation therapy alone (29).

Following radical hysterectomy, a subset of node-negative patients who have a constellation of primary risk factors (large tumors, depth of stromal infiltration, and lymphovascular space involvement) may be defined as having intermediate risk for relapse. For these patients, adjuvant pelvic radiation therapy provides clear therapeutic benefit, with significantly improved relapse-free survival rates when compared with those who had no further therapy. However, observation of improvement in overall survival favoring patients who had radiation therapy awaits further statistical confirmation following maturation of the data (30).

▶ *How is late-stage carcinoma (IIb or later) treated?*

Historically, primary radiation therapy has been used to treat patients with bulky or locally advanced cervical cancer. The approach generally consists of external beam radiation to achieve primary tumor reduction and provide coverage to the parametria and regional nodes at risk, supplemented by brachytherapy to increase radiation dose delivery to the central residual tumor. Earlier attempts to improve outcome results from primary radiation therapy by the addition of agents such as hydroxyurea or hypoxic cell sensitizers met with mixed success.

Results from five randomized trials on cervical cancer have established the role of concurrent cisplatin-based chemotherapy and radiation therapy for high-risk or locally advanced disease (29, 31–34). The various studies had different eligibility criteria, but in total included a broad spectrum of clinical presentations: 1) patients with locally advanced tumors for whom chemoradiation represented primary therapy (three studies [31, 32, 34]); 2) bulky early-stage cancers in which chemoradiation was delivered prior to adjuvant hysterectomy (one study [33]); and 3) postradical hysterectomy cases with high-risk pathologic factors (positive lymph nodes, positive parametria, positive margins) for whom adjuvant chemoradiation was given (one study [29]). In each of the five studies, a statistically significant survival advantage was observed among patients who received radiation therapy with a concurrent cisplatin-based regimen when compared with those who received radiation alone or radiation combined with hydroxyurea. The dramatic 30–50% reduction in the relative risk of death in the five trials prompted a rare clinical announcement from the National Cancer Institute stating that "strong consideration should be given to the incorporation of concurrent cisplatin-based chemotherapy with radiation therapy in women who require radiation therapy for treatment of cervical cancer" (35).

The five reported studies used cisplatin administered either weekly as a single agent or in combination with infusion 5-fluorouracil every 3–4 weeks (29, 31–34). Although the optimal cisplatin-based chemotherapeutic regimen has not yet been fully defined, many are choosing to use weekly cisplatin because of its ease of delivery and favorable toxicity profile (36). However, it is clear that the previously controversial use of hydroxyurea can be abandoned. Furthermore, it should be remembered that the advantages of chemoradiation are obtained only in the setting of concurrent therapy. Neoadjuvant chemotherapy prior to radiation therapy has shown no benefit and has even been detrimental in some cases.

The cumulative results from the recently reported randomized trials represent a major advance in the management of women with cervical cancer and have established a new paradigm for therapy. At present, women with locally advanced cervical cancer in North America should receive cisplatin-based chemotherapy concurrent with radiation therapy.

▶ *Should squamous cell cancer and adenocarcinoma be treated differently?*

Underlying this question is the continuing debate regarding the independent prognostic implications of adenocarcinoma versus squamous cell histologies in cervical cancer, especially in early-stage disease. Two large reviews reflect the ongoing controversy. In an analysis of 813 patients with stage Ib cervical cancer entered into a Gynecologic Oncology Group surgical–pathologic study, excluding patients with positive paraaortic nodes or gross extracervical disease, three specific cell types were identified (645 squamous cell, 104 adenocarcinoma, and 64 adenosquamous). No significant differences were found among the cell types with regard to the

patient's age at presentation, performance status, pelvic nodal metastases, depth of cervical invasion, uterine extension, surgical margins, or parametrial infiltration. Relapse-free survival rates were similar for all three histologies, but adenosquamous cell was associated with a small, statistically significant reduction in overall survival, even after adjusting for associated pathologic risk factors (37). In contrast, a retrospective review of 1,767 stage Ib cervical cancer patients who were clinically staged and treated with primary radiation therapy identified adenocarcinoma histology (including adenosquamous cell types) as an independent risk factor for disease recurrence and death, with distant metastases the primary site of failure (38, 39).

Despite the ongoing discussion regarding cell type and prognosis, there is no evidence to support differences in treatment of invasive squamous cell cancer versus adenocarcinoma of the cervix. The only exception to this is the management of microinvasive disease, where guidelines have been developed for more conservative management of patients with FIGO stage Ia1 squamous cell cancer, corresponding with the Society of Gynecologic Oncologists' working definition for minimally invasive tumors discussed previously. It should be emphasized that no definition for microinvasive adenocarcinoma of the cervix has been agreed upon; therefore, treatment algorithms for such patients remain undefined.

For patients with frankly invasive disease, regardless of squamous cell or adenocarcinoma histology, the primary options for treatment are radical hysterectomy with lymphadenectomy or definitive radiation therapy. In patients undergoing primary surgery who have positive nodes, positive margins, or parametrial infiltration, adjuvant radiation concurrent with cisplatin-based chemotherapy is indicated on the basis of positive results from a randomized trial (29). In this trial, the addition of chemotherapy to radiation appeared to overcome the worse prognosis associated with adenocarcinoma cell components, when compared with patients receiving adjuvant radiation therapy only (29). For more advanced disease in which primary radiation therapy is recommended, the addition of concurrent cisplatin-based chemotherapy provides clear therapeutic benefit (35).

▶ *How should patients be monitored over the long term?*

Surveillance after primary therapy for invasive carcinoma of the cervix is universally recommended. Approximately 35% of patients will have persistent or recurrent disease. The main goal of surveillance is early detection of recurrent disease so that patients can be offered potentially curative salvage therapy. The average

1-year survival for patients with recurrent cervical cancer is 10–20% (39, 40). Surveillance schedules should take into account the risk of recurrence, which is highest in the first 2 years following treatment (41). The potential benefit of salvage therapy depends on the stage of disease, type of treatment, and location of recurrence (ie, local, regional, or distant). In general, radical radiation therapy is used for recurrent cervical cancer after primary hysterectomy, while salvage surgery is required for those who relapse after primary radiation therapy. In selected patients with centralized pelvic recurrences, salvage may be achieved in about 50% of cases (42).

Few studies have specifically addressed the efficacy of routine surveillance follow-up after definitive cervical cancer therapy in asymptomatic and disease-free patients, as opposed to symptom-based reassessment. Schedules for posttherapy surveillance vary by practitioner and institution, although a common approach includes examinations and Pap tests every 3–4 months for the first 3 years, decreasing to twice yearly in the fourth and fifth years (4).

Investigators recently attempted to develop an optimal surveillance program based on outcome analysis following primary therapy for stage-Ib cervical cancer (43). Detection of asymptomatic recurrences, whether locally in the pelvis or with isolated pulmonary metastases, led to significantly better salvage options and survival when compared with detection only in patients presenting with symptomatic recurrences. The authors concluded this subset of patients may benefit from careful posttherapy surveillance and proposed a schedule involving thrice-yearly follow-up visits for the first 2 years, and twice-yearly visits subsequently to year 5, with Pap tests and chest X-rays on a yearly basis.

Posttreatment follow-up also is beneficial for reasons other than the diagnosis of recurrence. The psychologic support and reassurance of continued contact with the treating team is vitally important. Annual health maintenance visits for mammography, blood pressure, and evaluation of other medical problems are important. Many of these patients undergo bilateral salpingo-oophorectomy or radiation therapy, and hormone replacement therapy should be considered in such patients. Cervical adenocarcinoma is not a contraindication to hormone replacement therapy.

▶ *How should patients with invasive cancer diagnosed during pregnancy be treated?*

Between 2.7% and 3.5% of cases of cervical cancer occur in pregnant women (44). The diagnosis of invasive carcinoma during pregnancy presents a therapeutic dilemma. Fortunately, cervical cancer rarely causes maternal mortality (45). The survival rate of patients with stage I cervical cancer is excellent regardless of the time of diagnosis during pregnancy, with recent reported survival rates of 85% and 95% (46, 47). The overall survival rate for women who were pregnant and had invasive cervical cancer is 80% (48).

This clinical problem requires attention to the health of the woman as well as the safety of the fetus. The appropriate treatment is influenced by ethical concerns, cultural and religious issues, and whether the patient wishes to continue the pregnancy after being informed of the potential risks and benefits of treatment. Optimal counseling and therapy require an interdisciplinary approach.

Therapeutic recommendations for a patient with invasive cervical carcinoma are individualized according to the patient's presenting stage, lesion size, and desire to continue the pregnancy. Pregnant women are 3.1 times more likely than nonpregnant women to have diagnosed Stage I disease, probably because of regular examinations (48). A summary of the current literature confirmed that most patients with cervical cancer diagnosed during pregnancy have stage I cancer (49). Seventy-six percent have stage Ib, and 78% have squamous cell histology.

Pregnancy offers an ideal opportunity for cervical cytologic screening. Figure 1 provides a general algorithm for the evaluation of abnormal cervical cytology in pregnancy (50). A pregnant patient with carcinoma in situ and microinvasive squamous carcinoma of 3 mm or less can deliver vaginally and be reevaluated and treated at 6 weeks postpartum.

Pregnant patients with invasive carcinoma of the cervix may choose early termination or choose to continue the pregnancy. Those who have a mature fetus at the time of diagnosis also may wish to delay treatment. If the patient opts to continue the pregnancy, predelivery assessment of fetal lung maturity by amniotic fluid analysis should be strongly considered, taking into account the availability of neonatal support to optimize fetal outcome and to avoid the potentially severe complications of prematurity, both in the neonatal period and in long-term development (51–54). Even those patients with early-stage disease should be aware that delaying treatment carries an undefined, but likely small, risk of disease progression. However, delaying treatment to optimize fetal maturity provides a major, quantifiable benefit for the infant. All of the studies reporting outcome when treatment is intentionally delayed to optimize fetal outcome suggest no measurable increased maternal risk (49). The studies included 77 patients with early-stage cervical cancers who opted to delay treatment for 1–40 weeks. The recurrence rate was 5% (4 of 77), which is similar to that in nonpregnant patients.

Abnormal cervical cytology
|
Colposcopy
Directed biopsy
No endocervical curettage

Cervical intraepithelial neoplasia | Microinvasive squamous carcinoma | Invasive carcinoma

Abnormal cytology without suggesting invasion | Malignant cytology suggesting invasion | Diagnostic conization or wedge biopsy of cervix | Appropriate therapy

Papanicolaou test and colposcopy every 8 weeks | Microinvasion ≤ 3 mm | Invasive carcinoma

Anticipate vaginal delivery | Appropriate therapy

Reevaluate 6 weeks postpartum

Figure 1. Evaluation of the patient with abnormal cytology during pregnancy. (Hannigan EV. Cervical cancer in pregnancy. Clin Obstet Gynecol 1990;33: 837–845)

The mode of delivery for those patients who choose to delay treatment to allow fetal maturation remains controversial. Patients with small-volume, early-stage lesions may be candidates for vaginal delivery. Whether vaginal delivery promotes disease progression is not clear. If possible, the patient should give birth by cesarean delivery at the time of planned radical surgery, and vaginal delivery should be reserved for those patients with preinvasive disease or stage Ia invasive disease with planned postpartum fertility-sparing therapy. Intuitively, it is prudent not to attempt vaginal delivery of women with large or friable tumors, given the risk of obstructing the progress of labor or the risk of bleeding with potentially life-threatening hemorrhage that might require emergency hysterectomy under less than optimal circumstances.

The available literature includes reports of 10 cases of implantation of malignancy at the episiotomy site (55–57). Posttreatment follow-up should include inspection and palpation of the episiotomy site. Treatment of recurrent disease in the episiotomy consists of excision followed by radiation.

For early-stage cervical cancer during pregnancy, radical surgery and radiation therapy offer similar cure rates. Radical hysterectomy with lymphadenectomy for stage Ia2 to IIa cervical cancer during pregnancy has demonstrated low associated morbidity, high survival rates, and an opportunity for preservation of ovarian function (49). Gestational edema and more pronounced cleavage planes facilitate the dissection.

When radical cesarean hysterectomy is performed, a classical uterine incision is preferred. Bilateral ovariopexy is a reasonable consideration at the time of surgery in the event that adjuvant radiation might be indicated for patients with high-risk histopathologic features. Results of a case–control study comparing radical surgery outcomes in pregnant and nonpregnant patients demonstrated a higher blood loss in pregnant patients, but this did not translate into a significant increase in blood transfusion, operative morbidity, or major complication rates (58). Survival was 97% in the pregnant patients and 90% in the controls, with mean follow-up over 140 months.

Most pregnant patients who are candidates for radical surgery will benefit from surgery rather than radiation therapy, given the advantage of ovarian preservation and the avoidance of radiation-associated vaginal fibrosis. Pregnant patients with stage IIb or more advanced invasive cervical cancer and patients either not medically fit or not interested in primary surgical treatment should undergo definitive radiation therapy. Patients with advanced disease who elect to delay treatment should have documented fetal pulmonary maturity prior to classic cesarean delivery and should start their radiation therapy postdelivery following uterine involution. Pelvic and paraaortic lymph node dissection can be performed at the time of cesarean delivery to aid treatment planning.

Planning radiation treatment for pregnant patients with cervical cancer requires careful adaptation to adjust for the anatomic distortion created by the gravid state. Patients opting for primary radiation therapy with the intent of pregnancy termination should begin with external-beam therapy. It is common for the pregnancy to abort spontaneously when the woman is irradiated with less than 4,000 cGy of external-beam radiation. In one series, however, 27% of 45 patients did not abort and required subsequent surgical uterine evacuation (58).

Summary

The following recommendations are based on good and consistent scientific evidence (Level A):

▶ For stage Ib and selected IIa carcinomas of the cervix, either radical hysterectomy and lymph node dissection or radiation therapy with cisplatin-based chemotherapy should be considered. Adjuvant radiation therapy may be required in those treated surgically, based on pathologic risk factors, especially in those with stage Ib2 carcinoma.

▶ Stage IIb and greater should be treated with external-beam and brachytherapy radiation and concurrent cisplatin-based chemotherapy.

The following recommendations are based on limited or inconsistent scientific evidence (Level B):

▶ For stage Ia1 microinvasive squamous carcinoma of the cervix, treatment with conization of the cervix or simple extrafascial hysterectomy may be considered.

▶ Stage Ia2 invasive squamous carcinoma of the cervix should be treated with radical hysterectomy with lymph node dissection or radiation therapy, depending on clinical circumstances.

▶ Stage Ib1 should be distinguished from stage Ib2 carcinoma of the cervix because the distinction predicts nodal involvement and overall survival and may, therefore, affect treatment and outcome.

▶ Patients with squamous cell cancers and those with adenocarcinomas should be managed similarly, except for those with microinvasive disease. Criteria for microinvasive adenocarcinomas have not been established.

The following recommendations are based primarily on expert opinion and consensus (Level C):

▶ Following treatment for cervical carcinoma, patients should be monitored regularly, for example, with thrice-yearly follow-up examinations for the first 2 years and twice-yearly visits subsequently to year 5, with Pap tests annually and chest X-rays annually for up to 5 years.

▶ Treatment for pregnant patients with invasive carcinoma of the cervix should be individualized on the basis of evaluation of maternal and fetal risks.

References

1. Parkin DM, Pisani P, Ferlay J. Global cancer statistics. CA Cancer J Clin 1999;49:33–64,1 (Level II-3)

2. Greenlee RT, Hill-Harmon MB, Murray T, Thun M. Cancer statistics, 2001. CA Cancer J Clin 2001;51:15–36 (Level II-3)

3. Anttila T, Saikku P, Koskela P, Bloigu A, Dillner J, Ikaneimo I, et al. Serotypes of Chlamydia trachomatis and risk for development of cervical squamous cell carcinoma. JAMA 2001;285:47–51 (Level II-2)

4. National Comprehensive Cancer Network. NCCN practice guidelines for cervical cancer. In: The complete library of NCCN oncology practice guidelines (CD-ROM), Version 2000, Revision date: June 1, 2000 (Level III)

5. Benedet JL, Odicino F, Maisonneuve P, Beller U, Creasman WT, Heintz AP, et al. Carcinoma of the cervix uteri. J Epidemiol Biostat 2001;6:7–43 (Level II-3)

6. Heller PB, Maletano JH, Bundy BN, Barnhill DR, Okagaki T. Clinical-pathologic study of stage IIB, III and IVA carcinoma of the cervix: extended diagnostic evaluation for paraaortic node metastasis—a Gynecologic Oncology Group study. Gynecol Oncol 1990;38:425–430 (Level II-3)

7. Scheidler J, Hricak H, Yu KK, Subak L, Segal MR. Radiological evaluation of lymph node metastases in patients with cervical cancer. A meta-analysis. JAMA 1997;278:1096–1101 (Meta-analysis)

8. Rose PG, Adler LP, Rodriguez M, Faulhaber PF, Abdul-Karim FW, Miraldi F. Positron emission tomography for evaluating para-aortic nodal metastasis in locally advanced cervical cancer before surgical staging: a surgicopathologic study. J Clin Oncol 1999;17:41–45 (Level III)

9. Alvarez RD, Soong SJ, Kinney WK, Reid GC, Schray MF, Podratz KC, et al. Identification of prognostic factors and risk groups in patients found to have nodal metastasis at the time of radical hysterectomy for early-stage squamous carcinoma of the cervix. Gynecol Oncol 1989;35:130–135 (Level II-2)

10. Fuller AF Jr, Elliott N, Kosloff C, Hoskins WJ, Lewis JL Jr. Determinants of increased risk for recurrence in patients undergoing radical hysterectomy for stage IB and IIA carcinoma of the cervix. Gynecol Oncol 1989;33: 34–39 (Level II-2)

11. Delgado G, Bundy B, Zaino R, Sevin BU, Creasman WT, Major F. Prospective surgical-pathological study of disease-free interval in patients with stage IB squamous cell carcinoma of the cervix: a Gynecologic Oncology Group study. Gynecol Oncol 1990;38:352–357 (Level II-3)

12. Eifel PJ, Morris M, Wharton JT, Oswald MJ. The influence of tumor size and morphology on the outcome of patients with FIGO stage IB squamous cell carcinoma of the uterine cervix. Int J Radiat Oncol Biol Phys 1994; 29:9–16 (Level II-3)

13. Grigsby PW. Primary radiotherapy for stage IB or IIA cervical cancer. J Natl Cancer Inst Monogr 1996;(21):61–64 (Level III)

14. Finan MA, DeCesare S, Fiorica JV, Chambers R, Hoffman MS, Kline RC, et al. Radical hysterectomy for stage IB1 vs IB2 carcinoma of the cervix: does the new staging system predict morbidity and survival? Gynecol Oncol 1996;62:139–147 (Level II-3)

15. Cosin JA, Fowler JM, Chen MD, Paley PJ, Carson LF, Twiggs LB. Pretreatment surgical staging of patients with cervical carcinoma: the case for lymph node debulking. Cancer 1998;82:2241–2248 (Level II-2)

16. Goff BA, Muntz HG, Paley PJ, Tamimi HK, Koh WJ, Greer BE. Impact of surgical staging in women with locally advanced cervical cancer. Gynecol Oncol 1999;74: 436–442 (Level II-3)

17. Mestwerdt G. Probeexzision und Kolposkopie Frühdiagnose des Portiokarzinoms. Zentralb Gynaekol. 1947;69: 326–332 (German)

18. Burghardt E, Holzer E. Diagnosis and treatment of microinvasive carcinoma of the cervix uteri. Obstet Gynecol 1977;49:641–653 (Level III)

19. Greer BE, Figge DC, Timimi HK, Cain JC, Lee RB. Stage IA2 squamous carcinoma of the cervix: difficult diagnosis and therapeutic dilemma. Am J Obstet Gynecol 1990;162:1406–1409; discussion 1409–1411 (Level III)

20. Kolstad P. Follow-up study of 232 patients with stage [Ia1] and 411 patients with stage Ia2 squamous cell carcinoma of the cervix (microinvasive carcinoma). Gynecol Oncol 1989;33:265–272 (Level III)

21. Morgan PR, Anderson MC, Buckley CH, Murdoch JB, Lopes A, Duncan ID, et al. The Royal College of Obstetricians and Gynaecologists micro-invasive carcinoma of the cervix study: preliminary results. Br J Obstet Gynaecol 1993;100:664–668 (Level III)

22. Benedet JL, Anderson GH. Stage IA carcinoma of the cervix revisited. Obstet Gynecol 1996;87:1052–1059 (Level III)

23. Sevin BU, Nadji M, Averette HE, Hilsenbeck S, Smith D, Lampe B. Microinvasive carcinoma of the cervix. Cancer 1992;70:2121–2128 (Level III)

24. Covens A, Shaw P, Murphy J, DePetrillo D, Lickrish G, Laframboise S, et al. Is radical trachelectomy a safe alternative to radical hysterectomy for patients with stage IA-B carcinoma of the cervix? Cancer 1999;86: 2273–2279 (Level II-2)

25. Dargent D, Martin X, Sacchetoni A, Mathevet P. Laparoscopic vaginal radical trachelectomy: a treatment to preserve the fertility of cervical carcinoma patients. Cancer 2000;88:1877–1882 (Level II-3)

26. Averette HE, Method MW, Sevin B-U, Penalver MA. Radical abdominal hysterectomy in the primary management of invasive cervical cancer. In: Rubin SC, Hoskins WJ, eds. Cervical cancer and preinvasive neoplasia. Philadelphia: Lippincott–Raven Publishers, 1996: 189–106 (Level III)

27. Landoni F, Maneo A, Colombo A, Placa F, Milani R, Perego P, et al. Randomised study of radical surgery versus radiotherapy for stage Ib-IIa cervical cancer. Lancet 1997;350:535–540 (Level I)

28. Koh WJ, Panwala K, Greer B. Adjuvant therapy for high-risk, early stage cervical cancer. Semin Radiat Oncol 2000;10:51–60 (Level III)

29. Peters WA 3rd, Liu PY, Barrett RJ 2nd, Stock RJ, Monk BJ, Berek JS, et al. Concurrent chemotherapy and pelvic radiation therapy compared with pelvic radiation therapy alone as adjuvant therapy after radical surgery in high-risk early-stage cancer of the cervix. J Clin Oncol 2000; 18:1606–1613 (Level I)

30. Sedlis A, Bundy BN, Rotman MZ, Lentz SS, Muderspach LI, Zaino RJ. A randomized trial of pelvic radiation therapy versus no further therapy in selected patients with stage IB carcinoma of the cervix after radical hysterectomy and pelvic lymphadenectomy: a Gynecologic Oncology Study Group Study. Gynecol Oncol 1999;73: 177–183 (Level I)

31. Morris M, Eifel PJ, Lu J, Grigsby PW, Levenback C, Stevens RE, et al. Pelvic radiation with concurrent chemotherapy compared with pelvic and para-aortic radiation for high-risk cervical cancer. N Engl J Med 1999;340:1137–1143 (Level I)

32. Rose PG, Bundy BN, Watkins EB, Thigpen JT, Deppe G, Maiman MA, et al. Concurrent cisplatin-based radiotherapy and chemotherapy for locally advanced cervical cancer. N Engl J Med 1999;340:1144–1153 (Level I)

33. Keys HM, Bundy BN, Stehman FB, Muderspach LI, Chafe WE, Suggs CL 3rd, et al. Cisplatin, radiation, and adjuvant hysterectomy compared with radiation and adjuvant hysterectomy for bulky stage IB cervical carcinoma. N Engl J Med 1999;340:1154–1161 (Level I)

34. Whitney CW, Sause W, Bundy BN, Malfetano JH, Hannigan EV, Fowler WC Jr, et al. Randomized comparison of fluorouracil plus cisplatin versus hydroxyurea as an adjunct to radiation therapy in stage IIB-IVA carcinoma of the cervix with negative para-aortic lymph nodes: a Gynecologic Oncology Group and Southwest Oncology Group Study. J Clin Oncol 1999;17:1339–1348 (Level I)

35. National Cancer Institute. PDQ treatment summary for health professionals. Cervical cancer. Bethesda, Maryland: National Institutes of Health, 2002. Available at http://cancernet.nci.nih.gov/cgi-bin/srchcgi.exe?DBID =pdq&TYPE=search&SFMT=pdq_statement/1/0/0&Z20 8=208_00103H. Retrieved January 8, 2002 (Level III)

36. Thomas GM. Improved treatment for cervical cancer—concurrent chemotherapy and radiotherapy. N Engl J Med 1999;340:1198–1200 (Level III)

37. Look KY, Brunetto VL, Clarke-Pearson DL, Averette HE, Major FJ, Alvarez RD, et al. An analysis of cell type in patients with surgically staged stage IB carcinoma of the cervix: a Gynecologic Oncology Group study. Gynecol Oncol 1996;63:304–311 (Level II-3)

38. Eifel PJ, Burke TW, Morris M, Smith TL. Adenocarcinoma as an independent risk factor for disease recurrence in patients with stage IB cervical carcinoma. Gynecol Oncol 1995;59:38–44 (Level II-3)

39. Burke TW, Hoskins WJ, Heller PB, Shen MC, Weiser EB, Park RC. Clinical patterns of tumor recurrence after radical hysterectomy in stage IB cervical carcinoma. Obstet Gynecol 1987;69:382–385 (Level III)

40. Adcock LL, Potish RA, Julian TM, Okagaki T, Prem KA, Twiggs LB, et al. Carcinoma of the cervix, FIGO Stage IB: treatment failures. Gynecol Oncol 1984;18:218–225 (Level II-3)

41. Naumann RW, Shingleton HM. Posttreatment surveillance and patterns of recurrence. In: Rubin SC, Hoskins WJ, eds. Cervical cancer and preinvasive neoplasia. Philadelphia: Lippincott–Raven Publishers, 1996:361–369 (Level III)

42. Koh WJ, Paley PJ, Comsia ND, Greer BE. Radical management of recurrent cervical cancer. In: Eifel PJ, Levenback C, eds. American Cancer Society atlas of clinical oncology: neoplasms of the female genital tract. Hamilton, Ontario: BC Decker; 2001 (Level III)

43. Bodurka-Bevers D, Morris M, Eifel PJ, Levenback C, Bevers MW, Lucas KR, et al. Posttherapy surveillance of women with cervical cancer: an outcomes analysis. Gynecol Oncol 2000;78:187–193 (Level II-3)

44. Donegan WL. Cancer and pregnancy. CA Cancer J Clin 1983;33:194–214. Review (Level III)

45. Landis SH, Murray T, Bolden S, Wingo PA. Cancer statistics, 1998. CA Cancer J Clin 1998;48:6–29 (Level II-3)

46. Hopkins MP, Morley GW. The prognosis and management of cervical cancer associated with pregnancy. Obstet Gynecol 1992;80:9–13 (Level II-2)

47. Monk BJ, Montz FJ. Invasive cervical cancer complicating intrauterine pregnancy: treatment with radical hysterectomy. Obstet Gynecol 1992;80:199–203 (Level III)

48. Zemlickis D, Lishner M, Degendorfer P, Panzarella T, Sutcliffe SB, Koren G. Maternal and fetal outcome after invasive cervical cancer in pregnancy. J Clin Oncol 1991;9:1956–1961 (Level II-2)

49. Goff BA, Paley PJ, Koh WJ, Petersdorf SH, Douglas JG, Greer BE. Cancer in the pregnant patient. In: Hoskins WJ, Perez CA, Young RC, eds. Principles and practice of gynecologic oncology. Philadelphia: Lippincott Williams & Wilkins, 2000:501–528 (Level III)

50. Hannigan EV. Cervical cancer in pregnancy. Clin Obstet Gynecol 1990;33:837–845 (Level III)

51. Greer BE, Easterling TR, McLennan DA, Benedetti TJ, Cain JM, Figge DC, et al. Fetal and maternal considerations in the management of Stage I-B cervical cancer during pregnancy. Gynecol Oncol 1989;34:61–65 (Level III)

52. Vohr BR, Garcia Coll CT. Neurodevelopmental and school performance of very low-birth-weight infants: a seven-year longitudinal study. Pediatrics 1985;76:345–350 (Level II-2)

53. Papile LA, Munsick-Bruno G, Schaefer A. Relationship of cerebral intraventricular hemorrhage and early childhood neurologic handicaps. J Pediatr 1983;103:273–277 (Level III)

54. Halsey CL, Collin MF, Anderson CL. Extremely low birth weight children and their peers: a comparison of preschool performance. Pediatrics 1993;91:807–811 (Level II-2)

55. Cliby WA, Dodson MK, Podratz KC. Cervical cancer complicated by pregnancy: episiotomy site recurrences following vaginal delivery. Obstet Gynecol 1994;84:179–182 (Level III)

56. Copeland LJ, Saul PB, Sneige N. Cervical adenocarcinoma: tumor implantation in the episiotomy sites of two patients. Gynecol Oncol 1987;28:230–235 (Level III)

57. Gordon AN, Jensen R, Jones HW 3rd. Squamous carcinoma of the cervix complicating pregnancy: recurrence in episiotomy after vaginal delivery. Obstet Gynecol 1989;73:850–852 (Level III)

58. Sood AK, Sorosky JI, Krogman S, Anderson B, Benda J, Buller RE. Surgical management of cervical cancer complicating pregnancy: a case-control study. Gynecol Oncol 1996;63:294–298 (Level II-2)

The MEDLINE database, the Cochrane Library, and ACOG's own internal resources and documents were used to conduct a literature search to locate relevant articles published between January 1985 and December 2000. Priority was given to articles reporting results of original research, although review articles and commentaries also were consulted. Abstracts of research presented at symposia and scientific conferences were not considered adequate for inclusion in this document. Guidelines published by organizations or institutions such as the National Institutes of Health and the American College of Obstetricians and Gynecologists were reviewed, and additional studies were located by reviewing bibliographies of identified articles. When reliable research was not available, expert opinions from obstetrician–gynecologists were used.

Studies were reviewed and evaluated for quality according to the method outlined by the U.S. Preventive Services Task Force:

I   Evidence obtained from at least one properly designed randomized controlled trial.

II-1   Evidence obtained from well-designed controlled trials without randomization.

II-2   Evidence obtained from well-designed cohort or case–control analytic studies, preferably from more than one center or research group.

II-3   Evidence obtained from multiple time series with or without the intervention. Dramatic results in uncontrolled experiments also could be regarded as this type of evidence.

III   Opinions of respected authorities, based on clinical experience, descriptive studies, or reports of expert committees.

Based on the highest level of evidence found in the data, recommendations are provided and graded according to the following categories:

Level A—Recommendations are based on good and consistent scientific evidence.

Level B—Recommendations are based on limited or inconsistent scientific evidence.

Level C—Recommendations are based primarily on consensus and expert opinion.

ISSN 1099-3630

The American College of Obstetricians and Gynecologists
409 12th Street, SW, PO Box 96920
Washington, DC 20090-6920

12345/65432

Diagnosis and treatment of cervical carcinomas. ACOG Practice Bulletin No. 35. American College of Obstetricians and Gynecologists. Obstet Gynecol 2002;99:855-867

ACOG PRACTICE BULLETIN

CLINICAL MANAGEMENT GUIDELINES FOR
OBSTETRICIAN–GYNECOLOGISTS

NUMBER 53, JUNE 2004

This Practice Bulletin was developed by the ACOG Committee on Practice Bulletins— Gynecology and the SGO Education Committee with the assistance of John Soper, MD, Julian Schink, MD, and David Mutch, MD. The information is designed to aid practitioners in making decisions about appropriate obstetric and gynecologic care. These guidelines should not be construed as dictating an exclusive course of treatment or procedure. Variations in practice may be warranted based on the needs of the individual patient, resources, and limitations unique to the institution or type of practice.

Diagnosis and Treatment of Gestational Trophoblastic Disease

Gestational trophoblastic disease comprises a spectrum of interrelated conditions originating from the placenta. Other terms often used to refer to these conditions include gestational trophoblastic neoplasia and gestational trophoblastic tumor. Histologically distinct disease entities encompassed by this general terminology include complete and partial hydatidiform moles, invasive moles, gestational choriocarcinomas, and placental site trophoblastic tumors. Before the advent of sensitive assays for human chorionic gonadotropin (hCG) and efficacious chemotherapy, the morbidity and mortality from gestational trophoblastic disease were substantial. At present, with sensitive quantitative assays for β-hCG and current approaches to chemotherapy, most women with malignant gestational trophoblastic disease can be cured and their reproductive function preserved. The purpose of this document is to address current evidence regarding the diagnosis, staging, and management of gestational trophoblastic disease.

Background

Estimates for the incidence of various forms of gestational trophoblastic disease vary. In the United States, hydatidiform moles are observed in approximately 1 in 600 therapeutic abortions and 1 in 1,500 pregnancies (1). Approximately 20% of patients will develop malignant sequelae requiring administration of chemotherapy after evacuation of hydatidiform moles (2, 3). Most patients with postmolar gestational trophoblastic disease will have nonmetastatic molar proliferation or invasive moles, but gestational choriocarcinomas and metastatic disease can develop in this setting. Gestational choriocarcinoma occurs in approximately 1 in 20,000–40,000 pregnancies: approximately 50% after term pregnancies, 25% after molar pregnancies, and the remainder after other gestational events (4). Although much rarer than hydatidiform moles or gestational chorocarcinomas, placental site trophoblastic tumors can develop after any type of pregnancy (5, 6). To allow optimal management, practicing obstetrician–gynecologists should be able to diagnose and manage primary molar pregnancies, diagnose and stage malignant gestational trophoblastic disease, and assess risk in women with malignant gestational trophoblastic disease to allow referral for appropriate initial treatment. Experience, such as that found at regional gestational trophoblastic disease treatment centers, improves outcomes in the management of malignant gestational trophoblastic disease. Any woman for whom initial therapy for invasive mole has failed or who has a choriocarcinoma diagnosis should be referred to a physician or facility with training, expertise, and experience in managing gestational trophoblastic disease.

Hydatidiform Mole

Classification

Partial and complete hydatidiform moles are distinct disease processes with characteristic cytogenetic, histologic, and clinical features (4). The distinct pathologic features and clinical presentation of these 2 entities are outlined in Table 1. Despite the cytogenetic, pathologic, and clinical differences between the 2 diagnoses, the management of patients with complete and partial moles is similar.

The volume and amount of trophoblastic proliferation in complete moles generally exceed that observed in partial moles and are reflected in the different clinical presentations (see Table 1). The average initial serum hCG levels usually are higher in patients with complete moles than in patients with partial moles (7). Although an increasing proportion of moles are diagnosed as missed abortions on the basis of an early ultrasound examination in the absence of symptoms (8), most patients with complete moles have a clinical or ultrasonographic diagnosis of hydatidiform mole. Uterine enlargement beyond the expected gestational age is observed in up to 50% of patients with complete moles (1). These patients may present with vaginal bleeding or expulsion of molar vesicles. Medical complications of molar pregnancy, including pregnancy-induced hypertension, hyperthyroidism, anemia, and hyperemesis gravidarum, are more frequently seen among patients with complete moles (9). Approximately 15–25% of patients with complete moles will have theca lutein cysts with ovarian enlargement of more than 6 cm (10). Malignant sequelae occur in less than 5% of patients with partial moles, compared with approximately 20% after evacuation of complete hydatidiform moles (see Table 1) (4).

Diagnosis

Hydatidiform moles usually are diagnosed during the first trimester of pregnancy (8, 11). The most common symptom is abnormal bleeding. Other signs and symptoms include uterine enlargement greater than expected for gestational age, absent fetal heart tones, cystic enlargement of the ovaries, hyperemesis gravidarum, and an abnormally high level of hCG for gestational age (4). Presence of these features in the first trimester should

Table 1. Features of Partial and Complete Hydatidiform Moles

Feature	Partial Mole	Complete Mole
Karyotype	Most commonly 69,XXX or 69,XXY	Most commonly 46,XX or 46,XY
Pathology		
Fetus	Often present	Absent
Amnion, fetal red blood cells	Usually present	Absent
Villous edema	Variable, focal	Diffuse
Trophoblastic proliferation	Focal, slight to moderate	Diffuse, slight to severe
Clinical presentation		
Diagnosis	Missed abortion	Molar gestation
Uterine size	Small for gestational age	50% larger for gestational age
Theca lutein cysts	Rare	15–25%
Medical complications	Rare	Less than 25%
Postmolar malignant sequelae	<5%	6–32%

Modified from Soper JT, Lewis Jl. Jr, Hammond CB. Gestational trophoblastic disease. In: Hoskins WJ, Perez CA, Young RC, editors. Principals and practice of gynecologic oncology, 2nd ed. Philadelphia (PA): Lippincott-Raven; 1997. p. 1040.

alert the clinician to the possibility of a molar gestation. Pregnancy-induced hypertension in the first half of pregnancy, although uncommon, is suggestive of hydatidiform mole. Ultrasonography has replaced all other noninvasive means of establishing the diagnosis (4, 8). Molar tissue typically is identified as a diffuse mixed echogenic pattern replacing the placenta, produced by villi and intrauterine blood clots, but these findings may be subtle or lacking in cases of early complete or partial moles (8, 11).

Management After Evacuation of Hydatidiform Mole

As long as hCG values are decreasing after molar evacuation, there is no role for chemotherapy. However, if hCG levels increase or plateau over several weeks, immediate evaluation and treatment for malignant postmolar gestational trophoblastic disease are indicated. Occasionally, the plateauing or increasing hCG levels are a result of a false-positive laboratory test result caused by heterophilic antibodies cross-reacting with the hCG test. Such false-positive test results, also known as "phantom hCG," are discussed later.

The diagnosis of malignant sequelae as indicated by the need for chemotherapy include the plateau or increase of hCG levels after evacuation of hydatidiform moles as mentioned previously, the histologic diagnosis of choriocarcinoma or invasive mole on the basis of findings from uterine curettage, or identification of clinical or radiographic evidence of metastases. Repeat curettage is not recommended because it does not often induce remission or influence treatment and may result in uterine perforation and hemorrhage (12).

A variety of hCG criteria have been used to diagnose postmolar gestational trophoblastic disease (1–3, 13, 14). Recently, the International Federation of Gynecologists and Obstetricians (FIGO) standardized hCG criteria for the diagnosis of postmolar gestational trophoblastic disease (14). Based on consensus committee recommendations from the Society of Gynecologic Oncology, the International Society for the Study of Trophoblastic Disease, and the International Gynecologic Cancer Society, the following criteria were proposed by FIGO (14):

1. An hCG level plateau of 4 values plus or minus 10% recorded over a 3-week duration (days 1, 7, 14, and 21)

2. An hCG level increase of more than 10% of 3 values recorded over a 2-week duration (days 1, 7, and 14)

3. Persistence of detectable hCG for more than 6 months after molar evacuation

A new intrauterine pregnancy should be ruled out on the basis of hCG levels and ultrasonography, especially when there has been a long delay in follow-up of serial hCG levels and noncompliance with contraception.

Malignant Gestational Trophoblastic Disease

Histologic Considerations

The clinical presentation of malignant gestational trophoblastic disease is more important in determining treatment and outcome than the precise histologic diagnosis (4). Postmolar gestational trophoblastic disease is only one of many forms of malignant gestational trophoblastic disease; it comprises noninvasive trophoblastic proliferation, invasive moles, and gestational choriocarcinoma. Gestational choriocarcinomas are derived from term pregnancies in one half of cases, with equal portions of the remaining half from histologically normal gestations and hydatidiform moles. The rarest form of malignant gestational trophoblastic disease, placental site trophoblastic tumor, can follow any pregnancy.

The term invasive mole is used to describe disease confined to the uterus and is characterized by the presence of edematous chorionic villi with trophoblastic proliferation that invade directly into the myometrium. Most cases are clinically diagnosed and are not determined histologically. Dilation and curettage (D&C) should be avoided to prevent morbidity and mortality caused by uterine perforation. Gestational choriocarcinoma is a malignancy, comprising both neoplastic syncytiotrophoblast and cytotrophoblast elements without chorionic villi (4). Gestational choriocarcinomas tend to develop early systemic metastasis (the vagina, lung, liver, and brain are the most common sites), and chemotherapy is indicated when it is diagnosed histologically. When indicated, chemotherapy should be initiated in a timely manner to avoid bleeding complications at metastatic sites.

Placental site trophoblastic tumors are relatively rare (5, 6). They are characterized by absence of villi with proliferation of intermediate trophoblast cells. The number of syncytiotrophoblast cells observed is decreased in placental site trophoblastic tumors, with relatively lower levels of hCG secreted by these tumors. Generally, placental site trophoblastic tumors are not as sensitive to chemotherapy as other forms of malignant gestational trophoblastic disease; therefore, it is important to distinguish these tumors histologically (4). Surgery assumes a critical role in the management of placental site trophoblastic tumors (5, 6). Fortunately, most patients have disease confined to the uterus and are cured by hysterectomy.

Clinical Diagnosis of Malignant Gestational Trophoblastic Disease

Postmolar gestational trophoblastic disease is most frequently diagnosed on the basis of increasing or plateauing hCG values. Women with malignant gestational trophoblastic disease following nonmolar pregnancies may have subtle signs and symptoms of disease, which make the diagnosis difficult (15). Abnormal bleeding for more than 6 weeks following any pregnancy should be evaluated with hCG testing to exclude a new pregnancy or gestational trophoblastic disease. Metastases of gestational choriocarcinoma have been reported in virtually every body site, most commonly the vagina, liver, lung, and brain; however, biopsy of these sites is rarely necessary and may cause excessive bleeding. Central nervous system metastases may produce neurologic symptoms, intracranial hemorrhage, or mass lesions. Gestational choriocarcinoma should be considered in any woman of reproductive age with metastatic disease from an unknown primary site (15). A serum hCG determination and exclusion of pregnancy are all that are required to diagnose metastatic gestational trophoblastic disease in these circumstances.

Clinical Considerations and Recommendations

▶ *How are patients with hydatidiform moles managed?*

With increasing frequency, the diagnosis of complete or partial moles usually is made after performing a D&C for a suspected incomplete spontaneous abortion (8, 11). In these cases, patients should be monitored with serial determinations of quantitative hCG values. A baseline postevacuation chest X-ray should be considered.

For patients in whom hydatidiform moles are suspected before evacuation, the following tests are recommended (4):

- Complete blood count with platelet determination
- Clotting function studies
- Renal and liver function studies
- Blood type with antibody screen
- Determination of hCG level
- Preevacuation chest X-ray

Medical complications of hydatidiform moles are observed in approximately 25% of patients with uterine enlargement of more than 14–16 weeks' gestational size and are seen less frequently among patients with lesser degrees of uterine enlargement (9). Common medical complications include anemia, infection, hyperthyroidism, pregnancy-induced hypertension, and coagulopathy. Women with signs and symptoms of these complications will need more intensive evaluation (ie, thyroid-stimulating hormones and coagulopathy studies). Moles should be evacuated as soon as possible after stabilization of any medical complications.

To manage potential complications of molar evacuation in a woman with a large uterus, consideration should be given to performing the evacuation in a facility with an intensive care unit, a blood bank, and anesthesia services. For most patients, the preferred method of evacuation is suction D&C (1, 9). Medical induction of labor with oxytocin or prostaglandin and hysterotomy are not recommended for evacuation because they increase blood loss and may increase the risk for malignant sequelae when compared with suction D&C (3, 4, 9, 16). Furthermore, patients most often require D&C to complete the evacuation of moles after medical induction of labor (9). Evacuation usually is performed with the patient under general anesthesia, but local or regional anesthesia may be used for a cooperative patient who has a small uterus. After serial dilation of the cervix, uterine evacuation is accomplished with the largest cannula that can be introduced through the cervix. In some cases, ultrasound guidance may facilitate complete evacuation of the uterus. Intravenous oxytocin is administered after the cervix is dilated and is continued for several hours postoperatively. Rh-negative patients should be treated with anti-D immune globulin after the evacuation even though fetal red blood cells should not be present in a complete mole.

Pulmonary complications are frequently observed around the time of molar evacuation among patients with marked uterine enlargement (9, 17, 18). Although the syndrome of trophoblastic embolization (deportation) has been emphasized as an underlying cause of respiratory distress syndrome following molar evacuation, there are many other potential causes of pulmonary complications in these women. Respiratory distress syndrome can be caused by high-output congestive heart failure caused by anemia or hyperthyroidism, preeclampsia, or iatrogenic fluid overload (17, 18). Generally, these complications should be treated aggressively with therapy directed by central venous or Swan-Ganz catheter monitoring and assisted ventilatory support, as required. Hyperthyroidism and pregnancy-induced hypertension usually abate promptly after evacuation of the mole and may not require specific therapy. Theca lutein cysts are associated with hCG stimulation of the ovaries (10). These may take several months to resolve after molar evacuation but rarely need to be removed. Surgical intervention should be reserved for rupture or torsion, which is rare (10).

Hysterectomy with preservation of the adnexa is an alternative to suction D&C for molar evacuation in selected patients who do not wish to preserve childbearing. Hysterectomy reduces the risk of malignant postmolar sequelae when compared with evacuation by D&C. However, the risk of postmolar gestational trophoblastic disease after hysterectomy remains approximately 3–5%, and these patients should be monitored postoperatively with serial hCG determinations (3, 4).

▶ *How are patients monitored after evacuation of hydatidiform moles, and what are the considerations regarding contraception and future pregnancies?*

After molar evacuation, it is important to monitor all patients carefully to diagnose and treat malignant sequelae promptly. Serial quantitative serum hCG determinations should be performed using commercially available assays capable of detecting β-hCG to baseline values (<5 mIU/mL). Ideally, serum hCG levels should be obtained within 48 hours of evacuation, every 1–2 weeks while elevated, and then at monthly intervals for an additional 6 months (4). Use of reliable hormonal contraception is recommended while hCG values are being monitored. Frequent pelvic examinations are performed while hCG values are elevated to monitor the involution of pelvic structures and to aid in the early identification of vaginal metastases.

The rationale for an interval of monitoring after normalization of the hCG level is to identify patients who develop malignant postmolar gestational trophoblastic disease. Although rare instances of long latent periods have been reported, most episodes of malignant sequelae after hydatidiform moles occur within approximately 6 months of evacuation (2, 3). Although pregnancies after molar evacuation usually are normal gestations, pregnancy obscures the value of monitoring hCG levels during this interval and may result in a delayed diagnosis of postmolar malignant gestational trophoblastic disease.

Oral contraceptives do not increase the incidence of postmolar gestational trophoblastic disease or alter the pattern of regression of hCG values (13, 19). In a randomized study, patients treated with oral contraceptives had one half as many intercurrent pregnancies as those using barrier methods, and the incidence of postmolar trophoblastic disease was lower in patients using oral contraceptives (20). After completion of documented remission for 6–12 months, women who desire pregnancy may discontinue contraception, and hCG monitor-

ing may be discontinued. Patients with prior partial or complete moles have a 10-fold increased risk (1–2% incidence) of a second hydatidiform mole in a subsequent pregnancy (20). Therefore, all future pregnancies should be evaluated by early obstetric ultrasonography.

▶ *Which patients should be considered for prophylactic chemotherapy to reduce the risk of postmolar trophoblastic disease after molar evacuation?*

Two randomized studies have evaluated prophylactic chemotherapy after molar evacuation. In one study, a single course of methotrexate and folinic acid reduced the incidence of postmolar trophoblastic disease from 47.4% to 14.3% (P <.05) in patients with high-risk moles (as defined by hCG levels greater than 100,000 mIU/mL, uterine size greater than gestational age, and ovarian size greater than 6 cm), but the incidence was not reduced in patients with low-risk moles (21). Patients who received prophylactic chemotherapy but developed postmolar trophoblastic disease required more chemotherapy than those who had not been exposed to prophylactic chemotherapy (21). In the second study, a single course of prophylactic dactinomycin was given to patients after evacuation of high-risk moles (22). Postmolar trophoblastic disease occurred in 50% of the control group, compared with 13.8% of the treatment group. In both studies, there were no deaths in the treatment or control groups caused by gestational trophoblastic disease or treatment toxicity (21, 22). However, there are anecdotal cases of fatalities caused by prophylactic chemotherapy (3, 4), and prophylactic chemotherapy does not eliminate the need for postevacuation follow-up. In compliant patients, the low morbidity and mortality achieved by monitoring patients with serial hCG determinations and instituting chemotherapy only in patients with postmolar gestational trophoblastic disease outweighs the potential risk and small benefit of routine prophylactic chemotherapy.

▶ *What are the considerations for a patient with both a hydatidiform mole and a co-existent fetus?*

Co-existence of a fetus with molar changes of the placenta is relatively rare, occurring in 1 in 22,000–100,000 pregnancies (23). Most of the literature covering this entity consists of case reports, small case series, and reviews of cases reported in the literature. Both complete and partial moles with co-existent fetuses have been reported (24). A variety of criteria have been used to evaluate these pregnancies. Many of the reports that antedated the histologic and cytogenetic distinction between complete and partial moles likely included partial moles and twin gestations with co-existent fetuses and molar gestations. There may be an increased incidence of co-existing mole and fetus related to an increase in multifetal pregnancies associated with ovulation induction, but this may reflect reporting bias (25).

Most of these twin pregnancies are diagnosed antepartum by ultrasound findings of a complex, cystic placental component distinct from the fetoplacental unit (23, 24); however, in a few cases, the diagnosis is not suspected until examination of the placenta following delivery (25). Medical complications of hydatidiform mole with a co-existent fetus appear to be increased and include hyperthyroidism, hemorrhage, and pregnancy-induced hypertension (23, 24, 26).

Compared with singleton hydatidiform moles, twin pregnancies with a fetus and a mole carry an increased risk for postmolar gestational trophoblastic disease, with a higher proportion of patients having metastatic disease and requiring multiagent chemotherapy (23–26). Among patients with co-existent moles and fetuses who continue pregnancy, a subset develops early complications leading to termination of the pregnancy before fetal viability, with a markedly increased risk of postmolar gestational trophoblastic disease, when compared with patients whose pregnancies continue into the third trimester (23, 24). Among 72 patients identified by a national survey of physicians in Japan in 1997, 24 underwent first-trimester evacuation, with 20.8% subsequently developing postmolar gestational trophoblastic disease (26). In comparison, 45.2% of 31 patients who required evacuation during the second trimester and 17.6% of the 17 who gave birth in the third trimester developed postmolar gestational trophoblastic disease. Nine (50%) of the 18 patients with proved complete hydatidiform moles in association with a fetus subsequently were treated for postmolar gestational trophoblastic disease (26), but it is not certain whether this increased risk resulted from selection bias. Major congenital abnormalities have not been reported in surviving infants.

For patients with co-existing hydatidiform moles and fetuses suspected on the basis of ultrasound findings, there are no clear guidelines for management. The ultrasound examination should be repeated to exclude retroplacental hematoma, other placental abnormalities, or degenerating myoma and to fully evaluate the fetoplacental unit for evidence of a partial mole or gross fetal malformations. If the diagnosis is still suspected and continuation of the pregnancy is desired, fetal karyotype should be obtained, a chest X-ray performed to screen for metastases, and serial serum hCG values monitored. These patients are at an increased risk for medical complications of pregnancy requiring evacuation, including bleeding, preterm labor, and pregnancy-induced hypertension. They should be counseled about these risks and the increased risk of postmolar trophoblastic disease after evacuation or delivery. If the fetal karyotype is normal, major fetal malformations are excluded by ultrasound examination, and there is no evidence of metastatic disease, it is reasonable to allow the pregnancy to continue unless pregnancy-related complications force delivery. After delivery, the placenta should be histologically evaluated and the patient followed closely with serial hCG values, similar to management of a woman with a singleton hydatidiform mole.

▶ *What are the characteristics of false-positive hCG values, also known as "phantom hCG"?*

Rarely, women have persistently elevated hCG levels but are subsequently found to have a false-positive hCG assay result, sometimes after receiving chemotherapy or surgery for presumed malignant gestational trophoblastic disease. Most patients with false-positive hCG values have low-level hCG elevations (27–29), but occasionally values higher than 300 mIU/mL have been recorded. False-positive hCG values result from interference with the hCG immunometric sandwich assays, most often caused by nonspecific heterophilic antibodies in the patient's sera (27). Many of these patients have an undefined previous pregnancy event and do not have radiographic evidence of metastatic disease.

False-positive hCG values also may appear after evacuation of a hydatidiform mole or following a clearly defined pregnancy event, such as an ectopic pregnancy, and a urine pregnancy test may be considered to differentiate between the two (30). False-positive test results should be suspected if hCG values plateau at relatively low levels and do not respond to therapeutic maneuvers, such as methotrexate given for a presumed persistent mole or ectopic pregnancy. Evaluation should include evaluation of serum hCG levels using a variety of assay techniques at different dilutions of patient serum, combined with a urinary hCG level if the serum level is higher than the threshold for the urinary assay, usually more than 50–60 mIU/mL (27–29). False-positive hCG assays usually will not be affected by serial dilution of patient sera and will have marked variability using different assay techniques, with most assays reflecting undetectable hCG levels (27, 29). Heterophilic antibodies are not excreted in the urine; therefore, urinary hCG values will not be detectable if they are the cause of serum hCG level elevation (27). Other techniques also are available to inactivate or strip the patient's serum of heterophilic antibodies. It is important to exclude the possibility of false-positive hCG values before subjecting these patients to hysterectomy or chemotherapy for gestational trophoblastic disease.

▶ *How are patients with malignant gestational trophoblastic disease classified and staged?*

Three systems have been used to categorize patients with malignant gestational trophoblastic disease: 1) the World Health Organization (WHO) prognostic index score, 2) the Clinical Classification system developed from early experience with chemotherapy for patients treated at the National Institutes of Health (NIH), and 3) the FIGO staging system, which was revised in 2000. The original anatomic FIGO staging system did not take into account other factors that might reflect disease outcome, such as hCG level, duration of disease, or type of antecedent pregnancy (14). The revised FIGO staging system includes a modification of the WHO prognostic index score for risk assessment (Table 2). All systems correlate with clinical outcomes of patients treated for malignant gestational trophoblastic disease and identify patients at risk for failure to respond to chemotherapy (4, 31–33).

The WHO prognostic index score assigned a weighted value to several individual clinical variables (4, 14). The total prognostic index score used a sum of the individual component scores to generate 3 risk categories. The 2000 FIGO modification of the WHO prognostic index score eliminated the determination of patient and consort blood types because these are not uniformly available and consolidated the risk categories into low-risk (total score less than 7) and high-risk (total score of 7 or higher) categories (14). The new FIGO risk index also standardized the radiologic studies to be used for determining the number and size of metastases. In one retrospective analysis, the new FIGO risk index correlated with outcome better than previous modifications of the WHO prognostic index score (32), and several other studies have correlated outcome to WHO prognostic index risk categories (4, 31, 33).

The original analyses of patients treated for metastatic gestational trophoblastic disease at the NIH led to the current Clinical Classification system that is frequently used in the United States (Table 3) (4). This system segregates patients with nonmetastatic disease from those with metastatic disease because virtually all patients with nonmetastatic disease can be cured using initial single-agent chemotherapy, regardless of other risk factors (33, 34). Patients with metastatic disease are further subdivided depending on the presence or absence of factors that correlate with response to initial single-agent chemotherapy (34, 35). Those who lack any of the high-risk clinical factors are likely to respond to initial single-agent therapy and are classified as having good-prognosis metastatic gestational trophoblastic disease. Patients who have any single high-risk clinical factor are classified as having poor-prognosis disease. These patients are not only at an increased risk of failure of single-agent chemotherapy but also have an increased risk of death if treated with single-agent therapy followed by multiagent regimens when compared with patients receiving initial multiagent regimens (35).

Although the WHO prognostic index score may provide a more precise definition of prognosis among patients with high-risk disease, the Clinical Classification system is less complicated and allows easy identification of patients for whom initial single-agent chemotherapy is likely to fail (33). Virtually all deaths from malignant gestational trophoblastic disease occur

---

Table 2. Revised FIGO Scoring System

FIGO Score	0	1	2	4
Age (y)	≤39	>39	—	—
Antecedent pregnancy	Hydatidiform mole	Abortion	Term pregnancy	—
Interval from index pregnancy (mo)	<4	4–6	7–12	>12
Pretreatment human chorionic gonadotropin level (mIU/mL)	<1,000	1,000–10,000	>10,000–100,000	>100,000
Largest tumor size including uterus (cm)	3–4	5	—	—
Site of metastases	Lung, vagina	Spleen, kidney	Gastrointestinal tract	Brain, liver
Number of metastases identified	0	1–4	4–8	>8
Previous failed chemotherapy	—	—	Single drug	2 or more drugs

The total score for a patient is obtained by adding the individual scores for each prognostic factor. Total score 0–6 = low risk; ≥7 = high risk.

Kohorn EI. The new FIGO 2000 staging and risk factor scoring system for gestational trophoblastic disease: description and clinical assessment. Int J Gynecol Cancer 2001;11:73–7.

Table 3. Clinical Classification System for Patients With Malignant Gestational Trophoblastic Disease

Category	Criteria
Nonmetastatic gestational trophoblastic disease	No evidence of metastases; not assigned to prognostic category
Metastatic gestational trophoblastic disease	Any extrauterine metastases
Good-prognosis metastatic gestational trophoblastic disease	No risk factors: Short duration (<4 mo) Pretherapy hCG level <40,000 mIU/mL No brain or liver metastases No antecedent term pregnancy No prior chemotherapy
Poor-prognosis metastatic gestational trophoblastic disease	Any risk factor: Long duration (≥4 mo since last pregnancy) Pretherapy hCG level ≥40,000 mIU/mL Brain or liver metastases Antecedent term pregnancy Prior chemotherapy

Abbreviation: hCG, human chorionic gonadotropin.

Soper JT, Lewis JL Jr, Hammond CB. Gestational trophoblastic disease. In: Hoskins WJ, Perez CA, Young RC, editors. Principals and practice of gynecologic oncology, 2nd ed. Philadelphia (PA): Lippincott-Raven; 1997. p. 1055.

among women who fall into the poor-prognostic disease category, and these patients should be considered to have high-risk disease (33). All patients with high-risk malignant gestational trophoblastic disease should be referred for management in consultation with individuals who are experienced in the treatment of this disease.

▶ *What are the general considerations for the evaluation and treatment of malignant gestational trophoblastic disease?*

Once the diagnosis of malignant gestational trophoblastic disease is suspected or established, immediate evaluation for metastases and risk factors is mandatory. Along with history and physical examinations, the following laboratory studies should be performed: complete blood count with platelet determinations, clotting function studies, renal and liver function studies, blood type and antibody screen, and determination of baseline (pretherapy) hCG level. Recommended radiographic studies include chest X-ray or computerized tomography (CT) scan of the chest, pelvic ultrasonography, brain magnetic resonance imaging or CT scan, and abdominopelvic

CT with contrast or magnetic resonance imaging scans (14). Systemic venous metastasis of malignant gestational trophoblastic disease results in pulmonary or occasional vaginal lesions. Systemic arterial metastasis usually occurs only after pulmonary metastases have been established; therefore, the minimum evaluation of a patient with postmolar gestational trophoblastic disease is a chest X-ray. If lung lesions are detected, further imaging of the abdomen and brain should be performed to identify possible liver or brain metastasis.

Because of the relative rarity of malignant gestational trophoblastic disease, there are few randomized trials of therapy, and only one completed trial has been reported to date (13). Most studies have been retrospective analyses of single-institution experiences, but these confirm high activity for a variety of agents in the treatment of malignant gestational trophoblastic disease, including methotrexate, dactinomycin, etoposide, 5-fluorouracil, and cisplatin (4, 36).

▶ *How is nonmetastatic gestational trophoblastic disease treated? In a patient with nonmetastatic gestational trophoblastic disease, which is better: hysterectomy alone or in combination with chemotherapy?*

Primary remission rates of patients treated with a variety of chemotherapy regimens for nonmetastatic gestational trophoblastic disease are similar (4). Essentially all patients with this condition can be cured, usually without hysterectomy. Randomized comparisons of these regimens have not been completed. A prospective phase-II trial by the Gynecologic Oncology Group reported a 70–80% primary remission rate for patients with nonmetastatic gestational trophoblastic disease treated with weekly intramuscular methotrexate at a dose of 30–50 mg/m^2 (37). There was no apparent benefit of increasing the dose to 50 mg/m^2. It was concluded that the weekly methotrexate regimen was the preferred choice of several methotrexate or dactinomycin schedules when efficacy, toxicity, and cost were taken into consideration (37, 38). Chemotherapy is continued until hCG values have reached normal levels; an additional course is administered after the first normal hCG value has been recorded (37, 39). Hematologic indices should be monitored carefully during chemotherapy, but significant hematologic toxicity is infrequent among patients treated with weekly methotrexate (37). Patients should have normal renal and liver functions before each treatment because methotrexate is excreted entirely by the kidney and can produce hepatic toxicity.

In patients with nonmetastatic gestational trophoblastic disease, early hysterectomy will shorten the duration and amount of chemotherapy required to produce remission (34, 40). Therefore, each patient's desire for future fertility should be evaluated at the onset of treatment. Many experts prefer to perform hysterectomy during the first cycle of chemotherapy and continue administration of chemotherapy for 2 cycles after a negative hCG measurement has been obtained. Chemotherapy after hysterectomy is needed until hCG values become normal.

Patients whose hCG levels reach a plateau or increase during therapy should be switched to an alternative single-agent regimen. If metastases appears or alternative single-agent chemotherapy fails, the patient should be treated with multiagent regimens (4). Hysterectomy should be considered for the treatment of nonmetastatic disease that is refractory to chemotherapy and remains confined to the uterus (34, 41).

The overall cure rate for patients with nonmetastatic disease is nearly 100% (1, 33, 34, 37, 42). When chemotherapy is given for an additional 1–2 cycles after the first normal hCG value, recurrence rates are less than 5% (39).

▶ How is low-risk metastatic gestational trophoblastic disease treated?

Patients with metastatic gestational trophoblastic disease who lack any of the clinical high-risk factors (33–35) or have a FIGO risk score less than 7 (14) have low-risk disease. They can be treated successfully with initial single-agent regimens. Most often, this consists of 5-day treatment using methotrexate or intravenous dactinomycin recycled at 14-day intervals (33, 42, 43). Approximately 40% of these patients will require alternative therapy to achieve remission (43); however, essentially all patients with low-risk metastatic gestational trophoblastic disease can be cured with conventional chemotherapy (31, 33, 34, 42). Hysterectomy in conjunction with chemotherapy also may decrease the amount of chemotherapy required to achieve remission in these patients (34). Similar to the treatment of women with nonmetastatic gestational trophoblastic disease, 1–2 cycles of chemotherapy should be given after the first normal hCG level. Recurrence rates are less than 5% among patients successfully treated for low-risk metastatic disease (39).

▶ How is high-risk metastatic gestational trophoblastic disease treated?

Patients with 1 or more of the Clinical Classification system risk factors (33–35) or a FIGO risk score of 7 or higher (14) have high-risk disease. They will require multiagent chemotherapy with additional surgery or radiation often incorporated into treatment (34). Survival rates reported by trophoblastic disease centers have been reported as high as 84% (31–34, 36, 44). In contrast to patients with nonmetastatic or low-risk metastatic gestational trophoblastic disease, early hysterectomy does not appear to improve the outcome in women with high-risk metastatic disease (34).

Aggressive treatment with multiagent chemotherapy is an important component for management of these patients. Triple therapy with methotrexate, dactinomycin, and either chlorambucil or cyclophosphamide was the standard regimen for many years in the United States (4, 35, 44). In a randomized trial, a more complex multiagent regimen was not proved to be superior to triple therapy with methotrexate, dactinomycin, and either chlorambucil or cyclophosphamide (44, 45). More recent regimens have incorporated etoposide with or without cisplatin into combination chemotherapy (4, 36, 46–48) with high rates of success but with an increased risk for leukemia in survivors. A randomized comparison of the newer combinations with triple therapy with methotrexate, dactinomycin, and either chlorambucil or cyclophosphamide would provide helpful information.

Management of cerebral metastases is controversial. Radiation therapy has been used concurrently with chemotherapy in an attempt to limit acute hemorrhagic complications from these metastases. Brain irradiation combined with systemic chemotherapy is successful in controlling brain metastases with cure rates up to 75% in patients with brain metastases (49). However, a similar primary remission rate also has been reported among patients treated with combination regimens that incorporated high-dose systemic methotrexate combined with intrathecal methotrexate infusions without brain irradiation (46). The best treatment for liver or other high-risk sites of metastases has not been established. Even with intense chemotherapy, additional surgery may be necessary to control hemorrhage from metastases, remove chemoresistant disease, or treat other complications to stabilize high-risk patients during therapy (34, 41).

Chemotherapy is continued until hCG values have normalized, followed by at least 2 or 3 courses of maintenance chemotherapy in the hope of eradicating all viable tumors. Despite the use of sensitive hCG assays and maintenance chemotherapy, up to 13% of patients with high-risk disease will develop recurrence after achieving an initial remission (39).

▶ What is the recommended surveillance following completion of chemotherapy for malignant gestational trophoblastic disease?

After hCG remission has been achieved, patients with malignant gestational trophoblastic disease should undergo serial determinations of hCG levels at 2-week intervals for the first 3 months of remission and then at 1-month intervals until monitoring has shown 1 year of normal hCG levels. The risk of recurrence after 1 year of remission is less than 1% (39), but late recurrences have been observed rarely.

Patients should be counseled to use a reliable form of hormonal contraception during the first year of remission. Because of the 1–2% risk for a second mole in subsequent pregnancies (20), early ultrasound examination is recommended for all future pregnancies. There does not appear to be an increase in the risk of congenital malformations or other complications related to pregnancy (20).

Summary of Recommendations

The following recommendations are based on good and consistent scientific evidence (Level A):

▶ In women of reproductive age with abnormal bleeding or symptoms that could be caused by a malignancy, β-hCG levels should be evaluated to facilitate early diagnosis and treatment of gestational trophoblastic disease.

▶ In patients with molar pregnancy, the preferred method of evacuation is suction D&C. After molar evacuation, all patients should be monitored with serial hCG determinations to diagnose and treat malignant sequelae promptly.

▶ Oral contraceptives have been demonstrated to be safe and effective during posttreatment monitoring based on randomized controlled trials.

▶ Women with nonmetastatic gestational trophoblastic disease should be treated with single-agent chemotherapy.

▶ For women with nonmetastatic gestational trophoblastic disease, weekly doses of 30–50 mg/m² of intramuscular methotrexate has been found to be the most cost-effective treatment when taking efficacy, toxicity, and cost into consideration.

▶ Women with metastatic gestational trophoblastic disease should be referred to specialists with experience treating this disease.

▶ Women with high-risk metastatic disease should be treated with multiagent chemotherapy. This includes triple therapy with methotrexate, dactinomycin, and either chlorambucil or cyclophosphamide. More recent regimens further incorporate etoposide with or without cisplatin into combination chemotherapy.

The following recommendations are based on limited or inconsistent scientific evidence (Level B):

▶ False-positive test results should be suspected if hCG values plateau at relatively low levels and do not respond to therapeutic maneuvers, such as methotrexate given for a presumed persistent mole or ectopic pregnancy.

▶ Serial quantitative serum hCG determinations should be performed using a commercially available assay capable of detecting β-hCG to baseline values (<5 mIU/mL). Ideally, serum hCG levels should be obtained within 48 hours of evacuation, every 1–2 weeks while elevated, and then at 1–2 month intervals for an additional 6–12 months.

The following recommendations are based primarily on consensus and expert opinion (Level C):

▶ Abnormal bleeding for more than 6 weeks following any pregnancy should be evaluated with hCG testing to exclude a new pregnancy or gestational trophoblastic disease.

▶ In compliant patients, the low morbidity and mortality achieved by monitoring patients with serial hCG determinations and instituting chemotherapy only in patients with postmolar gestational trophoblastic disease outweighs the potential risk and small benefit of routine prophylactic chemotherapy after evacuation of a molar pregnancy.

▶ Serious complications are not uncommon in women with a uterus size greater than a 16-week gestation, so they should be managed by physicians experienced in the prevention and management of complications.

▶ Patients for whom initial therapy for nonmetastatic or low-risk metastatic disease fails and those with high-risk malignant gestational trophoblastic disease should be managed in consultation with individuals or facilities with expertise in the complex, multimodality treatment of these patients.

References

1. Berkowitz RS, Goldstein DP. Gestational trophoblastic diseases. In: Hoskins WJ, Perez CA, Young RC, editors. Principals and practice of gynecologic oncology. 3rd ed. Philadelphia (PA): Lippincott Williams & Wilkins; 2000. p. 1117–37. (Level III)

2. Lurain JR, Brewer JI, Torok EE, Halpern B. Natural history of hydatidiform mole after primary evacuation. Am J Obstet Gynecol 1983;145:591–5. (Level III)

3. Curry SL, Hammond CB, Tyrey L, Creasman WT, Parker RT. Hydatidiform mole: diagnosis, management, and long-term follow-up of 347 patients. Obstet Gynecol 1975;45:1–8. (Level II-3)

4. Soper JT, Lewis JL Jr, Hammond CB. Gestational trophoblastic disease. In: Hoskins WJ, Perez CA, Young RC, editors. Principals and practice of gynecologic oncology. 2nd ed. Philadelphia (PA): Lippincott-Raven; 1997. p. 1039–77. (Level III)

5. Feltmate CM, Genest DR, Wise L, Bernstein MR, Goldstein DP, Berkowitz RS. Placental site trophoblastic tumor: a 17-year experience at the New England Trophoblastic Disease Center. Gynecol Oncol 2001;82:415–9. (Level II-2)

6. Papadopoulos AJ, Foskett M, Seckl MJ, McNeish I, Paradinas FJ, Rees H, et al. Twenty-five years' clinical experience with placental site trophoblastic tumors. J Reprod Med 2002;47:460–4. (Level III)

7. Szulman AE, Surti U. The syndromes of hydatidiform mole. I. Cytogenetic and morphologic correlations. Am J Obstet Gynecol 1978;131:665–71. (Level III)

8. Soto-Wright V, Bernstein M, Goldstein DP, Berkowitz RS. The changing clinical presentation of complete molar pregnancy. Obstet Gynecol 1995;86:775–9. (Level II-3)

9. Schlaerth JB, Morrow CP, Montz FJ, d'Abling G. Initial management of hydatidiform mole. Am J Obstet Gynecol 1988;158:1299–306. (Level III)

10. Montz FJ, Schlaerth JB, Morrow CP. The natural history of theca lutein cysts. Obstet Gynecol 1988;72:247–51. (Level II-2)

11. Coukos G, Makrigiannakis A, Chung J, Randall TC, Rubin SC, Benjamin I. Complete hydatidiform mole: a disease with a changing profile. J Reprod Med 1999;44:698–704. (Level III)

12. Schlaerth JB, Morrow CP, Rodriguez M. Diagnostic and therapeutic curettage in gestational trophoblastic disease. Am J Obstet Gynecol 1990;162:1465–70; discussion 1470–1. (Level III)

13. Curry SL, Schlaerth JB, Kohorn EI, Boyce JB, Gore H, Twiggs LB, et al. Hormonal contraception and trophoblastic sequelae after hydatidiform mole. A Gynecologic Oncology Group study. Am J Obstet Gynecol 1989;160:805–9; discussion 809–11. (Level I)

14. Kohorn EI. The new FIGO 2000 staging and risk factor scoring system for gestational trophoblastic disease: description and clinical assessment. Int J Gynecol Cancer 2001;11:73–7. (Level III)

15. Tidy JA, Rustin GJ, Newlands ES, Foskett M, Fuller S, Short D, et al. Presentation and management of choriocarcinoma after nonmolar pregnancy. Br J Obstet Gynaecol 1995;102:715–9. (Level II-3)

16. Tidy JA, Gillespie AM, Bright N, Radstone CR, Coleman RE, Hancock BW. Gestational trophoblastic disease: a study of the mode of evacuation and subsequent need for treatment with chemotherapy. Gynecol Oncol 2000;78:309–12. (Level II-3)

17. Orr JW Jr, Austin JM, Hatch KD, Shingleton HM, Younger JB, Boots LR. Acute pulmonary edema associated with molar pregnancies: a high-risk factor for development of persistent trophoblastic disease. Am J Obstet Gynecol 1980;136:412–5. (Level III)

18. Twiggs LB, Morrow CP, Schlaerth JB. Acute pulmonary complications of molar pregnancy. Am J Obstet Gynecol 1979;135:189–94. (Level III)

19. Morrow P, Nakamura R, Schlaerth J, Gaddis O Jr, Eddy G. The influence of oral contraceptives on the postmolar human chorionic gonadotropin regression curve. Am J Obstet Gynecol 1985;151:906–14. (Level II-2)

20. Berkowitz RS, Im SS, Bernstein MR, Goldstein DP. Gestational trophoblastic disease: subsequent pregnancy outcome, including repeat molar pregnancy. J Reprod Med 1998;43:81–6. (Level III)

21. Kim DS, Moon H, Kim KT, Moon YJ, Hwang YY. Effects of prophylactic chemotherapy for persistent trophoblastic disease in patients with complete hydatidiform mole. Obstet Gynecol 1986;67:690–4. (Level I)

22. Limpongsanurak S. Prophylactic actinomycin D for high-risk complete hydatidiform mole. J Reprod Med 2001;46:110–6. (Level I)

23. Bristow RE, Shumway JB, Khouzami AN, Witter FR. Complete hydatidiform mole and surviving coexistent twin. Obstet Gynecol Surv 1996;51:705–9. (Level III)

24. Steller MA, Genest DR, Bernstein MR, Lage JM, Goldstein DP, Berkowitz RS. Clinical features of multiple conception with partial or complete molar pregnancy and coexisting fetuses. J Reprod Med 1994;39:147–54. (Level III)

25. Bruchim I, Kidron D, Amiel A, Altaras M, Fejgin MD. Complete hydatidiform mole and a coexistent viable fetus: report of two cases and review of the literature. Gynecol Oncol 2000;77:197–202. (Level III)

26. Matsui H, Sekiya S, Hando T, Wake N, Tomoda Y. Hydatidiform mole coexistent with a twin live fetus: a national collaborative study in Japan. Human Reprod 2000;15:608–11. (Level II-2)

27. Cole LA. Phantom hCG and phantom choriocarcinoma. Gynecol Oncol 1998;71:325–9. (Level III)

28. Cole LA, Shahabi S, Butler SA, Mitchell H, Newlands ES, Behrman HR, et al. Utility of commonly used commercial human chorionic gonadotropin immunoassays in the diagnosis and management of trophoblastic diseases. Clin Chem 2001;47:308–15. (Level III)

29. Rotmensch S, Cole LA. False diagnosis and needless therapy of presumed malignant disease in women with false-positive human chorionic gonadotropin concentrations [published erratum appears in Lancet 2000;356:600]. Lancet 2000;355:712–5. (Level III)

30. Avoiding inappropriate clinical decisions based on false-positive human chorionic gonadotropin test results. ACOG Committee Opinion No. 278. American College of Obstetricians and Gynecologists. Obstet Gynecol 2002;100:1057–9. (Level III)

31. DuBeshter B, Berkowitz RS, Goldstein DP, Cramer DW, Bernstein MR. Metastatic gestational trophoblastic disease: experience at the New England Trophoblastic

Disease Center, 1965 to 1985. Obstet Gynecol 1987;69: 390–5. (Level II-3)

32. Hancock BW, Welch EM, Gillespie AM, Newlands ES. A retrospective comparison of current and proposed staging and scoring systems for persistent gestational trophoblastic disease. Int J Gynecol Cancer 2000;10:318–22. (Level III)

33. Soper JT, Evans AC, Conaway MR, Clarke-Pearson DL, Berchuck A, Hammond CB. Evaluation of prognostic factors and staging in gestational trophoblastic tumor. Obstet Gynecol 1994;84:969–73. (Level II-2)

34. Hammond CB, Weed JC Jr, Currie JL. The role of operation in the current therapy of gestational trophoblastic disease. Am J Obstet Gynecol 1980;136:844–58. (Level III)

35. Hammond CB, Borchert LG, Tyrey L, Creasman WT, Parker RT. Treatment of metastatic trophoblastic disease: good and poor prognosis. Am J Obstet Gynecol 1973; 115:451–7. (Level III)

36. Schink JC, Singh DK, Rademaker AW, Miller DS, Lurain JR. Etoposide, methotrexate, actinomycin D, cyclophosphamide, and vincristine for the treatment of metastatic, high-risk gestational trophoblastic disease. Obstet Gynecol 1992;80:817–20. (Level III)

37. Homesley HD, Blessing JA, Rettenmaier M, Capizzi RL, Major FJ, Twiggs LB. Weekly intramuscular methotrexate for nonmetastatic gestational trophoblastic disease. Obstet Gynecol 1988;72:413–8. (Level III)

38. Homesley HD, Blessing JA, Schlaerth J, Rettenmaier M, Major FJ. Rapid escalation of weekly intramuscular methotrexate for nonmetastatic gestational trophoblastic disease. A Gynecologic Oncology Group study. Gynecol Oncol 1990;39:305–8. (Level II-2)

39. Mutch DG, Soper JT, Babcock CJ, Clarke-Pearson DL, Hammond CB. Recurrent gestational trophoblastic disease: experience of the Southeastern Regional Trophoblastic Disease Center Cancer 1990;66:978–82. (Level II-3)

40. Suzuka K, Matsui H, Iitsuka Y, Yamazawa K, Seki K, Sekiya S. Adjuvant hysterectomy in low-risk gestational trophoblastic disease. Obstet Gynecol 2001;97:431–4. (Level II-2)

41. Lehman E, Gershenson DM, Burke TW, Levenback C, Silva EG, Morris M. Salvage surgery for chemorefactory gestational trophoblastic disease. J Clin Oncol 1994;12: 2737–42. (Level II-2)

42. Roberts JP, Lurain JR. Treatment of low-risk metastatic gestational trophoblastic tumors with single-agent chemotherapy. Am J Obstet Gynecol 1996;174:1917–23; discussion 1923–4. (Level II-2)

43. Soper JT, Clarke-Pearson DL, Berchuck A, Rodriguez G, Hammond CB. 5-day methotrexate for women with metastatic gestational trophoblastic disease. Gynecol Oncol 1994;54:76–9. (Level II-2)

44. Curry SL, Blessing JA, DiSaia PJ, Soper JT, Twiggs LB. A prospective randomized comparison of methotrexate, dactinomycin and chlorambucil versus methotrexate, dactinomycin, cyclophosphamide, doxorubicin, melphalan, hydroxyurea, and vincristine in "poor prognosis" metastatic gestational trophoblastic disease. A Gynecologic Oncology Group study. Obstet Gynecol 1989; 73:357–62. (Level I)

45. Bagshawe KD, Dent J, Newlands ES, Begent RH, Rustin GJ. The role of low-dose methotrexate and folinic acid in gestational trophoblastic tumours (GTT). Br J Obstet Gynaecol 1989;96:795–802. (Level III)

46. Rustin GJ, Newlands ES, Begent RH, Dent J, Bagshawe KD. Weekly alternating etoposide, methotrexate, and actinomycin/vincristine and cyclophosphamide chemotherapy for the treatment of CNS metastases of choriocarcinoma. J Clin Oncol 1989;7:900–3. (Level III)

47. Soper JT, Evans AC, Clarke-Pearson DL, Berchuck A, Rodriguez G, Hammond CB. Alternating weekly chemotherapy with etoposide-methotrexate-dactinomycin/cyclophosphamide-vincristine for high-risk gestational trophoblastic disease. Obstet Gynecol 1994;83:113–7. (Level III)

48. Soto-Wright V, Goldstein DP, Bernstein MR, Berkowitz RS. The management of gestational trophoblastic tumors with etoposide, methotrexate, and actinomycin D. Gynecol Oncol 1997;64:156–9. (Level II-2)

49. Evans AC Jr, Soper JT, Clarke-Pearson DL, Berchuck A, Rodriguez GC, Hammond CB. Gestational trophoblastic disease metastatic to the central nervous system. Gynecol Oncol 1995;59:226–30. (Level II-2)

The MEDLINE database, the Cochrane Library, and ACOG's own internal resources and documents were used to conduct a literature search to locate relevant articles published between January 1985 and February 2004. The search was restricted to articles published in the English language. Priority was given to articles reporting results of original research, although review articles and commentaries also were consulted. Abstracts of research presented at symposia and scientific conferences were not considered adequate for inclusion in this document. Guidelines published by organizations or institutions such as the National Institutes of Health and the American College of Obstetricians and Gynecologists were reviewed, and additional studies were located by reviewing bibliographies of identified articles. When reliable research was not available, expert opinions from obstetrician–gynecologists were used.

Studies were reviewed and evaluated for quality according to the method outlined by the U.S. Preventive Services Task Force:

I   Evidence obtained from at least 1 properly designed randomized controlled trial.

II-1   Evidence obtained from well-designed controlled trials without randomization.

II-2   Evidence obtained from well-designed cohort or case–control analytic studies, preferably from more than 1 center or research group.

II-3   Evidence obtained from multiple time series with or without the intervention. Dramatic results in uncontrolled experiments also could be regarded as this type of evidence.

III   Opinions of respected authorities, based on clinical experience, descriptive studies, or reports of expert committees.

Based on the highest level of evidence found in the data, recommendations are provided and graded according to the following categories:

Level A—Recommendations are based on good and consistent scientific evidence.

Level B—Recommendations are based on limited or inconsistent scientific evidence.

Level C—Recommendations are based primarily on consensus and expert opinion.

ISSN 1099-3630

**The American College of
Obstetricians and Gynecologists
409 12th Street, SW
PO Box 96920
Washington, DC 20090-6920**

12345/87654

Diagnosis and treatment of gestational trophoblastic disease. ACOG Practice Bulletin No. 53. American College of Obstetricians and Gynecologists. Obstet Gynecol 2004;103:1365–77.

ACOG PRACTICE BULLETIN

CLINICAL MANAGEMENT GUIDELINES FOR
OBSTETRICIAN–GYNECOLOGISTS

NUMBER 49, DECEMBER 2003

(Replaces Technical Bulletin Number 218, December 1995)

This Practice Bulletin was developed by the ACOG Committee on Practice Bulletins— Obstetrics with the assistance of Andrew Satin, MD. The information is designed to aid practitioners in making decisions about appropriate obstetric and gynecologic care. These guidelines should not be construed as dictating an exclusive course of treatment or procedure. Variations in practice may be warranted based on the needs of the individual patient, resources, and limitations unique to the institution or type of practice.

Dystocia and Augmentation of Labor

Dystocia, characterized by the slow, abnormal progression of labor, is the leading indication for primary cesarean delivery in the United States. Currently, 1 in every 10 women who give birth in the United States has had a previous cesarean delivery (1). Because many repeat cesarean deliveries are performed after primary operations for dystocia, an estimated 60% of all cesarean deliveries in the United States are attributable to the diagnosis of dystocia (2). Thus, with decreasing rates of vaginal birth after cesarean delivery, dystocia is the leading cause of both operative vaginal delivery and cesarean delivery and their accompanying complications.

Despite the high prevalence of labor disorders, considerable variability exists in the diagnosis, management, and criteria for dystocia that requires intervention. The purpose of this document is to provide a review of the definition of dystocia, risk factors associated with dystocia, the criteria that require delivery, and approaches to clinical management of labor complicated by dystocia.

Background

Definitions

The definition of labor is the presence of uterine contractions of sufficient intensity, frequency, and duration to bring about demonstrable effacement and dilation of the cervix. At present, there is much uncertainty about the definition of the latent phase of labor, but there is agreement that women in labor enter the active phase when cervical dilatation is between 3 cm and 4 cm (3). The active phase is characterized by the most rapid changes in cervical dilatation as plotted against time. The active phase of labor includes both an increased rate of cervical dilation and, ultimately, descent of the presenting fetal part. This document focuses on labor subsequent to entering the active phase, diagnosis of active-phase abnormalities, clinical considerations, and management recommendations for the active phase and the second stage of labor.

Dystocia is defined as abnormal labor that results from what have been categorized classically as abnormalities of the power (uterine contractions or maternal expulsive forces), the passenger (position, size, or presentation of the fetus), or the passage (pelvis or soft tissues). The term "cephalopelvic disproportion" has been used to describe a disparity between the size of the maternal pelvis and the fetal head that precludes vaginal delivery. Because dystocia can rarely be diagnosed with certainty, the relatively imprecise term "failure to progress" has been used, which includes lack of progressive cervical dilation or lack of descent of the fetal head or both. The diagnosis of dystocia should not be made before an adequate trial of labor has been achieved. A more practical classification is to categorize labor abnormalities as slower-than-normal (protraction disorders) or complete cessation of progress (arrest disorders).

Augmentation refers to stimulation of uterine contractions when spontaneous contractions have failed to result in progressive cervical dilation or descent of the fetus. Augmentation should be considered if the frequency of contractions is less than 3 contractions per 10 minutes or the intensity of contractions is less than 25 mm Hg above baseline or both. Before augmentation, an assessment of the maternal pelvis and cervix and fetal position, station, and well-being should be performed. Contraindications to augmentation are similar to those for labor induction and may include placenta or vasa previa, umbilical cord presentation, prior classical uterine incision, active genital herpes infection, pelvic structural deformities, or invasive cervical cancer.

Second-Stage Arrest

In a retrospective review of nearly 7,000 women with minimal intervention, the mean length of the second stage of labor was 19 minutes for multiparous women and 54 minutes for nulliparous women, without regard for anesthesia (4). The use of conduction anesthesia increased the mean duration of the second stage by 20–30 minutes (4, 5). In a nulliparous woman, the diagnosis of a prolonged second stage should be considered when the second stage exceeds 3 hours if regional anesthesia has been administered or 2 hours if no regional anesthesia is used. In multiparous women, the diagnosis can be made when the second stage exceeds 2 hours with regional anesthesia or 1 hour without. A prolonged second stage of labor warrants clinical reassessment of the woman, fetus, and expulsive forces. These statistical parameters are useful for defining when labor becomes prolonged and intervention should be considered.

Criteria for Arrest that Require Delivery

Oxytocin administration should be considered when a patient has a protraction or arrest disorder. The goal of oxytocin administration is to effect uterine activity sufficient to produce cervical change and fetal descent while avoiding uterine hyperstimulation and fetal compromise. Minimally effective uterine activity has been defined as 3 contractions per 10 minutes averaging greater than 25 mm Hg above baseline. However, adequate labor encompasses a wide range of uterine activity, as previously noted. The amplitude of each contraction may vary from 25 mm Hg to 75 mm Hg, and contractions may occur for a total of 2–4.5 minutes in every 10-minute window, achieving 95–395 Montevideo units (the peak of contractions in millimeters of mercury multiplied by the frequency per 10 minutes). Typically, a goal of a maximum of 5 contractions in a 10-minute period with resultant cervical dilation is considered adequate. As a general guideline, hyperstimulation may be defined as a persistent pattern of more than 5 contractions in 10 minutes, contractions lasting 2 minutes or more, or contractions of normal duration occurring within 1 minute of each other, and may or may not include nonreassuring fetal heart rate measurements. The term "tachysystole" has been used to define hyperstimulation without corresponding fetal heart rate abnormalities to distinguish this complication from hyperstimulation with fetal heart rate changes.

In a retrospective report of induction of labor with oxytocin, 91% of women achieved at least 200–224 Montevideo units, and 40% achieved at least 300 Montevideo units (6). Accordingly, it has been suggested that before an arrest disorder can be diagnosed in the first stage of labor, the following 2 criteria should be met: 1) the latent phase is completed, and 2) a uterine contraction pattern exceeds 200 Montevideo units for 2 hours without cervical change. However, there is no convincing evidence to demonstrate a reduction in the rate of cesarean deliveries or improvement in perinatal outcome attributable to the use of the sophisticated measurements of uterine activity as compared with external tocodynamometry.

The "2-hour rule" for the diagnosis of arrest in active labor has recently been challenged. In a clinical trial, 542 women were managed by a protocol in which, after active-phase arrest was diagnosed, oxytocin was initiated with the intent to achieve a sustained uterine contraction pattern of greater that 200 Montevideo units (7). Cesarean delivery was not performed for labor arrest until there were at least 4 hours of a sustained uterine contraction pattern of greater than 200 Montevideo units, or a minimum of 6 hours of oxytocin augmentation if the contraction pattern could not be achieved. The protocol resulted in a high rate of vaginal delivery (92%) with no severe adverse maternal or fetal outcomes. Thus, extending the minimum period of oxytocin augmentation for active-phase arrest from 2 hours to 4 hours appears effective.

Reassessment of the fetus may identify those that are not tolerating labor. Intervention is not necessary for all factors solely based on time (8). Contemporary practice patterns may be associated with more variation in duration of the second stage of labor (5). If progress is being made, the duration of the second stage alone does not mandate intervention by operative delivery. Once a second-stage arrest disorder is diagnosed, the obstetrician has 3 options: 1) continued observation, 2) operative vaginal delivery, or 3) cesarean delivery. The decision to perform an operative delivery in the second stage versus continued observation should be made on the basis of clinical assessment of the woman and the fetus and the skill and training of the obstetrician.

Risk Factors for Dystocia

Cesarean delivery for dystocia or arrest of labor that requires delivery may occur in either the first or second stage of labor. Cesarean delivery rates for dystocia are similar but are associated with different factors when performed in the first or second stage (9, 10). In a retrospective review of nearly 150,000 deliveries, patients with nonprogressive labor in the first stage were significantly older and more likely to have complications, such as previous perinatal death, diabetes, hypertension, infertility treatment, premature rupture of membranes, and amniotic fluid abnormalities, when compared with patients experiencing second-stage arrest (9). Labors that failed to progress during the first stage were significantly associated with nonreassuring fetal heart rate patterns when compared with pregnancies with dystocia in the second stage. The significant increase in cesarean deliveries during the first stage of labor among women at high risk can reflect exaggerated concern of caregivers. A variety of labor interventions and complications have been associated with slow progress in labor, including epidural analgesia, chorioamnionitis, pelvic contractions, and macrosomia (11, 12). Several factors have been shown to be associated with longer duration of the second stage, including epidural analgesia, occiput posterior position, longer first stage of labor, nulliparity, short maternal stature, birth weight, and high station at complete cervical dilation (13).

Relationship of Dystocia to Other Adverse Outcomes

Dystocia may be associated with serious complications for both the woman and the fetus. Infection, namely chorioamnionitis, is a consequence of prolonged labor, especially in the setting of ruptured membranes (14). In one report analyzing more than 500 women, labor was 4.7 hours longer on average when chorioamnionitis was diagnosed late in labor (12). Fetal infection and bacteremia, including pneumonia caused by aspiration of infected amniotic fluid, is linked to prolonged labor. There is debate whether a prolonged second stage may be associated with injuries of the pelvic floor (15, 16). In cases of neglected, obstructed labors (more likely to be seen in developing countries), pressure necrosis after very prolonged second stages may result in vesicovaginal, vesicocervical, or rectovaginal fistulas (17, 18).

In the past, labor, particularly the second stage, was thought to be a time of asphyxial risk for the fetus. In one large study of more than 6,000 women with normal fetal heart rate monitoring tracings in labor, duration in and of itself was not associated with low 5-minute Apgar scores, neonatal seizures, or admission to the neonatal intensive care unit (8).

Role of Allied Personnel

Continuous support during labor from caregivers, including nurses, midwives, or lay individuals, has a number of benefits for women and their newborns, with no apparent harmful effects (19). The continuous presence of a support person may reduce the likelihood of the use of medication for pain relief, operative delivery, and patient dissatisfaction (19–21).

Clinical Considerations and Recommendations

▶ *Can dystocia be predicted?*

The ability to accurately predict which women or fetuses will ultimately benefit from operative delivery has been disappointing (13). Generally, orderly, spontaneous progression to full dilation indicates that vaginal delivery most likely will be successful. Abnormal labor or dystocia in the first or second stage of labor can be associated with 1 or more abnormalities of the cervix, uterus, maternal pelvis, or fetus. In addition, advanced maternal age, nulliparity, maternal anxiety, multiple gestation, and intrauterine infections have been reported to be associated with longer active labors (12, 22). Epidural analgesia, prolonged first stage of labor, nulliparity, large fetuses, and high station at complete cervical dilation are associated with a longer second stage (13).

In an attempt to identify risk factors for difficult delivery among nulliparous women in the second stage of labor, investigators used a multivariate analysis of 1,862 women and found that the risk of difficult delivery was increased for women of short stature (less than 150 cm), age greater than 35 years, gestational age greater than 41 weeks, interval between epidural induction and full cervical dilation of greater than 6 hours, fetal station above +2 cm at full cervical dilation, or occiput posterior fetal position (23). Importantly, a multivariable predictive model of difficult delivery found a sensitivity of only 57%, specificity of 75%, and positive predicative value of 35%.

▶ How does epidural analgesia affect the progress of labor?

In a systematic review of 11 randomized trials involving 3,157 women, epidural analgesia was associated with increases in the duration of the first and second stages of labor, incidence of fetal malpositions, use of oxytocin, and operative vaginal delivery (11). Nevertheless, epidural analgesia was not shown to increase the cesarean delivery rate for dystocia.

Less controversial is the causal role epidural analgesia plays in prolonging labor by 40–90 minutes (24–27) and in the approximate 2-fold increased need for oxytocin augmentation (27, 28). These findings are supported by most prospective studies as well as meta-analyses (11, 25). An increased risk of a second stage of labor longer than 2 hours (24, 26) in women with epidural analgesia likely contributes to the higher rates of operative vaginal delivery seen in most prospective studies. The 4 best prospective studies, in which elective forceps use was not permitted (24, 26–28), yielded a combined relative risk (RR) of 1.9 (95% confidence interval [CI] 1.4, 2.5) of forceps delivery in women who received epidural analgesia. Some investigators have found a decreased risk of operative vaginal delivery with combined spinal epidural when compared with low-dose epidural (29). This finding is difficult to interpret because elective forceps were not excluded in this study, and the rate of forceps use was high (28–40%). High rates of operative vaginal deliveries have been implicated in the increased rate of third- and fourth-degree lacerations seen in women who had epidural analgesia (30).

▶ Is there a role for intrauterine pressure catheters in diagnosing dystocia?

Uterine activity can be monitored by palpation, external tocodynamometry, or internal pressure catheters. Current evidence does not support routine use of intrauterine pressure catheters for labor management. In a randomized trial of 250 patients undergoing labor augmentation with contractions monitored by either external tocotransducers or intrauterine catheters, there were no significant differences between the groups regarding length of labor, dose of oxytocin, hyperstimulation, cesarean delivery, or neonatal outcomes (31). Nevertheless, intrauterine pressure catheters may be beneficial for women when the evaluation of contractions is difficult because of such factors as obesity or lack of one-on-one nursing care or when response to oxytocin is limited.

▶ Does ambulation affect the course of labor?

Women experiencing normal labor should be encouraged to assume a position in which they are most comfortable. Walking during labor has not been shown to enhance or impair progress in labor. Investigators who randomized more than 1,000 women in active labor at term to either walking or no walking found no differences in the duration of labor, need for oxytocin, use of analgesia, operative vaginal delivery, or cesarean delivery between study groups (32). Neonatal outcomes also were similar, and walking was not harmful to the women or their newborns. Ambulatory epidural analgesia with walking or sitting does not appear to shorten labor duration. In a randomized trial, 160 nulliparous women were assigned to receive epidural either with or without ambulation (33). There was no difference in time from epidural placement to complete dilation between the groups. Thus, ambulation in labor is not harmful, and mobility may result in greater comfort and ability to tolerate labor (34).

▶ Is there a role for pelvimetry in the management of dystocia?

A systematic review that included more than 1,000 women in 4 trials found that women undergoing X-ray pelvimetry were more likely to undergo cesarean delivery (odds ratio [OR], 2.17; 95% CI 1.63, 2.88) without any significant impact on perinatal outcome (35). Although the reasons for the increase in cesarean delivery rates are not clearly defined, the author concluded there is not enough evidence to support the use of X-ray pelvimetry in women whose fetuses have cephalic presentations. Other investigators expanded the use of X-ray pelvimetry by developing the fetal-pelvic index as a predictor of the likelihood of vaginal delivery in women at high risk for cesarean delivery (36). The test incorporates the determination of fetal weight by ultrasonography compared with the size of the pelvis as determined by X-ray pelvimetry. Initial studies in patients at risk for cesarean delivery demonstrated significant diagnostic ability of the test

(37). However, further prospective studies are necessary to establish the usefulness of this diagnostic modality to predict dystocia.

Clinical pelvimetry can be useful to qualitatively identify the general architectural features of the pelvis and identify patients at risk for dystocia. Researchers correlated pelvimetry data from postpartum magnetic resonance imaging (MRI) with fetal and neonatal dimensions to evaluate criteria for diagnosis of cephalopelvic disproportion (38). Fetal head volume estimates exceeded MRI-measured capacity in nearly 90% of nulliparous women who underwent cesarean delivery because of cephalopelvic disproportion. A prospective investigation of MRI has not been performed, and the use of MRI to measure pelvic capacity remains investigational.

▶ *Are there data supporting the benefits of caregivers providing continuous support during labor?*

Continuous support during labor from caregivers (nurses, midwives, or lay individuals) may have a number of benefits for women and their newborns. A randomized trial of 413 nulliparous women compared one-on-one nursing care with usual care (1 nurse monitoring 2 or 3 laboring women) and found a reduction in the need for oxytocin stimulation (RR, 0.83%; 95% CI 0.67, 1.04) (21). There were no differences in labor duration, cesarean deliveries, epidural analgesia, or neonatal intensive care admissions. A comparison of continuous support of a doula with an inconspicuous observer found that continuous labor support was associated with a reduction in cesarean deliveries (8% versus 13%) and forceps deliveries (8% versus 21%) (20). A systematic review that included more than 12,000 women in 15 trials found that the continuous presence of a support person reduced the likelihood of medication for pain relief, operative vaginal delivery, cesarean delivery, and 5-minute Apgar scores less than 7 (19, 39). Few data compare differences in benefits on the basis of level of training of support personnel—that is, whether the caregivers were nurses, midwives, or doulas. Continuous support during labor has several benefits without any evidence of harmful effects.

▶ *Does the degree of hydration affect the course of labor?*

In many obstetric centers, establishing an intravenous infusion of fluids in early labor has become routine. Although not necessary in all normally laboring women, intravenous fluids are beneficial before epidural analgesia, and the practice provides intravenous access and the ability to administer oxytocin prophylaxis for postpartum hemorrhage. On the basis of knowledge that increased fluids improve skeletal muscle performance during prolonged exercise, scientists speculated that increased intravenous fluids may affect labor progress (40). Nearly 200 nulliparous women with uncomplicated pregnancies in spontaneous active labor were randomized to receive either 125 mL or 250 mL of intravenous fluid per hour. The frequency of labor lasting longer than 12 hours was higher in the 125-mL group (26% versus 13%). Furthermore, there was a lower frequency of oxytocin administration for dystocia in the higher fluid rate group (49% versus 65%). The potential of natural hydration status to affect the course of labor warrants further investigation.

▶ *Is there a role for active management of labor?*

A system of labor management for nulliparous women, termed "active management of labor," was developed in Ireland (41). Although many obstetricians have focused on the use of high-dose oxytocin as the principal component of the active management of labor, it is important to emphasize that high-dose oxytocin is just one part of this approach. In fact, most women undergoing active management of labor do not receive oxytocin.

Active management of labor is confined to nulliparous women with singleton, cephalic presentations at term that show no evidence of fetal compromise. Active management of labor, as developed and practiced in Ireland, involves several distinct entities: patient education, strict criteria for the diagnosis of labor, strict criteria for the determination of abnormal progress of labor, high-dose oxytocin infusion, one-to-one nursing support in labor, strict criteria for interpretation of fetal compromise, and peer review of operative deliveries.

The safety of active management of labor has been demonstrated by several randomized trials involving more than 3,000 patients (10, 42–44). Active management of labor has not been associated with an increase in maternal or neonatal morbidity and mortality (44, 45). Unfortunately, success in decreasing cesarean delivery rates with active management of labor has not been uniform. One large randomized trial reported a statistically significant reduction in cesarean deliveries only after controlling for numerous confounding variables (43). A meta-analysis of 4 randomized trials failed to show a reduction in cesarean deliveries related to active management of labor (RR, 0.93; 95% CI 0.8, 1.08) (44).

Active management of labor is not associated with untoward maternal or neonatal outcomes. It may lead to shortened labor in nulliparous women but has not consistently led to a reduction in cesarean deliveries.

▶ *Is low-dose oxytocin superior to high-dose regimens for augmentation?*

Hypocontractile uterine activity is treated with oxytocin, the only medication approved by the U.S. Food and Drug Administration for labor stimulation. Numerous protocols for initial dose, incremental increases, and time intervals between doses have been studied. Regardless of whether a low-dose or high-dose oxytocin regimen is used, oxytocin is infused to titrate dose to effect because prediction of a woman's response to a particular dose is not possible (46). In a blinded, randomized study comparing a high-dose (4.5 mU/min every 30 minutes) with a low-dose (1.5 mU/min every 30 minutes) oxytocin protocol for augmentation, high-dose oxytocin was associated with a significant shortening of labor without a significant difference in cesarean delivery rates (47). No differences in neonatal outcomes were noted between groups. In another randomized trial of more than 300 women, use of high-dose oxytocin for augmentation benefited both nulliparous women and parous women by decreasing the mean time to correct the labor abnormality by nearly 2 hours and decreasing the need for cesarean delivery (10.4% versus 25.7%) (48).

In a prospective trial involving 1,676 women, comparing high-dose (6 mU/min every 20 minutes) with low-dose (1–2 mU/min every 20 minutes) oxytocin regimens for augmentation, the high-dose regimen was associated with fewer cesarean deliveries for dystocia (9% versus 12%), a 3-hour reduction in mean time to delivery, fewer incidences of chorioamnionitis (8% versus 12%), and fewer cases of neonatal sepsis (0.3% versus 2%) (49). The high-dose regimen was associated with an increase in hyperstimulation, but no adverse fetal effects were observed. In another small randomized trial, a high-dose regimen was associated with a shorter second stage of labor without measurable differences in neonatal outcomes (50). Thus, the current data available do not support the notion that low-dose oxytocin regimens are superior to high-dose regimens for augmentation of labor. Low-dose regimens are associated with less uterine hyperstimulation and lower maximum doses. High-dose regimens may be used for multiparous women, but there are no data available to support the use of high-dose oxytocin regimens for augmentation in a woman with a previously scarred uterus. Importantly, a wide variety of oxytocin regimens may be used for labor augmentation provided proper precautions are met (Table 1).

▶ *Should women with twin gestations undergo augmentation of labor?*

Twin gestation is not a contraindication to augmentation of labor, but it does warrant special attention. In a retrospective report, 62 women with twin gestations were

Table 1. Labor Augmentation with Oxytocin: Examples of Low-Dose and High-Dose Regimens

Regimen	Starting Dose (mU/min)	Incremental Increase (mU/min)	Dosage Interval (min)	Maximum Dose (mU/min)
Low-Dose	0.5–1*	1	30–40	20
	1–2†	2	15	40
High-Dose	≈6‡	≈6	15	≈40
	6§	6, 3, 1	20–40	42

*Seitchik J, Amico JA, Castillo M. Oxytocin augmentation of dysfunctional labor. V. An alternative oxytocin regimen. Am J Obstet Gynecol 1985;151:757–61.

†Hauth JC, Hankins GD, Gilstrap LC 3rd, Strickland DM, Vance P. Uterine contraction pressures with oxytocin induction/augmentation. Obstet Gynecol 1986;68:305–9.

‡O'Driscoll K, Foley M, MacDonald D. Active management of labor as an alternative to cesarean section for dystocia. Obstet Gynecol 1984;63:485–90.

§Satin AJ, Maberry MC, Leveno KJ, Sherman ML, Kline DM. Chorioamnionitis: a harbinger of dystocia. Obstet Gynecol 1992;79:913–5.

matched by parity, cervical dilatation at initiation of oxytocin, gestational age, oxytocin dosage regimen, and indications for oxytocin with controls with singleton pregnancies (51). Twenty-seven women received oxytocin for augmentation and 35 for induction. Women with twin pregnancies responded similarly to those with singleton pregnancies regarding the maximum oxytocin dosage, time to delivery, and successful vaginal delivery. The authors concluded that twin gestation has no adverse impact on the effectiveness or efficacy of oxytocin used for labor stimulation. In a small study of women with twin gestations undergoing labor induction and oxytocin augmentation, no adverse neonatal outcomes were observed (52). In a retrospective review of 134 women with twin gestations who underwent a trial of labor, 49 women required augmentation (53). Augmentation was not found to be a significant risk factor for cesarean delivery or adverse outcomes. Thus, twin gestation does not preclude the use of oxytocin for labor augmentation.

▶ *How does amniotomy affect labor?*

Amniotomy is commonly performed to induce or augment labor. Surprisingly few studies exist focusing on the impact of amniotomy on augmentation. A recent systematic review primarily addressed the effect of amniotomy on the rate of cesarean delivery (54). This review included controlled trials of amniotomy during the first stage of labor. Amniotomy was associated with a reduction in labor duration of 1–2 hours and a decrease in the use of oxytocin (OR, 0.79; 95% CI 0.67, 0.92). In a trial of 459 women randomized to undergo either elective amniotomy (amniotomy group) or no amniotomy unless there were specific indications (intact group), analysis of fetal heart rate patterns revealed more mild or moderate variable decelerations in the active phase of labor in the amniotomy group (55). Importantly, there was no difference in nonreassuring heart rates or operative deliveries. Amniotomy was associated with a decreased need for oxytocin augmentation (36% versus 76%) and a shorter active phase of labor (4 hours, 35 minutes, versus 5 hours, 56 minutes).

Another randomized trial addressed the impact of amniotomy after an arrest disorder was diagnosed in the active phase (14). Women with an active phase arrest were randomized to receive either oxytocin with intact membranes or oxytocin with amniotomy and internal monitoring. A trend toward longer labor (44 minutes longer) was seen in the intact group with no differences in cesarean deliveries. The amniotomy group had a higher incidence of fever. Thus, amniotomy may enhance progress in the active phase and negate the need for oxytocin augmentation but may increase the risk of chorioamnionitis.

▶ *Should electronic fetal monitoring be used during oxytocin augmentation?*

No overwhelming evidence has identified the most effective method of fetal heart rate surveillance when oxytocin is used for augmentation. A systematic review of continuous electronic heart rate monitoring for fetal assessment during labor identified 13 randomized trials addressing efficacy and safety of electronic fetal monitoring (56). Routine electronic fetal monitoring was associated with a statistically significant decrease in neonatal seizures. (RR, 0.51; 95% CI 0.32, 0.82). No differences were seen in low Apgar scores, neonatal intensive care unit admissions, perinatal deaths, or cerebral palsy. Electronic fetal monitoring was associated with an increase in cesarean deliveries (RR, 1.41; 95% CI 1.23, 1.61) and operative vaginal deliveries (RR, 1.2; 95% CI 1.11, 1.3). Well-controlled studies of intermittent auscultation of the fetal heart rate have shown it to be equivalent to continuous electronic fetal monitoring when performed at specific intervals with a one-to-one nurse-to-patient ratio (57–61). There are no comparative data indicating the optimal frequency at which intermittent auscultation should be performed in the absence of risk factors.

Summary of Recommendations

The following recommendations are based on good and consistent scientific evidence (Level A):

▶ Patients should be counseled that walking during labor does not enhance or improve progress in labor nor is it harmful.

▶ Continuous support during labor from caregivers should be encouraged because it is beneficial for women and their newborns.

The following recommendations are based on limited or inconsistent scientific evidence (Level B):

▶ Active management of labor may shorten labor in nulliparous women, although it has not consistently been shown to reduce the rate of cesarean delivery.

▶ Amniotomy may be used to enhance progress in active labor, but may increase the risk of maternal fever.

▶ X-ray pelvimetry alone as a predictor of dystocia has not been shown to have benefit, and, therefore, is not recommended.

The following recommendations are based primarily on consensus and expert opinion (Level C):

▶ Intrauterine pressure catheters may be helpful in the management of dystocia in selected patients, such as those who are obese.

▶ Women with twin gestations may undergo augmentation of labor.

References

1. Martin JA, Hamilton BE, Ventura SJ, Menacker F, Park MM, Sutton PD. Births: final data for 2001. Natl Vital Stat Rep 2002;51(2):1–102. (Level II-3)

2. Gifford DS, Morton SC, Fiske M, Keesey J, Keeler E, Kahn KL. Lack of progress in labor as a reason for cesarean. Obstet Gynecol 2000;95:589–95. (Level II-3)

3. Cunningham FG, Gant NF, Leveno KJ, Gilstrap LC 3rd, Hauth JC, Wenstrom KD. Dystocia: abnormal labor and fetopelvic disproportion. In: Williams Obstetrics. 21st ed. New York (NY): McGraw-Hill; 2001. p. 425–50. (Level III)

4. Kilpatrick SJ, Laros RK Jr. Characteristics of normal labor. Obstet Gynecol 1989;74:85–7. (Level II-3)

5. Zhang J, Yancey MK, Klebanoff MA, Schwarz J, Schweitzer D. Does epidural analgesia prolong labor and increase risk of cesarean delivery? A natural experiment. Am J Obstet Gynecol 2001;185:128–34. (Level II-2)

6. Hauth JC, Hankins GD, Gilstrap LC 3rd, Strickland DM, Vance P. Uterine contraction pressures with oxytocin induction/augmentation. Obstet Gynecol 1986;68:305–9. (Level II-2)

7. Rouse DJ, Owen J, Goldenberg RL, Cliver SP. The effectiveness and costs of elective cesarean delivery for fetal macrosomia diagnosed by ultrasound. JAMA 1996;276:1480–6. (Decision analysis)

8. Menticoglou SM, Manning F, Harman C, Morrison I. Perinatal outcome in relation to second-stage duration. Am J Obstet Gynecol 1995;173:906–12. (Level II-3)

9. Sheiner E, Levy A, Feinstein U, Hershkovitz R, Hallak M, Mazor M. Obstetric risk factors for failure to progress in the first versus the second stage of labor. J Matern Fetal Neonatal Med 2002;11:409–13. (Level II-2)

10. Frigoletto FD Jr, Lieberman E, Lang JM, Cohen A, Barss V, Ringer S, et al. A clinical trial of active management of labor [published erratum appears in N Engl J Med 1995;333:1163]. N Engl J Med 1995;333:745–50. (Level I)

11. Howell CJ. Epidural versus non-epidural analgesia for pain relief in labour (Cochrane Review). In: The Cochrane Library, Issue 3, 2003. Oxford: Update Software. (Meta-analysis)

12. Satin AJ, Maberry MC, Leveno KJ, Sherman ML, Kline DM. Chorioamnionitis: a harbinger of dystocia. Obstet Gynecol 1992;79:913–5. (Level II-2)

13. Piper JM, Bolling DR, Newton ER. The second stage of labor: factors influencing duration. Am J Obstet Gynecol 1991;165:976–9. (Level II-3)

14. Rouse DJ, McCullough C, Wren AL, Owen J, Hauth JC. Active-phase labor arrest: a randomized trial of chorioamnion management. Obstet Gynecol 1994;83:937–40. (Level I)

15. Fitzpatrick M, Harkin R, McQuillan K, O'Brien C, O'Connell PR, O'Herlihy C. A randomised clinical trial comparing the effects of delayed versus immediate pushing with epidural analgesia on mode of delivery and faecal continence. BJOG 2002;109:1359–65. (Level I)

16. Donnelly V, Fynes M, Campbell D, Johnson H, O'Connell PR, O'Herlihy C. Obstetric events leading to anal sphincter damage. Obstet Gynecol 1998;92:955–61. (Level II-2)

17. Hilton P, Ward A. Epidemiological and surgical aspects of urogenital fistulae: a review of 25 years' experience in southeast Nigeria. Int Urogynecol J Pelvic Floor Dysfunct 1998;9:189–94. (Level II-3)

18. Kelly J. Vesico-vaginal and recto-vaginal fistulae. J R Soc Med 1992;85:257–8. (Level III)

19. Hodnett ED, Gates S, Hofmeyr GJ, Sakala C. Continuous support for women during childbirth (Cochrane Review). In: The Cochrane Library, Issue 3, 2003. Oxford: Update Software. (Meta-analysis)

20. Kennell J, Klaus M, McGrath S, Robertson S, Hinkley C. Continuous emotional support during labor in a US hospital. A randomized controlled trial. JAMA 1991;265: 2197–201. (Level I)

21. Gagnon AJ, Waghorn K, Covell C. A randomized trial of one-to-one nurse support of woman in labor. Birth 1997;24:71–7. (Level I)

22. Albers LL, Schiff M, Gorwoda JG. The length of active labor in normal pregnancies. Obstet Gynecol 1996;87: 355–9. (Level II-3)

23. Fraser WD, Cayer M, Soeder BM, Turcot L, Marcoux S; PEOPLE (Pushing Early or Pushing Late with Epidural) Study Group. Risk factors for difficult delivery in nulli-paras with epidural analgesia in second stage of labor. Obstet Gynecol 2002;99:409–18. (Level II-2)

24. Gambling DR, Sharma SK, Ramin SM, Lucas MJ, Leveno KJ, Wiley J, et al. A randomized study of combined spinal-epidural analgesia versus intravenous meperidine during labor: impact on cesarean delivery rate. Anesthesiology 1998;89:1336–44. (Level I)

25. Halpern SH, Leighton BL, Ohlsson A, Barrett JF, Rice A. Effect of epidural vs. parenteral opioid analgesia on the progress of labor: a meta-analysis. JAMA 1998;280: 2105–10. (Meta-analysis)

26. Ramin SM, Gambling DR, Lucas MJ, Sharma SK, Sidawi JE, Leveno KJ. Randomized trial of epidural versus intravenous analgesia during labor. Obstet Gynecol 1995;86: 783–9. (Level I)

27. Sharma SK, Sidawi JE, Ramin SM, Lucas MJ, Leveno KJ, Cunningham FG. Cesarean delivery: a randomized trial of epidural versus patient-controlled meperidine analgesia during labor. Anesthesiology 1997;87:487–94. (Level I)

28. Thorp JA, Hu DH, Albin RM, McNitt J, Meyer BA, Cohen GR, et al. The effect of intrapartum epidural analgesia on nulliparous labor: a randomized, controlled, prospective trial. Am J Obstet Gynecol 1993;169:851–8. (Level I)

29. Nageotte MP, Larson D, Rumney PJ, Sidhu M, Hollenbach K. Epidural analgesia compared with combined spinal-epidural analgesia during labor in nulliparous women. N Engl J Med 1997;337:1715–9. (Level I)

30. Robinson JN, Norwitz ER, Cohen AP, McElrath TF, Lieberman ES. Epidural analgesia and third- or fourth-degree lacerations in nulliparas. Obstet Gynecol 1999; 94:259–62. (Level II-2)

31. Chua S, Kurup A, Arulkumaran S, Ratnam SS. Augmentation of labor: does internal tocography result in better obstetric outcome than external tocography? Obstet Gynecol 1990;76:164–7. (Level I)

32. Bloom SL, McIntire DD, Kelly MA, Beimer HL, Burpo RH, Garcia MA, et al. Lack of effect of walking on labor and delivery. N Engl J Med 1998;339:76–9. (Level I)

33. Vallejo MC, Firestone LL, Mandell GL, Jamie F, Makishima S, Ramanathan S. Effect of epidural analgesia with ambulation on labor duration. Anesthesiology 2001; 95:857–61. (Level I)

34. Lupe PJ, Gross TL. Maternal upright posture and mobility in labor—a review. Obstet Gynecol 1986;67:727–34. (Level III)

35. Pattinson RC. Pelvimetry for fetal cephalic presentations at term (Cochrane Review). In: The Cochrane Library, Issue 3, 2003. Oxford: Update Software. (Meta-analysis)

36. Morgan MA, Thurnau GR, Fishburne JI Jr. The fetal-pelvic index as an indicator of fetal-pelvic disproportion: a preliminary report. Am J Obstet Gynecol 1986;155: 608–13. (Level II-3)

37. Morgan MA, Thurnau GR. Efficacy of the fetal-pelvic index in nulliparous women at high risk for fetal-pelvic

disproportion. Am J Obstet Gynecol 1992;166:810–4. (Level II-2)

38. Sporri S, Hanggi W, Braghetti A, Vock P, Schneider H. Pelvimetry by magnetic resonance imaging as a diagnostic tool to evaluate dystocia. Obstet Gynecol 1997;89: 902–8. (Level II-2)

39. Thornton JG, Lilford RJ. Active management of labour: current knowledge and research issues [published erratum appears in BMJ 1994;309:704]. BMJ 1994;309:366–9. (Level III)

40. Garite TJ, Weeks J, Peters-Phair K, Pattillo C, Brewster WR. A randomized controlled trial of the effect of increased intravenous hydration on the course of labor in nulliparous women. Am J Obstet Gynecol 2000;183: 1544–8. (Level I)

41. O'Driscoll K, Foley M, MacDonald D. Active management of labor as an alternative to cesarean section for dystocia. Obstet Gynecol 1984;63:485–90. (Level II-3)

42. Rogers R, Gilson GJ, Miller AC, Izquierdo LE, Curet LB, Qualls CR. Active management of labor: does it make a difference? Am J Obstet Gynecol 1997;177:599–605. (Level I)

43. Lopez-Zeno JA, Peaceman AM, Adashek JA, Socol ML. A controlled trial of a program for the active management of labor. N Engl J Med 1992;326:450–4. (Level I)

44. Sadler LC, Davison T, McCowan LM. A randomised controlled trial and meta-analysis of active management of labour. BJOG 2000;107:909–15. (Level II-1)

45. Cahill DJ, Boylan PC, O'Herlihy C. Does oxytocin augmentation increase perinatal risk in primigravid labor? Am J Obstet Gynecol 1992;166:847–50. (Level II-2)

46. Satin AJ, Leveno KJ, Sherman ML, McIntire DD. Factors affecting the dose response to oxytocin for labor stimulation. Am J Obstet Gynecol 1992;166:1260–1. (Level II-2)

47. Merrill DC, Zlatnik FJ. Randomized, double-masked comparison of oxytocin dosage in induction and augmentation of labor. Obstet Gynecol 1999;94:455–63. (Level I)

48. Xenakis EM, Langer O, Piper JM, Conway D, Berkus MD. Low-dose versus high-dose oxytocin augmentation of labor—a randomized trial. Am J Obstet Gynecol 1995; 173:1874–8. (Level I)

49. Satin AJ, Leveno KJ, Sherman ML, Brewster DS, Cunningham FG. High- versus low-dose oxytocin for labor stimulation. Obstet Gynecol 1992;80:111–6. (Level II-2)

50. Bidgood KA, Steer PJ. A randomized control study of oxytocin augmentation of labour. 1. Obstetric outcome. Br J Obstet Gynaecol 1987;94:512–7. (Level I)

51. Fausett MB, Barth WH Jr, Yoder BA, Satin AJ. Oxytocin labor stimulation of twin gestations: effective and efficient. Obstet Gynecol 1997;90:202–4. (Level II-2)

52. Manor M, Blickstein I, Ben-Arie A, Weissman A, Hagay Z. Case series of labor induction in twin gestations with an intrauterine balloon catheter. Gynecol Obstet Invest 1999;47:244–6. (Level III)

53. Grobman WA, Dooley SL, Peaceman AM. Risk factors for cesarean delivery in twin gestations near term. Obstet Gynecol 1998;92:940–4. (Level II-2)

54. Fraser WD, Turcot L, Krauss I, Brisson-Carrol G. Amniotomy for shortening spontaneous labour (Cochrane Review). In: The Cochrane Library, Issue 3, 2003. Oxford: Update Software. (Meta-analysis)

55. Garite TJ, Porto M, Carlson NJ, Rumney PJ, Reimbold PA. The influence of elective amniotomy on fetal heart rate patterns and the course of labor in term patients: a randomized study. Am J Obstet Gynecol 1993;168: 1827–31; discussion 1831–2. (Level I)

56. Thacker SB, Stroup D, Chang M. Continuous electronic heart rate monitoring for fetal assessment during labor (Cochrane Review). In: The Cochrane Library, Issue 3, 2003. Oxford: Update Software. (Meta-analysis)

57. Haverkamp AD, Orleans M, Langendoerfer S, McFee J, Murphy J, Thompson HE. A controlled trial of the differential effects of intrapartum fetal monitoring. Am J Obstet Gynecol 1979;134:399–412. (Level I)

58. Renou P, Chang A, Anderson I, Wood C. Controlled trial of fetal intensive care. Am J Obstet Gynecol 1976;126: 470–6. (Level I)

59. Kelso IM, Parsons RJ, Lawrence GF, Arora SS, Edmonds DK, Cooke ID. An assessment of continuous fetal heart rate monitoring in labor. A randomized trial. Am J Obstet Gynecol 1978;131:526–32. (Level I)

60. Wood C, Renou P, Oats J, Farrell E, Beischer N, Anderson I. A controlled trial of fetal heart rate monitoring in a low-risk obstetric population. Am J Obstet Gynecol 1981; 141:527–34. (Level I)

61. MacDonald D, Grant A, Sheridan-Pereira M, Boylan P, Chalmers I. The Dublin randomized controlled trial of intrapartum fetal heart rate monitoring. Am J Obstet Gynecol 1985;152:524–39. (Level I)

The MEDLINE database, the Cochrane Library, and ACOG's own internal resources and documents were used to conduct a literature search to locate relevant articles published between January 1985 and August 2003. The search was restricted to articles published in the English language. Priority was given to articles reporting results of original research, although review articles and commentaries also were consulted. Abstracts of research presented at symposia and scientific conferences were not considered adequate for inclusion in this document. Guidelines published by organizations or institutions such as the National Institutes of Health and the American College of Obstetricians and Gynecologists were reviewed, and additional studies were located by reviewing bibliographies of identified articles. When reliable research was not available, expert opinions from obstetrician–gynecologists were used.

Studies were reviewed and evaluated for quality according to the method outlined by the U.S. Preventive Services Task Force:

I   Evidence obtained from at least 1 properly designed randomized controlled trial.

II-1 Evidence obtained from well-designed controlled trials without randomization.

II-2 Evidence obtained from well-designed cohort or case–control analytic studies, preferably from more than 1 center or research group.

II-3 Evidence obtained from multiple time series with or without the intervention. Dramatic results in uncontrolled experiments also could be regarded as this type of evidence.

III   Opinions of respected authorities, based on clinical experience, descriptive studies, or reports of expert committees.

Based on the highest level of evidence found in the data, recommendations are provided and graded according to the following categories:

Level A—Recommendations are based on good and consistent scientific evidence.

Level B—Recommendations are based on limited or inconsistent scientific evidence.

Level C—Recommendations are based primarily on consensus and expert opinion.

ISSN 1099-3630

**The American College of
Obstetricians and Gynecologists
409 12th Street, SW
PO Box 96920
Washington, DC 20090-6920**

12345/76543

Dystocia and augmentation of labor. ACOG Practice Bulletin No. 49. American College of Obstetricians and Gynecologists. Obstet Gynecol 2003;102:1445–54.

ACOG PRACTICE BULLETIN

CLINICAL MANAGEMENT GUIDELINES FOR
OBSTETRICIAN–GYNECOLOGISTS
NUMBER 69, DECEMBER 2005

(Replaces Practice Bulletin Number 25, March 2001)

This Practice Bulletin was developed by the ACOG Committee on Practice Bulletins— Gynecology with the assistance of Elizabeth Raymond, MD, MPH. The information is designed to aid practitioners in making decisions about appropriate obstetric and gynecologic care. These guidelines should not be construed as dictating an exclusive course of treatment or procedure. Variations in practice may be warranted based on the needs of the individual patient, resources, and limitations unique to the institution or type of practice.

Emergency Contraception

Emergency contraception, also called the morning-after pill *and* postcoital contraception, *is therapy used to prevent pregnancy after an unprotected or inadequately protected act of sexual intercourse. Women seeking emergency contraception typically are younger than 25 years, have never been pregnant, and have used some form of contraception in the past (1–3). Common indications for emergency contraception include contraceptive failure (eg, condom breakage, missed doses of oral contraceptives) and failure to use any form of contraception (2, 4, 5). Although oral emergency contraception was first described in the medical literature decades ago, this therapy is still not widely used in the United States to reduce unintended pregnancy. The results of a 2003 survey of 800 U.S. women aged 18–49 years indicate that only 6% reported having ever used emergency contraception (1). Many women are unaware of the existence of emergency contraception, misunderstand its use and safety, do not have convenient and prompt access to it, or do not use it when a need arises. Increasing emergency contraception awareness, knowledge, and access are important priorities in the effort to reduce the incidence of unintended pregnancy.*

Methods of emergency contraception include administration of progestin-only or combination estrogen–progestin oral contraceptives, synthetic estrogens and conjugated estrogens, or antiprogestins and the insertion of a copper intrauterine device (IUD). This bulletin addresses the progestin-only and combined oral contraceptive medical methods, which are the most frequently used and the only methods currently approved by the U.S. Food and Drug Administration (FDA) specifically for emergency contraception, and briefly addresses the IUD because of its use as long-term contraception in addition to emergency contraception.

Background

Research on the postcoital use of contraceptive steroids began in the 1960s. The first oral regimen, which used a widely available brand of combined estrogen–progestin oral contraceptive pills, was published in 1974 by Yuzpe and colleagues (6). Research on progestin-only regimens for occasional postcoital use by women having infrequent intercourse also began about that time (7).

Regimens

The two most commonly used oral emergency contraception regimens are the progestin-only regimen, which consists of a total of 1.5 mg levonorgestrel, and the combined estrogen–progestin regimen, which consists of two doses—each containing 100 µg of ethinyl estradiol plus 0.5 mg of levonorgestrel—taken 12 hours apart. Both regimens are available in many countries as products labeled specifically for use as emergency contraception, but the levonorgestrel-only product (Plan B) is the only dedicated emergency contraception product currently marketed in the United States. Both regimens also can be made from a variety of standard oral contraceptives (Table 1), although data exist only for regimens containing levonorgestrel, norgestrel (levonorgestrel plus an equal amount of the inactive enantiomer dextronorgestrel), and norethindrone.

The package insert of Plan B instructs patients to take one 0.75-mg levonorgestrel pill as soon as possible after unprotected intercourse and to take the second 0.75-mg pill 12 hours after the first dose. However, randomized trials have shown that taking both pills at the same time (8, 9) or taking each 0.75-mg pill 24 hours apart (10) is as effective as taking them 12 hours apart and does not increase the risk of side effects.

Method of Action

No single mechanism of action has been established for emergency contraception; rather, the mode of action varies according to the day of the menstrual cycle on which intercourse occurs and emergency contraception is administered (11–14). Both the combined regimen and the levonorgestrel-only regimen have been shown to inhibit or delay ovulation (15–21). Earlier studies documented histologic and biochemical changes in the endometrium after administration of the combined regimen, suggesting that emergency contraception may alter the receptiveness of the endometrium and inhibit implantation of a fertilized egg (6, 18, 22–24). However, several more recent studies have not supported these findings (16, 19, 21, 25–28), and the endometrial changes that have been observed may not be sufficient to prevent implantation. Interference with sperm transport or penetration (7, 29) and impairment of corpus luteum function (18, 30) have been proposed as other possible mechanisms of action, but there is no direct clinical evidence to support these theories. However, it is statistically unlikely that emergency contraception could be as effective as it is for preventing pregnancy if interference with ovulation is its only method of action (31).

Emergency contraception is sometimes confused with medical abortion (32). However, whereas medical abortion is used to terminate an existing pregnancy, emergency contraception is effective only before a pregnancy is established. Emergency contraception can prevent pregnancy during the 5 or more days between intercourse and implantation of a fertilized egg, but it is ineffective after implantation. Studies of high-dose oral contraceptives indicate that emergency contraception confers no increased risk to an established pregnancy or harm to a developing embryo (33).

Side Effects

Plan B is available only by prescription. However, in 2003 a combined panel of the FDA's Advisory Committee on Reproductive Health Drugs and the Advisory Committee on Nonprescription Drugs concluded that the safety of the levonorgestrel-only emergency contraception regimen has been sufficiently demonstrated to warrant approval for nonprescription status.

No deaths or serious complications have been causally linked to emergency contraception (34). Short-term side effects include the following:

- Nausea and vomiting: The levonorgestrel-only regimen is associated with significantly lower incidences of nausea and vomiting than the combined regimen (35, 36). Nausea and vomiting, respectively, occur in about 18% and 4% of women using levonorgestrel-only emergency contraception (8, 9, 36) and in approximately 43% and 16% of women using the combined regimen (37).

- Irregular bleeding: After emergency contraception use, the menstrual period usually occurs within 1 week before or after the expected time (36). Some patients experience irregular bleeding or spotting in the week or month after treatment; one recent trial of the levonorgestrel-only regimen found that 16% of women reported nonmenstrual bleeding in the first week after use (9). Irregular bleeding associated with emergency contraception resolves without treatment.

- Other side effects: Some patients have reported experiencing short-term side effects, such as breast tenderness, abdominal pain, dizziness, headache, and fatigue (38).

Table 1. Twenty-one Brands of Oral Contraceptives That Can Be Used for Emergency Contraception in the United States

Brand	Company	Pills per Dose*	Ethinyl Estradiol per Dose (µg)	Levonorgestrel per Dose (mg)[†]
Plan B[‡]	Barr	1 white pill	0	0.75
Ovral	Wyeth-Ayerst	2 white pills	100	0.50
Ogestrel	Watson	2 white pills	100	0.50
Cryselle	Barr	4 white pills	120	0.60
Levora	Watson	4 white pills	120	0.60
Lo/Ovral	Wyeth-Ayerst	4 white pills	120	0.60
Low-Ogestrel	Watson	4 white pills	120	0.60
Levlen	Berlex	4 light orange pills	120	0.60
Nordette	Wyeth-Ayerst	4 light orange pills	120	0.60
Portia	Barr	4 pink pills	120	0.60
Seasonale	Barr	4 pink pills	120	0.60
Trivora	Watson	4 pink pills	120	0.50
Tri-Levlen	Berlex	4 yellow pills	120	0.50
Triphasil	Wyeth-Ayerst	4 yellow pills	120	0.50
Enpresse	Barr	4 orange pills	120	0.50
Alesse	Wyeth-Ayerst	5 pink pills	100	0.50
Lessina	Barr	5 pink pills	100	0.50
Levlite	Berlex	5 pink pills	100	0.50
Lutera	Watson	5 white pills	100	0.50
Aviane	Barr	5 orange pills	100	0.50
Ovrette	Wyeth-Ayerst	20 yellow pills	0	0.75

*The treatment schedule is one dose as soon as possible after unprotected intercourse, and another dose 12 hours later. However, recent research has found that both doses of Plan B or Ovrette can be taken at the same time.

[†]The progestin in Cryselle, Lo/Ovral, Low-Ogestrel, Ogestrel, Ovral, and Ovrette is norgestrel, which contains two isomers, only one of which (levonorgestrel) is bioactive; the amount of norgestrel in each tablet is twice the amount of levonorgestrel. Levonorgestrel regimens also can be formulated by substituting double the amount of norgestrel as is indicated for levonorgestrel.

[‡]Plan B is the only dedicated product specifically marketed for emergency contraception in the United States. Preven, a combined emergency contraception pill, is no longer available on the U.S. market.

NOT-2-LATE.com: the emergency contraception website. Princeton University Office of Population Research. Princeton (NJ): Office of Population Research; 2005. Available at: http://ec.princeton.edu/questions/dose.html. Retrieved October 13, 2005.

Effects on Pregnancy

No studies have specifically investigated adverse effects of exposure to emergency contraception during early pregnancy. However, numerous studies of the teratogenic risk of conception during daily use of oral contraceptives (including older, higher-dose preparations) have found no increase in risk to either the pregnant woman or the developing fetus (39).

Existing data indicate that use of emergency contraception does not increase the chance that a subsequent pregnancy will be ectopic. Emergency contraception, like all other contraceptives, actually reduces the absolute risk of ectopic pregnancy by preventing pregnancy overall (40).

Drug Interactions

Although no evidence exists regarding the interaction between emergency contraception and other medications, it is biologically plausible that any drug interactions involving emergency contraception would be similar to those interactions observed with use of combined estrogen–progestin oral contraceptives. A detailed discussion of adverse interactions involving oral contraceptives is beyond the scope of this bulletin, but several resources are available on this topic (41–45). Medications and herbal supplements that may decrease the effectiveness of oral contraceptives (including but not limited to rifampicin, St. John's wort, certain anticonvulsants, and certain antiretrovirals) also may reduce the efficacy of emergency contraception.

Awareness and Access

Recent surveys have documented that a large number of women are unaware of the existence of emergency contraception or have insufficient knowledge to allow them to use it effectively (46–50). The results of a 2003 survey of Californians between the ages of 15 and 44 years indicate that 35% did not know of any way to prevent becoming pregnant after sex, and 43% were not aware that emergency contraception is available in the United States (1). Many health care providers are poorly informed about this method (51–53), and access to emergency contraception through health care providers, pharmacies, student health centers, urgent care centers, and other sources is limited (54, 55). A study of 320 pharmacies in Pennsylvania found that only 35% could fill a prescription for emergency contraception on the same day it was requested (56). Data from a nationally representative sample of female sexual assault victims seen in U.S. emergency departments in 2002 indicated that only 21% of eligible women received emergency contraception (57).

A prominent concern among both women and health care providers is that making emergency contraception more readily available could encourage irresponsible sexual behavior, which would increase the risks of both unintended pregnancy and sexually transmitted diseases (58). However, numerous studies have shown that this concern is unfounded. At least seven published randomized trials have evaluated the policy of providing emergency contraception to women at the time of a routine gynecologic visit, so that they will have the medication immediately available if a contraceptive mishap occurs (4, 59–64). These trials compared this policy of advance provision with a policy of instructing women to contact a clinician if emergency contraception is needed. All but one (63) of these trials showed no difference between groups regarding self-reported frequency of either unprotected intercourse or use of contraception. In all the trials, use of emergency contraception was substantially more common in the group that was provided emergency contraception in advance, and one trial found that providing emergency contraception in advance of need resulted in earlier use of the treatment (4).

Clinical Considerations and Recommendations

▶ Who are candidates for emergency contraception?

Emergency contraception should be offered to women who have had unprotected or inadequately protected sexual intercourse and who do not desire pregnancy. Some emergency contraception studies have excluded women with specific contraindications to oral contraceptives, but no evidence demonstrates that emergency contraception is unsafe for women with these contraindications or for those with any particular medical conditions. Similarly, although some product package inserts list contraindications similar to those accepted for regular use of oral contraceptives, these precautions likely do not apply to emergency contraception because of the short duration of use. The World Health Organization's "Medical Eligibility Criteria for Contraceptive Use" include no conditions in which the risks of emergency contraception use outweigh the benefits (65). These criteria note specifically that women with previous ectopic pregnancy, cardiovascular disease, migraines, or liver disease and women who are breastfeeding may use emergency contraception. No data specifically examine the risk of using hormonal methods of emergency contraception among women with contraindications to the use of conventional oral contraceptive preparations; nevertheless, emergency contraception may be made available to such women. In addition, no rationale exists for denying emergency contraception to women with undiagnosed genital bleeding. Although existing pregnancy is not a contraindication for emergency contraception use in terms of risk of adverse effects, emergency contraception is not indicated in women with confirmed pregnancy because it will have no effect.

▶ What screening procedures are needed before provision of emergency contraception?

No clinical examination or testing is required before emergency contraception is provided. Emergency contraception should not be withheld or delayed in order to test for pregnancy, nor should it be denied because the unprotected coital act may not have occurred on a fertile day of the menstrual cycle. Emergency contraception generally should be provided any time unprotected or inadequately protected intercourse occurs and the patient is concerned that she is at risk for unwanted pregnancy.

▶ When should emergency contraception be initiated?

Treatment should be initiated as soon as possible after unprotected or inadequately protected intercourse, because efficacy seems to decline substantially with time (9, 66). Several studies have shown that both combined and progestin-only regimens are more effective the closer dosing is to the time of intercourse (9, 35, 36, 67). However, a few studies have not observed this time effect with the combined regimen (68, 69). Because earlier studies demonstrated that both regimens are effective when initiated up to 72 hours after intercourse (6, 36), some product package instructions advise use only within that time frame. More recent studies have shown that emergency contraception is still moderately effective when the first dose is taken up to 120 hours after intercourse. Therefore, emergency contraception should be made available to patients who request it up to 120 hours after intercourse (9, 59, 69–72). There currently are no data evaluating the efficacy of emergency contraception when treatment is initiated more than 120 hours after intercourse.

▶ *How effective is emergency contraception in preventing pregnancy?*

In the ideal setting, the effectiveness of a preventive therapy is best measured by comparing the probability that the condition will occur if the therapy is used with the probability that it will occur without treatment. For emergency contraception, efficacy is defined as the number of pregnancies observed after treatment divided by the estimated number of pregnancies that would occur without treatment. When this proportion is subtracted from one, the resulting statistic is the "prevented fraction," which represents the estimated percentage of cases averted by the treatment. Calculation of this statistic in clinical observation involves many assumptions that are difficult to validate. The numerator may become artificially inflated because preexisting pregnancies and those resulting from subsequent acts of intercourse are difficult to distinguish from pregnancies resulting from emergency contraception treatment failure. In addition, calculation of the denominator requires that estimates of the timing of ovulation be compared with data about the daily probability of conception that may not be appropriate for the study populations. Therefore, reported figures on the efficacy of emergency contraception vary considerably and are imprecise.

Six studies comprising a total of more than 8,000 women who used the levonorgestrel-only regimen calculated prevented fractions ranging from 60% to 94%, meaning that the regimen reduced women's chances of pregnancy by that amount (8–10, 35, 36, 73). Similarly, eight studies including a total of more than 3,800 women who used the combined regimen yielded prevented fractions ranging from 56% to 89%; a meta-analysis of pooled data from these studies concluded that the regimen prevents at least 74% of expected pregnancies (74).

Other data suggest that the levonorgestrel-only regimen is more effective than the combined regimen. The first of two randomized trials that directly compared the two regimens found no statistically significant difference in efficacy between failure rates of the levonorgestrel-only regimen and the combined regimen (2.4% versus 2.7%, respectively) (35). However, a second larger trial reported that the levonorgestrel-only regimen was significantly more effective for preventing pregnancy than the combined regimen (85% versus 57%, respectively) (36). Estimates based on combined data from these two studies show a reduced relative risk of pregnancy (0.51, 95% confidence interval, 0.31–0.83) with the levonorgestrel-only regimen (75). Therefore, the levonorgestrel-only regimen is preferred to the combined estrogen–progestin regimen, if available.

▶ *Are antiemetics useful as an adjunct to treatment?*

Because the incidence of nausea and vomiting is low with the levonorgestrel-only regimen, prophylactic antiemetics are probably not necessary. With the combined regimen, antiemetic pretreatment may be beneficial because the incidence of nausea is reported to be 30–60% (76). A single dose of an antiemetic taken 1 hour before the first dose of emergency contraception has been shown to decrease the incidence or severity of nausea (37, 77). Taking emergency contraception with food does not appear to affect the risk of nausea (37, 78). No evidence exists that vomiting within 3 hours of taking the dose is associated with an increased failure rate; however, no studies were designed specifically to measure this effect. Many experts recommend that the dose should be repeated if vomiting occurs within 2 hours of taking a dose. If severe vomiting occurs, emergency contraception may be administered vaginally. Studies of vaginally administered combined oral contraceptive pills suggest that the hormones are effectively absorbed through the vaginal epithelium (79, 80).

▶ *Is emergency contraception safe if used repeatedly?*

Data are not available on the safety of current regimens of emergency contraception if used frequently over a long period. However, experience with similar regimens (81) and with high-dose oral contraceptives suggests that the likelihood of serious harm from at least moderate repeat use is low. Therefore, emergency contraception may be used even if the woman has used it before, even within the same menstrual cycle. Information about other forms of contraception and counseling about how to avoid future contraceptive failures should be made available to women who use emergency contraception, especially those who use it repeatedly.

Emergency contraception is less effective than most other available methods for long-term contraception. In addition, continued use would result in exposure to higher total levels of hormones than those of either combined or progestin-only oral contraceptives, and frequent use also would result in more side effects, including menstrual irregularities. Therefore, emergency contraception should not be used as long-term contraception.

▶ *What clinical follow-up is needed after use of emergency contraception?*

No scheduled follow-up is required after use of emergency contraception. However, the woman should be advised that if her menstrual period is delayed by a week or more, she should consider the possibility that she may be pregnant and seek clinical evaluation. A woman also should seek follow-up care for persistent irregular bleeding or lower abdominal pain because these symptoms could indicate a spontaneous abortion or an ectopic pregnancy. Women also should be advised about available resources if they need ongoing contraceptive or other services, such as testing for sexually transmitted diseases, at the time emergency contraception is provided or at some convenient time thereafter.

▶ *When should regular contraception be initiated or resumed after use of emergency contraception?*

Treatment with emergency contraception may not protect against pregnancy in subsequent coital acts (9); in fact, because emergency contraception may work by delaying ovulation, women who have taken emergency contraception are at risk for becoming pregnant later in the same menstrual cycle. Therefore, all women should begin using barrier contraceptives to prevent pregnancy (eg, condoms, diaphragms, and spermicides) immediately after taking emergency contraception. Short-term hormonal contraceptives (eg, pills, patches, and rings) may be started either immediately (with a backup barrier method) or after the next menstrual period. Long-term hormonal methods should be started after the next menstrual period, when it is clear that the patient is not pregnant.

▶ *How can access to emergency contraception be facilitated?*

To maximize the effectiveness of treatment, women should be able to obtain emergency contraception quickly when the need arises. Providing an advance prescription or sup-

ply of emergency contraception, educating staff who may be in contact with the patient about its availability, and prescribing it by phone without requiring an office visit will facilitate access (82).

▶ *When is an intrauterine device appropriate for emergency contraception?*

Use of a copper IUD for emergency contraception, first reported in 1976 (83), has been studied in prospective cohort trials with pregnancy rates of 0–0.1% (84). In these trials, the IUD was inserted up to 5 days after unprotected intercourse. A more recent report of 1,013 women who underwent insertion of a copper IUD for emergency contraception, including 170 nulliparous women, found a pregnancy rate of 0.2% (85). One advantage of the copper IUD for emergency contraception is that it can be retained for continued long-term contraception. The same study found 86% of parous women and 80% of nulliparous women maintained the IUD for contraception. No randomized controlled trials have compared IUD insertion with medical regimens for emergency contraception. A recent meta-analysis concluded that the IUD is very effective for emergency contraception but that further comparative studies are needed (86).

The copper T380A is appropriate for emergency contraception in women who meet standard criteria for IUD insertion and is most effective if inserted within 5 days after unprotected intercourse. This method is particularly useful for women who desire long-term contraception and who are otherwise appropriate candidates for IUD use.

Summary of Recommendations and Conclusions

The following recommendations are based on good and consistent scientific evidence (Level A):

▶ Emergency contraception should be offered or made available to women who have had unprotected or inadequately protected sexual intercourse and who do not desire pregnancy.

▶ The levonorgestrel-only regimen is more effective and is associated with less nausea and vomiting; therefore, if available, it should be used in preference to the combined estrogen–progestin regimen.

▶ The 1.5-mg levonorgestrel-only regimen can be taken as a single dose.

▶ The two 0.75-mg doses of the levonorgestrel-only regimen are equally effective if taken 12–24 hours apart.

▶ To reduce the chance of nausea with the combined estrogen–progestin regimen, an antiemetic agent may be taken 1 hour before the first emergency contraception dose.

▶ Prescription or provision of emergency contraception in advance of need can increase availability and use.

The following recommendations are based on limited or inconsistent scientific evidence (Level B):

▶ Treatment with emergency contraception should be initiated as soon as possible after unprotected or inadequately protected intercourse to maximize efficacy.

▶ Emergency contraception should be made available to patients who request it up to 120 hours after unprotected intercourse.

▶ No clinician examination or pregnancy testing is necessary before provision or prescription of emergency contraception.

The following recommendations are based primarily on consensus and expert opinion (Level C):

▶ No data specifically examine the risk of using hormonal methods of emergency contraception among women with contraindications to the use of conventional oral contraceptive preparations; nevertheless, emergency contraception may be made available to such women.

▶ Clinical evaluation is indicated for women who have used emergency contraception if menses are delayed by a week or more after the expected time or if lower abdominal pain or persistent irregular bleeding develops.

▶ Information regarding effective contraceptive methods should be made available either at the time emergency contraception is prescribed or at some convenient time thereafter.

▶ Emergency contraception may be used even if the woman has used it before, even within the same menstrual cycle.

Additional Resources

Emergency Contraception Hotline: 1-888-NOT-2-LATE

World Wide Web Pages:

- The American College of Obstetricians and Gynecologists: http://www.acog.org
- Emergency Contraception: http://www.not-2-late. com
- International Consortium for Emergency Contraception: http://www.cecinfo.org
- Pastillas Anticonceptivas de Emergencia: http://www.en3dias.org.mx

References

1. Henry J. Kaiser Family Foundation. Emergency contraception in California. Findings from a 2003 Kaiser Family Foundation survey. Menlo Park (CA): KFF; 2004. Available at: http://www.kff.org/womenshealth/upload/Emergency-Contraception-in-California.pdf. Retrieved August 18, 2005. (Level III)

2. Lete I, Cabero C, Alvarez D, Olle C. Observational study on the use of emergency contraception in Spain: results of a national survey. Eur J Contracept Reprod Health Care 2003;8:203–9. (Level II-2)

3. Tyden T, Wetterholm M, Odlind V. Emergency contraception: the user profile. Adv Contracept 1998;14:171–8. (Level III)

4. Gold MA, Wolford JE, Smith KA, Parker AM. The effects of advance provision of emergency contraception on adolescent women's sexual and contraceptive behaviors. J Pediatr Adolesc Gynecol 2004;17:87–96. (Level I)

5. Harvey SM, Beckman LJ, Sherman C, Petitti D. Women's experience and satisfaction with emergency contraception. Fam Plann Perspect 1999;31:237–40, 260. (Level III)

6. Yuzpe AA, Thurlow HJ, Ramzy I, Leyshon JI. Post coital contraception—A pilot study. J Reprod Med 1974;13:53–8. (Level II-3)

7. Kesseru E, Garmendia F, Westphal N, Parada J. The hormonal and peripheral effects of d-norgestrel in postcoital contraception. Contraception 1974;10:411–24. (Level III)

8. Arowojolu AO, Okewole IA, Adekunle AO. Comparative evaluation of the effectiveness and safety of two regimens of levonorgestrel for emergency contraception in Nigerians [published erratum appears in Contraception 2003;67:165]. Contraception 2002;66:269–73. (Level I)

9. von Hertzen H, Piaggio G, Ding J, Chen J, Song S, Bartfai G, et al. Low dose mifepristone and two regimens of levonorgestrel for emergency contraception: a WHO multicentre randomised trial. WHO Research Group on Post-Ovulatory Methods of Fertility Regulation. Lancet 2002;360:1803–10. (Level I)

10. Ngai SW, Fan S, Li S, Cheng L, Ding J, Jing X, et al. A randomized trial to compare 24 h versus 12 h double dose regimen of levonorgestrel for emergency contraception. Hum Reprod 2005;20:307–11. (Level I)

11. Croxatto HB, Devoto L, Durand M, Ezcurra E, Larrea F, Nagle C, et al. Mechanism of action of hormonal preparations used for emergency contraception: a review of the literature. Contraception 2001;63:111–21. (Level III)

12. Croxatto HB, Ortiz ME, Muller AL. Mechanisms of action of emergency contraception. Steroids 2003;68:1095–8. (Level III)

13. Gemzell-Danielsson K, Marions L. Mechanisms of action of mifepristone and levonorgestrel when used for emergency contraception. Hum Reprod Update 2004;10: 341–8. (Level III)

14. Grimes DA, Raymond EG. Emergency contraception. Ann Intern Med 2002;137:180–9. (Level III)

15. Croxatto HB, Fuentealba B, Brache V, Salvatierra AM, Alvarez F, Massai F, et al. Effects of the Yuzpe regimen, given during the follicular phase, on ovarian function. Contraception 2002;65:121–8. (Level II-3)

16. Durand M, del Carmen Cravioto M, Raymond EG, Duran-Sanchez O, De la Luz Cruz-Hinojosa M, Castell-Rodriguez A, et al. On the mechanisms of action of short-term levonorgestrel administration in emergency contraception. Contraception 2001;64:227–34. (Level I)

17. Hapangama D, Glasier AF, Baird DT. The effects of peri-ovulatory administration of levonorgestrel on the menstrual cycle. Contraception 2001;63:123–9. (Level II-3)

18. Ling WY, Robichaud A, Zayid I, Wrixon W, MacLeod SC. Mode of action of DL-norgestrel and ethinylestradiol combination in postcoital contraception. Fertil Steril 1979;32:297–302. (Level II-3)

19. Marions L, Hultenby K, Lindell I, Sun X, Stabi B, Gemzell-Danielsson K. Emergency contraception with mifepristone and levonorgestrel: mechanism of action. Obstet Gynecol 2002;100:65–71. (Level II-3)

20. Marions L, Cekan SZ, Bygdeman M, Gemzell-Danielsson K. Effect of emergency contraception with levonorgestrel or mifepristone on ovarian function. Contraception 2004;69:373–7. (Level II-2)

21. Swahn ML, Westlund P, Johannisson E, Bygdeman M. Effect of post-coital contraceptive methods on the endometrium and the menstrual cycle. Acta Obstet Gynecol Scand 1996;75:738–44. (Level II-2)

22. Kubba AA, White JO, Guillebaud J, Elder MG. The biochemistry of human endometrium after two regimens of postcoital contraception: a dl-norgestrel/ethinylestradiol combination or danazol. Fertil Steril 1986;45:512–6. (Level III)

23. Ling WY, Wrixon W, Zayid I, Acorn T, Popat R, Wilson E. Mode of action of dl-norgestrel and ethinylestradiol combination in postcoital contraception. II. Effect of postovulatory administration on ovarian function and endometrium. Fertil Steril 1983;39:292–7. (Level II-3)

24. Young DC, Wiehle RD, Joshi SG, Poindexter AN 3rd. Emergency contraception alters progesterone-associated endometrial protein in serum and uterine luminal fluid. Obstet Gynecol 1994;84:266–71. (Level III)

25. Muller AL, Llados CM, Croxatto HB. Postcoital treatment with levonorgestrel does not disrupt postfertilization events in the rat. Contraception 2003;67:415–9. (Level III)

26. Ortiz ME, Ortiz RE, Fuentes MA, Parraguez VH, Croxatto HB. Post-coital administration of levonorgestrel does not interfere with post-fertilization events in the new-world monkey Cebus apella. Hum Reprod 2004; 19:1352–6. (Level III)

27. Raymond EG, Lovely LP, Chen-Mok M, Seppala M, Kurman RJ, Lessey BA. Effect of the Yuzpe regimen of emergency contraception on markers of endometrial receptivity. Hum Reprod 2000;15:2351–5. (Level II-2)

28. Taskin O, Brown RW, Young DC, Poindexter AN, Wiehle RD. High doses of oral contraceptives do not alter endometrial alpha 1 and alpha v beta 3 integrins in the late implantation window. Fertil Steril 1994;61:850–5. (Level III)

29. Kesseru E, Camacho-Ortega P, Laudahn G, Schopflin G. In vitro action of progestogens on sperm migration in human cervical mucus. Fertil Steril 1975;26:57–61. (Level II-3)

30. Ling WY, Wrixon W, Acorn T, Wilson E, Collins J. Mode of action of dl-norgestrel and ethinylestradiol combination in postcoital contraception. III. Effect of preovulatory administration following the luteinizing hormone surge on ovarian steroidogenesis. Fertil Steril 1983;40:631–6. (Level II-3)

31. Trussell J, Raymond EG. Statistical evidence about the mechanism of action of the Yuzpe regimen of emergency contraception. Obstet Gynecol 1999;93:872–6. (Level III)

32. Conard LA, Gold MA. Emergency contraceptive pills: a review of the recent literature. Curr Opin Obstet Gynecol 2004;16:389–95. (Level III)

33. Bacic M, Wesselius de Casparis A, Diczfalusy E. Failure of large doses of ethinyl estradiol to interfere with early embryonic development in the human species. Am J Obstet Gynecol 1970;107:531–4. (Level III)

34. Vasilakis C, Jick SS, Jick H. The risk of venous thromboembolism in users of postcoital contraceptive pills. Contraception 1999;59:79–83. (Level II-2)

35. Ho PC, Kwan MS. A prospective randomized comparison of levonorgestrel with the Yuzpe regimen in post-coital contraception. Hum Reprod 1993;8:389–92. (Level I)

36. Randomised controlled trial of levonorgestrel versus the Yuzpe regimen of combined oral contraceptives for emergency contraception. Task Force on Postovulatory Methods of Fertility Regulation. Lancet 1998;352:428–33. (Level I)

37. Raymond EG, Creinin MD, Barnhart KT, Lovvorn AE, Rountree RW, Trussell J. Meclizine for prevention of nausea associated with use of emergency contraceptive pills: a randomized trial. Obstet Gynecol 2000;95:271–7. (Level I)

38. Van Santen MR, Haspels AA. Interception II: postcoital low-dose estrogens and norgestrel combination in 633 women. Contraception 1985;31:275–93. (Level II-3)

39. Prescription drug products; certain combined oral contraceptives for use as postcoital emergency contraception; notice. Fed Regist 1997;62:8609–12. (Level III)

40. Trussell J, Hedley A, Raymond E. Ectopic pregnancy following use of progestin-only ECPs. J Fam Plann Reprod Health Care 2003;29:249. (Level III)

41. Breckenridge AM, Back DJ, Orme M. Interactions between oral contraceptives and other drugs. Pharmacol Ther 1979;7:617–26. (Level III)

42. Dickinson BD, Altman RD, Nielsen NH, Sterling ML. Drug interactions between oral contraceptives and antibi-

otics. Council on Scientific Affairs, American Medical Association. Obstet Gynecol 2001;98:853–60. (Level III)

43. Geurts TB, Goorissen EM, Sitsen JM. Summary of drug interactions with oral contraceptives. Carnforth, Lancs (UK); Pearl River (NY): Parthenon Publishing Group; 1993.

44. Shenfield GM. Drug interactions with oral contraceptive preparations. Med J Aust 1986;144:205–11. (Level III)

45. Szoka PR, Edgren RA. Drug interactions with oral contraceptives: compilation and analysis of an adverse experience report database. Fertil Steril 1988;49:31S–8S. (Level III)

46. Abbott J, Feldhaus KM, Houry D, Lowenstein SR. Emergency contraception: what do our patients know? Ann Emerg Med 2004;43:376–81. (Level III)

47. Foster DG, Harper CC, Bley JJ, Mikanda JJ, Indunia M, Saviano EC, et al. Knowledge of emergency contraception among women aged 18 to 44 in California. Am J Obstet Gynecol 2004;191:150–6. (Level III)

48. Isaacs JN, Creinin MD. Miscommunication between healthcare providers and patients may result in unplanned pregnancies. Contraception 2003;68:373–6. (Level III)

49. Romo LF, Berenson AB, Wu ZH. The role of misconceptions on Latino women's acceptance of emergency contraceptive pills. Contraception 2004;69:227–35. (Level III)

50. Spence MR, Elgen KK, Harwell TS. Awareness, prior use, and intent to use emergency contraception among Montana women at the time of pregnancy testing. Matern Child Health J 2003;7:197–203. (Level III)

51. Golden NH, Seigel WM, Fisher M, Schneider M, Quijano E, Suss A, et al. Emergency contraception: pediatricians' knowledge, attitudes, and opinions. Pediatrics 2001;107:287–92. (Level III)

52. Khan Y, Sbrocca N, Stanojevic S, Penava D. Exposure to emergency contraception in an undergraduate medical curriculum. J Obstet Gynaecol Can 2003;25:391–5. (Level III)

53. Sherman CA, Harvey SM, Beckman LJ, Petitti DB. Emergency contraception: knowledge and attitudes of health care providers in a health maintenance organization [published erratum appears in Womens Health Issues 2001;11:503]. Womens Health Issues 2001;11:448–57. (Level III)

54. Brening RK, Dalve-Endres AM, Patrick K. Emergency contraception pills (ECPs): current trends in United States college health centers. Contraception 2003;67:449–56. (Level III)

55. Wallace JL, Wu J, Weinstein J, Gorenflo DW, Fetters MD. Emergency contraception: knowledge and attitudes of family medicine providers. Fam Med 2004;36:417–22. (Level III)

56. Bennett W, Petraitis C, D'Anella A, Marcella S. Pharmacists' knowledge and the difficulty of obtaining emergency contraception. Contraception 2003;68:261–7. (Level III)

57. Rovi S, Shimoni N. Prophylaxis provided to sexual assault victims seen at US emergency departments. J Am Med Womens Assoc 2002;57:204–7. (Level II-3)

58. Karasz A, Kirchen NT, Gold M. The visit before the morning after: barriers to preprescribing emergency contraception. Ann Fam Med 2004;2:345–50. (Level III)

59. Ellertson C, Ambardekar S, Hedley A, Coyaji K, Trussell J, Blanchard K. Emergency contraception: randomized comparison of advance provision and information only. Obstet Gynecol 2001;98:570–5. (Level I)

60. Glasier A, Baird D. The effects of self-administering emergency contraception. N Engl J Med 1998;339:1–4. (Level II-1)

61. Jackson RA, Bimla Schwarz E, Freedman L, Darney P. Advance supply of emergency contraception. Effect on use and usual contraception—a randomized trial. Obstet Gynecol 2003;102:8–16. (Level I)

62. Lo SS, Fan SY, Ho PC, Glasier AF. Effect of advanced provision of emergency contraception on women's contraceptive behaviour: a randomized controlled trial. Hum Reprod 2004;19:2404–10. (Level I)

63. Raine T, Harper C, Leon K, Darney P. Emergency contraception: advance provision in a young, high-risk clinic population. Obstet Gynecol 2000;96:1–7. (Level II-1)

64. Raine TR, Harper CC, Rocca CH, Fischer R, Padian N, Klausner JD, et al. Direct access to emergency contraception through pharmacies and effect on unintended pregnancy and STIs: a randomized controlled trial. JAMA 2005;293:54–62. (Level I)

65. World Health Organization. Medical eligibility criteria for contraceptive use. 3rd ed. Geneva: WHO; 2004. Available at: http://www.who.int/reproductive-health/publications/med/mec.pdf. Retrieved August 18, 2005. (Level III)

66. Piaggio G, von Hertzen H, Grimes DA, Van Look PF. Timing of emergency contraception with levonorgestrel or the Yuzpe regimen. Task Force on Postovulatory Methods of Fertility Regulation. Lancet 1999;353:721. (Level III)

67. Kane LA, Sparrow MJ. Postcoital contraception: a family planning study. N Z Med J 1989;102:151–3. (Level II-3)

68. Trussell J, Ellertson C, von Hertzen H, Bigrigg A, Webb A, Evans M, et al. Estimating the effectiveness of emergency contraceptive pills. Contraception 2003;67:259–65. (Level III)

69. Trussell J, Ellertson C, Rodriguez G. The Yuzpe regimen of emergency contraception: how long after the morning after? Obstet Gynecol 1996;88:150–4. (Meta-analysis)

70. Ellertson C, Evans M, Ferden S, Leadbetter C, Spears A, Johnstone K, et al. Extending the time limit for starting the Yuzpe regimen of emergency contraception to 120 hours. Obstet Gynecol 2003;101:1168–71. (Level II-3)

71. Grou F, Rodrigues I. The morning-after pill—how long after? Am J Obstet Gynecol 1994;171:1529–34. (Meta-analysis)

72. Rodrigues I, Grou F, Joly J. Effectiveness of emergency contraceptive pills between 72 and 120 hours after unprotected sexual intercourse. Am J Obstet Gynecol 2001;184:531–7. (Level II-2)

73. Hamoda H, Ashok PW, Stalder C, Flett GM, Kennedy E, Templeton A. A randomized trial of mifepristone (10 mg)

and levonorgestrel for emergency contraception. Obstet Gynecol 2004;104:1307–13. (Level I)

74. Trussell J, Rodriguez G, Ellertson C. Updated estimates of the effectiveness of the Yuzpe regimen of emergency contraception. Contraception 1999;59:147–51. (Level III)

75. Raymond E, Taylor D, Trussell J, Steiner MJ. Minimum effectiveness of the levonorgestrel regimen of emergency contraception. Contraception 2004;69:79–81. (Level III)

76. Rowlands S, Guillebaud J, Bounds W, Booth M. Side effects of danazol compared with an ethinyloestradiol/norgestrel combination when used for postcoital contraception. Contraception 1983;27:39–49. (Level I)

77. Ragan RE, Rock RW, Buck HW. Metoclopramide pretreatment attenuates emergency contraceptive-associated nausea. Am J Obstet Gynecol 2003;188:330–3. (Level II-1)

78. Ellertson C, Webb A, Blanchard K, Bigrigg A, Haskell S, Shochet T, et al. Modifying the Yuzpe regimen of emergency contraception: a multicenter randomized controlled trial. Obstet Gynecol 2003;101:1160–7. (Level I)

79. Alvarez F, Faundes A, Johansson E, Coutinho E. Blood levels of levonorgestrel in women following vaginal placement of contraceptive pills. Fertil Steril 1983;40:120–3. (Level III)

80. Back DJ, Grimmer SF, Rogers S, Stevenson PJ, Orme ML. Comparative pharmacokinetics of levonorgestrel and ethinyloestradiol following intravenous, oral and vaginal administration. Contraception 1987;36:471–9. (Level II-3)

81. Efficacy and side effects of immediate postcoital levonorgestrel used repeatedly for contraception. United Nations Development Programme/United Nations Population Fund/World Health Organization/World Bank Special Programme of Research, Development and Research Training in Human Reproduction, Task Force on Post-Ovulatory Methods of Fertility Regulation. Contraception 2000;61:303–8. (Level II-3)

82. Raymond EG, Spruyt A, Bley K, Colm J, Gross S, Robbins LA. The North Carolina DIAL EC project: increasing access to emergency contraceptive pills by telephone. Contraception 2004;69:367–72. (Level III)

83. Lippes J, Malik T, Tatum HJ. The postcoital copper-T. Adv Plan Parent 1976;11:24–9. (Level III)

84. Trussell J, Leveque JA, Koenig JD, London R, Borden S, Henneberry J, et al. The economic value of contraception: a comparison of 15 methods. Am J Public Health 1995;85:494–503. (Level III)

85. Zhou L, Xiao B. Emergency contraception with Multiload Cu-375 SL IUD: a multicenter clinical trial. Contraception 2001;64:107–12. (Level I)

86. Cheng L, Gülmezoglu AM, Van Oel CJ, Piaggio G, Ezcurra E, Van Look PF. Interventions for emergency contraception. The Cochrane Database of Systematic Reviews 2004, Issue 3. Art. No.: CD001324. DOI: 10.1002/14651858.CD001324.pub2. (Meta-analysis)

The MEDLINE database, the Cochrane Library, and the American College of Obstetricians and Gynecologists' own internal resources and documents were used to conduct a literature search to locate relevant articles published between January 1985 and January 2005. The search was restricted to articles published in the English language. Priority was given to articles reporting results of original research, although review articles and commentaries also were consulted. Abstracts of research presented at symposia and scientific conferences were not considered adequate for inclusion in this document. Guidelines published by organizations or institutions such as the National Institutes of Health and ACOG were reviewed, and additional studies were located by reviewing bibliographies of identified articles. When reliable research was not available, expert opinions from obstetrician–gynecologists were used.

Studies were reviewed and evaluated for quality according to the method outlined by the U.S. Preventive Services Task Force:

I   Evidence obtained from at least one properly designed randomized controlled trial.

II-1 Evidence obtained from well-designed controlled trials without randomization.

II-2 Evidence obtained from well-designed cohort or case–control analytic studies, preferably from more than one center or research group.

II-3 Evidence obtained from multiple time series with or without the intervention. Dramatic results in uncontrolled experiments also could be regarded as this type of evidence.

III Opinions of respected authorities, based on clinical experience, descriptive studies, or reports of expert committees.

Based on the highest level of evidence found in the data, recommendations are provided and graded according to the following categories:

Level A—Recommendations are based on good and consistent scientific evidence.

Level B—Recommendations are based on limited or inconsistent scientific evidence.

Level C—Recommendations are based primarily on consensus and expert opinion.

ISSN 1099-3630

The American College of Obstetricians and Gynecologists
409 12th Street, SW, PO Box 96920, Washington, DC 20090-6920

12345/98765

Emergency contraception. ACOG Practice Bulletin No. 69. American College of Obstetricians and Gynecologists. Obstet Gynecol 2005; 106:1443–52.

ACOG PRACTICE BULLETIN

CLINICAL MANAGEMENT GUIDELINES FOR
OBSTETRICIAN–GYNECOLOGISTS

NUMBER 13, FEBRUARY 2000

(Replaces Practice Pattern Number 4, July 1997)

This Practice Bulletin was developed by the ACOG Committee on Practice Bulletins—Obstetrics. The information is designed to aid practitioners in making decisions about appropriate obstetric and gynecologic care. These guidelines should not be construed as dictating an exclusive course of treatment or procedure. Variations in practice may be warranted based on the needs of the individual patient, resources, and limitations unique to the institution or type of practice.

External Cephalic Version

In the United States, there is a widespread belief that the overall cesarean delivery rate is higher than necessary. Efforts are being directed toward decreasing the number of these procedures, in part by encouraging physicians to make changes in their management practices. Because breech presentations are associated with a high rate of cesarean delivery, there is renewed interest in techniques such as external cephalic version (ECV) and vaginal breech delivery. The purpose of this document is to provide information about ECV by summarizing the relevant evidence presented in published studies and to make recommendations regarding its use in obstetric practice.

Background

Breech presentation occurs in 3–4% of term pregnancies. In 1997, 84.5% of all malpresentations, including breech presentation, resulted in cesarean deliveries (1). External cephalic version involves applying pressure to the mother's abdomen to turn the fetus in either a forward or backward somersault to achieve a vertex presentation. The goal of ECV is to increase the proportion of vertex presentations among fetuses that were formerly in the breech position near term. Once a vertex presentation is achieved, the chances for a vaginal delivery increase.

Clinical Considerations and Recommendations

▶ *Which patients are candidates for external cephalic version?*

Patients who have completed 36 weeks of gestation are preferred candidates for ECV for several reasons. First, if spontaneous version is going to occur, it is likely to have taken place by 36 completed weeks of gestation (2, 3). Second, risk of a spontaneous reversion is decreased after external cephalic version at term compared with earlier gestations. Preterm version attempts are associated with high initial success rates but also with higher reversion rates, necessitating additional procedures (4, 5). Third, if complications arise during an attempted version, emergency delivery of a term infant can be accomplished (6). Finally, most of the evidence pertaining to ECV comes from recent studies that selected patients near term.

There is scant information concerning ECV attempts among women who have a preexisting uterine scar or who undergo the procedure during the early stages of labor. For women with a previous cesarean delivery, compared with those who had not experienced cesarean delivery, results from one small randomized controlled trial indicate that they experience comparable success rates (7). Although no serious adverse events occurred in a small series (8), larger studies would be needed to establish the risk of uterine rupture. There are scattered reports of successful ECV performed during early labor; to date, however, no large study has been published (4, 5, 9, 10).

Contraindications to ECV are based on a common-sense approach designed to minimize the risks of an adverse outcome and to maximize the chances for success. Clearly any indication for a cesarean delivery in a patient, such as placenta previa, would be a contraindication to ECV (4, 9, 11–20), but there is insufficient evidence to construct a comprehensive list.

▶ *What are the benefits and risks of external cephalic version?*

The immediate benefit of successful version is an increased probability that the fetus will be in a vertex presentation for delivery. The ultimate goal is an uncomplicated vaginal delivery. Reports from published studies indicate there are fewer cesarean deliveries among women who have undergone successful version compared with women who have not undergone attempted version (4, 6, 18, 21–24). One randomized trial found no significant difference between the cesarean delivery rates of patients with an ECV attempt and controls who did not undergo ECV (25). In this study, however, the majority of patients undergoing ECV were between 33 and 36 weeks of gestation rather than closer to term as in the other reports. An additional randomized trial reported similar rates of cesarean delivery for women who underwent ECV and for those who did not, but the rate of breech vaginal deliveries was very high; approximately 80% of breech presentations in each group was delivered vaginally, resulting in an unusually low cesarean delivery rate (4).

Fetal heart rate changes during attempted versions are not uncommon but usually stabilize when the procedure is discontinued (4, 21, 23, 26, 27). Serious adverse effects associated with ECV do not occur often, but there have been a few reported cases of placental abruption and preterm labor. A report from Copenhagen described two cases of intrauterine death 2 and 5 weeks after version among 316 women and one instance of premature partial separation of the placenta 2 days following an unsuccessful version attempt, but the two deaths could not be causally linked to ECV with certainty (16). In the study including mothers at 36 weeks of gestation or less, two placental abruptions and one premature labor occurred shortly after version, resulting in one neonatal and two fetal deaths (25). Subsequently, there has been a follow-up study at the same institution, but changes in management practices and selection criteria had been made (18). Only term gestations were selected, and tocolytic agents as well as fetal monitoring were used during version attempts. There were no fetal deaths causally linked to ECV. The authors concluded that ECV can substantially decrease breech presentations and the cesarean delivery rate for these patients (18). A more recent study reported a placental abruption during an ECV attempt requiring emergency cesarean delivery of a viable but depressed infant (28). It was the only major complication attributed to ECV among 113 women. Although the incidence of serious complications associated with ECV is low, the potential is present, making it prudent to perform ECV in a facility that has ready access to cesarean delivery services.

▶ *What are the success rates for external cephalic version, and what factors are predictive of either success or failure?*

A review of 20 studies indicates that success rates for ECV range from 35% to 86%, with an average success rate of 58% (4, 6, 9, 12–14, 16–18, 21–25, 27, 29–31). Most authors report a positive association between parity and successful version (4, 6, 13, 21–25, 30, 31). A transverse or oblique lie is associated with higher immediate success rates (13, 29, 30). Opinion is divided about the predictiveness of other factors, including amniotic fluid volume, location of placenta, and maternal weight. Some reports indicate an association between normal or increased amounts of amniotic fluid and successful ECV (12, 13, 24, 32), whereas other reports do not (20). Two authors reported an association between successful ECV and placenta location (20, 24), whereas others failed to find an association (12, 13, 29). Two authors found obesity to be associated with a higher failure rate (23, 30), whereas others found maternal weight not to be a significant predictor of success (12, 13, 19, 20).

Although scoring systems have been developed to predict which candidates will have a successful version attempt, these have not been validated by multiple studies. One system considered parity, dilatation, estimated fetal weight, placenta location, and station. Nulliparity, advanced dilatation, fetal weight of less than 2,500 g, anterior placenta, and low station were less likely to be associated with success (20). Such variables may provide useful clinical information for obtaining informed consent from individuals for ECV; no single system, however, has been shown to have complete accuracy.

▶ How does the use of tocolysis affect the success rate of external cephalic version?

Two of six randomized controlled trials failed to find a significant advantage in using tocolytics during ECV attempts (19, 27). One third reported significantly greater success associated with hexoprenaline but not with ritodrine (33). An additional randomized study reported an initial advantage associated with the use of ritodrine, specifically among nulliparous women. However, as the physicians became proficient at the ECV technique, the advantage diminished (34). The largest randomized study using a ritodrine infusion found significant improvement only among nulliparous patients (35). Finally, a randomized study of terbutaline found the success rate of version associated with use of this tocolytic to be almost double the rate without its use (36). In the vast majority of published studies, a tocolytic agent was used routinely (6, 11–18, 20–23, 27–29, 37). Several studies used tocolytics selectively (5, 7, 9, 34), and some used no tocolytic agents (4, 25). Existing evidence may support the use of a tocolytic agent during ECV attempts, particularly in nulliparous patients.

▶ Does successful version translate into lower cesarean delivery rates?

Whether ECV results in a lower cesarean delivery rate for women with breech presentation who elect this procedure compared with those women who do not depends upon several factors. Obviously, the first factor is whether the version is successful. Clearly, women who have successful version have lower cesarean delivery rates than those who do not (6, 9, 12–14, 21–24, 26, 29, 30). Two randomized studies also have shown a significant decrease in cesarean delivery rates among patients assigned to version compared with those not assigned to version (18, 23). Factors that tend to lessen overall differences between version and nonversion groups include spontaneous conversion of presentation from breech to vertex or vice versa and the willingness of providers to perform vaginal breech deliveries. Clearly, cesarean delivery rates

for version and nonversion groups will be less when there is a greater willingness to attempt a vaginal breech delivery. The need to perform a cesarean delivery for other indications in women who have had a successful version also may lessen the overall impact of version on the cesarean delivery rate. One author has reported that women who have had successful ECV have higher cesarean delivery rates due to fetal distress and dystocia compared with matched controls who never required the procedure (31).

Although ECV may not lead to a substantial reduction in the national cesarean delivery rate, it is nonetheless a valuable management technique. In a properly selected population, this procedure poses little risk to either mother or fetus. If successful, ECV provides a clear benefit to the individual woman by allowing her an opportunity for a successful vertex vaginal delivery.

▶ How does the use of anesthesia affect the success rate of external cephalic version?

A randomized study found a significantly greater success rate associated with the use of epidural anesthesia, although the success rate was unusually low for the women who did not receive epidural anesthesia (32%) (38). Two studies reported results for women in whom ECV was performed while using epidural anesthesia (10, 15). In one study, use of epidural anesthesia was associated with a significantly greater success rate compared with no use of epidural anesthesia (15). However, the procedure was administered selectively to patients according to physician preference, raising the potential for selection bias. The other study merely noted that ECV was performed without difficulty on three women undergoing epidural anesthesia (10). It also has been suggested that epidural anesthesia be considered for women who failed a previous version attempt (39). Another randomized trial addressed the use of spinal anesthesia before the version attempt and found no significant difference between treatment groups (40). Currently, there is not enough consistent evidence to make a recommendation favoring spinal or epidural anesthesia during ECV attempts.

▶ What is an example of a standard protocol for performing an external cephalic version attempt?

Prior to attempting ECV, patients must provide informed consent and should undergo an ultrasound examination. The ultrasound examination is necessary to confirm the breech position of the fetus and rule out the presence of any anomalies that would complicate a vaginal delivery.

Fetal well-being should be assessed by a prior nonstress test or concurrent biophysical profile (see Fig. 1).

Because there is a chance that an expedient delivery may become necessary, patients should have ready access to a facility that is equipped to perform emergency cesarean deliveries. One version technique involves lifting the breech upward from the pelvis with one hand and providing pressure on the head with the other hand to produce a forward roll. If the forward roll fails, a backward somer-

sault may be attempted. Version may be performed by one person or two. A version attempt will be abandoned if there is significant fetal bradycardia, if there is discomfort to the patient, or if the attempt cannot be completed easily or is unsuccessful after a brief period. Following the attempt, fetal evaluation is repeated and the patient is monitored until stable. Rh-negative patients may receive anti-D immune globulin. There is no support for routine practice of immediate induction of labor to minimize reversion.

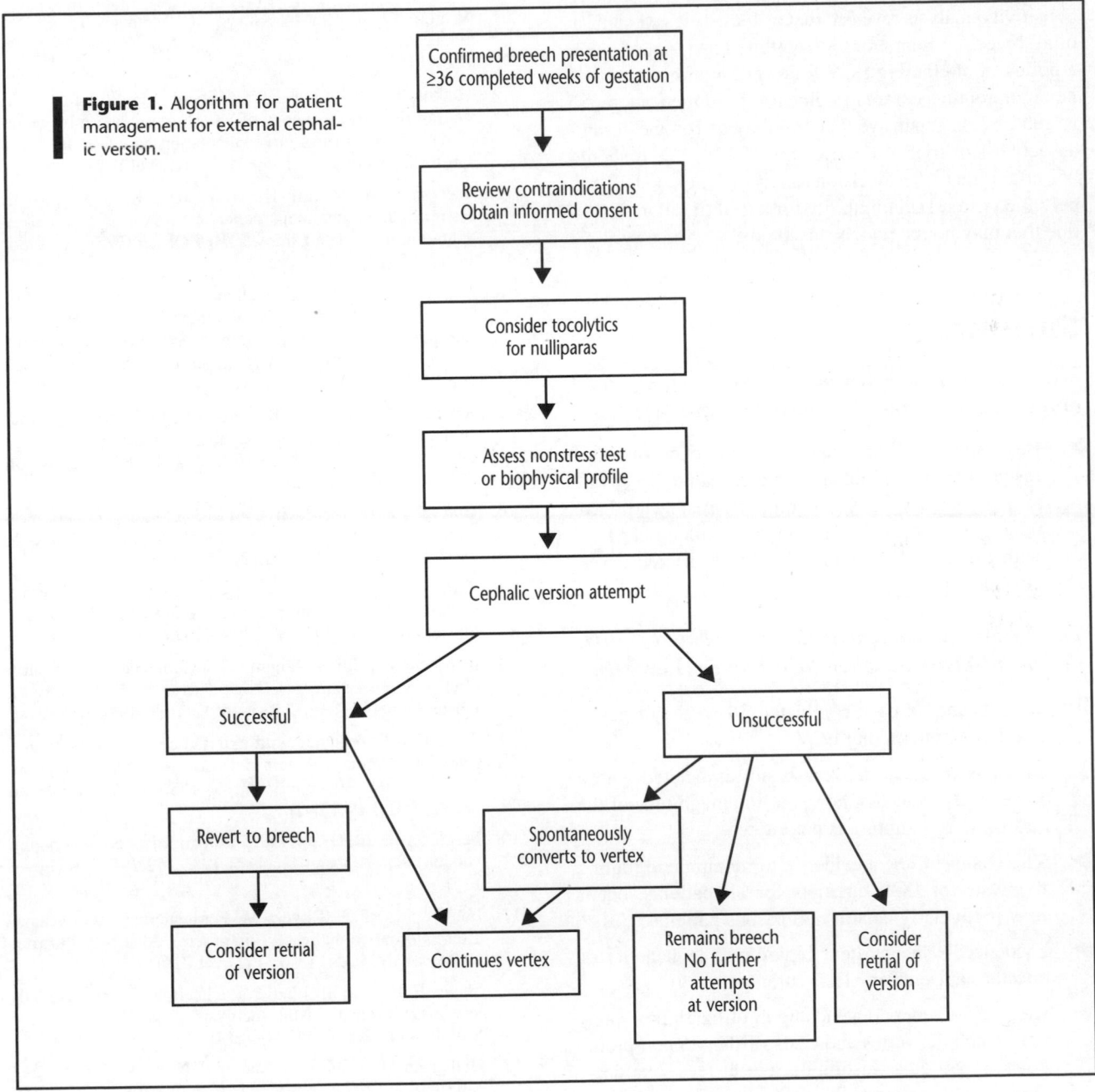

Figure 1. Algorithm for patient management for external cephalic version.

▶ *What are the cost implications of external cephalic version?*

A recent decision analysis measuring cost implications associated with four potential methods of managing term pregnancies with breech presentations predicted that use of ECV would result in fewer cesarean deliveries and lower costs than either scheduled cesarean delivery or trial of labor without an ECV attempt (41). Even if failed ECV attempts were followed by routine cesarean delivery, the overall cesarean delivery rate would be lower than that of a trial of labor without an ECV attempt. Sensitivity analysis revealed that as long as less than 52% of all breech presentations are eligible for a trial of labor, a policy of attempting ECV followed by either a trial of labor or routine cesarean delivery (for failed attempts) would be less expensive than a policy of routine cesarean delivery or trial of labor without ECV (41). It should be noted that the decision analysis included X-ray pelvimetry to assess eligibility for a trial of labor, a practice that may not be widely accepted.

Summary

The following recommendation is based on good and consistent scientific evidence (Level A):

▶ Because the risk of an adverse event occurring as a result of ECV is small and the cesarean delivery rate is significantly lower among women who have undergone successful version, all women near term with breech presentations should be offered a version attempt.

The following recommendations are based on limited or inconsistent scientific evidence (Level B):

▶ Patients should have completed 36 weeks of gestation before attempting ECV.

▶ Previous cesarean delivery is not associated with a lower rate of success; however, the magnitude of the risk of uterine rupture is not known.

▶ There is insufficient evidence to recommend routine tocolysis for ECV attempts for all patients, but it may particularly benefit nulliparous patients.

▶ Evidence is inconsistent regarding the benefits of anesthesia use during ECV attempts.

▶ Cost-effectiveness depends upon utilization of vaginal breech deliveries and costs of the version protocol at a particular institution, but at least one decision analysis suggests the policy is cost effective.

The following recommendations are based primarily on consensus and expert opinion (Level C):

▶ Fetal assessment before and after the procedure is recommended.

▶ External cephalic version should be attempted only in settings in which cesarean delivery services are readily available.

References

1. Ventura SJ, Martin JA, Curtin SC, Mathews TJ. Births: final data for 1997. Natl Vital Stat Rep 1999;47(18):1–96 (Level II-3)

2. Hickok DE, Gordon DC, Milberg JA, Williams MA, Daling JR. The frequency of breech presentation by gestational age at birth: a large population-based study. Am J Obstet Gynecol 1992;166:851–852 (Level II-2)

3. Westgren M, Edvall H, Nordstrom L, Svalenius E, Ranstam J. Spontaneous cephalic version of breech presentation in the last trimester. Br J Obstet Gynaecol 1985; 92:19–22 (Level II-3)

4. Van Veelen AJ, Van Cappellen AW, Flu PK, Straub MJ, Wallenburg HC. Effect of external cephalic version in late pregnancy on presentation at delivery: a randomized controlled trial. Br J Obstet Gynaecol 1989;96:916–921 (Level I)

5. Kornman MT, Kimball KT, Reeves KO. Preterm external cephalic version in an outpatient environment. Am J Obstet Gynecol 1995;172:1734–1738; discussion 1738–1741 (Level II-2)

6. Goh JT, Johnson CM, Gregora MG. External cephalic version at term. Aust N Z J Obstet Gynaecol 1993;33:364–366 (Level II-2)

7. Flamm BL, Fried MW, Lonky NM, Giles WS. External cephalic version after previous cesarean section. Am J Obstet Gynecol 1991;165;370–372 (Level I)

8. de Meeus JB, Ellia F, Magnin G. External cephalic version after previous cesarean section: a series of 38 cases. Eur J Obstet Gynecol Reprod Biol 1998;81:65–68 (Level III)

9. Cook HA. Experience with external cephalic version and selective vaginal breech delivery in private practice. Am J Obstet Gynecol 1993;168:1886–1889; discussion 1889–1890 (Level II-3)

10. Ferguson JE 2d, Dyson DC. Intrapartum external cephalic version. Am J Obstet Gynecol 1985;152:297–298 (Level II-3)

11. Lau TK, Stock A, Rogers M. Fetomaternal haemorrhage after external cephalic version at term. Aust N Z J Obstet Gynaecol 1995;35:173–174 (Level III)

12. Shalev E, Battino S, Giladi Y, Edelstein S. External cephalic version at term—using tocolysis. Acta Obstet Gynecol Scand 1993;72:455–457 (Level II-3)

13. Hellstrom AC, Nilsson B, Stange L, Nylund L. When does external cephalic version succeed? Acta Obstet Gynecol Scand 1990;69:281–285 (Level II-3)

14. Morrison JC, Myatt RE, Martin JN Jr, Meeks GR, Martin RW, Bucovaz ET, et al. External cephalic version of the breech presentation under tocolysis. Am J Obstet Gynecol 1986;154:900–903 (Level II-3)

15. Carlan SJ, Dent JM, Huckaby T, Whittington EC, Shaefer D. The effect of epidural anesthesia on safety and success of external cephalic version at term. Anesth Analg 1994;79:525–528 (Level II-3)

16. Thunedborg P, Fischer-Rasmussen W, Tollund L. The benefit of external cephalic version with tocolysis as a routine procedure in late pregnancy. Eur J Obstet Gynecol Reprod Biol 1991;42:23–27 (Level II-3)

17. Bewley S, Robson SC, Smith M, Glover A, Spencer JA. The introduction of external cephalic version at term into routine clinical practice. Eur J Obstet Gynecol Reprod Biol 1993;52:89–93 (Level II-3)

18. Mahomed K, Seeras R, Coulson R. External cephalic version at term. A randomized controlled trial using tocolysis. Br J Obstet Gynaecol 1991;98:8–13 (Level I)

19. Tan GW, Jen SW, Tan SL, Salmon YM. A prospective randomised controlled trial of external cephalic version comparing two methods of uterine tocolysis with a non-tocolysis group. Singapore Med J 1989;30:155–158 (Level I)

20. Newman RB, Peacock BS, VanDorsten JP, Hunt HH. Predicting success of external cephalic version. Am J Obstet Gynecol 1993;169:245–249; discussion 249–250 (Level II-3)

21. Dyson DC, Ferguson JE 2d, Hensleigh P. Antepartum external cephalic version under tocolysis. Obstet Gynecol 1986;67:63–68 (Level II-2)

22. Marchick R. Antepartum external cephalic version with tocolysis: a study of term singleton breech presentations. Am J Obstet Gynecol 1988;158:1339–1346 (Level II-2)

23. Brocks V, Philipsen T, Secher NJ. A randomized trial of external cephalic version with tocolysis in late pregnancy. Br J Obstet Gynaecol 1984;91:653–656 (Level II-1)

24. Hofmeyr GJ, Sadan O, Myer IG, Galal KC, Simko G. External cephalic version and spontaneous version rates: ethnic and other determinants. Br J Obstet Gynaecol 1986;93:13–16 (Level II-2)

25. Kasule J, Chimbira TH, Brown IM. Controlled trial of external cephalic version. Br J Obstet Gynaecol 1985;92:14–18 (Level I)

26. Stine LE, Phelan JP, Wallace R, Eglinton GS, Van Dorsten JP, Schifrin BS. Update on external cephalic version performed at term. Obstet Gynecol 1985;65:642–646 (Level II-3)

27. Robertson AW, Kopelman JN, Read JA, Duff P, Magelssen DJ, Dashow EE. External cephalic version at term: is a tocolytic necessary? Obstet Gynecol 1987;70:896–899 (Level I)

28. Calhoun BC, Edgeworth D, Brehm W. External cephalic version at a military teaching hospital: predictors of success. Aust N Z J Obstet Gynaecol 1995;35:277–279 (Level II-3)

29. Donald WL, Barton JJ. Ultrasonography and external cephalic version at term. Am J Obstet Gynecol 1990;162:1542–1545; discussion 1545–1547 (Level II-3)

30. Mauldin JG, Mauldin PD, Feng TI, Adams EK, Durkalski VL. Determining the clinical efficacy and cost savings of successful external cephalic version. Am J Obstet Gynecol 1996;175:1639–1644 (Level II-3)

31. Lau TK, Lo KW, Wan D, Rogers MS. Predictors of successful external cephalic version at term: a prospective study. Br J Obstet Gynaecol 1997;104:798–802 (Level II-3)

32. Healey M, Porter R, Galimberti A. Introducing external cephalic version at 36 weeks or more in a district general hospital: a review and an audit. Br J Obstet Gynaecol 1997;104:1073–1079 (Level II-3)

33. Stock A, Chung T, Rogers M, Ming WW. Randomized, double blind, placebo controlled comparison of ritodrine and hexoprenaline for tocolysis prior to external cephalic version at term. Aust N Z J Obstet Gynaecol 1993;33:265–268 (Level I)

34. Chung T, Neale E, Lau TK, Rogers M. A randomized, double blind, controlled trial of tocolysis to assist external cephalic version in late pregnancy. Acta Obstet Gynecol Scand 1996;75:720–724 (Level I)

35. Marquette GP, Boucher M, Theriault D, Rinfret D. Does the use of a tocolytic agent affect the success rate of external cephalic version? Am J Obstet Gynecol 1996;175:859–861 (Level I)

36. Fernandez CO, Bloom SL, Smulian JC, Ananth CV, Wendel GD Jr. A randomized placebo-controlled evaluation of terbutaline for external cephalic version. Obstet Gynecol 1997;90:775–779 (Level I)

37. Hanss JW Jr. The efficacy of external cephalic version and its impact on the breech experience. Am J Obstet Gynecol 1990;162:1459–1463; discussion 1463–1464 (Level II-3)

38. Schorr SJ, Speights SE, Ross EL, Bofill JA, Rust OA, Norman PF, et al. A randomized trial of epidural anesthesia to improve external cephalic version success. Am J Obstet Gynecol 1997;177:1133–1137 (Level I)

39. Neiger R, Hennessey MD, Patel M. Reattempting failed external cephalic version under epidural anesthesia. Am J Obstet Gynecol 1998;179:1136–1139 (Level III)

40. Dugoff L, Stamm CA, Jones OW 3rd, Mohling SI, Hawkins JL. The effect of spinal anesthesia on the success rate of external cephalic version: a randomized trial. Obstet Gynecol 1999;93:345–349 (Level I)

41. Gifford DS, Keeler E, Kahn KL. Reductions in cost and cesarean rate by routine use of external cephalic version: a decision analysis. Obstet Gynecol 1995;85:930–936 (Level III)

The MEDLINE database, the Cochrane Library, and ACOG's own internal resources and documents were used to conduct a literature search to locate relevant articles published between January 1981 and May 1999. The search was restricted to articles published in the English language. Priority was given to articles reporting results of original research, although review articles and commentaries also were consulted. Abstracts of research presented at symposia and scientific conferences were not considered adequate for inclusion in this document. Guidelines published by organizations or institutions such as the National Institutes of Health and the American College of Obstetricians and Gynecologists were reviewed, and additional studies were located by reviewing bibliographies of identified articles. When reliable research was not available, expert opinions from obstetrician–gynecologists were used.

Studies were reviewed and evaluated for quality according to the method outlined by the U.S. Preventive Services Task Force:

I   Evidence obtained from at least one properly designed randomized controlled trial.
II-1 Evidence obtained from well-designed controlled trials without randomization.
II-2 Evidence obtained from well-designed cohort or case–control analytic studies, preferably from more than one center or research group.
II-3 Evidence obtained from multiple time series with or without the intervention. Dramatic results in uncontrolled experiments could also be regarded as this type of evidence.
III   Opinions of respected authorities, based on clinical experience, descriptive studies, or reports of expert committees.

Based on the highest level of evidence found in the data, recommendations are provided and graded according to the following categories:

Level A—Recommendations are based on good and consistent scientific evidence.

Level B—Recommendations are based on limited or inconsistent scientific evidence.

Level C—Recommendations are based primarily on consensus and expert opinion.

ISSN 1099-3630

The American College of
Obstetricians and Gynecologists
409 12th Street, SW
PO Box 96920
Washington, DC 20090-6920

12345/43210

ACOG PRACTICE BULLETIN

CLINICAL MANAGEMENT GUIDELINES FOR
OBSTETRICIAN–GYNECOLOGISTS

NUMBER 22, NOVEMBER 2000

(Replaces Technical Bulletin Number 159, September 1991)

This Practice Bulletin was developed by the ACOG Committee on Practice Bulletins — Obstetrics with the assistance of William H. Barth, Jr, MD. The information is designed to aid practitioners in making decisions about appropriate obstetric and gynecologic care. These guidelines should not be construed as dictating an exclusive course of treatment or procedure. Variations in practice may be warranted based on the needs of the individual patient, resources, and limitations unique to the institution or type of practice.

Fetal Macrosomia

Suspected fetal macrosomia is a common obstetric condition. As birth weight increases, the likelihood of labor abnormalities, shoulder dystocia, birth trauma, and permanent injury to the neonate increases. The purpose of this document is to quantify those risks, address the accuracy and limitations of methods for estimating fetal weight, and suggest clinical management for the pregnancy with suspected fetal macrosomia.

Background

Definition

Two terms identify excessive fetal growth: *large for gestational age* and *macrosomia*. The term large for gestational age generally implies a birth weight equal to or greater than the 90th percentile for a given gestational age. For years, clinicians have relied on popular fetal growth curves to identify weight cutoffs for the 90th percentile for a given gestational age (1–3). A national reference for fetal growth is now available. A study using the 1991 U.S. Live Birth File of the National Center for Health Statistics reported data for fetal growth based on more than 3.8 million births (4). The 50th, 90th, and 95th percentiles for birth weight from 37 to 42 completed weeks of gestation are shown in Table 1.

The term *fetal macrosomia* implies growth beyond a specific weight, usually 4,000 g or 4,500 g, regardless of the gestational age. Although the risks of morbidity for infants and mothers when birth weight is between 4,000 g and 4,500 g are greater than those of the general obstetric population, these risks increase sharply beyond 4,500 g (5–10). Recent large cohort studies (11–14) further support the continued use of 4,500 g as an appropriate estimated weight beyond which the fetus should be considered macrosomic.

Rather than assigning a different minimum estimated fetal weight for macrosomia among infants of women with diabetes, understanding that maternal diabetes is an independent predictor of fetal morbidity will help avoid confusion. Regardless of their birth weight, infants of women with diabetes have

Table 1. Percentiles for Birth Weight for Gestational Age: U.S. 1991 Single Live Births to Resident Mothers 37–42 Completed Weeks

	Birth Weight (g)		
Gestational Age	50th Percentile	90th Percentile	95th Percentile
37	3,117	3,755	3,956
38	3,263	3,867	4,027
39	3,400	3,980	4,107
40	3,495	4,060	4,185
41	3,527	4,094	4,217
42	3,522	4,098	4,213

Modified from Alexander GR, Himes JH, Kaufman RB, Mor J, Kogan M. A United States national reference for fetal growth. Obstet Gynecol 1996;87:163–168

an increased risk of shoulder dystocia, clavicular fracture, and brachial plexus injury (14, 15–17).

Frequency of Occurrence

Information from the National Center for Health Statistics shows that 10% of all liveborn infants in the United States weigh more than 4,000 g (18). In contrast, only 1.5% weigh more than 4,500 g. The most serious complication of fetal macrosomia is shoulder dystocia. Fortunately, shoulder dystocia is rare, complicating only 1.4% of all vaginal deliveries (19). When birth weight exceeds 4,500 g, however, the risk of shoulder dystocia is increased, with rates reported from 9.2% to 24% (8, 11–14). In the presence of maternal diabetes, birth weights greater than 4,500 g have been associated with rates of shoulder dystocia from 19.9% to 50% (8, 12, 14). Figure 1 shows the relationship between birth weight, maternal diabetes status, spontaneous or assisted vaginal delivery, and the mean frequency of shoulder dystocia based on a study of more than 175,000 deliveries in California in 1992 (14).

Several issues complicate attempts to define precisely the incidence of shoulder dystocia among macrosomic infants. First, clinicians tend to underreport the occurrence of shoulder dystocia (20, 21). Second, the incidence of shoulder dystocia and the likelihood of subsequent fetal injury vary depending on the criteria used to render a diagnosis of dystocia (22). Studies requiring the use of auxiliary maneuvers other than gentle downward traction and episiotomy to effect delivery (16) report a lower overall incidence of shoulder dystocia—but greater proportional fetal morbidity—than those studies with less precise definitions (11). Finally, although macrosomia clearly increases risk, it is important to note that most instances of shoulder dystocia occur unpredictably among infants of normal birth weight (19, 23).

Risk Factors for Macrosomia

A number of factors predispose to newborn macrosomia. A large case–control study examined the relative contributions of proposed risk factors for macrosomia, excluding preexisting diabetes (24). In decreasing order of importance, these risk factors included a prior history of macrosomia, maternal prepregnancy weight, weight gain during pregnancy, multiparity, male fetus, gestational age greater than 40 weeks, ethnicity, maternal birth weight, maternal height, maternal age younger than 17 years, and a positive 50-g glucose screen with a negative result on the 3-hour glucose tolerance test. Although maternal smoking decreases the likelihood of newborn macrosomia (25), it should not be recommended as a protective measure for obvious reasons.

Both pregestational diabetes and gestational diabetes are associated with fetal macrosomia. Even in patients without diabetes, observational cohort studies and case–control studies demonstrate that graded increases in the level of maternal glycemia are associated with increases in newborn birth weight (26, 27). A study reported that 6% of mothers with untreated borderline gestational diabetes delivered infants exceeding 4,500 g, compared with only 2% of women with normal glucose tolerance (28). If gestational diabetes is unrecognized and untreated, the risk of macrosomia may be as high as 20% (29).

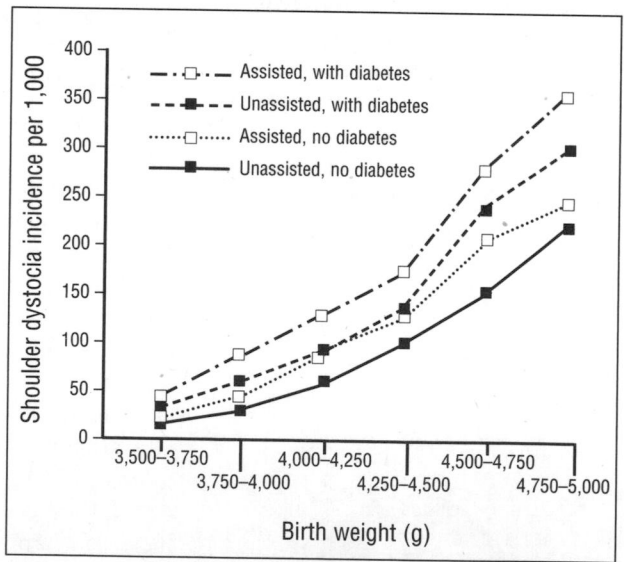

Figure 1. Frequency of shoulder dystocia for increasing birth weight by maternal diabetes status and method of vaginal delivery—spontaneous or assisted. (Nesbitt TS, Gilbert WM, Herrchen B. Shoulder dystocia and associated risk factors with macrosomic infants born in California. Am J Obstet Gynecol 1998;179:476–480)

Anthropometric studies suggest that the macrosomia produced by maternal glucose intolerance is different from that associated with other predisposing factors (30, 31). These macrosomic infants tend to have greater total body fat, greater shoulder and upper-extremity circumferences, greater upper-extremity skin-fold measurements, and smaller head-to-abdominal-circumference ratios than macrosomic infants of mothers without diabetes. Some have suggested that it is this altered fetal body shape that is responsible for the higher incidence of shoulder dystocia seen among infants of women with diabetes (31).

The relative contributions of maternal diabetes and obesity to fetal macrosomia remain controversial. One study reported that the risk for fetal macrosomia associated with unrecognized gestational diabetes persisted after controlling for both maternal body mass index and maternal weight gain (29). In a study among women with diet-controlled gestational diabetes, adjusting for maternal weight decreased the relative risk for large infants (greater than the 90th percentile) from 2.5 to 1.5 (32). Although both diabetes and maternal obesity increase the risk of fetal macrosomia, most agree that maternal obesity plays a greater role (7, 24, 33).

The interaction of maternal weight, weight gain during pregnancy, and newborn macrosomia is complex. There is little doubt that birth weight, in general, increases with maternal body mass index (34–36). Almost all authors report that obese women are more likely than women of normal weight to have large infants (35, 37). However, several issues confound this observation. First, obese women are more likely to have diabetes mellitus. One study demonstrated that morbidly obese women (>300 lb) are eight times more likely to deliver an infant exceeding 4,500 g (38). Second, high weight gain during pregnancy is itself a risk factor for excessive fetal growth (39). The risk of newborn macrosomia associated with excessive maternal weight gain is greater for obese women than for nonobese women (35, 37).

Understandably, gestational age influences birth weight and the risk of macrosomia. Among all races in the United States, the risk of macrosomia increases from 1.6% at term to 2.5% if gestational age exceeds 42 weeks (18). However, as Table 1 shows, there is little additional weight gain after 41 weeks of gestation.

A number of maternal historic factors and habits also influence infant birth weight. Women who have previously delivered an infant weighing more than 4,000 g are five to 10 times more likely to deliver an infant exceeding 4,500 g than women without such a history (5, 24, 40). To a degree, maternal birth weight may predict newborn weight. Women whose own birth weight exceeded 8 lb (approximately 3,600 g) are twice as likely to deliver infants greater than 4,000 g than are women whose birth weight was between 6 lb and 7.9 lb (approximately 2,700–3,500 g) (41). Finally, three cohort studies show that multiparity and grand-multiparity (≥ 5 deliveries) increase the risk of macrosomia (42–44).

Genetic, racial, and ethnic factors also influence birth weight and the risk of macrosomia. Male infants typically weigh more than female infants at any gestational age and, therefore, constitute a greater proportion of infants with birth weights exceeding 4,500 g (12, 45). The risk of macrosomia varies with race and ethnicity as well. Two reports, both of which controlled for diabetes, have demonstrated that Hispanic women have a higher risk of fetal macrosomia than do white, black, or Asian women (46, 47). Genetic factors such as parental height and race play a role in determining newborn birth weight, but these factors interact in a complex manner with environmental factors during pregnancy (48, 49). No combination of these risk factors predicts macrosomia well enough to be used clinically. Much of the variation in birth weights remains unexplained, and most infants greater than 4,500 g do not have identifiable risk factors (6).

Diagnosis

An accurate diagnosis of macrosomia can be made only by weighing the newborn after delivery. Unfortunately, the prenatal diagnosis of fetal macrosomia remains imprecise. Methods used to predict birth weight include assessment of maternal risk factors, clinical examination, and ultrasound measurement of the fetus. Although ultrasonography enables the direct measurement of various fetal body parts, its accuracy in predicting macrosomia has been unreliable (50–52). Furthermore, the superiority of ultrasound-derived estimates of fetal weight over clinical estimates has not been established (53–55). Indeed, parous women are able to predict the weight of their newborns as well as clinicians who use ultrasound measurements or Leopold's maneuvers (56).

Risks Associated with Macrosomia

Maternal Morbidity

The primary maternal risk associated with macrosomia is an increased risk of cesarean delivery. With birth weights greater than 4,500 g, cohort studies show that the risk of cesarean delivery for women attempting a vaginal delivery is at least double that of controls (5, 7, 13, 40). Almost all the increased risk is attributed to labor abnormalities

(5, 11). Not surprisingly, a study has demonstrated that the inaccurate ultrasonographic prediction of macrosomia predisposes to the diagnosis of labor abnormalities and cesarean delivery independent of actual birth weight (57). The risks of postpartum hemorrhage and significant vaginal lacerations also are elevated with macrosomia. A case–control study of risk factors for major obstetric hemorrhage (estimated blood loss >1 L) reported that a birth weight greater than 4,000 g doubled the odds of significant maternal blood loss (odds ratio [OR]: 1.9, 95% confidence interval [CI]: 1.38–2.6) (58). Although the risk of third- and fourth-degree lacerations is slightly increased with macrosomia (12), this is especially true if delivery is complicated by shoulder dystocia (59). Maternal infectious morbidity generally is limited to urinary tract infection in women undergoing elective cesarean delivery (60) and puerperal fever in women undergoing cesarean delivery after a trial of labor (12).

Fetal Morbidity and Mortality

The fetal injuries most commonly associated with macrosomia and shoulder dystocia are fracture of the clavicle and damage to the nerves of the brachial plexus, specifically C5 and C6, producing Erb-Duchenne paralysis. Fracture of the clavicle complicates 0.3–0.7% of all deliveries and usually resolves without permanent sequelae (61–63). For macrosomic infants, the risk of clavicular fracture is increased approximately 10-fold (63).

Brachial plexus injury is rare, with an incidence reported between 0.5 and 1.89 injuries per 1,000 vaginal deliveries (9, 15, 17, 63–65). Case–control studies demonstrate that the risk of brachial plexus injury among infants delivered vaginally is increased 18- to 21-fold when birth weight exceeds 4,500 g (9, 17, 63). Recent reports place the occurrence of brachial plexus injury for macrosomic infants delivered vaginally between 4% and 8% (12, 13, 65). Even though shoulder dystocia is underreported (20), the occurrence of brachial plexus injury in the absence of documented shoulder dystocia is well described (14, 21). Brachial plexus injury has been associated with cesarean delivery (66). As with clavicular fracture, most brachial plexus injuries resolve without permanent handicap. Among 59 confirmed brachial plexus injuries described in the Collaborative Perinatal Project, only 6 (12%) were still evident by age 4 months (64). By age 2 years, all but 4 (7%) had resolved. Other large case series confirm that 80–90% of brachial plexus injuries will resolve by age 1 year (23, 67). However, persistent injury may be more common with birth weights greater than 4,500 g (68). Nonetheless, as with shoulder dystocia, most brachial plexus injuries occur in nonmacrosomic infants (65).

Macrosomia is associated with a number of other risks to the newborn. These infants face an increased risk of depressed 5-minute Apgar scores and increased rates of admission to a neonatal intensive care unit (65). However, most of this risk likely is the result of complications of the birth process, because macrosomic infants do not have higher rates of fetal heart rate abnormalities in labor (5). Finally, overweight newborns are more likely to be overweight later in life than are normal-weight newborns (69).

Clinical Considerations and Recommendations

▶ How accurate are clinical estimates of fetal weight?

The two primary methods for clinical estimation of fetal weight are Leopold's maneuvers (abdominal palpation) and measurement of the height of the uterine fundus above the maternal symphysis pubis. In a prospective study of 602 term patients, clinical palpation alone predicted macrosomia as accurately as any reported ultrasonographic method (53). A study of more than 1,700 women concluded that although ultrasound-derived estimates are more accurate for newborns weighing between 2,500 g and 4,000 g, above this level, ultrasound measurement and clinical palpation have similar accuracy (70).

Measurement of the symphysis–fundal height alone is a poor predictor of fetal macrosomia. Although the average fundal height measurement is greater for fetuses exceeding 4,500 g (71), the utility of this measurement alone is questionable (72). To be useful, measurement of the uterine fundal height must be combined with clinical palpation or Leopold's maneuvers. Prospective studies designed to evaluate Leopold's maneuvers with fundal height measurement for the detection of macrosomia report sensitivities of 10–43%, specificities of 99.0–99.8%, and positive predictive values between 28% and 53% (55, 73). Ultrasound measurements of those women with suspected fetal macrosomia on the basis of clinical examination alone decreased sensitivity and positive predictive value without measurably affecting specificity (73). Prospective studies among women with diabetes also have shown that clinical estimates of macrosomia are as predictive as those derived with ultrasonography (54).

Finally, simply asking a parous woman her estimate of the fetal weight may provide an estimate as accurate as any other. In one study, a parous woman's ability to predict birth weight greater than 4,000 g was as accurate as that of clinicians using Leopold's maneuvers alone (56).

▶ How accurate is ultrasound measurement in determining fetal weight?

Ultrasound-derived estimates of fetal weight are obtained by entering the measurements of various fetal body parts, usually including the abdominal circumference, into one of several popular regression equations (74, 75). Most commercially available ultrasound units have one or more of these equations already programmed into the software of the system, allowing immediate calculation of estimated fetal weights. Unfortunately, most of the regression formulas currently in use are associated with significant errors when the fetus is macrosomic. For example, Hadlock's formula to predict fetal weight has a mean absolute percent error of 13% for infants greater than 4,500 g, compared with 8% for nonmacrosomic infants (76).

Ultrasound-derived diagnosis of an estimated fetal weight exceeding 4,500 g is not as accurate as many believe it to be. Among women without diabetes, ultrasound biometry used to detect macrosomia has a sensitivity of 22–44%, a specificity of 99%, a positive predictive value of 30–44%, and a negative predictive value of 97–99% (77, 78). Reports demonstrating greater accuracy generally rely on less stringent criteria for macrosomia, such as birth weight greater than 4,000 g or that exceeding the 90th percentile for a given gestational age. However, when birth weight exceeds 4,500 g, only 50% of fetuses weigh within 10% of the ultrasound-derived estimate (79). Using existing formulas, an estimated fetal weight would have to exceed 4,800 g for the fetus to have more than a 50% chance of being macrosomic (77, 80). These observations suggest that the usefulness of ultrasonography for obtaining estimated weights is limited, and these limitations are neither operator-dependent nor equipment-dependent (79).

As with clinical estimates of fetal weight, the true value of ultrasonography in the management of expected fetal macrosomia may be its ability to rule out the diagnosis, which may help avoid maternal morbidity. One study revealed that clinicians who suspected fetal macrosomia on the basis of an ultrasonogram were more likely to diagnose labor abnormalities and were more likely to perform cesarean deliveries despite normal birth weights (57).

▶ Are interventions for treating suspected macrosomia available?

For mothers without diabetes, no clinical interventions designed to treat or curb fetal growth when macrosomia is suspected have been reported. For pregnancies that are complicated by diabetes mellitus, one clinical trial suggests that the addition of insulin to diet therapy may treat early macrosomia diagnosed between 29 and 33 weeks of gestation (81). This study randomized 98 women with a fetal abdominal circumference exceeding the 75th percentile for gestational age to either diet therapy alone or diet therapy with twice-daily insulin. The addition of insulin therapy decreased the likelihood of birth weight greater than the 90th percentile from 45% among those treated with diet only to 13% among those receiving insulin (P <0.01) (81).

Three large cohort studies confirm that excessive weight gain during pregnancy is associated with fetal macrosomia, suggesting a possible role for caloric restriction (35, 37, 39). One of these studies demonstrated that for most women, excessive weight gain doubled the risk of delivering an infant weighing more than 4,500 g. Although this relationship held true for average, obese, and very obese women, the actual incidence of macrosomia was still low (between 2.7% and 5.6%). Although dietary regulation has long been a mainstay of therapy for gestational diabetes, a recent meta-analysis of four randomized clinical trials examining primary diet therapy for women with impaired glucose tolerance showed no significant reduction in the number of newborns weighing more than 4,000 g (OR: 0.73, 95% CI: 0.45–1.35) (82). Although maternal obesity and weight gain during pregnancy are two of the strongest birth weight predictors, no randomized clinical trials have investigated dietary intervention to prevent macrosomia among obese women without diabetes.

▶ When is cesarean delivery appropriate for suspected macrosomia at a particular estimated fetal weight?

Controversy surrounds the question of cesarean delivery for suspected fetal macrosomia. First, the risk of birth trauma associated with vaginal delivery increases with birth weight (9, 17, 63). Second, cesarean delivery reduces—but does not eliminate—the risk of birth trauma and brachial plexus injury associated with fetal macrosomia (7, 9, 17, 83). The protective effect of cesarean delivery is large. Using a multivariate analysis to investigate risk factors for brachial plexus injury, investigators reported an odds ratio for cesarean delivery of 0.01–0.20 (17). It thus seems logical that for each woman, there must be a fetal weight beyond which the risks of vaginal delivery to the fetus are high enough to warrant cesarean delivery.

Despite such reasoning, the clinical effectiveness of offering prophylactic cesarean delivery to women with any specific estimated fetal weight has not been established in randomized clinical trials. Currently, only one observational study has evaluated a policy of using ultrasound-derived fetal weight estimates to determine the route of delivery (84). The use of historic controls, the nonrandomized design of the study, the use of multiple interventions, and the small sample size severely limit the usefulness of conclusions from the study. In this study, 1,337 women with diabetes were offered elective cesarean delivery based on ultrasound-derived fetal weight estimates beyond 4,250 g and induction of labor if ultrasound measurements resulted in a prediction of a large-for-gestational-age infant with an estimated fetal weight less than 4,250 g (84). The study cohort was compared with a historic control group of 1,227 women with diabetes who were managed without intervention for accelerated fetal growth during the 3 years preceding implementation of the study protocol. Implementation of the study protocol was associated with a nonsignificant reduction in the risk of shoulder dystocia from 2.4% in controls to 1.1% in the intervention group. In addition, a significant increase in the institutional cesarean delivery rate from 21.7% in controls to 25.1% in the intervention group was reported. Although the sample size was insufficient for comparison, the risk of birth trauma was not eliminated (2 versus 1 brachial plexus injury, 12 versus 6 fractures).

Currently, no prospective studies have assessed the true risk of either shoulder dystocia or brachial plexus injury in conjunction with estimated fetal weight alone. Until well-designed randomized clinical trials of sufficient sample size are available, clinicians must rely on retrospective data to make clinical management decisions.

In addition, recent large cohort and case–control studies demonstrate the safety of allowing a trial of labor for estimated birth weights of more than 4,000 g (12, 13). Among the 2,924 infants previously identified with birth weights greater than 4,000 g in utero, only 48 injuries (1.6%) related to shoulder dystocia were noted. Among the 22 brachial plexus injuries with documented follow-up, only 5 (17%) were clinically evident at 6 months (68). A second study reported 27 episodes (11.4%) of shoulder dystocia and 3 instances (1.3%) of brachial plexus paralysis in a group of 236 neonates weighing at least 4,200 g (85). In an additional series of 87 infants with birth weights greater than 4,500 g who were delivered vaginally, investigators reported only 5 cases (5.7%) of Erb-Duchenne paralysis. By 3 months of age, all affected infants were without evidence of brachial plexus paralysis (13). A fourth study reported that of the 157 infants delivered vaginally with birth weights greater than

4,500 g, no permanent sequelae were identified by age 2 months (12). The risks of short-term morbidity associated with vaginal delivery in this group are low, and those of permanent injury are even lower.

In conjunction with published cost-effectiveness data, the sum of these reports does not support a policy of prophylactic cesarean delivery for suspected fetal macrosomia with estimated weights less than 5,000 g (86). Along with a description of the limitations of estimating fetal weight, the obstetrician should present accurate statistics for the short- and long-term risks of maternal and fetal morbidity for both vaginal and cesarean delivery as discussed previously.

Despite the poor predictive value of an estimated fetal weight beyond 5,000 g and a lack of evidence supporting cesarean delivery at any estimated fetal weight, most, but not all, authors agree that consideration should be given to cesarean delivery in this situation (7, 13, 65). Among infants with birth weights exceeding 5,000 g, there are reports of cesarean delivery rates of 35–60%, brachial paralysis rates of 7–11%, and a perinatal death rate as high as 2.4% (7). In contrast, despite reporting an OR of 45 (95% CI: 16–129) for brachial plexus injury among vaginally delivered infants exceeding 5,000 g, some investigators suggest that ultrasound-derived fetal weight estimates alone should not be used to determine the route of delivery (17, 52).

▶ *Is there a role for induction of labor in the management of term patients with suspected fetal macrosomia?*

Current evidence from cohort studies does not support a policy of early induction of labor in term patients with suspected fetal macrosomia. Three recent reports show that induction of labor at least doubles the risk of cesarean delivery without reducing shoulder dystocia or newborn morbidity (87–89). Although the increased risk of cesarean delivery with induction of labor is clear, on the basis of these reports, one cannot rule out the possibility of a small beneficial effect on fetal outcome. These studies, however, are affected by small sample size and possible bias introduced by their retrospective nature.

One randomized clinical trial of women without diabetes has addressed the role of induction of labor for suspected fetal macrosomia at term. A total of 273 women with ultrasound-derived estimated fetal weights between 4,000 g and 4,500 g were randomized to either planned induction of labor or expectant management (90). Inductions were performed with oxytocin or prostaglandins followed by oxytocin, depending on the condition of the cervix. The cesarean delivery rates were similar: 19.4% for the induction group and 21.6% for the expectant group. There were 11 cases of shoulder dystocia, 5 in the induction group and 6 in the expectant group. All were managed without brachial plexus injury or other trauma.

▶ *How many elective cesarean deliveries for suspected fetal macrosomia would have to be performed to prevent one case of brachial plexus injury?*

The cost-effectiveness of elective cesarean delivery for fetal macrosomia usually is expressed as the number of cesarean deliveries required to prevent one brachial plexus injury or the cost, in dollars, of each brachial plexus injury avoided. A case–control study of brachial plexus paralysis demonstrated that 51 cesarean deliveries would be needed to prevent one case of brachial plexus paralysis if the cutoff for cesarean delivery were 4,500 g among patients without diabetes (17). For a cutoff of 5,000 g, this number decreased to 19. Assuming persistent rates for brachial plexus impairment are between 5% and 22%, the authors suggested that to prevent a single permanent injury, the number of cesarean deliveries increases to between 233 and 1,026 for a birth weight cutoff of 4,500 g, and from 85 to 373 for a cutoff of 5,000 g. Another study using similar methods concluded that 155–588 cesarean deliveries are needed to prevent a single permanent injury using a cutoff of 4,500 g for infants of women without diabetes (65). However, because the authors did not consider the imperfect predictive values of ultrasonography for macrosomia, they underestimated the number of cesarean deliveries that would be needed to implement such a policy.

In two reports analyzing a policy of prophylactic cesarean delivery for macrosomia, which took into account the reported sensitivity and specificity of ultrasonography for the detection of macrosomia (4,500 g), it was calculated that 3,695 cesarean deliveries would be required to prevent one permanent injury at a cost of $8.7 million for each injury avoided (86, 91). For pregnancies complicated by diabetes, these figures were still high at 443 cesarean deliveries to prevent a single permanent injury. In summary, because of the lack of well-designed and well-executed randomized clinical trials, a policy of prophylactic cesarean delivery for suspected fetal macrosomia less than 5,000 g may not be effective for pregnancies without diabetes. Furthermore, even for pregnancies complicated by diabetes, the cost-effectiveness of such a policy is doubtful.

▶ *How should a diagnosis of suspected fetal macrosomia affect the management of labor and vaginal delivery?*

Perhaps the most important consideration for labor and delivery with suspected fetal macrosomia is the decision to conduct a midpelvic operative vaginal delivery. As depicted in Figure 1, the risk of shoulder dystocia is associated with assisted vaginal delivery. Case–control and cohort studies consistently demonstrate an increased risk of shoulder dystocia when the macrosomic fetus is delivered by forceps, especially midforceps for a prolonged second stage (8, 10, 14, 19, 92). Rates of shoulder dystocia with midforceps deliveries of infants greater than 4,500 g have been reported to be above 50%. Barring extreme emergencies, cesarean delivery should be performed for midpelvic arrest of the fetus with suspected macrosomia. If a decision is made to proceed with cesarean delivery in the presence of suspected macrosomia, the incision should be large enough to avoid a difficult abdominal delivery.

Suspected fetal macrosomia is not a contraindication to attempt vaginal birth after prior cesarean delivery. A cohort study compared maternal and fetal outcomes associated with a trial of labor for infants suspected to be macrosomic and with documented birth weights less than 4,000 g versus those greater than 4,000 g (93). The success rate for vaginal delivery was 58% for birth weights between 4,000 g and 4,499 g and 43% for birth weights of 4,500 g and higher. Maternal and newborn morbidities were equal. A case–control study examining risk factors for uterine rupture during a trial of labor found no association between rupture and birth weight greater than 4,000 g (94).

Summary

The following recommendation is based on good and consistent scientific evidence (Level A):

▶ The diagnosis of fetal macrosomia is imprecise. For suspected fetal macrosomia, the accuracy of estimated fetal weight using ultrasound biometry is no better than that obtained with clinical palpation (Leopold's maneuvers).

The following recommendations are based on limited or inconsistent scientific evidence (Level B):

▶ Suspected fetal macrosomia is not an indication for induction of labor, because induction does not improve maternal or fetal outcomes.

▶ Labor and vaginal delivery are not contraindicated for women with estimated fetal weights up to 5,000 g in the absence of maternal diabetes.

▶ With an estimated fetal weight greater than 4,500 g, a prolonged second stage of labor or arrest of descent in the second stage is an indication for cesarean delivery.

The following recommendations are based primarily on consensus and expert opinion (Level C):

▶ Although the diagnosis of fetal macrosomia is imprecise, prophylactic cesarean delivery may be considered for suspected fetal macrosomia with estimated fetal weights greater than 5,000 g in women without diabetes and greater than 4,500 g in women with diabetes.

▶ Suspected fetal macrosomia is not a contraindication to attempted vaginal birth after a previous cesarean delivery.

References

1. Lubchenco LO, Hansman C, Dressler M, Boyd E. Intrauterine growth as estimated from liveborn birth-weight data at 24 to 42 weeks of gestation. Pediatrics 1963;32:793–800 (Level III)

2. Williams RL. Intrauterine growth curves: intra- and international comparisons with different ethnic groups in California. Prev Med 1975;4:163–172 (Level III)

3. Brenner WE, Edelman DA, Hendricks CH. A standard of fetal growth in the United States of America. Am J Obstet Gynecol 1976;126:555–564 (Level III)

4. Alexander GR, Himes JH, Kaufman RB, Mor J, Kogan M. A United States national reference for fetal growth. Obstet Gynecol 1996;87:163–168 (Level III)

5. Modanlou HD, Dorchester WL, Thorosian A, Freeman RK. Macrosomia—maternal, fetal and neonatal implications. Obstet Gynecol 1980;55:420–424 (Level II-2)

6. Boyd ME, Usher RH, McLean FH. Fetal macrosomia: prediction, risks, proposed management. Obstet Gynecol 1983;61:715–722 (Level II-2)

7. Spellacy WN, Miller S, Winegar A, Peterson PQ. Macrosomia—maternal characteristics and infant complications. Obstet Gynecol 1985;66:158–161 (Level II-2)

8. Acker DB, Sachs BP, Friedman EA. Risk factors for shoulder dystocia. Obstet Gynecol 1985;66:762–768 (Level II-3)

9. McFarland LV, Raskin M, Daling JR, Benedetti TJ. Erb/Duchenne's palsy: a consequence of fetal macrosomia and method of delivery. Obstet Gynecol 1986;68:784–788 (Level II-2)

10. Gross TL, Sokol RJ, Williams T, Thompson K. Shoulder dystocia: a fetal-physician risk. Am J Obstet Gynecol 1987;156:1408–1418 (Level II-2)

11. Menticoglou SM, Manning FA, Morrison I, Harman CR. Must macrosomic fetuses be delivered by a cesarean section? A review of outcome for 786 babies ≥ 4,500 g. Aust N Z J Obstet Gynaecol 1992;32:100–103 (Level III)

12. Lipscomb KR, Gregory K, Shaw K. The outcome of macrosomic infants weighing at least 4500 grams: Los Angeles county + University of Southern California experience. Obstet Gynecol 1995;85:558–564 (Level II-3)

13. Bérard J, Dufour P, Vinatier D, Subtil D, Vanderstichèle S, Monnier JC, et al. Fetal macrosomia: risk factors and outcome. A study of the outcome concerning 100 cases >4500 g. Eur J Obstet Gynecol Reprod Biol 1998; 77:51–59 (Level II-3)

14. Nesbitt TS, Gilbert WM, Herrchen B. Shoulder dystocia and associated risk factors with macrosomic infants born in California. Am J Obstet Gynecol 1998;179:476–480 (Level II-3)

15. Acker DB, Gregory KD, Sachs BP, Friedman EA. Risk factors for Erb-Duchenne palsy. Obstet Gynecol 1988; 71:389–392 (Level II-3)

16. Bahar AM. Risk factors and fetal outcome in cases of shoulder dystocia compared with normal deliveries of a similar birth weight. Br J Obstet Gynaecol 1996;103: 68–872 (Level II-2)

17. Ecker JL, Greenberg JA, Norwitz ER, Nadel AS, Repke JT. Birth weight as a predictor of brachial plexus injury. Obstet Gynecol 1997;89:643–647 (Level II-2)

18. Ventura SJ, Martin JA, Curtin SC, Mathews TJ, Park MM. Births: final data for 1998. Natl Vital Stat Rep 2000;48: 1–100 (Level II-3)

19. Nocon JJ, McKenzie DK, Thomas LJ, Hansell RS. Shoulder dystocia: an analysis of risks and obstetric maneuvers. Am J Obstet Gynecol 1993;168:1732–1739 (Level II-2)

20. Gonik B, Hollyer L, Allen R. Shoulder dystocia recognition: differences in neonatal risks for injury. Am J Perinatol 1991;8:31–34 (Level II-3)

21. Jennett RJ, Tarby TJ, Kreinick CJ. Brachial plexus palsy: an old problem revisited. Am J Obstet Gynecol 1992;166: 1673–1677 (Level II-2)

22. Gross SJ, Shime J, Farine D. Shoulder dystocia: predictors and outcome. A five-year review. Am J Obstet Gynecol 1987;156:334–336 (Level II-3)

23. Morrison JC, Sanders JR, Magann EF, Wiser WL. The diagnosis and management of dystocia of the shoulder. Surg Gynecol Obstet 1992;175:515–522 (Level II-3)

24. Okun N, Verma A, Mitchell BF, Flowerdew G. Relative importance of maternal constitutional factors and glucose intolerance of pregnancy in the development of newborn macrosomia. J Matern Fetal Med 1997;6:285–290 (Level II-2)

25. Hellerstedt WL, Himes JH, Story M, Alton IR, Edwards LE. The effects of cigarette smoking and gestational weight change on birth outcomes in obese and normal-

weight women. Am J Public Health 1997;87:591–596 (Level II-2)

26. Sermer M, Naylor CD, Gare DJ, Kenshole AB, Ritchie JW, Farine D, et al. Impact of increasing carbohydrate intolerance on maternal-fetal outcomes in 3637 women without gestational diabetes. The Toronto Tri-Hospital Gestational Diabetes Project. Am J Obstet Gynecol 1995; 173:146–156 (Level II-2)

27. Verma A, Mitchell BF, Demianczuk N, Flowerdew G, Okun NB. Relationship between plasma glucose levels in glucose-intolerant women and newborn macrosomia. J Matern Fetal Med 1997;6:187–193 (Level II-2)

28. Naylor CD, Sermer M, Chen E, Sykora K. Cesarean delivery in relation to birth weight and gestational glucose tolerance: pathophysiology or practice style? Toronto Trihospital Gestational Diabetes Investigators. JAMA 1996;275:1165–1170 (Level II-2)

29. Adams KM, Li H, Nelson RL, Ogburn PL Jr, Danilenko-Dixon DR. Sequelae of unrecognized gestational diabetes. Am J Obstet Gynecol 1998;178:1321–1332 (Level II-2)

30. Nasrat H, Abalkhail B, Fageeh W, Shabat A, el Zahrany F. Anthropometric measurements of newborns of gestational diabetic mothers: does it indicate disproportionate fetal growth? J Matern Fetal Med 1997;6:291–295 (Level II-2)

31. McFarland MB, Trylovich CG, Langer O. Anthropometric differences in macrosomic infants of diabetic and nondiabetic mothers. J Matern Fetal Med 1998;7:292–295 (Level II-2)

32. Casey BM, Lucas MJ, McIntire DD, Leveno KJ. Pregnancy outcomes in women with gestational diabetes compared with the general obstetric population. Obstet Gynecol 1997;90:869–873 (Level II-2)

33. Lucas MJ, Lowe TW, Bowe L, McIntire DD. Class A1 gestational diabetes: a meaningful diagnosis? Obstet Gynecol 1993;82:260–265 (Level II-2)

34. Larsen CE, Serdula MK, Sullivan KM. Macrosomia: Influence of maternal overweight among a low-income population. Am J Obstet Gynecol 1990;162:490–494 (Level II-3)

35. Cogswell ME, Serdula MK, Hungerford DW, Yip R. Gestational weight gain among average-weight and overweight women—what is excessive? Am J Obstet Gynecol 1995;172:705–712 (Level II-2)

36. Ogunyemi D, Hullett S, Leeper J, Risk A. Prepregnancy body mass index, weight gain during pregnancy, and perinatal outcome in a rural black population. J Matern Fetal Med 1998;7:190–193 (Level II-3)

37. Bianco AT, Smilen SW, Davis Y, Lopez S, Lapinski R, Lockwood CJ. Pregnancy outcome and weight gain recommendations for the morbidly obese woman. Obstet Gynecol 1998;91:97–102 (Level II-2)

38. Perlow JH, Morgan MA, Montgomery D, Towers CV, Porto M. Perinatal outcome in pregnancy complicated by massive obesity. Am J Obstet Gynecol 1992;167:958–962 (Level II-2)

39. Parker JD, Abrams B. Prenatal weight gain advice: an examination of the recent prenatal weight gain recommendations of the Institute of Medicine. Obstet Gynecol 1992;79:664–669 (Level II-3)

40. Lazer S, Biale Y, Mazor M, Lewenthal H, Insler V. Complications associated with the macrosomic fetus. J Repro Med 1986;31:501–505 (Level II-2)

41. Klebanoff MA, Mills JL, Berendes HW. Mother's birth weight as a predictor of macrosomia. Am J Obstet Gynecol 1985;153:253–257 (Level II-2)

42. Toohey JS, Keegan KA Jr, Morgan MA, Francis J, Task S, deVeciana M. The "dangerous multipara": fact or fiction? Am J Obstet Gynecol 1995;172:683–686 (Level II-2)

43. Juntunen K, Kirkinen P, Kauppila A. The clinical outcome in pregnancies of grand grand multiparous women. Acta Obstet Gynecol Scand 1997;76:755–759 (Level II-3)

44. Babinszki A, Kerenyi T, Torok O, Grazi V, Lapinski RH, Berkowitz RL. Perinatal outcome in grand and great-grand multiparity: effects of parity on obstetric risk factors. Am J Obstet Gynecol 1999;181:669–674 (Level II-3)

45. Brunskill AJ, Rossing MA, Connel FA, Daling J. Antecedents of macrosomia. Paediatr Perinat Epidemiol 1991;5:392–401 (Level II-2)

46. Dooley SL, Metzger BE, Cho NH. Gestational diabetes mellitus. Influence of race on disease prevalence and perinatal outcome in a U.S. population. Diabetes 1991;40:25–29 (Level II-3)

47. Homko CJ, Sivan E, Nyirjesy P, Reece EA. The interrelationship between ethnicity and gestational diabetes in fetal macrosomia. Diabetes Care 1995;18:1442–1445 (Level II-3)

48. Little RE, Sing CF. Genetic and environmental influences on human birth weight. Am J Hum Genet 1987;40: 512–526 (Level III)

49. Wilcox MA, Newton CS, Johnson IR. Paternal influences on birth weight. Acta Obstet Gynecol Scand 1995;74: 15–18 (Level II-3)

50. Deter RL, Hadlock FP. Use of ultrasound in the detection of macrosomia: a review. J Clin Ultrasound 1985;13: 519–524 (Level III)

51. Rossavik IK, Joslin GL. Macrosomatia and ultrasonography: what is the problem? South Med J 1993; 86:1129–1132 (Level II-3)

52. Sandmire HF. Whither ultrasonic prediction of fetal macrosomia? Obstet Gynecol 1993;82:860–862 (Level III)

53. Chauhan SP, Cowan BD, Magann EF, Bradford TH, Roberts WE, Morrison JC. Intrapartum detection of a macrosomic fetus: clinical versus 8 sonographic models. Aust N Z J Obstet Gynaecol 1995;35:3:266–270 (Level II-2)

54. Johnstone FD, Prescott RJ, Steel JM, Mao JH, Chambers S, Muir N. Clinical and ultrasound prediction of macrosomia in diabetic pregnancy. Br J Obstet Gynaecol 1996; 103:747–754 (Level II-3)

55. Chauhan SP, Hendrix NW, Magann EF, Morrison JC, Kenney SP, Devoe LD. Limitations of clinical and sonographic estimates of birth weight: experience with 1034 parturients. Obstet Gynecol 1998;91:72–77 (Level II-2)

56. Chauhan SP, Sullivan CA, Lutton TD, Magann EF, Morrison JC. Parous patients' estimate of birth weight in postterm pregnancy. J Perinatol 1995;15:192–194 (Level II-2)

57. Levine AB, Lockwood CJ, Brown B, Lapinski R, Berkowitz RL. Sonographic diagnosis of the large for gestational age fetus at term: does it make a difference? Obstet Gynecol 1992;79:55–58 (Level II-2)

58. Stones RW, Paterson CM, Saunders NJ. Risk factors for major obstetric haemorrhage. Eur J Obstet Gynecol Reprod Biol 1993;48:15–18 (Level II-2)

59. el Madany AA, Jallad KB, Radi FA, el Hamdan H, O'deh HM. Shoulder dystocia: anticipation and outcome. Int J Gynaecol Obstet 1990;34:7–12 (Level II-2)

60. Irion O, Hirsbrunner Almagbaly P, Morabia A. Planned vaginal delivery versus elective caesarean section: a study of 705 singleton term breech presentations. Br J Obstet Gynaecol 1998;105:710–717 (Meta-analysis)

61. Oppenheim WL, Davis A, Growdon WA, Dorey FJ, Davlin LB. Clavicle fractures in the newborn. Clin Orthop 1990;250:176–180 (Level II-2)

62. Chez RA, Carlan S, Greenberg SL, Spellacy WN. Fractured clavicle is an unavoidable event. Am J Obstet Gynecol 1994;171:797–798 (Level II-2)

63. Perlow JH, Wigton T, Hart J, Strassner HT, Nageotte MP, Wolk BM. Birth trauma. A five-year review of incidence and associated perinatal factors. J Reprod Med 1996;41:754–760 (Level II-2)

64. Gordon M, Rich H, Deutschberger J, Green M. The immediate and long-term outcome of obstetric birth trauma. I. Brachial plexus paralysis. Am J Obstet Gynecol 1973;117:51–56 (Level II-2)

65. Bryant DR, Leonardi MR, Landwehr JB, Bottoms SF. Limited usefulness of fetal weight in predicting neonatal brachial plexus injury. Am J Obstet Gynecol 1998;179:686–689 (Level II-3)

66. Gherman RB, Goodwin TM, Ouzounian JG, Miller DA, Paul RH. Brachial plexus palsy associated with cesarean section: an in utero injury? Am J Obstet Gynecol 1997;177:1162–1164 (Level III)

67. Hardy AE. Birth injuries of the brachial plexus: incidence and prognosis. J Bone Joint Surg Br 1981;63-B:98–101 (Level III)

68. Kolderup LB, Laros RK Jr, Musci TJ. Incidence of persistent birth injury in macrosomic infants: association with mode of delivery. Am J Obstet Gynecol 1997;177:37–41 (Level II-2)

69. Seidman DS, Laor A, Stevenson DK, Sivan E, Gale R, Shemer J. Macrosomia does not predict overweight in late adolescence in infants of diabetic mothers. Acta Obstet Gynecol Scand 1998;77:58–62 (Level II-2)

70. Sherman DJ, Arieli S, Tovbin J, Siegel G, Caspi E, Bukovsky I. A comparison of clinical and ultrasonic estimation of fetal weight. Obstet Gynecol 1998;91:212–217 (Level II-3)

71. Wikstrom I, Bergstrom R, Bakketeig L, Jacobsen G, Lindmark G. Prediction of high birth weight from maternal characteristics, symphysis fundal height and ultrasound biometry. Gynecol Obstet Invest 1993;35:27–33 (Level II-2)

72. Neilson JP. Symphysis-fundal height measurement in pregnancy. Cochrane Database Syst Rev 2000; 2: CD000944. Review (Meta-analysis)

73. Gonen R, Spiegel D, Abend M. Is macrosomia predictable, and are shoulder dystocia and birth trauma preventable? Obstet Gynecol 1996;88:526–529 (Level II-3)

74. Shepard MJ, Richards VA, Berkowitz RL, Warsof SL, Hobbins JC. An evaluation of two equations for predicting fetal weight by ultrasound. Am J Obstet Gynecol 1982;142: 47–54 (Level II-3)

75. Hadlock FP, Harrist RB, Carpenter RJ, Deter RL, Park SK. Sonographic estimation of fetal weight. The value of femur length in addition to head and abdomen measurements. Radiology 1984;150:535–540 (Level II-3)

76. Alsulyman OM, Ouzounian JG, Kjos SL. The accuracy of intrapartum ultrasonographic fetal weight estimation in diabetic pregnancies. Am J Obstet Gynecol 1997;177:503–506 (Level II-2)

77. Smith GC, Smith MF, McNay MB, Fleming JE. The relation between fetal abdominal circumference and birth weight: findings in 3512 pregnancies. Br J Obstet Gynaecol 1997;104:186–190 (Level II-3)

78. O'Reilly-Green CP, Divon MY. Receiver operating characteristic curves of sonographic estimated fetal weight for prediction of macrosomia in prolonged pregnancies. Ultrasound Obstet Gynecol 1997;9:403–408 (Level II-3)

79. Benacerraf BR, Gelman R, Frigoletto FD Jr. Sonographically estimated fetal weights: accuracy and limitation. Am J Obstet Gynecol 1988;159:1118–1121 (Level II-2)

80. McLaren RA, Puckett JL, Chauhan SP. Estimators of birth weight in pregnant women requiring insulin: a comparison of seven sonographic models. Obstet Gynecol 1995;85:565–569 (Level II-2)

81. Buchanan TA, Kjos SL, Montoro MN, Wu PY, Madrilejo NG, Gonzalez M, et al. Use of fetal ultrasound to select metabolic therapy for pregnancies complicated by mild gestational diabetes. Diabetes Care 1994;17:275–283 (Level II-1)

82. Walkinshaw SA. Dietary regulation for 'gestational diabetes.' Cochrane Database Syst Rev 2000;2:CD000070. Review (Meta-analysis)

83. Gregory KD, Henry OA, Ramicone E, Chan LS, Platt LD. Maternal and infant complications in high and normal weight infants by method of delivery. Obstet Gynecol 1998;92:507–513 (Level II-2)

84. Conway DL, Langer O. Elective delivery of infants with macrosomia in diabetic women: reduced shoulder dystocia versus increased cesarean deliveries. Am J Obstet Gynecol 1998;178:922–925 (Level II-2)

85. Blickstein I, Ben-Arie A, Hagay ZJ. Antepartum risks of shoulder dystocia and brachial plexus injury for infants weighing 4,200 g or more. Gynecol Obstet Invest 1998;45:77–80 (Level II-2)

86. Rouse DJ, Owen J, Goldenberg RL, Cliver SP. The effectiveness and costs of elective cesarean delivery for fetal macrosomia diagnosed by ultrasound. JAMA 1996;276:1480–1486 (Level III)

87. Combs CA, Singh NB, Khoury JC. Elective induction versus spontaneous labor after sonographic diagnosis of fetal macrosomia. Obstet Gynecol 1993;81:492–496 (Level II-2)

88. Friesen CD, Miller AM, Rayburn WF. Influence of spontaneous or induced labor on delivering the macrosomic fetus. Am J Perinatol 1995;12:63–66 (Level II-2)

89. Leaphart WL, Meyer MC, Capeless EL. Labor induction with a prenatal diagnosis of fetal macrosomia. J Matern Fetal Med 1997;6:99–102 (Level II-2)

90. Gonen O, Rosen DJ, Dolfin Z, Tepper R, Markow S, Fejgin MD. Induction of labor versus expectant management in macrosomia: a randomized study. Obstet Gynecol 1997;89:913–917 (Level I)

91. Rouse DJ, Owen J. Prophylactic cesarean delivery for fetal macrosomia diagnosed by means of ultrasonography—a Faustian bargain? Am J Obstet Gynecol 1999;181:332–338 (Level III)

92. Benedetti TJ, Gabbe SG. Shoulder dystocia. A complication of fetal macrosomia and prolonged second stage of labor with midpelvic delivery. Obstet Gynecol 1978;52:526–529 (Level III)

93. Flamm BL, Goings JR. Vaginal birth after cesarean section: is suspected fetal macrosomia a contraindication? Obstet Gynecol 1989;74:694–697 (Level II-2)

94. Leung AS, Farmer RM, Leung EK, Medearis AL, Paul RH. Risk factors associated with uterine rupture during trial of labor after cesarean delivery: a case-control study. Am J Obstet Gynecol 1993;168:1358–1363 (Level II-2)

The MEDLINE database, the Cochrane Library, and ACOG's own internal resources and documents were used to conduct a literature search to locate relevant articles published between January 1985 and May 1999. The search was restricted to articles published in the English language. Priority was given to articles reporting results of original research, although review articles and commentaries also were consulted. Abstracts of research presented at symposia and scientific conferences were not considered adequate for inclusion in this document. Guidelines published by organizations or institutions such as the National Institutes of Health and the American College of Obstetricians and Gynecologists were reviewed, and additional studies were located by reviewing bibliographies of identified articles. When reliable research was not available, expert opinions from obstetrician–gynecologists were used.

Studies were reviewed and evaluated for quality according to the method outlined by the U.S. Preventive Services Task Force:

I   Evidence obtained from at least one properly designed randomized controlled trial.
II-1 Evidence obtained from well-designed controlled trials without randomization.
II-2 Evidence obtained from well-designed cohort or case–control analytic studies, preferably from more than one center or research group.
II-3 Evidence obtained from multiple time series with or without the intervention. Dramatic results in uncontrolled experiments also could be regarded as this type of evidence.
III Opinions of respected authorities, based on clinical experience, descriptive studies, or reports of expert committees.

Based on the highest level of evidence found in the data, recommendations are provided and graded according to the following categories:

Level A—Recommendations are based on good and consistent scientific evidence.

Level B—Recommendations are based on limited or inconsistent scientific evidence.

Level C—Recommendations are based primarily on consensus and expert opinion.

ISSN 1099-3630

The American College of Obstetricians and Gynecologists
409 12th Street, SW, PO Box 96920
Washington, DC 20090-6920

12345/43210

ACOG PRACTICE BULLETIN

CLINICAL MANAGEMENT GUIDELINES FOR
OBSTETRICIAN–GYNECOLOGISTS
NUMBER 30, SEPTEMBER 2001

(Replaces Technical Bulletin Number 200, December 1994)

This Practice Bulletin was developed by the ACOG Committee on Practice Bulletins— Obstetrics with the assistance of Donald R. Coustan, MD. The information is designed to aid practitioners in making decisions about appropriate obstetric and gynecologic care. These guidelines should not be construed as dictating an exclusive course of treatment or procedure. Variations in practice may be warranted based on the needs of the individual patient, resources, and limitations unique to the institution or type of practice.

Gestational Diabetes

Gestational diabetes mellitus (GDM) is one of the most common clinical issues facing obstetricians and their patients. A lack of data from well-designed studies has contributed to the controversy surrounding the diagnosis and management of this condition. The purpose of this document is to provide a brief overview of our understanding of GDM and provide management guidelines that have been validated by appropriately conducted clinical research. When outcomes-based research is not available, expert opinion is provided to aid the practitioner.

Background

Definition and Prevalence

Diabetes is classified as type 1 or type 2 according to whether the patient requires insulin injections to avoid ketoacidosis. Gestational diabetes mellitus has been characterized as carbohydrate intolerance that begins or is first recognized during pregnancy. The prevalence of GDM varies in direct proportion to the prevalence of type-2 diabetes in a given population or ethnic group. Reported prevalence in the United States ranges from 1% to 14%, with 2–5% being the most common figure (1).

Maternal and Fetal Complications

Women with GDM are more likely to develop hypertensive disorders than women without GDM (2). Some of this additional risk may be related to the underlying risk factors for GDM (eg, increased maternal age and obesity). The diagnosis of GDM may prompt health care providers to intervene more readily for perceived problems (3). In women without GDM, there is a significant association between increasing carbohydrate intolerance and both preeclampsia and cesarean delivery (4). Women with GDM in Korea have a higher incidence of preeclampsia and primary cesarean delivery, yet only 10% of the women are obese (5). Whether the relationship with GDM is causal or not, clinicians should be aware of these risks. In addition, women with GDM have an increased risk of developing diabetes later in life.

The offspring of women with GDM are prone to such adverse events as macrosomia with its potential complications and hyperbilirubinemia. Infants of women with GDM are at increased risk for operative delivery, shoulder dystocia, and birth trauma. Because the risk factors for GDM (particularly obesity) are independent risk factors for fetal macrosomia, the role of maternal hyperglycemia has been widely debated. Although controlling for maternal obesity eliminated the apparent relationship between hyperglycemia and macrosomia in some studies (6, 7), these results may have been confounded because the women with GDM were treated. The relationship between GDM, fetal macrosomia, and other adverse outcomes has been confirmed in cohort studies in which maternal obesity and other potential confounders were controlled (8, 9), in a study of Korean women among whom only 10% were obese (5), and in another study of women whose abnormal glucose tolerance tests (GTTs) went clinically unrecognized (10). In women without GDM, there is an independent relationship between GTT levels and macrosomia (4, 11). When data were corrected for maternal weight, age, parity, and race, the 12% risk of macrosomia was independently attributable to GDM (9). A number of studies also have linked maternal hyperglycemia with long-term obesity and diabetes in the offspring (12–14). Nevertheless, considerable contro-versy remains regarding the exact relationship of these complications to maternal hyperglycemia.

Controversy of Current Screening Practices and Treatment Benefits

At one time, screening for GDM consisted of taking the patient's history. In 1973, O'Sullivan and Mahan proposed the 50-g, 1-hour laboratory screening test. This test has become widely used—94% of obstetric groups surveyed reported universal testing (15)—despite the absence of data to demonstrate a benefit to the population as a whole. However, as noted previously, maternal hyperglycemia is related to at least some of the adverse perinatal outcomes seen with GDM. Available evidence does not support the concept that women with GDM who do not have risk factors are of less concern than are those who do (16).

The use of traditional historic risk factors (family or personal history of diabetes, previous adverse pregnancy outcome, glycosuria, obesity) to identify GDM will miss approximately half of women with GDM (17, 18). If the risks of adverse outcomes are related to the presence or absence of confounding risk factors, rather than the GDM, then limited screening based on risk may be rea-

sonable. The U.S. Preventive Services Task Force has concluded that although there is insufficient evidence to recommend universal screening, screening high-risk women may be beneficial (19).

Despite the lack of population-derived data supporting the benefit of making the diagnosis of GDM, clinical recommendations often must be made without unassailable epidemiologic evidence. Older, admittedly flawed, studies suggested an increased perinatal mortality rate among undiagnosed or untreated women with GDM (20, 21). More recent studies that did not demonstrate an increase in perinatal mortality risk all included interventions of diet or insulin, antepartum testing, or merely making the diagnosis, which has been shown to be a powerful intervention in and of itself (3). If the perinatal mortality rate in undiagnosed and untreated GDM were double the background rate, as suggested in earlier studies, and GDM occurs in 2–5% of the population, any increase in overall perinatal loss attributable to discontinuing screening programs would likely go unnoticed.

Another important issue to consider is the possibility that some patients diagnosed with GDM may have preexisting type-2 diabetes, which can only be confirmed postpartum. One study found such patients to have a perinatal mortality rate 6 times higher than those with milder forms of GDM (22). Another study found mothers with GDM who had infants with birth defects were more likely to have high fasting glucose values, suggesting the presence of undiagnosed preexisting diabetes (23).

For the population to benefit from the diagnosis of GDM, there should be an effective treatment for the condition. Although a number of comparative studies of various treatments are available, there is little information regarding the effectiveness of treatment versus no treatment. In a pilot randomized trial comparing strict metabolic control with routine obstetric care in 300 women with GDM, there was no difference in the rate of macrosomia or other pregnancy outcomes (24). However, even the control subjects monitored their own glucose levels 1 day each week, and 10% were removed from the study and treated for hyperglycemia.

The first consideration in selecting a therapy for GDM is a determination of the treatment goals. Although the degree, if any, of excess perinatal mortal-ity associated with milder GDM has not been established, management plans typically include some type of fetal surveillance. A second goal of treatment may be the prevention of adverse pregnancy outcomes, such as macrosomia and its attendant consequences of operative delivery, shoulder dystocia, and birth trauma. Potential treatments toward this goal include diet, exercise, and insulin; oral agents also have been suggested. Safety, efficacy, and patient acceptance should be considered in choosing a treatment.

The goal of treatment is to lower the likelihood of macrosomia and its consequences; neonatal hypoglycemia also may be reduced (25). Although the quality of the information varies, evidence is available to confirm these benefits. However, there has been no demonstrated treatment benefit on long-term outcomes for the offspring such as obesity and the development of diabetes. It should be emphasized that although the evidence is inconclusive that treating GDM can prevent maternal and fetal complications, universal screening and treatment are widely practiced.

Clinical Considerations and Recommendations

▶ *How should screening for GDM be accomplished?*

All pregnant patients should be screened for GDM, whether by patient's history, clinical risk factors, or a laboratory screening test to determine blood glucose levels. The optimal method of screening is controversial, and there are insufficient data from which to draw firm conclusions.

A number of clinical risk factors have been demonstrated to be associated with an increased likelihood of GDM, including age, ethnicity, obesity, family history of diabetes, and past obstetric history (26). In one study, more than 3,000 pregnant women underwent both the 50-g, 1-hour screening test and the diagnostic oral GTT (27). Using a complex scoring system of weighted risk factors, the study found test thresholds for the 1-hour screening test varied depending on individual risk status. Sensitivity rates were similar to those of universal screening, and one third of the subjects avoided the glucose screening test. Thus, it appears it is possible to use historic risk factors to identify individuals who may have such a low risk for GDM that glucose challenge testing may not be worthwhile. Conversely, there may be groups of individuals at such high risk for GDM that it may be more convenient and cost-effective to proceed directly to the diagnostic GTT without obtaining the laboratory screening test.

Specific risk factors and the degree of their influence on GDM prevalence are difficult to quantify across populations. For example, in one Canadian study, African race was not associated with an increased risk of GDM (27), whereas in another large, observational study African race was found to be an independent predictor of the likelihood of GDM, even when investigators controlled for obesity (28). Because no single study can be generalized to the entire population, it seems reasonable

to base the definition of high and low risk for GDM on the prevalence of type-2 diabetes in each ethnic group. The relationship between obesity and GDM is most likely a continuum, so that the definition of the upper limit of normal weight suggested by the Institute of Medicine (ie, a body mass index ≤25) (29) should reasonably serve to identify individuals who are not obese. A low-risk individual meets all of the following criteria (30):

1. Age younger than 25 years
2. Not a member of an ethnic group with an increased risk for the development of type-2 diabetes (examples of high-risk ethnic groups include women of Hispanic, African, Native American, South or East Asian, or Pacific Islands ancestry)
3. Body mass index of 25 or less
4. No previous history of abnormal glucose tolerance
5. No previous history of adverse obstetric outcomes usually associated with GDM
6. No known diabetes in first degree relative

When the 1997 criteria, similar to those listed previously for low risk, were applied to data from more than 18,000 pregnancies in a predominantly Caucasian population, researchers determined that only 3% of women with GDM would not have been diagnosed (31). However, only 10% of the population would have been exempted from screening. For this reason, many physicians elect to screen all pregnant patients as a practical matter.

▶ *At what gestational age should laboratory screening be performed?*

A number of studies have demonstrated that the prevalence of GDM increases with advancing gestation (32–36). It has been customary to recommend the 50-g, 1-hour oral glucose challenge test be administered at 24–28 weeks of gestation. This arbitrary recommendation results from an attempt to balance two competing interests. Insulin resistance increases as pregnancy progresses, therefore, testing later in pregnancy will result in a higher yield of abnormal tests. However, the later the abnormality is diagnosed, the less time will be available for intervention. Although many practitioners choose to screen high-risk patients early in pregnancy, the benefit of early treatment of women with GDM identified early in pregnancy has not been demonstrated but rather has been accepted on a theoretical basis.

Patients who had GDM in a previous pregnancy have a 33–50% likelihood of recurrence in a subsequent pregnancy (37–39). If such patients were not tested between pregnancies, some of these recurrences may represent preexisting diabetes undetected between pregnancies. In such individuals there should still be a benefit to making the diagnosis of diabetes during the first half of pregnancy. Unlike typical patients with GDM, patients with abnormal glucose tolerance in the first half of pregnancy may manifest severe degrees of hyperglycemia.

▶ *How is laboratory screening accomplished?*

Although the use of random glucose measurements or fasting glucose measurements have been advocated to screen for GDM, inadequate data are available to evaluate the relative effectiveness of these approaches. Random glucose screening does not appear to be adequately sensitive (40). The screening test most commonly used in the United States is the 50-g, 1-hour glucose challenge, using a pure glucose load of 50 g in 150 mL of fluid. Glucose polymer solutions, which provide a lower osmotic load for a given glucose load, appear to be associated with fewer gastrointestinal symptoms and have been demonstrated to yield fair correlation with monomeric glucose solutions (41–43). The use of jelly beans instead of a pure glucose challenge has been shown to be better tolerated, but this method has poor sensitivity (40%) when compared with glucose polymer solutions (80–90%) (44).

Among subjects with GDM, for whom the function of the screening test is most critical, either higher (45) or similar (46) values were reported when the test was administered in the fasting state. Therefore, given the lack of evidence that fasting improves the accuracy of the screening test and the fact that fasting may pose significant logistic problems, the 50-g, 1-hour screening test may be administered without regard to the time elapsed since the last meal.

▶ *Should venous or capillary blood be used?*

The original description of the screening test used venous whole blood (17), but laboratories have switched from whole blood to plasma or serum samples. Studies of the screening test have generally used venous plasma. Convenient and relatively inexpensive meters for measuring glucose in capillary blood samples raise the possibility of performing the screening test in an office setting without expensive and complicated laboratory equipment. During fasting, capillary and venous blood have similar glucose concentrations, but after a meal or glucose challenge, capillary glucose is higher than venous glucose. Laboratory instruments are generally checked for quality against standard samples at regular intervals to ensure accuracy. Precision is an important factor. Two studies of various meters used in pregnancy demonstrated inadequate precision for all but one or two meter systems tested (47, 48). Therefore, if capillary blood samples are to be used for GDM screening, the precision of the meter should be known, and its correlation with

simultaneously obtained venous samples should be ascertained. Appropriate thresholds can then be derived. Office-based glucose testing is not recommended because of the difficulty in complying with required federal standards for testing. However, if used, it may be most practical to continue to use venous plasma samples and published thresholds for further testing.

▶ *Is there an appropriate threshold value for the laboratory screening test?*

The screening test threshold at which a diagnostic GTT is recommended will be arbitrary. The higher the threshold, the lower the sensitivity but the better the specific-ity and the lower the likelihood of a false-positive test result. The lower the threshold, the higher the sensitivity but the higher the likelihood of a false-positive test result and thus the performance of an unnecessary diagnostic GTT. O'Sullivan and Mahan (17) used venous whole blood samples and the Somogyi-Nelson method of glucose analysis. At the recommended threshold of 130 mg/dL, the screening test had a sensitivity of 79% and a specificity of 87%. When venous plasma and specific enzymatic methods of glucose analysis were used, 10% of women with GDM manifested screening test values between 130–139 mg/dL (18). Absolute sensitivity levels could not be determined because women with screening test values below 130 mg/dL did not undergo oral GTTs. When the threshold was lowered from 140 mg/dL to 130 mg/dL, the number of women requiring glucose tolerance testing increased from 14% to 23%, or approximately one quarter of patients.

Although a threshold of 140 mg/dL was recommended in the past, the most recent position statement of the American Diabetes Association ascribes a sensitivity of approximately 80% to this cutoff and 90% sensitivity with a threshold of 130 mg/dL and leaves the choice open (49). Because the precise cost-benefit ratio of diagnosing GDM remains unresolved, either threshold is acceptable.

▶ *How is GDM diagnosed?*

The diagnostic test specific for pregnancy and about which the greatest body of data exists is the 100-g, 3-hour oral GTT. Diagnostic criteria were originally derived by O'Sullivan and Mahan (50). Cutoff levels two standard deviations above the mean were found to be the best predictors for developing diabetes later in life. There are no well-designed studies that demonstrate whether these diagnostic criteria are optimal to identify pregnancies at risk for maternal or perinatal morbidity. The relationship between maternal glucose intolerance and adverse pregnancy outcomes appears to be more or less continuous with no absolute threshold (4). Two sets of criteria were adapted from the original O'Sullivan and Mahan values when laboratories switched to venous plasma or serum. These samples yield results approximately 14% higher than does whole blood. The National Diabetes Data Group published conversions derived by adding 15% to each of the four thresholds (51). Lower thresholds were subsequently derived by also correcting for the change to enzymatic methods of glucose analysis (52). Expert panels have supported both criteria, but there are no data from clinical trials to determine which is superior (Table 1) (53).

A positive diagnosis requires that two or more thresholds be met or exceeded. The test is administered in the morning after an overnight fast. Patients should not smoke before the test and should remain seated during the test. Patients should be instructed to follow an unrestricted diet, consuming at least 150 g of carbohydrate per day for at least 3 days prior to the test. This should avoid carbohydrate depletion, which could cause spuriously high values on the GTT.

Patients with only one abnormal value have been demonstrated to manifest increased risk for macrosomic infants and other morbidities (54, 55). However, because the relationship between carbohydrate metabolism, macrosomia, and other morbidity is a continuum (4, 56), and because not all of this morbidity arises from carbohydrate intolerance, it should be anticipated that no threshold will identify all patients at risk.

▶ *How should blood glucose be monitored in a woman with GDM?*

The optimal frequency of blood glucose testing in patients with GDM has not been established. Whether daily testing is essential for women with GDM has not been proven. One large, prospective trial compared seven-times-daily self-glucose monitoring using memory-based reflectance meters with weekly fasting and 2-hour laboratory glucose determinations supplemented by four-times-daily self-monitoring with only test strips and no meters (57). The more intensively monitored group had fewer primary cesarean deliveries and fewer macrosomic neonates, and their infants were less likely to experience shoulder dystocia and neonatal hypoglycemia than the more conventionally monitored group. Other centers have reported similar results with four-times-daily glucose monitoring (25, 58). Although daily self-glucose monitoring has not been demonstrated to reduce perinatal mortality in women with GDM, it appears to be useful in reducing potentially adverse outcomes such as macrosomia. However, evidence from well-designed, randomized trials that compare daily self-glucose monitoring with less frequent assessment in women with GDM is still needed.

Further uncertainty surrounds the timing of glucose determinations and the selection of appropriate thresholds for intervention. In nonpregnant individuals, diabetes is most often managed using preprandial glucose determinations. However, the fetus may be more sensitive to glucose excesses than to the nadirs of glucose values at various times of the day. In studies of preexisting diabetes, 1-hour postprandial glucose values were found to be more predictive of fetal macrosomia than were fasting values (59), and a 1-hour value of 130 mg/dL or more was found to be an appropriate threshold (60). A randomized trial compared preprandial with 1-hour postprandial glucose measurements in 66 women whose GDM was severe enough to require insulin treatment by 30 weeks of gestation (25). Macrosomia, neonatal hypoglycemia, and cesarean deliveries for shoulder dystocia were significantly lower among those who had postprandial monitoring, and their glycohemoglobin levels also decreased more markedly than did the levels of the subjects who used preprandial monitoring. No studies are available to compare the efficacy of 1-hour postprandial versus the more traditional 2-hour postprandial glucose determinations.

Table 1. Two Diagnostic Criteria for Gestational Diabetes Mellitus

Status	Plasma or Serum Glucose Level Carpenter/Coustan Conversion		Plasma Level National Diabetes Data Group Conversion	
	mg/dL	mmol/L	mg/dL	mmol/L
Fasting	95	5.3	105	5.8
One hour	180	10.0	190	10.6
Two hours	155	8.6	165	9.2
Three hours	140	7.8	145	8.0

Adapted from Expert Committee on the Diagnosis and Classification of Diabetes Mellitus. Report of the Expert Committee on the Diagnosis and Classification of Diabetes Mellitus. Diab Care 2000;23(suppl 1):S4–S19

Because these studies only included individuals with preexisting diabetes or those with GDM severe enough to require insulin treatment by 30 weeks of gestation, it remains to be established whether fasting or preprandial glucose measurements will suffice for individuals with milder forms of GDM. One study demonstrated a moderate correlation between fasting and 2-hour postprandial glucose values in GDM; if the fasting value was below 105 mg/dL, then only 17% of the 2-hour values exceeded 120 mg/dL (61). Given the available data, postprandial glucose values appear to be most effective at determining the likelihood of macrosomia and other adverse pregnancy outcomes in patients with GDM.

▶ Is there a role for diet therapy in the treatment of GDM?

Although there are no available data comparing medical nutrition therapy (diet) with no treatment in women with GDM, there is one such randomized trial of women who had abnormal glucose challenge test results but normal oral GTT results (62). Those on the prescribed diet delivered fewer macrosomic infants. Nutritional intervention in women with GDM should be designed to achieve normal glucose levels and avoid ketosis, while maintaining appropriate nutrition and weight gain. The American Diabetes Association recommends nutritional counseling, if possible by a registered dietitian, with individualization of the nutrition plan based on height and weight (49). The American Diabetes Association also recommends an average of 30 kcal/kg/d based on prepregnant body weight for nonobese individuals (49). The most appropriate diet for women with GDM has yet to be established.

The American Diabetes Association suggests that obese women (body mass index >30) may do well with moderate caloric restriction (30–33%) (49). Caloric restriction of 30% in obese women with GDM was associated with pregnancy outcomes (birth weight and macrosomia) similar to those of a group of matched controls who had normal values on the glucose challenge screening tests (63). One concern about caloric restriction is that, although glucose levels may decrease, there is the possibility that it may cause starvation ketosis (64). Levels of glucose, free fatty acids, and ketone bodies have been assessed during each trimester in long-term follow-up studies of infants of women with and without diabetes. These studies have reported an inverse association between maternal circulating levels of ketone acids in the second and third trimesters and psychomotor development and intelligence in the offspring at 3–5 years of age and through 9 years of age (65, 66). Even when investigators reevaluated their findings by taking into account socioeconomic status, race or ethnicity, and

the presence of gestational or preexisting diabetes, this association persisted. Although the correlation between IQ and ketone levels was weak (r = 0.2), it was statistically significant (P = 0.02); therefore, it would be prudent to avoid excessive ketonemia or ketonuria during pregnancy. When obese women with GDM were placed on moderate caloric restriction (25 kcal/kg of ideal nonpregnant weight per day), no ketonuria was detected during weekly clinic visits (67). Serum ketones were not reported. Available evidence does not support a recommendation for or against moderate caloric restriction in obese women with GDM. However, if caloric restriction is used, the diet should be restricted by no more than 33%, and ketonuria should be avoided.

Supplemental dietary fiber may improve glycemic control in women with type-2 diabetes. In a cohort study, increasing dietary fiber enrichment did not improve glucose control in patients with GDM (68). Available evidence does not support the prescription of fiber supplements for GDM.

▶ Is there a role for insulin in the treatment of GDM?

Some (69–71) but not all (72) prospective trials have demonstrated that insulin treatment of all women with GDM can reduce the likelihood of delivering a macrosomic baby. However, using such a paradigm would require that 100% of individuals be treated although less than half (between 9% and 40%) would benefit. It would be preferable to select the most appropriate patients for treatment.

One traditional approach has been to add insulin if medical nutrition therapy does not maintain fasting plasma glucose below 105 mg/dL or 2-hour values below 120 mg/dL or both. These thresholds have been extrapolated from recommendations for managing pregnancy in women with preexisting diabetes. A randomized trial demonstrated that using a 1-hour postmeal goal of 140 mg/dL was effective in preventing adverse outcomes in women with GDM severe enough to require insulin (25). It would be logical, although unproven, that similar thresholds should be used for initiating insulin treatment. A study of individuals with preexisting diabetes found the most appropriate target 1-hour postprandial glucose level for preventing macrosomia was 130 mg/dL (60). It may be reasonable to apply these data to women with GDM. Women with higher fasting glucose levels are more likely to require insulin therapy to achieve optimal glucose control than women with lower fasting glucose levels. Thirty-eight percent of women with GDM with an initial fasting plasma glucose level of 95 mg/dL or less required insulin to achieve "optimized control" (mean of seven daily values <100 mg/dL), whereas 70% required insulin when the initial fasting value was 95–104 mg/dL (73). Although each fasting glucose group delivered a similar, low proportion of babies with birth weights above the 90th percentile, large-for-gestational-age (LGA) babies were born to 29% of those treated with diet and 10% of those treated with insulin. All subjects with fasting values above 105 mg/dL were treated with insulin, and 14% had LGA offspring. These data suggest that insulin therapy should be considered for patients treated with medical nutrition therapy when 1-hour postprandial values exceed 130–140 mg/dL or 2-hour postprandial values exceed 120 mg/dL or fasting glucose exceeds 95 mg/dL.

Early third-trimester ultrasonography may help in identifying women with GDM who would benefit from insulin therapy despite relatively good metabolic control on diet. In a randomized trial of women with mild gestational diabetes, ultrasound abdominal circumference greater than the 75th percentile at 29–33 weeks of gestation was effective in selecting patients among whom the LGA rate was reduced to 13% with insulin therapy compared with 45% in those randomized to diet alone (74).

A frequent question is how long to attempt dietary management before adding insulin. One study suggested diet be tried for 2 weeks before adding insulin if the initial fasting plasma glucose was 95 mg/dL or less (75). In women with GDM with initial fasting values above 95 mg/dL, the results of diet therapy alone were less salutary. The available evidence does not support a clear recommendation as to the number of times glucose values should exceed targets before insulin is added or the dosage increased.

No particular insulin regimen or insulin dose has been demonstrated to be superior for GDM. Generally, it is easiest for the patient to start with the simplest regimen and work up to a more complex regimen as needed. Regardless of the starting dosage, subsequent dosage adjustments should be based on the blood glucose levels at particular times of day. Because free insulin apparently does not cross the placenta, all types of insulin have been used in patients with GDM. Insulin lispro (Humalog), an analog of human insulin with a single amino acid substitution, has a more rapid onset of action than regular insulin and may be useful in improving postprandial glucose concentrations. It has been used in GDM and has been demonstrated not to cross the placenta (76).

Is there a role for exercise in the treatment of GDM?

Exercise often is recommended for individuals with diabetes, both as a way to achieve weight reduction and as a treatment to improve glucose metabolism. At least three randomized trials have explored exercise as an adjunct to, or substitute for, insulin in GDM. When women with GDM who needed intervention were randomly assigned to insulin or an exercise program, there was no difference in the likelihood of macrosomic infants, although glucose levels were not reported (77). A randomized trial of diet and exercise versus diet alone found improvement in both fasting plasma glucose and the response to a 50-g challenge in those who exercised (78) while a third study found improvement in cardiorespiratory fitness but no differences in glucose control with exercise (79). A regular exercise program has clear benefits for all women and may offer additional advantages for women with GDM. Women with GDM who lead an active lifestyle should be encouraged to continue a program of exercise approved for pregnancy.

▶ Is there a role for oral antidiabetic agents in the treatment of GDM?

Oral antidiabetic agents have been contraindicated in pregnancy. The early-generation sulfonylureas crossed the placenta and had the potential to stimulate the fetal pancreas, leading to fetal hyperinsulinemia. There also was concern about the potential for teratogenicity, although diabetes itself is teratogenic, and it is difficult to distinguish the effects of the treatment from those of the disease. Glyburide, a second-generation sulfonylurea, was compared with insulin in a randomized trial among patients with GDM who failed to achieve adequate glycemic control with diet alone (80). Glucose control was similar, and the glyburide group had pregnancy outcomes similar to those of the insulin group, including rates of cesarean delivery, preeclampsia, macrosomia (>4 kg), and neonatal hypoglycemia. Cord serum analyses showed no detectable glyburide in the infants. At this time, no other oral agent has been shown to be safe and effective in GDM, and this study has not been confirmed. Further study is recommended before the use of newer oral hypoglycemic agents can be supported for use in pregnancy.

▶ Is fetal assessment indicated in pregnancies complicated by GDM?

Antepartum fetal testing is recommended for patients with preexisting diabetes (81). If the increased risk of fetal demise in patients with preexisting diabetes is related to suboptimal metabolic control, it would be expected that patients with GDM who have poor metabolic control also would be at risk and thus merit antepartum fetal surveillance. Patients with well-controlled GDM are presumably at lower risk for fetal death than are those whose condition is not well controlled or who require insulin therapy, but there is no consensus regarding antepartum testing in women with well-controlled GDM. There are no data available from randomized trials of antepartum testing in patients with GDM. Most case series report good outcomes with a given testing protocol and conclude the protocol used is appropriate. Twice-weekly nonstress tests and amniotic fluid volume determinations were associated with no stillbirths and a 4.9% rate of cesarean delivery for nonreassuring fetal status in a cohort of women with GDM who had fasting glucose levels below 105 mg/dL (82).

Another cohort study of women with GDM who required only diet therapy and were monitored by daily fetal movement determinations beginning at 28 weeks of gestation and who underwent nonstress testing beginning at 40 weeks of gestation found no stillbirths or neonatal deaths (83). Patients requiring insulin or who had previous stillbirths, chronic hypertension, or pregnancy-induced hypertension underwent earlier fetal testing as did patients with preexisting diabetes. Because this latter study lacked sufficient power to evaluate perinatal mortality, it is not possible to make an unequivocal recommendation. Despite the lack of conclusive data, it would seem reasonable that women whose GDM is not well controlled, who require insulin, or have other risk factors such as hypertension or adverse obstetric history should be managed the same as individuals with preexisting diabetes. The particular antepartum test selected, whether nonstress test, contraction stress test, or biophysical profile, may be chosen according to local practice.

Ultrasonography has been used to estimate fetal weight, especially to predict macrosomia prior to delivery. However, the reliability of these measures has not been established (84–86). Regression formulas using combined fetal measures for weight estimates are associated with systematic errors. Using existing formulas, an estimated fetal weight would have to exceed 4,800 g for the fetus to have more than a 50% chance of being macrosomic (87, 88). In addition, the use of ultrasound-derived measures of fetal weight have not been shown to be superior to clinical measures.

▶ *When and how should delivery occur in pregnancies complicated by GDM?*

The timing of delivery in patients with GDM remains relatively open. When glucose control is good and no other complications supervene, there is no good evidence to support routine delivery before 40 weeks of gestation. In a study in which women with insulin-treated GDM and fetuses believed to be of appropriate weight for gestational age were randomized at 38 weeks of gestation to induction of labor within 1 week or expectant management, there was no difference in cesarean delivery rates (89). However, the induction group delivered a smaller proportion of LGA babies. In a cohort multiple time series study, a policy of induction of labor at 38–39 weeks of gestation for women with insulin-treated GDM was compared with the results in expectantly managed historic controls (90). There was no significant difference in macrosomia or cesarean delivery rates, but shoulder dystocia was experienced by 10% of the expectant management group beyond 40 weeks of gestation versus 1.4% in the group induced at 38–39 weeks of gestation. Although significant, these data have not been confirmed by additional studies.

Available data do not address women with GDM not treated with insulin or those believed to have macrosomic fetuses. Individuals whose metabolic control does not meet the goals described earlier, or is undocumented, or those with risk factors such as hypertensive disorders or previous stillbirth should be managed the same as those with preexisting diabetes.

When GDM is well controlled and dates are well documented, respiratory distress syndrome at or beyond 39 weeks of gestation is rare enough that routine amniocentesis for pulmonary maturity is not necessary (91). At earlier gestational ages, or when control is poor or undocumented, pulmonary maturity should be assessed before induction. However, when early delivery is planned because of maternal or fetal compromise, the urgency of the indication should be considered in the decision to perform amniocentesis.

Cesarean delivery rates are higher in women with GDM compared with controls, and the difference is not entirely attributable to fetal macrosomia (3, 9). It may be that caregivers are more prone to perform cesarean deliveries in patients with GDM because of concern about the likelihood of shoulder dystocia. There are no data to support a policy of cesarean delivery purely on the basis of GDM. However, macrosomia is distinctly more common in women with GDM, and shoulder dystocia is more likely at a given birth weight in pregnancies complicated by diabetes than in nondiabetic pregnancies (92, 93). It may be reasonable, therefore, to recommend cesarean delivery without a trial of labor at some particular threshold of fetal weight.

One of the problems in trying to apply such a threshold is the poor accuracy of ultrasound prediction of birth weight. In particular, a study reported that when birth weight exceeds 4,500 g, only 50% of the fetuses weigh within 10% of the ultrasound-derived estimate (94). A decision analytic model was developed to estimate the potential effectiveness and costs of a policy of elective cesarean delivery for fetal macrosomia diagnosed by ultrasonography (95). Investigators factored in such considerations as the poor predictive accuracy of ultrasonography, the background cesarean delivery rates at various fetal weights, and the effect of maternal diabetes. The analysis predicted that in women with diabetes it would be necessary to perform 489 cesarean deliveries to prevent one permanent brachial plexus injury at a threshold of 4,000 g estimated fetal weight, or 443 cesarean deliveries at a threshold of 4,500 g estimated fetal weight. These figures are one fifth to one eighth of the figures developed for pregnancies of women without diabetes. The authors concluded such a policy may be tenable, although the merits are debatable. On the basis of available data, it is not possible to determine whether the potential benefits of cesarean delivery without labor at a given estimated fetal weight are similar for patients with GDM and those with preexisting diabetes. It would appear reasonable to recommend that patients with GDM be counseled regarding possible cesarean delivery without labor when the estimated fetal weight is 4,500 g or greater. When the estimated weight is 4,000–4,500 g, additional factors such as the patient's past delivery history, clinical pelvimetry, and the progress of labor may be helpful to consider in determining mode of delivery.

With an estimated fetal weight greater than 4,500 g, prolonged second stage of labor or arrest of descent in the second stage is an indication for cesarean delivery. Because of the higher likelihood of shoulder dystocia at a given birth weight in the pregnancies of women with diabetes, it may be best to apply the above recommendation to an estimated fetal weight greater than 4,000 g for GDM. Operative deliveries from the midpelvis should be avoided, if possible, in patients with GDM who have an estimated fetal weight of 4,000 g or more and a prolonged second stage of labor (92, 96).

▶ *Should women with a history of GDM be screened postpartum?*

Women with a history of GDM are at increased risk for developing diabetes (generally type-2 diabetes) later in life (97, 98). Diabetes will be diagnosed in some women soon after pregnancy, suggesting they had preexisting diabetes that was not diagnosed prior to pregnancy. Populations with a high prevalence of type-2 diabetes who do not have access to screening when not pregnant are at particularly high risk for this phenomenon (99). Current recommendations for the diagnosis and classification of diabetes in the nonpregnant state are based on the recommendations of an expert committee of the American Diabetes Association and are depicted in Table 2 (100). Diagnostic testing for diabetes may be performed after the immediate effects of pregnancy on glucose metabolism have dissipated and is most convenient at around the time of the postpartum checkup. However, there are no long-term follow-up studies that verify the benefit of postpartum diagnostic testing.

Although the American Diabetes Association advocates the use of a fasting plasma glucose determination as being less cumbersome than the oral GTT, the oral GTT will more accurately identify those women who had GDM and now have impaired glucose tolerance (101). Because the presence of such a condition may be important in counseling for future pregnancies, there may be advantages to performing the oral GTT as the initial diagnostic test after pregnancy complicated by GDM. If the results of both the fasting plasma glucose and the oral GTT are normal, subsequent follow-up tests may use the fasting plasma glucose.

The estimate of long-term risk for developing diabetes among women who had GDM depends on the diagnostic test used, the duration of follow-up, age, and other characteristics of the population studied; reported rates vary widely (102). In follow-up studies up to 28 years on the cohort of patients used to derive the O'Sullivan and Mahan criteria for GDM, diabetes was found in 50% of women who had GDM compared with 7% of controls (103). Factors identifiable during or shortly after pregnancy that increase the risk for subsequent diabetes

Table 2. Criteria for the Diagnosis of Diabetes Mellitus in the Nonpregnant State*

Normal Values	Impaired Fasting Glucose or Impaired Glucose Tolerance	Diabetes Mellitus
FPG <110 mg/dL	FPG 110–125 mg/dL	FPG ≥126 mg/dL
75-g, 2-h OGTT	75-g, 2-h OGTT	75-g, 2-h OGTT
2-h PG <140 mg/dL	2-h PG 140–199 mg/dL	2-h PG ≥200 mg/dL
		Symptoms of diabetes and PG (without regard to time since last meal) ≥ 200 mg/dL

*Abbreviations: FPG, fasting plasma glucose; OGTT, oral glucose tolerance test; PG, plasma glucose. The diagnosis of diabetes mellitus should be confirmed on a separate day by any of these three tests.

Data from Expert Committee on the Diagnosis and Classification of Diabetes Mellitus. Report of the Expert Committee on the Diagnosis and Classification of Diabetes Mellitus. Diab Care 2000;23(suppl 1):S4–S19 include the degree of abnormality of the diagnostic GTT, the presence or absence of obesity, the gestational age at diagnosis of GDM, and the degree of abnormality of the postpartum oral GTT (104, 105). Individuals at increased risk should be counseled regarding diet, exercise, and weight reduction or maintenance to forestall or prevent the onset of type-2 diabetes.

Summary of Recommendations

The following recommendations are based on limited or inconsistent scientific evidence (Level B):

▶ The laboratory screening test should consist of a 50-g, 1-hour oral glucose challenge at 24–28 weeks of gestation, which may be administered without regard to the time of the last meal.

▶ A screening test threshold of 140 mg/dL has 10% less sensitivity than a threshold of 130 mg/dL but fewer false-positive results; either threshold is acceptable.

▶ The screening test generally should be performed on venous plasma or serum samples using well-calibrated and well-maintained laboratory instruments.

▶ Available evidence does not support a recommendation for or against moderate caloric restriction in obese women with GDM. However, if caloric restriction is used, the diet should be restricted by no more than 33% of calories.

▶ For women with GDM and an estimated fetal weight of 4,500 g or more, cesarean delivery may be considered because it may reduce the likelihood of permanent brachial plexus injury in the infant.

▶ When medical nutritional therapy has not resulted in fasting glucose levels less than 95 mg/dL or 1-hour postprandial values less than 130–140 mg/dL or 2-hour postprandial values less than 120 mg/dL, insulin should be considered.

The following recommendations are based primarily on consensus and expert opinion (Level C):

▶ Although universal glucose challenge screening for GDM is the most sensitive approach, there may be pregnant women at low risk who are less likely to benefit from testing. Such low-risk women should have all of the following characteristics:

1. Age younger than 25 years
2. Not a member of a racial or ethnic group with high prevalence of diabetes (eg, Hispanic, African, Native American, South or East Asian, or Pacific Islands ancestry)
3. Body mass index of 25 or less
4. No history of abnormal glucose tolerance
5. No previous history of adverse pregnancy outcomes usually associated with GDM
6. No known diabetes in first degree relative

▶ There is insufficient evidence to determine the optimal antepartum testing regimen for women with GDM with relatively normal glucose levels on diet therapy and no other risk factors.

▶ Either the plasma or serum glucose level established by Carpenter and Coustan or the plasma level designated by the National Diabetes Data Group conversions are appropriate to use in the diagnosis of GDM.

References

1. Coustan DR. Gestational diabetes. In: National Institutes of Diabetes and Digestive and Kidney Diseases. Diabetes in America. 2nd ed. Bethesda, Maryland: NIDDK, 1995; NIH Publication No. 95-1468:703–717 (Level III)

2. Cousins L. Obstetric complications. In: EA Reece, DR Coustan, eds. Diabetes mellitus in pregnancy. 2nd ed. New York: Churchill Livingstone, 1995:287–302 (Level III)

3. Naylor CD, Sermer M, Chen E, Sykora K. Cesarean delivery in relation to birth weight and gestational glucose tolerance: pathophysiology or practice style? Toronto Trihospital Gestational Diabetes Investigators. JAMA 1996;275:1165–1170 (Level II-2)

4. Sermer M, Naylor CD, Gare DJ, Kenshole AB, Ritchie JW, Farine D, et al. Impact of increasing carbohydrate intolerance on maternal-fetal outcomes in 3637 women without gestational diabetes. The Toronto Tri-Hospital Gestational Diabetes Project. Am J Obstet Gynecol 1995;173:146–156 (Level II-3)

5. Jang HC, Cho NH, Min YK, Han IK, Jung KB, Metzger BE. Increased macrosomia and perinatal morbidity independent of maternal obesity and advanced age in Korean women with GDM. Diabetes Care 1997;20:1582–1588 (Level II-2)

6. Cundy T, Gamble G, Manuel A, Townend K, Roberts A. Determinants of birth-weight in women with established and gestational diabetes. Aust NZJ Obstet Gynaecol 1993;33:249–254 (Level II-2)

7. Dang K, Homko C, Reece EA. Factors associated with fetal macrosomia in offspring of gestational diabetic women. J Matern Fetal Med 2000;9:114–117 (Level II-2)

8. Langer O, Levy J, Brustman L, Anyaegbunam A, Merkatz R, Divon M. Glycemic control in gestational diabetes mellitus—how tight is tight enough: small for gestational age versus large for gestational age? Am J Obstet Gynecol 1989;161:646–653 (Level II-2)

9. Casey BM, Lucas MJ, McIntire DD, Leveno KJ. Pregnancy outcomes in women with gestational diabetes compared with the general obstetric population. Obstet Gynecol 1997;90:869–873 (Level II-2)

10. Adams KM, Li H, Nelson RL, Ogburn PL Jr, Danilenko-Dixon DR. Sequelae of unrecognized gestational diabetes. Am J Obstet Gynecol 1998;178:1321–1332 (Level II-2)

11. Tallarigo L, Giampietro O, Penno G, Miccoli R, Gregori G, Navalesi R. Relation of glucose tolerance to complications of pregnancy in nondiabetic women. N Engl J Med 1986;315:989–992 (Level II-3)

12. Pettitt DJ, Bennett PH, Saad MF, Charles MA, Nelson RG, Knowler WC. Abnormal glucose tolerance during pregnancy in Pima Indian women. Long-term effects on offspring. Diabetes 1991;40(suppl 2):126–130 (Level II-2)

13. Vohr BR, McGarvey ST, Tucker R. Effects of maternal gestational diabetes on offspring adiposity at 4–7 years of age. Diabetes Care 1999;22:1284–1291 (Level II-2)

14. Silverman BL, Metzger BE, Cho NH, Loeb CA. Impaired glucose tolerance in adolescent offspring of diabetic mothers. Relationship to fetal hyperinsulinism. Diabetes Care 1995;18:611–617 (Level II-2)

15. Wilkins-Haug L, Horton JA, Cruess DF, Frigoletto FD. Antepartum screening in the office-based practice: findings from the collaborative Ambulatory Research Network. Obstet Gynecol 1996;88:483–489 (Level III)

16. Weeks, JW, Major CA, de Veciana M, Morgan MA. Gestational diabetes: does the presence of risk factors influence perinatal outcome? Am J Obstet Gynecol 1994; 171:1003–1007 (Level II-2)

17. O'Sullivan JB, Mahan CM, Charles D, Dandrow R. Screening criteria for high-risk gestational diabetic patients. Am J Obstet Gynecol 1973;116:895–900 (Level II-2)

18. Coustan DR, Nelson C, Carpenter MW, Carr SR, Rotondo L, Widness JA. Maternal age and screening for gestational diabetes: a population-based study. Obstet Gynecol 1989;73:557–561 (Level II-2)

19. Screening for diabetes mellitus. In: United States Preventive Services Task Force. Guide to clinical preventive services. 2nd ed. Baltimore: Williams & Wilkins, 1996:193–208 (Level III)

20. O'Sullivan JB, Charles D, Mahan CM, Dandrow RV. Gestational diabetes and perinatal mortality rate. Am J Obstet Gynecol 1973;116:901–904 (Level II-2)

21. Pettitt DJ, Knowler WC, Baird MR, Bennett PH. Gestational diabetes: infant and maternal complications of pregnancy in relation to third-trimester glucose tolerance in the Pima Indians. Diabetes Care 1980;3:458–464 (Level II-2)

22. Cundy T, Gamble G, Townend K, Henley PG, MacPherson P, Roberts AB. Perinatal mortality in type 2 diabetes. Diabet Med 2000;17:33–39 (Level II-2)

23. Schaefer-Graf UM, Buchanan TA, Xiang A, Songster G, Montoro M, Kjos SL. Patterns of congenital anomalies and relationship to initial maternal fasting glucose levels in pregnancies complicated by type 2 and gestational diabetes. Am J Obstet Gynecol 2000;182:313–320 (Level II-2)

24. Garner P, Okun N, Keely E, Wells G, Perkins S, Sylvain J, et al. A randomized controlled trial of strict glycemic control and tertiary level obstetric care versus routine obstetric care in the management of gestational diabetes: a pilot study. Am J Obstet Gynecol 1997;177:190–195 (Level I)

25. de Veciana M, Major CA, Morgan MA, Asrat T, Toohey JS, Lien JM, et al. Postprandial versus preprandial blood glucose monitoring in women with gestational diabetes mellitus requiring insulin therapy. N Engl J Med 1995;333:1237–1241 (Level I)

26. Solomon CG, Willett WC, Carey VJ, Rich-Edwards J, Hunter DJ, Colditz GA, et al. A prospective study of pregravid determinants of gestational diabetes mellitus. JAMA 1997;278:1078–1083 (Level II-3)

27. Naylor CD, Sermer M, Chen E, Farine D. Selective screening for gestational diabetes mellitus. Toronto Trihospital Gestational Diabetes Investigators. N Engl J Med 1997;337:1591–1596 (Level II-3)

28. Dooley SL, Metzger BE, Cho NH. Gestational diabetes mellitus. Influence of race on disease prevalence and perinatal outcome in a US population. Diabetes 1991; 40(suppl 2):25–29 (Level III)

29. The nature and problem of obesity. In: Insitute of Medicine. Committee to Develop Criteria for Evaluating the Outcomes of Approaches to Prevent and Treat Obesity. Food and Nutrition Board. Weighing the options: criteria for evaluating weight-management programs. Washington, DC: National Academy Press, 1995:37–63 (Level III)

30. American Diabetes Association. Gestational diabetes mellitus. Diabetes Care 2001;24(suppl 1):S77–S79 (Level III)

31. Danilenko-Dixon DR, Van Winter JT, Nelson RL, Ogburn PL Jr. Universal versus selective gestational diabetes screening: application of 1997 American Diabetes Association recommendations. Am J Obstet Gynecol 1999;181:798–802 (Level II-2)

32. Jovanovic L, Peterson CM. Screening for gestational diabetes. Optimum timing and criteria for retesting. Diabetes 1985;34(suppl 2):21–23 (Level II-3)

33. Benjamin F, Wilson SJ, Deutsch S, Seltzer VL, Droesch K, Droesch J. Effect of advancing pregnancy on the glucose tolerance test and on the 50-g oral glucose load screening test for gestational diabetes. Obstet Gynecol 1986;68:362–365 (Level II-2)

34. Watson WJ. Serial changes in the 50-g oral glucose test in pregnancy: implications for screening. Obstet Gynecol 1989;74:40–43 (Level II-2)

35. Nahum GG, Huffaker, BJ. Correlation between first- and early third-trimester glucose screening test results. Obstet Gynecol 1990;76:709–713 (Level II-2)

36. Super DM, Edelberg SC, Philipson EH, Hertz RH, Kalhan SC. Diagnosis of gestational diabetes in early pregnancy. Diabetes Care 1991;14:288–294 (Level II-2)

37. Philipson EH, Super DM. Gestational diabetes mellitus: does it recur in subsequent pregnancy? Am J Obstet Gynecol 1989;160:1324–1331 (Level II-2)

38. Gaudier FL, Hauth JC, Poist M, Corbet D, Cliver SP. Recurrence of gestational diabetes mellitus. Obstet Gynecol 1992;80:755–758 (Level II-2)

39. Moses RG. The recurrence rate of gestational diabetes in subsequent pregnancies. Diabetes Care 1996;19:1348–1350 (Level II-2)

40. McElduff A, Goldring J, Gordon P, Wyndham L. A direct comparison of the measurement of a random plasma glucose and a post-50 g glucose load glucose, in the detection of gestational diabetes. Aust NZJ Obstet Gynecol 1994;34:28–30 (Level II-2)

41. Reece EA, Holford T, Tuck S, Bargar M, O'Connor T, Hobbins JC. Screening for gestational diabetes: one-hour carbohydrate tolerance test performed by a virtually tasteless polymer of glucose. Am J Obstet Gynecol 1987;156:132–134 (Level II-2)

42. Murphy NJ, Meyer BA, O'Kell RT, Hogard ME. Carbohydrate sources for gestational diabetes mellitus screening. A comparison. J Reprod Med 1994;39:977–981 (Level I)

43. Bergus GR, Murphy NJ. Screening for gestational diabetes mellitus: comparison of a glucose polymer and a glucose monomer test beverage. J Am Board Fam Pract 1992;5:241–247 (Level II-1)

44. Lamar ME, Kuehl TJ, Cooney AT, Gayle LJ, Holleman S, Allen SR. Jelly beans as an alternative to a fifty gram glucose beverage for gestational diabetes screening. Am J Obstet Gynecol 1999;181:1154–1157 (Level I)

45. Coustan DR, Widness JA, Carpenter MW, Rotondo L, Pratt DC, Oh W. Should the fifty-gram, one-hour plasma glucose screening test for gestational diabetes be administered in the fasting or fed state? Am J Obstet Gynecol 1986;154:1031–1035 (Level I)

46. Lewis GF, McNally C, Blackman JD, Polonsky KS, Barron WM. Prior feeding alters the response to the 50-g glucose challenge test in pregnancy. The Staub Traugott effect revisited. Diabetes Care 1993;16:1551–1556 (Level II-3)

47. Carr S, Coustan DR, Martelly P, Brosco F, Rotondo L. Precision of reflectance meters in screening for gestational diabetes. Obstet Gynecol 1989;73:727–731 (Level II-2)

48. Carr SR, Slocum J, Tefft L, Haydon B, Carpenter M. Precision of office-based blood glucose meters in screening for gestational diabetes. Am J Obstet Gynecol 1995;173:1267–1272 (Level II-2)

49. Nutritional management during pregnancy in preexisting diabetes. In: American Diabetes Association. Medical management of pregnancy complicated by diabetes. 3rd ed Alexandria, Virginia: ADA, 2000:70–86 (Level III)

50. O'Sullivan JB, Mahan CM. Criteria for the oral glucose tolerance test in pregnancy. Diabetes 1964;13:278–285 (Level II-3)

51. National Diabetes Data Group. Classification and diagnosis of diabetes mellitus and other categories of glucose intolerance. Diabetes 1979;28:1039–1057 (Level III)

52. Carpenter MW, Coustan DR. Criteria for screening tests for gestational diabetes. Am J Obstet Gynecol 1982;144:768–773 (Level II-3)

53. Expert Committee on the Diagnosis and Classification of Diabetes Mellitus. Report of the Expert Committee on the Diagnosis and Classification of Diabetes Mellitus. Diab Care 2000;23(suppl 1):S4–S19 (Level III)

54. Langer O, Brustman L, Anyaegbunam A, Mazze R. The significance of one abnormal glucose tolerance test value on adverse outcome in pregnancy. Am J Obstet Gynecol 1987;157:758–763 (Level II-2)

55. Lindsay MK, Graves W, Klein L. The relationship of one abnormal glucose tolerance test value and pregnancy complications. Obstet Gynecol 1989;73:103–106 (Level II-2)

56. Sacks DA, Greenspoon JS, Abu-Fadil S, Henry HM, Wolde-Tsadik G, Yao JF. Toward universal criteria for gestational diabetes: the 75-gram glucose tolerance test in pregnancy. Am J Obstet Gynecol 1995;172:607–614 (Level II-3)

57. Langer O, Rodriguez DA, Xenakis EM, McFarland MB, Berkus MD, Arrendondo F. Intensified versus conventional management of gestational diabetes. Am J Obstet Gynecol 1994;170:1036–1047 (Level II-1)

58. Goldberg JD, Franklin B, Lasser D, Jornsay DL, Hausknecht RU, Ginsberg-Fellner F, et al. Gestational diabetes: impact of home glucose monitoring on neonatal birth weight. Am J Obstet Gynecol 1986;154:546–550 (Level II-2)

59. Jovanovic-Peterson L, Peterson CM, Reed GF, Metzger BE, Mills JL, Knopp RH, et al. Maternal postprandial glucose levels and infant birth weight: the Diabetes in Early Pregnancy Study. The National Institute of Child Health and Human Development-Diabetes in Early Pregnancy Study. Am J Obstet Gynecol 1991;164: 103–111 (Level II-2)

60. Combs CA, Gunderson E, Kitzmiller JL, Gavin LA, Main EK. Relationship of fetal macrosomia to maternal postprandial glucose control during pregnancy. Diabetes Care 1992;15:1251–1257 (Level II-2)

61. Huddleston JF, Cramer MK, Vroon DH. A rationale for omitting two-hour postprandial glucose determinations in gestational diabetes. Am J Obstet Gynecol 1993;169:257–264 (Level II-2)

62. Bevier WC, Fischer R, Jovanovic L. Treatment of women with an abnormal glucose challenge test (but a normal oral glucose tolerance test) decreases the prevalence of macrosomia. Am J Perinatol 1999;16:269–275 (Level II-1)

63. Dornhorst A, Nicholls JSD, Probst F, Paterson CM, Hollier KL, Elkeles RS, et al. Calorie restriction for treatment of gestational diabetes. Diabetes 1991;40(suppl 2):161–164 (Level II-2)

64. Knopp RH, Magee MS, Raisys V, Benedetti T, Bonet B. Hypocaloric diets and ketogenesis in the management of obese gestational diabetic women. J Amer Coll Nutr 1991;10:649–667 (Level II-2)

65. Rizzo T, Metzger BE, Burns WJ, Burns K. Correlations between antepartum maternal metabolism and child intelligence. N Engl J Med 1991;325:911–916 (Level II-2)

66. Rizzo TA, Dooley SL, Metzger BE, Cho NH, Ogata ES, Silverman BL. Prenatal and perinatal influences on long-term psychomotor development in offspring of diabetic mothers. Am J Obstet Gynecol 1995;173:1753–1758 (Level II-2)

67. Algert S, Shragg P, Hollingsworth DR. Moderate caloric restriction in obese women with gestational diabetes. Obstet Gynecol 1985;65:487–491 (Level II-2)

68. Reece EA, Hagay Z, Caseria D, Gay LJ, DeGennaro N. Do fiber-enriched diabetic diets have glucose-lowering effects in pregnancy? Am J Perinatol 1993;10:272–274 (Level II-2)

69. O'Sullivan JB, Gellis SS, Dandrow RV, Tenney BO. The potential diabetic and her treatment in pregnancy. Obstet Gynecol 1966;27:683–689 (Level I)

70. Coustan DR, Lewis SB. Insulin therapy for gestational diabetes. Obstet Gynecol 1978;51:306–310 (Level I)

71. Thompson DJ, Porter KB, Gunnells DJ, Wagner PC, Spinnato JA. Prophylactic insulin in the management of gestational diabetes. Obstet Gynecol 1990;75:960–964 (Level I)

72. Persson B, Stangenberg M, Hansson U, Nordlander E. Gestational diabetes mellitus (GDM). Comparative evaluation of two treatment regimens, diet versus insulin and diet. Diabetes 1985;34(suppl 2):101–105 (Level I)

73. Langer O, Berkus M, Brustman L, Anyaegbunam A, Mazze R. Rationale for insulin management in gestational diabetes mellitus. Diabetes 1991;40(suppl 2):186–190 (Level II-3)

74. Buchanan TA, Kjos SL, Montoro MN, Wu PY, Madrilejo NG, Gonzalez M. Use of fetal ultrasound to select metabolic therapy for pregnancies complicated by mild gestational diabetes. Diabetes Care 1994;17:275–283 (Level II-1)

75. McFarland MB, Langer O, Conway DL, Berkus MD. Dietary therapy for gestational diabetes: how long is long enough? Obstet Gynecol 1999;93:978–982 (Level II-3)

76. Jovanovic L, Ilic S, Pettitt DJ, Hugo K, Gutierrez M, Bowsher RR, et al. Metabolic and immunologic effects of insulin lispro in gestational diabetes. Diabetes Care 1999;22:1422–1427 (Level I)

77. Bung P, Bung C, Artal R, Khodiguian N, Fallenstein F, Spätling L. Therapeutic exercise for insulin-requiring gestational diabetics: effects on the fetus—results of a randomized prospective longitudinal study. J Perinat Med 1993;21:125–137 (Level II-2)

78. Jovanovic-Peterson L, Durak EP, Peterson CM. Randomized trial of diet versus diet plus cardiovascular conditioning on glucose levels in gestational diabetes. Am J Obstet Gynecol 1989;161:415–419 (Level II-1)

79. Avery MD, Leon AS, Kopher RA. Effects of a partially home-based exercise program for women with gestational diabetes. Obstet Gynecol 1997;89:10–15 (Level I)

80. Langer O, Conway DL, Berkus MD, Xenakis EM, Gonzales O. A comparison of glyburide and insulin in women with gestational diabetes mellitus. New Engl J Med 2000;343:1134–1138 (Level I)

81. American College of Obstetricians and Gynecologists. Antepartum fetal surveillance. ACOG Practice Bulletin 9. Washington, DC: ACOG, 1999 (Level III)

82. Kjos SL, Leung A, Henry OA, Victor MR, Paul RH, Medearis AL. Antepartum surveillance in diabetic pregnancies: predictors of fetal distress in labor. Am J Obstet Gynecol 1995;173:1532–1539 (Level II-3)

83. Landon MB, Gabbe SG. Antepartum fetal surveillance in gestational diabetes mellitus. Diabetes 1985;34(suppl 2):50–54 (Level II-2)

84. Deter RL, Hadlock FP. Use of ultrasound in the detection of macrosomia: a review. J Clin Ultrasound 1985;13:519–524 (Level III)

85. Rossavik IK, Joslin GL. Macrosomatia and ultrasonography: what is the problem? South Med J 1993;86:1129–1132 (Level II-3)

86. Sandmire HF. Whither ultrasonic prediction of fetal macrosomia? Obstet Gynecol 1993;82:860–862 (Level III)

87. Smith GC, Smith MF, McNay MB, Fleming JE. The relation between fetal abdominal circumference and birthweight: findings in 3512 pregnancies. Br J Obstet Gynaecol 1997;104:186–190 (Level II-3)

88. McLaren RA, Puckett JL, Chauhan SP. Estimators of birth weight in pregnant women requiring insulin: a comparison of seven sonographic models. Obstet Gynecol 1995;85:565–569 (Level II-2)

89. Kjos SL, Henry OA, Montoro M, Buchanan TA, Mestman JH. Insulin-requiring diabetes in pregnancy: a randomized trial of active induction of labor and expectant management. Am J Obstet Gynecol 1993;169:611–615 (Level II-1)

90. Lurie S, Insler V, Hagay ZJ. Induction of labor at 38 to 39 weeks of gestation reduces the incidence of shoulder dystocia in gestational diabetic patients Class A2. Am J Perinatol 1996;13:293–296 (Level II-2)

91. Kjos SL, Walther FJ, Montoro M, Paul RH, Diaz F, Stabler M. Prevalence and etiology of respiratory distress in infants of diabetic mothers: predictive values of fetal lung maturation tests. Am J Obstet Gynecol 1990;163: 898–903 (Level II-3)

92. Acker DB, Sachs BP, Friedman EA. Risk factors for shoulder dystocia. Obstet Gynecol 1985;66:762–768 (Level II-2)

93. Langer O, Berkus MD, Huff RW, Samueloff A. Shoulder dystocia: should the fetus weighing greater than or equal to 4000 grams be delivered by cesarean section? Am J Obstet Gynecol 1991;165:831–837 (Level II-2)

94. Benacerraf BR, Gelman R, Frigoletto FD Jr. Sonographically estimated fetal weights: accuracy and limitation. Am J Obstet Gynecol 1988;159;1118–1121 (Level II-2)

95. Rouse DJ, Owen J, Goldenberg RL, Cliver SP. The effectiveness and costs of elective cesarean delivery for fetal macrosomia diagnosed by ultrasound. JAMA 1996;276:1480–1486 (Level III)

96. Benedetti TJ, Gabbe SG. Shoulder dystocia. A complication of fetal macrosomia and prolonged second stage of labor with midpelvic delivery. Obstet Gynecol 1978;52:526–529 (Level II-2)

97. Dornhorst A, Rossi M. Risk and prevention of type 2 diabetes in women with gestational diabetes. Diabetes Care 1998;21 suppl:B43–B49 (Level III)

98. Buchanan TA, Xiang A, Kjos SL, Lee WP, Trigo E, Nader I, et al. Gestational diabetes: antepartum characteristics that predict postpartum glucose intolerance and type 2 diabetes in Latino women. Diabetes 1998;47:1302–1310 (Level II-3)

99. Kjos SL, Buchanan TA, Greenspoon JS, Montoro M, Bernstein GS, Mestman JH. Gestational diabetes mellitus: the prevalence of glucose intolerance and diabetes mellitus in the first two months post partum. Am J Obstet Gynecol 1990;163:93–98 (Level II-2)

100. Report of the Expert Committee on the Diagnosis and Classification of Diabetes Mellitus. American Diabetes Association. Expert Committee on the Diagnosis and Classification of Diabetes Mellitus. Diabetes Care 2001;4(suppl 1):S5–S20 (Level III)

101. Conway DL, Langer O. Effects of the new criteria for type 2 diabetes on the rate of postpartum glucose intolerance in women with gestational diabetes. Am J Obstet Gynecol 1999;181:610–614 (Level II-2)

102. O'Sullivan JB. Diabetes mellitus after GDM. Diabetes 1991;29(suppl 2):131–135 (Level III)

103. O'Sullivan JB. Subsequent morbidity among gestational diabetic women. In: Sutherland HW, Stowers JM, eds. Carbohydrate metabolism in pregnancy and the newborn. New York: Churchill Livingstone, 1984:174–180 (Level I)

104. Coustan DR, Carpenter MW, O'Sullivan PS, Carr SR. Gestational diabetes: predictors of subsequent disordered glucose metabolism. Am J Obstet Gynecol 1993;168:1139–1145 (Level II-2)

105. Kjos SL, Peters RK, Xiang A, Henry OA, Montoro M, Buchanan TA. Predicting future diabetes in Latino women with gestational diabetes. Utility of early postpartum glucose testing. Diabetes 1995;44:586–591 (Level II-3)

The MEDLINE database, the Cochrane Library, and ACOG's own internal resources and documents were used to conduct a literature search to locate relevant articles published between January 1985 and June 2000. The search was restricted to articles published in the English language. Priority was given to articles reporting results of original research, although review articles and commentaries also were consulted. Abstracts of research presented at symposia and scientific conferences were not considered adequate for inclusion in this document. Guidelines published by organizations or institutions such as the National Institutes of Health and the American College of Obstetricians and Gynecologists were reviewed, and additional studies were located by reviewing bibliographies of identified articles. When reliable research was not available, expert opinions from obstetrician–gynecologists were used.

Studies were reviewed and evaluated for quality according to the method outlined by the U.S. Preventive Services Task Force:

I   Evidence obtained from at least one properly designed randomized controlled trial.
II-1 Evidence obtained from well-designed controlled trials without randomization.
II-2 Evidence obtained from well-designed cohort or case–control analytic studies, preferably from more than one center or research group.
II-3 Evidence obtained from multiple time series with or without the intervention. Dramatic results in uncontrolled experiments could also be regarded as this type of evidence.
III Opinions of respected authorities, based on clinical experience, descriptive studies, or reports of expert committees.

Based on the highest level of evidence found in the data, recommendations are provided and graded according to the following categories:

Level A—Recommendations are based on good and consistent scientific evidence.

Level B—Recommendations are based on limited or inconsistent scientific evidence.

Level C—Recommendations are based primarily on consensus and expert opinion.

ISSN 1099-3630

The American College of Obstetricians and Gynecologists
409 12th Street, SW, PO Box 96920
Washington, DC 20090-6920

12345/54321

Gestational Diabetes. ACOG Practice Bulletin No. 30. American College of Obstetricians and Gynecologists. Obstet Gynecol 2001;98:525–538

ACOG PRACTICE BULLETIN

CLINICAL MANAGEMENT GUIDELINES FOR
OBSTETRICIAN–GYNECOLOGISTS

NUMBER 57, NOVEMBER 2004

This Practice Bulletin was developed by the ACOG Committee on Practice Bulletins—Gynecology with the assistance of Anna Wald, MD, and Zane Brown, MD. The information is designed to aid practitioners in making decisions about appropriate obstetric and gynecologic care. These guidelines should not be construed as dictating an exclusive course of treatment or procedure. Variations in practice may be warranted based on the needs of the individual patient, resources, and limitations unique to the institution or type of practice.

Gynecologic Herpes Simplex Virus Infections

Both herpes simplex virus (HSV) type 1 and HSV type 2 can cause genital herpes. Because the infection is chronic, genital herpes has become the most common sexually transmitted disease among women (1). The prevalence of the HSV-2 antibody among women in the United States is 26%, although genital herpes has been diagnosed in only a small proportion (10–25%) of individuals with HSV-2 antibodies (2). Herpes simplex virus type 1 is becoming a more frequent cause of genital herpes, especially among young women (3). Overall, HSV-1 seroprevalence in the United States is estimated at 67%, although serologic data do not provide information about site of infection (4). Recent advances in diagnostic methods and therapeutic options are likely to change the management of genital herpes.

Background

Serologic surveys show that 26% of women aged 12 years and older have antibodies to HSV-2. This represents a substantial increase in prevalence since the 1970s and suggests that more than 910,000 new infections with HSV-2 occur annually in women (5). The increase in the HSV-2 seroprevalence has been mirrored by a continual increase in the reported number of cases of first episode genital herpes seen in physician offices, with approximately 150,000 cases reported in 2000 (6). Correlates of HSV-2 antibodies include markers of high levels of sexual activity, such as reported number of sexual partners and age of first sexual contact (7). However, these risk factors do not reliably identify women with HSV-2 because the infection has reached such high levels that even women without these risk factors may be HSV-2 seropositive.

The reported HSV-2 seroprevalence underestimates the frequency of genital herpes because an increasing proportion of first episode genital herpes is caused by HSV-1 infection (8, 9). Although the initial presentation of genital herpes is the same for HSV-1 and HSV-2, the rate of recurrence is much lower for HSV-1, and most recurrences are caused by HSV-2 (10). Women with genital HSV-2 will have an average of 4 recurrences in the first year of infection compared with 1 recurrence for genital HSV-1. After the first year, the rate of recurrences decreases very slowly for HSV-2, but recurrences are rare for HSV-1 after the first year of infection. As such, the type of genital herpes has prognostic significance for frequency of recurrences and should be determined in every patient (1). In addition, although the acquisition of a new HSV-1 infection in an individual with HSV-2 antibodies is unusual, women with genital HSV-1 infection are still at risk for HSV-2 acquisition (11).

Genital HSV infection can cause a large spectrum of disease. First episode infections, which represent new acquisition of HSV, usually are most severe, and recurrent infections may be milder (12). However, serologic studies show that up to 25% of first clinical episodes are in reality first recognized recurrences; its presentation often is surprising to the patient and the provider (13, 14). First episode infections often are accompanied by systemic symptoms, including prominent flulike syndrome and frequent neurologic involvement, with aseptic meningitis reported in up to 25% of patients. However, as many as 75% of primary infections are unrecognized by either patient or provider (15). Recurrences usually are limited to the genital area. Most women with HSV-2 do not know they have genital herpes because their recurrences are mild and infrequent (16, 17). Such women may have nonspecific genital conditions and may have been receiving treatment for other genital conditions, such as recurrent yeast infections, urinary tract infections, or allergic rashes in the genital area (18).

An important feature of HSV infection is intermittent reactivation, with or without accompanying symptoms, and resultant shedding of the virus in the genital tract (19). DNA from HSV can be detected in the genital tract 10–50% of the time among HSV-2 seropositive women (20). Women close to the time of acquisition or with severe clinical disease have a higher risk of viral shedding between symptomatic recurrences (19, 21). For example, in a study of women with genital HSV-2 infection within 2 years of HSV-2 acquisition, HSV-2 was isolated in culture from the genital area on 9.9% of days overall and on 6.9% of days without genital lesion (19). At those times, the virus can be transmitted sexually or perinatally (22). For many patients, the most bothersome aspect of genital herpes is the unpredictable nature of viral shedding.

An accurate diagnosis enables appropriate treatment for the woman with genital herpes. In addition, it can reduce the risk of transmission of HSV to a sexual partner and reduce the risk of HSV transmission to a neonate.

Clinical Considerations and Recommendations

▶ How is the diagnosis established?

It is difficult to make the diagnosis of genital herpes on clinical grounds alone (1). The classic presentation of a painful cluster of vesicles and ulcers occurs in a small proportion of women, and most women will have atypical lesions, such as abrasions, fissures, or itching without obvious lesions. Conversely, even in at-risk women with a presentation compatible with genital herpes, up to 20% of women will not have genital herpes (15). Thus, a definitive diagnosis should be confirmed by a laboratory test, even if the infection was established in the past on clinical grounds.

Traditionally, the laboratory test used most often has been viral culture (23) because it is highly specific, widely available, and relatively inexpensive. Viral culture can be useful in women presenting with new or recurrent genital ulcer disease. However, viral culture is insensitive, even with a primary infection, with a false-negative rate up to 25%. In recurrent disease, the rate of viral isolation is less than 50%. This low rate of viral isolation results in the need for repeat visits or leaves the impression that the patient does not have genital herpes. Antigen detection tests also are available. They have comparable performance characteristics to viral culture but do not distinguish between HSV-1 and HSV-2 infection.

Polymerase chain reaction (PCR) testing has become more available, and several studies have demonstrated that its sensitivity is 1.5–4 times greater than viral culture (24–26). Thus, PCR is the test of choice in the diagnosis of herpes-related infections of the central nervous system (meningitis and encephalitis) (27–29). Because samples for PCR testing are easier to obtain and more stable than samples for viral culture, PCR testing is likely to replace viral culture for the diagnosis of HSV genital infections in the future (30).

In addition to viral detection methods, the detection of type-specific antibodies to HSV-1 and HSV-2 also can help to establish the diagnosis. The incubation period for HSV is short (approximately 4 days), and infection of the ganglia with establishment of latency has occurred by the time the patient is evaluated for symptomatic disease. Antibodies to HSV-2 are detected 2–12 weeks after acquisition of infection and persist indefinitely (31). Only tests that are based on the detection of antibody response to glycoprotein G-2 for HSV-2 and glycoprotein G-1 for HSV-1 are type specific because much of the immune response is type-common for both HSV types. Many serologic tests on the market are not type specific, despite labeling claims to the contrary (32). Currently, there are only 3 commercially available, FDA-approved type-specific tests (Herpes Select ELISA, Herpes Select Immunoblot, Captia ELISA) for serologic diagnosis of genital herpes, although other tests are in development. When compared with the Western blot test, the sensitivity of these tests range from 96% to 100%, and specificity is 97–98% (31). Caution should be used in populations with low HSV-2 prevalence because the positive predictive value could be low, and a confirmatory test, such as Western blot, may be required. The serologic test results are likely to be negative with newly acquired genital herpes because the median time to seroconversion is 22 days by enzyme-linked immunosorbent assay with approximately 20% still remaining seronegative after 3 months, particularly if the patient has received antiviral chemotherapy (33).

▶ Is there a role for testing an asymptomatic patient who reports possible exposure?

Most women with genital HSV-1 or genital HSV-2 infection are asymptomatic. A small proportion may recall symptoms or lesions compatible with genital herpes when they receive a diagnosis of HSV-2. Because HSV is so prevalent among women, infection rates are very high among sexually active women, even if the number of sexual partners is not very high. Therefore, type-specific antibody testing is more accurate than assessment of infection based on symptoms or past sexual behavior (15). Such testing is especially important in women who are in relationships with partners who have genital herpes. In this setting, knowledge of infection may result in decreased distress because the relationship is no longer discordant, and confirmation of seronegativity may precipitate increased adherence to interventions to reduce transmission.

▶ Is there a role for postexposure prophylaxis in an asymptomatic patient?

No data are available on the efficacy of postexposure prophylaxis in an asymptomatic patient. Chronic or intermittent antiviral therapy is not recommended for women who lack HSV-2 infection and whose partners have HSV-2. However, some physicians offer antiviral therapy in the setting of unanticipated known high-risk exposure (for example, rape or intercourse without a condom with a partner who had an unnoticed recurrence). Although the effectiveness of this approach is unlikely ever to be documented, the safety of antiviral medication for HSV suggests this approach carries very low risk.

▶ How are first clinical episodes of infection treated?

Acyclovir, famciclovir, and valacyclovir are antiviral drugs approved for treatment of genital herpes (1, 34). They interrupt viral DNA synthesis and have excellent safety profiles. They require viral thymidine kinase for the initial activation step; that is, the drug is not activated unless HSV is actively replicating. Comparative trials of these medications suggest they have comparable clinical efficacy and result in a comparable decrease in viral shedding. Because acyclovir is available in generic form, it generally is the least expensive product. Valacyclovir, a prodrug of acyclovir, can be taken less frequently than acyclovir and famciclovir for some indications, which may be an advantage for some patients. Table 1 lists the antiviral regimens recommended for genital herpes in nonpregnant women.

Treatment should be offered for first episodes of genital herpes, even if they appear to be mild initially. Treatment of first episodes of genital herpes decreases lesions, viral shedding, and symptoms but does not affect the long-term natural history of the infection (35). Newly acquired HSV infections can have a prolonged course, with systemic and neurologic involvement that can be substantially ameliorated by using antiviral therapy (36). Oral therapy is recommended, except in severe cases in which a woman is unable to tolerate oral intake or has prominent neurologic involvement. Such patients should be hospitalized and treated with intravenous acyclovir. Topical antiviral medication is not effective therapy and does not add to the benefit of the oral medication; its use is discouraged.

Antiviral medication is the best intervention for severe symptoms. In addition, analgesics should be provided as needed (ie, acetaminophen or ibuprofen). Warm water baths often are helpful during the first few days. Topical lidocaine also is occasionally beneficial, but it can result in local allergic reactions.

▶ How are recurrent episodes treated?

Recurrent episodes of genital herpes can be managed effectively either with daily suppressive or episodic antiviral drugs. The choice of approach should be made in consultation with the patient; the frequency of recurrences should be one, but not the only, consideration in deciding whether to use suppressive therapy.

▶ When is treatment to prevent recurrence indicated, and which regimens are effective?

Episodic therapy decreases the duration of the episode (lesion, pain, and viral shedding) and is most effective when the patient initiates the therapy at prodrome or at the beginning of the episode. This form of therapy is most effective for a patient with infrequent symptomatic recurrences. Therefore, women who choose this approach should be encouraged to fill their prescriptions and have the medications available.

Suppressive therapy (in which the medication is taken daily) for genital herpes prevents approximately 80% of recurrences. Studies indicate many patients prefer this treatment (37, 38). Breakthrough recurrences are short, and in some patients, this approach may eliminate recurrences for several years. In those taking daily antiviral therapy, viral shedding from the genital area is markedly decreased, and the breakthrough shedding contains reduced amounts of viral DNA (21). This reduction in shedding translates into a 48% reduction in transmission between sexual partners (39).

▶ How are severe episodes treated?

Some patients have severe disease or complications, such as disseminated infection, pneumonitis, hepatitis, or complications of the central nervous system (eg, meningitis, encephalitis), that require hospitalization. They should receive intravenous acyclovir therapy (see Table 1) (1).

▶ How should patients be counseled about living with genital herpes?

Management of women with genital herpes may be complicated by psychologic distress, especially at the time of initial diagnosis (40). Counseling them about the disease may decrease the distress (41). Therefore, women who present with a first clinical episode of genital herpes and are overwhelmed by the diagnosis and the clinical illness may require a separate visit for counseling. Many materials, both printed and web-based, are available to complement counseling, and their use is encouraged.

Women in whom a first episode genital HSV infection is diagnosed should be told they are likely to have recurrences and that these will be milder than the first episode. Women without a history of genital herpes are

Table 1. Recommended Antiviral Regimens for Genital Herpes

Indication	Drug	Dose	Duration of Therapy
First episode of genital herpes	Acyclovir	400 mg PO tid	7–10 d; longer if new lesions persist
	Acyclovir	200 mg PO 5 times per day	
	Valacyclovir	1,000 mg PO bid	
	Famciclovir	250 mg PO tid	
Recurrent genital herpes			
Episodic therapy	Acyclovir	400 mg PO tid	5 d
	Acyclovir	200 mg PO 5 times per day	5 d
	Acyclovir	800 mg PO bid	2 d*
	Valacyclovir	500 mg PO bid	3–5 d
	Valacyclovir	1,000 mg PO sid	5 d
	Famciclovir	125 mg PO bid	5 d
Suppressive therapy	Acyclovir	400 mg PO bid	Suppressive therapy can be continued for several years†
	Valacyclovir	500–1,000 mg PO sid	
	Famciclovir	250 mg PO bid	
Severe disease/concurrent complications	Acyclovir	5–10 mg/kg of body weight intravenously every 8 h	2–7 d or until clinical improvement is observed, followed by oral antiviral therapy to complete at least 10 days of total therapy

Abbreviations: bid, twice per day; PO, orally; sid, once per day; tid, 3 times per day.

*Thrice-daily acyclovir, 800 mg, has been shown to be effective when given for 2 days (Wald A, Carrell D, Remington M, Kexel E, Zeh J, Corey L. Two-day regimen of acyclovir for treatment of recurrent genital herpes simplex virus type 2 infection. Clin Infect Dis 2002;34:944–8.).

†Annual discussions with patients about continuation are recommended, but the medication does not need to be discontinued. Antiviral resistance has not emerged in immunocompetent individuals (Fife KH, Crumpacker CS, Mertz GJ, Hill EL, Boone GS. Recurrence and resistance patterns of herpes simplex virus following cessation of > or = 6 years of chronic suppression with acyclovir. Acyclovir Study Group. J Infect Dis 1994;169:1338–41.).

Data from Sexually transmitted diseases treatment guidelines 2002. Centers for Disease Control and Prevention. MMWR Recomm Rep 2002;51(RR-6):1–82.

likely to recognize recurrences once they know they have HSV-2 infection. Women should be told they may have viral shedding with or without symptoms and that they are infectious at that time. It is important to reassure women that they can have healthy children despite the infection and that the risk of perinatal transmission of herpes is low if the infection is acquired before or during the first half of pregnancy.

Often, the most difficult part of having genital herpes is telling a partner about the infection. However, this should be encouraged, ideally before the initiation of sexual activity. If the partner is known to have the same type of genital herpes (ie, HSV-1 or HSV-2 concordance), transmission of a different strain of the same type of virus is thought to occur infrequently, and safer sex practices specifically to avoid HSV are not necessary.

▶ *What are appropriate methods for preventing the acquisition of genital herpes by women whose partners have genital herpes?*

Women who have partners with genital herpes should be tested with type-specific serology to assess the woman's risk of infection. A finding of concordant HSV types may be reassuring to the couple. If the partners have discordant HSV types, the couple should be counseled about consistent use of condoms or dental dams, although condoms do not offer total protection from acquisition of HSV-2 infection (42). If the couple is discordant with the woman being at risk for acquiring genital HSV-1 or HSV-2 from her partner, the risk of new HSV infection during late pregnancy should be explained together with its consequences, such as a 40–50% rate of infection of the newborn (43). Finally, use of suppressive antiviral therapy in the potential source partner has been shown to decrease transmission of HSV-2 by 48% to susceptible partners (39). However, this trial did not evaluate prevention of HSV-1 transmission or transmission of HSV-2 to pregnant women.

A preventive vaccine with recombinant glycoprotein D for genital herpes currently is being developed. In early trials, the vaccine protected seronegative women from genital herpes disease (73% reduction) and showed partial protection from HSV-2 infection (40% reduction) (44). The effect of the vaccine on subclinical shedding in women who acquire HSV-2 after vaccination is unknown. An ongoing trial is evaluating this vaccine in more than 7,000 seronegative young women. The vaccine lacked efficacy in men and in women with previous HSV-1 infection.

Summary of Recommendations

The following recommendations are based on good and consistent scientific evidence (Level A):

▶ Antiviral therapy should be prescribed at the first clinical episode to reduce the duration of symptoms and viral shedding.

▶ Women should be offered antiviral treatment for recurrent episodes at prodrome or at the beginning of an episode of genital herpes.

▶ Women with frequent recurrences should be offered suppressive therapy.

▶ For couples in which one partner has HSV-2 infection, suppressive antiviral therapy should be recommended for the partner with HSV-2 to reduce the rate of transmission.

▶ Topical antivirals are not effective in the treatment of genital herpes and should not be used.

The following recommendations are based on limited or inconsistent scientific evidence (Level B):

▶ Clinical suspicion of genital herpes should be confirmed using reliable laboratory testing.

▶ Discordant couples should be counseled that consistent use of condoms decreases but does not eliminate the risk of transmission.

References

1. Sexually transmitted diseases treatment guidelines 2002. Centers for Disease Control and Prevention. MMWR Recomm Rep 2002;51(RR-6):1–78. (Level II–3)

2. Fleming DT, McQuillan GM, Johnson RE, Nahmias AJ, Aral SO, Lee FK, et al. Herpes simplex virus type 2 in the United States, 1976 to 1994. N Engl J Med 1997;337: 1105–11. (Level II–3)

3. Cowan FM, Copas A, Johnson AM, Ashley R, Corey L, Mindel A. Herpes simplex virus type 1 infection: a sexually transmitted infection of adolescence? Sex Transm Infect 2002;78:346–8. (Level II–3)

4. Xu F, Schillinger JA, Sternberg MR, Johnson RE, Lee FK, Nahmias AJ, et al. Seroprevalence and coinfection with herpes simplex virus type 1 and type 2 in the United States, 1988–1994. J Infect Dis 2002;185:1019–24. (Level II–3)

5. Armstrong GL, Schillinger J, Markowitz L, Nahmias AJ, Johnson RE, McQuillan GM, et al. Incidence of herpes simplex virus type 2 infection in the United States. Am J Epidemiol 2001;153:912–20. (Level II–3)

6. Centers for Disease Control and Prevention. Sexually transmitted disease surveillance 2002. Atlanta (GA): CDC; 2003. (Level II-3)

7. Cowan FM, Johnson AM, Ashley R, Corey L, Mindel A. Antibody to herpes simplex virus type 2 as serological marker of sexual lifestyle in populations. BMJ 1994; 309:1325–9. (Level II–3)

8. Lafferty WE, Downey L, Celum C, Wald A. Herpes simplex virus type 1 as a cause of genital herpes: impact on surveillance and prevention. J Infect Dis 2000;181: 1454–7. (Level II–2)

9. Roberts CM, Pfister JR, Spear SJ. Increasing proportion of herpes simplex virus type 1 as a cause of genital herpes infection in college students. Sex Transm Dis 2003;30: 797–800. (Level II–3)

10. Benedetti J, Corey L, Ashley R. Recurrence rates in genital herpes after symptomatic first-episode infection. Ann Intern Med 1994;121:847–54. (Level II–2)

11. Sucato G, Wald A, Wakabayashi E, Vieira J, Corey L. Evidence of latency and reactivation of both herpes simplex virus (HSV)-1 and HSV-2 in the genital region. J Infect Dis 1998;177:1069–72. (Level III)

12. Corey L, Adams HG, Brown ZA, Holmes KK. Genital herpes simplex virus infections: clinical manifestations, course, and complications. Ann Intern Med 1983;98: 958–72. (Level III)

13. Bernstein DI, Lovett MA, Bryson YJ. Serologic analysis of first-episode nonprimary genital herpes simplex virus infection. Presence of type 2 antibody in acute serum samples. Amer J Med 1984;77:1055–60. (Level III)

14. Diamond C, Selke S, Ashley R, Benedetti J, Corey L. Clinical course of patients with serologic evidence of recurrent genital herpes presenting with signs and symptoms of first episode disease. Sex Transm Dis 1999; 26:221–5. (Level II-2)

15. Langenberg AG, Corey L, Ashley RL, Leong WP, Straus SE. A prospective study of new infections with herpes simplex virus type 1 and type 2. Chiron HSV Vaccine Study Group. N Engl J Med 1999;341:1432–8. (Level I)

16. Langenberg A, Benedetti J, Jenkins J, Ashley R, Winter C, Corey L. Development of clinically recognizable genital lesions among women previously identified as having "asymptomatic" herpes simplex virus type 2 infection. Ann Intern Med 1989;110:882–7. (Level II–3)

17. Wald A, Zeh J, Selke S, Warren T, Ryncarz A, Ashley R, et al. Reactivation of genital herpes simplex virus type 2 infection in asymptomatic seropositive persons. N Engl J Med 2000;342:844–50. (Level II–2)

18. Ashley RL, Wald A. Genital herpes: review of the epidemic and potential use of type-specific serology. Clin Microbiol Rev 1999;12:1–8. (Level III)

19. Wald A, Zeh J, Selke S, Ashley RL, Corey L. Virologic characteristics of subclinical and symptomatic genital herpes infections. N Engl J Med 1995;333:770–5. (Level II–2)

20. Wald A, Corey L, Cone R, Hobson A, Davis G, Zeh J. Frequent genital herpes simplex virus 2 shedding in immunocompetent women. Effect of acyclovir treatment. J Clin Invest 1997;99:1092–7. (Level II–2)

21. Wald A, Zeh J, Barnum G, Davis LG, Corey L. Suppression of subclinical shedding of herpes simplex virus type 2 with acyclovir. Ann Intern Med 1996;124: 8–15. (Level II–3)

22. Mertz GJ, Benedetti J, Ashley R, Selke SA, Corey L. Risk factors for the sexual transmission of genital herpes. Ann Intern Med 1992;116:197–202. (Level I)

23. Ashley RL. Laboratory techniques in the diagnosis of herpes simplex infection. Genitourin Med 1993;69:174–83. (Level III)

24. Slomka MJ, Emery L, Munday PE, Moulsdale M, Brown DW. A comparison of PCR with virus isolation and direct antigen detection for diagnosis and typing of genital herpes. J Med Virol 1998;55:177–83. (Level II–3)

25. Cone RW, Hobson AC, Palmer J, Remington M, Corey L. Extended duration of herpes simplex virus DNA in genital lesions detected by the polymerase chain reaction. J Infect Dis 1991;164:757–60. (Level III)

26. Wald A, Huang ML, Carrell D, Selke S, Corey L. Polymerase chain reaction for detection of herpes simplex virus (HSV) DNA on mucosal surfaces: comparison with HSV isolation in cell culture. J Infect Dis 2003;188: 1345–51. (Level III)

27. Whitley RJ, Lakeman F. Herpes simplex virus infections of the central nervous system: therapeutic and diagnostic considerations. Clin Infect Dis 1995;20:414–20. (Level III)

28. Kimura H, Futamura M, Kito H, Ando T, Goto M, Kuzushima K, et al. Detection of viral DNA in neonatal herpes simplex virus infections: frequent and prolonged presence in serum and cerebrospinal fluid. J Infect Dis 1991;164:289–93. (Level III)

29. Kimberlin DW, Lin CY, Jacobs RF, Powell DA, Frenkel LM, Gruber WC, et al. Natural history of neonatal herpes simplex virus infections in the acyclovir era. National Institute of Allergy and Infectious Diseases Collaborative Antiviral Study Group. Pediatrics 2001;108:223–9. (Level II–3)

30. Jerome KR, Huang ML, Wald A, Selke S, Corey L. Quantitative stability of DNA after extended storage of clinical specimens as determined by real-time PCR. J Clin Microbiol 2002;40:2609–11. (Level III)

31. Ashley RL. Sorting out the new HSV type specific antibody tests. Sex Transm Infect 2001;77:232–7. (Level III)

32. Ashley RL, Cent A, Maggs V, Nahmias AJ, Corey L. Inability of enzyme immunoassays to discriminate between infections with herpes simplex virus types 1 and 2. Ann Intern Med 1991;115(7):520–6. (Level II–3)

33. Ashley-Morrow R, Krantz E, Wald A. Time course of seroconversion by HerpeSelect ELISA after acquisition of genital herpes simplex virus type 1 (HSV-1) or HSV-2. Sex Transm Dis 2003;30:310–4. (Level II–3)

34. Whitley RJ, Gnann JW Jr. Acyclovir: a decade later [published erratum appears in N Engl J Med 1993;328:671. N Engl J Med 1997;337:1703]. N Engl J Med 1992;327: 782–9. (Level III)

35. Corey L, Mindel A, Fife KH, Sutherland S, Benedetti J, Adler MW. Risk of recurrence after treatment of first episode genital herpes with intravenous acyclovir. Sex Transm Dis 1985;12:215–8. (Level I)

36. Corey L, Benedetti J, Critchlow C, Mertz G, Douglas J, Fife K, et al. Treatment of primary first-episode genital herpes simplex virus infections with acyclovir: results of topical, intravenous and oral therapy. J Antimicrob Chemother 1983;12 (suppl B):79–88. (Level I)

37. Romanowski B, Marina RB, Roberts JN. Patients' preference of valacyclovir once-daily suppressive therapy versus twice-daily episodic therapy for recurrent genital herpes: a randomized study. Valtrex HS23oo17 Study Group. Sex Transm Dis 2003;30:226–31. (Level II–3)

38. Patel R, Tyring S, Strand A, Price MJ, Grant DM. Impact of suppressive antiviral therapy on the health related quality of life of patients with recurrent genital herpes infection. Sex Transm Infect 1999;75:398–402. (Level II–3)

39. Corey L, Wald A, Patel R, Sacks SL, Tyring SK, Warren T, et al. Once-daily valacyclovir to reduce the risk of transmission of genital herpes. Valacyclovir HSV Transmission Study Group. N Engl J Med 2004;350:11–20. (Level I)

40. Carney O, Ross E, Bunker C, Ikkos G, Mindel A. A prospective study of the psychological impact on patients with a first episode of genital herpes. Genitourin Med 1994;70:40–5. (Level II–3)

41. Melville J, Sniffen S, Crosby R, Salazar L, Whittington W, Dithmer-Schreck D, et al. Psychosocial impact of serological diagnosis of herpes simplex virus type 2: a qualitative assessment. Sex Transm Infect 2003;79:280–5. (Level III)

42. Wald A, Langenberg AG, Link K, Izu AE, Ashley R, Warren T, et al. Effect of condoms on reducing the transmission of herpes simplex virus type 2 from men to women. JAMA 2001;285:3100–6. (Level II–2)

43. Brown ZA, Selke SA, Zeh J, Kopelman J, Maslow A, Ashley RL, et al. The acquisition of herpes simplex virus during pregnancy. N Engl J Med 1997;337:509–15. (Level II–2)

44. Stanberry LR, Spruance SL, Cunningham AL, Bernstein DI, Mindel A, Sacks S, et al. Glycoprotein-D-adjuvant vaccine to prevent genital herpes. GlaxoSmithKline Herpes Vaccine Efficacy Study Group. N Engl J Med 2002;347:1652–61. (Level I)

The MEDLINE database, the Cochrane Library, and ACOG's own internal resources and documents were used to conduct a literature search to locate relevant articles published between January 1985 and June 2004. The search was restricted to articles published in the English language. Priority was given to articles reporting results of original research, although review articles and commentaries also were consulted. Abstracts of research presented at symposia and scientific conferences were not considered adequate for inclusion in this document. Guidelines published by organizations or institutions such as the National Institutes of Health and the American College of Obstetricians and Gynecologists were reviewed, and additional studies were located by reviewing bibliographies of identified articles. When reliable research was not available, expert opinions from obstetrician–gynecologists were used.

Studies were reviewed and evaluated for quality according to the method outlined by the U.S. Preventive Services Task Force:

I Evidence obtained from at least 1 properly designed randomized controlled trial.

II-1 Evidence obtained from well-designed controlled trials without randomization.

II-2 Evidence obtained from well-designed cohort or case–control analytic studies, preferably from more than 1 center or research group.

II-3 Evidence obtained from multiple time series with or without the intervention. Dramatic results in uncontrolled experiments also could be regarded as this type of evidence.

III Opinions of respected authorities, based on clinical experience, descriptive studies, or reports of expert committees.

Based on the highest level of evidence found in the data, recommendations are provided and graded according to the following categories:

Level A—Recommendations are based on good and consistent scientific evidence.

Level B—Recommendations are based on limited or inconsistent scientific evidence.

Level C—Recommendations are based primarily on consensus and expert opinion.

ISSN 1099-3630

The American College of Obstetricians and Gynecologists
409 12th Street, SW, PO Box 96920, Washington, DC 20090-6920

12345/87654

Gynecologic herpes simplex virus infections. ACOG Practice Bulletin No. 57. American College of Obstetricians and Gynecologists. Obstet Gynecol 2004;104:1111–7.

ACOG PRACTICE BULLETIN

CLINICAL MANAGEMENT GUIDELINES FOR
OBSTETRICIAN–GYNECOLOGISTS

NUMBER 64, JULY 2005

(Replaces Committee Opinion Number 238, July 2000)

This Practice Bulletin was developed by the ACOG Committee on Practice Bulletins— Obstetrics with the assistance of John Williams III, MD. The information is designed to aid practitioners in making decisions about appropriate obstetric and gynecologic care. These guidelines should not be construed as dictating an exclusive course of treatment or procedure. Variations in practice may be warranted based on the needs of the individual patient, resources, and limitations unique to the institution or type of practice.

Hemoglobinopathies in Pregnancy

The hemoglobinopathies are a heterogeneous group of single-gene disorders that includes the structural hemoglobin variants and the thalassemias. More than 270 million people worldwide are heterozygous carriers of hereditary disorders of hemoglobin, and at least 300,000 affected homozygotes or compound heterozygotes are born each year (1). The purpose of this document is to review the most common hemoglobinopathies and to provide recommendations for screening and clinical management of hemoglobinopathies during pregnancy.

Background

Hemoglobin Structure

Hemoglobin consists of four interlocking polypeptide chains, each of which has an attached heme molecule. The polypeptide chains are called alpha (α), beta (β), gamma (γ), delta (δ), epsilon (ϵ), and zeta (ζ). Adult hemoglobins consist of two α-chains and either two β-chains (hemoglobin A), two γ-chains (hemoglobin F), or two δ-chains (hemoglobin A_2). Hemoglobin F (fetal hemoglobin, Hb F) is the primary hemoglobin of the fetus from 12 to 24 weeks of gestation. In the third trimester, production of Hb F decreases as production of β-chains and Hb A begins. The genes that code for α-globin chains are located on the short arm of chromosome 16, and the β-globin gene is located on the short arm of chromosome 11.

Sickle Cell Disease

Sickle cell disease refers to a group of autosomal recessive disorders involving abnormal hemoglobin (hemoglobin S). Hemoglobin S differs from the normal Hb A because of a single nucleotide substitution of thymine for adenine in the β-globin gene; this alteration causes a substitution of valine for glutamic acid in the number six position of the β-globin polypeptide. Asymptomatic individuals with heterozygous Hb S genotypes (carriers) are said to have sickle cell trait. The most severe form of the disease, Hb SS (homozygous Hb S), is called sickle cell anemia.

Sickle cell disorders are found not only in patients who have the hemoglobin genotype SS, but also in those who have Hb S and one other abnormality of β-globin structure or β-globin production. The most common of these are Hb SC disease and Hb S/β-thalassemia. In Hb C, the same nucleotide involved in the Hb S mutation is altered with the substitution of adenine for guanine, which results in the amino acid substitution of lysine for glutamic acid. This and other abnormal hemoglobins, when inherited with Hb S, may cause clinically significant vasoocclusive phenomena and hemolytic anemia similar to Hb SS.

Sickle cell disease occurs most commonly in people of African origin. Approximately 1 in 12 African Americans has sickle cell trait (2). One in every 300 African-American newborns has some form of sickle cell disease, and approximately 1 in 600 has sickle cell anemia. Hemoglobin S also is found in high frequency in other populations such as Greeks, Italians (particularly Sicilians), Turks, Arabs, Southern Iranians, and Asian Indians (3).

The classical clinical feature of patients with sickle cell disease is seen under conditions of decreased oxygen tension, in which the red blood cells become distorted into various shapes, some of which resemble sickles. The distorted red cells lead to increased viscosity, hemolysis, and anemia and a further decrease in oxygenation. When sickling occurs within small blood vessels, it can cause "logjams" that can interrupt blood supply to vital organs (vasoocclusive crisis). Repeated vasoocclusive crises result in widespread microvascular obstruction with interruption of normal perfusion and function of several organs, including the spleen, lungs, kidneys, heart, and brain. Adults with Hb SS are functionally asplenic, having undergone autosplenectomy by adolescence. Absence of the spleen contributes to the increased incidence and severity of infection in patients with sickle cell disease.

The most significant threat to patients with sickle cell disease is acute chest syndrome. Chest syndrome is characterized by a pulmonary infiltrate with fever that leads to hypoxemia and acidosis. The infiltrates are not infectious in origin but rather are due to vasoocclusion from sickling or embolization of marrow from long bones affected by sickling (4).

The diagnosis of hemoglobinopathies, including sickle cell disorders, is made by hemoglobin electrophoresis. In the homozygous form, nearly all the hemoglobin is Hb S with small amounts of Hb A_2 and Hb F. Heterozygous sickle cell trait (Hb AS) is identified by a larger percentage of Hb A and an asymptomatic course. Solubility tests (Sickledex) alone are inadequate for diagnosis of sickle cell disorders because they cannot distinguish between the heterozygous AS and homozygous SS

genotypes. In addition, they fail to detect other pathologic variants such as Hb C trait, β-thalassemia trait, Hb E trait, Hb B trait, and Hb D trait.

The Thalassemias

The thalassemias represent a wide spectrum of hematologic disorders that are characterized by a reduced synthesis of globin chains, resulting in microcytic anemia. Thalassemias are classified according to the globin chain affected, with the most common types being α-thalassemia and β-thalassemia. Many different molecular mechanisms lead to thalassemia in populations from different areas of the world (5).

Alpha-Thalassemia

Alpha-thalassemia usually results from a gene deletion of two or more copies of the four α-globin genes. Deletion of one α-globin gene (α-/αα) is clinically unrecognizable, and laboratory testing yields normal results. Deletion of two α-globin genes causes α-thalassemia trait, a mild asymptomatic microcytic anemia. The deletions can be on the same chromosome or in *cis* (αα/--), or on each chromosome or in *trans* (α-/α-). These individuals are referred to as carriers and are at an increased risk for having a child with a more severe form of thalassemia caused by deletions of three or four copies of the α-globin gene (α-thalassemia major). The possible genetic combinations are summarized in Table 1.

Alpha-thalassemia trait (α-thalassemia minor) is common among individuals of Southeast Asian, African, and West Indian descent. It also is common in individuals with Mediterranean ancestry. Individuals with Southeast Asian ancestry are more likely to carry two gene deletions in *cis* or on the same chromosome (--/αα) and are at an increased risk for offspring with Hb Bart's or Hb H disease. Hemoglobin H disease, which is caused by the deletion of three α-globin genes, usually is associated with mild to moderate hemolytic anemia. Alpha-thalassemia major (Hb Bart's) results in the absence of α-globin (--/--); this is associated with hydrops fetalis, intrauterine death, and preeclampsia (3).

In individuals of African descent, α-thalassemia usually is due to a deletion of a single α-globin gene on each chromosome 16 (α-/α-). This is in contrast to the common Asian genotype, which is a deletion of both α-globin genes on one chromosome 16 (*cis*) (αα/--). Hemoglobin Bart's disease does not typically develop in fetuses of α-thalassemia carriers of African origin.

Because Hb S results from an abnormality of the β-chain, both heterozygous (AS) and homozygous (SS) forms can be inherited with heterozygous or homozygous α+-thalassemia. In individuals with sickle cell trait (Hb AS), α-thalassemia lowers the proportion of Hb S, and in those with Hb SS, it lessens the severity of sickle cell disease.

Table 1. Classification of Alpha-Thalassemias

Number of Globin Genes	Genotype	Description	Clinical Features
4	$\alpha\alpha/\alpha\alpha$	Normal	Normal
3	$\alpha-/\alpha\alpha$	Heterozygous α^+-thalassemia	Asymptomatic
2	$\alpha-/\alpha-$	Homozygous α^+-thalassemia	Mild anemia
	$\alpha\alpha/--$	Heterozygous α^0-thalassemia	
1	$\alpha-/--$	α^+-Thalassemia/ α^0-thalassemia	Hb H disease hemolytic anemia
0	$--/--$	Homozygous α^0-thalassemia	Hb Bart's disease hydrops fetalis

Alpha-thalassemia also may occur as a result of a gene mutation. In this case, the genes are present but not functioning normally. This may result from mutation in the stop codon leading to synthesis of a longer and unstable α-chain (Hb Constant Spring), from substitutions impairing αβ dimer formation (Hb Qong Sze), and from point substitutions in the poly A region at the 3' end of the gene (α^{TSaudi}).

Beta-Thalassemia

Beta-thalassemia is caused by a mutation in the β-globin gene that causes deficient or absent β-chain production, which results in absence of Hb A. Classification of β-thalassemias is based on a description of the molecular mutation or by clinical manifestations. Individuals who are heterozygous for this mutation have β-thalassemia minor. Those who are homozygous have β-thalassemia major (Cooley's Anemia) or a milder form called thalassemia intermedia. Beta-thalassemia major is characterized by severe anemia with resultant extramedullary erythropoesis, delayed sexual development, and poor growth. Elevated levels of Hb F in individuals with β-thalassemia major partially compensate for the absence of Hb A; however, death usually occurs by age 10 years unless treatment is begun early with periodic blood transfusions. With transfusion, the severe anemia is reversed and extramedullary erythropoesis is suppressed. In homozygotes with the less severe β⁺-thalassemia mutations, often referred to as β-thalassemia intermedia, variable but decreased amounts of β-chains are produced and, as a result, variable amounts of Hb A are produced. The genes for Hb S and β-thalassemia usually behave as alleles, with only one gene inherited from each parent. The expression of the resulting Hb S/β-thalassemia is determined by the type of β-thalassemia mutation (6).

Beta-thalassemia minor, common in individuals of Mediterranean, Asian, Middle Eastern, Hispanic, and West Indian descent, varies in severity of disease. Depending on the amount of β-chain production, it usually is associated with asymptomatic mild anemia. Beta-thalassemia minor often occurs in association with Hb S. In the most severe form, no normal β-globin chains are produced. This results in a clinically severe syndrome called sickle cell–β⁰-thalassemia, in which no Hb A is produced.

Clinical Considerations and Recommendations

▶ *Who should be screened for hemoglobinopathies and how should this be accomplished?*

Genetic screening can identify couples at risk for offspring with hemoglobinopathies and allow them to make informed decisions regarding reproduction and prenatal diagnosis (3). Individuals of African, Southeast Asian, and Mediterranean ancestry are at a higher risk for being carriers of hemoglobinopathies and should be offered carrier screening. Ethnic groups considered to be at low risk for hemoglobinopathies include northern Europeans, Japanese, Native Americans, Inuit (Eskimo), and Koreans. If both parents are determined to be carriers, genetic counseling is recommended. It should be noted that ethnicity is not always a good predictor of risk because individuals from at-risk groups may marry outside their ethnic group (3).

A combination of laboratory tests may be required to provide the information necessary to counsel couples who are carriers of one of the thalassemias or sickle cell disease (Fig. 1). To ensure accurate hemoglobin identification, which is essential for genetic counseling, a complete blood count (CBC) and Hb electrophoresis are the appropriate initial laboratory tests for individuals at risk for a hemoglobinopathy. Several tests, including solubility testing such as a test for the presence of Hb S (Sickledex), isoelectric focusing, and high-performance liquid chromatography (HPLC), have been used for primary screening. However, solubility tests alone are inadequate for screening and fail to identify important transmissible hemoglobin gene abnormalities affecting fetal outcome (eg, Hb C trait, β-thalassemia trait, Hb E trait, Hb B trait, Hb D trait). Many individuals with these genotypes are asymptomatic, but if their partners have the sickle cell trait or other hemoglobinopathies, they may produce offspring with more serious hemoglobinopathies, such as Hb S/β-thalassemia and Hb SC disease. Solubility testing may be valuable, however, for rapid screening for sickling when this information is critical for immediate patient care.

Determination of mean corpuscular volume (MCV) is recommended for patients who are at risk for α- or β-thalassemia. Patients who have a low MCV (<80 μ^3) may have one of the thalassemia traits and are candidates for hemoglobin electrophoresis. These individuals

also may have iron deficiency anemia, and measurement of serum ferretin levels is recommended. Beta-thalassemia is associated with elevated Hb F and elevated Hb A_2 levels (>3.5%). Neither hemoglobin electrophoresis nor solubility testing can identify individuals with α-thalassemia trait; only molecular genetic testing can identify this condition. If the MCV is below normal, iron deficiency anemia has been excluded, and the hemoglobin electrophoresis is not consistent with β-thalassemia trait (ie, there is no elevation of Hb A_2 or Hb F), then DNA-based testing should be used to detect α-globin gene deletions characteristic of α-thalassemia.

The hematologic features of some of the common hemoglobinopathies are shown in Table 2. If both partners are identified as carriers of a gene for abnormal hemoglobins, genetic counseling is recommended.

▶ *For couples with an increased risk for having an affected offspring, what methods are available for genetic diagnosis of the fetus or embryo?*

Couples at risk for having a child with a hemoglobinopathy may benefit from genetic counseling to review the

Figure 1. Specialized antepartum evaluation for hematologic assessment of patients of African, Southeast Asian, or Mediterranean descent. Patients of Southeast Asian or Mediterranean descent should undergo electrophoresis if their blood test results reveal anemia. Abbreviations: CBC, complete blood count; Hb, hemoglobin; MCV, mean corpuscular volume; RBC, red blood cell.

Table 2. Hematologic Features of Main Hemoglobinopathies

Disorder	Heterozygous State	Homozygous State	DNA Analysis
α^+ Thalassemia (-α)	0–2% Hb Bart's at birth	5–10% Hb Bart's in the neonatal period, low MCV	S. blot: α-gene probe, abnormal band with Bam H1
α° Thalassemia (--)	5–10% Hb Bart's in the neonatal period, low MCV, normal Hb A_2	Hb Bart's hydrops fetalis	S. blot or PCR: absence of: α-gene band in homozygote
β° Thalassemia	Low MCH & MCV, Hb A_2 3.5–7.0%	Thalassemia major: Hb F 98% Hb A_2 2%	PCR, ASO – dot blot, S. blot β-gene probe
β^+ Thalassemia (severe)	Low MCH & MCV, Hb A_2 3.5–7.0%	Thalassemia major: Hb F 70–95%	PCR, ASO – dot blot, S. blot β-gene probe
β^+ Thalassemia (mild)	Low MCH & MCV, Hb A_2 3.5–7.0%	Thalassemia intermedia: Hb F 20–40%	PCR, ASO – dot blot, S. blot β-gene probe
Hb S	Hb A, Hb S, Hb A_2	Hb S, Hb F (1–15%), Hb A_2	PCR: Dde 1 digestion PCR, ASO – dot blot
Hb S/β-Thalassemia	—	If β° thalassemia, severe sickle cell anemia; if β^+ thalassemia, less severe	PCR,: Dde 1 digestion PCR, ASO – dot blot
Hb E/β-Thalassemia	—	Thalassemia major or intermedia: Hb E 60–70%, Hb F 30–40%	PCR: Hb E by Mnl 1 digestion

Abbreviations: ASO, allele specific oligonucleotide; Hb, hemoglobin; MCH, mean corpuscular hemoglobin; MCV, mean corpuscular volume; PCR, polymerase chain reaction; S. blot, Southern blot.

Modified from Old JM. Prenatal diagnosis of hemoglobinopathies. In: Milunsky A, editor. Genetic disorders and the fetus: diagnosis, prevention, and treatment. 5th ed. Baltimore (MD): Johns Hopkins University Press; 2004. p. 665.

natural history of these disorders, prospects for treatment and cure, their risk, availability of prenatal genetic testing, and reproductive options. Prenatal diagnostic testing for the single mutation responsible for sickle cell disease is widely available. Testing for α- and β-thalassemia is possible if the mutations and deletions have been previously identified in both parents. These DNA-based tests can be performed using chorionic villi obtained by chorionic villus sampling (CVS) at 10–12 weeks of gestation or using cultured amniotic fluid cells obtained by amniocentesis after 15 weeks of gestation. For some couples, preimplantation genetic diagnosis in combination with in vitro fertilization may be a desirable alternative to avoid termination of an affected pregnancy. Preimplantation genetic diagnosis has been successfully performed for sickle cell disease and most cases of β-thalassemia.

Although the advances in prenatal diagnosis of hemoglobinopathies have been impressive, use of the technology has been somewhat limited because of ethical, social, and cultural concerns. Prenatal diagnosis is most commonly requested by families who have had a child with sickle cell disease and who wish to be certain that their next child is not affected. In many respects, these families are "self counseled." The difficulty in counseling families who have not had an affected child lies in the variable severity of the disease and the inability to predict its course (6). One investigator found that nearly 70% of families in whom prenatal diagnosis confirmed that the fetus was affected with Hb SS elected to continue the pregnancy (7).

▶ How is sickle cell disease in pregnancy managed?

Pregnancy in women with sickle cell disease is associated with an increased risk of morbidity and mortality, because of the combination of underlying hemolytic anemia and multiorgan dysfunction associated with this disorder. Morbidity and mortality have decreased markedly over the past 3 decades because of improvements in general medical care for patients with sickle cell disease, improvements in transfusion medicine, and advancements in neonatal care (8, 9). In spite of the decline in maternal and perinatal mortality rates, however, pregnancy is still a significant clinical risk for many patients with sickle cell disease. The magnitude of the risk varies with genotype and severity of anemia. When compared with Hb AA patients, women with Hb SS have increased risk for maternal complications, such as preterm labor, premature rupture of membranes, antepartum hospitalization, and postpartum infection. In addition, patients with Hb SS are at higher risk for fetal complications, such as intrauterine growth restriction (IUGR), low birth weight, and preterm delivery (9, 10). Patients with Hb SC disease also are at risk for the aforementioned complications but to a lesser extent than patients with Hb SS disease (10).

Pregnant patients with sickle cell disease need increased prenatal folic acid supplementation. The standard 1 mg of folate in prenatal vitamins is not adequate for patients with hemoglobinopathies; 4 mg per day of folic acid should be prescribed due to the continual turnover of red blood cells.

Routine cesarean delivery for women with sickle cell disease is not indicated and should be performed only for obstetric indications. Epidural analgesia usually is well tolerated as long as care is taken to avoid hypotension and hypoxemia. Pregnant patients should, if possible, be cared for at institutions that are able to manage both the complications of sickle cell disease and high-risk pregnancies. They also should have regular prenatal care by or in consultation with obstetricians who are experienced in the management of sickle cell disease.

The most common cause of recurrent morbidity in Hb SS disease is painful crisis. If possible, precipitating factors such as cold environment, heavy physical exertion, dehydration, and stress should be avoided. Hydroxyurea has been shown to reduce the frequency of painful crises in nonpregnant patients with severe sickle cell disease (11). However, the use of hydroxyurea is not recommended during pregnancy because it is teratogenic.

Painful crises in pregnancy as well as in the nonpregnant patient are managed with rapid assessment of the level of pain and prompt administration of analgesia. Pain, respiratory rate, and level of sedation should be assessed until pain is controlled. Opiates can be given orally or parenterally by the intravenous, intramuscular, or subcutaneous route. Oxygen should be given if the O_2 saturation is less than 95% by pulse oximetry. The initial clinical assessment also should focus on detection of serious medical complications requiring specific therapy, such as acute chest syndrome (fever tachypnea, chest pain, and hypoxia), infection, dehydration, severe anemia, cholecystitis, and hypersplenism. A multidisciplinary approach should be used involving obstetricians, hematologists, and anesthesiologists (12). Painful crises in the third trimester may have a prolonged course and may not resolve until after delivery.

▶ *What is the role of transfusion or prophylactic exchange transfusion for pregnancies complicated by sickle cell anemia?*

Controversy exists regarding the role of prophylactic blood transfusion in the management of sickle cell disease in pregnancy (13–15). By limiting transfusion to situations in which it is clinically indicated, patients are not subjected to the increased risk for alloimmunization (16), viral infections, and iron overload. Major complications (eg, worsening anemia; intrapartum complications such as hemorrhage, septicemia, and cesarean delivery; painful crisis; and chest syndrome) may require intervention with an exchange transfusion. There is no consensus regarding the exact hematocrit value below which transfusion should be considered. However, when a transfusion is clinically indicated in the patient with sickle cell

disease, the objective is to lower the percentage of Hb S to approximately 40% while simultaneously raising the total hemoglobin concentration to about 10 g/dL. Hemoglobin levels and the percentage of Hb S should be monitored serially during the remainder of the pregnancy to determine the need for subsequent transfusions.

Prophylactic exchange transfusion was first proposed by Ricks in 1965, who recommended exchange transfusion 4–6 weeks before the delivery date (17). Preliminary results appeared to show a benefit in that all women and infants survived (18). Subsequently, several studies have shown improvement in maternal and fetal outcome with prophylactic transfusion (15, 19). However, the evidence is not conclusive that transfusion is responsible for the improvement; similar improvement has been observed in programs that do not use prophylactic transfusion. In the only randomized controlled trial published to date, prophylactic transfusion was associated with a decreased risk for painful crisis and severe anemia, but no difference was observed for pregnancy outcome (14). It appears from the available evidence that the reduction in morbidity and mortality of sickle cell disease in pregnancy is attributable to improvements in general management of pregnancy rather than prophylactic transfusion per se.

▶ *Is fetal surveillance useful in pregnancies complicated by sickle cell anemia?*

Pregnancies in women with sickle cell disease are at increased risk for spontaneous abortion, preterm labor, IUGR, and stillbirth (20). For this reason, a plan for serial ultrasound examinations and antepartum fetal testing is reasonable. Published data on antenatal fetal surveillance in women with sickle cell disease are limited. In a retrospective review of 58 pregnancies in women with sickle cell disease undergoing prophylactic transfusion, no patients had a nonreactive nonstress test result or positive contraction stress test (21). All pregnancy outcomes were normal. The investigators concluded that placental reserve and fetal reactivity were uncompromised and that these tests were as sensitive for assessment of fetal well-being in women with sickle cell disease as for women with other indications for antenatal testing.

Because patients with sickle cell crisis usually require narcotics for pain control, the results of abnormal antepartum testing should be interpreted with caution. One small study has shown that nonstress test results and biophysical profiles may be abnormal during an episode of crisis but revert back to normal with resolution of the episode (22). The clinical significance of this is unclear.

▶ *How is thalassemia in pregnancy managed?*

The course of pregnancy in women with the α-thalassemia trait is not significantly different from that of women with normal hemoglobin. Pregnancy in women with Hb H disease has been reported, and with the exception of mild to moderate chronic anemia, outcomes have been favorable. However, the number of reports is too few to draw definite conclusions regarding pregnancy outcome in all women with Hb H disease (23).

Until recently, pregnancy in women with β-thalassemia major was extremely rare. Initially, this was because delay of growth and sexual development and early death in untreated patients prevented reproduction. After the introduction of transfusion therapy in the 1960s, pregnancy was still uncommon because of infertility (secondary to hypothalamic dysfunction and anovulation caused by hemosiderin deposition). Since the introduction of hypertransfusion and iron chelation therapy with deferoxamine in the late 1970s, several reports and case series have documented favorable pregnancy outcomes in women with β-thalassemia major (24, 25). Pregnancy in women with β-thalassemia major is recommended only for those with normal cardiac function who have had prolonged hypertransfusion therapy to maintain hemoglobin levels at 10 g/dL and iron chelation therapy with deferoxamine (25). During pregnancy, hemoglobin levels should be maintained at or near 10 g/dL with transfusions. Deferoxamine usually is discontinued because the safety of iron chelation therapy during pregnancy has not been established. Fetal growth should be monitored with serial ultrasonography. In cases in which fetal growth is suboptimal, patients should have fetal surveillance. The mode of delivery should be individualized, with cesarean delivery reserved for obstetric indications.

Beta-thalassemia minor usually causes mild asymptomatic anemia. In the absence of documented iron deficiency, replacement beyond prophylactic doses of iron is not indicated. Studies involving fairly small numbers of patients suggest that pregnancy outcome is favorable in women with β-thalassemia minor. A study of 261 pregnant women with β-thalassemia minor found a significantly higher rate of IUGR and oligohydramnios than is found in nonthalassemic patients (26). No differences were noted in perinatal outcomes such as low Apgar scores, congenital malformations, or perinatal mortality (26).

Summary of Recommendations and Conclusions

The following recommendations are based on good and consistent scientific evidence (Level A):

▶ Individuals of African, Southeast Asian, and Mediterranean descent are at increased risk for

being carriers of hemoglobinopathies and should be offered carrier screening and, if both parents are determined to be carriers, genetic counseling.

▶ A complete blood count and hemoglobin electrophoresis are the appropriate laboratory tests for screening for hemoglobinopathies. Solubility tests alone are inadequate for screening because they fail to identify important transmissible hemoglobin gene abnormalities affecting fetal outcome.

▶ Couples at risk for having a child with sickle cell disease or thalassemia should be offered genetic counseling to review prenatal testing and reproduction options. Prenatal diagnosis of hemoglobinopathies is best accomplished by DNA analysis of cultured amniocytes or chorionic villi.

References

1. Angastiniotis M, Modell B. Global epidemiology of hemoglobin disorders. Ann N Y Acad Sci 1998;850:251–69. (Level II-3)

2. Motulsky AG. Frequency of sickling disorders in U.S. blacks. N Engl J Med 1973;288:31–3. (Level III)

3. Davies SC, Cronin E, Gill M, Greengross P, Hickman M, Normand C. Screening for sickle cell disease and thalassemia: a systematic review with supplementary research. Health Technol Assess 2000;4:i–v, 1–99. (Level III)

4. Duffy TP. Hematologic aspects of pregnancy. In: Burrow GN, Duffy TP, Copel JA, editors. Medical complications during pregnancy. 6th ed. Philadelphia (PA): Elsevier Saunders; 2004. p. 69–86. (Level III)

5. Kazazian HH Jr. The thalassemia syndromes: molecular basis and prenatal diagnosis in 1990. Semin Hematol 1990;27:209–28. (Level III)

6. Serjeant GR, Serjeant BE. Sickle cell disease. 3rd ed. New York (NY): Oxford University Press; 2001. (Level III)

7. Alter BP. Prenatal diagnosis of hematologic diseases, 1986 update. Acta Haematol 1987;78:137–41. (Level II-3)

8. Smith JA, Espeland M, Bellevue R, Bonds D, Brown AK, Koshy M. Pregnancy in sickle cell disease: experience of the Cooperative Study of Sickle Cell Disease. Obstet Gynecol 1996;87:199–204. (Level II-2)

9. Sun PM, Wilburn W, Raynor BD, Jamieson D. Sickle cell disease in pregnancy: twenty years of experience at Grady Memorial Hospital, Atlanta, Georgia. Am J Obstet Gynecol 2001;184:1127–30. (Level II-2)

10. Powars DR, Sandhu M, Niland-Weiss J, Johnson C, Bruce S, Manning PR. Pregnancy in sickle cell disease. Obstet Gynecol 1986;67:217–28. (Level II-3)

11. Charache S. Mechanism of action on hydroxyurea in the management of sickle cell anemia in adults. Semin Hematol 1997;34(suppl 3):15–21. (Level I)

12. Rees DC, Olujohungbe AD, Parker NE, Stephens AD, Telfer P, Wright J. Guidelines for the management of the

acute painful crisis in sickle cell disease. British Committee for Standards in Haematology General Haematology Task Force by the Sickle Cell Working Party. Br J Haematol 2003;120:744–52. (Level III)

13. Tuck SM, James CE, Brewster EM, Pearson TC, Studd JW. Prophylactic blood transfusion in maternal sickle cell syndromes. Br J Obstet Gynaecol 1987;94:121–5. (Level III)

14. Koshy M, Burd L, Wallace D, Moawad A, Baron J. Prophylactic red-cell transfusions in pregnant patients with sickle cell disease. A randomized cooperative study. N Engl J Med 1988;319:1447–52. (Level I)

15. Morrison JC, Schneider JM, Whybrew WD, Bucovaz ET, Menzel DM. Prophylactic transfusions in pregnant patients with sickle cell hemoglobinopathies: benefit versus risk. Obstet Gynecol 1980;56:274–80. (Level III)

16. Brumfield CG, Huddleston JF, DuBois LB, Harris BA Jr. A delayed hemolytic transfusion reaction after partial exchange transfusion for sickle cell disease in pregnancy: a case report and review of literature. Obstet Gynecol 1984;63(suppl):13s–15s. (Level III)

17. Ricks P Jr. Exchange transfusion in sickle cell anemia in pregnancy. Obstet Gynecol 1965;25:117–9. (Level III)

18. Ricks P Jr. Further experience with exchange transfusion in sickle cell anemia in pregnancy. Am J Obstet Gynecol 1968;100:1087–90. (Level III)

19. Morrison JC, Wiser WL. The use of prophylactic partial exchange transfusion in pregnancies associated with sickle cell hemoglobinopathies. Obstet Gynecol 1976;48: 516–20. (Level III)

20. Serjeant GR, Loy LL, Crowther M, Hambleton IR, Thame M. Outcome of pregnancy in homozygous sickle cell disease. Obstet Gynecol 2004;103:1278–85. (Level II–2)

21. Morrison JC, Blake PG, McCoy C, Martin JN Jr, Wiser WL. Fetal health assessment in pregnancies complicated by sickle hemoglobinopathies. Obstet Gynecol 1983;61: 22–4. (Level III)

22. Anyaegbunam A, Morel MI, Merkatz IR. Antepartum fetal surveillance tests during sickle cell crisis. Am J Obstet Gynecol 1991;165:1081–3. (Level II-2)

23. Ong HC, White JC, Sinnathuray TA. Haemoglobin H disease and pregnancy in a Malaysian woman. Acta Haematol 1977;58:229–33. (Level III)

24. Jensen CE, Tuck SM, Wonke B. Fertility in beta thalassemia major: a report of 16 pregnancies, preconceptual evaluation and a review of the literature. Br J Obstet Gynaecol 1995;102:625–9. (Level III)

25. Aessopos A, Karabatsos F, Farmakis D, Katsantoni A, Hatziliami A, Youssef J, et al. Pregnancy in patients with well-treated beta-thalassemia: outcome for mothers and newborn infants. Am J Obstet Gynecol 1999;180:360–5. (Level III)

26. Sheiner E, Levy A, Yerushalmi R, Katz M. Beta-thalassemia minor during pregnancy. Obstet Gynecol 2004;103:1273–7. (Level II-2)

The MEDLINE database, the Cochrane Library, and ACOG's own internal resources and documents were used to conduct a literature search to locate relevant articles published between January 1985 and March 2005. The search was restricted to articles published in the English language. Priority was given to articles reporting results of original research, although review articles and commentaries also were consulted. Abstracts of research presented at symposia and scientific conferences were not considered adequate for inclusion in this document. Guidelines published by organizations or institutions such as the National Institutes of Health and the American College of Obstetricians and Gynecologists were reviewed, and additional studies were located by reviewing bibliographies of identified articles. When reliable research was not available, expert opinions from obstetrician–gynecologists were used.

Studies were reviewed and evaluated for quality according to the method outlined by the U.S. Preventive Services Task Force:

I   Evidence obtained from at least one properly designed randomized controlled trial.

II-1   Evidence obtained from well-designed controlled trials without randomization.

II-2   Evidence obtained from well-designed cohort or case–control analytic studies, preferably from more than one center or research group.

II-3   Evidence obtained from multiple time series with or without the intervention. Dramatic results in uncontrolled experiments also could be regarded as this type of evidence.

III   Opinions of respected authorities, based on clinical experience, descriptive studies, or reports of expert committees.

Based on the highest level of evidence found in the data, recommendations are provided and graded according to the following categories:

Level A—Recommendations are based on good and consistent scientific evidence.

Level B—Recommendations are based on limited or inconsistent scientific evidence.

Level C—Recommendations are based primarily on consensus and expert opinion.

ISSN 1099-3630

**The American College of
Obstetricians and Gynecologists
409 12th Street, SW
PO Box 96920
Washington, DC 20090-6920**

12345/98765

Hemoglobinopathies in pregnancy. ACOG Practice Bulletin No. 64. American College of Obstetricians and Gynecologists. Obstet Gynecol 2005;106:203–11.

ACOG PRACTICE BULLETIN

CLINICAL MANAGEMENT GUIDELINES FOR
OBSTETRICIAN–GYNECOLOGISTS

NUMBER 61, APRIL 2005

This Practice Bulletin was developed by the ACOG Committee on Practice Bulletins— Gynecology with the assistance of Mark Spitzer, MD and Robert D. Burk, MD. The information is designed to aid practitioners in making decisions about appropriate obstetric and gynecologic care. These guidelines should not be construed as dictating an exclusive course of treatment or procedure. Variations in practice may be warranted based on the needs of the individual patient, resources, and limitations unique to the institution or type of practice.

Human Papillomavirus

More than 15 years ago, a relationship between human papillomavirus (HPV) infection and cervical cancer was recognized. Since then, important strides in understanding the virus have been made, particularly in the following areas: modes of transmission and risk factors associated with transmission; the oncogenic potential of specific viral types and the mechanism by which they cause cancer; and the spectrum of infection, ranging from asymptomatic carrier states to overt warts, preneoplastic lesions, and invasive cancer. Sophisticated new tests for the detection of HPV that hold great promise for improved screening for cervical cancer precursors and invasive cancer and for the triage of abnormal cervical cytology also have been developed. Understanding the immunology of HPV has allowed the development of new and more effective treatment modalities for HPV infection and the preliminary development of primary prevention modalities, including HPV vaccines.

Background

Epidemiology

Although most infections with HPV are not clinically detectable, the most commonly recognized visible HPV-induced lesion of the female lower genital tract is genital or venereal warts (condylomata acuminata). The lesions typically are multiple, well-circumscribed, papillomatous growths that may involve the vaginal introitus, the vulva, the perineum, the anus, and the cervix. The true prevalence and incidence of genital warts in the United States is unknown because it is not a reportable disease. However, the occurrence of genital warts can be measured indirectly by surveys of first office visits to physicians compiled annually by the Centers for Disease Control and Prevention. Between 1966 and 1987, the number of consultations for genital warts increased from approximately 70,000 to 360,000 per year; the number then decreased to approximately 150,000 visits in 1997 (1). The prevalence of genital warts varies with the age and population being studied. Among women seen for an annual gynecologic examination at a health maintenance organization between 1984 and 1987, the prevalence of genital warts was 0.8% for women between ages 21 and 29 years and 0.6% for women between ages 29 and 39 years (2). The prevalence of genital warts is higher in individuals visiting sexually transmitted disease clinics. In a study of patients seen at the Seattle & Kings County sexually transmitted disease clinic in 1986, 13% of men and 9% of women had genital warts (2).

Most HPV infections of the genital tract are subclinical, but in many cases they can be diagnosed cytologically. The cytologic effects of HPV infection include a spectrum of abnormalities. The mildest abnormalities usually are called condylomatous atypia or koilocytotic atypia. The more severe abnormalities correspond to the traditional classification of precursor lesions of invasive cervical cancer, namely, mild, moderate, or severe cervical intraepithelial neoplasia (low-grade and high-grade squamous intraepithelial lesions).

The most recent available data for U.S. women come from the National Breast and Cervical Cancer Early Detection Program (3). The overall rate of abnormal cervical cytology was 3.8%. The rates for low-grade and high-grade squamous lesions and squamous cancer were 2.9%, 0.8%, and less than 0.1%, respectively. Rates in the United States are higher than in other developed countries. The true ratio of subclinical to clinical HPV infection may be even higher. In three studies of unselected college-aged women evaluated by both cervical cytology and HPV DNA detection by polymerase chain reaction (PCR), the prevalence of cytologic abnormalities ranged from 1% to 3.6%, whereas the prevalence of cervical HPV DNA was 28–35%, indicating that subclinical HPV infections may be 10–30 times more common than cytologically apparent infections (4–6). It was estimated that the number of new cases of invasive cervical cancer in the United States for 2004 would be 10,520 and the estimated number of deaths that would occur because of this disease would be 3,900 (7). The lifetime risk for U.S. women of being diagnosed with cervical cancer and the lifetime risk of dying from cervical cancer are 0.78% and 0.26%, respectively.

Estimates of the prevalence of cervical HPV infection vary greatly depending on the method of diagnosis and the demographic and behavioral characteristics of the study population. Infection can be diagnosed clinically (genital warts), cytologically (Pap test), or virologically (DNA detection). The point prevalence of cervical HPV infection varies from 14% to 35% (4, 5, 8–10). Studies in which women have been sampled repeatedly suggest that exposure to genital HPV is much higher than indicated by point prevalence studies (10–12). In a study of 608 female university students with an average age of 20 years at recruitment who were monitored at 6-month intervals for an average of 2.2 years, the baseline prevalence of HPV infection was 26%, but approximately 60% of the women tested positive for HPV at some time during the 3-year period of study (9). Within individuals, the detection of HPV DNA also is highly variable, indicating the limitations of single-point measurements of cervical HPV infection for calculating prevalence. In studies in which the interval between samplings has been longer, the reported cumulative HPV prevalence has been lower (8, 13, 14). The best estimates of incident infection are provided by the previously mentioned studies conducted in New Brunswick, New Jersey, and Brazil (8, 9). In these studies, estimates of incident HPV infection were 1.2% and 1.3% new infections per month. In both studies the incidence rates generally were higher for younger women.

Transmission of Human Papillomavirus

Human papillomavirus is a sexually transmitted infection. As many as three quarters of individuals sexually exposed to genital warts have been reported to develop genital warts subsequently (15, 16). The predominant risk factor for a genital HPV infection is the number of lifetime sexual partners (6, 17–22). The other risk factor identified in most studies of HPV infection is young age (23). The maximum prevalence occurs between ages 20 and 24 years (21%), followed by a decrease until age 35 years. The prevalence remains stable through age 50 years and then gradually decreases again (23). The age trend is consistent with an epidemic curve of a sexually acquired infection (24). The prevalence increases as newly, sexually active young women are exposed for the first time and then decreases among older women because of decreased exposure or acquisition of protective immunity.

Male sexual behavior has been shown to be an independent risk factor for infection in women. Evidence suggests that the male partners of women infected with HPV tend to be more sexually promiscuous (6). Similarly, in a case–control study of cervical cancer in Spain, a woman's risk of cervical cancer was strongly related to her husband's number of extramarital partners (25).

A recent study noted differences in the risk factors for high-risk oncogenic HPV types and low-risk nononcogenic types (22). The main risk factors for high-risk types were younger age and measures of lifetime sexual activity, such as number of partners. In contrast, the most important determinants for nononcogenic types were contraceptive variables related to the physical protection of the cervix, such as the use of a condom or a diaphragm, and the number of partners in the past

4–12 months. One explanation for this difference is that infections with low-risk HPV types are transient and, thus, correlate with recent sexual behavior, whereas some infections with oncogenic types may be more persistent and, therefore, correlate with measures of lifetime sexual exposure. Genito-oral transmission is rare (26).

Genital HPV types appear to be infrequently transmitted in the neonatal period, although published studies are conflicting. Some studies (27, 28) have shown limited transmission to infants of women infected with HPV (<1.5%), whereas others reported HPV DNA prevalence in neonates and young children ranging from 32% to 72% in children born to women with an HPV infection and from 5% to 29% in children born to women without an HPV infection (29–33). The estimates of prevalence may vary widely because of differences in populations, sampling methods, or the specificity of laboratory assays, or might simply indicate contamination with infected maternal cells.

Natural History of Human Papillomavirus

Most cervical HPV infections diagnosed by PCR and other nucleic acid detection methods appear to be transient. In one study, the proportion of women who cleared their infections increased with younger age, had a longer interval between sampling, and were infected with low-risk as compared to high-risk HPV types (13). Only one third of women aged 30 years and older cleared their infections, compared with two thirds of those aged 24 years and younger. Slightly more than one half of the initially infected women who had a follow-up visit within 12 months had lost the HPV type detected at entry, and nearly 75% of those who returned after more than 18 months had resolved their initial infections. Three quarters of the women infected with low-risk HPV types at entry no longer harbored the initial HPV type in their genital tracts at the second visit. In contrast, among women infected with high-risk HPV types, only one half had cleared their infections by the second visit. In other studies, the proportion of women with a transient cervical HPV infection has been even higher (14, 34).

In longitudinal studies, the time interval required for 50% of prevalent cases to become HPV DNA negative for the HPV type detected at enrollment was 4.8 months for nononcogenic types and 8.1 months for oncogenic types (8). However, this is not a true measure of the duration of infections because it is unknown how long the women had been infected by the time they were found to be positive at enrollment. In another longitudinal study, the duration of infection was determined for incident infection (9). The median duration of HPV DNA was 8 months.

Nomenclature and Taxonomy

Human papillomaviruses are a group of closed-circular, double-stranded DNA viruses that are now recognized as the necessary but insufficient cause of cervical cancer (35). Human papillomaviruses are classified by the homology of their genomes. More than 100 putative HPVs have been described; approximately 40 HPV types can be found in the cervicovaginal area. Classification of HPV types into clinically relevant categories, such as cancer causing and noncancer causing or cutaneous and mucosal, has been accomplished based on sequence information alone (36). The development of cervical carcinoma is restricted to a subset of viruses that increase the risk of cervical cancer in infected women (high-risk), of which HPV16 and HPV18 together account for approximately two thirds of observed cervical cancer cases (37). In contrast, infections with low-risk HPVs rarely lead to cancer.

The ability of HPV infections to progress to malignancies is caused in large part by the biochemical activities of E6 and E7, the primary oncoproteins encoded by HPV genomes. Although other oncoproteins, such as E4 and E5, are thought to complement their activity, E6 and E7 from high-risk types manipulate cell cycle regulators, induce chromosomal abnormalities, and block apoptosis (38–42). Their expression is sufficient to immortalize primary human keratinocytes in tissue culture systems. In addition to their phenotypic distinction, members of high-risk types share up to 60% sequence similarity in E6, whereas comparisons across low-risk and high-risk types show only 35–40% similarity, implying that E6 oncogenicity may have evolved early, remaining largely conserved and successful.

Use in Screening

Oncogenic HPV types are now recognized as the cause of cervical cancer (35), but very few individuals with an HPV infection will develop cancer. Despite the success of cytology screening, which has been responsible for a 70% decrease in cervical cancer mortality in the United States over the past five decades (7), the sensitivity of a single conventional cytology has been estimated to be approximately 50–60% (43, 44). More recent well-controlled clinical trials with verification of positive and some negative results have found sensitivities of 70–80% for conventional cervical cytology and 85–95% for liquid-based cytology (45, 46). With such a low sensitivity for a single cervical cytology test, the reduction in cervical cancer incidence is dependent on regular serial screening. Even newer liquid-based cytology techniques may miss 15–35% of cervical intraepithelial neoplasia (CIN) 3 or cancer (47, 48). This carries important medical implications and has stimulated substantial interest in the development of more sensitive screening tools.

Because of its relationship to cervical cancer, several potential uses have been suggested for HPV DNA testing. These include primary screening; triage of patients with cytology showing atypical squamous cells of undetermined significance (ASC-US); follow-up after treatment for a test of cure; follow-up for patients with abnormal cytology in whom no lesions or only minor lesions have been identified by colposcopy; and resolution of discordant cytology, colposcopy, or histology findings.

Clinical Considerations and Recommendations

▶ When is HPV testing recommended?

Every year in the United States, between two and three million women are identified with cervical cytology showing ASC-US, and 1.25 million women are identified with low-grade squamous intraepithelial lesions (LSIL) (49). In 2001, the National Cancer Institute completed a large multicenter randomized trial called the Atypical Squamous Cells of Undetermined Significance/Low Grade Squamous Intraepithelial Lesion Triage Study (ALTS) (50). The study compared immediate colposcopy, HPV DNA testing by Hybrid Capture 2, and repeat cytology in the management of women with ASC-US and LSIL cytology. The study showed that 83% of women with LSIL cytology tested positive for high-risk HPV DNA, limiting the usefulness and the cost-effectiveness of HPV testing in differentiating which women with LSIL cytology should undergo colposcopy. However, the age distribution in ALTS did not permit assessment of postmenopausal women with LSIL separate from the overall population. These women may have a lower rate of HPV positivity, allowing for the use of HPV triage in this group. In women with ASC-US cervical cytology screening results, ALTS found that triage using liquid-based cytology alone had a sensitivity of 85% for CIN 2 and CIN 3 lesions while referring 59% of women to colposcopy following the first repeat cervical cytology screening and 67% following the second repeat cervical cytology screening. Human papillomavirus testing detected more than 90% of CIN 2 and CIN 3 while referring only 56% of the patients to colposcopy. Both HPV testing and repeat cytology referred more women younger than 30 years to colposcopy than older women, but HPV testing was significantly more sensitive for CIN 2 and CIN 3 at all ages (51).

In 2001, the American Society for Colposcopy and Cervical Pathology (ASCCP), in conjunction with the American College of Obstetricians and Gynecologists and 28 other participating professional and health organi-

zations and federal agencies, hosted a consensus conference to develop comprehensive evidence-based guidelines for the management of women with cervical cytologic abnormalities and cervical cancer precursors. Among repeat cytology, immediate colposcopy, and HPV DNA testing, the consensus conference concluded that all three options were acceptable for managing women with ASC-US cytology. However, the preferred option was reflex HPV DNA testing for high-risk types when liquid-based cytology was used at the time of the initial visit. This approach eliminates the need for a repeat office visit, is the most sensitive of the triage tools, and results in the referral of fewer women to colposcopy than the other options at all age groups. Human papillomavirus testing was not recommended for triage of women with LSIL, atypical squamous cells that cannot exclude high-grade squamous intraepithelial lesions, or atypical glandular cells cytology. These women should undergo immediate colposcopy, and the use of HPV testing is not cost-effective in this population (52).

A particularly challenging clinical problem is the management of women with high-risk HPV-positive ASC-US or LSIL cytology who are not found to have CIN 2 or CIN 3 at their initial colposcopy. In ALTS, only 10% of these women were found to have CIN 2 or CIN 3 after a follow-up period of 2 years (53). There was no difference in the risk of CIN 2 or CIN 3 between women in this group with CIN 1 at their initial colposcopy (12.5%), those with a normal colposcopy (12.8%), and those with a negative biopsy (10.6%) (54). Using the triage strategies studied by ALTS, HPV testing at 12 months was 95% sensitive for detection of CIN 3+ while referring 55% of patients for colposcopy, whereas repeat cytology at 6 and 12 months cumulatively detected 88% of the lesions while referring 64% of patients for colposcopy (53). For the follow-up of these women, the ASCCP consensus guidelines recommended either HPV testing at 12 months (with women with high-risk HPV referred for colposcopy) or cytology at 6 and 12 months (with women referred for colposcopy if either cervical cytology screening result shows ASC-US or greater) (52).

The ASCCP consensus conference recommended that HPV DNA testing could be used as a test of cure for women with CIN 2 or CIN 3 at least 6 months following excision or ablation of the transformation zone (52). Those women with high-risk HPV would be referred for colposcopy.

▶ Should women older than 30 years be routinely screened for HPV with cervical cytology screening?

Several large studies have used a combination of HPV DNA testing and cervical cytology to detect cervical cancer and its precursors (45, 52, 55–61). These studies were performed in populations where cervical cancer risk varied widely. These ranged from unscreened populations in China with a prevalence of CIN 2 and CIN 3 of 4.3% (55, 56) to a low-risk population in the United Kingdom whose prevalence of CIN 2 and CIN 3 was 1.4% (61). In each of these studies, HPV DNA testing had greater sensitivity but lower specificity than cervical cytology.

One study detected 100% of CIN 2 and CIN 3 lesions using HPV DNA testing compared with 58% using conventional cytology and 84% using liquid-based cytology (45). Another study, using Hybrid Capture 2 for HPV DNA testing, detected 88.4% of CIN 2 and CIN 3 lesions and cancers with a specificity of 89%, whereas liquid-based cytology detected 77.7% of CIN 2 and CIN 3 with a specificity of 94.2% (57). Studies using combined HPV testing with cervical cytology reported a negative predictive value for CIN 2 and CIN 3 of 99–100% (52, 55, 57–60). In addition, most studies found that the specificity of the combination of two tests was lower than cytology alone.

One difficult clinical issue has been the significance of a positive HPV DNA test result in the face of negative cytology result and a negative colposcopy result. Three studies provided longitudinal data that shed light on this question. Kjaer et al (62) performed PCR testing for HPV DNA in more than 10,000 women. Women who had positive test results for HPV DNA and were cytologically normal at baseline were monitored for 2 years. Compared with the group of women who had negative test results for HPV DNA at both time points, the odds ratios for CIN 2 or CIN 3 for patients who demonstrated persistence of any high-risk HPV type was extremely high (692 and 813, respectively) for those who demonstrated persistence of the same high-risk HPV type (62).

In February 2003, the U.S. Food and Drug Administration approved HPV DNA testing by Hybrid Capture 2 in combination with cervical cytology as a screening tool for cervical cancer in women older than 30 years. Because HPV DNA testing is more sensitive than cervical cytology, women with negative concurrent test results (negative cytology and negative HPV DNA) can be reassured that their risk of unidentified CIN 2 and CIN 3 or cervical cancer is approximately 1 in 1,000. The natural history of the disease and several large longitudinal studies (63, 64) suggest that women with negative concurrent test results could avoid rescreening for 3 years even if they have new sexual partners.

In February 2003, the National Cancer Institute, ASCCP, and the American Cancer Society held a workshop to discuss the use of HPV DNA testing for screening (65). They issued interim guidelines recommending that the use of a combination of cervical cytology and

HPV DNA screening is appropriate for women aged 30 years and older. If this combination is used, women who receive negative results on both tests should be rescreened no more frequently than every 3 years. Those with negative cytology results but have high-risk HPV DNA positive test results should have both tests repeated in 6–12 months. Those with persistent high-risk HPV (on repeat testing) should undergo colposcopy regardless of the cytology result. Those with cytologic abnormalities should be managed according to published guidelines (52).

The target population for cervical cytology screening with HPV DNA testing is women older than 30 years. At younger ages, the prevalence of HPV is very high, whereas the prevalence of cervical cancer is relatively low. Screening young women would lead to unnecessary testing and worry because most positive test results would spontaneously revert to normal. The decreasing prevalence of HPV DNA positivity in women older than 30 years (61) and the improved specificity of HPV DNA testing in predicting CIN 2 and CIN 3 makes it a more practical screening test, combined with cervical cytology screening, in that age group.

▶ Can transmission or sequela of HPV be prevented or decreased?

Genital HPV infection is transmitted sexually. Transmission occurs through contact with infected genital skin, mucous membranes, or body fluids from a partner with either overt or subclinical HPV infections. Studies have demonstrated that the most effective way to prevent HPV transmission is to abstain from all sexual contact (26). Long-term monogamy with a single partner is likely to be the next most effective prevention strategy. Other factors that may decrease the risk of infection include limiting the number of sexual partners (66), limiting sexual contact to men who have been abstinent for a longer period (possibly allowing prevalent HPV infections to resolve spontaneously) (26), or having a circumcised partner (66, 67). Genital HPV types also have been isolated from skin and nail samples of individuals with genital warts (68); therefore, transmission also may be possible by oral–genital, manual–genital, and nonpenetrative genital–genital contact (26, 69–71). Covering infected areas with a latex condom provides theoretical protection from infection. Particles the size of HPV virions do not penetrate an intact latex condom (72), and many HPV infections in men are located in anatomical locations that would be covered by a male condom (73–76). However, areas not covered by the condom (because the area is not intended to be covered, the condom was used incorrectly, or it broke or slipped) can transmit HPV infection (76).

Because HPV infection is intermittently detectable, it is difficult to distinguish between existing and new HPV infections. Many of the epidemiological studies of condom use were not designed or conducted in ways that allow the accurate assessment of the effectiveness of condoms against HPV infection. The effectiveness of male condoms in preventing sexually transmitted diseases was the subject of a recent National Institute of Allergy and Infectious Diseases report (77). The report concluded that, although evidence is lacking that condoms offer complete protection from HPV infection, condom use may reduce the risk of HPV-related disease, such as genital warts and cervical neoplasia (77). In a meta-analysis (78), most studies found that self-reported use of condoms did not protect against acquiring HPV infection (79–83). One study showed a statistically significant protective effect for condom use, but this only applied to nononcogenic HPV types (84). Only one study examined the effect of condom use on genital warts in women. It found that condom use significantly reduces the risk of acquiring genital warts (85).

Studies that looked at the relationship of condom use to CIN 1 or unspecified CIN showed conflicting results. Three showed no significant effect after adjustment for confounding factors (82, 86, 87) and one other reported an increased risk (88). Several studies evaluated the protective effects of condoms for CIN 2 and CIN 3. Some showed a significant reduction in risk (80, 87, 89–92) whereas the others did not (86, 93–96). Five studies evaluated the effect of condoms as a risk factor for invasive cervical cancer. Two found a significant protective effect (89, 91), whereas three found no significant effect (86, 90, 95). Three studies evaluated the effectiveness of condoms on the clearance of HPV or HPV-associated lesions and all found a benefit (97–99). Women whose partners were randomized to use condoms were more likely to clear an HPV infection and resolve abnormal cervical cytology than those whose partners did not use condoms (99).

Another strategy for preventing HPV infection is the use of a prophylactic vaccine. The ideal prophylactic vaccine would be safe; easily administered in all settings, including those with poor resources; inexpensive to produce; and fully effective after a single dose. The protection should last for many years and be effective against most HPV types related to cervical cancer. Most of the prophylactic vaccines currently under development are based on purified viruslike particles composed of the viral L1 protein. Animal models have shown that systemic vaccination with L1 viruslike particles can induce high titers of neutralizing antibodies and can protect against high-dose experimental infections with the homologous virus (100–102). This was confirmed in early phase trials of L1 viruslike particles. A recent double-blind placebo-controlled trial of an HPV16 L1 viruslike particle vaccine demonstrated substantial protection against transient HPV16 infection and complete protection against persistent HPV16 infection, defined as two or more samples positive for HPV DNA during the 17-month follow-up period (103). In these studies, none of the cytologic abnormalities that occurred in the study group was attributable to HPV16, the infection the vaccine was intended to prevent.

Current vaccines have several shortcomings. They are expensive, they require multiple injections, and the protection is specific for HPV16. New trials are evaluating viruslike particle vaccines that are either bivalent against HPV16 and HPV 18 or quadrivalent against HPV6, HPV11, HPV16, and HPV18. It is estimated that a vaccine against HPV16 would prevent one half of the cases of cervical cancer, a vaccine against HPV16 and HPV18 would prevent two thirds of cases, and a vaccine against the six most prevalent types would prevent four fifths of cervical cancer cases (104). Because the incidence of HPV infection peaks at age 19 years in the United States (105) and one half of sexually transmitted HPV infections are contracted within 3 years after the initiation of sexual intercourse (106), future vaccines would be most effective if administered to young adolescents who are not yet sexually active. In addition, those who had sexual contact before vaccination may not be protected.

Regardless of the success of these phase three trials, it is unlikely that any vaccine will significantly decrease the incidence of cervical cancer in the near future. Completion of the trials is likely to take several years, and wide acceptance and use is unlikely for several years after that. Because the peak incidence of high-grade cervical dysplasia is 10–20 years after the initiating HPV infection and cervical cancer as much as 10 years after that, a reduction in the incidence of cervical dysplasia and cancer attributed to a prophylactic HPV vaccine may not be seen for several decades.

▶ *When should patient-applied therapies for genital warts be considered?*

Left untreated, visible genital warts often resolve spontaneously, but some remain unchanged or increase in size and number (1, 107). In placebo-controlled studies, genital warts resolve spontaneously in 20–30% of women in 3 months (108). Existing data cannot determine whether any available treatment for genital warts reduces or eradicates their infectiousness. Successful treatment requires a thorough evaluation. Many treatment failures actually are a failure to identify and treat all lesions. The Centers for Disease Control and Prevention guidelines divide the treatment regimens for external genital warts into patient-applied and provider-administered therapies (1). Treatment for genital warts should be guided by the preference of the patient and the experience of the heath care provider. There is no current evidence to suggest that any one treatment is superior to any other, and no single treatment is ideal for all patients and all types of warts. The patient's cognitive, emotional, and physical state influences whether self-applied therapies can be used safely and effectively. Patient-applied agents may be best suited for the needs of those patients who want to be in control of their own care. However, providers should be careful to offer such self-applied agents only to patients who can understand how to use them properly, who can successfully identify where to apply the medication, and who are physically able to reach the warts that need treatment.

Warts that are small in size and few in number will respond to almost any treatment or no treatment at all. Many patients require a course of therapy rather than a single treatment. Generally, warts on moist or mucosal surfaces are more responsive to topical treatment than are warts on drier surfaces. Warts that do not respond to a particular treatment modality after three provider-administered treatments and warts that are not cleared completely after six treatments should be re-evaluated (1). All treatment modalities result in local inflammation or discomfort, and the patient should be warned that ablation modalities might be associated with persistent hypopigmentation or hyperpigmentation and rarely in disabling chronic pain syndromes, such as vulvodynia.

Two patient-applied therapies that may be used for the treatment of genital warts are podofilox (0.5% solution or gel) and imiquimod (5% cream). Podofilox is a purified derivative of podophyllin that the patient can apply. The mechanism of action includes antimitosis, inhibition of nucleoside transport, damage to vessels within the wart, stimulation of macrophage proliferation, and production of interleukin-1 and interleukin-2. Podofilox is applied twice daily for 3 consecutive days followed by 4 days of no therapy. If possible, the health care provider should apply the initial treatment to demonstrate the proper application technique and to identify the warts that should be treated. The total area of warts that should be treated should be limited to 10 cm². Although 45–90% of warts are cleared following podofilox therapy, posttreatment recurrence is 30–60% (109, 110).

Imiquimod acts by inducing a local immune response. Imiquimod activates macrophages and dendritic cells to release α interferon and other proinflammatory cytokines. These cytokines activate HPV-specific T cells that then kill HPV-infected cells. Imiquimod is applied once daily at bedtime, three times per week for up to 16 weeks. The treatment area should be washed with soap and water 6–10 hours after application. The treatment area should be limited to no more than 20 cm². Imiquimod results in clearance rates of 70–85% with recurrence rates of 5–20% (109–111).

Because of a similar risk of recurrence, no single treatment for external genital warts can be recommended over another. In addition, neither podofilox nor imiquimod should be used during pregnancy.

▶ *When should provider-applied medication or procedures for genital warts be considered?*

No single provider-applied treatment has been found to be ideal for all patients or all warts, and most treatments appear to have comparable efficacy. The anatomic location of the warts and the number and character of the external genital warts will affect treatment decisions, as will co-existing medical conditions, such as pregnancy and immune deficiency. Commonly used provider-administered treatments include cryosurgery, trichloroacetic acid or bichloracetic acid, surgical removal (including excision with a scissor, scalpel or electrosurgical loop), electrocautery, and laser vaporization or excision.

Cryotherapy destroys tissue by causing cytolysis that results in sloughing of the wart and other affected tissues. Efficacy studies have shown clearance rates of up to 90% with a recurrence rate of up to 40% (109). Although there are no real patient-related contraindications to cryotherapy, proper training is required to avoid overtreatment or undertreatment. Pain and necrosis and occasional blistering follow the application of liquid nitrogen. Cryotherapy is effective for both dry and moist warts; however, when treating large warts or large areas, wound care problems can occasionally be encountered.

Trichloroacetic acid and bichloracetic acid in concentrations of 80–90% are caustic agents that destroy warts by the chemical coagulation of proteins. Because these solutions have a very low viscosity, they can run onto adjacent normal tissue if over-applied, causing damage. They should be applied sparingly and allowed to dry before the patient is allowed to sit or stand. This modality is more appropriate for small warts on moist surfaces. The few studies on the effectiveness of trichloroacetic acid and bichloracetic acid show clearance rates between 60% and 80%, but their use requires several weekly applications, and large and keratinized warts are more refractory to trichloroacetic acid and bichloracetic acid. Recurrence rates are unclear (109, 110).

Surgical removal of external genital warts may be advantageous because the patient often is cured in one visit. Although surgical treatment is relatively expensive, the ability to avoid multiple visits saves both the patient and the physician time and money and adds to the cost-effectiveness of the technique. Surgical removal is probably most appropriate when the patient has only a few small warts or large numbers of warts over a large surface area that require surgical debulking. The former generally is done in the office using a local anesthetic, whereas the latter requires general anesthesia.

Laser ablation requires specialized training and equipment and generally is reserved for extensive and recalcitrant disease. It can effectively treat both large and small warts, and when properly applied, scarring is rare. Clearance rates of approximately 90% have been reported; however, the efficacy of all these treatments depends on the time lapse between treatment and assessment, the number of treatments required, the initial cure of the lesions, the type and volume of warts treated, and the immune status of the patients being treated (109). Pain following laser vaporization is dependent on the area being treated. Treatment of large areas can result in severe pain that peaks after 5–7 days and can last up to 3 weeks. Vitiligo and hyperpigmentation are possible, and scarring is a potential complication of laser vaporization that is very extensive or too deep. However, in experienced hands, laser surgery provides better depth control than any of the other surgical modalities. Because of the cost of the equipment and because laser surgery usually is performed in an operating room with general anesthesia, it is the most expensive modality for the treatment of genital warts.

▶ *What are common patient questions, and how should a patient be counseled about the diagnosis of HPV?*

How did I get HPV? Any individual who is sexually active can get HPV except those in a mutually monogamous lifelong relationship. At least 75% of all sexually active women will have HPV in their lifetime (112). Genital HPV usually is spread by direct skin-to-skin contact, including vaginal, anal, or more rarely, oral sex, with someone who has the overt or subclinical HPV infection. Human papillomavirus is site-specific so that genital warts do not spread to other parts of the body, such as the hands, and warts from other parts of the body do not spread to the genital area. However, the hands can act as a vector for the spread of genital HPV.

How can I reduce the risk of getting genital HPV? Because HPV is so common, especially in young women who have recently become sexually active, every sexual encounter with a new partner carries the risk of HPV infection. Limiting those encounters limits the risk of infection. Latex condoms may provide some protection from HPV-related disease, such as genital warts and cervical neoplasia, but only if they are used consistently and only for the area that they cover. However, because HPV can affect areas of the genital skin that are not covered by condoms, they do not provide complete protection from HPV infection.

If I am treated for an HPV infection, can my partner reinfect me? As long as a couple remains mutually monogamous and does not introduce new strains of HPV into the relationship, the risk of a "ping-pong" effect is minimal. Each partner will have developed (or failed to develop) an immune response to the HPV types prevalent in the relationship. If the immune response of one of the partners is able to eradicate the HPV, that individual will maintain the immunity to that HPV type even if re-exposed by the partner. However, this immunity does not confer protection against new HPV types introduced into the relationship by the same or a different partner. Furthermore, if either partner subsequently becomes immune deficient because of disease, advanced age, or medication, HPV may re-manifest itself.

Because I am in a monogamous relationship, does the diagnosis of HPV mean that my partner has cheated? Until recently, physicians did not screen women with normal cervical cytology for the presence of HPV. Human papillomavirus testing was performed only in some women who were found to have abnormal cervical cytology. Because most patients with high-risk HPV have no overt manifestations of the disease, they may have had high-risk HPV for many months or years without knowing it. Also, HPV positivity may fluctuate between consecutive tests. Patients who previously had negative test results for HPV may have latent HPV at a level below the threshold of detection for commercially available tests. Furthermore, it is impossible to determine how long a particular infection has been present or to trace it back to a particular partner unless one of the partners was a virgin (including nonpenetrating sexual contact and digital–genital contact) at the beginning of the relationship. It is impossible to say whether one or the other partner or both partners introduced HPV into the relationship.

What about pregnancy and genital warts? Most pregnant women with a history of HPV or genital warts are unlikely to have any HPV-related complications during pregnancy or childbirth. During pregnancy, genital warts may proliferate because of relative immune suppression. Treatment may be delayed until postpartum to evaluate the degree of spontaneous resolution. Most children born to women with a history of genital warts have no HPV-related complications. Rarely, infants exposed to HPV may develop warty growths in the throat called laryngeal papillomatosis. Cesarean delivery is not useful in preventing the transmission of HPV (1).

Summary of Recommendations and Conclusions

The following recommendations are based on good and consistent scientific evidence (Level A):

▶ Because HPV DNA testing is more sensitive than cervical cytology in detecting CIN 2 and CIN 3, women with negative concurrent test results can be reassured that their risk of unidentified CIN 2 and CIN 3 or cervical cancer is approximately 1 in 1,000.

▶ Studies using combined HPV testing with cervical cytology have reported a negative predictive value for CIN 2 and CIN 3 of 99–100%.

▶ Human papillomavirus DNA testing is not recommended in women with LSIL, atypical squamous cells that cannot exclude high-grade squamous intraepithelial lesions, or atypical glandular cell cytology.

▶ The triage of women with ASC-US cytology using reflex HPV DNA testing for high-risk types when liquid-based cytology was used at the time of the initial visit eliminates the need for a repeat office visit and is a more sensitive triage tool than repeat cytology while referring fewer women to colposcopy.

▶ Women with high-risk HPV who have ASC-US or LSIL cytology but are not found to have CIN 2 or CIN 3 at their initial colposcopy have approximately a 10% risk of having CIN 2 or CIN 3 within 2 years.

The following recommendations are based on limited or inconsistent scientific evidence (Level B):

▶ Although evidence is lacking that condoms offer complete protection from HPV infection, condom use may reduce the risk of HPV-related disease, such as genital warts and cervical neoplasia.

▶ Studies show that condoms may be effective in the clearance of HPV or HPV-associated lesions.

▶ Use of a combination of cervical cytology and HPV DNA screening is appropriate for women aged 30 years and older. If this combination is used,

women who receive negative results on both tests should be rescreened no more frequently than every 3 years.

▶ Because of a similar risk of recurrence, no single treatment for external genital warts can be recommended over another.

The following recommendations are based primarily on consensus and expert opinion (Level C):

▶ Women older than 30 years with a negative cytology result who have high-risk HPV DNA positive test results should have both tests repeated in 6–12 months. Those with persistent high-risk HPV (on repeat testing) should undergo colposcopy regardless of the cytology result.

▶ Human papillomavirus DNA testing could be used as a test of cure for women with CIN 2 or CIN 3 at 6–12 months following excision or ablation of the transformation zone. Those with high-risk HPV should be referred for colposcopy.

▶ Treatment for genital warts should be guided by the preference of the patient and the experience of the heath care provider.

References

1. Sexually transmitted diseases treatment guidelines 2002. Centers for Disease Control and Prevention. MMWR Recomm Rep 2002;51(RR–6):1–78. (Level III)

2. Koutsky LA, Galloway DA, Holmes KK. Epidemiology of genital human papillomavirus infection. Epidemiol Rev 1988;10:122–63. (Level III)

3. Lawson HW, Lee NC, Thames SF, Henson R, Miller DS. Cervical cancer screening among low-income women: results of a national screening program, 1991–1995. Obstet Gynecol 1998;92:745–52. (Level II-2)

4. Kotloff KL, Wasserman SS, Russ K, Shapiro S, Daniel R, Brown W, et al. Detection of genital human papillomavirus and associated cytological abnormalities among college women. Sex Transm Dis 1998;25:243–50. (Level II-2)

5. Bauer HM, Ting Y, Greer CE, Chambers JC, Tashiro CJ, Chimera J, et al. Genital human papillomavirus infection in female university students as determined by a PCR-based method. JAMA 1991;265:472–7. (Level II-3)

6. Burk RD, Ho GY, Beardsley L, Lempa M, Peters M, Bierman R. Sexual behavior and partner characteristics are the predominant risk factors for genital human papillomavirus infection in young women. J Infect Dis 1996; 174:679–89. (Level II-3)

7. Jemal A, Tiwari RC, Murray T, Ghafoor A, Samuels A, Ward E, et al. Cancer statistics, 2004. American Cancer Society. CA Cancer J Clin 2004;54:8–29. (Level II-3)

8. Franco EL, Villa LL, Sobrinho JP, Prado JM, Rousseau MC, Desy M, et al. Epidemiology of acquisition and clearance of cervical human papillomavirus infection in women from a high-risk area for cervical cancer. J Infect Dis 1999;180:1415–23. (Level II-3)

9. Ho GY, Bierman R, Beardsley L, Chang CJ, Burk RD. Natural history of cervicovaginal papillomavirus infection in young women. N Engl J Med 1998;338:423–8. (Level II-2)

10. Wheeler CM, Greer CE, Becker TM, Hunt WC, Anderson SM, Manos MM. Short-term fluctuations in the detection of cervical human papillomavirus DNA. Obstet Gynecol 1996;88:261–8. (Level II-3)

11. Schneider A, Kirchhoff T, Meinhardt G, Gissmann L. Repeated evaluation of human papillomavirus 16 status in cervical swabs of young women with a history of normal Papanicolaou smears. Obstet Gynecol 1992;79:683–8. (Level III)

12. Moscicki AB, Palefsky J, Smith G, Siboshski S, Schoolnik G. Variability of human papillomavirus DNA testing in a longitudinal cohort of young women. Obstet Gynecol 1993;82:578–85. (Level II-2)

13. Hildesheim A, Schiffman MH, Gravitt PE, Glass AG, Greer CE, Zhang T, et al. Persistence of type-specific human papillomavirus infection among cytologically normal women. J Infect Dis 1994;169:235–40. (Level II-2)

14. Evander M, Edlund K, Gustafsson A, Jonsson M, Karlsson R, Rylander E, et al. Human papillomavirus infection is transient in young women: a population-based cohort study. J Infect Dis 1995;171:1026–30. (Level II-2)

15. Oriel JD. Natural history of genital warts. Br J Vener Dis 1971;47:1–13. (Level III)

16. Campion MJ, Singer A, Clarkson PK, McCance DJ. Increased risk of cervical neoplasia in consorts of men with penile condylomata acuminata. Lancet 1985;1:943–6. (Level II-2)

17. Ley C, Bauer HM, Reingold A, Schiffman MH, Chambers JC, Tashiro CJ, et al. Determinants of genital human papillomavirus infection in young women. J Natl Cancer Inst 1991;83:997–1003. (Level III)

18. Hildesheim A, Gravitt P, Schiffman MH, Kurman RJ, Barnes W, Jones S, et al. Determinants of genital human papillomavirus infection in low-income women in Washington, D.C. Sex Transm Dis 1993;20:279–85. (Level III)

19. Bauer HM, Hildesheim A, Schiffman MH, Glass AG, Rush BB, Scott DR, et al. Determinants of genital human papillomavirus infection in low-risk women in Portland, Oregon. Sex Transm Dis 1993;20:274–8. (Level II-3)

20. Wheeler CM, Parmenter CA, Hunt WC, Becker TM, Greer CE, Hildesheim A, et al. Determinants of genital human papillomavirus infection among cytologically normal women attending the University of New Mexico student health center. Sex Transm Dis 1993;20:286–9. (Level II-2)

21. Karlsson R, Jonsson M, Edlund K, Evander M, Gustavsson A, Boden E, et al. Lifetime number of part-

ners as the only independent risk factor for human papillomavirus infection: a population-based study. Sex Transm Dis 1995;22:119–27. (Level II-2)

22. Kjaer SK, van den Brule AJ, Bock JE, Poll PA, Engholm G, Sherman ME, et al. Determinants for genital human papillomavirus (HPV) infection in 1000 randomly chosen young Danish women with normal Pap smear: are there different risk profiles for oncogenic and nononcogenic HPV types? Cancer Epidemiol Biomarkers Prev 1997;6:799–805. (Level II-2)

23. Melkert PW, Hopman E, van den Brule AJ, Risse EK, van Diest PJ, Bleker OP, et al. Prevalence of HPV in cytomorphologically normal cervical smears, as determined by the polymerase chain reaction, is age-dependent. Int J Cancer 1993;53:919–23. (Level III)

24. Schiffman MH. Epidemiology of cervical human papillomavirus infections. Curr Top Microbiol Immunol 1994;186:55–81. (Level III)

25. Bosch FX, Castellsague X, Munoz N, de Sanjose S, Ghaffari AM, Gonzalez LC, et al. Male sexual behavior and human papillomavirus DNA: key risk factors for cervical cancer in Spain. J Natl Cancer Inst 1996;88:1060–7. (Level II-3)

26. Winer RL, Lee SK, Hughes JP, Adam DE, Kiviat NB, Koutsky LA. Genital human papillomavirus infection: incidence and risk factors in a cohort of female university students [published erratum appears in Am J Epidemiol 2003;157:858]. Am J Epidemiol 2003;157:218–26. (Level II-2)

27. Watts DH, Koutsky LA, Holmes KK, Goldman D, Kuypers J, Kiviat NB, et al. Low risk of perinatal transmission of human papillomavirus: results from a prospective cohort study. Am J Obstet Gynecol 1998;178:365–73. (Level II-2)

28. Kashima HK, Shah F, Lyles A, Glackin R, Muhammad N, Turner L, et al. A comparison of risk factors in juvenile-onset and adult-onset recurrent respiratory papillomatosis. Laryngoscope 1992;102:9–13. (Level II-2)

29. Pakarian F, Kaye J, Cason J, Kell B, Jewers R, Derias NW, et al. Cancer associated human papillomaviruses: perinatal transmission and persistence. Br J Obstet Gynaecol 1994;101:514–7. (Level III)

30. Cason J, Kaye JN, Jewers RJ, Kambo PK, Bible JM, Kell B, et al. Perinatal infection and persistence of human papillomavirus types 16 and 18 in infants. J Med Virol 1995;47:209–18. (Level III)

31. Puranen M, Yliskoski M, Saarikoski S, Syrjanen K, Syrjanen S. Vertical transmission of human papillomavirus from infected mothers to their newborn babies and persistence of the virus in childhood. Am J Obstet Gynecol 1996;174:694–9. (Level II-2)

32. Fredericks BD, Balkin A, Daniel HW, Schonrock J, Ward B, Frazer IH. Transmission of human papillomaviruses from mother to child. Aust N Z J Obstet Gynaecol 1993;33:30–2. (Level III)

33. Tenti P, Zappatore R, Migliora P, Spinillo A, Belloni C, Carnevali L. Perinatal transmission of human papillomavirus from gravidas with latent infections. Obstet Gynecol 1999;93:475–9. (Level II-2)

34. Moscicki AB, Shiboski S, Hills NK, Powell KJ, Jay N, Hanson EN, et al. Regression of low-grade squamous intra-epithelial lesions in young women. Lancet 2004; 364:1678–83. (Level II-2)

35. Bosch FX, Lorincz A, Munoz N, Meijer CJ, Shah KV. The causal relation between human papillomavirus and cervical cancer. J Clin Pathol 2002;55:244–65. (Level III)

36. Van Ranst M, Kaplan JB, Burk RD. Phylogenetic classification of human papillomaviruses: correlation with clinical manifestations. J Gen Virol 1992;73:2653–60. (Level III)

37. Munoz N, Bosch FX, de Sanjose S, Herrero R, Castellsague X, Shah KV, et al. Epidemiologic classification of human papillomavirus types associated with cervical cancer. International Agency for Research on Cancer Multicenter Cervical Cancer Study Group. N Engl J Med 2003;348:518–27. (Level II-2)

38. Duensing S, Munger K. Mechanisms of genomic instability in human cancer: insights from studies with human papillomavirus oncoproteins. Int J Cancer 2004;109: 157–62. (Level III)

39. Munger K, Howley PM. Human papillomavirus immortalization and transformation functions. Virus Res 2002; 89:213–28. (Level III)

40. Fehrmann F, Laimins LA. Human papillomaviruses: targeting differentiating epithelial cells for malignant transformation. Oncogene 2003;22:5201–7. (Level III)

41. Finzer P, Aguilar-Lemarroy A, Rosl F. The role of human papillomavirus oncoproteins E6 and E7 in apoptosis. Cancer Lett 2002;188:15–24. (Level III)

42. zur Hausen H. Papillomaviruses and cancer: from basic studies to clinical application. Nat Rev Cancer 2002;2: 342–50. (Level III)

43. Fahey MT, Irwig L, Macaskill P. Meta-analysis of Pap test accuracy. Am J Epidemiol 1995;141:680–9. (Meta-analysis)

44. Agency for Health Care Policy and Research. Evaluation of cervical cytology. Evidence report/technology assessment 5. Available at: http://www.ncbi.nlm.nih.gov/books/bv.fcgi?rid=hstat1.chapter.6794. Retrieved December 6, 2004. (Level III)

45. Clavel C, Masure M, Bory JP, Putaud I, Mangeonjean C, Lorenzato M, et al. Human papillomavirus testing in primary screening for the detection of high-grade cervical lesions: a study of 7932 women. Br J Cancer 2001;84: 1616–23. (Level II-3)

46. Hutchinson ML, Zahniser DJ, Sherman ME, Herrero R, Alfaro M, Bratti MC, et al. Utility of liquid-based cytology for cervical carcinoma screening: results of a population-based study conducted in a region of Costa Rica with a high incidence of cervical carcinoma. Cancer 1999;87:48–55. (Level II-2)

47. Kulasingam SL, Hughes JP, Kiviat NB, Mao C, Weiss NS, Kuypers JM, et al. Evaluation of human papillomavirus testing in primary screening for cervical abnormalities: comparison of sensitivity, specificity, and frequency of referral. JAMA 2002;288:1749–57. (Level II-3)

48. Solomon D, Schiffman M, Tarone B. Comparison of three management strategies for patients with atypical squamous cells of undetermined significance: baseline results from a randomized trial. ASCUS-LSIL Triage Study (ALTS) Group. J Natl Cancer Inst 2001;93:293–9. (Level I)

49. Schiffman M, Adrianza ME. ASCUS-LSIL Triage Study. Design, methods and characteristics of trial participants. Acta Cytol 2000;44:726–42. (Level I)

50. Human papillomavirus testing for triage of women with cytologic evidence of low-grade squamous intraepithelial lesions: baseline data from a randomized trial. The Atypical Squamous Cells of Undetermined Significance/Low-Grade Squamous Intraepithelial Lesions Triage Study (ALTS) Group. J Natl Cancer Inst 2000; 92:397–402. (Level I)

51. Sherman ME, Schiffman M, Cox JT. Effects of age and human papilloma viral load on colposcopy triage: data from the randomized Atypical Squamous Cells of Undetermined Significance/Low-Grade Squamous Intraepithelial Lesion Triage Study (ALTS). J Natl Center Inst 2002;94:102–7. (Level II-3)

52. Wright TC Jr, Cox JT, Massad JS, Twiggs LB, Wilkinson EJ. 2001 Consensus Guidelines for the management of women with cervical cytological abnormalities. 2001 ASCCP-Sponsored Consensus Conference. JAMA 2002; 287:2120–9. (Level III)

53. Guido R, Schiffman M, Solomon D, Burke L. Postcolposcopy management strategies for women referred with low-grade squamous intraepithelial lesions or human papillomavirus DNA-positive atypical squamous cells of undetermined significance: a two-year prospective study. ASCUS-LSIL Triage Study (ALTS) Group. Am J Obstet Gynecol 2003;188:1401–5. (Level II-3)

54. Cox JT, Schiffman M, Solomon D. Prospective follow-up suggests similar risk of subsequent cervical intraepithelial neoplasia grade 2 or 3 among women with cervical intraepithelial neoplasia grade 1 or negative colposcopy and directed biopsy. ASCUS-LSIL Triage Study (ALTS) Group. Am J Obstet Gynecol 2003;188:1406–12. (Level II-3)

55. Belinson J, Qiao YL, Pretorius R, Zhang WH, Elson P, Li L, et al. Shanxi Province Cervical Cancer Screening Study: a cross-sectional comparative trial of multiple techniques to detect cervical neoplasia [published erratum appears in Gynecol Oncol 2002;84:355]. Gynecol Oncol 2001;83:439–44. (Level II-3)

56. Belinson JL, Qiao YL, Pretorius RG, Zhang WH, Rong SD, Huang MN, et al. Shanxi Province Cervical Cancer Screening Study II: self-sampling for high-risk human papillomavirus compared to direct sampling for human papillomavirus and liquid based cervical cytology. Int J Gynecol Cancer 2003;13:819–26. (Level II-3)

57. Schiffman M, Herrero R, Hildesheim A, Sherman ME, Bratti M, Wacholder S, et al. HPV DNA testing in cervical cancer screening: results from women in a high-risk province of Costa Rica. JAMA 2000;283:87–93. (Level II-3)

58. Ratnam S, Franco EL, Ferenczy A. Human papillomavirus testing for primary screening of cervical cancer precursors. Cancer Epidemiol Biomarkers Prev 2000;9: 945–51. (Level II-3)

59. Salmeron J, Lazcano-Ponce E, Lorincz A, Hernandez M, Hernandez P, Leyva A, et al. Comparison of HPV-based assays with Papanicolaou smears for cervical cancer screening in Morelos State, Mexico. Cancer Causes Control 2003;14:505–12. (Level II-3)

60. Petry KU, Menton S, Menton M, van Loenen-Frosch F, de Carvalho Gomes H, Holz B, et al. Inclusion of HPV testing in routine cervical cancer screening for women above 29 years in Germany: results for 8466 patients. Br J Cancer 2003;88:1570–7. (Level II-2)

61. Cuzick J, Beverley E, Ho L, Terry G, Sapper H, Mielzynska I, et al. HPV testing in primary screening of older women. Br J Cancer 1999;81:554–8. (Level II-3)

62. Kjaer SK, van den Brule AJ, Paull G, Svare EI, Sherman ME, Thomsen BL, et al. Type specific persistence of high risk human papillomavirus (HPV) as indicator of high grade cervical squamous intraepithelial lesions in young women: population based prospective follow up study. BMJ 2002;325:572–6. (Level II-2)

63. Sherman ME, Lorincz AT, Scott DR, Wacholder S, Castle PE, Glass AG, et al. Baseline cytology, human papillomavirus testing, and risk for cervical neoplasia: a 10-year cohort analysis. J Natl Cancer Inst 2003;95:46–52. (Level II-2)

64. Bory JP, Cucherousset J, Lorenzato M, Gabriel R, Quereux C, Birembaut P, et al. Recurrent human papillomavirus infection detected with the hybrid capture II assay selects women with normal cervical smears at risk for developing high grade cervical lesions: a longitudinal study of 3,091 women. Int J Cancer 2002;102:519–25. (Level II-2)

65. Wright TC Jr, Schiffman M, Solomon D, Cox JT, Garcia F, Goldie S, et al. Interim guidance on use of human papillomavirus DNA testing as an adjunct to cervical cytology for screening. Obstet Gynecol 2004;103:304–9. (Level III)

66. Svare EI, Kjaer SK, Worm AM, Osterlind A, Meijer CJ, van den Brule AJ. Risk factors for genital HPV DNA in men resemble those found in women: a study of male attendees at a Danish STD clinic. Sex Transm Infect 2002;78:215–8. (Level II-2)

67. Castellsague X, Bosch FX, Munoz N, Meijer CJ, Shah KV, de Sanjose S, et al. Male circumcision, penile human papillomavirus infection, and cervical cancer in female partners. International Agency for Research on Cancer Multicenter Cervical Cancer Study Group. N Engl J Med 2002;346:1105–12. (Level II-2)

68. Sonnex C, Strauss S, Gray JJ. Detection of human papillomavirus DNA on the fingers of patients with genital warts. Sex Transm Infect 1999;75:317–9. (Level III)

69. Coutlee F, Trottier AM, Ghattas G, Leduc R, Toma E, Sanche G, et al. Risk factors for oral human papillomavirus in adults infected and not infected with human immunodeficiency virus. Sex Transm Dis 1997;24:23–31. (Level II-2)

70. Fairley CK, Gay NJ, Forbes A, Abramson M, Garland SM. Hand-genital transmission of genital warts? An analysis of prevalence data. Epidemiol Infect 1995;115:169–76. (Level III)

71. Marrazzo JM, Stine K, Koutsky LA. Genital human papillomavirus infection in women who have sex with women: a review. Am J Obstet Gynecol 2000;183:770–4. (Level III)

72. Lytle CD, Routson LB, Seaborn GB, Dixon LG, Bushar HF, Cyr WH. An in vitro evaluation of condoms as barriers to a small virus. Sex Transm Dis 1997;24:161–4. (Level II-3)

73. Kennedy L, Buntine DW, O'Connor D, Frazer IH. Human papillomavirus—a study of male sexual partners. Med J Aust 1988;149:309–11. (Level II-2)

74. Krebs HB, Schneider V. Human papillomavirus-associated lesions of the penis: colposcopy, cytology, and histology. Obstet Gynecol 1987;70:299–304. (Level II-3)

75. Schultz RE, Miller JW, MacDonald GR, Auman JR, Peterson NR, Ward BE, et al. Clinical and molecular evaluation of acetowhite genital lesions in men. J Urol 1990;143:920–3. (Level II-3)

76. van Doornum GJ, Hooykaas C, Juffermans LH, van der Lans SM, van der Linden MM, Coutinho RA, et al. Prevalence of human papillomavirus infections among heterosexual men and women with multiple sexual partners. J Med Virol 1992;37:13–21. (Level III)

77. National Institute of Allergy and Infectious Diseases. Workshop summary: scientific evidence on condom effectiveness for sexually transmitted disease (STD) prevention. Available at: http://www.niaid.nih.gov/dmid/stds/condomreport.pdf. Retrieved December 3, 2004. (Level III)

78. Manhart LE, Koutsky LA. Do condoms prevent genital HPV infection, external genital warts or cervical neoplasia? A meta-analysis. Sex Transm Dis 2002;29:725–35. (Meta-analysis)

79. Davidson M, Schnitzer PG, Bulkhow LR, Parkinson AJ, Schloss ML, Fitzgerald MA, et al. The prevalence of cervical infection with human papillomaviruses and cervical dysplasia in Alaska native women. J Infect Dis 1994;169:792–800. (Level III)

80. Ho GY, Kadish AS, Burk RD, Basu J, Palan PR, Mikhail M, et al. HPV 16 and cigarette smoking as risk factors for high-grade cervical intra-epithelial neoplasia. Int J Cancer 1998;78:281–5. (Level II-2)

81. Jamison JH, Kaplan DW, Hamman R, Eagar R, Beach R, Douglas JM Jr. Spectrum of genital human papillomavirus infection in a female adolescent population. Sex Transm Dis 1995;22:236–43. (Level II-3)

82. Kataja V, Syrjanen S, Yliskoski M, Hippelinen M, Vayrynen M, Saarikoski S, et al. Risk factors associated with cervical human papillomavirus infections: a case–control study. Am J Epidemiol 1993;138:735–45. (Level II-2)

83. Young TK, McNicol P, Beauvais J. Factors associated with human papillomavirus infection detected by polymerase chain reaction among urban Canadian aboriginal and non-aboriginal women. Sex Transm Dis 1997;24:293–8. (Level II-3)

84. Kjaer SK, Svare EI, Worm AM, Walboomers JM, Meijer CJ, van den Brule AJ. Human papillomavirus infection in

Danish female sex workers. Decreasing prevalence with age despite continuously high sexual activity. Sex Transm Dis 2000;27:438–45. (Level II-2)

85. Wen LM, Estcourt CS, Simpson JM, Mindel A. Risk factors for the acquisition of genital warts: are condoms protective? Sex Transm Infect 1999;75:312–6. (Level II-2)

86. Zondervan KT, Carpenter LM, Painter R, Vessey MP. Oral contraceptives and cervical cancer—further findings from the Oxford Family Planning Association contraceptive study. Br J Cancer 1996;73:1291–7. (Level II-2)

87. Adam E, Berkova Z, Daxnerova Z, Icenogle J, Reeves WC, Kaufman RH. Papillomavirus detection: demographic and behavioral characteristics influencing the identification of cervical disease. Am J Obstet Gynecol 2000;182:257–64. (Level II-3)

88. Syrajanen K, Vayrynen M, Castren O, Yliskoski M, Mantyjarvi R, Pyrhonen S, et al. Sexual behavior of women with human papillomavirus (HPV) lesions of the uterine cervix. Br J Vener Dis 1984;60:243–8. (Level II-2)

89. Kjaer SK, de Villiers EM, Dahl C, Engholm G, Bock JE, Vestergaard BF, et al. Case-control study of risk factors for cervical neoplasia in Denmark. I: role of the "male factor" in women with one lifetime sexual partner. Int J Cancer 1991;48:39–44. (Level II-2)

90. Slattery ML, Overall JC Jr, Abbott TM, French TK, Robison LM, Gardner J. Sexual activity, contraception, genital infections, and cervical cancer: support for a sexually transmitted disease hypothesis. Am J Epidemiol 1989;130:248–58. (Level II-2)

91. Thomas DB, Ray RM, Pardthaisong T, Chutivongse S, Koetsawang S, Silpisornkosol S, et al. Prostitution, condom use, and invasive squamous cell cervical cancer in Thailand. Am J Epidemiol 1996;143:779–86. (Level II-2)

92. Wang PD, Lin RS. Risk factors for cervical intraepithelial neoplasia in Taiwan. Gynecol Oncol 1996;62:10–8. (Level II-2)

93. Becker TM, Wheeler CM, McGough NS, Stidley CA, Parmenter CA, Dorin MH, et al. Contraceptive and reproductive risks for cervical dysplasia in southwestern Hispanic and non-Hispanic white women. Int J Epidemiol 1994;23:913–22. (Level II-2)

94. Deschamps MM, Pape JW, Hafner A, Johnson WD Jr. Heterosexual transmission of HIV in Haiti. Ann Intern Med 1996;125:324–30. (Level II-2)

95. Hildesheim A, Brinton LA, Mallin K, Lehman HF, Stolley P, Savitz DA, et al. Barrier and spermicidal contraceptive methods and risk of invasive cervical cancer. Epidemiology 1990;1:266–72. (Level II-2)

96. Munoz N, Bosch FX, de Sanjose S, Vergara A, del Moral A, Munoz MT, et al. Risk factors for cervical intraepithelial neoplasia grade III/carcinoma in situ in Spain and Colombia. Cancer Epidemiol Biomarkers Prev 1993;2: 423–31. (Level II-2)

97. Bleeker MC, Hogewoning CJ, Voorhorst FJ, van den Brule AJ, Snijders PJ, Starink TM, et al. Condom use promotes regression of human papillomavirus-associated penile lesions in male sexual partners of women with cer-

vical intraepithelial neoplasia. Int J Cancer 2003;107: 804–10. (Level I)

98. Hippelainen MI, Hippelainen M, Saarikoski S, Syrjanen K. Clinical course and prognostic factors of human papillomavirus infections in men. Sex Transm Dis 1994;21: 272–9. (Level II-3)

99. Hogewoning CJ, Bleeker MC, van den Brule AJ, Voorhorst FJ, Snijders PJ, Berkhof J, et al. Condom use promotes regression of cervical intraepithelial neoplasia and clearance of human papillomavirus: a randomized clinical trial. Int J Cancer 2003;107:811–6. (Level I)

100. Breitburd P, Kirnbauer R, Hubbert NL, Nonnenmacher B, Trin-Dinh-Desmarquet C, Orth G, et al. Immunization with viruslike particles from cottontail rabbit papillomavirus (CRPV) can protect against experimental CRPV infection. J Virol 1995;69:3959–63. (Level III)

101. Kirnbauer R, Chandrachud LM, O'Neil BW, Wagner ER, Grindlay GJ, Armstrong A, et al. Virus-like particles of bovine papillomavirus type 4 in prophylactic and therapeutic immunization. Virology 1996;219:37–44. (Level III)

102. Suzich JA, Ghim SJ, Palmer-Hill FJ, White WI, Tamura JK, Bell JA, et al. Systemic immunization with papillomavirus L1 protein completely prevents the development of viral mucosal papillomas. Proc Natl Acad Sci U S A 1995;92:11553–7. (Level III)

103. Koutsky LA, Ault KA, Wheeler CM, Brown DR, Barr E, Alvarez FB, et al. A controlled trial of a human papillomavirus type 16 vaccine. Proof of Principle Study Investigators. N Engl J Med 2002;347:1645–51. (Level I)

104. Monsonego J, Bosch FX, Coursaget P, Cox JT, Franco E, Frazer I, et al. Cervical cancer control, properties and new directions [published erratum appears in Int J Cancer 2004;108:945]. Int J Cancer 2004;108:329–33. (Level III)

105. Myers ER, McCrory DC, Nanda K, Bastien L, Matchar DB. Mathematical model for the natural history of human papillomavirus infection and cervical carcinogenesis. Am J Epidemiol 2000;151:1158–71. (Level III)

106. Collins S, Mazloomzadeh S, Winter H, Blomfield P, Baily A, Young LS, et al. High incidence of cervical human papillomavirus infection in women during their first sexual relationship. BJOG 2002;109:96–8. (Level II-3)

107. Beutner KR, Reitano MV, Richwald GA, Wiley DJ. External genital warts: report of the American Medical Association Consensus Conference. AMA Expert Panel on External Genital Warts. Clin Infect Dis 1998;27: 796–806. (Level III)

108. 1993 sexually transmitted diseases treatment guidelines. Centers for Disease Control and Prevention. MMWR Recomm Rep 1993;42(RR–14):1–102. (Level III)

109. Gunter J. Genital and perianal warts: new treatment opportunities for human papillomavirus infection. Am J Obstet Gynecol 2003;189:S3–11. (Level III)

110. Wiley DJ, Douglas J, Beutner K, Cox T, Fife K, Moscicki AB, et al. External genital warts: diagnosis, treatment, and prevention. Clin Infect Dis 2002;35:S210–24. (Level III)

111. Moore RA, Edwards JE, Hopwood J, Hicks D. Imiquimod for the treatment of genital warts: a quantitative systematic review. BMC Infect Dis 2001;1:3. (Level III)

112. Koutsky LA. Epidemiology of genital human papillomavirus infection. Am J Med 1997;102(5A):3–8. (Level III)

The MEDLINE database, the Cochrane Library, and ACOG's own internal resources and documents were used to conduct a literature search to locate relevant articles published between January 1985 and December 2004. The search was restricted to articles published in the English language. Priority was given to articles reporting results of original research, although review articles and commentaries also were consulted. Abstracts of research presented at symposia and scientific conferences were not considered adequate for inclusion in this document. Guidelines published by organizations or institutions such as the National Institutes of Health and the American College of Obstetricians and Gynecologists were reviewed, and additional studies were located by reviewing bibliographies of identified articles. When reliable research was not available, expert opinions from obstetrician–gynecologists were used.

Studies were reviewed and evaluated for quality according to the method outlined by the U.S. Preventive Services Task Force:

I   Evidence obtained from at least one properly designed randomized controlled trial.

II-1   Evidence obtained from well-designed controlled trials without randomization.

II-2   Evidence obtained from well-designed cohort or case–control analytic studies, preferably from more than one center or research group.

II-3   Evidence obtained from multiple time series with or without the intervention. Dramatic results in uncontrolled experiments also could be regarded as this type of evidence.

III   Opinions of respected authorities, based on clinical experience, descriptive studies, or reports of expert committees.

Based on the highest level of evidence found in the data, recommendations are provided and graded according to the following categories:

Level A—Recommendations are based on good and consistent scientific evidence.

Level B—Recommendations are based on limited or inconsistent scientific evidence.

Level C—Recommendations are based primarily on consensus and expert opinion.

ISSN 1099-3630

The American College of Obstetricians and Gynecologists
409 12th Street, SW, PO Box 96920, Washington, DC 20090-6920

12345/98765

Human papillomavirus. ACOG Practice Bulletin No. 61. American College of Obstetricians and Gynecologists. Obstet Gynecol 2005; 105:905–18.

ACOG PRACTICE BULLETIN

CLINICAL MANAGEMENT GUIDELINES FOR
OBSTETRICIAN–GYNECOLOGISTS

NUMBER 10, NOVEMBER 1999

(Replaces Technical Bulletin Number 217, December 1995)

This Practice Bulletin was developed by the ACOG Committee on Practice Bulletins—Obstetrics with the assistance of Susan M. Ramin, MD. The information is designed to aid practitioners in making decisions about appropriate obstetric and gynecologic care. These guidelines should not be construed as dictating an exclusive course of treatment or procedure. Variations in practice may be warranted based on the needs of the individual patient, resources, and limitations unique to the institution or type of practice.

Induction of Labor

The goal of induction of labor is to achieve vaginal delivery by stimulating uterine contractions before the spontaneous onset of labor. According to the National Center for Health Statistics, the overall rate of induction of labor in the United States has increased from 90 per 1,000 live births in 1989 to 184 per 1,000 live births in 1997 (1). Generally, induction of labor has merit as a therapeutic option when the benefits of expeditious delivery outweigh the risks of continuing the pregnancy. The benefits of labor induction must be weighed against the potential maternal or fetal risks associated with this procedure. The purpose of this bulletin is to review current methods for cervical ripening and induction of labor and to summarize the effectiveness of these approaches based on appropriately conducted outcomes-based research. These practice guidelines classify the indications for and contraindications to induction of labor, describe the various agents used for cervical ripening, cite methods used to induce labor, and outline the requirements for the safe clinical use of the various methods of inducing labor.

Background

In 1948, Theobald and associates described their use of the posterior pituitary extract, oxytocin, by intravenous drip for labor induction (2). Five years later, oxytocin was the first polypeptide hormone synthesized by du Vigneaud and associates (3). This synthetic polypeptide hormone has since been used to stimulate uterine contractions. Other methods used for induction of labor include membrane stripping, amniotomy, and administering prostaglandin E (PGE) analogues.

Cervical Ripening

If induction is indicated and the status of the cervix is unfavorable, agents for cervical ripening may be used. The status of the cervix can be determined by the Bishop pelvic scoring system (Table 1) (4). If the total score is more than 8,

Table 1. Bishop Scoring System

Score	Factor				
	Dilation (cm)	Effacement (%)	Station*	Cervical Consistency	Position of Cervix
0	Closed	0–30	–3	Firm	Posterior
1	1–2	40–50	–2	Medium	Midposition
2	3–4	60–70	–1, 0	Soft	Anterior
3	5–6	80	+1, +2	—	—

*Station reflects a –3 to +3 scale.

Modified from Bishop EH. Pelvic scoring for elective induction. Obstet Gynecol 1964;24:267

the probability of vaginal delivery after labor induction is similar to that after spontaneous labor.

Acceptable methods for cervical ripening include mechanical cervical dilators and administration of synthetic prostaglandin E_1 (PGE_1) and prostaglandin E_2 (PGE_2) (5-9). Mechanical dilation methods are effective in ripening the cervix and include hygroscopic dilators, osmotic dilators (*Laminaria japonicum*), the 24-French Foley balloon, and the double balloon device (Atad Ripener Device) (10-15). Laminaria ripen the cervix but may be associated with increased peripartum infections (6, 16).

Misoprostol, a synthetic PGE_1 analogue, can be administered intravaginally or orally and is used for both cervical ripening and induction. It currently is available as a 100-mcg or 200-mcg tablet, and can be broken to provide 25-mcg or 50-mcg doses. Misoprostol currently is approved by the U.S. Food and Drug Administration (FDA) for the prevention of peptic ulcers, but not for cervical ripening or induction of labor.

Two PGE_2 preparations are commercially available: a gel available in a 2.5-mL syringe containing 0.5 mg of dinoprostone and a vaginal insert containing 10 mg of dinoprostone. Both are approved by the FDA for cervical ripening in women at or near term. The vaginal insert releases prostaglandin (PG) at a slower rate (0.3 mg/h) than the gel. Both the gel and the vaginal insert have been reported to increase the probability of successful initial induction, shorten the interval from induction to delivery, and decrease the total and maximal doses of oxytocin needed to induce contractions (17).

Other pharmacologic methods for cervical ripening include continuous intravenous oxytocin drip, extraamniotic saline infusion, vaginal recombinant human relaxin, and intracervical purified porcine relaxin. The safety and efficacy of these latter methods are unclear.

Methods of Labor Induction

In addition to oxytocin and misoprostol, other agents can be used for induction of labor. The progesterone antagonist mifepristone (RU 486) is one such suitable and effective induction agent (18). Nonpharmacologic methods of labor induction include stripping the amniotic membranes, amniotomy, and nipple stimulation.

Oxytocin

Oxytocin, an octapeptide, is one of the most commonly used drugs in the United States. The physiology of oxytocin-stimulated labor is similar to that of spontaneous labor, although individual patients vary in sensitivity and response to oxytocin. Based on pharmacokinetic studies of synthetic oxytocin, uterine response ensues after 3–5 minutes of infusion, and a steady state of oxytocin is achieved in plasma by 40 minutes (19). The uterine response to oxytocin depends on the duration of the pregnancy; there is a gradual increase in response from 20 to 30 weeks of gestation, followed by a plateau from 34 weeks of gestation until term, when sensitivity increases (20). Cervical dilation, parity, and gestational age are predictors of the dose response to oxytocin for labor stimulation (21).

Membrane Stripping

Stripping the amniotic membranes is commonly practiced to induce labor. However, several studies have yielded conflicting results regarding the efficacy of membrane stripping (22–24). Significant increases in phospholipase A_2 activity and prostaglandin $F_{2\alpha}$ ($PGF_{2\alpha}$) levels occur from membrane stripping (25). Stripping membranes appears to be associated with a greater frequency of spontaneous labor and fewer inductions for postterm pregnancy. In a randomized trial of 195 normal pregnancies beyond 40 weeks of gestation, two thirds of the patients who underwent membrane stripping labored spontaneously within 72 hours, compared with one third of the patients who underwent examination only (26).

Amniotomy

Artificial rupture of the membranes may be used as a method of labor induction, especially if the condition of the cervix is favorable. Used alone for inducing labor, amniotomy can be associated with unpredictable and sometimes long intervals before the onset of contractions. However, in a trial of amniotomy combined with early oxytocin infusion compared with amniotomy alone, the induction-to-delivery interval was shorter with the amniotomy-plus-oxytocin method (27).

Clinical Considerations and Recommendations

▶ *What are the indications and contraindications to induction of labor?*

Indications for induction of labor are not absolute but should take into account maternal and fetal conditions, gestational age, cervical status, and other factors. Following are examples of maternal or fetal conditions that may be indications for induction of labor:

- Abruptio placentae
- Chorioamnionitis
- Fetal demise
- Pregnancy-induced hypertension
- Premature rupture of membranes
- Postterm pregnancy
- Maternal medical conditions (eg, diabetes mellitus, renal disease, chronic pulmonary disease, chronic hypertension)
- Fetal compromise (eg, severe fetal growth restriction, isoimmunization)
- Preeclampsia, eclampsia

Labor also may be induced for logistic reasons, for example, risk of rapid labor, distance from hospital, or psychosocial indications. In such circumstances, at least one of the criteria in the box should be met or fetal lung maturity should be established (28).

Generally, the contraindications to labor induction are the same as those for spontaneous labor and vaginal delivery. They include, but are not limited to, the following situations:

- Vasa previa or complete placenta previa
- Transverse fetal lie
- Umbilical cord prolapse
- Previous transfundal uterine surgery

Confirmation of Term Gestation

- Fetal heart tones have been documented for 20 weeks by nonelectronic fetoscope or for 30 weeks by Doppler.
- It has been 36 weeks since a positive serum or urine human chorionic gonadotropin pregnancy test was performed by a reliable laboratory.
- An ultrasound measurement of the crown–rump length, obtained at 6–12 weeks, supports a gestational age of at least 39 weeks.
- An ultrasound obtained at 13–20 weeks confirms the gestational age of at least 39 weeks determined by clinical history and physical examination.

However, the individual patient and clinical situation should be considered in determining when induction of labor is contraindicated. Several obstetric situations are not contraindications to the induction of labor but do necessitate special attention. These include, but are not limited to, the following:

- One or more previous low-transverse cesarean deliveries
- Breech presentation
- Maternal heart disease
- Multifetal pregnancy
- Polyhydramnios
- Presenting part above the pelvic inlet
- Severe hypertension
- Abnormal fetal heart rate patterns not necessitating emergent delivery

▶ *What criteria should be met before the cervix is ripened or labor is induced?*

Assessment of gestational age and consideration of any potential risks to the mother or fetus are of paramount importance for appropriate evaluation and counseling before initiating cervical ripening or labor induction. The patient should be counseled regarding the indications for induction, the agents and methods of labor stimulation, and the possible need for repeat induction or cesarean delivery.

Additional requirements for cervical ripening and induction of labor include cervical assessment, pelvic assessment, assessment of fetal size and presentation, and personnel familiar with the effects of uterine stimulants on the mother and fetus because uterine hyperstimulation may occur with induction of labor. Monitoring fetal heart rate and uterine contractions is recommended as for any high-risk patient in active labor. Although trained nursing personnel can monitor labor induction, a physician capable of performing a cesarean delivery should be readily available.

▶ *What is the relative effectiveness of available pharmacologic methods for cervical ripening?*

Intracervical or intravaginal PGE_2 (dinoprostone) commonly is used and is superior to placebo or no therapy in promoting cervical ripening (29). Several prospective randomized clinical trials and a meta-analysis have demonstrated that PGE_1 (misoprostol) is an effective method for cervical ripening (30-34). Misoprostol administered intravaginally has been reported to be either superior to or as efficacious as dinoprostone gel (9, 32, 34, 35). It is difficult, however, to compare the results of studies on misoprostol because of differences in endpoints, including Bishop score, duration of labor, total oxytocin use, successful induction, and cesarean delivery rate. The rates of operative vaginal delivery and cesarean delivery are inconsistent between trials. The cesarean delivery rate has been reported to be higher with dinoprostone compared with misoprostol (31); however, further studies are needed. The results of cesarean delivery rate with dinoprostone use are inconsistent; some have shown a reduction but most have not shown a significant decrease.

▶ *How should prostaglandin be administered?*

If there is inadequate cervical change with minimal uterine activity after one dose of intracervical PGE_2, a second dose may be given 6–12 hours later. The manufacturers recommend a maximum cumulative dose of 1.5 mg of dinoprostone (three doses or 7.5 mL of gel) within a 24-hour period. A minimum safe time interval between PG administration and initiation of oxytocin has not been determined. According to the manufacturers' guidelines, after use of 1.5 mg of dinoprostone in the cervix or 2.5 mg in the vagina, oxytocin induction should be delayed for 6–12 hours because the effect of PG may be heightened with oxytocin. After use of dinoprostone in sustained-release form, delaying oxytocin induction for 30–60 minutes after removal is sufficient. One quarter of one 100-mcg tablet (approximately 25-mcg) of misoprostol should be considered for cervical ripening and labor induction.

▶ *What are the potential complications with each method of cervical ripening, and how are they managed?*

Hyperstimulation may occur with the use of the PGE analogues. There is no uniform definition of uterine hyperstimulation. In some studies hyperstimulation is never defined. In others, uterine hyperstimulation has been defined as either a series of single contractions lasting 2 minutes or more or a contraction frequency of five or more in 10 minutes (36). Another definition of hyperstimulation is uterine contractions lasting 2 minutes or more or a contraction frequency of 5 or more in 10 minutes with evidence that the fetus is not tolerating this contraction pattern, as demonstrated by late deceleration, or fetal bradycardia (37). Fortunately, most women and their fetuses tolerate uterine hyperstimulation without adverse outcome.

The intracervical PGE_2 gel (0.5 mg) has a 1% rate of uterine hyperstimulation, while the intravaginal PGE_2 gel (2–5 mg) or vaginal insert is associated with a 5% rate (29, 36–38). Uterine hyperstimulation typically begins within 1 hour after the gel or insert is placed but may occur up to 9 1/2 hours after the vaginal insert has been placed (36–38).

Removing the PGE_2 vaginal insert usually will help reverse the effect of hyperstimulation. Irrigation of the cervix and vagina is not beneficial. Maternal side effects from low-dose PGE_2 (fever, vomiting, and diarrhea) are quite uncommon (17). Prophylactic antiemetics, antipyretics, and antidiarrheal agents usually are not needed. The manufacturers recommend that caution be exercised when using PGE_2 in patients with glaucoma, severe hepatic or renal dysfunction, or asthma. However, PGE_2 is a bronchodilator, and there are no reports of bronchoconstriction or significant blood pressure changes after the administration of the low-dose gel.

In several studies of misoprostol, the term tachysystole was used to define hyperstimulation without corresponding fetal heart rate abnormalities in order to distinguish this complication from hyperstimulation with fetal heart rate changes. Data indicate that both tachysystole (defined in some studies as six or more uterine contractions in 10 minutes in consecutive 10-minute intervals) and hyperstimulation (with and without fetal heart rate changes) are increased with a 50-mcg or greater dose of misoprostol (9, 30, 39, 40). There seems to be a trend toward lower rates of uterine hyperstimulation with fetal heart rate changes with lower dosages of misoprostol (25 mcg every 6 hours versus every 3 hours) (40). Although in studies of misoprostol there were no differences in perinatal outcome, the studies have been insufficient in size to exclude the possibility of uncommon serious adverse effects (40). The use of misoprostol in women with prior cesarean birth has been associated with an increase in uterine rupture (41). Misoprostol use for second-trimester pregnancy termination also has been associated with uterine rupture, especially when used with oxytocin infusion (40). An increase in meconium-stained amniotic fluid also has been reported with misoprostol use (34). Although misoprostol appears to be safe and effective in inducing labor in women with unfavorable cervices, further studies are needed to determine the optimal dosage, timing interval, and pharmacokinetics of misoprostol. Moreover, data are needed on the management of complications related to misoprostol and when it should be discontinued. If uterine hyperstimulation and a nonreassuring fetal heart rate pattern occur with misoprostol use and there is no response to routine corrective measures (maternal repositioning and supplemental oxygen administration), cesarean delivery should be considered. Subcutaneous terbutaline also can be used in an attempt to correct the nonreassuring fetal heart rate tracing or the abnormal contraction pattern or both.

Increased maternal and neonatal infection have been reported in connection with the use of laminaria and hygroscopic dilators when compared with the PGE_2 analogues (6, 12, 16).

What are the recommended guidelines for fetal surveillance for each type of prostaglandin preparation?

The PG preparations should be administered at or near the labor and delivery suite, where uterine activity and fetal heart rate can be monitored continuously. The patient should remain recumbent for at least 30 minutes. The fetal heart rate and uterine activity should be monitored continuously for a period of 30 minutes to 2 hours after administration of the PGE_2 gel (42). The patient may be transferred elsewhere if there is no increase in uterine activity and the fetal heart rate is unchanged after this period of observation. Uterine contractions usually are evident in the first hour and exhibit peak activity in the first 4 hours (42, 43). Fetal heart rate monitoring should be continued if regular uterine contractions persist; maternal vital signs should be recorded as well.

Because uterine hyperstimulation can occur as late as 9 1/2 hours after placement of the PGE_2 vaginal insert, fetal heart rate and uterine activity should be monitored electronically from the time the device is placed until at least 15 minutes after it is removed (44). This controlled-release PGE_2 vaginal pessary should be removed at the onset of labor (37).

Patients treated with misoprostol should receive fetal heart rate and uterine activity monitoring in a hospital setting until further studies evaluate the safety of outpatient therapy.

▶ Are cervical ripening methods restricted to inpatient use only?

One small, randomized trial found that sequential outpatient administration of low-dose (2-mg) PGE_2 gel was no better than placebo in ripening the cervix in postterm patients (45). Larger controlled studies are needed to establish an effective and safe dose and vehicle for PGE_2 before application on an outpatient basis can be recommended. However, outpatient use may be appropriate in carefully selected patients.

▶ What are the potential complications of various methods of induction?

The side effects of oxytocin use are principally dose related; uterine hyperstimulation and subsequent fetal heart rate deceleration are the most common side effects. Hyperstimulation may result in abruptio placentae or uterine rupture. Fortunately, uterine rupture secondary to oxytocin use is rare even in parous women (46). Water intoxication can occur with high concentrations of oxytocin infused with large quantities of hypotonic solutions. The antidiuretic effect usually is observed only after prolonged administration with at least 40mU of oxytocin per minute (47).

Misoprostol appears to be safe and beneficial for inducing labor in a woman with an unfavorable cervix. Although the exact incidence of uterine tachysystole is unknown and the criteria used to define this complication are not always clear in the various reports, there are reports of uterine tachysystole occurring more frequently in women given misoprostol (30–32). There does not appear to be a significant increase in adverse fetal outcomes from tachysystole (31, 35); however, one also must consider the possibility of uterine rupture as a rare complication of induction of labor with misoprostol (40). The occurrence of complications does appear to be dose-dependent (9, 40). Oral misoprostol administration is associated with fewer abnormal fetal heart rate patterns and episodes of uterine hyperstimulation when compared with vaginal administration (48), but there are not yet enough data to support oral administration as an alternative method.

The potential risks associated with amniotomy include prolapse of the umbilical cord, chorioamnionitis, significant umbilical cord compression, and rupture of vasa previa. The physician should palpate for an umbili-

Table 2. Labor Stimulation with Oxytocin: Examples of Low- and High-Dose Oxytocin

Regimen	Starting Dose	Incremental Increase (mU/min)	Dosage Interval (min)
Low-Dose	0.5–1	1	30–40
	1–2	2	15
High-Dose	~6	~6	15
	6	6*, 3, 1	20–40

*The incremental increase is reduced to 3 mU/min in presence of hyperstimulation and reduced to 1 mU/min with recurrent hyperstimulation.

cal cord and avoid dislodging the fetal head. The fetal heart rate should be assessed before and immediately after amniotomy.

Stripping the amniotic membranes is associated with bleeding from undiagnosed placenta previa or low-lying placenta, and accidental amniotomy. Uterine hyperactivity and fetal heart rate decelerations have been reported in association with nipple stimulation (49).

▶ *When oxytocin is used for induction of labor, what dosage should be used and what precautions should be taken?*

Any of the low- or high-dose oxytocin regimens outlined in Table 2 are appropriate for labor induction (50–56). Most women attain normal progression of labor with 150–350 Montevideo units of uterine activity (50). Low-dose regimens and less frequent increases in dose are associated with decreased uterine hyperstimulation (52). High-dose regimens and more frequent dose increases are associated with shorter labor and less frequent cases of chorioamnionitis and cesarean delivery for dystocia, but increased rates of uterine hyperstimulation (52).

Each hospital's obstetrics and gynecology department should develop guidelines for the preparation and administration of oxytocin. Synthetic oxytocin generally is diluted 10 U in 1,000 mL of an isotonic solution for an oxytocin concentration of 10 mU/mL. Oxytocin should be administered by infusion using a pump that allows precise control of the flow rate and permits accurate minute-to-minute control. Bolus administration of oxytocin can be avoided by piggybacking the infusion into the main intravenous line near the venipuncture site. Oxytocin also can be administered by pulsatile infusion, which may better simulate spontaneous labor (53). The total amount of oxytocin given may be decreased by administering oxytocin in 10-minute pulse infusions (53, 57).

A numeric value for the maximum dose of oxytocin has not been established. The fetal heart rate and uterine contractions should be monitored closely. Oxytocin should be administered by trained personnel who are familiar with its effects.

▶ *How should complications associated with oxytocin use be managed?*

If hyperstimulation with a nonreassuring fetal heart rate occurs, intravenous infusion of oxytocin should be decreased or discontinued to correct the pattern. Additional measures may include turning the woman on her side and administering oxygen or more intravenous fluid. If hyperstimulation persists, use of terbutaline or other tocolytics may be considered.

Hypotension may occur following a rapid intravenous injection of oxytocin; therefore, it is imperative that a dilute oxytocin infusion be used even in the immediate puerperium. Although amniotic fluid embolism was once thought to be associated with oxytocin-induced labor, there is no causal relationship between oxytocin use or antecedent hyperstimulation and amniotic fluid embolism (58, 59).

▶ *Are the various methods of labor induction equally applicable to patients with intact or ruptured membranes?*

The same precautions should be exercised when prostaglandins are used for induction of labor with ruptured membranes as for intact membranes. Intravaginal PGE_2 for induction of labor in women with premature rupture of membranes appears to be safe and effective, although it has not been approved by the FDA for this indication (60). In a meta-analysis of labor induction in women with premature rupture of membranes at term, only one dose of intravaginal misoprostol was necessary for successful labor induction in 86% of the patients (61). There is no evidence that use of either of these prostaglandins increases the risk of infection in women with ruptured membranes (60, 61).

▶ *What methods can be used for induction of labor with intrauterine fetal demise in the late second or third trimester?*

Intravenous oxytocin usually is a safe and effective method of inducing labor for a fetal death near term but is less effective remote from term (62). Laminaria or hygroscopic cervical dilators may be beneficial before the use of oxytocin or PGE for induction (63, 64). High-dose PGE_2 vaginal suppositories and more concentrated intravenous oxytocin are effective for achieving delivery, particularly when the gestational age is 28 weeks or less (62, 65, 66). Reported side-effects associated with higher doses of PGE_2 include nausea, vomiting, and diarrhea, which may be ameliorated with pretreatment medications. Although PGE_2 vaginal suppositories have been used safely in the third trimester (67), the risk of uterine rupture is increased. Vaginal misoprostol, intramuscular or extraamniotic infusion of $PGF_{2\alpha}$, and mifepristone also have been used safely and effectively; however, studies are few. In one study, mifepristone (600 mg per day for 48 hours) was effective in achieving delivery within 72 hours after the initial dose in 63% of women (68). In another study using intravaginal misoprostol, the mean time from induction to delivery was 12.6 hours, and all women delivered by 48 hours (69).

▶ *What is the cost effectiveness of these agents?*

There is a significant cost difference for induction of labor between misoprostol and dinoprostone. The approximate cost of a 100-mcg tablet of misoprostol ranges from $0.36 to $1.20, whereas a dinoprostone gel kit ranges from $65 to $75, and the dinoprostone vaginal insert is $165 (34, 35, 39, 70). The cost would be increased further if oxytocin augmentation were needed. Moreover, dinoprostone is an unstable compound that requires refrigeration to maintain its potency, whereas misoprostol is stable at room temperature.

Summary

The following recommendations are based on good and consistent scientific evidence (Level A):

▶ Prostaglandin E analogues are effective in promoting cervical ripening and inducing labor.

▶ Women in whom induction of labor is indicated may be appropriately managed with either a low- or high-dose oxytocin regimen.

▶ Fetal heart rate and uterine activity should be continuously monitored from the time the PGE_2 vaginal insert is placed until at least 15 minutes after it is removed.

▶ High-dose PGE_2 vaginal suppositories may be used in the management of intrauterine fetal demise in the second trimester of pregnancy.

▶ Although the optimal dose and timing interval of misoprostol is unknown, lower doses (25 mcg every 3–6 hours) are effective for cervical ripening and induction of labor.

▶ With term premature rupture of membranes, labor may be induced with prostaglandins.

The following recommendations are based on evidence that may be limited or inconsistent (Level B):

▶ Misoprostol use in women with prior cesarean birth should be avoided because of the possibility of uterine rupture.

▶ The use of higher doses of misoprostol (50 mcg every 6 hours) to induce labor may be appropriate in some situations, although there are reports of increased risk of complications, including uterine hyperstimulation.

The following recommendations are based primarily on consensus and expert opinion (Level C):

▶ For women with third-trimester intrauterine fetal demise, intravaginal misoprostol can be used to induce labor.

▶ Fetal heart rate and uterine activity should be continuously monitored from 30 minutes to 2 hours after administration of PGE_2 gel.

References

1. Ventura SJ, Martin JA, Curtin SC, Mathews TJ. Births: Final data for 1997. National Center for Health Statistics, National Vital Statistics Reports, 1999;47(18):1–96 (Level II-3)

2. Theobald GW, Graham A, Campbell J, Gange PD, Driscoll WJ. The use of post-pituitary extract in physiological amounts in obstetrics. BMJ 1948;2:123–127 (Level III)

3. du Vigneaud V, Ressler C, Swan JM, Roberts CW, Katsoyannis PG, Gordon S. The synthesis of an octapeptide amide with the hormonal activity of oxytocin. J Am Chem Soc 1953;75:4879–4880 (Level III)

4. Bishop EH. Pelvic scoring for elective induction. Obstet Gynecol 1964;24:266–268 (Level III)

5. Cross WG, Pitkin RM. Laminaria as an adjunct in induction of labor. Obstet Gynecol 1978;51:606–608 (Level I)

6. Krammer J, Williams MC, Sawai SK, O'Brien WF. Preinduction cervical ripening: a randomized comparison of two methods. Obstet Gynecol 1995;85:614–618 (Level I)

7. Fletcher HM, Mitchell S, Simeon D, Frederick J, Brown D. Intravaginal misoprostol as a cervical ripening agent. Br J Obstet Gynaecol 1993;100:641–644 (Level I)

8. Porto M. The unfavorable cervix: methods of cervical priming. Clin Obstet Gynecol 1989;32:262–268 (Level III)

9. Wing DA, Rahall A, Jones MM, Goodwin TM, Paul RH. Misoprostol: an effective agent for cervical ripening and labor induction. Am J Obstet Gynecol 1995;172: 1811–1816 (Level I)

10. Atad J, Hallak M, Ben-David Y, Auslender R, Abramovici H. Ripening and dilatation of the unfavourable cervix for induction of labour by a double balloon device: experience with 250 cases. Br J Obstet Gynaecol 1997;104:29–32 (Level III)

11. Blumenthal PD, Ramanauskas R. Randomized trial of Dilapan and Laminaria as cervical ripening agents before induction of labor. Obstet Gynecol 1990;75:365–368 (Level I)

12. Chua S, Arulkumaran S, Vanja K, Ratnam SS. Preinduction cervical ripening: prostaglandin E$_2$ gel vs. hygroscopic mechanical dilator. J Obstet Gynaecol Res 1997;23: 171–177 (Level I)

13. Gilson GJ, Russell DJ, Izquierdo LA, Qualls CR, Curet LB. A prospective randomized evaluation of a hygroscopic cervical dilator, Dilapan, in the preinduction ripening of patients undergoing induction of labor. Am J Obstet Gynecol 1996;175:145–149 (Level I)

14. Lin A, Kupferminc M, Dooley SL. A randomized trial of extra-amniotic saline infusion versus laminaria for cervical ripening. Obstet Gynecol 1995;86:545–549 (Level I)

15. Lyndrup J, Nickelsen C, Weber T, Molnitz E, Guldbaek E. Induction of labour by balloon catheter with extra-amniotic saline infusion (BCEAS): a randomized comparison with PGE$_2$ vaginal pessaries. Eur J Obstet Gynecol Reprod Biol 1994;53:189–197 (Level I)

16. Kazzi GM, Bottoms SF, Rosen MG. Efficacy and safety of laminaria digitata for preinduction ripening of the cervix. Obstet Gynecol 1982;60:440–443 (Level II-2)

17. Brindley BA, Sokol RJ. Induction and augmentation of labor: basis and methods for current practice. Obstet Gynecol Surv 1988;43:730–743 (Level III)

18. Frydman R, Lelaidier C, Baton-Saint-Mleux C, Fernandez H, Vial, M, Bourget P. Labor induction in women at term with mifepristone (RU 486): a double-blind, randomized, placebo-controlled study. Obstet Gynecol 1992;80: 972–975 (Level I)

19. Seitchik J, Amico J, Robinson AG, Castillo M. Oxytocin augmentation of dysfunctional labor. IV. Oxytocin pharmacokinetics. Am J Obstet Gynecol 1984;150:225–228 (Level III)

20. Caldeyro-Barcia R, Poseiro JJ. Physiology of the uterine contraction. Clin Obstet Gynecol 1960;3:386–408 (Level III)

21. Satin AJ, Leveno KJ, Sherman ML, McIntire DD. Factors affecting the dose response to oxytocin for labor stimulation. Am J Obstet Gynecol 1992;166:1260–1261 (Level II-3)

22. Crane J, Bennett K, Young D, Windrim R, Kravitz H. The effectiveness of sweeping membranes at term: a randomized trial. Obstet Gynecol 1997;89:586–590 (Level I)

23. Goldenberg M, Dulitzky M, Feldman B, Zolti M, Bider D. Stretching of the cervix and stripping of the membranes at term: a randomised controlled study. Eur J Obstet Gynecol Reprod Biol 1996;66:129–132 (Level I)

24. Wiriyasirivaj B, Vutyavanich T, Ruangsri RA. A randomized controlled trial of membrane stripping at term to promote labor. Obstet Gynecol 1996;87:767–770 (Level I)

25. McColgin SW, Bennett WA, Roach H, Cowan BD, Martin JN Jr, Morrison JC. Parturitional factors associated with membrane stripping. Am J Obstet Gynecol 1993;169: 71–77 (Level I)

26. Allott HA, Palmer CR. Sweeping the membranes: a valid procedure in stimulating the onset of labour? Br J Obstet Gynaecol 1993;100:898–903 (Level I)

27. Moldin PG, Sundell G. Induction of labour: a randomised clinical trial of amniotomy versus amniotomy with oxytocin infusion. Br J Obstet Gynaecol 1996;103:306–312 (Level I)

28. American College of Obstetricians and Gynecologists. Assessment of fetal lung maturity. ACOG Educational Bulletin 230. Washington DC: ACOG, 1996 (Level III)

29. Rayburn WF. Prostaglandin E$_2$ gel for cervical ripening and induction of labor: a critical analysis. Am J Obstet Gynecol 1989;160:529–534 (Level III)

30. Buser D, Mora G, Arias F. A randomized comparison between misoprostol and dinoprostone for cervical ripening and labor induction in patients with unfavorable cervices. Obstet Gynecol 1997;89:581–585 (Level I)

31. Sanchez-Ramos L, Kaunitz AM, Wears RL, Delke I, Gaudier FL. Misoprostol for cervical ripening and labor induction: a meta-analysis. Obstet Gynecol 1997;89: 633–642 (Meta-analysis)

32. Sanchez-Ramos L, Peterson DE, Delke I, Gaudier FL, Kaunitz AM. Labor induction with prostaglandin E$_1$ misoprostol compared with dinoprostone vaginal insert: a randomized trial. Obstet Gynecol 1998;91:401–405 (Level I)

33. Srisomboon J, Piyamongkol W, Aiewsakul P. Comparison of intracervical and intravaginal misoprostol for cervical ripening and labour induction in patients with an unfavorable cervix. J Med Assoc Thai 1997;80:189–194 (Level I)

34. Wing DA, Jones MM, Rahall A, Goodwin TM, Paul RH. A comparison of misoprostol and prostaglandin E$_2$ gel for preinduction cervical ripening and labor induction. Am J Obstet Gynecol 1995;172:1804–1810 (Level I)

35. Wing DA, Ortiz-Omphroy G, Paul RH. A comparison of intermittent vaginal administration of misoprostol with continuous dinoprostone for cervical ripening and labor induction. Am J Obstet Gynecol 1997;177:612–618 (Level I)

36. Rayburn WF, Wapner RJ, Barss VA, Spitzberg E, Molina RD, Mandsageer N, Yonekura ML. An intravaginal controlled-release prostaglandin E$_2$ pessary for cervical ripening and initiation of labor at term. Obstet Gynecol 1992;79:374–379 (Level I)

37. Witter FR, Rocco LE, Johnson TR. A randomized trial of prostaglandin E₂ in a controlled-release vaginal pessary for cervical ripening at term. Am J Obstet Gynecol 1992; 166:830–834 (Level I)

38. Witter FR, Mercer BM. Improved intravaginal controlled-release prostaglandin E₂ insert for cervical ripening at term. The Prostaglandin E₂ Insert Study Group. J Matern Fetal Med 1996;5:64–69 (Level I)

39. Magtibay PM, Ramin KD, Harris DY, Ramsey PS, Ogburn PL Jr. Misoprostol as a labor induction agent. J Matern Fetal Med 1998;7:15–18 (Level I)

40. Hofmeyr GJ. Vaginal misoprostol for cervical ripening and labour induction in late pregnancy. The Cochrane Library 1999; Issue 2:1–18 (Meta-analysis)

41. Wing DA, Lovett K, Paul RH. Disruption of prior uterine incision following misoprostol for labor induction in women with previous cesarean section. Obstet Gynecol 1998;91:828–830 (Level III)

42. Bernstein P. Prostaglandin E₂ gel for cervical ripening and labour induction: a multicentre placebo-controlled trial. CMAJ 1991;145:1249–1254 (Level I)

43. Miller AM, Rayburn WF, Smith CV. Patterns of uterine activity after intravaginal prostaglandin E₂ during preinduction cervical ripening. Am J Obstet Gynecol 1991; 165:1006–1009 (Level II-1)

44. American College of Obstetricians and Gynecologists. Monitoring during induction of labor with dinoprostone. ACOG Committee Opinion 209. Washington DC: ACOG, 1998 (Level III)

45. Sawai SK, Williams MC, O'Brien WF, Angel JL, Mastrogiannis DS, Johnson L. Sequential outpatient application of intravaginal prostaglandin E₂ gel in the management of postdates pregnancies. Obstet Gynecol 1991;78: 19–23 (Level I)

46. Flannelly GM, Turner MJ, Rassmussen MJ, Stronge JM. Rupture of the uterus in Dublin; An update. J Obstet Gynaecol 1993;13:440–443 (Level II-3)

47. Whalley PJ, Pritchard JA. Oxytocin and water intoxication. JAMA 1963;186;601–603

48. Toppozada MK, Anwar MY, Hassan HA, El-Gazaerly WS. Oral or vaginal misoprostol for induction of labor. Int J Gynaecol Obstet 1997;56:135–139 (Level I)

49. Schellpfeffer MA, Hoyle D, Johnson JWC. Antepartal uterine hypercontractility secondary to nipple stimulation. Obstet Gynecol 1985;65:588–591 (Level III)

50. Hauth JC, Hankins GD, Gilstrap LC III, Strickland DM, Vance P. Uterine contraction pressures with oxytocin induction/augmentation. Obstet Gynecol 1986;68: 305–309 (Level II-2)

51. Satin AJ, Leveno KJ, Sherman ML, Brewster DS, Cunningham FG. High- versus low-dose oxytocin for labor stimulation. Obstet Gynecol 1992;80:111–116 (Level II-1)

52. Crane JM, Young DC. Meta-analysis of low-dose versus high-dose oxytocin for labour induction. J Soc Obstet Gynaecol Can 1998;20:1215–1223 (Meta-analysis)

53. Cummiskey KC, Dawood MY. Induction of labor with pulsatile oxytocin. Am J Obstet Gynecol 1990;163: 1868–1874 (Level I)

54. Blakemore KJ, Qin NG, Petrie RH, Paine LL. A prospective comparison of hourly and quarter-hourly oxytocin dose increase intervals for the induction of labor at term. Obstet Gynecol 1990;75:757–761 (Level I)

55. Mercer B, Pilgrim P, Sibai B. Labor induction with continuous low-dose oxytocin infusion: a randomized trial. Obstet Gynecol 1991;77:659–663 (Level I)

56. Muller PR, Stubbs TM, Laurent SL. A prospective randomized clinical trial comparing two oxytocin induction protocols. Am J Obstet Gynecol 1992;167:373–380; discussion 380–381 (Level I)

57. Willcourt RJ, Pager D, Wendel J, Hale RW. Induction of labor with pulsatile oxytocin by a computer-controlled pump. Am J Obstet Gynecol 1994;170:603–608 (Level I)

58. Clark SL, Hankins GD, Dudley DA, Dildy GA, Porter TF. Amniotic fluid embolism: analysis of the national registry. Am J Obstet Gynecol 1995;172:1158–1169 (Level III)

59. Morgan M. Amniotic fluid embolism. Anaesthesia 1979; 34:20–32 (Level III)

60. Ray DA, Garite TJ. Prostaglandin E₂ for induction of labor in patients with premature rupture of membranes at term. Am J Obstet Gynecol 1992;166:836–843 (Level I)

61. Sanchez-Ramos L, Chen AH, Kaunitz AM, Gaudier FL, Delke I. Labor induction with intravaginal misoprostol in term premature rupture of the membranes: a randomized study. Obstet Gynecol 1997;89:909–912 (Level I)

62. Pitkin RM. Fetal death: diagnosis and management. Am J Obstet Gynecol 1987;157:583–589 (Level III)

63. Berkus MD, Laufe LE, Castillo M. Lamicel for induction of labor. J Reprod Med 1990;35:219–221 (Level II-2)

64. Sanchez-Ramos L, Kaunitz AM, Connor PM. Hygroscopic cervical dilators and prostaglandin E₂ gel for preinduction cervical ripening. A randomized, prospective comparison. J Reprod Med 1992;37:355–359 (Level I)

65. Kochenour NK. Management of fetal demise. Clin Obstet Gynecol 1987;30:322–330 (Level III)

66. American College of Obstetricians and Gynecologists. Diagnosis and management of fetal death. ACOG Technical Bulletin 176. Washington DC: ACOG, 1993 (Level III)

67. Kent DR, Goldstein AI, Linzey EM. Safety and efficacy of vaginal prostaglandin E₂ suppositories in the management of third-trimester fetal demise. J Reprod Med 1984;29: 101–102 (Level III)

68. Cabrol D, Dubois C, Cronje H, Gonnet JM, Guillot M, Maria B, et al. Induction of labor with mifepristone (RU 486) in intrauterine fetal death. Am J Obstet Gynecol 1990;163:540–542 (Level I)

69. Bugalho A, Bique C, Machungo F, Faaundes A. Induction of labor with intravaginal misoprostol in intrauterine fetal death. Am J Obstet Gynecol 1994;171:538–541 (Level III)

70. Chuck FJ, Huffaker BJ. Labor induction with intravaginal misoprostol versus intracervical prostaglandin E₂ gel (Prepidil gel): randomized comparison. Am J Obstet Gynecol 1995;173:1137–1142 (Level I)

The MEDLINE database, the Cochrane Library, and ACOG's own internal resources and documents were used to conduct a literature search to locate relevant articles published between January 1985 and February 1999. The search was restricted to articles published in the English language. Priority was given to articles reporting results of original research, although review articles and commentaries also were consulted. Abstracts of research presented at symposia and scientific conferences were not considered adequate for inclusion in this document. Guidelines published by organizations or institutions such as the National Institutes of Health and the American College of Obstetricians and Gynecologists were reviewed, and additional studies were located by reviewing bibliographies of identified articles. When reliable research was not available, expert opinions from obstetrician–gynecologists were used.

Studies were reviewed and evaluated for quality according to the method outlined by the U.S. Preventive Services Task Force:

I   Evidence obtained from at least one properly designed randomized controlled trial.

II-1 Evidence obtained from well-designed controlled trials without randomization.

II-2 Evidence obtained from well-designed cohort or case–control analytic studies, preferably from more than one center or research group.

II-3 Evidence obtained from multiple time series with or without the intervention. Dramatic results in uncontrolled experiments could also be regarded as this type of evidence.

III   Opinions of respected authorities, based on clinical experience, descriptive studies, or reports of expert committees.

Based on the highest level of evidence found in the data, recommendations are provided and graded according to the following categories:

Level A—Recommendations are based on good and consistent scientific evidence.

Level B—Recommendations are based on limited or inconsistent scientific evidence.

Level C—Recommendations are based primarily on consensus and expert opinion.

ISSN 1099-3630

**The American College of
Obstetricians and Gynecologists
409 12th Street, SW
PO Box 96920
Washington, DC 20090-6920**

12345/32109

ACOG PRACTICE BULLETIN

CLINICAL MANAGEMENT GUIDELINES FOR
OBSTETRICIAN–GYNECOLOGISTS
NUMBER 70, DECEMBER 2005

(Replaces Practice Bulletin Number 62, May 2005)

This Practice Bulletin was developed by the ACOG Committee on Practice Bulletins—Obstetrics with the assistance of Suneet P. Chauhan, MD and George A. Macones, MD. The information is designed to aid practitioners in making decisions about appropriate obstetric and gynecologic care. These guidelines should not be construed as dictating an exclusive course of treatment or procedure. Variations in practice may be warranted based on the needs of the individual patient, resources, and limitations unique to the institution or type of practice.

Intrapartum Fetal Heart Rate Monitoring

In 2002, approximately 3.4 million fetuses (85% of approximately 4 million live births) in the United States were assessed with electronic fetal monitoring (EFM), making it the most common obstetric procedure (1). Despite its widespread use, there is controversy about the efficacy of EFM, interpretation of fetal heart rate (FHR) patterns, reproducibility of its interpretation, and management algorithms for abnormal or nonreassuring patterns. Moreover, there is evidence that the use of EFM increases the rate of cesarean and operative vaginal deliveries. The purpose of this document is to review nomenclature for FHR assessment, review the data on the efficacy of EFM, delineate the strengths and shortcomings of EFM, and describe the management of nonreassuring FHR patterns.

Background

Even though the fetus is efficient at extracting oxygen from the maternal compartment, a complex interplay of antepartum complications, suboptimal uterine perfusion, placental dysfunction, and intrapartum events may be associated with adverse outcome. Known obstetric conditions, such as hypertensive disease, fetal growth restriction, and preterm birth, predispose fetuses to poor outcomes, but they account for a fraction of asphyxial injury. In a study of term pregnancies with fetal asphyxia, 63% had no known risk factors (2).

Monitoring the FHR is a modality intended to determine if a fetus is well oxygenated because the brain modulates the heart rate. It was used among 45% of parturients in 1980, 62% in 1988, 74% in 1992 (3), and 85% in 2002 (1). Despite the frequency of its use, issues with EFM include poor interobserver and intraobserver reliability, uncertain efficacy, and a high false-positive rate.

Fetal heart rate monitoring may be performed externally or internally. Most external monitors use a Doppler device with computerized logic to interpret and count the Doppler signals. Internal FHR monitoring is accomplished with a fetal electrode, which is a spiral wire placed directly on the fetal scalp or other presenting part.

Guidelines for Interpretation of Electronic Fetal Heart Rate Monitoring

In 1997, the National Institute of Child Health and Human Development Research Planning Workshop gathered investigators with expertise in the field and proposed definitions for intrapartum FHR tracing (4). The underlying assumptions of the definitions included that the FHR patterns, obtained either from a direct fetal electrode or an external Doppler device, are for visual interpretation, and that no a priori assumptions were made about the putative etiology of patterns or their relationship to hypoxemia or metabolic acidosis. The guidelines did not differentiate between short- and long-term variability because they are visually determined as one entity; however, they did encourage clinicians to take gestational age, medications, prior fetal assessment, and obstetric and medical conditions into account when interpreting the FHR patterns during labor.

A complete clinical understanding of the FHR necessitates discussion of baseline rate, variability, presence of accelerations, periodic or episodic decelerations, and the changes in these characteristics over time. Table 1 provides

Table 1. Definitions of Fetal Heart Rate Patterns

Pattern	Definition
Baseline	• The mean FHR rounded to increments of 5 beats per min during a 10 min segment, excluding: —Periodic or episodic changes —Periods of marked FHR variability —Segments of baseline that differ by more than 25 beats per min • The baseline must be for a minimum of 2 min in any 10-min segment
Baseline variability	• Fluctuations in the FHR of two cycles per min or greater • Variability is visually quantitated as the amplitude of peak-to-trough in beats per min —Absent—amplitude range undetectable —Minimal—amplitude range detectable but 5 beats per min or fewer —Moderate (normal)—amplitude range 6–25 beats per min —Marked—amplitude range greater than 25 beats per min
Acceleration	• A visually apparent increase (onset to peak in less than 30 sec) in the FHR from the most recently calculated baseline • The duration of an acceleration is defined as the time from the initial change in FHR from the baseline to the return of the FHR to the baseline • At 32 weeks of gestation and beyond, an acceleration has an acme of 15 beats per min or more above baseline, with a duration of 15 sec or more but less than 2 min • Before 32 weeks of gestation, an acceleration has an acme of 10 beats per min or more above baseline, with a duration of 10 sec or more but less than 2 min • Prolonged acceleration lasts 2 min or more but less than 10 min • If an acceleration lasts 10 min or longer, it is a baseline change
Bradycardia	• Baseline FHR less than 110 beats per min
Early deceleration	• In association with a uterine contraction, a visually apparent, gradual (onset to nadir 30 sec or more) decrease in FHR with return to baseline • Nadir of the deceleration occurs at the same time as the peak of the contraction
Late deceleration	• In association with a uterine contraction, a visually apparent, gradual (onset to nadir 30 sec or more) decrease in FHR with return to baseline • Onset, nadir, and recovery of the deceleration occur after the beginning, peak, and end of the contraction, respectively
Tachycardia	• Baseline FHR greater than 160 beats per min
Variable deceleration	• An abrupt (onset to nadir less than 30 sec), visually apparent decrease in the FHR below the baseline • The decrease in FHR is 15 beats per min or more, with a duration of 15 sec or more but less than 2 min
Prolonged deceleration	• Visually apparent decrease in the FHR below the baseline • Deceleration is 15 beats per min or more, lasting 2 min or more but less than 10 min from onset to return to baseline

Abbreviation: FHR, fetal heart rate.

FHR pattern definitions and descriptions based on National Institute of Child Health and Human Development Working Group findings. Decelerations are quantified by the depth of the nadir in beats per minute, as well as the duration in minutes and seconds from the beginning to the end of the deceleration. Accelerations are quantified similarly, whereas bradycardia and tachycardia are quantitated by the actual FHR. Decelerations generally are defined as recurrent if they occur with at least one half of the contractions.

Guidelines for Review of Electronic Fetal Heart Rate Monitoring

When EFM is used during labor, the nurses or physicians should review it frequently. In a patient without complications, the FHR tracing should be reviewed approximately every 30 minutes in the first stage of labor and every 15 minutes during the second stage. The corresponding frequency for patients with complications (eg, fetal growth restriction, preeclampsia) is approximately every 15 minutes in the first stage of labor and every 5 minutes during the second stage. Health care providers should periodically document that they have reviewed the tracing. The FHR tracing, as part of the medical record, should be labeled and available for review if the need arises. Computer storage of the FHR tracing that does not permit overwriting or revisions is reasonable, as is microfilm recording.

Clinical Considerations and Recommendations

▶ *How efficacious is electronic fetal heart rate monitoring?*

The efficacy of EFM during labor is judged by its ability to decrease complications, such as neonatal seizures, cerebral palsy, or intrapartum fetal death, while minimizing the need for unnecessary obstetric interventions, such as operative vaginal or cesarean delivery. There are no randomized clinical trials to compare the benefits of EFM with no form of monitoring during labor (5). Thus, the benefits of EFM are gauged from reports comparing it with intermittent auscultation.

A meta-analysis synthesizing the findings of nine randomized clinical trials comparing the modalities had the following conclusions (6):

- The use of EFM compared with intermittent auscultation increased the overall cesarean delivery rate (odds ratio [OR] 1.53, 95% confidence interval [CI], 1.17–2.01) and the cesarean rate for suspected fetal distress (OR 2.55, 95% CI, 1.81–3.53).

- The use of EFM increased the use of both vacuum (OR 1.23, 95% CI, 1.02–1.49) and forceps (OR 2.4, 95% CI, 1.97–3.18) operative vaginal deliveries.

- The use of EFM did not reduce overall perinatal mortality (OR 0.87, 95% CI, 0.57–1.33) although perinatal mortality caused by fetal hypoxia appeared to be reduced (OR 0.41, 95% CI, 0.17–0.98). It is important to recognize that for the comparison of perinatal mortality between EFM and intermittent auscultation, the results presented are based on a small number of events; thus, the findings are statistically unstable. For example, for perinatal deaths caused by hypoxia, there were 17 deaths out of a total of 9,163 fetuses in the intermittent auscultation group and seven out of 9,398 in the EFM group. If there had been one fewer case of perinatal death in the intermittent auscultation group, the results of the meta-analysis for this outcome would not be statistically significant.

There is an unrealistic expectation that a nonreassuring FHR tracing is predictive of cerebral palsy. The positive predictive value of a nonreassuring pattern to predict cerebral palsy among singleton newborns with birth weights of 2,500 g or more is 0.14%, meaning that out of 1,000 fetuses with a nonreassuring FHR pattern, only one or two will develop cerebral palsy (7). The false-positive rate is extremely high, at greater than 99%.

Available data, although limited in size, suggest that EFM does not result in a reduction in cerebral palsy (3). This is consistent with data that suggest that the occurrence of cerebral palsy has been stable over time, despite the widespread introduction of EFM (8). The principal explanation for why the prevalence of cerebral palsy has not diminished despite the use of EFM is that 70% of cases occur before the onset of labor; only 4% of encephalopathies can be attributed solely to intrapartum events (9, 10).

Given that the available data do not clearly support EFM over intermittent auscultation, either option is acceptable in a patient without complications. Logistically, it may not be feasible to adhere to guidelines for how frequently the heart rate should be auscultated. One prospective study noted that the protocol for intermittent auscultation was successfully completed in only 3% of the cases (11). The most common reasons for unsuccessful intermittent auscultation included the frequency of recording and the requirements for recording.

Intermittent auscultation may not be appropriate for all pregnancies. Most of the clinical trials that compare EFM with intermittent auscultation have excluded subjects at high risk for adverse outcomes, and the relative safety of intermittent auscultation in such cases is uncertain. Those with high-risk conditions (eg, suspected fetal growth restriction, preeclampsia, and type 1 diabetes) should be monitored continuously.

There are no comparative data indicating the optimal frequency at which intermittent auscultation should be performed in the absence of risk factors. One method is to evaluate and record the FHR at least every 15 minutes in the active phase of the first stage of labor and at least every 5 minutes in the second stage (12).

▶ *What is the interobserver and intraobserver variability of electronic fetal heart rate monitoring assessment?*

There is a wide variation in the way obstetricians interpret and respond to EFM tracings. When four obstetricians, for example, examined 50 cardiotocograms, they agreed in only 22% of the cases (13). Two months later, during the second review of the same 50 tracings, the clinicians interpreted 21% of the tracings differently than they did during the first evaluation (14). In another study, five obstetricians independently interpreted 150 cardiotocograms (15). The obstetricians interpreted the tracings similarly in 29% of the cases, suggesting poor interobserver reliability.

An important factor that influences the interpretation of cardiotocograms is whether the tracing is normal, equivocal, or ominous, with greater agreement if the tracing is reassuring (16). With retrospective reviews, the foreknowledge of neonatal outcome may alter the reviewer's impressions of the tracing. Given the same intrapartum tracing, a reviewer is more likely to find evidence of fetal hypoxia and criticize the obstetrician's management if the outcome was supposedly poor versus good (17).

▶ *Should the very preterm fetus be monitored?*

The decision of whether to monitor the very preterm fetus is complicated. It requires a discussion between the obstetrician, pediatrician, and patient concerning the likelihood of survival or severe morbidity of the preterm child (based on gestational age, estimated fetal weight, and other factors) and issues related to mode of delivery.

If a patient would undergo a cesarean delivery for fetal indications for a very preterm fetus, monitoring should be achieved continuously rather than intermittently auscultated. The earliest gestational age that this will occur may vary by the institution. Nonreassuring FHR patterns may occur with up to 60% of preterm parturients, with the most common abnormality being deceleration and bradycardia, followed by tachycardia and a flat tracing (18). Variable decelerations are more common among preterm (55–70%) than term (20–30%)

deliveries (19). Because preterm fetuses may be more susceptible to intrapartum hypoxemia, they should be monitored. If FHR abnormalities are persistent, intrauterine resuscitation, ancillary tests to ensure fetal well-being, and possibly delivery should be undertaken (20).

▶ *What medications affect the fetal heart rate?*

Fetal heart rate patterns can be influenced by the medications administered in the intrapartum period. Most often, these changes are transient, although they sometimes lead to obstetric interventions.

Epidural analgesia with local anesthetic agents (lidocaine, bupivacaine) can lead to sympathetic blockade, maternal hypotension, transient uteroplacental insufficiency, and alterations in the FHR. Parenteral narcotics also may affect the FHR. A randomized trial comparing epidural anesthesia with 0.25% of bupivacaine and intravenous meperidine reported that the beat-to-beat variability was decreased, and FHR accelerations were significantly less common with parenteral analgesia compared with regional analgesia (21). The rates of decelerations and cesarean delivery for nonreassuring FHR tracings were similar for the two groups. A systematic review of five randomized trials and seven observational studies also noted that the rate of cesarean delivery for nonreassuring FHR was similar between those who did and those who did not receive epidural analgesia during labor (22).

Concern has been raised about combined spinal–epidural anesthesia during labor. An intent-to-treat analysis of 1,223 parturients randomized to combined spinal–epidural anesthesia (10 µg intrathecal sufentanil, followed by epidural bupivacaine and fentanyl at the next request for analgesia) or intravenous meperidine (50 mg on demand, maximum 200 mg in 4 hours) noted a significantly higher rate of bradycardia and emergent cesarean delivery for nonreassuring abnormal FHR in the group randomized to combined spinal–epidural anesthesia (23). Neonatal outcome, however, was not significantly different between the two groups. There are methodologic concerns with this study, and additional trials are necessary to determine the potential safety and efficacy of the combined spinal–epidural technique (22).

The effect of corticosteroids, to enhance pulmonary maturity of fetuses during preterm labor, on FHR has been studied (Table 2). Among twins (24) and singletons (25, 26), the use of betamethasone transiently decreased the FHR variability, which returned to pretreatment status by the fourth (25) to seventh (26) day. There also may be a decrease in the rate of accelerations with the use of betamethasone. These changes, however, were not associated with increased obstetric interventions or with adverse outcomes (24). The biologic mechanism of this is

Table 2. Effects of Medications on Fetal Heart Rate Patterns

Medications	Reference	Study Design	Effect on Fetal Heart Rate
Butorphanol	Hatjis 1986[1]	Case–control	Transient sinusoidal FHR pattern
Cocaine	Chazotte 1991[2]	Case–control	No characteristic changes in FHR pattern
Corticosteroid	Senat 1998[3]	Randomized clinical trial	Decrease in FHR variability with betamethasone but not dexamethasone
Magnesium sulfate	Hallak 1999[4] and Wright 1996[5]	Randomized clinical trial and retrospective	A significant decrease in the FHR baseline and variability; inhibits the increase in accelerations with advancing gestational age
Meperidine	Giannina 1995[6]	Randomized clinical trial	No characteristic changes in FHR pattern
Morphine	Kopecky 2000[7]	Case–control	Decreased number of accelerations
Nalbuphine	Giannina 1995[6]	Randomized clinical trial	Decreased the number of accelerations, long- and short-term variation
Terbutaline	Tejani 1983[8]	Retrospective	Abolishment or decrease in frequency of late and variable decelerations
Zidovudine	Blackwell 2001[9]	Case–control	No difference in the FHR baseline, variability, number of accelerations or decelerations

Abbreviation: FHR, fetal heart rate.

[1]Hatjis CG, Meis PJ. Sinusoidal fetal heart rate pattern associated with butorphanol administration. Obstet Gynecol 1986;67:377–80.

[2]Chazotte C, Forman L, Gandhi J. Heart rate patterns in fetuses exposed to cocaine. Obstet Gynecol 1991;78:323–5.

[3]Senat MV, Minoui S, Multon O, Fernandez H, Frydman R, Ville Y. Effect of dexamethasone and betamethasone on the fetal heart rate variability in preterm labour: a randomised study. Br J Obstet Gynaecol 1998;105:749–55.

[4]Hallak M, Martinez-Poyer J, Kruger ML, Hassan S, Blackwell SC, Sorokin Y. The effect of magnesium sulfate on fetal heart rate parameters: a randomized, placebo-controlled trial. Am J Obstet Gynecol 1999;181:1122–7.

[5]Wright JW, Ridgway LE, Wright BD, Covington DL, Bobitt JR. Effect of MgSO4 on heart rate monitoring in the preterm fetus. J Reprod Med 1996;41:605–8.

[6]Giannina G, Guzman ER, Lai YL, Lake MF, Cernadas M, Vintzileos AM. Comparison of the effects of meperidine and nalbuphine on intrapartum fetal heart rate tracings. Obstet Gynecol 1995;86:441–5.

[7]Kopecky EA, Ryan ML, Barrett JF, Seaward PG, Ryan G, Koren G, et al. Fetal response to maternally administered morphine. Am J Obstet Gynecol 2000;183:424–30.

[8]Tejani NA, Verma UL, Chatterjee S, Mittelmann S. Terbutaline in the management of acute intrapartum fetal acidosis. J Reprod Med 1983;28:857–61.

[9]Blackwell SC, Sahai A, Hassan SS, Treadwell MC, Tomlinson MW, Jones TB, et al. Effects of intrapartum zidovudine therapy on fetal heart rate parameters in women with human immunodeficiency virus infection. Fetal Diagn Ther 2001;16:413–6.

unknown. Computerized analysis of the cardiotocograms indicates that use of dexamethasone is not associated with a decrease in the FHR variability (26).

Other medications that influence FHR tracing have been studied (see Table 2). Pseudosinusoidal FHR patterns occurred in 75% of patients who received butorphanol during labor, but this was not associated with adverse outcomes (27). Fetuses exposed to cocaine did not exhibit any characteristic changes in the heart rate pattern, although they did have frequent contractions even when labor was unstimulated (28). Multiple regression analysis indicated that decreased variability associated with the use of magnesium sulfate was related to early gestational age but not the serum magnesium level (29). As determined by computer analysis of cardiotocograms, a randomized trial reported that compared with meperidine, nalbuphine used for intrapartum analgesia decreased the likelihood of two 15-second accelerations over 20 minutes (30). In antepartum patients, administration of morphine decreased not only the fetal breathing movement but also the number of accelerations (31).

▶ *What findings on EFM reassure fetal status?*

The presence of FHR accelerations generally ensures that the fetus is not acidemic and provides reassurance of fetal status. The data relating FHR variability to clinical outcomes, however, are sparse. One study reported that in the presence of late or variable decelerations, the umbilical arterial pH was higher than 7 in 97% of the cases if the FHR tracing had normal variability (32). In another retrospective study, most cases of adverse neonatal outcome demonstrated normal FHR variability (33). This study is limited because it did not consider other characteristics of the FHR tracing, such as the presence of accelerations or decelerations. Thus, in most cases, normal FHR variability provides reassurance about fetal status.

▶ *How is a nonreassuring EFM tracing initially assessed?*

A persistently nonreassuring FHR tracing requires evaluation of the possible causes. Initial evaluation and treatment may include:

- Discontinuation of any labor stimulating agent
- Cervical examination to assess for umbilical cord prolapse or rapid cervical dilation or descent of the fetal head
- Changing maternal position to left or right lateral recumbent position, reducing compression of the vena cava and improving uteroplacental blood flow
- Monitoring maternal blood pressure level for evidence of hypotension, especially in those with regional anesthesia (if present, treatment with ephedrine or phenylephrine may be warranted)
- Assessment of patient for uterine hyperstimulation by evaluating uterine contraction frequency and duration

▶ *Are there ancillary tests that reassure fetal status?*

The false-positive rate of EFM is high. There are some ancillary tests available that help to ensure fetal well-being in the face of a nonreassuring FHR tracing, thereby reducing the false-positive rate of EFM.

In the case of an EFM tracing with decreased or absent variability without spontaneous accelerations, an effort should be made to elicit one. A meta-analysis of 11 studies of intrapartum fetal stimulation noted that four techniques are available to stimulate the fetus: 1) fetal scalp sampling, 2) Allis clamp scalp stimulation, 3) vibroacoustic stimulation, and 4) digital scalp stimulation (34). Each of these tests is a reliable method to exclude acidosis if accelerations are noted after stimulation. Because vibroacoustic stimulation and scalp stimulation are less invasive than the other two methods, they are the preferred methods. When there is an acceleration following stimulation, acidosis is unlikely and labor can continue.

When a nonreassuring FHR tracing persists and neither spontaneous nor stimulated accelerations are present, a scalp blood sample for the determination of pH or lactate can be considered. However, the use of scalp pH has decreased (35), and it may not even be available at some tertiary hospitals (36). The sensitivity and positive predictive value of a low scalp pH (defined in the study as less than 7.21 because it is the 75th percentile) to predict umbilical arterial pH less than 7 were 36% and 9%, respectively. More importantly, the sensitivity and positive predictive value of a low scalp pH to identify a new-

born with hypoxic–ischemic encephalopathy were 50% and 3%, respectively (37).

The use of pulse oximetry has been suggested as a modality to reduce the false-positive rate of a nonreassuring FHR tracing. A multicenter randomized clinical trial reported that among term singleton fetuses with nonreassuring FHR patterns, the use of fetal pulse oximetry along with electronic tracing was associated with a significantly lower rate (4.5%) of cesarean delivery for presumed nonreassuring tracing than the controls (10%), who were managed with FHR monitoring alone (38). However, before proceeding with emergent cesarean delivery, most of the patients had not undergone ancillary tests to assess fetal well-being or intrauterine resuscitation, both of which could have decreased the need to proceed with cesarean delivery. Moreover, the randomized trial decreased neither the overall rate of cesarean delivery nor the rate of umbilical arterial pH less than 7. Because of the uncertain benefit of pulse oximetry and concerns about falsely reassuring fetal oxygenation, use of the fetal pulse oximeter in clinical practice cannot be supported at this time. Additional studies to test the efficacy and safety of fetal pulse oximetry are underway.

▶ *Are there methods of intrauterine resuscitation that can be used for persistently nonreassuring patterns?*

Maternal oxygen commonly is used in cases of a persistently nonreassuring pattern. Unfortunately, there are no data on the efficacy or safety of this therapy. Often, the nonreassuring FHR patterns persist and do not respond to change in position or oxygenation. In such cases, the use of tocolytic agents has been suggested to abolish uterine contractions and perhaps avoid umbilical cord compression. A meta-analysis reported the pooled results of three randomized clinical trials that compared tocolytic therapy (terbutaline, hexoprenaline, or magnesium sulfate) with untreated controls in the management of a suspected nonreassuring FHR tracing (39). Compared with no treatment, tocolytic therapy more commonly improved the FHR tracing. However, there were no differences in rates of perinatal mortality, low 5-minute Apgar score, or admission to the neonatal intensive care unit between the groups (possibly because of the small sample size). Thus, although tocolytic therapy appears to reduce the number of FHR abnormalities, there is insufficient evidence to recommend it.

Hyperstimulation (six or more contractions in 10 minutes) or hypertonus (single contraction lasting more than 2 minutes) in conjunction with a nonreassuring FHR pattern can be successfully treated with β_2-adrenergic drugs (hexoprenaline or terbutaline). A retrospective study suggested that 98% of cases of uterine hyperstimulation respond to treatment with a β-agonist (40).

When the FHR abnormality is recurrent variable decelerations, amnioinfusion to relieve umbilical cord compression should be considered (41). A meta-analysis of 12 randomized trials that allocated patients to no treatment or transcervical amnioinfusion noted that placement of fluid in the uterine cavity significantly reduced the rate of decelerations (relative risk 0.54, 95% CI, 0.43–0.68) and cesarean delivery for suspected fetal distress (relative risk 0.35, 95% CI, 0.24–0.52) (42). Because of the lower rate of cesarean delivery, amnioinfusion also decreased the likelihood that either the patient or the newborn will stay in the hospital more than 3 days (42). Amnioinfusion can be done by bolus or continuous infusion technique. A randomized trial compared the two techniques of amnioinfusion and concluded that both have a similar ability to relieve recurrent variable decelerations (43).

Another common cause of nonreassuring FHR patterns is maternal hypotension secondary to regional anesthesia. If maternal hypotension is identified and suspected to be secondary to regional anesthesia, treatment with intravenous ephedrine is warranted.

Summary of Recommendations and Conclusions

The following recommendations are based on good and consistent scientific evidence (Level A):

▶ The false-positive rate of EFM for predicting adverse outcomes is high.

▶ The use of EFM is associated with an increase in the rate of operative interventions (vacuum, forceps, and cesarean delivery).

▶ The use of EFM does not result in a reduction of cerebral palsy rates.

▶ With persistent variable decelerations, amnioinfusion reduces the need to proceed with emergent cesarean delivery and should be considered.

The following recommendations are based on limited or inconsistent scientific evidence (Level B):

▶ The labor of parturients with high-risk conditions should be monitored continuously.

▶ Reinterpretation of the FHR tracing, especially knowing the neonatal outcome, is not reliable.

▶ The use of fetal pulse oximetry in clinical practice cannot be supported at this time.

References

1. Martin JA, Hamilton BE, Ventura SJ, Menacker F, Park MM, Sutton PD. Births: final data for 2002. Natl Vital Stat Rep 2003;52(10):1–113. (Level II-3)

2. Low JA, Pickersgill H, Killen H, Derrick EJ. The prediction and prevention of intrapartum fetal asphyxia in term pregnancies. Am J Obstet Gynecol 2001;184:724–30. (Level II-2)

3. Thacker SB, Stroup D, Chang M. Continuous electronic heart rate monitoring for fetal assessment during labor. The Cochrane Database of Systematic Reviews 2001, Issue 2. Art. No.: CD000063. DOI: 10.1002/14651858. CD000063. (Meta-analysis)

4. Electronic fetal heart rate monitoring: research guidelines for interpretation. National Institute of Child Health and Human Development Research Planning Workshop. Am J Obstet Gynecol 1997;177:1385–90. (Level III)

5. Freeman RK. Problems with intrapartum fetal heart rate monitoring interpretation and patient management. Obstet Gynecol 2002;100:813–26. (Level III)

6. Vintzileos AM, Nochimson DJ, Guzman EF, Knuppel RA, Lake M, Schifrin BS. Intrapartum electronic fetal heart rate monitoring versus intermittent auscultation: a meta-analysis. Obstet Gynecol 1995;85:149–55. (Meta-analysis)

7. Nelson KB, Dambrosia JM, Ting TY, Grether JK. Uncertain value of electronic fetal monitoring in predicting cerebral palsy. N Engl J Med 1996,324:613–8. (Level II-2)

8. Clark SL, Hankins GD. Temporal and demographic trends in cerebral palsy—fact and fiction. Am J Obstet Gynecol 2003;188:628–33. (Level III)

9. Hankins GD, Speer M. Defining the pathogenesis and pathophysiology of neonatal encephalopathy and cerebral palsy. Obstet Gynecol 2003;102:628–36. (Level III)

10. Badawi N, Kurinczuk JJ, Keogh JM, Alessandri LM, O'Sullivan F, Burton PR, et al. Antepartum risk factors for newborn encephalopathy: the Western Australian case-control study. BMJ 1998;317:1549–53. (Level II-2)

11. Morrison JC, Chez BF, Davis ID, Martin RW, Roberts WE, Martin JN Jr, et al. Intrapartum fetal heart rate assessment: monitoring by auscultation or electronic means. Am J Obstet Gynecol 1993;168:63–6. (Level III)

12. Vintzileos AM, Nochimson DJ, Antsaklis A, Varvarigos I, Guzman EF, Knuppel RA. Comparison of intrapartum electronic fetal heart rate monitoring versus intermittent auscultation in detecting fetal acidemia at birth. Am J Obstet Gynecol 1995;173:1021–4. (Level I)

13. Helfand M, Marton K, Ueland K. Factors involved in the interpretation of fetal monitor tracings. Am J Obstet Gynecol 1985;151:737–44. (Level III)

14. Nielsen PV, Stigsby B, Nickelsen C, Nim J. Intra- and inter-observer variability in the assessment of intrapartum

cardiotocograms. Acta Obstet Gynecol Scand 1987;66: 421–4. (Level III)

15. Beaulieu MD, Fabia J, Leduc B, Brisson J, Bastide A, Blouin D, et al. The reproducibility of intrapartum cardiotocogram assessments. Can Med Assoc J 1982;127: 214–6. (Level III)

16. Blix E, Sviggum O, Koss KS, Oian P. Inter-observer variation in assessment of 845 labour admission tests: comparison between midwives and obstetricians in the clinical setting and two experts. BJOG 2003;110:1–5. (Level III)

17. Zain HA, Wright JW, Parrish GE, Diehl SJ. Interpreting the fetal heart rate tracing. Effect of knowledge of neonatal outcome. J Reprod Med 1998;43:367–70. (Level III)

18. Ayoubi JM, Audibert F, Vial M, Pons JC, Taylor S, Frydman R. Fetal heart rate and survival of the very premature newborn. Am J Obstet Gynecol 2002;187: 1026–30. (Level II-2)

19. Westgren M, Holmquist P, Svenningsen NW, Ingemarsson I. Intrapartum fetal monitoring in preterm deliveries: prospective study. Obstet Gynecol 1982;60:99–106. (Level II-2)

20. Westgren M, Holmquist P, Ingemarsson I, Svenningsen N. Intrapartum fetal acidosis in preterm infants: fetal monitoring and long-term morbidity. Obstet Gynecol 1984; 63:355–9. (Level II-2)

21. Hill JB, Alexander JM, Sharma SK, McIntire DD, Leveno KJ. A comparison of the effects of epidural and meperidine analgesia during labor on fetal heart rate. Obstet Gynecol 2003;102:333–7. (Level I)

22. Lieberman E, O'Donoghue C. Unintended effects of epidural analgesia during labor: a systematic review. Am J Obstet Gynecol 2002;186:S31–68. (Level III)

23. Gambling DR, Sharma SK, Ramin SM, Lucas MJ, Leveno KJ, Wiley J, et al. A randomized study of combined spinal-epidural analgesia versus intravenous meperidine during labor: impact on cesarean delivery rate. Anesthesiology 1998;89:1336–44. (Level I)

24. Ville Y, Vincent Y, Tordjman N, Hue MV, Fernandez H, Frydman R. Effect of betamethasone on the fetal heart rate pattern assessed by computerized cardiotocography in normal twin pregnancies. Fetal Diagn Ther 1995;10: 301–6. (Level II-3)

25. Subtil D, Tiberghien P, Devos P, Therby D, Leclerc G, Vaast P, et al. Immediate and delayed effects of antenatal corticosteroids on fetal heart rate: a randomized trial that compares betamethasone acetate and phosphate, betamethasone phosphate, and dexamethasone. Am J Obstet Gynecol 2003;188:524–31. (Level I)

26. Senat MV, Minoui S, Multon O, Fernandez H, Frydman R, Ville Y. Effect of dexamethasone and betamethasone on the fetal heart rate variability in preterm labour: a randomised study. Br J Obstet Gynaecol 1998;105:749–55. (Level I)

27. Hatjis CG, Meis PJ. Sinusoidal fetal heart rate pattern associated with butorphanol administration. Obstet Gynecol 1986;67:377–80. (Level II-2)

28. Chazotte C, Forman L, Gandhi J. Heart rate patterns in fetuses exposed to cocaine. Obstet Gynecol 1991;78: 323–5. (Level II-3)

29. Wright JW, Ridgway LE, Wright BD, Covington DL, Bobitt JR. Effect of MgSO4 on heart rate monitoring in the preterm fetus. J Reprod Med 1996;41:605–8. (Level II-2)

30. Giannina G, Guzman ER, Lai YL, Lake MF, Cernadas M, Vintzileos AM. Comparison of the effects of meperidine and nalbuphine on intrapartum fetal heart rate tracings. Obstet Gynecol 1995;86:441–5. (Level I)

31. Kopecky EA, Ryan ML, Barrett JF, Seaward PG, Ryan G, Koren G, et al. Fetal response to maternally administered morphine. Am J Obstet Gynecol 2000;183:424–30. (Level II-2)

32. Williams KP, Galerneau F. Intrapartum fetal heart rate patterns in the prediction of neonatal acidemia. Am J Obstet Gynecol 2003;188:820–3. (Level II-3)

33. Samueloff A, Langer O, Berkus M, Field N, Xenakis E, Ridgway L. Is fetal heart rate variability a good predictor of fetal outcome? Acta Obstet Gynecol Scand 1994;73; 39–44. (Level II-2)

34. Skupski DW, Rosenberg CR, Eglinton GS. Intrapartum fetal stimulation tests: a meta-analysis. Obstet Gynecol 2002;99:129–34. (Meta-analysis)

35. Goodwin TM, Milner-Masterson L, Paul RH. Elimination of fetal scalp blood sampling on a large clinical service. Obstet Gynecol 1994;83:971–4. (Level II-3)

36. Hendrix NW, Chauhan SP, Scardo JA, Ellings JM, Devoe LD. Managing nonreassuring fetal heart rate patterns before cesarean delivery. Compliance with ACOG recommendations. J Reprod Med 2000;45:995–9. (Level III)

37. Kruger K, Hallberg B, Blennow M, Kublickas M, Westgren M. Predictive value of fetal scalp blood lactate concentration and pH markers of neurologic disability. Am J Obstet Gynecol 1999;181:1072–8. (Level II-3)

38. Garite TJ, Dildy GA, McNamara H, Nageotte MP, Boehm FH, Dellinger EH, et al. A multicenter controlled trial of fetal pulse oximetry in the intrapartum management of nonreassuring fetal heart rate patterns. Am J Obstet Gynecol 2000;183:1049–58. (Level I)

39. Kulier R, Hofmeyr GJ. Tocolytics for suspected intrapartum fetal distress. The Cochrane Database of Systematic Reviews 1998, Issue 1. Art. No.: CD000035. DOI: 10.1002/14651858.CD000035. (Meta-analysis)

40. Egarter CH, Husslein PW, Rayburn WF. Uterine hyperstimulation after low-dose prostaglandin E2 therapy: tocolytic treatment in 181 cases. Am J Obstet Gynecol 1990;163:794–6. (Level II-2)

41. Miyazaki FS, Taylor NA. Saline amnioinfusion for relief of variable or prolonged decelerations: a preliminary report. Am J Obstet Gynecol 1983;146:670–8. (Level III)

42. Hofmeyr GJ. Amnioinfusion for umbilical cord compression in labour. The Cochrane Database of Systematic Reviews 1998, Issue 1. Art. No.: CD000013. DOI: 10.1002/14651858.CD000013. (Meta-analysis)

43. Rinehart BK, Terrone DA, Barrow JH, Isler CM, Barrilleaux PS, Roberts WE. Randomized trial of intermittent or continuous amnioinfusion for variable decelerations. Obstet Gynecol 2000;96:571–4. (Level I)

The MEDLINE database, the Cochrane Library, and ACOG's own internal resources and documents were used to conduct a literature search to locate relevant articles published between January 1985 and December 2004. The search was restricted to articles published in the English language. Priority was given to articles reporting results of original research, although review articles and commentaries also were consulted. Abstracts of research presented at symposia and scientific conferences were not considered adequate for inclusion in this document. Guidelines published by organizations or institutions such as the National Institutes of Health and the American College of Obstetricians and Gynecologists were reviewed, and additional studies were located by reviewing bibliographies of identified articles. When reliable research was not available, expert opinions from obstetrician–gynecologists were used.

Studies were reviewed and evaluated for quality according to the method outlined by the U.S. Preventive Services Task Force:

I   Evidence obtained from at least one properly designed randomized controlled trial.

II-1   Evidence obtained from well-designed controlled trials without randomization.

II-2   Evidence obtained from well-designed cohort or case–control analytic studies, preferably from more than one center or research group.

II-3   Evidence obtained from multiple time series with or without the intervention. Dramatic results in uncontrolled experiments also could be regarded as this type of evidence.

III   Opinions of respected authorities, based on clinical experience, descriptive studies, or reports of expert committees.

Based on the highest level of evidence found in the data, recommendations are provided and graded according to the following categories:

Level A—Recommendations are based on good and consistent scientific evidence.

Level B—Recommendations are based on limited or inconsistent scientific evidence.

Level C—Recommendations are based primarily on consensus and expert opinion.

ISSN 1099-3630

The American College of Obstetricians and Gynecologists
409 12th Street, SW
PO Box 96920
Washington, DC 20090-6920

12345/98765

Intrapartum fetal heart rate monitoring. ACOG Practice Bulletin No. 70. American College of Obstetricians and Gynecologists. Obstet Gynecol 2005;106:1453–61.

ACOG PRACTICE BULLETIN

CLINICAL MANAGEMENT GUIDELINES FOR
OBSTETRICIAN–GYNECOLOGISTS
NUMBER 59, JANUARY 2005

This Practice Bulletin was developed by the ACOG Committee on Practice Bulletins— Gynecology with the assistance of Eve Espey, MD. The information is designed to aid practitioners in making decisions about appropriate obstetric and gynecologic care. These guidelines should not be construed as dictating an exclusive course of treatment or procedure. Variations in practice may be warranted based on the needs of the individual patient, resources, and limitations unique to the institution or type of practice.

Intrauterine Device

Intrauterine devices (IUDs) offer safe, effective, long-term contraception and should be considered for all women who seek a reliable, reversible contraception that is effective before coitus. Two IUDs currently are available in the United States: 1) the copper T380A, and 2) the levonorgestrel intrauterine system. A growing body of evidence attests to the safety and effectiveness of IUDs and to their potential role in decreasing rates of unintended pregnancy. Only a very small proportion of women in the United States, however, currently use an IUD.

This document presents evidence regarding the safety and efficacy of the copper T380A and the levonorgestrel intrauterine system. To achieve more widespread use of IUDs among women who are appropriate candidates, clinicians should understand the risks, benefits, indications, and contraindications to IUD use.

Background

Historical Perspective

Intrauterine contraception became popular in the United States in the 1960s and 1970s. Prospective trials demonstrated its safety and efficacy (1). At the height of its popularity, the IUD was used by approximately 11% of women using contraception in the United States (2). In 1970, the Dalkon Shield was first marketed in the United States. Soon after, reports of septic abortion and pelvic infection contributed to class action lawsuits against IUD manufacturers. By 1988, all but 1 IUD had been removed from the U.S. market by manufacturers because of economic considerations, including product liability concerns. Among some providers, concern remains about the safety of IUDs as a result of the Dalkon Shield controversy despite reassuring evidence about modern IUDs and the correction of a design flaw unique to the Dalkon Shield. In 1995, the National Survey of Family Growth reported that fewer than 1% of women who use contraception use an IUD (3). Providers remain concerned about product liability and the risk of infection associated with IUDs and, therefore, apply restrictive criteria in selecting candidates for IUD use (4). Worldwide, IUDs are the most common reversible method of contraception and are used by more than 90 million women. The largest number of IUD users resides in China, where 40% of women who use contraception use the IUD. Other countries with high rates of IUD use include Vietnam, Norway, Finland, and Sweden (5, 6).

Overview of Currently Available Intrauterine Devices

The copper T380A is a T-shaped device of polyethylene wrapped with copper wire around the stem and arms. The U.S. Food and Drug Administration (FDA) has approved its use for 10 continuous years, during which it remains highly effective, with a 10-year cumulative pregnancy rate comparable to that of sterilization. Its major advantage over other reversible methods of contraception is that it requires only a single act of motivation for long-term use. Typical-use pregnancy rates (0.1–0.8% for levonorgestrel intrauterine system and copper T380A) are lower than with oral contraceptives, and continuation rates are higher (78–81%) (7). The copper IUD also may be used for postcoital contraception. It has a failure rate of less than 1% when inserted within 5 days after unprotected intercourse (8). The IUD may then be retained for use as long-term contraception (9).

The levonorgestrel intrauterine system also is T-shaped and contains a polydimethylsiloxane sleeve containing 52 mg of levonorgestrel on the stem. The IUD releases 20 μg of levonorgestrel daily. This small amount of steroid confers minimal systemic side effects, although some women may experience hormone-related effects, such as headache, nausea, breast tenderness, and depression. Most women ovulate normally but experience diminished menstrual bleeding because of the local effect of levonorgestrel on the endometrium. In an economic analysis, the levonorgestrel intrauterine system was shown to be the most cost-effective reversible method of contraception after 5 years of continuous use (10). As with the copper T380A, return to fertility is rapid after removal of the device (11). Table 1 compares the copper IUD and the levonorgestrel intrauterine system.

Mechanism of Action

A number of different mechanisms of action have been proposed for copper-containing IUDs. These include inhibition of sperm migration and viability, change in transport speed of the ovum, and damage to or destruction of the ovum. The evidence suggests these prefertilization

Table 1. Comparison of Levonorgestrel Intrauterine System and Copper Intrauterine Device

| Characteristic | Termination Rates at 7 Years per 100 Women | |
	Levonorgestrel Intrauterine System	Copper Intrauterine Device
Pregnancy	0.2	0.3
Expulsion	2.9	1.8
Pelvic inflammatory disease	0.7	0.7
Amenorrhea	4.4	0.1
Other menstrual problems	1.5	2.9
Pain	1.4	1.5
Ectopic pregnancy	0	0
Perforation	0.1	0
Continuation	22.8	27.2

Reprinted from Fertility & Sterility, Vol 61, Sivin I, Stern J. Health during prolonged use of levonorgestrel 20 micrograms/d and the copper TCu 380Ag intrauterine contraceptive devise: a multicenter study, 70–7, copyright 1994, with permission from The American Society for Reproductive Medicine.

effects constitute the primary mechanism of action for pregnancy prevention in the copper IUD (12). Postfertilization effects, including damage to or destruction of the fertilized ovum, also may occur (13). In addition to these effects, the levonorgestrel intrauterine system causes endometrial suppression and changes the amount and viscosity of cervical mucus. All effects, both prefertilization and postfertilization, occur before implantation.

Intrauterine Device Candidate Selection

Candidates for IUD use and contraindications to IUD use are shown in the boxes. Women considering an IUD should be counseled about its advantages and side effects as well as other family planning methods. They should understand when to return for follow-up evaluation and should be instructed in checking for the strings of the IUD. Generally, women should be reevaluated 1–4 weeks after IUD placement. For women who use the copper T380A, a missed period should prompt a pregnancy test; a positive pregnancy test result should prompt an immediate visit to a provider to rule out ectopic pregnancy. Amenorrhea in women using the levonorgestrel intrauterine system is common. However, in a woman who misses a period and experiences pain, ectopic pregnancy should be ruled out. Women should be instructed about warning signs of pelvic infection, particularly in the first month after insertion of the device, when the risk of pelvic infection is increased.

Candidates for Intrauterine Device Use

- Multiparous and nulliparous women at low risk for sexually transmitted diseases
- Women who desire long-term reversible contraception
- Women with the following medical conditions, for which an intrauterine device may be an optimal method:
  - Diabetes*
  - Thromboembolism[†]
  - Menorrhagia/dysmenorrhea[‡]
  - Breastfeeding[§]
  - Breast cancer[‖]
  - Liver disease[¶]

*Limited data suggest no increased complications in women with diabetes. (Kimmerle R, Weiss R, Berger M, Kurz KH. Effectiveness, safety and acceptability of a copper intrauterine device [Cu safe 300] in type 1 diabetic women. Diabetes Care 1993;16:1227–30.)

[†]Consider the levonorgestrel intrauterine system for women with bleeding disorders or those taking anticoagulants because it decreases menstrual bleeding. (Siegel JE, Kouides PA. Menorrhagia from a haematologist's point of view. Part II: management. Haemophilia 2002;8:339–47.)

[‡]Consider the levonorgestrel intrauterine system for women with menorrhagia or dysmenorrhea. (Lethaby AE, Cooke I, Rees M. Progesterone/progestogen releasing intrauterine systems for heavy menstrual bleeding [Cochrane Review]. In: The Cochrane Library, Issue 3, 2004. Chichester, UK: John Wiley & Sons, Ltd.)

[§]Copper only until 4–6 weeks postpartum.

[‖]Copper only for current breast cancer.

[¶]The levonorgestrel intrauterine system is not recommended for current liver disease.

Data from World Health Organization. Medical eligibility criteria for contraceptive use. 3rd ed. Geneva: WHO; 2004.

Contraindications to Intrauterine Device Use

- Pregnancy
- Pelvic inflammatory disease (current or within the past 3 months)
- Sexually transmitted diseases (current)
- Puerperal or postabortion sepsis (current or within the past 3 months)
- Purulent cervicitis
- Undiagnosed abnormal vaginal bleeding
- Malignancy of the genital tract
- Known uterine anomalies or fibroids distorting the cavity in a way incompatible with intrauterine device (IUD) insertion
- Allergy to any component of the IUD or Wilson's disease (for copper-containing IUDs)

Data from The intra-uterine device. Canadian Consensus Conference on Contraception. J SOGC 1998;20:769–73; IMAP statement on intrauterine devices. International Planned Parenthood Federation (IPPF). International Medical Advisory Panel (IMAP). IPPF Med Bull 1995;29:1–4; and World Health Organization. Medical eligibility criteria for contraceptive use. 3rd ed. Geneva: WHO; 2004

Clinical Considerations and Recommendations

▶ *Does the IUD increase the risk of pelvic inflammatory disease (PID)? Are nulliparous women with an IUD at higher risk of PID or infertility?*

The concern about a causal association of IUDs with PID has been arguably the most important barrier to increased IUD use. A recent meta-analysis examined the large body of evidence regarding this association (15). The review concluded that the risk of PID after the first month following insertion is small. The increased risk of upper genital tract infection seen in the first month after IUD insertion is related to the contamination of the uterus with vaginal bacteria, despite aseptic technique (16). Although the relative risk of PID is increased by a factor of 6 in the first month after insertion, the absolute risk is still low. In 22,908 IUD insertions, investigators found a risk of PID after 20 days of 1.4 cases per 1,000 woman-years of use, compared with 9.7 cases per 1,000 woman-years in the first 20 days after IUD insertion (16).

Intrauterine Device Insertion

For the treatment of pain during IUD insertion, a randomized nonblinded study compared pretreatment with 2% intracervical lignocaine gel versus an inert gel versus no treatment and found significantly lower pain scores in those who received the active gel (14). Many clinicians use ibuprofen or nonsteroidal antiinflammatory drugs for pain control on insertion, but there are limited data of their efficacy. No reports about other modalities, such as paracervical block, have appeared in the literature.

Additionally, rates of PID remained low and stable for up to 8 years of follow-up monitoring, which demonstrates that PID is an uncommon event in IUD users after the first 20 days following insertion.

The appropriateness of IUD use in nulliparous women is controversial, largely because of fears of PID with subsequent infertility. Initial case–control studies from 1985 showed an increased risk of tubal infertility associated with certain IUDs but not with copper IUDs and not when controlling for the number of sexual partners (17, 18). In 2001, in a case–control study of 1,895 women with primary tubal infertility using several control groups to minimize bias, previous copper IUD use was not found to be associated with an increased risk of tubal occlusion in nulliparous women at low risk of sexually transmitted diseases (STDs) (19). Although some reports document higher rates of expulsion and lower rates of continuation in nulliparous IUD users (20, 21), others show rates of these complications similar to those found in parous women (22, 23). Contraception counseling should include information about risk factors for STDs and PID. Nulliparous and multiparous women at low risk of STDs are not at increased risk of PID and are good candidates for IUD use.

▶ *What are the difficulties associated with IUD insertion and removal, and how are they best addressed?*

Difficulties that may occur at IUD insertion include vasovagal reaction, the need for cervical dilation, severe pain, inability to insert the IUD, and uterine perforation. Overall, these conditions rarely occur. Uterine perforation, the most concerning complication, is estimated to occur in approximately 1 in 1,000 insertions (24). Adherence to insertion guidelines included with IUD packaging may help avoid uterine perforation; the risk of perforation appears to decrease with increasing experience. If either the copper T380A or the levonorgestrel intrauterine system perforates into the peritoneal cavity, the location of the IUD should be confirmed by ultrasonography, and the IUD should be removed by laparoscopy or laparotomy (25, 26).

A common challenge when removing IUDs is the lack of visible strings. A Cytobrush may be placed in the endocervix and gently swept downward to locate strings curled up in the canal (26, 27). If this maneuver is not helpful, ultrasonography should be performed to ensure intrauterine location of the IUD. The clinician may then attempt to remove the IUD with an "IUD hook" under sterile conditions in the outpatient setting or may elect to remove the IUD in the operating room, where hysteroscopic guidance may be helpful.

▶ *Is routine screening for STDs (eg, gonorrhea and chlamydia) required before insertion of an IUD?*

Current data do not support routine screening in women at low risk for STDs. However, because the rate of endometritis in women with gonorrhea and chlamydia is 25–75%, and because endometritis may be asymptomatic (28), women at high risk of STDs may benefit from screening. The prevalence of STDs is a more important predictor of subsequent upper genital tract infection than is IUD insertion (29). In a study of 4,031 women at low risk for STDs who had an IUD inserted, no cases of PID were reported (16). In contrast, 8 cases of PID were noted in 1,292 woman-years of follow-up in a study in which the prevalence of STDs was higher (30). Some case reports suggest that women with positive cultures for chlamydia performed at the time of IUD insertion are unlikely to develop PID if the chlamydia is treated with the IUD remaining in situ (31, 32). Clinical judgment should be used to determine whether the IUD should be removed.

▶ *Is the presence of bacterial vaginosis a contraindication to IUD insertion?*

The association between bacterial vaginosis and IUD use remains controversial. Studies have not addressed whether the presence of bacterial vaginosis at the time of IUD insertion leads to adverse effects. Although several early reports documented higher rates of bacterial vaginosis in IUD users (33, 34), these reports were hampered by methodological flaws. Two recent studies reexamined the association between IUD use and bacterial vaginosis and reached opposing conclusions. A case–control study comparing women with and without bacterial vaginosis showed no association between bacterial vaginosis and IUD use and a protective effect of oral contraceptives and condoms against bacterial vaginosis (35). However, a cross-sectional study of IUD users and nonusers did show a significant association between IUD use and bacterial vaginosis (relative risk: 2.78) (36). Despite this association, IUD users were no more likely to have STDs or PID than nonusers.

▶ *Does antibiotic prophylaxis before IUD insertion decrease the risk of subsequent pelvic infection?*

Four randomized controlled trials have examined the benefit of prophylactic doxycycline or azithromycin given at the time of IUD insertion (30, 37–39). Outcome measures included PID, unscheduled visits to the clinician, and removal of the IUD within the first 90 days of use. A meta-analysis concluded that prophylactic antibiotics conferred little benefit (15). Antibiotics did not reduce the risk of PID, which was a rare outcome in both the antibiotic and placebo groups. In a U.S. trial, the rate of PID was 1 per 1,000 in both groups. Prophylaxis did not reduce the likelihood of IUD removal within the first 90 days. Use of antibiotics did, however, result in a small but significant decrease in unscheduled provider visits in some trials. Overall, use of prophylactic antibiotics is unlikely to be cost-effective in populations with a low prevalence of STDs.

Studies of prophylactic antibiotics for IUD insertion did not examine women at risk for subacute bacterial endocarditis. However, bacteremia is uncommon in clinically well women who undergo IUD insertion and removal. Therefore, on the basis of expert opinion, the American Heart Association does not recommend subacute bacterial endocarditis antibiotic prophylaxis for IUD insertion and removal (40).

▶ What treatment options are appropriate for an asymptomatic patient with an IUD who has actinomyces identified on a Pap test?

Actinomyces israelii, a gram-positive anaerobic bacterium normally found in the human gastrointestinal tract, may be a normal component of vaginal flora. This organism may be more prevalent in the genital tract of IUD users than in nonusers. The likelihood of colonization appears to increase with increasing duration of IUD use (41). Recent studies demonstrated that colonization may be lower in levonorgestrel intrauterine system users than in copper IUD users (2.9% versus 5–10%) (41–43). However, actinomyces found via a Pap test is not diagnostic of actinomycosis infection, nor is it predictive of future disease. Pelvic actinomycosis is a very rare but serious condition characterized by granulomatous pelvic abscesses. Its prevalence has been estimated to be less than 0.001%; because of its rarity, the relationship between actinomyces found on a Pap test in an asymptomatic IUD user and the eventual development of this infection is unclear.

Studies of pelvic actinomycosis are limited to case reports, so management of the asymptomatic IUD user whose Pap test shows actinomyces is not clearly established. A recent review of pelvic actinomycosis underlines the ubiquity of *Actinomyces israelii* in both IUD users and nonusers and the lack of an association between the finding of this organism on a Pap test and adverse outcomes when no treatment is offered (44). A single randomized controlled trial has looked at management of asymptomatic IUD users with actinomyces identified on a Pap test (45). Women were randomized to undergo either removal of the IUD and receive oral

antibiotics or receive oral antibiotics alone. One month after treatment, the Pap test was repeated. No Pap tests revealed actinomyces in the women whose IUDs were removed. Thirty-three percent of Pap tests still showed actinomyces in the group of women who received antibiotics alone. However, the importance of clearing the actinomyces colonization is still not established. The options for management of asymptomatic IUD users with actinomyces on Pap test are expectant management, an extended course of oral antibiotics, removal of the IUD, and both antibiotic use and IUD removal.

▶ Do IUDs cause ectopic pregnancy?

A history of ectopic pregnancy has traditionally been considered a contraindication to use of an IUD because IUDs were thought to increase the risk of ectopic pregnancy. Both case–control studies and randomized controlled trials have addressed the question of IUDs and the risk of ectopic pregnancy. Findings from case–control studies have been inconsistent, and discrepancies in the choice of control groups have made accurate conclusions difficult to reach. The complexity of ascertaining an appropriate control group has been the major impediment to these studies. A recent meta-analysis of 16 case–control studies concluded that IUDs do not increase the risk of ectopic pregnancy because they generally prevent pregnancy effectively (46). However, if pregnancy does occur with an IUD in place, the pregnancy is more likely to be ectopic. The authors also concluded that past IUD use may slightly increase the risk of ectopic pregnancy.

Although case–control studies express relative risk, prospective data from randomized controlled trials describe the absolute risk of ectopic pregnancy associated with IUD use, a measure that is more useful clinically. U.S. cohort data with both the copper T380A and the levonorgestrel intrauterine system have shown an ectopic pregnancy rate of 0–0.5 per 1,000 woman-years, compared with an ectopic pregnancy rate of 3.25–5.25 per 1,000 woman-years among women who do not use contraception (47, 48). Given this very low risk, a history of ectopic pregnancy should not be considered a contraindication to IUD use. The most recent World Health Organization guidelines for appropriate candidates for an IUD support the routine use of IUDs (both copper T380A and the levonorgestrel intrauterine system) in women with a past history of ectopic pregnancy (49).

▶ In a pregnant woman, does removal of the IUD affect pregnancy outcome?

Complications that may occur in IUD users who become pregnant include an increased risk of spontaneous abortion and an increased risk of septic abortion. Several reports suggest a higher rate of pregnancy loss in women who conceive an intrauterine pregnancy with an IUD in situ. The loss rate may be higher if the IUD is retained (50, 51) than if it is removed (52). Several cases of death associated with septic abortion from retained Dalkon Shields were reported shortly after distribution of these IUDs in the early 1970s (53). As a direct result of these cases, the FDA recommends that IUDs be removed from pregnant women when possible without an invasive procedure (54). No IUD-related deaths among pregnant women in the United States have been reported since that time.

▶ *What impact does IUD use have on menstrual blood loss in a woman with normal flow?*

The copper IUD and the levonorgestrel intrauterine system have different effects on menstrual bleeding. Long-term follow-up evaluation of a randomized trial of the 2 devices found that copper IUD users were more likely to discontinue the device because of heavy menstrual bleeding and dysmenorrhea, whereas levonorgestrel intrauterine system users were more likely to discontinue the device because of amenorrhea and spotting (55). The levonorgestrel released from the levonorgestrel intrauterine system concentrates in the endometrium and produces a thin decidualized endometrial lining, despite the presence of endogenous estrogen. Although most women continue to ovulate while using the levonorgestrel intrauterine system, the amount and duration of bleeding is reduced because of levonorgestrel's direct effect on the endometrium. Several randomized controlled trials comparing the levonorgestrel intrauterine system with copper devices demonstrate a mean increase in hemoglobin levels in levonorgestrel intrauterine system users of 0.5 g/dL at 2 years up to 1.5 g/dL at 5 years of use (56–58). Although women with a copper IUD initially demonstrate a slight decrease in hemoglobin levels, continuing users over a period of 5–7 years experience an increase over levels at insertion. In the largest trial comparing the levonorgestrel intrauterine system with a copper device, one third of women immediately and 70% of women at the end of 2 years developed oligomenorrhea (ie, no more than 1 episode of bleeding in a 90-day interval) or amenorrhea (58). Similarly, symptoms of dysmenorrhea were reduced in levonorgestrel intrauterine system users. Patients should be advised that menstrual bleeding and cramping may initially increase with the copper IUD and may decrease with the levonorgestrel intrauterine system. The number of bleeding days as well as the amount of bleeding decreases with use of the levonorgestrel intrauterine system. Approximately 8–10% of women discontinue the levonorgestrel intrauterine system over

2 years of use because of oligomenorrhea or amenorrhea; therefore, all women considering this form of contraception should be informed of the likelihood of these effects (59).

▶ *What is the efficacy of the levonorgestrel intrauterine system in treating menorrhagia?*

Five randomized controlled trials have compared the levonorgestrel intrauterine system with other treatments, including the oral progestin norethindrone and transcervical resection of the endometrium, for women with menorrhagia (60–64). A meta-analysis concluded that the levonorgestrel intrauterine system was significantly more effective than oral cyclical norethindrone as a treatment for heavy menstrual bleeding (59). Also, the levonorgestrel intrauterine system resulted in a smaller mean reduction in menstrual blood loss than transcervical resection of the endometrium although the decrease in blood loss was large in both groups and resulted in similar high rates of satisfaction. Several case series (65–67) also suggest a substantial reduction in menstrual blood loss, averaging 74–97%, with use of the levonorgestrel intrauterine system in women with idiopathic menorrhagia. Two recent clinical trials randomized women with menorrhagia who were scheduled to undergo hysterectomy to either treatment with the levonorgestrel intrauterine system or their previous medical treatment (60, 68). In these 2 trials, 64% and 80% of women with the levonorgestrel intrauterine system, respectively, canceled their surgery, compared with 14% and 9%, respectively, in the normal medical care groups. Therefore, the levonorgestrel intrauterine system may be an acceptable alternative to hysterectomy in women with menorrhagia.

▶ *When should an IUD be removed in a menopausal woman?*

An IUD placed for contraception should be removed in a woman who has become menopausal. Awaiting 1 year of amenorrhea to ensure menopausal status is advisable before removing the device. Many women experience dysfunctional bleeding in the perimenopausal period, and unexpected bleeding should prompt an endometrial biopsy in women with an IUD to evaluate the possibility of endometrial pathology (69). Although no clinical trials have been performed that document risks from prolonged IUD retention in asymptomatic menopausal women, several case reports discuss pelvic infection (eg, pelvic actinomycosis) in women with IUDs (70–72). In the absence of data, it seems prudent to remove the IUD placed for contraception from a menopausal woman.

▶ *When is an IUD appropriate for emergency contraception?*

Use of a copper IUD for postcoital contraception, first reported in 1976 (73), has been studied in prospective cohort trials with pregnancy rates of 0–0.1% (74). In these trials, the IUD was inserted up to 5 days after unprotected intercourse. A more recent report of 1,013 women who underwent insertion of a copper IUD for postcoital contraception, including 170 nulliparous women, found a pregnancy rate of 0.2% (8). One advantage of the copper IUD for postcoital contraception is that it can be retained for continued long-term contraception. The same study found 86% of parous women and 80% of nulliparous women maintained the IUD for contraception. No randomized controlled trials have compared IUD insertion with medical regimens for emergency contraception. A recent meta-analysis concluded that the IUD is very effective for emergency contraception but that further comparative studies are needed (9).

The copper T380A is appropriate for emergency contraception in women who meet standard criteria for IUD insertion and is most effective if inserted within 5 days after unprotected intercourse. This method is particularly useful for women who desire long-term contraception and who are otherwise appropriate candidates for IUD use.

Conclusions

▶ Pelvic inflammatory disease complicating IUD insertion is uncommon, and the risk of PID decreases to the background risk after the first 20 days after insertion.

▶ Nulligravid and multiparous women at low risk of STDs who desire long-term reversible contraception are good candidates for IUDs.

Summary of Recommendations

The following recommendations are based on good and consistent scientific evidence (Level A):

▶ Routine use of prophylactic antibiotics at the time of IUD insertion confers little benefit.

▶ The copper T380A is very effective for postcoital emergency contraception and is most effective if inserted within 5 days after unprotected intercourse.

The following recommendations are based on limited or inconsistent scientific evidence (Level B):

▶ Intrauterine devices may be offered to women with a history of ectopic pregnancy.

▶ The levonorgestrel intrauterine system may be an acceptable alternative to hysterectomy in women with menorrhagia.

The following recommendations are based primarily on consensus and expert opinion (Level C):

▶ The FDA recommends that IUDs be removed from pregnant women when possible without an invasive procedure.

▶ An IUD placed for contraception should be removed in a woman who has become menopausal.

▶ Contraception counseling should include information about risk factors for STDs and PID.

References

1. Tietze C, Lewit S. Evaluation of intrauterine devices: ninth progress report of the Cooperative Statistical Program. Stud Fam Plann 1970;1(55):1–40. (Level II-3)

2. Piccinino LJ, Mosher WD. Trends in contraceptive use in the United States: 1982–1995. Fam Plann Perspect 1998; 30:4–10, 46. (Level II-3)

3. Abma JC, Chandra A, Mosher WD, Peterson L, Piccinino LJ. Fertility, family planning, and women's health: new data from the 1995 National Survey of Family Growth. Vital Health Stat 23 1997;(19):1–114. (Level II-3)

4. Stanwood NL, Garrett JM, Konrad TR. Obstetrician–gynecologists and the intrauterine device: a survey of attitudes and practice. Obstet Gynecol 2002;99:275–80. (Level III)

5. Farley TM, Meirik O, Rowe PJ. Safety and efficacy of existing methods of fertility regulation. Ann Tech Rep 1999:181–93. (Level II-2)

6. Mauldin WP, Segal SJ. IUD use throughout the world: past, present, and future. In: Bardin CW, Mishell DR Jr, editors. Proceedings from the Fourth International Conference on IUDs. Boston (MA): Butterworth-Heinemann; 1994. p. 1–10. (Level III)

7. Trussell J. Contraceptive failure in the United States. Contraception 2004;70:89–96. (Level III)

8. Zhou L, Xiao B. Emergency contraception with Multiload Cu-375 SL IUD: a multicenter clinical trial. Contraception 2001;64:107–12. (Level II-3)

9. Cheng L, Gulmezoglu AM, Oel CJ, Piaggio G, Ezcurra E, Van Look PF. Interventions for emergency contraception (Cochrane Review). In: The Cochrane Library, Issue 3, 2004. Chichester, UK: John Wiley & Sons, Ltd. (Meta-analysis)

10. Chiou CF, Trussell J, Reyes E, Knight K, Wallace J, Udani J, et al. Economic analysis of contraceptives for women. Contraception 2003;68:3–10. (Cost-effectiveness analysis)

11. Andersson K, Batar I, Rybo G. Return to fertility after removal of a levonorgestrel-releasing intrauterine device and Nova-T. Contraception 1992;46:575–84. (Level I)

12. Rivera R, Yacobson I, Grimes D. The mechanism of action of hormonal contraceptives and intrauterine contraceptive devices. Am J Obstet Gynecol 1999;181:1263–9. (Level III)

13. Stanford JB, Mikolajczyk RT. Mechanisms of action of intrauterine devices: update and estimation of postfertilization effects. Am J Obstet Gynecol 2002;187:1699–708. (Level III)

14. Oloto EJ, Bromham DR, Murty JA. Pain and discomfort perception at IUD insertion—effect of short-duration, low-volume, intracervical application of two per cent lignocaine gel (Instillagel (TM))—a preliminary study. Br J Fam Plann 1997;22:177–80. (Level I)

15. Grimes DA, Schulz KF. Antibiotic prophylaxis for intrauterine contraceptive device insertion (Cochrane Review). In: The Cochrane Library, Issue 3, 2004. Chichester, UK: John Wiley & Sons, Ltd. (Meta-analysis)

16. Farley TM, Rosenberg MJ, Rowe PJ, Chen JH, Meirik O. Intrauterine devices and pelvic inflammatory disease: an international perspective. Lancet 1992;339:785–8. (Level II-2)

17. Daling JR, Weiss NS, Metch BJ, Chow WH, Soderstrom RM, Moore DE, et al. Primary tubal infertility in relation to the use of an intrauterine device. N Engl J Med 1985; 312:937–41. (Level II-2)

18. Cramer DW, Schiff I, Schoenbaum SC, Gibson M, Belisle S, Albrecht B, et al. Tubal infertility and the intrauterine device. N Engl J Med 1985;312:941–7. (Level II-2)

19. Hubacher D, Lara-Ricalde R, Taylor DJ, Guerra-Infante F, Guzman-Rodriguez R. Use of copper intrauterine devices and the risk of tubal infertility among nulligravid women. N Engl J Med 2001;345:561–7. (Level II-2)

20. Petersen KR, Brooks L, Jacobsen N, Skoby SO. Clinical performance of intrauterine devices in nulligravidae: is the length of the endometrial cavity of significance? Acta Eur Fertil 1991;22:225–8. (Level I)

21. Weiner E, Berg AA, Johanson I. Copper intrauterine contraceptive devices in adolescent nulliparae. Br J Obstet Gynaecol 1978;85:204–6. (Level III)

22. Duenas JL, Albert A, Carrasco F. Intrauterine contraception in nulligravid vs parous women. Contraception 1996; 53:23–4. (Level III)

23. Wildemeersch D, Van Kets H, Vrijens M, Delbarge W, Van Trappen Y, Temmerman M, et al. Intrauterine contraception in adolescent women. The GyneFix intrauterine implant. Ann N Y Acad Sci 1997;816:440–50. (Level III)

24. Long-term reversible contraception. Twelve years of experience with the TCU380A and TCU220C. Contraception 1997;56:341–52. (Level I)

25. World Health Organization. Mechanism of action, safety and efficacy of intrauterine devices. Geneva: WHO; 1997. (Level III)

26. Speroff L, Darney PD. A clinical guide for contraception. 3rd ed. Philadelphia (PA): Lippincott, Williams and Wilkins; 2001. (Level III)

27. Ben-Rafael Z, Bider D. A new procedure for removal of a "lost" intrauterine device. Obstet Gynecol 1996;87: 785–6. (Level III)

28. Eckert LO, Thwin SS, Hillier SL, Kiviat NB, Eschenbach DA. The antimicrobial treatment of subacute endometritis: a proof of concept study. Am J Obstet Gynecol 2003; 190:305–13. (Level I)

29. Grimes DA. Intrauterine device and upper-genital-tract infection. Lancet 2000;356:1013–9. (Level III)

30. Sinei SK, Schulz KF, Lamptey PR, Grimes DA, Mati JK, Rosenberg MJ, et al. Preventing IUCD-related pelvic infection: the efficacy of prophylactic doxycycline at insertion. Br J Obstet Gynaecol 1990;97:412–9. (Level I)

31. Skjeldestad FE, Halvorsen LE, Kahn H, Nordbo SA, Saake K. IUD users in Norway are at low risk for genital C. trachomatis infection. Contraception 1996;54:209–12. (Level III)

32. Faundes A, Telles E, Cristofoletti ML, Faundes D, Castro S, Hardy E. The risk of inadvertent intrauterine device insertion in women carriers of endocervical Chlamydia trachomatis. Contraception 1998;58:105–9. (Level II-3)

33. Avonts D, Sercu M, Heyerick P, Vandermeeren I, Meheus A, Piot P. Incidence of uncomplicated genital infections in women using oral contraception or an intrauterine device: a prospective study. Sex Transm Dis 1990;17: 23–9. (Level II-2)

34. Moi H. Prevalence of bacterial vaginosis and its association with genital infections, inflammation, and contraceptive methods in women attending sexually transmitted disease and primary health clinics. Int J STD AIDS 1990; 1:86–94. (Level III)

35. Shoubnikova M, Hellberg D, Nilsson S, Mardh PA. Contraceptive use in women with bacterial vaginosis. Contraception 1997;55:355–8. (Level II-2)

36. Hodoglugil NN, Aslan D, Bertan M. Intrauterine device use and some issues related to sexually transmitted disease screening and occurrence. Contraception 2000;61: 359–64. (Level II-2)

37. Walsh T, Grimes D, Frezieres R, Nelson A, Bernstein L, Coulson A, et al. Randomised controlled trial of prophylactic antibiotics before insertion of intrauterine devices. IUD Study Group. Lancet 1998;351:1005–8. (Level I)

38. Ladipo OA, Farr G, Otolorin E, Konje JC, Sturgen K, Cox P, et al. Prevention of IUD-related pelvic infection: the efficacy of prophylactic doxycycline at IUD insertion. Adv Contracept 1991;7:43–54. (Level I)

39. Zorlu CG, Aral K, Cobanoglu O, Gurler S, Gokmen O. Pelvic inflammatory disease and intrauterine devices: prophylactic antibiotics to reduce febrile complications. Adv Contracept 1993;9:299–302. (Level II-2)

40. Dajani AS, Taubert KA, Wilson W, Bolger AF, Bayer A, Ferrieri P, et al. Prevention of bacterial endocarditis. Recommendations by the American Heart Association. JAMA 1997;277:1794–801. (Level III)

41. Evans DT. Actinomyces israelii in the female genital tract: a review. Genitourin Med 1993;69:54–9. (Level III)

42. Merki-Feld GS, Lebeda E, Hogg B, Keller PJ. The incidence of actinomyces-like organisms in Papanicolaou-stained smears of copper- and levonorgestrel-releasing intrauterine devices. Contraception 2000;61:365–8. (Level III)

43. Valicenti JF Jr, Pappas AA, Graber CD, Williamson HO, Willis NF. Detection and prevalence of IUD-associated Actinomyces colonization and related morbidity. A prospective study of 69,925 cervical smears. JAMA 1982;247:1149–52. (Level II-2)

44. Lippes J. Pelvic actinomycosis: a review and preliminary look at prevalence. Am J Obstet Gynecol 1999;180: 265–9. (Level III)

45. Bonacho I, Pita S, Gomez-Besteiro MI. The importance of the removal of the intrauterine device in genital colonization by actinomyces. Gynecol Obstet Invest 2001;52: 119–23. (Level I)

46. Xiong X, Buekens P, Wollast E. IUD use and the risk of ectopic pregnancy: a meta-analysis of case-control studies. Contraception 1995;52:23–34. (Meta-analysis)

47. Sivin I. Dose- and age-dependent ectopic pregnancy risks with intrauterine contraception. Obstet Gynecol 1991;78: 291–8. (Level III)

48. Sivin I, Stern J. Health during prolonged use of levonorgestrel 20 micrograms/d and the copper TCu 380Ag intrauterine contraceptive devise: a multicenter study. International Committee for Contraception Research (ICCR). Fertil Steril 1994;61:70–7. (Level I)

49. World Health Organization. Medical eligibility criteria for contraceptive use. 3rd ed. Geneva: WHO; 2004. (Level III)

50. Foreman H, Bruce SV, Schlesselman S. Intrauterine device usage and fetal loss. Obstet Gynecol 1981;58: 669–77. (Level II-2)

51. Tatum HJ, Schmidt FH, Jain AK. Management and outcome of pregnancies associated with the Copper T intrauterine contraceptive device. Am J Obstet Gynecol 1976;126:869–79. (Level II-3)

52. Skjeldestad FE, Hammervold R, Peterson DR. Outcomes of pregnancy with an IUD in situ—a population based case-control study. Adv Contracept 1988;4:265–70. (Level II-2)

53. Christian CD. Maternal deaths associated with an intrauterine device. Am J Obstet Gynecol 1974;119:441–4. (Level III)

54. Food and Drug Administration. Second report on intrauterine contraceptive devices. Washington, DC: FDA; 1978. (Level III)

55. Andersson K, Odlind V, Rybo G. Levonorgestrel-releasing and copper-releasing (Nova T) IUDs during five years of use: a randomized comparative trial. Contraception 1994;49:56–72. (Level I)

56. Sivin I, Stern J, Coutinho E, Mattos CE, el Mahgoub S, Diaz S, et al. Prolonged intrauterine contraception: a seven-year randomized study of the levonorgestrel 20

57. Ronnerdag M, Odlind V. Health effects of long-term use of the intrauterine levonorgestrel-releasing system. A follow-up study over 12 years of continuous use. Acta Obstet Gynccol Scand 1999;78:716–21. (Level III)

58. Sivin I, Stern J, Diaz J, Diaz MM, Faundes A, el Mahgoub S, et al. Two years of intrauterine contraception with levonorgestrel and with copper: a randomized comparison of the TCU 380Ag and levonorgestrel 20 mcg/day devices. Contraception 1987;35:245–55. (Level I)

59. Lethaby AE, Cooke I, Rees M. Progesterone/progestogen releasing intrauterine systems for heavy menstrual bleeding (Cochrane Review). In: The Cochrane Library, Issue 3, 2004. Chichester, UK: John Wiley & Sons, Ltd. (Meta-analysis)

60. Istre O, Trolle B. Treatment of menorrhagia with the levonorgestrel intrauterine system versus endometrial resection. Fertil Steril 2001;76:304–9. (Level I)

61. Lahteenmaki P, Haukkamaa M, Puolakka J, Riikonen U, Sainio S, Suvisaari, et al. Open randomised study of use of levonorgestrel releasing intrauterine system as alternative to hysterectomy. BMJ 1998;316:1122–6. (Level I)

62. Crosignani PG, Vercellini P, Mosconi P, Oldani S, Cortesi I, De Giorgi O. Levonorgestrel-releasing intrauterine device versus hysteroscopic endometrial resection in the treatment of dysfunctional uterine bleeding. Obstet Gynecol 1997;90:257–63. (Level I)

63. Irvine GA, Campbell-Brown MB, Lumsden MA, Heikkila A, Walker JJ, Cameron IT. Randomised comparative trial of the levonorgestrel intrauterine system and norethisterone for the treatment of idiopathic menorrhagia. Br J Obstet Gynaecol 1998;105:592–8. (Level I)

64. Kittelsen N, Istre O. A randomized study comparing levonorgestrel intrauterine system (LNG IUS) and transcervical resection of the endometrium (TCRE) in the treatment of menorrhagia: preliminary results. Gynaecol Endosc 1998;7:61–5. (Level I)

65. Barrington JW, Bowen-Simpkins P. The levonorgestrel intrauterine system in the management of menorrhagia. Br J Obstet Gynaecol 1997;104:614–6. (Level II-2)

66. Tang GW, Lo SS. Levonorgestrel intrauterine device in the treatment of menorrhagia in Chinese women: efficacy versus acceptability. Contraception 1995;51:231–5. (Level III)

67. Andersson JK, Rybo G. Levonorgestrel-releasing intrauterine device in the treatment of menorrhagia. Br J Obstet Gynaecol 1990;97:690–4. (Level II-2)

68. Hurskainen R, Teperi J, Rissanen P, Aalto AM, Grenman S, Kivela A, et al. Quality of life and cost-effectiveness of levonorgestrel-releasing intrauterine system versus hysterectomy for treatment of menorrhagia: a randomised trial. Lancet 2001;357:273–7. (Level I)

69. Ozalp S, Kabukcuoglu S, Tanir HM. Should endometrial hyperplasia be regarded as a reason for abnormal uterine bleeding in users of the intrauterine contraceptive device? Eur J Contracept Reprod Health Care 2003;8:17–20. (Level II-3)

70. Yeguez JF, Martinez SA, Sands LR, Hellinger MD. Pelvic actinomycosis presenting as malignant large bowel obstruction: a case report and a review of the literature. Am Surg 2000;66:85–90. (Level III)

71. Laurent T, de Grandi P, Schnyder P. Abdominal actinomycosis associated with intrauterine device: CT features. Eur Radiol 1996;6:670–3. (Level III)

72. Nugteren SK, Ouwendijk RJ, Jonkman JG, Straub M, Dees A. Colitis and lower abdominal mass by Actinomyces israelii in a patient with an IUD. Neth J Med 1996; 49:73–6. (Level III)

73. Lippes J, Malik T, Tatum HJ. The post-coital copper-T. Adv Plan Parent 1976;11:24–9. (Level III)

74. Trussell J, Leveque JA, Koenig JD, London R, Borden S, Henneberry J, et al. The economic value of contraception: a comparison of 15 methods. Am J Public Health 1995;85: 494–503. (Level III)

The MEDLINE database, the Cochrane Library, and ACOG's own internal resources and documents were used to conduct a literature search to locate relevant articles published between January 1985 and September 2004. The search was restricted to articles published in the English language. Priority was given to articles reporting results of original research, although review articles and commentaries also were consulted. Abstracts of research presented at symposia and scientific conferences were not considered adequate for inclusion in this document. Guidelines published by organizations or institutions such as the National Institutes of Health and the American College of Obstetricians and Gynecologists were reviewed, and additional studies were located by reviewing bibliographies of identified articles. When reliable research was not available, expert opinions from obstetrician–gynecologists were used.

Studies were reviewed and evaluated for quality according to the method outlined by the U.S. Preventive Services Task Force:

I   Evidence obtained from at least 1 properly designed randomized controlled trial.

II-1   Evidence obtained from well-designed controlled trials without randomization.

II-2   Evidence obtained from well-designed cohort or case–control analytic studies, preferably from more than 1 center or research group.

II-3   Evidence obtained from multiple time series with or without the intervention. Dramatic results in uncontrolled experiments also could be regarded as this type of evidence.

III   Opinions of respected authorities, based on clinical experience, descriptive studies, or reports of expert committees.

Based on the highest level of evidence found in the data, recommendations are provided and graded according to the following categories:

Level A—Recommendations are based on good and consistent scientific evidence.

Level B—Recommendations are based on limited or inconsistent scientific evidence.

Level C—Recommendations are based primarily on consensus and expert opinion.

ISSN 1099-3630

The American College of Obstetricians and Gynecologists
409 12th Street, SW, PO Box 96920, Washington, DC 20090-6920

12345/98765

Intrauterine device. ACOG Practice Bulletin No. 59. American College of Obstetricians and Gynecologists. Obstet Gynecol 2005;105:223–32.

ACOG PRACTICE BULLETIN

CLINICAL MANAGEMENT GUIDELINES FOR
OBSTETRICIAN–GYNECOLOGISTS

NUMBER 12, JANUARY 2000

This Practice Bulletin was developed by the ACOG Committee on Practice Bulletins—Obstetrics with the assistance of Susan M. Cox, MD. The information is designed to aid practitioners in making decisions about appropriate obstetric and gynecologic care. These guidelines should not be construed as dictating an exclusive course of treatment or procedure. Variations in practice may be warranted based on the needs of the individual patient, resources, and limitations unique to the institution or type of practice.

Intrauterine Growth Restriction

Intrauterine growth restriction (IUGR) is one of the most common and complex problems in modern obstetrics. Diagnosis and management are complicated by the use of ambiguous terminology and a lack of uniform diagnostic criteria. In addition, some authors do not make a clear distinction between suspected prenatal growth restriction and confirmed IUGR in the perinatal period. Furthermore, size alone is not an indication of a complication. As a result of this confusion, underintervention and overintervention can occur. This bulletin will focus on the etiology, diagnosis, and management of intrauterine growth restriction.

Background

Definitions

Several factors have contributed to the confusion in terminology associated with IUGR:

- By definition, 10% of infants in any population will have birth weights at or below the 10th percentile. Intrauterine growth restriction could be manifest at a weight above the population determined at the 10th percentile (eg, an undernourished infant born at the 15th percentile whose genetic makeup would have placed it at the 90th percentile). Distinctions between normal and pathologic growth often cannot reliably be made in clinical practice, especially prior to birth.

- Although defining a pathologic condition using a 10th percentile cutoff makes statistical sense, it may not be clinically relevant. One study suggests that adverse perinatal outcome generally is confined to those infants with birth weights below the 5th percentile, and in most cases below the 3rd percentile (1).

- Although specific ethnic- and geographic-based growth curves are increasingly used to evaluate birth weight, it remains unclear whether this is appropriate. These distinctions become even more difficult in ethnically heterogeneous and geographically mobile populations, such as those in the United States. Birth weight also is related to maternal height, parity, paternal height, and the fetus' sex.

The use of the terms "small for gestational age" (SGA) and "intrauterine growth restriction" has been confusing, and the terms often are used interchangeably. For the purpose of this document, SGA will be used only in reference to the infant and IUGR to the fetus.

Small for Gestational Age

Infants with a birth weight at the lower extreme of the normal birth weight distribution are termed SGA. In the United States, the most commonly used definition of SGA is a birth weight below the 10th percentile for gestational age (2, 3).

Intrauterine Growth Restriction

Intrauterine growth restriction is a term used to describe a fetus whose estimated weight appears to be less than expected, usually less than the 10th percentile, which is the convention this document will adopt. The term IUGR includes normal fetuses at the lower end of the growth spectrum, as well as those with specific clinical conditions in which the fetus fails to achieve its inherent growth potential as a consequence of either pathologic extrinsic influences (such as maternal smoking) or intrinsic genetic defects (such as aneuploidy).

Etiology

Several conditions have been found to be associated with IUGR (see the box). These antecedents can be divided into several broad categories: maternal, fetal, or placental. Maternal behavioral conditions include substance use (including smoking and alcohol use) (4–6), extremes of reproductive age (younger than 16 years and older than 35 years), little maternal weight gain (7), malnutrition, and low prepregnancy weight (7). In addition, low socioeconomic status is associated with IUGR (7).

Maternal Medical Conditions

Medical complications that affect the microcirculation causing fetal hypoxemia or vasoconstriction or a reduction in fetal perfusion also are significantly associated with IUGR (8). These include hypertension, both chronic and acute (as in preeclampsia) (9), and severe chronic diseases, such as renal insufficiency (10), systemic lupus

---

Risk Factors for Intrauterine Growth Restriction

- Maternal medical conditions
  - Hypertension
  - Renal disease
  - Restrictive lung disease
  - Diabetes (with microvascular disease)
  - Cyanotic heart disease
  - Antiphospholipid syndrome
  - Collagen-vascular disease
  - Hemoglobinopathies
- Smoking and substance use and abuse
- Severe malnutrition
- Primary placental disease
- Multiple gestation
- Infections (viral, protozoal)
- Genetic disorders
- Exposure to teratogens

---

erythematosus, antiphospholipid antibody syndrome, chronic anemia, and pregestational diabetes (especially White's classifications C, D, F, and R). Growth restriction may be preceded by defective maternal volume adaptation in early pregnancy (11, 12).

Placental association with IUGR is unique in that it can be the primary cause (eg, mosaicism) or merely involved in an adaptive process of a pregnancy complication. The placenta and impaired placental perfusion are the most common cause of SGA in nonanomalous infants (13), as seen in early-onset preeclampsia, which produces the most severe IUGR (14). Intrauterine growth restriction also is related to other placental abnormalities, including partial abruptions, previa, infarcts, and hematomas (15). In unexplained IUGR, placental mosaicism may be identified in up to 25% of patients (16). Factors not associated with IUGR include caffeine use in nonsmokers (6, 17) and passive smoking (18).

Substance Use and Abuse

Maternal alcohol abuse is associated with impaired fetal growth; virtually all neonates with fetal alcohol syndrome will exhibit significant growth restriction (6, 19). It is unknown whether a threshold effect exists for alcohol, but effects on the fetus are related to the amount consumed.

Women who smoke have a 3.5-fold increase of SGA infants, compared with nonsmokers (9). Newborns of smokers are smaller at every gestational age. Women who stop smoking before 16 weeks of gestation have infants with birth weights similar to those of babies of women who never smoked (20), and women who quit as late as the seventh month have mean birth weights higher than those who smoked during the entire pregnancy (21).

The incidence of IUGR is markedly increased in pregnant women who use illicit drugs, but it is difficult to differentiate the drug effect from the effects of other behaviors associated with drug use. The incidence of SGA infants in mothers with heroin addiction is as high as 50% (22) and is reported to be as high as 35% in patients managed with methadone (23). Cocaine abuse in pregnancy is associated with delivery of an SGA neonate in 30% or more of cases (24).

Malnutrition

There is a common belief that severe maternal malnutrition will result in fetal growth restriction. The data from studies of the Siege of Leningrad during World War II (25) and the Dutch famine of the same period (26) suggest that maternal intake must be reduced to below 1,500 kilocalories per day before a measurable effect on birth weight becomes evident. In these studies, it is not entirely clear, however, how much of the effect on birth weight was the result of IUGR and how much the result of preterm delivery.

Although low prepregnancy weight and low maternal weight gain have been positively associated with an increase in IUGR (7, 27, 28), and increased weight gain has been associated with decreased IUGR in some populations (29), there is as yet no demonstration that altering dietary recommendations or habits can affect birth weight in a positive manner. Rather, although there are associations between maternal prepregnancy weight, maternal weight gain, and birth weight, there has been no trial showing that any intervention to alter pregnancy weight gain has a beneficial effect on fetal weight gain.

Placental Disease

Primary placental disease (such as chorioangioma) is a rare but recognized cause of growth restriction (30). Placenta previa has been associated with an increase in growth restriction, presumably secondary to abnormal placental implantation. Confined placental mosaicism has been identified three times more frequently from placentas of SGA infants than in infants of normal growth (16).

Multiple Gestation

Intrauterine growth restriction is a common complication of multiple gestation. It is more pronounced in higher order multiple gestations when compared with twin gestations (31). Investigators have reported a greater likelihood of IUGR among surviving fetuses after multifetal reduction (32, 33). The growth restriction is a result of placental reserve inadequate to sustain the normal growth of more than one fetus. Growth restriction can occur in dizygotic twin gestations but is more common and severe in monozygotic twins. It is evident that equal sharing of functional placental mass is not the norm; rather, one twin is more likely to have a larger share of functional placental mass than the other (31).

Infections

Viral infections have been estimated to be etiologic in less than 5% of all growth-restricted fetuses (34). However, when evaluated in documented cases of in utero viral infection, the frequency of IUGR can be strikingly high. Fetal rubella infection is associated with growth restriction in up to 60% of cases (35). Cytomegalovirus also is a recognized cause of growth restriction (36). In one study, approximately 40% of fetuses with varicella syndrome exhibited growth restriction (37). Bacterial infections have not been shown to cause growth restriction. Some protozoal infections, such as *Toxoplasma gondii, Trypanosoma cruzi* (Chagas disease), and syphilis, are associated with growth restriction (38, 39).

Genetic Disorders

Chromosome anomalies are a major cause of IUGR (40, 41). Many fetal structural anomalies also are associated with an increased risk of growth restriction, with a relative risk ranging from as high as 24.7 with anencephaly to as low as 1.2 with pyloric stenosis (42).

Exposure to Teratogens

Maternal ingestion of certain medications is a recognized cause of growth restriction; the incidence and severity vary by substance, gestational age at exposure, duration of exposure, and dosage. Therapeutic agents known to be associated with growth restriction include anticonvulsants (eg, trimethadione, phenytoin) (43–45), folic acid antagonists (eg, methotrexate) (46), and warfarin (47, 48).

Morbidity and Mortality

Fetal Morbidity and Mortality

Perinatal morbidity and mortality is significantly increased in the presence of low birth weight for gestational age, especially with weights below the 3rd percentile for gestational age (1). One study found that 26% of all stillbirths were SGA (49). The risk of death in the presence of IUGR also is affected by gestational age and the primary etiology and may be further modified by the severity and progression of associated maternal etiologic factors (eg, hypertension) (50) (see Table 1).

Both intrapartum and neonatal complications are increased in the presence of IUGR. During labor, up to 50% of growth-restricted fetuses exhibit abnormal heart rate patterns, most often variable decelerations, and such fetuses have an increased cesarean delivery rate (51, 52). Oligohydramnios is a common finding in growth-restricted fetuses and may render the umbilical cord vulnerable to compression (53–55). Sustained antepartum cord compression in growth-restricted fetuses is a presumed cause of sudden fetal death (51, 55). Incidences of low Apgar scores and cord blood acidemia increase significantly in SGA neonates (56).

Neonatal Morbidity

Neonatal complications in the SGA infant include polycythemia, hyperbilirubinemia, hypoglycemia, hypothermia, and apneic episodes (57, 58), as well as low Apgar scores, umbilical artery pH less than 7.0, need for intubation in the delivery room, seizures, sepsis, and neonatal death (1). It is uncertain whether IUGR accelerates fetal pulmonary maturity. One study found a decreased incidence of both respiratory distress syndrome and intraventricular hemorrhage in infants with SGA compared with a control group of infants of appropriate size for their gestational age (59). In contrast, other studies failed to document a difference in lung profile in a matched series (60) and found no difference in the need for ventilatory support in newborns with SGA when compared with controls. The use of glucocorticoids in fetuses with IUGR has not been studied, but current recommendations are to give glucocorticoids to women with

complicated pregnancies who are likely to deliver before 34 weeks of gestation (61).

Long-term development of infants born with SGA depends in part on the cause of the growth failure. In infants with karyotype abnormalities or viral infection, the etiology rather than the weight percentile ultimately will determine the outcome. There are conflicting data on whether infants catch up in growth. Most otherwise normal infants with SGA secondary to placental insufficiency will exhibit normal catch-up growth by the age of 2 years, although this pattern may not be seen universally in severely affected infants (58, 62–64) or in preterm growth-restricted infants (65). A comparison of 714 neonates of appropriate size for age with 347 SGA neonates, derived from several studies, indicated a twofold increase of major neurologic sequelae among SGA infants (54). There is no evidence to suggest that any specific management scheme or delivery route prevents neurologic injury in such fetuses. Long-term follow-up of infants with SGA shows that they are more prone to develop adult-onset hypertension and cardiovascular complications (66). It is important to note that IUGR and SGA both have a multitude of etiologies, and there is a danger in grouping them. There may be no consequences of low birth weight under some circumstances; under others, it may be devastating.

Antenatal Diagnosis of Intrauterine Growth Restriction

There are two essential steps involved in the antenatal recognition of growth restriction. The first step involves the elucidation of maternal risk factors associated with growth restriction and the clinical assessment of uterine size in relation to gestational age. The second step involves the ultrasonographic assessment of fetal size and growth, supplemented by invasive fetal testing for aneuploidy or viral infection in select cases.

Clinical Evaluation

The key physical finding in IUGR is a uterine size that is smaller than expected for gestational age. Several methods are available for clinical determination of uterine size, the most common of which is an objective measurement of fundal height. Such techniques, however, are prone to considerable inaccuracy and should be used for screening only, not as a sole guide to obstetric management in the presence of risk factors for or suspicions of IUGR. These inaccuracies are revealed in clinical studies suggesting that growth restriction is undetected in about one third of cases and is incorrectly diagnosed about 50% of the time (3, 67).

Table 1. Corrected Perinatal Mortality Rates (Excluding Lethal Anomaly) Among Low-risk and High-risk (Screened/Unscreened) Pregnancies and Among SGA Fetuses (Screened/Unscreened), Manitoba Experience

Category	Number of Cases	Corrected Perinatal Mortality Rates (per 1,000 live births)
All cases	144,786	5.6
All low risk	101,350	3.8
All high risk	43,436	9.8
Screened high risk	31,740	2.2
All SGA (7% total population)	10,135	17.8
Unscreened SGA	7,460	21.3
Screened SGA*	2,675	8.4

* Serial fetal assessment management by fetal biophysical profile score.

Manning FA. Intrauterine growth retardation, etiology, pathophysiology, diagnosis, and treatment. In: Fetal medicine: principles and practice. Norwalk, Connecticut: Appleton & Lange, 1995:372

Prior to birth, the diagnosis of IUGR is not precise. Currently, the use of ultrasonographically estimated fetal weight, head- or femur-to-abdomen ratios, or serial observation of biometric growth patterns (growth velocity) are all acceptable and widely used methods to diagnose IUGR (68–72). This document does not address the concept of asymmetrical versus symmetrical IUGR, because it is unclear whether the distinction is important with respect to etiology or neonatal outcome.

Four standard fetal measurements generally are obtained as part of any complete obstetric ultrasound examination after the first trimester: 1) fetal abdominal circumference, 2) head circumference, 3) biparietal diameter, and 4) femur length (73). Fetal morphologic parameters can be converted to fetal weight estimates using published formulas and tables (74). An abdominal circumference within the normal range reliably excludes growth restriction with a false-negative rate of less than 10% (71). A small abdominal circumference or fetal weight estimate below the 10th percentile suggests the possibility of growth restriction, with the likelihood increasing as the percentile rank decreases (71). When IUGR is suspected, serial measurements of fetal biometric parameters provide an estimated growth rate. Such serial measurements are of considerable clinical value in confirming or excluding the diagnosis and assessing the progression and severity of growth restriction. Given the high incidence of genetic and structural defects associated with IUGR, a detailed ultrasound survey for the presence of fetal structural and functional defects may be indicated.

Amniotic fluid volume is an important diagnostic and prognostic parameter in fetuses with IUGR (75, 76). Oligohydramnios is highly suggestive of growth failure and indicates an increased risk of fetal death. Oligohydramnios is diagnosed ultrasonographically in approximately 77–83% of pregnancies with growth-restricted fetuses (75–77). In contrast, amniotic fluid volume often is normal even in a fetus with significant growth restriction; thus, the absence of oligohydramnios should not detract from the diagnosis of IUGR.

Although Doppler velocimetry of the umbilical arteries is not useful as a screening technique for IUGR (78, 79), it has been demonstrated to be useful once IUGR has been diagnosed. Not only are Doppler velocimetry findings normal in growth-restricted fetuses with chromosomal or other structural etiologies (80) but Doppler velocimetry has been shown to both reduce interventions and improve fetal outcome in pregnancies at risk for IUGR (81). Thus, once IUGR is suspected or diagnosed, Doppler velocimetry may be useful as a part of fetal evaluation. Fetuses with normal flow patterns seem less likely to benefit from consideration of early delivery than do their counterparts with abnormal studies.

Clinical Considerations and Recommendations

▶ *Which pregnancies should be screened for intrauterine growth restriction, and how is screening accomplished?*

Unfortunately, approximately one half of growth-restricted fetuses are not diagnosed until delivery. In essence, all pregnancies are screened for IUGR using serial fundal height measurements. A single measurement at 32–34 weeks of gestation is approximately 70–85% sensitive and 96% specific for detecting the growth-restricted fetus (82). A third-trimester ultrasound examination, with a single measurement of abdominal circumference, detects about 80% of IUGR fetuses (70). Even so, this does not justify ultrasonography as a screening tool, because fundal height measurement performs comparably (70). All pregnancies should be screened with serial fundal height assessments, reserving ultrasonography for those with risk factors, lagging growth, or no growth (69, 83, 84).

Women who have previously given birth to an SGA infant are at an increased risk for this condition in subsequent pregnancies (9). Physicians should consider an early ultrasound examination to confirm gestational age, as well as subsequent ultrasonography to evaluate sequential fetal growth, in women with significant risk factors.

▶ *What are the best ways to evaluate and monitor a pregnancy complicated by suspected intrauterine growth restriction?*

Once IUGR is suspected (ie, lagging fundal height), it should be confirmed using multiple ultrasonographic parameters, such as estimated weight percentile, amniotic fluid volume, elevated head circumference and abdominal circumference ratio, and possibly Doppler criteria (ie, elevated systolic–diastolic ratio or reversed or absent enddiastolic flow) (85). Identification of IUGR is improved by recording growth velocity or through two sets of examinations generally 2–4 weeks apart.

The diagnosis of IUGR as the fetus approaches term may be an indication for delivery (86). If pregnancy is remote from term or if delivery is not elected, the optimal mode of monitoring has not been established. Periodic fetal assessment (approximately weekly) using Doppler velocimetry, contraction stress test, traditional biophysical profile (BPP), modified BPP, or nonstress test (NST) are all accepted monitoring techniques. Randomized controlled trials have demonstrated that monitoring with Doppler velocimetry reduces the risk of perinatal morbidity (81). Comparable studies for the other methods have not been done.

Serial ultrasonograms to determine the rate of growth should be obtained approximately every 2–4 weeks. Measurements at shorter intervals (<2 weeks) may overlap with measurement errors. If any test result is abnormal (decreased amniotic fluid volume or low BPP scores), more frequent testing, possibly daily, may be indicated. An abnormal result from fetal heart rate testing (decreased variability) coupled with abnormal results from Doppler velocimetry suggests poor fetal well-being and a potential need for delivery, despite prematurity (72).

▶ *What interventions improve pregnancy outcome in cases of intrauterine growth restriction or suspected intrauterine growth restriction?*

Evidence from randomized controlled trials finds few interventions beneficial in preventing or treating IUGR. Avoidance of smoking during pregnancy has been shown to have a positive effect on birth weight (20). Treatment of infections such as malaria in endemic areas has been shown to be of some benefit (87, 88).

A number of interventions have been suggested for which there is insufficient evidence from randomized clinical trials to conclude either benefit or harm. Among them are bed rest, which demonstrated no benefit in one small study (89), and early delivery in the presence of pulsatile flow in waveforms from the umbilical vein, which remains to be assessed in a randomized control trial. Other interventions of questionable efficacy and safety include nutrient treatment or supplementation (90), zinc supplementation (91), calcium supplementation (92), plasma volume expansion (93), maternal oxygen therapy (94), heparin (47), and low-dose aspirin (95–99). Thus, such interventions should be used only in experimental protocols.

▶ *Is there any evidence that prenatal diagnosis or suspicion of intrauterine growth restriction with antenatal surveillance alters outcome?*

The nonanomalous fetus with IUGR should be monitored serially for risk of perinatal mortality and morbidity. Risk to the fetus can be determined by several methods: traditional or modified BPP, contraction stress test, NST, amniotic fluid volume, or Doppler velocimetry of fetal vessels. Unfortunately, these tests are performed to determine the optimal time for delivery and are not predictive of individual fetuses at greatest risk for a complicated neonatal course (100).

There are no randomized trials of interventions in a fetus with abnormal heart rate tracings. Thus, in the case of a very premature infant, delivery or expectant manage-

ment are the usual courses of action at present. Overall experience with the NST confirms that with a reactive NST the fetus is not likely to die in utero immediately. In several studies, nonreactive or abnormal NSTs were found in fetuses with acidosis, hypoxemia, or both (101, 102). In four randomized clinical trials comparing BPP with conventional fetal monitoring in high-risk pregnancies (including those with IUGR), there was no obvious benefit for pregnancy outcome using BPP for surveillance (103), although different results might have been obtained in an IUGR-only population.

Doppler ultrasound has been shown to be useful in the assessment of the growth-restricted fetus (104). Absent or reversed end-diastolic flow velocities in the umbilical arteries have a poor positive predictive value but are associated with poor perinatal outcome and high perinatal mortality (105–107). In contrast, a normal systolic–diastolic ratio in a growth-restricted fetus has excellent negative predictive value and may be used as a rationale to delay delivery with some reassurance. Currently, there are not enough data to warrant cordocentesis in the management of IUGR.

With the exception of Manning's data, which includes IUGR among other high-risk conditions, there is no evidence that antenatal surveillance in fetuses with suspected IUGR alters perinatal outcome. Instead, it is used to predict which fetuses are at risk for in utero demise and thus may potentially benefit from preterm delivery. Currently, there are no intrauterine therapies available for affected fetuses; therefore, delivery is the optimal treatment in the mature fetus, but must be weighed against gestational age for the immature fetus.

▶ *How does knowledge of the etiology of intrauterine growth restriction alter management?*

If maternal medical conditions are thought to be the cause of IUGR, there is no evidence that changes in maternal medical management other than delivery alter outcome. For example, antihypertensive therapy has not been shown to have a benefit with respect to IUGR (108). However, it is still important to optimize maternal treatment.

Although the etiology and manifestations of IUGR are numerous, a concerted effort should be made to determine the underlying cause. If a lethal anomaly is identified, one would not usually undertake antepartum surveillance.

A detailed ultrasound survey should be performed to detect fetal structural defects. Fetal karyotype determinations are not routinely indicated in the assessment of growth-restricted fetuses, but should be considered when early or severe IUGR is detected or when the fetus has a recognized structural anomaly. It is estimated that about 10% of structurally abnormal fetuses with fetal growth restriction will have a karyotype anomaly.

Prenatal diagnosis of in utero infections also can be accomplished via amniotic fluid or fetal blood analyses. Viral infections associated with IUGR, such as rubella, cytomegalovirus, or varicella, can be diagnosed by polymerase chain reaction or by measuring viral-specific immunoglobulin M antibodies. There are, however, no in utero treatments for these infections. However, if toxoplasmosis is identified, medication taken by the mother may prevent the spread of maternal infection to the fetus (38).

▶ *When should a growth-restricted fetus be delivered?*

The fetus should be delivered if the risk of fetal death exceeds that of neonatal death, although in many cases these risks are difficult to assess. The timing of delivery in the growth-restricted fetus should be individualized. Early delivery may yield an infant with all the serious sequelae of prematurity, whereas delaying delivery may yield a hypoxic, acidotic infant with long-term neurologic sequelae. Gestational age and the findings of antenatal surveillance should be taken into account. The decision to deliver is based often on nonreassuring fetal assessment or a complete cessation of fetal growth assessed ultrasonographically over a 2–4-week interval. When extrauterine survival is likely despite significantly abnormal antenatal testing, delivery should be seriously considered.

Summary

The general approach to management of the fetus with ultrasonographically suspected IUGR involves risk factor modification when possible and the initiation of antepartum fetal surveillance, ultrasonography, and delivery when the risks of continued in utero development outweigh the benefits.

The risks to the growth-impaired fetus are well documented. Currently, although the incidence of IUGR has not changed appreciably, the prognosis for SGA infants has improved dramatically. It must be emphasized, however, that perinatal morbidity and mortality will continue to occur despite optimal management of the fetus with suspected IUGR. In those fetuses managed expectantly, antepartum injury or death may occur because current methods of fetal surveillance are less than perfect in the prediction of fetal outcome.

The following recommendations are based on good and consistent scientific evidence (Level A):

▶ The use of Doppler ultrasonography to measure umbilical artery waveforms in the management of IUGR is associated with a reduction in perinatal death, and may be considered a part of fetal evaluation once IUGR is suspected or diagnosed.

▶ Nutrient treatment or supplementation, zinc or calcium supplementation, plasma volume expansion, maternal oxygen therapy, antihypertensive therapy, heparin, and aspirin therapy have not been shown to be effective for prevention or treatment of IUGR.

The following recommendations are based primarily on consensus and expert opinion (Level C):

▶ Antepartum surveillance should be instituted once the possibility of extrauterine survival for the growth-restricted fetus has been determined. This may include Doppler velocimetry, contraction stress testing, NST with amniotic fluid volume assessment, and BPP.

▶ Routine screening for IUGR in low-risk patients should comprise classical clinical monitoring techniques. Ultrasound evaluation of the fetus is appropriate in patients determined to be at high risk.

References

1. McIntire DD, Bloom SL, Casey BM, Leveno KJ. Birth weight in relation to morbidity and mortality among newborn infants. N Engl J Med 1999;340:1234–1238 (Level II-2)
2. Battaglia FC, Lubchenco LO. A practical classification of newborn infants by weight and gestational age. J Pediatr 1967;71:159–163 (Level III)
3. Jahn A, Razum O, Berle P. Routine screening for intrauterine growth retardation in Germany: low sensitivity and questionable benefit for diagnosed cases. Acta Obstet Gynecol Scand 1998;77:643–648 (Level II-2)
4. Spinillo A, Capuzzo E, Nicola SE, Colonna L, Egbe TO, Zara C. Factors potentiating the smoking-related risk of fetal growth retardation. Br J Obstet Gynaecol 1994;101:954–958 (Level II-2)
5. Lieberman E, Gremy I, Lang JM, Cohen AP. Low birth weight at term and the timing of fetal exposure to maternal smoking. Am J Public Health 1994;84:1127–1131 (Level II-2)
6. Shu XO, Hatch MC, Mills J, Clemens J, Susser M. Maternal smoking, alcohol drinking, caffeine consumption, and fetal growth: results from a prospective study. Epidemiology 1995;6:115–120 (Level II-3)
7. Nieto A, Matorras R, Serra M, Valenzuela P, Molero J. Multivariate analysis of determinants of fetal growth retardation. Eur J Obstet Gynecol Reprod Biol 1994;53:107–113 (Level II-2)

8. Rotmensch S, Liberati M, Luo JS, Kliman HJ, Gollin Y, Bellati U, et al. Color Doppler flow patterns and flow velocity waveforms of the intraplacental fetal circulation in growth-retarded fetuses. Am J Obstet Gynecol 1994; 171:1257–1264 (Level II-2)

9. Ounsted M, Moar VA, Scott A. Risk factors associated with small-for-dates and large-for-dates infants. Br J Obstet Gynaecol 1985;92:226–232 (Level II-2)

10. Cunningham FG, Cox SM, Harstad TW, Mason RA, Pritchard JA. Chronic renal disease and pregnancy outcome. Am J Obstet Gynecol 1990;163:453–459 (Level II-3)

11. Duvekot JJ, Cheriex EC, Pieters FA, Menheere PP, Schouten HJ, Peeters LL. Maternal volume homeostasis in early pregnancy in relation to fetal growth restriction. Obstet Gynecol 1995;85:361–367 (Level III)

12. Duvekot JJ, Cheriex EC, Pieters FA, Peeters LL. Severely impaired fetal growth is preceded by maternal hemodynamic maladaptation in very early pregnancy. Acta Obstet Gynecol Scand 1995;74:693–697 (Level III)

13. Salafia CM, Minior VK, Pezzullo JC, Popek EJ, Rosenkrantz TS, Vintzileos AM. Intrauterine growth restriction in infants of less than thirty-two weeks' gestation: associated placental pathologic features. Am J Obstet Gynecol 1995;173:1049–1057 (Level III)

14. Ounsted M, Moar V, Scott WA. Perinatal morbidity and mortality in small-for-dates babies: the relative importance of some maternal factors. Early Hum Dev 1981;5:367–375 (Level II-2)

15. Laurini R, Laurin J, Marsal K. Placental histology and fetal blood flow in intrauterine growth retardation. Acta Obstet Gynecol Scand 1994;73:529–534 (Level II-3)

16. Wilkins-Haug L, Roberts DJ, Morton CC. Confined placental mosaicism and intrauterine growth retardation: a case-control analysis of placentas at delivery. Am J Obstet Gynecol 1995;172:44–50 (Level II-2)

17. Cook DG, Peacock JL, Feyerabend C, Carey IM, Jarvis MJ, Anderson HR, et al. Relation of caffeine intake and blood caffeine concentrations during pregnancy to fetal growth: prospective population based study. BMJ 1996; 313:1358–1362 (Level II-3)

18. Fortier I, Marcoux S, Brisson J. Passive smoking during pregnancy and the risk of delivering a small-for-gesta-tion-al-age infant. Am J Epidemiol 1994;139:294–301 (Level II-3)

19. Virji SK. The relationship between alcohol consumption during pregnancy and infant birthweight. An epidemiologic study. Acta Obstet Gynecol Scand 1991;70:303–308 (Level II-3)

20. MacArthur C, Knox EG. Smoking in pregnancy: effects of stopping at different stages. Br J Obstet Gynaecol 1988; 95:551–555 (Level II-2)

21. Rush D, Cassano P. Relationship of cigarette smoking and social class to birth weight and perinatal mortality among all births in Britain, 5-11 April 1970. J Epidemiol Community Health 1983;37:249–255 (Level II-2)

22. Naeye RL, Blanc W, Leblanc W, Khatamee MA. Fetal complications of maternal heroin addiction: abnormal growth, infections and episodes of stress. J Pediatr 1973;83:1055–1061 (Level III)

23. Newman RG, Bashkow S, Calko D. Results of 313 consecutive live births of infants delivered to patients in the New York City Methadone Maintenance Treatment Program. Am J Obstet Gynecol 1975;121:233–237 (Level III)

24. Fulroth R, Phillips B, Durand DJ. Perinatal outcome of infants exposed to cocaine and/or heroin in utero. Am J Dis Child 1989;143:905–910 (Level II-3)

25. Anatov AN. Children born during the siege of Leningrad in 1942. J Pediatr 1947;30:250–259 (Level III)

26. Smith CA. Effect of maternal undernutrition upon the newborn infant in Holland (1944-1945). J Pediatr 1947; 30:229–243 (Level III)

27. Neggers YH, Goldenberg RL, Tamura T, Cliver SP, Hoffman HJ. The relationship between maternal dietary intake and infant birthweight. Acta Obstet Gynecol Scand 1997;165:71–75 (Level II-3)

28. Wen SW, Goldenberg RL, Cutter GR, Hoffman HJ, Cliver SP. Intrauterine growth retardation and preterm delivery: prenatal risk factors in an indigent population. Am J Obstet Gynecol 1990;162:213–218 (Level II-3)

29. Hickey CA, Cliver SP, Goldenberg RL, Kohatsu J, Hoffman HJ. Prenatal weight gain, term birth weight, and fetal growth retardation among high-risk multiparous black and white women. Obstet Gynecol 1993;81: 529–535 (Level II-2)

30. Pollack RN, Divon MY. Intrauterine growth retardation: definition, classification, and etiology. Clin Obstet Gynecol 1992;35:99–107 (Level III)

31. Sassoon DA, Castro LC, Davis JL, Hobel CJ. Perinatal outcome in triplet versus twin gestations. Obstet Gynecol 1990;75:817–820 (Level II-2)

32. Alexander JM, Hammond KR, Steinkampf MP. Multifetal reduction of high-order multiple pregnancy: comparison of obstetrical outcome with nonreduced twin gestations. Fertil Steril 1995;64:1201–1203 (Level II-2)

33. Silver RK, Helfand BT, Russell TL, Ragin A, Sholl JS, MacGregor SN. Multifetal reduction increases the risk of preterm delivery and fetal growth restriction in twins: a case-control study. Fertil Steril 1997;67:30–33 (Level II-2)

34. Klein JO, Remington JS. Current concepts of infections of the fetus and newborn infant. In: Remington JS, Klein JO, eds. Infectious diseases of the fetus & newborn infant. 4th ed. Philadelphia: W.B. Saunders, 1995:1–19 (Level III)

35. Peckham CS. Clinical and laboratory study of children exposed in utero to maternal rubella. Arch Dis Child 1972;47:571–577 (Level II-3)

36. Donner C, Liesnard C, Content J, Busine A, Aderca J, Rodesch F. Prenatal diagnosis of 52 pregnancies at risk for congenital cytomegalovirus infection. Obstet Gynecol 1993;82:481–486

37. Alkalay AL, Pomerance JJ, Rimoin DL. Fetal varicella syndrome. J Pediatr 1987;111:320–323 (Level III)

38. Daffos F, Forestier F, Capella-Pavlovsky M, Thulliez P, Aufrant C, Valenti D, et al. Prenatal management of 746 pregnancies at risk for congenital toxoplasmosis. N Engl J Med 1988;318:271–275 (Level III)

39. Ricci JM, Fojaco RM, O'Sullivan MJ. Congenital syphilis: The University of Miami/Jackson Memorial Medical Center experience, 1986-1988. Obstet Gynecol 1989;74:687–693 (Level II-2)

40. Nicolaides KH, Economides DL, Soothill PW. Blood gases, pH, and lactate in appropriate- and small-for-gestational-age fetuses. Am J Obstet Gynecol 1989;161:996–1001 (Level II-3)

41. van Vugt JM, Karsdorp VH, van Zalen-Sprock RM, van Geijn HP. Fetal growth retardation and structural anomalies. Eur J Obstet Gynecol Reprod Biol 1991;42 Suppl:S79–S83 (Level III)

42. Khoury MJ, Erickson JD, Cordero JF, McCarthy BJ. Congenital malformations and intrauterine growth retardation: a population study. Pediatrics 1988;82:83–90 (Level II-3)

43. Battino D, Granata T, Binelli S, Caccamo ML, Canevini MP, Canger R, et al. Intrauterine growth in the offspring of epileptic mothers. Acta Neurol Scand 1992;86:555–557 (Level III)

44. Hiilesmaa VK, Teramo K, Granstrom ML, Bardy AH. Fetal head growth retardation associated with maternal antiepileptic drugs. Lancet 1981;2:165–167 (Level II-2)

45. Mastroiacovo P, Bertollini R, Licata D. Fetal growth in the offspring of epileptic women: results of an Italian multicentric cohort study. Acta Neurol Scand 1988;78:110–114 (Level II-2)

46. Aviles A, Diaz-Maqueo JC, Talavera A, Guzman R, Garcia EL. Growth and development of children of mothers treated with chemotherapy during pregnancy: current status of 43 children. Am J Hematol 1991;36:243–248 (Level III)

47. Hall JG, Pauli RM, Wilson KM. Maternal and fetal sequelae of anticoagulation during pregnancy. Am J Med 1980;68:122–140 (Level III)

48. Stevenson RE, Burton OM, Ferlauto GJ, Taylor HA. Hazards of oral anticogulants during pregnancy. JAMA 1980;243:1549–1551 (Level III)

49. Morrison I, Olsen J. Weight-specific stillbirths and associated causes of death: an analysis of 765 stillbirths. Am J Obstet Gynecol 1985;152:975–980 (Level III)

50. Piper JM, Langer O, Xenakis EM, McFarland M, Elliott BD, Berkus MD. Perinatal outcome in growth-restricted fetuses: do hypertensive and normotensive pregnancies differ? Obstet Gynecol 1996;88:194–199 (Level II-2)

51. Druzin ML, Gratacos J, Keegan KA, Paul RH. Antepartum fetal heart rate testing. VII. The significance of fetal bradycardia. Am J Obstet Gynecol 1981;139:194–198 (Level III)

52. Bekedam DJ, Visser GH. Effects of hypoxemic events on breathing, body movements, and heart rate variation: a study in growth-retarded human fetuses. Am J Obstet Gynecol 1985;153:52–56 (Level III)

53. Magann EF, Bass JD, Chauham SP, Young RA, Whitworth NS, Morrison JC. Amniotic fluid volume in normal singleton pregnancies. Obstet Gynecol 1997;90:524–528 (Level III)

54. Manning FA, Morrison I, Harman CR, Lange IR, Menticoglou S. Fetal assessment based on the fetal biophysical profile scoring: experience in 19,221 referred high-risk pregnancies. II. An analysis of false-negative fetal deaths. Am J Obstet Gynecol 1987;157:880–884 (Level III)

55. Peipert JF, Donnenfeld AE. Oligohydramnios: a review. Obstet Gynecol Surv 1991;46:325–339 (Level III)

56. Kramer MS, Olivier M, McLean FH, Willis DM, Usher RH. Impact of intrauterine growth retardation and body proportionality on fetal and neonatal outcome. Pediatrics 1990;86:707–713 (Level II-3)

57. Jones RA, Robertson NR. Problems of the small-for-dates baby. Clin Obstet Gynaecol 1984;11:499–524 (Level III)

58. Alkalay AL, Graham JM Jr, Pomerance JJ. Evaluation of neonates born with intrauterine growth retardation: review and practice guidelines. J Perinatol 1998;18:142–151 (Level III)

59. Procianoy RS, Garcia-Prats JA, Adams JM, Silvers A, Rudolph AJ. Hyaline membrane disease and intraventricular haemorrhage in small for gestational age infants. Arch Dis Child 1980;55:502–505 (Level II-2)

60. Piper JM, Langer O. Is lung maturation related to fetal growth in diabetic or hypertensive pregnancies? Eur J Obstet Gynecol Reprod Biol 1993;51:15–19 (Level II-3)

61. Effect of cortiscosteroids for fetal maturation on perinatal outcomes. NIH Consens Statement 1994;12:1–24 (Level III)

62. Fay RA, Ellwood DA. Categories of intrauterine growth retardation. Fetal Matern Med Rev 1993;5:203–212 (Level III)

63. Bergsjo P. Why are some children stunted at birth, and do they catch up with their peers in infancy? Acta Obstet Gynecol Scand Suppl 1997;165:1–2 (Level III)

64. Hadders-Algra M, Touwen BC. Body measurements, neurological and behavioural development in six-year-old children born preterm and/or small-for-gestational-age. Early Hum Dev 1990;22:1–13 (Level II-2)

65. Smedler C, Faxelius G, Bremme K, Lagerstrom M. Psychological development in children born with very low birth weight after severe intrauterine growth retardation: a 10-year follow-up study. Acta Paediatr 1992;81:197–203 (Level III)

66. Barker DJ, Osmond C, Golding J, Kuh D, Wadsworth ME. Growth in utero, blood pressure in childhood and adult life, and mortality from cardiovascular diseases. BMJ 1989;298:564–567 (Level II-3)

67. Kean LH, Liu DT. Antenatal care as a screening tool for the detection of small for gestational age babies in the low risk population. J Obstet Gynaecol 1996;16:77–82 (Level III)

68. Harding K, Evans S, Newnham J. Screening for the small fetus: a study of the relative efficacies of ultrasound biometry and symphysiofundal height. Aust N Z J Obstet Gynaecol 1995;35:160–164 (Level I)

69. Neilson JP, Munjanja SP, Whitfield CR. Screening for small for dates fetuses: a controlled trial. BMJ 1984; 289:1179–1182 (Level II-2)

70. Pearce JM, Campbell S. A comparison of symphysis-fundal height and ultrasound as screening tests for light-for-gestational age infants. Br J Obstet Gynaecol 1987;94: 100–104 (Level II-3)

71. Warsof SL, Cooper DJ, Little D, Campbell R. Routine ultrasound screen for antenatal detection of intrauterine growth restriction. Obstet Gynecol 1986;67:33–39 (Level II-2)

72. Weiner Z, Farmakides G, Schulman H, Lopresti S, Schneider E. Surveillance of growth-retarded fetuses with computerized fetal heart rate monitoring combined with Doppler velocimetry of the umbilical and uterine arteries. J Reprod Med 1996;41:112–118 (Level III)

73. Hadlock FP, Deter RL, Harrist RB, Park SK. Estimating fetal age: computer-assisted analysis of multiple fetal growth parameters. Radiology 1984;152:497–501 (Level II-3)

74. Shepard MJ, Richards VA, Berkowitz RL, Warsof SL, Hobbins JC. An evaluation of two equations for predicting fetal weight by ultrasound. Am J Obstet Gynecol 1982; 142:47–54 (Level III)

75. Chamberlain PF, Manning FA, Morrison I, Harman CR, Lange IR. Ultrasound evaluation of amniotic fluid volume. I. The relationship of marginal and decreased amniotic fluid volumes to perinatal outcome. Am J Obstet Gynecol 1984:150:245–249 (Level II-3)

76. Varma TR. Bateman S, Patel RH, Chamberlain GV, Pillai U. Ultrasound evaluation of amniotic fluid: outcome of pregnancies with severe oligohydramnios. Int J Gynaecol Obstet 1988;27:185–192 (Level II-2)

77. Philipson EH, Sokol RJ, Williams T. Oligohydraminios: clinical associations and predictive value for intrauterine growth retardation. Am J Obstet Gynecol 1983;146: 271–278 (Level II-2)

78. Davies JA, Gallivan S, Spencer JA. Randomised controlled trial of Doppler ultrasound screening of placental perfusion during pregnancy. Lancet 1992;340:1299–1303 (Level I)

79. Low JA. The current status of maternal and fetal blood flow velocimetry. Am J Obstet Gynecol 1991;164: 1049–1063 (Level III)

80. Wladimiroff JW, v.d.Wijngaard JA, Degani S, Noordam MJ, van Eyck J, Tonge HM. Cerebral and umbilical arterial blood flow velocity waveforms in normal and growth-retarded pregnancies. Obstet Gynecol 1987;69:705–709 (Level II-2)

81. Alfirevic Z, Neilson JP. Doppler ultrasonography in high-risk pregnancies: systemic review with meta-analysis. Am J Obstet Gynecol 1995;172:1379–1387 (Meta-analysis)

82. Leeson S, Aziz N. Customised fetal growth assessment. Br J Obstet Gynaecol 1997;104:648–651 (Level III)

83. Ewigman BG, Crane JP, Frigoletto FD, LeFevre ML, Bain RP, McNellis D. Effect of prenatal ultrasound screening on perinatal outcome. RADIUS Study Group. N Engl J Med 1993;329:821–827 (Level I)

84. Newnham JP, Evans SF, Michael CA, Stanley FJ, Landau LI. Effect of frequent ultrasound during pregnancy: a randomised conrolled trial. Lancet 1993;342:887–891 (Level I)

85. Doubilet PM, Benson CB. Sonographic evaluation of intrauterine growth retardation. AJR Am J Roentgenol 1995;164:709–717 (Level III)

86. Snijders R, Hyett J. Fetal testing in intra-uterine growth retardation. Curr Opin Obstet Gynecol 1997;9:91–95 (Level III)

87. Garner P, Brabin B. A review of randomized controlled trials of routine antimalarial drug prophylaxis during pregnancy in endemic malarious areas. Bull World Health Organ 1994;72:89–99 (Level III)

88. Taha Tel T, Gray RH, Mohamedani AA. Malaria and low birth weight in central Sudan. Am J Epidemiol 1993; 138:318–325 (Level II-2)

89. Laurin J, Persson PH. The effect of bedrest in hospital on fetal outcome in pregnancies complicated by intra-uterine growth retardation. Acta Obstet Gynecol Scand 1987; 66:407–411 (Level II-1)

90. Gulmezoglu AM, Hofmeyr GJ. Maternal nutrient supplementation for suspected impaired fetal growth (Cochrane Review). In: The Cochrane Library, Issue 2, 1999. Oxford: Update Software (Meta-analysis)

91. Mahomed K. Zinc supplementation in pregnancy (Cochrane Review). In: The Cochrane Library, Issue 2, 1999. Oxford: Update Software (Meta-analysis)

92. Carroli G, Duley L, Belizan JM, Villar J. Calcium supplementation during pregnancy: a systematic review of randomised controlled trials. Br J Obstet Gynaecol 1994; 101:753–758 (Meta-analysis)

93. Gulmezoglu AM, Hofmeyr GJ. Plasma volume expansion for suspected impaired fetal growth (Cochrane Review). In: The Cochrane Library, Issue 2, 1999. Oxford: Update Software (Level III)

94. Gulmezoglu AM, Hofmeyr GJ. Maternal oxygen administration for suspected impaired fetal growth. (Cochrane Review). In: The Cochrane Library, Issue 2, 1999. Oxford: Update Software (Level III)

95. Bar J, Hod M, Pardo J, Fisch B, Rabinerson D, Kaplan B, et al. Effect on fetal circulation of low-dose aspirin for prevention and treatment of pre-eclampsia and intrauterine growth restriction: Doppler flow study. Ultrasound Obstet Gynecol 1997;9:262–265

96. CLASP: a randomised trial of low-dose aspirin for the prevention and treatment of pre-eclampsia among 9364 pregnant women. CLASP (Collaborative Low-Dose Aspirin Study in Pregnancy) Collaborative Group. Lancet 1994; 343:619–629 (Level I)

97. Golding J. A randomised trial of low dose aspirin for primiparae in pregnancy. The Jamaica Low Dose Aspirin Study Group. Br J Obstet Gynaecol 1998;105:293–299 (Level I)

98. Leitich H, Egarter C, Husslein P, Kaider A, Schemper M. A meta-analysis of low dose aspirin for the prevention of intrauterine growth retardation. Br J Obstet Gynaecol 1997;104:450–459 (Meta-analysis)

99. Newnham JP, Godfrey M, Walters BJ, Phillips J, Evans SF. Low dose aspirin for the treatment of fetal growth restriction: a randomized controlled trial. Aust N Z J Obstet Gynaecol 1995;35:370–374 (Level I)

100. Craigo SD, Beach ML, Harvey-Wilkes KB, D'Alton ME. Ultrasound predictors of neonatal outcome in intrauterine growth restriction. Am J Perinatol 1996;13:465–471 (Level II-3)

101. Visser GH, Sandovsky G, Nicolaides KH. Antepartum fetal heart rate patterns in small-for-gestational-age third-trimester fetuses: correlations with blood gas values obtained at cordocentesis. Am J Obstet Gynecol 1990; 162:698–703 (Level II-2)

102. Donner C, Vermeylen D, Kirkpatrick C, de Maertelaer V, Rodesch F. Management of the growth-restricted fetus: the role of noninvasive tests and fetal blood sampling. Obstet Gynecol 1995;85:965–970 (Level II-3)

103. Alfirevic Z, Neilson JP. Biophysical profile for fetal assessment in high risk pregnancies (Cochrane review). In: The Cochrane Library, Issue 2, 1999. Oxford: Update Software (Meta-analysis)

104. Arduini D, Rizzo G. Doppler studies of deteriorating growth-retarded fetuses. Curr Opin Obstet Gynecol 1993;5:195–203 (Level III)

105. Kingdom JC, Burrell SJ, Kaufmann P. Pathology and clinical implications of abnormal umbilical artery Doppler waveforms. Ultrasound Obstet Gynecol 1997;9:271–286 (Level III)

106. Karsdorp VH, van Vugt JM, van Geijn HP, Kostense PJ, Arduini D, Montenegro N, et al. Clinical significance of absent or reversed end diastolic velocity waveforms in umbilical artery. Lancet 1994;344:1664–1668 (Level II-3)

107. Pardi G, Cetin I, Marconi AM, Lanfranchi A, Bozzetti P, Ferrazzi E, et al. Diagnostic value of blood sampling in fetuses with growth retardation. N Engl J Med 1993; 328:692–696 (Level III)

108. Redman CW. Fetal outcome in trial of antihypertensive treatment in pregnancy. Lancet 1976;2:753–756 (Level II-1)

The MEDLINE database, the Cochrane Library, and ACOG's own internal resources were used to conduct a literature search to locate relevant articles published between January 1985 and March 1999. The search was restricted to articles published in the English language. Priority was given to articles reporting results of original research, although review articles and commentaries also were consulted. Abstracts of research presented at symposia and scientific conferences were not considered adequate for inclusion in this document. Guidelines published by organizations or institutions such as the National Institutes of Health and the American College of Obstetricians and Gynecologists were reviewed, and additional studies were located by reviewing bibliographies of identified articles. When reliable research was not available, expert opinions from obstetrician–gynecologists were used.

Studies were reviewed and evaluated for quality according to the method outlined by the U.S. Preventive Services Task Force:

I   Evidence obtained from at least one properly designed randomized controlled trial.

II-1   Evidence obtained from well-designed controlled trials without randomization.

II-2   Evidence obtained from well-designed cohort or case–control analytic studies, preferably from more than one center or research group.

II-3   Evidence obtained from multiple time series with or without the intervention. Dramatic results in uncontrolled experiments could also be regarded as this type of evidence.

III   Opinions of respected authorities, based on clinical experience, descriptive studies, or reports of expert committees.

Based on the highest level of evidence found in the data, recommendations are provided and graded according to the following categories:

Level A—Recommendations are based on good and consistent scientific evidence.

Level B—Recommendations are based on limited or inconsistent scientific evidence.

Level C—Recommendations are based primarily on consensus and expert opinion.

ISSN 1099-3630

**The American College of
Obstetricians and Gynecologists
409 12th Street, SW
PO Box 96920
Washington, DC 20090-6920**

12345/43210

ACOG PRACTICE BULLETIN

CLINICAL MANAGEMENT GUIDELINES FOR
OBSTETRICIAN–GYNECOLOGISTS

NUMBER 66, SEPTEMBER 2005

This Practice Bulletin was developed by the ACOG Committee on Practice Bulletins— Gynecology with the assistance of Walter Kinney, MD. The information is designed to aid practitioners in making decisions about appropriate obstetric and gynecologic care. These guidelines should not be construed as dictating an exclusive course of treatment or procedure. Variations in practice may be warranted based on the needs of the individual patient, resources, and limitations unique to the institution or type of practice.

Management of Abnormal Cervical Cytology and Histology

Cervical cytology screening has been associated with a dramatic reduction in cervical cancer incidence and mortality. However, screening techniques are fraught with the potential for unnecessary visits, procedures, and patient anxiety (1); conversely, the value of accurate screening results can be reduced by loss to follow-up or undertreatment of significant lesions that may progress to invasive cancer (2). The purpose of this document is to define strategies for diagnosis and management of abnormal cervical cytology and histology. These strategies reflect new information concerning the natural history of cervical carcinogenesis and the performance of screening and diagnostic tests, and they take into account the cost and efficacy of various treatment and follow-up options.

Background

Cytologic and Histologic Findings and Interpretation

Effective cervical cancer prevention requires recognition and treatment of the precursors of invasive cancer and includes standardized terminology to report cervical cytology results. The 2001 Bethesda System of nomenclature (see box) is used throughout this document to describe the categories of epithelial cell abnormalities, including atypical squamous cells (ASC), atypical glandular cells (AGC), and low-grade or high-grade squamous intraepithelial lesions (LSIL or HSIL). Histologic diagnoses of abnormalities are reported as cervical intraepithelial neoplasia (CIN) grades 1–3 (3).

The Bethesda System should be used to communicate accurately the risk of CIN 2, CIN 3, adenocarcinoma in situ (AIS), or cancer (collectively referred to in this document as CIN 2/3+). This is necessary both for the clinician to treat

---

The 2001 Bethesda System Categorizing of Epithelial Cell Abnormalities

Squamous cell

- Atypical squamous cells (ASC)
  - Of undetermined significance (ASC-US)
  - Cannot exclude HSIL (ASC-H)
- Low-grade squamous intraepithelial lesions (LSIL)
  - Encompassing human papillomavirus (HPV), mild dysplasia, and cervical intraepithelial neoplasia (CIN) 1
- High-grade squamous intraepithelial lesions (HSIL)
  - Encompassing moderate and severe dysplasia, carcinoma in situ, CIN 2, and CIN 3
- Squamous cell carcinoma

Glandular cell

- Atypical glandular cells (AGC) (specify endocervical, endometrial, or not otherwise specified)
- Atypical glandular cells, favor neoplastic (specify endocervical or not otherwise specified)
- Endocervical adenocarcinoma in situ (AIS)
- Adenocarcinoma

---

the patient and for the patient to benefit from cytologic screening. If the cytologic result does not define that risk clearly because of the use of categories not found in the Bethesda System, the clinician may wish to request from the interpreting laboratory or cytopathologist an interpretation that falls within the Bethesda System.

The clinical management of cytologic abnormalities has been modified based on the results of several large studies. Of particular importance is the National Cancer Institute's Atypical Squamous Cells of Undetermined Significance–Low-Grade Squamous Intraepithelial Lesion Triage Study (ALTS), a large, randomized study that compared follow-up and triage strategies for the less severe cytologic abnormalities in the Bethesda System (4). The study provided information about the natural history of CIN, cervical cytology test performance and reproducibility, and the relationship of abnormal cytology, histology, and human papillomavirus (HPV) test results to the risk of diagnosis of CIN 2 or CIN 3 at enrollment and during observation of up to 24 months. Strengths of this study include 2-year follow-up, cytologic and histologic quality control by individuals who participated in drafting the

Bethesda systems, and loop electrosurgical excision procedure (LEEP) for patients who have persistent abnormalities consistent with CIN (5, 6).

Natural History of Cervical Intraepithelial Neoplasia

The natural history of CIN is linked to the presence of high-risk HPV, also called "oncogenic" HPV. High-risk HPV types can be distinguished from low-risk types by the function of their E6 and E7 proteins, which interfere with the cell's growth regulatory mechanisms to a degree sufficient for immortalization of infected cell lines (7). In this document, use of the term HPV refers to the high-risk types of the virus unless otherwise noted.

Carriage of HPV DNA is extremely common in the general population, reported in one study to occur at least once over a 3-year period in 60% of young women (8). Infection with HPV occurs at a reported rate of 1.2–1.3% per month (9, 10). Extrapolating from these reported acquisition rates, the lifetime cumulative risk is at least 80% (11). The vast majority of women clear the virus or suppress it to levels not associated with CIN 2/3+, and for most women this occurs promptly (9, 12). The duration of HPV positivity is shorter and the likelihood of clearance is higher in younger women (13–15).

The presence of HPV is a marker for the risk of diagnosis of CIN 2/3+; only 1 in 10 to 1 in 30 HPV infections are associated with abnormal cervical cytology results (16–18), with an even smaller proportion associated with CIN 2/3+ (19). Among women with negative cytology test results and a positive HPV test result, only 15% will have abnormal cytology results within 5 years (20). However, HPV is necessary for the development and maintenance of CIN 3 (21). Persistent high-risk HPV is a necessary but not sufficient condition for the development of almost all invasive cancers (22, 23). Conversely, the risk of cervical cancer in women who do not harbor oncogenic HPV is extremely low (24). The longer HPV is present and the older the patient, the greater the risk of CIN (25). When HPV is present, smoking doubles the risk of progression to CIN 3 (26).

From a clinical perspective, it is important to distinguish which intraepithelial neoplasias will progress to invasive cancer if left untreated. However, the diagnostic categories currently available have only modest predictive value, and that value decreases as the lesions become less severe. Cancer precursors include CIN 3, AIS, and to a lesser extent CIN 2. The likelihood of progression to cancer is higher and the time to progression is shorter as the grade of dysplasia increases (27). Although expression of the presence of HPV as CIN can occur within months of viral acquisition (28), the time course from CIN 3 to invasive cancer averages between 8.1 and 12.6 years (29–31). The leisurely pace of these changes in immunocompetent women means that accurate estimates of progression risk require long follow-up times. Perhaps more relevant for clinical practice are estimates of regression to normal. A review of the literature from 1950 to 1992 noted the likelihood of regression to be 60% for CIN 1 and 40% for CIN 2 (4, 32).

Cervical intraepithelial neoplasia 1 is the histologic appearance of cells producing HPV (11), usually high-risk HPV. The goals of cervical cancer screening are not to prevent CIN but to prevent and detect early invasive cervical cancer and to reduce mortality. The detection of CIN 2 or CIN 3 is not a screening failure but rather the goal of the screening system.

Cervical screening test results measure the risk that CIN 2/3+ is present, as well as the risk that CIN 2/3+ subsequently will be diagnosed. These risks define the intensity of initial evaluation required and the interval and intensity of follow-up. Results that convey equivalent risk are managed in similar fashion. For example, the risk that CIN 2/3+ will be diagnosed in the 2 years following an ASC HPV-positive or LSIL cytology result is the same whether the results of colposcopic biopsy are negative or CIN 1; hence, the management of cases with these results is similar (33).

Cervical Cytology

Cervical cytology screening is associated with a reduction in the incidence of and mortality from invasive squamous cancer. Conventional cytology is reported to be 30–87% sensitive for dysplasia (34). A meta-analysis of cervical cytology studies suggested a sensitivity of 58% in a screening population (35). Treatment based on conventional cytology results does not seem to decrease the incidence of glandular invasive cancers, suggesting that sensitivity for glandular precursors is less than that observed for squamous lesions (36).

Because the range of sensitivity (30–87%) is so broad, all abnormal cytology results must be evaluated, although the vast majority do not represent underlying CIN 2/3+ (19). Reproducibility among observers and among multiple readings by the same observer is quite modest, even under optimal research conditions (6, 37–39). In ALTS, the quality control reviewer at the National Cancer Institute and the university-based cytopathologist at the study site agreed on an ASC result in 43% of 1,473 cases, on an LSIL result in 68% of 1,335 slides, and on an HSIL result in 47% of 433 cases (6). Therefore, when cytologic testing is selected for follow-up of previous abnormal results, repeat testing at 6–12 month intervals is recommended.

Human Papillomavirus Testing

Testing for low-risk HPV types has no role in cervical cancer prevention. The low-risk HPV types are associated with genital warts and low-grade intraepithelial lesions of the cervix, vagina, and vulva (40). Testing for high-risk HPV at the 1 pg/mL cutoff is uniformly more sensitive for CIN 2/3+ than cytology (regardless of method), and in most studies, HPV testing is less specific than cytology (41–53). The results of using both tests on a screening population of 11,085 women are listed in Table 1 (45).

For women aged 30 years and older, HPV testing can help predict whether CIN 2/3+ will be diagnosed in women with a normal cytology result in the next few years (9, 28, 45, 54, 55). Results are similar between hybridization and polymerase chain reaction methods if the positive cutoff and viral types tested for are similar (56). As new tests are introduced, decisions about clinical practice implementation must be based on clinical sensitivity (relationship of the test result to CIN 2/3+), not analytic sensitivity (ability of the test to detect low levels of HPV). In addition to a high sensitivity for detecting CIN 2/3+, HPV test results obtained by hybridization are reproducible, in contrast to cytology. Masked testing of 200 pairs from the same specimen using hybridization demonstrated "97% exact agreement" (57). Testing for HPV DNA, therefore, has clinical relevance for predicting the risk of the presence of CIN 2/3+ and the risk of the development of CIN 2/3+.

Colposcopy With and Without Directed Biopsy

Colposcopy with directed biopsy has been the criterion of disease detection and remains the technique of choice for treatment decisions. Evaluation of colposcopic sensitivity has, until recently, focused on populations with identified lesions sufficient to produce abnormal cytology.

A realistic assessment of the sensitivity of directed colposcopic biopsies for the detection of CIN 2/3+ is essential to clinical practice recommendations. Older studies have been hampered by bias, such as expert colposcopists evaluating only women with abnormal cytology results or with lesions severe enough to undergo excision. A review of these studies indicates that in 1–10% of cases, lesions more severe than anticipated by biopsy are

Table 1. Sensitivity and Specificity of Tests for Detection of Cervical Intraepithelial Neoplasia 2+

Detection of CIN 2+	Sensitivity	Specificity
Human papillomavirus testing	97.1%	93.3%
Cytology	76.6%	95.8%

Data from Cuzick J, Szarewski A, Cubie H, Hulman G, Kitchener H, Luesley D, et al. Management of women who test positive for high-risk types of human papillomavirus: the HART study. Lancet 2003;362:1871–6.

found at excision, including 16 missed invasive cancers among 1,975 patients (58). The risk of undiagnosed cancer is the major reason for the recommendation of excision for women with unexplained high-grade abnormal cytology results.

In recent studies, colposcopy with endocervical curettage and blind four-quadrant ectocervical biopsies or LEEP have been used as the diagnostic criteria (4, 41). This approach permits a more realistic evaluation of the sensitivity of colposcopy with directed biopsies. The presence of CIN 2/3+ was missed on directed biopsy and detected only on the random four-quadrant biopsies in 18.6–31.6% of CIN 2/3+ cases (41, 42). These figures may underestimate the prevalence of CIN 2/3+ not diagnosed on colposcopic-directed biopsy; excisions were not performed in the entire population because many women had normal screening test results. Comparing directed biopsy to conization also demonstrates a significant rate of underdiagnosis of CIN 2 and CIN 3 (59, 60).

Similar conclusions are reported in ALTS (4) in which women with CIN 1 after 2 years of follow-up and a previous LSIL or ASC HPV-positive test result were offered LEEP. Of the 189 cases of CIN 2/3+ diagnosed during the 2-year study in the "immediate colposcopy" arm of the trial, only 106 (56%) were diagnosed on the initial colposcopy. The others were identified after HSIL cytology or an exit colposcopy or LEEP. In the research setting, where LEEP is the criterion, the sensitivity of a single colposcopic examination is poor.

Results of these studies indicate that biopsies of all visible lesions are warranted regardless of colposcopic impression and that follow-up should include multiple colposcopies over time for those women with abnormal cytology or histology results who have persistent low-grade abnormalities or persistently test positive for HPV.

Clinical Considerations and Recommendations

▶ *When the results of cervical cytology screening are normal but a concurrent HPV test result is positive, what is the appropriate follow-up?*

The use of high-risk HPV testing as an adjunct to cervical cytology in women aged 30 years and older was recently introduced. (Combined testing is contraindicated in women who are immunosuppressed or who have had a total hysterectomy.) If both test results are negative, combined testing should not be repeated more often than every 3 years (61). Women with a normal cytology result who test positive for HPV on routine screening have a risk of CIN 2/3+ of approximately 4% (43), which is

lower than the risk for women with ASC cytology results. For this reason, colposcopy is not recommended as further testing after a single HPV-positive, cytology-negative result. Current expert consensus recommendations include a repeat cytology and HPV test in 6–12 months to allow for resolution of transient HPV carriage and a colposcopy only if test results remain abnormal (HPV-positive or ASC or higher-grade cytology results) (62).

▶ *When the results of cervical cytology are reported as atypical squamous cells, how should the patient be treated?*

A cytology result of ASC is used to describe "cellular abnormalities that were more marked than those attributable to reactive changes but that fell short of a definitive diagnosis of 'squamous intraepithelial lesion' (SIL)" (63). This interpretation is by far the most common cytologic abnormality, and as a consequence, it precedes the diagnoses of CIN 2/3+ more frequently than any other cytology result (19). However, aggressive investigation should be avoided because the ASC diagnosis is poorly reproducible between observers (38), the risk of cancer is very low (0.1–0.2%) (64, 65), and the risk of CIN 2/3+ for any individual patient is also low (6.4–11.9%) (4, 66, 67).

Options for evaluation include immediate colposcopy, triage to colposcopy by HPV DNA testing, or repeat cytology tests at 6 and 12 months. Colposcopy provides a rapid diagnosis with the least possible loss to follow-up, but it is expensive and unpleasant for patients. Testing for oncogenic HPV and referral to colposcopy only for those women who test positive has the advantage of prompt diagnosis and the ability to reassure 44–69% of patients without colposcopy that their risk of a significant lesion is very low (4, 66, 67). Reflex testing for HPV if liquid cytology was used, or from a separate sample collected at the time of the initial cervical cytology test, is preferred for patient convenience and cost-effectiveness (68). If HPV testing is elected, those women whose test results are HPV positive have a 15–27% chance of having a CIN 2/3+ and should be referred for colposcopy (4, 66, 67). Those women who test negative for HPV can be reassured that their risk of harboring CIN 2/3+ is less than 2%, and they can be scheduled for repeat cytology testing in 1 year (4, 67).

The exception to this recommendation for HPV follow-up is the adolescent, for whom the risk of invasive cancer approaches zero and the likelihood of HPV clearance is very high (12, 69). As an alternative to immediate colposcopy, adolescents with ASC HPV-positive test results may be monitored with cytology tests at 6 and 12 months or with a single HPV test at 12 months, with colposcopy for any abnormal cytology result or positive HPV test result. The recommendation and the rationale are similar for follow-up of LSIL in adolescents.

At least two consecutive follow-up cytology tests, with referral to colposcopy for an ASC or higher-grade result, are required to reach the sensitivity of a single HPV test for the detection of CIN 2/3+ (5). Although follow-up cytology tests may allow some women to avoid colposcopy, waiting 6–12 months for a definitive diagnosis can create anxiety (70) and will delay the possible diagnosis of cancer. In addition, the rate of loss to follow-up is substantial, with 15–25% reported in the research setting (71, 72) and 54–81% noncompliance in clinical practice settings (73–76). A randomized trial demonstrates that loss to follow-up is almost twice as great with cytology rescreening as with recall for HPV testing (32.7% versus 17.1%, $P = .009$) (77). In addition, ALTS reported that a larger number of women who completed both follow-up cytology examinations were referred to colposcopy (67%) than those undergoing triage with HPV testing (56%) (3).

▶ *When the results of cervical cytology are reported as LSIL or atypical squamous cells cannot exclude HSIL (ASC-H), how should the patient be treated?*

A cytology result of LSIL is the second most common abnormal cytology result and is more frequent in younger populations with larger numbers of recent partners (64). It is also the most reproducible of the SIL diagnoses (78), representing (when correctly interpreted) the appearance of cells that are actively engaged in HPV replication (79). An LSIL diagnosis is associated with a positive test result for high-risk HPV in most women (83% of the women with LSIL cytology in ALTS); therefore, HPV testing is of limited value in triage to colposcopy.

The risk of CIN 2/3+ at initial colposcopy following an LSIL result is between 15% and 30% in most studies (64, 65, 80–83). This level of risk of CIN 2/3+ is similar to results of initial colposcopy associated with an ASC HPV-positive cytology result in other studies (17.8% versus 17.9%) (4, 67). Therefore, colposcopy is recommended for evaluation of LSIL. For adolescents with LSIL results, it may be reasonable to follow up without immediate colposcopy. Low-grade squamous intraepithelial lesions are very common in sexually active adolescents because of the recent onset of sexual activity in this group (84), but clearance of HPV is high and cancer rates are extremely low (12, 69). Therefore, follow-up recommendations are similar to those for adolescents with ASC HPV-positive results.

The cytology result "atypical squamous cells—cannot exclude HSIL" (ASC-H) is intended to include 5–10% of ASC cases overall. Findings of CIN 2/3+ in 24–94% of patients with ASC-H cytology results suggest that colposcopy is an appropriate initial diagnostic intervention (85). This terminology is used to alert clinicians that the risk of CIN 3 or cancer exceeds that of ASC findings but

lacks the certainty required for the patient to be given an HSIL interpretation, which would prompt an excision if colposcopic evaluation was negative. The presence of HPV in 86% of women with ASC-H monolayer cytology and in 70% of women with ASC-H conventional cytology in the ALTS experience suggests that HPV testing defines a population at low risk, but it may not be cost-effective for triage in younger women (86). In women aged 30 years or older with ASC-H cytology results, HPV-positive test results decrease dramatically, and triage to colposcopy using HPV testing may be considered as with other ASC findings. Otherwise, women with ASC-H should be cared for in a fashion similar to women with LSIL; follow-up of a colposcopy result of CIN 1 or normal should include either cytology tests at 6 and 12 months or an HPV DNA test at 12 months, rather than excision.

▶ *When the results of colposcopy performed for the evaluation of ASC, ASC-H, or LSIL reveal no dysplasia or CIN 1, how should the patient be treated?*

In women with ASC cytology results who have had primary triage with colposcopy without HPV testing, the risk of CIN 2/3+ is reported to be approximately 6–12% before the colposcopic examination (4, 67). Risk of harboring CIN 2/3+ after an ASC test result (with HPV status unknown) and a negative satisfactory colposcopy result should be less than the risk for women with an ASC cytology result and a negative HPV test result. Hence the recommended follow-up is the same: repeat cytology in 1 year.

A negative colposcopy result following an ASC-H cytology result should be managed identically to a case with LSIL and similar colposcopy results. Because HSIL and ASC-H do not carry the same risk of CIN 2/3+, recommendations for follow-up differ. Excision generally is recommended for women with HSIL cytology results and a negative initial colposcopic evaluation. Detection of CIN 2/3+ by colposcopy for ASC-H was 27% and 40% (conventional versus monolayer cytology) in ALTS (86). One study reported that 49% of women evaluated for ASC-H had no dysplastic lesion identified (87). This suggests that for women with ASC-H, excision is not warranted in those with an initial negative colposcopy result.

In ALTS, follow-up with two cervical cytology screenings 6 months apart and subsequent colposcopy for a diagnosis of ASC or higher-grade cytology was 88% sensitive for CIN 2/3+ and required 64% of women to undergo a second colposcopy (88). A single HPV test at 12 months was 92% sensitive and required 55% of women to undergo a second colposcopy examination. All other schemes evaluated indicated colposcopy for more women, with minimal or no gain in sensitivity, or were less sensitive for CIN 2/3+. For women with an ASC HPV-positive, ASC-H, or LSIL cytology result and a negative initial colposcopy examination or a histologic result of CIN 1, optimal follow-up is repeat cervical cytology screening tests at 6 and 12 months or an HPV test at 12 months. If the follow-up cytology result is ASC or higher-grade cytology or a positive HPV test, colposcopy should be repeated.

▶ *When the results of cervical cytology tests are reported as HSIL, how should the patient be treated?*

Among women with HSIL cytology results, CIN 2 or CIN 3 have been reported in 70% or more, and 1–2% harbor invasive cancer (19, 64). Given the level of risk, colposcopy and biopsy of visible lesions are recommended. Endocervical assessment should be performed in the nonpregnant patient, and the entire vagina should be examined, especially when a lesion corresponding to the cytology result is not found. An alternative "see and treat" management plan may be used in this patient population in the event that a lesion consistent with CIN 2 or CIN 3 is seen. In women who have such a lesion and are not pregnant, LEEP may be performed at the same visit as the colposcopy. In these cases, the cervical biopsy is omitted and an endocervical assessment after the LEEP may be considered.

▶ *When the initial evaluation of an HSIL cytology result is a diagnosis of CIN 1 or less, how should the patient be treated?*

Interpretations of HSIL and CIN 2 or CIN 3 are poorly reproducible (6, 78, 89, 90). One study reported that less than half of HSIL results and 77% of CIN 2 or CIN 3 results were confirmed on quality control review (6). As a consequence, experts have recommended review of the cytology and histology results in cases with HSIL diagnoses and discrepancies in colposcopic results (85), although this approach has not been tested in clinical studies. If review is not undertaken or colposcopy results are not satisfactory, excision is recommended. This approach is favored because (as discussed previously) a single colposcopy can miss CIN 2 or CIN 3, particularly small lesions (91), and because reports have documented CIN 2/3+ when examining excision specimens in up to 35% of women with HSIL cytology results and either negative or noncorrelating (CIN 1) colposcopy results (92–94).

Adolescents are exceptions to this recommendation because interobserver variability is most pronounced in younger women (95), the risk of invasive cancer is extremely low, and the likelihood of spontaneous resolution of CIN 1 or CIN 2 is high. Therefore, follow-up with colposcopy and cytology tests at 4–6 months may be undertaken (96), as long as the colposcopy results are adequate and the endocervical curettage is negative.

▶ *When the results of cervical cytology tests are reported as AGC or AIS, how should the patient be treated?*

The 2001 Bethesda System expanded the categories of cytology results associated with AGC to include "atypical glandular cells not otherwise specified" (AGC, or AGC-NOS), "AGC favor neoplasia," and endocervical AIS. These categories were defined with the intention of providing additional information about the patient's risk of underlying high-grade dysplasia. In a review of 1,869 AGC results with histologic correlation, 33.7% were found to harbor SIL, 2.5% AIS, and 1% cervical adenocarcinoma (97), indicating that the most common significant lesions associated with AGC are actually squamous (98). The risk of CIN 2/3+ in women with AGC cytology results is 9–41%, in contrast to 27–96% with AGC favor neoplasia (85). At least half of AIS and adenocarcinoma results will be accompanied by squamous CIN (99). An AIS cytology result is associated with a 48–69% risk of histologic AIS and a 38% risk of invasive adenocarcinoma of the cervix (100, 101). The balance between adequate disease detection and overly aggressive evaluation in women with AGC results is particularly challenging. Endocervical curettage and colposcopy are both relatively insensitive for AIS and adenocarcinoma (100–105), but most women with AGC cytology results do not have significant lesions (11).

The initial evaluation of women with AGC results is dictated by the risk of CIN 2/3+ noted previously, by the possibility that the source of the abnormality may be the endometrium, and by the recognition that the entire endocervix is at risk for AIS, mandating endocervical sampling. As a consequence, colposcopy and endocervical sampling should be included in the initial evaluation of all women with AGC results, except for those with results that specify "atypical endometrial cells." Women with atypical endometrial cells and a normal endometrial sampling should undergo colposcopy and endocervical sampling. Endometrial sampling is indicated in women with atypical endometrial cells and all women with AGC results who are aged 35 years or older (106), as well as those younger than 35 years with abnormal bleeding, morbid obesity, oligomenorrhea, or clinical evaluation suggesting endometrial cancer (107, 108).

▶ *When the results of the initial evaluation of AGC or AIS do not reveal intraepithelial neoplasia or cancer, how should the patient be treated?*

Treatment of women with AGC and negative initial evaluations is determined by the risk that significant disease is present but was not detected. The category AGC-NOS is associated with a sufficiently low risk of missed disease that follow-up with repeat cytology testing and endocervical sampling four times at 6-month intervals is recommended. Although untested in a clinical trial, this prolonged follow-up scheme is recommended because of the recognized insensitivity of cytology testing and endocervical sampling for glandular neoplasia.

Like squamous CIN, HPV is found in more than 95% of AIS and 90–100% of invasive adenocarcinomas of the cervix (109–111). The largest published series of AGC results uniformly evaluated with cervical histology and HPV testing found that 40 of 137 women (29%) were HPV positive, including 11 of 12 women with CIN 2 or CIN 3 and all 5 women with AIS (112). Similar reports (113, 114) suggest that it is reasonable to monitor women with AGC cytology test results, a negative initial evaluation, and a negative HPV test result with a repeat cytology and endocervical sampling in 1 year rather than requiring four visits at 6-month intervals.

For women with reports of 1) AGC favor neoplasia or an AIS cytology result and a negative initial evaluation, or 2) a second AGC-NOS result and a second negative evaluation, the risk of missing a significant lesion is sufficient that an excision is warranted (85). Cold-knife conization is a good choice in this situation because of the prognostic importance in AIS of the pathologic evaluation of margins, which may be obscured by thermal artifact in some LEEP specimens (115, 116). The rarity of this diagnosis and the difficulty with management may require consultation with a practitioner with expertise in this area, such as a gynecologic oncologist.

▶ **When should endocervical curettage be used in the colposcopic examination?**

Endocervical sampling may be conducted either with vigorous endocervical brushing or by traditional endocervical curettage with a sharp curette. Compared with curettage, the brush technique is at least as sensitive for endocervical dysplasia (117–121) and returns fewer reports of insufficient specimens (120, 121). The disadvantage is that the result can be equivocal, such as ASC, in which case the patient must be recalled for sharp curettage.

Endocervical sampling is not indicated in the pregnant patient. The following discussion of indications applies to the nonpregnant patient. In the evaluation of an ASC or LSIL cytology result with a satisfactory colposcopy result, endocervical sampling may be considered, although the identification of cancer cases is low (122, 123). Sampling should be performed if colposcopy results are unsatisfactory (124, 125) or if ablative treatment, such as cryotherapy or laser ablation, is contemplated. Higher rates of postablation CIN 2 or

CIN 3 and cancer have been reported if pretreatment endocervical assessment is not done (126). Studies of the contribution of endocervical curettage to diagnosis of CIN 2/3+ at colposcopy suggest that its addition to directed biopsy may be expected to add 5–9% to the total number of CIN 2/3+ diagnoses (125, 127–129). This percentage becomes more important as the risk of CIN 2/3+ increases with higher-grade abnormal cytology results. As a consequence, in women with ASC-H, HSIL, AGC, or AIS cytology results, endocervical sampling should be considered as part of the initial colposcopic evaluation (130), unless excision is planned. If an excision is planned, endocervical sampling may be omitted (124), although it may be performed at the time of the procedure following the excision to assess the completeness of the procedure.

▶ *If the results of colposcopy are adequate and consistent with the results of cervical cytology, is biopsy necessary?*

A review of eight studies of colposcopic impression with histologic endpoints found that a colposcopic impression of CIN 1 was associated with CIN 1 histology an average of 42.8% of the time (131). Another study included women with LSIL cytology results who were believed not to have CIN 2 or CIN 3 on colposcopic impression and directed biopsies and who underwent excision. In 49 of the 233 cases (21%), CIN 2 or CIN 3 was diagnosed in the excision specimen (129). In a review of 510 cases of CIN 2 and CIN 3 preceded by ASC, AGC, or LSIL test results, colposcopic impression indicated CIN 2 or CIN 3 in 60 of the 510 cases (12%) (91). A meta-analysis comparing colposcopic impression to colposcopic biopsies reported an average 48% sensitivity of colposcopic impression for separation of CIN 2/3+ from other diagnoses (132). Use of colposcopic impression alone could have caused 18–60% of patients to be treated incorrectly. Therefore, biopsy of any visible lesion is an important component of a colposcopic examination, regardless of colposcopic impression.

▶ *How should CIN 1 be managed?*

Untreated CIN 1 signifies a risk of 13% for diagnosis of CIN 2 or CIN 3 at 2-year follow-up, which is the same as the risk for ASC HPV-positive or LSIL cytology results following a negative colposcopy (33) and consistent with reports from other populations of 9–16% risk (133, 134).

Another predictable consequence of this new understanding is recognition that most cases of CIN 1 will remit spontaneously over time. One study reported spontaneous regression in 57% of 4,504 patients with CIN 1 (32), and spontaneous regression at 36 months of follow-up was noted in 91% of women aged 13–23 years (69).

The decision for treatment or observation should be based on the preferences of the patient and the physician. For most women, especially younger women, observation provides the best balance between risk and benefit and should be encouraged. The recommendation for follow-up of untreated CIN 1 is appropriate to the level of risk described previously, including two cytology screening tests 6 months apart with colposcopy for an ASC or higher-grade result, or a single HPV test at 12 months, with colposcopy if the test result is positive (33).

▶ *How should CIN 2 and CIN 3 be managed?*

In contrast to CIN 1, CIN 2 and CIN 3 are recognized potential cancer precursors, although CIN 2 is associated with significant spontaneous regression. Evidence from ALTS suggests that approximately 40% of CIN 2 cases regressed over 2 years, whereas regression of CIN 3, if present, was too rare to measure accurately during the study (5). Reports of significant regression of CIN 3 generally are based on cytology and not histology or are associated with multiple follow-up biopsies, which influence the natural history of the disease (135). Even when histology is assessed, only 77% of CIN 2 and CIN 3 diagnoses were verified on quality control review in ALTS, making assertions about regression more difficult to interpret in studies without rigorous pathology review (6). In addition, histologic differentiation between CIN 2 and CIN 3 is not sufficiently reliable to permit clear stratification of risk (136). As a consequence, immediate treatment of CIN 2 and CIN 3 with excision or ablation in the nonpregnant patient is recommended. The only exception to this recommendation is that follow-up similar to CIN 1 may be considered in the adolescent with CIN 2, whose likelihood of spontaneous clearance is substantial and whose risk of cancer approaches zero (137). Therefore, care of the adolescent with CIN 2 may be individualized.

▶ *Does management of CIN 2 or CIN 3 differ for women who are HIV positive?*

Effective treatment of CIN requires immunologic clearance or suppression of HPV to avoid recurrence (138). Women who are HIV positive have difficulty clearing the virus and, therefore, are at increased risk of progressive and recurrent disease in direct relation to their level of immunosuppression (139–142). Treatment of CIN should be pursued despite high recurrence rates (>50% recurrence rate after standard treatment) because it can effectively interrupt progression to invasive cancer (139, 143–146). Women who are HIV positive also appear more likely to have positive surgical margins, which may contribute to increased recurrence rates (147). Standard ablative or excisional treatment is recommended for women who are HIV positive with documented CIN 2 or CIN 3, regardless of HIV viral load.

The role of highly active antiretroviral therapy in the management of precancerous cervical lesions remains unclear (148). Therefore, CIN 2 and CIN 3 should be treated similarly in women who are HIV positive regardless of their use of antiretroviral therapy.

▶ *Is excision or ablation the better treatment for CIN?*

A large body of evidence (149–153), including a meta-analysis (154) and a randomized trial (155), indicates that rates for the clearance of squamous dysplasia of all grades are the same for laser therapy, LEEP, and cryotherapy. Endocervical sampling before ablation is recommended to avoid treatment of unrecognized invasive cancer (126, 156). Ablation should not be performed in patients with dysplasia on endocervical curettage. Rates of cervical stenosis were comparable among modalities in the randomized trial (155). Excision offers the advantage of a specimen for histologic examination and the disadvantage of increased surgical complications, primarily bleeding (155). Reports that as many as 2–3% of patients with CIN 2 or CIN 3 diagnosed on colposcopic biopsy harbor unrecognized AIS or invasive cancer found in the specimens from excision have discouraged some practitioners from using ablative techniques for patients with high-grade abnormalities diagnosed by biopsies (157).

▶ *How should AIS be managed? How should patients with AIS be monitored after treatment?*

Because AIS of the cervix is sufficiently rare, most of the literature consists of case reports or small retrospective series; no trials have compared management strategies. However, similarities in reports can provide some guidance in approaching this disorder (130, 158–174). Expert consultation may be desirable for pathologic diagnosis, treatment, and follow-up.

For the patient with a colposcopic biopsy diagnosis of AIS, exclusion of invasive cancer and the removal of all affected tissue is the primary goal. Hysterectomy is not appropriate until invasive cancer has been excluded. Excision is required to accomplish these goals. Cold-knife conization is recommended to preserve specimen orientation and permit optimal interpretation of histology and margin status, which are important to inform decisions about the risks of conservative management. Ablation does not permit recognition of invasive cancer, if present, or assessment of the treatment margins (175) and should not be used. Use of LEEP in this situation is associated with an increase in positive cone margins over cold-knife conization (115, 176) and is not recommended (173, 177). Endocervical sampling immediately after conization has been reported to have better positive and negative predictive value for residual disease than cone margins (178).

If the margins of the cone specimen are involved, conization should be repeated. The risk of residual AIS at subsequent conization or hysterectomy has been reported to be as high as 80% in patients with positive margins (179), and most of the women found to have undiagnosed invasive cancer at hysterectomy are in this group (176, 179). Repeat conization is preferred to immediate hysterectomy so that if invasive cancer is found, the appropriate surgical or radiotherapeutic treatment can be recommended.

If the margins of the cone specimen are not involved, risk of residual disease is still substantial (170, 180). In a review of 14 studies involving 157 women with AIS and negative conization margins who underwent a subsequent conization or hysterectomy, 41 (26%) harbored additional AIS and 3 (1.9%) were found to have unsuspected invasive cancer (179). This is of concern because both cytology and endocervical curettage have substantial false-negative rates for glandular lesions, and there are multiple reports of the diagnosis of invasive adenocarcinoma after long periods of regular follow-up with negative screening test results (161, 163, 165, 181). This level of risk and the insensitivity of screening tests supports a recommendation for hysterectomy when fertility is no longer desired.

When fertility is desired and cervical conization margins are clear, conservative follow-up may be undertaken with cytology tests and endocervical sampling every 6 months, provided that the patient understands the risk of subsequent recognition or development of invasive cancer. There are series supporting this practice (176, 177, 182, 183), but only one series to date had a mean follow-up longer than 5 years, and the small series and case reports suggest that follow-up in excess of 10 years will be required to assess the risk accurately. Recognizing that the vast majority of AIS and invasive adenocarcinomas are HPV positive, some experts use the combination of HPV testing and cytology to further stratify risk and assist women with decisions regarding continued fertility.

▶ *How should a colposcopic biopsy with inconclusive results for early invasive cancer be managed?*

A colposcopic biopsy with inconclusive results for cancer should be followed by excision to define whether cancer is present and to permit treatment planning. The management of early invasive cervical cancer depends on the depth of invasion and the presence or absence of lymph-vascular space invasion. Biopsy alone does not adequately provide this information. Cold-knife conization is favored for this purpose because it maintains tissue orientation in a single specimen, which is essential to permit pathologic evaluation of depth of invasion and other variables that define stage and treatment (184).

▶ *How should a patient's condition be monitored after treatment for CIN? If LEEP or cone biopsy reveals a positive margin, how should management proceed?*

Most of the literature concerning risk of invasive cancer after treatment of CIN pertains to CIN 2 and CIN 3. Long-term follow-up of untreated CIN 1 with minimal occurrence of invasive cancer suggests that the risk of cancer after treatment should be considerably lower than that for CIN 2 and CIN 3. For CIN 1 with positive margins, cytology screening at 6 and 12 months or HPV testing at 12 months is a reasonable choice before reestablishing routine screening.

Risk of invasive cancer after treatment of CIN 2 or CIN 3 remains 10–15 times greater than that of the general population and is constant over time (185–187). Positive margins on a specimen excised for squamous CIN (188–192) or endocervical curettage positive for squamous CIN performed after excision (126, 193) indicates a risk of persistent disease. Risk of recurrence was 2–3% in women with negative margins (194, 195) and 5–12% in women with positive margins (196, 197). This finding necessitates follow-up, including endocervical sampling until routine screening is reestablished, but it does not require reexcision (188, 190, 198–201). Reexcision may be elected but should be undertaken with the knowledge that the most common outcome is the absence of residual dysplasia. In one large series, 84% of women with margins that were positive at conization who underwent follow-up cytology without reexcision remained disease-free at 5 years (191). Another study found similar results at a mean follow-up of 19 years (202). Excision technique also may influence the decision. Sparing the endocervical mucosa from cautery after the excision increases subsequent satisfactory colposcopy results and decreases cervical stenosis, but it also may reasonably be expected to increase recurrence rates in the event of positive margins (203).

Human papillomavirus testing is a powerful predictor of the risk of recurrent CIN 2 or CIN 3 after treatment of CIN. Multiple large series support a recommendation for HPV testing as an alternative to cytology screening after treatment of CIN 2 or CIN 3, provided that it is conducted at least 6 months after treatment (204–211).

After treatment of CIN 2 or CIN 3, women may be monitored with cytology screening three to four times at 6-month intervals or undergo a single Pap and HPV test at 6 months before annual follow-up is reestablished. The addition of colposcopy to cytology follow-up has not been shown to significantly increase detection of persistent or recurrent disease (212) and is not recommended.

▶ *When is hysterectomy appropriate in women with CIN 2/3+?*

In the absence of other indications, hysterectomy is not the initial treatment of choice for CIN 2 and CIN 3. Hysterectomy may be considered for treatment of persistent or recurrent CIN 2 or CIN 3 or when a repeat excision is indicated but technically unfeasible (137). If excision is indicated, it should be performed (where possible) before hysterectomy to rule out invasive cancer. If hysterectomy is performed, the choice of either vaginal or abdominal approach should be dictated by other indications and patient characteristics and preferences.

▶ *How does care and follow-up differ for women during pregnancy?*

In pregnancy, the only diagnosis that may alter management is invasive cancer. The presence of cancer may change treatment goals or change the route and timing of delivery. Therefore, colposcopic examination during pregnancy should have as its primary goal the exclusion of invasive cancer. Women with cytology results that are not likely to be associated with cancer, such as ASC and LSIL, may undergo colposcopic evaluation either during pregnancy or at 6–12 weeks postpartum.

Pregnant women with ASC-H, HSIL, AGC, or AIS test results should undergo colposcopy without endocervical sampling, reserving biopsy for those with visible lesions consistent with CIN 3, AIS, or cancer. The purpose of biopsy in these women is only to exclude invasive cancer (213, 214). Although many women with colposcopic impressions of CIN 1 harbor either normal histology or CIN 2 or CIN 3, the risk of invasive cancer with a colposcopic impression of CIN 1 is low. Accordingly, pregnant women may be spared biopsy if the colposcopic impression is CIN 1 (85).

Excisions should be considered for pregnant women only if a lesion detected at colposcopy is suggestive of invasive cancer. Those with unsatisfactory colposcopy results, and those with satisfactory colposcopy results who are not found to have invasive cancer, should be reevaluated with colposcopy and cytology tests in each trimester until delivery (85). Repeat biopsy is indicated only for colposcopic evidence of progression or cytology suggestive of invasive cancer (85). Reassessment by colposcopy and cytology tests and endocervical assessment if indicated should be undertaken 6–12 weeks postpartum. Obtaining expert assistance with difficult management decisions or procedures is encouraged.

Summary of Recommendations

The following recommendations are based on good and consistent scientific evidence (Level A):

▶ Women with ASC cytology results may undergo immediate colposcopy, triage to colposcopy by high-risk HPV DNA testing, or repeat cytology screening at 6 and 12 months. Triage to colposcopy should occur after positive HPV test results or ASC or higher-grade diagnosis. Women with ASC who test negative for HPV or whose HPV status is unknown and test negative for abnormalities using colposcopy should have a repeat cytology test in 1 year.

▶ Most women with ASC who are HPV positive or women with ASC-H, LSIL, or HSIL test results should undergo colposcopy.

▶ For women with an ASC HPV-positive test result or ASC-H or LSIL cytology result and a negative initial colposcopy or a histologic result of CIN 1, optimal follow-up is repeat cervical cytology tests (not screening) at 6 and 12 months or an HPV test at 12 months; a repeat colposcopy is indicated for a cytology result of ASC or higher-grade abnormality or a positive high-risk HPV test.

▶ The recommendation for follow-up of untreated CIN 1 includes cytology tests at 6 and 12 months with colposcopy for an ASC or higher-grade result, or a single HPV test at 12 months, with colposcopy if the test result is positive.

The following recommendations are based on limited and inconsistent scientific evidence (Level B):

▶ Endocervical sampling using a brush or curette may be undertaken as part of the evaluation of ASC and LSIL cytology results and should be considered as part of the evaluation of AGC, AIS, and HSIL cytology results.

  — Endocervical sampling is recommended at the time of an unsatisfactory colposcopy or if ablative treatment is contemplated.

  — Endocervical sampling is not indicated in pregnancy.

▶ Endometrial sampling is indicated in women with atypical endometrial cells and in all women aged 35 years or older who have AGC cytology results, as well as in women younger than 35 years with abnormal bleeding, morbid obesity, oligomenorrhea, or clinical results suggesting endometrial cancer.

▶ Women with HSIL cytology results and negative or unsatisfactory colposcopy results should undergo excision unless they are pregnant or adolescent.

▶ Women with AGC favor neoplasia or AIS cytology results and negative or unsatisfactory colposcopy results should undergo excision unless they are pregnant. A colposcopic examination negative for abnormalities after two AGC-NOS cytology results is also an indication for excision in the absence of pregnancy.

▶ Pregnant women with CIN 2 or CIN 3 may undergo follow-up with colposcopy during each trimester and should be reevaluated with cytology and colposcopy examinations at 6–12 weeks postpartum or thereafter. Treatment of CIN 2 and CIN 3 in pregnancy is not indicated.

▶ Women with CIN 2 or CIN 3 should be treated (in the absence of pregnancy) with excision or ablation. Management of CIN 2 in adolescents may be individualized.

▶ Women treated for CIN 2 or CIN 3 with a positive margin on excision may be followed by repeat cytology testing, including endocervical sampling every 6 months for 2 years or HPV DNA testing at 6 months; if these test results are negative, annual screening may be reestablished.

▶ Women with a cervical biopsy diagnosis of AIS should undergo excision to exclude invasive cancer. Cold-knife conization is recommended to preserve specimen orientation and permit optimal interpretation of histology and margin status.

▶ After treatment of CIN 2 or CIN 3, women may be monitored with cytology screening three to four times at 6-month intervals or undergo a single HPV test at 6 months before returning to annual follow-up.

The following recommendations are based primarily on consensus and expert opinion (Level C):

▶ Colposcopic examination during pregnancy should have as its primary goal the exclusion of invasive cancer. Excisions in pregnant women should be considered only if a lesion detected at colposcopy is suggestive of invasive cancer.

▶ Cervical cytology screening lacking endocervical cells may be repeated in 1 year when testing was performed for routine screening. Cytology screening performed for a specific indication (ie, AGC follow-up or posttreatment follow-up after LEEP with a positive margin) may need to be repeated.

▶ Adolescents with ASC who are HPV positive or with LSIL results may be monitored with repeat cytology tests at 6 and 12 months or a single HPV test at 12 months, with colposcopy for a cytology result of ASC or higher-grade abnormality or a positive HPV test result.

▶ After treatment of AIS, when future fertility is desired and cervical conization margins are clear, conservative follow-up may be undertaken with cytology and endocervical sampling every 6 months.

▶ Women should not be treated with ablative therapy unless endocervical sampling test results are negative for abnormalities and the lesion seen and histologically evaluated explains the cytologic finding.

▶ In the absence of other indications for hysterectomy, excisional or ablative therapy for CIN 2 or CIN 3 is preferred.

References

1. Sawaya GF, McConnell KJ, Kulasingam SL, Lawson HW, Kerlikowske K, Melnikow J, et al. Risk of cervical cancer associated with extending the interval between cervical-cancer screenings. N Engl J Med 2003;349: 1501–9. (Level II-3)

2. Robertson JH, Woodend BE, Crozier EH, Hutchinson J. Risk of cervical cancer associated with mild dyskaryosis. BMJ 1988;297:18–21. (Level II-3)

3. Solomon D, Davey D, Kurman R, Moriarty A, O'Connor D, Prey M, et al. The 2001 Bethesda System: terminology for reporting results of cervical cytology. Forum Group Members; Bethesda 2001 Workshop. JAMA 2002;287:2114–9. (Level III)

4. Solomon D, Schiffman M, Tarone R. Comparison of three management strategies for patients with atypical squamous cells of undetermined significance: baseline results from a randomized trial. ALTS Study Group. J Natl Cancer Inst 2001;93:293–9. (Level I)

5. Results of a randomized trial on the management of cytology interpretations of atypical squamous cells of undetermined significance. ASCUS–LSIL Triage Study (ALTS) Group. Am J Obstet Gynecol 2003;188: 1383–92. (Level I)

6. Stoler MH, Schiffman M. Interobserver reproducibility of cervical cytologic and histologic interpretations: realistic estimates from the ASCUS-LSIL Triage Study. Atypical Squamous Cells of Undetermined Significance—Low-Grade Squamous Intraepithelial Lesion Triage Study (ALTS) Group. JAMA 2001;285:1500–5. (Level III)

7. zur Hausen H. Papillomaviruses and cancer: from basic studies to clinical application. Nat Rev Cancer 2002;2: 342–50. (Level III)

8. Einstein MH, Burk RD. Persistent human papillomavirus infection: definitions and clinical implications. Papillomavirus Rep 2001;12:119–23. (Level III)

9. Ho GY, Bierman R, Beardsley L, Chang CJ, Burk RD. Natural history of cervicovaginal papillomavirus infection in young women. N Engl J Med 1998;338:423–8. (Level II-2)

10. Franco EL, Villa LL, Sobrinho JP, Prado JM, Rousseau MC, Desy M, et al. Epidemiology of acquisition and clearance of cervical human papillomavirus infection in women from a high-risk area for cervical cancer. J Infect Dis 1999;180:1415–23. (Level II-2)

11. Ferris DG, Cox JT, O'Connor DM, Wright VC, Foerster J, editors. Modern colposcopy: textbook and atlas. 2nd ed. Dubuque (IA): Kendall Hunt; 2004. (Level III)

12. Hildesheim A, Schiffman MH, Gravitt PE, Glass AG, Greer CE, Zhang T, et al. Persistence of type-specific human papillomavirus infection among cytologically normal women. J Infect Dis 1994;169:235–40. (Level II-2)

13. Moscicki AB, Shiboski S, Broering J, Powell K, Clayton L, Jay N, et al. The natural history of human papillomavirus infection as measured by repeated DNA testing in adolescent and young women. J Pediatr 1998;132: 277–84. (Level II-2)

14. Evander M, Edlund K, Gustafsson A, Jonsson M, Karlsson R, Rylander E, et al. Human papillomavirus infection is transient in young women: a population-based cohort study. J Infect Dis 1995;171:1026–30. (Level II-2)

15. Herrero R, Munoz N. Human papillomavirus and cancer. Cancer Surv 1999;33:75–98. (Level III)

16. Burk RD, Ho GY, Beardsley L, Lempa M, Peters M, Bierman R. Sexual behavior and partner characteristics are the predominant risk factors for genital human papillomavirus infection in young women. J Infect Dis 1996; 174:679–89. (Level II-2)

17. Kotloff KL, Wasserman SS, Russ K, Shapiro S, Daniel R, Brown W, et al. Detection of genital human papillomavirus and associated cytological abnormalities among college women. Sex Transm Dis 1998;25:243–50. (Level II-2)

18. Bauer HM, Ting Y, Greer CE, Chambers JC, Tashiro CJ, Chimera J, et al. Genital human papillomavirus infection in female university students as determined by a PCR-based method. JAMA 1991;265:472–7. (Level II-3)

19. Kinney WK, Manos MM, Hurley LB, Ransley JE. Where's the high-grade cervical neoplasia? The importance of minimally abnormal Papanicolaou diagnoses. Obstet Gynecol 1998;91:973–6. (Level III)

20. Castle PE, Wacholder S, Sherman ME, Lorincz AT, Glass AG, Scott DR, et al. Absolute risk of a subsequent abnormal pap among oncogenic human papillomavirus DNA-positive, cytologically negative women. Cancer 2002;95:2145–51. (Level II-2)

21. Nobbenhuis MA, Walboomers JM, Helmerhorst TJ, Rozendaal L, Remmink AJ, Risse EK, et al. Relation of human papillomavirus status to cervical lesions and consequences for cervical-cancer screening: a prospective study. Lancet 1999;354:20–5. (Level II-2)

22. Walboomers JM, Jacobs MV, Manos MM, Bosch FX, Kummer JA, Shah KV, et al. Human papillomavirus is a necessary cause of invasive cervical cancer worldwide. J Pathol 1999;189:12–9. (Level II-3)

23. Munoz N, Bosch FX, de Sanjose S, Herrero R, Castellsague X, Shah KV, et al. Epidemiologic classification of human papillomavirus types associated with cervical cancer. International Agency for Research on Cancer Multicenter Cervical Cancer Study Group. N Engl J Med 2003;348:518–27. (Level II-2)

24. Wright TC Jr, Schiffman M. Adding a test for human papillomavirus DNA to cervical-cancer screening. N Engl J Med 2003;348:489–90. (Level III)

25. Hopman EH, Rozendaal L, Voorhorst FJ, Walboomers JM, Kenemans P, Helmerhorst TJ. High risk human papillomavirus in women with normal cervical cytology prior to the development of abnormal cytology and colposcopy. BJOG 2000;107:600–4. (Level II-2)

26. Castle PE, Wacholder S, Lorincz AT, Scott DR, Sherman ME, Glass AG, et al. A prospective study of high-grade cervical neoplasia risk among human papillomavirus-infected women. J Natl Cancer Inst 2002;94:1406–14. (Level II-2)

27. Barron BA, Richart RM. A statistical model of the natural history of cervical carcinoma based on a prospective study of 557 cases. J Natl Cancer Inst 1968;41:1343–53. (Level III)

28. Koutsky LA, Holmes KK, Critchlow CW, Stevens CE, Paavonen J, Beckmann AM, et al. A cohort study of the risk of cervical intraepithelial neoplasia grade 2 or 3 in relation to papillomavirus infection. N Engl J Med 1992;327:1272–8. (Level II-2)

29. Boyes DA, Fidler HK, Lock DR. Significance of in situ carcinoma of the uterine cervix. Br Med J 1962;5273: 203–5. (Level III)

30. Dunn JE Jr, Martin PL. Morphogenesis of cervical cancer. Findings from San Diego County Cytology Registry. Cancer 1967;20:1899–906. (Level III)

31. Fidler HK, Boyes DA, Worth AJ. Cervical cancer detection in British Columbia. A progress report. J Obstet Gynaecol Br Commonw 1968;75:392–404. (Level II-3)

32. Ostor AG. Natural history of cervical intraepithelial neoplasia: a critical review. Int J Gynecol Pathol 1993; 12:186–92. (Level III)

33. Cox JT, Schiffman M, Solomon D. Prospective follow-up suggests similar risk of subsequent cervical intraepithelial neoplasia grade 2 or 3 among women with cervical intraepithelial neoplasia grade 1 or negative colposcopy and directed biopsy. ASCUS–LSIL Triage Study (ALTS) Group. Am J Obstet Gynecol 2003; 188:1406–12. (Level II-2)

34. Nanda K, McCrory DC, Myers ER, Bastian LA, Hasselblad V, Hickey JD, et al. Accuracy of the Papanicolaou test in screening for and follow-up of cervical cytologic abnormalities: a systematic review. Ann Intern Med 2000;132:810–9. (Level III)

35. Fahey MT, Irwig L, Macaskill P. Meta-analysis of Pap test accuracy. Am J Epidemiol 1995;141:680–9. (Meta-analysis)

36. Kinney W, Sawaya GF, Sung HY, Kearny KA, Miller M, Hiatt RA. Stage at diagnosis and mortality in patients with adenocarcinoma and adenosquamous carcinoma of the uterine cervix diagnosed as a consequence of cytologic screening. Acta Cytol 2003;47:167–71. (Level II-3)

37. Sherman ME, Schiffman MH, Lorincz AT, Manos MM, Scott DR, Kuman RJ, et al. Toward objective quality assurance in cervical cytopathology. Correlation of

cytopathologic diagnoses with detection of high-risk human papillomavirus types. Am J Clin Pathol 1994; 102:182–7. (Level III)

38. Smith AE, Sherman ME, Scott DR, Tabbara SO, Dworkin L, Olson J, et al. Review of the Bethesda System atlas does not improve reproducibility or accuracy in the classification of atypical squamous cells of undetermined significance smears. Cancer 2000;90: 201–6. (Level II-3)

39. Quddus MR, Sung CJ, Steinhoff MM, Lauchlan SC, Singer DB, Hutchinson ML. Atypical squamous metaplastic cells: reproducibility, outcome, and diagnostic features on ThinPrep Pap test. Cancer 2001;93:16–22. (Level III)

40. Lowy DR, Howley PM. Papillomaviruses. In: Knipe DM, Howley PM, editors. Fields virology. 4th ed. Philadelphia (PA): Lippincott Williams & Wilkins; 2001. p. 2231–64. (Level III)

41. Belinson J, Qiao YL, Pretorius R, Zhang WH, Elson P, Li L, et al. Shanxi Province Cervical Cancer Screening Study: a cross-sectional comparative trial of multiple techniques to detect cervical neoplasia [published erratum appears in: Gynecol Oncol 2002;84:355]. Gynecol Oncol 2001;83:439–44. (Level II-3)

42. Belinson JL, Qiao YL, Pretorius RG, Zhang WH, Rong SD, Huang MN, et al. Shanxi Province cervical cancer screening study II: self-sampling for high-risk human papillomavirus compared to direct sampling for human papillomavirus and liquid based cervical cytology. Int J Gynecol Cancer 2003;13:819–26. (Level II-3)

43. Clavel C, Masure M, Bory JP, Putaud I, Mangeonjean C, Lorenzato M, et al. Human papillomavirus testing in primary screening for the detection of high-grade cervical lesions: a study of 7932 women. Br J Cancer 2001; 84:1616–23. (Level II-3)

44. Cuzick J, Beverley E, Ho L, Terry G, Sapper H, Mielzynska I, et al. HPV testing in primary screening of older women. Br J Cancer 1999;81:554–8. (Level III)

45. Cuzick J, Szarewski A, Cubie H, Hulman G, Kitchener H, Luesley D, et al. Management of women who test positive for high-risk types of human papillomavirus: the HART study. Lancet 2003;362:1871–6. (Level I)

46. Kjaer SK, van den Brule AJ, Paull G, Svare EI, Sherman ME, Thomsen BL, et al. Type specific persistence of high risk human papillomavirus (HPV) as indicator of high grade cervical squamous intraepithelial lesions in young women: population based prospective follow up study. BMJ 2002;325:572. (Level II-2)

47. Kulasingam SL, Hughes JP, Kiviat NB, Mao C, Weiss NS, Kuypers JM, et al. Evaluation of human papillomavirus testing in primary screening for cervical abnormalities: comparison of sensitivity, specificity, and frequency of referral. JAMA 2002;288:1749–57. (Level II-3)

48. Petry KU, Menton S, Menton M, van Loenen-Frosch F, de Carvalho Gomes H, Holz B, et al. Inclusion of HPV testing in routine cervical cancer screening for women above 29 years in Germany: results for 8466 patients. Br J Cancer 2003;88:1570–7. (Level II-3)

49. Salmeron J, Lazcano-Ponce E, Lorincz A, Hernandez M, Hernandez P, Leyva A, et al. Comparison of HPV-based assays with Papanicolaou smears for cervical cancer screening in Morelos State, Mexico. Cancer Causes Control 2003;14:505–12. (Level II-3)

50. Schiffman M, Herrero R, Hildesheim A, Shenman ME, Bratti M, Wacholder S, et al. HPV DNA testing in cervical cancer screening: results from women in a high-risk province of Costa Rica. JAMA 2000;283:87–93. (Level II-3)

51. Schneider A, Hoyer H, Lotz B, Leistritza S, Kuhne-Heid R, Nindl I, et al. Screening for high-grade cervical intraepithelial neoplasia and cancer by testing for high-risk HPV, routine cytology or colposcopy. Int J Cancer 2000; 89:529–34. (Level II-3)

52. Sherman ME, Lorincz AT, Scott DR, Wacholder S, Castle PE, Glass AG, et al. Baseline cytology, human papillomavirus testing, and risk for cervical neoplasia: a 10-year cohort analysis. J Natl Cancer Inst 2003; 95:46–52. (Level II-2)

53. Wright TC Jr, Denny L, Kuhn L, Pollack A, Lorincz A. HPV DNA testing of self-collected vaginal samples compared with cytologic screening to detect cervical cancer. JAMA 2000;283:81–6. (Level II-3)

54. Schlecht NF, Kulaga S, Robitaille J, Ferreira S, Santos M, Miyamura RA, et al. Persistent human papillomavirus infection as a predictor of cervical intraepithelial neoplasia. JAMA 2001;286:3106–14. (Level II-2)

55. Woodman CB, Collins S, Winter H, Bailey A, Ellis J, Prior P, et al. Natural history of cervical human papillomavirus infection in young women: a longitudinal cohort study. Lancet 2001;357:1831–6. (Level II-2)

56. Morin C, Bairati I, Bouchard C, Fortier M, Roy M, Moore L, et al. Managing atypical squamous cells of undetermined significance in Papanicolaou smears. J Reprod Med 2001;46:799–805. (Level II-3)

57. Castle PE, Lorincz AT, Mielzynska-Lohnas I, Scott DR, Glass AG, Sherman ME, et al. Results of human papillomavirus DNA testing with the hybrid capture 2 assay are reproducible. J Clin Microbiol 2002;40:1088–90. (Level II-3)

58. Sze EH, Rosenzweig BA, Birenbaum DL, Silverman RK, Baggish MS. Excisional conization of the cervix uteri: a five-part review. J Gynecol Surg 1989;5:325–41. (Level III)

59. Bonardi R, Cecchini S, Grazzini G, Ciatto S. Loop electrosurgical excision procedure of the transformation zone and colposcopically directed punch biopsy in the diagnosis of cervical lesions. Obstet Gynecol 1992; 80:1020–2. (Level III)

60. Buxton EJ, Luesley DM, Shafi MI, Rollason M. Colposcopically directed punch biopsy: a potentially misleading investigation. Br J Obstet Gynaecol 1991; 98:1273–6. (Level III)

61. Saslow D, Runowicz CD, Solomon D, Moscicki AB, Smith RA, Eyre HJ, et al. American Cancer Society guideline for the early detection of cervical neoplasia and cancer. CA Cancer J Clin 2002;52:342–62. (Level III)

62. Wright TC Jr, Schiffman M, Solomon D, Cox JT, Garcia F, Goldie S, et al. Interim guidance for the use of human papillomavirus DNA testing as an adjunct to cervical cytology for screening. Obstet Gynecol 2004;103: 304–9. (Level III)

63. The 1988 Bethesda System for reporting cervical/vaginal cytologic diagnoses. National Cancer Institute Workshop. JAMA 1989;262:931–4. (Level III)

64. Jones BA, Davey DD. Quality management in gynecologic cytology using interlaboratory comparison. Arch Pathol Lab Med 2000;124:672–81. (Level III)

65. Lonky NM, Sadeghi M, Tsadik GW, Petitti D. The clinical significance of the poor correlation of cervical dysplasia and cervical malignancy with referral cytologic results. Am J Obstet Gynecol 1999;181:560–6. (Level II-3)

66. Cox JT, Lorincz AT, Schiffman MH, Sherman ME, Cullen A, Kurman RJ. Human papillomavirus testing by hybrid capture appears to be useful in triaging women with a cytologic diagnosis of atypical squamous cells of undetermined significance. Am J Obstet Gynecol 1995; 172:946–54. (Level II-3)

67. Manos MM, Kinney WK, Hurley LB, Sherman ME, Shieh-Ngai J, Kurman RJ, et al. Identifying women with cervical neoplasia: using human papillomavirus DNA testing for equivocal Papanicolaou results. JAMA 1999; 281:1605–10. (Level II-3)

68. Kim JJ, Wright TC, Goldie SJ. Cost-effectiveness of alternative triage strategies for atypical squamous cells of undetermined significance. JAMA 2002;287: 2382–90. (Level III)

69. Moscicki AB, Shiboski S, Hills NK, Powell KJ, Jay N, Hanson EN, et al. Regression of low-grade squamous intra-epithelial lesions in young women. Lancet 2004;364:1678–83. (Level II-2)

70. Bell S, Porter M, Kitchener H, Fraser C, Fisher P, Mann E. Psychological response to cervical screening. Prev Med 1995;24:610–6. (Level II-2)

71. Flannelly G, Anderson D, Kitchener HC, Mann EM, Campbell M, Fisher P, et al. Management of women with mild and moderate cervical dyskaryosis. BMJ 1994;308:1399–403. (Level I)

72. Montz FJ, Monk BJ, Fowler JM, Nguyen L. Natural history of the minimally abnormal Papanicolaou smear. Obstet Gynecol 1992;80:385–8. (Level II-2)

73. Bucchi L, Zani J, Pierri C, Amadori A, Ghidoni D, Folicaldi S, et al. Cervical screening behavior of women with atypical squamous cells of undetermined significance (ASCUS). Diagn Cytopathol 2001;24:21–7. (Level II-3)

74. Engelstad LP, Stewart SL, Nguyen BH, Bedeian KL, Rubin MM, Pasick RJ, et al. Abnormal Pap smear follow-up in a high-risk population. Cancer Epidemiol Biomarkers Prev 2001;10:1015–20. (Level I)

75. Hunt JM, Irwig LM, Towler BP. The management of women with initial minor Pap smear abnormalities. Med J Aust 1994;160:558–63. (Level III)

76. Massad LS, Anoina D. Colposcopic and cytologic findings among adolescents referred to two urban teaching hospitals. J Pediatr Adolesc Gynecol 1996;9:190–4. (Level III)

77. Lytwyn A, Sellors JW, Mahony JB, Daya D, Chapman W, Ellis N, et al. Comparison of human papillomavirus DNA testing and repeat Papanicolaou test in women with low-grade cervical cytologic abnormalities: a randomized trial. HPV Effectiveness in Lowgrade Paps (HELP) Study No. 1 Group. CMAJ 2000;163:701–7. (Level I)

78. Renshaw AA, Davey DD, Birdsong GG, Walsh M, Styer PE, Mody DR, et al. Precision in gynecologic cytologic interpretation: a study from the College of American Pathologists Interlaboratory Comparison Program in Cervicovaginal Cytology. Arch Pathol Lab Med 2003;127:1413–20. (Level III)

79. Moscicki AB, Hills N, Shiboski S, Powell K, Jay N, Hanson E, et al. Risks for incident human papillomavirus infection and low-grade squamous intraepithelial lesion development in young females. JAMA 2001;285:2995–3002. (Level II-2)

80. Law KS, Chang TC, Hsueh S, Jung SM, Tseng CJ, Lai CH. High prevalence of high grade squamous intraepithelial lesions and microinvasive carcinoma in women with a cytologic diagnosis of low grade squamous intraepithelial lesions. J Reprod Med 2001;46:61–4. (Level III)

81. Spitzer M, Brennessel D, Seltzer VL, Silver L, Lox MS. Is human papillomavirus-related disease an independent risk factor for human immunodeficiency virus infection? Gynecol Oncol 1993;49:243–6. (Level II-3)

82. Takezawa K, Bennett BB, Wilkinson EJ, Drew PA, Hardt NS. Squamous intraepithelial lesions of the cervix in a high risk population. J Lower Genital Tract Dis 1998;2:136–40. (Level II-3)

83. Wright TC, Sun XW, Koulos J. Comparison of management algorithms for the evaluation of women with low-grade cytologic abnormalities. Obstet Gynecol 1995; 85:202–10. (Level II-3)

84. Simsir A, Brooks S, Cochran L, Bourquin P, Ioffe OB. Cervicovaginal smear abnormalities in sexually active adolescents. Implications for management. Acta Cytol 2002;46:271–6. (Level II-3)

85. Wright TC Jr, Cox JT, Massad LS, Twiggs LB, Wilkinson EJ. 2001 Consensus Guidelines for the management of women with cervical cytological abnormalities. ASCCP-Sponsored Consensus Conference. JAMA 2002;287:2120–9. (Level III)

86. Sherman ME, Solomon D, Schiffman M. Qualification of ASCUS. A comparison of equivocal LSIL and equivocal HSIL cervical cytology in the ASCUS LSIL Triage Study. ASCUS LSIL Triage Study Group. Am J Clin Pathol 2001;116:386–94. (Level II-2)

87. Alli PM, Ali SZ. Atypical squamous cells of undetermined significance—rule out high-grade squamous intraepithelial lesion: cytopathologic characteristics and clinical correlates. Diagn Cytopathol 2003;28:308–12. (Level III)

88. Guido R, Schiffman M, Solomon D, Burke L. Postcolposcopy management strategies for women referred with low-grade squamous intraepithelial lesions or human papillomavirus DNA-positive atypical squamous cells of undetermined significance: a two-year prospective study. ASCUS LSIL Triage Study (ALTS) Group. Am J Obstet Gynecol 2003;188:1401 5. (Level II 2)

89. Grenko RT, Abendroth CS, Frauenhoffer EE, Ruggiero FM, Zaino RJ. Variance in the interpretation of cervical biopsy specimens obtained for atypical squamous cells

of undetermined significance. Am J Clin Pathol 2000;114:735–40. (Level III)

90. Joste NE, Rushing L, Granados R, Zitz JC, Genest DR, Crum CP, et al. Bethesda classification of cervicovaginal smears: reproducibility and viral correlates. Hum Pathol 1996;27:581–5. (Level III)

91. Pretorius RG, Belinson JL, Zhang WH, Burchette RJ, Elson P, Qiao YL. The colposcopic impression. Is it influenced by the colposcopist's knowledge of the findings on the referral Papanicolaou smear? J Reprod Med 2001;46:724–8. (Level II-3)

92. Brown FM, Faquin WC, Sun D, Crum CP, Cibas ES. LSIL biopsies after HSIL smears. Correlation with high-risk HPV and greater risk of HSIL on follow-up. Am J Clin Pathol 1999;112:765–8. (Level III)

93. Chappatte OA, Byrne DL, Raju KS, Nayagam M, Kenney A. Histological differences between colposcopic-directed biopsy and loop excision of the transformation zone (LETZ): a cause for concern. Gynecol Oncol 1991;43:46–50. (Level II-3)

94. Ramirez EJ, Hernandez E, Miyazawa K. Cervical conization findings in women with dysplastic cervical cytology and normal colposcopy. J Reprod Med 1990;35:359–61. (Level III)

95. Kato I, Santamaria M, De Ruiz PA, Aristizabal N, Bosch FX, De Sanjose S, et al. Inter-observer variation in cytological and histological diagnoses of cervical neoplasia and its epidemiologic implication. J Clin Epidemiol 1995;48:1167–74. (Level III)

96. Hellberg D, Nilsson S, Valentin J. Positive cervical smear with subsequent normal colposcopy and histology—frequency of CIN in a long-term follow-up. Gynecol Oncol 1994;53:148–51. (Level II-3)

97. Eddy GL, Strumpf KB, Wojtowycz MA, Piraino PS, Mazur MT. Biopsy findings in five hundred thirty-one patients with atypical glandular cells of uncertain significance as defined by the Bethesda system. Am J Obstet Gynecol 1997;177:1188–95. (Level II-3)

98. Raab SS. Can glandular lesions be diagnosed in pap smear cytology? Diagn Cytopathol 2000;23:127–33. (Level III)

99. Mayeaux EJ Jr, Harper MB, Abreo F, Pope JB, Phillips GS. A comparison of the reliability of repeat cervical smears and colposcopy in patients with abnormal cervical cytology. J Fam Pract 1995;40:57–62. (Level II-3)

100. Laverty CR, Farnsworth A, Thurloe J, Bowditch R. The reliability of a cytological prediction of cervical adenocarcinoma in situ. Aust N Z J Obstet Gynaecol 1988;28:307–12. (Level III)

101. Lee KR, Manna EA, St John T. Atypical endocervical glandular cells: accuracy of cytologic diagnosis. Diagn Cytopathol 1995;13:202–8. (Level III)

102. Kim TJ, Kim HS, Park CT, Park IS, Hong SR, Park JS, et al. Clinical evaluation of follow-up methods and results of atypical glandular cells of undetermined significance (AGUS) detected on cervicovaginal Pap smears. Gynecol Oncol 1999;73:292–8. (Level III)

103. Krane JF, Granter SR, Trask CE, Hogan CL, Lee KR. Papanicolaou smear sensitivity for the detection of adenocarcinoma of the cervix: a study of 49 cases. Cancer 2001;93:8–15. (Level III)

104. Lee KR, Minter LJ, Granter SR. Papanicolaou smear sensitivity for adenocarcinoma in situ of the cervix. A study of 34 cases. Am J Clin Pathol 1997;107:30–5. (Level III)

105. Mitchell H, Medley G, Gordon I, Giles G. Cervical cytology reported as negative and risk of adenocarcinoma of the cervix: no strong evidence of benefit. Br J Cancer 1995;71:894–7. (Level II-2)

106. Parellada CI, Schivartche PL, Pereyra EA, Chuery AC, Mioni SM, Carvalho FM. Atypical glandular cells on cervical smears. Int J Gynaecol Obstet 2002;78:227–34. (Level III)

107. Chhieng DC, Elgert P, Cohen JM, Cangiarella JF. Clinical significance of atypical glandular cells of undetermined significance in postmenopausal women. Cancer 2001;93:1–7. (Level III)

108. Obenson K, Abreo F, Grafton WD. Cytohistologic correlation between AGUS and biopsy-detected lesions in postmenopausal women. Acta Cytol 2000;44:41–5. (Level III)

109. Bosch FX, Manos MM, Munoz N, Sherman M, Jansen AM, Peto J, et al. Prevalence of human papillomavirus in cervical cancer: a worldwide perspective. International biological study on cervical cancer (IBSCC) Study Group. J Natl Cancer Inst 1995;87:796–802. (Level II-3)

110. Madeleine MM, Daling JR, Schwartz SM, Shera K, McKnight B, Carter JJ, et al. Human papillomavirus and long-term oral contraceptive use increase the risk of adenocarcinoma in situ of the cervix. Cancer Epidemiol Biomarkers Prev 2001;10:171–7. (Level II-2)

111. Pirog EC, Kleter B, Olgac S, Bobkiewicz P, Lindeman J, Quint WG, et al. Prevalence of human papillomavirus DNA in different histological subtypes of cervical adenocarcinoma. Am J Pathol 2000;157:1055–62. (Level III)

112. Ronnett BM, Manos MM, Ransley JE, Fetterman BJ, Kinney WK, Hurley LB, et al. Atypical glandular cells of undetermined significance (AGUS): cytopathologic features, histopathologic results, and human papillomavirus DNA detection. Hum Pathol 1999;30:816–25. (Level III)

113. Krane JF, Lee KR, Sun D, Yuan L, Crum CP. Atypical glandular cells of undetermined significance: outcome predictions based on human papillomavirus testing. Am J Clin Pathol 2004;121:87–92. (Level III)

114. Oliveira ER, Derchain SF, Rabelo-Santos SH, Westin MC, Zeferino LC, Campos EA, et al. Detection of high-risk human papillomavirus (HPV) DNA by Hybrid Capture II in women referred due to atypical glandular cells in the primary screening. Diagn Cytopathol 2004;31:19–22. (Level III)

115. Azodi M, Chambers SK, Rutherford TJ, Kohorn EI, Schwartz PE, Chambers JT. Adenocarcinoma in situ of the cervix: management and outcome. Gynecol Oncol 1999;73:348–53. (Level III)

116. Goldstein NS. Management of adenocarcinoma in situ of the cervix [letter]. Gynecol Oncol 1999;75:520. (Level III)

117. Andersen W, Frierson H, Barber S, Tabbarah S, Taylor P, Underwood P. Sensitivity and specificity of endocervi-

cal curettage and the endocervical brush for the evaluation of the endocervical canal. Am J Obstet Gynecol 1988;159:702–7. (Level II-3)

118. Hoffman MS, Sterghos S Jr, Gordy LW, Gunasekaran S, Cavanagh D. Evaluation of the cervical canal with the endocervical brush. Obstet Gynecol 1993;82:573–7. (Level II-3)

119. Klam S, Arseneau J, Mansour N, Franco E, Ferenczy A. Comparison of endocervical curettage and endocervical brushing. Obstet Gynecol 2000;96:90–4. (Level I)

120. Mogensen ST, Bak M, Dueholm M, Frost L, Knoblauch NO, Praest J, et al. Cytobrush and endocervical curettage in the diagnosis of dysplasia and malignancy of the uterine cervix. Acta Obstet Gynecol Scand 1997;76:69–73. (Level I)

121. Tate KM, Strickland JL. A randomized controlled trial to evaluate the use of the endocervical brush after endocervical curettage. Obstet Gynecol 1997;90:715–7. (Level I)

122. Naumann RW, Crispens MA, Alvarez RD, Partridge EE, Shingleton HM, Kilgore LC. Treatment of cervical dysplasia with large loop excision of the transformation zone: is endocervical curettage necessary? South Med J 1996;89:961–5. (Level III)

123. Williams DL, Dietrich C, McBroom J. Endocervical curettage when colposcopic examination is satisfactory and normal. Obstet Gynecol 2000;95:801–3. (Level III)

124. Drescher CW, Peters WA 3rd, Roberts JA. Contribution of endocervical curettage in evaluating abnormal cervical cytology. Obstet Gynecol 1983;62:343–7. (Level III)

125. Moniak CW, Kutzner S, Adam E, Harden J, Kaufman RH. Endocervical curettage in evaluating abnormal cervical cytology. J Reprod Med 2000;45:285–92. (Level III)

126. Fine BA, Feinstein GI, Sabella V. The pre- and postoperative value of endocervical curettage in the detection of cervical intraepithelial neoplasia and invasive cervical cancer. Gynecol Oncol 1998;71:46–9. (Level II-3)

127. Massad LS, Collins YC. Using history and colposcopy to select women for endocervical curettage. Results from 2,287 cases. J Reprod Med 2003;48:1–6. (Level II-3)

128. Pretorius RG, Zhang WH, Belinson JL, Huang MN, Wu LY, Zhang X, et al. Colposcopically directed biopsy, random cervical biopsy, and endocervical curettage in the diagnosis of cervical intraepthelial neoplasia II or worse. Am J Obstet Gynecol 2004;191:430–4. (Level II-3)

129. Spitzer M, Chernys AE, Shifrin A, Ryskin M. Indications for cone biopsy: pathologic correlation. Am J Obstet Gynecol 1998;178:74–9. (Level III)

130. Denehy TR, Gregori CA, Breen JL. Endocervical curettage, cone margins, and residual adenocarcinoma in situ of the cervix. Obstet Gynecol 1997;90:1–6. (Level III)

131. Hopman EH, Kenemans P, Helmerhorst TJ. Positive predictive rate of colposcopic examination of the cervix uteri: an overview of literature. Obstet Gynecol Surv 1998;53:97–106. (Level III)

132. Mitchell MF, Schottenfeld D, Tortolero-Luna G, Cantor SB, Richards-Kortum R. Colposcopy for the diagnosis of squamous intraepithelial lesions: a meta-analysis. Obstet Gynecol 1998;91:626–31. (Meta-analysis)

133. Nasiell K, Roger V, Nasiell M. Behavior of mild cervical dysplasia during long-term follow-up. Obstet Gynecol 1986;67:665–9. (Level II-3)

134. Weaver MG, Abdul-Karim FW, Dale G, Sorensen K, Huang YT. Outcome in mild and moderate cervical dysplasias related to the presence of specific human papillomavirus types. Mod Pathol 1990;3:679–83. (Level III)

135. Mitchell MF, Schottenfeld D. The natural history of cervical intraepithelial neoplasia and management of the abnormal Papanicolau smear. In: Rubin SC, Hoskins WJ, editors. Cervical cancer and preinvasive neoplasia. Philadelphia (PA): Lippincott Raven; 1996. p. 103–13. (Level III)

136. Ismail SM, Colclough AB, Dinnen JS, Eakins D, Evans DM, Gradwell E, et al. Observer variation in histopathological diagnosis and grading of cervical intraepithelial neoplasia. BMJ 1989;298:707–10. (Level III)

137. Wright TC Jr, Cox JT, Massad LS, Carlson J, Twiggs LB, Wilkinson EJ. 2001 consensus guidelines for the management of women with cervical intraepithelial neoplasia. American Society for Colposcopy and Cervical Pathology. Am J Obstet Gynecol 2003;189:295–304. (Level III)

138. Ahdieh L, Munoz A, Vlahov D, Trimble CL, Timpson LA, Shah K. Cervical neoplasia and repeated positivity of human papillomavirus infection in human immunodeficiency virus-seropositive and -seronegative women. Am J Epidemiol 2000;151:1148–57. (Level II-3)

139. Maiman M, Fruchter RG, Serur E, Levine PA, Arrastia CD, Sedlis A. Recurrent cervical intraepithelial neoplasia in human immunodeficiency virus-seropositive women. Obstet Gynecol 1993;82:170–4. (Level II-2)

140. Maiman M, Watts DH, Andersen J, Clax P, Merino M, Kendall MA. Vaginal 5-fluorouracil for high-grade cervical dysplasia in human immunodeficiency virus infection: a randomized trial. Obstet Gynecol 1999;94:954–61. (Level I)

141. Massad LS, Ahdieh L, Benning L, Minkoff H, Greenblatt RM, Watts H, et al. Evolution of cervical abnormalities among women with HIV-1: evidence from surveillance cytology in the women's interagency HIV study. J Acquir Immune Defic Syndr 2001;27:432–42. (Level II-2)

142. Tate DR, Anderson RJ. Recrudescence of cervical dysplasia among women who are infected with the human immunodeficiency virus: a case-control analysis. Am J Obstet Gynecol 2002;186:880–2. (Level II-2)

143. Adachi A, Fleming I, Burk RD, Ho GY, Klein RS. Women with human immunodeficiency virus infection and abnormal Papanicolaou smears: a prospective study of colposcopy and clinical outcome. Obstet Gynecol 1993;81:372–7. (Level II-3)

144. Holcomb K, Matthews RP, Chapman JE, Abulafia O, Lee YC, Borges A, et al. The efficacy of cervical conization in the treatment of cervical intraepithelial neoplasia in HIV-positive women. Gynecol Oncol 1999;74:428–31. (Level II-3)

145. Fruchter RG, Maiman M, Sedlis A, Bartley L, Camilien L, Arrastia CD. Multiple recurrences of cervical intraepithelial neoplasia in women with the human immunodeficiency virus. Obstet Gynecol 1996;87:338–44. (Level II-2)

146. Wright TC Jr, Koulos J, Schnoll F, Swanbeck J, Ellerbrock TV, Chiasson MA, et al. Cervical intraepithelial neoplasia in women infected with the human immunodeficiency virus: outcome after loop electrosurgical excision. Gynecol Oncol 1994;55:253–8. (Level II-3)

147. Boardman LA, Peipert JF, Hogan JW, Cooper AS. Positive cone biopsy specimen margins in women infected with the human immunodeficiency virus. Am J Obstet Gynecol 1999;181:1395–9. (Level II-2)

148. Heard I, Palefsky JM, Kazatchkine MD. The impact of HIV antiviral therapy on human papillomavirus infections (HPV) and HPV-related diseases. Antivir Ther 2004;9:13–22. (Level II-2)

149. Berget A, Andreasson B, Bock JE. Laser and cryo surgery for cervical intraepithelial neoplasia. A randomized trial with longterm follow-up. Acta Obstet Gynecol Scand 1991;70:231–5. (Level I)

150. Kirwan PH, Smith IR, Naftalin NJ. A study of cryosurgery and the CO2 laser in treatment of carcinoma in situ (CIN III) of the uterine cervix. Gynecol Oncol 1985;22:195–200. (Level III)

151. Kwikkel HJ, Helmerhorst TJ, Bezemer PD, Quaak MJ, Stolk JG. Laser or cryotherapy for cervical intraepithelial neoplasia: a randomized study to compare efficacy and side effects. Gynecol Oncol 1985;22:23–31. (Level I)

152. Ostergard DR. Cryosurgical treatment of cervical intraepithelial neoplasia. Obstet Gynecol 1980;56: 231–3. (Level II-3)

153. Wright VC, Davies EM. The conservative management of cervical intraepithelial neoplasia: the use of cryosurgery and the carbon dioxide laser. Br J Obstet Gynaecol 1981;88:663–8. (Level II-3)

154. Martin-Hirsch PL, Paraskevaidis E, Kitchener H. Surgery for cervical intraepithelial neoplasia. The Cochrane Database of Systematic Reviews 1999, Issue 3. Art. No.: CD001318. DOI: 10.1002/14651858. CD001318. (Meta-analysis)

155. Mitchell MF, Tortolero-Luna G, Cook E, Whittaker L, Rhodes-Morris H, Silva E. A randomized clinical trial of cryotherapy, laser vaporization, and loop electrosurgical excision for treatment of squamous intraepithelial lesions of the cervix. Obstet Gynecol 1998;92:737–44. (Level I)

156. Townsend DE, Richart RM, Marks E, Nielsen J. Invasive cancer following outpatient evaluation and therapy for cervical disease. Obstet Gynecol 1981;57: 145–9. (Level III)

157. Ferenczy A, Choukroun D, Arseneau J. Loop electrosurgical excision procedure for squamous intraepithelial lesions of the cervix: advantages and potential pitfalls. Obstet Gynecol 1996;87:332–7. (Level II-3)

158. Anderson MC. Glandular lesions of the cervix: diagnostic and therapeutic dilemmas. Baillieres Clin Obstet Gynaecol 1995;9:105–19. (Level III)

159. Boddington MM, Spriggs AI, Cowdell RH. Adenocarcinoma of the uterine cervix: cytological evidence of a long preclinical evolution. Br J Obstet Gynaecol 1976;83:900–3. (Level III)

160. Boon ME, Baak JP, Kurver PJ, Overdiep SH, Verdonk GW. Adenocarcinoma in situ of the cervix: an under-diagnosed lesion. Cancer 1981;48:768–73. (Level III)

161. Chang T, Bova C, Wong F. Re: Adenocarcinoma in situ of the uterine cervix progressing to invasive adenocarcinoma. Aust N Z J Obstet Gynaecol 1997;37:132–3. (Level III)

162. Goldstein NS, Mani A. The status and distance of cone biopsy margins as a predictor of excision adequacy for endocervical adenocarcinoma in situ. Am J Clin Pathol 1998;109:727–32. (Level III)

163. Hocking GR, Hayman JA, Ostor AG. Adenocarcinoma in situ of the uterine cervix progressing to invasive adenocarcinoma. Aust N Z J Obstet Gynaecol 1996; 36:218–20. (Level III)

164. Hopkins MP, Roberts JA, Schmidt RW. Cervical adenocarcinoma in situ. Obstet Gynecol 1988;71:842–4. (Level III)

165. Kashimura M, Shinohara M, Oikawa K, Hamasaki K, Sato H. An adenocarcinoma in situ of the uterine cervix that developed into invasive adenocarcinoma after 5 years. Gynecol Oncol 1990;36:128–33. (Level III)

166. Luesley DM, Jordan JA, Woodman CB, Watson N, Williams DR, Waddell C. A retrospective review of adenocarcinoma-in-situ and glandular atypia of the uterine cervix. Br J Obstet Gynaecol 1987;94:699–703. (Level III)

167. Muntz HG, Bell DA, Lage JM, Goff BA, Feldman S, Rice LW. Adenocarcinoma in situ of the uterine cervix. Obstet Gynecol 1992;80:935–9. (Level III)

168. Nicklin JL, Wright RG, Bell JR, Samaratunga H, Cox NC, Ward BG. A clinicopathological study of adenocarcinoma in situ of the cervix. The influence of cervical HPV infection and other factors, and the role of conservative surgery. Aust N Z J Obstet Gynaecol 1991; 31:179–83. (Level III)

169. Ostor AG, Pagano R, Davoren RA, Fortune DW, Chanen W, Rome R. Adenocarcinoma in situ of the cervix. Int J Gynecol Pathol 1984;3:179–90. (Level III)

170. Poynor EA, Barakat RR, Hoskins WJ. Management and follow-up of patients with adenocarcinoma in situ of the uterine cervix. Gynecol Oncol 1995;57:158–64. (Level III)

171. Qizilbash AH. In-situ and microinvasive adenocarcinoma of the uterine cervix. A clinical, cytologic and histologic study of 14 cases. Am J Clin Pathol 1975;64: 155–70. (Level III)

172. Weisbrot IM, Stabinsky C, Davis AM. Adenocarcinoma in situ of the uterine cervix. Cancer 1972;29:1179–87. (Level III)

173. Widrich T, Kennedy AW, Myers TM, Hart WR, Wirth S. Adenocarcinoma in situ of the uterine cervix: management and outcome. Gynecol Oncol 1996;61:304–8. (Level III)

174. Wolf JK, Levenback C, Malpica A, Morris M, Burke T, Mitchell MF. Adenocarcinoma in situ of the cervix: significance of cone biopsy margins. Obstet Gynecol 1996;88:82–6. (Level III)

175. Hopkins MP. Adenocarcinoma in situ of the cervix—the margins must be clear [editorial]. Gynecol Oncol 2000;79:4–5. (Level III)

176. Kennedy AW, Biscotti CV. Further study of the management of cervical adenocarcinoma in situ. Gynecol Oncol 2002;86:361–4. (Level III)

177. Shin CH, Schorge JO, Lee KR, Sheets EE. Conservative management of adenocarcinoma in situ of the cervix. Gynecol Oncol 2000;79:6–10. (Level III)

178. Lea JS, Shin CH, Sheets EE, Coleman RL, Gehrig PA, Duska LR, et al. Endocervical curettage at conization to predict residual cervical adenocarcinoma in situ. Gynecol Oncol 2002;87:129–32. (Level III)

179. Krivak TC, Rose GS, McBroom JW, Carlson JW, Winter WE 3rd, Kost ER. Cervical adenocarcinoma in situ: a systematic review of therapeutic options and predictors of persistent or recurrent disease. Obstet Gynecol Surv 2001;56:567–75. (Level III)

180. Im DD, Duska LR, Rosenshein NB. Adequacy of conization margins in adenocarcinoma in situ of the cervix as a predictor of residual disease. Gynecol Oncol 1995;59:179–82. (Level III)

181. McHale MT, Le TD, Burger RA, Gu M, Rutgers JL, Monk BJ. Fertility sparing treatment for in situ and early invasive adenocarcinoma of the cervix. Obstet Gynecol 2001;98:726–31. (Level III)

182. Andersen ES, Nielsen K. Adenocarcinoma in situ of the cervix: a prospective study of conization as definitive treatment. Gynecol Oncol 2002;86:365–9. (Level III)

183. Ostor AG, Duncan A, Quinn M, Rome R. Adenocarcinoma in situ of the uterine cervix: an experience with 100 cases. Gynecol Oncol 2000;79:207–10. (Level III)

184. Orr JW Jr, Orr PJ. Cervical cancer: staging. In: Rubin SC, Hoskins WJ, editors. Cervical cancer and preinvasive neoplasia. Philadelphia (PA): Lippincott Raven; 1996. p. 171–82. (Level III)

185. Anderson MC. Invasive carcinoma of the cervix following local destructive treatment for cervical intraepithelial neoplasia. Br J Obstet Gynaecol 1993;100:657–63. (Level III)

186. Boyes DA, Worth AJ, Fidler HK. The results of treatment of 4389 cases of preclinical cervical squamous carcinoma. J Obstet Gynaecol Br Commonw 1970;77: 769–80. (Level II-3)

187. Draeby-Kristiansen J, Garsaae M, Bruun M, Hansen K. Ten years after cryosurgical treatment of cervical intraepithelial neoplasia. Am J Obstet Gynecol 1991;165:43–5. (Level III)

188. Chang DY, Cheng WF, Torng PL, Chen RJ, Huang SC. Prediction of residual neoplasia based on histopathology and margin status of conization specimens. Gynecol Oncol 1996;63:53–6. (Level II-3)

189. Felix JC, Muderspach LI, Duggan BD, Roman LD. The significance of positive margins in loop electrosurgical cone biopsies. Obstet Gynecol 1994;84:996–1000. (Level III)

190. Gardeil F, Barry-Walsh C, Prendiville W, Clinch J, Turner MJ. Persistent intraepithelial neoplasia after excision for cervical intraepithelial neoplasia grade III. Obstet Gynecol 1997;89:419–22. (Level II-3)

191. Vedel P, Jakobsen H, Kryger-Baggesen N, Rank F, Bostofte E. Five-year follow up of patients with cervical intra-epithelial neoplasia in the cone margins after conization. Eur J Obstet Gynecol Reprod Biol 1993; 50:71–6. (Level II-2)

192. Zaitoun AM, McKee G, Coppen MJ, Thomas SM, Wilson PO. Completeness of excision and follow up cytology in patients treated with loop excision biopsy. J Clin Pathol 2000;53:191–6. (Level II-2)

193. Kobak WH, Roman LD, Felix JC, Muderspach LI, Schlaerth JB, Morrow CP. The role of endocervical curettage at cervical conization for high-grade dysplasia. Obstet Gynecol 1995;85:197–201. (Level II-2)

194. Ahlgren M, Ingemarsson I, Lindberg LG, Nordqvist RB. Conization as treatment of carcinoma in situ of the uterine cervix. Obstet Gynecol 1975;46:135–9. (Level III)

195. Kolstad P, Klem V. Long term followup of 1121 cases of carcinoma in situ. Obstet Gynecol 1976;48:125–9. (Level III)

196. Anderson ES, Nielsen K, Larsen G. Laser conization: follow-up in patients with cervical intraepithelial neoplasia in the cone margin. Gynecol Oncol 1990;39: 328–31. (Level III)

197. Lopes A, Morgan P, Murdoch J, Piura B, Monaghan JM. The case of conservative management of "incomplete excision" of CIN after laser conization. Gynecol Oncol 1993;49:247–9. (Level III)

198. Buxton EJ, Luesley DM, Wade-Evans T, Jordan JA. Residual disease after cone biopsy: completeness of excision and follow-up cytology as predictive factors. Obstet Gynecol 1987;70:529–32. (Level II-2)

199. Jansen FW, Trimbos JB, Hermans J, Fleuren GJ. Persistent cervical intraepithelial neoplasia after incomplete conization: predictive value of clinical and histological parameters. Gynecol Obstet Invest 1994;37: 270–4. (Level II-2)

200. Lapaquette TK, Dinh TV, Hannigan EV, Doherty MG, Yandell RB, Buchanan VS. Management of patients with positive margins after cervical conization. Obstet Gynecol 1993;82:440–3. (Level III)

201. Monk A, Pushkin SF, Nelson AL, Gunning JE. Conservative management of options for patients with dysplasia involving endocervical margins of cervical cone biopsy specimens. Am J Obstet Gynecol 1996; 174:1695–9; discussion 1699–700. (Level III)

202. Reich O, Lahousen M, Pickel H, Tamussino K, Winter R. Cervical intraepithelial neoplasia III: long-term follow-up after cold-knife conization with involved margins. Obstet Gynecol 2002;99:193–6. (Level II-3)

203. Paraskevaidis E, Koliopoulos G, Paschopoulos M, Stefanidis K, Navrozoglou I, Lolis D. Effects of ball cauterization following loop excision and follow-up colposcopy. Obstet Gynecol 2001;97:617–20. (Level II-1)

204. Bodner K, Bodner-Adler B, Wierrani F, Kimberger O, Denk C, Grunberger W. Is therapeutic conization sufficient to eliminate a high-risk HPV infection of the uterine cervix? A clinicopathological analysis. Anticancer Res 2002;22:3733–6. (Level III)

205. Chua KL, Hjerpe A. Human papillomavirus analysis as a prognostic marker following conization of the cervix uteri. Gynecol Oncol 1997;66:108–13. (Level II-2)

206. Cruickshank ME, Sharp L, Chambers G, Smart L, Murray G. Persistent infection with human papillomavirus following the successful treatment of high grade cervical intraepithelial neoplasia. BJOG 2002; 109:579–81. (Level II-2)

207. Jain S, Tseng CJ, Horng SG, Soong YK, Pao CC. Negative predictive value of human papillomavirus test following conization of the cervix uteri. Gynecol Oncol 2001;82:177–80. (Level II-2)

208. Kucera E, Sliutz G, Czerwenka K, Breitenecker G, Leodolter S, Reinthaller A. Is high-risk human papillomavirus infection associated with cervical intraepithelial neoplasia eliminated after conization by large-loop excision of the transformation zone? Eur J Obstet Gynecol Reprod Biol 2001;100:72–6. (Level II-2)

209. Nagai Y, Maehama T, Asato T, Kanazawa K. Persistence of human papillomavirus infection after therapeutic conization for CIN 3: is it an alarm for disease recurrence? Gynecol Oncol 2000;79:294–9. (Level II-3)

210. Nobbenhuis MA, Meijer CJ, van den Brule AJ, Rozendaal L, Voorhorst FJ, Risse EK, et al. Addition of high-risk HPV testing improves the current guidelines on follow-up after treatment for cervical intraepithelial neoplasia. Br J Cancer 2001;84:796–801. (Level II-2)

211. Strand A, Wilander E, Zehbe I, Rylander E. High risk HPV persists after treatment of genital papillomavirus infection but not after treatment of cervical intraepithelial neoplasia. Acta Obstet Gynecol Scand 1997;76: 140–4. (Level II-2)

212. Lopes A, Mor-Yosef S, Pearson S, Ireland D, Monaghan JM. Is routine colposcopic assessment necessary following laser ablation of cervical intraepithelial neoplasia? Br J Obstet Gynaecol 1990;97:175–7. (Level III)

213. Demeter A, Sziller I, Csapo Z, Szantho A, Papp Z. Outcome of pregnancies after cold-knife conization of the uterine cervix during pregnancy. Eur J Gynaecol Oncol 2002;23:207–10. (Level II-3)

214. Takushi M, Moromizato H, Sakumoto K, Kanazawa K. Management of invasive carcinoma of the uterine cervix associated with pregnancy: outcome of intentional delay in treatment. Gynecol Oncol 2002;87: 185–9. (Level III)

The MEDLINE database, the Cochrane Library, and ACOG's own internal resources and documents were used to conduct a literature search to locate relevant articles published between January 1985 and April 2005. The search was restricted to articles published in the English language. Priority was given to articles reporting results of original research, although review articles and commentaries also were consulted. Abstracts of research presented at symposia and scientific conferences were not considered adequate for inclusion in this document. Guidelines published by organizations or institutions such as the National Institutes of Health and the American College of Obstetricians and Gynecologists were reviewed, and additional studies were located by reviewing bibliographies of identified articles. When reliable research was not available, expert opinions from obstetrician–gynecologists were used.

Studies were reviewed and evaluated for quality according to the method outlined by the U.S. Preventive Services Task Force:

I   Evidence obtained from at least one properly designed randomized controlled trial.

II-1   Evidence obtained from well-designed controlled trials without randomization.

II-2   Evidence obtained from well-designed cohort or case–control analytic studies, preferably from more than one center or research group.

II-3   Evidence obtained from multiple time series with or without the intervention. Dramatic results in uncontrolled experiments also could be regarded as this type of evidence.

III   Opinions of respected authorities, based on clinical experience, descriptive studies, or reports of expert committees.

Based on the highest level of evidence found in the data, recommendations are provided and graded according to the following categories:

Level A—Recommendations are based on good and consistent scientific evidence.

Level B—Recommendations are based on limited or inconsistent scientific evidence.

Level C—Recommendations are based primarily on consensus and expert opinion.

ISSN 1099-3630

The American College of
Obstetricians and Gynecologists
409 12th Street, SW
PO Box 96920
Washington, DC 20090-6920

12345/98765

Management of abnormal cervical cytology and histology. ACOG Practice Bulletin No. 66. American College of Obstetricians and Gynecologists. Obstet Gynecol 2005;106:645–64.

ACOG PRACTICE BULLETIN

CLINICAL MANAGEMENT GUIDELINES FOR
OBSTETRICIAN–GYNECOLOGISTS
NUMBER 14, MARCH 2000

This Practice Bulletin was developed by the ACOG Committee on Practice Bulletins—Gynecology with the assistance of Dale Stovall, MD. The information is designed to aid practitioners in making decisions about appropriate obstetric and gynecologic care. These guidelines should not be construed as dictating an exclusive course of treatment or procedure. Variations in practice may be warranted based on the needs of the individual patient, resources, and limitations unique to the institution or type of practice.

Management of Anovulatory Bleeding

Anovulatory bleeding, the most common form of noncyclic uterine bleeding, is a condition for which women frequently seek gynecologic care and accounts for considerable patient anxiety and inconvenience. Over the past decade, significant advances have been made in the evaluation and management of women with anovulatory bleeding. The choice of treatment for anovulatory bleeding depends on several factors, including the woman's age, the severity of her bleeding, and her desire for future fertility. The purpose of this document is to provide management guidelines for the treatment of patients with menstrual irregularities associated with anovulation based on the best available evidence.

Background

Definition and Nomenclature

The terms menses, menstrual flow, and menstruation will be used in this document interchangeably, and each of these terms simply refer to the presence of menstrual effluent irrespective of whether the effluent is normal or abnormal. Anovulatory uterine bleeding is defined as noncyclic menstrual blood flow that may range from spotty to excessive, is derived from the uterine endometrium, and is due to anovulatory sex steroid production specifically excluding an anatomic lesion. Several terms have been used to describe anovulatory bleeding, including dysfunctional, irregular, and abnormal. In this bulletin, the term *anovulatory uterine bleeding* will be used as the standard terminology to describe menstrual bleeding arising from anovulation or oligo-ovulation.

Several descriptive terms also are used to describe menstrual bleeding patterns, including menorrhagia, metrorrhagia, polymenorrhea, and menometrorrhagia. Menorrhagia is defined as prolonged or excessive uterine bleeding that occurs at regular intervals, or more strictly, the loss of 80 mL or more of blood per menstrual cycle or bleeding that lasts for more than 7 days (1). Metrorrhagia is defined as irregular menstrual bleeding or bleeding between periods. Polymenorrhea is defined as frequent menstrual bleeding or, more strictly, menstrual bleeding that occurs every 21 days or less. Menometrorrhagia is defined as frequent menstrual bleeding that is excessive and irregular in amount and duration.

Ovulatory Cycle

During a normal ovulatory cycle—including follicular development, ovulation, corpus luteal function, and luteolysis—the endometrium is sequentially exposed to ovarian production of estrogen alone, followed by a combination of estrogen and progesterone; the cycle is culminated by estrogen and progesterone withdrawal. Ovulation is associated with a cyclic pattern of endometrial histology commencing with proliferation followed by secretion change, desquamation, and repair. Normal ovarian steroid production is important for nidation and pregnancy. From a clinical perspective, the result is cyclic, predictable, and relatively consistent menstrual blood loss (2).

Pathophysiology

With anovulation, a corpus luteum is not produced, and the ovary fails to secrete progesterone, although estrogen production continues. This condition results in continual endometrial proliferation without progesterone-induced desquamation and bleeding. The clinical result is bleeding that is noncyclic, unpredictable, and inconsistent in volume.

Continuous, unopposed estrogen stimulation of the endometrium results in unsustainable endometrial growth. The endometrium becomes excessively vascular without sufficient stromal support and becomes fragile, resulting in variable endometrial bleeding. Unlike the uniform, synchronized endometrial sloughing and bleeding that occurs with normal cyclic estrogen and progesterone stimulation, endometrial loss during continuous estrogen stimulation is irregular. As one area of bleeding begins to heal, another area begins to slough, resulting in irregular and prolonged menstrual flow.

Alterations in endometrial prostaglandin (PG) synthesis and release appear to occur in women with anovulatory uterine bleeding. In particular, lower concentrations of $PGF_{2\alpha}$ have been found in the endometrium of women with anovulatory bleeding as compared with women with ovulatory menstrual cycles (3). Furthermore, these investigators found a reverse correlation between the endometrial $PGF_{2\alpha}/PGE_2$ ratio and the amount of menstrual blood lost. Therefore, abnormal vasoconstriction produced by altered endometrial prostaglandins may enhance blood loss in women with chronic anovulation.

Establishing the Diagnosis

The diagnosis of anovulatory uterine bleeding is made after the exclusion of anatomic pathology. Diagnostic techniques to exclude anatomic pathology include physical examination supplemented by endometrial sampling, transvaginal ultrasonography, sonohysterography, hysterosalpingography, hysteroscopy, curettage, endometrial cultures, and timed tests for determining progesterone levels in serum. Recognized causes of anovulation are given in the box below and should be considered when evaluating the medical history and results of the physical examination. There are numerous other causes of noncyclic vaginal bleeding. The differential diagnosis of abnormal bleeding is listed in the box on the next page. In this document, recommendations are based on the assumption that the diagnosis of anovulatory bleeding has been firmly established.

The physical examination should include an assessment for obesity and hirsutism, because these findings are associated with chronic anovulation (4, 5). Thyroid disease may cause anovulation as well as hyperprolactinemia. Approximately one third of all women with hyperprolactinemia will have galactorrhea (6). In women of reproductive age with noncyclic uterine bleeding, pregnancy must be ruled out. If medical therapy fails to resolve bleeding thought to be the result of anovulation, an anatomic cause, including a malignant or premalignant lesion or a coagulopathy, should be reconsidered and the patient reevaluated.

Causes of Anovulation

Physiologic

    Adolescence

    Perimenopause

    Lactation

    Pregnancy

Pathologic

    Hyperandrogenic anovulation (eg, polycystic ovary syndrome, congenital adrenal hyperplasia, androgen-producing tumors)

    Hypothalamic dysfunction (eg, secondary to anorexia nervosa)

    Hyperprolactinemia

    Hypothyroidism

    Primary pituitary disease

    Premature ovarian failure

    Iatrogenic (eg, secondary to radiation or chemotherapy)

Differential Diagnosis of Noncyclic Uterine Bleeding

- Anovulation
- Uterine leiomyoma
- Endometrial polyp
- Endometrial hyperplasia or carcinoma
- Cervical or vaginal neoplasia
- Endometritis
- Adenomyosis
- Bleeding associated with pregnancy
  - –threatened or incomplete abortion
  - –trophoblastic disease
  - –ectopic pregnancy
- Bleeding associated with the puerperium
  - –retained products of conception
  - –placental polyp
  - –subinvolution of the uterus
- Coagulopathies (von Willebrand's disease, platelet abnormalities, thrombocytopenic purpura)
- Iatrogenic causes and medications
- Systemic diseases

Age Considerations of Anovulatory Bleeding

Adolescents (13–18 Years)

Anovulatory bleeding is a normal physiologic process in the perimenarchal years of the reproductive cycle. Ovulatory menstrual cycles may not be established until a year or more after menarche. This phenomenon is attributed to the immaturity of the hypothalamic–pituitary– gonadal axis. Anovulatory bleeding at this age can be excessive, resulting in anemia and requiring emergency care. Occasionally, adolescents with blood dyscrasias, including von Willebrand's disease and prothrombin deficiency, have heavy vaginal bleeding beginning at menarche. Disorders such as leukemia, idiopathic thrombocytopenic purpura, and hypersplenism can all produce platelet dysfunction and cause excessive bleeding. Studies have demonstrated a wide variation in the prevalence of blood dyscrasias ranging from 5% to 20% of hospitalized adolescents (7, 8). Because the prevalence of blood dyscrasias in the adolescent population is significant, routine screening for coagulation disorders is warranted in these patients, including a partial thromboplastin time, prothrombin time, and assessment of platelet

function. Physical examination should include an assessment for petechiae or ecchymoses.

Women of Reproductive Age (19–39 Years)

Between 6% and 10% of women have hyperandrogenic chronic anovulation (eg, polycystic ovary syndrome), which includes noncyclic menstrual bleeding, hirsutism, and obesity (body mass index ≥ 25 kg/m^2). As many as 65% of hirsute, chronically anovulatory women are obese (4). Numerous underlying biochemical abnormalities exist, including noncyclic estrogen production, elevated serum testosterone levels, hypersecretion of luteinizing hormone, and hyperinsulinemia (9). A history of rapidly progressing hirsutism accompanied by virilization suggests a tumor. In most cases, tumors can be ruled out by testing testosterone and dehydroepiandrosterone sulfate levels in serum.

Although anovulation may be considered physiologic in adolescents, adult women of reproductive age who have menorrhagia, metrorrhagia, or amenorrhea require evaluation for a specific cause. The laboratory assessment of these women should include a pregnancy test, a fasting serum prolactin level, and determination of levels of thyroid-stimulating hormone (TSH). When the diagnosis of ovarian failure is suspected, levels of follicle-stimulating hormone (FSH) also should be determined. Anovulation was found to be the most common cause of amenorrhea in a series of 262 women who experienced adult-onset amenorrhea (10). Chronic anovulation that results from hypothalamic dysfunction, as diagnosed by a low FSH level, may be the result of excessive psychologic stress, exercise, or weight loss (10). Both hyperthyroidism and hypothyroidism can be excluded using the sensitive TSH assay. In patients with amenorrhea who have a negative pregnancy test result and normal FSH, TSH, and prolactin levels, the diagnosis of anovulation can be made.

Women of Later Reproductive Age (40 Years to Menopause)

The incidence of anovulatory uterine bleeding increases as women approach the end of their reproductive years. In this regard, perimenopausal women are not unlike their perimenarchal counterparts. In perimenopausal women, the onset of anovulatory cycles represents a continuation of declining ovarian function. These patients need to be educated regarding the specific health risks associated with menopause so that an early proactive approach toward the prevention of menopause-associated conditions, such as osteoporosis, can be initiated. In addition to the use of hormone replacement therapy for cycle control, important lifestyle changes include exercise, dietary modification, and smoking cessation.

Clinical Considerations and Recommendations

▶ *In women of each age group with anovulatory bleeding, when is endometrial evaluation indicated?*

Adolescents (13–18 Years). In 1995, the incidence of endometrial cancer in women between the ages of 15 and 19 years was 0.1 per 100,000 (11). In one report of endometrial carcinoma in adolescents, the patients experienced 2–3 years of anovulatory uterine bleeding (12). One patient experienced precocious puberty, which extended the number of years of unopposed estrogen exposure for someone of her age. All of the adolescents were obese. Because obesity is associated with conversion of androgens to estrogens and chronic anovulation, obese patients may be at an increased risk for developing endometrial hyperplasia and carcinoma. Therefore, one should consider endometrial assessment particularly for those adolescents who have a history of 2–3 years of untreated anovulatory bleeding and especially for those who are obese.

Women of Reproductive Age (19–39 Years). The incidence of endometrial carcinoma increases with age. However, the incidence of endometrial carcinoma is still very low in women between the ages of 19 and 39 years, reported as 9.5 per 100,000 in 1995 (11). However, there is a distinct increase in the incidence of endometrial carcinoma from ages 30–34 years (2.3/100,000 in 1995) to ages 35–39 years (6.1/100,000 in 1995) (11). Therefore, based on age alone, endometrial assessment to exclude cancer is indicated in any woman older than 35 years who is suspected of having anovulatory uterine bleeding.

Although endometrial carcinoma is rare in women younger than 35 years, patients between the ages of 19 and 35 years who do not respond to medical therapy or have prolonged periods of unopposed estrogen stimulation secondary to chronic anovulation are candidates for endometrial assessment.

Women of Later Reproductive Age (40 Years to Menopause). The incidence of endometrial carcinoma in women ages 40–49 years was 36.2 per 100,000 in 1995 (11). Therefore, all women older than 40 years who present with suspected anovulatory uterine bleeding should be evaluated with endometrial assessment (after pregnancy has been excluded).

▶ *What medical therapies are most appropriate for each age group?*

Because anovulatory uterine bleeding is by definition an endocrinologic abnormality, medical management is the preferred method of therapy. The goals of medical treatment for anovulatory bleeding are to alleviate acute bleeding, prevent future episodes of noncyclic bleeding, decrease the patient's risk of long-term complications from anovulation, and improve the patient's overall quality of life. To encourage compliance with medical therapy, it is important to counsel patients that treatment may cause initial heavy menstrual bleeding secondary to endometrial buildup, but will lighten over time (within three cycles).

Adolescents (13–18 Years). Most adolescents who experience anovulatory bleeding can be treated with medical therapy. Occasionally, adolescents may have acute, profuse menstrual bleeding. High-dose estrogen therapy is an appropriate treatment to control acute bleeding episodes because it promotes rapid endometrial growth to cover denuded endometrial surfaces. Patients with blood dyscrasias need to be treated for their specific disease, and leukemia needs to be ruled out in this population. Conjugated equine estrogens can be administered orally up to 10 mg/d in four divided doses or intravenously at 25 mg every 4 hours for up to 24 hours (13). In a retrospective study, most adolescent patients with acute bleeding (93%) responded to medical therapy (8). After acute bleeding has been treated, recurrent anovulatory bleeding should be prevented with either a cyclic progestogen or an oral contraceptive.

Women with chronic anovulation can be treated successfully using either a cyclic progestogen or an oral contraceptive. Oral contraceptives suppress both ovarian and adrenal androgen production and increase sex hormone binding globulin, further reducing bioavailable androgens (14, 15). They also may inhibit 5α-reductase activity in the skin of adults (16). Treatment with a low-dose combination oral contraceptive (≤35 μg ethinyl estradiol) is appropriate, and maintenance oral contraceptives are the treatment of choice in women with chronic anovulation, especially if they are hyperandrogenic and hirsute (17).

Women of Reproductive Age (19–39 Years). Adult women of reproductive age with anovulatory uterine bleeding can be treated safely with either a cyclic progestogen or oral contraceptives similar to those prescribed for adolescent patients. However, estrogen-containing oral contraceptives are relatively contraindicated in some women (eg, those with hypertension or diabetes). Estrogen-containing oral contraceptives are contraindicated for women older than 35 years who smoke or have a history of thromboembolic disease.

If pregnancy is desired, induction of ovulation with clomiphene citrate is the initial treatment of choice (18). Patients can have withdrawal bleeding induced with progestogen followed by initiation of therapy with clomiphene citrate, 50 mg/d for 5 days, beginning between days 3 and 5 of the menstrual cycle.

Women of Later Reproductive Age (40 Years to Menopause). Women who are older than 40 years and who have anovulatory uterine bleeding can be treated with cyclic progestogen, low-dose oral contraceptives, or cyclic hormone replacement therapy. Not unlike younger women, these patients usually have adequate estrogen production. However, women older than 40 years with oligomenorrhea may have reduced estrogen production. Women with hot flashes secondary to declining estrogen production can obtain symptomatic relief with estrogen replacement therapy in combination with continuous or cyclic progestogen. Up to 90% of perimenopausal women receiving continuous estrogen and cyclic progestogen therapy will respond with predictable progesterone withdrawal bleeding (19).

▶ *In patients who have completed childbearing, what is the benefit of treating anovulatory bleeding surgically rather than medically?*

Currently, there are few randomized trials comparing medical versus surgical therapy for anovulatory uterine bleeding. One randomized trial that compared endometrial resection with medical management for women with menorrhagia found that women who underwent medical therapy were less likely to be satisfied with their therapy (20). However, because of its reduced cost and risks, medical therapy should be offered before surgical intervention unless it is otherwise contraindicated. Surgical therapy is indicated for women with excessive anovulatory bleeding in whom medical management has failed and who have completed their childbearing. Avoidance of anemia, reduction of excessively heavy bleeding, and increased, though imperfect, predictability of bleeding are appropriate goals to attempt to achieve with medical therapy. Success and failure of medical therapy should be defined in partnership with the patient, to better achieve the therapeutic goal.

▶ *In women who have completed childbearing, what is the evidence of efficacy among surgical techniques?*

The surgical options include hysterectomy and endometrial ablation. Recent studies have reported morbidity rates of 7% (21) and 15% (22) for women undergoing hysterectomy for various indications. The overall mortality rate for hysterectomy is 12 deaths per 10,000 procedures, for all surgical indications (23). A surgical alternative to hysterectomy is endometrial ablation. Endometrial ablation can be performed with or without the assistance of hysteroscopy.

Hysteroscopic-assisted endometrial ablation can be performed with the resectoscope. Using the resectoscope, the endometrium can be removed or resected with an electrocautery loop or ablated with the rollerball. Endometrial ablation also can be accomplished with the YAG laser. An alternative to hysteroscopic-assisted endometrial ablation is thermal balloon ablation in which the endometrium is ablated by heating saline inside an intrauterine balloon to approximately 85°C. The most frequently reported complications of hysteroscopy are uterine perforation, which occurs in approximately 14 per 1,000 procedures (24) and fluid overload, which occurs in approximately 2 per 1,000 cases.

Studies evaluating the effectiveness of endometrial ablation have been performed in a group of women who were diagnosed with menorrhagia and who were not necessarily anovulatory. However, women with anovulatory uterine bleeding are candidates for endometrial ablation if they have failed medical therapy and have completed their childbearing. The proportion of women who are amenorrheic after undergoing an endometrial resection using the resectoscope or endometrial laser ablation is approximately 45%, and the percentage of women at 12 months postoperatively who are satisfied with their therapy approaches 90% (25, 26). This high degree of satisfaction indicates that reduction of flow is adequate symptom control for most women, and achievement of amenorrhea is not as important. Endometrial ablation with the thermal balloon yields an amenorrhea rate of approximately 15% and a 12-month postoperative satisfaction rate of approximately 90% (27, 28).

Patient satisfaction with hysterectomy and endometrial ablation performed for dysfunctional uterine bleeding has been compared. One study demonstrated a higher satisfaction rate in women who underwent hysterectomy as compared with women who underwent hysteroscopic-assisted endometrial ablation (29). Furthermore, the long-term satisfaction of women who have undergone endometrial ablation has been questioned. In a 3-year follow-up study, 8.5% of women who had undergone endometrial ablation later underwent repeat ablation, and an additional 8.5% had undergone hysterectomy (30). In a 5-year follow-up study, 34% of women who had undergone hysteroscopic ablation subsequently had a hysterectomy (31). Because women who undergo endometrial ablation can have residual active endometrium, these women should receive progestogen if they are prescribed estrogen replacement therapy.

Numerous studies have compared costs and surgical outcomes between endometrial resection or ablation and hysterectomy. The evidence suggests that hysteroscopic endometrial ablation results in less morbidity and shorter recovery periods and is more cost-effective than hysterectomy (32–37). However, if as many as one third of women who undergo endometrial ablation undergo hysterectomy within the following 5 years, that would have a significant impact on these cost analyses.

Evidence from randomized trials supports the use of either a gonadotropin-releasing hormone agonist or danazol prior to endometrial ablation or resection with regard to improved intrauterine operating environment and short-term postoperative outcome (38). The choice of agents should be based on cost, efficacy, and side effects. There are insufficient data to assess the value of progestogen therapy prior to endometrial ablation.

▶ *What is the role of high-dose estrogen in acute vaginal bleeding?*

Women who experience acute, profuse anovulatory bleeding are candidates for estrogen therapy. In approximately 90% of cases, acute bleeding does not require surgical intervention, but it can be treated with medical therapy (8). In a large series of 61 adolescents (mean age, 13.8 ± 2.1 years) with acute anovulatory uterine bleeding, only five (8.2%) failed medical therapy and required dilation and curettage to stop their bleeding. Conjugated equine estrogen therapy can be administered intravenously (25 mg every 4 hours for 24 hours). However, oral conjugated estrogen therapy at 10–20 mg per day in four divided doses can be substituted for intravenous estrogen administration. In a randomized trial of intravenous conjugated equine estrogen therapy versus placebo, conjugated estrogens were effective in stopping vaginal bleeding in a significantly greater proportion of women (72%) than those who received a placebo (38%)

(13). Although this study included women with biopsy-proven pathology, it is one of the few studies performed to assess the efficacy of intravenous estrogen therapy for the treatment of women with anovulatory uterine bleeding. Patients who do not respond to 1–2 doses of estrogen with a significant decline in blood loss or are not hemodynamically stable should undergo dilation and curettage. Furthermore, as high-dose estrogen therapy is commonly associated with nausea, concomitant medical therapy with antiemetics should be considered.

After the acute episode of bleeding has been controlled, amenorrhea should be maintained for several weeks to allow for resolution of anemia. The best method of therapy is a combination oral contraceptive. To extend the interval before the next menses, continuous oral contraceptives (without the use of placebo pills) can be given for several months; however, over time the patient will be susceptible again to breakthrough bleeding. Once the patient's anemia has resolved, cyclic oral contraceptives can be prescribed. All anemic patients should be given iron therapy.

Summary

The following recommendations are based on good and consistent scientific evidence (Level A):

▶ The treatment of choice for anovulatory uterine bleeding is medical therapy with oral contraceptives. Cyclic progestins also are effective.

▶ Women who have failed medical therapy and no longer desire future childbearing are candidates for endometrial ablation, which appears to be an efficient and cost-effective alternative treatment to hysterectomy for anovulatory uterine bleeding. However, endometrial ablation may not be definitive therapy.

The following recommendations are based primarily on consensus and expert opinion (Level C):

▶ An underlying coagulopathy, such as von Willebrand's disease, should be considered in all patients (particularly adolescents) with abnormal uterine bleeding, especially when bleeding is not otherwise easily explained or does not respond to medical therapy.

▶ Although there is limited evidence evaluating the efficacy of conjugated equine estrogen therapy in anovulatory bleeding, it is effective in controlling abnormal uterine bleeding.

References

1. Hallberg L, Hogdahl AM, Nilsson L, Rybo G. Menstrual blood loss—a population study. Variation at different ages and attempts to define normality. Acta Obstet Gynecol Scand 1966;45:320–351 (Level III)

2. Hallberg L, Nilsson L. Constancy of individual menstrual blood loss. Acta Obstet Gynecol Scand 1964;43:352–359 (Level III)

3. Smith SK, Abel MH, Kelly RW, Baird DT. The synthesis of prostaglandins from persistent proliferative endometrium. J Clin Endocrinol Metab 1982;55:284–289 (Level II-2)

4. Singh KB, Mahajan DK, Wortsman J. Effect of obesity on the clinical and hormonal characteristics of the polycystic ovary syndrome. J Reprod Med 1994;39:805–808 (Level II-2)

5. Falsetti L, Eleftheriou G. Hyperinsulinemia in the polycystic ovary syndrome: a clinical, endocrine and echographic study in 240 patients. Gynecol Endocrinol 1996;10:319–326 (Level II-2)

6. Schlechte J, Sherman B, Halmi N, VanGilder J, Chapler F, Dolan K, et al. Prolactin-secreting pituitary tumors in amenorrheic women: a comprehensive study. Endocr Rev 1980;1:295–308

7. Claessens EA, Cowell CL. Acute adolescent menorrhagia. Am J Obstet Gynecol 1981;139:277–280 (Level III)

8. Falcone T, Desjardins C, Bourque J, Granger L, Hemmings R, Quiros E. Dysfunctional uterine bleeding in adolescents. J Reprod Med 1994;39:761–764 (Level II-2)

9. Goudas VT, Dumesic DA. Polycystic ovary syndrome. Endocrinol Metab Clin North Am 1997;26:893–912 (Level III)

10. Reindollar RH, Novak M, Tho SP, McDonough PG. Adult-onset amenorrhea: a study of 262 patients. Am J Obstet Gynecol 1986;155:531–543 (Level III)

11. SEER cancer statistics review, 1973–1996 [serial online]. Available at <http://www-seer.ims.nci.nih.gov/Publications/CSR1973_1996>. Retrieved February 1, 2000 (Level II-3)

12. Stovall DW, Anderson RJ, De Leon FD. Endometrial adenocarcinoma in teenagers. Adolesc Pediatr Gynecol 1989; 2:157–159 (Level III)

13. DeVore GR, Owens O, Kase N. Use of intravenous Premarin in the treatment of dysfunctional uterine bleeding—a double-blind randomized controlled study. Obstet Gynecol 1982;59:285–291 (Level I)

14. Wild RA, Umstot ES, Andersen RN, Givens JR. Adrenal function in hirsutism. II. Effect of an oral contraceptive. J Clin Endocrinol Metab 1982;54:676–681 (Level III)

15. Wiebe RH, Morris CV. Effect of an oral contraceptive on adrenal and ovarian androgenic steroids. Obstet Gynecol 1984;63:12–14 (Level III)

16. Cassidenti DL, Paulson RJ, Serafini P, Stanczyk FZ, Lobo RA. Effects of sex steroids on skin 5 alpha-reductase activity in vitro. Obstet Gynecol 1991;78:103–107 (Level III)

17. Rittmaster RS. Clinical review 73: Medical treatment of androgen-dependent hirsutism. J Clin Endocrinol Metab 1995;80:2559–2563 (Level III)

18. Hughes E, Collins J, Vandekerckhove P. Clomiphene citrate for unexplained subfertility in women (Cochrane review). In: The Cochrane Library, Issue 4, 1999. Oxford: Update Software. (Meta-analysis)

19. Strickland DM, Hammond TL. Postmenopausal estrogen replacement in a large gynecologic practice. Am J Gynecol Health 1988;2(1):26–31 (Level III)

20. Cooper KG, Parkin DE, Garratt AM, Grant AM. Two-year follow up of women randomised to medical management or transcervical resection of the endometrium for heavy menstrual loss: clinical and quality of life outcomes. Br J Obstet Gynaecol 1999;106:258–265 (Level I)

21. Carlson KJ, Miller BA, Fowler FJ Jr. The Maine Women's Health Study: I. Outcomes of hysterectomy. Obstet Gynecol 1994;83:556–565 (Level II-3)

22. Summitt RL Jr, Stovall TG, Steege JF, Lipscomb GH. A multicenter randomized comparison of laparoscopically assisted vaginal hysterectomy and abdominal hysterectomy in abdominal hysterectomy candidates. Obstet Gynecol 1998;92:321–326 (Level I)

23. Bachmann GA. Hysterectomy: A critical review. J Reprod Med 1990;35:839–862 (Level III)

24. Hulka JF, Peterson HA, Phillips JM, Surrey MW. Operative hysteroscopy: American Association of Gynecologic Laparoscopists' 1993 membership survey. J Am Assoc Gynecol Laparosc 1995;2:131–132 (Level II-3)

25. Bhattacharya S, Cameron IM, Parkin DE, Abramovich DR, Mollison J, Pinion SB, et al. A pragmatic randomised comparison of transcervical resection of the endometrium with endometrial laser ablation for the treatment of menorrhagia. Br J Obstet Gynaecol 1997;104:601–607 (Level I)

26. A randomized trial of endometrial ablation versus hysterectomy for the treatment of dysfunctional uterine bleeding: outcome at four years. Aberdeen Endometrial Ablation Trials Group. Br J Obstet Gynaecol 1999;106: 360–366 (Level I)

27. Amso NN, Stabinsky SA, McFaul P, Blanc B, Pendley L, Neuwirth R. Uterine thermal balloon therapy for the treatment of menorrhagia: the first 300 patients from a multi-centre study. International Collaborative Uterine Thermal Balloon Working Group. Br J Obstet Gynaecol 1998;105: 517–523 (Level 1)

28. Meyer WR, Walsh BW, Grainger DA, Peacock LM, Loffer FD, Steege JF. Thermal balloon and rollerball ablation to treat menorrhagia: a multicenter comparison. Obstet Gynecol 1998;92:98–103 (Level I)

29. Pinion SB, Parkin DE, Abramovich DR, Naji A, Alexander DA, Russell IT, et al. Randomised trial of hysterectomy, endometrial laser ablation, and transcervical endometrial resection for dysfunctional uterine bleeding. BMJ 1994; 309:979–983 (Level I)

30. Chullapram T, Song JY, Fraser IS. Medium-term follow-up of women with menorrhagia treated by rollerball

endometrial ablation. Obstet Gynecol 1996;88:71–76 (Level II-3)

31. Unger JB, Meeks GR. Hysterectomy after endometrial ablation. Am J Obstet Gynecol 1996;175:1432–1436; discussions 1436–1437 (Level II-3)

32. Gannon MJ, Holt EM, Fairbank J, Fitzgerald M, Milne MA, Crystal AM, et al. A randomised trial comparing endometrial resection and abdominal hysterectomy for the treatment of menorrhagia. BMJ 1991;303:1362–1364 (Level I)

33. Brooks PG, Clouse J, Morris LS. Hysterectomy vs. resectoscopic endometrial ablation for the control of abnormal uterine bleeding. A cost-comparative study. J Reprod Med 1994;39:755–760 (Level II-2)

34. Goldenberg M, Sivan E, Bider D, Mashiach S, Seidman DS. Endometrial resection vs. abdominal hysterectomy for menorrhagia. Correlated sample analysis. J Reprod Med 1996;41:333–336 (Level II-2)

35. Cameron IM, Mollison J, Pinion SB, Atherton-Naji A, Buckingham K, Torgerson D. A cost comparison of hysterectomy and hysteroscopic surgery for the treatment of menorrhagia. Eur J Obstet Gynecol Reprod Biol 1996;70:87–92 (Level I)

36. Vilos GA, Pispidikis JT, Botz CK. Economic evaluation of hysteroscopic endometrial ablation versus vaginal hysterectomy for menorrhagia. Obstet Gynecol 1996;88:241–245 (Level II-2)

37. Brumsted JR, Blackman JA, Badger GJ, Riddick DH. Hysteroscopy versus hysterectomy for the treatment of abnormal uterine bleeding: a comparison of cost. Fertil Steril 1996;65:310–316 (Level II-2)

38. Fraser IS, Healy DL, Torode H, Song JY, Mamers P, Wilde F. Depot goserelin and danazol pre-treatment before rollerball endometrial ablation for menorrhagia. Obstet Gynecol 1996;87:544–550 (Level I)

The MEDLINE database, the Cochrane Library, and ACOG's own internal resources and documents were used to conduct a literature search to locate relevant articles published between January 1985 and May 1999. The search was restricted to articles published in the English language. Priority was given to articles reporting results of original research, although review articles and commentaries also were consulted. Abstracts of research presented at symposia and scientific conferences were not considered adequate for inclusion in this document. Guidelines published by organizations or institutions such as the National Institutes of Health and the American College of Obstetricians and Gynecologists were reviewed, and additional studies were located by reviewing bibliographies of identified articles. When reliable research was not available, expert opinions from obstetrician–gynecologists were used.

Studies were reviewed and evaluated for quality according to the method outlined by the U.S. Preventive Services Task Force:

I   Evidence obtained from at least one properly designed randomized controlled trial.

II-1   Evidence obtained from well-designed controlled trials without randomization.

II-2   Evidence obtained from well-designed cohort or case–control analytic studies, preferably from more than one center or research group.

II-3   Evidence obtained from multiple time series with or without the intervention. Dramatic results in uncontrolled experiments could also be regarded as this type of evidence.

III   Opinions of respected authorities, based on clinical experience, descriptive studies, or reports of expert committees.

Based on the highest level of evidence found in the data, recommendations are provided and graded according to the following categories:

Level A—Recommendations are based on good and consistent scientific evidence.

Level B—Recommendations are based on limited or inconsistent scientific evidence.

Level C—Recommendations are based primarily on consensus and expert opinion.

**The American College of
Obstetricians and Gynecologists
409 12th Street, SW
PO Box 96920
Washington, DC 20090-6920**

12345/43210

ACOG PRACTICE BULLETIN

CLINICAL MANAGEMENT GUIDELINES FOR
OBSTETRICIAN–GYNECOLOGISTS

NUMBER 65, AUGUST 2005

This Practice Bulletin was developed by the ACOG Committee on Practice Bulletins—Gynecology and the Society of Gynecologic Oncologists member contributors James Orr Jr, MD, Donald Chamberlain, MD, Larry Kilgore, MD, and Wendal Naumann, MD, and the editorial assistance of Joan Walker, MD, and Jonathan Berek, MD. The information is designed to aid practitioners in making decisions about appropriate obstetric and gynecologic care. These guidelines should not be construed as dictating an exclusive course of treatment or procedure. Variations in practice may be warranted based on the needs of the individual patient, resources, and limitations unique to the institution or type of practice.

Management of Endometrial Cancer

Endometrial carcinoma is the most common gynecologic malignancy that will be encountered by almost every gynecologist. A thorough understanding of the epidemiology, pathophysiology, and management strategies allows the obstetrician–gynecologist to identify women at increased risk, to contribute toward risk reduction, and to facilitate early diagnosis of this cancer. The purpose of this document is to review the risks and benefits of current treatment options to optimize treatment for women with endometrial cancer.

Background

Epidemiology

Endometrial cancer is the most common female genital tract malignancy, with more than 40,000 cases estimated to be diagnosed in 2005 in the United States (1). Most women (90%) with endometrial cancer develop symptomatic bleeding or discharge, facilitating early diagnosis and resulting in an increased opportunity for cure. Currently, most endometrial cancers (72%) are diagnosed while in stage I; however, a significant number are in stage II (12%), stage III (13%), or stage IV (3%) (2). Despite this favorable stage distribution, endometrial cancer is responsible for 7,310 deaths each year, making it the eighth leading site of cancer-related death among American women (1).

It is estimated that 2.62% of women in the United States will develop uterine cancer during their lifetime, with a 0.5% lifetime mortality risk (whites 2.8%, 0.48%; blacks 1.7%, 0.73% respectively for risk of disease and death) (3). The 5-year survival rate for white women older than 65 years is 80.8% and for black women in the same age group is 53.3%. It is unclear whether the high mortality in black women is a result of delayed treatment, lack of access to care, or a higher likelihood of cancers with more serious prognostic characteristics. It is known that of women with endometrial cancer, only 52% of black women older than 50 years have disease confined to the uterus at the time of original surgery, compared with 73% of white women older than 50 years. The overall incidence of endometrial cancer likely will increase in the future secondary to increasing obesity and the aging of the population.

Etiology

The etiology of most endometrial cancers has been well described (4). The most common cause is an excess of endogenous or exogenous estrogen unopposed by progestin leading to endometrial hyperplasia followed by cancer. This cause allows for prevention and early detection of the most common and most indolent form of endometrial cancer (type I or estrogen dependent). Type I endometrial cancer typically has lower grade nuclei, endometrioid histologic cell type, phosphatase and tensin homologue mutation, and a good prognosis.

The more lethal variety of endometrial cancer, type II, accounts for approximately 10% of cases. It has aggressive high-grade nuclei or serous and clear cell histology and P53 tumor suppression mutation. In contrast to type I, the background underlying endometrium generally is atrophic or associated with polyps. There is no clear epidemiologic profile for type II cancers (Table 1). Carcinosarcoma of the

Table 1. Risk Factors for Uterine Corpus Cancer

Factors Influencing Risk	Estimated Relative Risk
Older age	2–3
Residency in North America or Northern Europe	3–18
Higher level of education or income	1.5–2
White race	2
Nulliparity	3
History of infertility	2–3
Menstrual irregularities	1.5
Late age at natural menopause	2–3
Early age at menarche	1.5–2
Long-term use of high dosages of menopausal estrogens	10–20
Long-term use of high dosages of combination oral contraceptives	0.3–0.5
High cumulative doses of tamoxifen	3–7
Obesity	2–5
Stein-Leventhal disease or estrogen-producing tumor	>5
History of diabetes, hypertension, gallbladder disease, or thyroid disease	1.3–3
Cigarette smoking	0.5

*Relative risks depend on the study and referent group employed.

Reprinted from Gynecologic cancer: controversies in management, Gershenson DM, McGuire WP, Gore M, Quinn MA, Thomas G, editors. Copyright 2004, with permission from Elsevier.

endometrium is the most aggressive form of endometrial cancer, and the classification of this lesion as a sarcoma or dedifferentiated carcinoma is controversial. Using endometrial sampling, carcinosarcoma may be interpreted preoperatively as adenocarcinoma, thereby making unexpected intraoperative findings more common.

Obtaining a family history may alert the gynecologist to women at increased risk for genetically linked cancers (eg, hereditary nonpolyposis colorectal cancer) in which young age at presentation of colon cancer is important. The most common manifestation of hereditary nonpolyposis colorectal cancer in women is endometrial cancer (40–60% lifetime risk), followed by colon cancer, then ovarian cancer. It is important to identify women at risk in order to provide them with appropriate screening, prophylactic surgery, and counseling (5). In addition, women with anovulatory disorders should be counseled about their long-term risk of endometrial cancer and modalities available for prevention.

Histologic Considerations

Endometrioid adenocarcinoma is the most common histologic cell type of endometrial cancer, making up more than three fourths of the cases. Benign or malignant squamous differentiation can coexist with the adenocarcinoma; however, the grade and prognosis are currently determined based only on the glandular component (6, 7). The ultimate prognosis depends on both the depth of myometrial invasion and the grade determined by glandular and nuclear cellular differentiation (8).

The precursor lesion of the endometrioid adenocarcinoma is endometrial hyperplasia, which produces a continuum of lesions that are difficult to differentiate by standard histologic characteristics. The classification of endometrial hyperplasias by the World Health Organization is shown in the box. An additional classification system is accepted by the International Society of Gynecologic Pathologists.

Atypical endometrial hyperplasia is commonly found coexisting with undiagnosed cancer in the uterus,

---

World Health Organization's Classification of Endometrial Hyperplasia

1. Simple hyperplasia
2. Complex hyperplasia (adenomatous)
3. Simple atypical hyperplasia
4. Complex atypical hyperplasia (adenomatous with atypia)

Data from Scully RE, Bonfiglio TA, Kurman RJ, Silverberg SG, Wilkinson ED, editors. Histological typing of female genital tract tumours. 2nd ed. New York (NY): Springer-Verlag; 1994.

or if found alone, it may progress to endometrial cancer in untreated women (9). A prospective trial was conducted to identify the prevalence of underlying cancer and to define more clearly the diagnostic criteria for atypical endometrial hyperplasia compared with cancer (10). In this study, 306 women had diagnosed atypical endometrial hyperplasia, established by community pathologists on preoperative biopsy, followed immediately, without medical treatment, by hysterectomy. More than 42% of women were found to have invasive cancer, and some even had high-grade lesions and deep myometrial invasion. The results demonstrate the futility of trying to make a "true" diagnosis before hysterectomy until protein or molecular biomarkers have been established (11, 12).

Papillary serous histology portends an increased risk of extrauterine disease and carries a poor prognosis. Although this cell type accounts for only about 10% of all cases, it represents most recurrent endometrial cancers (13). Clear cell histology is rare but also is associated with a poor prognosis (14). Carcinosarcoma, also known as malignant mixed müllerian tumor of the uterus, is another histologic cell type with a poor prognosis and may represent a subset of adenocarcinoma. This lesion is high grade and spreads intraperitoneally, through lymphatics and by hematogenous routes.

Prognosis

The 1988 International Federation of Gynecology and Obstetrics (FIGO) surgical staging system (Table 2) incorporates important pathologic risk factors associated with prognosis and recurrent disease, including histologic (FIGO) grade, nuclear grade, depth of myometrial invasion, cervical glandular or stromal invasion, vaginal and adnexal metastases, positive cytology, metastatic disease in pelvic or paraaortic lymph nodes, and the presence of intraabdominal or distant metastases (15–17). Other prognostic factors not included in this system are DNA ploidy and the presence of lymph–vascular space involvement (18–20). The latter has been associated with a worsened prognosis, even in the absence of documented lymph node metastasis (21).

The FIGO system emphasizes the overriding prognostic value of surgical staging information as well as its use in postoperative treatment planning. The prognosis of women with endometrial cancer is dictated primarily by the site of metastatic disease (Fig. 1). When disease has been systematically documented to be confined to the uterine fundus, the prognosis is based on grade, histologic cell type, and depth of invasion. The degree of lymph–vascular space invasion and the patient's race and age are important independent prognostic factors. Recently, the American Joint Committee on Cancer (AJCC) joined FIGO in recommending the use of surgical staging in order to adequately evaluate regional lymph nodes and to sample paraaortic and bilateral obturators and at least one other bilateral pelvic node group (22). These organizations recommend that findings be documented in the pathology or operative reports, or both. The AJCC further defined the difference between pathologic staging (p T, p N, p M) and clinical staging (c T, c N, c M).

Survival data generally are obtained from population-based registries such as those maintained by the American Cancer Society, the American College of Surgeons, and the Surveillance, Epidemiology and End Results (SEER) Program of the National Cancer Institute. However, these data are limited by the diversity of interventions used, including surgical staging. In addition, clinical trial research organizations—Postoperative Radiation Therapy in Endometrial Carcinoma (PORTEC) study group in the Netherlands and Gynecologic Oncology Group in the United States—provide data that are not population based but are quality controlled for patients treated with a standardized surgery as well as prescribed postoperative therapy.

Clinical Considerations and Recommendations

▶ *What elements of preoperative evaluation are useful for women with endometrial cancer?*

Patients with endometrial cancer often have comorbidities, including obesity, hypertension, diabetes, and, frequently, cardiac and pulmonary dysfunction, making them high-risk or poor surgical candidates. Careful attention to functional status and medical history will assist in optimizing perioperative outcome. Perioperative risk assessment also serves as the basis for appropriate patient counseling of the risks and benefits of available treatment options.

Only a physical examination and a chest radiograph are required for preoperative staging of the usual (type I endometrioid grade 1) histology, clinical stage I patient. All other preoperative testing should be directed toward optimizing the surgical outcome. The use of computed tomography or magnetic resonance imaging is not necessary because the surgeon should be prepared to resect metastatic disease commonly found in patients with endometrial cancer.

A preoperative physical examination provides information that may affect the surgical approach and subsequent risks, and it assists with developing a therapeutic plan. For example, supraclavicular lymph node metastasis may make chemotherapy an appropriate first line of treatment. If the cervix appears to be enlarged (suggest-

Table 2. International Federation of Gynecology and Obstetrics and Tumor–Node–Metastases Surgical Staging Systems for Endometrial Cancer

TNM Categories	FIGO Stages*	Surgical–Pathologic Findings
Primary Tumor (T)		
TX		Primary tumor cannot be assessed
T0		No evidence of primary tumor
Tis	0	Carcinoma in situ
T1	I	Tumor confined to corpus uteri
T1a	IA	Tumor limited to endometrium
T1b	IB	Tumor invades less than one half of the myometrium
T1c	IC	Tumor invades one half or more of the myometrium
T2	II	Tumor invades cervix but does not extend beyond uterus
T2a	IIA	Tumor limited to the glandular epithelium of the endocervix; there is no evidence of connective tissue stromal invasion
T2b	IIB	Invasion of the stromal connective tissue of the cervix
T3	III	Local and/or regional spread
T3a	IIIA	Tumor involves serosa and/or adnexa (direct extension or metastasis) and/or cancer cells in ascites or peritoneal washings
T3b	IIIB	Vaginal involvement (direct extension or metastasis)
T4	IVA	Tumor invades bladder mucosa and/or bowel mucosa (bullous edema is not sufficient to classify a tumor as T4)
Regional Lymph Nodes (N)		
NX		Regional lymph nodes cannot be assessed
N0		No regional lymph node metastasis
N1	IIIC	Regional lymph node metastasis to pelvic and/or paraaortic nodes
Distant Metastasis (M)		
MX		Distant metastasis cannot be assessed
M0		No distant metastasis
M1	IVB	Distant metastasis (includes metastasis to abdominal lymph nodes other than paraaortic, and/or inguinal lymph nodes; excludes metastasis to vagina, pelvic serosa, or adnexa)

FIGO indicates International Federation of Gynecology and Obstetrics; TNM, tumor–node–metastases.

*All cases of FIGO Stage I–IVA should be subclassified by histologic grade as follows: GX, grade cannot be assessed; G1, well differentiated; G2, moderately differentiated; G3, poorly differentiated or undifferentiated.

Used with the permission of the American Joint Committee on Cancer (AJCC), Chicago, Illinois. The original source for this material is the AJCC Cancer Staging Manual, Sixth edition (2002), published by Springer-Verlag New York, www.springeronline.com.

ing possible tumor involvement), the differential diagnosis of cervical adenocarcinoma should be considered. If cervical involvement is confirmed, treatment options may include radical hysterectomy or preoperative radiation therapy. The finding of vaginal, parametrial, or adnexal extension of disease also can complicate treatment planning, and special skills may be required for complete surgical resection.

Preoperative measurement of the CA 125 level may be appropriate because it is frequently elevated in women with advanced-stage disease. Elevated levels of CA 125 may assist in predicting treatment response or in post-treatment surveillance (23, 24).

▶ *What constitutes appropriate staging for women with endometrial cancer?*

Most women with endometrial cancer benefit from systematic surgical staging, including pelvic washings, bilateral pelvic and paraaortic lymphadenectomy, and complete resection of all disease. Appropriate surgical staging is prognostic and facilitates targeted therapy to maximize survival and to minimize the effects of under-treatment (eg, recurrent disease or increased mortality) and potential morbidity (eg, radiation injury) associated with overtreatment. Exceptions to the need for surgical staging include young or perimenopausal women with

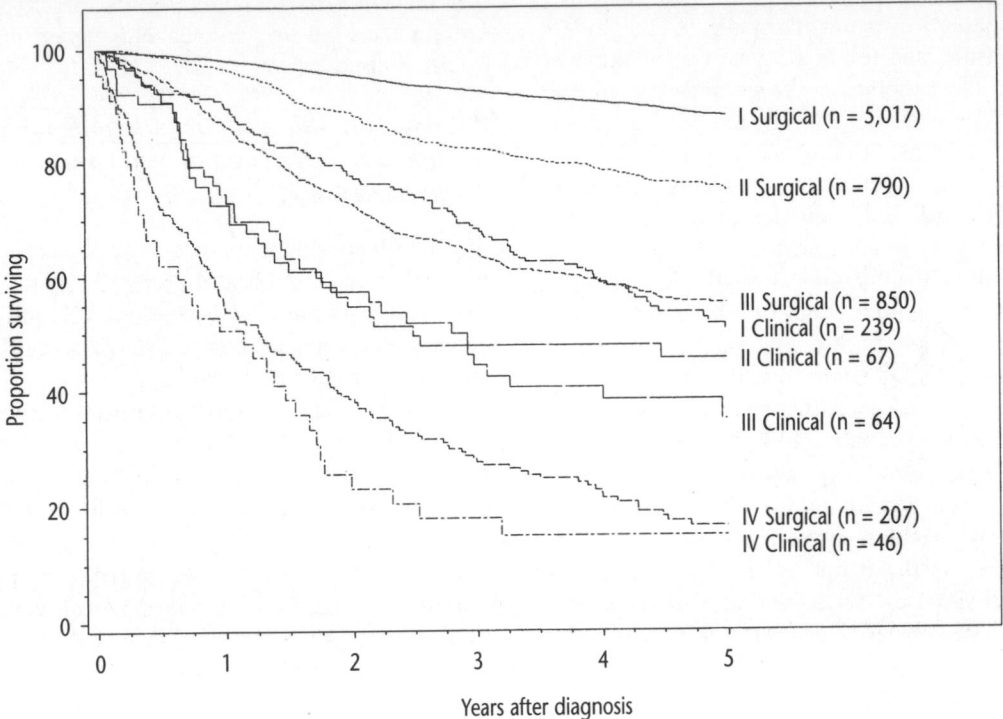

Figure 1. Carcinoma of the corpus uteri, patients treated 1996–1998. Survival by mode of staging, N = 7,280. (Reprinted from Int J Gynaecol Obstet, Vol. 83 (Suppl 1), Creasman WT, Odicino F, Maisonneuve P, Beller U, Benedet JL, Heintz AP, et al. Carcinoma of the corpus uteri. p. 79–118. Copyright 2003, with permission from the International Federation of Gynecology and Obstetrics.)

grade 1 endometrioid adenocarcinoma associated with atypical endometrial hyperplasia and women at increased risk of mortality secondary to comorbidities.

Retroperitoneal lymph node assessment is a critical component of surgical staging and is associated with improved survival. Women testing negative for disease of the pelvic and paraaortic lymph nodes and for abnormal pelvic cytology have better survival rates than women with matched uterine histologic factors and positive results of testing of nodes or cytology (25). These negative results allow the adjuvant radiotherapy to be withheld and change the survival estimates from that of a clinical stage I patient to a surgical stage I. Palpation of the retroperitoneum is an inaccurate measure and cannot substitute for surgical dissection of nodal tissue for histopathology. Sampling of pelvic lymph nodes alone ignores the fact that 62% of women with any positive lymph nodes have paraaortic metastasis, and 17% have paraaortic disease alone (16, 26–29).

The incidence and severity of complications associated with extensive surgical staging of women with endometrial cancer frequently are related to the effects of existing medical comorbidities (ie, obesity, diabetes, coronary artery disease) (30, 31). The average hospital stay for abdominal staging is similar to that for benign hysterectomy (32).

In specific situations, hysterectomy, bilateral salpingo-oophorectomy, and bilateral pelvic and paraaortic lymphadenectomy can be completed successfully and safely with less perioperative morbidity by using a laparoscopic approach (33–35).

▶ *How are women with endometrial cancer treated postoperatively?*

The use of adjuvant radiation therapy in women with disease limited to the uterus based on systematic surgical staging is controversial. Many practitioners have abandoned teletherapy (whole pelvic radiation therapy) and replaced it with vaginal brachytherapy for selected patients (36). One study reported a 5-year survival rate of 92% for systematically staged IC patients treated with postoperative whole pelvic radiation, compared with 90% for those treated with surgery alone (37). The authors concluded that radiation should be tailored to sites of known metastatic disease or reserved for recurrence.

The large, randomized controlled PORTEC trial was conducted to determine the value of postoperative whole pelvic radiation therapy in women after hysterectomy and bilateral salpingo-oophorectomy without comprehensive surgical staging and lymphadenectomy. The initial report included women with grade 1 deep myometrial invasion, grade 2 invasion of any depth, and grade 3 superficial invasion, and found a 5-year overall survival rate of 81% in the radiotherapy group and 85% for the controls (38). These results confirm the conclusions of another large randomized prospective study of 540 patients that there is no benefit to whole pelvic radiation therapy, except local control in the vagina and pelvis (39). Deaths generally result from disease recurrence outside the radiation field. Of patients treated with radiation, 2% have major complications, and 20% have minor complaints that affected quality of life.

The second PORTEC report focused on women with grade 3 histology with deep myometrial invasion, all women receiving whole pelvic radiotherapy (40). The 5-year survival rate for this group of women without comprehensive surgical staging was 58%. In contrast, when stage IIIC patients are appropriately staged, metastatic disease in the lymph nodes is removed, and treatment is delivered to the known sites of metastatic spread, the overall 5-year survival rate is 70–85%, demonstrating that radiation cannot overcome poor surgical treatment (29, 41, 42).

Women who do not receive postoperative radiation with surgical stage I endometrial cancer may have isolated recurrent disease in the vagina. Treatment of these recurrences demonstrated 60–75% survival (38). Another randomized trial also indicates that radiation does not improve survival or reduce distant metastases; it prevents only vaginal recurrences. These recurrences can be treated subsequently, avoiding the unnecessary exposure of radiation toxicity (39). Therefore, for patients with surgical stage I disease, postoperative radiation therapy can reduce the risk of local recurrence. In deciding whether to use radiation, the cost and toxicity should be balanced with the evidence that the therapy does not improve survival or reduce distant metastasis.

Evidence for the treatment of metastatic endometrial cancer has advanced significantly in the past decade. Recognition in multiple reports that most deaths are from distant failure secondary to hematogenous spread makes optimizing chemotherapy, possibly in combination with local brachytherapy, the foundation for future research.

A cost analysis of treatment options of intermediate-risk patients (surgical stage I, grade 2–3, deep myometrial invasion) who underwent complete staging made the following assumptions: 1) lymph node status is the most important prognostic factor, 2) removal of lymph nodes testing negative for disease improves survival, 3) lymphadenectomy has minimal morbidity, 4) lymphadenectomy improves the cost effectiveness, and 5) teletherapy can be eliminated for stage I–II disease (36). The analysis demonstrated a 12% cost reduction with routine lymphadenectomy by avoiding teletherapy and substituting brachytherapy (43). The same analysts also report a 31%

cost reduction by avoiding routine brachytherapy and treating the high-risk women only when they develop recurrent disease.

▶ *What are the recommendations for women found to have endometrial cancer after a hysterectomy?*

To counsel the patient appropriately on her risk of metastases, recurrence, and death, a multidisciplinary review of pathologic material is important (2, 15). In this clinical situation, therapeutic options include no further therapy and surveillance only, reoperation to complete the surgical staging, or radiotherapy to prevent local recurrence. The acceptable level of risk that determines the need for reoperation or radiation varies among individuals. The survival advantages of surgical staging must be weighed against the complications from a new major surgical procedure. This risk of additional surgery contrasts with the minimal difference in risk with planned, combined procedures of surgical staging with hysterectomy, bilateral pelvic and paraaortic lymphadenectomy, and peritoneal cytology tests. The advent of laparoscopic surgical restaging has resulted in less morbidity using this approach. One study on the use of laparoscopic restaging for endometrial cancer reported a hospital stay of 1.5 days and less than 100 mL estimated blood loss (44). Treatment decisions with endometrial cancer following hysterectomy are best made in consultation with a specialist with advanced training and demonstrated competence, such as a gynecologic oncologist.

▶ *What is the mode of therapy for patients with positive pelvic or paraaortic nodes?*

Every patient found to have extrauterine disease (stage III, IV) is at significant risk for developing persistent or recurrent disease and should be considered a candidate for additional therapy (45). Factors influencing postoperative treatment decisions may include tumor histology, extent of disease, the presence of medical comorbidities, and the availability of research protocols. Regional or systemic therapeutic modalities may be considered.

Despite the potential therapeutic role of lymphadenectomy, most women with nodal metastases should receive adjuvant therapy. The addition of therapeutic pelvic radiation for the treatment of women with stage IIIC disease (and testing negative for disease of the paraaortic nodes) results in disease-free survival rates from 57% to 72% (42, 46).

Women with paraaortic nodal disease should have the tumor completely resected and should have postoperative imaging studies (eg, chest computed tomography or positron emission tomography scans) to detect or exclude the presence of occult extraabdominal disease (41, 47).

The addition of paraaortic radiation is associated with improved survival (median survival, 27–43 months) and is of significant benefit, particularly for those with microscopic nodal metastases (48–51).

Patterns of failure in women with stage IIIC disease suggest the possible benefit of concomitant or sequential systemic therapy. Retrospective studies of concomitant chemotherapy also support the benefit of systemic chemotherapy (29, 47, 50).

▶ *What is the mode of therapy for patients with intraperitoneal disease?*

The primary mode of therapy for women with intraperitoneal disease includes an attempt at optimal tumor cytoreduction and the addition of systemic chemotherapy or radiation therapy or both (52). Optimal cytoreduction can be completed with limited morbidity and likely offers a survival benefit (53–56). The ability to resect isolated metastases when combined with additional therapy can result in long-term survival similar to the treatment of women with ovarian cancer (31).

Postoperatively, progestational agents or systemic cytotoxic therapy may be used alone or in combination with directed radiation. A randomized trial showed the superiority of the combination of doxorubicin, cisplatin, and paclitaxel systemic chemotherapy for advanced and recurrent endometrial cancer (57). The use of carboplatin and paclitaxel in combination, similar to use for ovarian cancer, is favored by some because of the combination's more favorable toxicity profile.

▶ *What is the mode of therapy for patients with cervical involvement?*

In the absence of macroscopic cervical involvement, the preoperative diagnosis of stage II disease is difficult to establish. Endocervical curettage is notoriously imprecise for such use, with a reported accuracy of 50% (58). It is challenging to differentiate primary cervical adenocarcinoma from stage II endometrial cancer. Patients may benefit from HPV testing and immunohistochemistry or cone biopsy for further evaluation. The treatment plan for each diagnosis is markedly different. When the diagnosis is unclear, radical hysterectomy and lymphadenectomy can be performed, followed by tailored adjuvant therapy based on the pathologic findings.

Treatment of women with cervical involvement may include preoperative radiation combined with total hysterectomy, or radical hysterectomy with lymphadenectomy followed by the addition of adjuvant chemotherapy or radiation therapy directed toward known sites of disease (59, 60). The use of radical hysterectomy has been associated with improved local control and survival when compared with total hysterectomy at 5 years (94%

versus 79%) and 10 years (94% versus 74%) (61, 62). It would appear that grade is more predictive of survival than depth of cervical invasion (63). Optimal treatment of women with stage II disease has resulted in survival rates approaching or exceeding 80% (64–66).

▶ *Is there a role for radiotherapy as an alternative to surgery?*

The primary treatment of endometrial cancer typically involves hysterectomy. In the unusual instance (<3.5%) when a patient is deemed an exceptionally poor surgical candidate, primary therapeutic radiation may be considered for treating the uterine disease (67). Although primary therapeutic radiation is suboptimal, the use of brachytherapy to control disease offers reasonable results in this ultra-high-risk surgical population (68). The additional benefit of teletherapy remains unclear.

Radiation therapy alone does not allow for directed therapy and fails to eradicate the uterine cancer in 10–15% of cases. The cancer-specific 5-year survival rates in stage I inoperable patients (80%) are less than that of stage I operable patients (98%) (67) and are related to tumor grade (69). Others have reported lower survival rates of approximately 50% (69, 70). A significant number of these patients die of intercurrent disease (71). These results suggest that a careful preoperative evaluation and appropriate consultation be undertaken before denying any woman the benefits of hysterectomy.

▶ *Is there a role for progestin therapy in the treatment of atypical endometrial hyperplasia and endometrial cancer?*

Atypical endometrial hyperplasia and endometrial cancer should be considered part of a continuum. The diagnosis remains uncertain as long as the uterus is in situ. For women who do not desire fertility, hysterectomy should be recommended for treatment of atypical endometrial hyperplasia because of the high risk of an underlying cancer. Women who desire to maintain fertility, whether they have a diagnosis of atypical endometrial hyperplasia or grade 1 endometrioid adenocarcinoma, may be treated with progestins in an attempt to reverse the lesion.

Progestational agents have been evaluated as a primary treatment modality of early grade 1 disease in women who wish to maintain their fertility or in those who are extremely poor operative candidates. Oral, parenteral, or intrauterine device delivery of progestin (72) has been successful, with response rates ranging from 58% to 100% (73–75). Although long-term outcomes are uncertain, the disease will likely recur in most patients. There is controversy about whether progestin should be prescribed continuously or cyclically, and these regimens are currently under investigation. Other hormonal therapies have been reported to be effective but are less well studied (76).

Continued histologic monitoring is vital both to assure medication response and to exclude recurrence, which may approach 50% (73). Following therapy, patients should undergo serial complete intrauterine evaluation approximately every 3 months to document response. Progestin therapy may successfully reverse atypical endometrial hyperplasia as well as an early endometrial carcinoma; conception may then be attempted (76). A review of the literature found a 76% response rate for progestin therapy in 81 patients with a median age of 30.5 years (77). The median response time was 12 weeks, with a median treatment duration of 24 weeks. Of the 62 responders, 47 did not experience recurrence. Twenty patients became pregnant, and 12 required assisted reproductive technologies for conception.

▶ *What is the mode of treatment for patients with endometrial cancer and morbid obesity or other high-risk medical problems?*

Operative intervention should be considered for all women with uterine cancer; however, many of these women will have significant coexisting conditions that place them at higher risk of perioperative morbidity. Additionally, the staging procedure may predispose to some specific morbidities (eg, thromboembolism). Therefore, care for women with coexisting conditions should be individualized, with appropriate perioperative consultation sought. With disease-specific preoperative medical and intraoperative intervention undertaken, most of this population can undergo an appropriate surgical procedure.

Specialized long instrumentation is available for operative procedures in the obese patient; however, additional considerations such as incision placement (eg, upper abdomen), thromboembolic prophylaxis, and attention to recovery of postoperative pulmonary function are important in reducing morbidity. Panniculectomy has been advocated in women with a specific body habitus (large panniculus adiposus) (78).

Laparoscopy and vaginal hysterectomy may be of benefit for some patients. In a study of 125 elderly women (average age, 75 years), laparoscopic staging was successfully completed in 77.6% (79). The average hospital stay was 3 days, which compares favorably to the average 5.6-day hospital stay for total abdominal hysterectomy, bilateral salpingo-oophorectomy, and bilateral pelvic and paraaortic lymphadenectomy. Thirteen patients underwent only vaginal hysterectomy because of medical conditions and were in the hospital an average of 2.1 days (79). In many cases, the ovaries are not removed to decrease the risk of requiring laparotomy. Conversion to laparotomy is advised when a) the uterus is too large to

remove intact, b) adhesions or obesity impair visualization, and c) metastatic disease is encountered, to facilitate optimal surgical resection. Vaginal hysterectomy usually can be accomplished in even nulliparous obese patients by experienced surgeons (80).

▶ *What is the appropriate follow-up for women after treatment of endometrial cancer?*

The pattern of recurrent disease depends on the original sites of metastasis in patients with advanced stage disease, as well as the treatment received. In women in whom the disease is confined to the uterus, the types of recurrence depend on histologic cell type, lymph–vascular invasion, depth of invasion, and the use of radiation therapy. Investigators reported on 379 patients in whom recurrence sites were local in 50%, distant in 29%, and combined in 21% (81). The median time to detection of recurrence was 14 months for vaginal disease and 19 months for distant disease. Thirty-four percent of recurrences were diagnosed in the first year of follow-up, 76% were found within 3 years, and 10% did not recur until more than 5 years of follow-up. The recurrent disease was found on physical examination in 32% of cases, when the patients were asymptomatic. Only 37% reported vaginal bleeding. The patients who received postoperative radiotherapy had a decreased risk of vaginal recurrence (2–4%). In addition, they have few therapeutic options to treat recurrence and, therefore, would benefit less from frequent surveillance with cervical cytology screening and pelvic examinations for detection of recurrent disease.

The follow-up strategy in the nonirradiated patient is based on the knowledge that recurrent disease in the pelvis, particularly in the vaginal cuff, can be treated successfully with radiotherapy (37, 38, 82). Vaginal or pelvic recurrence can be detected and treated successfully in 68–88% of women who have not received radiation therapy (38, 82). Most studies cited monitored patients every 3–4 months for 2–3 years, then twice yearly with a speculum and rectovaginal examination at each visit. The use of cervical cytology testing for detection of recurrent disease is mostly anecdotal. The identification of asymptomatic distant recurrence is unlikely to have a survival benefit; treatment is primarily palliative chemotherapy. The use of periodic chest radiographic evaluation cannot be supported outside a research setting.

▶ *Which patients may benefit from referral to a gynecologic oncologist?*

Physicians with advanced training and expertise in the treatment of women with endometrial cancer, such as gynecologic oncologists, understand the nuances of uterine cancer management, including the selection and sequencing of treatment modalities likely to benefit the individual patient. When it is practical and feasible, preoperative consultation with a physician with advanced training and demonstrated competence such as a gynecologic oncologist may be recommended. Consultation may be particularly beneficial in the following situations:

- The ability to completely and adequately surgically stage the patient is not readily available at the time of her initial procedure.
- Preoperative histology (grade 3, papillary serous, clear cell, carcinosarcoma) suggests a high risk for extrauterine spread.
- The final pathology test result reveals an unexpected endometrial cancer following hysterectomy performed for other indications.
- There is evidence of cervical or extrauterine disease.
- The pelvic washings are positive for malignant cells.
- Recurrent disease is diagnosed or suspected.
- Nonoperative therapy is contemplated.

Summary of Recommendations and Conclusions

The following recommendations are based on limited or inconsistent scientific evidence (Level B):

▶ Most women with endometrial cancer should undergo systematic surgical staging, including pelvic washings, bilateral pelvic and paraaortic lymphadenectomy, and complete resection of all disease. Exceptions to this include young or perimenopausal women with grade 1 endometrioid adenocarcinoma associated with atypical endometrial hyperplasia and those at increased risk of mortality secondary to comorbidities.

▶ Women with atypical endometrial hyperplasia and endometrial cancer who desire to maintain their fertility may be treated with progestin therapy. Following therapy they should undergo serial complete intrauterine evaluation approximately every 3 months to document response. Hysterectomy should be recommended for women who do not desire future fertility.

▶ Patients with surgical stage I disease may be counseled that postoperative radiation therapy can reduce the risk of local recurrence, but the cost and toxicity should be balanced with the evidence that it does not improve survival or reduce distant metastasis.

▶ For those women who have not received radiation therapy, pelvic examinations every 3–4 months for 2–3 years, then twice yearly following surgical treatment of endometrial cancer are recommended for detection and treatment of recurrent disease.

The following recommendations are based primarily on consensus and expert opinion (Level C):

▶ Women who cannot undergo systematic surgical staging because of comorbidities may be candidates for vaginal hysterectomy.

▶ Only a physical examination and a chest radiograph are required for preoperative staging of the usual (type I endometrioid grade 1) histology, clinical stage I patient. All other preoperative testing should be directed toward optimizing the surgical outcome.

References

1. Jemal A, Murray T, Ward E, Samuels A, Tiwari RC, Ghafoor A, et al. Cancer statistics, 2005. CA Cancer J Clin 2005;55:10–30. (Level II-3)

2. Creasman WT, Odicino F, Maisonneuve P, Beller U, Benedet JL, Heintz AP, et al. Carcinoma of the corpus uteri. Int J Gynaecol Obstet 2003;83(Suppl 1):79–118. (Level II-3)

3. Ries LA, Eisner MP, Kosary CL, Hankey BF, Miller BA, Clegg L, et al, editors. SEER Cancer Statistics Review, 1975–2001, National Cancer Institute. Bethesda (MD): 2004. Available at: http://seer.cancer.gov/csr/1975_2001/. Retrieved November 9, 2004. (Level II-3)

4. Gershenson DM, McGuire WP, Gore M, Quinn MA, Thomas G, editors. Gynecologic cancer: controversies in management. Philadephia (PA): Elsevier; 2004. (Level III)

5. Boyd J. Hereditary gynecology cancer syndromes. In: Gershenson DM, McGuire WP, Gore M, Quinn MA, Thomas G, editors. Gynecologic cancer: controversies in management. Philadephia (PA): Elsevier; 2004. p. 833–45. (Level III)

6. Alberhasky RC, Connelly PJ, Christopherson WM. Carcinoma of the endometrium. IV. Mixed adenosquamous carcinoma. A clinical-pathological study of 68 cases with long-term follow-up. Am J Clin Pathol 1982;77:655–64. (Level III)

7. Pekin T, Yildizhan B, Eren F, Pekin O, Yildizhan R. Adenocarcinoma, adenoacanthoma, and mixed adenosquamous carcinoma of the endometrium. Eur J Gynaecol Oncol 2001;22:151–3. (Level III)

8. Zaino RJ, Kurman R, Herbold D, Gliedman J, Bundy BN, Voet R, et al. The significance of squamous differentiation in endometrial carcinoma. Data from a Gynecologic Oncology Group study. Cancer 1991;68:2293–302. (Level II-2)

9. Kurman RJ, Kaminski PF, Norris HJ. The behavior of endometrial hyperplasia. A long-term study of "untreated" hyperplasia in 170 patients. Cancer 1985;56:403–12. (Level III)

10. Trimble CL. Atypical endometrial hyperplasia: a tough call. Int J Gynecol Cancer 2005;15:401.

11. Mutter GL, Lin MC, Fitzgerald JT, Kum JB, Baak JP, Lees JA, et al. Altered PTEN expression as a diagnostic marker for the earliest endometrial precancers. J Natl Cancer Inst 2000;92:924–30. (Level III)

12. Maxwell GL, Risinger JI, Gumbs C, Shaw H, Bentley RC, Barrett JC, et al. Mutation of the PTEN tumor suppressor gene in endometrial hyperplasias. Cancer Res 1998;58: 2500–3. (Level III)

13. Hendrickson M, Ross J, Eifel P, Martinez A, Kempson R. Uterine papillary serous carcinoma: a highly malignant form of endometrial adenocarcinoma. Am J Surg Pathol 1982;6:93–108. (Level III)

14. Christopherson WM, Alberhasky RC, Connelly PJ. Carcinoma of the endometrium: I. A clinicopathologic study of clear-cell carcinoma and secretory carcinoma. Cancer 1982;49:1511–23. (Level III)

15. Morrow CP, Bundy BN, Kurman RJ, Creasman WT, Heller P, Homesley HD, et al. Relationship between surgical-pathological risk factors and outcome in clinical stage I and II carcinoma of the endometrium: a Gynecologic Oncology Group study. Gynecol Oncol 1991;40:55–65. (Level II-2)

16. Creasman WT, Morrow CP, Bundy BN, Homesley HD, Graham JE, Heller PB. Surgical pathologic spread patterns of endometrial cancer. A Gynecologic Oncology Group Study. Cancer 1987;60(Suppl 8):2035–41. (Level II-2)

17. Boronow RC, Morrow CP, Creasman WT, Disaia PJ, Silverberg SG, Miller A, et al. Surgical staging in endometrial cancer: clinical-pathologic findings of a prospective study. Obstet Gynecol 1984;63:825–32. (Level III)

18. Kodama S, Kase H, Tanaka K, Matsui K. Multivariate analysis of prognostic factors in patients with endometrial cancer. Int J Gynaecol Obstet 1996;53:23–30. (Level II-3)

19. Baak JP, Snijders WP, Van Diest PJ, Armee-Horvath E, Kenemans P. Confirmation of the prognostic value of the ECPI-1 score (myometrial invasion, DNA-ploidy and mean shortest nuclear axis) in FIGO stage I endometrial cancer patients with long follow-up. Int J Gynecol Cancer 1995;5:112–6. (Level II-2)

20. Ambros RA, Kurman RJ. Identification of patients with stage I uterine endometrioid adenocarcinoma at high risk of recurrence by DNA ploidy, myometrial invasion, and vascular invasion. Gynecol Oncol 1992;45:235–9. (Level II-3)

21. Gal D, Recio FO, Zamurovic D, Tancer ML. Lymphvascular space involvement—a prognostic indicator in endometrial adenocarcinoma. Gynecol Oncol 1991; 42:142–5. (Level II-3)

22. American Joint Committee on Cancer. AJCC cancer staging manual. 6th ed. New York (NY): Springer-Verlag; 2002. (Level III)

23. Patsner B, Tenhoppen DJ, Mann WJ. Use of serum CA-125 levels to monitor therapy of patients with advanced or recurrent endometrial carcinoma. Eur J Gynaecol Oncol 1989;10:322–5. (Level III)

24. Patsner B, Orr JW Jr, Mann WJ Jr. Use of serum CA 125 measurement in posttreatment surveillance of early-stage endometrial carcinoma. Am J Obstet Gynecol 1990;162: 427–9. (Level II-2)

25. Kilgore LC, Partridge EE, Alvarez RD, Austin JM, Shingleton HM, Noojin F 3rd, et al. Adenocarcinoma of the endometrium: survival comparisons of patients with and without pelvic node sampling. Gynecol Oncol 1995; 56:29–33. (Level II-3)

26. Giradi F, Petru E, Heydarfadai M, Haas J, Winter R. Pelvic lymphadenectomy in the surgical treatment of endometrial cancer. Gynecol Oncol 1993;49:177–80. (Level III)

27. Chuang L, Burke TW, Tornos C, Marino BD, Mitchell MF, Tortolero-Luna G, et al. Staging laparotomy for endometrial carcinoma: assessment of retroperitoneal lymph nodes. Gynecol Oncol 1995;58:189–93. (Level II-3)

28. Arango HA, Hoffman MS, Roberts WS, DeCesare SL, Fiorica JV, Drake J. Accuracy of lymph node palpation to determine need for lymphadenectomy in gynecologic malignancies. Obstet Gynecol 2000;95:553–6. (Level II-3)

29. McMeekin DS, Lashbrook D, Gold M, Johnson G, Walker JL, Mannel R. Analysis of FIGO Stage III endometrial cancer patients. Gynecol Oncol 2001;81:273–8. (Level II-3)

30. Geisler JP, Geisler HE, Melton ME, Wiemann MC. What staging surgery should be performed on patients with uterine papillary serous carcinoma? Gynecol Oncol 1999;74:465–7. (Level II-3)

31. Orr JW Jr, Orr PF, Taylor PT. Surgical staging endometrial cancer. Clin Obstet Gynecol 1996;39:656–68. (Level III)

32. Kennedy AW, Austin JM Jr, Look KY, Munger CB. The Society of Gynecologic Oncologists Outcomes Task Force. Study of endometrial cancer: initial experiences. Gynecol Oncol 2000;79:379–98. (Level III)

33. Holub Z, Jabor A, Bartos P, Eim J, Urbanek S, Pivovarnikova R. Laparoscopic surgery for endometrial cancer: long-term results of a multicentric study. Eur J Gynaecol Oncol 2002;23:305–10. (Level II-2)

34. Eltabbakh GH, Shamonki MI, Moody JM, Garafano LL. Laparoscopy as the primary modality for the treatment of women with endometrial carcinoma. Cancer 2001;91: 378–87. (Level II-2)

35. Malur S, Possover M, Michels W, Schneider A. Laparoscopic-assisted vaginal versus abdominal surgery in patients with endometrial cancer—a prospective randomized trial. Gynecol Oncol 2001;80:239–44. (Level I)

36. Fanning J, Hoffman ML, Andrews SJ, Harrah AW, Feldmeier JJ. Cost-effectiveness analysis of the treatment for intermediate risk endometrial cancer: postoperative brachytherapy vs. observation. Gynecol Oncol 2004; 93:632–6. (Level III)

37. Straughn JM, Huh WK, Orr JW Jr, Kelly FJ, Roland PY, Gold MA, et al. Stage IC adenocarcinoma of the endometrium: survival comparisons of surgically staged patients with and without adjuvant radiation therapy. Gynecol Oncol 2003;89:295–300. (Level II-3)

38. Creutzberg CL, van Putten WL, Koper PC, Lybeert ML, Jobsen JJ, Warlam-Rodenhuis CC, et al. Surgery and post-operative radiotherapy versus surgery alone for patients with stage-1 endometrial carcinoma: multicentre randomised trial. PORTEC Study Group. Post Operative Radiation Therapy in Endometrial Carcinoma. Lancet 2000;355:1404–11. (Level I)

39. Aalders J, Abeler V, Kolstad P, Onsrud M. Postoperative external irradiation and prognostic parameters in stage I endometrial carcinoma: clinical and histopathologic study of 540 patients. Obstet Gynecol 1980;56:419–27. (Level II-2)

40. Creutzberg CL, van Putten WL, Warlam-Rodenhuis CC, van den Bergh AC, de Winter KA, Koper PC, et al. Outcome of high-risk stage IC, grade 3, compared with stage I endometrial carcinoma patients: the Postoperative Radiation Therapy in Endometrial Carcinoma Trial. J Clin Oncol 2004;22:1234–41. (Level II-2)

41. Mariani A, Webb MJ, Keeney GL, Aletti G, Podratz KC. Predictors of lymphatic failure in endometrial cancer. Gynecol Oncol 2002;84:437–42. (Level II-3)

42. Nelson G, Randall M, Sutton G, Moore D, Hurteau J, Look K. FIGO stage IIIC endometrial carcinoma with metastases confined to pelvic lymph nodes: analysis of treatment outcomes, prognostic variables, and failure patterns following adjuvant radiation therapy. Gynecol Oncol 1999;75:211–4. (Level II-3)

43. Fanning J. Treatment for early endometrial cancer. Cost-effectiveness analysis. J Reprod Med 1999;44:719–23. (Level III)

44. Childers JM, Spirtos NM, Brainard P, Surwit EA. Laparoscopic staging of the patient with incompletely staged early adenocarcinoma of the endometrium. Obstet Gynecol 1994;83:597–600. (Level III)

45. Mundt AJ, McBride R, Rotmensch J, Waggoner SE, Yamada SD, Connell PP. Significant pelvic recurrence in high-risk pathologic stage I–IV endometrial carcinoma patients after adjuvant chemotherapy alone: implications for adjuvant radiation therapy. Int J Radiat Oncol Biol Phys 2001;50:1145–53. (Level II-3)

46. Ayhan A, Taskiran C, Celik C, Aksu T, Yuce K. Surgical stage III endometrial cancer: analysis of treatment outcomes, prognostic factors and failure patterns. Eur J Gynaecol Oncol 2002;23:553–6. (Level II-3)

47. Bristow RE, Zahurak ML, Alexander CJ, Zellars RC, Montz FJ. FIGO stage IIIC endometrial carcinoma: resection of macroscopic nodal disease and other determinants of survival. Int J Gynecol Cancer 2003;13:664–72. (Level II-3)

48. Rose PG, Cha SD, Tak WK, Fitzgerald T, Reale F, Hunter RE. Radiation therapy for surgically proven para-arotic node metastasis in endometrial carcinoma. Int J Radiat Oncol Biol Phys 1992;24:229–33. (Level II-3)

49. Husseinzadeh N, Shrake P, DeEulis T, Rowley K, Aron B. Chemotherapy and extended-field radiation therapy to para-aortic area in patients with histologically proven metastatic cervical cancer to para-artic nodes: a phase II pilot study. Gynecol Oncol 1994;52:326–31. (Level I)

50. Katz LA, Andrews SJ, Fanning J. Survival after multimodality treatment for stage IIIC endometrial cancer. Am J Obstet Gynecol 2001;184:1071–3. (Level II-2)

51. McMeekin DS, Tillmanns T. Endometrial cancer: treatment of nodal metastases. Curr Treat Options Oncol 2003;4:121–30. (Level III)

52. Memarzadeh S, Holschneider CH, Bristow RE, Jones NL, Fu YS, Karlan BY, et al. FIGO stage III and IV uterine papillary serous carcinoma: impact of residual disease on survival. Int J Gynecol Cancer 2002;12:454–8. (Level II-3)

53. Ayhan A, Taskiran C, Celik C, Yuce K, Kucukali T. The influence of cytoreductive surgery on survival and morbidity in stage IVB endometrial cancer. Int J Gynecol Cancer 2002;12:448–53. (Level II-3)

54. Bristow RE, Zerbe MJ, Rosenshein NB, Grumbine FC, Montz FJ. Stage IVB endometrial carcinoma: the role of cytoreductive surgery and determinants of survival. Gynecol Oncol 2000;78:85–91. (Level II-3)

55. Chi DS, Welshinger M, Venkatraman ES, Barakat RR. The role of surgical cytoreduction in Stage IV endometrial carcinoma. Gynecol Oncol 1997;67:56–60. (Level II-3)

56. Goff BA, Goodman A, Muntz HG, Fuller AF Jr, Nikrui N, Rice LW. Surgical stage IV endometrial carcinoma: a study of 47 cases. Gynecol Oncol 1994;52:237–40. (Level II-3)

57. Fleming GF, Brunetto VL, Cella D, Look KY, Reid GC, Munkarah AR, et al. Phase III trial of doxorubicin plus cisplatin with or without paclitaxel plus filgrastim in advanced endometrial carcinoma: a Gynecologic Oncology Group Study. J Clin Oncol 2004;22:2159–66. (Level I)

58. Leminen A, Forss M, Lehtovirta P. Endometrial adenocarcinoma with clinical evidence of cervical involvement: accuracy of diagnostic procedures, clinical course, and prognostic factors. Acta Obstet Gynecol Scand 1995;74:61–6. (Level II-3)

59. Boente MP, Orandi YA, Yordan EL, Miller A, Graham JE, Kirshner C, et al. Recurrence patterns and complications in endometrial adenocarcinoma with cervical involvement. Ann Surg Oncol 1995;2:138–44. (Level II-3)

60. Maggino T, Romagnolo C, Landoni F, Sartori E, Zola P, Gadducci A. An analysis of approaches to the management of endometrial cancer in North America: a CTF study. Gynecol Oncol 1998;68:274–9. (Level III)

61. Mariani A, Webb MJ, Kenney GL, Calori G, Podratz KC. Role of wide/radical hysterectomy and pelvic lymph node dissection in endometrial cancer with cervical involvement. Gynecol Oncol 2001;83:72–80. (Level II-3)

62. Sartori E, Gadducci A, Landoni F, Lissoni A, Maggino T, Zola P, et al. Clinical behavior of 203 stage II endometrial cancer cases: the impact of primary surgical approach and of adjuvant radiation therapy. Int J Gynecol Cancer 2001;11:430–7. (Level II-3)

63. Reisinger SA, Staros EB, Mohiuddin M. Survival and failure analysis in stage II endometrial cancer using the revised 1988 FIGO staging system. Int J Radiat Oncol Biol Phys 1991;21:1027–32. (Level II-3)

64. Maingon P, Horiot JC, Fraisse J, Salas S, Collin F, Bone-Lepinoy MC, et al. Preoperative radiotherapy in stage I/II endometrial adenocarcinoma. Radiother Oncol 1996;39:201–8. (Level II-3)

65. Eltabbakh GH, Moore AD. Survival of women with surgical stage II endometrial cancer. Gynecol Oncol 1999; 74:80–5. (Level II-3)

66. Calvin DP, Connell PP, Rotmensch J, Waggoner S, Mundt AJ. Surgery and postoperative radiation therapy in stage II endometrial carcinoma. Am J Clin Oncol 1999;22: 338–43. (Level II-3)

67. Fishman DA, Roberts KB, Chambers JT, Kohorn EI, Schwartz PE, Chambers SK. Radiation therapy as exclusive treatment for medically inoperable patients with stage I and II endometrioid carcinoma with endometrium. Gynecol Oncol 1996;61:189–96. (Level II-2)

68. Kucera H, Knocke TH, Kucera E, Potter R. Treatment of endometrial carcinoma with high-dose-rate brachytherapy alone in medically inoperable stage I patients. Acta Obstet Gynecol Scand 1998;77:1008–12. (Level II-3)

69. Rouanet P, Dubois JB, Gely S, Pourquier H. Exclusive radiation therapy in endometrial carcinoma. Int J Radiat Oncol Biol Phys 1993;26:223–8. (Level II-3)

70. Knocke TH, Kucera H, Weidinger B, Holler W, Potter R. Primary treatment of endometrial carcinoma with high-dose rate brachytherapy: results of 12 years of experience with 280 patients. Int J Radiat Oncol Biol Phys 1997; 37:359–65. (Level II-3)

71. Kupelian PA, Eifel PJ, Tornos C, Burke TW, Delclos L, Oswald MJ. Treatment of endometrial carcinoma with radiation therapy alone. Int J Radiat Oncol Biol Phys 1993;27:817–24. (Level II-3)

72. Montz FJ, Bristow RE, Bovicelli A, Tomacruz R, Kurman RJ. Intrauterine progesterone treatment of early endometrial cancer. Am J Obstet Gynecol 2002;186:651–7. (Level III)

73. Gotlieb WH, Beiner ME, Shalmon B, Korach Y, Segal Y, Zmira N, et al. Outcome of fertility-sparing treatment with progestins in young patients with endometrial cancer. Obstet Gynecol 2003;102:718–25. (Level III)

74. Imai M, Jobo T, Sato R, Kawaguchi M, Kuramoto H. Medroxyprogesterone acetate therapy for patients with adenocarcinoma of the endometrium who wish to preserve the uterus—usefulness and limitations. Eur J Gynaecol Oncol 2001;22:217–20. (Level III)

75. Kaku T, Yoshikawa H, Tsuda H, Sakamoto A, Fukunaga M, Kuwabara Y, et al. Conservative therapy for adenocarcinoma and atypical endometrial hyperplasia of the endometrium in young women: central pathologic review and treatment outcome. Cancer Lett 2001;167:39–48. (Level III)

76. Wang CB, Wang CJ, Huang HJ, Hsueh S, Chou HH, Soong YK, et al. Fertility-preserving treatment in young patients with endometrial adenocarcinoma. Cancer 2002; 94:2192–8. (Level III)

77. Ramirez PT, Frumovitz M, Bodurka DC, Sun CC, Levenback C. Hormonal therapy for the management of grade 1 endometrial adenocarcinoma: a literature review. Gynecol Oncol 2004;95:133–8. (Level III)

78. Tillmanns TD, Kamelle SA, Abudayyeh I, McMeekin SD, Gold MA, Korkos TG, et al. Panniculectomy with simultaneous gynecologic oncology surgery. Gynecol Oncol 2001;83:518–22. (Level III)

79. Scribner DR Jr, Walker JL, Johnson GA, McMeekin SD, Gold MA, Mannel RS. Surgical management of early-stage endometrial cancer in the elderly: is laparoscopy feasible? Gynecol Oncol 2001;83:563–8. (Level II-3)

80. Bloss JD, Berman ML, Bloss LP, Buller RE. Use of vaginal hysterectomy for the management of stage I endometrial cancer in the medically compromised patient. Gynecol Oncol 1991;40:74–7. (Level II-3)

81. Aalders JG, Abeler V, Kolstad P. Recurrent adenocarcinoma of the endometrium: a clinical and histopathological study of 379 patients. Gynecol Oncol 1984;17:85–103. (Level II-2)

82. Keys HM, Roberts JA, Brunetto VL, Zaino RJ, Spirtos NM, Bloss JD, et al. A phase III trial of surgery with or without adjunctive external pelvic radiation therapy in intermediate risk endometrial adenocarcinoma: a Gynecologic Oncology Group study [published erratum appears in Gynecol Oncol 2004;94:241–2]. Gynecol Oncol 2004;92:744–51. (Level I)

The MEDLINE database, the Cochrane Library, and ACOG's own internal resources and documents were used to conduct a literature search to locate relevant articles published between January 1985 and April 2005. The search was restricted to articles published in the English language. Priority was given to articles reporting results of original research, although review articles and commentaries also were consulted. Abstracts of research presented at symposia and scientific conferences were not considered adequate for inclusion in this document. Guidelines published by organizations or institutions such as the National Institutes of Health and the American College of Obstetricians and Gynecologists were reviewed, and additional studies were located by reviewing bibliographies of identified articles. When reliable research was not available, expert opinions from obstetrician–gynecologists were used.

Studies were reviewed and evaluated for quality according to the method outlined by the U.S. Preventive Services Task Force:

I   Evidence obtained from at least one properly designed randomized controlled trial.

II-1   Evidence obtained from well-designed controlled trials without randomization.

II-2   Evidence obtained from well-designed cohort or case–control analytic studies, preferably from more than one center or research group.

II-3   Evidence obtained from multiple time series with or without the intervention. Dramatic results in uncontrolled experiments also could be regarded as this type of evidence.

III   Opinions of respected authorities, based on clinical experience, descriptive studies, or reports of expert committees.

Based on the highest level of evidence found in the data, recommendations are provided and graded according to the following categories:

Level A—Recommendations are based on good and consistent scientific evidence.

Level B—Recommendations are based on limited or inconsistent scientific evidence.

Level C—Recommendations are based primarily on consensus and expert opinion.

ISSN 1099-3630

**The American College of
Obstetricians and Gynecologists
409 12th Street, SW
PO Box 96920
Washington, DC 20090-6920**

12345/98765

Management of endometrial cancer. ACOG Practice Bulletin No. 65. American College of Obstetricians and Gynecologists. Obstet Gynecol 2005;106:413–25.

ACOG PRACTICE BULLETIN

CLINICAL MANAGEMENT GUIDELINES FOR
OBSTETRICIAN–GYNECOLOGISTS

NUMBER 8, OCTOBER 1999

This Practice Bulletin was developed by the ACOG Committee on Practice Bulletins— Obstetrics with the assistance of David A. Baker, MD. The information is designed to aid practitioners in making decisions about appropriate obstetric and gynecologic care. These guidelines should not be construed as dictating an exclusive course of treatment or procedure. Variations in practice may be warranted based on the needs of the individual patient, resources, and limitations unique to the institution or type of practice.

Management of Herpes in Pregnancy

Genital herpes simplex virus (HSV) infection during pregnancy poses a significant risk to the developing fetus and newborn. In the United States, the incidence of this sexually transmitted disease (STD) has increased significantly since 1970 (1). Because many women of childbearing age are infected or are becoming infected, the risk of maternal transmission of this virus to the fetus or newborn is a major health concern. The purpose of this document is to define the stages of herpetic infection, outline the spectrum of maternal and neonatal infection, including rates of transmission and risks, and provide management guidelines that have been validated by appropriately conducted outcome-based research. Additional guidelines based on consensus and expert opinion also are presented to permit a review of most clinical aspects of HSV.

Background

Etiology

Two types of HSV, herpes simplex virus type 1 (HSV-1) and herpes simplex virus type 2 (HSV-2), can be identified on the basis of divergent biologic properties. They also can be differentiated by minor differences in antigenic composition and biochemical characteristics. Although they are distinct types, the degree of sharing of antigenic determinants between HSV-1 and HSV-2 results in cross-reacting antibodies capable of neutralizing the other virus type (2).

Initial contact with HSV usually occurs early in childhood and involves HSV-1. Less than 10% of primary infections with HSV-1 are clinically overt. Herpes simplex virus type 1 causes most nongenital herpetic lesions: eg, herpes labialis, gingivostomatitis, and keratoconjunctivitis. The female genital tract can be infected with HSV-1 or HSV-2. In the United States, most genital infection is from HSV-2.

Incidence

Herpes simplex virus infection of the genital tract is one of the most common viral STDs. Approximately 45 million adolescent and adult Americans have been infected with genital herpes based on positive serology test results for HSV-2 and estimates of genital HSV-1 infection (1). The greatest incidence of overt HSV-2 infection occurs in women in their late teens and early twenties. In one study, 5% of reproductive-aged women indicated a history of genital herpes virus infection (3). However, approximately 30% of the female population in the United States have antibodies to HSV-2 (1). Factors that influence the incidence of genital infection with HSV are age of the patient, duration of sexual activity, race, previous genital infections, family income, and number of sex partners (4). The number of initial visits to physicians' offices as a result of genital HSV infection increased from approximately 75,000 per year in 1978 to more than 150,000 per year in the early 1990s (1).

The last available data from the mid-1980s indicated that, in the United States, approximately 1,500–2,000 newborns contracted neonatal herpes each year (5). Most infections occur in the perinatal period from contact with infected maternal secretions. Most newborns acquire the virus from asymptomatic mothers without identified lesions (3, 6).

Presentation of Infection

There are three stages of HSV infection based on clinical presentation and serology (see the box). Primary infections are those in which no HSV-1 or HSV-2 antibodies are present. In nonprimary first-episode disease, HSV-1 antibodies are present in the woman who has HSV-2 infection or HSV-2 antibodies are present in the woman who has HSV-1 infection. In recurrent infections, homologous antibodies are present.

Clinical Designation of HSV Infection

Primary genital HSV: Antibodies to both HSV-1 and HSV-2 are absent at the time the patient acquires genital HSV due to HSV-1 or HSV-2.

Nonprimary first-episode genital HSV: Acquisition of genital HSV (due to HSV-1) with preexisting antibodies to HSV-2 or acquisition of genital HSV (due to HSV-2) with preexisting antibodies to HSV-1.

Recurrent genital HSV: Reactivation of genital HSV where the HSV type recovered from the lesion is the same type as the antibody in the sera.

Riley LE. Herpes simplex virus. Sem Perinatol 1998;22:284–292.

In the absence of systemic symptoms, the distinction between first-episode and recurrent herpetic infections is difficult. In one study, women with severe first-recognized clinical outbreaks of genital herpes in the second and third trimesters of pregnancy were evaluated serologically and virologically (7). Of these 23 women with clinical illnesses consistent with primary genital HSV infections, only one had serologically verified primary infection. This primary infection was caused by HSV-1. Three women had nonprimary HSV-2 infections, and 19 women had recurrent infections.

Primary Infection

Initial genital infection due to herpes may be either asymptomatic or associated with severe symptoms. With symptomatic primary infection, lesions may occur on the vulva, vagina, or cervix, or on all three between 2 and 14 days following exposure to infectious virus. These lesions are larger in number and size than those observed in patients with recurrent disease and patients who have had prior infection with HSV-1. The initial vesicles rupture and subsequently appear as shallow and eroded ulcers. Inguinal lymphadenopathy is demonstrated readily as the consequence of virus replication in the sites of lymphatic drainage (2).

When systemic symptoms (malaise, myalgia, and fever) occur, they are most commonly restricted to presumed primary herpetic infections. These symptoms reflect the viremia that occurs more likely with primary infection. Local symptoms of pain, dysuria, and soreness of the vulva and vagina are common in both primary and recurrent infections. The lesions of primary infection tends to resolve within 3 weeks without therapy. However, when secondary bacterial or mycotic infection is present and not treated, the lesions may persist up to 6 weeks.

Increased symptomatic and subclinical shedding from the lower genital tract of women occurs during the first 3 months after primary genital HSV-2 lesions have healed. Subclinical cervical and vulvar shedding occur at a rate of approximately 2.3% in women with HSV-2 infection and 0.65% in women with HSV-1 infection (8).

Nonprimary First Episode

Prior infection with HSV-1 does not fully protect a patient from initial infection with HSV-2 in the genital tract. It may be difficult for a physician to differentiate primary disease from nonprimary first-episode disease based only on clinical findings and patient symptoms (9); serologic confirmation would be required for definitive diagnosis.

A nonprimary first episode can be identified as a first clinically recognized genital HSV infection that does not behave clinically like a symptomatic primary infection. There are fewer systemic manifestations, less pain, a briefer duration of viral shedding, and a more rapid resolution of the clinical lesions in the nonprimary infection. These episodes usually are thought to be the result of an initial HSV-2 infection in the presence of partially protective HSV-1 antibodies.

Recurrent Infection

Recurrences of genital HSV infection can be symptomatic or subclinical, and there is significant variation from patient to patient in the frequency, severity, and duration of symptoms and amount of viral shedding (8, 10–12). Confinement of the ulcers to the genital area is more common in recurrent forms of the disease. The ulcers tend to be limited in size, number, and duration. Local symptoms predominate over systemic symptoms, with many patients indicating increased vaginal discharge or pain (13).

Shedding of the virus from the genital tract without symptoms or signs of clinical lesions (subclinical shedding) is episodic and lasts an average of 1.5 days (11). During this time, the virus quantity is lower than when a lesion is present; however, a susceptible partner can acquire the infection. Subclinical shedding makes this viral STD difficult to control and prevent.

Neonatal Herpes

Most neonatal HSV infection is the consequence of delivery of a neonate through an infected birth canal. There are three categories of neonatal disease: localized disease of the skin, eye, and mouth; central nervous system (CNS) disease with or without skin, eye, and mouth disease; or disseminated disease. Most infected neonates have localized skin, eye, and mouth disease, which generally is a mild illness. Localized disease may progress to encephalitis or disseminated disease. Subtle signs, such as poor feeding, listlessness, and irritability, may indicate CNS disease. One study of the predictors of mortality and morbidity of neonatal HSV showed no mortality with skin, eye, and mouth disease, 15% mortality with CNS disease, and 57% mortality with disseminated disease (14).

Transmission

Sexual and Direct Contact

Herpes simplex virus is transmitted via direct contact with an individual who is infected. Genital-to-genital contact or contact of the genital tract with an area that is infected with HSV, such as oral-to-genital contact, can result in transmission. One study showed that among sexual partners who were discordant for HSV infection, the annual risk of acquisition of genital HSV infection was 31.9% among women who were HSV-1-negative and HSV-2-negative versus 9.1% among women who were HSV-1-positive (4). Furthermore, most of the transmission between discordant couples occurs when there is no evidence of active lesions, which suggests that asymptomatic shedding is the source of more than half of all cases of transmission (15). In one study, about 10% of pregnant women were at risk of contracting primary HSV-2 infection from their HSV-2-seropositive husbands (16).

Maternal–Fetal Transmission

The vertical transmission of HSV appears to be related to gestational age and whether the disease is primary, nonprimary first episode, or recurrent. Investigators prospectively obtained HSV cultures on 15,923 women in early labor who were without signs or symptoms of genital HSV infection (17). Herpes simplex virus was isolated from 56 women (0.35%) with serum samples for HSV antibody testing available from 52 women. Eighteen women (35%) had serologic evidence of recently acquired, subclinical first-episode HSV, and 34 (65%) had asymptomatic recurrent disease. Herpes simplex virus infection developed in six (33%) of 18 neonates born to women with subclinical first-episode disease and in one (3%) of 34 infants born to women with recurrent HSV. This study also showed that preexisting antibody to HSV-2 but not to HSV-1 reduced the vertical transmission of HSV-2. In a more recent study, 8,538 women were prospectively evaluated during pregnancy and at delivery with HSV cultures. Investigators found that 94 (1.3%) of 7,046 women who were susceptible to either HSV-1 or HSV-2 seroconverted during pregnancy. Nine women acquired HSV at or near the time of delivery. Of these nine women, four delivered neonates who developed HSV (one died, and one had developmental delay). In this cohort, there were no cases of neonates with HSV-2 born to women with recurrent HSV (18). Vertical transmission rates at the time of vaginal delivery based on the type of maternal disease may be summarized as follows: primary HSV resulted in approximately 50% transmission; nonprimary first-episode HSV resulted in approximately 33% transmission; and recurrent HSV resulted in 0–3% transmission (17).

During Pregnancy

A threefold increase in the rate of spontaneous abortion following primary maternal genital infection with HSV early in pregnancy has been reported (17). However, this finding was not confirmed in a more recent study (18).

Primary infection in the second or third trimesters increases the risk for preterm delivery as well as the risk of HSV transmission to the newborn (17). Asymptomatic genital shedding of herpes from a subclinical primary genital infection may be associated with preterm delivery (18).

During pregnancy, primary maternal herpetic infection, in the absence of cross-protecting antibodies, theoretically may result in hematogenous dissemination of the virus to the fetus. Isolated case reports have associated in utero infection during the first 12–14 weeks of gestation with a variety of anomalies, such as microcephaly, microphthalmia, intracranial calcifications, and chorioretinitis (19–21).

Clinical Considerations and Recommendations

▶ *How can the diagnosis of HSV be confirmed?*

Herpes simplex virus infection may be documented in several ways. The standard and most sensitive test for detecting HSV from clinical specimens continues to be isolation of the virus by cell culture. Because HSV is a DNA virus, it produces cytopathic effects in cells indicative of virus replication. However, the sensitivity of this technique is affected by numerous factors related to sampling and transporting the specimen. Cytologic tests have a maximum sensitivity of 60–70% when dealing with overt clinical disease (22); thus, both the Papanicolaou and Tzanck tests are poor HSV screening procedures. Newer, more sensitive techniques are increasingly available, such as polymerase chain reaction and hybridization methods (23–25).

Early primary and nonprimary first-episode ulcers yield the virus in 80% of patients, whereas ulcers from recurrent infections are less likely to be culture-positive; only 40% of crusted lesions contain recoverable virus (26). When testing for HSV, overt lesions that are not in the ulcerated state should be unroofed and the fluid sampled.

Commercially available serologic tests designed to detect antibodies to genital herpes infection cannot reliably distinguish between HSV-1 and HSV-2. Serologic diagnosis of primary infection is possible by documenting seroconversion from a negative to a positive antibody titer. The usual time for obtaining a second specimen is 2–3 weeks after the onset of infection. The presence of an antibody titer in the initial specimen, obtained at the onset of disease, strongly suggests nonprimary first-episode or recurrent infection. Newer tests to differentiate between HSV-1 and HSV-2 antibodies are currently in development.

▶ *What is the optimal medical management of women with primary HSV infection during pregnancy?*

Antiviral therapy for primary infection is recommended for women with primary HSV infection during pregnancy to reduce viral shedding and enhance lesion healing. It is important to recognize that primary HSV cannot be distinguished from nonprimary first-episode disease unless serology is performed. Primary infection during pregnancy constitutes a higher risk for vertical transmission than does recurrent infection. The absence of episodes of symptomatic genital HSV infection throughout pregnancy does not eliminate the risk of asymptomatic shedding at delivery (27). Furthermore, suppressive therapy for the duration of the pregnancy needs to be considered to reduce the potential of continued viral shedding (8) and the likelihood of recurrent episodes (28).

Data are limited concerning prevention of disease in the fetus with maternal antiviral therapy. In one randomized study, 21 women received acyclovir and 25 did not to determine whether suppressive therapy started at 36 weeks of gestation could decrease viral shedding, prevent neonatal herpes, and reduce the need for cesarean delivery (29). Although the study did not differentiate between primary and nonprimary first episodes, it did show a significant reduction in cesarean delivery. There were no cases of neonatal herpes in either group, a finding that is compatible with a maximum 14% risk of infection with either therapy.

Significant benefits of acyclovir antiviral therapy using acyclovir have been shown in cases of pregnant women with disseminated HSV, herpes pneumonitis, herpes hepatitis, and herpes encephalitis (30–32).

▶ *What is the optimal medical management of women with recurrent HSV infection during pregnancy?*

A randomized trial of acyclovir given after 36 weeks of gestation in women with recurrent genital herpes infection demonstrated a significant decrease in clinical recurrences. The trial also showed a reduction in the number of cesarean deliveries performed for active infection, although this finding was not statistically significant (33).

▶ *What medications are available for treatment of HSV infection during pregnancy?*

Numerous compounds are available for the treatment of genital herpes (34), although none of these antiviral compounds has received approval for use in pregnancy by the U.S. Food and Drug Administration. These compounds are nucleoside analogues that selectively inhibit viral replication and produce minimal effect on the cell. Research in antiviral therapy has focused on improving bioavailability, which improves absorption and increases plasma levels of the compound while decreasing the number of daily doses of medication.

Acyclovir, a class-C medication, has selective activity against HSV-1 and HSV-2. In the treatment of primary genital herpes infections, oral acyclovir reduces viral shedding, reduces pain, and heals lesions faster when compared with a placebo (35). Acyclovir has been shown to be safe and has minimal side effects (36). However, only approximately 20% of each oral dose is absorbed.

The newer antiherpetic drugs valacyclovir and famciclovir are class-B medications. Their increased bio-availability means that they may require less frequent dosing to achieve the same therapeutic benefits as acyclovir. The U.S. Food and Drug Administration has approved both valacyclovir and famciclovir for the treatment of primary genital herpes, the treatment of episodes of recurrent disease, and the daily treatment for suppression of outbreaks of recurrent genital herpes.

Daily treatment with oral acyclovir significantly reduces symptomatic recurrences and suppresses subclinical viral shedding (28, 37). One study showed that 6 years of continuous daily acyclovir suppressive therapy did not produce the emergence of acyclovir-resistant isolates in immunocompetent patients (36). Valacyclovir therapy, 500 mg once daily, is effective in suppressing recurrent genital herpes (38). Suppressive famciclovir therapy requires a twice daily, 250 mg dosage (38). See Table 1.

Numerous studies have demonstrated the safety of acyclovir use during pregnancy (29, 32, 39). Neither medically indicated nor inadvertent use in the first trimester of pregnancy demonstrated any increased risk to the developing fetus. When acyclovir is given orally or intravenously, it crosses the placenta, concentrates in amniotic fluid and breast milk, and reaches therapeutic levels in the fetus (40). An acyclovir pregnancy registry has been maintained since 1984. In 1993, the Centers for Disease Control and Prevention published data showing no increase in fetal problems in women who received acyclovir during the first trimester of pregnancy (39).

▶ *Is there a role for universal screening during pregnancy or at delivery?*

Viral cultures are costly and imprecise. The correlation between asymptomatic viral shedding and ensuing neonatally acquired disease is poor. Negative cultures do not preclude the possibility of subsequent neonatal infection because the culture sensitivity is well below 100%, and infection may occur in the interim. Virologic monitoring is not recommended for pregnant women whose onset of disease antedated pregnancy or for those whose sexual partners have had herpetic lesions (27). Similarly, there are no data to support the value of culturing asymptomatic patients with a history of recurrent disease (11).

Table 1. Antiviral Treatment for Herpes Simplex Virus

Indication	Valacyclovir	Acyclovir	Famciclovir
First clinical episode	1,000 mg twice a day for 7–14 days	200 mg five times a day or 400 mg three times a day for 7–14 days	250 mg three times a day for 7–14 days
Recurrent episodes	500 mg twice a day for 5 days	200 mg five times a day or 400 mg three times a day for 5 days	125 mg twice a day for 5 days
Daily suppressive therapy	500 mg once a day (≤9 recurrences per year) or 1,000 mg once a day or 250 mg twice a day (>9 recurrences per year)	400 mg twice a day	250 mg twice a day

Baker DA. Antiviral therapy for genital herpes in nonpregnant and pregnant women. Int J Fertil 1998;43:243–248

▶ *In which situations should cesarean delivery be considered?*

Cesarean delivery is indicated in women with active genital lesions or symptoms of vulvar pain or burning, which may indicate an impending outbreak. The incidence of infection in infants whose mothers have recurrent infections is low, but cesarean delivery is warranted because of the potentially serious nature of the disease. The low incidence of neonatal HSV has raised concern that cesarean delivery is unwarranted for recurrent genital herpes (41). The extent to which maternal antibodies will protect a neonate from infection during a recurrence has not been determined with certainty. Cesarean delivery is not warranted in women with a history of HSV infection but with no active genital disease during labor (42).

▶ *Is cesarean delivery recommended for women with recurrent HSV lesions on areas distant from the vulva, vagina, or cervix (eg, thigh or buttock)?*

Among women with recurrent HSV and genital lesions at the time of labor, the risk of neonatal HSV infection associated with vaginal birth is low, estimated to be no more than 3% (17). In part, this low risk is probably attributable to preexisting maternal type-specific antibodies. When infection occurs among neonates of women with recurrent HSV, it is due either to shedding of the virus from the genital lesion itself or to shedding from the cervix. In patients with recurrent genital HSV and nongenital lesions at the time of labor, the only viral exposure faced by the infant during vaginal delivery is that of cervical shedding, which occurs in approximately 2% of such cases (43). Thus, the risk of neonatal HSV associated with vaginal delivery in a woman with recurrent HSV and nongenital lesions would appear to be very low. Cesarean delivery is not recommended for these women. Nongenital lesions should be covered with an occlusive dressing; the patient then can deliver vaginally.

▶ *In a patient with active HSV infection and ruptured membranes, is there any length of time at which vaginal delivery remains appropriate?*

In patients with active HSV infection and ruptured membranes at or near term, a cesarean delivery should be performed as soon as the necessary personnel and equipment can be readied. There is no evidence that there is a duration of premature rupture of membranes beyond which the fetus does not benefit from cesarean delivery (44).

▶ *How should a woman with active HSV and preterm premature rupture of membranes be managed?*

In the decision to deliver a patient with preterm premature rupture of membranes and active HSV, the risk of prematurity versus the potential risk of neonatal disease should be considered. In pregnancies remote from term, especially in women with recurrent disease, there is increasing support for continuing the pregnancy to gain benefit from time and glucocorticoids (45). If this expectant management plan is followed, treatment with an antiviral agent is indicated. Concern has been raised about the potential effects of glucocorticoids on patients with viral infection, but there is no conclusive evidence that this is a concern in this setting. The decision to perform a cesarean delivery depends on whether active lesions are present at the time of delivery.

The utility of suppressive antiviral therapy to prevent ascending infection has not been proven. The lack of evidence complicates the situation, because it is clear that premature neonates are at the greatest risk of infection. In such situations, it may be appropriate to consult personnel well versed in the management of such complicated cases.

▶ *Are invasive procedures contraindicated in women with HSV?*

In patients with recurrent HSV, invasive procedures, such as amniocentesis, percutaneous umbilical cord blood sampling, or transabdominal chorionic villus sampling may be performed; however, transcervical procedures should be delayed until lesions appear to have resolved. In a patient with primary HSV and systemic symptoms, it seems prudent to delay invasive procedures until symptoms appear to resolve.

Local neonatal infection may result from the use of fetal scalp electrode monitoring in patients with a history of herpes, even when lesions are not present (46–48). However, if there are indications for fetal scalp monitoring, it may be appropriate in a woman who has a history of recurrent HSV and no active lesions. If vesicular or vesiculopustular lesions develop at the site of the electrode, it is important to make a quick and accurate diagnosis and start systemic antiviral therapy.

▶ *Should women with active HSV breastfeed or handle their infants?*

Postnatally acquired disease can be as lethal as that acquired during delivery through an infected birth canal. Oropharyngeal or cutaneous lesions can be an effective source of virus. It is unlikely that breastfeeding will lead to neonatal infection; however, if the mother has an obvious lesion on the breast, breastfeeding is contraindicated. Because the herpes virus is transmitted through direct contact (eg, hand-to-mouth), neonatal infection may be acquired from family members other than the mother and from sites other than the genital tract (49, 50). Most strains of HSV responsible for nosocomial neonatal disease are HSV-1 rather than HSV-2. Mothers with active lesions should use caution when handling their babies.

Summary

The following recommendations are based on limited or inconsistent scientific evidence (Level B):

▶ Women with primary HSV during pregnancy should be treated with antiviral therapy.

▶ Cesarean delivery should be performed on women with first-episode HSV who have active genital lesions at delivery.

▶ For women at or beyond 36 weeks of gestation with a first episode of HSV occurring during the current pregnancy, antiviral therapy should be considered.

The following recommendations are based primarily on consensus and expert opinion (Level C):

▶ Cesarean delivery should be performed on women with recurrent HSV infection who have active genital lesions or prodromal symptoms at delivery.

▶ Expectant management of patients with preterm labor or preterm premature rupture of membranes and active HSV may be warranted.

▶ For women at or beyond 36 weeks of gestation who are at risk for recurrent HSV, antiviral therapy also may be considered, although such therapy may not reduce the likelihood of cesarean delivery.

▶ In women with no active lesions or prodromal symptoms during labor, cesarean delivery should not be performed on the basis of a history of recurrent disease.

References

1. Fleming DT, McQuillan GM, Johnson RE, Nahmias AJ, Aral SO, Lee FK. Herpes simplex virus type 2 in the United States, 1976 to 1994. N Engl J Med 1997;337: 1105–1111 (Level II-3)

2. Corey L, Spear PG. Infections with herpes simplex viruses. N Engl J Med 1986;314:686–691 (Level III)

3. Prober C, Corey L, Brown ZA, Hensleigh PA, Frenkel LM, Bryson YJ. The management of pregnancies complicated by genital infections with herpes simplex virus. Clin Infect Dis 1992;15:1031–1038 (Level III)

4. Mertz GL, Benedetti J, Ashley R, Selke SA, Corey L. Risk factors for the sexual transmission of genital herpes. Ann Intern Med 1992;116:197–202 (Level II-3)

5. Whitley RJ, Hutto C. Neonatal herpes simplex virus infections. Pediatr Rev 1985;7:119–126 (Level III)

6. Frenkel LM, Garratty EM, Shen JP, Wheeler N, Clark O, Bryson YJ. Clinical reactivation of herpes simplex virus type 2 infection in seropositive pregnant women with no history of genital herpes. Ann Intern Med 1993;118: 414–418 (Level II-3)

7. Hensleigh PA, Andrews WW, Brown Z, Greenspoon J, Yasukawa L, Prober CG. Genital herpes during pregnancy: inability to distinguish primary and recurrent infections clinically. Obstet Gynecol 1997;89:891–895 (Level III)

8. Koelle DM, Benedetti J, Langenberg A, Corey L. Asymptomatic reactivation of herpes simplex virus in women after the first episode of genital herpes. Ann Intern Med 1992;116:433–437 (Level II-3)

9. Mertz GL. Epidemiology of genital herpes infections. Infect Dis Clin North Am 1993;7:825–839 (Level III)

10. Brock BV, Selke S, Benedetti J, Douglas JM Jr, Corey L. Frequency of asymptomatic shedding of herpes simplex virus in women with genital herpes. JAMA 1990;263:418–420 (Level III)

11. Prober CG. Herpetic vaginitis in 1993. Clin Obstet Gynecol 1993;36:177–187 (Level III)

12. Wald A, Zeh J, Selke S, Ashley RL, Corey L. Virologic characteristics of subclinical and symptomatic genital herpes infections. N Engl J Med 1995;333:770–775 (Level II-3)

13. Hirsch MS. Herpes simplex virus. In: Mandell GL, Bennett JE, Dolin R, eds. Mandell, Douglas and Bennett's principles and practice of infectious diseases. 4th ed. New York: Churchill Livingstone, 1995:1336–1345 (Level III)

14. Whitley R, Arvin A, Prober C, Corey L, Burchett S, Plotkin S. Predictors of morbidity and mortality in neonates with herpes simplex infections. The National Institute of Allergy and infectious Diseases Collaborative Antiviral Study Group. N Engl J Med 1991;324:450–454 (Level III)

15. Mertz GJ, Schmidt O, Jourden JL, Guinan ME, Remington ML, Fahnlander A. Frequency of acquisition of first-episode genital infection with herpes simplex virus from symptomatic and asymptomatic source contacts. Sex Transm Dis 1985;12:33–39 (Level III)

16. Kulhanjian JA, Soroush V, Au DS, Bronzan RN, Yasukawa LL, Weylman LE. Identification of women at unsuspected risk of primary infection with herpes simplex virus type 2 during pregnancy. N Engl J Med 1992;326: 916–920 (Level II-3)

17. Brown ZA, Benedetti J, Ashley R, Burchett S, Selke S, Berry S. Neonatal herpes simplex virus infection in relation to asymptomatic maternal infection at the time of labor. N Engl J Med 1991;324:1247–1252 (Level II-3)

18. Brown ZA, Selke S, Zeh J, Kopelman J, Maslow A, Ashley RL. The acquisition of herpes simplex virus during pregnancy. N Engl J Med 1997;337:509–515 (Level II-3)

19. Altshuler G. Pathogenesis of congenital herpesvirus infection: case report including a description of the placenta. Am J Dis Child 1974;127:427–429 (Level III)

20. Chalhub EG, Baenziger J, Feigen RD, Middlekamp JN, Shackelford GD. Congenital herpes simplex type II infection with extensive hepatic calcification bone lesions and cataracts: complete postmortem examination. Dev Med Child Neurol 1977;19:527–534 (Level III)

21. Monif GR, Kellner KR, Donnelly WH Jr. Congenital herpes simplex type II infection. Am J Obstet Gynecol 1985;152:1000–1002 (Level III)

22. Woods GL. Update on laboratory diagnosis of sexually transmitted diseases. Clin Lab Med 1995;15:665–684 (Level III)

23. Hardy DA, Arvin AM, Yasukawa LL, Bronzan RN, Lewinsohn DM, Hensleigh PA. Use of polymerase chain reaction for successful identification of asymptomatic genital infection with herpes simplex virus in pregnant women at delivery. J Infect Dis 1990;162:1031–1035 (Level III)

24. Boggess KA, Watts DH, Hobson AC, Ashley RL, Brown ZA, Corey L. Herpes simplex type 2 detection by culture and polymerase chain reaction and relationship to genital symptoms and cervical antibody status during the third trimester of pregnancy. Am J Obstet Gynecol 1997;176:443–451 (Level III)

25. Cone RW, Hobson AC, Palmer J, Remington M, Corey L. Extended duration of herpes simplex virus DNA in genital lesions detected by the polymerase chain reaction. J Infect Dis 1991;164:757–760 (Level III)

26. Mosely RC, Corey L, Benjamin D, Winter C, Remington ML. Comparison of viral isolation, direct immunofluorescence, and indirect immunoperoxidase techniques for detection of genital herpes simplex virus infection. J Clin Microbiol 1981;13:913–918 (Level II-2)

27. Arvin AM, Hensleigh PA, Prober CG, Au DS, Yasukawa LL, Wittek AE. Failure of antepartum maternal cultures to predict the infant's risk of exposure to herpes simplex virus at delivery. N Engl J Med 1986;315:796–800 (Level II-3)

28. Goldberg LK, Kaufman R, Kurtz TO, Conant MA, Eron LJ, Batenhorst RL. Long-term suppression of recurrent genital herpes with acyclovir. A 5-year benchmark. Acyclovir Study Group. Arch Dermatol 1993;129:582–587 (Level I)

29. Scott LL, Sanchez PJ, Jackson GL, Zeray F, Wendel GD Jr. Acyclovir suppression to prevent cesarean delivery after first-episode genital herpes. Obstet Gynecol 1996;87:69–73 (Level I)

30. Grover L, Kane J, Kravitz J, Cruz A. Systemic acyclovir in pregnancy: a case report. Obstet Gynecol 1985;65:284–287 (Level III)

31. Lagrew DC Jr, Furlow TG, Hager WD, Yarrish RL. Disseminated herpes simplex virus infection in pregnancy. Successful treatment with acyclovir. JAMA 1984;252:2058–2059 (Level III)

32. Brown ZA, Baker DA. Acyclovir therapy during pregnancy. Obstet Gynecol 1989;3:526–531 (Level III)

33. Brockelhurst P, Kinghorn G, Carney O, Helsen K, Ross E, Ellis E, et al. A randomised placebo controlled trial of suppressive acyclovir in late pregnancy in women with recurrent genital herpes infection. Br J Obstet Gynaecol 1998;105:275–280 (Level I)

34. Lavoie SR, Kaplowitz LG. Management of genital herpes infection. Semin Dermatol 1994;13:248–255 (Level III)

35. Mertz GJ, Critchlow CW, Benedetti J, Reichman RC, Dolin R, Connor J. Double-blind placebo-controlled trial of oral acyclovir in first-episode genital herpes simplex virus infections. JAMA 1984;252:1147–1151 (Level I)

36. Fife KII, Crumpacker CS, Mertz GJ, Hill EL, Boone GS. Recurrence and resistance patterns of herpes simplex virus following cessation of > or = 6 years of chronic suppression with acyclovir. Acyclovir Study Group. J Infect Dis 1994;169:1338–1341 (Level II-3)

37. Wald A, Zeh J, Barnum G, Davis LG, Corey L. Suppression of subclinical shedding of herpes simplex virus type 2 with acyclovir. Ann Intern Med 1996;124:8–15 (Level I)

38. Centers for Disease Control and Prevention. 1998 guidelines for treatment of sexually transmitted diseases. MMWR Morb Mortal Wkly Rep 1998;47(RR-1):20–24 (Level III)

39. Pregnancy outcomes following systemic acyclovir exposure. June 1, 1984–June 30, 1993. MMWR Morb Mortal Wkly Rep 1993;42:806–809 (Level III)

40. Frenkel LM, Brown ZA, Bryson YJ, Corey L, Unadkat JD, Hensleigh PA, et al. Pharmacokinetics of acyclovir in the term human pregnancy and neonate. Am J Obstet Gynecol 1991;164:569–576 (Level II-2)

41. Randolph AG, Washington E, Prober CG. Cesarean delivery for women presenting with genital herpes lesions. Efficacy, risks, and costs. JAMA 1993;270:77–82 (Decision Analysis)

42. Roberts SW, Cox SM, Dax J, Wendel GD Jr, Leveno KJ. Genital herpes during pregnancy: no lesions, no cesarean. Obstet Gynecol 1995;85:261–264 (Level II-2)

43. Wittek AE, Yeager AS, Au DS, Hensleigh PA. Asymptomatic shedding of herpes simplex virus from the cervix and lesion site during pregnancy. Correlation of antepartum shedding with shedding at delivery. Am J Dis Child 1984;138:439–442 (Level II-3)

44. Nahmias AJ, Josey WE, Naib ZM, Freeman MG, Fernandez RJ, Wheeler JH. Perinatal risk associated with maternal genital herpes simplex virus infection. Am J Obstet Gynecol 1971;110:825–837 (Level II-3)

45. National Institutes of Health. Consensus Development Conference Statement. Effect of corticoids for fetal maturation on perinatal outcomes, February 28–March 2, 1994. Am J Obstet Gynecol 1995;173:246–252 (Level III)

46. Amann ST, Fagnant RJ, Chartrand SA, Monif GR. Herpes simplex infection with short-term use of a fetal scalp electrode. A case report. J Reprod Med 1992;37:372–374 (Level III)

47. Golden SM, Merenstein GB, Todd WA, Hill JM. Disseminated herpes simplex neonatorum: a complication of fetal monitoring. Am J Obstet Gynecol 1977;129:917–918 (Level III)

48. Goldkrand JW. Intrapartum inoculation of herpes simplex virus by fetal scalp electrode. Obstet Gynecol 1982;59:263–265 (Level III)

49. Douglas J, Schmidt O, Corey L. Acquisition of neonatal HSV-1 infection from a paternal source contact. J Pediatr 1983;103:908–910 (Level III)

50. Hammerberg O, Watts J, Chernesky M, Luchsinger I, Rawls W. An outbreak of herpes simplex virus type 1 in an intensive care nursery. Pediatr Infect Dis J 1983;2:290–294 (Level III)

The MEDLINE database was used to conduct a literature search to locate relevant articles published between January 1985 and December 1998. The search was restricted to articles published in the English language. Priority was given to articles reporting results of original research, although review articles and commentaries also were consulted. Abstracts of research presented at symposia and scientific conferences were not considered adequate for inclusion in this document. Guidelines published by organizations or institutions such as the National Institutes of Health and the American College of Obstetricians and Gynecologists were reviewed, and additional studies were located by reviewing bibliographies of identified articles. When reliable research was not available, expert opinions from obstetrician–gynecologists were used.

Studies were reviewed and evaluated for quality according to the method outlined by the U.S. Preventive Services Task Force:

I   Evidence obtained from at least one properly designed randomized controlled trial.
II-1 Evidence obtained from well-designed controlled trials without randomization.
II-2 Evidence obtained from well-designed cohort or case–control analytic studies, preferably from more than one center or research group.
II-3 Evidence obtained from multiple time series with or without the intervention. Dramatic results in uncontrolled experiments also could be regarded as this type of evidence.
III   Opinions of respected authorities, based on clinical experience, descriptive studies, or reports of expert committees.

Based on the highest level of evidence found in the data, recommendations are provided and graded according to the following categories:

Level A—Recommendations are based on good and consistent scientific evidence.

Level B—Recommendations are based on limited or inconsistent scientific evidence.

Level C—Recommendations are based primarily on consensus and expert opinion.

ISSN 1099-3630

The American College of Obstetricians and Gynecologists
409 12th Street, SW
PO Box 96920
Washington, DC 20090-6920

12345/32109

ACOG PRACTICE BULLETIN

CLINICAL MANAGEMENT GUIDELINES FOR
OBSTETRICIAN–GYNECOLOGISTS
NUMBER 34, FEBRUARY 2002

This Practice Bulletin was developed by the ACOG Committee on Practice Bulletins— Gynecology with the assistance of Robert Barbieri, MD. The information is designed to aid practitioners in making decisions about appropriate obstetric and gynecologic care. These guidelines should not be construed as dictating an exclusive course of treatment or procedure. Variations in practice may be warranted based on the needs of the individual patient, resources, and limitations unique to the institution or type of practice.

Management of Infertility Caused by Ovulatory Dysfunction

Approximately 20% of infertile women have ovulatory disorders (1, 2). In infertile women with ovulatory disorders, the cause of anovulation will guide the selection of an appropriate treatment plan. Advances in reproductive endocrinology allow the generalist obstetrician–gynecologist to provide treatment that results in successful ovulatory stimulation and pregnancy in most women with ovulatory disorders.

Background

Etiology

Ovulatory dysfunction is likely to be present in women with polymenorrhea or oligomenorrhea and is almost always present in women with amenorrhea (except in patients with uterine disease, such as uterine synechiae or Asherman's syndrome). Regular menstrual cycles, with a cycle length between 22 and 35 days, and the presence of premenstrual bloating, dysmenorrhea, and breast tenderness suggest the presence of ovulatory cycles.

Laboratory methods for determining ovulation include the basal body temperature chart, urine testing for the luteinizing hormone (LH) surge, properly timed measurement of serum progesterone, and endometrial biopsy. Serial pelvic ultrasonography also may be able to identify the growth and rupture of a follicle, suggesting that ovulation has occurred. Basal body temperature charts are inexpensive but may be a burden to the patient to complete and only document ovulation retrospectively. The pulsatile ovarian secretion of progesterone in the luteal phase may decrease the sensitivity of a single measurement of progesterone, but a serum progesterone level higher than 3 ng/mL is highly specific for detecting ovulation. (These tests also can detect ovulation in induced cycles.)

If anovulation or clinically significant oligo-ovulation has been documented, a complete physical examination and selected laboratory testing are important to identify the etiology of the ovulatory dysfunction. The most common causes of ovulatory dysfunction are 1) polycystic ovary syndrome (PCOS) (approximately 70% of cases of ovulatory dysfunction) (3), 2) hypothalamic amenorrhea, also known as hypogonadotropic hypogonadism (approximately 10% of cases), 3) hyperprolactinemia (approximately 10% of cases), and 4) premature ovarian failure, also known as hypergonadotropic hypoestrogenic anovulation (approximately 10% of cases) (4).

During the physical examination, the practitioner should note the presence of galactorrhea, thyromegaly or other evidence of hypothyroidism or hyperthyroidism, acanthosis nigricans, hirsutism, acne, or signs of virilization. In addition, the patient's body mass index (BMI) should be calculated. A BMI less than 20 may indicate hypothalamic ovulatory dysfunction (low gonadotropin-releasing hormone [GnRH] secretion, low LH and follicle-stimulating hormone [FSH] secretion, low endogenous estrogen secretion) (5). The combination of amenorrhea and galactorrhea strongly correlates with hyperprolactinemia. The presence of acanthosis nigricans suggests the patient has a marked degree of insulin resistance.

In general, clinicians should first recommend the least resource-intensive ovulation induction regimens that are appropriate for each cause of ovulatory dysfunction. For example, for women with hypogonadotropic hypogonadism and a BMI less than 20, weight gain may be associated with the resumption of normal menses.

Polycystic Ovary Syndrome

Polycystic ovary syndrome is defined as the presence of oligomenorrhea or amenorrhea and hyperandrogenism in the absence of other hyperandrogenic disorders, such as androgen-secreting tumors or nonclassical adrenal hyperplasia. Clinical evidence of hyperandrogenism includes hirsutism and acne. Laboratory evidence of hyperandrogenism includes an elevated total, bioavailable, or free testosterone concentration. Elevated serum dehydroepiandrosterone sulfate (DHEAS) or androstenedione levels also are evidence of hyperandrogenism. The morphologic characteristics of "polycystic ovaries" as demonstrated on pelvic ultrasonography are not essential for the diagnosis of PCOS but support the diagnosis. In women of reproductive age, the prevalence of PCOS is approximately 5%, making it one of the most common reproductive disorders (3). Among women with ovulatory dysfunction, about 70% have PCOS (3).

In women with PCOS, many therapies are available to treat anovulatory infertility, including weight loss, clomiphene, clomiphene plus metformin, clomiphene plus glucocorticoid, gonadotropin injections, ovarian surgery, and in vitro fertilization-embryo transfer (IVF-ET). Using the principle of progressing from the least resource-intensive treatments to the most resource-intensive treatments, one potential strategy for organizing the care of women with PCOS is presented in the box.

Hypothalamic Anovulation

Hypothalamic anovulation (hypogonadotropic hypogonadism) usually is associated with low levels of GnRH secretion, low or normal levels of LH and FSH secretion, and low levels of endogenous estrogen secretion. Diseases associated with hypothalamic anovulation include anorexia nervosa, Kallmann's syndrome, and hypothalamic tumors and cysts. Factors associated with hypogonadotropic hypogonadism include a low BMI (<20); high-intensity exercise; certain dietary patterns, including high-fiber, low-fat diets; and excessive stress. One approach to treating this condition is to reverse the lifestyle factors that contribute to the anovulation. For example, in one study of 26 underweight women who practiced strict dieting and were infertile, the subjects were counseled by a dietitian and given physician-directed advice to increase their BMI (5). After the intervention, the women gained a mean 3.7 kg, and 73% of the women became pregnant. Decreasing the intensity of

---

A Step-by-Step Approach to Ovulation Induction in Women with PCOS

The least resource-intensive interventions are recommended in the early steps in the protocol, while the most resource-intensive interventions are reserved for later treatment.

Step 1.   If the BMI is higher than 30, recommend weight loss of at least 10% of body weight.

Step 2.   Prescribe clomiphene to induce ovulation.

Step 3.   If DHEAS is higher than 2 μg/mL, consider combining clomiphene with a glucocorticoid to induce ovulation.

Step 4.   If clomiphene does not result in ovulation, consider a combination of metformin plus clomiphene.

Step 5.   Initiate low-dose FSH injections.

Step 6.   Initiate low-dose FSH injections plus metformin.

Step 7.   Consider laparoscopic ovarian surgery or in vitro fertilization.

exercise and stress also may help improve the rate of ovulation in some of these women. However, no well-designed clinical trials testing these recommendations have been reported.

In the past, one option for ovulation induction for hypogonadotropic hypogonadism was the parenteral administration of GnRH in pulses using a portable programmable pump. It was associated with monofollicular ovulation and a high rate of singleton pregnancy but the pump is not commercially available in the United States (6, 7).

Hyperprolactinemia

The most common causes of hyperprolactinemia are a prolactin-secreting pituitary gland tumor and the use of psychiatric medications. The presence of hyperprolactinemia should be confirmed if there is any question about the timing of the blood test or the quality of the assay; blood should be drawn after the patient has fasted and preferably not after a breast examination or breast stimulation (8). All women with hyperprolactinemia should be tested for hypothyroidism (a thyroid-stimulating hormone screening or additional thyroid hormone testing as clinically indicated) and pregnancy (9). An imaging study (magnetic resonance imaging or computed tomography) of the central nervous system and the pituitary gland should be obtained in all women with hyperprolactinemia unless there is an obvious cause, such as hypothyroidism, that makes a pituitary gland tumor unlikely (10). If the imaging study reveals a macroadenoma of the pituitary gland (tumor diameter ≥10 mm), the patient should be referred to a physician with expertise in endocrinology or pituitary gland disease for consultation. Induction of ovulation in women with large pituitary gland tumors is associated with a high risk of neurosurgical complications during pregnancy (11–13). In addition, women with large pituitary gland tumors may have undiagnosed adrenal insufficiency, a condition that poses significant health risks. For women with microadenomas (tumor diameter <10 mm) that secrete prolactin, the risk of pituitary insufficiency and neurosurgical complications during pregnancy is very low (<1%) (11–13). Observational studies indicate that during 4–6 years of observation, 95% of microadenomas do not increase in size (14, 15).

Age-Related Ovulation Dysfunction and Premature Ovarian Failure

As the ovarian follicular pool depletes with age, the remaining follicles appear to be less capable of fertilization and establishing a successful pregnancy. Inhibin B production by the small follicles decreases with age, the inhibin suppression of FSH secretion decreases, and pituitary gland secretion of FSH increases. An elevated random FSH level in amenorrheic or severely oligomenorrheic women or an elevated day-3 FSH level in women with menses is highly sensitive and specific for identifying women with a depleted ovarian follicular pool (16). If initial attempts at ovulation induction do not result in a pregnancy in women older than 37 years, consultation with an infertility specialist may be advisable to develop a plan for when assisted reproductive procedures, such as IVF-ET or oocyte donation should be pursued.

Treatments proposed to induce ovulation in women with premature ovarian failure include 1) oral contraceptive suppression of gonadotropins followed by discontinuation of the oral contraceptive to allow a rebound in gonadotropin secretion and ovarian function, 2) GnRH-agonist suppression of gonadotropin secretion followed by high-dose gonadotropin injections, and 3) glucocorticoid suppression of the immune system. None of these treatments has demonstrated efficacy in randomized clinical trials for inducing ovulation in women with premature ovarian failure (17). Women with infertility, ovulatory dysfunction, and an elevated FSH level should be referred to a physician with specialized expertise in treating infertility.

Luteal Phase Deficiency

Luteal phase deficiency is a theoretical disorder in which ovulation occurs, but there is insufficient progesterone production by the corpus luteum to allow for successful implantation. Luteal phase deficiency is thought to cause recurrent pregnancy loss, especially in the first trimester, and is believed to be responsible for a subset of cases of infertility. Studies that have attempted to establish luteal phase deficiency as a cause of infertility have not included control groups of fertile women. However, women who have regular menstrual cycles may have luteal phase abnormalities in as many as 31% of their cycles (18). Methods to diagnose and treat luteal phase deficiencies, therefore, are largely speculative. Because current infertility treatment often includes empiric treatment for unexplained infertility, most women who have luteal phase deficiencies and are infertile will receive treatment that includes controlled ovarian hyperstimulation. Therefore, a therapy specific to luteal phase deficiency is not being aggressively pursued.

Treatment Options

Clomiphene Citrate

The precise mechanism of action of clomiphene citrate is not completely understood. The administration of clomiphene to anovulatory women with endogenous estrogen secretion often is followed by an increase in both hypothalamic GnRH secretion and pituitary LH and FSH secretion, which causes follicle growth, triggering the LH surge and ovulation.

Clomiphene treatment is most effective in women with normal FSH levels and adequate endogenous production of estrogen and is least effective in women with hypothalamic amenorrhea or in women with an elevated basal FSH concentration (19). In women with PCOS, the presence of obesity, elevated testosterone concentration, and severe insulin resistance decreases the efficacy of clomiphene citrate (20). Most women with hypogonadotropic hypogonadism do not ovulate in response to treatment with clomiphene.

Most clomiphene-induced pregnancies occur within the first three menstrual cycles, and the vast majority occur within 6 months. There is no benefit to increasing the dosage once ovulation has occurred or to continuing beyond 6 months of treatment (21). Clomiphene administration in anovulatory women differs from superovulation, or controlled ovarian hyperstimulation, which is frequently attempted in couples with unexplained infertility. With clomiphene, monofolliculogenesis is the goal, and adjunctive treatments, such as intensive follicle monitoring and intrauterine insemination, do not have a defined role. With superovulation, women are already ovulatory; clomiphene, if administered, is typically given with human chorionic gonadotropin (hCG) to ensure ovulation, and intrauterine insemination also is appropriate.

Gonadotropin Injection

Gonadotropins can be administered using human urinary menopausal gonadotropins, which contain both LH and FSH, or by using recombinant FSH. Both types of gonadotropins are effective in treating anovulation in women with PCOS. The use of gonadotropin injections to induce ovulation in women with PCOS is resource intensive and is associated with a high risk of adverse outcomes, such as ovarian hyperstimulation and high-order multiple pregnancy.

Gonadotropin injections are effective in the treatment of hypothalamic anovulation. Women with hypothalamic anovulation who have a baseline serum LH level lower than 0.5 IU/L should be treated with both FSH and LH because they have a deficiency in both gonadotropins. Women with hypothalamic amenorrhea and a baseline LH level higher than 0.5 IU/L can be successfully treated with FSH alone (22). In most circumstances, the use of FSH injections to induce ovulation should be performed by physicians with advanced training in treating infertility.

Metformin

Metformin is an oral biguanide antihyperglycemic agent approved for the treatment of adult-onset diabetes mellitus. It is a category-B drug used by some clinicians to treat diabetes mellitus in pregnant women. Metformin decreases blood glucose levels by inhibiting hepatic glucose production and by enhancing peripheral glucose uptake. Metformin increases insulin sensitivity at the postreceptor level and stimulates insulin-mediated glucose disposal. Unlike sulfonylureas, metformin does not cause hypoglycemia because it does not increase insulin secretion. Unlike phenformin, metformin does not block mitochondrial metabolism of lactate unless the patient has renal failure (renal failure will cause lactate to accumulate to very high concentrations) or severe hypoxia (mitochondrial dysfunction). Metformin is not approved by the U.S. Food and Drug Administration (FDA) for ovulation induction.

Dopamine Agonists

Dopamine-agonist drugs (bromocriptine, pergolide, cabergoline) are the treatment of choice for ovulation induction in women with hyperprolactinemia (23). Dopamine-agonist drugs directly suppress prolactin production by the tumor and cause an increase in endogenous GnRH secretion, which stimulates pituitary gland secretion of LH and FSH and consequently induces follicle development and ovulation. In addition, dopamine agonists decrease the size of prolactin-secreting pituitary gland tumors.

With dopamine-agonist therapy, a near-maximal decrease in serum prolactin levels should be achieved after 4 weeks of treatment. Serum prolactin levels should be measured approximately 1 month after initiating therapy and about 1 month after a change in the dosage or drug. Normalization of prolactin levels is the therapeutic goal, as well as assuring that the tumor is responding to the dopamine agonists. If the serum prolactin concentration is normal and no side effects have occurred, the initial dosage should be continued. If the serum prolactin level has not decreased to normal and no side effects are present, the dosage should be gradually increased. The maximal dosage of bromocriptine is 5 mg twice daily; pergolide, 0.25 mg once daily. Cabergoline is the newest of these agents; it can be administered less frequently and may induce nausea less often. However, as a result of FDA approval, its use in pregnancy is extremely limited. Women who do not tolerate the side effects of bromocriptine may need to be referred to a practitioner with additional expertise in the field to discuss in detail the risks and benefits of newer therapies that have not been tested as thoroughly.

If the serum prolactin level does not decrease to normal, switching to a different dopamine agonist may be effective. If the patient cannot tolerate the dopamine agonist initially prescribed, a different dopamine agonist may be associated with fewer side effects. If the patient experiences side effects with all dopamine agonists, vaginal administration can be tried. If the patient cannot tolerate any of the dopamine agonists, transsphenoidal surgery may be effective in removing the tumor, returning prolactin secretion to normal, and causing the resumption of ovulatory menses.

Following correction of hyperprolactinemia, about 80% of women will ovulate, and cumulative pregnancy rates of 80% are commonly observed (24). Treatment usually is discontinued once pregnancy is diagnosed. However, in women with a macroprolactinoma, therapy should be continued throughout pregnancy to decrease the risk of tumor growth and neurosurgical complications, such as compression of the optic nerve.

In the small percentage of women with hyperprolactinemia who do not respond to dopamine-agonist therapy, standard ovulation induction therapy with clomiphene citrate may be considered. In rare cases, gonadotropin therapy may be considered.

Clinical Considerations and Recommendations

▶ *How is the diagnosis of ovulatory dysfunction established?*

If the patient is amenorrheic, the minimal laboratory evaluation should include measurement of serum levels of FSH, thyroid-stimulating hormone, and prolactin. If the patient has evidence of hyperandrogenism (eg, hirsutism, acne, signs of virilization), measurement of testosterone and DHEAS may have clinical value if ovulation induction is planned. Clinical evaluation may be used to determine if testing for Cushing's syndrome or Addison's disease should be performed. If the patient has a BMI higher than 30, testing for diabetes mellitus may be indicated before inducing ovulation (25). To decrease the risk of congenital malformations, diabetes mellitus should be treated before inducing pregnancy. In women with irregular menses, attempting to obtain a luteal-phase progesterone measurement may be cumbersome and unnecessary if menses are relatively infrequent. Documenting ovulation by basal body temperature evaluation or LH surge testing may be helpful. Women with regular menses can be assessed for ovulatory status by any of the techniques described previously.

Before using ovulation-inducing medications, it is useful to consider evaluating the couple for male factor infertility by performing a semen analysis. Routinely performing hysterosalpingography is unnecessary. However, if the woman has a history of sexually transmitted diseases, pelvic inflammatory disease, appendicitis with rupture, in utero exposure to diethylstilbestrol, or previous pelvic surgery, hysterosalpingography should be considered to establish tubal patency. Laparoscopy is not routinely necessary before ovulation induction. The age of the woman strongly influences the pregnancy rate with ovulation induction (see Fig. 1). In older women, this may lead to a greater sense of urgency and a rapid progression to more intensive treatments, with their greater associated risks (26, 27).

▶ *Does weight loss improve fertility in obese women?*

In women with a high BMI, abnormal hypothalamic GnRH secretion, pituitary gland LH and FSH secretion, insulin resistance, and anovulation are common (28). Women with a BMI greater than 30 and oligo-ovulation often have PCOS.

Epidemiologic studies have demonstrated that a BMI greater than 27 is associated with an increased risk of ovulatory infertility. For example, in one study of 597

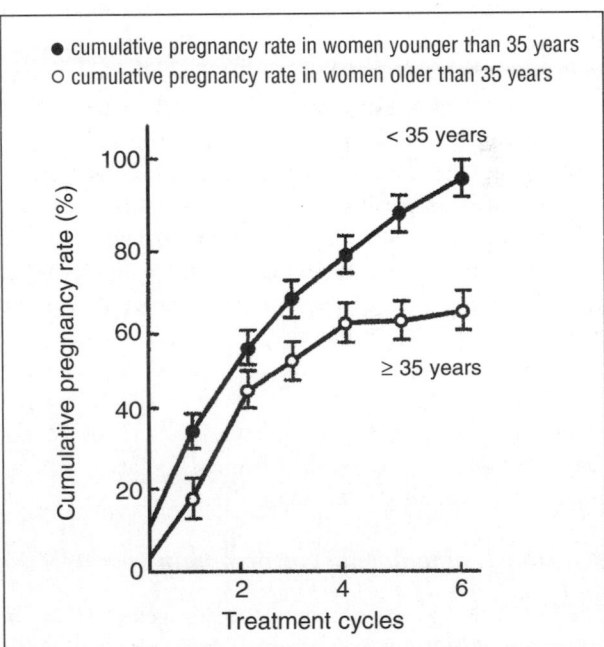

Figure 1. Cumulative pregnancy rates for hypogonadotropic anovulatory women treated with gonadotropins. (From Lunenfeld B, Insler V. Human gonadotropins. In: Wallach EE, Zacur HA, eds. Reproductive medicine and surgery. St. Louis: Mosby-Year Book, 1995:617)

women with ovulatory infertility and 1,695 controls, the women with a BMI higher than 27 had a relative risk of ovulatory infertility of 3.1 (95% confidence interval, 2.2–4.4) when compared with the control group with a BMI of 20–24.9 (29).

Many studies (most without a control group) have demonstrated that in women who have PCOS and are obese, weight loss often is associated with a decrease in serum testosterone concentration, resumption of ovulation, and, for infertile women, pregnancy. For example, in one study, 18 obese women with PCOS were treated with a hypocaloric diet (30). Before the diet, the mean weight of the women was 77 kg; after the diet, it was 57 kg. The plasma testosterone concentration was 0.75 ng/mL before the diet and 0.39 ng/mL after (P <0.001). Many of the women resumed ovulation after weight loss. Another study evaluated the effects of weight loss on 20 obese women with PCOS (31). Before the diet, the women had a mean BMI of 32, amenorrhea for more than 3 months, and increased plasma concentrations of androstenedione, testosterone, or DHEAS. Following a hypocaloric diet of 1,000–1,500 kcal per day, weight loss ranged from 4.8 kg to 15.2 kg. After weight loss, significant reductions in the concentration of LH (45% decrease), fasting insulin (40% decrease), and testosterone (35% decrease) were observed. After weight loss, most of the women ovulated, and many of the infertile women became pregnant.

In a small trial that examined the effect of weight loss on reproductive function in 12 obese women with PCOS, the women were randomized to either a weight reduction program or a "waiting list" observation control group (32). The six women randomized to the weight reduction program had a mean weight decrease of 16 kg, a significant decrease in circulating testosterone concentration, and a decrease in fasting insulin; four of the six women resumed ovulating. The women randomized to the observational control group had no weight change during the study. All of the women in the control group who were anovulatory before the study (five) remained anovulatory during the study.

Weight reduction is best achieved by a combination of diet and exercise. However, exercise at levels greater than 60 minutes per day has been associated with an increase in ovulatory infertility (33).

▶ *How is clomiphene citrate administered?*

The FDA has approved clomiphene dosages of 50 mg or 100 mg daily for a maximum of 5 days per cycle. After spontaneous menses or the induction of menses with a progestin withdrawal, clomiphene is started on cycle day 3, 4, or 5 at 50 mg daily for 5 days. Starting clomiphene on cycle day 3 or 5 does not appear to influence the preg-

nancy rate (34). It is important to give clomiphene only after menstrual bleeding to help ensure that the patient is not pregnant. In properly selected women, approximately 50% will ovulate using the 50-mg daily dosage, and another 25% will ovulate if the dosage is increased to 100 mg daily (35). If lower dosages are not successful in inducing ovulation, many clinicians will prescribe 150 mg daily for 5 days; a few have used dosages as high as 250 mg daily for 5 days. However, the pregnancy rates associated with the use of clomiphene at dosages higher than 150 mg daily for 5 days are very low (21). In general, if the 150-mg dosage is not successful, alternative approaches to ovulation induction should be considered. Of those women who ovulate while taking clomiphene, between 40% and 80% will become pregnant. In one study of 3,022 women taking clomiphene, the pregnancy rate per ovulatory cycle was 20% (36). The pregnancy rate decreases substantially after six cycles of clomiphene therapy (37).

Patients taking clomiphene should be monitored for ovulation, pregnancy, and ovarian enlargement, as clinically indicated. Ovulation can be determined by measuring serum progesterone levels (about 14 days after the last dose of clomiphene), basal body temperature charting, or properly timed endometrial biopsy. Detection of an LH surge in the urine suggests a preovulatory follicle has triggered the surge. Intense cycle monitoring with frequent measurement of serum estradiol levels and pelvic ultrasonography is generally not necessary with the use of clomiphene but is required for gonadotropin therapy. Clomiphene treatment can be associated with luteal phase defects and the suboptimal production of cervical mucus. Some clinicians recommend an endometrial biopsy in a test cycle of clomiphene treatment to assess whether clomiphene-induced ovulation is associated with luteal phase defect (38). A few authorities recommend a postcoital test be performed during the first clomiphene cycle to assess cervical mucus quality and quantity. However, little evidence exists to support either practice.

Of clomiphene-induced pregnancies, 7% are twin gestations and 0.3% are triplet gestations (39). The rate of spontaneous abortion after clomiphene-induced pregnancy is approximately 15%. The incidence of birth defects is similar to that seen in spontaneous pregnancy (40). The most common symptoms experienced by women taking clomiphene include vasomotor symptoms (20%), adnexal tenderness (5%), nausea (3%), headache (1%), and, rarely, blurring of vision or scotomata (21, 41). Many clinicians permanently discontinue clomiphene treatment in women with clomiphene-induced visual changes. The main contraindications to the use of clomiphene are pregnancy, hypersensitivity to the medication, and ovarian cysts.

▶ *In women who do not ovulate using clomi-*
phene alone, can the chances of ovulation be
improved by adding glucocorticoids?

Women with PCOS and a serum DHEAS concentration higher than the middle of the normal range (>2 µg/mL) appear to have decreased ovulation and pregnancy rates when they are treated with clomiphene. Some studies suggest treatment with clomiphene plus a glucocorticoid improves pregnancy rates in these women. One study randomized 64 anovulatory infertile women to receive either clomiphene, 50 mg daily on cycle days 5–9, or clomiphene plus 0.5 mg dexamethasone daily (42). If ovulation did not occur, the dosage of clomiphene was increased by 50-mg increments up to 150 mg daily for 5 days each cycle. The investigators observed significantly higher rates of ovulation and conception in women treated with clomiphene plus dexamethasone than with clomiphene alone. The impact of combined therapy was especially marked in the women with a DHEAS concentration higher than 2 µg/mL. Of the women with a DHEAS concentration higher than 2 µg/mL, 12 were randomized to receive clomiphene alone, and 13 were randomized to receive clomiphene plus dexamethasone. Among the 12 women receiving clomiphene alone, six (50%) ovulated and four (33%) became pregnant. Among the 13 women who received clomiphene plus dexamethasone, 13 (100%) ovulated and 11 (85%) became pregnant.

▶ *In women who do not ovulate using clomi-*
phene alone, can the chances of ovulation be
improved by adding an hCG injection?

The combination of clomiphene plus a single dose of hCG may increase the efficacy of clomiphene induction of ovulation when women fail to ovulate with standard dosages of clomiphene (43). After the last dose of clomiphene, pelvic ultrasonography can be used to monitor follicle size. When the mean diameter of the lead follicle reaches 18 mm, a single dose of hCG can be administered. Ovulation occurs approximately 36–44 hours after the injection. There are no randomized controlled clinical trials that document the efficacy of this approach.

It has been proposed that a regimen of 2 months of oral contraceptives before ovulation induction with clomiphene followed by an hCG injection when follicle ripening has occurred may improve the rate of ovulation and pregnancy. No randomized clinical trial supports this approach. However, a clinical trial without controls reported oral contraceptive treatment followed by clomiphene therapy (100 mg daily for 5 days) plus an

hCG injection was an inexpensive and potentially effective approach to treating women with PCOS who had failed to ovulate and become pregnant with standard clomiphene therapy (44). In that study, 38 infertile women with PCOS who had failed to ovulate when treated with clomiphene (150 mg daily for 5 days) and who had a DHEAS concentration lower than 2 µg/mL took oral contraceptives (ethinyl estradiol 0.03 mg, and desogestrel 0.15 mg daily) for 2 months followed by clomiphene. Instead of the usual 7-day pill-free interval between cycles, the investigators prescribed a regimen with a 3-day pill-free interval. On cycle days 5–9 after completion of the second month of oral contraceptives, clomiphene (100 mg daily for 5 days) was prescribed. Transvaginal ultrasonography was initiated on cycle day 12 and repeated every 1–2 days until hCG was administered. When the mean diameter of the lead follicle reached 20 mm, hCG (10,000 units) was administered. The 38 women completed 95 treatment cycles. Sixty-nine of the 95 cycles were ovulatory (73%), and 29 of the 38 women (76%) ovulated. Twenty-two pregnancies occurred. Most of the pregnancies (82%) occurred in one of the first three treatment cycles.

▶ *In women who do not respond to clomi-*
phene, does ovarian diathermy increase the
chances of ovulation more than FSH?

A number of surgical techniques have been described that may increase the rate of ovulation in women with PCOS. To date, no randomized, controlled clinical trial has demonstrated the efficacy of surgery in this setting, but case series totaling more than 1,000 subjects have been published. Although ovarian wedge resection was the initial surgical procedure reported to increase ovulation in women with PCOS, this procedure has been replaced by laparoscopic techniques that use electrosurgical or laser energy. Overall, the case series report ovulation rates of 80% and pregnancy rates of 50% (45). For women with PCOS, ovulation induction with FSH also is associated with pregnancy rates of 50% (46). Injections with FSH for ovulation induction are associated with a high rate of multiple gestations (approximately 20%), and it is not known if ovarian diathermy affects ovarian reserve. Thus, treatment should be individualized.

▶ *In women with hyperprolactinemia, which*
medical treatments stimulate the resumption
of ovulation?

Bromocriptine has been used for more than 25 years to induce ovulation in women with hyperprolactinemia. In one study of 280 women with hyperprolactinemia, bromocriptine normalized the circulating prolactin level in 82% of the women (47). The main side effects associated with bromocriptine are nausea, vomiting, and orthostatic hypotension. To minimize these potential side effects, it is recommended that bromocriptine be initiated at a dosage of 1.25 mg at bedtime. After 1 week, the dosage can be increased to 1.25 mg twice daily. The dosage can then be increased to 2.5 mg twice daily, a standard dosage that successfully decreases serum prolactin levels in most women with hyperprolactinemia (47).

Pergolide, an ergot dopamine agonist, is approved by the FDA for the treatment of Parkinson's disease but is not approved for the treatment of hyperprolactinemia. Unlike bromocriptine, pergolide can be given once per day. Pergolide is the least expensive of the dopamine agonists.

▶ In women with PCOS, what is the role of gonadotropins in inducing ovulation?

In one randomized clinical trial, low-dose FSH treatment appeared to improve outcomes and decrease adverse events when compared with standard-dose FSH treatment in women with PCOS (48). In this study, 50 infertile women with PCOS who had failed to conceive with clomiphene therapy were randomized to receive either conventional FSH treatment (75 IU daily, increasing by 75 IU every 5–6 days until follicular ripening occurred) or low-dose FSH treatment (75 IU daily for 14 days of treatment, increasing by 37.5 IU every 7 days thereafter until follicular ripening was complete). Compared with standard FSH treatment, women who received long-term, low-dose FSH treatment had more cycles with the development of a single dominant follicle (74% versus 27%), fewer high-order multiple gestations, and a higher pregnancy rate (40% versus 24%).

▶ When should metformin be added for the treatment of ovulatory infertility?

Insulin sensitizers can be used alone or in combination with clomiphene to induce ovulation in infertile women with oligo-ovulation, hyperandrogenism, and insulin resistance (49). To date, no large-scale clinical trials have been published that demonstrate the impact of metformin on live birth rates in women with PCOS and insulin resistance. A few small clinical trials have been published demonstrating that in women with PCOS the combination of clomiphene plus metformin is associated with higher rates of ovulation and pregnancy than clomiphene plus a placebo (50, 51). In one study, women with PCOS who did not ovulate when treated with clomiphene (150 mg daily for 5 days) were randomized

to receive either metformin (1,500 mg daily) or placebo for 7 weeks (51). During the initial 7-week treatment period, one of the 12 women in the metformin group ovulated, and none of the 15 women in the placebo group ovulated. After this initial treatment period, all of the women received clomiphene citrate, beginning at a dosage of 50 mg daily for 5 days, with dosage escalation if ovulation did not occur. Nine of the 12 women in the metformin-plus-clomiphene group ovulated, compared with four of the 15 women in the placebo-plus-clomiphene group (P <0.02). Of the women who completed the clinical trial, six (of 11) in the metformin-plus-clomiphene group became pregnant, and one (of 14) in the placebo-plus-clomiphene group became pregnant (P <0.02). Of the six pregnancies in the metformin-plus-clomiphene group, two resulted in spontaneous abortion and four resulted in live singleton births. The one pregnancy in the placebo-plus-clomiphene group resulted in a live singleton birth.

A commonly used dosage of metformin is 500 mg three times daily. The most common side effects of metformin are gastrointestinal disturbances, including diarrhea, nausea, vomiting, and abdominal bloating. To minimize gastrointestinal side effects, many clinicians recommend starting metformin at 500 mg daily for 1 week, increasing to 500 mg twice daily for 1 week, and then increasing to 500 mg three times daily. Once the full dosage is achieved, some clinicians switch to a dosing regimen of 850 mg twice daily to improve patient compliance. Progesterone measurements can be periodically obtained to determine whether ovulation has occurred, or the patient can keep a basal body temperature chart. If ovulation has not occurred after 4–8 weeks of metformin therapy, clomiphene (50 mg daily for 5 days) can be administered after progestin-induced menstrual withdrawal bleeding. If the patient becomes pregnant, the metformin therapy can be discontinued. Ovulation, if it is going to occur, can be expected to occur within 6–8 weeks.

In rare cases, metformin therapy has caused fatal lactic acidosis. In most of these cases, renal insufficiency or severe hypoxia (congestive heart failure, septic shock) was present. Before treatment with metformin is initiated, it is recommended that serum creatinine levels be demonstrated to be lower than 1.4 mg/dL. Women with liver dysfunction should not take metformin. Also, metformin should be discontinued 48 hours before—and not restarted for 72 hours after—any radiologic test involving intravenous contrast or before surgery.

Metformin appears to improve the ovulatory response in women with PCOS treated with FSH injections. A trial randomized 20 infertile women with PCOS and insulin resistance who had failed to ovulate when treated with clomiphene (150 mg daily for 5 days) to receive either FSH injections alone or FSH injections plus metformin (500 mg three times daily) (52). The mean BMI of the subjects was approximately 27. Compared with the women who received FSH alone, the women who received both FSH and metformin had fewer dominant follicles (2.4 versus 4.5, P <0.01), a lower peak estradiol concentration (450 pg/mL versus 720 pg/mL, P <0.001), and a lower cycle cancellation rate (0% versus 32%, P < 0.03). The investigators concluded a combination of FSH plus metformin is associated with an orderly follicular response that probably decreases the risk for ovarian hyperstimulation and multiple pregnancy.

▶ *Is a postcoital test useful in a patient taking clomiphene citrate?*

The postcoital test has low reproducibility and low interobserver reliability and has not been proved to help guide treatment recommendations (53–55). In addition, there is little consensus on what constitutes an abnormal postcoital test result. Given these limitations, there is little scientific rationale for performing a postcoital test. However, clinical experience suggests that clomiphene, acting as an antiestrogen in the cervix, can cause cervical mucus production that is abnormal in quantity and quality. Therefore, some clinicians recommend performing a postcoital test to assess the impact of clomiphene on cervical mucus production.

▶ *Can the risk of multiple gestation be minimized?*

Multiple gestation is a growing problem. Public awareness is increasing about the hazards associated with multiple births, as well as the long-term costs and consequences (56). Monofolliculogenesis is the goal of therapy in infertile patients.

To decrease the risk of multiple gestation, treatments associated with low rates of multiple gestation should be used. For example, in women with PCOS, ovulation induction with weight loss, clomiphene, clomiphene plus metformin, clomiphene plus glucocorticoid, and ovarian surgery are associated with low rates of triplet pregnancy. Gonadotropin injections and in vitro fertilization are associated with higher rates of multiple gestation (48). When using gonadotropin injections, the use of low-dose regimens appears to be associated with lower rates of multiple gestation than the use of standard dose regimens. In addition, the risk of multiple gestation with FSH injections can probably be decreased by withholding hCG and prescribing a barrier contraceptive whenever more than three follicles greater than 15 mm in diameter are detected with pelvic ultrasonography.

▶ *Is the risk of ovarian cancer increased with the use of induction agents, such as clomiphene or gonadotropin injections?*

The risk of ovarian cancer is increased in women who are nulligravid (voluntarily and involuntarily) and women with a strong family history of ovarian cancer. The risk of ovarian cancer is decreased by pregnancy, use of oral contraceptives for more than 6 months, surgical tubal ligation, and hysterectomy. Preliminary studies reported ovulation-inducing medications may be associated with a small increase in the risk of ovarian tumors (borderline tumors and cancer) and that the risk may increase with the extended use of ovulation-inducing agents for many months (57, 58). In one of these studies, the strongest risk occurred among 13 nulligravid women who had used infertility drugs and had never become pregnant. In this subset, the association was statistically significant, but the confidence interval was wide, suggesting a great deal of variation, and the sample size was small (n=13). Some practitioners believe infertility (involuntary childlessness) is a more powerful risk factor for ovarian tumors than treatment with an ovulation-inducing medication. However, given the low pregnancy rates observed after six cycles of ovulation induction with an induction agent (such as clomiphene) and the potential (although low) risk that 12 or more cycles of clomiphene may be associated with an increased risk of ovarian tumors, it is reasonable to limit clomiphene treatment to fewer than 12 cycles. There are no evidence-based guidelines about the appropriate duration of gonadotropin administration; however, given the possibility that such agents can cause harm, it seems appropriate to use them sparingly and only with clear-cut indications.

Summary of Recommendations

The following recommendations are based on limited or inconsistent scientific evidence (Level B):

▶ In obese women with PCOS, weight loss should be considered because it is associated with a decrease in circulating testosterone concentration, an increase in the frequency of ovulation, and in some women, pregnancy.

▶ In obese women with PCOS who did not ovulate when treated with clomiphene, the combination of clomiphene plus metformin may be considered because the rate of ovulation is greater than it is with clomiphene alone.

▶ In women with PCOS and a serum DHEAS level higher than 2 μg/mL, the combination of clomiphene plus glucocorticoid may be considered because the rate of ovulation is greater than it is with clomiphene alone.

▶ In women with hypothalamic amenorrhea and a BMI lower than 20, weight gain should be considered because it may be associated with the resumption of ovulation and pregnancy.

▶ In women with PCOS receiving gonadotropin injections for ovulation induction, low-dose FSH may be considered because it is associated with a higher rate of cycles with the development of a single dominant follicle and fewer high-order multiple gestations.

References

1. Collins JA. Unexplained infertility. In: Keye WR, Chang RJ, Rebar RW, Soules MR, eds. Infertility: evaluation and treatment. Philadelphia: WB Saunders, 1995:249–262 (Level III)

2. Hull MG, Glazener CM, Kelly NJ, Conway DI, Foster PA, Hinton RA, et al. Population study of causes, treatment, and outcome of infertility. Br Med J (Clin Res Ed) 1985;291:1693–1697 (Level II-3)

3. Knochenhauer ES, Key TJ, Kashar-Miller M, Waggoner W, Boots LR, Azziz R. Prevalence of the polycystic ovary syndrome in unselected black and white women of the southeastern United States: a prospective study. J Clin Endocrinol Metab 1998;83:3078–3082 (Level II-3)

4. Reindollar RH, Novak M, Tho SP, McDonough PG. Adult-onset amenorrhea: a study of 262 patients. Am J Obstet Gynecol 1986;155:531–543 (Level III)

5. Bates GW, Bates SR, Whitworth NS. Reproductive failure in women who practice weight control. Fertil Steril 1982;37:373–378 (Level II-3)

6. Santoro N. Efficacy and safety of intravenous pulsatile gonadotropin-releasing hormone: Lutrepulse for injection. Am J Obstet Gynecol 1990;163:1759–1764 (Level III)

7. Martin KA, Hall JE, Adams JM, Crowley WF Jr. Comparison of exogenous gonadotropins and pulsatile gonadotropin-releasing hormone for induction of ovulation in hypogonadotropic amenorrhea. J Clin Endocrinol Metab 1993;77:125–129 (Level II-3)

8. Reichlin S. Neuroendocrinology. In: Wilson JD, Foster DW, Kronenberg HM, Larsen PR, eds. Williams textbook of endocrinology. Philadelphia: WB Saunders, 1998: 165– 248 (Level III)

9. Grubb MR, Chakeres D, Malarkey WB. Patients with primary hypothyroidism presenting as prolactinomas. Am J Med 1987;83:765–769 (Level III)

10. Gsponer J, De Tribolet N, Deruaz JP, Janzer R, Uske A, Mirimanoff RO, et al. Diagnosis, treatment, and outcome of pituitary tumors and other abnormal intrasellar masses. Retrospective analysis of 353 patients. Medicine (Baltimore) 1999;78:236–269 (Level II-2)

11. Gemzell C, Wang CF. Outcome of pregnancy in women with pituitary adenoma. Fertil Steril 1979;31:363–372 (Level III)

12. Lamberts SW, Klijn JG, de Lange SA, Singh R, Stefanko SZ, Birkenhager JC. The incidence of complications during pregnancy after treatment of hyperprolactinemia with bromocriptine in patients with radiologically evident pituitary tumors. Fertil Steril 1979;31:614–619 (Level III)

13. Griffith RW, Turkalj I, Braun P. Pituitary tumors during pregnancy in mothers treated with bromocriptine. Br J Clin Pharmacol 1979;7:393–396 (Level III)

14. Sisam DA, Sheehan JP, Sheeler LR. The natural history of untreated microprolactinomas. Fertil Steril 1987;48: 67–71 (Level II-3)

15. Schlechte J, Dolan K, Sherman B, Chapler F, Luciano A. The natural history of untreated hyperprolactinemia: a prospective analysis. J Clin Endocrinol Metab 1989;68: 412–418 (Level III)

16. Scott RT Jr, Hofmann GE. Prognostic assessment of ovarian reserve. Fertil Steril 1995;63:1–11 (Level III)

17. van Kasteren YM, Hoek A, Schoemaker J. Ovulation induction in premature ovarian failure: a placebo-controlled randomized trial combining pituitary suppression with gonadotropin stimulation. Fertil Steril 1995;64: 273–278 (Level II-1)

18. Davis OK, Berkeley AS, Naus GJ, Cholst IN, Freedman KS. The incidence of luteal phase defect in normal, fertile women, determined by serial endometrial biopsy. Fertil Steril 1989;51:582–586 (Level III)

19. Hull MG, Knuth UA, Murray MA, Jacobs HS. The practical value of the progestogen challenge test, serum oestradiol estimation or clinical examination in assessment of the oestrogen state and response to clomiphene in amenorrhea. Br J Obstet Gynaecol 1979;86:799–805 (Level II-3)

20. Murakawa H, Hasegawa I, Kurabayashi T, Tanaka K. Polycystic ovary syndrome. Insulin resistance and ovulatory responses to clomiphene citrate. J Reprod Med 1999;44:23–27 (Level II-2)

21. Derman SG, Adashi EY. Induction of ovulation. Compr Ther 1995;21:583–589 (Level III)

22. Sills ES, Levy DP, Moomjy M, McGee M, Rosenwaks Z. A prospective, randomized comparison of ovulation induction using highly purified follicle-stimulating hormone alone and with recombinant human luteinizing hormone in in-vitro fertilization. Hum Reprod 1999;14: 2230–2235 (Level I)

23. Verhelst J, Abs R, Maiter D, van den Bruel A, vandeweghe M, Velkeniers B. Cabergoline in the treatment of hyperprolactinemia: a study in 455 patients. J Clin Endocrinol Metab 1999;84:2518–2522 (Level II-3)

24. Weil C. The safety of bromocriptine in hyperprolactinaemic female infertility: a literature review. Curr Med Res Opin 1986;10:172–195 (Level III)

25. Legro RS, Kunselman AR, Dodson WC, Dunaif A. Prevalence and predictors of risk for type 2 diabetes mellitus and impaired glucose tolerance in polycystic ovary syndrome: a prospective, controlled study in 254 affected women. J Clin Endocrinol Metab 1999;84:165–169 (Level II-2)

26. Gleicher N, Campbell DP, Chan CL, Karande V, Rao R, Balin M, et al. The desire for multiple births in couples with infertility problems contradicts present practice patterns. Hum Reprod 1995;10:1079–1085 (Level III)

27. Paulson RJ, Ory SJ, Giudice LC, Schlaff WD, Santoro NF, Coddington C 3rd. Multiple pregnancies: what action should we take? [comment] Fertil Steril 2001;75:14–15; discussion 16–17 (Level III)

28. Yen SS. Chronic anovulation due to CNS-hypothalamic-pituitary dysfunction. In: Yen SS, Jaffe RB, Barbieri RL, eds. Reproductive endocrinology: physiology, pathophysiology, and clinical management. 4th ed. Philadelphia: WB Saunders, 1999:516–561 (Level III)

29. Grodstein F, Goldman MB, Cramer DW. Body mass index and ovulatory infertility. Epidemiology 1994;5:247–250 (Level II-2)

30. Bates GW, Whitworth NS. Effect of body weight reduction on plasma androgens in obese, infertile women. Fertil Steril 1982;38:406–409 (Level II-2)

31. Pasquali R, Antenucci D, Casimirri F, Venturoli S, Paradisi R, Fabbri R, et al. Clinical and hormonal characteristics of obese amenorrheic hyperandrogenic women before and after weight loss. J Clin Endocrinol Metab 1989;68:173–179 (Level III)

32. Guzick DS, Wing R, Smith D, Berga SL, Winters SJ. Endocrine consequences of weight loss in obese, hyperandrogenic, anovulatory women. Fertil Steril 1994;61:598–604 (Level II-2)

33. Green BB, Daling JR, Weiss NS, Liff JM, Koepsell T. Exercise as a risk factor for infertility with ovulatory dysfunction. Am J Public Health 1986;76:1432–1436 (Level II-2)

34. Wu CH, Winkel CA. The effect of therapy initiation day on clomiphene citrate therapy. Fertil Steril 1989;52:564–568 (Level II-3)

35. Gysler M, March CM, Mishell DR Jr, Bailey EJ. A decade's experience with an individualized clomiphene treatment regimen including its effect on the postcoital test. Fertil Steril 1982;37:161–167 (Level II-3)

36. Macgregor AH, Johnson JE, Bunde CA. Further clinical experience with clomiphene citrate. Fertil Steril 1968;19:616–622 (Level II-3)

37. Hammond MG. Monitoring techniques for improved pregnancy rates during clomiphene ovulation induction. Fertil Steril 1984;42:499–509 (Level III)

38. Keenan JA, Herbert CM, Bush JR, Wentz AC. Diagnosis and management of out-of-phase endometrial biopsies among patients receiving clomiphene citrate for ovulation induction. Fertil Steril 1989;51:964–967 (Level II-2)

39. Dickey RP, Holtkamp DE. Development, pharmacology and clinical experience with clomiphene citrate. Hum Reprod Update 1996;2:483–506 (Level III)

40. Kurachi K, Aono T, Minagawa J, Miyuake A. Congenital malformations of newborn infants after clomiphene induced ovulation. Fertil Steril 1983;40:187–189 (Level II-2)

41. Clomid. In: Physicians' desk reference. 55th ed. Montvale, New Jersey: Medical Economics Company, 2001:700–702 (Level III)

42. Daly DC, Walters CA, Soto-Albors CE, Tohan N, Riddick DH. A randomized study of dexamethasone in ovulation induction with clomiphene citrate. Fertil Steril 1984;41:844–848 (Level I)

43. Swyer GI, Radwanska E, Mcgarrigle HH. Plasma oestradiol and progesterone estimation for the monitoring of induction of ovulation with clomiphene and chorionic gonadotrophin. Br J Obstet Gynaecol 1975;82:794–804 (Level II-2)

44. Branigan EF, Estes MA. Treatment of chronic anovulation resistant to clomiphene citrate (CC) by using oral contraceptive ovarian suppression followed by repeat CC treatment. Fertil Steril 1999;71:544–546 (Level III)

45. Donesky BW, Adashi EY. Surgically induced ovulation in the polycystic ovary syndrome: wedge resection revisted in the age of laparoscopy. Fertil Steril 1995;63:439–463 (Level III)

46. Lunenfeld B, Insler V. Human gonadotropins. In: Wallach EE, Zacur HA, eds. Reproductive medicine and surgery. St. Louis: Mosby-Year Book, 1995:611–638 (Level III)

47. Vance ML, Evans WS, Thorner MO. Drugs five years later. Bromocriptine. Ann Intern Med 1984;100:78–91 (Level III)

48. Homburg R, Levy T, Ben-Rafael Z. A comparative study of conventional regimen with chronic low-dose administration of follicle-stimulating hormone for anovulation associated with polycystic ovary syndrome. Fertil Steril 1995;63:729–733 (Level II-2)

49. Barbieri RL. Induction of ovulation in infertile women with hyperandrogenism and insulin resistance. Am J Obstet Gynecol 2000;183:1412–1418 (Level III)

50. Nestler JE, Jakubowicz DJ, Evans WS, Pasquali R. Effects of metformin on spontaneous and clomiphene-induced ovulation in the polycystic ovary syndrome. N Engl J Med 1998;38:1876–1880 (Level II-2)

51. Vandermolen DT, Ratts VS, Evans WS, Stovall DW, Kauma SW, Nestler JE. Metformin increases the ovulatory rate and pregnancy rate from clomiphene citrate in patients with polycystic ovary syndrome who are resistant to clomiphene citrate alone. Fertil Steril 2001;75:310–315 (Level I)

52. De Leo V, la Marca A, Ditto A, Morgante G, Cianci A. Effects of metformin on gonadotropin-induced ovulation in women with polycystic ovary syndrome. Fertil Steril 1999;72:282–285 (Level I)

53. Glatstein IZ, Best CL, Palumbo A, Sleeper LA, Friedman AJ, Hornstein MD. The reproducibility of the postcoital test: a prospective study. Obstet Gynecol 1995;85:396–400 (Level III)

54. Griffith CS, Grimes DA. The validity of the postcoital test. Am J Obstet Gynecol 1990;162:615–620 (Level III)

55. Oei SG, Helmerhorst FM, Bloemenkamp KW, Hollants FA, Meerpoel DE, Keirse MJ. Effectiveness of the post-coital test: randomised controlled trial. BMJ 1998;317: 502–505 (Level I)

56. Callahan TL, Hall JE, Ettner SL, Christiansen CL, Green MF, Crowley WF Jr. The economic impact of multiple-gestation pregnancies and the contribution of assisted-reproduction techniques to their incidence. N Engl J Med 1994;331:244–249 (Level III)

57. Rossing MA, Daling JR, Weiss NS, Moore DE, Self SG. Ovarian tumors in a cohort of infertile women. N Engl J Med 1994;331:771–776 (Level II-2)

58. Whittemore AS, Harris R, Itnyre J. Characteristics relating to ovarian cancer risk: collaborative analysis of 12 US case-control studies. II. Invasive epithelial ovarian cancers in white women. Collaborative Ovarian Cancer Group. Am J Epidemiol 1992;136:1184–1203 (Level II-2)

The MEDLINE database, the Cochrane Library, and ACOG's own internal resources and documents were used to conduct a literature search to locate relevant articles published between January 1985 and June 2001. The search was restricted to articles published in the English language. Priority was given to articles reporting results of original research, although review articles and commentaries also were consulted. Abstracts of research presented at symposia and scientific conferences were not considered adequate for inclusion in this document. Guidelines published by organizations or institutions such as the National Institutes of Health and the American College of Obstetricians and Gynecologists were reviewed, and additional studies were located by reviewing bibliographies of identified articles. When reliable research was not available, expert opinions from obstetrician–gynecologists were used.

Studies were reviewed and evaluated for quality according to the method outlined by the U.S. Preventive Services Task Force:

I   Evidence obtained from at least one properly designed randomized controlled trial.

II-1 Evidence obtained from well-designed controlled trials without randomization.

II-2 Evidence obtained from well-designed cohort or case–control analytic studies, preferably from more than one center or research group.

II-3 Evidence obtained from multiple time series with or without the intervention. Dramatic results in uncontrolled experiments could also be regarded as this type of evidence.

III   Opinions of respected authorities, based on clinical experience, descriptive studies, or reports of expert committees.

Based on the highest level of evidence found in the data, recommendations are provided and graded according to the following categories:

Level A—Recommendations are based on good and consistent scientific evidence.

Level B—Recommendations are based on limited or inconsistent scientific evidence.

Level C—Recommendations are based primarily on consensus and expert opinion.

ISSN 1099-3630

The American College of Obstetricians and Gynecologists
409 12th Street, SW, PO Box 96920
Washington, DC 20090-6920

12345/65432

Management of infertility caused by ovulatory dysfunction. ACOG Practice Bulletin No. 34. American College of Obstetricians and Gynecologists. Obstet Gynecol 2002;99:347–358

ACOG PRACTICE BULLETIN

CLINICAL MANAGEMENT GUIDELINES FOR
OBSTETRICIAN–GYNECOLOGISTS

NUMBER 55, SEPTEMBER 2004

(Replaces Practice Pattern Number 6, October 1997)

This Practice Bulletin was developed by the ACOG Committee on Practice Bulletins—Obstetrics with the assistance of Errol R. Norwitz, MD, PhD and Julian N. Robinson, MD. The information is designed to aid practitioners in making decisions about appropriate obstetric and gynecologic care. These guidelines should not be construed as dictating an exclusive course of treatment or procedure. Variations in practice may be warranted based on the needs of the individual patient, resources, and limitations unique to the institution or type of practice.

Management of Postterm Pregnancy

Postterm pregnancy, by definition, refers to a pregnancy that has extended to or beyond 42 weeks of gestation (294 days, or estimated date of delivery [EDD] +14 days). Accurate pregnancy dating is critical to the diagnosis. The term "postdates" is poorly defined and should be avoided. Although some cases of postterm pregnancy likely result from an inability to accurately define the EDD, many cases result from a true prolongation of gestation. The reported frequency of postterm pregnancy is approximately 7% (1).

Accurate assessment of gestational age and diagnosis of postterm gestation, as well as recognition and management of risk factors, may reduce the risk of adverse sequelae. Antenatal surveillance and induction of labor are 2 widely used strategies that theoretically may decrease the risk of an adverse fetal outcome; maternal risk factors for postterm pregnancy also should be considered. The purpose of this document is to examine the evidence and provide recommendations about these 2 management strategies.

Background

Etiologic Factors

The most frequent cause of an apparently prolonged gestation is an error in dating (2, 3). When postterm pregnancy truly exists, the cause usually is unknown. Primiparity and prior postterm pregnancy are the most common identifiable risk factors for prolongation of pregnancy (4, 5). Rarely, postterm pregnancy may be associated with placental sulfatase deficiency or fetal anencephaly. Male sex also has been associated with prolongation of pregnancy (6). Genetic predisposition may play a role in prolonging pregnancy (5, 7).

Assessment of Gestational Age

Accurate pregnancy dating is important for minimizing the false diagnosis of postterm pregnancy. The EDD is most reliably and accurately determined early in pregnancy. It may be determined on the basis of the known last menstrual period in women with regular, normal menstrual cycles.

Inconsistencies or concern about the accuracy of the estimated gestational age requires further assessment with ultrasonography. Useful measurements include the crown–rump length of the fetus during the first trimester and the biparietal diameter or head circumference and femur length during the second trimester. Because of the normal variations in size of infants in the third trimester, dating the pregnancy at that time is less reliable (±21 days). Although recent data have highlighted the accuracy of first trimester ultrasonography, the variation by ultrasonography generally is ±7 days up to 20 weeks of gestation, ±14 days between 20 and 30 weeks of gestation, and ±21 days beyond 30 weeks of gestation. If the estimated gestational age by a patient's last menstrual period differs from the ultrasound estimate by more than these accepted variations, the ultrasound estimate of gestational age should be used instead of the patient's menstrual cycle estimate.

Risks to the Fetus

Postterm pregnancy is associated with significant risks to the fetus. The perinatal mortality rate (stillbirths plus early neonatal deaths) at greater than 42 weeks of gestation is twice that at term (4–7 deaths versus 2–3 deaths per 1,000 deliveries) and increases 6-fold and higher at 43 weeks of gestation and beyond (8–10). Uteroplacental insufficiency, meconium aspiration, and intrauterine infection contribute to the increased rate of perinatal deaths (11). Postterm pregnancy also is an independent risk factor for low umbilical artery pH levels at delivery and low 5-minute Apgar scores (12). For these reasons, the trend has been toward delivery by 41 completed weeks of gestation (42 weeks, 294 days, EDD +14 days).

Although postterm infants are larger than term infants and have a higher incidence of fetal macrosomia (2.5–10% versus 0.8–1%) (13, 14), no evidence supports inducing labor as a preventive measure in such cases. Complications associated with fetal macrosomia include prolonged labor, cephalopelvic disproportion, and shoulder dystocia with resultant risks of orthopedic or neurologic injury.

Approximately 20% of postterm fetuses have dysmaturity syndrome, which refers to infants with characteristics resembling chronic intrauterine growth restriction from uteroplacental insufficiency (15, 16). These pregnancies are at increased risk of umbilical cord compression from oligohydramnios, meconium aspiration, and short-term neonatal complications (such as hypoglycemia, seizures, and respiratory insufficiency) and have an increased incidence of nonreassuring fetal testing, both antepartum and intrapartum (17). Whether such infants also are at risk of long-term neurologic sequelae is not clear. In a large, prospective, follow-up study of children at ages 1 and 2 years, the general intelligence quotient, physical milestones, and frequency of intercurrent illnesses were not significantly different between normal infants born at term and those born postterm (18).

Fetuses born postterm also are at increased risk of death within the first year of life (10, 19, 20). Although some of these infant deaths clearly result from peripartum complications (such as meconium aspiration syndrome), most have no known cause.

Risks to the Pregnant Woman

Postterm pregnancy also is associated with significant risks to the pregnant woman, including an increase in labor dystocia (9–12% versus 2–7% at term), an increase in severe perineal injury related to macrosomia (3.3% versus 2.6% at term), and a doubling in the rate of cesarean delivery (21–23). Cesarean delivery is associated with higher risks of complications, such as endometritis, hemorrhage, and thromboembolic disease. Finally, postterm pregnancy can be a source of substantial anxiety for the pregnant woman.

Clinical Considerations and Recommendations

▶ *Are there interventions that decrease the rate of postterm pregnancy?*

Accurate dating on the basis of ultrasonography performed early in pregnancy can reduce the incidence of pregnancies diagnosed as postterm (odds ratio [OR], 0.68; 95% confidence interval [CI], 0.57–0.82) (2) and thereby minimize unnecessary intervention (3, 24). However, routine early ultrasonography has not been recommended as a standard of prenatal care in the United States. Breast and nipple stimulation at term have not been shown to affect the incidence of postterm pregnancy (2). The data regarding sweeping of the membranes at term to reduce postterm pregnancy are conflicting: some studies show a benefit (25, 26), whereas others have found no difference in the incidence of postterm pregnancy (27).

▶ *When should antepartum fetal testing begin?*

Because of ethical and medicolegal considerations, no studies have included postterm patients who were not monitored; it is unlikely that any future studies will include an unmonitored control group. The published studies are of insufficient power to demonstrate a benefit of monitoring. However, there is no evidence that antenatal fetal monitoring adversely affects patients experiencing postterm pregnancy. Data suggest a gradual increase in perinatal morbidity and mortality during this period (Fig. 1) (10). Therefore, despite evidence that it does not decrease perinatal mortality, antenatal fetal surveillance for postterm pregnancies has become a common practice on the basis of universal acceptance.

Patients who have passed their EDD but who have not yet reached 42 weeks of gestation constitute another group for whom antenatal fetal surveillance has been proposed. Some studies report a greater complication rate among women giving birth during the latter half of this 2-week period (21–23, 28, 29). However, no randomized controlled trial has demonstrated an improvement in perinatal outcome attributable to fetal surveillance between 40 and 42 weeks of gestation (30). Despite the lack of evidence demonstrating a beneficial effect, antenatal fetal surveillance often is performed during this period. To further complicate matters, in most studies of postterm pregnancies, women are recruited and fetal monitoring initiated before 42 weeks of gestation

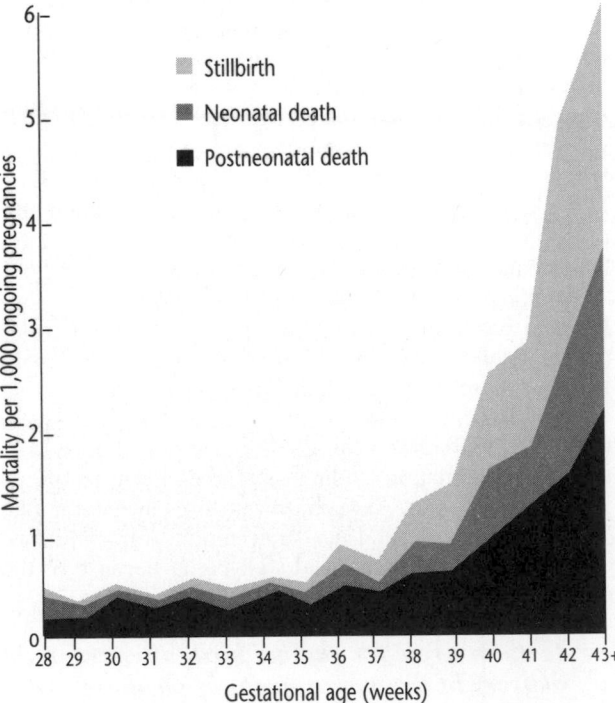

Figure 1. Perinatal mortality per 1,000 ongoing pregnancies. (Reproduced from BJOG Volume 105, Hilder L, Costeloe K, Thilaganathan B, Prolonged pregnancy: evaluating gestation-specific risks of fetal and infant mortality, 169–73, 1998, with the permission of the Royal College of Obstetricians and Gynaecologists.)

(31–36). Finally, there is insufficient evidence to indicate whether routine antenatal surveillance of low-risk patients between 40 and 42 weeks of gestation improves perinatal outcome (2, 28).

▶ *What form of antenatal surveillance should be performed, and how frequently should a postterm patient be reevaluated?*

The literature is inconsistent regarding both the type and frequency of antenatal surveillance among postterm patients (2, 31–42). Options for evaluating fetal well-being include nonstress testing, biophysical profile (BPP) or modified BPP (nonstress test plus amniotic fluid volume estimation), contraction stress testing, and a combination of these modalities, but practices vary widely. No single method has been shown to be superior (2). Assessment of amniotic fluid volume appears to be important. Delivery should be effected if there is evidence of fetal compromise or oligohydramnios (43, 44). Adverse pregnancy outcome (nonreassuring fetal heart rate tracing, neonatal intensive care unit admission, low Apgar score) is more common when oligohydramnios is present (45–47). However, a consistent definition of low amniotic fluid volume in the postterm pregnancy has not been established. Options include 1) no vertical fluid pocket that is measurable and more than 2–3 cm in depth or 2) amniotic fluid index less than 5 (43, 48). Of note, Doppler velocimetry has no proven benefit in monitoring the postterm fetus and is not recommended for this indication (49, 50). Although no firm recommendation can be made on the basis of published research regarding the frequency of antenatal surveillance among postterm patients, many practitioners use twice-weekly testing.

▶ *For a postterm patient with a favorable cervix, does the evidence support labor induction or expectant management?*

Management of low-risk postterm pregnancy is controversial. Because delivery cannot always be brought about readily, maternal risks and considerations may complicate this decision. Factors to consider include gestational age; results of antepartum fetal testing; the condition of the cervix; and maternal preference after discussion of the risks, benefits, and alternatives to expectant management with antepartum monitoring versus labor induction.

Many studies of postterm pregnancies comparing outcomes of labor induction with those of expectant management excluded women with favorable cervices (33–36, 39–41). Moreover, when women allocated to expectant management experienced a change in cervical status, expectant management ceased and labor induction was initiated (32, 33, 36, 37, 40). In studies on postterm pregnancy in which women with favorable cervices were managed expectantly, there was no indication that expectant management had a deleterious effect on the outcome, but results were not stratified according to the condition of the cervix (31, 32, 38, 42, 51, 52).

For women who are experiencing postterm pregnancies and have favorable cervices, data are insufficient to determine whether labor induction or expectant management yields a better outcome. However, labor generally is induced in postterm pregnancies in which the cervix is favorable because the risk of failed induction and subsequent cesarean delivery is low.

▶ *For a postterm patient with an unfavorable cervix, does the evidence support labor induction or expectant management?*

Both expectant management and labor induction are associated with low complication rates and good perinatal outcomes in low-risk postterm women with unfavorable cervices (24–36, 39, 40). However, there appears to be a small advantage to labor induction using cervical ripening agents, when indicated, regardless of parity or method of induction. The introduction of preinduction cervical maturation has resulted in fewer failed and serial inductions, reduced fetal and maternal morbidity, reduced medical cost, and possibly a reduced rate of cesarean delivery in the general obstetric population (2, 35, 36, 53–55).

Although postterm pregnancy is defined as a pregnancy of 42 weeks or more of gestation, several large multicenter randomized studies of management of pregnancy beyond 40 weeks of gestation reported favorable outcomes with routine induction as early as the beginning of 41 weeks of gestation (2, 35, 36). The largest study to date randomly assigned 3,407 low-risk women with uncomplicated singleton pregnancies at 41 weeks of gestation to labor induction (with or without cervical ripening agents) within 4 days of randomization or expectant management until 44 weeks of gestation (35). Elective induction resulted in a lower cesarean delivery rate (21.2% versus 24.5%), primarily related to fewer surgeries performed for nonreassuring fetal heart rate tracings. However, the authors could not identify a particular cause related to postterm pregnancy status. Patient satisfaction was significantly higher in women randomly assigned to labor induction.

A meta-analysis of 19 trials of routine versus selective labor induction in postterm patients found that routine induction after 41 weeks of gestation was associated with a lower rate of perinatal mortality (OR, 0.2; 95% CI, 0.06–0.7) and no increase in the cesarean delivery rate (OR, 1.02; 95% CI, 0.75–1.38) (2). Routine labor induction also had no effect on the instrumental delivery rate, use of analgesia, or incidence of fetal heart rate abnor-

mality. The risk of meconium-stained amniotic fluid was reduced, but the risks of meconium aspiration syndrome and neonatal seizures were unaffected (2). The actual risk of stillbirth during the 41st week of gestation is estimated at 1.04–1.27 per 1,000 undelivered women, compared with 1.55–3.1 per 1,000 women at or beyond 42 weeks of gestation (56). Taken together, these data suggest that routine induction at 41 weeks of gestation has fetal benefit without incurring the additional maternal risks of a higher rate of cesarean delivery (2, 20).

This conclusion has not been universally accepted. Smaller studies report mixed results regarding cesarean delivery rates; some show an increase (33, 38), and others show no difference in the cesarean delivery rate (31, 34, 36, 37, 39, 40). Two studies reported an increase in cesarean delivery rates only among certain subgroups of patients (eg, high-risk groups) (32, 42).

▶ *What is the role of prostaglandin preparations in managing a postterm pregnancy?*

Prostaglandin (PG) is a valuable tool for improving cervical ripeness and inducing labor. Several placebo-controlled clinical trials have reported significant changes in Bishop scores, shorter durations of labor, lower maximum doses of oxytocin, and a reduced incidence of cesarean delivery among postterm patients who received PGE_2 gel (57–59). In contrast, a National Institute of Child Health and Human Development study reported no reduction in the cesarean delivery rate or the induction-to-delivery interval among postterm patients who were randomized to receive PGE_2 gel as compared with those receiving placebo, although the gel was more effective in initiating persistent contractions in nulliparous women (36). Both PGE_2 (dinoprostone) (31, 33, 35, 36, 42, 59–62) and PGE_1 (misoprostol) preparations (63–65) have been used for labor induction in postterm pregnancies.

Although multiple studies have used PG to induce labor in postterm pregnancies, no standardized dose or dosing interval has been established. Overall, the medications were well tolerated with few reported side effects. Higher doses of PG (especially PGE_1) have been associated with an increased risk of uterine tachysystole and hyperstimulation leading to nonreassuring fetal testing results (55, 66). As such, lower doses are preferable. When PG is used, fetal heart rate monitoring should be done routinely to assess fetal well-being because of the risk of uterine hyperstimulation.

▶ *Is there a role for vaginal birth after cesarean delivery in the management of postterm pregnancy?*

Vaginal birth after cesarean delivery (VBAC) has been promoted as a reasonable alternative to elective repeat cesarean delivery for some women. The risk of uterine rupture does not appear to increase substantially after 40 weeks of gestation (67, 68), but the risk appears to be increased with labor induction with PG or pitocin regardless of gestational age (68, 69). In a population-based, retrospective cohort analysis, the risk of uterine rupture with VBAC was 1.6 per 1,000 women with repeat cesarean delivery without labor, 5.2 per 1,000 women with spontaneous onset of labor, 7.7 per 1,000 women whose labor was induced without PG, and 24.5 per 1,000 women who underwent a PG induction of labor (69). There is limited evidence on the efficacy or safety of VBAC after 42 weeks of gestation. As such, no firm recommendation can be made.

Summary of Recommendations

The following recommendations are based on good and consistent scientific evidence (Level A):

▶ Women with postterm gestations who have unfavorable cervices can either undergo labor induction or be managed expectantly.

▶ Prostaglandin can be used in postterm pregnancies to promote cervical ripening and induce labor.

▶ Delivery should be effected if there is evidence of fetal compromise or oligohydramnios.

The following recommendations are based primarily on consensus and expert opinion (Level C):

▶ Despite a lack of evidence that monitoring improves perinatal outcome, it is reasonable to initiate antenatal surveillance of postterm pregnancies between 41 weeks (287 days; EDD +7 days) and 42 weeks (294 days; EDD +14 days) of gestation because of evidence that perinatal morbidity and mortality increase as gestational age advances.

▶ Many practitioners use twice-weekly testing with some evaluation of amniotic fluid volume beginning at 41 weeks of gestation. A nonstress test and amniotic fluid volume assessment (a modified BPP) should be adequate.

▶ Many authorities recommend prompt delivery in a postterm patient with a favorable cervix and no other complications.

References

1. Martin JA, Hamilton BE, Sutton PD, Ventura SJ, Menacker F, Munson ML. Births: final data for 2002. Natl Vital Stat Rep 2003;52(10):1–113. (Level II-3)
2. Crowley P. Interventions for preventing or improving the outcome of delivery at or beyond term (Cochrane review). In: The Cochrane Library, Issue 2, 2004. Chicester, UK: John Wiley & Sons, Ltd. (Meta-analysis)
3. Neilson JP. Ultrasound for fetal assessment in early pregnancy (Cochrane Review). In: The Cochrane Library, Issue 2, 2004. Chicester, UK: John Wiley & Sons, Ltd. (Meta-analysis)
4. Alfirevic Z, Walkinshaw SA. Management of post-term pregnancy: to induce or not? Br J Hosp Med 1994;52:218–21. (Level III)
5. Mogren I, Stenlund H, Hogberg U. Recurrence of prolonged pregnancy. Int J Epidemiol 1999;28:253–7. (Level II-2)
6. Divon MY, Ferber A, Niscll H, Westgren M. Male gender predisposes to prolongation of pregnancy. Am J Obstet Gynecol 2002;187:1081–3. (Level II-3)
7. Olesen AW, Basso O, Olsen J. Risk of recurrence of prolonged pregnancy. BMJ 2003;326:476. (Level II-2)
8. Feldman GB. Prospective risk of stillbirth. Obstet Gynecol 1992;79:547–53. (Level II-3)
9. Smith GC. Life-table analysis of the risk of perinatal death at term and post term in singleton pregnancies. Am J Obstet Gynecol 2001;184:489–6. (Level III)
10. Hilder L, Costeloe K, Thilaganathan B. Prolonged pregnancy: evaluating gestation-specific risks of fetal and infant mortality. Br J Obstet Gynaecol 1998;105:169–73. (Level II-3)
11. Hannah ME. Postterm pregnancy: should all women have labour induced? A review of the literature. Fetal Maternal Med Review 1993;5:3–17. (Level III)
12. Kitlinski ML, Kallen K, Marsal K, Olofsson P. Gestational age-dependent reference values for pH in umbilical cord arterial blood at term. Obstet Gynecol 2003;102:338–45. (Level II-2)
13. Spellacy WN, Miller S, Winegar A, Peterson PQ. Macrosomia—maternal characteristics and infant complications. Obstet Gynecol 1985;66:158–61. (Level II-2)
14. Rosen MG, Dickinson JC. Management of post-term pregnancy. N Engl J Med 1992;326:1628–9. (Level III)
15. Vorherr H. Placental insufficiency in relation to postterm pregnancy and fetal postmaturity. Evaluation of fetoplacental function; management of the postterm gravida. Am J Obstet Gynecol 1975;123:67–103. (Level III)
16. Mannino F. Neonatal complications of postterm gestation. J Reprod Med 1988;33:271–6. (Level III)
17. Knox GE, Huddleston JF, Flowers CE Jr. Management of prolonged pregnancy: results of a prospective randomized trial. Am J Obstet Gynecol 1979;134:376–84. (Level II-2)

18. Shime J, Librach CL, Gare DJ, Cook CJ. The influence of prolonged pregnancy on infant development at one and two years of age: a prospective controlled study. Am J Obstet Gynecol 1986;154:341–5. (Level II-2)

19. Cotzias CS, Paterson-Brown S, Fisk NM. Prospective risk of unexplained stillbirth in singleton pregnancies at term: population based analysis. BMJ 1999;319:287–8. (Level III)

20. Rand L, Robinson JN, Economy KE, Norwitz ER. Postterm induction of labor revisited. Obstet Gynecol 2000;96:779–83. (Level III)

21. Alexander JM, McIntire DD, Leveno KJ. Forty weeks and beyond: pregnancy outcomes by week of gestation. Obstet Gynecol 2000;96:291–4. (Level II-2)

22. Alexander JM, McIntire DD, Leveno KJ. Prolonged pregnancy: induction of labor and cesarean births. Obstet Gynecol 2001;97:911–5. (Level II-2)

23. Treger M, Hallak M, Silberstein T, Friger M, Katz M, Mazor M. Post-term pregnancy: should induction of labor be considered before 42 weeks? J Matern Fetal Neonatal Med 2002;11:50–3. (Level II-2)

24. Savitz DA, Terry JW Jr, Dole N, Thorp JM Jr, Siega-Riz AM, Herring AH. Comparison of pregnancy dating by last menstrual period, ultrasound scanning, and their combination. Am J Obstet Gynecol 2002;187:1660–6. (Level II-3)

25. Magann EF, Chauhan SP, Nevils BG, McNamara MF, Kinsella MJ, Morrison JC. Management of pregnancies beyond forty-one weeks' gestation with an unfavorable cervix. Am J Obstet Gynecol 1998;178:1279–87. (Level I)

26. Magann EF, Chauhan SP, McNamara MF, Bass JD, Estes CM, Morrison JC. Membrane sweeping versus dinoprostone vaginal insert in the management of pregnancies beyond 41 weeks with an unfavorable cervix. J Perinatol 1999;19:88–91. (Level I)

27. Wong SF, Hui SK, Choi H, Ho LC. Does sweeping of membranes beyond 40 weeks reduce the need for formal induction of labour? BJOG 2002;109:632–6. (Level I)

28. Bochner CJ, Williams J 3rd, Castro L, Medearis A, Hobel CJ, Wade M. The efficacy of starting postterm antenatal testing at 41 weeks as compared with 42 weeks of gestational age. Am J Obstet Gynecol 1988;159:550–4. (Level II-2)

29. Guidetti DA, Divon MY, Langer O. Postdate fetal surveillance: is 41 weeks too early? Am J Obstet Gynecol 1989;161:91–3. (Level II-2)

30. Usher RH, Boyd ME, McLean FH, Kramer MS. Assessment of fetal risk in postdate pregnancies. Am J Obstet Gynecol 1988;158:259–64. (Level II-2)

31. Cardozo L, Fysh J, Pearce JM. Prolonged pregnancy: the management debate. Br Med J (Clin Res Ed) 1986;293:1059–63. (Level II-1)

32. Augensen K, Bergsjo P, Eikeland T, Askvik K, Carlsen J. Randomised comparison of early versus late induction of labour in post-term pregnancy. Br Med J (Clin Res Ed) 1987;294:1192–5. (Level I)

33. Dyson DC, Miller PD, Armstrong MA. Management of prolonged pregnancy: induction of labor versus antepartum fetal testing. Am J Obstet Gynecol 1987;156:928–34. (Level I)

34. Martin JN Jr, Sessums JK, Howard P, Martin RW, Morrision JC. Alternative approaches to the management of gravidas with prolonged-postterm-postdate pregnancies. J Miss State Med Assoc 1989;30:105–11. (Level I)

35. Hannah ME, Hannah WJ, Hellmann J, Hewson S, Milner R, Willan A. Induction of labor as compared with serial antenatal monitoring in post-term pregnancy. A randomized controlled trial. The Canadian Multicenter Post-term Pregnancy Trial Group [published erratum appears in N Engl J Med 1992;327:368]. N Engl J Med 1992;326:1587–92. (Level I)

36. A clinical trial of induction of labor versus expectant management in post-term pregnancy. The National Institute of Child Health and Human Development Network of Maternal–Fetal Medicine Units. Am J Obstet Gynecol 1994;170:716–23. (Level I)

37. Witter FR, Weitz CM. A randomized trial of induction at 42 weeks gestation versus expectant management for postdates pregnancies. Am J Perinatol 1987;4:206–11. (Level I)

38. Bergsjo P, Huang GD, Yu SQ, Gao ZZ, Bakketeig LS. Comparison of induced versus non-induced labor in post-term pregnancy. A randomized prospective study. Acta Obstet Gynecol Scand 1989;68:683–7. (Level I)

39. Heden L, Ingemarsson I, Ahlstrom H, Solum T. Induction of labor versus conservative management in prolonged pregnancy: controlled study. Int J Feto-Maternal Med 1991;4:231–6. (Level II-1)

40. Herabutya Y, Prasertsawat PO, Tongyai T, Isarangura NA, Ayudthya N. Prolonged pregnancy: the management dilemma. Int J Gynaecol Obstet 1992;37:253–8. (Level I)

41. Shaw KJ, Medearis AL, Horenstein J, Walla CA, Paul RH. Selective labor induction in postterm patients. Observations and outcomes. J Reprod Med 1992;37:157–61. (Level II-2)

42. Almstrom H, Granstrom L, Ekman G. Serial antenatal monitoring compared with labor induction in post-term pregnancies. Acta Obstet Gynecol Scand 1995;74:599–603. (Level II-2)

43. Crowley P, O'Herlihy C, Boylan P. The value of ultrasound measurement of amniotic fluid volume in the management of prolonged pregnancies. Br J Obstet Gynaecol 1984;91:444–8. (Level II-2)

44. Phelan JP, Platt LD, Yeh SY, Broussard P, Paul RH. The role of ultrasound assessment of amniotic fluid volume in the management of the postdate pregnancy. Am J Obstet Gynecol 1985;151:304–8. (Level II-2)

45. Bochner CJ, Medearis AL, Davis J, Oakes GK, Hobel CJ, Wade ME. Antepartum predictors of fetal distress in postterm pregnancy. Am J Obstet Gynecol 1987;157:353–8. (Level II-2)

46. Oz AU, Holub B, Mendilcioglu I, Mari G, Bahado-Singh RO. Renal artery Doppler investigation of the etiology of oligohydramnios in postterm pregnancy. Obstet Gynecol 2002;100:715–8. (Level II-2)

47. Tongsong T, Srisomboon J. Amniotic fluid volume as a predictor of fetal distress in postterm pregnancy. Int J Gynaecol Obstet 1993;40:213–7. (Level II-2)

48. Chamberlain PF, Manning FA, Morrison I, Harman CR, Lange IR. Ultrasound evaluation of amniotic fluid volume. I. The relationship of marginal and decreased amniotic fluid volumes to perinatal outcome. Am J Obstet Gynecol 1984;150:245–9. (Level II-2)

49. Guidetti DA, Divon MY, Cavalieri RL, Langer O, Merkatz IR. Fetal umbilical artery flow velocimetry in postdate pregnancies. Am J Obstet Gynecol 1987;157:1521–3. (Level II-2)

50. Stokes HJ, Roberts RV, Newnham JP. Doppler flow velocity waveform analysis in postdate pregnancies. Aust N Z J Obstet Gynaecol 1991;31:27–30. (Level II-2)

51. James C, George SS, Gaunekar N, Seshadri L. Management of prolonged pregnancy: a randomised trial of induction of labour and antepartum foetal monitoring. Natl Med J India 2001;14:270–3. (Level I)

52. Chanrachakul B, Herabutya Y. Postterm with favorable cervix: is induction necessary? Eur J Obstet Gynecol Reprod Biol 2003;106:154–7. (Level I)

53. Xenakis EM, Piper JM, Conway DL, Langer O. Induction of labor in the nineties: conquering the unfavorable cervix. Obstet Gynecol 1997;90:235–9. (Level II-2)

54. Poma PA. Cervical ripening. A review and recommendations for clinical practice. J Reprod Med 1999;44:657–68. (Level III)

55. Sanchez-Ramos L, Kaunitz AM, Delke I. Labor induction with 25 micro versus 50 micro intravaginal misoprostol: a systematic review. Obstet Gynecol 2002;99:145–51. (Meta-analysis)

56. Menticoglou SM, Hall PF. Routine induction of labour at 41 weeks gestation: nonsensus consensus. BJOG 2002; 109:485–91. (Level III)

57. Rayburn W, Gosen R, Ramadei C, Woods R, Scott J Jr. Outpatient cervical ripening with prostaglandin E2 gel in uncomplicated postdate pregnancies. Am J Obstet Gynecol 1988;158:1417–23. (Level II-1)

58. Papageorgiou I, Tsionou C, Minaretzis D, Michalas S, Aravantinos D. Labor characteristics of uncomplicated prolonged pregnancies after induction with intracervical prostaglandin E2 gel versus intravenous oxytocin. Gynecol Obstet Invest 1992;34:92–6. (Level II-1)

59. Sawai SK, O'Brien WF, Mastrogiannis DS, Krammer J, Mastry MG, Porter GW. Patient-administered outpatient intravaginal prostaglandin E2 suppositories in post-date pregnancies: a double-blind, randomized, placebo-controlled study. Obstet Gynecol 1994;84:807–10. (Level I)

60. Ekman G, Persson PH, Ulmsten U. Induction of labor in postterm pregnant women. Int J Gynaecol Obstet 1986;24: 47–52. (Level II-2)

61. Egarter C, Kofler E, Fitz R, Husslein P. Is induction of labor indicated in prolonged pregnancy? Results of a prospective randomized trial. Gynecol Obstet Invest 1989;27: 6–9. (Level I)

62. Doany W, McCarty J. Outpatient management of the uncomplicated postdate pregnancy with intravaginal prostaglandin E2 gel and membrane stripping. J Matern Fetal Med 1997;6:71–8. (Level I)

63. Lee HY. A randomised double-blind study of vaginal misoprostol vs dinoprostone for cervical ripening and labour induction in prolonged pregnancy. Singapore Med J 1997;38:292–4. (Level I)

64. Wing DA, Fassett MJ, Mishell DR. Mifepristone for preinduction cervical ripening beyond 41 weeks' gestation: a randomized controlled trial. Obstet Gynecol 2000;96: 543–8. (Level I)

65. Meydanli MM, Caliskan E, Burak F, Narin MA, Atmaca R. Labor induction post-term with 25 micrograms vs. 50 micrograms of intravaginal misoprostol. Int J Gynaecol Obstet 2003;81:249–55. (Level I)

66. How HY, Leaseburge L, Khoury JC, Siddiqi TA, Spinnato JA, Sibai BM. A comparison of various routes and dosages of misoprostol for cervical ripening and the induction of labor. Am J Obstet Gynecol 2001;185:911–5. (Level I)

67. Callahan C, Chescheir N, Steiner BD. Safety and efficacy of attempted vaginal birth after cesarean beyond the estimated date of delivery. J Reprod Med 1999;44:606–10. (Level II-2)

68. Zelop CM, Shipp TD, Cohen A, Repke JT, Lieberman E. Trial of labor after 40 weeks' gestation in women with prior cesarean. Obstet Gynecol 2001;97:391–3. (Level II-3)

69. Lydon-Rochelle M, Holt VL, Easterling TR, Martin DP. Risk of uterine rupture during labor among women with a prior cesarean delivery. N Engl J Med 2001;345:3–8. (Level II-2)

The MEDLINE database, the Cochrane Library, and ACOG's own internal resources and documents were used to conduct a literature search to locate relevant articles published between January 1985 and April 2004. The search was restricted to articles published in the English language. Priority was given to articles reporting results of original research, although review articles and commentaries also were consulted. Abstracts of research presented at symposia and scientific conferences were not considered adequate for inclusion in this document. Guidelines published by organizations or institutions such as the National Institutes of Health and the American College of Obstetricians and Gynecologists were reviewed, and additional studies were located by reviewing bibliographies of identified articles. When reliable research was not available, expert opinions from obstetrician–gynecologists were used.

Studies were reviewed and evaluated for quality according to the method outlined by the U.S. Preventive Services Task Force:

I   Evidence obtained from at least 1 properly designed randomized controlled trial.

II-1 Evidence obtained from well-designed controlled trials without randomization.

II-2 Evidence obtained from well-designed cohort or case–control analytic studies, preferably from more than 1 center or research group.

II-3 Evidence obtained from multiple time series with or without the intervention. Dramatic results in uncontrolled experiments also could be regarded as this type of evidence.

III   Opinions of respected authorities, based on clinical experience, descriptive studies, or reports of expert committees.

Based on the highest level of evidence found in the data, recommendations are provided and graded according to the following categories:

Level A—Recommendations are based on good and consistent scientific evidence.

Level B—Recommendations are based on limited or inconsistent scientific evidence.

Level C—Recommendations are based primarily on consensus and expert opinion.

ISSN 1099-3630

**The American College of
Obstetricians and Gynecologists
409 12th Street, SW
PO Box 96920
Washington, DC 20090-6920**

12345/87654

Management of postterm pregnancy. ACOG Practice Bulletin No. 55. American College of Obstetricians and Gynecologists. Obstet Gynecol 2004;104:639–46.

ACOG PRACTICE BULLETIN

CLINICAL MANAGEMENT GUIDELINES FOR
OBSTETRICIAN–GYNECOLOGISTS

Number 43, May 2003

This Practice Bulletin was developed by the ACOG Committee on Practice Bulletins— Obstetrics with the assistance of John M. Thorp Jr, MD. The information is designed to aid practitioners in making decisions about appropriate obstetric and gynecologic care. These guidelines should not be construed as dictating an exclusive course of treatment or procedure. Variations in practice may be warranted based on the needs of the individual patient, resources, and limitations unique to the institution or type of practice.

Management of Preterm Labor

Preterm birth is the leading cause of neonatal mortality in the United States, and preterm labor precedes 40–50% of preterm births (1–3). Preterm birth accounts for 35% of all U.S. health care spending for infants and 10% of all such spending for children (4). Approximately 467,000 live births annually (11.5% of all live births) occur before term in the United States, and preterm births are responsible for three quarters of neonatal mortality and one half of long-term neurologic impairments in children (1, 5–7). The purpose of this document is to present the various methods proposed to manage preterm labor and the evidence for their roles in clinical practice. Despite the numerous management methods proposed, the incidence of preterm birth has changed little over the past 40 years (Fig. 1) (1, 8, 9). Uncertainty persists about the best strategies for managing preterm labor.

Background

Preterm labor generally can be defined as regular contractions that occur before 37 weeks of gestation and are associated with changes in the cervix. Although the causes of preterm labor are not well understood, the incidence and burden of preterm births are more clear. Preterm labor is the most common cause of antenatal hospitalization (10). It is important to recognize that preterm labor is not the only mechanism leading to preterm birth; numerous preterm births are preceded by either rupture of membranes or other medical problems (Fig. 2) (10, 11).

Historically, nonpharmacologic treatments to prevent preterm births in women who have symptoms of preterm labor have included bed rest, abstention from intercourse and orgasm, and hydration, either orally or parenterally. The effectiveness of these interventions is uncertain.

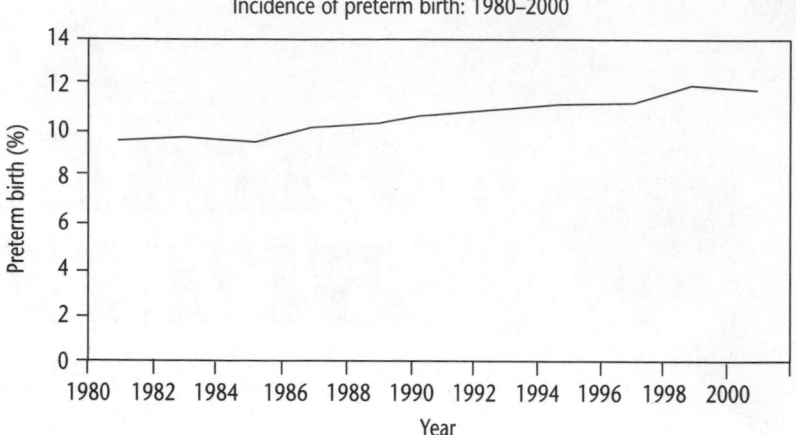

Figure 1. Incidence of preterm birth: 1980–2000. (Data from Martin JA, Hamilton BE, Ventura SJ, Menacker F, Park MM, Sutton PD. Births: final data for 2001. Natl Vital Stat Rep 2002;51:1–104; Ventura SJ, Martin JA, Curtin SC, Mathews TJ. Report of final natality statistics, 1996. Monthly vital statistics report; vol. 46, no. 11, supl. Hyattsville (MD): National Center for Health Statistics; 1998; and Ventura SJ, Martin JA, Taffel SM, Matthews ST, Clarke SC. Advance report of final natality statistics, 1992. Monthly vital statistics report; vol. 43, no. 5, suppl. Hyattsville (MD): National Center for Health Statistics; 1994.)

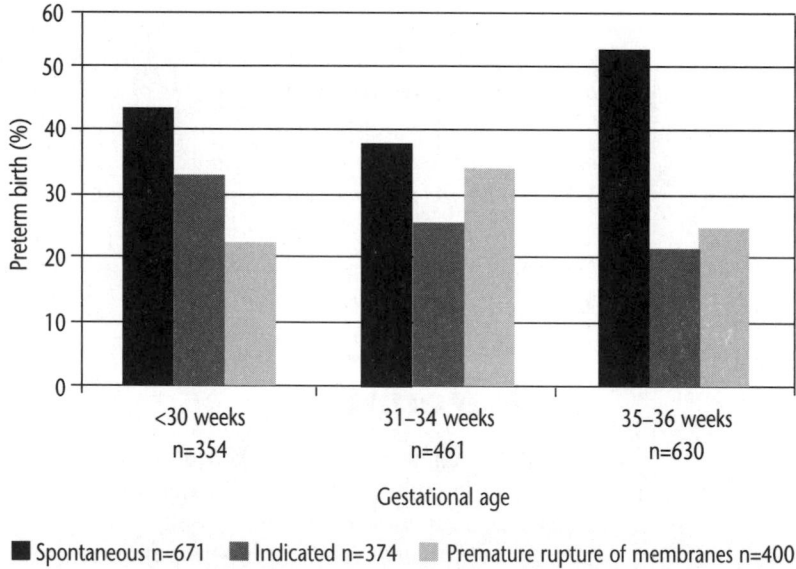

Figure 2. Gestational age distributions of spontaneous, indicated, and premature rupture of membranes preterm births. (Modified from Tucker JM, Goldenberg RL, Davis RO, Copper RL, Winkler CL, Hauth JC. Etiologies of preterm birth in an indigent population: is prevention a logical expectation? Obstet Gynecol 1991; 77:343–7.)

Tocolytic Drugs for Treatment of Preterm Labor

Tocolytic drugs inhibit myometrial contractions. Many agents have been used, including ethanol, magnesium sulfate, calcium channel blockers, oxytocin antagonists, nonsteroidal antiinflammatory drugs (NSAIDs), and beta-mimetic agonists. Tocolytics can be administered either parenterally or orally. Table 1 describes various tocolytic drugs, their mechanisms of action, and their side effects.

Antibiotics for Treatment of Preterm Labor

Women who present with symptoms of preterm labor may have infections of the upper genital tract (12, 13). It has been theorized that infections or inflammation are associated with contractions, and this theory provided the rationale for studies using antibiotics to decrease the risk of spontaneous preterm birth. Studies have shown mixed results, but most of the evidence has

Table 1. Tocolytics for Preterm Labor

Tocolytic Agent	Dosage and Administration	Contraindications	Maternal Side Effects	Fetal and Neonatal Side Effects
Beta-mimetic	Terbutaline, .25 mg subcutaneously every 20 min to 3 hr (hold for pulse >120 beats per minute)	Cardiac arrhythmias	Cardiac or cardiopulmonary arrhythmias, pulmonary edema, myocardial ischemia, hypotension, tachycardia	Fetal tachycardia, hyperinsulinemia, hyperglycemia, myocardial and septal hypertrophy, myocardial ischemia
	Ritodrine initial dose of 50–100 µg/min, increase 50 µg/min every 10 min until contractions cease or side effects develop	Poorly controlled thyroid disease	Metabolic hyperglycemia, hyperinsulinemia, hypokalemia, antidiuresis, altered thyroid function	Neonatal tachycardia, hypoglycemia, hypocalcemia, hyperbilirubinemia, hypotension, intraventricular hemorrhage
	Maximum dose = 350 µg/min	Poorly controlled diabetes mellitus	Physiologic tremor, palpitations, nervousness, nausea or vomiting, fever, hallucinations	—
Magnesium sulfate	4–6 g bolus for 20 min, then 2–3 g/hr	Myasthenia gravis	Flushing, lethargy, headache, muscle weakness, diplopia, dry mouth, pulmonary edema, cardiac arrest	Lethargy, hypotonia, respiratory depression, demineralization with prolonged use
Calcium channel blockers	30 mg loading dose, then 10–20 mg every 4–6 hr	Cardiac disease, use caution with renal disease, maternal hypotension (<90/50 mm Hg), avoid concomitant use with magnesium sulfate	Flushing, headache, dizziness, nausea, transient hypotension	None noted as yet
Prostaglandin synthetase inhibitors	Indomethacin loading dose of 50 mg rectally or 50–100 mg orally, then 25–50 mg orally every 6 hr × 48 hr	Significant renal or hepatic impairment	Nausea, heartburn	Constriction of ductus arteriosus, pulmonary hypertension, reversible decrease in renal function with oligohydramnios, intraventricular hemorrhage, hyperbilirubinemia, necrotizing enterocolitis
	Ketorolac loading dose of 60 mg intramuscularly, then 30 mg intramuscularly every 6 hr × 48 hr	Active peptic ulcer disease	—	—
	Sulindac, 200 mg orally every 12 hr × 48 hr	Coagulation disorders or thrombocytopenia, NSAID-sensitive asthma, other sensitivity to NSAIDs	—	—

Abbreviation: NSAIDs, nonsteroidal antiinflammatory drugs

Hearne AE, Nagey DA. Therapeutic agents in preterm labor: tocolytic agents. Clin Obstet Gynecol 2000;43:787–801.

failed to show a benefit from treatment with antibiotics (14–26).

Antenatal Corticosteroid Use

The most beneficial intervention for patients in true preterm labor is the administration of corticosteroids. A recent meta-analysis confirmed that antenatal corticosteroids significantly reduced the incidence and severity of neonatal respiratory distress syndrome (27). The incidence of intraventricular hemorrhage and necrotizing enterocolitis also are reduced by the use of antenatal corticosteroids. The administration of betamethasone has been shown to decrease neonatal mortality (28). All women who are at risk for preterm delivery between 24 weeks and 34 weeks of gestation are potential candidates for corticosteroid therapy. Treatment should consist of either two doses of betamethasone or four doses of dexamethasone, both administered intramuscularly.

Clinical Considerations and Recommendations

▶ Who are appropriate candidates for intervention?

In 80% of women with presumptive preterm labor, preterm delivery will not occur (29). Many factors influence the decision to intervene when women have symptoms of preterm labor, including the probability of progressive labor, gestational age, and the risks of treatment (30). Historically, the clinical criteria commonly suggested for determining when intervention is needed included regular uterine activity that does not diminish with bed rest or hydration, cervical change during an observation period, or a cervix that is dilated on presentation. However, all of these clinical conditions are inaccurate predictors of preterm delivery (31).

Gestational age is inversely proportional to the risk of neonatal morbidity and mortality. The upper limit of gestational age for the use of tocolytic drugs may be a function of the neonatal treatment capabilities in the hospital where a clinician practices. Examples of general contraindications for tocolysis may include severe preeclampsia, placental abruption, intrauterine infection, lethal congenital or chromosomal abnormalities, advanced cervical dilatation, and evidence of fetal compromise or placental insufficiency.

▶ Are there tests that can help identify patients at risk for progressing to preterm birth?

Many tests to identify women at risk of preterm birth have been proposed and evaluated; however, only ultra-sonography and fetal fibronectin testing have been shown to have benefit (32–37). Ultrasonography to determine cervical length, fetal fibronectin testing, or a combination of both may be useful in determining which women are at high risk for preterm delivery. However, their clinical usefulness may rest primarily with their ability to identify women who are least likely to deliver (ie, their negative predictive value) given the lack of proven treatment options to prevent preterm birth. Fetal fibronectin testing may be useful in women with symptoms of preterm labor to identify those with negative values and a reduced risk of preterm birth, thereby avoiding unnecessary intervention (38).

▶ Does tocolytic therapy improve neonatal outcome?

Tocolytic drugs may prolong gestation for 2–7 days, which can provide time for administration of steroids and maternal transport to a facility with a neonatal intensive care unit (26). The benefits of prolonging pregnancy for 2–7 days are otherwise unclear (39–44).

▶ Is there a clear "first-line" tocolytic drug?

Comparison studies of the effectiveness of different tocolytic drugs show conflicting results between beta-mimetics, magnesium sulfate, calcium channel blockers, and NSAIDs (45–58). However, all have demonstrated only limited benefit. Hence, there is no clear first-line tocolytic drug. If tocolytic drugs are used, the choice of drug should be individualized and based on maternal condition, potential drug side effects, and gestational age (see Table 1). Prolonged use of any tocolytic drug may potentially increase the maternal–fetal risk without offering a clear benefit.

Serious adverse events are rare but potentially life-threatening. Beta-mimetics, magnesium sulfate, and calcium channel blockers are all associated with an increased risk of pulmonary edema. Beta-mimetics are potent cardiovascular stimulants and can cause serious complications, such as maternal myocardial ischemia, metabolic derangements (eg, hyperglycemia and hypokalemia), and fetal cardiac effects. Magnesium sulfate may cause maternal lethargy, drowsiness, double vision, nausea, and vomiting. The NSAIDs appear to have the fewest maternal risks, but fetal effects include oligohydramnios and premature closure of the ductus arteriosus. Calcium channel blockers used as a single agent appear to have a good maternal and fetal safety profile. However, concomitant use of calcium channel blockers and magnesium sulfate is potentially harmful and has resulted in cardiovascular collapse (59). Combining tocolytic drugs potentially increases maternal morbidity and should be used with caution (60).

▶ *Is there a role for adjunctive antibiotics?*

An array of antibiotics and bacteriostatic drugs have been evaluated in randomized, controlled trials to determine if they can prevent preterm birth in women with preterm labor, but these studies have reported mixed results. A recent meta-analysis assessed eight randomized controlled trials comparing antibiotic treatment with placebo for patients with documented preterm labor (26). No difference was noted between the antibiotic treatment and placebo for prolonging pregnancy or preventing preterm delivery respiratory distress syndrome or neonatal sepsis. Treating women in preterm labor with antibiotics for the sole purpose of preventing preterm delivery is not recommended (61). At present, it seems prudent to follow protocols for antibiotic prophylaxis against early-onset group B streptococcal sepsis, but there is little evidence that this approach also will prolong gestation (62).

▶ *Is preventive treatment efficacious?*

Because of the large variations in symptoms of preterm labor and the inability of routine clinical tools to precisely determine a woman's risk, the assessment of preterm delivery risk is fraught with inaccuracy (29, 63, 64). Previously, when symptoms of preterm delivery were present, most clinicians handled this uncertainty by recommending reduced maternal activity and administering fluids with the aim of stopping the uterine activity. Most advocated awaiting clinical detection of cervical change before administering tocolytic drugs. Prophylactic therapy, including tocolytic drugs, bed rest, hydration, and sedation, in asymptomatic women at increased risk for preterm delivery has not been demonstrated to be effective (30, 61).

▶ *Should women with preterm contractions without cervical change be treated?*

Regular preterm contractions are common. However, their presence does not reliably predict who will have subsequent progressive cervical change (65). In a study of 763 women who had unscheduled visits for symptoms of preterm labor, only 18% delivered before 37 weeks of gestation, and only 3% delivered within 2 weeks of presenting with symptoms (29). Although bed rest, pelvic rest, and hydration are commonly recommended to women with symptoms of preterm labor to prevent preterm delivery, the effectiveness of these measures is not known, and their potential harms (eg, thrombosis from stasis in the lower extremities) or negative impacts (eg, loss of employment) should not be underestimated

(66). No evidence exists to support the use of tocolytic therapy (67), home uterine activity monitoring, elective cerclage, or narcotics to prevent preterm delivery in women with contractions but no cervical change.

▶ *Should women with multiple gestations be treated differently?*

Women with multiple gestations who have preterm contractions but no cervical change do not require tocolytic therapy. Although women with multiple gestations who are experiencing preterm labor may benefit from short-term tocolysis to allow for steroid administration, they have a greater risk of pulmonary edema when exposed to beta-mimetics or magnesium sulfate (68).

▶ *Is there a role for maintenance treatment after completing acute treatment?*

Studies of maintenance tocolytic therapy in women who present with symptoms of preterm labor and receive tocolysis acutely show no differences in effectiveness between treatment and control groups (30). Meta-analysis likewise fails to demonstrate any benefit of maintenance tocolysis in terms of gestational age at birth, pregnancy prolongation, or birth weight (30). Prolonged oral, subcutaneous, or intravenous tocolytic treatment is not effective. Two prospective randomized trials showed the terbutaline pump was no more effective than saline (69, 70).

▶ *Is tocolysis warranted for recurrent preterm labor?*

The role of repeated acute tocolytic therapy in women with recurring symptoms of preterm labor is unknown. Given the limited benefits of an initial course of treatment with a tocolytic drug and current recommendations that corticosteroids be administered only as a single course (71), the effectiveness of subsequent acute tocolysis is uncertain. Maternal transport is a potential rationale for a subsequent treatment course (72).

▶ *Is there a role for amniocentesis?*

Amniocentesis to determine fetal lung maturity may have some benefit in guiding clinical decision making in women with symptoms of preterm labor. There is no evidence to suggest that routine amniocentesis to check for infection in these women can provide information that could be used to improve perinatal outcomes (30). In a multicenter study in women with preterm labor and intact membranes, the overall prevalence of microbial invasion of the amniotic cavity as documented by amniocentesis was 5.8% (17). Both amniotic fluid Gram stain and glucose levels have been used as rapid diagnostic tests of intraamniotic infection (73, 74). The results of amniotic fluid cultures, the best method for diagnosing intraamniotic infection, are unlikely to be available quickly enough to affect decision making.

Summary of Recommendations

The following recommendations are based on good and consistent scientific evidence (Level A):

▶ There are no clear "first-line" tocolytic drugs to manage preterm labor. Clinical circumstances and physician preferences should dictate treatment.

▶ Antibiotics do not appear to prolong gestation and should be reserved for group B streptococcal prophylaxis in patients in whom delivery is imminent.

▶ Neither maintenance treatment with tocolytic drugs nor repeated acute tocolysis improve perinatal outcome; neither should be undertaken as a general practice.

▶ Tocolytic drugs may prolong pregnancy for 2–7 days, which may allow for administration of steroids to improve fetal lung maturity and the consideration of maternal transport to a tertiary care facility.

The following recommendations are based on limited or inconsistent scientific evidence (Level B):

▶ Cervical ultrasound examination and fetal fibronectin testing have good negative predictive value; thus, either approach or both combined may be helpful in determining which patients do not need tocolysis.

▶ Amniocentesis may be used in women in preterm labor to assess fetal lung maturity and intraamniotic infection.

▶ Bed rest, hydration, and pelvic rest do not appear to improve the rate of preterm birth and should not be routinely recommended.

References

1. Martin JA, Hamilton BE, Ventura SJ, Menacker F, Park MM, Sutton PD. Births: final data for 2001. Natl Vital Stat Rep 2002;51(2):1–104. (Level III)

2. Tucker JM, Goldenberg RL, Davis RO, Copper RL, Winkler CL, Hauth JC. Etiologies of preterm birth in an indigent population: is prevention a logical expectation? Obstet Gynecol 1991;77:343–7. (Level II-3)

3. Kramer MS. Preventing preterm birth: are we making any progress? Yale J Biol Med 1997;70:227–32. (Level III)

4. Lewit EM, Baker LS, Corman H, Shiono PH. The direct cost of low birth weight. Future Child 1995;5:35–56. (Level III)

5. Goldenberg RL, Rouse DJ. Prevention of premature birth. N Engl J Med 1998;339:313–20. (Level III)

6. Paneth NS. The problem of low birth weight. Future Child 1995;5:19–34. (Level II)

7. McCormick MC. The contribution of low birth weight to infant mortality and childhood morbidity. N Engl J Med 1985;312:82–90. (Level III)

8. Ventura SJ, Martin JA, Curtin SC, Mathews TJ. Report of final natality statistics, 1996. Monthly vital statistics report; vol. 46, no. 11, suppl. Hyattsville (MD): National Center for Health Statistics; 1998. (Level III)

9. Ventura SJ, Martin JA, Taffel SM, Mathews TJ, Clarke SC. Advance report of final natality statistics, 1992. Monthly vital statistics report; vol. 43, no. 5, suppl. Hyattsville (MD): National Center for Health Statistics; 1994. (Level III)

10. Savitz DA, Blackmore CA, Thorp JM. Epidemiologic characteristics of preterm delivery: etiologic heterogeneity. Am J Obstet Gynecol 1991;164:467–71. (Level III)

11. Berkowitz GS, Blackmore-Prince C, Lapinski RH, Savitz DA. Risk factors for preterm birth subtypes. Epidemiology 1998;9:279–85. (Level II-2)

12. Gibbs RS, Eschenbach DA. Use of antibiotics to prevent preterm birth. Am J Obstet Gynecol 1997;177:375–80. (Level III)

13. Andrews WW, Goldenberg RL, Hauth JC. Preterm labor: emerging role of genital tract infections. Infect Agents Dis 1995;4:196–211. (Level III)

14. Nadisauskiene R, Bergstrom S, Kilda A. Ampicillin in the treatment of preterm labor: a randomised, placebo-controlled study. Gynecol Obstet Invest 1996;41:89–92. (Level I)

15. Svare J, Langhoff-Roos J, Andersen LF, Kryger-Baggesen N, Borch-Christensen H, Heisterberg L, et al. Ampicillin-metronidazole treatment in idiopathic preterm labour: a randomised controlled multicentre trial. Br J Obstet Gynaecol 1997;104:892–7. (Level I)

16. Gordon M, Samuels P, Shubert P, Johnson F, Gebauer C, Iams J. A randomized, prospective study of adjunctive ceftizoxime in preterm labor. Am J Obstet Gynecol 1995;172:1546–52. (Level I)

17. Romero R, Sibai B, Caritis S, Paul R, Depp R, Rosen M, et al. Antibiotic treatment of preterm labor with intact membranes: a multicenter, randomized, double-blinded, placebo-controlled trial. Am J Obstet Gynecol 1993;169:764–74. (Level I)

18. Newton ER, Dinsmoor MJ, Gibbs RS. A randomized, blinded, placebo-controlled trial of antibiotics in idiopathic preterm labor. Obstet Gynecol 1989;74:562–6. (Level I)

19. Newton ER, Shields L, Ridgway LE 3rd, Berkus MD, Elliott BD. Combination antibiotics and indomethacin in idiopathic preterm labor: a randomized double-blind

clinical trial. Am J Obstet Gynecol 1991;165:1753–9. (Level I)

20. Cox SM, Bohman VR, Sherman ML, Leveno KJ. Randomized investigation of antimicrobials for the prevention of preterm birth. Am J Obstet Gynecol 1996; 174:206–10. (Level I)

21. Morales WJ, Angel JL, O'Brien WF, Knuppel RA, Finazzo M. A randomized study of antibiotic therapy in idiopathic preterm labor. Obstet Gynecol 1988;72:829–33. (Level I)

22. McGregor JA, French JI, Seo K. Adjunctive clindamycin therapy for preterm labor: results of a double-blind, placebo-controlled trial. Am J Obstet Gynecol 1991;165:867–75. (Level I)

23. Norman K, Pattinson RC, de Souza J, de Jong P, Moller G, Kirsten G. Ampicillin and metronidazole treatment in preterm labour: a multicentre, randomised controlled trial. Br J Obstet Gynaecol 1994;101:404–8. (Level I)

24. Nadisauskiene R, Bergstrom S. Impact of intrapartum intravenous ampicillin on pregnancy outcome in women with preterm labor: a randomised, placebo-controlled study. Gynecol Obstet Invest 1996;41:85–8. (Level I)

25. Winkler M, Baumann L, Ruckhaberle KE, Schiller EM. Erythromycin therapy for subclinical intrauterine infections in threatened preterm delivery—a preliminary report. J Perinat Med 1988;16:253–6. (Level I)

26. King J, Flenady V. Prophylactic antibiotics for inhibiting preterm labour with intact membranes (Cochrane Review). In: The Cochrane Library, Issue 1, 2003. Oxford: Update Software. (Level I)

27. Crowley P. Prophylactic corticosteroids for preterm birth (Cochrane Review). In: The Cochrane Library, Issue 1, 2003. Oxford: Update Software. (Level I)

28. Ballard PL, Ballard RA. Scientific basis and therapeutic regimens for use of antenatal glucocorticoids. Am J Obstet Gynecol 1995;173:254–62. (Level III)

29. Peaceman AM, Andrews WW, Thorp JM, Cliver SP, Lukes A, Iams JD, et al. Fetal fibronectin as a predictor of preterm birth in patients with symptoms: a multicenter trial. Am J Obstet Gynecol 1997;177:13–8. (Level II-2)

30. Agency for Healthcare Research and Quality. Management of preterm labor. Evidence Report/Technology Assessment No. 18. Rockville (MD): AHRQ; 2000. AHRQ Publication No. 01–E021. (Level III)

31. Creasy RK, Golbus MS, Laros RK Jr, Parer JT, Roberts JM. Oral ritodrine maintenance in the treatment of preterm labor. Am J Obstet Gynecol 1980;137:212–9. (Level I)

32. Iams JD, Goldenberg RL, Meis PJ, Mercer BM, Moawad A, Das A, et al. The length of the cervix and the risk of spontaneous premature delivery. NICHD Maternal Fetal Medicine Units Network. N Engl J Med 1996;334: 567–72. (Level II-2)

33. Lockwood CJ, Senyei AE, Dische MR, Casal D, Shah KD, Thung SN, et al. Fetal fibronectin in cervical and vaginal secretions as a predictor of preterm delivery. N Engl J Med 1991;325:669–74. (Level II-2)

34. Lockwood CJ, Wein R, Lapinski R, Casal D, Berkowitz G, Alvarez M, et al. The presence of cervical and vaginal fetal fibronectin predicts preterm delivery in an inner-city obstetric population. Am J Obstet Gynecol 1993;169: 798–804. (Level II-2)

35. Goldenberg RL, Thom E, Moawad AH, Johnson F, Roberts J, Caritis SN. The preterm prediction study: fetal fibronectin, bacterial vaginosis, and peripartum infection. NICHD Maternal Fetal Medicine Units Network. Obstet Gynecol 1996;87:656–60. (Level III)

36. Sonek JD, Iams JD, Blumenfeld M, Johnson F, Landon M, Gabbe S. Measurement of cervical length in pregnancy: comparison between vaginal ultrasonography and digital examination. Obstet Gynecol 1990;76:172–5. (Level II-2)

37. Iams JD, Newman RB, Thom EA, Goldenberg RL, Mueller-Heubach E, Moawad A, et al. Frequency of uterine contractions and the risk of spontaneous preterm delivery. N Engl J Med 2002;346:250–5. (Level II-1)

38. Assessment of risk factors for preterm birth. ACOG Practice Bulletin No. 31. American College of Obstetricians and Gynecologists. Obstet Gynecol 2001;98: 709–16. (Level III)

39. Larsen JF, Eldon K, Lange AP, Leegaard M, Osler M, Olsen JS, et al. Ritodrine in the treatment of preterm labor: second Danish Multicenter Study. Obstet Gynecol 1986;67:607–13. (Level I)

40. Holleboom CA, Merkus JM, van Elferen LW, Keirse MJ. Double-blind evaluation of ritodrine sustained release for oral maintenance of tocolysis after active preterm labour. Br J Obstet Gynaecol 1996;103:702–5. (Level I)

41. Guinn DA, Goepfert AR, Owen J, Brumfield C, Hauth JC. Management options in women with preterm uterine contractions: a randomized clinical trial. Am J Obstet Gynecol 1997;177:814–8. (Level I)

42. Merkatz IR, Peter JB, Barden TP. Ritodrine hydrochloride: a betamimetic agent for use in preterm labor. II. Evidence of efficacy. Obstet Gynecol 1980;56:7–12. (Level I)

43. Leveno KJ, Klein VR, Guzick DS, Young DC, Hankins GD, Williams ML. Single-centre randomised trial of ritodrine hydrochloride for preterm labour. Lancet 1986;1: 1293–6. (Level I)

44. Gyetvai K, Hannah ME, Hodnett ED, Ohlsson A. Tocolytics for preterm labor: a systematic review. Obstet Gynecol 1999;94:869–77. (Meta-analysis)

45. Jannet D, Abankwa A, Guyard B, Carbonne B, Marpeau L, Milliez J. Nicardipine versus salbutamol in the treatment of premature labor. A prospective randomized study. Eur J Obstet Gynecol Reprod Biol 1997;73:11–6. (Level I)

46. Koks CA, Brolmann HA, de Kleine MJ, Manger PA. A randomized comparison of nifedipine and ritodrine for suppression of preterm labor. Eur J Obstet Gynecol Reprod Biol 1998;77:171–6. (Level I)

47. Papatsonis DN, Van Geijn HP, Ader HJ, Lange FM, Bleker OD, Dekker GA. Nifedipine and ritodrine in the management of preterm labor: a randomized multicenter trial. Obstet Gynecol 1997;90:230–4. (Level I)

48. Eronen M, Pesonen E, Kurki T, Ylikorkala O, Hallman M. The effects of indomethacin and a beta-sympathomimetic agent on the fetal ductus arteriosus during treatment of premature labor: a randomized double-blind study. Am J Obstet Gynecol 1991;164:141–6. (Level I)

49. Bracero LA, Leikin E, Kirshenbaum N, Tejani N. Comparison of nifedipine and ritodrine for the treatment of preterm labor. Am J Perinatol 1991;8:365–9. (Level I)

50. Kurki T, Eronen M, Lumme R, Ylikorkala O. A randomized double-dummy comparison between indomethacin and nylidrin in threatened preterm labor. Obstet Gynecol 1991;78:1093–7. (Level I)

51. Caritis SN, Carson D, Greebon D, McCormick M, Edelstone DI, Mueller-Heubach E. A comparison of terbutaline and ethanol in the treatment of preterm labor. Am J Obstet Gynecol 1982;142:183–90. (Level I)

52. Meyer WR, Randall HW, Graves WL. Nifedipine versus ritodrine for suppressing preterm labor. J Reprod Med 1990;35:649–53. (Level I)

53. Kupferminc M, Lessing JB, Yaron Y, Peyser MR. Nifedipine versus ritodrine for suppression of preterm labour. Br J Obstet Gynaecol 1993;100:1090–4. (Level I)

54. Neldam S, Osler M. Premature rupture of the membranes and Ritodrine treatment. Acta Obstet Gynecol Scand 1983;62:135–9. (Level I-1)

55. Wilkins IA, Lynch L, Mehalek KE, Berkowitz GS, Berkowitz RL. Efficacy and side effects of magnesium sulfate and ritodrine as tocolytic agents. Am J Obstet Gynecol 1988;159:685–9. (Level I)

56. Morales WJ, Smith SG, Angel JL, O'Brien WF, Knuppel RA. Efficacy and safety of indomethacin versus ritodrine in the management of preterm labor: a randomized study. Obstet Gynecol 1989;74:567–72. (Level I)

57. Tchilinguirian NG, Najem R, Sullivan GB, Craparo FJ. The use of ritodrine and magnesium sulfate in the arrest of premature labor. Int J Gynaecol Obstet 1984;22:117–23. (Level I)

58. Garcia-Velasco JA, Gonzalez Gonzalez A. A prospective, randomized trial of nifedipine vs. ritodrine in threatened preterm labor. Int J Gynaecol Obstet 1998;61:239–44. (Level I)

59. Ben-Ami M, Giladi Y, Shalev E. The combination of magnesium sulphate and nifedipine: a cause of neuromuscular blockade. Br J Obstet Gynaecol 1994;101:262–3. (Level III)

60. Hatjis CG, Swain M, Nelson LH, Meis PJ, Ernest JM. Efficacy of combined administration of magnesium sulfate and ritodrine in the treatment of premature labor. Obstet Gynecol 1987;69:317–22. (Level I)

61. Goldenberg RL. The management of preterm labor. Obstet Gynecol 2002:100:1020–37. (Level III)

62. Scrag S, Gorwitz R, Fultz-Butts K, Schuchat A. Prevention of perinatal group B streptococcal disease. Revised guidelines for CDC. MMWR Recomm Rep 2002;51(RR–11):1–22. (Level III)

63. Main DM, Gabbe SG, Richardson D, Strong S. Can preterm deliveries be prevented? Am J Obstet Gynecol 1985;151:892–8. (Level I)

64. Dyson DC, Crites YM, Ray DA, Armstrong MA. Prevention of preterm birth in high-risk patients: the role of education and provider contact versus home uterine monitoring. Am J Obstet Gynecol 1991;164:756–62. (Level I)

65. Iams JD. Preterm birth. In: Gabbe SG, Niebyl JR, Simpson JL, eds. Obstetrics: normal and problem pregnancies. 4th ed. New York (NY): Churchill Livingstone; 2002. p. 755–826. (Level III)

66. Luke B, Mamelle N, Keith L, Munoz F, Minogue J, Papiernik E, et al. The association between occupational factors and preterm birth: a United States nurses' study. Research Committee of the Association of Women's Health, Obstetric, and Neonatal Nurses. Am J Obstet Gynecol 1995;173:849–62. (Level II-2)

67. Crowther CA, Hiller JE, Doyle LW. Magnesium sulphate for preventing preterm birth in threatened preterm labour (Cochrane Review). In: The Cochrane Library, Issue 4, 2002. Oxford: Update Software. (Level I)

68. Katz M, Robertson PA, Creasy RK. Cardiovascular complications associated with terbutaline treatment for preterm labor. Am J Obstet Gynecol 1981;139:605–8. (Level II-3)

69. Guinn DA, Goepfert AR, Owen J, Wenstrom KD, Hauth JC. Terbutaline pump maintenance therapy for prevention of preterm delivery: a double-blind trial. Am J Obstet Gynecol 1998;179:874–8. (Level I)

70. Lam F, Gill P, Smith M, Kitzmiller JL, Katz M. Use of the subcutaneous terbutaline pump for long-term tocolysis. Obstet Gynecol 1988;72:810–3. (Level I)

71. Antenatal corticosteroids revisited: repeat courses. NIH Consensus Statement 2000;17(2):1–10. (Level III)

72. Treatment of preterm labor with the beta-adrenergic agonist ritodrine. The Canadian Preterm Labor Investigators Group. N Engl J Med 1992;327:308–12. (Level I)

73. Greig PC, Ernest JM, Teot L. Low amniotic fluid glucose levels are a specific but not sensitive marker for subclinical intrauterine infections in patients in preterm labor with intact membranes. Am J Obstet Gynecol 1994;171:365–71. (Level II-3)

74. Hussey MJ, Levy ES, Pombar X, Meyer P, Strassner HT. Evaluating rapid diagnositic tests of intra-amniotic infection: Gram stain, amniotic fluid glucose level, and amniotic fluid to serum glucose level ratio. Am J Obstet Gynecol 1998;179:650–6. (Level II-2)

The MEDLINE database, the Cochrane Library, and ACOG's own internal resources and documents were used to conduct a literature search to locate relevant articles published between January 1985 and January 2003. The search was restricted to articles published in the English language. Priority was given to articles reporting results of original research, although review articles and commentaries also were consulted. Abstracts of research presented at symposia and scientific conferences were not considered adequate for inclusion in this document. Guidelines published by organizations or institutions such as the National Institutes of Health and the American College of Obstetricians and Gynecologists were reviewed, and additional studies were located by reviewing bibliographies of identified articles. When reliable research was not available, expert opinions from obstetrician–gynecologists were used.

Studies were reviewed and evaluated for quality according to the method outlined by the U.S. Preventive Services Task Force:

I Evidence obtained from at least one properly designed randomized controlled trial.

II-1 Evidence obtained from well-designed controlled trials without randomization.

II-2 Evidence obtained from well-designed cohort or case–control analytic studies, preferably from more than one center or research group.

II-3 Evidence obtained from multiple time series with or without the intervention. Dramatic results in uncontrolled experiments also could be regarded as this type of evidence.

III Opinions of respected authorities, based on clinical experience, descriptive studies, or reports of expert committees.

Based on the highest level of evidence found in the data, recommendations are provided and graded according to the following categories:

Level A—Recommendations are based on good and consistent scientific evidence.

Level B—Recommendations are based on limited or inconsistent scientific evidence.

Level C—Recommendations are based primarily on consensus and expert opinion.

ISSN 1099-3630

**The American College of
Obstetricians and Gynecologists
409 12th Street, SW
PO Box 96920
Washington, DC 20090-6920**

12345/76543

Management of preterm labor. ACOG Practice Bulletin No. 43. American College of Obstetricians and Gynecologists. Obstet Gynecol 2003;101:1039–47.

ACOG PRACTICE BULLETIN

CLINICAL MANAGEMENT GUIDELINES FOR
OBSTETRICIAN–GYNECOLOGISTS

NUMBER 24, FEBRUARY 2001

(Replaces Technical Bulletin Number 212, September 1995)

This Practice Bulletin was developed by the ACOG Committee on Practice Bulletins—Obstetrics with the assistance of Sandra A. Carson, MD, and D. Ware Branch, MD. The information is designed to aid practitioners in making decisions about appropriate obstetric and gynecologic care. These guidelines should not be construed as dictating an exclusive course of treatment or procedure. Variations in practice may be warranted based on the needs of the individual patient, resources, and limitations unique to the institution or type of practice.

Management of Recurrent Early Pregnancy Loss

Recurrent pregnancy loss is a common clinical problem in reproduction, occurring in approximately 1% of reproductive-aged women (1). A definite cause is established in no more than 50% of couples, and several alleged causes of recurrent pregnancy loss are controversial. Moreover, in the field of recurrent pregnancy loss, inappropriate emphasis often is given to unproven hypotheses and poorly designed clinical studies. Seeking a solution, some patients and physicians explore less-well-accepted etiologies and empirical or alternative treatments. This bulletin will provide the practitioner with a rational, modern approach to the management of recurrent pregnancy loss. New and controversial etiologies will be presented so that the practitioner can discuss them with couples who have a history of recurrent pregnancy loss.

Background

Broadly defined, pregnancy loss includes any type of loss of the conceptus from fertilized ovum to neonate. This bulletin covers the repetitive loss of recognized pregnancies in the first or early second trimester (<15 weeks of gestation). It usually is referred to as recurrent spontaneous abortion, miscarriage, or recurrent early pregnancy loss.

Recurrent abortion must be distinguished from sporadic spontaneous abortions that are nonconsecutive pregnancy losses occurring randomly during a woman's reproductive years. Sporadic pregnancy loss occurs in 10–15% of all clinically recognized pregnancies as first- or early second-trimester spontaneous abortions. Most of these pregnancy losses are clinically evident by the 12th week of gestation and are preembryonic or embryonic losses in which the demise of the conceptus precedes clinical features of pregnancy loss by one or more weeks.

Recurrent pregnancy loss typically is defined as two or three or more consecutive pregnancy losses. Most women with recurrent pregnancy loss have recurrent preembryonic or embryonic losses. Recurrent fetal loss is less common, and recurrent fetal loss at or beyond 14 weeks of gestation is infrequent.

Causes of Recurrent Pregnancy Loss

Genetic Abnormalities

Parental Structural Chromosome Abnormalities

In approximately 2–4% of couples with recurrent pregnancy loss, one partner will have a genetically balanced structural chromosome rearrangement. Balanced translocations account for the largest percentage of these karyotypic abnormalities. They can cause pregnancy loss because segregation during meiosis results in gametes with duplication or deficiency of chromosome segments. Other genetically balanced structural chromosome abnormalities, such as chromosome inversions, account for a small percentage of abnormal parental karyotypes among couples with recurrent pregnancy loss.

Molecular Genetic Abnormalities

In the past decade, the development of techniques for DNA analysis has resulted in identification of molecular genetic abnormalities as causes of various human diseases. One report indicated that highly skewed X-chromosome inactivation is associated with otherwise unexplained recurrent pregnancy loss (2). As yet, however, commercially available tests for this and other related molecular genetic abnormalities are not widely available.

Recurrent Preembryonic or Embryonic Aneuploidy

Analyses of karyotypes in consecutive abortions suggest that recurrent aneuploidy in the conceptus may be a cause of recurrent pregnancy loss. In one analysis of data, the karyotype of a second successive spontaneous abortion was abnormal in nearly 70% of cases when aneuploidy was found in the first abortus, but in only 20% of cases where the first abortus was chromosomally normal (3). However, these aneuploid losses may have been a result of the older age of the mothers, rather than a nonrandom event in predisposed couples (4). More recently, two groups of investigators using different techniques of analysis have shown that the next abortion in women with recurrent pregnancy loss was chromosomally abnor-

mal in 48% or more of cases (5, 6), raising the possibility of recurrent aneuploidy despite normal parental karyotypes. Supportive evidence comes from studies of preimplantation genetic studies of women with recurrent pregnancy loss in which more than 50% of embryos were found to have aneuploidy (7, 8).

Hormonal and Metabolic Disorders

Luteal Phase Defect

The luteal phase defect (LPD) has long been thought to be a cause of spontaneous abortion, but the evidence linking LPD to recurrent abortion is subject to criticism. Investigators initially hypothesized that with LPD, the corpus luteum failed to make enough progesterone to establish a mature endometrial lining suitable for placentation. This theory has evolved to implicate poor follicular-phase oocyte development, which results in disordered estrogen secretion and subsequent dysfunction of either the corpus luteum or progesterone effect. In turn, these effects could result from excess luteinizing hormone or hyperandrogenic states. Some investigators believe that LPD is a common cause of recurrent pregnancy loss, accounting for approximately 25–40% of cases. However, studies of this disorder have not included concurrently tested controls, a serious oversight given that normal women have endometrial histology suggestive of LPD in up to 50% of single menstrual cycles and 25% of sequential cycles (9). Thus, the association between LPD and recurrent pregnancy loss remains speculative.

Polycystic Ovary Syndrome

Investigators have found that 36–56% of women with recurrent pregnancy loss have polycystic ovary syndrome (PCOS) diagnosed by ultrasound examination of the ovaries (10–12). One group (11) demonstrated that more than half of women with ultrasonographic evidence of PCOS also had hypersecretion of luteinizing hormone. But ultrasonographic evidence of PCOS in women with recurrent pregnancy loss does not predict worse pregnancy outcome than in women with recurrent pregnancy loss without PCOS (10, 12, 13). However, it has been reported that women with PCOS who miscarry have higher levels of circulating androgens (10). There is no known therapy for reducing the risk of pregnancy loss in women with PCOS.

Other Metabolic Abnormalities

Maternal endocrinologic and metabolic disorders have been implicated as a cause of recurrent pregnancy loss. Women with poorly controlled type 1 (insulin-dependent) diabetes mellitus have an increased rate of abortion (14). However, there is no evidence that asymptomatic endocrinologic or metabolic disorders, such as mild thyroid disease or glucose intolerance, cause recurrent pregnancy loss.

Uterine Anatomic Abnormalities

Congenital uterine abnormalities have been associated most often with second-trimester pregnancy loss. However, 10–15% of women with recurrent early pregnancy loss have congenital uterine abnormalities. The most common malformations associated with pregnancy loss are variations of the double uterus (bicornuate, septate, or didelphic), with septate uterus predominating. The contribution of arcuate uterus to recurrent pregnancy loss is debated. A recent study using three-dimensional ultrasonography and hysteroscopy found that 15% of 61 women with recurrent pregnancy loss had an arcuate uterus, compared with only 3% of more than 1,000 women attending a gynecology clinic (15, 16). Other investigators doubt an association between an arcuate uterus and recurrent pregnancy loss (17, 18). Severe uterine synechiae (Asherman's syndrome) and uterine abnormalities associated with in utero exposure to diethylstilbestrol also may be associated with pregnancy loss. An association between submucosal leiomyoma and recurrent pregnancy loss is controversial.

Some investigators believe that poor vascularization of the uterine septum is a cause of spontaneous abortion, but studies provide mixed results. In one study of 12 pregnancies, all four successful pregnancies became implanted away from the uterine septum (19). However, the vascular density in uterine septa removed at the time of metroplasty is similar to that of the normal uterine wall (20).

Infectious Causes

Certain infectious agents, such as *Listeria monocytogenes,* are known to cause sporadic pregnancy loss, but no infectious agent has been proven to cause recurrent pregnancy loss. In addition, *Toxoplasma gondii* and some viruses (eg, rubella, herpes simplex, and measles viruses; cytomegalovirus; and coxsackieviruses) have been linked to sporadic abortion. However, none has been convincingly associated with recurrent pregnancy loss.

Environmental Factors, Occupational Factors, and Personal Habits

Although a common concern of patients, environmental factors rarely have been linked to sporadic pregnancy loss, and no associations between environmental factors and recurrent pregnancy loss have been established. Likewise, occupational exposures to certain products,

such as certain organic solvents, rarely have been linked to sporadic pregnancy loss (21). However, no associations between occupational exposure or working itself and recurrent pregnancy loss have been established.

Study results are conflicting on the association of smoking, use of alcohol, and use of caffeine with sporadic pregnancy loss. They may act in a dose-dependent fashion or synergistically to increase the rate of sporadic pregnancy loss. However, none of these habits has been associated with recurrent pregnancy loss. Exercise does not appear to increase the rate of sporadic pregnancy loss, particularly in women in good physical condition, and there are no studies of exercise effects in women with recurrent pregnancy loss.

Thrombophilia

The most common inherited thrombophilic disorders are factor V Leiden and prothrombin G20210A mutation, found in approximately 8% and 3%, respectively, of Caucasian women in the United States. These mutations are associated with approximately 25% of isolated thrombotic events and approximately 50% of familial thrombosis. Other less common thrombophilias include deficiencies of the anticoagulants protein C, protein S, and antithrombin III. Some investigators have (22–25), and some have not (13, 26–29), found that one or more of these thrombophilic mutations are associated with recurrent pregnancy loss. In two studies (22, 30), however, these heritable thrombophilias were associated with second- or third-trimester fetal loss, not with first-trimester loss. Also, one group has found that next pregnancy outcomes among women with recurrent pregnancy losses are no different with or without factor V Leiden (13).

Despite the recent interest in this field, no treatment trials have been performed. Thus, which therapy, if any, is effective in promoting successful pregnancy among women with recurrent pregnancy loss and thrombophilia is uncertain.

Autoimmune Disorders
Antiphospholipid Antibodies

Antiphospholipid syndrome (APS) is an autoimmune disorder characterized by the presence of significant levels of antiphospholipid antibodies and one or more clinical features, among which are recurrent pregnancy loss, fetal death, and thrombosis (31). Antiphospholipid syndrome may occur as a primary condition in women with no other recognizable autoimmune disease, or as a secondary condition in patients with underlying autoimmune disease (eg, systemic lupus erythematosus). The diagnosis of APS is made by demonstrating lupus anticoagulant, anticardiolipin antibodies, or both.

Some investigators have found that a small percentage of women with recurrent pregnancy loss who test negative for anticardiolipin antibodies have antibodies to other phospholipids, such as phosphatidylserine or phosphatidylethanolamine (32). Others have found that no such relationship exists (33) or that testing for antibodies other than lupus anticoagulant and anticardiolipin antibodies does not increase the rate of diagnosis of APS (34). In addition, assays for phospholipid-binding antibodies other than anticardiolipin are not standardized. Finally, there is no proven treatment for women with recurrent pregnancy loss and phospholipid-binding antibodies other than lupus anticoagulant and anticardiolipin antibodies.

Thyroid Antibodies

Autoantibodies to thyroid antigens (thyroglobulin and thyroid peroxidase) are associated with an increased rate of pregnancy loss if identified in early pregnancy or immediately before pregnancy (35, 36). However, current evidence does not allow a definite conclusion regarding the association of antithyroid antibodies and recurrent pregnancy loss, and no treatment options have been proven beneficial.

Antinuclear Antibodies

A significant percentage (approximately 15%) of women with recurrent pregnancy loss have detectable antinuclear antibodies (ANA) (37, 38). Without treatment, subsequent pregnancy outcomes among women with a positive ANA test result are similar to those among women with a negative ANA test result. More important, a randomized treatment trial of women with recurrent pregnancy loss and a positive autoantibody result, including ANA, found no difference in pregnancy outcomes between women treated with prednisone and low-dose aspirin and women treated with placebo (39). Thus, currently available data do not support testing women with recurrent pregnancy loss for ANA.

Alloimmune Disorders

Alloimmune traits—immunologic differences between individuals—have been proposed as factors between reproductive partners that cause otherwise unexplained recurrent pregnancy loss. The tendency for 1) partners with recurrent loss to share human leukocyte antigens, 2) the female partner to fail to produce serum "blocking factor," and 3) the female partner to produce antileukocytotoxic antibodies against paternal leukocytes have been described. Others have refuted the significance of each of these factors. In addition, no test for these traits provides results that predict the next pregnancy outcome in patients treated or untreated for recurrent pregnancy loss (40, 41). More recently, some researchers have claimed that flow cytometric assays for maternal antibodies to paternal leukocytes are useful in evaluating couples with recurrent pregnancy loss. However, studies of these assays have lacked appropriate controls and are of unproven value in terms of indicating an efficacious treatment.

More recent investigations of the maternal–fetal immunologic relationship suggest that pregnancy losses may result from dysregulation of normal immune mechanisms, probably operating at the maternal–fetal interface. It has been proposed that a predominance of Th-2 lymphocytic cytokines is crucial for successful pregnancy and that Th-1 lymphocytic cytokines, such as interferon-γ and tumor necrosis factor-α, adversely affect embryo and trophoblast viability (42–44). The presence of natural killer (NK)-like cells secreting a transforming growth factor at the maternal–fetal interface may be necessary for successful pregnancy (45). Clinical studies have found decreased (45, 46) or increased (47) numbers of these cells in the luteal phase endometria of women with recurrent pregnancy loss. Pregnancy outcomes may be worse in women with recurrent pregnancy loss found to have increased numbers of NK-like cells in the luteal phase endometria (48), but further studies are necessary before valid conclusions can be drawn. One group has found that an embryotoxic factor, similar to interferon-γ, generated by patient leukocytes in vitro predicted pregnancy failure in the next pregnancy attempt (44), but others have not been able to reproduce these findings (49). Others have found that an increased percentage of circulating NK cells in women with recurrent pregnancy loss predicts a relatively poor next pregnancy outcome (50, 51). There is, however, no proven treatment for women with recurrent pregnancy loss found to have increased percentages of circulating NK cells.

Unexplained Recurrent Pregnancy Loss

In 50% or more of couples with recurrent pregnancy loss, an evaluation, including parental karyotypes, hysterosalpingography or hysteroscopy, and antiphospholipid antibody testing will be negative. Therefore, a majority (approximately 50–75%) of couples with recurrent pregnancy loss will have no certain diagnosis. Informative and sympathetic counseling appears to serve an important role in this situation. Live birth rates between 35% and 85% are commonly reported in couples with unexplained recurrent pregnancy loss who undertake an untreated or placebo-treated subsequent pregnancy (12, 52–55). Meta-analysis of randomized, prospective studies suggests that 60–70% of women with unexplained recurrent pregnancy loss will have a successful next pregnancy (56), figures that many couples will view as optimistic.

Clinical Considerations and Recommendations

▶ *When is a diagnosis of recurrent pregnancy loss appropriate?*

Traditionally, recurrent pregnancy loss has been defined as three consecutive spontaneous abortions. However, the risk of abortion after two successive abortions (30%) is clinically similar to the risk of recurrence among women with three or more consecutive abortions (33%) (37, 57–66). Thus, patients with two or more consecutive spontaneous abortions are candidates for an evaluation to determine the etiology, if any, for their pregnancy losses.

The number of previous pregnancy losses influences the likelihood of successful pregnancy. One study reported recurrent pregnancy loss rates of 29%, 27%, 44%, and 53% after 3, 4, 5, and 6 or more recurrent pregnancy losses, respectively (67). In addition, maternal age influences the recurrent pregnancy loss rate (67, 68), with a recurrent pregnancy loss rate of approximately 25% in women aged 30 years or younger and a recurrent pregnancy loss rate of 50–60% in those 40 years or older. Some investigators have found the prognosis for a successful pregnancy is increased by 10–20% in women with at least one previous live birth (58, 69), but others did not (67).

▶ *Should all couples with recurrent pregnancy loss have chromosomal analysis performed?*

Parents with recurrent pregnancy loss should be analyzed for balanced chromosome abnormalities because: 1) couples would like to know why they are experiencing repetitive pregnancy loss; 2) a couple in which one partner carries a balanced chromosome abnormality is at increased risk for having a fetus with an unbalanced chromosome abnormality and may benefit from prenatal genetic testing; and 3) the apparently normal offspring of a couple in which one partner carries a balanced chromosome abnormality is at risk for carrying the same balanced chromosome abnormality and, thus, is at risk for reproductive complications.

Balanced chromosome abnormalities occurring in one partner are relatively infrequent among couples with only recurrent pregnancy loss but no other adverse perinatal outcomes (eg, stillborns, anomalous infants). One study reported that of couples with recurrent loss, only 2.4% of female partners and 1.6% of male partners with a history of stillbirths or anomalous infants had a balanced chromosome abnormality, compared with 4.6% of female partners and 1.7% of male partners with a history of adverse perinatal outcomes (70). However, no historic factor unequivocally allows the clinician to determine which couples may benefit from karyotype analyses. In addition, phenotypically normal offspring do not exclude the possibility of a balanced chromosome abnormality in a couple with recurrent pregnancy loss.

Parental cytogenetic analysis should be offered to all couples with recurrent pregnancy loss. In addition, all couples in which one partner has been found to have a balanced translocation or inversion should be offered prenatal genetic diagnosis because of the increased risk of a karyotypic abnormality in the conceptus.

In addition, many experts obtain a karyotype of the abortus tissue when a couple with recurrent pregnancy loss experiences a subsequent spontaneous abortion. The rationale is that if the abortus is aneuploid, the physician and patient may conclude that a maternal cause of pregnancy loss is excluded. Also, an abnormal abortus karyotype is a legitimate explanation for the loss that may provide a source of comfort to the couple. However, no published evidence supports these hypotheses, and definite recommendations for routinely obtaining abortus karyotypes cannot be made.

▶ *How should the uterine cavity be evaluated in a woman with recurrent pregnancy loss, and how should abnormal findings be treated?*

Uterine anatomic abnormalities are diagnosed by hysterosalpingography, hysteroscopy, or sonohysteroscopy. Three-dimensional ultrasonography, although not routinely available in the United States, also has been shown to be useful in the diagnosis of uterine abnormalities. Suspicious or confusing cases can be evaluated further by magnetic resonance imaging. However, the relationship between uterine abnormalities and recurrent pregnancy loss is uncertain, and some authorities do not recommend routinely evaluating the uterine cavity by hysterosalpingography, hysteroscopy, or sonohysteroscopy (71).

No prospective, controlled trials have proved that the correction of uterine anatomic abnormalities benefits the next pregnancy outcome. Retrospectively analyzed case series suggest that 70–85% of women with recurrent pregnancy loss with bicornuate and septate uteri who undergo surgical correction will deliver viable live born infants in their next pregnancies (72), but these seemingly excellent results are subject to criticism because of the methods of patient selection and the lack of controls.

Hysteroscopic resection has been used successfully for treatment of the uterine septum, and subsequent pregnancy results are comparable to those for metroplasty (72). It is preferable to abdominal surgery because it is an outpatient procedure with low morbidity and allows for labor with expected vaginal delivery. Uterine synechiae also may be treated hysteroscopically.

▶ *Should women with recurrent pregnancy loss be evaluated for luteal phase defect?*

Although assessment of luteal phase progesterone production or effect is firmly entrenched in the traditional evaluation of women with recurrent pregnancy loss, the evidence supporting this practice is scant. The endometrium is considered out of phase when the histologic dating lags behind the menstrual dating by 2 days or more. However, interobserver variation in the interpretation of the biopsies is considerable (73), and modest intraobserver variation occurs (74). Because of 1) such variation, 2) the frequent finding of out-of-phase endometrial histology in normal women, and 3) the inconsistent expression of luteal phase defect in affected women, luteal phase defect is diagnosed only when two consecutive biopsies are out of phase. The measurement of luteal phase progesterone concentrations is not an adequate method for diagnosing or excluding luteal phase defect.

No properly designed studies have evaluated the role of progesterone treatment in women with recurrent pregnancy loss with luteal phase defect. Two meta-analyses of studies from the 1950s and 1960s reached conflicting conclusions regarding the efficacy of progesterone treatment in variously selected women with recurrent abortion (75, 76). The studies included in these meta-analyses are difficult to interpret because they 1) did not assess patients for luteal phase defect using currently accepted criteria, 2) employed 17-OH progesterone caproate or medroxyprogesterone as treatment, 3) used various inclusion criteria, and 4) entered patients after pregnancy had progressed to at least 8 weeks of gestation. Also, these studies totaled only 130 patients, and one of them (77) was not randomized. In addition, in a more recent randomized trial, a subgroup of women with PCOS and three or more miscarriages were randomized to treatment with either progesterone or placebo pessaries (78). There was no difference in the pregnancy outcomes.

Human chorionic gonadotropin has been used in an attempt to stimulate the corpus luteum support of pregnancy in women with recurrent abortion. One international multicentered trial randomized 75 women to receive either placebo or 10,000 IU of human chorionic gonadotropin at the first diagnosis of pregnancy and 5,000 IU weekly thereafter (79). No significant difference in the successful pregnancy rates (83% versus 79%) between the groups was found.

In summary, the relationship between the luteal phase defect and recurrent pregnancy loss remains a subject of controversy. It has not been shown conclusively that progesterone treatment or corpus luteum support influences pregnancy outcome in women with recurrent pregnancy loss.

▶ *Should thyroid tests and tests for glucose intolerance be performed in women with recurrent pregnancy loss?*

An association between recurrent pregnancy loss and asymptomatic endocrinologic or metabolic disorders such as mild thyroid disease or glucose intolerance has not been established. Thus, tests for thyroid dysfunction or glucose intolerance are not required in the evaluation of otherwise normal women with recurrent pregnancy loss.

An association between antithyroid antibodies and recurrent pregnancy loss has been reported by some investigators (31, 80–83). Very few patients identified in these studies are clinically hypothyroid, and less than 20% have abnormal thyroid-stimulating hormone test results (80). In addition, no treatments have proved to benefit next pregnancy outcome in women found to have antithyroid antibodies. Thus, tests for antithyroid antibodies are not required in the evaluation of women with recurrent pregnancy loss.

▶ *Should women with recurrent pregnancy loss be evaluated for possible infectious causes, and should they be treated?*

Endocervical *Chlamydia* and *Mycoplasma* have been implicated as causes of recurrent pregnancy loss, but study results are conflicting. Bacterial vaginosis may be associated with midtrimester pregnancy loss (84, 85), and one study found an increased rate of pregnancy loss in women with bacterial vaginosis undergoing in vitro fertilization (86). However, there is no direct evidence (confirmed by cultures) of *Chlamydia*, *Mycoplasma*, and organisms causing bacterial vaginosis in systematically analyzed recurrent abortus specimens. These infectious agents are very common. *Mycoplasma* may be recovered from the endocervix of one third of sexually active adults. One group of investigators found that women with recurrent pregnancy loss have a significantly higher rate of endometrial colonization with *Ureaplasma urealyticum* compared with controls, raising the speculation that endometrial (but not endocervical) colonization with

Mycoplasma may play a role in recurrent pregnancy loss. Existing nonrandomized studies of the effects of antibiotic treatment on subsequent pregnancy outcome in women with endocervical *Mycoplasma* colonization have yielded conflicting results.

Currently, routine serologic or endocervical cultures for *Chlamydia* or *Mycoplasma* and vaginal evaluation for bacterial vaginosis are not useful in evaluating otherwise healthy women presenting with recurrent abortion. In addition, empiric treatment with antibiotics in the absence of documented infection is not warranted.

▶ *Should women with recurrent pregnancy loss be evaluated for antiphospholipid syndrome?*

Antiphospholipid syndrome is associated with pregnancy loss in 3–15% of women with recurrent pregnancy loss (33, 87–90). Some investigators have emphasized the relationship between APS and second- or early third-trimester fetal death (91), whereas others have found that a small percentage of women with recurrent first-trimester pregnancy loss have antiphospholipid antibodies (90). Women with a previous fetal death (33, 92) and high levels of anticardiolipin immunoglobulin G (IgG) antibodies (92) are at the greatest risk of fetal loss in subsequent pregnancies. Therefore, women with recurrent pregnancy loss should be tested for antiphospholipid syndrome using standard assays for anticardiolipin antibodies and lupus anticoagulant.

Antiphospholipid syndrome is identified in a woman with recurrent pregnancy loss by the detection of lupus anticoagulant, β_2-glycoprotein I–dependent anticardiolipin antibodies, or both on two occasions at least 6 weeks apart (31). The IgG isotype of anticardiolipin is most relevant clinically, but tests repeatedly positive for IgM anticardiolipin may be used to make the diagnosis. In individuals demonstrating only anticardiolipin antibodies, definite APS is diagnosed when the antibody levels are repeatedly 20 units or greater. Repeatedly positive test results for anticardiolipin antibodies with levels of less than 20 units are of uncertain significance.

Women with APS benefit from treatment with heparin and low-dose aspirin during pregnancy. Two studies have shown that women with recurrent early pregnancy loss and positive test results for antiphospholipid antibodies benefit from treatment with low-dose aspirin and heparin. Successful pregnancy rates for these women are 70–75%, compared with less than 50% for the untreated patients (93, 94). These studies used heparin dosages in the range of 10,000–25,000 U/d, and neither study included women with a history of thrombosis or systemic lupus erythematosus.

▶ *Should women with recurrent pregnancy loss be evaluated for thrombophilias?*

The role of thrombophilia in recurrent pregnancy loss is a controversial subject of current research interest. Tests for factor V Leiden, the prothrombin G20210A mutation, or deficiencies of protein C, protein S, or antithrombin III should be considered in cases of otherwise unexplained fetal death in the second or third trimesters. However, the role of these heritable thrombophilias in recurrent early pregnancy loss is uncertain at present, and tests for these thrombophilias are not required as part of the evaluation. Whether antithrombotic treatment improves subsequent pregnancy outcomes in women with evidence of thrombophilia is uncertain.

▶ *Should women with recurrent pregnancy loss be evaluated for possible alloimmune causes?*

Results of tests for human leukocyte antigen types, maternal serum blocking factors, or maternal antileukocytic antibodies directed against the male partner's leukocytes have not been shown to predict subsequent pregnancy outcome. Therefore, testing is not recommended, and treatment is not warranted. Luteal phase biopsy to determine the status of NK-like cells is not recommended because of mixed results in the literature, the uncertainty of prognostic implications, and the lack of an effective treatment. Finally, in the absence of a proven effective treatment, tests for embryotoxic factor or determination of the percentage of circulating NK cells in women with recurrent pregnancy loss is not beneficial.

▶ *Is paternal lymphocyte immunization or intravenous immune globulin (IVIG) an effective treatment for recurrent pregnancy loss?*

The most widely used immunotherapeutic treatment regimen for women with unexplained recurrent loss involves immunizing the female partner with the male partner's leukocytes. Of several randomized, prospective studies (53, 54, 95), only one found a benefit to leukocyte immunization (96). The largest trial, and the only multicenter effort, found that women undergoing leukocyte immunization actually had a higher rate of pregnancy loss than placebo controls (55), suggesting that the treatment may be harmful. In addition, there is no consensus regarding patient selection or the dose, route, or timing of leukocyte immunization, and immunization using viable leukocytes carries risks similar to those of blood transfusion, including the transmission of viral diseases.

The second immunomodulatory therapy used as a treatment for recurrent pregnancy loss is IVIG (97). Initial interest in this therapy derives from the observation that IVIG contains antibodies that block antibody-mediated immune damage (98). Other known immunomodulating effects of IVIG include T cell receptor blockade, inhibition of NK-cell activity, inhibition of Th-1 cytokine secretion, Fc receptor blockade, complement inactivation, down-regulation of B cell responsiveness, and enhanced T cell suppressor cell function (99). However, only one of five randomized trials using IVIG treatment in women with recurrent pregnancy loss demonstrated a benefit (52); results of the others were negative (100–103). In addition, the results of two meta-analyses also were negative (104, 105).

Summary

The following recommendations are based on good and consistent scientific evidence (Level A):

▶ Women with recurrent pregnancy loss should be tested for lupus anticoagulant and anticardiolipin antibodies using standard assays. If test results are positive for the same antibody on two consecutive occasions 6–8 weeks apart, the patient should be treated with heparin and low-dose aspirin during her next pregnancy attempt.

▶ Mononuclear cell (leukocyte) immunization and IVIG are not effective in preventing recurrent pregnancy loss.

The following recommendations are based on limited or inconsistent scientific evidence (Level B):

▶ An association between the luteal phase defect and recurrent pregnancy loss is controversial. If a diagnosis of luteal phase defect is sought in a woman with recurrent pregnancy loss, it should be confirmed by endometrial biopsy.

▶ Luteal phase support with progesterone is of unproven efficacy.

The following recommendations are based primarily on consensus and expert opinion (Level C):

▶ Couples with recurrent pregnancy loss should be tested for parental balanced chromosome abnormalities.

▶ Women with recurrent pregnancy loss and a uterine septum should undergo hysteroscopic evaluation and resection.

▶ Cultures for bacteria or viruses and tests for glucose intolerance, thyroid abnormalities, antibodies to infectious agents, antinuclear antibodies, antithyroid antibodies, paternal human leukocyte antigen status, or maternal antipaternal antibodies are not beneficial and, therefore, are not recommended in the evaluation of otherwise normal women with recurrent pregnancy loss.

▶ Couples with otherwise unexplained recurrent pregnancy loss should be counseled regarding the potential for successful pregnancy without treatment.

References

1. Stirrat GM. Recurrent miscarriage. I: definition and epidemiology. Lancet 1990;336:673–675 (Level III)

2. Lanasa MC, Hogge WA, Kubic C, Blancato J, Hoffman EP. Highly skewed X-chromosome inactivation is associated with idiopathic recurrent spontaneous abortion. Am J Hum Genet 1999;65:252–254 (Level II-2)

3. Hassold TJ. A cytogenetic study of repeated spontaneous abortions. Am J Hum Genet 1980;32:723–730 (Level II-3)

4. Warburton D, Kline J, Stein Z, Hutzler M, Chin A, Hassold T. Does the karyotype of a spontaneous abortion predict the karyotype of a subsequent abortion? Evidence from 273 women with two karyotyped spontaneous abortions. Am J Hum Genet 1987;41:465–483 (Level II-3)

5. Stern JJ, Dorfmann AD, Gutierrez-Najar AJ, Cerrillo M, Coulam CB. Frequency of abnormal karyotypes among abortuses from women with and without a history of recurrent spontaneous abortion. Fertil Steril 1996;65:250–253 (Level II-2)

6. Daniely M, Aviram-Goldring A, Barkai G, Goldman B. Detection of chromosomal aberration in fetuses arising from recurrent spontaneous abortion by comparative genomic hybridization. Hum Reprod 1998;13:805–809 (Level II-3)

7. Vidal F, Gimenez C, Rubrio C, Simon C, Pellicer A, Santalo J, et al. FISH preimplantation diagnosis of chromosome aneuploidy in recurrent pregnancy wastage. J Assist Reprod Genet 1998;15:310–313 (Level III)

8. Simon C, Rubio C, Vidal F, Gimenez C, Moreno C, Parrilla JJ, et al. Increased chromosome abnormalities in human preimplantation embryos after in-vitro fertilization in patients with recurrent miscarriage. Reprod Fertil Dev 1998;10:87–92 (Level III)

9. Davis OK, Berkeley AS, Naus GJ, Cholst IN, Freedman KS. The incidence of luteal phase defect in normal, fertile women determined by serial endometrial biopsies. Fertil Steril 1989;51:582–586 (Level III)

10. Tulppala M, Stenman UH, Cacciatore B, Ylikorkala O. Polycystic ovaries and levels of gonadotropins and androgens in recurrent miscarriage: prospective study in 50 women. Br J Obstet Gynaecol 1993;100:348–352 (Level II-2)

11. Clifford K, Rai R, Watson H, Regan L. An informative protocol for the investigation of recurrent miscarriage: preliminary experience of 500 consecutive cases. Hum Reprod 1994;9:1328–1332 (Level III)

12. Liddell HS, Sowden K, Farquhar CM. Recurrent miscarriage: screening for polycystic ovaries and subsequent pregnancy outcome. Aust N Z J Obstet Gynaecol 1997;37:402–406 (Level II-2)

13. Rai R, Backos M, Rushworth F, Regan L. Polycystic ovaries and recurrent miscarriage—a reappraisal. Hum Reprod 2000:15;612–615 (Level II-2)

14. Dorman JS, Burke JP, McCarthy BJ, Norris JM, Steenkiste AR, Aarons JH, et al. Temporal trends in spontaneous abortion associated with Type 1 diabetes. Diabetes Res Clin Pract 1999;43:41–47 (Level II-3)

15. Jurkovic D, Geipel A, Gruboeck K, Jauniaux E, Natucci M, Campbell S. Three-dimensional ultrasound for the assessment of uterine anatomy and detection of congenital anomalies: a comparison with hysterosalpingography and two-dimensional sonography. Ultrasound Obstet Gynecol 1995;5:233–237 (Level II-3)

16. Jurkovic D, Gruboeck K, Tailor A, Nicolaides KH. Ultrasound screening for congenital uterine anomalies. Br J Obstet Gynaecol 1997;104:1320–1321 (Level II-3)

17. Maneschi F, Zupi E, Marconi D, Valli E, Romanini C, Mancuso S. Hysteroscopically detected asymptomatic mullerian anomalies. Prevalence and reproductive implications. J Reprod Med 1995;40:684–688 (Level II-2)

18. Sorensen SS, Trauelsen AG. Obstetric implications of minor mullerian anomalies in oligomenorrheic women. Am J Obstet Gynecol 1987;156:1112–1118 (Level II-2)

19. Fedele L, Dorta M, Brioschi D, Guidici MN, Candiani GB. Pregnancies in septate uteri: outcome in relation to site of uterine implantation as determined by sonography. AJR Am J Roentgenol 1989;152:781–784 (Level III)

20. Dabirashrafi H, Bahadori M, Mohammad K, Alavi M, Moghadami-Tabrizi N, Zandinejad K, et al. Septate uterus: new idea on the histologic features of the septum in this abnormal uterus. Am J Obstet Gynecol 1995;172:105–107 (Level II-3)

21. Sharara FI, Seifer DB, Flaws JA. Environmental toxicants and female reproduction. Fertil Steril 1998;70:613–622 (Level III)

22. Rai R, Regan L, Hadley E, Dave M, Cohen H. Second-trimester pregnancy loss is associated with activated C resistance. Br J Haematol 1996;92:489–490 (Level II-2)

23. Brenner B, Mandel H, Lanir N, Younis J, Rothbart H, Ohel G, et al. Activated protein C resistance can be associated with recurrent fetal loss. Br J Haematol 1997;97:551–554 (Level II-2)

24. Ridker PM, Miletich JP, Buring JE, Ariyo AA, Prince DT, Manson JE, et al. Factor V Leiden mutation and risks of recurrent pregnancy loss. Ann Intern Med 1998;128:1000–1003 (Level II-2)

25. Foka ZJ, Lambropoulos AF, Saravelos H, Karas GB, Karavida A, Agorastos T, et al. Factor V Leiden and prothrombin G20210A mutations, but not methylenetetrahydrofolate reductase C677T, are associated with recurrent miscarriages. Hum Reprod 2000;15:459–462 (Level II-2)

26. Balasch J, Reverter JC, Fabregues F, Tassies D, Rafel M, Creus M, et al. First-trimester repeated abortion is not associated with activated protein C resistance. Hum Reprod 1997;12:1094–1097 (Level II-2)

27. Dizon-Townson DS, Meline L, Nelson LM, Varner M, Ward K. Fetal carriers of the factor V Leiden mutation are prone to miscarriage and placental infarction. Am J Obstet Gynecol 1997;177:402–405 (Level II-2)

28. Kutteh WH. Report from the Society for Gynecologic Investigation, Atlanta, Georgia, March 11-14, 1998. J Reprod Immunol 1998;40:175–182 (Level III)

29. Pauer HU, Neesen J, Hinney B. Factor V Leiden and its relevance in patients with recurrent abortions. Am J Obstet Gynecol 1998;178:629 (Level III)

30. Preston FE, Rosendaal FR, Walker ID, Briët E, Berntorp E, Conard J, et al. Increased fetal loss in women with heritable thrombophilia. Lancet 1996;348:913–916 (Level II-2)

31. Wilson R, Ling H, MacLean MA, Mooney J, Kinnane D, McKillop JH, et al. Thyroid antibody titer and avidity in patients with recurrent miscarriage. Fertil Steril 1999;71:558–561 (Level II-3)

32. Yetman DL, Kutteh WH. Antiphospholipid antibody panels and recurrent pregnancy loss: prevalence of anticardiolipin antibodies compared with other antiphospholipid antibodies. Fertil Steril 1996;66:540–546 (Level II-2)

33. Branch DW, Silver R, Pierangeli S, van Leeuwen I, Harris EN. Antiphospholipid antibodies other than lupus anticoagulant and anticardiolipin antibodies in women with recurrent pregnancy loss, fertile controls, and antiphospholipid syndrome. Obstet Gynecol 1997;89:549–555 (Level II-2)

34. Bertolaccini ML, Roch B, Amengual O, Atsumi T, Khamashta MA, Hughes GR. Multiple antiphospholipid tests do not increase the diagnostic yield in antiphospholipid syndrome. Br J Rheumatol 1998;37:1229–1232 (Level II-2)

35. Stagnaro-Green A, Roman SH, Colin RH, el-Harazy E, Alvarez-Marfany M, Davies TF, et al. Detection of at-risk pregnancy by means of highly sensitive assays for thyroid autoantibodies. JAMA 1990;264:1422–1425 (Level II-2)

36. Lejeune B, Grun JP, de Nayer P, Servais G, Glinoer D. Antithyroid antibodies underlying thyroid abnormalities and miscarriage or pregnancy induced hypertension. Br J Obstet Gynaecol 1983;100:669–672 (Level II-2)

37. Harger JH, Archer DF, Marchese SG, Muracca-Clemens M, Garver KL. Etiology of recurrent pregnancy losses and outcome of subsequent pregnancies. Obstet Gynecol 1983;6:574–581 (Level II-3)

38. Ogasawara M, Kajiura S, Katano K, Aoyama T, Aoki K. Are serum progesterone levels predictive of recurrent miscarriage in future pregnancies? Fertil Steril 1997;68:806–809 (Level II-3)

39. Laskin CA, Bombardier C, Hannah ME, Mandel FP, Ritchie JW, Farewell V, et al. Prednisone and aspirin in

women with autoantibodies and unexplained recurrent fetal loss. N Engl J Med 1997;337:148–153 (Level I)

40. Coulam CB. Immunologic tests in the evaluation of reproductive disorders: a critical review. Am J Obstet Gynecol 1992;167:1844–1851 (Level II-2)

41. Cowchock FS, Reece EA, Balaban D, Branch DW, Plouffe L. Repeated fetal losses associated with antiphospholipid antibodies: a collaborative randomized trial comparing prednisone with low-dose heparin treatment. Am J Obstet Gynecol 1992;166:1318–1323 (Level I)

42. Hill JA, Polgar K, Harlow BL, Anderson DJ. Evidence of embryo- and trophoblast-toxic cellular immune response(s) in women with recurrent spontaneous abortion. Am J Obstet Gynecol 1992;166:1044–1052 (Level II-2)

43. Hill JA, Polgar K, Anderson DJ. T-helper 1-type immunity to trophoblast in women with recurrent spontaneous abortion. JAMA 1995;273:1933–1936 (Level II-2)

44. Ecker JL, Laufer MR, Hill JA. Measurement of embryotoxic factors is predictive of pregnancy outcome in women with a history of recurrent spontaneous abortion. Obstet Gynecol 1993;81:84–87 (Level II-3)

45. Clark DA, Vince G, Flanders KC, Hirte H, Starkey P. CD56+ lymphoid cells in human first trimester pregnancy decidua as a source of novel transforming growth factor-beta 2-related immunosuppressive factors. Hum Reprod 1994;9:2270–2277 [erratum Hum Reprod 1994:9;2270–2277] (Level III)

46. Lachapelle MH, Miron P, Hemmings R, Roy DC. Endometrial T, B and NK cells in patients with recurrent spontaneous abortion: altered profile and pregnancy outcome. J Immunol 1996;256:4027–4034 (Level II-2)

47. Clifford K, Flanagan AM, Regan L. Endometrial CD56+ natural killer cells in women with recurrent miscarriage: a histomorphometric study. Hum Reprod 1999;14:2727–2730 (Level II-2)

48. Quenby S, Bates M, Doig T, Brewster J, Lewis-Jones DI, Johnson PM, et al. Pre-implantation endometrial leukocytes in women with recurrent miscarriage. Hum Reprod 1999;14:2386–2391 (Level II-2)

49. Hewitt MJ, Pratten MK, Regan L, Quenby SM, Baker PN. The use of whole rat embryo culture as a technique for investigating potential serum toxicity in recurrent miscarriage patients. Hum Reprod 2000;15:2200–2204 (Level II-2)

50. Coulam CB, Goodman C, Roussev RG, Thomason EJ, Beaman KD. Systemic CD56+ cells can predict pregnancy outcome. Am J Reprod Immunol 1995;33:40–46 (Level II-3)

51. Aoki K, Kajiura S, Metsumoto Y, Ogasawara M, Okada S, Yagami Y, et at. Preconceptual natural-killer-cell activity as a predictor of miscarriage. Lancet 1995;345:1340–1342 (Level II-2)

52. Coulam CB, Krysa L, Stern JJ, Bustillo M. Intravenous immunoglobulin for treatment of recurrent pregnancy loss. Am J Reprod Immunol 1995;34:333–337 (Level I)

53. Ho HN, Gill TJ 3rd, Hsieh HJ, Jiang JJ, Lee TY, Hsieh CY. Immunotherapy for recurrent spontaneous abortion in a Chinese population. Am J Reprod Immunol 1991;25:10–15 (Level I)

54. Cauchi MN, Lim D, Young DE, Kloss M, Pepperell RJ. Treatment of recurrent aborters by immunization with paternal cells—controlled trials. Am J Reprod Immunol 1991;25:16–17 (Level I)

55. Ober C, Karrison T, Odem RR, Barnes RB, Branch DW, Stephenson MD, et al. Mononuclear-cell immunisation in prevention of recurrent miscarriages: a randomised trial. Lancet 1999;354:365–369 (Level I)

56. Jeng GT, Scott JR, Burmeister LF. A comparison of meta-analytic results using literature vs. individual patient data. Paternal cell immunization for recurrent miscarriage. JAMA 1995;274:830–836 (Meta-analysis)

57. Stevenson AC, Dudgeon MY, McClure H. Observations on the results of pregnancies in women resident in Belfast. II. Abortions, hydatidiform moles and ectopic pregnancies. Ann Hum Genet 1959;23:395–414 (Level II-3)

58. Warburton D, Fraser FC. Spontaneous abortion risks in man: data from reproductive histories collected in a medical genetics unit. Am J Hum Genet 1964;16:1–25 (Level II-3)

59. Leridon H. Facts and artifacts in the study of intra uterine mortality: a reconsideration from pregnancy histories. Popul Stud 1976;30:319–335 (Level III)

60. Poland BJ, Miller JR, Jones DC, Trimble BK. Reproductive counseling in patients who have had a spontaneous abortion. Am J Obstet Gynecol 1977;127:685–691 (Level II-3)

61. Naylor AF, Warburton D. Sequential analysis of spontaneous abortion. II. Collaborative study data show that gravidity determines a very substantial increase in risk. Fertil Steril 1979;31:282–286 (Level II-3)

62. Shapiro S, Levine HS, Abramivicz M. Factors associated with early and late fetal loss. Adv Plan Parenthood 1970; VI:45–63 (Level III)

63. Awan AK. Some biologic correlates of pregnancy wastage. Am J Obstet Gynecol 1974;119:525–532 (Level III)

64. Boue J, Bou A, Lazer P. Retrospective and prospective epidemiological studies of 1,500 karyotyped spontaneous human abortions. Teratology 1975;12:11–26 (Level II-3)

65. FitzSimmons J, Jackson D, Wapner R, Jackson L. Subsequent reproductive outcome in couples with repeated pregnancy loss. Am J Med Genet 1983;16:583–587 (Level II-3)

66. Regan L. A prospective study of spontaneous abortion. In: Beard RW, Sharp F, eds. Early pregnancy loss: mechanisms and treatment. London: Springer–Verlag, 1988: 23–37 (Level II-2)

67. Clifford K, Rai R, Regan L. Future pregnancy outcome in unexplained recurrent first trimester miscarriage. Hum Reprod 1997;12:387–389 (Level II-2)

68. Quenby S, Farquharson RG. Human chorionic gonadotropin supplementation in recurrent pregnancy loss: a controlled trial. Fertil Steril 1994;62:708–710 (Level I)

69. Roman EA, Alberman E, Pharoah PO. Pregnancy order and fetal loss. Br Med J 1980;280(6215):715 (Level III)

70. Simpson JL, Martin AO. Prenatal diagnosis of cytogenetic disorders. Clin Obstet Gynecol 1976;19:841–853 (Level III)

71. Royal College of Obstetrians and Gynaecologists. The management of recurrent miscarriage. RCOG Guideline 17. London: RCOG, 1998 (Level III)

72. March CM, Israel R. Hysteroscopic management of recurrent abortion caused by septate uterus. Am J Obstet Gynecol 1987;156:834–842 (Level II-3)

73. Scott RT, Snyder RR, Strickland DM, Tyburski CC, Bagnall JA, Reed KR, et al. The effect of interobserver variation in dating endometrial histology on the diagnosis of luteal phase defects. Fertil Steril 1988;50:888–892 (Level II-3)

74. Daya S. Efficacy of progesterone support for pregnancy in women with recurrent miscarriage. A meta-analysis of controlled trials. Br J Obstet Gynaecol 1989;96:275–280 (Meta-analysis)

75. Scott RT, Snyder RR, Bagnall JW, Reed KD, Adair CF, Hensley SD. Evaluation of the impact of intraobserver variability on endometrial dating and the diagnosis of luteal phase defects. Fertil Steril 1993;60:652–657 (Level II-3)

76. Goldstein P, Berrier J, Rosen S, Sacks HS, Chalmers TC. A meta-analysis of randomized control trials of progestational agents in pregnancy. Br J Obstet Gynaecol 1989; 96:265–274 (Meta-analysis)

77. Clifford K, Rai R, Watson H, Franks S, Regan L. Does suppressing luteinising hormone secretion reduce the miscarriage rate? Results of a randomised controlled trial. BMJ 1996;312:1508–1511 (Level I)

78. Levine L. Habitual abortion. A controlled study of progestational therapy. West J Surg 1964;72:30–36 (Level II-1)

79. Harrison RF. Human chorionic gonadotropin (hCG) in the management of recurrent abortion; results of a multi-centre placebo-controlled study. Eur J Obstet Gynecol Reprod Biol 1992;47:175–179 (Level I)

80. Kutteh WH, Yetman DL, Carr AC, Beck LA, Scott RT Jr. Increased prevalence of antithyroid antibodies identified in women with recurrent pregnancy loss but not in women undergoing assisted reproduction. Fertil Steril 1999;71: 843–848 (Level II-3)

81. Pratt D, Novotny M, Kaberlein G, Dudkiewicz A, Gleicher N. Antithyroid antibodies and the association with non-specific antibodies in recurrent pregnancy loss. Am J Obstet Gynecol 1993;168:837–841 (Level II-2)

82. Esplin MS, Branch DW, Silver R, Stagnaro-Green A. Thyroid autoantibodies are not associated with recurrent pregnancy loss. Am J Obstet Gynecol 1998;179: 1583–1586 (Level II-2)

83. Rushworth FH, Backos M, Rai R, Chilcott IT, Baxter N, Regan L. Prospective pregnancy outcome in untreated recurrent miscarriers with thyroid autoantibodies. Hum Reprod 2000;15:1637–1639 (Level II-3)

84. Kurki T, Sivonen A, Renkonen OV, Savia E, Ylikorkala O. Bacterial vaginosis in early pregnancy and pregnancy outcome. Obstet Gynecol 1992;80:173–177 (Level II-2)

85. Hay PE, Lamont RF, Taylor-Robinson D, Morgan DJ, Ison C, Pearson J. Abnormal bacterial colonisation of the genital tract and subsequent preterm delivery and late miscarriage. BMJ 1994;308:295–298 (Level II-2)

86. Ralph SG, Rutherford AJ, Wilson JD. Influence of bacterial vaginosis on conception and miscarriage in the first trimester: cohort study. BMJ 1999;319:220–223 (Level II-2)

87. Out HJ, Kooijman CD, Bruinse HW, Derksen RH. Histopathological findings in placentae from patients with intra-uterine fetal death and anti-phospholipid antibodies. Eur J Obstet Gynecol Reprod Biol 1991;41:179–186 (Level II-2)

88. Parazzini F, Acaia B, Faden D, Lovotti M, Marelli G, Cortelazzo S. Antiphospholipid antibodies and recurrent abortion. Obstet Gynecol 1991;77:854–858 (Level II-2)

89. Parke AL, Wilson D, Maier D. The prevalence of antiphospholipid antibodies in women with recurrent spontaneous abortion, women with successful pregnancies, and women who have never been pregnant. Arthritis Rheum 1991;34: 1231–1235 (Level II-2)

90. Rai RS, Regan L, Clifford K, Pickering W, Dave M, Mackie I, et al. Antiphospholipid antibodies and beta 2-glycoprotein-I in 500 women with recurrent miscarriage: results of a comprehensive screening approach. Hum Reprod 1995;10:2001–2005 (Level II-3)

91. Oshiro BT, Silver RM, Scott JR, Yu H, Branch DW. Antiphospholipid antibodies and fetal death. Obstet Gynecol 1996;87:489–493 (Level II-2)

92. Lockshin MD, Druzin ML, Goei S, Quamar T, Magid MS, Jovanovic L, et al. Antibody to cardiolipin as a predictor of fetal distress or death in pregnant patients with systemic lupus erythematosus. N Engl J Med 1985;313:152–156 (Level II-2)

93. Kutteh WH. Antiphospholipid antibody-associated recurrent pregnancy loss: treatment with heparin and low-dose aspirin is superior to low-dose aspirin alone. Am J Obstet Gynecol 1996;174:1584–1589 (Level I)

94. Rai R, Cohen H, Dave M, Regan L. Randomized controlled trial of aspirin and aspirin plus heparin in pregnant women with recurrent miscarriage associated with phospholipid antibodies (or antiphospholipid antibodies). BMJ 1997;314:253–257 (Level I)

95. Gatenby PA, Cameron K, Simes RJ, Adelstein S, Bennett MJ, Jansen RP, et al. Treatment of recurrent spontaneous abortion by immunization with paternal lymphocytes: results of a controlled trial. Am J Reprod Immunol 1993;29:88–94 (Meta-analysis)

96. Mowbray JF, Gibbings C, Liddell H, Reginald PW, Underwood JL, Beard RW. Controlled trial of treatment of recurrent spontaneous abortion by immunisation with paternal cells. Lancet 1985;1(8435):941–943 (Level I)

97. American Society for Reproductive Medicine. Intravenous immunoglobulin (IVIG) and recurrent spontaneous pregnancy loss. ASRM Practice Committee Report. Birmingham, Alabama: ASRM, 1998 (Level III)

98. Brand A, Witvliet M, Claas FH, Eernisse JG. Beneficial effect of intravenous gammaglobulin in a patient with complement-mediated autoimmune thrombocytopenia due to IgM-anti-platelet antibodies. Br J Haematol 1988:69; 507–511 (Level III)

99. Dwyer JM, Johnson C. The regulation of T cell responses by spontaneously active suppressor cells. Clin Exp Immunol 1982;50:406–415 (Level II-2)

100. Intravenous immunoglobulin in the prevention of recurrent miscarriage. The German RSA/IVIG Group. Br J Obstet Gynaecol 1994;101:1072–1077 (Level I)

101. Christiansen OB, Mathiesen O, Husth M, Rasmussen KL, Ingerslev HJ, Lauritsen JG, et al. Placebo-controlled trial of treatment of unexplained secondary recurrent spontaneous abortions and recurrent late spontaneous abortions with IVF immunoglobulin. Hum Reprod 1995;10:2690–2695 (Level I)

102. Stephenson MD, Dreher K, Houlihan E, Wu V. Prevention of unexplained recurrent spontaneous abortion using intravenous immunoglobulin: a prospective, randomized, double-blinded, placebo-controlled trial. Am J Reprod Immunol 1998;39:82–88 (Level I)

103. Perino A, Vassiliadis A, Vucetich A, Colacurci N, Menato G, Cignitti M, et al. Short-term therapy for recurrent abortion using intravenous immunoglobulins: results of a double-blind placebo-controlled Italian study. Hum Reprod 1997;12:2388–2392 (Level I)

104. Daya S, Gunby J, Clark DA. Intravenous immunoglobulin therapy for recurrent spontaneous abortion: a meta-analysis. Am J Reprod Immunol 1998;39:69–76 (Meta-analysis)

105. Daya S, Gunby J, Porter F, Scott J, Clark DA. Critical analysis of intravenous immunoglobulin therapy for recurrent miscarriage. Hum Reprod Update 1999;5:475–482 (Meta-analysis)

The MEDLINE database, the Cochrane Library, and ACOG's own internal resources and documents were used to conduct a literature search to locate relevant articles published between January 1985 and October 2000. The search was restricted to articles published in the English language. Priority was given to articles reporting results of original research, although review articles and commentaries also were consulted. Abstracts of research presented at symposia and scientific conferences were not considered adequate for inclusion in this document. Guidelines published by organizations or institutions such as the National Institutes of Health and the American College of Obstetricians and Gynecologists were reviewed, and additional studies were located by reviewing bibliographies of identified articles. When reliable research was not available, expert opinions from obstetrician–gynecologists were used.

Studies were reviewed and evaluated for quality according to the method outlined by the U.S. Preventive Services Task Force:

I Evidence obtained from at least one properly designed randomized controlled trial.

II-1 Evidence obtained from well-designed controlled trials without randomization.

II-2 Evidence obtained from well-designed cohort or case–control analytic studies, preferably from more than one center or research group.

II-3 Evidence obtained from multiple time series with or without the intervention. Dramatic results in uncontrolled experiments also could be regarded as this type of evidence.

III Opinions of respected authorities, based on clinical experience, descriptive studies, or reports of expert committees.

Based on the highest level of evidence found in the data, recommendations are provided and graded according to the following categories:

Level A—Recommendations are based on good and consistent scientific evidence.

Level B—Recommendations are based on limited or inconsistent scientific evidence.

Level C—Recommendations are based primarily on consensus and expert opinion.

ISSN 1099-3630

The American College of Obstetricians and Gynecologists
409 12th Street, SW, PO Box 96920
Washington, DC 20090-6920

12345/54321

ACOG PRACTICE BULLETIN

CLINICAL MANAGEMENT GUIDELINES FOR
OBSTETRICIAN–GYNECOLOGISTS

NUMBER 67, OCTOBER 2005

(Replaces Practice Bulletin Number 26, April 2001)

Medical Management of Abortion

Over the past two decades, medical methods of abortion have been developed throughout the world and are now used in the United States. Medical abortion, which involves the use of medications to induce an abortion rather than a surgical abortion, is an option for women who wish to terminate a pregnancy up to 63 days of gestation (calculated from the first day of the last menstrual period). Medical abortions currently account for 6% of all abortions in the United States (1). The purpose of this document is to present evidence of the effectiveness, benefits, and risks of medical abortion and provide a framework for the evaluation and counseling of women who are considering medical abortion.

Background

Medications Currently Used in Medical Abortion

Mifepristone

Mifepristone (RU-486), a derivative of norethindrone, binds to the progesterone receptor with an affinity greater than progesterone but does not activate the receptor, thereby acting as an antiprogestin (2). Mifepristone's known actions on a pregnant uterus include necrotizing the decidua, softening the cervix, and increasing both uterine contractility and prostaglandin sensitivity (3, 4). Human studies have suggested that uterine contractility does not increase until 24–36 hours after mifepristone administration (4). At this point, the myometrium is five times more sensitive to the stimulatory effects of exogenous prostaglandins (4).

Administration of mifepristone followed by a prostaglandin analogue, usually misoprostol, is the most commonly used medical abortion regimen throughout the world. As a progesterone receptor antagonist, mifepristone also has several other potential medical applications, including emergency contraception, cervical ripening for labor induction, and treatment of conditions

This Practice Bulletin was developed by the ACOG Committee on Practice Bulletins— Gynecology with the assistance of Mitchell D. Creinin, MD. The information is designed to aid practitioners in making decisions about appropriate obstetric and gynecologic care. These guidelines should not be construed as dictating an exclusive course of treatment or procedure. Variations in practice may be warranted based on the needs of the individual patient, resources, and limitations unique to the institution or type of practice.

such as symptomatic leiomyomata uteri, endometriosis, Cushing's syndrome, breast cancer, and glaucoma.

Misoprostol

Misoprostol is an inexpensive prostaglandin analogue in a tablet form that is stable at room temperature. Misoprostol is used clinically for prevention of gastric ulcers in individuals taking antiinflammatory drugs on a long-term basis, for abortion, and for labor induction. Pharmacokinetic evaluation of oral and vaginal administration of misoprostol demonstrates that oral misoprostol is absorbed more rapidly, resulting in a higher peak serum level (5, 6), but vaginal administration results in greater uterine contractility. Recent evaluations of sublingual administration show higher peak serum concentrations (7, 8), which may result in more unnecessary side effects (7). Further study of buccal administration may be warranted because its pharmacokinetic profile appears to be similar to vaginal administration (7).

Other Agents

Methotrexate is used less often today for medical abortion because of the greater availability of mifepristone. Methotrexate blocks dihydrofolate reductase, an enzyme involved in producing thymidine during DNA synthesis. Methotrexate exerts its action primarily on the cytotrophoblast rather than the developing embryo. Methotrexate has been used for more than 40 years to treat neoplastic diseases, rheumatoid arthritis, and psoriasis; other medical applications include treatment of systemic lupus erythematosus, dermatomyositis, severe asthma, Crohn's disease, and extrauterine pregnancy.

Tamoxifen has been used in combination with misoprostol in some studies of early abortion. However, randomized trials have demonstrated no benefit of using a tamoxifen–misoprostol regimen compared with a methotrexate–misoprostol regimen (9) or misoprostol alone (10).

Mifepristone Regimens

Protocol Approved by the U.S. Food and Drug Administration

Mifepristone regimens vary according to dosage, timing, and route of administration (see Table 1). The U.S. Food and Drug Administration (FDA) approved the protocol of mifepristone, 600 mg orally, followed approximately 48 hours later by misoprostol, 400 μg orally. This is safe and effective for medical abortion through 49 days of gestation (calculated from the first day of the last menstrual period [LMP]). A follow-up evaluation is scheduled approximately 14 days after administration of mifepristone. At that time, if clinical history and physical exami-

nation do not confirm expulsion, ultrasonography is performed. If a gestational sac is seen, aspiration is typically performed.

Efficacy with this regimen is approximately 92% in women with pregnancies up to 49 days of gestation (11, 12). Complete abortion rates are higher with earlier gestations: approximately 96–98% for pregnancies up to 42 days of gestation (13, 14), 91–95% from 43 to 49 days of gestation (13, 14), and less than 85% beyond 49 days of gestation (11, 13, 14).

Alternative Regimens

Other evidence-based medical abortion regimens have been developed in an effort to reduce side effects and to make medical abortion less expensive, safer, and more rapid. Regimens using 200-mg doses of mifepristone orally have efficacy rates comparable to the FDA-approved regimen (12, 15) at one third of the cost. Additionally, increasing the misoprostol dose to 800 μg and administering the medication vaginally decreases the time to expulsion (16), results in fewer side effects (16, 17), and improves complete abortion rates when compared with oral administration of a 400-μg dose of misoprostol (16, 18–20). Multiple large studies in the United States have demonstrated that a patient can safely and effectively self-administer the misoprostol (orally or vaginally) in her home (18, 19, 21–27).

Investigations also have demonstrated the flexibility in timing between the two medications. One study demonstrated that 800 μg of misoprostol may be administered either 24, 48, or 72 hours after 200 mg of mifepristone with equal efficacy in pregnancies up to 56 days of gestation (23); a follow-up study using a regimen with a 24-hour interval between medications yielded similar results in pregnancies up to 63 days of gestation (24). Moreover, the results of a randomized multicenter study indicated that 800 μg of misoprostol administered vaginally 6–8 hours after 200 mg of mifepristone resulted in significantly fewer side effects (and no decrease in efficacy) than regimens using a 24-hour interval (27).

Compared with the FDA-approved regimen, mifepristone–misoprostol regimens using mifepristone, 200 mg orally, and misoprostol, 800 μg vaginally, are associated with a decreased rate of continuing pregnancies, decreased time to expulsion, fewer side effects, improved complete abortion rates, and lower cost for women with pregnancies up to 63 days of gestation based on LMP.

Nonmifepristone Regimens

Methotrexate and Misoprostol

The combination of methotrexate and misoprostol is an alternative early medical abortion regimen. Among

Table 1. Comparison of Common Medical Abortion Regimens

Common Regimens	Overall Success Rate (%)	Advantages and Disadvantages	Gestational Age
Mifepristone, 600 mg orally + misoprostol, 400 µg orally (FDA-approved regimen)	92[a]	Must remain in office or clinic 4 hours after administration	Up to 49 days
Mifepristone, 200 mg orally + misoprostol, 800 µg vaginally (alternative evidence-based regimen)	95–99[b–f]	Compared with FDA-approved regimen: • More effective • Less time to expulsion • Fewer side effects • Requires vaginal administration of a medication	Up to 63 days
Methotrexate, 50 mg/m² IM or 50 mg vaginally, + misoprostol, 800 µg vaginally 3–7 days later	92–96[g–i]	Compared with mifepristone–misoprostol regimen: • Takes longer for expulsion in 20–30% of women • Readily available medications • Low drug cost	Up to 49 days
Misoprostol only, 800 µg vaginally repeated for up to three doses	88[j]	• Requires complicated dosing regimens • Significantly higher incidence of side effects than other regimens • Low drug cost	Up to 56 days

Abbreviations: FDA, U.S. Food and Drug Administration; IM, intramuscularly

[a]Spitz IM, Bardin CW, Benton L, Robbins A. Early pregnancy termination with mifepristone and misoprostol in the United States. N Engl J Med 1998;338:1241–7.

[b]Schaff EA, Eisinger SH, Stadalius LS, Franks P, Gore BZ, Poppema S. Low-dose mifepristone 200 mg and vaginal misoprostol for abortion. Contraception 1999;59:1–6.

[c]Schaff EA, Fielding SL, Westhoff C. Randomized trial of oral versus vaginal misoprostol at one day after mifepristone for early medical abortion. Contraception 2001;64:81–5.

[d]el-Refaey H, Rajasekar D, Abdalla M, Calder L, Templeton A. Induction of abortion with mifepristone (RU 486) and oral or vaginal misoprostol. N Engl J Med 1995;332:983–7.

[e]von Hertzen H, Honkanen H, Piaggio G, Bartfai G, Erdenetungalag R, Gemzell-Danielsson K, et al. WHO multinational study of three misoprostol regimens after mifepristone for early medical abortion. I: Efficacy. WHO Research Group on Post-Ovulatory Methods for Fertility Regulation. BJOG 2003;110:808–18.

[f]Creinin MD, Fox MC, Teal S, Chen A, Schaff EA, Meyn LA. A randomized comparison of misoprostol 6 to 8 hours versus 24 hours after mifepristone for abortion. MOD Study Trial Group. Obstet Gynecol 2004;103:851–9.

[g]Creinin MD, Vittinghoff E, Schaff E, Klaisle C, Darney PD, Dean C. Medical abortion with oral methotrexate and vaginal misoprostol. Obstet Gynecol 1997;90:611–6.

[h]Creinin MD, Carbonell JL, Schwartz JL, Varela L, Tanda R. A randomized trial of the effect of moistening misoprostol before vaginal administration when used with methotrexate for abortion. Contraception 1999;59:11–6.

[i]Wiebe E, Dunn S, Guilbert E, Jacot F, Lugtig L. Comparison of abortions induced by methotrexate or mifepristone followed by misoprostol. Obstet Gynecol 2002;99:813–9.

[j]Jain JK, Dutton C, Harwood B, Meckstroth KR, Mishell DR Jr. A prospective randomized, double-blinded, placebo-controlled trial comparing mifepristone and vaginal misoprostol to vaginal misoprostol alone for elective termination of early pregnancy. Hum Reprod 2002;17:1477–82.

women with pregnancies up to 49 days of gestation, this regimen results in a complete abortion rate of 92–96%. Between 50 days and 56 days of gestation, however, efficacy decreases to 82% (28). Although overall efficacy is equal to the standard regimen of mifepristone–misoprostol, approximately 15–25% of women using methotrexate regimens may wait up to 4 weeks for complete abortion to occur (25, 29, 30).

Methotrexate is most commonly administered intramuscularly at a dose based on body surface area (50 mg/m²), the same dose used for the management of ectopic pregnancy (31). However, regimens using 50 mg of methotrexate orally appear to be as effective as those using methotrexate, 50 mg/m² intramuscularly (29, 32, 33). Misoprostol (800 µg) is administered by the woman 3–7 days later at home. A follow-up examination is per-

formed approximately 1 week after methotrexate administration; a vaginal ultrasound examination is performed to confirm passage of the gestational sac. If abortion has not occurred, the misoprostol dose is repeated. Further follow-up for women requiring a second dose of misoprostol is performed in 4 weeks unless embryonic cardiac activity is still visible on ultrasound examination, in which case patients return in 1 week. If gestational cardiac activity is present 2 weeks after initiating treatment or expulsion has not occurred by the 4-week follow-up visit, aspiration is performed.

Misoprostol Alone

Misoprostol, 800 µg vaginally, when moistened with water, can result in complete abortion rates of 90% in women with pregnancies up to 56 days of gestation

(10, 34–38). Studies with nonmoistened vaginal misoprostol demonstrated lower rates of 50–67% (39–41). Studies showing that misoprostol alone is effective for abortion often involve complex dosing regimens or require clinician application of the tablets. Additionally, this treatment results in significantly higher rates of side effects (nausea, vomiting, diarrhea, and fever and chills) than those using misoprostol after pretreatment with either mifepristone or methotrexate (10, 34–37). Recent trials with sublingual misoprostol in repeated doses do not appear to improve outcome over vaginal misoprostol and may cause even more side effects (38, 42).

A recent randomized, double-blind trial in women with pregnancies up to 56 days of gestation compared a misoprostol-only regimen (800 µg vaginally) with a regimen of 200 mg of mifepristone orally followed 48 hours later by 800 µg of misoprostol vaginally (43). In both groups, misoprostol was repeated every 24 hours for up to three doses. Complete abortion rates for each regimen were 88.0% and 95.7%, respectively ($P < .05$). The women who received mifepristone aborted much more quickly and required fewer doses of misoprostol compared with women who received misoprostol alone.

Mifepristone–misoprostol regimens using 200 mg of mifepristone orally and 800 µg of misoprostol vaginally generally are preferred to regimens using methotrexate and misoprostol or misoprostol only for medical abortion.

Counseling Patients

Medical Versus Surgical Abortion

Patient counseling must first include discussion of pregnancy options to be sure that a woman is certain about her decision to have an abortion. If she is uncertain, the decision about abortion technique must be delayed until she has reached a firm decision, even if the delay means that she will be unable to choose a medical option. It is important to respect the patient's autonomy and to separate the decision to terminate the pregnancy from the decision about the method to be used.

After a woman has considered her options and has decided to have an abortion, the method must be selected. Most women seeking early abortion will be eligible for both medical and surgical methods. Medical abortion should be considered a medically acceptable alternative to surgical abortion in selected, carefully counseled, and informed women. The general advantages and disadvantages of each approach (Table 2) should be explained early in the counseling process because most women will have a clear preference (44, 45). Even among women who think they are unsure, most will have some preference after counseling (44).

Table 2. Features of Medical and Surgical Abortion

Medical Abortion	Surgical Abortion
• Usually avoids invasive procedure	• Involves invasive procedure
• Usually avoids anesthesia	• Allows use of sedation if desired
• Requires two or more visits	• Usually requires one visit
• Days to weeks to complete	• Complete in a predictable period of time
• Available during early pregnancy	• Available during early pregnancy
• High success rate (~95%)	• High success rate (99%)
• Bleeding moderate to heavy for short time	• Bleeding commonly perceived as light
• Requires follow-up to ensure completion of abortion	• Does not require follow-up in all cases
• Patient participation throughout a multiple-step process	• Patient participation in a single-step process

Adapted from Breitbart V. Counseling for medical abortion. Am J Obstet Gynecol 2000;183:S26–33.

Counseling and Symptom Management

Some degree of bleeding and uterine cramping are necessary for the medical abortion process to occur. Other potential side effects of medical abortion include nausea, vomiting, diarrhea, warmth or chills, headache, dizziness, and fatigue (Table 3). Counseling should emphasize that bleeding may be much heavier than menses, potentially with severe cramping. The woman should understand how much bleeding is considered too much. An easy reference for the patient to use is soaking of two pads per hour for 2 hours in a row (46). This is not necessarily a point at which intervention is needed but a time when the woman should call the health care provider. Whether or not it is imperative for the patient to seek emergency care depends on how she is feeling, her baseline hemoglobin, whether the bleeding seems to be slowing, and how far she is from an emergency treatment facility.

Pain management is especially important for the woman aborting at home. She should be sent home with appropriate instructions for analgesia with over-the-counter medications, as well as with prescriptions for oral narcotics to use if needed.

The incidence of each symptom will depend on the regimen used, the dose and route of administration of the prostaglandin analogue, and gestational age. Gastrointestinal side effects are less common when dry misoprostol is administered vaginally compared with regimens that use oral misoprostol or moistened vaginal misoprostol. Oral ulcers with methotrexate use, although rare, have been reported in the literature.

Table 3. Incidence of Side Effects in Selected North American Trials of Medical Abortion Regimens*

| Trial | Incidence of Side Effects (%) | | | | | | | | | | | |
| | Nausea | | Vomiting | | Diarrhea | | Headache | | Dizziness | | Thermoregulatory[†] | |
	Mife	Miso	Mife	Miso	Mife	Miso	Mife	Miso	Mife	Miso	Mife	Miso
Schaff et al (1997)[‡]	36	36	14	14	8	22	18	19	22	37	20	37
Schaff et al (1999)[§]	45	43	13	26	11	23	14	13	15	28	14	32
Wiebe et al (2002)[‖]	45	39	13	15	5	16	19	29	NR	NR	NR	23
Creinin (2004)[¶]	20	44	5	23	1	27	10	37	12	35	9	56
Creinin (2004)[#]	39	52	14	30	7	25	20	37	20	37	19	53

Abbreviations: Mife, mifepristone; Miso, misoprostol; NR, not reported

*Studies are included only if the incidences of side effects were differentiated between the medications.

[†]Fever, warmth, hot flashes, or chills

[‡]Mifepristone, 600 mg, followed by misoprostol, 800 µg vaginally, 36–48 hours later. (Schaff EA, Stadalius LS, Eisinger SH, Franks P. Vaginal misoprostol administered at home after mifepristone (RU486) for abortion. J Fam Pract 1997;44:353–60.)

[§]Mifepristone, 200 mg, followed by misoprostol, 800 µg vaginally, 48 hours later. (Schaff EA, Eisinger SH, Stadalius LS, Franks P, Gore BZ, Poppema S. Low-dose mifepristone 200 mg and vaginal misoprostol for abortion. Contraception 1999;59:1–6.)

[‖]Mifepristone, 600 mg, followed by misoprostol, 400 µg orally, 36–48 hours later. (Wiebe E, Dunn S, Guilbert E, Jacot F, Lugtig L. Comparison of abortions induced by methotrexate or mifepristone followed by misoprostol. Obstet Gynecol 2002;99:813–9.)

[¶]Mifepristone, 200 mg, followed by misoprostol, 800 µg vaginally, 6–8 hours later (first row). (Creinin MD, Fox MC, Teal S, Chen A, Schaff EA, Meyn LA. A randomized comparison of misoprostol 6 to 8 hours versus 24 hours after mifepristone for abortion. Obstet Gynecol 2004;103:851–9.)

[#]Mifepristone, 200 mg, followed by misoprostol, 800 µg vaginally, 23–25 hours later (second row). (Creinin MD, Fox MC, Teal S, Chen A, Schaff EA, Meyn LA. A randomized comparison of misoprostol 6 to 8 hours versus 24 hours after mifepristone for abortion. Obstet Gynecol 2004;103: 851–9.)

Need for Follow-up Dilation and Curettage

A failed medical abortion is defined as the presence of gestational cardiac activity on vaginal ultrasonography 2 weeks after the initiation of treatment. No studies have assessed the efficacy of additional doses of mifepristone, methotrexate, or misoprostol after a medical abortion failure. Continuing pregnancies, which should be terminated by surgical evacuation, are typically reported in less than 1% of women who begin treatment at 49 days of gestation or less regardless of regimen.

Intervention guidelines vary for women who have a persistent gestational sac seen on ultrasonography without evidence of embryonic cardiac activity or continuing development. Typically, protocols used in mifepristone studies define a retained sac 2 weeks after the administration of mifepristone as an indication for suction evacuation. However, medical abortion studies using methotrexate and misoprostol demonstrate that intervention for a nonviable pregnancy is unnecessary and that expulsion will occur, on average, between 22 and 29 days after the methotrexate is administered (28, 29, 40, 47, 48). With this understanding, the mifepristone studies performed in the United States over the past 6 years have allowed approximately 36 days to elapse after mifepristone administration before recommending surgical intervention (18, 19, 22–25, 27). Most commonly, a woman

who has not aborted and is awaiting delayed expulsion will no longer feel pregnant or have medication-induced symptoms; the patient will be waiting for the onset of bleeding or cramping similar to anticipating the start of menses (28). Providers must differentiate this scenario from women who have incomplete expulsion of the pregnancy tissue, for whom symptoms can include prolonged and irregular bleeding episodes. Early trials of methotrexate and misoprostol showed that serial β-hCG evaluations did not aid in the diagnosis of incomplete abortion. All women with an incomplete abortion presented clinically, and the incomplete abortion was not diagnosed by increasing or plateaued β-hCG levels (40, 49, 50).

Understanding the difference between incomplete abortion and the normal course of medical abortion is important. The sole purpose of ultrasound examination after misoprostol administration is to determine whether the gestational sac is present. After expulsion, the uterus will normally contain ultrasonographically hyperechoic tissue consisting of blood, blood clots, and decidua. Rarely does this finding during medical abortion indicate a need for intervention. In the absence of excessive bleeding, providers can follow such patients conservatively (51).

Overall, large studies demonstrate that less than 1% of women undergoing medical abortion will need emergent curettage because of excessive bleeding

(13, 22, 52–54). Moreover, the risk of clinically significant bleeding and transfusion may be lower in women with pregnancies up to 49 days of gestation compared with those beyond 49 days (11); this relative risk will vary depending on the regimen used. Still, just as for women undergoing surgical abortion, surgical curettage must be available on a 24-hour basis for cases of hemorrhage. Clinicians who wish to provide medical abortion services either should be trained in surgical abortion or should work in conjunction with a clinician who is trained in surgical abortion.

Clinical Considerations and Recommendations

▶ *What factors determine whether a woman is a candidate for medical abortion?*

Gestational Age

The upper limit of gestational age at which a medical abortion regimen is still an option varies depending on the types, dosages, and routes of administration of the medications. Outpatient treatment with mifepristone–misoprostol regimens up to 63 days of gestation and for methotrexate–misoprostol regimens up to 49 days of gestation are highly effective. Complete abortion rates among all regimens are highest for earlier gestations and are clinically similar in women with pregnancies up to 49 days of gestation. Between 50 and 63 days of gestation, the use of vaginal misoprostol in regimens with mifepristone results in complete abortion in 96–99% of women (18, 22–24, 26, 27, 43, 53, 55), whereas regimens using oral misoprostol demonstrate significantly lower success rates for these gestational ages.

Contraindications

Medical contraindications to abortion with mifepristone regimens include confirmed or suspected ectopic pregnancy or undiagnosed adnexal mass, intrauterine device in place, current long-term systemic corticosteroid therapy, chronic adrenal failure, severe anemia, known coagulopathy or anticoagulant therapy, and mifepristone intolerance or allergy. Most clinical trials also exclude women with severe liver, renal, or respiratory disease, uncontrolled hypertension, cardiovascular disease (angina, valvular disease, arrhythmia, or cardiac failure), or severe anemia. Misoprostol should not be used in women with an uncontrolled seizure disorder or those who have an allergy or intolerance to misoprostol or other prostaglandins. Asthma is not a contraindication because misoprostol is a weak bronchodilator.

Although medical contraindications are infrequent, social or psychologic contraindications to medical abortion are more common. Women are not good candidates for medical abortion if they do not wish to take responsibility for their care, are anxious to have the abortion over quickly, cannot return for follow-up visits, or cannot understand the instructions because of language or comprehension barriers. Other nonmedical criteria to be considered are access to a phone in case of an emergency and access to 24-hour emergency medical treatment (eg, surgical curettage for hemorrhage). Counseling should include a description of cramping and bleeding and should indicate that, rarely, the process may not be completed for several weeks.

▶ *Which pretreatment laboratory tests are needed?*

No special pretreatment laboratory tests are necessary for medical abortion beyond those for surgical abortion. Confirmation of pregnancy by ultrasonography or pregnancy testing is necessary before attempting abortion regardless of method. Pretreatment assessment of hemoglobin or hematocrit and blood typing are imperative, and anti-D immune globulin should be administered if indicated.

▶ *What is the risk of infection with medical abortion?*

Endometritis is a rare complication of medical abortion. In trials involving more than 500 participants, infection rates typically vary from 0.09% to 0.6% (11, 17, 18, 22, 23, 27, 56, 57). No data exist to support the universal use of prophylactic antibiotics for medical abortion. Five cases of death have been reported in women using mifepristone, 200 mg, followed by misoprostol, 800 µg vaginally, in North America since 2001; all appear to be infectious, with *Clostridium sordellii* identified in three of the cases (58). The cause of these infections and the relationship of the deaths to mifepristone and misoprostol are still under investigation. Even if related, the death rate would be less than 1 per 100,000 mifepristone procedures, a rate comparable to that for early surgical abortion and miscarriage (59).

▶ *Is ultrasonography useful in the medical management of abortion before treatment?*

Gestational age should be confirmed by clinical evaluation or ultrasonography. Only 85% of U.S. women are able to predict gestational age within 2 weeks of the gestational age assigned by the clinician using ultrasound examination (60). Additionally, medical abortion studies in U.S. women have found that the gestational age determined by LMP was confirmed for only 40–60% of study participants (14, 27, 61). Because efficacy for some regimens decreases significantly with increasing gestational age, the clinical relevance of erroneous gestational age assignment will vary according to the regimen used.

Although not required, all major U.S. trials of mifepristone or methotrexate have relied on transvaginal ultrasonography for dating and follow-up. In France, however, clinicians use ultrasonography for preabortion screening only when they find a discrepancy between uterine size and dating by LMP and when patients present with bleeding or symptoms suggestive of ectopic pregnancy. Pregnancy termination services in France are offered only by authorized abortion clinics staffed by highly experienced providers. The high efficacy and safety results in the French trials suggest that this selective use of ultrasonography suffices when medical abortion is provided by experienced clinicians.

A concern when providing early abortion services is the possibility of an undiagnosed extrauterine gestation. Although the ectopic pregnancy rate in the general population is currently around 19–21 per 1,000 pregnancies (62, 63), ectopic pregnancy rates in studies of women seeking abortion are consistently lower. A study of surgical abortion in women with pregnancies less than 42 days of gestation in the United States found the ectopic pregnancy rate to be 5.9 per 1,000 pregnancies (64). Similarly, the largest published study of medical abortion involved 16,369 women with pregnancies up to 49 days of gestation, 21 of whom were excluded from the analysis because of an ectopic pregnancy, yielding an ectopic pregnancy rate of 1.3 per 1,000 pregnancies (57). Although ectopic pregnancy in a population of women seeking early abortion is rare, women with significant medical risk factors or history (eg, unilateral pain and vaginal bleeding) should have pretreatment ultrasonography.

▶ What methods can be used to confirm complete abortion?

Transvaginal ultrasonography offers an efficient means of assessing outcome in patients who undergo medical abortion. Its primary objective is to determine if the gestational sac is absent (with or without the presence of other ultrasonographically hyperechoic tissue). However, French clinicians, who have extensive experience with medical abortion, use ultrasonography significantly less than American clinicians (65). One explanation for this difference may be less familiarity with the process by both American clinicians and patients; another reason could be liability concerns in the United States. A study of U.S. providers indicated that ultrasonography is perceived to be unnecessary to assess abortion outcome for most women (66). Researchers asked physicians if they felt

comfortable with their assessment without ultrasonography or if they would feel better in that situation with an ultrasound examination to confirm their impression based on the patient's history and physical examination. Physicians thought an ultrasound examination was not needed in 60% of the women who were ultimately found to have expelled the gestational sac. However, the gestational sac was still present in 29% of women for whom physicians believed ultrasonography was not indicated.

Methods to verify abortion include reports of bleeding combined with evidence of uterine involution on pelvic examination or hCG testing. When misoprostol is administered 2–5 days after methotrexate or mifepristone, β-hCG concentrations should decrease by at least 50% within 1 week of initiating the medication regimen. However, performing sensitive serum or urine hCG assays (detection threshold, 25–50 mIU/mL) too soon after the termination of a pregnancy may result in an erroneous diagnosis of failed medical abortion. Two trials using methotrexate and misoprostol found that the average time to disappearance of β-hCG is 33–34 days and may take as long as 90 days (40, 67). The utility of nonsensitive urine hCG assays in follow-up after mifepristone and misoprostol administration warrants investigation.

In clinical trials with methotrexate and misoprostol, only about half of the women who thought they had aborted actually had done so (28). Moreover, women may experience symptom resolution consistent with a complete medical abortion and still have a persistent gestational sac (28), or even an ectopic pregnancy (22). The importance of patient follow-up must be emphasized because failure rates for medical abortion are higher than those for surgical techniques.

However, recent data suggest that for most women having an abortion with mifepristone and misoprostol, no follow-up may be needed other than a telephone conversation. One report compared clinicians' and patients' impressions of whether or not expulsion occurred based solely on the patient's history with the results of vaginal ultrasonography performed approximately 1 week after initiating treatment (68). When the clinician and the patient both thought that expulsion had occurred, they were correct 99% of the time. Additional studies are needed to validate the premise that such women need only a home pregnancy test for follow-up and that office evaluation should be required only if either the clinician or the patient is not certain that expulsion has occurred.

▶ Do nonsteroidal antiinflammatory drugs affect the success rates for medical abortion?

Cramping pain for patients who are not undergoing abortion usually is treated with ibuprofen or other nonsteroidal antiinflammatory drugs (NSAIDs). Although NSAIDs inhibit the synthesis of new prostaglandins, they do not block the action of prostaglandin receptors; therefore, such agents should not inhibit the action of a prostaglandin used for medical abortion. The only report to evaluate the effects of analgesics on abortion outcome was a retrospective analysis of NSAIDs and complete abortion in 416 women who received misoprostol following methotrexate for medical abortion of pregnancies up to 56 days of gestation (69). The use of ibuprofen did not seem to interfere with the action of misoprostol to induce uterine contractions and pregnancy expulsion. Therefore, NSAIDs such as ibuprofen are not contraindicated for women undergoing a medical abortion.

▶ *How should a patient be counseled about potential teratogenicity if a medical method fails to lead to abortion?*

Because teratogenicity of medical abortifacients becomes an important issue if the pregnancy continues, patients must be informed of the need for a surgical abortion in the event of a continuing pregnancy. There is no evidence to date of a teratogenic effect of mifepristone. However, methotrexate is an antimetabolite that can cause fetal anomalies (70, 71). Evidence suggests that misoprostol also can result in congenital anomalies when used during the first trimester, possibly due to mild uterine contractions resulting in decreased blood flow during organogenesis (72). Anomalies associated with misoprostol use that have been described in the literature include defects in the frontal or temporal bones (73) and limb abnormalities with or without Möbius sequence (masklike facies with bilateral sixth and seventh nerve palsy and frequently coincident micrognathia) (74–77). No conclusions regarding teratogenicity can be drawn from these reports because of the extremely small sample sizes.

▶ *Does medical abortion affect future fertility?*

Future fertility following medical abortion has been evaluated only within a 1-year period after medical abortion in a group of 93 women who received methotrexate and misoprostol for abortion (78). Although none of the women were actively attempting to achieve pregnancy, 25% became pregnant, a rate higher than would be expected for a group of women using contraception. By comparison, another report indicated a pregnancy rate of 13% within 1 year after a first surgical abortion (79).

Summary of Recommendations and Conclusions

The following recommendations are based primarily on good and consistent scientific evidence (Level A):

▶ Medical abortion should be considered a medically acceptable alternative to surgical abortion in selected, carefully counseled, and informed women.

▶ The FDA-approved protocol of 600 mg of mifepristone orally followed approximately 48 hours later by 400 µg of misoprostol orally is safe and effective for medical abortion through 49 days of gestation (calculated from the first day of the LMP).

▶ Compared with the FDA-approved regimen, mifepristone–misoprostol regimens using 200 mg of mifepristone orally and 800 µg of misoprostol vaginally are associated with a decreased rate of continuing pregnancies, decreased time to expulsion, fewer side effects, improved complete abortion rates, and lower cost for women with pregnancies up to 63 days of gestation based on LMP.

▶ A methotrexate–misoprostol regimen is appropriate for medical abortion only in pregnancies up to 49 days of gestation. Women using this regimen may wait up to 4 weeks for complete abortion to occur.

▶ Mifepristone–misoprostol regimens using 200 mg of mifepristone orally and 800 µg of misoprostol vaginally are generally preferred to regimens using methotrexate and misoprostol or misoprostol only for medical abortion.

▶ A patient can administer misoprostol safely and effectively, orally or vaginally, in her home as part of a medical abortion regimen.

The following recommendations are based primarily on limited scientific evidence (Level B):

▶ Because teratogenicity of medical abortifacients becomes an important issue if the pregnancy continues, patients must be informed of the need for a surgical abortion in the event of a failed abortion.

▶ Gestational age should be confirmed by clinical evaluation or ultrasonography.

The following recommendations are based primarily on consensus and expert opinion (Level C):

▶ Surgical curettage must be available on a 24-hour basis for cases of hemorrhage, even though less than

1% of women having a medical abortion will need a curettage because of excessive bleeding.

▶ Pretreatment anti-D immune globulin should be administered if indicated.

▶ No data exist to support the universal use of prophylactic antibiotics for medical abortion.

References

1. Finer LB, Henshaw SK. Abortion incidence and services in the United States in 2000. Perspect Sex Reprod Health 2003;35:6–15. (Level II-3)

2. Gravanis A, Schaison G, George M, de Brux J, Satyaswaroop PG, Baulieu EE, et al. Endometrial and pituitary responses to the steroidal antiprogestin RU 486 in postmenopausal women. J Clin Endocrinol Metab 1985;60:156–63. (Level II-3)

3. Johannisson E, Oberholzer M, Swahn ML, Bygdeman M. Vascular changes in the human endometrium following the administration of the progesterone antagonist RU 486. Contraception 1989:39;103–17. (Level II-2)

4. Swahn ML, Bygdeman M. The effect of the antiprogestin RU 486 on uterine contractility and sensitivity to prostaglandin and oxytocin. Br J Obstet Gynaecol 1988:95;126–34. (Level II-2)

5. Danielsson KG, Marions L, Rodriguez A, Spur BW, Wong PY, Bygdeman M. Comparison between oral and vaginal administration of misoprostol on uterine contractility. Obstet Gynecol 1999;93:275–80. (Level II-2)

6. Zieman M, Fong SK, Benowitz NL, Banskter D, Darney PD. Absorption kinetics of misoprostol with oral or vaginal administration. Obstet Gynecol 1997;90:88–92. (Level II-1)

7. Schaff EA, DiCenzo R, Fielding SL. Comparison of misoprostol plasma concentrations following buccal and sublingual administration. Contraception 2005;71:22–5. (Level II-3)

8. Tang OS, Schweer H, Seyberth HW, Lee SW, Ho PC. Pharmacokinetics of different routes of administration of misoprostol. Hum Reprod 2002;17:332–6. (Level I)

9. Wiebe ER. Tamoxifen compared to methotrexate when used with misoprostol for abortion. Contraception 1999;59:265–70. (Level I)

10. Jain JK, Meckstroth KR, Park M, Mishell DR Jr. A comparison of tamoxifen and misoprostol to misoprostol alone for early pregnancy termination. Contraception 2000;60:353–6. (Level I)

11. Spitz IM, Bardin CW, Benton L, Robbins A. Early pregnancy termination with mifepristone and misoprostol in the United States. N Engl J Med 1998;338:1241–7. (Level II-3)

12. Comparison of two doses of mifepristone in combination with misoprostol for early medical abortion: a randomised trial. World Health Organisation Task Force on Post-ovulatory Methods of Fertility Regulation. BJOG 2000; 107:524–30. (Level I)

13. Aubény E, Peyron R, Turpin CL, Renault M, Targosz V, Silvestre L, et al. Termination of early pregnancy (up to 63 days of amenorrhea) with mifepristone and increasing doses of misoprostol [published erratum appears in Int J Fertil Menopausal Stud 1996;41:56]. Int J Fertil Menopausal Stud 1995;40 (suppl 2):85–91. (Level II-3)

14. Creinin MD, Spitz IM. Use of various ultrasound criteria to evaluate the efficacy of mifepristone and misoprostol for medical abortion. Am J Obstet Gynecol 1999; 181:1419–24. (Level II-3)

15. McKinley C, Thong KJ, Baird DT. The effect of dose of mifepristone and gestation on the efficacy of medical abortion with mifepristone and misoprostol. Hum Reprod 1993;8:1502–5. (Level I)

16. el-Refaey H, Rajasekar D, Abdalla M, Calder L, Templeton A. Induction of abortion with mifepristone (RU 486) and oral or vaginal misoprostol. N Engl J Med 1995;332:983–7. (Level I)

17. Honkanen H, Piaggio G, Hertzen H, Bartfai G, Erdenetungalag R, Gemzell-Danielsson K, et al. WHO multinational study of three misoprostol regimens after mifepristone for early medical abortion. WHO Research Group on Post-Ovulatory Methods for Fertility Regulation. BJOG 2004;111:715–25. (Level I)

18. Schaff EA, Fielding SL, Eisinger SH, Stadalius LS, Fuller L. Low-dose mifepristone followed by vaginal misoprostol at 48 hours for abortion up to 63 days. Contraception 2000;61:41–6. (Level II-3)

19. Schaff EA, Fielding SL, Westhoff C. Randomized trial of oral versus vaginal misoprostol 2 days after mifepristone 200 mg for abortion up to 63 days of pregnancy [published erratum appears in Contraception 2002;66:481]. Contraception 2002;66:247–50. (Level I)

20. von Hertzen H, Honkanen H, Piaggio G, Bartfai G, Erdenetungalag R, Gemzell-Danielsson K, et al. WHO multinational study of three misoprostol regimens after mifepristone for early medical abortion. I: Efficacy. WHO Research Group on Post-Ovulatory Methods for Fertility Regulation. BJOG 2003;110:808–18. (Level I)

21. Schaff EA, Stadalius LS, Eisinger SH, Franks P. Vaginal misoprostol administered at home after mifepristone (RU486) for abortion. J Fam Pract 1997;44:353–60. (Level II-3)

22. Schaff EA, Eisinger SH, Stadalius LS, Franks P, Gore BZ, Poppema S. Low-dose mifepristone 200 mg and vaginal misoprostol for abortion. Contraception 1999;59:1–6. (Level II-3)

23. Schaff EA, Fielding SL, Westhoff C, Ellertson C, Eisinger SH, Stadalius LS, et al. Vaginal misoprostol administered 1, 2, or 3 days after mifepristone for early medical abortion: a randomized trial [published erratum appears in JAMA 2000;284:2597]. JAMA 2000;284:1948–53. (Level I)

24. Schaff EA, Fielding SL, Westhoff C. Randomized trial of oral versus vaginal misoprostol at one day after mifepristone for early medical abortion. Contraception 2001;64: 81–5. (Level I)

25. Wiebe E, Dunn S, Guilbert E, Jacot F, Lugtig L. Comparison of abortions induced by methotrexate or mifepristone followed by misoprostol. Obstet Gynecol 2002;99:813–9. (Level I)

26. Creinin MD, Potter C, Holovanisin M, Janczukiewicz L, Pymar HC, Schwartz JL, et al. Mifepristone and misoprostol and methotrexate/misoprostol in clinical practice for abortion. Am J Obstet Gynecol 2003;188:664–9. (Level II-3)

27. Creinin MD, Fox MC, Teal S, Chen A, Schaff EA, Meyn LA. A randomized comparison of misoprostol 6 to 8 hours versus 24 hours after mifepristone for abortion. MOD Study Trial Group. Obstet Gynecol 2004;103:851–9. (Level I)

28. Creinin MD, Vittinghoff E, Keder L, Darney PD, Tiller G. Methotrexate and misoprostol for early abortion: a multicenter trial. I. Safety and efficacy. Contraception 1996;53:321–7. (Level II-3)

29. Creinin MD, Vittinghoff E, Schaff E, Klaisle C, Darney PD, Dean C. Medical abortion with oral methotrexate and vaginal misoprostol. Obstet Gynecol 1997;90:611–6. (Level II-3)

30. Creinin MD, Carbonell JL, Schwartz JL, Varela L, Tanda R. A randomized trial of the effect of moistening misoprostol before vaginal administration when used with methotrexate for abortion. Contraception 1999;59:11–6. (Level I)

31. Lipscomb GH, Bran D, McCord ML, Portera JC, Ling FW. Analysis of three hundred fifteen ectopic pregnancies treated with single-dose methotrexate. Am J Obstet Gynecol 1998;178:1354–8. (Level II-3)

32. Carbonell JL, Varela L, Velazco A, Cabezas E, Fernandez C, Sanchez C. Oral methotrexate and vaginal misoprostol for early abortion. Contraception 1998;57:83–8. (Level I)

33. Creinin MD. Oral methotrexate and vaginal misoprostol for early abortion. Contraception 1996;54:15–8. (Level I)

34. Carbonell JL, Varela L, Velazco A, Fernandez C. The use of misoprostol for termination of early pregnancy. Contraception 1997;55:165–8. (Level II-3)

35. Carbonell JL, Varela L, Velazco A, Fernandez C, Sanchez C. The use of misoprostol for abortion at ≤9 weeks' gestation. Eur J Contracept Reprod Health Care 1997;2:181–5. (Level II-3)

36. Esteve JL, Varela L, Velazco A, Tanda R, Cabezas E, Sanchez C. Early abortion with 800 micrograms of misoprostol by the vaginal route. Contraception 1999;59:219–25. (Level II-3)

37. Jain JK, Meckstroth KR, Mishell DR Jr. Early pregnancy termination with intravaginally administered sodium chloride solution-moistened misoprostol tablets: historical comparison with mifepristone and oral misoprostol. Am J Obstet Gynecol 1999;181:1386–91. (Level II-2)

38. Singh K, Fong YF, Dong F. A viable alternative to surgical vacuum aspiration: repeated doses of intravaginal misoprostol over 9 hours for medical termination of pregnancies up to eight weeks. BJOG 2003;110:175–80. (Level II-3)

39. Bugalho A, Faundes A, Jamisse L, Usfa M, Maria E, Bique C. Evaluation of the effectiveness of vaginal misoprostol to induce first trimester abortion. Contraception 1996;53:244–6. (Level II-1)

40. Creinin MD, Vittinghoff E. Methotrexate and misoprostol vs misoprostol alone for early abortion. A randomized controlled trial. JAMA 1994;272:1190–5. (Level I)

41. Koopersmith TB, Mishell DR Jr. The use of misoprostol for termination of early pregnancy. Contraception 1996;53:238–42. (Level I)

42. Tang OS, Miao BY, Lee SW, Ho PC. Pilot study on the use of repeated doses of sublingual misoprostol in termination of pregnancy up to 12 weeks gestation: efficacy and acceptability. Hum Reprod 2002;17:654–8. (Level II-3)

43. Jain JK, Dutton C, Harwood B, Meckstroth KR, Mishell DR Jr. A prospective randomized, double-blinded, placebo-controlled trial comparing mifepristone and vaginal misoprostol to vaginal misoprostol alone for elective termination of early pregnancy. Hum Reprod 2002;17:1477–82. (Level I)

44. Creinin MD. Randomized comparison of efficacy, acceptability and cost of medical versus surgical abortion. Contraception 2000;62:117–24. (Level I)

45. Henshaw RC, Naji SA, Russell IT, Templeton AA. Comparison of medical abortion with surgical vacuum aspiration: women's preferences and acceptability of treatment. BMJ 1993;307:714–7. (Level II-1)

46. Creinin MD, Aubény E. Medical abortion in early pregnancy. In: Paul M, Lichtenberg ES, Borgatta L, Grimes DA, Stubblefield PG, editors. A clinician's guide to medical and surgical abortion. New York (NY): Churchill Livingstone; 1999. p. 91–106. (Level III)

47. Creinin MD, Vittinghoff E, Galbraith S, Klaisle C. A randomized trial comparing misoprostol three and seven days after methotrexate for early abortion. Am J Obstet Gynecol 1995;173:1578–84. (Level I)

48. Creinin MD. Medical abortion with methotrexate 75 mg intramuscularly and vaginal misoprostol. Contraception 1997;56:367–71. (Level II-3)

49. Creinin MD, Darney PD. Methotrexate and misoprostol for early abortion [published erratum appears in Contraception 1994;49:99]. Contraception 1993;48:339–48. (Level II-3)

50. Creinin MD. Methotrexate for abortion at ≤42 days gestation. Contraception 1993;48:519–25. (Level II-3)

51. Harwood B, Meckstroth KR, Mishell DR, Jain JK. Serum beta-human chorionic gonadotropin levels and endometrial thickness after medical abortion. Contraception 2001;63:255–6. (Level III)

52. Allen RH, Westhoff C, De Nonno L, Fielding SL, Schaff EA. Curettage after mifepristone-induced abortion: frequency, timing, and indications. Obstet Gynecol 2001;98:101–6. (Level II-3)

53. Ashok PW, Penney GC, Flett GM, Templeton A. An effective regimen for early medical abortion: a report of 2000 consecutive cases. Hum Reprod 1998;13:2962–5. (Level II-3)

54. Winikoff B, Sivin I, Coyaji KJ, Cabezas E, Xiao B, Gu S, et al. Safety, efficacy, and acceptability of medical abortion in China, Cuba, and India: a comparative trial of mifepristone-misoprostol versus surgical abortion. Am J Obstet Gynecol 1997;176:431–7. (Level II-3)

55. Bartley J, Brown A, Elton R, Baird DT. Double-blind randomized trial of mifepristone in combination with vaginal gemeprost or misoprostol for induction of abortion up to 63 days gestation. Hum Reprod 2001;16:2098–102. (Level I)

56. Silvestre L, Dubois C, Renault M, Rezvani Y, Baulieu EE, Ulmann A. Voluntary interruption of pregnancy with mifepristone (RU 486) and a prostaglandin analogue. A large-scale French experience. N Engl J Med 1990;322: 645–8. (Level II-3)

57. Ulmann A, Silvestre L, Chemama L, Rezvani Y, Renault M, Aguillaume CJ, et al. Medical termination of early pregnancy with mifepristone (RU 486) followed by a prostaglandin analogue. Study in 16,369 women. Acta Obstet Gynecol Scand 1992;71:278–83. (Level II-3)

58. Centers for Disease Control and Prevention. Clostridium sordellii toxic shock syndrome after medical abortion with mifepristone and intravaginal misoprostol—United States and Canada, 2001–2005. MMWR Morb Mortal Wkly Rep 2005;54:724.

59. Grimes DA. Risk of mifepristone abortion in context. Contraception 2005;71:161.

60. Ellertson C, Elul B, Ambardekar S, Wood L, Carroll J, Coyaji K. Accuracy of assessment of pregnancy duration by women seeking early abortions. Lancet 2000;355: 877–81. (Level III)

61. Creinin MD, Jerald H. Success rates and estimation of gestational age for medical abortion vary with transvaginal ultrasonographic criteria. Am J Obstet Gynecol 1999; 180:35–41. (Level II-3)

62. Ectopic pregnancy—United States, 1988-1989. MMWR Morb Mortal Wkly Rep 1992;41:591–4. (Level II-3)

63. Van Den Eeden SK, Shan J, Bruce C, Glasser M. Ectopic pregnancy rate and treatment utilization in a large managed care organization. Obstet Gynecol 2005;105: 1052–7. (Level II-3)

64. Edwards J, Creinin MD. Surgical abortion for gestations of less than 6 weeks. Curr Probl Obstet Gynecol Fertil 1997;20:11–9. (Level II-3)

65. Paul M, Schaff E, Nichols M. The roles of clinical assessment, human chorionic gonadotropin assays, and ultrasonography in medical abortion practice. Am J Obstet Gynecol 2000;183(suppl 2):S34–43. (Level III)

66. Fielding SL, Schaff EA, Nam NY. Clinicians' perception of sonogram indication for mifepristone abortion up to 63 days. Contraception 2002;66:27–31. (Level III)

67. Schaff EA, Eisinger SH, Franks P, Kim SS. Combined methotrexate and misoprostol for early induced abortion. Arch Fam Med 1995;4:774–9. (Level II-3)

68. Rossi B, Creinin MD, Meyn LA. Ability of the clinician and patient to predict the outcome of mifepristone and misoprostol medical abortion. Contraception 2004;70: 313–7. (Level II-3)

69. Creinin MD, Shulman T. Effect of non-steroidal anti-inflammatory drugs on the action of misoprostol in a regimen for early abortion. Contraception 1997;56:165–8. (Level II-2)

70. Darab DJ, Minkoff R, Sciote J, Sulik KK. Pathogenesis of median facial clefts in mice treated with methotrexate. Teratology 1987;36:77–86. (Level III)

71. Kozlowski RD, Steinbrunner JV, MacKenzie AH, Clough JD, Wilke WS, Segal AM. Outcome of first-trimester exposure to low-dose methotrexate in eight patients with rheumatic disease. Am J Med 1990;88:589–92. (Level III)

72. Yip SK, Tse AO, Haines CJ, Chung TK. Misoprostol's effect on uterine arterial blood flow and fetal heart rate in early pregnancy. Obstet Gynecol 2000;95:232–5. (Level II-3)

73. Fonseca W, Alencar AJ, Mota FS, Coelho HL. Misoprostol and congenital malformations. Lancet 1991;338: 56. (Level III)

74. Gonzalez CH, Vargas FR, Perez AB, Kim CA, Brunoni D, Marques-Dias MJ, et al. Limb deficiency with or without Möbius sequence in seven Brazilian children associated with misoprostol use in the first trimester of pregnancy. Am J Med Genet 1993;47:59–64. (Level III)

75. Marques-Dias MJ, Gonzalez CH, Rosemberg S. Mobius sequence in children exposed in utero to misoprostol: neuropathological study of three cases. Birth Defects Res A Clin Mol Teratol 2003;67:1002–7. (Level III)

76. Pastuszak AL, Schuler L, Speck-Martins CE, Coelho KE, Cordello SM, Vargas F, et al. Use of misoprostol during pregnancy and Mobius' syndrome in infants. N Engl J Med 1998;338:1881–5. (Level II-2)

77. Wiebe ER. Abortion induced with methotrexate and misoprostol: a comparison of various protocols. Contraception 1997;55:159–63. (Level II-1)

78. Creinin MD. Conception rates after abortion with methotrexate and misoprostol. Int J Gynaecol Obstet 1999;65:183–8. (Level II-2)

79. Steinhoff PG, Smith RG, Palmore JA, Diamond M, Chung CS. Women who obtain repeat abortions: a study based on record linkage. Fam Plann Perspect 1979;11:30–8. (Level III)

The MEDLINE database, the Cochrane Library, and ACOG's own internal resources and documents were used to conduct a literature search to locate relevant articles published between January 1985 and June 2005. The search was restricted to articles published in the English language. Priority was given to articles reporting results of original research, although review articles and commentaries also were consulted. Abstracts of research presented at symposia and scientific conferences were not considered adequate for inclusion in this document. Guidelines published by organizations or institutions such as the National Institutes of Health and the American College of Obstetricians and Gynecologists were reviewed, and additional studies were located by reviewing bibliographies of identified articles. When reliable research was not available, expert opinions from obstetrician–gynecologists were used.

Studies were reviewed and evaluated for quality according to the method outlined by the U.S. Preventive Services Task Force:

I   Evidence obtained from at least one properly designed randomized controlled trial.

II-1   Evidence obtained from well-designed controlled trials without randomization.

II-2   Evidence obtained from well-designed cohort or case–control analytic studies, preferably from more than one center or research group.

II-3   Evidence obtained from multiple time series with or without the intervention. Dramatic results in uncontrolled experiments also could be regarded as this type of evidence.

III   Opinions of respected authorities, based on clinical experience, descriptive studies, or reports of expert committees.

Based on the highest level of evidence found in the data, recommendations are provided and graded according to the following categories:

Level A—Recommendations are based on good and consistent scientific evidence.

Level B—Recommendations are based on limited or inconsistent scientific evidence.

Level C—Recommendations are based primarily on consensus and expert opinion.

ISSN 1099-3630

**The American College of
Obstetricians and Gynecologists
409 12th Street, SW
PO Box 96920
Washington, DC 20090-6920**

12345/98765

Medical management of abortion. ACOG Practice Bulletin No. 67. American College of Obstetricians and Gynecologists. Obstet Gynecol 2005;106:871–82.

ACOG PRACTICE BULLETIN

CLINICAL MANAGEMENT GUIDELINES FOR
OBSTETRICIAN–GYNECOLOGISTS

NUMBER 11, DECEMBER 1999

(Replaces Technical Bulletin Number 184, September 1993)

This Practice Bulletin was developed by the ACOG Committee on Practice Bulletins— Gynecology with the assistance of Kamran S. Moghissi, MD and Craig A. Winkel, MD. The information is designed to aid practitioners in making decisions about appropriate obstetric and gynecologic care. These guidelines should not be construed as dictating an exclusive course of treatment or procedure. Variations in practice may be warranted based on the needs of the individual patient, resources, and limitations unique to the institution or type of practice.

Medical Management of Endometriosis

Endometriosis represents a significant health problem for women of reproductive age. Defined as the presence of endometrial-like glands and stroma in any extrauterine site, endometriosis continues to defy our complete understanding regarding etiology, the relationship between extent of disease and the degree of symptoms, its relationship to fertility, and the most appropriate means of therapy. The purpose of this document is to present the evidence, including risks and benefits, for the effectiveness of medical therapy for women who experience symptoms and problems believed to be secondary to endometriosis.

Background

Incidence

Endometriosis is a gynecologic condition that occurs in 7–10% of women in the general population and up to 50% of premenopausal women (1), with a prevalence of 38% (range, 20–50%) (2–4) in infertile women, and in 71–87% of women with chronic pelvic pain (5–7). Contrary to much speculation, there are no data to support the view that the incidence of endometriosis is increasing, although improved recognition of endometriosis lesions (8) may have led to an increase in the rate of detection. There also appears to be no particular racial predisposition to endometriosis.

A familial association of endometriosis has been documented (9), and patients with an affected first-degree relative have nearly a 10-fold increased risk of developing endometriosis. The proposed inheritance is characteristic of a polygenic-multifactorial mechanism.

Etiology

Although the pathogenesis of endometriosis remains unclear, leading theories include retrograde menstruation, hematogenous or lymphatogenous transport, and coelomic metaplasia. It has been suggested that virtually all women are potentially vulnerable to the development of the lesions of endometriosis, but appropriate immuno-competency in most eradicates such lesions in a timely fashion, preventing clinical sequelae (10). Menstrual flow that produces a greater volume of retrograde menstruation may increase the risk of developing endometriosis. Cervical or vaginal atresia with outflow obstruction also is linked with the development of endometriosis (11). Early menarche, regular cycles (especially without intervening pregnancy-induced amenorrhea), and a longer and heavier than normal flow are associated with this disease (12). Because endometriosis is an estrogen-dependent disease, factors that reduce estrogen levels, such as exercise-induced menstrual disorders, decreased body-fat content, and tobacco smoking, are associated with reduced risk of developing endometriosis (12).

Clinical Manifestations

The clinical manifestations of endometriosis are variable and unpredictable in both presentation and course. Dysmenorrhea, chronic pelvic pain, dyspareunia, uterosacral ligament nodularity, and adnexal mass (either symptomatic or asymptomatic) are among the most well-recognized manifestations (13–16). A significant number of women with endometriosis remain asymptomatic.

The association between endometriosis and infertility remains the subject of considerable debate. It is clear that endometriosis may induce infertility as a result of anatomic distortion secondary to invasive endometriosis and related adhesions. Although it was previously believed that patients with minimal and mild endometriosis displayed reduced monthly fecundity rates (17), a cause-and-effect relationship has not been proven, and more recent prospective controlled trials suggest that minimal to mild endometriosis is not associated with reduced fecundity (18) and may not be a direct cause of infertility (19).

Pelvic pain that is typical of endometriosis is characteristically described as secondary dysmenorrhea (with pain frequently commencing prior to the onset of menses), deep dyspareunia (exaggerated during menses), or sacral backache with menses. Endometriosis that involves specific organs may result in pain or physiologic dysfunction of those organs, such as perimenstrual tenesmus or diarrhea in cases of bowel involvement or dysuria and hematuria in cases of bladder involvement.

The pain associated with endometriosis has little relationship to the type or location of the lesions that are visible at laparoscopy (20). Surgical assessment is complicated by the varying, and subtle appearances of endometriosis (21, 22), and may be demonstrated histologically in a normal-appearing peritoneum (23, 24). It has been shown that the depth of infiltration of endometriosis lesions correlates best with pain severity (6, 25, 26). Systematic analysis of the source of pain in awake patients undergoing laparoscopy (sometimes referred to as "pain mapping") demonstrates that pain arises from stimulation of adjacent normal peritoneal surfaces that extend well beyond the visible lesions of endometriosis. This suggests that painful lesions are those involving peritoneal surfaces innervated by peripheral spinal nerves, rather than those innervated by the autonomic nervous system (20).

Diagnosis

Direct visualization confirmed by histologic examination, especially of lesions with nonclassical appearance (21, 22, 27), remains the standard for diagnosing endometriosis. The presence of two or more of the following histologic features is used as the threshold criteria for the diagnosis by a pathologist (28):

- Endometrial epithelium
- Endometrial glands
- Endometrial stroma
- Hemosiderin-laden macrophages

Visual inspection as the sole means for making the diagnosis of endometriosis requires an experienced surgeon who is familiar with the protean appearances of endometriosis. Experience is associated with increased diagnostic accuracy (8, 21, 22), but the correlation between visual inspection and histologic confirmation of the presence of endometriosis in biopsy specimens is imperfect (22). The finding of microscopic endometriosis in normal-appearing peritoneum (23, 24) exemplifies the inaccuracy of diagnosis by visualization alone. Peritoneal biopsy may be used for diagnosing questionable peritoneal lesions (22).

Because tissue confirmation of the diagnosis of endometriosis requires a surgical procedure, investigators have searched for a noninvasive alternative. The correlation between the presence of moderate and severe endometriosis and an increased concentration of CA 125 in serum has been known for more than 10 years (29). Although the specificity of CA 125 measurements had been reported to be greater than 85%, with sensitivities between 20% and 50% (30–33), the clinical utility of measuring CA 125 as a diagnostic marker for endometriosis appears to be limited. Determining the level of CA 125 in serum appears to be useful in detecting women with severe endometriosis but is of questionable value in detecting women with minimal or mild disease (34, 35).

Measurement of peritoneal fluid levels, however, appears to be better for detecting minimal and moderate disease (34).

Concentrations of CA 125 in serum also have been studied as a marker to determine the response to medical therapy for endometriosis. Although CA 125 levels may decrease during treatment when compared with pretreatment values (36–38), posttreatment values that are normal do not confirm the absence of endometriosis (36, 38), nor are they useful for predicting disease recurrence (37).

Imaging studies, such as ultrasonography, magnetic resonance imaging, and computed tomography, appear to be useful only in the presence of a pelvic or adnexal mass. Ovarian endometriomas, visualized ultrasonographically, typically appear as cysts that contain low-level, homogeneous internal echoes consistent with old blood. Imaging studies alone appear to have greater predictive accuracy in differentiating ovarian endometriomas from other adnexal masses than when used in combination with measurement of CA 125 levels in plasma (39). Magnetic resonance imaging may detect deeply infiltrating endometriosis that involves the uterosacral ligaments and the cul-de-sac, but lacks sensitivity in detecting rectal involvement (40).

American Society for Reproductive Medicine
Revised Classification of Endometriosis

Patient's name _____   Date _____

Stage I (minimal)   —   1–5
Stage II (mild)   —   6–15
Stage III (moderate)   —   16–40   Laparoscopy_____ Laparotomy _____ Photography _____
Stage IV (severe)   —   >40   Recommended treatment _____

Total _____   Prognosis _____

Peritoneum	Endometriosis	<1 cm	1–3 cm	>3 cm
	Superficial	1	2	4
	Deep	2	4	6
Ovary	R Superficial	1	2	4
	Deep	4	16	20
	L Superficial	1	2	4
	Deep	4	16	20

	Posterior cul-de-sac obliteration	Partial		Complete	
		4		40	

	Adhesions	<$^1/_3$ Enclosure	$^1/_3$ – $^2/_3$ Enclosure	>$^2/_3$ Enclosure
Ovary	R Filmy	1	2	4
	Dense	4	8	16
	L Filmy	1	2	4
	Dense	4	8	16
Tube	R Filmy	1	2	4
	Dense	4*	8*	16
	L Filmy	1	2	4
	Dense	4*	8*	16

*If the fimbriated end of the fallopian tube is completely enclosed, change the point assignment to 16. Denote appearance of superficial implant types as red [(R), red, red-pink, flamelike, vesicular blobs, clear vesicles], white [(W), opacifications, peritoneal defects, yellow-brown], or black [(B), black, hemosiderin deposits, blue]. Denote percent of total described as R___%, W___%, and B___%. Total should equal 100%.

Figure 1. Modified from the revised American Fertility Society classification of endometriosis. (Reprinted with permission from the American Society for Reproductive Medicine. Fertility and Sterility 1996;67(5):819–820)

Classification

Numerous classification schemas have been proposed to describe endometriosis by anatomic location and severity of disease. The American Society for Reproductive Medicine (ASRM [formerly the American Fertility Society]) classification, which is the most commonly used system, was revised for the third time in 1996 (41) (see Figure 1) but still has limitations and inherent defects. The system is not a good predictor of pregnancy following treatment despite adjustments to the point scores and cut-points for disease stage. The ASRM system does not correlate well with the symptoms of pain and dyspareunia (6). The true value of the ASRM 1996 revised system is in uniform recording of operative findings and perhaps for comparing the results of various therapies.

Clinical Considerations and Recommendations

▶ *In women with endometriosis-related pain who desire future fertility, how does medical therapy compare with no therapy for the treatment of pain and long-term preservation of fertility potential?*

Deeply infiltrating endometriosis, rather than surface noninfiltrating endometriosis, is commonly associated with pelvic pain (6). At present, evidence suggests that pain associated with endometriosis can be reduced with the use of a variety of medications (progestins, danazol, oral contraceptives, nonsteroidal antiinflammatory drugs, and gonadotropin-releasing hormone [GnRH] agonists) (42–47). There is also evidence that such medical therapies are likely to reduce the size of endometriosis lesions and, thus, the stage of disease (42, 48, 49). There are no data, however, showing that medical therapy eradicates the lesions. Although medical treatment may eliminate the symptoms associated with endometriosis, there is no evidence that such treatment has an impact on the future fertility of women with endometriosis. Because early-stage endometriosis is more likely to be associated with pain symptoms without associated alterations in fecundity, it is unlikely that such data will be forthcoming. Furthermore, whereas infiltrating lesions of endometriosis are associated with pain, studies are lacking that suggest the absence of treatment is associated with a progressive or future decline in fertility.

In a woman with normal or minor gynecologic findings suggesting mild disease (pelvic tenderness, uterosacral

nodularity), ovarian suppression with a combination oral contraceptive may be effective in reducing pain (50). The efficacy of continuous administration of oral contraceptives compared with cyclic administration has not been tested in a prospective fashion. Oral contraceptives probably should not be used for more than 3 months if the patient experiences no relief of symptoms. Furthermore, there is no reason to suspect that one oral contraceptive is better than another for suppression of pain symptoms. If recurrent symptoms do not respond to oral contraceptives, then therapy with medroxyprogesterone acetate (MPA), danazol, or a GnRH agonist may be appropriate.

Danazol, when used in doses of 600–800 mg per day appears to as effective as GnRH agonists for pain relief in most patients, but is associated with a significantly greater incidence of side effects (51). The cost of treatment with danazol is about one third less than treatment with a GnRH agonist but nearly twice as costly as treatment with oral contraceptives and oral or depot MPA.

▶ *In women with endometriosis-related pain who desire future fertility, how does medical therapy compare with surgical therapy alone for the management of pain and long-term preservation of fertility potential?*

The debate regarding medical treatment versus surgical treatment for the management of pain related to endometriosis continues despite of the lack of substantive data on either side of the argument. Surgical therapy for women with endometriosis is associated with a significant reduction in pain symptoms during the first 6 months following surgery (52). With continued follow-up, however, a substantial portion (44%) of women experience recurrence of symptoms within 1 year postoperatively (53). The cumulative recurrence rate of pain symptoms during the initial 5 years following discontinuation of therapy with a GnRH agonist is 53% (54). No evidence exists regarding the effectiveness of adjunctive treatment with danazol, oral contraceptives, or progestins in comparison with surgical treatment alone in the management of endometriosis-related pelvic pain. A major issue in considering comparisons of surgical treatment with medical treatment is the experience and expertise of the surgeon.

Likewise, debate continues over the best means of surgical therapy. One opinion considers vaporization or cautery of peritoneal implants adequate, whereas the other recommends surgical excision as necessary for adequate treatment (55). Currently, there are limited data to show that one method is better than the other. Moreover, there are no data regarding whether surgical therapy influences long-term fertility. Also, no data exist to indicate whether medical or surgical treatments result in the best fertility outcomes.

▶ *Following surgical diagnosis of endometriosis, what is the role of surgical destruction of lesions, or medical therapy in conjunction with surgery, for long-term pain relief in patients with minimal to moderate endometriosis that has been completely resected?*

It is probably impossible to completely resect all endometriosis lesions, if for no other reason than in up to 25% of biopsies of normal-appearing peritoneum one will find histologic evidence of endometriosis (23, 24). In addition, even when experienced surgeons attempt to resect completely a deeply infiltrating lesion, histologic study often reveals that the lesion is incompletely resected (26).

Operative laparoscopy for surgical treatment of pelvic pain related to endometriosis appears to have numerous advantages over laparotomy. These include more rapid recovery, the potential to decrease postoperative adhesion formation (56), and complication rates of 10% with laparoscopy (57). Although technical difficulties can be overcome partially through skill and experience, the efficacy of surgical therapy still depends heavily on the surgeon. Regardless of the technique employed—excision, endocoagulation, electrocautery, or laser vaporization—no study demonstrates the superiority of any one method, and recurrence rates average 19% (58). For successful surgical treatment, considering the varied appearances of endometriosis, the challenge lies in the surgeon's ability to recognize all visible lesions.

The only prospective, double-blind, randomized, controlled trial designed to evaluate the effectiveness of laparoscopic surgery for women with pelvic pain was reported in 1994 (52). Of the women who underwent laser ablation of endometriosis and laser uterosacral nerve ablation, 62% experienced pain relief 6 months after surgery, compared with 22% who underwent laparoscopic visualization only (52). If one considers the results of this study and a number of retrospective analyses, it appears that surgical treatment alone will confer pain relief in approximately two thirds of women for up to 1 year.

Postoperative medical treatment could be useful when residual disease is expected, when pain is not relieved, or to extend the pain-free interval following surgery. Although not demonstrated on the basis of clinical studies available at present, postoperative treatment should minimize the risk of recurrence. Two studies support the use of postoperative

GnRH agonists to extend the period of pain relief. In a randomized, controlled trial of an intranasal GnRH agonist, 31% of women who received the GnRH agonist following laparoscopy needed additional medical treatment 18 months following surgery, whereas 57% of the women who received placebo required additional medical suppression (59).

The efficacy of other hormonal therapy in conjunction with surgery for treating women with endometriosis remains unclear. Oral MPA has been shown to induce regression of endometriosis lesions. One study has demonstrated that depot MPA is safe and effective in reducing pain associated with endometriosis (45). Importantly, depot MPA confers contraception during therapy while the use of low-dose danazol (200–400 mg) to reduce the dose-related side effects may not prevent conception and thus exposes the patient to the potential for teratogenesis. A combination of low-dose danazol and oral contraceptives appears to offer a similar degree of efficacy while providing effective contraception (45).

Few reports have examined the use of danazol as an adjunct to surgical therapy. It appears that danazol treatment for 3 months following laparoscopic surgery for women with Stage III and Stage IV endometriosis offers no advantage over expectant management with regard to pain recurrence (60).

▶ *Following surgical diagnosis of endometriosis, what is the role of surgical destruction of lesions, or medical therapy in conjunction with surgery, for long-term pain relief in patients with severe endometriosis with residual disease present?*

The recurrence rates for endometriosis appear to correlate with severity of disease (54), with a recurrence rate over a 7-year period following medical treatment of 37% for women with mild disease and 74% for women with severe disease. Although one might conclude that postoperative medical treatment would make sense for the woman with severe endometriosis with residual disease, there are no data documenting the efficacy of this therapy. In most cases, studies of the efficacy of postoperative medical treatment specifically address those patients with minimal to moderate disease, excluding those with severe endometriosis. Treatment with a GnRH agonist prior to laparoscopic surgery was associated with a higher fecundity rate within the first year following surgery than with preoperative danazol or gestrinone (61). However, such therapy was not associated with a reduction in operating time or any decrease in recurrence rate 1 year after surgery for ovarian endometriomata (62). For women with severe endometriosis, with or without suspected residual disease, the efficacy of either preoperative or postoperative medical therapy has yet to be established.

▶ *In women receiving a 3–6-month regimen of GnRH analog therapy for treatment of endometriosis-related pelvic pain, what are the advantages and disadvantages of an "add-back" regimen?*

Gonadotropin-releasing hormone agonists have been shown to be efficacious and safe for treating women with endometriosis-related pelvic pain (47, 49, 63–66). However, because these agents create a state of relative estrogen deficiency, their use has been limited generally to a 6-month course of therapy, particularly because of the potential effects on bone density, as well as the side effects, most notably vasomotor symptoms.

To minimize both the loss of bone and side effects, add-back regimens (using either sex-steroid hormones or other specific bone-sparing agents) have been advocated for use in women undergoing long-term therapy (ie, >6 months). Such treatment strategies have included progestins alone (67–69), progestins and organic bisphosphonates (70), low-dose progestins and estrogens (71,72), pulsatile parathyroid hormone (73), and nasal calcitonin (74). Although there are no published studies specifically designed to compare the various add-back regimens, virtually all add-back regimens (except nasal calcitonin) have considerable efficacy in reducing the loss of bone mineral density associated with GnRH agonist treatment. Some regimens appear to reduce vasomotor symptoms better than others; parathyroid hormone therapy has little effect on such symptoms.

The potential advantages of add-back therapy for women undergoing short-term (3–6 months) GnRH agonist therapy are twofold. First, while it has been shown that the bone loss after 3 months of treatment with a GnRH agonist is less than that after 6 months of treatment (69, 70, 72), add-back therapy does reduce the bone loss observed after only 3 months of GnRH agonist therapy (72). Add-back treatment does not diminish the efficacy of pain relief observed during 3 months or 6 months of GnRH agonist therapy. Second, add-back regimens that employ progestins alone (67–72) or in combination with estrogens (71, 72, 75) reduce significantly the vasomotor symptoms associated with GnRH agonist treatment. There appear to be no disadvantages to the use of an add-back regimen in combination with a GnRH agonist other than the incremental cost associated with the additional medication.

▶ *In women who have had a good response to GnRH therapy and who may benefit from an extended duration of therapy with add-back therapy (>6 months), what is the safety and efficacy of such long-term treatment?*

There are few data available on the use of GnRH agonists for more than 6 months. The major concern with prolonged use of GnRH agonists is the loss of bone mineral density that is observed during 6 months of therapy with these drugs (76). The mean loss of bone mineral density during a 6-month course of therapy with GnRH agonists ranges from 5.9% to 15% and may depend on the dose, route, and particular agonist being used (77). Marked individual differences in susceptibility to bone loss have been noted. Bone loss during a 6-month course of intranasal GnRH agonist was less than that observed with the intramuscular form (3% versus 5%) (78). Gonadotropin-releasing hormone agonists do not have adverse effects on triglyceride or cholesterol metabolism (79), as may be seen with danazol (80) or MPA (81).

A 12-month course of GnRH agonist therapy was associated with approximately a 6% decrease in bone density. The addition of norethindrone acetate alone or in combination with conjugated equine estrogens had no adverse impact on pain relief but did prevent bone mineral loss (44); there was also an associated increase in low-density lipoprotein cholesterol, a decrease in high-density lipoprotein cholesterol, and an increase in triglycerides. The clinical significance of these latter changes is unclear. Currently, there are no data regarding extended treatment with GnRH agonists beyond 1 year. Patients receiving this treatment should be monitored regularly for physical findings, bone density, and serum lipid parameters.

If the woman has previously undergone therapy with a GnRH agonist, it appears safe to retreat with a GnRH agonist alone provided there has been suitable time for recovery of bone mineral density since the previous course of treatment (82). If bone mineral density has not recovered fully, or if bone density has not been evaluated, the use of either a potent progestin or danazol is recommended. No studies have been reported to evaluate bone density after progestin administration following initial GnRH agonist therapy. Finally, a GnRH agonist in combination with add-back treatment may be considered, especially if the add-back regimen is commenced coincidentally with the reinitiation of therapy with the GnRH agonist. The long-term effects of multiple courses of treatment with a GnRH agonist have yet to be assessed.

▶ *In a woman with symptoms consistent with endometriosis, is empiric medical therapy (without definitive surgical diagnosis) an efficacious and cost-effective approach to pain relief?*

The need for laparoscopy (or any other surgical procedure) for diagnosis or treatment of pelvic pain secondary to suspected endometriosis has been the subject of debate (83). Arguments against the requirement to perform surgery to definitively diagnose endometriosis include the imprecision of surgical diagnosis as well as the inherent risks of surgery. "Empiric" therapy is used commonly in clinical gynecology when the signs and symptoms support the particular diagnosis being entertained and the consequences of an inaccurate diagnosis are likely to be minimal (eg, mild cystitis, suspected pelvic infection, and bacterial vaginosis).

In a woman with pelvic pain, diagnostic evaluation should include a thorough history and physical examination to rule out other gynecologic causes of pain, such as chronic pelvic inflammatory disease, leiomyomata uteri, and ovarian cysts. Nongynecologic causes of pain, such as gastrointestinal and urinary tract problems, may be ruled out by appropriate testing. Consideration also should be given to pelvic ultrasonography, complete blood count, urinalysis, and endocervical sampling for gonococcal and chlamydial infection if signs and symptoms warrant.

Based on a well-designed, prospective, randomized, controlled, double-blind clinical trial, the following statement can be made (7). After an appropriate pretreatment evaluation (to exclude other conditions) and failure of initial treatment with oral contraceptives and nonsteroidal antiinflammatory drugs, empiric therapy with a 3-month course of a GnRH agonist is appropriate. This approach is associated with clinically and statistically significant improvement in dysmenorrhea, pelvic pain, and pelvic tenderness. Furthermore, if the diagnostic algorithm described is employed prior to the initiation of empiric GnRH therapy, the likelihood of endometriosis being present on posttreatment laparoscopy is 78–87%. Thus, it appears that empiric treatment with a GnRH agonist (ie, without surgical diagnosis) is efficacious.

Comparing costs of empiric medical management versus definitive surgical diagnosis is more difficult to address. Although there are a lack of well-designed studies that compare the actual costs between the two approaches, it has been estimated that the cost of 3 months of empiric therapy is less than that of a laparoscopic procedure. No trials comparing primary medical and surgical

therapies have been reported, nor have data been reported regarding the percentage of women who will still require surgical therapy following satisfactory empiric treatment.

▶ *In asymptomatic women in whom endometriosis is discovered incidentally, how does medical therapy compare with no intervention for long-term pain relief and preservation of fertility?*

The pathophysiology of endometriosis remains poorly understood. Largely because of failure to identify a suitable animal model, there is little systematic research regarding either the progression of the disease or the prediction of clinical outcomes. The presence of endometriosis among asymptomatic infertility patients varies between 20% and 50%, suggesting that it may not always be pathologic. In biopsies of apparently normal peritoneum, one can demonstrate the presence of endometrial glands and stroma in 25%, thus confirming the presence of endometriosis (23). In 50% of cases, endometriosis regresses spontaneously or remains constant (84). There are a number of obstacles, therefore, to predicting what the presence of endometriosis holds for a given woman. There are no data available regarding medical therapy for prevention of disease progression or for prevention of future pain.

Although preliminary data suggest that the destruction of all apparent lesions is associated with improved fecundity during the next 36 months (85), there are no data available on which to make a recommendation regarding medical therapy to prevent progression of disease or to prevent pain symptoms.

Endometriosis frequently is associated with infertility, although a cause-and-effect relationship between the two remains controversial. Essential steps in the development of endometriosis require a series of complex interactions between peritoneal leukocytes and endometrial cells, but the exact etiologic factor(s) remains unknown. In addition, both specific and nonspecific immunologic alterations are likely required. Whether these are the result or the cause of the disease also remains unclear. Although the pathophysiology of infertility arising from endometriosis that results in distortion of normal anatomy is relatively easy to understand, the mechanisms by which nonadhesive disease leads to infertility are still not clear.

There are no data to support the suggestion that medical treatment to prevent the progression of the disease will result in successful fertility in the future. It is not even clear whether fertility can be predicted based on the presence of endometriosis unless there is gross distortion of tubal and ovarian anatomy.

▶ *In women with endometriosis-related pain who have completed childbearing, how does medical management compare with no therapy for long-term pain relief?*

The rates for recurrence of pain symptoms following medical or surgical treatment for endometriosis do not differ greatly. Following surgical therapy, about two thirds of patients experience recurrence of pain symptoms within 2 years of surgery (52, 56). However, the recurrence of pain symptoms may be delayed by the addition of 3 months of treatment with a GnRH agonist (59).

Medical therapy alone is likely to result in a significant pain-free interval following treatment with a GnRH agonist (54, 86) in the absence of surgical treatment. In addition, treatment with either oral contraceptives, danazol, or progestins has been shown to reduce, at least in the short term, pain symptoms associated with endometriosis (43, 45, 46). Currently, there are no follow-up data beyond 7 years after medical treatment. The long-term impact of medical therapy on pain recurrence beyond this period remains unclear.

▶ *In a woman with pelvic pain arising from known endometriosis, does the presence of an ovarian endometrioma on ultrasound influence the efficacy or safety of employing medical therapy for pain relief?*

The reliability of ultrasonography for diagnosing endometriosis depends on the nature of the lesions. The endovaginal ultrasonographic approach appears to be superior to the transvesical approach for the evaluation of an ovarian mass. For the diagnosis of ovarian endometriomas, ultrasonography is reliable, with sensitivity up to 83% and specificity of 98% (87). Scattered internal echoes that tend to appear homogeneous are characteristic of endometriomas.

Gonadotropin-releasing hormone agonist treatment resulted in a greater than 25% reduction in the diameter of endometriomas for more than 80% of the women observed, compared with 30% of those treated with danazol (61). These authors did not report on the reduction in pain symptoms. Although it is theorized that preoperative medical treatment of the woman with an ovarian endometrioma might facilitate surgery by reducing inflammation and vascularity, there are no studies that address this practice. A 3-month preoperative course of a GnRH agonist has been reported to produce decreased cyst wall thickness and inflammation (88), but was not associated with either reduced operating time or reduced incidence of recurrence

1 year later (62). There is only anecdotal information regarding responses of suspected ovarian endometriomas to therapy with oral contraceptives or MPA. When medical treatment is used in a woman with an ovarian mass that is assumed to be an endometrioma, the potential for missed diagnosis or delay in diagnosis of a more serious condition (such as a malignant or borderline tumor) must always be kept in mind.

Because it is likely that the pain associated with endometriosis is most closely related to deeply infiltrating peritoneal disease rather than the ovarian endometrioma, medical therapy aimed at suppressing ovarian function is likely to result in a similar reduction in pain symptoms, whether or not there is a coincident ovarian endometrioma. There are no studies, however, of the efficacy of medical therapy for pain in the presence or absence of an endometrioma.

▶ *In patients with pain or bleeding arising from known endometriosis affecting nonreproductive organs, what is the evidence for the efficacy of medical therapy for these symptoms?*

Extrapelvic endometriosis has been reported in a variety of sites, including the upper abdomen, the diaphragm, the abdominal wall (particularly the umbilicus), the perineum (episiotomy scar), and the thorax (89, 90). In addition, endometriosis may invade the full thickness of the rectum, large and small bowel, ureters, or bladder. The symptoms that are associated with endometriosis at these sites vary depending on location and depths of infiltration, including women who experience cyclic episodes of gross hematuria, hematochezia, and hemoptysis. Although a number of therapeutic approaches have been employed for women with presumed extrapelvic endometriosis (91), the efficacy of ovarian suppression with a GnRH agonist appears to support it as the first line of therapy (92, 93). Based on current available evidence, medical treatment appears to be efficacious for women with signs and symptoms of extrapelvic endometriosis provided other, potentially serious diseases have been excluded.

▶ *In a woman who has undergone a total abdominal hysterectomy for definitive therapy for endometriosis, what is the risk of symptomatic recurrence with estrogen replacement therapy, and is there a role for suppressive therapy after total abdominal hysterectomy with bilateral salpingo-oophorectomy if there is residual disease?*

The rates of recurrence of endometriosis after initial conservative surgery tend to vary based on stage or extent of disease at the time of surgery. It is particularly difficult, however, to distinguish between recurrence and persistence of endometriosis. Recurrence rates range between 20% and 40% within 5 years after surgery for endometriosis (52, 53, 55, 94).

Hysterectomy, with or without bilateral oophorectomy, is often regarded as "definitive" therapy for the treatment of endometriosis associated with intractable pelvic pain, adnexal masses, or multiple previous conservative surgical procedures. Based on the results of a recently published retrospective analysis of women monitored for a mean duration of 58 months after hysterectomy, ovarian conservation was associated with a 62% likelihood of recurrent symptoms and a 31% chance of requiring additional surgical treatment (95). In women who underwent bilateral adnexectomy, there was a 10% chance of recurrence of symptoms with only a 4% likelihood of additional surgery (95). The relative risk for pain recurrence after total abdominal hysterectomy was found to be 6.1 (95% confidence interval: 2.5–14.6) with ovarian preservation when compared with women who have their ovaries removed. The relative risk of additional surgery was 8.1 (95% confidence interval: 2.1–31.3) with ovarian conservation (95).

Symptoms may recur in women even after hysterectomy and oophorectomy. Endometriosis may recur in up to 15% of women whether or not the patients are treated with estrogen replacement therapy following bilateral oophorectomy (96). Although the true rate of recurrence is unknown, among those patients in whom recurrent symptoms result in an additional surgical procedure, endometriosis lesions may be demonstrated. The most common site of recurrent lesions is the large and small bowel. It is not clear whether such lesions were present at the time of the oophorectomy and were overlooked or were not visualized because they were present only as microscopic disease in normal-appearing peritoneum.

After total abdominal hysterectomy with bilateral salpingo-oophorectomy, delayed initiation of estrogen replacement therapy has been thought to decrease the risk of recurrent symptoms. Furthermore, the possibility does exist that estrogen replacement therapy may support infiltration of endometriosis lesions and result in continued progression of the disease (97). Currently, there are limited data on which to base a recommendation. It appears there is no advantage, in terms of recurrence rate, in delaying introduction of estrogen treatment following surgery (96, 98). There is also a concern about the possibility of estrogen induced malignant transformation in residual endometriosis implants (99),

which has led some to recommend the routine addition of a progestin to the estrogen therapy, although there are no outcomes-based evidence to support this recommendation.

Although limited data indicate hormone replacement therapy may stimulate the growth of residual ovarian or endometrial tissue after total abdominal hysterectomy, the overall benefits of hormone replacement (cardiovascular benefits, reduced risk of osteoporosis, relief of vasomotor symptoms) may outweigh these risks, and the decision should be individualized.

Summary

The following recommendations are based on good and consistent scientific evidence (Level A):

▶ For pain relief, treatment with a GnRH agonist for at least 3 months or with danazol for at least 6 months appears to be equally effective in most patients.

▶ When relief of pain from treatment with a GnRH agonist supports continued therapy, the addition of add-back therapy reduces or eliminates GnRH-induced bone mineral loss without reducing the efficacy of pain relief.

The following recommendations are based on limited or inconsistent scientific evidence (Level B):

▶ Therapy with a GnRH agonist is an appropriate approach to the management of the woman with chronic pelvic pain, even in the absence of surgical confirmation of endometriosis, provided that a detailed initial evaluation fails to demonstrate some other cause of pelvic pain.

▶ For pain relief, oral contraceptives and oral or depot MPA are effective in comparison with placebo and may be equivalent to other more costly regimens.

▶ Hormone replacement therapy with estrogen is not contraindicated following hysterectomy and bilateral salpingo-oophorectomy for endometriosis.

The following recommendations are based primarily on consensus and expert opinion (Level C):

▶ For severe endometriosis, medical treatment alone may not be sufficient.

▶ Because endometriosis often is unpredictable and may regress, expectant management may be appropriate in asymptomatic patients.

References

1. Wheeler JM. Epidemiology of endometriosis-associated infertility. J Reprod Med 1989;34:41–46 (Level III)

2. Rawson JM. Prevalence of endometriosis in asymptomatic women. J Reprod Med 1991;36:513–515 (Level III)

3. Strathy JH, Molgaard CA, Coulam CB, Melton LJ 3d. Endometriosis and infertility: a laparoscopic study of endometriosis among fertile and infertile women. Fertil Steril 1982;38:667–672 (Level II-2)

4. Verkauf BS. Incidence, symptoms, and signs of endometriosis in fertile and infertile women. J Fla Med Assoc 1987;74:671–675 (Level II-2)

5. Carter JE. Combined hysteroscopic and laparoscopic findings in patients with chronic pelvic pain. J Am Assoc Gynecol Laparosc 1994;2:43–47 (Level III)

6. Koninckx PR, Meuleman C, Demeyere S, Lesaffre E, Cornillie FJ. Suggestive evidence that pelvic endometriosis is a progressive disease, whereas deeply infiltrating endometriosis is associated with pelvic pain. Fertil Steril 1991;55:759–765 (Level III)

7. Ling FW. Randomized controlled trial of depot leuprolide in patients with chronic pelvic pain and clinically suspected endometriosis. Pelvic Pain Study Group. Obstet Gynecol 1999;93:51–58 (Level I)

8. Ripps BA, Martin DC. Endometriosis and chronic pelvic pain. Obstet Gynecol Clin North Am 1993;20:709–717 (Level III)

9. Cramer DW. Epidemiology of endometriosis. In: Wilson EA, ed. Endometriosis. New York: Alan R. Liss Inc, 1987:5–22 (Level III)

10. Vigano P, Vercellini P, Di Blasio AM, Colombo A, Candiani GB, Vignali M. Deficient antiendometrium lymphocyte-mediated cytotoxicity in patients with endometriosis. Fertil Steril 1991;56:894–899 (Level II-2)

11. Keltz MD, Berger SB, Comite F, Olive DL. Duplicated cervix and vagina associated with infertility, endometriosis, and chronic pelvic pain. Obstet Gynecol 1994;84:701–703 (Level III)

12. Cramer DW, Wilson E, Stillman RJ, Berger MJ, Belisle S, Schiff I, et al. The relation of endometriosis to menstrual characteristics, smoking and exercise. JAMA 1986;255:1904–1908 (Level II-2)

13. Adamson GD. Diagnosis and clinical presentation of endometriosis. Am J Obstet Gynecol 1990;162:568–569 (Level III)

14. Management of endometriosis in the presence of pelvic pain. The American Fertility Society. Fertil Steril 1993;60:952–955 (Level III)

15. Luciano AA, Pitkin RM. Endometriosis: approaches to diagnosis and treatment. Surg Annu 1984;16:297–312 (Level III)

16. Muse K. Clinical manifestations and classification of endometriosis. Clin Obstet Gynecol 1988;31:813–822 (Level III)

17. Candiani GB, Vercellini P, Fedele L, Colombo A, Candiani M. Mild endometriosis and infertility: a critical review of epidemiologic data, diagnostic pitfalls, and classification limits. Obstet Gynecol Surv 1991;46:374–382 (Level III)

18. Berube S, Marcoux S, Langevin M, Maheux R. Fecundity of infertile women with minimal or mild endometriosis and women with unexplained infertility. Canadian Collaborative Group on Endometriosis. Fertil Steril 1998;69:1034–1041 (Level II-2)

19. Ronnberg L. Endometriosis and infertility. Ann Med 1990;22:91–96 (Level III)

20. Demco L. Mapping the source and character of pain due to endometriosis by patient-assisted laparoscopy. J Am Assoc Gynecol Laparosc 1998;5:241–245 (Level III)

21. Martin DC, Hubert GD, Vander Zwaag R, el-Zeky FA. Laparoscopic appearances of peritoneal endometriosis. Fertil Steril 1989;51:63–67 (Level III)

22. Stripling MC, Martin DC, Chatman DL, Zwaag RV, Poston WM. Subtle appearance of pelvic endometriosis. Fertil Steril 1988;49:427–431 (Level III)

23. Murphy AA, Green WR, Bobbie D, dela Cruz ZC, Rock JA. Unsuspected endometriosis documented by scanning electron microscopy in visually normal peritoneum. Fertil Steril 1986;46:522–524 (Level III)

24. Redwine DB, Yocum LB. A serial section study of visually normal pelvic peritoneum in patients with endometriosis. Fertil Steril 1990;54:648–651 (Level III)

25. Koninckx PR, Martin DC. Deep endometriosis: a consequence of infiltration or retraction or possibly adenomyosis externa? Fertil Steril 1992;58:924–928 (Level III)

26. Koninckx PR, Oosterlynck D, D'Hooghe T, Meuleman C. Deeply infiltrating endometriosis is a disease whereas mild endometriosis could be considered a non-disease. Ann NY Acad Sci 1994;734:333–341 (Level III)

27. Jansen RP, Russell P. Nonpigmented endometriosis: clinical, laparoscopic, and pathologic definition. Am J Obstet Gynecol 1986;155:1154–1159 (Level III)

28. Pittaway DE. CA-125 in women with endometriosis. Obstet Gynecol Clin North Am 1989;16:237–252 (Level II-1)

29. Barbieri RL, Niloff JM, Bast RC Jr, Scaetzl E, Kistner RW, Knapp RC. Elevated serum concentrations of CA-125 in patients with advanced endometriosis. Fertil Steril 1986;45:630–634 (Level II-2)

30. Barbati A, Cosmi EV, Spaziani R, Ventura R, Montanino G. Serum and peritoneal fluid CA-125 in patients with endometriosis. Fertil Steril 1994;61:438–442 (Level II-2)

31. Franchi M, Beretta P, Zanaboni F, Donadello N, Ghezzi F. Use of serum CA125 measurement in patients with endometriosis. Ital J Gynaecol Obstet 1993;5:149–152 (Level III)

32. Moretuzzo RW, DiLauro S, Jenison E, Chen SL, Reindollar RH, McDonough PG. Serum and peritoneal lavage fluid CA-125 levels in endometriosis. Fertil Steril 1988;50:430–433 (Level II-2)

33. Pittaway DE, Fayez JA. The use of CA-125 in the diagnosis and management of endometriosis. Fertil Steril 1986; 46:790–795 (Level II-2)

34. Colacurci N, Fortunato N, DeFranciscis P, Fratta M, Cioffi M, Zarcone R, et al. A. Serum and peritoneal CA-125 levels as diagnostic test for endometriosis. Eur J Obstet Gynecol Reprod Biol 1996;66:41–43 (Level III)

35. Mol BW, Bayram N, Lijmer JG, Wiegerinck MA, Bongers MY, van der Veen F, Bossuyt PM. The performance of CA-125 measurement in the detection of endometriosis: a meta-analysis. Fertil Steril 1998;70:1101–1108 (Meta-analysis)

36. Chen FP, Soong YK, Lee N, Lo SK. The use of serum CA-125 as a marker for endometriosis in patients with dysmenorrhea for monitoring therapy and for recurrence of endometriosis. Acta Obstet Gynecol Scand 1998;77: 665–670 (Level III)

37. Ozaksit G, Caglar T, Cicek N, Kuscu E, Batioglu S, Gokmen O. Serum CA 125 levels before, during and after treatment for endometriosis. Int J Gynaecol Obstet 1995; 50:269–273 (Level III)

38. Takahashi K, Kijima S, Yoshino K, Shibukawa T, Kitao M. Serum CA 125 as a marker for patients with external endometriosis. Int J Fertil 1989;34:143–148 (Level II-2)

39. Guerriero S, Mais V, Ajossa S, Paoletti AM, Angiolucci M, Melis GB. Transvaginal ultrasonography combined with CA-125 plasma levels in the diagnosis of endometrioma. Fertil Steril 1996;65:293–298 (Level II-2)

40. Kinkel K, Chapron C, Balleyguier C, Fritel X, Dubuisson JB, Moreau JF. Magnetic resonance imaging characteristics of deep endometriosis. Hum Reprod 1999;14: 1080–1086 (Level III)

41. Revised American Society for Reproductive Medicine classification of endometriosis: 1996. Fertil Steril 1997; 67:817–821 (Level III)

42. Bergqvist A, Bergh T, Hogstrom L, Mattson S, Nordenskjold F, Rasmussen C. Effects of triptorelin versus placebo on the symptoms of endometriosis. Fertil Steril 1998;69:702–708 (Level I)

43. Bulletti C, Flamigni C, Polli V, Giacomucci E, Albonetti A, Negrini V, et al. The efficacy of drugs in the management of endometriosis. J Am Assoc Gynecol Laprosc 1996;3:495–501 (Level II-2)

44. Hornstein MD, Surrey ES, Weisberg GW, Casino LA. Leuprolide acetate depot and hormonal add-back in endometriosis: a 12-month study. Lupron Add-Back Study Group Obstet Gynecol 1998;91:16–24 (Level I)

45. Vercellini P, De Giorgi O, Oldani S, Cortesi I, Panazza S, Crosignani PG. Depot medroxyprogesterone acetate versus an oral contraceptive combined with very-low-dose danazol for long-term treatment of pelvic pain associated with endometriosis. Am J Obstet Gynecol 1996;175: 396–401 (Level I)

46. Vercellini P, Cortesi I, Crosignani PG. Progestins for symptomatic endometriosis: a critical analysis of the evidence. Fertil Steril 1997;68:393–401 (Critical Analysis)

47. Rock JA, Truglia JA, Caplan RJ. Zoladex (goserelin acetate implant) in the treatment of endometriosis: a randomized comparison with danazol. The Zoladex Endometriosis Study Group Obstet Gynecol 1993;82: 198–205 (Level I)

48. Wheeler JM, Knittle JD, Miller JD. Depot leuprolide acetate versus danazol in the treatment of women with symptomatic endometriosis: a multicenter, double-blind, randomized clinical trial. II. Assessment of safety. The Lupron Endometriosis Study Group. Am J Obstet Gynecol 1993;169:26–33 (Level I)

49. Zorn JR, Mathieson J, Risquez F, Comaru-Schally AM, Schally AV. Treatment of endometriosis with delayed release preparation of the agonist D-Trp6-luteinizing hormone-releasing hormone: long-term follow-up in a series of 50 patients. Fertil Steril 1990;53:401–406 (Level II-3)

50. Vercellini P, Trespidi L, Colombo A, Vendola N, Marchini M, Crosignani PG. A gonadotropin-releasing hormone agonist versus a low-dose oral contraceptive for pelvic pain associated with endometriosis. Fertil Steril 1993; 60:75–79 (Level I)

51. Telimaa S, Puolakka J, Ronnberg L, Kauppila A. Placebo-controlled comparison of danazol and high-dose medroxy-progesterone acetate in the treatment of endometriosis. Gynecol Endocrinol 1987;1:13–23 (Level I)

52. Sutton CJ, Ewen SP, Whitelaw N, Haines P. Prospective, randomized, double-blind, controlled trial of laser laparoscopy in the treatment of pelvic pain associated with minimal, mild, and moderate endometriosis. Fertil Steril 1994;62:696–700 (Level I)

53. Sutton CJ, Pooley AS, Ewen SP, Haines P. Follow-up report on a randomized controlled trial of laser laparoscopy in the treatment of pelvic pain associated with minimal to moderate endometriosis. Fertil Steril 1997; 68:1070–1074 (Level I)

54. Waller KG, Shaw RW. Gonadotropin-releasing hormone analogues for the treatment of endometriosis: long-term follow-up. Fertil Steril 1993;59:511–515 (Level I)

55. Redwine DB. Conservative laparoscopic excision of endometriosis by sharp dissection: life table analysis of reoperation and persistent or recurrent disease. Fertil Steril 1991;56:628–634 (Level II-3)

56. Cook AS, Rock JA. The role of laparoscopy in the treatment of endometriosis. Fertil Steril 1991;55:663–680 (Level III)

57. Saidi MH, Vancaillie TG, White AJ, Sadler RK, Akright BD, Farhardt SA. Complications of major operative laparoscopy. A review of 452 cases. J Reprod Med 1996; 41:471–476 (Level III)

58. Revelli A, Modottii M, Ansaldi C, Massobrio M. Recurrent endometriosis: a review of biological and clinical aspects. Obstet Gynecol Surv 1995;50:747–754 (Level III)

59. Hornstein MD, Hemmings J, Yuzpe AA, Heinrichs WL. Use of nafarelin versus placebo after reductive laparoscopic surgery for endometriosis. Fertil Steril 1997;68: 860–864 (Level I)

60. Bianchi S, Busacca M, Agnoli B, Candiani M, Calia C, Vignali M. Effects of 3 month therapy with danazol after laparoscopic surgery for stage III/IV endometriosis: a randomized study. Hum Reprod 1999;14:1335–1337 (Level I)

61. Donnez J, Nisolle M, Clerckx F. Evaluation of preoperative use of danazol, gestrinone, lynestrenol, buserelin spray and buserelin implant, in the treatment of endometriosis associated infertility. In: Chadha DR, Buttram VC Jr eds. Current concepts in endometriosis. New York: Alan R. Liss, Inc, 1990:427–442 (Level II-2)

62. Muzii L, Marana R, Caruana P, Mancuso S. The impact of preoperative gonadotropin-releasing hormone agonist treatment in laparoscopic excision of ovarian endometriotic cysts. Fertil Steril 1996;65:1235–1237 (Level II-1)

63. Dlugi AM, Miller JD, Knittle J, Lupron Depot (leuprolide acetate for depot suspension) in the treatment of endometriosis: A randomized, placebo-controlled, double-blind study. Lupron Study Group. Fertil Steril 1990; 54:419–427 (Level I)

64. Henzl MR, Corson SL, Moghissi K, Buttram VC, Berqvist C, Jacobson J. Administration of nasal nafarelin as compared with oral danazol for endometriosis. A multicenter double-blind comparative clinical trial. N Engl J Med 1988;318:485–489 (Level I)

65. Hornstein MD, Yuzpe AA, Burry KA, Heinrichs LR, Buttram VC Jr, Orwoll ES. Prospective randomized double-blind trial of 3 versus 6 months of nafarelin therapy for endometriosis associated with pelvic pain. Fertil Steril 1995;63:955–962 (Level I)

66. Tummon IS, Pepping ME, Binor Z, Radwanska E, Dmowski WP. A randomized, prospective comparison of endocrine changes induced with intranasal leuprolide or danazol for treatment of endometriosis. Fertil Steril 1989;51:390–394 (Level I)

67. Cedars MI, Lu JK, Meldrum DR, Judd HL. Treatment of endometriosis with a long-acting gonadotropin-releasing hormone agonist plus medroxyprogesterone acetate. Obstet Gynecol 1990;75:641–645 (Level III)

68. Makarainen L, Ronnberg L, Kauppila A. Medroxyprogesterone acetate supplementation diminishes the hypoestrogenic side effects of gonadotropin-releasing hormone agonist without changing its efficacy in endometriosis. Fertil Steril 1996;65:29–34 (Level I)

69. Surrey ES, Judd HL. Reduction of vasomotor symptoms and bone mineral density loss with combined norethindrone and long-acting gonadotropin-releasing hormone agonist therapy of symptomatic endometriosis: a prospective randomized trial. J Clin Endocrinol Metab 1992; 75:558–563 (Level I)

70. Surrey ES, Fournet N, Voigt B, Judd HL. Effects of sodium etidronate in combination with low-dose norethindrone in patients administered a long-acting GnRH agonist. a preliminary report. Obstet Gynecol 1993;81: 581–586 (Level I)

71. Kiilholma P, Tuimala R, Kivinen S, Korhonen M, Hagman E. Comparison of the gonadotropin-releasing hormone agonist goserelin acetate alone versus goserelin combined with estrogen-progestin add-back therapy in the treatment of endometriosis. Fertil Steril 1995;64:903–908 (Level I)

72. Moghissi KS, Schlaff WD, Olive DL, Skinner MA, Yin H. Goserelin acetate (Zoladex) with or without hormone replacement therapy for the treatment of endometriosis. Fertil Steril 1998;69:1056–1062 (Level I)

73. Finkelstein JS, Klibanski A, Schaefer EH, Hornstein MD, Schiff I, Neer RM. Parathyroid hormone for the prevention of bone loss induced by estrogen deficiency. N Engl J Med 1994;331:1618–1623 (Level I)

74. Roux C, Pelissier C, Listrat V, Kolta S, Simonetta C, Guignard M, et al. Bone loss during gonadotropin releasing hormone agonist treatment and use of nasal calcitonin. Osteoporos Int 1995;5:185–190 (Level I)

75. Howell R, Edmonds DK, Dowsett M, Crook D, Lees B, Stevenson JC. Gonadotropin-releasing hormone analogue (goserelin) plus hormone replacement therapy for the treatment of endometriosis: a randomized controlled trial. Fertil Steril 1995;64:474–481 (Level I)

76. Fogelman I. Gonadotropin-releasing hormone agonists and the skeleton. Fertil Steril 1992;57:715–724 (Level III)

77. Dawood MY. Hormonal therapies for endometriosis: implications for bone metabolism. Acta Obstet Gynecol Scand 1994;159:22–34 (Level III)

78. Agarwal SK, Harmrang C, Henzl MR, Judd HL. Nafarelin vs. leuprolide acetate depot for endometriosis. Changes in bone mineral density and vasomotor symptoms. Nafarelin Study Group. J Reprod Med 1997;42:413–423 (Level I)

79. Lemay A, Brideau NA, Forest JC, Dodin S, Maheux R. Cholesterol fractions and apolipoproteins during endometriosis treatment by a gonadotrophin releasing hormone (GnRH) agonist implant or by danazol. Clin Endocrinol (Oxf)1991;35:305–310 (Level II-3)

80. Fahraeus L, Larsson-Cohn U, Ljungberg S, Wallentin L. Profound alterations of the lipoprotein metabolism during danazol treatment in premenopausal women. Fertil Steril 1984;42:52–57 (Level III)

81. Fahraeus L, Sydsjo A, Wallentin L. Lipoprotein changes during treatment of pelvic endometriosis with medroxyprogesterone acetate. Fertil Steril 1986;45:503–506 (Level III)

82. Hornstein MD, Yuzpe AA, Burry K, Buttram VC Jr, Heinrichs LR, Soderstrom RM, et al. Retreatment with nafarelin for recurrent endometriosis symptoms: efficacy, safety and bone mineral density. Fertil Steril 1997; 67:1013–1018 (Level III)

83. Howard FM. The role of laparoscopy in chronic pelvic pain: promises and pitfalls. Obstet Gynecol Surv 1993; 48:357–387 (Level III)

84. Wardle PG, Hull MG. Is endometriosis a disease? Baillieres Clin Obstet Gynaecol 1993;7:673–685 (Level III)

85. Marcoux S, Maheux R, Berube S. Laparoscopic surgery in infertile women with minimal or mild endometriosis. Canadian Collaborative Group on Endometriosis. N Engl J Med 1997;337:217–222 (Level I)

86. Canadian Consensus Conference on Endometriosis Chapter 2 Consensus Statements. J SOGC 1999;21: 471–473 (Level III)

87. Guerriero S, Mais V, Ajossa S, Paoletti AM, Angiolucci M, Labate F, et al. The role of endovaginal ultrasound in differentiating endometriomas from other ovarian cysts. Clin Exp Obstet Gynecol 1995;22:20–22 (Level III)

88. Donnez J, Nisolle M, Clerckx F, Casanas-Roux F, Saussoy P, Gillerot S. Advanced endoscopic techniques used in dysfunctional bleeding, fibroids and endometriosis, and the role of gonadotropin-releasing hormone agonist treatment. Br J Gynaecol 1994;101(Suppl 10):2–9 (Level III)

89. Shimizu I, Nakanishi R, Yoshino I, Yasumoto K. An endometrial nodule in the lung without pelvic endometriosis. J Cardiovasc Surg (Torino) 1998;39:867–868 (Level III)

90. Hughes ML, Bartholomew D, Paluzzi M. Abdominal wall endometriosis after amniocentesis. A case report. J Reprod Med 1997;42:597–599 (Level III)

91. Shek Y, De Lia JE, Pattillo RA. Endometriosis with a pleural effusion and ascites. Report of a case treated with nafarelin acetate. J Reprod Med 1995;40:540–542 (Level III)

92. Espaulella J, Armengol J, Bella F, Lain JM, Calaf J. Pulmonary endometriosis: conservative treatment with GnRH agonists. Obstet Gynecol 1991;78:535-537 (Level III)

93. Johnson WM 3d, Tyndal CM. Pulmonary endometriosis: treatment with danazol. Obstet Gynecol 1987;69:506–507 (Level III)

94. Wheeler JH, Malinak LR. Recurrent endometriosis: incidence, management, and prognosis. Am J Obstet Gynecol 1983;146:247–253 (Level III)

95. Namnoun AB, Hickman TN, Goodman SB, Gehlbach DL, Rock JA. Incidence of symptom recurrence after hysterectomy for endometriosis. Fertil Steril 1995;64:898–902 (Level III)

96. Redwine DB. Endometriosis persisting after castration: clinical characteristics and results of surgical management. Obstet Gynecol 1994;83:405–413 (Level III)

97. Lam AM, French M, Charnock FM. Bilateral ureteric obstruction due to recurrent endometriosis associated with hormone replacement therapy. Aust N Z J Obstet Gynaecol 1992;32:83–84 (Level III)

98. Hickman TN, Namnoun AB, Hinton EL, Zacur HA, Rock JA Timing of estrogen replacement therapy following hysterectomy with oophorectomy for endometriosis. Obstet Gynecol 1998;91:673–677 (Level II-3)

99. Gucer F, Pieber D, Arikan MG. Malignancy arising in extraovarian endometriosis during estrogen stimulation. Eur J Gynaecol Oncol 1998;19:39–41 (Level III)

The MEDLINE database, the Cochrane Library, and ACOG's own internal resources were used to conduct a literature search to locate relevant articles published between January 1985 and May 1999. The search was restricted to articles published in the English language. Priority was given to articles reporting results of original research, although review articles and commentaries also were consulted. Abstracts of research presented at symposia and scientific conferences were not considered adequate for inclusion in this document. Guidelines published by organizations or institutions such as the National Institutes of Health and the American College of Obstetricians and Gynecologists were reviewed, and additional studies were located by reviewing bibliographies of identified articles. When reliable research was not available, expert opinions from obstetrician–gynecologists were used.

Studies were reviewed and evaluated for quality according to the method outlined by the U.S. Preventive Services Task Force:

I   Evidence obtained from at least one properly designed randomized controlled trial.

II-1 Evidence obtained from well-designed controlled trials without randomization.

II-2 Evidence obtained from well-designed cohort or case–control analytic studies, preferably from more than one center or research group.

II-3 Evidence obtained from multiple time series with or without the intervention. Dramatic results in uncontrolled experiments could also be regarded as this type of evidence.

III   Opinions of respected authorities, based on clinical experience, descriptive studies, or reports of expert committees.

Based on the highest level of evidence found in the data, recommendations are provided and graded according to the following categories:

Level A—Recommendations are based on good and consistent scientific evidence.

Level B—Recommendations are based on limited or inconsistent scientific evidence.

Level C—Recommendations are based primarily on consensus and expert opinion.

ISSN 1099-3630

The American College of Obstetricians and Gynecologists 409 12th Street, SW PO Box 96920 Washington, DC 20090-6920

12345/32109

ACOG PRACTICE BULLETIN

CLINICAL MANAGEMENT GUIDELINES FOR
OBSTETRICIAN–GYNECOLOGISTS

NUMBER 3, December 1998

(Replaces Technical Bulletin Number 150, December 1990)

This Practice Bulletin was developed by the ACOG Committee on Practice Bulletins—Gynecology with the assistance of Steven J. Ory, MD. The information is designed to aid practitioners in making decisions about appropriate obstetric and gynecologic care. These guidelines should not be construed as dictating an exclusive course of treatment or procedure. Variations in practice may be warranted based on the needs of the individual patient, resources, and limitations unique to the institution or type of practice.

Medical Management of Tubal Pregnancy

Ectopic pregnancy is a major health problem for women of reproductive age and, in the United States, is the leading cause of pregnancy-related death during the first trimester. Diagnosis and treatment of tubal pregnancy before tubal rupture occurs decreases the risk of death. Early detection may make it possible for some patients to receive medical therapy instead of surgery. Methotrexate, a folinic acid antagonist, has been used to treat patients with small unruptured tubal pregnancies. The purpose of this document is to present evidence, including risks and benefits, about methotrexate as an alternative treatment for selected ectopic pregnancies.

Background

Incidence

The incidence of ectopic pregnancy has increased in the United States since 1970, the year the Centers for Disease Control (CDC; now the Centers for Disease Control and Prevention) first began collecting data, when the rate was 4.5 per 1,000 reported pregnancies. In 1992, there were an estimated 108,800 ectopic pregnancies, accounting for about 20 per 1,000 pregnancies and about 9% of all pregnancy-related deaths (1). Current data do not include conditions diagnosed and treated in physicians' offices; therefore, the true incidence of ectopic pregnancy is probably underestimated.

Etiology

Prior pelvic inflammatory disease, especially that caused by *Chlamydia trachomatis*, is the most important risk factor for ectopic pregnancy; observed odds ratios range from 2.0 to 7.5 (2). Other factors that appear to be associated with an increased risk of ectopic pregnancy include prior ectopic pregnancy, cigarette smoking, prior tubal surgery (especially for distal tubal disease), diethylstilbestrol exposure, and increasing age.

A history of infertility, independent of tubal disease, and ovulation induction also appear to be risk factors for ectopic pregnancy. Ectopic pregnancy is more likely to be diagnosed early in patients being treated for infertility. Such patients may be good candidates for medical therapy.

Effects of Therapy

Methotrexate is a folinic acid antagonist that inhibits dihydrofolic acid reductase, interfering with DNA synthesis, repair, and cellular replication. Actively proliferating tissue such as malignant cells, bone marrow, fetal cells, buccal and intestinal mucosa, and cells of the urinary bladder generally are more sensitive to these effects of methotrexate. Methotrexate has the potential for serious toxicity. Toxic effects usually are related to the amount and duration of therapy, but toxicity has been seen even with low doses. When methotrexate is used as a treatment for ectopic pregnancy, most reported side effects have been mild and self-limiting (3–12). This is probably a reflection of the lower dosage and shortened duration of treatment compared with dosages used in treating malignancies.

Diagnosis

Serial quantitative levels of the beta subunit of human chorionic gonadotropin (β-hCG) can be used in combination with transvaginal ultrasonography and, in some cases, suction curettage and serum progesterone measurements to differentiate failed intrauterine pregnancy, threatened abortion, and intrauterine or ectopic pregnancies. A presumptive diagnosis of unruptured tubal ectopic pregnancy is required before medical management can be considered.

Beta Subunit of Human Chorionic Gonadotropin

The mean plasma concentration of human chorionic gonadotropin (hCG) is significantly lower for an ectopic pregnancy than for a viable intrauterine pregnancy, but there is no definitive laboratory level permitting distinction between the two. A consistently declining hCG level indicates a nonviable pregnancy.

Conventionally, serial hCG testing to diagnose suspected ectopic pregnancy is performed at 48-hour intervals; a 66% or greater increase should be observed in a normal pregnancy. Approximately 15% of normal intrauterine pregnancies are associated with less than a 66% increase in hCG, and 17% of ectopic pregnancies have normal doubling times (13). Limitations of serial hCG testing include its inability to distinguish a failing intrauterine pregnancy from an ectopic pregnancy and the inherent 48-hour delay. A prospective study of asymptomatic patients described a 36% sensitivity and a 63–71% specificity (14). However, most reports and clin-

icians have found serial hCG testing useful in the early diagnosis of ectopic pregnancy. The rate of hCG doubling decreases from every 1.4–1.5 days in early pregnancy to every 3.3–3.5 days at 6–7 weeks of gestation, at which point the reliability of serial testing may be diminished.

The elimination of hCG after treatment of ectopic pregnancy follows a two-phase distribution. The major elimination has a half-life of 5–9 hours and a second, longer phase has a half-life of 22–32 hours.

The quantitation of hCG has been complicated by the existence of three different reference standards for hCG assays, the existence of multiple antibodies in commercial assays, and confusing nomenclature. These complicating factors can cause varying and inconsistent results, both from one laboratory to another and within the same laboratory, and affect interpretation of the results and clinical management.

Ultrasonography

Transvaginal ultrasonography often can detect intrauterine pregnancy within 5 weeks of the last menstrual period. The concept of the discriminatory hCG zone, originally applied to transabdominal ultrasonography, is the range of serum hCG concentration above which a normal intrauterine gestation can be visualized consistently. When the hCG level exceeds the discriminatory zone, the absence of an intrauterine gestational sac is suggestive of ectopic pregnancy, but this also can occur with multiple gestation or failed intrauterine pregnancy. The specific discriminatory zone varies with the hCG assay chosen, the reference standard with which it is calibrated, and the available ultrasound resolution. Findings also may be compromised by obesity, fibroids, and the axis of the uterus. An intrauterine gestational sac in a normal uterus usually can be seen with transvaginal ultrasonography when the hCG level is between 1,000 to 2,000 mIU/mL (1st and 2nd International Reference Preparation or IRP) (15, 16). If the precise gestational age is known, as in the case of patients receiving hCG for ovulation induction or oocyte retrieval, the failure to detect a gestational sac 24 days or later after conception is presumptive evidence of an abnormal pregnancy (13).

Historically, detection of an intrauterine sac has led to the presumptive exclusion of ectopic pregnancy, based on the estimate of the incidence of heterotopic pregnancy of 1 in 30,000. This figure was calculated almost 50 years ago by multiplying the incidence of ectopic pregnancy by that of dizygotic twinning, thus producing a hypothetical estimate. The incidence of heterotopic pregnancy appears to have increased with the use of assisted reproductive techniques. It has been reported to be as high as 1% in some series (17), although the overall incidence of heterotopic pregnancy is probably much lower.

The identification of an ectopic gestational sac is diagnostic of ectopic pregnancy, but it is not seen in all cases. Sensitivity and specificity of transvaginal ultrasonography to identify ectopic pregnancy vary according to criteria used for diagnosis. Reported sensitivity of transvaginal ultrasonography ranges from 20.1% to 84% and specificity from 98.9% to 100%, depending on the criteria applied (18). Color flow Doppler may aid in the diagnosis of ectopic pregnancy; however, it requires considerably greater technical expertise (19, 20).

Serum Progesterone

Some clinicians maintain that measurement of serum progesterone levels may be useful for distinguishing viable intrauterine pregnancies from spontaneous abortions and ectopic pregnancies, but serum progesterone levels cannot distinguish ectopic pregnancy from spontaneous abortion (21). There is no single progesterone value that will definitively confirm the viability or nonviability of an intrauterine pregnancy or the presence of an ectopic pregnancy. Serum progesterone levels increase during pregnancy (22). If the duration of the pregnancy is unknown, interpretation of the test results is less reliable. The use of ovulation-induction agents is associated with higher serum progesterone levels in intrauterine and ectopic pregnancies.

Of pregnant patients with serum progesterone values of less than 5 ng/mL, 85% have spontaneous abortions, 0.16% have viable intrauterine pregnancies, and 14% have ectopic pregnancies (23). Pregnant patients with serum progesterone levels between 20.0 and 24.9 ng/mL have ectopic pregnancies in 4% of cases; 2% of ectopic pregnancies occur with serum progesterone levels greater than 25 ng/mL. Most ectopic pregnancies (52%) are associated with serum progesterone levels between 10 and 20 ng/mL, thus limiting the clinical utility of this assessment (24).

The absence of products of conception on curettage in the presence of an elevated β-hCG level is evidence of a presumptive diagnosis of ectopic pregnancy. More rarely, gestational trophoblastic disease, nongestational choriocarcinoma, or an embryonal cell tumor may be the cause.

Success Rates

Success is defined as resolution of the ectopic pregnancy without surgical intervention. Reported success rates range from 67% to 100%, with a median of 84% for the single-dose methotrexate regimen (3–12). The largest study involved 120 women and had an overall success rate of 94.1% (10). Variation in success rates may be affected by the selection criteria and differences in management. Of those cases with successful outcome, as

many as 25% required more than one dose of methotrexate (3, 6, 8, 25).

Clinical Considerations and Recommendations

▶ *Who are candidates for medical management?*

General factors to consider in determining candidates for medical therapy include the size of the ectopic mass, whether it has ruptured, and the desire for future fertility. Patients should be hemodynamically stable without active bleeding or signs of hemoperitoneum. Furthermore, they should be willing and able to return for follow-up care.

Criteria for Receiving Methotrexate

Absolute indications

    Hemodynamically stable without active bleeding or signs of hemoperitoneum

    Nonlaparoscopic diagnosis

    Patient desires future fertility

    General anesthesia poses a significant risk

    Patient is able to return for follow-up care

    Patient has no contraindications to methotrexate

Relative indications

    Unruptured mass ≤3.5 cm at its greatest dimension

    No fetal cardiac motion detected

    Patients whose β-hCG level does not exceed a predetermined value (6,000–15,000 mIU/mL)

Contraindications to Medical Therapy

Absolute contraindications

    Breastfeeding

    Overt or laboratory evidence of immunodeficiency

    Alcoholism, alcoholic liver disease, or other chronic liver disease

    Preexisting blood dyscrasias, such as bone marrow hypoplasia, leukopenia, thrombocytopenia, or significant anemia

    Known sensitivity to methotrexate

    Active pulmonary disease

    Peptic ulcer disease

    Hepatic, renal, or hematologic dysfunction

Relative contraindications

    Gestational sac ≥3.5 cm

    Embryonic cardiac motion

Absolute and relative indications and contraindications to medical therapy are shown in the boxes.

▶ How is methotrexate used in the medical management of tubal ectopic pregnancy?

Because injected methotrexate is a relatively new treatment for ectopic pregnancy, a standardized protocol has yet to be defined. There are small variations among the published protocols, but all share a basic strategy. The differences are in the amount of methotrexate given, the frequency of follow-up visits, and the types of tests and procedures routinely used to monitor treatment response.

Before methotrexate is injected, blood is drawn to determine baseline laboratory values for renal, liver, and bone marrow function, as well as to measure the β-hCG level. Progesterone also may be measured. Blood type, Rh factor, and the presence of antibodies should be determined. Patients who are Rh negative receive Rh immune globulin. The methotrexate dose usually is calculated according to estimated body surface area (50 mg/m^2) and is given in one dose. Treatment with a standard 75 mg dose (11) and multiple serial doses with a folinic acid rescue on alternate days (four doses of methotrexate [1.0 mg/kg] on days 0, 2, 4, and 6 and four doses of leucovorin [0.1 mg/kg] on days 1, 3, 5, and 7) (26, 27) also have been successful. Methotrexate is given either in divided doses, half into each buttock, or in one intramuscular injection (3–12).

Follow-up care continues until β-hCG levels are nondetectable. Time to resolution is variable and can be protracted, taking a month or longer (3, 5, 6, 9, 10, 12). With the single-dose regimen, levels of β-hCG usually increase during the first several days following methotrexate injection and peak 4 days after injection. If a treatment response is observed, hCG levels should decline by 7 days after injection (4, 10, 11). If the β-hCG level does not decline by at least 15% from day 4 to day 7, the patient may require either surgery (4), or a second dose of methotrexate if no contraindications exist (3, 5, 10–12). If there is an adequate treatment response, hCG determinations are reduced to once a week. An additional dose of methotrexate may be given if β-hCG levels plateau or increase in 7 days (6–10). Surgical intervention may be required for patients who do not respond to medical therapy. Ultrasound examination may be repeated to evaluate significant changes in clinical status, such as increased pelvic pain, bleeding, or inadequate declines of β-hCG levels (5, 6, 9, 10).

▶ What are the potential problems associated with medical management of ectopic pregnancy?

Potential problems can be divided into three categories: 1) drug-related side effects, 2) treatment-related compli-

---

Side Effects Associated with Methotrexate Treatment

Drug side effects
- Nausea
- Vomiting
- Stomatitis
- Diarrhea
- Gastric distress
- Dizziness
- Severe neutropenia (rare)
- Reversible alopecia (rare)
- Pneumonitis

Treatment effects
- Increase in abdominal pain (occurs in up to two thirds of patients)
- Increase in β-hCG levels during first 1–3 days of treatment
- Vaginal bleeding or spotting

Signs of treatment failure and tubal rupture
- Significantly worsening abdominal pain, regardless of change in β-hCG levels
- Hemodynamic instability
- Levels of β-hCG that do not decline by at least 15% between day 4 and day 7 postinjection
- Increasing or plateauing β-hCG levels after the first week of treatment

---

cations, and 3) treatment failure (see the box). If medical therapy fails, additional treatment is required; in case of tubal rupture, rapid surgical intervention is necessary. It is important, therefore, to monitor patients for signs and symptoms of tubal rupture and treatment failure.

During treatment, patients should be counseled to discontinue folinic acid supplements, including prenatal vitamins. Because of its potential toxicity, patients receiving methotrexate should be monitored carefully. Physicians using this drug should be aware of potential side effects and signs of toxicity and be advised to avoid the use of nonsteroidal antiinflammatory drugs.

An initial increase in β-hCG levels often occurs by the third day and is not a cause for alarm (4, 10, 11). Most patients experience at least one episode of increased abdominal pain sometime during treatment (5, 6, 9–11). Because abdominal pain also is suggestive of tubal rupture, care should be taken to evaluate any significant change in discomfort. The pain associated with resolution of tubal pregnancy usually can be distinguished from tubal rupture. It generally is milder, of limited duration (24–48 hours), and not associated with signs of an acute abdomen or hemodynamic instability.

Medical treatment has failed when β-hCG levels either increase or plateau by day 7 postinjection, indicating a continuing ectopic pregnancy, or when the tube ruptures. Tubal rupture may occur despite declining β-hCG levels (6, 9, 10).

▶ *How should patients be counseled about immediate and long-term effects of medical therapy?*

Patients should receive information about the types of side effects they may experience and about activity restrictions during treatment. They should be informed of the ongoing risk of tubal rupture during treatment; it is important to educate patients about symptoms of tubal rupture and emphasize the need to seek immediate medical attention if these symptoms occur (see the box).

It is difficult to assess the impact of methotrexate treatment for ectopic pregnancy on a woman's ability to conceive. Published evidence regarding conception rates following methotrexate administration is limited. One study reported a 20% conception rate among 15 women, with a mean follow-up time of 11.8 months (5). Another study reported a significantly greater conception rate of 79.6%, with a mean time to conception of 3.2 months (10); 12.8% of the conceptions were recurrent ectopic pregnancies. The impact of methotrexate on future fertility requires further study.

▶ *How cost-effective is methotrexate treatment?*

There is evidence that methotrexate therapy is a cost-effective treatment for small unruptured ectopic pregnancies when compared with laparoscopic salpingostomy. The direct cost advantages are due to elimination of oper-ating room use, anesthesia services, and surgical fees. Indirect costs decrease as a result of quicker recovery times; however, the amount of savings depends on the proportion of patients eligible to receive medical therapy and the overall success rate. A study comparing direct costs of methotrexate with laparoscopic salpingostomy found there are significant savings if methotrexate is used as the primary therapy (28). An additional study looked retrospectively at patients treated for ectopic pregnancy and also found methotrexate was cost-effective (29).

▶ *Is there ever a role for expectant management?*

Distinguishing patients who are experiencing spontaneous resolution of their ectopic pregnancies from patients who have proliferating ectopic pregnancies and require active intervention is a clinical dilemma. In patients who are suspected to be undergoing spontaneous clinical resolution, expectant management is an option that has been used in the hope of avoiding therapy that might otherwise be unnecessary. Candidates for successful expectant management must be willing to accept the potential risks of tubal rupture and hemorrhage; they should be asymptomatic and have objective evidence of resolution (generally manifested by declining hCG levels). In general, patients with early, small tubal gestations with lower hCG levels are the best candidates for observant management. Approximately 20–30% of ectopic pregnancies are associated with declining hCG levels at the time of presentation (30). If the initial hCG level is less than 200 mIU/mL, 88% of patients experience spontaneous resolution. Lower success rates can be anticipated with higher hCG levels (31). Reasons for abandoning expectant management include intractable or significant increase in pain, failure of hCG levels to decrease, and tubal rupture with hemoperitoneum.

Summary

The following recommendations are based on limited or inconsistent scientific evidence (Level B):

▶ Intramuscular methotrexate is an appropriate method for treating selected patients with small, unruptured tubal pregnancies.*

▶ Successful treatment with methotrexate may require more than one dose of methotrexate.*

▶ Failure of β-hCG levels to decrease by at least 15% from day 4 to day 7 after methotrexate administration indicates the need for an additional dose of methotrexate or surgery.*

* Evidence is limited but consistent.

Counseling Patients

Patients should be instructed on the following points:

To expect to experience one or more side effects, including abdominal pain, vaginal bleeding or spotting, or medication side effects

To contact the physician in the presence of sudden onset of severe abdominal pain; substantial increase in abdominal pain; heavy vaginal bleeding; or dizziness, syncope, or tachycardia

To avoid alcoholic beverages, vitamins containing folic acid, nonsteroidal antiinflammatory drugs, and sexual intercourse until advised otherwise

The following recommendation is based primarily on consensus and expert opinion (Level C):

▶ There may be a role for expectant management of hemodynamically stable patients with presumptive ectopic pregnancy in whom β-hCG levels are low (<200 mIU/mL) and declining.

References

1. Centers for Disease Control and Prevention. Ectopic pregnancy—United States, 1990–1992. MMWR Morb Mortal Wkly Rep 1995;44:46–48 (Level II-3)

2. Chow WH, Daling JR, Cates W Jr, Greenberg RS. Epidemiology of ectopic pregnancy. Epidemiol Rev 1987;9: 70–94 (Level III)

3. Corsan GH, Karacan M, Qasim S, Bohrer MK, Ransom MX, Kemmann E. Identification of hormonal parameters for successful systemic single-dose methotrexate therapy in ectopic pregnancy. Hum Reprod 1995;10:2719–2722 (Level II-3)

4. Fernandez H, Bourget P, Ville Y, Lelaidier C, Frydman R. Treatment of unruptured tubal pregnancy with methotrexate: pharmacokinetic analysis of local versus intramuscular administration. Fertil Steril 1994;62:943–947 (Level I)

5. Glock JL, Johnson JV, Brumsted JR. Efficacy and safety of single-dose systemic methotrexate in the treatment of ectopic pregnancy. Fertil Steril 1994;62:716–721 (Level II-3)

6. Gross Z, Rodriguez JJ, Stalnaker BL. Ectopic pregnancy: nonsurgical, outpatient evaluation and single-dose methotrexate treatment. J Reprod Med 1995;40:371–374 (Level III)

7. Henry MA, Gentry WL. Single injection of methotrexate for treatment of ectopic pregnancies. Am J Obstet Gynecol 1994;171:1584–1587 (Level II-3)

8. Ransom MX, Garcia AJ, Bohrer M, Corsan GH, Kemmann E. Serum progesterone as a predictor of methotrexate success in the treatment of ectopic pregnancy. Obstet Gynecol 1994;83:1033–1037 (Level II-3)

9. Stika CS, Anderson L, Frederiksen MC. Single-dose methotrexate for the treatment of ectopic pregnancy: Northwestern Memorial Hospital three-year experience. Am J Obstet Gynecol 1996;174:1840–1846; discussion 1846–1848 (Level II-3)

10. Stovall TG, Ling FW. Single-dose methotrexate: an expanded clinical trial. Am J Obstet Gynecol 1993;168: 1759–1765 (Level II-3)

11. Wolf GC, Nickisch SA, George KE, Teicher JR, Simms TD. Completely nonsurgical management of ectopic pregnancies. Gynecol Obstet Invest 1994;37:232–235 (Level II-3)

12. Yao M, Tulandi T, Falcone T. Treatment of ectopic pregnancy by systemic methotrexate, transvaginal methotrexate, and operative laparoscopy. Int J Fertil 1996;41:470–475 (Level II-3)

13. Kadar N, Caldwell BV, Romero R. A method of screening for ectopic pregnancy and its indications. Obstet Gynecol 1981;58:162–166 (Level II-2)

14. Shepherd RW, Patton PE, Novy MJ, Burry KA. Serial beta-hCG measurements in the early detection of ectopic pregnancy. Obstet Gynecol 1990;75:417–420 (Level III)

15. Fossum GT, Davajan V, Kletzky OA. Early detection of pregnancy with transvaginal ultrasound. Fertil Steril 1988;49:788–791 (Level II-3)

16. Goldstein SR, Snyder JR, Watson C, Danon M. Very early pregnancy detection with endovaginal ultrasound. Obstet Gynecol 1988;72:200–204 (Level II-3)

17. Svare J, Norup P, Grove Thomsen S, Hornnes P, Maigaard S, Helm P, et al. Heterotopic pregnancies after in-vitro fertilization and embryo transfer—a Danish survey. Hum Reprod 1993;8:116–118 (Level III)

18. Brown DL, Doubilet PM. Transvaginal sonography for diagnosing ectopic pregnancy: positivity criteria and performance characteristics. J Ultrasound Med 1994;13:259–266 (Level III)

19. Kirchler HC, Seebacher S, Alge AA, Muller-Holzner E, Fessler S, Kolle D. Early diagnosis of tubal pregnancy: changes in tubal blood flow evaluated by endovaginal color Doppler sonography. Obstet Gynecol 1993;82:561– 565 (Level II-2)

20. Pellerito JS, Troiano RN, Quedens-Case C, Taylor KJ. Common pitfalls of endovaginal color Doppler flow imaging. Radiographics 1995;15:37–47 (Level III)

21. Stovall TG, Ling FW, Carson SA, Buster JE. Serum progesterone and uterine curettage in differential diagnosis of ectopic pregnancy. Fertil Steril 1992;57:456–457 (Level III)

22. Stern JJ, Voss F, Coulam CB. Early diagnosis of ectopic pregnancy using receiver-operator characteristic curves of serum progesterone concentrations. Hum Reprod 1993;8: 775–779 (Level III)

23. McCord ML, Muram D, Buster JE, Arheart KL, Stovall TG, Carson SA. Single serum progesterone as a screen for ectopic pregnancy: exchanging specificity and sensitivity to obtain optimal test performance. Fertil Steril 1996; 66:513–516 (Level II-3)

24. Gelder MS, Boots LR, Younger JB. Use of a single random serum progesterone value as a diagnostic aid for ectopic pregnancy. Fertil Steril 1991;55:497–500 (Level II-2)

25. Lipscomb GH, Bran D, McCord ML, Portera JC, Ling FW. Analysis of three hundred fifteen ectopic pregnancies treated with single-dose methotrexate. Am J Obstet Gynecol 1998;178:1354–1358 (Level II-3)

26. Hajenius PJ, Engelsbel S, Mol BW, Van der Veen F, Ankum WM, Bossuyt PM, et al. Randomised trial of systemic methotrexate versus laparoscopic salpingostomy in tubal pregnancy. Lancet 1997;350:774–779 (Level I)

27. Stovall TG, Ling FW, Gray LA, Carson SA, Buster JE. Methotrexate treatment of unruptured ectopic pregnancy: a report of 100 cases. Obstet Gynecol 1991;77:749–753 (Level II-3)

28. Alexander JM, Rouse DJ, Varner E, Austin JM Jr. Treatment of the small unruptured ectopic pregnancy: a

cost analysis of methotrexate versus laparoscopy. Obstet Gynecol 1996;88:123–127 (Level III)

29. Creinin MD, Washington AE. Cost of ectopic pregnancy management: surgery versus methotrexate. Fertil Steril 1993;60:963–969 (Level II-2)

30. Shalev E, Peleg D, Tsabari A, Romano S, Bustan M. Spontaneous resolution of ectopic tubal pregnancy: natural history. Fertil Steril 1995;63:15–19 (Level II-3)

31. Korhonen J, Stenman UH, Ylöstalo P. Serum human chorionic gonadotropin dynamics during spontaneous resolution of ectopic pregnancy. Fertil Steril 1994;61:632–636 (Level III)

The MEDLINE database, the Cochrane Library, and ACOG's own internal resources and documents were used to conduct a literature search to locate relevant articles published between January 1985 and June 1998. The search was restricted to articles published in the English language. Priority was given to articles reporting results of original research, although review articles and commentaries also were consulted. Abstracts of research presented at symposia and scientific conferences were not considered adequate for inclusion in this document. Guidelines published by organizations or institutions such as the National Institutes of Health and the American College of Obstetricians and Gynecologists were reviewed, and additional studies were located by reviewing bibliographies of identified articles. When reliable research was not available, expert opinions from obstetrician–gynecologists were used.

Studies were reviewed and evaluated for quality according to the method outlined by the U.S. Preventive Services Task Force:

I   Evidence obtained from at least one properly designed randomized controlled trial

II-1 Evidence obtained from well-designed controlled trials without randomization

II-2 Evidence obtained from well-designed cohort or case–control analytic studies, preferably from more than one center or research group

II-3 Evidence obtained from multiple time series with or without the intervention. Dramatic results in uncontrolled experiments could also be regarded as this type of evidence.

III Opinions of respected authorities, based on clinical experience, descriptive studies, or reports of expert committees

Based on the highest level of evidence found in the data, recommendations are provided and graded according to the following categories:

Level A—Recommendations are based on good and consistent scientific evidence.

Level B—Recommendations are based on limited or inconsistent scientific evidence.

Level C—Recommendations are based primarily on consensus and expert opinion.

ISSN 1099-3630   12345/21098

The American College of
Obstetricians and Gynecologists
409 12th Street, SW
PO Box 96920
Washington, DC 20090-6920

ACOG PRACTICE BULLETIN

CLINICAL MANAGEMENT GUIDELINES FOR
OBSTETRICIAN–GYNECOLOGISTS

NUMBER 56, OCTOBER 2004

(Replaces Educational Bulletin Number 253, November 1998)

This Practice Bulletin was developed by the ACOG Committee on Practice Bulletins—Obstetrics, the Society for Maternal-Fetal Medicine and ACOG Joint Editorial Committee with the assistance of Katharine Wenstrom, MD, and contributors John Elliot, MD; Roger Newman, MD; Alan Peaceman, MD; and Suneet Chahaun, MD. The information is designed to aid practitioners in making decisions about appropriate obstetric and gynecologic care. These guidelines should not be construed as dictating an exclusive course of treatment or procedure. Variations in practice may be warranted based on the needs of the individual patient, resources, and limitations unique to the institution or type of practice.

The Society for
Maternal-Fetal Medicine

Multiple Gestation: Complicated Twin, Triplet, and High-Order Multifetal Pregnancy

In 2002, more than 130,000 infants were born of multifetal gestations in the United States (1). Since 1980, there has been a 65% increase in the frequency of twins and a 500% increase in triplet and high-order births (1). Most of this increase results from increased use of ovulation induction agents and assisted reproductive technology (ART); the risk of multiple gestation associated with these therapies may be as high as 25% (2). Similar increases in multifetal gestation have occurred worldwide (3–6).

Although multifetal births account for only 3% of all live births, they are responsible for a disproportionate share of perinatal morbidity and mortality (Table 1). They account for 17% of all preterm births (before 37 weeks of gestation), 23% of early preterm births (before 32 weeks of gestation), 24% of low-birth-weight infants (<2,500 g), and 26% of very-low-birth-weight infants (<1,500 g) (1, 7–9). Although twins do have an increased risk of morbidity and mortality, a far greater proportion of triplet and high-order multiple gestations have poor outcomes. All survivors of preterm multifetal births have an increased risk of mental and physical handicap.

The purpose of this document is to address the risks associated with these pregnancies and present an evidence-based approach to management when possible. Because the literature on high-order multiple gestation is still largely composed of case reports or small series, experience is important in the decision-making process for complicated twin or high-order multiple gestations.

Background

Infant and Maternal Morbidity

One fifth of triplet pregnancies and one half of quadruplet pregnancies result in at least 1 child with a major long-term handicap, such as cerebral palsy (10). Cerebral palsy occurs 17 times more often in triplet pregnancies and more than 4 times more often in twin pregnancies than in singleton pregnancies (10, 11). This risk is not solely related to preterm birth. When matched for gestational age at delivery, infants from multifetal pregnancies have a nearly 3-fold greater risk of cerebral palsy (12, 13). One confounding factor may be growth restriction, which complicates approximately 50–60% of triplet and quadruplet pregnancies (14). Growth-restricted preterm infants, regardless of plurality, have a significantly higher risk of morbidity (including an excess of neurodevel-

opmental abnormalities) and mortality than appropriately grown infants of the same gestational age (15–19).

Multifetal gestations also are associated with significantly higher maternal morbidity and associated health care costs. Women with multiple gestations are nearly 6 times more likely to be hospitalized with complications, including preeclampsia, preterm labor, preterm premature rupture of membranes, placental abruption, pyelonephritis, and postpartum hemorrhage (20–26). Hospital costs for women with multiple gestations are on average 40% higher than for women with gestational-age-matched singleton pregnancies because of their longer length of stay and obstetric complications. Neonatal intensive care unit (NICU) admission is required for one fourth of twins, three fourths of triplets, and virtually all quadruplets, with average NICU stays of 18 days, 30 days, and 58 days, respectively (20, 23–25, 27–29).

Table 1. Morbidity and Mortality in Multiple Gestation

Characteristic	Twins	Triplets	Quadruplets
Average birth weight[1]	2,347 g	1,687 g	1,309 g
Average gestational age at delivery[1]	35.3 wk	32.2 wk	29.9 wk
Percentage with growth restriction[2]	14–25	50–60	50–60
Percentage requiring admission to neonatal intensive care unit[3]	25	75	100
Average length of stay in neonatal intensive care unit[3–9]	18 days	30 days	58 days
Percentage with major handicap[9,10]	—	20	50
Risk of cerebral palsy[9,10]	4 times more than singletons	17 times more than singletons	—
Risk of death by age 1 year[11–13]	7 times higher than singletons	20 times higher than singletons	—

[1]Martin JA, Hamilton BE, Sutton PD, Ventura SJ, Menacker F, Munson ML. Births: final data for 2002. Natl Vital Stat Rep 2003;52(10):1–102.

[2]Mauldin JG, Newman RB. Neurologic morbidity associated with multiple gestation. Female Pat 1998;23(4):27–8, 30, 35–6, passim.

[3]Ettner SL, Christiansen CL, Callahan TL, Hall JE. How low birthweight and gestational age contribute to increased inpatient costs for multiple births. Inquiry 1997–98;34:325–39.

[4]McCormick MD, Brooks-Gunn J, Workman-Daniels K, Turner J, Peckham GJ. The health and developmental status of very low-birth-weight children at school age. JAMA 1992;267:2204–8.

[5]Luke B, Bigger HR, Leurgans S, Sietsema D. The cost of prematurity: a case-control study of twins vs singletons. Am J Public Health 1996;86:809–14.

[6]Albrecht JL, Tomich PG. The maternal and neonatal outcome of triplet gestations. Am J Obstet Gynecol 1996;174:1551–6.

[7]Newman RB, Hamer C, Miller MC. Outpatient triplet management: a contemporary review. Am J Obstet Gynecol 1989;161:547–53; discussion 553–5.

[8]Seoud MA, Toner JP, Kruithoff C, Muasher SJ. Outcome of twin, triplet, and quadruplet in vitro fertilization pregnancies: the Norfolk experience. Fertil Steril 1992;57:825–34.

[9]Elliott JP, Radin TG. Quadruplet pregnancy: contemporary management and outcome. Obstet Gynecol 1992;80:421–4.

[10]Grether JK, Nelson KB, Cummins SK. Twinning and cerebral palsy: experience in four northern California counties, births 1983 through 1985. Pediatrics 1993;92:854–8.

[11]Luke B, Minogue J. The contribution of gestational age and birth weight to perinatal viability in singletons versus twins. J Mat-Fetal Med 1994;3:263–74.

[12]Kiely JL, Kleinman JC, Kiely M. Triplets and higher order multiple births: time trends and infant mortality. Am J Dis Child 1992;146:862–8.

[13]Luke B, Keith LG. The contribution of singletons, twins, and triplets to low birth weight, infant mortality, and handicap in the United States. J Reprod Med 1992;37:661–6.

Role of Assisted Reproductive Technology

In 1980, there were 37 pregnancies delivered of triplets or more for every 100,000 live births; by 2002, this number had increased to 184 pregnancies per 100,000 live births (1). This marked increase in the number of high-order multiple gestations was a result of the increased use of ART and ovulation-induction agents during this period. A similar proportion of triplet and high-order gestations result from ART procedures and ovulation induction (43% and 38%, respectively), whereas spontaneous conception accounts for the remainder (19%) (30). Major morbidity in these pregnancies results from the associated high rates of preterm birth and low birth weight (see Table 1), although the characteristics of women seeking these therapies also may be a factor.

One unexpected complication of ART is the high incidence of monochorionic twins. One group evaluated 218 ART pregnancies and found the incidence of monochorionicity was 3.2%, compared with the background rate of 0.4% (31). Other studies have reported an incidence of monochorionicity ranging from 1% to 5% in association with both ART and ovulation induction (32). Both animal and human data indicate that manipulation of the zona pellucida or slowed movement through the fallopian tube can provoke monozygotic twinning (33–35), and both of these may occur during fertility treatments. Monozygotic twinning not only increases the incidence of high-order multiple gestations (ie, 3 embryos are implanted but 4 fetuses result), but also complicates fetal growth and development and can lead to rare complications, such as twin–twin transfusion syndrome or acardiac twinning. It also increases the morbidity of a pregnancy reduction procedure.

Maternal Age

The a priori risk of a poor perinatal outcome in a high-order multiple gestation is further increased by the woman's age. The growing proportion of older women successfully undergoing fertility treatment has resulted in an increase in pregnancies complicated by adult-onset diseases, such as hypertension and diabetes, labor abnormalities, and cesarean delivery.

Multifetal gestations in older women also complicates prenatal genetic screening and diagnosis. Increased maternal age alone increases the risk of fetal trisomies, such as Down syndrome. The presence of multiple fetuses increases the mathematical probability that 1 or more fetuses will be affected and, thus, results in a higher risk for the pregnancy than that attributed to maternal age alone. For example, because either 1 or both fetuses in a twin pair could have Down syndrome, the ultimate risk

of Down syndrome in a twin pregnancy carried by a 33-year-old woman is the same as the risk in a singleton pregnancy carried by a 35-year-old woman (36). Accordingly, a Down syndrome risk equivalent to that of a 35-year-old woman will occur at successively younger maternal ages as the number of fetuses increases.

Prenatal Diagnosis

Amniocentesis or chorionic villous sampling may be technically difficult to accomplish in patients with multiple gestations (37–42). Technical problems unique to high-order multiple gestation include the need to traverse another fetus' sac to reach a different fetus for sampling, incorrect fetal karyotype caused by cross contamination with other sacs, difficulty in accurately mapping the fetuses and determining which fetus is being sampled, difficulty in accurately determining whether any of the fetuses are monochorionic twins, and difficulty in locating and reducing only the affected fetus in the event an aneuploidy is diagnosed and termination chosen.

Complications of Pregnancy

Gestational Diabetes

The incidence of gestational diabetes in twin pregnancies is higher than in singleton pregnancies (43), and the incidence in triplet pregnancies is higher than in twin pregnancies; up to 22–39% of triplet pregnancies are complicated by gestational diabetes, compared with 3–6% of twin pregnancies (44, 45). One study of 95 twin and 26 triplet pregnancies, which controlled for other factors that influence the incidence of gestational diabetes, such as maternal age, weight, and parity, estimated that each additional fetus increases the risk of gestational diabetes by a factor of 1.8 (45). Another study has shown that pregnancy reduction significantly reduces the incidence of gestational diabetes from 22% in triplet pregnancies to 6% in reduced twin pregnancies (44).

Many aspects of the diagnosis and management of gestational diabetes in multiple gestation remain unexamined. The best time for testing, the ideal number of daily calories, the optimal weight gain, whether women treated with oral hypoglycemic agents for polycystic ovary syndrome should continue taking them, the best form of insulin to use, the best method of fetal surveillance, and the ideal time for delivery are all currently unknown. Consultation with an obstetrician–gynecologist who has expertise in the management of pregnant women with diabetes, such as a maternal–fetal medicine specialist, and with a dietitian would be helpful.

Hypertension and Preeclampsia

Multiple gestations are at higher risk than singleton gestations of developing gestational hypertension. The incidence of preeclampsia is 2.6 times higher in twin gestations than in singleton gestations (46) and is higher in triplet gestations than in twin gestations (47). In addition, when multiple gestation is complicated by preeclampsia, it is significantly more likely to occur earlier and to be severe (46, 48, 49). Gestational hypertension before 35 weeks of gestation, preeclampsia before 35 weeks of gestation, and hypertension with a diastolic blood pressure level greater than 110 mm Hg occur 12.4 times, 6.7 times, and 2.2 times more often, respectively, in twin gestations compared with singleton gestations (48). Placental abruption also is 8.2 times more likely (48). Multiple gestations as a result of ART seem to be at greater risk of developing hypertensive complications than spontaneous multiple gestations, for reasons that are not entirely known. One study of 198 ART multiple gestations compared with 330 spontaneous multiple gestations found that the ART pregnancies were at increased risk (relative risk, 2.1) of developing mild or severe preeclampsia even after controlling for maternal age and parity (50). High-order multiple gestations also are more likely to develop atypical preeclampsia (51). One study of women with triplet or quadruplet pregnancies and preeclampsia found that only 50% had hypertension, only 38% had edema, and only 19% had proteinuria before delivery, whereas 60% had epigastric pain and 56% had hemolysis, elevated liver enzymes, and low platelets (HELLP) syndrome (52). Multifetal reduction may decrease the risk of preeclampsia. One study reported that 14% of 59 twin pregnancies remaining after multifetal reduction developed preeclampsia compared with 30% of 54 triplet pregnancies (53).

The management of hypertensive complications in high-order multiple gestations has not been studied prospectively. Although many women with high-order multiple gestations are placed on bed rest, this therapy has been associated with increased fetal weight but not with prolongation of pregnancy or avoidance of hypertensive complications (54). If severe preeclampsia, HELLP syndrome, or another serious hypertensive complication develops before term, transfer to a tertiary care center may improve outcome for both the woman and her fetuses. It is unclear whether the risks associated with postponing delivery to administer steroids are outweighed by the benefits of antenatal steroid exposure in multifetal pregnancies.

Other Pregnancy Complications

Multiple gestations also are disproportionately affected by more serious pregnancy complications, such as acute fatty liver (55). Acute fatty liver, which is marked by severe coagulopathy, hypoglycemia, and hyperammonemia, can lead to fetal or maternal death (55). Although delivery usually halts the disease process, the postpartum period can be complicated by pancreatitis or diabetes insipidus or both. The coagulopathy makes delivery itself difficult in high-order multiple gestations because cesarean delivery usually is required. Diagnosis is frequently delayed because the symptoms, which typically include anorexia, nausea and vomiting, and malaise beginning late in pregnancy and developing over several days or weeks, are vague and nonspecific, and there is concurrent evidence of preeclampsia in at least one third of affected women (56).

Acute fatty liver is rare, occurring in 1 in 10,000 singleton gestations. However, 14% of reported cases have occurred in twin gestations even though they represent fewer than 2% of all pregnancies, and recent reports indicate that the rate may be as high as 7% in triplet pregnancies (55, 57). Many cases are associated with an autosomal recessive disorder, long-chain 3-hydroxyacyl-CoA dehydrogenase deficiency (58, 59). Disease occurs only when both the woman and the fetus are carrying at least 1 affected gene; multiple gestations are disproportionately affected with this and other genetic conditions because the more fetuses there are, the greater the chance that at least 1 of them has inherited the woman's gene mutation.

Pulmonary embolism is a leading cause of maternal death in the United States and around the world (60, 61), and thromboembolism is 6 times more likely during pregnancy or the puerperium than in the nonpregnant state. The factors most commonly associated with thromboembolism are multiple pregnancy, cesarean delivery, delivery before 36 weeks of gestation, a body mass index of 25 or higher, and maternal age of 35 years or older; all are more common in multiple gestation (62). In addition, women with multiple gestation frequently are placed on bed rest, and the enlarged uterus mechanically obstructs venous return and contributes to lower extremity stasis. One study of more than 395,000 births found that multiple gestation was associated with significantly increased risk of thromboembolism even after controlling for all other associated risks (62).

Prompt and sustained anticoagulation is needed for confirmed thrombosis or thromboembolism. Because the volume of distribution is increased to a much greater degree in multiple gestations than in singleton gestations, it may be difficult to achieve a therapeutic level of anticoagulation. In addition, because high-order multiple gestations are at significantly increased risk of preterm labor, cesarean delivery, and bleeding complications, such as abruption, the form of anticoagulation chosen should be readily reversible. Consultation with an individual with expertise in maternal–fetal medicine or hematology may be helpful.

Other less common pregnancy complications occur more frequently in multiple gestations than in singleton gestations. A recent study of 142 multiple gestations found that 3% of twin gestations and 14% of triplet gestations were complicated by pruritic urticarial papules and pustules of pregnancy, compared with only 0.5% of singleton gestations (63). Pruritic urticarial papules and pustules of pregnancy is a dermatosis that most commonly affects primigravid women in the third trimester (63). It usually starts in abdominal striae, and striae are common in multiple gestations because of excessive weight gain and rapid abdominal distention. Recently, fetal DNA has been detected in the dermis of affected women, which suggests that fetal–maternal cell trafficking and immune phenomena play a role (64).

Multifetal Reduction and Selective Fetal Termination

High-order multiple gestation creates a medical and ethical dilemma. If a pregnancy with 4 or more fetuses is continued, the probability is high that not all fetuses will survive intact and that the woman will experience serious morbidity. However, fetal reduction to triplet or twin gestations is associated with a significant risk of losing either another fetus or the whole pregnancy. Most studies have concluded that the risks associated with a quadruplet or higher pregnancy clearly outweigh the risks associated with fetal reduction.

The largest report of perinatal outcome after fetal reduction, which included 1,789 reduction procedures over a period of 9 years, noted an overall postprocedure pregnancy loss rate of 11.7% and a very early preterm (ie, between 25 and 28 weeks of gestation) delivery rate of 4.5% (65). The chance of losing either an additional fetus or the whole pregnancy, and the chance of early preterm delivery, increased according to the starting number of fetuses; 23% of pregnancies that started with 6 or more fetuses were lost before 24 weeks of gestation, and only 20% were delivered at 37 weeks of gestation or later. Whether to reduce high-order multiple gestations to twin or triplet gestations and whether to reduce triplet gestations at all are both areas of controversy.

Fetal reduction of a high-order multiple pregnancy has been associated with an increased risk of intrauterine fetal growth restriction (IUGR) in the remaining twins in some studies but not in others (66–69). One study found the incidence of IUGR was 36% in twins reduced from triplets, 42% in twins reduced from quadruplets, and 50% in twins reduced from quintuplets or greater, compared with 19% in twins who had not been reduced (67). Another study found a significant risk of IUGR in the

remaining twins only when the starting number of fetuses was 5 or more (70).

Monochorionicity can complicate the reduction procedure; if one fetus of a monochorionic twin pair is inadvertently reduced, sudden hypotension and thrombotic phenomena could result in death or damage of the remaining twin fetus. This is illustrated by one series of high-order multiple gestations (quadruplets and quintuplets) in which every pregnancy included a monochorionic twin pair (71). In each case, although the authors selectively reduced only 1 of the monochorionic twins by injection of potassium chloride, subsequent demise of all the co-twins was confirmed.

Selective fetal termination is the application of the fetal reduction technique to the selective termination of an anomalous or aneuploid fetus that is part of a multiple gestation. The risks of this procedure are higher than those associated with multifetal reduction (72). The pregnancy usually is more advanced by the time the anomaly is diagnosed (ie, 18–22 weeks of gestation compared with 10–12 weeks of gestation), and the location of the anomalous fetus may be associated with increased risk. The risk of losing the whole pregnancy, having a preterm birth, or having an infant with a birth weight less than 2,500 g is highest when the reduced fetus overlies the cervix and when the pregnancy is at or beyond 20 weeks of gestation (73).

Clinical Considerations and Recommendations

▶ *Can preterm labor be predicted in multiple gestation?*

Cervical Length Measurement by Ultrasonography

A shortened cervix identified by endovaginal ultrasonography is strongly predictive of preterm delivery in twin pregnancies (74–76). A large multicenter study of cervical length in twin pregnancies found that a cervix shorter than 25 mm at 24 weeks of gestation was the best predictor of delivery before 32, 35, and 37 weeks of gestation (74) and was significantly more common in twin gestations than in singleton gestations at both 24 and 28 weeks of gestation. One study of 32 triplet pregnancies reported similar data, with cervical measurements comparable to those reported for twin pregnancies (77).

Cervical Length Measurement by Digital Examination

Serial digital examinations by an experienced examiner, assessing both cervical length and dilation, have been reported to have positive predictive values of 60–70% in twin and triplet gestations (77–79). However, digital examination may be less objective than ultrasonographic measurement and does not allow assessment of the internal os.

Fetal Fibronectin

Fetal fibronectin is a high-molecular-weight extracellular matrix glycoprotein that is normally found in fetal membranes, placental tissues, and amniotic fluid. Its presence in cervical–vaginal fluids at concentrations higher than 50 ng/mL is abnormal and has been shown to predict preterm delivery in singleton gestations. Four studies examining the utility of measuring fetal fibronectin in twin or triplet gestations showed that a single fetal fibronectin test had a high negative predictive value, and serial tests had a fairly high positive predictive value (range: 38–53%) (74, 80–82). However, at least 1 study found that fetal fibronectin levels were not predictive of preterm delivery in twin gestations after controlling for cervical length (74).

Home Uterine Activity Monitoring

Although initially presented as a potentially effective tool for identifying preterm labor early enough to allow for treatment, several studies have now cast considerable doubt on the utility of home uterine activity monitoring for this purpose. In one large randomized prospective trial, 2,422 pregnant women, including 844 twin pregnancies, were randomly assigned to weekly contact with a perinatal nurse, daily contact with a perinatal nurse, or daily contact with a perinatal nurse and home uterine activity monitoring (83). There was no difference in outcome among the twin gestations in the 3 groups.

▶ *Are there interventions that can prolong pregnancy in multiple gestation?*

Current data from U.S. birth records indicate that 55–57% of all multiple gestations are delivered preterm, and 49–63% of these infants weigh less than 2,500 g (84). Twelve percent of twin pregnancies, 36% of triplet pregnancies, and 60% of quadruplet pregnancies are born before 32 weeks of gestation, when perinatal morbidity and mortality are greatest. The same factors that contribute to preterm birth in singleton pregnancies affect multiple gestations and may be more common: lower and upper genital tract infection; uterine overdistension; cervical incompetence; maternal medical complications; maternal stress; and fetal, placental, or uterine abnormalities. However, the identification of these risk factors has not lead to the development of effective protocols or therapies to prevent preterm delivery, although many different therapies have been investigated.

Prophylactic Cerclage

The value of prophylactic cerclage in prolonging high-order multiple gestation has not been assessed, but its use in twin pregnancy has been studied in at least 2 prospective trials, including 50 and 74 sets of twins, respectively; cerclage did not prolong gestation or improve perinatal outcome in either study (85, 86). The studies of cerclage in triplet pregnancies are all retrospective, making bias in assignment of this therapy highly likely.

Routine Hospitalization

No trials of routine hospitalization of high-order multiple gestations have been published. Four prospective randomized trials and one retrospective study have shown that bed rest in the hospital does not prolong twin gestation (54, 87–90). Retrospective series assessing the value of elective hospitalization for triplet pregnancies also have failed to identify any significant differences in perinatal outcome after hospitalization (91, 92).

Restriction of Activities and Rest at Home

Although this is the most commonly prescribed therapy for multiple gestation, it has not been evaluated in a prospective randomized manner. Most of the retrospective analyses of bed rest for multiple gestation are strongly biased by the indications for bed rest, and some studies were performed so long ago that bed rest was not instituted until the third trimester because the multiple pregnancy was not diagnosed until then (93–95).

▶ *How is preterm labor managed in multiple gestation?*

Tocolytics

If effective tocolytic therapy were available, identifying women at risk of preterm delivery could reduce the incidence of preterm birth. The use of prophylactic tocolysis in twin gestations has been examined in at least 7 prospective studies (96–102). These trials showed no consistent effect on preterm birth, birth weight, or neonatal mortality. Importantly, the risks associated with each tocolytic are amplified in multiple gestations. Beta-mimetics are associated with increased maternal and fetal cardiac stress and gestational diabetes; these complications occur more frequently in multiple gestations even without β-mimetic therapy (103, 104). In addition, women with multiple gestations are at increased risk of developing pulmonary edema resulting in severe respiratory distress when tocolytic agents, steroids, and intravenous fluids are administered together (105, 106).

Therefore, because of the associated risks of tocolytics in high-order pregnancies, they should be used judiciously.

Corticosteroids

The effect of antenatal steroid administration and the possible effects of steroid dose on efficacy in multiple gestations have not been examined. Nevertheless, the National Institutes of Health recommends that all women in preterm labor who have no contraindications to steroid use be given one course of steroids, regardless of the number of fetuses (107).

▶ *How should growth restriction or discordant growth be diagnosed and managed in multiple gestation?*

Fetuses of a multiple gestation generally do not grow at the same rate as singleton fetuses. One obvious etiology is placental pathology; multiple gestations are at increased risk to include at least 1 fetus with a suboptimal placental implantation site or abnormal umbilical cord morphology. For example, one study of 39 sets of triplets found that 28% included at least 1 fetus with a velamentous cord insertion site that was likely to be growth restricted as a result (108). Depending on the number of fetuses, a diminution in fetal growth may be discernible as early as 22 weeks of gestation (68). The long held theory that low-birth-weight infants from a multiple gestation do better than low-birth-weight singleton infants is not correct. Because infants of multiple gestations are likely to be both preterm and low birth weight, their outcome may actually be worse (109).

Abnormally slow fetal growth in a multiple gestation may be easier to recognize when not all of the fetuses are affected equally. Discordant fetal growth is common in multiple gestation and usually is defined by a 15–25% reduction in the estimated fetal weight of the smaller fetus when compared with the largest (110). Most published studies examine discordance in twins; twin weight discordance is associated with structural malformations, stillbirth, IUGR, preterm delivery, cesarean delivery for nonreassuring fetal heart tracing, umbilical arterial pH less than 7.1, admission to the NICU, respiratory distress syndrome, and neonatal death within 7 days of delivery (6, 8, 9). The threshold at which discordant growth is most strongly associated with adverse outcomes is still a matter of debate, even in twin gestations (1, 6, 7).

Some discordance is expected in multiple gestations, especially those resulting from ovulation induction or the implantation of 3 or more embryos, when the fetuses are not genetically identical and may be of different sexes. They would not be expected to be more similar in weight than any other siblings. If 2 fetuses are discordant but both have normal estimated weights and grow appropriately on their own growth curves, the discordance may not indicate a pathologic process (111). Conversely, concordance would not be desirable if both fetuses are growth restricted. One study of 279 twin pairs showed that when birth weight and gestational age at delivery were evaluated separately, discordance itself was not a strong predictor of neonatal outcome (112). However, attribution of fetal weight differences to zygosity should only be considered once other more serious etiologies have been ruled out.

Discordance can be caused by structural or genetic fetal anomalies; discordant infection; an unfavorable placental implantation or umbilical cord insertion site; placental damage (ie, partial abruption); or complications related to monochorionic placentation, such as twin–twin transfusion syndrome. All of these complications occur more frequently in high-order multiple gestations. The workup should include a review of all prenatal exposures, a specialized ultrasound examination, and, depending on the gestational age, a test of fetal well-being.

Because of the inherent difficulty in fully evaluating each fetus, the ultrasound examination should be performed by someone with skill and experience in scanning multiple gestations. If an anomaly is identified, the patient should receive counseling, and testing should be offered, if applicable. In rare cases (for example, twin–twin transfusion syndrome), therapy may be available. Before performing a preterm delivery to benefit the growth-restricted fetus, the well-being of the other fetuses needs to be considered. A consultation with an obstetrician–gynecologist with expertise in the management of high-risk pregnancies, such as a maternal–fetal medicine specialist, may be helpful.

▶ *How is the death of one fetus managed?*

Multiple gestations, especially high-order multiple gestations, are at increased risk of losing 1 or more fetuses remote from delivery. One report described the outcome of every twin, triplet, and higher order multiple gestation delivered at one perinatal center during a 5-year period (113). Of 310 twin and 45 triplet or higher pregnancies, 19 were complicated by the spontaneous demise of one fetus, a loss rate of 6%. Six losses occurred in the first trimester and 13 in the second or third trimester; an additional 9 pregnancies underwent fetal reduction, and one of these pregnancies was miscarried afterward. The causes of the first-trimester losses could not be determined, but the later losses were caused by twin–twin transfusion syndrome (n = 4), severe IUGR (n = 3), placental insufficiency (n = 4), and placental abruption (n = 1); the cause of 1 loss was unknown. Because high-order multiple gestations are significantly more likely to sustain the complications causing fetal demise in this study and others, the loss rates for high-order multiple gestations may be considerably higher than 6%.

No fetal monitoring protocol has been shown to predict most of these losses. In addition, authorities disagree about the preferred antepartum surveillance method and management once a demise has occurred. Some investigators have advocated immediate delivery of the remaining fetuses (114). However, if the death is the result of an abnormality of the fetus itself rather than maternal or uteroplacental pathology, and the pregnancy is remote from term, expectant management may be appropriate. The most difficult cases are those in which the fetal demise occurs in 1 fetus of a monochorionic twin pair. Because virtually 100% of monochorionic placentas contain vascular anastomoses that link the circulations of the 2 fetuses, the surviving fetus is at significant risk of sustaining damage caused by the sudden, severe, and prolonged hypotension that occurs at the time of the demise or by embolic phenomena that occurs later (115, 116). By the time the demise is discovered, the greatest harm has most likely already been done, and there may not be any benefit in immediate delivery, especially if the surviving fetuses are very preterm and otherwise healthy. In such cases, allowing the pregnancy to continue may provide the most benefit.

Although maternal disseminated intravascular coagulopathy (DIC) remains a theoretical risk, it rarely occurs. One series of 28 multiple gestations complicated by the demise of one fetus remote from term included no cases of DIC (113). Fibrinogen and fibrin degradation product levels can be monitored serially until delivery, and delivery can be expedited if DIC develops.

▶ *Is there a role for routine antepartum fetal surveillance?*

Multiple gestations are at increased risk of stillbirth. The risk in multifetal pregnancies is higher than the risk in singleton pregnancies at each week of gestation, and the loss is likely to occur at a much earlier gestational age than in singleton or twin pregnancies (117). The most effective fetal surveillance system for such pregnancies is not known. Because of the increased risk, clinicians frequently initiate fetal heart rate testing. Both the nonstress test and the fetal biophysical profile have been shown to be effective in identifying the compromised twin or triplet gestation (118–122). However, none of these data are based on prospective study and none per-

tain to high-order multiple gestations. Additionally, several issues have not been resolved. For example, it is not known at what gestational age testing should be initiated, whether testing should be performed once or twice per week, or whether there is a need to test normally growing dichorionic twins. At present, antepartum fetal surveillance in multiple gestations is recommended in all situations in which surveillance would ordinarily be performed in a singleton pregnancy (eg, IUGR, maternal disease, decreased fetal movement). Further studies are needed to determine whether routine antepartum fetal surveillance provides objective benefit in the absence of other high-risk conditions.

▶ *How is delayed delivery of the second twin managed?*

Rarely, preterm labor results in expulsion of a single fetus followed by cessation of uterine contractions and uterine quiescence. Often, the placenta remains in situ, with the umbilical cord visibly protruding through the cervical os. Whether such an event should prompt delivery of the remaining fetuses is controversial. In view of the paucity of objective, prospective, randomized data and the risk involved, consultation with individuals with training, experience, and expertise in maternal–fetal medicine and neonatology is indicated.

▶ *How are problems caused by monochorionic placentation managed?*

Twin–Twin Transfusion Syndrome

Twin–twin transfusion syndrome is believed to occur as the result of uncompensated arteriovenous anastomoses in a monochorionic placenta, which lead to greater net blood flow going to one twin at the expense of the other (123). The donor twin usually is anemic and growth restricted and appears "stuck" to one spot in the uterus because the lack of amniotic fluid in its sac precludes movement; the recipient twin usually is plethoric and much larger, and hydramnios is evident. The syndrome usually becomes apparent in the second trimester and can rapidly lead to premature rupture of membranes, preterm labor, or early mortality because of heart failure in either of the fetuses (124–126). A variety of therapies have been attempted, but serial therapeutic amniocenteses of the recipient twin's amniotic sac is most frequently used. This therapy is believed to work by favorably changing intraamniotic pressure and, thus, placental intravascular pressure, allowing redistribution of placental blood flow and normalization of amniotic fluid volumes in each sac (123–127). More aggressive therapies, which usually are considered only for very early, severe cases, include abolishing the placental anastomoses by endoscopic laser coagulation or selective feticide by umbilical cord occlusion (128–131). Because both twins are at significantly increased risk of sudden death resulting from either hypovolemic or hypervolemic heart failure, these pregnancies should be monitored closely. Death of one fetus has been reported to result in the sudden transfusion of blood from the viable fetus to the low pressure system of the dead fetus, resulting in exsanguination of the viable twin (132, 133). If the gestational age is such that survival is likely, immediate delivery should be considered, recognizing that damage to the remaining viable fetus may already have occurred.

Rare Complications

An acardiac or acephalus twin is a monozygotic fetus without a normally developed heart or brain, respectively, as the result of abnormal division of the zygote at the time of twinning. These "fetuses" are nonviable and survive antenatally only because they receive blood flow from their monochorionic co-twin. Because the "pump" twin is supplying blood flow to both its own body and that of its abnormal twin, death from heart failure is a common complication (134). Such pregnancies require close monitoring, with consideration of early delivery or selective feticide of the abnormal co-twin by umbilical cord occlusion if heart failure develops (135).

When division of the embryonic disc is not complete, twins can be joined at the head, thorax, abdomen, or spine and often share organs. Management of conjoined twins is directed by their chance of long-term survival. If postnatal separation or survival without separation is possible, the twins should be monitored closely for heart failure or other signs of stress and be delivered atraumatically, usually by cesarean delivery (136). Pregnancies in which survival of either fetus is unlikely can be managed expectantly but also may require cesarean delivery for dystocia.

▶ *Are there special considerations for timing of delivery in multiple gestations?*

The nadir of perinatal mortality for twin pregnancies occurs at approximately 38 completed weeks of gestation and at 35 completed weeks of gestation for triplets; the nadir for quadruplet and other high-order multiple gestations is not known (137). Fetal and neonatal morbidity and mortality begin to increase in twin and triplet pregnancies extended beyond 37 and 35 weeks of gestation, respectively (137, 138). However, no prospective randomized trials have tested the hypothesis that elective delivery at these gestational ages improves outcomes in these pregnancies. If the fetuses are appropriate in size

for gestational age with evidence of sustained growth and there is normal amniotic fluid volume and reassuring antepartum fetal testing in the absence of maternal complications, such as preeclampsia or gestational diabetes, the pregnancy can be continued. Alternatively, if the woman is experiencing morbidities that would improve with delivery but do not necessarily mandate delivery (eg, worsening dyspnea, inability to sleep, severe dependent edema, painful superficial varicosities), delivery may be considered at these gestational ages.

Determination of fetal pulmonary maturity before delivery may be necessary for twin and other multiple gestations if prenatal care was late, if the woman desires a scheduled delivery, or if the pregnancy is complicated by preterm labor or preterm premature rupture of membranes. Several reports have noted that beyond 31–32 weeks of gestation, the biochemical markers of pulmonary maturity (lecithin/sphingomyelin ratio or fluorescence polarization immunoassay) are higher in twin pregnancies than in singleton pregnancies at comparable gestational ages (139, 140). Recent publications note that asynchronous pulmonary maturity occurs in more than 5% of twins, regardless of fetal sex and size. Before 32 weeks of gestation, 25% of twin pairs have a significant disparity, usually resulting from one twin having a lecithin/sphingomyelin ratio that is more mature than expected for gestational age (141). Accordingly, some authorities recommend that the gestational sac of each twin be sampled if technically feasible. There are insufficient data to make a similar recommendation for pregnancies with 3 or more fetuses.

▶ *Are there special considerations for route of delivery for multiple gestations?*

The route of delivery for twins should be determined by the position of the fetuses, the ease of fetal heart rate monitoring, and maternal and fetal status. Data are insufficient to determine the best route of delivery for high-order multiple gestations. There are retrospective case series that validate vaginal delivery as a potential mode of delivery, especially for triplet gestations. However, most such pregnancies are delivered by cesarean delivery.

Summary of Recommendations

The following recommendations are based on limited or inconsistent scientific evidence (Level B):

▶ Tocolytic agents should be used judiciously in multiple gestations.

▶ Women with high-order multiple gestations should be queried about nausea, epigastric pain, and other unusual third-trimester symptoms because they are at increased risk to develop HELLP syndrome, in many cases before symptoms of preeclampsia have appeared.

▶ The higher incidence of gestational diabetes and hypertension in high-order multiple gestations warrants screening and monitoring for these complications.

The following recommendations are based primarily on consensus and expert opinion (Level C):

▶ The National Institutes of Health recommends that women in preterm labor with no contraindication to steroid use be given one course of steroids, regardless of the number of fetuses.

▶ Cerclage, hospitalization, bed rest, or home uterine activity monitoring have not been studied in high-order multiple gestations, and, therefore, should not be ordered prophylactically. There currently is no evidence that their prophylactic use improves outcome in these pregnancies.

▶ Because the risks of invasive prenatal diagnosis procedures, such as amniocentesis and chorionic villus sampling, are inversely proportional to the experience of the operator, only experienced clinicians should perform these procedures in high-order multiple gestations.

▶ Women should be counseled about the risks of high-order multiple gestation before beginning ART.

▶ Management of discordant growth restriction or death of one fetus in a high-order multiple gestation should be individualized, taking into consideration the welfare of the other fetus(es).

References

1. Martin JA, Hamilton BE, Sutton PD, Ventura SJ, Menacker F, Munson ML. Births: final data for 2002. Natl Vital Stat Rep 2003;52(10):1–102. (Level II-3)

2. Jewell SE, Yip R. Increasing trends in plural births in the United States. Obstet Gynecol 1995;85:229–32. (Level III)

3. Ho ML, Chen JY, Ling UP, Chen JH, Huang CM, Chang CC, et al. Changing epidemiology of triplet pregnancy: etiology and outcome over twelve years. Am J Perinatol 1996;13:269–75. (Level III)

4. Westergaard T, Wohlfahrt J, Aaby P, Melbye M. Population based study of rates of multiple pregnancies in Denmark, 1980–94. BMJ 1997;314:775–9. (Level II-3)

5. Platt MJ, Marshall A, Pharoah PO. The effects of assisted reproduction on the trends and zygosity of multiple births in England and Wales 1974–99. Twin Res 2001;4:417–21. (Level II-2)

6. Roberts CL, Raynes-Greenow CH, Algert CS, Peat B. Higher order multiple pregnancies in New South Wales 1990–1999. Aust N Z J Obstet Gynaecol 2002;42:51–4. (Level III)

7. Stevenson DK, Wright LL, Lemons JA, Oh W, Korones SB, Papile LA, et al. Very low birth weight outcomes of the National Institute of Child Health and Human Development Neonatal Research Network, January 1993 through December 1994. Am J Obstet Gynecol 1998; 179:1632–9. (Level II-3)

8. Powers WF, Kiely JL. The risk confronting twins: a national perspective. Am J Obstet Gynecol 1994;170: 456–61. (Level II-2)

9. Donovan EF, Ehrenkranz RA, Shankaran S, Stevenson DK, Wright LL, Younes N, et al. Outcomes of very low birth weight twins cared for in the National Institute of Child Health and Human Development Neonatal Research Network's intensive care units. Am J Obstet Gynecol 1998;179:742–9. (Level II-2)

10. Yokoyama Y, Shimizu T, Hayakawa K. Incidence of handicaps in multiple births and associated factors. Acta Genet Med Gemellol (Roma) 1995;44:81–91. (Level II-2)

11. Petterson B, Nelson KB, Watson L, Stanley F. Twins, triplets, and cerebral palsy in births in Western Australia in the 1980's. BMJ 1993;307:1239–43 (Level II-3)

12. Grether JK, Nelson KB, Cummins SK. Twinning and cerebral palsy: experience in four northern California counties, births 1983 through 1985. Pediatrics 1993;92: 854–8. (Level II-3)

13. Mauldin JG, Newman RB. Neurologic morbidity associated with multiple gestation. Female Pat 1998;23(4): 27–8, 30, 35–6, passim. (Level III)

14. Skrablin S, Kuvacic I, Pavicic D, Kalafatic D, Goluza T. Maternal neonatal outcome in quadruplet and quintuplet versus triplet gestations. Eur J Obstet Gynecol Reprod Biol 2000;88:147–52. (Level II-2)

15. Kilpatrick SJ, Jackson R, Croughan-Minihane MS. Perinatal mortality in twins and singletons matched for gestational age at delivery at > or = 30 weeks. Am J Obstet Gynecol 1996;174:66–71. (Level II-2)

16. Luke B, Minogue J, Witter FR. The role of fetal growth restriction in gestational age on length of hospital stay in twin infants. Obstet Gynecol 1993;81:949–53. (Level II-2)

17. Wolf EJ, Vintzileos AM, Rosenkrantz TS, Rodis JF, Lettieri L, Mallozzi A. A comparison of pre-discharge survival and morbidity in singleton and twin very low birth weight infants. Obstet Gynecol 1992;80:436–9. (Level II-2)

18. Low JA, Handley-Derry MH, Burke SO, Peters RD, Pater EA, Killen HL, et al. Association of intrauterine fetal growth retardation and learning deficits at age 9 to 11 years. Am J Obstet Gynecol 1992;167:1499–505. (Level II-2)

19. McCormick MD, Brooks-Gunn J, Workman-Daniels K, Turner J, Peckham GJ. The health and developmental status of very low-birth-weight children at school age. JAMA 1992;267:2204–8. (Level II-2)

20. Chelmow D, Penzias AS, Kaufman G, Cetrulo C. Costs of triplet pregnancy. Am J Obstet Gynecol 1995;172:677–82. (Level III)

21. Peaceman AM, Dooley SL, Tamura RK, Socol ML. Antepartum management of triplet gestations. Am J Obstet Gynecol 1992;167:1117–20. (Level II-3)

22. Haas JS, Berman S, Goldberg AB, Lee LW, Cook EF. Prenatal hospitalization and compliance with guidelines for prenatal care. Am J Public Health 1996;86:815–9. (Level II-2)

23. Luke B, Bigger HR, Leurgans S, Sietsema D. The cost of prematurity: a case-control study of twins vs singletons. Am J Public Health 1996;86:809–14. (Level II-2)

24. Albrecht JL, Tomich PG. The maternal and neonatal outcome of triplet gestations. Am J Obstet Gynecol 1996;174:1551–6. (Level III)

25. Newman RB, Hamer C, Miller MC. Outpatient triplet management: a contemporary review. Am J Obstet Gynecol 1989;161:547–53; discussion 553–5. (Level III)

26. Gardner MO, Goldenberg RL, Cliver SP, Tucker JM, Nelson KG, Copper RL. The origin and outcome of preterm twin pregnancies. Obstet Gynecol 1995;85:553–7. (Level II-2)

27. Seoud MA, Toner JP, Kruithoff C, Muasher SJ. Outcome of twin, triplet, and quadruplet in vitro fertilization pregnancies: the Norfolk experience. Fertil Steril 1992;57:825–34. (Level II-2)

28. Elliott JP, Radin TG. Quadruplet pregnancy: contemporary management and outcome. Obstet Gynecol 1992;80:421–4. (Level III)

29. Ettner SL, Christiansen CL, Callahan TL, Hall JE. How low birthweight and gestational age contribute to increased inpatient costs for multiple births. Inquiry 1997–98;34:325–39. (Level II-2)

30. Contribution of assisted reproductive technology and ovulation-inducing drugs to triplet and higher-order multiple births—United States, 1980–1997. MMWR Morb Mortal Wkly Rep 2000;49:535–8. (Level II-3)

31. Wenstrom KD, Syrop CH, Hammitt DG, van Voorhis BJ. Increased risk of monochorionic twinning associated with assisted reproduction. Fertil Steril 1993;60:510–4. (Level III)

32. Sutcliffe AG, D'Souza SW, Cadman J, Richards B, McKinlay IA, Lieberman B. Outcome in children from cryopreserved embryos. Arch Dis Child 1995;72:290–3. (Level II-2)

33. Schachter M, Raziel A, Friedler S, Strassburger D, Bern O, Ron-El R. Monozygotic twinning after assisted reproductive techniques: a phenomenon independent of micromanipulation. Hum Reprod 2001;16:1264–9. (Level III)

34. Edwards RG, Mettler L, Walters DE. Identical twins and in vitro fertilization. J In Vitro Fert Embryo Transf 1986;3:114–7. (Level III)

35. Bressers WM, Eriksson AW, Kostense PJ, Parisi P. Increasing trend in the monozygotic twinning rate. Acta Genet Med Gemellol (Roma) 1987;36:397–408. (Level II-3)

36. Meyers C, Adam R, Dungan J, Prenger V. Aneuploidy in twin gestations: when is maternal age advanced? Obstet Gynecol 1997;89:248–51. (Level II-2)

37. van den Berg C, Braat AP, van Opstal D, Halley DJ, Kleijer WJ, den Hollander NS, et al. Amniocentesis or chorionic villus sampling in multiple gestations? Experience with 500 cases. Prenat Diagn 1999;19:234–44. (Level II-2)

38. Wapner RJ, Johnson A, Davis G, Urban A, Morgan P, Jackson L. Prenatal diagnosis in twin gestations: a comparison between second-trimester amniocentesis and first-trimester chorionic villus sampling. Obstet Gynecol 1993:82:49–56. (Level II-2)

39. Pergament E, Schulman JD, Copeland K, Fine B, Black SH, Ginsberg NA, et al. The risk and efficacy of chorionic villus sampling in multiple gestations. Prenat Diagn 1992;12:377–84. (Level III)

40. Brambati B, Tului L, Guercilena S, Alberti E. Outcome of first-trimester chorionic villus sampling for genetic investigation in multiple pregnancy. Ultrasound Obstet Gynecol 2001;17:209–16. (Level II-2)

41. De Catte L, Liebaers I, Foulon W, Bonduelle M, Van Assche E. First trimester chorionic villus sampling in twin gestations. Am J Perinatol 1996;13:413–7. (Level II-2)

42. Casals G, Borrell A, Martinez JM, Soler A, Cararach V, Fortuny A. Transcervical chorionic villus sampling in multiple pregnancies using a biopsy forceps. Prenat Diagn 2002;22:260–5. (Level II-2)

43. Schwartz DB, Daoud Y, Zazula P, Goyert G, Bronsteen R, Wright D, et al. Gestational diabetes mellitus: metabolic and blood glucose parameters in singleton versus twin pregnancies. Am J Obstet Gynecol 1999;181:912–4. (Level II-2)

44. Sivan E, Maman E, Homko CJ, Lipitz S, Cohen S, Schiff E. Impact of fetal reduction on the incidence of gestational diabetes. Obstet Gynecol 2002;99:91–4. (Level II-1)

45. Roach VJ, Lau TK, Wilson D, Rogers MS. The incidence of gestational diabetes in multiple pregnancy. Aust N Z J Obstet Gynaecol 1998;38:56–7. (Level II-3)

46. Sibai BM, Hauth J, Caritis S, Lindheimer MD, Mac Pherson C, Klebanoff M, et al. Hypertensive disorders in twin versus singleton gestations. National Institute of Child Health and Human Development Network of Maternal-Fetal Medicine Units. Am J Obstet Gynecol 2000;182:938–42. (Level I)

47. Mastrobattista JM, Skupski DW, Monga M, Blanco JD, August P. The rate of severe preeclampsia is increased in triplet as compared to twin gestations. Am J Perinatol 1997;14:263–5. (Level II-2)

48. Krotz S, Fajardo J, Ghandi S, Patel A, Keith LG. Hypertensive disease in twin pregnancies: a review. Twin Res 2002;5:8–14. (Level III)

49. Long PA, Oats JN. Preeclampsia in twin pregnancy—severity and pathogenesis. Aust N Z J Obstet Gynaecol 1987;27:1–5. (Level II-2)

50. Lynch A, McDuffie R Jr, Murphy J, Faber K, Orleans M. Preeclampsia in multiple gestation: the role of assisted reproductive technologies. Obstet Gynecol 2002;99: 445–51. (Level II-2)

51. Heller CS, Elliott JP. High-order multiple pregnancies complicated by HELLP syndrome. A report of four cases with corticosteroid therapy to prolong gestation. J Reprod Med 1997;42:743–6. (Level III)

52. Hardardottir H, Kelly K, Bork MD, Cusick W, Campbell WA, Rodis JF. Atypical presentation of preeclampsia in high-order multifetal gestations. Obstet Gynecol 1996; 87:370–4. (Level III)

53. Smith-Levitin M, Kowalik A, Birnholz J, Skupski DW, Hutson JM, Chervenak FA, et al. Selective reduction of multifetal pregnancies to twins improves outcome over nonreduced triplet gestations. Am J Obstet Gynecol 1996;175:878–82. (Level II-2)

54. Andrews WW, Leveno KJ, Sherman ML, Mutz J, Gilstrap LC 3rd, Whalley PJ. Elective hospitalization in the management of twin pregnancies. Obstet Gynecol 1991;77:826–31. (Level II-1)

55. Davidson KM, Simpson LL, Knox TA, D'Alton ME. Acute fatty liver of pregnancy in triplet gestation. Obstet Gynecol 1998;91:806–8. (Level III)

56. Castro MA, Fassett MJ, Reynolds TB, Shaw KJ, Goodwin TM. Reversible peripartum liver failure: a new perspective on the diagnosis, treatment, and cause of acute fatty liver of pregnancy, based on 28 consecutive cases. Am J Obstet Gynecol 1999;181:389–95. (Level III)

57. Malone FD, Kaufman GE, Chelmow D, Athanassiou A, Nores JA, D'Alton ME. Maternal morbidity associated with triplet pregnancy. Am J Perinatol 1998;15:73–7. (Level II-2)

58. Sims HF, Brackett JC, Powell CK, Treem WR, Hale DE, Bennett MJ, et al. The molecular basis of pediatric long chain 3-hydroxyacyl-CoA dehydrogenase deficiency associated with maternal acute fatty liver of pregnancy. Proc Natl Acad Sci U S A 1995;92:841–5. (Level III)

59. Isaacs JD Jr, Sims HF, Powell CK, Bennett MJ, Hale DE, Treem WR, et al. Maternal acute fatty liver of pregnancy associated with fetal trifunctional protein deficiency: molecular characterization of a novel maternal mutant allele. Pediatr Res 1996;40:393–8. (Level III)

60. Chang J, Elam-Evans LD, Berg DJ, Herndon J, Flowers L, Seed KA, et al. Pregnancy-related mortality surveillance—United States, 1991–1999. MMWR 2003;52(SS-2):1–8. (Level II-3)

61. de Swiet M. Maternal mortality: confidential enquiries into maternal deaths in the United Kingdom. Am J Obstet Gynecol 2000;182:760–6. (Level II-3)

62. Simpson EL, Lawrenson RA, Nightingale AL, Farmer RD. Venous thromboembolism in pregnancy and the puerperium: incidence and additional risk factors from a London perinatal database. BJOG 2001;108:56–60. (Level II-2)

63. Elling SV, McKenna P, Powell FC. Pruritic urticarial papules and plaques of pregnancy in twin and triplet pregnancies. J Eur Acad Dermatol Venereol 2000;14: 378–81. (Level III)

64. Bianchi DW. Fetal cells in the mother: from genetic diagnosis to diseases associated with fetal cell microchimerism. Euro J Obstet Gynecol Reprod Biol 2000;92: 103–8. (Level III)

65. Evans MI, Dommergues M, Wapner RJ, Goldberg JD, Lynch L, Zador IE, et al. International, collaborative experience of 1789 patients having multifetal pregnancy reduction: a plateauing of risks and outcomes. J Soc Gynecol Investig 1996;3:23–6. (Level II-3)

66. Kadhel P, Olivennes F, Fernandez H, Vial M, Frydman R. Are there still obstetric and perinatal benefits for selective embryo reduction of triplet pregnancies? Hum Reprod 1998;13:3555–9. (Level II-2)

67. Depp R, Macones GA, Rosenn MF, Turzo E, Wapner RJ, Weinblatt VJ. Multifetal pregnancy reduction: evaluation of fetal growth in the remaining twins. Am J Obstet Gynecol 1996;174:1233–8; discussion 1238–40. (Level II-2)

68. Alexander GR, Kogan M, Martin J, Papiernik E. What are the fetal growth patterns of singletons, twins, and triplets in the United States? Clin Obstet Gynecol 1998; 41:114–25. (Level III)

69. Berkowitz RL, Lynch L, Lapinski R, Bergh P. First trimester transabdominal multifetal pregnancy reduction: a report of two hundred completed cases. Am J Obstet Gynecol 1993;169:17–21. (Level II-3)

70. Torok O, Lapinski R, Salafia CM, Bernasko J, Berkowitz RL. Multifetal pregnancy reduction is not associated with an increased risk of intrauterine growth restriction, except for very-high-order multiples. Am J Obstet Gynecol 1998;179:221–5. (Level II-2)

71. Benson CB, Doubilet PM, Acker D, Heffner LJ. Multifetal pregnancy reduction of both fetuses of a monochorionic pair by intrathoracic potassium chloride injection of one fetus. J Ultrasound Med 1998;17:447–9. (Level II-3)

72. Berkowitz RL, Lynch L, Stone J, Alvarez M. The current status of multifetal pregnancy reduction. Am J Obstet Gynecol 1996;174:1265–72. (Level III)

73. Lynch L, Berkowitz RL, Stone J, Alvarez M, Lapinski R. Preterm delivery after selective termination in twin pregnancies. Obstet Gynecol 1996;87:366–9. (Level II-2)

74. Goldenberg RL, Iams JD, Miodovnik M, Van Dorsten JP, Thurnau G, Bottoms S, et al. The preterm prediction study: risk factors in twin gestations. National Institute of Child Health and Human Development Maternal-Fetal Medicine Units Network. Am J Obstet Gynecol 1996; 175:1047–53. (Level II-2)

75. Souka AP, Heath V, Flint S, Sevastopoulou I, Nicolaides KH. Cervical length at 23 weeks in twins in predicting spontaneous preterm delivery. Obstet Gynecol 1999;94: 450–4. (Level II-2)

76. Imseis HM, Albert TA, Iams JD. Identifying twin gestations at low risk for preterm birth with a transvaginal

ultrasonographic cervical measurement at 24 to 26 weeks' gestation. Am J Obstet Gynecol 1997;177:1149–55. (Level II-2)

77. Ramin KD, Ogburn PL Jr, Mulholland TA, Breckle RJ, Ramsey PS. Ultrasonographic assessment of cervical length in triplet pregnancies. Am J Obstet Gynecol 1999;180:1442–5. (Level II)

78. Houlton MC, Marivate M, Philpott RH. Factors associated with preterm labour and changes in the cervix before labour in twin pregnancy. Br J Obstet Gynaecol 1982; 89:190–4. (Level II-2)

79. Neilson JP, Verkuyl DA, Crowther CA, Bannerman C. Preterm labor in twin pregnancies: prediction by cervical assessment. Obstet Gynecol 1988;72:719–23. (Level II-2)

80. Wennerholm UB, Holm B, Mattsby-Baltzer I, Nielsen T, Platz-Christensen J, Sundell G, et al. Fetal fibronectin, endotoxin bacterial vaginosis, and cervical length as predictors of preterm birth and neonatal morbidity in twin pregnancies. Br J Obstet Gynaecol 1997;104:1398–404. (Level II-2)

81. Oliveira T, de Souza E, Mariani-Neto C, Camano L. Fetal fibronectin as a predictor of preterm delivery in twin gestations. Int J Gynaecol Obstet 1998;62:135–9. (Level II-2)

82. Tolino A, Ronsini S, Zullo F, Pellicano M, Regine V, Nappi C. Fetal fibronectin as a screening test for premature delivery in multiple pregnancies. Int J Gynaecol Obstet 1996;52:3–7. (Level II-2)

83. Dyson DC, Crites YM, Ray DA, Armstrong MA. Prevention of preterm birth in high-risk patients: the role of education and provider contact versus home uterine monitoring. Am J Obstet Gynecol 1991;164:756–62. (Level I)

84. Branum AM, Schoendorf KC. Changing patterns of low birthweight and preterm birth in the United States, 1981-98. Paediatr Perinat Epidemiol 2002;16:8–15. (Level II-2)

85. Dor J, Shalev J, Mashiach S, Blankstein J, Serr DM. Elective cervical suture of twin pregnancies diagnosed ultrasonically in the first trimester following induced ovulation. Gynecol Obstet Invest 1982;13:55–60. (Level I)

86. Interim report of the Medical Research Council/Royal College of Obstetricians and Gynaecologists multicenter randomized trial of cervical cerclage. MRC/RCOG Working Party on Cervical Cerclage. Br J Obstet Gynaecol 1988;95:437–45. (Level I)

87. Crowther CA, Verkuyl DA, Neilson JP, Bannerman C, Ashurst HM. The effects of hospitalization for rest on fetal growth, neonatal morbidity and length of gestation in twin pregnancy. Br J Obstet Gynaecol 1990;97:872–7. (Level I)

88. MacLennan AH, Green RC, O'Shea R, Brookes C, Morris D. Routine hospital admission in twin pregnancy between 26 and 30 weeks' gestation. Lancet 1990;335: 267–9. (Level I)

89. Saunders MC, Dick JS, Brown IM, McPherson K, Chalmers I. The effects of hospital admission for bed rest on duration of twin pregnancy: a randomised trial. Lancet 1985;2:793–5. (Level I)

90. Hartikainen-Sorri AL, Jouppila P. Is routine hospitalization needed in antenatal care of twin pregnancy? J Perinat Med 1984;12:31–4. (Level II-1)

91. Crowther CA, Verkuyl DA, Ashworth MF, Bannerman C, Ashurst HM. The effects of hospitalization for bed rest on duration of gestation, fetal growth and neonatal morbidity in triplet pregnancy. Acta Genet Med Gemellol (Roma) 1991;40:63–8. (Level II-1)

92. Adams DM, Sholl JS, Haney EI, Russell TL, Silver RK. Perinatal outcome associated with outpatient management of triplet pregnancy. Am J Obstet Gynecol 1998; 178:843–7. (Level II-2)

93. Jeffrey RL, Bowes WA Jr, Delaney JJ. Role of bed rest in twin gestation. Obstet Gynecol 1974;43:822–6. (Level II-3)

94. Syrop CH, Varner MW. Triplet gestation: maternal and neonatal implications. Acta Genet Med Gemellol (Roma) 1985;34:81–8. (Level III)

95. Ron-el R, Caspi E, Schreyer P, Weintraub Z, Arieli S, Goldberg MD. Triplet and quadruplet pregnancies and management. Obstet Gynecol 1981;57:458–63. (Level III)

96. O'Connor MC, Murphy H, Dalrymple IJ. Double blind trial of ritodrine and placebo in twin pregnancy. Br J Obstet Gynaecol 1979;86:706–9. (Level I)

97. Marivate M, de Vilhers KQ, Fairbrother P. The effect of prophylactic outpatient administration of fenoterol on the time of onset of spontaneous labor and fetal growth rate in twin pregnancy. Am J Obstet Gynecol 1977;128: 707–8. (Level I)

98. Skjaerris J, Aberg A. Prevention of prematurity in twin pregnancy by orally administered terbutaline. Acta Obstet Gynecol Scand Suppl 1982;108:39–40. (Level I)

99. O'Leary JA. Prophylactic tocolysis of twins. Am J Obstet Gynecol 1986;154:904–5. (Level II-1)

100. Mathews DD, Friend JB, Michael CA. A double-blind trial of oral isoxuprine in the prevention of premature labour. J Obstet Gynaecol Br Commonw 1967;74:68–70. (Level I)

101. Cetrulo CL, Freeman RK. Ritodrine HCL for the prevention of premature labor in twin pregnancies. Acta Genet Med Gemellol (Roma) 1976;25:321–4. (Level I)

102. Ashworth MF, Spooner SF, Verkuyl DA, Waterman R, Ashurst HM. Failure to prevent preterm labour in twin pregnancy using prophylactic oral salbutamol. Br J Obstet Gynaecol 1990;97:878–82. (Level I)

103. Fletcher SE, Fyfe DA, Case CL, Wiles HB, Upshur JK, Newman RB. Myocardial necrosis in a newborn after long-term subcutaneous terbutaline infusion for suppression of preterm labor. Am J Obstet Gynecol 1991; 165:1401–4. (Level III)

104. Gabriel R, Harika G, Saniez D, Durot S, Quereux C, Wahl P. Prolonged intravenous ritodrine therapy: a comparison between multiple and singleton pregnancies. Eur J Obstet Gynecol Reprod Biol 1994;57:65–71. (Level II-1)

105. Perry KG Jr, Morrison JC, Rust OA, Sullivan CA, Martin RW, Naef RW 3rd. Incidence of adverse cardiopulmonary effects with low-dose continuous terbutaline infusion. Am J Obstet Gynecol 1995;173:1273–7. (Level II-3)

106. Katz M, Robertson PA, Creasy RK. Cardiovascular complications associated with terbutaline treatment for preterm labor. Am J Obstet Gynecol 1981;139:605–8. (Level II-3)

107. Effect of corticosteroids for fetal maturation on perinatal outcomes. NIH Consens Statement 1994;12:1–24. (Level III)

108. Feldman DM, Borgida AF, Trymbulak WP, Barsoom MJ, Sanders MM, Rodis JF. Clinical implications of velamentous cord insertion in triplet gestations. Am J Obstet Gynecol 2002;186:809–11. (Level III)

109. Kaufman GE, Malone FD, Harvey-Wilkes KB, Chelmau D, Penzias AS, D'Alton MD. Neonatal morbidity and mortality associated with triplet pregnancy. Obstet Gynecol 1998;91:342–8. (Level II-2)

110. Talbot GT, Goldstein RF, Nesbitt T, Johnson JL, Kay HH. Is size discordancy an indication for delivery of preterm twins? Am J Obstet Gynecol 1997;177:1050–4. (Level II-2)

111. Warner BB, Kiely JL, Donovan EF. Multiple births and outcome. Clin Perinatal 2000;27:347–61, ix. (Level III)

112. Hsieh TT, Chang TC, Chiu TH, Hsu JJ, Chao A. Growth discordancy, birth weight and neonatal adverse events in third trimester twin gestations. Gynecol Obstet Invest 1994;38:36–40. (Level III)

113. Petersen IR, Nyholm HC. Multiple pregnancies with single intrauterine demise. Description of twenty-eight pregnancies. Acta Obstet Gynecol Scand 1999;78:202–6. (Level III)

114. D'Alton ME, Newton ER, Cetrulo CL. Intrauterine fetal demise in multiple gestation. Acta Genet Med Gemellol (Roma) 1984;33:43–9. (Level III)

115. Robertson EG, Neer KJ. Placental injection studies in twin gestation. Am J Obstet Gynecol 1983;147:170–4. (Level III)

116. Langer B, Boudier E, Gasser B, Christmann D, Messer J, Schlaeder G. Antenatal diagnosis of brain damage in the survivor after the second trimester death of a monochorionic monoamniotic co-twin: case report and literature review. Fetal Diagn Ther 1997;12:286–91. (Level III)

117. Sairam S, Costeloe K, Thilaganathan B. Prospective risk of stillbirth in multiple-gestation pregnancies: a population-based analysis. Obstet Gynecol 2002;100:638–41. (Level III)

118. Bailey D, Flynn AM, Kelly J, O'Conor M. Antepartum fetal heart rate monitoring in multiple pregnancy. Br J Obstet Gynaecol 1980;87:561–4. (Level II-3)

119. Blake GD, Knuppel RA, Ingardia CJ, Lake M, Aumann G, Hanson M. Evaluation of nonstress fetal heart rate testing in multiple gestations. Obstet Gynecol 1984;63:528–32. (Level II-3)

120. Devoe LD, Azor H. Simultaneous nonstress fetal heart rate testing in twin pregnancy. Obstet Gynecol 1981;58:450–5. (Level II-3)

121. Knuppel RA, Rattan PK, Scerbo JC, O'Brien WF. Intrauterine fetal death in twins after 32 weeks of gestation. Obstet Gynecol 1985;65:172–5. (Level III)

122. Lodeiro JG, Vintzileos AM, Feinstein SJ, Campbell WA, Nochimson DJ. Fetal biophysical profile in twin gestation. Obstet Gynecol 1986;67:824–7. (Level II-3)

123. Talbert DG, Bajoria R, Sepulveda W, Bower S, Fisk NM. Hydrostatic and osmotic pressure gradients produce manifestations of fetofetal transfusion syndrome in a computerized model of monochorial twin pregnancy. Am J Obstet Gynecol 1996;174:598–608. (Level III)

124. De Lia J, Fisk N, Hecher K, Machin G, Nicolaides K, Hyett J, et al. Twin-to-twin transfusion syndrome—debates on the etiology, natural history and management. Ultrasound Obstet Gynecol 2000;16:210–3. (Level III)

125. Mahony BS, Petty CN, Nyberg DA, Luthy DA, Hickok DE, Hirsch JH. The "stuck twin" phenomenon: ultrasonographic findings, pregnancy outcome, and management with serial amniocenteses. Am J Obstet Gynecol 1990;163:1513–22. (Level III)

126. Urig MA, Clewell WH, Elliott JP. Twin-twin transfusion syndrome. Am J Obstet Gynecol 1990;163:1522–6. (Level III)

127. Dickinson JE. Severe twin-twin transfusion syndrome: current management concepts. Aust N Z J Obstet Gynaecol 1995;35:16–21. (Level III)

128. De Lia JE, Kuhlmann RS, Harstad TW, Cruikshank DP. Fetoscopic laser ablation of placental vessels in severe previable twin-twin transfusion syndrome. Am J Obstet Gynecol 1995;172:1202–8; discussion 1208–11. (Level II-3)

129. Quintero RA, Comas C, Bornick PW, Allen MH, Kruger M. Selective versus non-selective laser photocoagulation of placental vessels in twin-to-twin transfusion syndrome. Ultrasound Obstet Gynecol 2000;16:230–6. (Level II-1)

130. Quintero RA, Bornick PW, Allen MH, Johnson PK. Selective laser photocoagulation of communicating vessels in severe twin-twin transfusion syndrome in women with an anterior placenta. Obstet Gynecol 2001;97:477–81. (Level II-1)

131. Tanawattanacharoen S, Tantivatana J, Charoenvidhya D, Wisawasukmongchol W, Uerpairojkit B, Wacharaprechanont T, et al. Occlusion of umbilical artery using a Guglielmi detachable coil for the treatment of TRAP sequence. Ultrasound Obstet Gynecol 2002; 19:313–5. (Level III)

132. Fusi L, Gordon H. Twin pregnancy complicated by single intrauterine death. Problems and outcome with conservative management. Br J Obstet Gynaecol 1990; 97:511–6. (Level III)

133. Ohkuchi A, Minakami H, Shiraishi H, Suzuki I, Ohki T, Sato I. Intrauterine death of one twin, with rescue of the other, in twin-twin transfusion syndrome. Ultrasound Obstet Gynecol 2002;19:293–6. (Level III)

134. Moore TR, Gale S, Bernirschke K. Perinatal outcome of forty-nine pregnancies complicated by acardiac twinning. Am J Obstet Gynecol 1990;163:907–12. (Level III)

135. Quintero RA, Reich H, Puder KS, Bardicef M, Evans MI, Cotton DB, et al. Brief report: umbilical-cord ligation of an acardiac twin by fetoscopy at 19 weeks of gestation. N Engl J Med 1994;330:469–71. (Level III)

136. van den Brand SF, Nijhuis JG, van Dongen PW. Prenatal ultrasound diagnosis of conjoined twins. Obstet Gynecol Surv 1994;49:656–62. (Level III)

137. Luke B. Reducing fetal deaths in multiple births: optimal birthweights and gestational ages for infants of twin and triplet births. Acta Genet Med Gemellol (Roma) 1996; 45:333–48. (Level II-3)

138. Minakami H, Sato I. Reestimating date of delivery in multifetal pregnancies [published erratum appears in JAMA 1996;276:452]. JAMA 1996;275:1432–4. (Level II-3)

139. Leveno KJ, Quirk JG, Whalley PJ, Herbert WN, Trubey R. Fetal lung maturation in twin gestation. Am J Obstet Gynecol 1984;148:405–11. (Level II-2)

140. McElrath TF, Norwitz ER, Robinson JN, Tanasijevic MJ, Lieberman ES. Differences in TDx fetal lung maturity assay values between twin and singleton gestations. Am J Obstet Gynecol 2000;182:1110–2. (Level II-2)

141. Whitworth NS, Magann EF, Morrison JC. Evaluation of fetal lung maturity in diamniotic twins. Am J Obstet Gynecol 1999;180:1438–41. (Level II-2)

The MEDLINE database, the Cochrane Library, and ACOG's own internal resources and documents were used to conduct a literature search to locate relevant articles published between January 1985 and March 2004. The search was restricted to articles published in the English language. Priority was given to articles reporting results of original research, although review articles and commentaries also were consulted. Abstracts of research presented at symposia and scientific conferences were not considered adequate for inclusion in this document. Guidelines published by organizations or institutions such as the National Institutes of Health and the American College of Obstetricians and Gynecologists were reviewed, and additional studies were located by reviewing bibliographies of identified articles. When reliable research was not available, expert opinions from obstetrician–gynecologists were used.

Studies were reviewed and evaluated for quality according to the method outlined by the U.S. Preventive Services Task Force:

I   Evidence obtained from at least 1 properly designed randomized controlled trial.

II-1   Evidence obtained from well-designed controlled trials without randomization.

II-2   Evidence obtained from well-designed cohort or case–control analytic studies, preferably from more than 1 center or research group.

II-3   Evidence obtained from multiple time series with or without the intervention. Dramatic results in uncontrolled experiments also could be regarded as this type of evidence.

III   Opinions of respected authorities, based on clinical experience, descriptive studies, or reports of expert committees.

Based on the highest level of evidence found in the data, recommendations are provided and graded according to the following categories:

Level A—Recommendations are based on good and consistent scientific evidence.

Level B—Recommendations are based on limited or inconsistent scientific evidence.

Level C—Recommendations are based primarily on consensus and expert opinion.

ISSN 1099-3630

The American College of Obstetricians and Gynecologists
409 12th Street, SW, PO Box 96920, Washington, DC 20090-6920

12345/87654

Multiple gestation: complicated twin, triplet, and high-order multifetal pregnancy. ACOG Practice Bulletin No. 56. American College of Obstetricians and Gynecologists. Obstet Gynecol 2004;104:869–83.

ACOG PRACTICE BULLETIN

CLINICAL MANAGEMENT GUIDELINES FOR
OBSTETRICIAN–GYNECOLOGISTS
NUMBER 52, APRIL 2004

This Practice Bulletin was developed by the ACOG Committee on Practice Bulletins— Obstetrics with the assistance of T. Murphy Goodwin, MD. The information is designed to aid practitioners in making decisions about appropriate obstetric and gynecologic care. These guidelines should not be construed as dictating an exclusive course of treatment or procedure. Variations in practice may be warranted based on the needs of the individual patient, resources, and limitations unique to the institution or type of practice.

Nausea and Vomiting of Pregnancy

Nausea and vomiting of pregnancy is a common condition that affects the health of both the pregnant woman and her fetus. It can diminish the woman's quality of life and also contributes significantly to health care costs and time lost from work (1). Because "morning sickness" is common in early pregnancy, the presence of nausea and vomiting of pregnancy may be minimized by health care providers and by pregnant women (1) and, thus, undertreated. One investigator found that fewer than 50% of women who called a nausea and vomiting of pregnancy hotline and who subsequently terminated their pregnancies because of severe nausea and vomiting of pregnancy had been offered any sort of antiemetic therapy (2, 3). Of those offered treatment, 90% were offered regimens that were not likely to be effective. Furthermore, some women do not seek treatment because of concerns about safety (4). Yet, once symptoms of nausea and vomiting of pregnancy progress, treatment can become more difficult; treatment in the early stages may prevent more serious complications, including hospitalization (5). Mild cases of nausea and vomiting of pregnancy may be resolved with lifestyle and dietary changes, and safe and effective treatments are available for more severe cases. The woman's perception of the severity of her symptoms plays a critical role in the decision of whether, when, and how to treat nausea and vomiting of pregnancy. In addition, nausea and vomiting of pregnancy should be distinguished from nausea and vomiting related to other causes. The purpose of this document is to review the best available evidence about the diagnosis and management of nausea and vomiting of pregnancy.

Definition and Incidence

Nausea and vomiting of pregnancy is a common condition that affects 70–85% of pregnant women (6). Fifty percent of pregnant women have both nausea and vomiting, 25% have nausea only, and 25% are unaffected (7, 8). One study has attempted to categorize nausea and vomiting of pregnancy into degrees of severity by assessing the duration of nausea and vomiting each day (from less than 1 hour in mild cases to more than 6 hours in severe cases) and the amount of vomiting and retching per day (up to twice for mild and moderate nausea and vomiting of pregnancy; more than 5 times in severe cases) (1). However, although these categories recognize nausea and vomiting of pregnancy as a continuum, they may not be clinically useful. The woman's perception of the severity of her symptoms and her desire for treatment are more likely to influence clinical decision making.

From an epidemiologic perspective, hyperemesis gravidarum appears to represent the extreme end of the spectrum of nausea and vomiting of pregnancy (9). The incidence of hyperemesis gravidarum is approximately 0.5–2% of pregnancies. The reported incidence varies because of different diagnostic criteria and ethnic variation in study populations. There is no single accepted definition of hyperemesis gravidarum; it is a clinical diagnosis of exclusion based on a typical presentation in the absence of other diseases that could explain the findings (10). The most commonly cited criteria include persistent vomiting not related to other causes, a measure of acute starvation (usually large ketonuria), and some discrete measure of weight loss, most often at least 5% of prepregnancy weight (11). Electrolyte, thyroid, and liver abnormalities also may be present. Hyperemesis gravidarum is the most common indication for admission to the hospital during the first part of pregnancy and is second only to preterm labor as the most common reason for hospitalization during pregnancy (12, 13).

Differential Diagnosis

The timing of the onset of nausea and vomiting is important: symptoms of nausea and vomiting of pregnancy manifest before 9 weeks of gestation in virtually all affected women. When a patient experiences nausea and vomiting for the first time after 9 weeks of gestation, other conditions should be carefully considered in the differential diagnosis (see box). A history of a chronic condition associated with nausea and vomiting that predates pregnancy should be sought (eg, cholelithiasis or diabetic autonomic dysfunction). Rare cases of hyperemesis gravidarum related to a mendelian disorder of hormone-receptor interaction (14) and mitochondrial disorders (15) suggest that at least some portion of hyperemesis is caused by discrete disease states unmasked or exacerbated in pregnancy.

A number of physical findings point to conditions other than nausea and vomiting of pregnancy as the cause

---

Differential Diagnosis of Nausea and Vomiting of Pregnancy

Gastrointestinal Conditions
- Gastroenteritis
- Gastroparesis
- Achalasia
- Biliary tract disease
- Hepatitis
- Intestinal obstruction
- Peptic ulcer disease
- Pancreatitis
- Appendicitis

Genitourinary Tract Conditions
- Pyelonephritis
- Uremia
- Ovarian torsion
- Kidney stones
- Degenerating uterine leiomyoma

Metabolic Disease
- Diabetic ketoacidosis
- Porphyria
- Addison's disease
- Hyperthyroidism

Neurologic Disorders
- Pseudotumor cerebri
- Vestibular lesions
- Migraines
- Tumors of the central nervous system

Miscellaneous
- Drug toxicity or intolerance
- Psychologic

Pregnancy-Related Conditions
- Acute fatty liver of pregnancy
- Preeclampsia

Modified from Goodwin TM. Hyperemesis gravidarum. Clin Obstet Gynecol 1998;41:597–605.

---

of the nausea and vomiting. Abdominal pain is not a prominent characteristic of nausea and vomiting of pregnancy; abdominal pain or tenderness other than mild epigastric discomfort after retching is not seen with nausea and vomiting of pregnancy. Fever is not present in nausea and vomiting of pregnancy but is characteristic of many other diseases associated with nausea and vomiting. Headache is not characteristic of nausea and vomiting of pregnancy. An abnormal neurologic examination suggests a primary neurologic disorder as the cause of the nausea and vomiting, although it may rarely be encountered as a consequence of severe nausea and vomiting of pregnancy (eg, thiamine-deficient encephalopathy or central pontine myelinolysis). Although biochemical hyperthyroidism may be seen with hyperemesis gravidarum, goiter is not found with nausea and vomiting of pregnancy. If a goiter is present, primary thyroid disease should be suspected.

Etiology and Risk Factors

The etiology of nausea and vomiting of pregnancy is unknown. Various theories have been proposed, including a psychologic predisposition (16), evolutionary adaptation (17), and hormonal stimulus. The question of whether certain personality types or specific psychologic disorders predispose to hyperemesis gravidarum has been raised in the literature for many years. Two general hypotheses have been proposed to explain nausea and vomiting of pregnancy as a manifestation of psychopathology: 1) psychoanalytic theories describing hyperemesis gravidarum as a conversion or somatization disorder and 2) inability of the woman to respond to excessive life stress. There have been no controlled studies to support these hypotheses.

A recent review of psychologic theories proposed to explain the etiology of nausea and vomiting of pregnancy concluded that the evidence that nausea and vomiting of pregnancy is caused by a conversion disorder or an abnormal response to stress is "questionable at best" (18). It is likely that the concept that nausea and vomiting of pregnancy reflects a psychologic disorder has impeded progress toward a greater understanding of the true etiology of the condition (19).

It also has been posited that nausea and vomiting of pregnancy is an evolutionary adaptation that developed to protect the woman and her fetus from foods that might be potentially dangerous (20). This theory may explain the temporary aversions to tastes and smells that pregnant women experience. Proponents of the adaptation theory suggest nausea and vomiting of pregnancy is a healthy, protective response to pregnancy. Clinical application of this theory, however, may lead to undertreatment of women whose quality of life is diminished by nausea and vomiting of pregnancy.

Hormones

Human Chorionic Gonadotropin

Because of the close temporal relationship between peak human chorionic gonadotropin (hCG) concentrations and peak symptoms of nausea and vomiting of pregnancy, hCG has been considered a likely candidate for the emetogenic stimulus arising from the placenta. A role for hCG also is suggested by the fact that almost all studies of thyroid hormones in pregnancy show an association between transient hyperthyroidism and nausea and vomiting of pregnancy. It has been shown conclusively that hCG is the thyroid stimulator of pregnancy (21); because hyperthyroidism itself rarely causes vomiting, this finding has focused attention back on hCG and its relationship to nausea and vomiting of pregnancy. Among the many studies comparing nonthyroidal hormone concentrations in women with and without vomiting, only hCG and estradiol have been found to have an association. The failure of some studies to show an association of nausea and vomiting of pregnancy with hCG may be related to the varying biologic activity of different hCG isoforms as well as variation in the susceptibility of the individual woman to any emetogenic stimulus. The extent of the hCG stimulus may be modified by placental conditions that increase its concentration (eg, multiple gestation, molar gestation) and by hormone-receptor interactions modifying the effect of the hormone.

Estrogen

Another hormone known to influence nausea and vomiting of pregnancy is estrogen. Nausea and vomiting of pregnancy is more common when estradiol levels are increased and less common when estradiol levels are decreased (22, 23). Cigarette smoking is associated with lower levels of both hCG and estradiol (24), and numerous studies have shown that smokers are less likely to have hyperemesis gravidarum. Estrogens in the combined oral contraceptive pill were shown to induce nausea and vomiting in a dose-related fashion (25). Women with nausea and vomiting after estrogen exposure were more likely to have nausea and vomiting of pregnancy than women who did not demonstrate such sensitivity to estrogens (26).

Risk Factors

Women with increased placental mass (eg, advanced molar gestation, multiple gestation) are at risk for hyperemesis gravidarum. Other risk factors include family history (genetics) or a history of hyperemesis gravidarum in a previous pregnancy. One study found that approximately two thirds of women who described their vomiting as severe in one pregnancy had similar symptoms in the next pregnancy; one half of women who described their symptoms as mild in one pregnancy found that the symptoms worsened in the next (7). Daughters and sisters of women who had hyperemesis gravidarum are more likely to have the same problem, as are women carrying a female fetus (27). Other risk factors include a history of motion sickness or migraines (26).

Maternal Effects of Nausea and Vomiting of Pregnancy

Until 60 years ago, nausea and vomiting of pregnancy was an important cause of maternal mortality. In the 1930s in the United States, 7 deaths were reported among 85 women with severe vomiting (28). Although death from nausea and vomiting of pregnancy is reported rarely today, significant morbidity, such as Wernicke's encephalopathy, splenic avulsion, esophageal rupture, pneumothorax, and acute tubular necrosis, have been reported in recent years (29–36). Thirty-three cases of Wernicke's encephalopathy (caused by a vitamin B_1 deficiency) related to hyperemesis gravidarum have been reported in the past 20 years. It often is associated with maternal death or permanent neurological disability (29–31). In addition to increased hospital admissions (37, 38), some women experience significant psychosocial morbidity caused by nausea and vomiting of pregnancy, resulting in pregnancy termination.

A number of reversible responses to subacute disease states have been described in nausea and vomiting of pregnancy, including depression, somatization, and hypochondriasis (16). Poor support by their partners was reported by 85% of women who called a hotline for nausea and vomiting of pregnancy (3).

Fetal Effects of Nausea and Vomiting of Pregnancy

The effect of maternal vomiting on the embryo and fetus depends on the severity of the condition. With mild or moderate vomiting, there is little apparent effect on pregnancy outcome. The outcome most frequently examined is the incidence of low birth weight (LBW). Seven studies have identified no increase in LBW with nausea and vomiting of pregnancy (9, 10, 39–43). Three of these studies found a higher incidence of LBW among women who did not have nausea and vomiting of pregnancy (41–43). Among women with hyperemesis gravidarum, however, a higher incidence of LBW has been reported (44–49).

Numerous studies have documented a lower rate of miscarriage among women with nausea and vomiting of pregnancy and hyperemesis gravidarum when compared with controls. This result is thought to be related to robust placental synthesis in a healthy pregnancy rather than a protective effect of vomiting. It is unlikely that hyperemesis gravidarum is associated with a significantly increased risk of malformations in offspring (50). Little is known about the long-term health of children or women after pregnancies complicated by hyperemesis gravidarum. Although some cases of fetal death are still reported, they are very rare and usually are limited to cases of extreme hyperemesis gravidarum. It is appropriate to reassure patients that the presence of nausea and vomiting of pregnancy and even hyperemesis gravidarum most often portends well for pregnancy outcome.

Clinical Considerations and Recommendations

Many studies mix patients with hyperemesis gravidarum and those with other degrees of nausea and vomiting of pregnancy. Because it is likely that hyperemesis gravidarum is part of the continuum of nausea and vomiting of pregnancy and because evidence indicates that failure to treat early manifestations of nausea and vomiting of pregnancy increases the likelihood of hospital admission for hyperemesis gravidarum (37, 38), the following discussion focuses on treatment for all stages of nausea and vomiting of pregnancy.

▶ *Are nonpharmacologic therapies effective for the treatment of nausea and vomiting of pregnancy?*

Treatment of nausea and vomiting of pregnancy begins with prevention. Two studies found that women who were taking a multivitamin at the time of conception were less likely to need medical attention for vomiting (51, 52). Therefore, it is reasonable to advise women with a history of nausea and vomiting or hyperemesis gravidarum in a previous pregnancy to take a multivitamin at the time of the next conception.

The woman's perception of the severity of her symptoms and her desire for treatment are influential in clinical decision making. Common recommendations to alleviate initial signs of nausea and vomiting of pregnancy include rest and avoidance of sensory stimuli that may provoke symptoms. Frequent, small meals often are recommended. Obstetrician–gynecologists often suggest avoiding spicy or fatty foods; eliminating pills with iron; and eating bland or dry foods, high-protein snacks, and crackers in the morning before arising (53). However, there is little published evidence regarding the efficacy of dietary changes for prevention or treatment of nausea and vomiting of pregnancy. A small study showed that protein meals were more likely to alleviate nausea and vomiting of pregnancy than carbohydrate or fatty meals (54).

A study comparing powdered ginger capsules, 250 mg, with placebo in 27 women with hyperemesis gravidarum found the ginger reduced episodes of vomiting (55). Another study using a similar ginger regimen in 70 women with nausea and vomiting of pregnancy of varying severity found significant improvement in nausea and vomiting (56).

Pressure or electrical stimulation at the P6 (or Neguian) point on the inside of the wrist has been studied for nausea and vomiting of pregnancy with conflicting results. The preponderance of the literature does show a benefit, but many of the studies had significant methodologic flaws, and the 2 largest, best-designed studies showed no benefit over sham stimulation (57). Interestingly, the findings in both of these studies were consistent with a large placebo effect. A randomized, controlled trial of acustimulation with a commercial transcutaneous electrical stimulation device for varying degrees of nausea and vomiting of pregnancy found that acustimulation improved nausea and vomiting symptoms in the first trimester (58).

▶ *Are pharmacologic therapies effective for treatment of nausea and vomiting of pregnancy?*

Effective pharmacologic therapy is available, but agreement on the appropriate timing of antiemetic therapy has changed in recent years. Two randomized controlled trials have evaluated pyridoxine (vitamin B_6) for treatment of varying degrees of severity of nausea and vomiting of pregnancy. One compared pyridoxine, 25 mg every 8 hours, with placebo and found a significant reduction in severe vomiting but minimal effect on mild vomiting (59). A larger study (n = 342) used pyridoxine, 10 mg every 8 hours, and found a reduction in both nausea and vomiting compared with placebo (60). When the combination of vitamin B_6, 10 mg, plus doxylamine, 10 mg, was available in the United States from 1958 to 1983, it is estimated that 25–30% of all pregnant women received this agent. Analysis of hospital admissions during this period suggests that the ready availability of vitamin B_6 and doxylamine for the treatment of the spectrum of nausea and vomiting of pregnancy was associated with fewer hospital admissions for hyperemesis gravidarum (38). After the combination was removed from the U.S. market in 1983, use of antiemetics to treat nausea and vomit-

ing of pregnancy diminished considerably, and hospitalization rates for nausea and vomiting of pregnancy increased (38).

Figure 1 depicts a hierarchy of therapeutic interventions that balances safety and efficacy. Despite the fact that the combination of doxylamine and vitamin B_6 is no longer commercially available in the United States, it remains among the first-line therapies. Individual compounding pharmacies in many communities will make up the combination of 10 mg of pyridoxine and 10 mg of doxylamine on request. The only randomized, placebo-controlled trials have shown a 70% reduction in nausea and vomiting (61–63). Several case–control and cohort studies involving more than 170,000 exposures have found the combination to be safe with regard to fetal effects (64).

Many other conventional antiemetics have been described in the literature for treatment of nausea and vomiting of pregnancy (Table 1). Data that suggest safety and efficacy are available on several classes of these medications. The safety of antihistamine H_1 receptor blockers (eg, doxylamine) is supported by a review of more than 200,000 first-trimester exposures (65). Phenothiazines were identified as a possible cause of malformations in one study (66), but the aggregate of studies attest to their safety (67). Three studies attest to the safety of trimethobenzamide (68–70).

Medications for which there are some safety data but no conclusive evidence of efficacy include anticholinergics and metoclopramide. Additionally, evidence is limited on the safety or efficacy of the 5-hydroxytryptamine 3 inhibitors (eg, ondansetron) for nausea and vomiting of pregnancy; however, because of their effectiveness in reducing chemotherapy-induced emesis, their use appears to be increasing. Although the evidence is not strong, doses of droperidol greater than 25 mg were associated with a prolonged Q-T interval that in some cases has led to the potentially fatal arrhythmia torsades de pointes. This drug should be used with caution.

Several case series in the past 10 years have suggested a benefit of corticosteroids in the treatment of hyperemesis gravidarum. A randomized trial comparing methylprednisolone (16 mg, 3 times per day for 3 days, followed by a 2-week taper) with oral promethazine showed equal rates of improvement among hospitalized patients; however, readmission to the hospital within 2 weeks of discharge occurred significantly less frequently in those taking steroids (71). In contrast, a later randomized controlled trial of intravenous methylprednisolone followed by a tapered dose of an oral prednisone among women hospitalized for hyperemesis gravidarum found the use of corticosteroids did not reduce the need for rehospitalization (72).

*This algorithm assumes other causes of nausea and vomiting have been ruled out. At any step, consider parenteral nutrition if dehydration or persistent weight loss is noted. Alternative therapies may be added at any time during the sequence depending on patient acceptance and clinician familiarity; consider P6 acupressure with wrist bands or acustimulation or ginger capsules, 250 mg 4 times daily.

†In the United States, doxylamine is available as the active ingredient in some over-the-counter sleep aids; one half of a scored 25-mg tablet can be used to provide a 12.5-mg dose of doxylamine.

‡Thiamine, intravenously, 100 mg daily for 2–3 days (followed by intravenous multivitamins), is recommended for every woman who requires intravenous hydration and has vomited for more than 3 weeks. No study has compared different fluid replacements for nausea and vomiting of pregnancy.

§Corticosteroids appear to increase risk for oral clefts in the first 10 weeks of gestation.

‖Safety, particularly in the first trimester of pregnancy, not yet determined; less effect on nausea.

Figure 1. Pharmacologic treatment of nausea and vomiting of pregnancy. (Adapted from Levichek Z, Atanackovic G, Oepkes D, Maltepe C, Einarson A, Magee L, et al. Nausea and vomiting of pregnancy. Evidence-based treatment algorithm. Can Fam Physician 2002;48:267–8, 277.)

Table 1. Summary of Drugs Used to Treat Nausea and Vomiting of Pregnancy

Agent	Randomized Controlled Trial*	Comments on Efficacy	Comments on Safety
H₁ blockers		Effective in reducing nausea and vomiting of pregnancy	No increased risk of malformations
Doxylamine	√		
Dimenhydrinate	√		
Cetirizine			
Meclizine	√		
Buclizine	√		
Hydroxyzine	√		
Diphenhydramine			
Anticholinergics		No effectiveness trials for nausea and vomiting of pregnancy	No increased risk of malformations
Scopolamine			
Dopamine Antagonists			
Benzamides			
Trimethobenzamide	√	Effective in reducing nausea and vomiting of pregnancy	No known malformations
Metoclopramide		No trials regarding efficacy	No known malformations
Butyrophenones			
Droperidol			One study of limited power identified no known malformations Maternal risk of prolonged Q-T interval
Haloperidol			
Phenothiazines			
Promethazine	√	Effective in reducing nausea and vomiting of pregnancy	Bulk of evidence indicates no teratogenicity (isolated case report† discounted in meta-analysis)
Prochlorperazine			
Chlorpromazine			
Perphenazine			
Benzodiazepines			
Diazepam			
5-Hydroxytryptamine 3 receptor agonists			
Ondansetron	√	One trial found equal effectiveness to promethazine	No malformations noted
Steroids		Pooled results do not suggest benefit in decreasing nausea and vomiting of pregnancy	
Adrenocorticotropic hormone	√		
Corticosteroids	√		Small increased risks of clefts

*The drug has been evaluated in at least 1 randomized, controlled trial.

†Rumeau-Rouquette C, Goujard J, Huel G. Possible teratogenic effect of phenothiazines in human beings. Teratology 1977;15:57–64.

Data from Jewell D, Young G. Interventions for nausea and vomiting in early pregnancy (Cochrane Review). In: The Cochrane Library, Issue 4, 2003. Chichester, UK: John Wiley & Sons, Ltd.; and Magee LA, Mazzotta P, Koren G. Evidence-based view of safety and effectiveness of pharmacologic therapy for nausea and vomiting of pregnancy (NVP). Am J Obstet Gynecol 2002;186:S256–61.

Three recent studies have confirmed an association between oral clefts and methylprednisolone use in the first trimester (73–75). The teratogenic effect is weak, probably accounting for no more than 1 or 2 cases per 1,000 treated women (76). Nevertheless, in view of this probable association, corticosteroid use for hyperemesis gravidarum should be used with caution and avoided before 10 weeks of gestation.

Corticosteroids may be considered as a last resort in patients who will require enteral or parenteral nutrition because of weight loss. The most commonly described regimen is methylprednisolone, 48 mg daily for 3 days, given orally or intravenously. Patients who do not respond within 3 days are not likely to respond, and treatment should be stopped. For those who do respond, the dose may be tapered over a period of 2 weeks. For recurrent vomiting, the tapered dose may be stopped and the patient continued on the effective dose for up to 6 weeks. To limit serious maternal side effects, corticosteroids should not be continued beyond this period for the treatment of hyperemesis gravidarum (77).

▶ Is there a role for laboratory or radiologic assessment in the diagnosis of hyperemesis gravidarum?

Most patients with nausea and vomiting of pregnancy do not require laboratory evaluation, but in those with nausea and vomiting of pregnancy that is severe, prolonged, or extended, laboratory assessment may help in the differential diagnosis of hyperemesis gravidarum and to assess the severity of the condition. Common laboratory abnormalities in hyperemesis gravidarum include increased liver enzymes (usually <300 U/L), serum bilirubin (<4 mg/dL), and serum amylase or lipase concentrations (up to 5 times greater than normal levels). Primary hepatitis as a cause of nausea and vomiting of pregnancy results in increased liver enzyme levels, often in the thousands; bilirubin concentrations usually are greatly increased as well. Acute pancreatitis may cause vomiting and elevated amylase concentrations, but serum amylase concentrations usually are 5–10 times greater than the elevations associated with nausea and vomiting of pregnancy. A hypochloremic metabolic alkalosis can be seen with severe vomiting of any cause. Serum concentrations of hCG are not helpful in determining whether vomiting is caused by hyperemesis gravidarum. Urinalysis may show elevated specific gravity or ketonuria or both. Patients with persistent hyperemesis gravidarum that is unresponsive to standard therapy may have an ulcer; treatment with antibiotics and H_2 receptor antagonists is safe (78, 79) and has been reported to be beneficial in case reports (80).

Up to 70% of patients with hyperemesis gravidarum will have suppressed thyroid-stimulating hormone levels or elevated free thyroxine concentrations (81). For the patient who has no history of hyperthyroidism before pregnancy and no goiter, the hyperthyroidism of hyperemesis gravidarum can be expected to resolve by 20 weeks of gestation without specific antithyroid therapy. Hyperthyroidism itself rarely may present with significant vomiting (82), but in the patient who has no goiter, thyroid tests are not needed routinely to clarify the differential diagnosis. To confirm the diagnosis of hyperthyroidism in the setting of nausea and vomiting of pregnancy, measurement of free thyroxine and free triiodothyronine concentrations should be obtained.

An ultrasound evaluation may be useful in cases of severe presumed nausea and vomiting of pregnancy. It may identify a predisposing factor, such as multiple gestation or molar gestation.

▶ When is enteral or parenteral nutrition recommended?

The principal criterion for introducing additional nutritional strategies is persistent weight loss. Serious complications of hyperemesis gravidarum for the woman and fetus arise in the group of women who cannot maintain their weight despite antiemetic therapy. Intravenous hydration should be used for the patient who cannot tolerate oral liquids for a prolonged period or if clinical signs of dehydration are present. Correction of ketosis and vitamin deficiency should be strongly considered. Dextrose and vitamins, especially thiamine, should be included in the therapy when prolonged vomiting is present.

No randomized trials compare enteral with parenteral nutrition in women with nausea and vomiting of pregnancy who continue to lose weight despite antiemetic therapy. Several case reports and a small series (83) suggest that enteral tube feeding is well tolerated in pregnancy. Because life-threatening complications of parenteral nutrition have been described (35, 36, 84), it is reasonable to attempt enteral tube feeding initially. Peripheral parenteral nutrition using a high-lipid formula can be used for patients whose calorie requirements are not great and those whose length of treatment is anticipated to be no more than several days. For women who need longer-term support and who cannot tolerate enteral tube feedings, the use of total parenteral nutrition has been described for hyperemesis gravidarum in case reports and 2 small series (35, 85). A peripherally inserted central catheter can be used to avoid some of the complications of central access (86), but it is still associated with significant morbidity (87).

▶ When is hospitalization indicated?

No controlled trials compare hospitalization with outpatient management of hyperemesis gravidarum. When a woman cannot tolerate liquids without vomiting and has not responded to outpatient management, hospitalization for evaluation and treatment is recommended. After the patient has been hospitalized on one occasion and a workup for other causes of severe vomiting has been undertaken, intravenous hydration, nutritional support, and modification of antiemetic therapy often can be accomplished at home. Nevertheless, the option of hospitalization for observation and further assessment should be preserved for patients who experience a change in vital signs or a change in affect or who continue to lose weight.

▶ *Is there a role for psychotherapy in treatment?*

There is little evidence for a therapeutic effect of traditional psychotherapy in hyperemesis gravidarum. No controlled trials have evaluated behavioral therapy in nausea and vomiting of pregnancy, but there are data to indicate that delayed and anticipatory nausea and vomiting after chemotherapy is diminished by systematic desensitization (88) and relaxation therapy (89).

It has been suggested that hypnotized women with severe nausea and vomiting of pregnancy are more easily influenced by suggestion than controls, and at least one controlled study supports this hypothesis (90). In a limited number of studies, all lacking controls, hypnosis has been shown to decrease vomiting in patients undergoing chemotherapy (91, 92) and those with hyperemesis gravidarum (93, 94).

Summary of Recommendations

The following recommendations are based on good and consistent scientific evidence (Level A):

▶ Taking a multivitamin at the time of conception may decrease the severity of nausea and vomiting of pregnancy.

▶ Treatment of nausea and vomiting of pregnancy with vitamin B_6 or vitamin B_6 plus doxylamine is safe and effective and should be considered first-line pharmacotherapy.

▶ In patients with hyperemesis gravidarum who also have suppressed thyroid-stimulating hormone levels, treatment of hyperthyroidism should not be undertaken without evidence of intrinsic thyroid disease (including goiter and/or thyroid autoantibodies).

The following recommendations are based on limited or inconsistent scientific evidence (Level B):

▶ Treatment of nausea and vomiting of pregnancy with ginger has shown beneficial effects and can be considered as a nonpharmacologic option.

▶ In refractory cases of nausea and vomiting of pregnancy, the following medications have been shown to be safe and efficacious in pregnancy: antihistamine H_1 receptor blockers, phenothiazines, and benzamides.

Early treatment of nausea and vomiting of pregnancy is recommended to prevent progression to hyperemesis gravidarum.

▶ Treatment of severe nausea and vomiting of pregnancy or hyperemesis gravidarum with methylprednisolone may be efficacious in refractory cases; however, the risk profile of methylprednisolone suggests it should be a treatment of last resort.

The following recommendations are based primarily on consensus and expert opinion (Level C):

▶ Intravenous hydration should be used for the patient who cannot tolerate oral liquids for a prolonged period or if clinical signs of dehydration are present. Correction of ketosis and vitamin deficiency should be strongly considered. Dextrose and vitamins, especially thiamine, should be included in the therapy when prolonged vomiting is present.

▶ Enteral or parenteral nutrition should be initiated for any patient who cannot maintain her weight because of vomiting.

References

1. Attard CL, Kohli MA, Coleman S, Bradley C, Hux M, Atanackovic G, et al. The burden of illness of severe nausea and vomiting of pregnancy in the United States. Am J Obstet Gynecol 2002;186:S220–7. (Level II-2)

2. Mazzota P, Magee L, Koren G. Therapeutic abortions due to severe morning sickness. Unacceptable combination. Can Fam Physician 1997;43:1055–7. (Level III)

3. Mazzotta P, Stewart D, Atanackovic G, Koren G, Magee LA. Psychosocial morbidity among women with nausea and vomiting of pregnancy: prevalence and association with anti-emetic therapy. J Psychosom Obstet Gynaecol 2000;21:129–36. (Level II-3)

4. O'Brien B, Naber S. Nausea and vomiting during pregnancy: effects on the quality of women's lives. Birth 1992;19:138–43. (Level III)

5. Brent R. Medical, social, and legal implications of treating nausea and vomiting of pregnancy. Am J Obstet Gynecol 2002;186:S262–6. (Level III)

6. Jewell D, Young G. Interventions for nausea and vomiting in early pregnancy (Cochrane Review). In: The Cochrane Library, Issue 4, 2003. Chichester, UK: John Wiley & Sons, Ltd. (Meta-analysis)

7. Gadsby R, Barnie-Adshead AM, Jagger C. A prospective study of nausea and vomiting during pregnancy [published erratum appears in Br J Gen Pract 1993;43:325]. Br J Gen Pract 1993;43:245–8. (Level II-2)

8. Vellacott ID, Cooke EJ, James CE. Nausea and vomiting in early pregnancy. Int J Gynaecol Obstet 1988;27:57–62. (Level II-2)

9. Klebanoff MA, Koslowe PA, Kaslow R, Rhoads GG. Epidemiology of vomiting in early pregnancy. Obstet Gynecol 1985;66:612–6. (Level II-2)

10. Gadsby R, Barnie-Adshead AM, Jagger C. Pregnancy nausea related to women's obstetric and personal histories. Gynecol Obstet Invest 1997;43:108–11. (Level II-2)

11. Goodwin TM, Montoro M, Mestman JH. Transient hyperthyroidism and hyperemesis gravidarum: clinical aspects. Am J Obstet Gynecol 1992;167:648–52. (Level II-2)

12. Adams MM, Harlass FE, Sarno AP, Read JA, Rawlings JS. Antenatal hospitalization among enlisted servicewomen, 1987–1990. Obstet Gynecol 1994;84:35–9. (Level II-3)

13. Gazmararian JA, Petersen R, Jamieson DJ, Schild L, Adams MM, Deshpande AD, et al. Hospitalizations during pregnancy among managed care enrollees. Obstet Gynecol 2002;100:94–100. (Level II-2)

14. Rodien P, Bremont C, Sanson ML, Parma J, Van Sande J, Costagliola S, et al. Familial gestational hyperthyroidism caused by a mutant thyrotropin receptor hypersensitive to human chorionic gonadotropin. N Engl J Med 1998;339: 1823–6. (Level III)

15. Innes AM, Seargeant LE, Balachandra K, Roe CR, Wanders RJ, Ruiter JP, et al. Hepatic carnitine palmitoyltransferase I deficiency presenting as maternal illness in pregnancy. Pediatr Res 2000;47:43–5. (Level III)

16. Simpson SW, Goodwin TM, Robins SB, Rizzo AA, Howes RA, Buckwalter DK, et al. Psychological factors and hyperemesis gravidarum. J Women Health Gend Based Med 2001;10:471–7. (Level II-2)

17. Flaxman SM, Sherman PW. Morning sickness: a mechanism for protecting mother and embryo. Q Rev Biol 2000; 75:113–48. (Level III)

18. Buckwalter JG, Simpson SW. Psychological factors in the etiology and treatment of severe nausea and vomiting in pregnancy. Am J Obstet Gynecol 2002;186:S210–4. (Level III)

19. Bogen JT. Neurosis: a Ms-diagnosis. Perspect Biol Med 1994;37:263–74. (Level III)

20. Sherman PW, Flaxman SM. Nausea and vomiting of pregnancy in an evolutionary perspective. Am J Obstet Gynecol 2002;186:S190–7. (Level III)

21. Yoshimura M, Hershman JM. Thyrotropic action of human chorionic gonadotropin. Thyroid 1995;5:425–34. (Level III)

22. Bernstein L, Pike MC, Lobo RA, Depue RH, Ross RK, Henderson BE. Cigarette smoking in pregnancy results in marked decrease in maternal hCG and oestradiol levels. Br J Obstet Gynaecol 1989;96:92–6. (Level II-2)

23. Depue RH, Bernstein L, Ross RK, Judd HL, Henderson BE. Hyperemesis gravidarum in relation to estradiol levels, pregnancy outcome, and other maternal factors: a seroepidemiologic study. Am J Obstet Gynecol 1987;156: 1137–41. (Level II-2)

24. Goodwin TM. Nausea and vomiting of pregnancy: an obstetric syndrome. Am J Obstet Gynecol 2002;186: S184–9. (Level III)

25. Goldzieher JW, Moses LE, Averkin E, Scheel C, Taber BZ. A placebo-controlled double-blind crossover investigation of the side effects attributed to oral contraceptives. Fertil Steril 1971;22:609–23. (Level I)

26. Whitehead SA, Andrews PL, Chamberlain GV. Characterisation of nausea and vomiting in early pregnancy: a survey of 1,000 women. J Obstet Gynaecol 1992;12:364–9. (Level II-2)

27. Basso O, Olsen J. Sex ratio and twinning in women with hyperemesis or pre-eclampsia. Epidemiology 2001;12: 747–9. (Level II-2)

28. Reid DE, Teel HM. The treatment of the vomiting of early pregnancy. N Engl J Med 1938;218:109–13. (Level III)

29. Togay-Isikay C, Yigit A, Mutluer N. Wernicke's encephalopathy due to hyperemesis gravidarum: an under-recognised condition. Aust N Z J Obstet Gynecol 2001;41: 453–6. (Level III)

30. Spruill SC, Kuller JA. Hyperemesis gravidarum complicated by Wernicke's encephalopathy. Obstet Gynecol 2002;99:875–7. (Level III)

31. Kim YH, Lee SJ, Rah SH, Lee JH. Wernicke's encephalopathy in hyperemesis gravidarum. Can J Ophthalmol 2002;37:37–8. (Level III)

32. Eroglu A, Kurkcuoglu C, Karaoglanoglu N, Tekinbas C, Cesur M. Spontaneous esophageal rupture following severe vomiting in pregnancy. Dis Esophagus 2002;15: 242–3. (Level III)

33. Liang SG, Ooka F, Santo A, Kaibara M. Pneumomediastinum following esophageal rupture associated with hyperemesis gravidarum. J Obstet Gynaecol Res 2002; 28:172–5. (Level III)

34. Nguyen N, Deitel M, Lacy E. Splenic avulsion in a pregnant patient with vomiting. Can J Surg 1995;38:464–5. (Level III)

35. Russo-Stieglitz KE, Levine AB, Wagner BA, Armenti VT. Pregnancy outcome in patients requiring parenteral nutrition. J Matern Fetal Med 1999;8:164–7. (Level III)

36. Katz VL, Farmer R, York J, Wilson JD. Mycobacterium chelonae sepsis associated with long-term use of an intravenous catheter for treatment of hyperemesis gravidarum: a case report. J Reprod Med 2000;45:581–4. (Level III)

37. Lamm SH. The epidemiological assessment of the safety and efficacy of Bendectin. In: Koren G, Bishai R, editors. Nausea and vomiting of pregnancy: state of the art 2000. Toronto: Motherisk; 2000. p. 100–3. (Level III)

38. Neutel CI, Johansen HL. Measuring drug effectiveness by default: the case of Bendectin. Can J Public Health 1995; 86:66–70. (Level III)

39. Jarnfelt-Samsioe A, Eriksson B, Waldenstrom J, Samsioe G. Some new aspects on emesis gravidarum. Relations to clinical data, serum electrolytes, total protein and creatinine. Gynecol Obstet Invest 1985;19:174–86. (Level II-2)

40. Weigel MM, Weigel RM. Nausea and vomiting of early pregnancy and pregnancy outcome: an epidemiological study. Br J Obstet Gynaecol 1989;96:1304–11. (Level II-2)

41. Brandes JM. First-trimester nausea and vomiting as related to outcome of pregnancy. Obstet Gynecol 1967;30: 427–31. (Level II-2)

42. Little RE. Maternal alcohol and tobacco use and nausea and vomiting during pregnancy: relation to infant birthweight. Acta Obstet Gynecol Scand 1980;59:495–7. (Level II-3)

43. Tierson FD, Olsen CL, Hook EB. Nausea and vomiting of pregnancy and association with pregnancy outcome [published erratum appears in Am J Obstet Gynecol 1989; 160:518–9]. Am J Obstet Gynecol 1986;155:1017–22. (Level II-2)

44. Chin RK, Lao TT. Low birth weight and hyperemesis gravidarum. Eur J Obstet Gynecol Reprod Biol 1988;28: 179–83. (Level II-2)

45. Godsey RK, Newman RB. Hyperemesis gravidarum. A comparison of single and multiple admissions. J Reprod Med 1991;36:287–90. (Level II-3)

46. Gross S, Librach C, Cecutti A. Maternal weight loss associated with hyperemesis gravidarum: a predictor of fetal outcome. Am J Obstet Gynecol 1989;160:906–9. (Level II-3)

47. Kallen B. Hyperemesis during pregnancy and delivery outcome: a registry study. Eur J Obstet Gynecol Reprod Biol 1987;26:291–302. (Level II-2)

48. O'Brien B, Zhou Q. Variables related to nausea and vomiting during pregnancy. Birth 1995;22:93–100. (Level II-2)

49. Vilming B, Nesheim BI. Hyperemesis gravidarum in a contemporary population in Oslo. Acta Obstet Gynecol Scand 2000;79:640–3. (Level II-2)

50. Boneva RS, Moore CA, Botto L, Wong LY, Erickson JD. Nausea during pregnancy and congenital heart defects: a population-based case-control study. Am J Epidemiol 1999;149:717–25. (Level II-2)

51. Czeizel AE, Dudas I, Fritz G, Tecsoi A, Hanck A, Kunovits G. The effect of periconceptional multivitamin-mineral supplementation on vertigo, nausea and vomiting in the first trimester of pregnancy. Arch Gynecol Obstet 1992;251:181–5. (Level I)

52. Emelianova S, Mazzotta P, Einarson A, Koren G. Prevalence and severity of nausea and vomiting of pregnancy and effect of vitamin supplementation. Clin Invest Med 1999;22:106–10. (Level II-2)

53. Power ML, Holzman GB, Schulkin J. A survey on the management of nausea and vomiting in pregnancy by obstetrician/gynecologists. Prim Care Update Ob Gyns 2001;8:69–72. (Level III)

54. Jednak MA, Shadigian EM, Kim MS, Woods ML, Hooper FG, Owyang C, et al. Protein meals reduce nausea and gastric slow wave dysrhythmic activity in first trimester pregnancy. Am J Physiol 1999;277:G855–61. (Level II-3)

55. Fischer-Rasmussen W, Kjaer SK, Dahl C, Asping U. Ginger treatment of hyperemesis gravidarum. Eur J Obstet Gynecol Reprod Biol 1991;38:19–24. (Level II-2)

56. Vutyavanich T, Kraisarin T, Ruangsri R. Ginger for nausea and vomiting in pregnancy: randomized, double-masked, placebo-controlled trial. Obstet Gynecol 2001; 97:577–82. (Level I)

57. Roscoe JA, Matteson SE. Acupressure and acustimulation bands for control of nausea: a brief review. Am J Obstet Gynecol 2002;186:S244–7. (Level III)

58. Rosen T, de Veciana M, Miller HS, Stewart L, Rebarber A, Slotnick RN. A randomized controlled trial of nerve stimulation for relief of nausea and vomiting in pregnancy. Obstet Gynecol 2003;102:129–35. (Level I)

59. Sahakian V, Rouse D, Sipes S, Rose N, Niebyl J. Vitamin B6 is effective therapy for nausea and vomiting of pregnancy: a randomized, double-blind placebo-controlled study. Obstet Gynecol 1991;78:33–6. (Level I)

60. Vutyavanich T, Wongtra-ngan S, Ruangsri R. Pyridoxine for nausea and vomiting of pregnancy: a randomized, double-blind, placebo-controlled trial. Am J Obstet Gynecol 1995;173:881–4. (Level I)

61. Geiger CJ, Fahrenbach DM, Healey FJ. Bendectin in the treatment of nausea and vomiting in pregnancy. Obstet Gynecol 1959;14:688–90. (Level II-1)

62. Wheatley D. Treatment of pregnancy sickness. Br J Obstet Gynaecol 1977;84:444–7. (Level II-1)

63. McGuinness BW, Binns DT. 'Debendox' in pregnancy sickness. J R Coll Gen Pract 1971;21:500–3. (Level II-3)

64. McKeigue PM, Lamm SH, Linn S, Kutcher JS. Bendectin and birth defects: I. A meta-analysis of the epidemiologic studies. Teratology 1994;50:27–37. (Meta-analysis)

65. Seto A, Einarson T, Koren G. Pregnancy outcome following first trimester exposure to antihistamines: meta-analysis. Am J Perinatol 1997;14:119–24. (Meta-analysis)

66. Rumeau-Rouquette C, Goujard J, Huel G. Possible teratogenic effect of phenothiazines in human beings. Teratology 1977;15:57–64. (Level II-2)

67. Magee LA, Mazzotta P, Koren G. Evidence-based view of safety and effectiveness of pharmacologic therapy for nausea and vomiting of pregnancy (NVP). Am J Obstet Gynecol 2002;186:S256–61. (Level III)

68. Aselton P, Jick H, Milunsky A, Hunter JR, Stergachis A. First-trimester drug use and congenital disorders. Obstet Gynecol 1985;65:451–5. (Level II-2)

69. Heinonen OP, Slone D, Shapiro S. Birth defects and drugs in pregnancy. Littleton (MA): Publishing Sciences Group; 1977. (Level III)

70. Mitchell AA, Schwingl PJ, Rosenberg L, Louik C, Shapiro S. Birth defects in relation to Bendectin use in pregnancy. II. Pyloric stenosis. Am J Obstet Gynecol 1983;147:737–42. (Level II-2)

71. Safari HR, Fassett MJ, Souter IC, Alsulyman OM, Goodwin TM. The efficacy of methylprednisolone in the treatment of hyperemesis gravidarum: a randomized, double-blind, controlled study. Am J Obstet Gynecol 1998; 179:921–4. (Level I)

72. Yost NP, McIntire DD, Wians FH Jr, Ramin SM, Balko JA, Leveno KJ. A randomized, placebo-controlled trial of corticosteroids for hyperemesis due to pregnancy. Obstet Gynecol 2003;102:1250–4. (Level I)

73. Carmichael SL, Shaw GM. Maternal corticosteroid use and risk of selected congenital anomalies. Am J Med Genet 1999;86:242–4. (Level II-2)

74. Park-Wyllie L, Mazzotta P, Pastuszak A, Moretti ME, Beique L, Hunnisett L, et al. Birth defects after maternal exposure to corticosteroids: prospective cohort study and meta-analysis of epidemiological studies. Teratology 2000;62:385–92. (Meta-analysis)

75. Rodriguez-Pinilla E, Martinez-Frias ML. Corticosteroids during pregnancy and oral clefts: a case-control study. Teratology 1998;58:2–5. (Level II-2)

76. Shepard TH, Brent RL, Friedman JM, Jones KL, Miller RK, Moore CA, et al. Update on new developments in the study of human teratogens. Teratology 2002;65:153–61. (Level III)

77. Chan GC, Wilson AM. Complications of the use of corticosteroids for the treatment of hyperemesis gravidarum [Letter]. Br J Obstet Gynaecol 1995;102:507–8; author reply 508–9. (Level III)

78. Kallen BA. Use of omeprazole during pregnancy—no hazard demonstrated in 955 infants exposed during pregnancy. Eur J Obstet Gynecol Reprod Biol 2001;96:63–8. (Level II-2)

79. Ruigomez A, Garcia Rodriguez LA, Cattaruzzi C, Troncon MG, Agostinis L, Wallander MA, et al. Use of cimetidine, omeprazole, and ranitidine in pregnant women and pregnancy outcomes. Am J Epidemiol 1999;150:476–81. (Level II-2)

80. Jacoby EB, Porter KB. Helicobacter pylori infection and persistent hyperemesis gravidarum. Am J Perinatol 1999; 16:85–8. (Level III)

81. Goodwin TM, Montoro M, Mestman JH, Pekary AE, Hershman JM. The role of chorionic gonadotropin in transient hyperthyroidism of hyperemesis gravidarum. J Clin Endocrinol Metab 1992;75:1333–7. (Level II-2)

82. Rosenthal FD, Jones C, Lewis SI. Thyrotoxic vomiting. Br Med J 1976;2:209–11. (Level III)

83. Hsu JJ, Clark-Glena R, Nelson DK, Kim CH. Nasogastric enteral feeding in the management of hyperemesis gravidarum. Obstet Gynecol 1996;88:343–6. (Level III)

84. Greenspoon JS, Masaki DI, Kurz CR. Cardiac tamponade in pregnancy during central hyperalimentation. Obstet Gynecol 1989;73:465–6. (Level III)

85. Zibell-Frisk D, Jen KL, Rick J. Use of parenteral nutrition to maintain adequate nutritional status in hyperemesis gravidarum. J Perinatol 1990;10:390–5. (Level II-2)

86. Ogura JM, Francois KG, Perlow JH, Elliott JP. Complications associated with peripherally inserted central catheter use during pregnancy. Am J Obstet Gynecol 2003;188:1223–5. (Level III)

87. Greenspoon JS, Rosen DJ, Ault M. Use of peripherally inserted central catheter for parenteral nutrition during pregnancy. Obstet Gynecol 1993;81:831–4. (Level III)

88. Morrow GR, Asbury R, Hammon S, Dobkin P, Caruso L, Pandya K, et al. Comparing the effectiveness of behavioral treatment for chemotherapy-induced nausea and vomiting when administered by oncologists, oncology nurses, and clinical psychologists. Health Psychol 1992; 11:250–6. (Level I)

89. Burish TG, Jenkins RA. Effectiveness of biofeedback and relaxation training in reducing the side effects of cancer chemotherapy. Health Psychol 1992;11:17–23. (Level I)

90. Apfel RJ, Kelly SF, Frankel FH. The role of hypnotizability in the pathogenesis and treatment of nausea and vomiting of pregnancy. J Psychosom Obstet Gynaecol 1986;5: 179–86. (Level II-3)

91. Torem MS. Hypnotherapeutic techniques in the treatment of hyperemesis gravidarum. Am J Clin Hypn 1994;37: 1–11. (Level III)

92. Smith BJ. Management of the patient with hyperemesis gravidarum in family therapy with hypnotherapy as an adjunct. J N Y State Nurses Assoc 1982;13:17–26. (Level III)

93. Simon EP, Schwartz J. Medical hypnosis for hyperemesis gravidarum. Birth 1999;26:248–54. (Level III)

94. Fuchs K, Paldi E, Abramovici H, Peretz BA. Treatment of hyperemesis gravidarum by hypnosis. Int J Clin Exp Hypn 1980;28:313–23. (Level III)

The MEDLINE database, the Cochrane Library, and ACOG's own internal resources and documents were used to conduct a literature search to locate relevant articles published between January 1985 and December 2003. The search was restricted to articles published in the English language. Priority was given to articles reporting results of original research, although review articles and commentaries also were consulted. Abstracts of research presented at symposia and scientific conferences were not considered adequate for inclusion in this document. Guidelines published by organizations or institutions such as the National Institutes of Health and the American College of Obstetricians and Gynecologists were reviewed, and additional studies were located by reviewing bibliographies of identified articles. When reliable research was not available, expert opinions from obstetrician–gynecologists were used.

Studies were reviewed and evaluated for quality according to the method outlined by the U.S. Preventive Services Task Force:

I   Evidence obtained from at least 1 properly designed randomized controlled trial.

II-1   Evidence obtained from well-designed controlled trials without randomization.

II-2   Evidence obtained from well-designed cohort or case–control analytic studies, preferably from more than 1 center or research group.

II-3   Evidence obtained from multiple time series with or without the intervention. Dramatic results in uncontrolled experiments also could be regarded as this type of evidence.

III   Opinions of respected authorities, based on clinical experience, descriptive studies, or reports of expert committees.

Based on the highest level of evidence found in the data, recommendations are provided and graded according to the following categories:

Level A—Recommendations are based on good and consistent scientific evidence.

Level B—Recommendations are based on limited or inconsistent scientific evidence.

Level C—Recommendations are based primarily on consensus and expert opinion.

ISSN 1099-3630

The American College of Obstetricians and Gynecologists
409 12th Street, SW, PO Box 96920, Washington, DC 20090-6920

12345/87654

Nausea and vomiting of pregnancy. ACOG Practice Bulletin No. 52. American College of Obstetricians and Gynecologists. Obstet Gynecol 2004;103:803–15

ACOG PRACTICE BULLETIN

CLINICAL MANAGEMENT GUIDELINES FOR
OBSTETRICIAN–GYNECOLOGISTS

NUMBER 44, JULY 2003

(Replaces Committee Opinion Number 252, March 2001)

Neural Tube Defects

Neural tube defects (NTDs) are congenital structural abnormalities of the brain and vertebral column that occur either as an isolated malformation, along with other malformations, or as part of a genetic syndrome. Isolated (ie, nonsyndromic) NTDs occur in 1.4–2 per 1,000 pregnancies and are the second most common major congenital anomaly worldwide (cardiac malformations are first) (1). In the United States, approximately 4,000 fetuses are affected each year, of which one third are either aborted or spontaneously lost (2). Anencephaly accounts for one half of all cases of NTDs and is incompatible with life; with treatment, 80–90% of infants with spina bifida survive with varying degrees of disability (2, 3). Most importantly, NTDs are among the few birth defects for which primary prevention is possible; prenatal screening and diagnosis are widely available, and prenatal therapy is being investigated.

Background

Embryology

The neural plate appears during the third week of gestation and gives rise to the neural folds that fuse in the midline to form the neural tube. Recent animal and human data suggest that neural tube closure occurs in multiple regions, which then fuse (4, 5). Defects result either from failure of closure of one site or failure of two sites to meet. Neural tube closure is normally complete by the end of the fourth week after conception (6 weeks after the last period), a time when many women do not yet realize they are pregnant.

Pathophysiology

Neural tube defects can be categorized as either cranial or spinal defects (see Table 1). Cranial defects include abnormalities in skull, scalp, and brain tissue formation. These conditions, with the exception of small encephaloceles, are lethal. Abnormalities of the caudal portion of the neural tube generally are known as spina bifida. The various types of spina bifida include malformations

This Practice Bulletin was developed by the ACOG Committee on Practice Bulletins— Obstetrics with the assistance of Nancy Cheschier, MD. The information is designed to aid practitioners in making decisions about appropriate obstetric and gynecologic care. These guidelines should not be construed as dictating an exclusive course of treatment or procedure. Variations in practice may be warranted based on the needs of the individual patient, resources, and limitations unique to the institution or type of practice.

Table 1. Neural Tube Defect Pathophysiology

Neural Tube Defect	Malformation
Cranial	
Anencephaly	Failure of fusion of cephalic portion of neural folds; absence of all or part of brain, neurocranium, and skin
Exencephaly	Failure of scalp and skull formation; exteriorization of abnormally formed brain
Encephalocele	Failure of skull formation; extrusion of brain tissue into membranous sac
Iniencephaly	Defect of cervical and upper thoracic vertebrae; abnormally formed brain tissue and extreme retroflexion of upper spine
Spinal	
Spina bifida	Failure of fusion of caudal portion of neural tube, usually of 3–5 contiguous vertebrae; spinal cord or meninges or both exposed to amniotic fluid
Meningocele	Failure of fusion of caudal portion of neural tube; meninges exposed
Meningomyelocele	Failure of fusion of caudal portion of neural tube; meninges and neural tissue exposed
Myeloschisis	Failure of fusion of caudal portion of neural tube; flattened mass of neural tissue exposed
Holorachischisis	Failure of fusion of vertebral arches; entire spinal cord exposed
Craniorachischisis	Co-existing anencephaly and rachischisis

of the spinal cord, meninges, and vertebrae, and most of these conditions are compatible with life. The majority of NTDs affecting the spine are associated with ventriculomegaly, or enlargement of the cerebral ventricles, usually the result of an Arnold-Chiari type II malformation (3, 6, 7).

Clinical Consequences of Neural Tube Defects

The increased intracranial pressure caused by ventriculomegaly usually is relieved by placement of a ventricular-peritoneal shunt. Most infants with spina bifida and ventriculomegaly require shunting in their first year, and at least two thirds require several nonelective shunt revisions over the course of their lifetime (8, 9). Worsening of the Arnold-Chiari malformation, due in part to the small size of the posterior fossa, can cause severe or even lethal neurologic dysfunction, leading to respiratory and swallowing abnormalities. Surgical decompression of the posterior fossa involves significant risk.

With aggressive therapy at birth, including surgical closure of the defect within the first 48 hours of life, the degree of motor and sensory handicap associated with spina bifida is predicted most accurately by the level of the lesion: the higher the lesion, the worse the prognosis. Most individuals with thoracic lesions are wheelchair-bound, while 90% of those with sacral lesions can ambulate (10, 11). In one study reporting long-term follow-up of 101 children with meningomyelocele, 85% of those with quadriceps function (L2, L3, and L4 intact) ambulated independently, and another 8% walked at home and used a wheelchair only in public (11). In contrast, only 9% of those without quadriceps function were ambulatory even occasionally.

Most individuals with spina bifida, even those with low lesions, have some impairment of bowel and bladder function; urinary tract infections and stones are a common cause of chronic morbidity and even mortality caused by sepsis or renal failure (12). Sexual function may be affected by lack of genital sensation and difficulty achieving erection and ejaculation (13). Endocrine abnormalities, tethered cord, kyphosis, syringomyelia, and syringobulbia may develop as a result of the neurologic defect or its repair (14). At least one third of individuals with an NTD have a severe allergy to latex and can have life-threatening reactions after exposure (3).

Although most children with spina bifida have a normal intelligence quotient, intelligence may be affected (6). Several investigators have reported that in the absence of increased intracranial pressure, no correlation exists between ventricular size and intellectual performance in children with spina bifida (8,15). However, a reduction in mental functioning may occur as a result of central nervous system infection or increased intracranial pressure caused by shunt malfunction. One study of 167 children with myelodysplasia found an average intelligence quotient of 102 in children without hydrocephalus, 95 in those with hydrocephalus requiring a shunt, and 73 in those with a shunt and a history of shunt infection (15). Intellectual decline also may be associated with intraoperative complications during repair of an Arnold-Chiari malformation or another neurosurgical procedure.

Etiology

Isolated (nonsyndromic) NTDs are believed to be the result of a combination of genetic predisposition and environmental influences (16). Genetic predisposition is illustrated by the fact that NTDs tend to occur more frequently in certain families, and parents who have had one child with an NTD are at significantly increased risk of having another child with the same or similar defect (Table 2) (17). However, only 5% of NTDs occur in families with a positive family history (18). More than 90%

Table 2. Recurrence Risk of Neural Tube Malformations

Affected Relatives	Risk of Anencephaly and Spina Bifida (%)
No siblings	
Neither parent	0.3
One parent	4.5
Both parents	30
One sibling	
Neither parent	4
One parent	12
Both parents	38
Two siblings	
Neither parent	10
One parent	20
Both parents	43
One sibling and one second-degree relative	
Neither parent	7
One parent	18
Both parents	42
One sibling and one third-degree relative	
Neither parent	5.5
One parent	16
Both parents	42

Nussbaum RL, McInnes RR, Willard HF. Genetics of disorders with complex inheritance. In: Thompson & Thompson genetics in medicine. 6th ed. Philadelphia (PA): WB Saunders; 2001. p. 289–310 (reprinted with permission from Elsevier Science).

occur in families with no prior history, possibly because genetically susceptible individuals had not been exposed to the environmental influences necessary to produce a defect in their offspring. Thus, most individuals at increased risk do not realize it until they have an affected child.

Any environmental influence must be present during the first 28 days of gestation, when the neural tube is forming, to produce a defect. Factors known to be associated with NTDs include geographic region, ethnicity, diet, teratogen exposure, maternal diabetes, and high maternal core temperature (19–23). Regions with the highest NTD incidence include the British Isles, China, Egypt, and India. Certain ethnic and racial groups also appear to be at high risk. For example, a study using 5 years of population-based data from California found that Hispanic women (1.12 per 1,000, 95% confidence interval [CI], 1.04–1.21), and Caucasian women (0.96 per 1,000, 95% CI, 0.89–1.04) were at highest risk. African-American women (0.75 per 1,000, 95% CI,

0.59–0.91) and Asian women (0.75 per 1,000, 95% CI, 0.60–0.90) were at lower risk (24). Some of the ethnic differences observed may reflect geography and diet in addition to genetic predisposition. For example, Sikhs living in India have more than twice the incidence of NTDs as Sikhs living in Canada (17).

Most isolated NTDs occur in association with abnormal folate metabolism, discussed as follows. Genetic syndromes that can include an NTD and are likely to have a genetic etiology other than abnormal folate metabolism include Meckel-Gruber, Roberts, Jarcho-Levin, and HARD syndromes, as well as trisomy 13, trisomy 18, and triploidy. Cloacal exstrophy and sacrococcygeal teratoma may be associated with spina bifida, and amniotic bands may cause spina bifida or anencephaly (25).

Role of Folic Acid

The most important environmental influence on NTD formation appears to be diet or, more specifically, the intake of folic acid. It has long been known that women with pregnancies complicated by fetal NTDs have lower plasma levels of vitamin B_{12} and folate than women whose pregnancies are unaffected. Many of the medications known to cause fetal NTDs, such as diphenylhydantoin, aminopterin, or carbamazepine, interfere with folic acid metabolism. Several clinical studies showed that folic acid supplementation before conception reduces the recurrence of fetal NTDs (26–29). However, the benefits of folic acid were not widely accepted until 1991, when the Medical Research Council Vitamin Study Research Group published the results of a large, prospective, randomized, double-blind study of folic acid supplementation conducted at 33 centers in seven countries (30). A total of 1,817 women at high risk by virtue of a previously affected pregnancy were enrolled in the study and randomly assigned to receive folic acid, other vitamins, both, or neither. Women assigned to take 4 mg of folic acid per day before pregnancy and through the 12th week of gestation experienced a 72% reduction in their recurrence risk (odds ratio, 0.28; 95% CI, 0.15–0.53).

The Medical Research Council study included only women who already had an affected pregnancy, which accounts for only 5% of cases of NTDs. However, a double-blind, placebo-controlled, randomized trial subsequently showed that periconceptional folic acid supplementation decreased the risk of a first occurrence of an NTD as well (31). The efficacy of periconceptional folic acid supplementation for preventing both recurrence and occurrence of NTDs has since been confirmed by many other studies (32, 33).

The genetic basis for the relationship between folate metabolism and NTDs is now being investigated. The most important metabolic reaction that requires folate is the conversion of homocysteine to methionine; evidence indicates that this pathway is critically involved in the genesis of NTDs. Several studies have shown that parents who have had a pregnancy complicated by an NTD and their affected offspring are more likely to carry a mutation in the gene encoding the enzyme methylenetetrahydrofolate reductase (MTHFR) than the unaffected population. For example, in the Netherlands, 14–16% of mothers, 10–15% of fathers, and 13–18% of children with spina bifida are homozygous for the MTHFR mutation compared with 5% of the general population (34–36). Other mutations in this enzyme with similar effects also have been reported (36). Therefore, it seems possible that folic acid supplementation helps to overcome the effects of this enzyme mutation, resulting in more normal levels of homocysteine and adequate production of methionine (21). Methionine is important because it provides the methyl group necessary for gene regulation and for a wide variety of metabolic reactions essential for tissue growth and development.

Clinical Considerations and Recommendations

▶ *Is folic acid supplementation useful in preventing NTDs?*

Although folic acid is now widely acknowledged as beneficial in preventing isolated nonsyndromic NTDs, it must be ingested before conception and at least through the first 4 weeks of fetal development to be effective. Because the neural tube is nearly formed by the time of the first missed period, initiating folic acid supplementation at that time is not sufficient. Although women of reproductive age should be advised to ingest a diet that includes folate-rich foods, several studies have shown that diet alone is not effective in increasing serum folate levels. Folic acid supplementation should, therefore, be encouraged. Specific recommendations regarding the dose are evolving.

In 1991, the Centers for Disease Control and Prevention recommended that all women with a previous pregnancy complicated by a fetal NTD ingest 4 mg of folic acid daily before conception and through the first trimester (37). The following year, the U.S. Public Health Service recommended that all women capable of becoming pregnant take 400 µg of folic acid daily, and many groups, including the American College of Obstetricians and Gynecologists, subsequently endorsed these recommendations.

Few women actually take a folic acid supplement routinely. Even though women might take folic acid during a pregnancy, more than one half of all pregnancies are unplanned (38), and in these cases, the neural tube has already formed before pregnancy is recognized and before folic acid supplementation has been initiated. Therefore, most pregnancies in this country have not benefited from this preventive measure. Since January 1, 1998, the U.S. Food and Drug Administration has required folic acid fortification of cereal grains (39). Because of this requirement, the average woman eating a standard diet now ingests an extra 200 µg of folic acid each day (40).

Although grain fortification has improved the folate intake of all Americans, many authorities feel the current level of fortification is inadequate to prevent NTDs. An analysis of 13 published studies clarified the dose-response relationship of folic acid for NTD prevention (41). Women in western countries typically have a baseline serum folate level of approximately 5 ng/mL (normal range 6–20 ng/mL). This analysis determined that ingestion of an additional 200 µg of folic acid each day would reduce the incidence of NTDs by only approximately 20% (41). These calculations are supported by data from the U.S. Public Health Service that confirm since grain fortification began, the incidence of NTDs in the United States has decreased by only 19% (42).

It currently is recommended that women of reproductive age take a 400 µg folic acid supplement daily. Calculations based on existing data predict that the 400 µg dose recommended for women at low risk would reduce the incidence of NTDs by 36%. In this same analysis, the 4 mg dose, currently recommended only for women at high risk, was predicted to reduce the incidence by 82%, and a 5 mg dose was predicted to reduce the incidence by 85% (41).

The risks of higher levels of folic acid supplementation are believed to be minimal. Folic acid is considered nontoxic even at very high doses and is rapidly excreted in the urine. There have been concerns that supplemental folic acid could mask the symptoms of pernicious anemia and thus delay treatment. However, folic acid cannot mask the neuropathy typical of this diagnosis. Currently, 12% of patients with pernicious anemia present with neuropathy alone (43). With folic acid supplementation, this proportion may be increased, but there is no evidence that initiating treatment after the development of a neuropathy results in irreversible damage (44). A small number of women taking seizure medication (diphenylhydantoin, aminopterin, carbamazepine) may have lower serum drug levels and experience an associated increase in seizure frequency while taking folic acid supplements (45). Monitoring drug levels and increasing the dosage as needed may help to avert this complication.

Some over-the-counter multivitamin supplements and most prenatal vitamins contain 400 µg of folic acid.

Higher levels of supplementation should be achieved by taking an additional folic acid supplement and not by taking excess multivitamins. In particular, vitamin A is potentially teratogenic at high doses, and pregnant women should not take more than the 5,000 IU per day, which is typically found in one multivitamin/mineral supplement (46).

▶ Which NTDs may not be affected by folic acid?

There is limited evidence to indicate that folic acid supplementation may not decrease the risk of NTDs in women with high first-trimester blood glucose levels, or high first-trimester maternal temperature, or in women who take valproic acid. In women with high glucose levels, the exact mechanism is unknown but may involve inhibition of fetal glycolysis, a functional deficiency of arachidonic acid or myoinositol in the developing embryo, or alterations in the yolk sac (23). First-trimester maternal fever and sauna use both increase the relative risk of NTDs (to 2.6–6.2), although the duration and intensity necessary to produce an effect and the embryologic mechanism are unknown (47). First-trimester valproic acid use results in a 1–2% risk of having a fetus with spina bifida, but the mechanism may be different from that of other antiepileptic agents (19). Fetuses with aneuploidy or genetic syndromes may have NTDs as a result of their specific genetic abnormality. These NTDs are not prevented by folic acid.

▶ Is maternal serum alpha-fetoprotein testing useful in screening for NTDs?

Amniotic fluid and maternal serum alpha-fetoprotein (MSAFP) levels are elevated in 89–100% of pregnancies complicated by fetal NTDs (47). Many large prospective trials of MSAFP screening have shown that most affected pregnancies can be identified by an elevated MSAFP level, usually defined as more than 2.5 times the normal median for singleton pregnancies (48–51).

Because more than 90% of all children with NTDs are born to women with no family history of NTD and no obvious risk factors, MSAFP screening—which usually is performed as part of broader screening for aneuploidy—makes it possible to identify affected fetuses in such women. Most screening programs strive to identify most cases of NTDs without unduly increasing the false-positive rate, which requires a trade-off between sensitivity and specificity. When the screen-positive cutoff is set at 2.5 multiples of the median (MoM), the screen-positive rate is typically 5% or less, and approximately 85% of all NTDs in singleton pregnancies and 80% in twin pregnancies will be identified (48–51). The false-positive rate can

be decreased by performing an ultrasound examination before MSAFP screening to verify gestational age and identify multiple gestations and cases of intrauterine fetal demise.

▶ How should the diagnosis of NTDs be established?

Maternal serum alpha-fetoprotein evaluation is an effective screening test for NTDs and should be offered to all pregnant women unless they plan to have amniotic fluid alpha-fetoprotein (AFP) measurement as part of prenatal diagnosis for chromosomal abnormalities or other genetic diseases. The MSAFP test is a screening test and, therefore, has a high false-positive rate. Only 2% of all women with a positive test result are carrying a fetus with an NTD, and these affected pregnancies can only be identified by performing a diagnostic test. Women with MSAFP levels higher than a predetermined cutoff (usually 2–2.5 MoM) should, therefore, be referred for genetic counseling and consideration of a diagnostic test. Women already known to be at high risk of having a fetus with an NTD because of a previously affected pregnancy, a positive family history, medication exposure, diabetes, or another risk factor, can be offered a diagnostic test directly. Although MSAFP does not function as a screening test in these women because they will be offered a diagnostic test regardless of the results, it still may be helpful in evaluating the fetus.

The traditional diagnostic test offered to women with a positive MSAFP test result is genetic amniocentesis. If the amniotic fluid AFP level is elevated, an assay is performed to determine the presence or absence of acetylcholinesterase. Elevated amniotic fluid AFP together with the presence of acetylcholinesterase is considered diagnostic for a fetal NTD. In a study of almost 10,000 singleton pregnancies at 14–23 weeks of gestation with known outcomes, the amniotic fluid acetylcholinesterase level identified 100% of cases of anencephaly, 100% of cases of open spina bifida, and 20% of ventral wall defects, with a false-positive rate of 2.2 per 1,000 amniocenteses (52).

One advantage of amniocentesis is that amniotic fluid also can be obtained for determination of the fetal karyotype. Several studies suggest that elevated MSAFP levels independently increase the risk of fetal aneuploidy (53). In pregnancies complicated by an elevated MSAFP level, the incidence of fetal aneuploidy is 0.61% in ultrasonographically determined normal fetuses and 16% in abnormal fetuses (54, 55). Performing a genetic amniocentesis in all women at increased risk of an NTD would result in a 98% detection rate for NTDs and a 100% detection rate for aneuploidy. However, based on the high false-positive rate of the MSAFP screening test, a policy of universal amniocentesis for all high-risk women would mean many would undergo amniocentesis unnecessarily. Although second-trimester amniocentesis is a relatively safe procedure, it is associated with a postprocedure pregnancy loss rate of approximately 1 in 200 (56).

Ultrasound technology has improved remarkably since MSAFP screening was adopted. Centers with special expertise in obstetric ultrasonography report excellent sensitivity and specificity in detecting fetal NTDs, especially in high-risk patients, and many now offer specialized ultrasound examination as a diagnostic test for women at high risk of NTDs (57). In the hands of experienced operators, ultrasonography alone has up to 97% sensitivity and 100% specificity in the diagnosis of NTDs (57). In less experienced hands, however, ultrasonography is only a screening test that can have a high false-negative rate. In a large multicenter trial of ultrasound screening in low-risk women, only 35% of major anomalies were detected in tertiary hospital settings and only 13% in non-tertiary settings; 7 of 8 NTDs were identified (58).

To take advantage of both types of testing and to minimize risk, many centers now offer specialized ultrasound examinations initially to all high-risk women, and perform amniocenteses only in a subset of patients. If a high-quality ultrasound examination is performed and no fetal defects are identified, the risks and benefits of both amniocentesis and specialized ultrasound examination can be discussed with the patient. A decision about invasive testing can then be made that takes into account the degree of risk associated with the MSAFP level or the patient's history, the quality and findings of the specialized ultrasound examination, the patient's age, and the patient's wishes. Many high-risk patients decide against amniocentesis after a reassuring specialized ultrasound examination. Alternatively, amniocentesis is offered for confirmation to those patients in whom a fetal defect is identified or for reassurance to those in whom visualization of the fetus is suboptimal and the ultrasound examination is not helpful in making a diagnosis (59). Women with a very high MSAFP level also may be offered amniocentesis because there is a direct relationship between the degree of MSAFP elevation and the incidence of anomalies. With an MSAFP of 2.5 MoM, there is a 3.4% risk of anomalies; at 7 MoM, the risk increases to 40.3% (Table 3) (60). Some women at high risk for a fetal NTD may choose amniocentesis because they also are at increased risk for fetal aneuploidy. Some authorities dispute the use of ultrasonography as a diagnostic test and recommend that amniocentesis be offered to all women with elevated MSAFP levels (61–63).

Table 3. Relative Risk of Poor Pregnancy Outcomes with Elevated Maternal Serum Alpha-fetoprotein Level

Condition	Relative Risk
Open neural tube defect	225
Other anomalies	4.7
Fetal death	8.1
Neonatal death	4.7
Low birth weight	4.0
Newborn complications	3.6
Oligohydramnios	3.4
Abruption	3.0
Preeclampsia	2.3

Milunsky A, Jick SS, Bruell CL, MacLaughlin DS, Tsung YK, Jick H, et al. Predictive values, relative risks, and overall benefits of high and low maternal serum alpha-fetoprotein screening in singleton pregnancies: new epidemiologic data. Am J Obstet Gynecol 1989;161:291–7 (reprinted with permission from Elsevier Science).

▶ *Are there special considerations in the obstetric management and route of delivery of a fetus with an NTD?*

Most pregnancies complicated by fetal spina bifida will result in delivery at term unless there is obstetric intervention. Fetal spina bifida does not increase the risk of uteroplacental insufficiency or oligohydramnios; anencephaly can be associated with hydramnios as a result of decreased fetal swallowing. There is no evidence that antenatal testing for the sole indication of a fetal NTD improves outcome. Furthermore, the structurally abnormal fetus frequently has an abnormal fetal heart rate pattern, which can be difficult to interpret (64). Serial ultrasound examinations to monitor fetal growth and ventricular size may be helpful in planning delivery.

The fetus with spina bifida should be delivered at a hospital with neonatal intensive care facilities and personnel capable of managing the spine defect and any immediate complications; evidence suggests that outcomes are better in such settings (65). Because individuals with an NTD are at risk of developing a severe, potentially life-threatening allergy to latex (3), clinicians handling the infant should wear wear latex-free gloves. Generally, delivery at term is preferred. However, once fetal lung maturity has been documented, rapidly increasing ventriculomegaly may prompt delivery before term so that a ventriculo-peritoneal shunt can be placed. Each case should be managed individually in consultation with personnel with experience and knowledge of such complications and personnel from the neurosurgical and neonatal services.

Breech presentation, resulting from fetal neurologic dysfunction or hydrocephalus with an enlarged head, is common in pregnancies complicated by fetal spina bifida. For the breech fetus with an NTD, cesarean delivery is standard (66). The best delivery route for the vertex fetus remains controversial. No prospective randomized trial of vaginal delivery versus cesarean delivery for vertex fetuses with spina bifida has been performed. All studies in the current literature are retrospective with various biases. At least five studies representing a total of 400 patients suggest that vaginal delivery does not adversely affect neonatal outcome, while one large study of 200 patients suggests the opposite (66–71).

Most studies on this subject also are limited by lack of long-term follow-up, which is essential in evaluating medical care for these infants because loss of function and other neurologic reversals are common even when surgery is performed early to correct an NTD. Because it is still not clear whether or how the method of delivery significantly affects neurologic outcome in these infants, decisions about the timing and route of delivery should be made individually in consultation with personnel with experience and knowledge of such complications, which may include maternal–fetal medicine specialists, neonatologists, and pediatric neurosurgeons.

▶ *Is there a role for fetal surgery for NTDs?*

The "two-hit hypothesis" describes the likely cause of neurologic damage that occurs with NTDs: the "first hit" is the developmental abnormality that caused the open spina bifida, and the "second hit" is the inflammation and damage to the neural tissues possibly caused by chronic exposure to amniotic fluid, fetal movement, contact with the uterine wall, or pressure from labor and delivery. Although no prenatal intervention can eliminate the effects of the first hit once it has occurred, researchers investigating in utero surgical closure of fetal spina bifida theorize that fetal surgery might prevent the kind of trauma characterized as the second hit (72).

Approximately 220 in utero closures of fetal spina bifida were performed in four centers in the United States between 1997 and 2002. These procedures were not performed as part of a randomized study and generally were offered to women whose fetuses had lesions at or below the lower thoracic spine. Data gathered from this cohort suggest no improvement in bowel or bladder function or ambulatory ability beyond the degree of impairment predicted by the level of the lesion (73, 74). However, these children appear to require shunt placement less frequently or at least later in life. They also seem to experience an improvement in the degree of hindbrain herniation after

in utero surgery, which, if confirmed, might help to prevent serious morbidity or mortality from worsening Arnold-Chiari type II malformation (75, 76). Because of selection bias in the cohort and the nonstandard neurosurgical follow-up, it is difficult to know whether the medical need for shunting truly decreases or whether decreased herniation corresponds to improved function.

Maternal–fetal surgery is a risky procedure. The woman incurs the risks attendant with any surgical procedure (anesthetic complications, hemorrhage, bladder injury, chorioamnionitis) twice during the index pregnancy. First, a hysterotomy is placed in the muscular portion of the uterus during the late second trimester to provide access to the fetus. Because the hysterotomy confers an increased risk of uterine rupture, the woman then must undergo cesarean delivery for the index and all future pregnancies (77).

One of the most significant potential risks to the fetus is preterm delivery and its secondary complications (76). A fetus that has undergone in utero neurosurgical repair is delivered at approximately 33 weeks of gestation, with up to 40% being delivered before 32 weeks of gestation (75, 76, 78). One study of 29 infants who underwent in utero neurosurgery reported preterm labor in 50%, preterm premature rupture of the membranes in 28%, and oligohydramnios in 48% of the women who had fetal surgery, while only 4% of the controls had these complications (78). A study of 33 infants with known neurologic outcome after undergoing a variety of fetal surgery procedures found that additional central nervous system injuries occurred in 21% (79). Contributing factors included intraoperative fetal bradycardia, significant maternal blood loss, maternal respiratory failure or hypotension, neonatal hypotension, uterine contractions, and exposure to terbutaline and nitroglycerin.

Information on long-term complications for women and fetuses who undergo maternal–fetal surgery is only starting to accrue. Data from one large fetal surgery center documented no long-term effects on fertility in 70 women who underwent maternal–fetal surgery (80). However, an increased incidence of early tethered cord has been reported in fetuses undergoing in utero meningomyelocele repair (81). The parent(s) must understand these risks and recognize the potential for additional complications before undergoing such a procedure.

The ethical issues relevant to maternal–fetal surgery for fetal spina bifida are complex, and maternal–fetal surgery for repair of fetal spina bifida currently is considered investigational. A National Institutes of Health-supported prospective randomized trial of prenatal surgical closure of fetal spina bifida began in January 2003 and is expected to resolve many of these issues.

Summary of Recommendations

The following recommendations are based on good and consistent scientific evidence (Level A):

▶ Periconceptional folic acid supplementation is recommended because it has been shown to reduce the occurrence and recurrence of NTDs.

▶ For low-risk women, folic acid supplementation of 400 µg per day currently is recommended because nutritional sources alone are insufficient. Higher levels of supplementation should not be achieved by taking excess multivitamins because of the risk of vitamin A toxicity.

▶ For women at high risk of NTDs or who have had a previous pregnancy with an NTD, folic acid supplementation of 4 mg per day is recommended.

▶ Maternal serum alpha-fetoprotein evaluation is an effective screening test for NTDs and should be offered to all pregnant women.

The following recommendations are based on limited or inconsistent scientific evidence (Level B):

▶ Women with elevated serum AFP levels should have a specialized ultrasound examination to further assess the risk of NTDs.

▶ The fetus with an NTD should be delivered at a facility that has personnel capable of handling all aspects of neonatal complications.

The following recommendations are based primarily on consensus and expert opinion (Level C):

▶ The ideal dose for folic acid supplementation has not been appropriately evaluated in prospective clinical studies. A 400 µg supplement currently is recommended for women capable of becoming pregnant.

▶ The route of delivery for the fetus with an NTD should be individualized because data are lacking that any one route provides a superior outcome.

References

1. Cragan JD, Roberts HE, Edmonds LD, Khoury MJ, Kirby RS, Shaw GM, et al. Surveillance for anencephaly and spina bifida and the impact of prenatal diagnosis—United States, 1985–1994. MMWR CDC Surveill Summ 1995; 44(4):1–13. (Level III)

2. Botto LD, Moore CA, Khoury MJ, Erickson JD. Neural-tube defects. N Engl J Med 1999;341:1509–19. (Level III)

3. Bowman RM, McLone DG, Grant JA, Tomita T, Ito JA. Spina bifida outcome: a 25-year prospective. Pediatr Neurosurg 2001;34:114–20. (Level III)

4. Van Allen MI, Kalousek DK, Chernoff GF, Juriloff D, Harris M, McGillivray BC, et al. Evidence for multi-site closure of the neural tube in humans. Am J Med Genet 1993;47:723–43. (Level III)

5. Seller MJ. Sex, neural tube defects, and multisite closure of the human neural tube. Am J Med Genet 1995;58: 332–6. (Level II-2)

6. Steinbok P, Irvine B, Cochrane DD, Irwin BJ. Long-term outcome and complications of children born with meningomyelocele. Childs Nerv Syst 1992;8:92–6. (Level II-2)

7. Hunt GM. The Casey Holter lecture. Non-selective intervention in newborn babies with open spina bifida: the outcome 30 years on for the complete cohort. Eur J Pediatr Surg 1999;9(suppl 1):5–8. (Level II-2)

8. Storrs BB. Ventricular size and intelligence in myelodysplastic children. In: Martin AE, editor. Concepts in pediatric neurosurgery. Vol 8. Basel: Karger; 1988. p. 51–6. (Level II-3)

9. Rolle U, Grafe G. About the rate of shunt complications in patients with hydrocephalus and myelomeningocele. Eur J Pediatr Surg 1999;9(suppl 1):51–2. (Level III)

10. Nelson MD Jr, Bracchi M, Naidich TP, McLone DG. The natural history of repaired myelomeningocele. Radiographics 1988;8:695–706. (Level III)

11. Selber P, Dias L. Sacral-level myelomeningocele: long-term outcome in adults. J Pediatr Orthop 1998;18:423–7. (Level II-3)

12. McDonnell GV, McCann JP. Why do adults with spina bifida and hydrocephalus die? A clinic-based study. Eur J Pediatr Surg 2000;10(suppl 1):31–2. (Level III)

13. Joyner BD, McLorie GA, Khoury AE. Sexuality and reproductive issues in children with myelomeningocele. Eur J Pediatr Surg 1998;8:29–34. (Level III)

14. Caldarelli M, Di Rocco C, Colosimo C Jr, Fariello G, Di Gennaro M. Surgical treatment of late neurological deterioration in children with myelodysplasia. Acta Neurochir (Wien) 1995;137:199–206. (Level III)

15. McLone DG, Czyzewski D, Raimondi AJ, Sommers RC. Central nervous system infections as a limiting factor in the intelligence of children with myelomeningocele. Pediatrics 1982;70:338–42. (Level III)

16. Hall JG, Friedman JM, Kenna BA, Popkin J, Jawanda M, Arnold W. Clinical, genetic, and epidemiological factors in neural tube defects. Am J Hum Genet 1988;43:827–37. (Level II-3)

17. Nussbaum RL, McInnes RR, Willard HF. Genetics of disorders with complex inheritance. In: Thompson & Thompson genetics in medicine. 6th ed. Philadelphia (PA): W.B. Saunders; 2001. p. 289–310. (Level III)

18. Aitken DA, Crossley JA, Spencer K. Prenatal screening for neural tube defects and aneuploidy. In: Rimoin DL, Connor JM, Pyeritz RE, Korf BR, editors. Emery and Rimoin's principles and practice of medical genetics 4th

ed. New York: Churchill & Livingstone; 2002. p. 763–801. (Level III)

19. Lindhout D, Omtzigt JG, Cornel MC. Spectrum of neural-tube defects in 34 infants prentally exposed to antiepileptic drugs. Neurology 1992;42(4 suppl 5):111–8. (Level III)

20. Shaw GM, Todoroff K, Velie EM, Lammer EJ. Maternal illness, including fever and medication use as risk factors for neural tube defects. Teratology 1998;57:1–7. (Level II-2)

21. van der Put NM, van Straaten HW, Trijbels FJ, Blom HJ. Folate, homocysteine and neural tube defects: an overview. Exp Biol Med (Maywood) 2001;226:243–70. (Level III)

22. Lammer EJ, Sever LE, Oakley GP Jr. Teratogen update: valproic acid. Teratology 1987;35:465–73. (Level III)

23. Reece EA, Hobbins JC. Diabetic embryopathy: pathogenesis, prenatal diagnosis and prevention. Obstet Gynecol Surv 1986;41:325–35. (Level III)

24. Feuchtbaum LB, Currier RJ, Riggle S, Roberson M, Lorey FW, Cunningham GC. Neural tube defect prevalence in California (1990–1994): eliciting patterns by type of defect and maternal race/ethnicity. Genet Test 1999;3:265–72. (Level II-3)

25. Jones KL, editor. Smith's recognizable patterns of human malformation. 5th ed. Philadelphia (PA): W B Saunders; 1997. (Level III)

26. Hibbard ED, Smithells RW. Folic acid metabolism and human embryopathy. Lancet 1965;1:1254. (Level III)

27. Smithells RW, Nevin NC, Seller MJ, Sheppard S, Harris R, Read AP, et al. Further experience of vitamin supplementation for prevention of neural tube defect recurrences. Lancet 1983;1:1027–31. (Level II-2)

28. Laurence KM, James N, Miller MH, Tennant GB, Campbell H. Double-blind randomised controlled trial of folate treatment before conception to prevent recurrence of neural-tube defects. Br Med J (Clin Res Ed) 1981; 282:1509–11. (Level I)

29. Mulinare J, Cordero JF, Erickson JD, Berry RJ. Periconceptional use of multivitamins and the occurrence of neural tube defects. JAMA 1988;260:3141–5. (Level II-2)

30. Prevention of neural tube defects: results of the Medical Research Council Vitamin Study. MRC Vitamin Study Research Group. Lancet 1991;338:131–7. (Level I)

31. Czeizel AE, Dudas I. Prevention of the first occurrence of neural-tube defects by periconceptional vitamin supplementation. N Engl J Med 1992;327:1832–5. (Level I)

32. Berry RJ, Li Z, Erickson JD, Li S, Moore CA, Wang H, et al. Prevention of neural-tube defects with folic acid in China. China–U.S. Collaborative Project for Neural Tube Defect Prevention [corrected; erratum N Engl J Med 1999;341:24 and N Engl J Med 2000;342:7]. N Engl J Med 1999;341:1485–90. (Level II-2)

33. Lumley J, Watson L, Watson M, Bower C. Periconceptional supplementation with folate and/or multivitamins for preventing neural tube defects (Cochrane Review). In: The Cochrane Library, Issue 1, 2003. Oxford: Update Software. (Level I)

34. van der Put MN, Steegers-Theunissen RP, Frosst P, Trijbels FJ, Eskes TK, van den Heuvel LP, et al. Mutated methylenetetrahydrofolate reductase as a risk factor for spina bifida. Lancet 1995;346:1070–1. (Level II-2)

35. van der Put MN, Eskes TK, Blom HJ. Is the common 677 C→T mutation in the methylenetetrahydrofolate reductase gene a risk factor for neural tube defects? A meta-analysis. QJM 1997;90:111–5. (Meta-analysis)

36. van der Put MN, Blom HJ. Neural tube defects and a disturbed folate dependent homocysteine metabolism. Eur J Obstet Gynecol Reprod Biol 2000;92:57–61. (Level III)

37. Use of folic acid for prevention of spina bifida and other neural tube defects—1983–1991. MMWR Morb Mortal Wkly Rep 1991;40:513–6. (Level III)

38. Knowledge and use of folic acid by women of childbearing age—United States, 1995 and 1998. MMWR Morb Mortal Wkly Rep 1999;48:325–7. (Level III)

39. Food standards: amendment of standards of identity for enriched grain products to require addition of folic acid—FDA. Final rule. Fed Regist 1996;61:8781–97. (Level III)

40. Rader J, Weaver CM, Angyal G. Advances in the analysis of folates in foods. Food Test Anal 1999;5:14–32. (Level III)

41. Wald NJ, Law MR, Morris JK, Wald DS. Quantifying the effect of folic acid. Lancet 2001;358:2069–73. (Level III)

42. Honein MA, Paulozzi LJ, Mathews TJ, Erickson JD, Wong LY. Impact of folic acid fortification of the US food supply on the occurrence of neural tube defects. JAMA 2001;285:2981–6. (Level II-2)

43. Lindenbaum J, Healton EB, Savage DG, Brust JC, Garrett TJ, Podell ER, et al. Neuropsychiatric disorders caused by cobalamin deficiency in the absence of anemia or macrocytosis. N Engl J Med 1988;318:1720–8. (Level II-3)

44. Wald NJ, Bower C. Folic acid, pernicious anemia, and prevention of neural tube defects. Lancet 1994;343:307. (Level III)

45. Biale Y, Lewenthal H. Effect of folic acid supplementation on congenital malformations due to anticonvulsive drugs. Eur J Obstet Gynecol Reprod Biol 1984;18:211–6. (Level II-2)

46. Rothman KJ, Moore LL, Singer MR, Nguyen US, Mannino S, Milunsky A. Teratogenicity of high vitamin A intake. N Engl J Med 1995;333:1369–73. (Level III)

47. Milunsky A. Maternal serum screening for neural tube and other defects. In: Genetic disorders and the fetus: diagnosis, prevention, and treatment. 4th ed. Baltimore (MD): Johns Hopkins University Press; 1998. p. 635–701. (Level III)

48. Wald NJ, Cuckle H, Brock JH, Peto R, Polani PE, Woodford FR. Maternal serum-alpha-fetoprotein measurement in antenatal screening for anencephaly and spina bifida in early pregnancy. Report of U.K. collaborative study on alpha-fetoprotein in relation to neural-tube defects. Lancet 1977;1:1323–32. (Level II-2)

49. Haddow JE, Kloza EM, Smith DE, Knight GJ. Data from an alpha-fetoprotein pilot screening program in Maine. Obstet Gynecol 1983;62:556–60. (Level III)

50. Burton BK, Sowers SG, Nelson LH. Maternal serum alpha-fetoprotein screening in North Carolina: experience with more than twelve thousand pregnancies. Am J Obstet Gynecol 1983;146:439–44. (Level III)

51. Milunsky A. Prenatal detection of neural tube defects. VI. Experience with 20,000 pregnancies. JAMA 1980;244: 2731–5. (Level II-2)

52. Loft AG, Hogdall E, Larsen SO, Norgaard-Pedersen B. A comparison of amniotic fluid alpha-fetoprotein and acetylcholinesterase in the prenatal diagnosis of open neural tube defects and anterior abdominal wall defects. Prenat Diagn 1993;13:93–109. (Level II-2)

53. James SJ, Pogribna M, Pogribny IP, Melnyk S, Hine RJ, Gibson JB, et al. Abnormal folate metabolism and mutation in the methylenetetrahydrofolate reductase gene may be maternal risk factors for Down syndrome. Am J Clin Nutr 1999;70:495–501. (Level II-2)

54. Watson WJ, Chescheir NC, Katz VL, Seeds JW. The role of ultrasound in evaluation of patients with elevated maternal serum alpha-fetoprotein: a review. Obstet Gynecol 1991;78:123–8. (Level III)

55. Harmon JP, Hiett AK, Palmer CG, Golichowski AM. Prenatal ultrasound detection of isolated neural tube defects: is cytogenetic evaluation warranted? Obstet Gynecol 1995;86:595–9. (Level II-3)

56. Gardner RJ, Sutherland GR. Prenatal diagnostic procedures. In: Chromosome abnormalities and genetic counseling. Oxford monographs on medical genetics no. 29. 2nd ed. New York: Oxford University Press; 1996. p. 336–44. (Level III)

57. Lennon CA, Gray DL. Sensitivity and specificity of ultrasound for the detection of neural tube and ventral wall defects in a high-risk population. Obstet Gynecol 1999; 94:562–6. (Level II-2)

58. Crane JP, LeFevre ML, Winborn RC, Evans JK, Ewigman BG, Bain RP, et al. A randomized trial of prenatal ultrasonographic screening: impact on the detection, management, and outcome of anomalous fetuses. The RADIUS Study Group. Am J Obstet Gynecol 1994;171:392–9. (Level I)

59. Nadel AS, Green JK, Holmes LB, Frigoletto FD Jr, Benacerraf BR. Absence of need for amniocentesis in patients with elevated levels of maternal serum alpha-fetoprotein and normal ultrasonographic examinations. N Engl J Med 1990;323:557–61. (Level II-3)

60. Reichler A, Hume RF Jr, Drugan A, Bardicef M, Isada NB, Johnson MP, et al. Risk of anomalies as a function of level of elevated maternal serum alpha-fetoprotein. Am J Obstet Gynecol 1994;171:1052–5. (Level III)

61. Platt LD, Feuchtbaum L, Filly R, Lustig L, Simon M, Cunningham GC. The California Maternal Serum Alpha-Fetoprotein Screening Program: the role of ultrasonography in the detection of spina bifida. Am J Obstet Gynecol 1992;166:1328–9. (Level II-2)

62. Hogge WA, Thiagarajah S, Ferguson JE 2nd, Schnatterly PT, Harbert GM Jr. The role of ultrasonography and amniocentesis in the evaluation of pregnancies at risk for neural tube defects. Am J Obstet Gynecol 1989;161: 520–3; discussion 523–4. (Level II-2)

63. Drugan A, Zador IE, Syner FN, Sokol RJ, Sacks AJ, Evans MI. A normal ultrasound does not obviate the need for amniocentesis in patients with elevated serum alpha-fetoprotein. Obstet Gynecol 1988;72:627–30. (Level II-2)

64. Vindla S, Sahota DS, Coppens M, James DK. Computerized analysis of behavior in fetuses with congenital abnormalities. Ultrasound Obstet Gynecol 1997;9: 302–9. (Level II-3)

65. Wilkins-Haug L. Considerations for delivery of infants with congenital abnormalities. Obstet Gynecol Clin North Am 1999;26:399–412. (Level III)

66. Cochrane D, Aronyk K, Sawatzky B, Wilson D, Steinbok P. The effects of labor and delivery on spinal cord function and ambulation in patients with meningomyelocele. Childs Nerv Syst 1991;7:312–5. (Level II-2)

67. Bensen JT, Dillard RG, Burton BK. Open spina bifida: does cesarean section delivery improve prognosis? Obstet Gynecol 1988;71:532–4. (Level II-3)

68. Sakala EP, Andree I. Optimal route of delivery for meningomyelocele. Obstet Gynecol Surv 1990;45:209–12. (Level II-3)

69. Hill AE, Beattie F. Does caesarean section delivery improve neurological outcome in open spina bifida? Eur J Pediatr Surg 1994;4(suppl 1):32–4. (Level III)

70. Merrill DC, Goodwin P, Burson JM, Sato Y, Williamson R, Weiner CP. The optimal route of delivery for fetal meningomyelocele. Am J Obstet Gynecol 1998;179: 235–40. (Level II-3)

71. Luthy DA, Wardinsky T, Shurtleff DB, Hollenbach KA, Hickok DE, Nyberg DA, et al. Cesarean section before the onset of labor and subsequent motor function in infants with meningomyelocele diagnosed antenatally. N Engl J Med 1991;324:662–6. (Level II-3)

72. Meuli M, Meuli-Simmen C, Hutchins GM, Seller MJ, Harrison MR, Adzick NS. The spinal cord lesion in human fetuses with myelomeningocele: implications for fetal surgery. J Pediatr Surg 1997;32:448–52. (Level III)

73. Holzbeierlein J, Pope JC IV, Adams MC, Bruner J, Tulipan N, Brock JW 3rd. The urodynamic profile of myelodysplasia in childhood with spinal closure during gestation. J Urol 2000;164:1336–9. (Level III)

74. Hirose S, Farmer DL, Albanese CT. Fetal surgery for myelomeningocele. Curr Opin Obstet Gynecol 2001;13: 215–22. (Level III)

75. Tulipan N, Hernanz-Schulman M, Lowe LH, Bruner JP. Intrauterine myelomeningocele repair reverses preexisting hindbrain herniation. Pediatr Neurosurg 1999;31: 137–42. (Level III)

76. Sutton LN, Adzick NS, Bilaniuk LT, Johnson MP, Crombelholme TM, Flake AW. Improvement in hindbrain herniation demonstrated by serial fetal magnetic resonance imaging following fetal surgery for myelomeningocele. JAMA 1999;282:1826–31. (Level III)

77. Ranzini AC, White M, Guzman ER, Scorza WE. Prenatal sonographic diagnosis of uterine rupture following open fetal surgery. Obstet Gynecol 1999;93:826–7. (Level III)

78. Bruner JP, Tulipan N, Paschall RL, Boehm FH, Walsh WF, Silva SR, et al. Fetal surgery for myelomeningocele

and the incidence of shunt-dependent hydrocephalus. JAMA 1999;282:1819–25. (Level II-2)

79. Bealer JF, Raisanen J, Skarsgard ED, Long SR, Wong K, Filly RA, et al. The incidence and spectrum of neurological injury after open fetal surgery. J Pediatr Surg 1995;30:1150–4. (Level III)

80. Farrell JA, Albanese CT, Jennings RW, Kilpatrick SJ, Bratton BJ, Harrison MR. Maternal fertility is not affected by fetal surgery. Fetal Diagn and Ther 1999;14:190–2. (Level III)

81. Mazzola CA, Albright AL, Sutton LN, Tuite GF, Hamilton RL, Pollack IF. Dermoid inclusion cysts and early spinal cord tethering after fetal surgery for myelomeningocele. N Engl J Med 2002;347:256–9. (Level III)

The MEDLINE database, the Cochrane Library, and ACOG's own internal resources and documents were used to conduct a literature search to locate relevant articles published between January 1985 and January 2003. The search was restricted to articles published in the English language. Priority was given to articles reporting results of original research, although review articles and commentaries also were consulted. Abstracts of research presented at symposia and scientific conferences were not considered adequate for inclusion in this document. Guidelines published by organizations or institutions such as the National Institutes of Health and the American College of Obstetricians and Gynecologists were reviewed, and additional studies were located by reviewing bibliographies of identified articles. When reliable research was not available, expert opinions from obstetrician–gynecologists were used.

Studies were reviewed and evaluated for quality according to the method outlined by the U.S. Preventive Services Task Force:

I Evidence obtained from at least one properly designed randomized controlled trial.

II-1 Evidence obtained from well-designed controlled trials without randomization.

II-2 Evidence obtained from well-designed cohort or case–control analytic studies, preferably from more than one center or research group.

II-3 Evidence obtained from multiple time series with or without the intervention. Dramatic results in uncontrolled experiments also could be regarded as this type of evidence.

III Opinions of respected authorities, based on clinical experience, descriptive studies, or reports of expert committees.

Based on the highest level of evidence found in the data, recommendations are provided and graded according to the following categories:

Level A—Recommendations are based on good and consistent scientific evidence.

Level B—Recommendations are based on limited or inconsistent scientific evidence.

Level C—Recommendations are based primarily on consensus and expert opinion.

ISSN 1099-3630

**The American College of Obstetricians and Gynecologists
409 12th Street, SW, PO Box 96920
Washington, DC 20090-6920**

12345/76543

Neural tube defects. ACOG Practice Bulletin No. 44. American College of Obstetricians and Gynecologists. Obstet Gynecol 2003; 102:203–13.

ACOG PRACTICE BULLETIN

CLINICAL MANAGEMENT GUIDELINES FOR
OBSTETRICIAN–GYNECOLOGISTS
NUMBER 36, JULY 2002

This Practice Bulletin was developed by the ACOG Committee on Practice Bulletins—Obstetrics with the assistance of Laura M. Goetzl, MD, MPH. The information is designed to aid practitioners in making decisions about appropriate obstetric and gynecologic care. These guidelines should not be construed as dictating an exclusive course of treatment or procedure. Variations in practice may be warranted based on the needs of the individual patient, resources, and limitations unique to the institution or type of practice.

Obstetric Analgesia and Anesthesia

Labor results in severe pain for many women. There is no other circumstance in which it is considered acceptable for a person to experience untreated severe pain, amenable to safe intervention, while under a physician's care. In the absence of a medical contraindication, maternal request is a sufficient medical indication for pain relief during labor. Pain management should be provided whenever it is medically indicated. The purpose of this document is to help obstetrician–gynecologists understand the available methods of pain relief to facilitate communication with their colleagues in the field of anesthesia, thereby, optimizing patient comfort while minimizing the potential for maternal and neonatal morbidity and mortality.

Background

Labor Pain

Uterine contractions and cervical dilation result in visceral pain (T-10 through L-1). As labor progresses, the descent of the fetal head and subsequent pressure on the pelvic floor, vagina, and perineum generate somatic pain transmitted by the pudendal nerve (S2–4). Ideally, methods of obstetric pain relief will ameliorate both sources of pain in the patient in labor.

Available Methods of Anesthesia and Analgesia

Parenteral

Various opioid agonists and opioid agonist–antagonists are available for systemic analgesia (Table 1). These agents can be given in intermittent doses on patient request or via patient-controlled administration. Recent reports suggest that the analgesic effect of parenteral agents used in labor is limited, and the primary mechanism of action is heavy sedation (1). In randomized trials compar-

Table 1. Parenteral Agents for Labor Pain

Agent	Usual Dose	Frequency	Onset	Neonatal Half-Life
Meperidine	25–50 mg (IV)	Q 1–2 h	5 min (IV)	13–22.4 h
	50–100 mg (IM)	Q 2–4 h	30–45 min (IM)	63 h for active metabolites
Fentanyl	50–100 µg (IV)	Q 1 h	1 min	5.3 h
Nalbuphine	10 mg (IV or IM)	Q 3 h	2–3 min (IV)	4.1 h
			15 min (IM)	
Butorphanol	1–2 mg (IV or IM)	Q 4 h	1–2 min (IV)	Not known
			10–30 min (IM)	Similar to nalbuphine in adults
Morphine	2–5 mg (IV)	Q 4 h	5 min (IV)	7.1 h
	10 mg (IM)		30–40 min (IM)	

Abbreviations: IM, intramuscularly; IV, intravenously; Q, every.

Data from Lieberman BA, Rosenblatt DB, Belsey E, Packer M, Redshaw M, Mills M, et al. The effects of maternally administered pethidine or epidural bupivacaine on the fetus and newborn. B J Obstet Gynaecol 1979;86:598–606; Koehntop DE, Rodman JH, Brundage DM, Hegland MG, Buckley JJ. Pharmacokinetics of fentanyl in neonates. Anesth Analg 1986;65:227–232; Kuhnert BR, Kuhnert PM, Philipson EH, Syracuse CD. Disposition of meperidine and normeperidine following multiple doses in labor. II. Fetus and neonate. Am J Obstet Gynecol 1985;151:410–415; Nicolle E, Devillier P, Delanoy B, Durand C, Bessard G. Therapeutic monitoring of nalbuphine: transplacental transfer and estimated pharmacokinetics in the neonate. Eur J Clin Pharmacol 1996;49:485–489; Chay PC, Duffy BJ, Walker JS. Pharmacokinetic-pharmacodynamic relationships of morphine in neonates. Clin Pharmacol Ther 1992;51:334–342; Lynn AM, Slattery JT. Morphine pharmacokinetics in early infancy. Anesthesiology 1987;66:136–139

ing intermittent intravenous meperidine (2, 3), intermittent nalbuphine (4, 5), intermittent butorphanol (6), or patient-controlled administration of meperidine (7) with regional analgesia, parenteral agents resulted in significantly higher visual analog pain scores. Except when large doses of meperidine are used via patient-controlled administration (mean dose: 139 mg; 24% >200 mg) (7), administration of parenteral agents results in absent-to-minimal reductions in pain scores (2–6). However, when women receive high doses of meperidine, the number of infants requiring naloxone therapy increases fourfold when compared with women receiving epidural analgesia (7).

Although regional analgesia provides superior pain relief, some women are satisfied with the level of analgesia provided by narcotics when large enough doses are used (7). However, patients exposed to doses of this magnitude are at increased risk of aspiration and respiratory arrest. The use of shorter-acting agents, such as patient-controlled administration of fentanyl, may decrease some of the neonatal risks posed by meperidine. The decision to use parenteral agents to manage labor pain should be made in collaboration with the patient after a careful discussion of the risks and benefits.

The American Society of Anesthesiologists (ASA) and the American College of Obstetricians and Gynecologists (ACOG) have received reports that some third-party payers have denied reimbursement for regional analgesia and anesthesia during labor unless a physician has documented the presence of a "medical indication" for regional analgesia and anesthesia (8). Of the various pharmaco-

logic methods of pain relief during labor and delivery, regional analgesia techniques—spinal, epidural, and combined spinal epidural—are the most flexible, effective, and least depressing to the central nervous system, allowing for an alert, participating woman and an alert neonate. It is the opinion of the ASA and ACOG that third-party payers who provide reimbursement for obstetric services should not deny reimbursement for regional analgesia and anesthesia because of an absence of other medical indications.

Regional Analgesia

In obstetric patients, regional analgesia refers to a partial to complete loss of pain sensation below the T8 to T10 level. In addition, a varying degree of motor blockade may be present, depending on the agents used.

Epidural. Epidural analgesia offers the most effective form of pain relief (2–7) and is used by most women in the United States (9). In most obstetric patients, the primary indication for epidural analgesia is the patient's desire for pain relief. Medical indications for epidural analgesia during labor may include anticipated difficulty in intubation, a history of malignant hyperthermia, selected forms of cardiovascular and respiratory disease, and prevention or treatment of autonomic hyperreflexia in parturients with a high spinal cord lesion. A catheter is placed in the epidural space, allowing for continuous epidural infusion of local anesthetic agents or narcotics. The advantage of this method is that medication can be titrated over the course of labor as needed. In addition, epidural catheters placed for

labor analgesia can be used for cesarean delivery or postpartum tubal ligation. Modern epidural preparations that combine a low-dose local anesthetic, such as bupivacaine, levobupivacaine, or ropivacaine, with an opioid agonist are preferred because they decrease motor blockade and result in an increased rate of spontaneous vaginal delivery (10). Some women who receive epidural analgesia may be candidates for ambulation.

Spinal. Single-shot spinal analgesia provides excellent pain relief for procedures of limited duration, such as cesarean delivery, the second stage of labor, rapidly progressing labor, and postpartum tubal ligation. A long-acting local anesthetic often is used, with or without an opioid agonist. The duration of anesthesia is approximately 30–250 minutes depending on the drugs used (11). However, because of its inability to extend the duration of action, single-shot spinal analgesia is of limited use for the management of labor.

Combined Spinal Epidural. Combined spinal epidural offers the rapid onset of spinal analgesia combined with the ability to use the epidural catheter to prolong the duration of analgesia with a continuous epidural infusion for labor, to convert to anesthesia for cesarean delivery, or to provide postcesarean delivery pain control. This method of obstetric analgesia is increasing in popularity, especially with the advent of needle-through-needle techniques that eliminate the need for more than one skin puncture. In addition, the use of newer "atraumatic" spinal needles is associated with a dramatically decreased risk of spinal headache (12). The spinal component of combined spinal epidural may be an intrathecal narcotic plus a small amount of a local anesthetic. In one randomized, prospective study, intrathecal use of the short-acting, lipid-soluble narcotic sufentanil was associated with a small but increased incidence of profound fetal bradycardia within 60 minutes of the administration of the combined spinal epidural and an increased risk of cesarean delivery for nonreassuring fetal status (13). Emergency cesarean delivery for fetal bradycardia also occurred in 1.5% of cases in which combined spinal epidural was used, compared with none in cases using only epidural analgesia; the outcomes were the same in both groups. Increased fetal bradycardia after the use of intrathecal fentanyl also was seen in a retrospective study (14) but it was not significant because of the small sample size of the study. Failure of the spinal component occurs at a rate of 4% with combined spinal epidural (12, 15), but the block can be supplemented with the epidural catheter.

Side Effects of Regional Analgesia. Common side effects of regional analgesia are described in Table 2. The most common side effect is hypotension, which cannot be wholly prevented with prehydration with crystalloid or the use of prophylactic ephedrine (16, 17). It is common practice, however, to prehydrate women with 500–1,000 mL of nonglucose-containing isotonic crystalloid. Uterine perfusion also should be maximized at the time of cesarean delivery by maintaining left uterine displacement before delivery. Although prophylactic ephedrine is not commonly administered before epidural analgesia for labor pain, obstetrician–gynecologists should be prepared for the frequent occurrence of hypotension that should be treated with intravenous ephedrine to prevent decreased uterine perfusion. There is a reported 8% incidence of transient fetal heart rate deceleration, which often is related to epidural analgesia and is responsive to conservative management techniques, such as hydration, discontinuation of the epidural infusion, repositioning the woman so she is lying on her side, administration of oxygen, or administration of ephedrine (14).

Postdural puncture headache is possible with spinal analgesia but also can occur with combined spinal epidural and epidural analgesia (12, 15). Early conservative therapy for headache includes analgesics, supine positioning, and hydration. However, in 36% of cases, postdural puncture headache after spinal or combined spinal epidural is severe enough to require an autologous epidural blood patch (12). This rate is higher after unanticipated dural puncture during epidural analgesia (wet tap) because of the larger needle size. The initial blood patch procedure is approximately 61–75% effective in the treatment of postdural puncture headache (18, 19).

Transient neurologic symptoms—painful sensations in the buttocks or lower extremities—can occur with spinal anesthesia, although the incidence is low, occurring in approximately 3–7% of cases (20). Pruritus is extremely common after intrathecal or epidural opioids but it can be treated, as needed, with either naloxone or nalbuphine (10, 21). Approximately 10% of patients will have inadequate anesthesia with an epidural block but this often can be managed with further epidural boluses (22). Because a portion of an epidural narcotic enters the systemic circulation, close attention to the patient's total narcotic dosage over the course of parturition is important. Total spinal blockade, epidural or spinal hematoma, abscess, and neurotoxicity are all rare complications of regional analgesia. Fever (temperature >100.4°F) is one of the most common side effects of epidural analgesia; it occured in 24% of nulliparous women randomized to epidural analgesia compared with 5% of nulliparous women receiving parenteral narcotics (23). Although the overall risk of fever in multiparous women is not significantly higher than in controls (4% versus 3%), the risk of fever increases with the duration of labor; therefore, multiparous women who experience prolonged labor are at increased risk (23, 24).

Table 2. Complications of Regional Analgesia

Complication	Incidence (%)
Hypotension (in prehydrated women undergoing cesarean delivery)	
Spinal	25–67[1,2]
Epidural (in prehydrated women in labor)	28–31[3–5]
Epidural	8.5–9[6,7]
Fever >100.4° (excess rate over women treated with narcotics)	
Nulliparous women	19[8]
Multiparous women	1[8]
Postdural puncture headache	
Spinal	1.5–3[9,10]
Epidural	2[11]
Combined spinal epidural	1–2.77[11–13]
Transient fetal heart decelerations	8[14]
Pruritus (with added opioid only)	
Epidural	1.3–26[11,15]
Spinal and combined spinal epidural	41–85[16,17,11,18]
Inadequate pain relief: epidural	9–15[19,6]

[1]Vercauteren MP, Coppejans HC, Hoffmann VH, Mertens E, Adriaensen HA. Prevention of hypotension by a single 5-mg dose of ephedrine during small-dose spinal anesthesia in prehydrated cesarean delivery patients. Anesth Analg 2000;90:324–327

[2]Park GE, Hauch MA, Curlin F, Datta S, Bader AM. The effects of varying volumes of crystalloid administration before cesarean delivery on maternal hemodynamics and colloid osmotic pressure. Anesth Analg 1996;83:299–303

[3]Fong J, Gurewitsch ED, Press RA, Gomillion MC, Volpe L. Prevention of maternal hypotension by epidural administration of ephedrine sulfate during lumbar epidural anesthesia for cesarean section. Am J Obstet Gynecol 1996;175:985–990

[4]Sharma SK, Sidawi JE, Ramin SM, Lucas MJ, Leveno KJ, Cunningham FG. Cesarean delivery: a randomized trial of epidural versus patient-controlled meperidine analgesia during labor. Anesthesiology 1997;87:487–494

[5]Brizgys RV, Dailey PA, Shnider SM, Kotelko DM, Levinson G. The incidence and neonatal effects of maternal hypotension during epidural anesthesia for cesarean section. Anesthesiology 1987;67:782–786

[6]Eberle RL, Norris MC, Eberle AM, Naulty JS, Arkoosh VA. The effect of maternal position on fetal heart rate during epidural or intrathecal labor analgesia. Am J Obstet Gynecol 1998;179:150–155

[7]Collis RE, Davies DW, Aveling W. Randomized comparison of combined spinal-epidural and standard epidural analgesia in labour. Lancet 1995;345:1413–1416

[8]Philip J, Alexander JM, Sharma SK, Leveno KJ, McIntire DD, Wiley J. Epidural analgesia during labor and maternal fever. Anesthesiology 1999;90:1271–1275

[9]Sears DH, Leeman MI, Jassy LJ, O'Donnell LA, Allen SG, Reisner LS. The frequency of postdural puncture headache in obstetric patients: a prospective study comparing the 24-gauge versus the 22-gauge Sprotte needle. J Clin Anesth 1994;6:42–46

[10]Vallejo MC, Mandell GL, Sabo DP, Ramanathan S. Postdural puncture headache: a randomized comparison of five spinal needles in obstetric patients. Anesth Analg 2000;91:916–920

[11]Norris MC, Grieco WM, Borkowski M, Leighton BL, Arkoosh VA, Huffnagle HJ, et al. Complications of labor analgesia: epidural versus combined spinal epidural techniques. Anesth Analg 1994;79:529–537

[12]Collis RE, Plaat FS, Morgan BM. Comparison of midwife top-ups, continuous infusion and patient-controlled epidural analgesia for maintaining mobility after a low-dose combined spinal-epidural. Br J Anaesth 1999;82:233–236

[13]Herbstman CH, Jaffee JB, Tuman KJ, Newman LM. An in vivo evaluation of four spinal needles used for the combined spinal-epidural technique. Anesth Analg 1998;86:520–522

[14]Palmer CM, Maciulla JE, Cork RC, Nogami WM, Gossler K, Alves D. The incidence of fetal heart rate changes after intrathecal fentanyl labor analgesia. Anesth Analg 1999;88:577–581

[15]Vertommen JD, Vandermeulen E, Van Aken H, Vaes L, Soetens M, Van Steenberge A, et al. The effects of the addition of sufentanil to 0.125% bupivacaine on the quality of analgesia during labor and on the incidence of instrumental deliveries. Anesthesiology 1991;74:809–814

[16]Gambling DR, Sharma SK, Ramin SM, Lucas MJ, Leveno KJ, Wiley J, et al. A randomized study of combined spinal-epidural analgesia versus intravenous meperidine during labor: impact on cesarean delivery rate. Anesthesiology 1998;89:1336–1344

[17]Dahl JB, Jeppesen IS, Jorgensen H, Wetterslev J, Moiniche S. Intraoperative and postoperative analgesic efficacy and adverse effects of intrathecal opioids in patients undergoing cesarean section with spinal anesthesia: a qualitative and quantitative systematic review of randomized controlled trials. Anesthesiology 1999;91:1919–1927

[18]Shah MK, Sia AT, Chong JL. The effect of the addition of ropivacaine or bupivacaine upon pruritus induced by intrathecal fentanyl in labour. Anaesthesia 2000;55:1008–1013

[19]Beilin Y, Zahn J, Bernstein HH, Zucker-Pinchoff B, Zenzen WJ, Andres LA. Treatment of incomplete analgesia after placement of an epidural catheter and administration of local anesthetic for women in labor. Anesthesiology 1998;88:1502–1506

General Anesthesia

Because general anesthesia results in a loss of maternal consciousness, it must be accompanied by airway management by trained anesthesia personnel. Nitrous oxide may be supplemented with halogenated hydrocarbons, such as isoflurane, desflurane, and sevoflurane, at low concentrations. The use of intravenous agents, such as sodium pentothal, followed by rapid sequence induction is used to minimize the risk of aspiration. All inhaled anesthetic agents readily cross the placenta and have been associated with neonatal depression. Ideally, induction-to-delivery time should be minimized when general anesthesia is used. One study reported that fetal exposure of more than 8 minutes was associated with increased neonatal depression (25).

Halogenated agents are potent uterine relaxants when administered in high inhalation concentrations. This property can be useful to obstetricians in circumstances in which uterine relaxation is desirable, such as management of uterine inversion, internal podalic version, or fetal entrapment (either during vaginal or cesarean delivery), although intravenous nitroglycerin and terbutaline may achieve the same goal with fewer side effects. Increased uterine relaxation, however, is a concern because of its potential for increasing blood loss during cesarean delivery. Although some investigators have reported increased blood loss (26), especially with higher dosages (27), others have found no increased risk when women at high risk were excluded (28).

Local

Various local anesthetic agents are available for local infiltration of the perineum and vagina to provide analgesia before episiotomy and during repair of lacerations. Common rapidly acting agents include lidocaine (1–2%) and 2-chloroprocaine (1–3%), which provide local anesthesia for a duration of 20–40 minutes. Toxic effects of local anesthetic agents are rare and include seizures, hypotension, and cardiac arrhythmias. Toxicity is highest with intravascular injection; therefore, it is critical to aspirate for blood before injecting a local anesthetic into the vascular tissues of the vagina and perineum. The total dosage of plain lidocaine should not exceed the recommended dosage because of the increased incidence of lidocaine toxicity.

Local anesthetic agents also can be used by an obstetrician–gynecologist to perform a pudendal block (a type of regional block), an adequate form of temporary pain relief that can aid outlet operative vaginal deliveries in women not using regional analgesia. Complications from pudendal block include intravascular injection of anesthetic agents, hematoma, and infection. Paracervical blocks have been strongly associated with fetal bradycardia (29).

Infiltration of local anesthesia, although time consuming, has been used for cesarean delivery in rare circumstances when adequate general or regional anesthesia is unavailable (30). In slightly more common but still rare situations, practitioners have initiated a cesarean delivery under local anesthesia until the regional anesthesia has taken effect.

Maternal Mortality

Complications of anesthesia remain an important and often preventable cause of pregnancy-related mortality (31), accounting for more than 5% of maternal deaths (32). Anesthesia-related maternal mortality has decreased with time and is currently estimated at 1.7 per 1,000,000 live births (33). The removal from the market of 0.75% bupivacaine by the U.S. Food and Drug Administration in 1984 coupled with the increase in popularity of fractionated dosing of local anesthetics led to a sharp decrease in deaths from local anesthetic toxicity. The increased safety of regional analgesia has increased the relative risk of general anesthesia; the case fatality rate of general anesthesia for cesarean delivery is estimated to be approximately 32 per 1,000,000 live births compared with 1.9 per 1,000,000 live births for regional anesthesia (33). Failed intubation occurs in 1 out of 250 cases of general anesthesia administered to pregnant patients (34). This rate is approximately 10-fold higher than it is in the nonpregnant population. The significant added morbidity of general anesthesia over regional anesthesia for cesarean delivery suggests that regional anesthesia is the preferred method of pain control and should be used unless a contraindication to regional anesthesia is present (see box). Although general anesthesia may be indicated in some cases of fetal heart rate abnormality, the severity of the abnormality should be considered before incurring the excess risk of maternal mortality associated with general anesthesia. In patients with an increased risk of urgent cesarean delivery (eg, severe intrauterine growth restriction), it is reasonable to encourage early regional analgesia during labor. This approach has the potential benefit of reducing the need for emergent general anesthesia and its attendant risks.

Absolute Contraindications to Regional Anesthesia

- Refractory maternal hypotension
- Maternal coagulopathy
- Maternal use of once-daily dose of low-molecular-weight heparin within 12 hours
- Untreated maternal bacteremia
- Skin infection over site of needle placement
- Increased intracranial pressure caused by a mass lesion

Clinical Considerations and Recommendations

▶ *What factors should be considered in the choice of parenteral agent for labor pain?*

Historically, meperidine has been the most widely used systemic opioid. However, the use of drugs in the opioid agonist–antagonist class has become more popular because they are associated with less nausea and vomiting (35, 36) and respiratory depression is less likely, even when higher doses of nalbuphine are used (37). Conversely, nalbuphine has been associated with increased maternal sedation (35, 36). Fentanyl also has been used during labor as an alternative drug because of its relatively short half-life; it is associated with significantly less nausea, vomiting, and sedation than meperidine (38). Butorphanol may increase blood pressure levels and should be avoided in patients with chronic hypertension or preeclampsia (39).

There is significant transplacental passage of all parenteral drugs. A recent meta-analysis of several randomized trials revealed that parenteral analgesia is associated with a twofold to threefold increased risk of Apgar scores lower than 7 at 5 minutes and a fourfold increased need for neonatal naloxone (40), although the overall incidence of both was low. Although most neonatal depression is short-lived and can be treated as needed with naloxone, the long neonatal half-life of normeperidine (63 hours), an active metabolite of meperidine, has raised concerns regarding the prolonged duration of neonatal sedation following the administration of parenteral meperidine during labor (41, 42). Infants exposed to meperidine during labor demonstrate dose-dependent neurobehavioral depression that can be demonstrated on day 2 (43) and day 3 (44, 45) of life. Unlike other parenteral drugs, the neonatal effects of meperidine increase with a prolonged drug-to-delivery interval because of the accumulation of normeperidine (44, 45). Neonates exposed to transplacental nalbuphine are demonstrated to have a decreased response to sound and decreased tone and alertness for more than 24 hours after birth (35). Fentanyl also crosses the placenta but has not been associated with neonatal neurobehavioral depression (38).

All parenteral drugs can have a significant effect on intrapartum fetal heart rate tracing. Meperidine (46, 47), fentanyl (38), and nalbuphine (48) have all been associated with decreased heart rate variability. Nalbuphine and fentanyl also have been associated with transient sinusoidal fetal heart rate tracings (49, 50). Caution should be used in administering these drugs in the setting of diminished short- or long-term fetal heart rate variability. Naloxone is a pure opioid antagonist that is the drug of choice in the treatment of maternal respiratory and neurobehavioral depression secondary to opioid agonist drugs. Studies have suggested that naloxone may be associated with neonatal withdrawal seizures, especially in women who are opioid dependent (51). Because it is a pure antagonist, it does not cause additional respiratory depression. Naloxone should be given intravenously when possible; intramuscular or subcutaneous administration may delay absorption in the neonate who is stressed and vasoconstricted. Because naloxone has a relatively short duration of action, it may be necessary to repeat the dose.

▶ *What is the role of patient-controlled epidural analgesia during labor?*

The goal of epidural analgesia is to provide satisfactory pain control for labor with the lowest dose of analgesic drugs needed to minimize motor blockade and simultaneously reduce the potential side effects of epidural analgesia during the course of labor. Patient-controlled epidural analgesia provides pain control similar to that of standard epidural analgesia (52–54). Intermittent bolus patient-controlled epidural analgesia results in lower total dosages of anesthetic agents than continuous infusion epidural (52, 53, 55) and results in less motor blockade (53). When compared with practitioner-administered intermittent bolus techniques, some studies have found an increased use of anesthetic agents with patient-controlled epidural analgesia (53), while others have found no difference (55, 56). Motor blockade appears to be similar between patient-controlled epidural analgesia and intermittent bolus epidural analgesia (53, 54). Patient-controlled epidural analgesia is an acceptable alternative method of labor analgesia but does not appear to have additional benefits over standard epidural techniques. Patient satisfaction with all epidural techniques is high and is not significantly improved with patient-controlled epidural analgesia in most studies (53–55).

▶ *Is chronic back pain associated with epidural use?*

Retrospective studies have found an association between epidural analgesia and chronic back pain (57–59). One proposed explanation is that motor block of the lower back and legs leads to prolonged periods of poor posture and decreased perception of muscle strain. However, retrospective studies are plagued by recall bias and patients' perceptions of an association between epidural analgesia and chronic back pain. Prospective cohort studies and one small, randomized controlled trial have found no significant association between epidural analgesia and chronic back pain (60–62).

▶ *What is the effect of epidural analgesia on maternal fever?*

No well-designed, randomized trial has specifically addressed the issue of epidural-associated fever. However, studies in which women were randomized to receive epidural analgesia or parenteral drugs for other objectives have consistently shown an increased rate of fever in the epidural group (2, 7, 23). In three randomized studies with mixed populations of nulliparous and multiparous women, the relative risk for fever in the epidural group was between 4.0 and 4.6 (2, 7, 23). In the one randomized study in which logistic regression was performed to control for potential confounders, the risk of fever in the population receiving epidural was four-fold higher (95% confidence interval, 2.0–7.7) (23).

The mechanism for fever is not known. Theories include thermoregulation and chorioamnionitis. In one study, placental inflammation was more common with epidural analgesia (63). Epidural-related fever is not benign. Although there is no increased risk of neonatal sepsis, there is a statistically significant increase in neonatal sepsis evaluations (23, 24). Epidural-related fever results in a statistically significant risk of maternal antibiotic treatment (64, 65) and a statistically significant increase in neonatal antibiotic treatment (23).

▶ *Does epidural analgesia increase the rate of operative delivery?*

Although neuraxial techniques (epidural, spinal, and combined spinal epidural) provide the most effective and least depressant analgesia for labor, the question of whether their use is associated with an increased risk of cesarean delivery remains controversial. Several randomized prospective studies have shown an increased risk of cesarean delivery with epidural analgesia (2, 3), while others have shown no increased risk with epidural analgesia (7) or combined spinal epidural analgesia (13). Limitations to analysis of these studies include high crossover rates between study populations, substantial bias, and small numbers of patients.

Less controversial is the causal role epidural analgesia plays in prolonging labor by 40–90 minutes (2, 7, 13, 40) and in the approximate twofold increased need for oxytocin augmentation (3, 7). These findings are supported by most prospective studies as well as meta-analysis (40, 59). An increased risk of a second stage of labor longer than 2 hours (2, 13) in women with epidural analgesia likely contributes to the higher rates of operative vaginal delivery seen in most prospective studies. The four best prospective studies, in which elective forceps use was not permitted (2, 3, 7, 13), yielded a combined relative risk of 1.9 (95% confidence interval,

1.4–2.5) of forceps delivery in women who received epidural analgesia. Some investigators have found a decreased risk of operative delivery with combined spinal epidural when compared with low-dose epidural (66). This finding is difficult to interpret, because elective forceps were not excluded in this study, and the rate of forceps use was high (28–40%). Excessive operative vaginal deliveries have been implicated in the increased rate of third- and fourth-degree lacerations seen in women with epidural analgesia (67).

▶ *What is the effect of the timing of epidural analgesia on the course of labor and the risk of cesarean delivery?*

Reports regarding the effect of the timing of epidural analgesia on the course of labor offer conflicting results. Several retrospective studies have shown an increased risk of cesarean delivery in nulliparous women in whom epidural analgesia was administered before cervical dilatation of 4 cm (68) or 5 cm (69). Another retrospective study found an increased risk of cesarean delivery with higher station at epidural placement—but not related to cervical dilatation—after using logistic regression to control for potential confounders (70). A prospective trial comparing laboring women who were randomized to either an epidural group or an intravenous meperidine group, reported a 25% cesarean delivery rate in the epidural group and a 2.2% cesarean delivery rate in the narcotic group ($P<0.05$) (3). Limitations of this study included the small number of patients randomized in each group, as well as the small number of patients who required cesarean delivery. Another prospective randomized trial of 334 nulliparous women found no difference in the cesarean delivery rate for early (10%) compared with late (8%) epidural placement (4). This study was limited by only a small difference in timing and cervical dilatation between both groups, a median of 4 cm cervical dilatation for early administration and 5 cm for late administration. Other studies have shown conflicting results, and further studies are needed to identify whether early placement of epidural analgesia significantly increases the risk of cesarean delivery and to prospectively determine the risk at each level of cervical dilatation.

At this time, it appears to be possible that very early placement of epidural analgesia may increase the risk of cesarean delivery and that the risk decreases with delayed epidural placement. After weighing this conflicting data, the ACOG Task Force on Cesarean Delivery Rates recommended that, when feasible, obstetric practitioners should delay the administration of epidural analgesia in nulliparous women until cervical dilatation reaches 4–5 cm and that other forms of analgesia be used until that time (71). However, 4 cm of dilatation is an arbitrary cutoff because decreased risk with increased cervical dilatation is a continuum. Therefore, the decision of when to place epidural analgesia should be made individually with each patient, with other factors, such as parity, taken into consideration. Women in labor should not be required to reach 4–5 cm of cervical dilatation before receiving epidural analgesia.

▶ *How can the risks of epidural or spinal hematoma be minimized?*

Epidural or spinal hematoma is a rare but morbid complication of regional analgesia. Patients at higher risk include those with underlying bleeding dyscrasias or thrombocytopenia and those taking medications that may affect coagulation. Although it is not necessary to obtain a platelet count before using regional analgesia in healthy women experiencing normal labor (72), certain groups of patients may benefit from such evaluations, including those with severe preeclampsia, idiopathic thrombocytopenic purpura, known placental abruption, or other risk factors for disseminated intravascular coagulation.

Most anesthesiologists will administer regional analgesia to a patient with a platelet count higher than 100,000/μL. However, the management of patients with platelet counts lower than 100,000/μL is controversial. Several studies reported no complications in women who received epidural analgesia with platelet counts between 50,000–99,000/μL (73–75).

Patients who are taking anticoagulants also are at risk for epidural or spinal hematoma. Patients on unfractionated heparin therapy should be able to receive regional analgesia if they have a normal activated partial thromboplastin time (aPTT). Patients taking prophylactic doses of unfractionated heparin or low-dose aspirin are not at increased risk (76, 77) and can be offered regional analgesia. Low-molecular-weight heparin has been associated with multiple case reports of epidural and spinal hematoma, and the U.S. Food and Drug Administration has issued a public health advisory on this issue (78). Low-molecular-weight heparin has a longer half-life than standard heparin, and its anticoagulant activity is not reflected in the aPTT. In patients receiving once-daily, low-dose low-molecular-weight heparin, regional anesthesia should not be offered until 12 hours after the last injection of low-molecular-weight heparin (79). In addition, low-molecular-weight heparin should be withheld for at least 2 hours after the removal of an epidural catheter. The safety of regional analgesia in patients receiving twice-daily low-molecular-weight heparin has not been studied sufficiently, and it is not known whether delaying regional analgesia for 24 hours after the last injection is adequate. Because the onset of labor often is difficult to predict, it may be reasonable to convert patients to unfractionated heparin as they approach term.

▶ *How does preeclampsia influence the choice of analgesia or anesthesia?*

Regional anesthesia is preferred for women with preeclampsia and eclampsia—both for labor and delivery (80). A secondary analysis of women with severe preeclampsia in the National Institute of Child Health and Human Development's Maternal–Fetal Medicine Units Network trial of low-dose aspirin reported epidural anesthesia was not associated with an increased rate of cesarean delivery, pulmonary edema, or renal failure (81). Moreover, general anesthesia carries more risk to pregnant women than does regional anesthesia (33).

Regional analgesia in women with preeclampsia is associated with an overall 15–25% reduction in systemic mean arterial pressure (82–84). Although the peripheral vasodilation seen with regional analgesia may be helpful in decreasing severe hypertension, hypotension that requires cautious treatment with ephedrine may occur (83, 84). In addition, prehydration with crystalloid combined with intraoperative fluid boluses for hypotension results in an average additional fluid challenge of 600–800 mL in women with preeclampsia receiving regional analgesia (82, 84).

▶ *How can the risk of maternal aspiration be minimized?*

There is insufficient evidence to address the safest level of maternal oral intake during labor. The ASA Task Force on Obstetric Anesthesia recommends allowing a modest intake of clear liquids in patients experiencing normal labor (72). However, a fasting period of 6–8 hours for solids is preferable before elective cesarean delivery.

For both elective and indicated cesarean delivery, agents to decrease gastric acidity should be used. Sodium citrate with citric acid has been shown to neutralize the gastric contents of 88.5% of women undergoing cesarean delivery (85) and should be administered when the decision is made to perform cesarean delivery.

▶ *What are the potential negative effects of analgesia and anesthesia on breastfeeding?*

Although it is clear that both maternally administered opioids and local anesthetics used either parenterally

(45, 86) or in epidural analgesia (87–89) enter the fetal bloodstream, the effects on breastfeeding have not been well studied. Intrapartum opioid use may decrease neonatal rooting reflexes and delay initiation of breastfeeding (86, 90); however, there is limited evidence that these delays affect the ultimate success of breastfeeding. Few studies have examined the more clinically relevant outcomes of short- or long-term breastfeeding success. More recently, a study that controlled for potential confounders found no relationship between either parenteral opioids or epidural analgesia and breastfeeding success of neonates at age 6 weeks (91).

Postdelivery analgesia also has the potential to affect breastfeeding success because of the ongoing delivery of narcotics to breast milk (41). Postcesarean patient-controlled analgesia with morphine results in less neurobehavioral depression than meperidine (42), possibly because of the accumulation of the slowly metabolized active metabolite of meperidine (normeperidine) in the neonatal bloodstream. Postoperative analgesia via the epidural route decreases maternal opioid requirements (42). Additionally, continuous bupivacaine epidural analgesia results in significantly increased milk production and greater infant weight gain when compared with diclofenac suppositories alone for postcesarean pain management (92). Further studies are needed to address the effect of postoperative pain control on breastfeeding success, milk production, and infant weight gain.

▶ *What are the optimal agents for postoperative analgesia?*

Opioid therapy is the mainstay of postoperative pain management. Various routes of administration are available, including intravenous, intrathecal, and epidural (with or without local anesthetics). For patients undergoing cesarean delivery with spinal or epidural anesthesia, the most cost-effective regimen of pain management for the first 24 hours is preservative-free morphine hydrochloride placed in the intrathecal space at the time of the initial spinal anesthesia (93, 94) or after delivery when using epidural anesthesia. This method provides effective pain control in the first 12–24 hours following cesarean delivery (95, 96) without the added cost associated with an infusion pump. Initial concerns regarding the possibility of delayed respiratory depression with intrathecal morphine have led to a lowering of the standard dosage to 100–250 µg (95–98).

In patients undergoing cesarean delivery under epidural anesthesia, patient-controlled epidural analgesia for the first 24 hours is a reasonable choice. This strategy minimizes the dosage of maternally administered opioids (99, 100) and maternal sedation (99) compared with intravenously administered opioids (patient-controlled administration) and uses the preexisting catheter. Although patient-controlled epidural analgesia using a combination of opioid and local anesthesia reduces the cumulative opioid dosage, it results in increased motor weakness (101, 102), which may inhibit patient mobilization. Even low concentrations of local anesthesia result in significant motor weakness and can make ambulation difficult in up to 43% of patients (103). Consideration should be given to removing the epidural catheter after 24 hours to reduce side effects, such as urinary retention (100) pruritus and infection risk, as well as to minimize costs. All intrathecal and epidural opioid administration is accompanied by a dose-dependent, 35–56% incidence of maternal pruritus severe enough to require treatment (104–107). Effective treatment includes intravenous nalbuphine (105, 108, 109), prophylactic oral naltrexone (110), and intravenous ondansetron (111, 112).

In institutions where patient-controlled epidural analgesia is not available or in patients who received general anesthesia intraoperatively, intravenous patient-controlled administration is a reasonable choice because it is associated with increased patient satisfaction (113) and decreased sedation levels compared with intramuscular narcotics (113, 114). Morphine, hydromorphone hydrochloride, and fentanyl are all acceptable drugs for intravenous patient-controlled administration. Meperidine should be avoided because of the accumulation of its slowly metabolized active metabolite normeperidine in the neonate and its subsequent neurobehavioral effects (42).

An important goal of postoperative pain management should be minimizing the cumulative maternal opioid dosage to reduce maternal sedation and neonatal side effects. Maternal nonsteroidal antiinflammatory drugs are useful in achieving this goal and are effective at reducing maternal opioid consumption by 30–39% (115, 116).

▶ *When is it appropriate to obtain an anesthesia consultation?*

Failed intubation and pulmonary aspiration remain the leading causes of anesthesia-related maternal morbidity and mortality (34). Identifying women with risk factors for failed intubation or other complications of anesthesia and referring them for antepartum anesthesia consultation may reduce this risk, although this has not been studied (see box).

Risk Factors that May Prompt Anesthetic Consultation

Anesthetic consultation may be considered when any of the following risk factors are present:

- Marked obesity
- Severe edema or anatomical abnormalities of the face or neck or spine, including trauma or surgery
- Abnormal dentition, small mandible, or difficulty opening the mouth
- Extremely short stature, short neck, or arthritis of the neck
- Goiter
- Serious maternal medical problems, such as cardiac, pulmonary, or neurologic disease
- Bleeding disorders
- Severe preeclampsia
- Previous history of anesthetic complications
- Obstetric complications likely to lead to operative delivery, eg, placenta previa or high-order multiple gestation

American Academy of Pediatrics, American College of Obstetricians and Gynecologists. Guidelines for perinatal care. 4th ed. Elk Grove Village, Illinois: AAP; Washington DC: ACOG, 1997

Summary of Recommendations

The following recommendations are based on good and consistent scientific evidence (Level A):

▶ Regional analgesia provides a superior level of pain relief during labor when compared with systemic drugs and, therefore, should be available to all women.

▶ Parenteral pain medications for labor pain decrease fetal heart rate variability and may limit the obstetrician–gynecologist's ability to interpret the fetal heart rate tracing. Consideration should be given to other drugs in the setting of diminished short- or long-term fetal heart rate variability.

The following recommendations are based on limited or inconsistent scientific evidence (Level B):

▶ Patients with platelet counts of 50,000–100,000/µL may be considered potential candidates for regional analgesia.

▶ Regional analgesia is preferred in women with preeclampsia unless a contraindication to regional analgesia is present.

▶ Breastfeeding does not appear to be affected by the choice of anesthesia; therefore, the choice should be based on other considerations.

The following recommendations are based primarily on consensus and expert opinion (Level C):

▶ It is not necessary to routinely obtain a platelet count before administration of regional analgesia or anesthesia in a pregnant patient without complications.

▶ Clear liquid intake may be allowed in patients in labor without complications.

▶ Sodium citrate should be administered promptly to neutralize gastric contents following the decision to perform a cesarean delivery.

▶ Identifying women with risk factors for failed intubation or other complications of anesthesia and referring them for antepartum anesthesia consultation may reduce this risk.

▶ To avoid respiratory depression, close monitoring of the cumulative narcotic dosage given to a patient antepartum, intrapartum, and postpartum is essential.

▶ The decision of when to place epidural analgesia should be made individually with each patient, with other factors, such as parity, taken into consideration. Women in labor should not be required to reach 4–5 cm of cervical dilatation before receiving epidural analgesia.

References

1. Olofsson C, Ekblom A, Ekman-Ordeberg G, Hjelm A, Irestedt L. Lack of analgesic effect systemically administered morphine or pethidine on labour pain. Br J Obstet Gynaecol 1996;103:968–972 (Level II-1)

2. Ramin SM, Gambling DR, Lucas MJ, Sharma SK, Sidawi JE, Leveno KJ. Randomized trial of epidural versus intravenous analgesia during labor. Obstet Gynecol 1995;86:783–789 (Level I)

3. Thorp JA, Hu DH, Albin RM, McNitt J, Meyer BA, Cohen GR, et al. The effect of intrapartum epidural analgesia on nulliparous labor: a randomized, controlled, prospective trial. Am J Obstet Gynecol 1993;169:851–858 (Level I)

4. Chestnut DH, McGrath JM, Vincent RD Jr, Penning DH, Choi WW, Bates JN, et al. Does early administration of epidural analgesia affect obstetric outcome in nulliparous women who are in spontaneous labor? Anesthesiology 1994;80:1201–1208 (Level I)

5. Chestnut DH, Vincent RD Jr, McGrath JM, Choi WW, Bates JN. Does early administration of epidural analgesia

affect obstetric outcome in nulliparous women who are receiving intravenous oxytocin? Anesthesiology 1994;80: 1193–2000 (Level I)

6. Bofill JA, Vincent RD, Ross EL, Martin RW, Norman PF, Werhan CF, et al. Nulliparous active labor, epidural analgesia, and cesarean delivery for dystocia. Am J Obstet Gynecol 1997;177:1465–1470 (Level I)

7. Sharma SK, Sidawi JE, Ramin SM, Lucas MJ, Leveno KJ, Cunningham FG. Cesarean delivery: a randomized trial of epidural versus patient-controlled meperidine analgesia during labor. Anesthesiology 1997;87:487–494 (Level I)

8. American College of Obstetricians and Gynecologists. Pain relief during labor. ACOG Committee Opinion 231. Washington, DC: 2000 (Level III)

9. Hawkins JL, Gibbs CP, Orleans M, Martin-Salvaj G, Beaty B. Obstetric anesthesia workforce survey, 1981 versus 1992. Anesthesiology 1997;87:135–143 (Level II-3)

10. Collis RE, Baxandall ML, Srikantharajah ID, Edge G, Kadim MY, Morgan BM. Combined spinal-epidural (CSE) analgesia: technique, management, and outcome of 300 mothers. Int J Obstet Anesth 1994;3:75–81 (Level III)

11. Yeh HM, Chen LK, Shyu MK, Lin CJ, Sun WZ, Wang MJ, et al. The addition of morphine prolongs fentanyl-bupivacaine spinal analgesia for the relief of labor pain. Anesth Analg 2001;92:665–668 (Level I)

12. Vallejo MC, Mandell GL, Sabo DP, Ramanathan S. Postdural puncture headache: a randomized comparison of five spinal needles in obstetric patients. Anesth Analg 2000;91:916–920 (Level I)

13. Gambling DR, Sharma SK, Ramin SM, Lucas MJ, Leveno KJ, Wiley J, et al. A randomized study of combined spinal-epidural analgesia versus intravenous meperidine during labor: impact on cesarean delivery rate. Anesthesiology 1998;89:1336–1344 (Level I)

14. Palmer CM, Maciulla JE, Cork RC, Nogami WM, Gossler K, Alves D. The incidence of fetal heart rate changes after intrathecal fentanyl labor analgesia. Anesth Analg 1999; 88:577–581 (Level II-3)

15. Herbstman CH, Jaffee JB, Tuman KJ, Newman LM. An in vivo evaluation of four spinal needles used for the combined spinal-epidural technique. Anesth Analg 1998;86: 520–522 (Level II-2)

16. Fong J, Gurewitsch ED, Press RA, Gomillion MC, Volpe L. Prevention of maternal hypotension by epidural administration of ephedrine sulfate during lumbar epidural anesthesia for cesarean section. Am J Obstet Gynecol 1996; 175:985–990 (Level I)

17. Brizgys RV, Dailey PA, Shnider SM, Kotelko DM, Levinson G. The incidence and neonatal effects of maternal hypotension during epidural anesthesia for cesarean section. Anesthesiology 1987;67:782–786 (Level II-2)

18. Duffy PJ, Crosby ET. The epidural blood patch. Resolving the controversies. Can J Anaesth 1999;46:878–886 (Level III)

19. Safa-Tisseront V, Thormann F, Malassine P, Henry M, Riou B, Coriat P, et al. Effectiveness of epidural blood patch in the management of post-dural puncture headache. Anesthesiology 2001;95:334–339 (Level II-2)

20. Philip J, Sharma SK, Gottumukkala VN, Perez BJ, Slaymaker EA, Wiley J. Transient neurologic symptoms after spinal anesthesia with lidocaine in obstetric patients. Anesth Analg 2001;92:405–409 (Level I)

21. Dahl JB, Jeppesen IS, Jorgensen H, Wetterslev J, Moiniche S. Intraoperative and postoperative analgesic efficacy and adverse effects of intrathecal opioids in patients undergoing cesarean section with spinal anesthesia: a qualitative and quantitative systematic review of randomized controlled trials. Anesthesiology 1999;91: 1919–1927 (Level III)

22. Beilin Y, Zahn J, Bernstein HH, Zucker-Pinchoff B, Zenzen WJ, Andres LA. Treatment of incomplete analgesia after placement of an epidural catheter and administration of local anesthetic for women in labor. Anesthesiology 1998;88:1502–1506 (Level I)

23. Philip J, Alexander JM, Sharma SK, Leveno KJ, McIntire DD, Wiley J. Epidural analgesia during labor and maternal fever. Anesthesiology 1999;90:1271–1275 (Level I)

24. Lieberman E, Lang JM, Frigoletto F Jr, Richardson DK, Ringer SA, Cohen A. Epidural analgesia, intrapartum fever, and neonatal sepsis evaluation. Pediatrics 1997;99: 415–419 (Level II-2)

25. Datta S, Ostheimer GW, Weiss JB, Brown WU Jr, Alper MH. Neonatal effect of prolonged anesthetic induction for cesarean section. Obstet Gynecol 1981;58:331–335 (Level II-3)

26. Andrews WW, Ramin SM, Maberry MC, Wallace DH, Shearer V, Black S. Effect of type of anesthesia on blood loss at elective repeat cesarean section. Am J Perinatal 1992;9:197–200 (Level II-3)

27. Gilstrap LC 3rd, Hauth JC, Hankins GD, Patterson AR. Effect of type of anesthesia on blood loss at cesarean section. Obstet Gynecol 1987;69:328–332 (Level II-2)

28. Camann WR, Datta S. Red cell use during cesarean delivery. Transfusion 1991;31:12–15 (Level II-3)

29. LeFevre ML. Fetal heart rate pattern and postparacervical fetal bradycardia. Obstet Gynecol 1984;64:343–346 (Level II-2)

30. Cunningham FG, Gant NF, Leveno KJ, Gilstrap LC, Hauth JC, Wenstrom KD. Analgesia and anesthesia. In: Williams obstetrics. 21st ed. New York: McGraw-Hill, 2001:361– 383 (Level III)

31. Koonin LM, MacKay AP, Berg CJ, Atrash HK, Smith JC. Pregnancy-related mortality surveillance—United States, 1987–1990. Mor Mortal Wkly Rep CDC Surveill Summ 1997;46:17–36 (Level II-3)

32. Panchal S, Arria AM, Labhsetwar SA. Maternal mortality during hospital admission for delivery: a retrospective analysis using a state-maintained database. Anesth Analg 2001;93:134–141 (Level II-3)

33. Hawkins JL, Koonin LM, Palmer SK, Gibbs CP. Anesthesia-related deaths during obstetric delivery in the United States, 1979–1990. Anesthesiology 1997;86: 277–284 (Level II-3)

34. Barnardo PD, Jenkins JG. Failed tracheal intubation in obstetrics: a 6-year review in the UK region. Anaesthesia 2000;55:690–694 (Level II-3)

35. Wilson CM, McClean E, Moore J, Dundee JW. A double-blind comparison of intramuscular pethidine and nalbuphine in labour. Anaesthesia 1986;41:1207–1213 (Level I)

36. Dan U, Rabinovici Y, Barkai G, Modan M, Etchin A, Mashinach S. Intravenous pethidine and nalbuphine during labour: a prospective double-blind comparative study. Gynecol Obstet Invest 1991;32:39–43 (Level I)

37. Romagnoli A, Keats AS. Ceiling effect for respiratory depression by nalbuphine. Clin Pharmacol Ther 1980;27:478–485 (Level III)

38. Rayburn WF, Smith CV, Parriot JE, Wood RE. Randomized comparison of merperidine and fentanyl during labor. Obstet Gynecol 1989;74:604–606 (Level I)

39. Stadol. In: Physicians' desk reference. 56th ed. Montvale, New Jersey: Medical Economics Company, 2002:1108–1110 (Level III)

40. Halpern SH, Leighton BL, Ohlsson A, Barrett JF, Rice A. Effect of epidural vs. parenteral opioid analgesia on the progress of labor: a meta-analysis. JAMA 1998;280:2105–2110 (Meta-analysis)

41. Wittels B, Scott DT, Sinatra RS. Exogenous opioids in human breast milk and acute neonatal neurobehaviour: a preliminary study. Anesthesiology 1990;73:864–869 (Level II-3)

42. Wittels B, Glosten B, Faure EA, Moawad AH, Ismail M, Hibbard J, et al. Postcesarean analgesia with both epidural morphine and intravenous patient-controlled analgesia: neurobehavioral outcomes among nursing neonates. Anesth Analg 1997;85:600–606 (Level II-3)

43. Hodgkinson R, Bhatt M, Wang CN. Double-blind comparison of the neurobehaviour of neonates following the administration of different doses of meperidine to the mother. Can Anaesth Soc J 1978;25:405–411 (Level II-3)

44. Kuhnert BR, Kuhnert PM, Philipson EH, Syracuse CD. Disposition of meperidine and normeperidine following multiple doses in labor. II. Fetus and neonate. Am J Obstet Gynecol 1985;151:410–415 (Level III)

45. Kuhnert BR, Linn PL, Kennard MJ, Kuhnert PM. Effects of low doses of meperidine on neonatal behavior. Anesth Analg 1985;64:335–342 (Level II-2)

46. Zimmer EZ, Divon MY, Vadasz A. Influence of meperidine on fetal movements and heart rate beat-to-beat variability in the active phase of labor. Am J Perinatol 1988;5:197–200 (Level II-2)

47. Wheble AM, Dawes GS, Gillmer MD, Sykes GS. A double blind quantitative study of the effects of meptazinol and pethidine on the fetal heart rate in labour. J Obstet Gynaecol 1988;8:248–252 (Level I)

48. Giannina G, Guzman ER, Lai YL, Lake MF, Cernadas M, Vintzileos AM. Comparison of the effects of meperidine and nalbuphine on intrapartum fetal heart rate tracings. Obstet Gynecol 1995;86:441–445 (Level I)

49. Smith CV, Rayburn WF, Allen KV, Bane TM, Livezey GT. Influence of intravenous fentanyl on fetal biophysical parameters during labor. J Matern Fetal Med 1996;5:89–92 (Level II-2)

50. Feinstein SJ, Lodeiro JG, Vintzileos AM, Campbell WA, Montgomery JT, Nochimson DJ. Sinusoidal fetal heart rate pattern after administration of nalbuphine hydrochloride: a case report. Am J Obstet Gynecol 1986;154:159–160 (Level III)

51. Neonatal drug withdrawal. American Academy of Pediatrics Committee on Drugs. Pediatrics 1998;101:1079–1088 [erratum in Pediatrics 1998;102:660] (Level III)

52. Gambling DR, Yu P, Cole C, McMorland GH, Palmer L. A comparative study of patient controlled epidural analgesia (PCEA) and continuous infusion epidural analgesia (CIEA) during labour. Can J Anaesth 1988;35:249–254 (Level I)

53. Collis RE, Plaat FS, Morgan BM. Comparison of midwife top-ups, continuous infusion and patient-controlled epidural analgesia for maintaining mobility after a low-dose combined spinal-epidural. Br J Anaesth 1999;82:233–236 (Level I)

54. Vandermeulen EP, Van Aken H, Vertommen JD. Labor pain relief using bupivacaine and sufentanil: patient controlled epidural analgesia versus intermittent injections. Eur J Obstet Gynecol 1995;59:S47–S54 (Level II-1)

55. Purdie J, Reid J, Thorburn J, Asbury AJ. Continuous extradural analgesia: comparison of midwife top-ups, continuous infusions and patient controlled administration. Br J Anaesth 1992;68:580–584 (Level II-3)

56. Gambling DR, McMorland GH, Yu P, Laszlo C. Comparison of patient-controlled epidural analgesia and conventional intermittent "top up" injections during labor. Anesth Analg 1990;70:256–261 (Level II-3)

57. MacArthur C, Lewis M, Knox EG. Investigation of long term problems after obstetric epidural anaesthesia. BMJ 1992;304:1279–1282 (Level II-2)

58. Russell R, Groves P, Taub N, O'Dowd J, Reynolds F. Assessing long term backache after childbirth. BMJ 1993;306:1299–1303 (Level II-2)

59. Howell CJ. Epidural versus non-epidural analgesia for pain relief in labour. (Cochrane Review). In: The Cochrane Library, Issue 2, 2002. Oxford: Update Software (Meta-analysis)

60. Russell R, Dundas R, Reynolds F. Long term backache after childbirth: prospective search for causative factors. BMJ 1996;312:1384–1388 (Level II-2)

61. Macarthur AJ, Macarthur C, Weeks SK. Is epidural anesthesia in labor associated with chronic low back pain? A prospective cohort study. Anesth Analg 1997;85:1066–1070 (Level II-2)

62. Howell CJ, Kidd C, Roberts W, Upton P, Lucking L, Jones PW, et al. A randomised controlled trial of epidural compared with non-epidural analgesia in labour. BJOG 2001;108:27–33 (Level I)

63. Dashe JS, Rogers BB, McIntire DD, Leveno KJ. Epidural analgesia and intrapartum fever: placental findings. Obstet Gynecol 1999;93:341–344 (Level II-2)

64. Yancey MK, Zhang J, Schwarz J, Dietrich CS 3rd, Klebanoff M. Labor epidural analgesia and intrapartum

maternal hyperthermia. Obstet Gynecol 2001;98:763–770 (Level II-2)

65. Mayer DC, Chescheir NC, Spielman FJ. Increased intrapartum antibiotic administration associated with epidural analgesia in labor. Am J Perinaol 1997;14:83–86 (Level II-3)

66. Nageotte MP, Larson D, Rumney PJ, Sidhu M, Hollenbach K. Epidural analgesia compared with combined spinal-epidural analgesia during labor in nulliparous women. N Engl J Med 1997;337:1715–1719 (Level I)

67. Robinson JN, Norwitz ER, Cohen AP, McElrath TF, Lieberman ES. Epidural Analgesia and third- or fourth-degree lacerations in nulliparas. Obstet Gynecol 1999; 94:259–262 (Level II-2)

68. Thorp JA, Eckert LO, Ang MS, Johnston DA, Peaceman AM, Parisi VM. Epidural analgesia and cesarean section for dystocia: risk factors in nulliparas. Am J Perinatol 1991;8:402–410 (Level II-2)

69. Lieberman E, Lang JM, Cohen A, D'Agostino R Jr, Datta S, Frigoletto FD Jr. Association of epidural analgesia with cesarean delivery in nulliparas. Obstet Gynecol 1996;88: 993–1000 (Level II-2)

70. Traynor JD, Dooley SL, Seyb S, Wong CA, Shadron A. Is the management of epidural analgesia associated with an increased risk of cesarean delivery? Am J Obstet Gynecol 2000;182:1058–1062 (Level II-2)

71. American College of Obstetricians and Gynecologists. Task Force on Cesarean Delivery Rates. Evaluation of cesarean delivery. Washington, DC: ACOG, 2000 (Level III)

72. Practical guidelines for obstetrical anesthesia: a report by the American Society of Anesthesiologists Task Force on Obstetrical Anesthesia. Anesthesiology 1999;90:600–611 (Level III)

73. Beilin Y, Zahn J, Comerford M. Safe epidural analgesia in thirty parturients with platelet counts between 69,000 and 98,000 mm(-3). Anesth Analg 1997;85:385–388 (Level III)

74. Sharma SK, Philip J, Whitten CW, Padakandla UB, Landers DF. Assessment of changes in coagulation in parturients with preeclampsia using thromboelastography. Anesthesiology 1999;90:385–390 (Level II-2)

75. Rasmus KT, Rottman RL, Kotelko DM, Wright WC, Stone JJ, Rosenblatt RM. Unrecognized thrombocytopenia and regional anesthesia in parturients: a retrospective review. Obstet Gynecol 1989;73:943–946 (Level III)

76. Horlocker TT, Wedel DJ, Offord KP. Does preoperative antiplatelet therapy increase the risk of hemorrhagic complications associated with regional anesthesia? Anesth Analg 1990;70:631–634 (Level II-2)

77. Sibai BM, Caritis SN, Thom E, Shaw K, McNellis D. Low-dose aspirin in nulliparous women: safety of continuous epidural block and correlation between bleeding time and maternal-neonatal bleeding complications. National Institute of Child Health and Human Development Maternal-Fetal Medicine Network. Am J Obstet Gynecol 1995;172:1553–1557 (Level II-2)

78. Center for Drug Evaluation and Research. FDA Public Health Advisory: reports of epidural or spinal hematomas with the concurrent use of low molecular weight heparin and spinal/epidural anesthesia or spinal puncture. December 15, 1997. Available at http://www.fda.gov/ medwatch/safety/1997/antico.htm. Retrieved March 8, 2002 (Level III)

79. American Society of Regional Anesthesia and Pain Medicine (ASRA). Recommendations for neuraxial anesthesia and anticoagulation. Richmond, Virginia: ASRA, 1998. Available at http://www.asra.com/items_of_interest/consensus_statements/. Retrieved April 18, 2002 (Level III)

80. Report of the National High Blood Pressure Education Program Working Group on High Blood Pressure in Pregnancy. Am J Obstet Gynecol 2000;183:S1–S22 (Level III)

81. Hogg B, Hauth JC, Caritis SN, Sibai BM, Lindheimer M, Van Dorsten JP, et al. Safety of labor epidural anesthesia for women with severe hypertensive disease. National Institute of Child Health and Human Development Maternal-Fetal Medicine Units Network. Am J Obstet Gynecol 1999;181:1096–1101 (Level II-2)

82. Ramanthan J, Coleman P, Sibai B. Anesthetic modification of homodynamic and neuroendocrine stress responses to cesarean delivery in women with severe preeclampsia. Anesth Analg 1991;73:772–779 (Level II-3)

83. Hood DD, Curry R. Spinal versus epidural anesthesia for cesarean section in severely preeclamptic patients: a retrospective survey. Anesthesiology 1999;90:1276–1282 (Level II-3)

84. Wallace DH, Leveno KJ, Cunningham FG, Giesecke AH, Shearer VE, Sidawi JE. Randomized comparison of general and regional anesthesia for cesarean delivery in pregnancies complicated by severe preeclampsia. Obstet Gynecol 1995;86:193–199 (Level I)

85. Gibbs CP, Banner TC. Effectiveness of Bicitra as a preoperative antacid. Anesthesiology 1984;61:97–99 (Level II-3)

86. Nissen E, Widstrom AM, Lilja G, Matthiesen AS, Uvnas-Moberg K, Jacobsson G, et al. Effects of routinely given pethidine during labour on infants' developing breastfeeding behaviour. Effects of dose-delivery time interval and various concentrations of pethidine/norpethidine in cord plasma. Acta Paediatr 1997;86:201–208 (Level II-3)

87. Datta S, Camann W, Bader A, VanderBurgh L. Clinical effects and maternal and fetal plasma concentrations of epidural ropivacaine versus bupivacaine for cesarean section. Anesthesiology 1995;82:1346–1352 (Level I)

88. Loftus JR, Hill H, Cohen SE. Placental transfer and neonatal effects of epidural sufentanil and fentanyl administered with bupivacaine during labor. Anesthesiology 1995;83:300–308 (Level I)

89. Sepkoski CM, Lester BM, Ostheimer GW, Brazelton TB. The effects of maternal epidural anasthesia on neonatal behaviour during the first month. Dev Med Child Neurol 1992;34:1072–1080 (Level II-2)

90. Righard L, Aldade MO. Effect of delivery room routines on success of first breast-feed. Lancet 1990;336: 1105–1107 (Level II-3)

91. Halpern SH, Levine T, Wilson DB, MacDonell J, Katsiris SE, Leighton BL. Effect of labor analgesia on breastfeeding success. Birth 1999;26:83–88 (Level II-2)

92. Hirose M, Hara Y, Hosokawa T, Tanaka Y. The effect of postoperative analgesia with continuous epidural bupivacaine after cesarean section on the amount of breast feeding and infant weight gain. Anesth Analg 1996;82:1166–1169 (Level II-1)

93. Gerancher JC, Floyd H, Eisenach J. Determination of an effective dose of intrathecal morphine for pain relief after cesarean delivery. Anesth Analg 1999;88:346–351 (Level II-3)

94. Cohen SE, Subak LL, Brose WG, Halpern J. Analgesia after cesarean delivery: patient evaluations and cost of five opioid techniques. Reg Anesth 1991;16:141–149 (Level II-3)

95. Abboud TK, Dror A, Mosaad P, Zhu J, Mantilla M, Swart F, et al. Mini-dose intrathecal morphine for the relief of post-cesarean pain: safety, efficacy, and ventilatory responses to carbon dioxide. Anesth Analg 1988;67:137–143 (Level I)

96. Abouleish E, Rawal N, Fallon K, Hernandez D. Combined intrathecal morphine and bupivacaine for cesarean section. Anesth Analg 1988;67:370–374 (Level II-1)

97. Yang T, Breen TW, Archer D, Fick G. Comparison of 0.25 mg and 0.1 mg intrathecal morphine for analgesia after Cesarean section. Can J Anaesth 1999;46:856–860 (Level II-1)

98. Milner AR, Bogod DG, Harwood RJ. Intrathecal administration of morphine for elective Caesarean section. A comparison between 0.1 mg and 0.2 mg. Anaesthesia 1996;51:871–873 (Level I)

99. Paech MJ, Moore JS, Evans SF. Meperidine for patient-controlled analgesia after cesarean section. Intravenous versus epidural administration. Anesthesiology 1994;80:1268–1276 (Level I)

100. Parker RK, White PF. Epidural patient-controlled analgesia: an alternative to intravenous patient-controlled analgesia for pain relief after cesarean delivery. Anesth Analg 1992;75:245–251 (Level I)

101. Cooper DW, Ryall DM, McHardy FE, Lindsay SL, Eldabe SS. Patient-controlled extradural analgesia with bupivacaine, fentanyl, or a mixture of both, after cesarean section. Br J Anaesth 1996;76:611–615 (Level II-1)

102. Parker RK, Sawaki Y, White PF. Epidural patient-controlled analgesia: influence of bupivacaine and hydromorphone basal infusion on pain control after cesarean delivery. Anesth Analg 1992;75:740–746 (Level I)

103. Cohen S, Amar D, Pantuck CB, Pantuck EJ, Weissman AB. Adverse effects of epidural 0.03% bupivacaine during analgesia after cesarean section. Anesth Analg 1992;75:753–756 (Level II-1)

104. Charuluxananan S, Kyokong O, Somboonviboon W, Lertmaharit S, Ngamprasertwong P, Nimcharoendee K. Nalbuphine versus propofol for treatment of intrathecal morphine-induced pruritus after cesarean delivery. Anesth Analg 2001;93:162–165 (Level I)

105. Alhashemi JA, Crosby ET, Grodecki W, Duffy PJ, Hull KA, Gallant C. Treatment of intrathecal morphine-induced Pruritus following cesarean section. Can J Anaesth 1997;44:1060–1065 (Level I)

106. Rapp-Zingraff N, Bayoumeu F, Baka N, Hamon I, Virion JM, Laxenaire MC. Analgesia after caesarean section: patient-controlled intravenous morphine vs epidural morphine. Int J Obstet Anesth 1997;6:87–92 (Level II-1)

107. Harrison DM, Sinatra R, Morgese L, Chung JH. Epidural narcotic and patient-controlled analgesia for post-cesarean section pain relief. Anesthesiology 1988;68:454–457 (Level I)

108. Cohen SE, Ratner EF, Kreitzman TR, Archer JH, Mignano LR. Nalbuphine is better than naloxone for treatment of side effects after epidural morphine. Anesth Analg 1992;75:747–752 (Level II-1)

109. Somrat C, Oranuch K, Ketchada U, Siriprapa S, Thipawan R. Optimal dose of nalbuphine for treatment of intrathecal-morphine induced pruritus after caesarean section. J Obstet Gynaecol Res 1999;25:209–213 (Level I)

110. Abboud TK, Lee K, Zhu J, Reyes A, Afrasiabi A, Mantilla M, et al. Prophylactic oral naltrexone with intrathecal morphine for cesarean section: effects on adverse reactions and analgesia. Anesth Analg 1990;71:367–370 (Level I)

111. Borgeat A, Stirnemann HR. Ondansetron is effective to treat spinal or epidural morphine-induced pruritus. Anesthesiology 1999;90:432–436 (Level I)

112. Charuluxananan S, Somboonviboon W, Kyokong O, Nimcharoendee K. Ondansetron for treatment of intrathecal morphine-induced pruritus after cesarean delivery. Reg Anesth Pain Med 2000;25:535–539 (Level I)

113. Perez-Woods R, Grohar JC, Skaredoff M, Rock SG, Tse AM, Tomich P, et al. Pain control after cesarean birth. Efficacy of patient-controlled analgesia vs. traditional therapy (IM Morphine). J Perinatol 1991;11:174–181 (Level II-1)

114. Rayburn WF, Geranis BJ, Ramadei CA, Woods RE, Patil KD. Patient-controlled analgesia for post-cesarean section pain. Obstet Gynecol 1988;72:136–139 (Level II-1)

115. Olofsson CI, Legeby MH, Nygards EB, Ostman KM. Diclofenac in the treatment of pain after caesarean delivery. An opioid-saving strategy. Eur J Obstet Gynecol Reprod Biol 2000;88:143–146 (Level I)

116. Lim NL, Lo WK, Chong JL, Pan AX. Single dose diclofenac suppository reduces post-Cesarean PCEA requirements. Can J Anaesth 2001;48:383–386 (Level II-1)

The MEDLINE database, the Cochrane Library, and ACOG's own internal resources and documents were used to conduct a literature search to locate relevant articles published between January 1985 and April 2001. The search was restricted to articles published in the English language. Priority was given to articles reporting results of original research, although review articles and commentaries also were consulted. Abstracts of research presented at symposia and scientific conferences were not considered adequate for inclusion in this document. Guidelines published by organizations or institutions such as the National Institutes of Health and the American College of Obstetricians and Gynecologists were reviewed, and additional studies were located by reviewing bibliographies of identified articles. When reliable research was not available, expert opinions from obstetrician–gynecologists were used.

Studies were reviewed and evaluated for quality according to the method outlined by the U.S. Preventive Services Task Force:

I   Evidence obtained from at least one properly designed randomized controlled trial.

II-1   Evidence obtained from well-designed controlled trials without randomization.

II-2   Evidence obtained from well-designed cohort or case–control analytic studies, preferably from more than one center or research group.

II-3   Evidence obtained from multiple time series with or without the intervention. Dramatic results in uncontrolled experiments could also be regarded as this type of evidence.

III   Opinions of respected authorities, based on clinical experience, descriptive studies, or reports of expert committees.

Based on the highest level of evidence found in the data, recommendations are provided and graded according to the following categories:

Level A—Recommendations are based on good and consistent scientific evidence.

Level B—Recommendations are based on limited or inconsistent scientific evidence.

Level C—Recommendations are based primarily on consensus and expert opinion.

ISSN 1099-3630

**The American College of
Obstetricians and Gynecologists
409 12th Street, SW
PO Box 96920
Washington, DC 20090-6920**

12345/65432

Obstetric analgesia and anesthesia. ACOG Practice Bulletin No. 36. American College of Obstetricians and Gynecologists. Obstet Gynecol 2002;100:177–191

ACOG PRACTICE BULLETIN

CLINICAL MANAGEMENT GUIDELINES FOR
OBSTETRICIAN–GYNECOLOGISTS

NUMBER 17, JUNE 2000

(Replaces Technical Bulletin Number 196, August 1994)

This Practice Bulletin was developed by the ACOG Committee on Practice Bulletins—Obstetrics with the assistance of Michael Belfort, MD. The information is designed to aid practitioners in making decisions about appropriate obstetric and gynecologic care. These guidelines should not be construed as dictating an exclusive course of treatment or procedure. Variations in practice may be warranted based on the needs of the individual patient, resources, and limitations unique to the institution or type of practice.

Operative Vaginal Delivery

The incidence of operative vaginal delivery in the United States is estimated to be 10–15% (1), and although these procedures are safe in appropriate circumstances, controversy about them persists. Recent reports have highlighted the potential for maternal and neonatal complications associated with operative vaginal delivery, although the risks associated with alternative procedures also must be considered. This document will address specific controversial issues about the use of forceps and vacuum extractors for operative vaginal delivery and present the available information on which to base decisions concerning their use. The technical aspects of the use of forceps and vacuum extractors are beyond the scope of this publication.

Background

Clinical studies performed before the 1970s suggested that the risk of fetal morbidity and mortality was higher when the second stage of labor exceeded 2 hours. Currently, more intensive intrapartum surveillance provides the ability to identify the fetus that may not be tolerating labor well. Thus, the length of the second stage of labor is not in itself an absolute or even strong indication for operative termination of labor. When other obstetric factors prevail, however, there is a place for forceps or vacuum-assisted operations.

Operative vaginal deliveries are accomplished by applying direct traction on the fetal skull with forceps, or by applying traction to the fetal scalp by means of a vacuum extractor. The indications for operative vaginal delivery performed with either the vacuum extractor or forceps are the same (see the box, "Indications for Operative Vaginal Delivery").

The rate of cesarean deliveries in the United States has declined from 22.8% in 1987 to 20.8% in 1997 (2). During the same period, the percentage of births delivered by forceps or vacuum extraction increased slightly, from 9.0% to 9.4% (2). Of this number, the percentage of forceps deliveries has decreased

---

Indications for Operative Vaginal Delivery

No indication for operative vaginal delivery is absolute. The following indications apply when the fetal head is engaged and the cervix is fully dilated.

- Prolonged second stage:

  −Nulliparous women: lack of continuing progress for 3 hours with regional anesthesia, or 2 hours without regional anesthesia

  −Multiparous women: lack of continuing progress for 2 hours with regional anesthesia, or 1 hour without regional anesthesia

- Suspicion of immediate or potential fetal compromise.

- Shortening of the second stage for maternal benefit.

---

and the percentage of vacuum extraction deliveries has increased. Although some authors have suggested that operative vaginal deliveries have been replaced by cesarean deliveries, the relationship remains unclear. Geographic differences in operative delivery rates have been reported, with the lowest rate in the northeast United States and the highest rate in the South.

In 1988, ACOG redefined the classification of station and types of forceps deliveries. The revised classification uses the level of the leading bony point of the fetal head in centimeters at or below the level of the maternal ischial spines to define station (0–5 cm), instead of the previously used method of describing the birth canal in terms of thirds (0–3+).

The definitions of types of forceps deliveries also were refined to avoid the inclusion of either trivial or extremely difficult deliveries under the category of midforceps (see the box, "Criteria for Types of Forceps Deliveries"). Before this reclassification, a rotational delivery from occiput posterior at 0 station was classified the same as a delivery from left occiput anterior on the perineum. In a validation of ACOG's reclassification, investigators demonstrated that the lower the fetal head and the less rotation required, the less the risk of injury to the mother and the child (3). Assessment of clinical pelvimetry and fetal position is important in predelivery evaluation (see the box, "Predelivery Considerations").

Clinical Issues

Complications of Operative Vaginal Delivery

General statements about the applicability of operative vaginal delivery and the procedures for implementation in a particular situation are difficult. Selection of the appropriate instrument and decisions about the potential maternal and fetal consequences should be based on clinical findings at the time of delivery. Research into the complications of operative vaginal delivery is hampered by a number of potential biases, including the level of experience of the operators, the small numbers of patients studied under similar circumstances, changes in practice and definition, and the inability to achieve statistical power to answer relevant questions. The following discussion is based on currently available evidence and attempts to address maternal and fetal complications associated with operative vaginal delivery.

In a randomized trial comparing elective low-forceps delivery with spontaneous vaginal delivery in 50 term patients, there were no significant immediate differences in maternal or neonatal outcome variables. The researchers did show that in the forceps group, the mean time to delivery was shorter (10.2 minutes versus 18 minutes) and the cord arterial pH was higher (7.27 versus 7.23) (4). However, a larger randomized study comparing outlet forceps delivery with spontaneous vaginal delivery in 333 women at term showed that, although the use of forceps had no immediate adverse effects on the neonate, there was no significant shortening of the second stage of labor. However, the incidence of maternal perineal trauma increased in primiparous women (5).

Criteria for Types of Forceps Deliveries

Outlet forceps

1. Scalp is visible at the introitus without separating labia.

2. Fetal skull has reached pelvic floor.

3. Sagittal suture is in anteroposterior diameter or right or left occiput anterior or posterior position.

4. Fetal head is at or on perineum.

5. Rotation does not exceed 45°.

Low forceps

Leading point of fetal skull is at station ≥ +2 cm and not on the pelvic floor.

Rotation is 45° or less (left or right occiput anterior to occiput anterior, or left or right occiput posterior to occiput posterior).

Rotation is greater than 45°.

Midforceps

Station is above +2 cm but head is engaged.

High forceps

Not included in classification.

Predelivery Considerations

Position: the relationship of the fetal presenting part to the maternal pelvis. In a cephalic presentation the designated point is the occiput, while in a breech presentation it is the sacrum. The position always is described in relation to the maternal left and right sides of the pelvis.

Presentation: the relationship between the leading fetal part and the maternal pelvic inlet. The fetus may have a cephalic, breech, or shoulder presentation.

Lie: the relationship between the fetal and maternal longitudinal axes, which may be longitudinal, oblique, or transverse.

Engagement: the relationship that is present when the widest diameter of the fetal presenting part (biparietal diameter in a cephalic presentation, and bitrochanteric diameter in a breech presentation) has passed beyond the plane of the maternal pelvic brim. In a cephalic presentation the head usually is engaged when the leading point of the skull is at or below the maternal ischial spines.

Asynclitism: the relationship between the anterior and posterior parietal bones and the sagittal suture with the maternal pelvis. When neither of the parietal bones precedes the sagittal suture, the head is synclitic; if the anterior parietal bone precedes the sagittal suture, there is anterior asynclitism; and when the posterior parietal bone precedes the sagittal suture, there is posterior asynclitism.

Clinical Pelvimetry: assessment of the maternal pelvis before performing midpelvic delivery.

A meta-analysis comparing vacuum extraction to forceps delivery showed that vacuum extraction was associated with significantly less maternal trauma and less need for general and regional anesthesia. Overall, fewer cesarean deliveries were carried out in the vacuum extractor group (6). Other studies comparing vacuum extraction to forceps delivery indicate that more maternal morbidity (soft tissue injury, discomfort) occurs with forceps delivery (7, 8).

Both forceps delivery and vacuum extraction have been associated with the development of maternal hematomas, (9) and possibly linked to pelvic floor injury. However, other factors associated with pelvic floor injury include normal spontaneous vaginal delivery, episiotomy, prolonged second stage of labor, and increased fetal size (10).

To evaluate the risk of operative vaginal delivery with suspected fetal macrosomia, one study compared 2,924 macrosomic infants (birth weight >4,000 g) to those with a birth weight between 3,000 g and 3,999 g. Macrosomic infants delivered by forceps had a sixfold higher rate of significant injury (relative risk = 6.7; confidence interval, 6.5–6.9). Forceps delivery in this situation also was associated with a fourfold risk of clinically persistent neurologic abnormalities when compared with spontaneous vaginal delivery or cesarean delivery. The overall incidence of persistent injury was low (0.3%), and the authors calculated that as many as 258 elective cesarean deliveries would have to be performed for macrosomia to prevent a single case of persistent injury (11). In addition, a randomized study of forceps and vacuum-assisted vaginal delivery identified three factors associated with the development of shoulder dystocia: use of vacuum device ($P = 0.04$), time required for delivery ($P = 0.03$), and birth weight ($P = 0.0001$) (12). Therefore, a trial of labor and judicious use of operative vaginal delivery techniques for macrosomic infants are not contraindicated, although caution should be used given the possibility of shoulder dystocia.

Potential Newborn Complications of Vacuum-Assisted Deliveries

With forceps, almost unlimited compression and traction can be applied to the fetal head and cervical spine. Vacuum extractors are designed to limit the amount of traction on the fetal skull because detachment can occur. Nevertheless, traction achieved with vacuum extraction is substantial (up to 50 lb) (13) and can result in significant fetal injury if misused. The vacuum cup can cause scalp lacerations if torsion is excessive. In addition, separation of the scalp from the underlying structures can lead to cephalohematoma, which is more common in infants delivered by vacuum extractor (14–16%) than in those delivered with forceps (2%) (6, 7). The incidence of subgaleal hematomas (collections of blood occurring in the potential space between the cranial periosteum and the epicranial aponeurosis) following vacuum deliveries is estimated to range from 26 to 45 per 1,000 vacuum deliveries (14, 15).

Other potential neonatal complications associated with vacuum deliveries include intracranial hemorrhage, hyperbilirubinemia, and retinal hemorrhage. The higher rates of neonatal jaundice associated with vacuum delivery may be related to the higher rate of cephalohematoma (16). There is a higher rate of retinal hemorrhages (38%) with vacuum delivery than with forceps delivery (17%) (6, 7, 17, 18). However, corneal abrasions and external ocular trauma are more common with forceps delivery than with normal spontaneous delivery and are rare with vacuum extraction unless the cup is inadvertently placed over the eye. Long-term sequelae are extremely rare, and ophthalmologic screening should be reserved for specific cases (18). Overall, the incidence of serious complications with vacuum extraction is approximately 5% (19). Given the maternal and neonatal risks associated with operative vaginal delivery, it is important that the patient be made aware of the potential complications of the proposed procedure.

In 1998, the U.S. Food and Drug Administration (FDA) released a Public Health Advisory to alert individuals that vacuum extractors may cause serious or fatal complications, including subgaleal (subaponeurotic) hematoma and intracranial hemorrhage (20). The FDA indicated that between 1994 and 1998, 12 deaths and nine serious injuries were reported among neonates on whom vacuum-assisted devices had been used. This rate was greater than five times the rate for the preceding 11 years. According to the advisory, data collected from 1989 to 1995 showed that use of the vacuum cup had increased from 3.5% to 5.9% of all deliveries. Among the FDA recommendations for use of the vacuum device, two are particularly useful:

1. Rocking movements or torque should not be applied to the device; only steady traction in the line of the birth canal should be used.

2. Clinicians caring for the neonate should be alerted that a vacuum device has been used so that they can adequately monitor the neonate for the signs and symptoms of device-related injuries.

A recent study evaluating the incidence of severe birth trauma following operative deliveries assessed the outcome of 83,340 singleton infants born to nulliparous women between 1992 and 1994 in California (21). A database was created linking birth and death certificates with hospital discharge records of maternal and neonatal outcomes. The lowest risk of fetal injury was found in infants delivered spontaneously. An intermediate risk was observed for those infants delivered by forceps or vacuum alone or by cesarean delivery during labor. The highest risk of fetal injury was reported for those infants who were delivered with combined forceps and vacuum extraction or who were delivered by cesarean following failed operative vaginal delivery. There was no difference in outcome between vacuum and forceps delivery versus cesarean delivery during labor (Table 1). The morbidity that previously had been thought to be due to operative vaginal delivery actually may have resulted from the process of abnormal labor that led to the need for intervention. The study population was large, but data were collected retrospectively from medical records and hospital discharge reports. Therefore, detailed information on the operative vaginal delivery, frequency of congenital anom-

Table 1. Effect of Delivery on Neonatal Injury

Delivery Method	Death	Intracranial Hemorrhage	Other*
Spontaneous vaginal delivery	1/5,000	1/1,900	1/216
Cesarean delivery during labor	1/1,250	1/952	1/71
Cesarean delivery after vacuum/forceps	N/R	1/333	1/38
Cesarean delivery with no labor	1/1,250	1/2,040	1/105
Vacuum alone	1/3,333	1/860	1/122
Forceps alone	1/2,000	1/664	1/76
Vacuum and forceps	1/1,666	1/280	1/58

Abbreviation: N/R indicates not reported.

*Facial nerve/brachial plexus injury, convulsions, central nervous system depression, mechanical ventilation

Data from Towner D, Castro MA, Eby-Wilkens E, Gilbert WM. Effect of mode of delivery in nulliparous women on neonatal intracranial injury. N Engl J Med 1999;341:1709–1714

alies, or number of infants readmitted following the initial discharge was not available. Despite its limitations, this study confirms that injury can occur before operative delivery as a result of abnormal labor forces and that not all neonatal injuries are the result of poor operative technique.

Long-Term Infant Consequences

One randomized comparison of vacuum versus forceps delivery that evaluated children at 9 months of age found no statistically significant differences between the two groups regarding head circumference, weight, head-circumference-to-weight ratio, hearing, or vision (22). The study did note that infants delivered with the vacuum device were more likely to have been readmitted with jaundice than were those delivered with forceps.

In another study, the effects of forceps delivery on cognitive development were examined in a cohort of 3,413 children. No significant differences were seen in the 1,192 children delivered with forceps (114 were midforceps), compared with the 1,499 delivered spontaneously (23). A 10-year matched follow-up evaluation of 295 children delivered by vacuum extractor and 302 control patients who had been delivered spontaneously at the same hospital revealed no differences between the two groups in terms of scholastic performance, speech, ability of self-care, or neurologic abnormality (24).

Clinical Considerations and Recommendations

▶ *What are contraindications to operative vaginal delivery?*

Under certain circumstances, operative vaginal delivery should be avoided or, at the least, carefully considered in terms of relative maternal and fetal risk. Most authorities consider vacuum extraction inappropriate in pregnancies before 34 weeks of gestation because of the risk of fetal intraventricular hemorrhage. Operative delivery also is contraindicated if a live fetus is known to have a bone demineralization condition (eg, osteogenesis imperfecta), a bleeding disorder (eg, alloimmune thrombocytopenia, hemophilia, or von Willebrand's disease) is present, the fetal head is unengaged, or the position of the fetal head is unknown.

Operative vaginal delivery should be performed only by individuals with privileges for such procedures and in settings in which personnel are readily available to perform a cesarean delivery in the event the operative vaginal delivery is unsuccessful. One study showed that in cases in which the vacuum extractor was used to deliver fetuses with nonreassuring fetal heart rate patterns, blood gas parameters did not differ from those in cases with normal spontaneous deliveries. The authors concluded that the use of vacuum extraction is not contraindicated in cases of nonreassuring fetal heart rate patterns (25).

▶ *Is there a role for a trial of operative vaginal delivery?*

Few studies address the issue of maternal and neonatal outcome after an unsuccessful attempt at operative delivery. Earlier published reports were small retrospective studies that suggested outcome was no worse after failed operative delivery (26, 27). In a recent report of 102 cases of failed instrument delivery, almost half (43%) of cases where a trial of operative vaginal delivery was attempted resulted in the need for cesarean delivery. Of those where success was expected, only 3% went on to cesarean delivery (28). In addition, the California study previously discussed demonstrated significantly higher incidences of intracranial hemorrhage and other birth trauma following a failed operative vaginal delivery (21). Unless the preoperative assessment is highly suggestive of a successful outcome, trial of operative vaginal delivery is best avoided.

▶ *Is there a role for the use of alternative instruments after a failed attempt?*

Persistent efforts to obtain a vaginal delivery using different instruments may increase the potential for maternal and fetal injury and often indicates cephalopelvic disproportion. Although studies are limited, the weight of available evidence appears to be against attempting multiple efforts at operative vaginal delivery with different instruments, unless there is a compelling and justifiable reason (28). The California study reported that the incidence of intracranial hemorrhage was highest in infants delivered by combined vacuum and forceps compared with other reported methods of delivery (21). The incidences of other injuries also were increased with combined methods of operative vaginal delivery.

▶ *What special equipment and techniques should be considered with the use of a vacuum extractor?*

Vacuum extractors differ substantially from the original metal cup and currently vary by material, cup size and shape, and the method of vacuum application to the fetal scalp (manual or automatic). The proliferation and increased use of these instruments have resulted in the development of a number of different techniques. Randomized trials comparing soft vacuum cups to the original metal cup indicate that the pliable cup is associated with decreased fetal scalp trauma but increased rates of detachment from the fetal head (29–32). However, there are no differences between Apgar scores, cord pH, neurologic outcome, retinal hemorrhage, maternal trauma, and blood loss (32). These findings support those of another study, which found a 22% incidence of significant fetal scalp trauma with the soft cup, as opposed to a 37% incidence with the metal cup. This study also concluded the soft cup was more likely to fail than the metal cup when excessive caput was present (29).

Data show that the use of rapid vacuum application leads to a reduction in time to delivery (33, 34). No differences in detachment from the fetal scalp or in maternal or neonatal morbidity between the two techniques have been noted (33, 34). Specifically, one randomized study of 94 women comparing a one-step rapid application of vacuum with conventional stepwise application of vacuum found a significant reduction in the time from application to delivery (6 minutes) in the rapid application group without any differences in maternal or neonatal morbidity (33).

Cephalohematoma has been shown to be more likely to develop as the duration of vacuum application increases. One study demonstrated that 28% of neonates in whom the application-to-delivery time exceeded 5 minutes developed cephalohematoma (35). A further technical issue that has raised questions is whether the vacuum should be reduced between contractions to prevent fetal scalp injury. A randomized controlled trial involving 322 patients at 34 weeks or more of gestation highlighted factors involved in the development of fetal cephalohematoma from vacuum extraction using the M-cup (a semirigid plastic cup, modeled after the Malmstrom cup). To prevent fetal loss of station, 164 patients had continuous vacuum application (600 mm Hg) during and between contractions as well as during active efforts at delivery. In the comparison group, 158 patients had intermittent suction (reduction of vacuum application to 100 mm Hg between contractions) and no effort to prevent loss of station between contractions. Time to delivery, method failure, maternal lacerations, episiotomy extension, incidence of cephalohematoma, and neonatal outcome were similar between the two groups. Overall, the efficacy of the vacuum cup was 93.5%, and the cephalohematoma rate was 11.5%. The authors concluded that there are no differences in maternal or fetal outcome with intermittent reduction in vacuum or attempts to prevent loss of station. They also concluded that the results obtained with the M-cup are comparable to those reported with the stainless-steel Malmstrom cup (36).

▶ *Is there a role for midforceps rotational deliveries in current practice?*

The decrease in experienced teachers and the increase in medical–legal concerns have reduced the number of current practitioners skilled in the art of midcavity rotational delivery. Studies comparing midforceps and cesarean deliveries indicate that midforceps delivery is not associated with worse neonatal outcome (Apgar score, cord blood gas, neonatal intensive care admissions, birth trauma) than is cesarean delivery (37, 38). In addition, outcome appeared no worse for those infants in whom Kielland's forceps rotation was attempted but was unsuccessful (38). One retrospective analysis compared 358 midforceps deliveries with 486 cesarean deliveries and found maternal morbidity (intraoperative and postoperative complications, blood loss, and length of stay) to be higher in the cesarean delivery group (37). Another study reported similar findings in a 5-year retrospective study involving 253 patients (38).

A retrospective study compared 552 deliveries with Kielland's forceps rotation, 95 cases using Scanzoni maneuver with a different type of forceps, and 160 cases using manual rotation and forceps. Investigators found no significant differences in maternal or neonatal outcomes between the groups regardless of whether the indication was relative dystocia or nonreassuring fetal status (39). An earlier study found that Kielland's forceps rotation was associated with a higher incidence of neonatal trauma, although the analysis did not specify the indications for operative delivery (40).

There are no randomized controlled studies of long-term follow-up from which to draw conclusions. However, retrospective case–control analyses seem to indicate no differences in outcome between midforceps delivery and cesarean delivery or vacuum extraction (41, 42). A matched-pairs analysis of patients 2 years after a midforceps delivery compared with a group delivered via cesarean delivery (matched for the immediate indication for operative delivery, birth weight, gestational age, sex, and race) found no difference in abnormal outcomes between the groups (41). An 18-year follow-up study of males delivered by midcavity Kielland's forceps rotation did not show any late adverse effects when subjects were compared with males delivered by vacuum extractor (42). Thus, there appears to be a role for midforceps rotational deliveries in current practice. However, given the potential complications, this procedure is only for practitioners skilled in midforceps delivery and for cases where maternal and fetal assessment prior to the operation suggest a high chance of success.

Summary

The following recommendations are based on good and consistent scientific evidence (Level A):

▶ Both forceps and vacuum extractors are acceptable and safe instruments for operative vaginal delivery. Operator experience should determine which instrument should be used in a particular situation.

▶ The vacuum extractor is associated with an increased incidence of neonatal cephalohematomata, retinal hemorrhages, and jaundice when compared with forceps delivery.

The following recommendations are based on limited or inconsistent scientific evidence (Level B):

▶ Operators should attempt to minimize the duration of vacuum application, because cephalohematoma is more likely to occur as the interval increases.

▶ Midforceps operations should be considered an appropriate procedure to teach and to use under the correct circumstances by an adequately trained individual.

▶ The incidence of intracranial hemorrhage is highest among infants delivered by cesarean following a failed vacuum or forceps delivery. The combination of vacuum and forceps has a similar incidence of intracranial hemorrhage. Therefore, an operative vaginal delivery should not be attempted when the probability of success is very low.

786   COMPENDIUM OF SELECTED PUBLICATIONS

The following recommendations are based primarily on consensus and expert opinion (Level C):

▶ Operative vaginal delivery is not contraindicated in cases of suspected macrosomia or prolonged labor; however, caution should be used because the risk of shoulder dystocia increases with these conditions.

▶ Neonatal care providers should be made aware of the mode of delivery in order to observe for potential complications associated with operative vaginal delivery.

References

1. Bofill JA, Rust OA, Perry KG, Roberts WE, Martin RW, Morrison JC. Operative vaginal delivery: a survey of fellows of ACOG. Obstet Gynecol 1996;88:1007–1010 (Level III)

2. Ventura SJ, Martin JA, Curtin SC, Mathews TJ. Births: final data for 1997. Natl Vital Stat Rep 1999;47(18):1–96 (Level II-3)

3. Hagadorn-Freathy AS, Yeomans ER, Hankins GD. Validation of the 1988 ACOG forceps classification system. Obstet Gynecol 1991;77:356–360 (Level II-2)

4. Carmona F, Martinez-Roman S, Manau D, Cararach V, Iglesias X. Immediate maternal and neonatal effects of low-forceps delivery according to the new criteria of The American College of Obstetricians and Gynecologists compared with spontaneous vaginal delivery in term pregnancies. Am J Obstet Gynecol 1995;173:55–59 (Level I)

5. Yancey MK, Herpolsheimer A, Jordan GD, Benson WL, Brady K. Maternal and neonatal effects of outlet forceps delivery compared with spontaneous vaginal delivery in term pregnancies. Obstet Gynecol 1991;78:646–650 (Level I)

6. Johanson RB, Menon BKV. Vacuum extraction versus forceps for assisted vaginal delivery (Cochrane Review). In: The Cochrane Library, Issue 4, 1999. Oxford: Update Software (Meta-analysis)

7. Dell DL, Sightler SE, Plauche WC. Soft cup vacuum extraction: a comparison of outlet delivery. Obstet Gynecol 1985;66:624–628 (Level I)

8. Johanson R, Pusey J, Livera N, Jones P. North Staffordshire/Wigan assisted delivery trial. Br J Obstet Gynaecol 1989;96:537–544 (Level I)

9. Gei AF, Belfort MA. Forceps-assisted vaginal delivery. Obstet Gynecol Clin North Am 1999;26:345–370 (Level III)

10. Handa VL, Harris TA, Ostergard DR. Protecting the pelvic floor: obstetric management to prevent incontinence and pelvic organ prolapse. Obstet Gynecol 1996;88:470–478 (Level III)

11. Kolderup LB, Laros RK Jr, Musci TJ. Incidence of persistent birth injury in macrosomic infants: association with mode of delivery. Am J Obstet Gynecol 1997;177:37–41 (Level II-2)

12. Bofill JA, Rust OA, Devidas M, Roberts WE, Morrison JC, Martin JN Jr. Shoulder dystocia and operative vaginal delivery. J Matern Fetal Med 1997;6:220–224 (Level I)

13. Moolgaoker AS, Ahamed SOS, Payne PR. A comparison of different methods of instrumental delivery based on electronic measurements of compression and traction. Obstet Gynecol 1979;54:299–309 (Level II-3)

14. Boo NY. Subaponeurotic haemorrhage in Malaysian neonates. Singapore Med J 1990;31:207–210 (Level II-3)

15. Govaert P, Defoort P, Wigglesworth JS. Cranial haemorrhage in the term newborn infant. Clin Dev Med 1993;129:1–223 (Level III)

16. Vacca A, Grant A, Wyatt G, Chalmers I. Portsmouth operative delivery trial: a comparison of vacuum extraction and forceps delivery. Br J Obstet Gynaecol 1983;90:1107–1112 (Level I)

17. Williams MC, Knuppel RA, O'Brien WF, Weiss A, Kanarek KS. A randomized comparison of assisted vaginal delivery by obstetric forceps and polyethylene vacuum cup. Obstet Gynecol 1991;78:789–794 (Level I)

18. Holden R, Morsman DG, Davidek GM, O'Connor GM, Coles EC, Dawson AJ. External ocular trauma in instrumental and normal deliveries. Br J Obstet Gynaecol 1992;99:132–134 (Level II-2)

19. Robertson PA, Laros RK Jr, Zhao RL. Neonatal and maternal outcome in low-pelvic and midpelvic operative deliveries. Am J Obstet Gynecol 1990;162:1436–1442; discussion 1442–1444 (Level II-2)

20. Center for Devices and Radiological Health. FDA Public Health Advisory: need for caution when using vacuum assisted delivery devices. May 21, 1998. Available at http://www.fda.gov/cdrh/fetal598.html. Retrieved December 31, 1999 (Level III)

21. Towner D, Castro MA, Eby-Wilkens E, Gilbert WM. Effect of mode of delivery in nulliparous women on neonatal intracranial injury. N Engl J Med 1999; 341:1709–1714 (Level II-2)

22. Carmody F, Grant A, Mutch L, Vacca A, Chalmers I. Follow up of babies delivered in a randomized controlled comparison of vacuum extraction and forceps delivery. Acta Obstet Gynecol Scand 1986;65:763–766 (Level I)

23. Wesley BD, van den Berg BJ, Reece EA. The effect of forceps delivery on cognitive development. Am J Obstet Gynecol 1993;169:1091–1095 (Level II-2)

24. Ngan HY, Miu P, Ko L, Ma HK. Long-term neurological sequelae following vacuum extractor delivery. Aust N Z J Obstet Gynaecol 1990;30:111–114 (Level II-2)

25. Vintzileos AM, Nochimson DJ, Antsaklis A, Varvarigos I, Guzman ER, Knuppel RA. Effect of vacuum extraction on umbilical cord blood acid-base measurements. J Matern Fetal Med 1996;5:11–17 (Level II-2)

26. Revah A, Ezra Y, Farine D, Ritchie K. Failed trial of vacuum or forceps—maternal and fetal outcome. Am J Obstet Gynecol 1997;176:200–204 (Level II-3)

27. Boyd ME, Usher RH, McLean FH, Norman BE. Failed forceps. Obstet Gynecol 1986;68:779–783 (Level II-3)

28. Edozien LC, Williams JL, Chattopadhyay I, Hirsch PJ. Failed instrumental delivery: how safe is the use of a second instrument? J Obstet Gynaecol 1999;19:460–462 (Level III)

29. Chenoy R, Johanson R. A randomized prospective study comparing delivery with metal and silicone rubber vacuum extractor cups. Br J Obstet Gynaecol 1992;99:360–363 (Level I)

30. Cohn M, Barclay C, Fraser R, Zaklama M, Johanson R, Anderson D, et al. A mulitcentre randomized trial comparing delivery with a silicone rubber cup and rigid metal vacuum extractor cups. Br J Obstet Gynaecol 1989;96:545–551 (Level I)

31. Hofmeyr GJ, Gobetz L, Sonnendecker EW, Turner MJ. New design rigid and soft vacuum extractor cups: a preliminary comparison of traction forces. Br J Obstet Gynaecol 1990;97:681–685 (Level I)

32. Kuit JA, Eppinga HG, Wallenburg HC, Huikeshoven FJ. A randomized comparison of vacuum extraction delivery with a rigid and a pliable cup. Obstet Gynecol 1993;82:280–284 (Level I)

33. Lim FT, Holm JP, Schuitemaker NW, Jansen FH, Hermans J. Stepwise compared with rapid application of vacuum in ventouse extraction procedures. Br J Obstet Gynaecol 1997;104:33–36 (Level I)

34. Svenningsen L. Birth progression and traction forces developed under vacuum extraction after slow or rapid application of suction. Eur J Obstet Gynecol Reprod Biol 1987;26:105–112 (Level II-2)

35. Bofill JA, Rust OA, Devidas M, Roberts WE, Morrison JC, Martin JN Jr. Neonatal cephalohematoma from vacuum extraction. J Reprod Med 1997;42:565–569 (Level I)

36. Bofill JA, Rust OA, Schorr SJ, Brown RC, Roberts WE, Morrison JC. A randomized trial of two vacuum extraction techniques. Obstet Gynecol 1997;89:758–762 (Level I)

37. Bashore RA, Phillips WH Jr, Brinkman CR 3rd. A comparison of the morbidity of midforceps and cesarean delivery. Am J Obstet Gynecol 1990;162:1428–1434; discussion 1434–1435 (Level II-2)

38. Traub AI, Morrow RJ, Ritchie JW, Dornan KJ. A continuing use for Kielland's forceps? Br J Obstet Gynaecol 1984;91:894–898 (Level II-2)

39. Healy DL, Quinn MA, Pepperell RJ. Rotational delivery of the fetus: Kielland's forceps and two other methods compared. Br J Obstet Gynaecol 1982;89:501–506 (Level II-2)

40. Chiswick ML, James DK. Kielland's forceps: association with neonatal morbidity and mortality. Br Med J 1979;1:7–9 (Level II-3).

41. Dierker LJ Jr, Rosen MG, Thompson K, Lynn P. Midforceps deliveries: long-term outcome of infants. Am J Obstet Gynecol 1986;154:764–768 (Level II-2)

42. Nilsen ST. Boys born by forceps and vacuum extraction examined at 18 years of age. Acta Obstet Gynecol Scand 1984;63:549–554 (Level II-2)

The MEDLINE database, the Cochrane Library, and ACOG's own internal resources and documents were used to conduct a literature search to locate relevant articles published between January 1985 and November 1999. The search was restricted to articles published in the English language. Priority was given to articles reporting results of original research, although review articles and commentaries also were consulted. Abstracts of research presented at symposia and scientific conferences were not considered adequate for inclusion in this document. Guidelines published by organizations or institutions such as the National Institutes of Health and the American College of Obstetricians and Gynecologists were reviewed, and additional studies were located by reviewing bibliographies of identified articles. When reliable research was not available, expert opinions from obstetrician–gynecologists were used.

Studies were reviewed and evaluated for quality according to the method outlined by the U.S. Preventive Services Task Force:

I   Evidence obtained from at least one properly designed randomized controlled trial.

II-1   Evidence obtained from well-designed controlled trials without randomization.

II-2   Evidence obtained from well-designed cohort or case–control analytic studies, preferably from more than one center or research group.

II-3   Evidence obtained from multiple time series with or without the intervention. Dramatic results in uncontrolled experiments also could be regarded as this type of evidence.

III   Opinions of respected authorities, based on clinical experience, descriptive studies, or reports of expert committees.

Based on the highest level of evidence found in the data, recommendations are provided and graded according to the following categories:

Level A—Recommendations are based on good and consistent scientific evidence.

Level B—Recommendations are based on limited or inconsistent scientific evidence.

Level C—Recommendations are based primarily on consensus and expert opinion.

ISSN 1099-3630

The American College of
Obstetricians and Gynecologists
409 12th Street, SW
PO Box 96920
Washington, DC 20090-6920   12345/43210

ACOG PRACTICE BULLETIN

CLINICAL MANAGEMENT GUIDELINES FOR
OBSTETRICIAN–GYNECOLOGISTS

NUMBER 50, JANUARY 2004

*(Replaces Committee Opinion Number 270, March 2002,
and Educational Bulletin Number 246, April 1998)*

This Practice Bulletin was developed by the ACOG Committee on Practice Bulletins— Gynecology with the assistance of James A. Simon, MD. The information is designed to aid practitioners in making decisions about appropriate obstetric and gynecologic care. These guidelines should not be construed as dictating an exclusive course of treatment or procedure. Variations in practice may be warranted based on the needs of the individual patient, resources, and limitations unique to the institution or type of practice.

Osteoporosis

Osteoporosis is a systemic skeletal disease characterized by microarchitectural deterioration of bone tissue with a resultant increase in fragility. This leads to an increased risk of fractures, which may occur even in the absence of significant trauma. Approximately 13–18% of U.S. women aged 50 years and older have osteoporosis while another 37–50% have low bone mass (osteopenia) (1). Both osteopenia and osteoporosis increase the risk of fracture. Although hip fracture has been properly emphasized as a source of significant morbidity and mortality (15–20%), the more common thoracic spine fracture accounts for significant morbidity, including pain; deformity; loss of independence; and reduced cardiovascular, respiratory, and even digestive function. Osteoporosis is a largely preventable complication of menopause. Appropriate screening strategies and significant pharmacologic interventions are available to prevent and treat osteoporosis.

Background

Definitions

The World Health Organization (WHO) has defined low bone mass (osteopenia) and osteoporosis on the basis of axial skeleton measurements of bone density to facilitate screening and identification of individuals at risk (Table 1) (2). These definitions apply specifically to T scores derived from the use of dual-energy X-ray absorptiometry (DXA) of the lumbar spine or hip.

Bone mineral density testing is the preferred method to establish the diagnosis of osteoporosis. Bone mineral density is a strong predictor of fracture risk because bone mass accounts for 75–85% of the variation in bone strength (3). To standardize values from different bone densitometry tests, results are reported as standard deviations, either as a Z score or a T score, compared with a reference population stratified by age, sex, and race. The Z score is based on the standard deviation from the mean bone mineral density of a reference popula-

Table 1. World Health Organization Definition of Osteoporosis Based on Bone Mineral Density of Total Hip*

Bone Classification	T Score†
Normal	Greater than or equal to –1
Osteopenia (low bone mass)	–1 to –2.5
Osteoporosis	Less than or equal to –2.5

*These definitions were used to describe a Caucasian cohort to define risk. This classification was not intended to be applicable to non-Caucasians and men or to peripheral bone density screening devices. The use of the World Health Organization guidelines/definitions nonetheless has become generalized.

†Standard deviations from the average value of the mean peak bone mineral density of a normal, young adult population.

Data from World Health Organization. Assessment of fracture risks and its application to screening for postmenopausal osteoporosis. WHO Technical Report Series 843. Geneva: WHO; 1994.

tion of the same sex, race, and age. The T score is based on the mean peak bone mineral density of a normal, young adult population and is expressed in terms of standard deviations from the average value of this reference population. Both the T score and the Z score can refer to either spine or hip bone mass measurement.

The WHO defines osteopenia as a bone mineral density between 1 and 2.5 standard deviations below the young adult mean and osteoporosis as a bone mineral density 2.5 standard deviations or more below the young adult peak mean (2). Other authorities define osteoporosis as a bone mineral density more than 2 standard deviations below the young adult peak mean (4). At the spine and hip, a decrease of 1 standard deviation in bone mass is associated with approximately a 2-fold increase in fracture risk.

T score discrepancies exist between different central and peripheral bone density devices. Because few data correlate peripheral device-derived T scores (other than the wrist) and lifetime fracture risk T scores, peripheral technologies currently cannot be used for true WHO classification. These devices do predict fracture, however, and have a role in osteoporosis screening (5). Standard definitions for osteoporosis that apply to peripheral technologies are in development.

Pathophysiology

The bone-remodeling unit is the site on the surface of the bone where osteoblasts and osteoclasts act to form and resorb bone. Bone is constantly being remodeled to provide optimal support and to repair damage occurring from daily activities. The remodeling cycle can be divided into 4 phases: 1) resting, 2) resorption, 3) reversal, and 4) formation. Each remodeling cycle may take several months to complete.

During the resting phase, stem cells from the bone marrow are attracted to the bone surface and differentiate

into osteoclasts. During the resorption phase, the osteoclasts remove bone using an acid pH to dissolve the minerals and proteolytic enzymes to digest the bone proteins. During the reversal phase, the osteoclasts cease removing the bone, and mesenchymal stem cells are attracted to the bone surface and differentiate into osteoblasts. During the formation phase, osteoblasts make new bone by first laying down a protein matrix (osteoid), which is then mineralized. Type I collagen constitutes 90% of the osteoid. The protein matrix accounts for much of the tensile strength, while the mineral component provides compressional strength. Cytokines (interleukin-1, -3, -6, and -11) and growth factors (transforming growth factor [β], platelet-derived growth factor, and insulinlike growth factors I and II) may modulate osteoclast and osteoblast function and mediate the coordination of these 2 cell types.

Bone can be divided into 2 major types: 1) cortical and 2) trabecular. Cortical bone forms the outer shell of all bones and accounts for 75% of total bone mass. Trabecular bone is the spongy, interlacing network of struts that forms the internal support within the cortical bone. Trabecular bone is concentrated in the vertebral bodies and pelvis and at the ends of the long bones. Trabecular bone accounts for 25% of total bone mass, but because of its spongy, open architectural structure, it accounts for most of the volume in bone. Bone remodeling units are limited to the bone surface. Because trabecular bone has a larger surface area, it has a higher turnover rate than cortical bone. Trabecular bone is most likely to show early bone loss, but it also is the first to show response to therapy.

Bone formation and resorption are ongoing processes that usually are "in balance" in young adults who have adequate nutrition and exercise and experience normal puberty (6). Bone mass peaks at approximately age 30 years in both men and women. After reaching peak bone mass, approximately 0.4% of bone is lost per year in both sexes. In addition to this loss, women lose approximately 2% of cortical bone and 5% of trabecular bone per year for the first 5–8 years after menopause. With menopause and aging, the coordinated "balance" between osteoclasts and osteoblasts may be disturbed, resulting in excessive bone resorption and loss of both bone density and structure. In women who are recently menopausal, excess bone loss commonly is caused by excessive osteoclast-mediated resorption. In later postmenopausal years, suppressed osteoblast activity and inadequate formation of bone may play a major role in the progression of osteoporosis, providing an opportunity for new therapeutic approaches, such as stimulating bone formation. Osteoporosis is more common in women than men in part because of the accelerated loss of bone that occurs after menopause.

Factors Affecting Bone Mass

Bone mass is influenced by numerous factors (see box). Some of these factors are modifiable (eg, cigarette smoking) while others are not (eg, family history of hip fracture). Other factors may affect the risk for fracture but not necessarily the predisposition to osteoporosis (eg, propensity to fall).

The single largest factor influencing a woman's maximal or peak bone mass is genetics. Up to 80% of the variability in peak bone mass is attributable to genetic factors alone (7, 8). Female children of women with osteoporotic fractures have lower bone mass than would be expected for their age when compared with unrelated individuals (9, 10). First-degree relatives of women with osteoporosis have lower bone mass than those with no family history of osteoporosis (11).

Many studies have shown that the risk of osteoporosis is greater for Caucasian and Asian women than for African-American women. This is likely because African-American women have approximately a 6% higher bone mineral density than Caucasian women, a difference that further suggests a genetic influence (12). Mexican-American women have an intermediate risk of osteoporosis. These differences in risk are probably caused, in part, by genetic determinants of body size, body composition, and bone metabolism.

There is general agreement that weight-bearing exercise confers a positive effect on the skeleton, but during early menopause, weight-bearing exercise alone is insufficient to prevent bone loss. However, weight-bearing exercise will slow the rate of bone loss. Growing evidence suggests that impact-loading exercises (ie, weight-lifting in contrast to water aerobics) provide the greatest osteogenic stimulus (13–15). Exercise also appears to reduce the risk of falls, although it is unclear if exercise affects the risk for fracture from falls that do occur (16). Lack of physical activity, such as prolonged bed rest, extended space travel, or hemiplegia, are associated with rapid and significant bone loss (17, 18). The effects of exercise on bone mass are attributed to a stimulation of osteoblastic activity (19).

Certain diseases or medical conditions (see box) and certain drugs (see box) are known to be associated with bone loss. For example, a dose of prednisone or an equivalent corticosteroid that is less than 7.5 mg is associated with minimal bone loss. At high doses, corticosteroids are associated with bone loss in the range of 10% in the first year of treatment, putting women at increased risk. It is in this and similar subgroups that frequent bone mineral density testing, even twice in the first year on this therapy, may be warranted. Chronic heparin therapy (12,000–50,000 U/d) is associated with bone loss in approximately one third of women.

Hyperthyroidism, whether naturally occurring or iatrogenic from excessive therapy (thyroxine at doses of 200 μg or more daily is associated with osteopenia), is associated with decreased bone mass. The effect may persist for many years after the hyperthyroidism is successfully treated. Thyroxine therapy that normalizes thyroid-stimulating hormone levels but does not completely suppress them appears to be associated with normal bone density (20).

Screening Methods

Several tests to measure bone mineral density are available, either radiation-based or radiation-free. Dual-energy X-ray absorptiometry is the technical standard for measuring bone mineral density. Most of the recent large, randomized, controlled clinical trials have used DXA of the hip and spine to determine therapeutic efficacy. Dual-energy X-ray absorptiometry is preferred because it measures bone mineral density at the important sites of osteoporotic fractures (especially the hip), is relatively inexpensive, has high precision and accuracy, and has modest radiation exposure (21).

Risk Factors for Osteoporotic Fracture in Postmenopausal Women

- History of prior fracture
- Family history of osteoporosis
- Caucasian race
- Dementia
- Poor nutrition
- Smoking
- Low weight and body mass index
- Estrogen deficiency*
  - Early menopause (age younger than 45 years) or bilateral oophorectomy
  - Prolonged premenopausal amenorrhea (>1 year)
- Long-term low calcium intake
- Alcoholism
- Impaired eyesight despite adequate correction
- History of falls
- Inadequate physical activity

*A patient's current use of hormone therapy does not preclude estrogen deficiency.

Data from Osteoporosis prevention, diagnosis, and therapy. NIH Consens Statement 2000;17(1):1–45.

Medical Conditions That May Be Associated With an Increased Risk of Osteoporosis in Adults

- Acquired immunodeficiency syndrome or human immunodeficiency virus
- Amyloidosis
- Ankylosing spondylitis
- Chronic obstructive pulmonary disease
- Congenital porphyria
- Cushing's disease
- Eating disorders
- Female athlete triad
- Gastrectomy
- Gaucher's disease
- Hemochromatosis
- Hemophilia
- Hyperparathyroidism
- Hypogonadism, primary and secondary
- Hypophosphatasia
- Idiopathic scoliosis
- Inadequate diet
- Inflammatory bowel disease
- Insulin-dependent diabetes mellitus
- Lymphoma and leukemia
- Malabsorption syndromes
- Mastocytosis
- Multiple myeloma
- Multiple sclerosis
- Pernicious anemia
- Rheumatoid arthritis
- Severe liver disease, especially primary biliary cirrhosis
- Spinal cord transsection
- Sprue
- Stroke (cerebrovascular accident)
- Thalassemia
- Thyrotoxicosis
- Tumor secretion of parathyroid hormone-related peptide
- Weight loss

Drugs Associated With an Increased Risk of Generalized Osteoporosis in Adults

- Aluminum
- Anticonvulsants (phenobarbitol, phenytoin)
- Cytotoxic drugs
- Glucocorticosteroids and adrenocorticotropin
- Gonadotropin-releasing hormone agonists
- Immunosuppressants
- Lithium
- Long-term heparin use
- Progesterone, parenteral, long-acting
- Supraphysiologic thyroxine doses
- Tamoxifen (premenopausal use)
- Total parenteral nutrition

Although tests at peripheral sites (eg, wrist, calcaneus) can identify women with low bone mass, they may not be as useful as central-site tests (eg, hip, spine) because the results may not be as precise. Peripheral site measurements should be limited to the assessment of fracture risk when DXA is not available and lower-risk populations are being screened. These devices have been shown to predict fracture (5) and are less costly than axial devices. They should not be used for definitive diagnosis of osteoporosis or to monitor response to therapy (22).

Clinical Considerations and Recommendations

▶ *When should screening for osteoporosis be initiated?*

Testing of bone mineral density should be performed on the basis of an individual woman's risk profile and is not indicated unless the results will influence a treatment or management decision. Although not all experts or organizations agree, the following guidelines can be recommended:

- Bone mineral density testing should be recommended to all postmenopausal women aged 65 years or older.

- Bone mineral density testing may be recommended to postmenopausal women younger than 65 years who have 1 or more risk factors for osteoporosis (see box "Risk Factors for Osteoporotic Fracture in Postmenopausal Women").
- Bone mineral density testing should be performed on all postmenopausal women with fractures to confirm the diagnosis of osteoporosis and determine disease severity.

Bone mineral density testing may be useful for premenopausal and postmenopausal women with certain diseases or medical conditions (see box "Medical Conditions That May Be Associated With an Increased Risk of Osteoporosis in Adults") and those who take certain drugs associated with an increased risk of osteoporosis (see box "Drugs Associated With an Increased Risk of Generalized Osteoporosis in Adults"). In the absence of new risk factors, subsequent screening should not be performed more frequently than every 2 years. The usefulness of repeated screening will be greater in older women, those with lower baseline bone mineral density, and those with numerous risk factors.

For older women who have experienced an osteoporotic vertebral fracture, treatment may be given without bone mineral density measurement, although baseline bone mineral density testing may be useful to follow the effects of therapy. A nonvertebral fracture (eg, hip or wrist) is, by itself, not an indication for treatment in the absence of low bone mineral density. Testing of bone mineral density in early postmenopausal women may be of value in helping women make a decision about preventive therapy; however, it cannot be justified on the basis of fracture reduction in the short term.

Analyses performed by the National Osteoporosis Foundation support that bone mineral density testing is cost-effective when performed on postmenopausal women aged 50–60 years with risk factors or in those older than 60–65 years with or without risk factors (23).

▶ *Under what circumstances are screening tests other than DXA useful?*

Peripheral bone densitometry devices use a variety of techniques, which include quantitative ultrasonography, single-energy X-ray absorptiometry, peripheral DXA, and peripheral quantitative computed tomography. These devices have the advantages of less expense, portable equipment, reasonable precision, and low radiation exposure. Their use is limited to the evaluation of the peripheral skeleton. These peripheral devices are used as screening tools in the evaluation of bone loss, but presently cannot replace DXA scans for the prediction of

hip fractures and the diagnosis of osteoporosis or osteopenia. The T scores from these devices do not always correlate with the T scores of DXA.

Quantitative Ultrasonography

The use of quantitative ultrasonography to screen for osteoporosis and assess fracture risk has increased. Using the speed of sound and broadband ultrasonic attenuation measurements, ultrasound densitometry provides information on bone elasticity and structure in peripheral sites (eg, heel, tibia, patella). Advantages of this method include low cost and lack of ionizing radiation. Normative databases are being developed to compare the ability of quantitative ultrasonography to predict fracture risk at the hip and spine. Prospective studies comparing quantitative ultrasonography with axial measurements suggest that quantitative ultrasonography of the heel is able to predict hip fractures using other bone parameters, such as speed of sound and bone attenuation measurements, that are independent of bone density changes in older women (24, 25). Further clinical experience and research are needed to compare this technique with DXA (26–28).

Peripheral Quantitative Computed Tomography

Peripheral quantitative computed tomography measures bone mineral density using computerized tomography. Its main advantage is the ability to distinguish cortical from trabecular bone at a particular location. Because trabecular bone changes more quickly than cortical bone, it is suggested that peripheral quantitative computed tomography allows an earlier and more precise assessment of skeletal changes. Generally, these devices are more expensive and emit more radiation than do peripheral DXA or ultrasound devices. Bone mineral density measurements using peripheral quantitative computed tomography have less robust data correlating this technique with fracture than some of the other peripheral methods.

Biochemical Markers of Bone Turnover

Biochemical markers of bone turnover cannot diagnose osteoporosis, predict bone density, or predict fracture risk (see box). Biochemical markers can be useful to help identify women with high bone turnover. These tests have been studied as a means of assessment that could be used earlier in the course of therapy to show therapeutic response. Bone turnover changes can provide evidence of osteoporosis therapy efficacy much earlier than bone mineral density changes (sometimes within weeks).

Biochemical Markers

Markers of Bone Formation
- Serum bone specific alkaline phosphatase
- Serum osteocalcin
- Serum procollagen I extension peptides

Markers of Bone Resorption
- Urinary N-telopeptide
- Serum C-telopeptide
- Collagen cross-links
- Urinary deoxypyridinoline
- Urinary hydroxyproline

However, the value of such markers in routine clinical practice has not been established (29, 30). Generally, serum tests, when available, are preferable to urinary tests because of their lower assay coefficient of variation and lower propensity to diurnal variation. The technology for measurement of bone biochemical markers is evolving rapidly, but these tests are not universally available and can be very expensive.

▶ *Can lifestyle changes prevent osteoporosis and osteoporosis-related fractures?*

Sedentary lifestyle is associated with reduced bone mass. Weight-bearing exercise (eg, aerobic fitness, strength training) stimulates osteoblasts to form new bone (19). Observational studies suggest that exercise stimulates an increase in muscle mass and that exercise and increased muscle mass both contribute to the development of increased bone mass. The benefits of exercise can be demonstrated into the ninth decade of life but persist only when the exercise is continued (31). In menopausal women, weight-bearing exercise for 22 months was shown to result in a 6.1% increase in bone density of the lumbar spine (32). The benefits of physical exercise include maintenance of bone mass and an increase in muscle strength and coordination.

The risk of falling increases substantially with aging. Diseases and sensory impairments that can cause falling should be evaluated and treated (eg, a history of falls, fainting, or loss of consciousness; muscle weakness, dizziness, or balance problems; problems with muscle coordination; and impaired vision). Medications that reduce strength and balance (such as sedatives, narcotic analgesics, anticholinergics, and antihypertensives) should be avoided, if possible. Most falls that result in hip fractures occur indoors. The living environment should be monitored to reduce the risk of falling. Safety hazards in the home and at work, such as loose rugs and carpets; obstacles, especially to stairs; and poor lighting, should be assessed to reduce the risks of falls. Individuals at risk should consider installing handrails in and around the home.

Cessation of smoking and reducing alcohol intake may contribute to a decreased risk of developing a fracture. Heavy alcohol consumption (defined as 7 oz or more per week) has been shown to increase the risk for both falls and hip fracture (33). Excessive alcohol consumption also has detrimental effects on bone mineral density. However, moderate alcohol consumption in women aged 65 years and older is associated with increased bone mineral density (34) and lower risk for hip fracture (35). It is not clear why this occurs; however, an impact on the cardiovascular system as well as an estrogenic effect of some alcoholic beverages have been postulated.

▶ *Is there a role for estrogen and progestin for the prevention or treatment of osteoporosis?*

The Women's Health Initiative initial study results demonstrated a statistically significant reduction in fractures, including hip fractures, in a large group of otherwise healthy women using hormone therapy (36). A detailed analysis of the data from this study has not been published to date, so it is not clear whether this was truly a prevention or a treatment population. However, the preliminary results showed that conjugated equine estrogen (0.625 mg/d) along with medroxyprogesterone acetate (2.5 mg/d) reduced the risk of hip and clinical vertebral fractures by 34% and reduced overall fractures by 24%. The hip fracture reduction amounted to 5 fewer hip fractures per 10,000 women per year.

Recently, lower-dose combinations of conjugated equine estrogen (0.45 mg and 0.3 mg) and medroxyprogesterone acetate (1.5 mg) were shown to prevent bone loss in a randomized, placebo-controlled, 2-year clinical trial of early menopausal women (37). This study also demonstrated an additive effect of this nonandrogenic progestin that had not been demonstrated previously. Bone mineral density increased after 2 years of treatment by 1–2% for both dosages of conjugated equine estrogen alone, and in combination with medroxyprogesterone acetate. In another study, low-dose conjugated equine estrogen (0.3 mg/d), in a continuous-combined formulation, including medroxyprogesterone acetate (2.5 mg/d), increased spinal bone density 3.5–5.2% in postmenopausal women (older than 65 years) with low bone mass (38).

In another study of postmenopausal women, 0.3 mg per day of oral esterified estrogens, administered unopposed by progestogen for 24 months, resulted in positive bone changes without inducing endometrial hyperplasia (39). A randomized, controlled clinical trial of unopposed transdermal 17β-estradiol found that doses ranging from 0.025 to 0.1 mg per day significantly increased bone mineral density of the spine and hip when compared with placebo (40).

The optimal time to initiate therapy and the optimal duration of therapy have not been determined. Generally, estrogen or hormone therapy is believed to work best if it is started in the first 5–10 years after menopause. Even if it is started long after menopause, estrogen or hormone therapy produces substantial gains in bone mass (41–43). A study of older women (mean age 76 years) who had taken estrogen or hormone therapy for 7 or more years found they had significantly higher bone mineral densities than nonusers, although the effect diminished somewhat in those older than 75 years (44). When estrogen or hormone therapy is discontinued, however, bone turnover increases and bone loss tends to accelerate (45). Over time, bone mass approaches that of women who have not used hormones; fracture rates increase in proportion to both increasing bone turnover and decreasing bone density.

Although the risks of long-term use of estrogen or hormone therapy are small, many recommend such therapy be used for the shortest period at the lowest possible dose. The Women's Health Initiative study indicated a significantly increased risk of cardiovascular events and breast cancer for women taking combined estrogen and progestin therapy (36). Thus, the use of hormone therapy for osteoporosis prevention or fracture reduction should be evaluated based on an individual woman's history and risk factors, including the need for treatment of vasomotor symptoms.

▶ *When estrogen therapy is discontinued, how should a woman be monitored for osteoporosis risk?*

When a woman discontinues estrogen therapy, risk assessment and screening should follow the same criteria as for a woman who is in the early stages of menopause. It also should take into account the need for bone mineral density measurements based on age and other risk factors for osteoporosis.

▶ *Is other pharmacotherapy beneficial for the prevention and treatment of osteoporosis?*

In addition to estrogens, there are a number of agents available for the prevention of osteoporosis. These can be broadly grouped into 2 categories: 1) bisphosphonates (ie, alendronate, risedronate) and 2) selective estrogen

receptor modulators (SERMs) (ie, raloxifene, tibolone, tamoxifen).

Bisphosphonates reduce bone resorption and bone loss by inhibiting osteoclast activity. These agents increase bone mineral density at both the spine and hip and reduce fractures in women with established osteoporosis at all assessed locations by approximately 30–50% (16). Bisphosphonates may cause upper gastrointestinal side effects and are contraindicated in individuals with reflux, gastroesophageal reflux disease, and other esophageal abnormalities. This class of agents has very poor absorption, typically less than 1% of the administered dose. It is, therefore, very important that they be taken on an empty stomach only with plain water, that the patient remain upright for at least 30 minutes, and that no additional food or drink be ingested during this period.

Alendronate and risedronate also can be used to treat osteoporosis in individuals with established disease. Fracture reduction in this treatment population has been demonstrated for both of these agents (46–53).

Selective estrogen receptor modulators, sometimes called tissue selective estrogens, have mixed estrogenic and antiestrogenic properties depending on the tissue studied. These agents were specifically developed to have estrogenlike effects on skeleton bone density and to reduce fracture without stimulating endometrial or breast tissue, which can potentially result in endometrial and breast malignancies. The Food and Drug Administration (FDA) has determined that raloxifene and tibolone are safe and effective for the prevention of osteoporosis. Only raloxifene currently is marketed while the endometrial protective effects of tibolone are being investigated. In postmenopausal women, raloxifene significantly reduces bone resorption (54), increases bone mineral density (55), and reduces vertebral fractures 35–50% in women with established osteoporosis (56). Hip fracture reduction has not been demonstrated.

Raloxifene also has been shown to have estrogenlike activity in the prevention of bone loss. In a randomized trial (MORE trial), it was shown to significantly reduce the risk of vertebral fracture relative to placebo (56). Raloxifene does not appear to stimulate the endometrium, and preliminary results suggest breast cancer reduction (57, 58). Although generally well tolerated, side effects of raloxifene include vasomotor symptoms (hot flashes and night sweats). It also has risks (deep vein thrombosis and pulmonary embolism) similar to those of estrogens (58, 59).

Tibolone also has androgenic and progestogenic properties and has demonstrated efficacy in the prevention of postmenopausal bone loss with doses as low as 0.625 mg (42). Its impact on fracture reduction, its androgenic effects on sexual function, and the efficacy of its progestational impact on the endometrium are the subjects of ongoing research.

Tamoxifen, a SERM used as adjuvant therapy in estrogen receptor positive breast cancer and for chemoprevention of breast cancer in women at high risk of disease, also has demonstrated slight but statistically significant reductions in fracture risk. Side effects include triggering or increasing vasomotor symptoms, stimulating the endometrium (hyperplasias and adenocarcinomas), and increasing venous thromboembolism. Its use as a primary bone antiresorptive therapy is thereby limited (60).

Although not approved for the prevention of osteoporosis, both nasal salmon calcitonin and human recombinant parathyroid hormone (PTH) are available for osteoporosis treatment. Salmon calcitonin, available as both a subcutaneous injection and as a nasal spray, is approved for the treatment of osteoporosis in women 5 or more years after menopause. The more commonly used nasal spray has demonstrated efficacy in the reduction of lumbar spine fractures (36%) at a dose of 200 IU per day, but did not reduce hip fractures in a 5-year clinical trial of postmenopausal women with established osteoporosis (61). This agent appears to work primarily by its effects on reducing bone turnover, but bone density changes are small (approximately 1%). Calcitonin also has been found to reduce bone pain from osteoporotic vertebral compression fractures (62) and other pain syndromes. Calcitonin generally is well tolerated. Its side effects are nausea, local inflammation (injection), flushing of the face or hands (injection), and nasal irritation (nasal spray).

Daily subcutaneous injections of recombinant human PTH activate bone formation and result in substantial increases in trabecular bone density and connectivity in women with postmenopausal osteoporosis, regardless of whether they are receiving estrogen therapy (63–65). Parathyroid hormone is approved for the treatment of osteoporosis particularly in cases of failed response to other therapies. In postmenopausal women with prior vertebral fracture, 19 months of PTH therapy (20–40 µg daily) reduced the incidence of new vertebral fractures by 65% and 69%, respectively, and new nonvertebral fractures by 53% and 54%, respectively (65). This therapy should be limited to patients who have not responded to antiresorptive therapies, those with very severe disease, and those for whom therapeutic alternatives are limited. The medication is expensive and requires daily injections. A recent randomized controlled study has shown that the impact of PTH is significantly reduced when co-administered with bisphosphonates; therefore, they should not be combined (66).

Although fluoride supplements have been used for many years to "harden" permanent teeth, this compound increases bone brittleness and propensity to fracture; thus, its use for osteoporosis prevention should be discouraged. Testosterone currently may be a useful adjunct for increasing bone mass for the rare patient who has responded poorly to antiresorptive therapies, but it has not been shown to reduce fractures and requires prior estrogen therapy.

Combinations of Antiresorptive Therapies

It has long been known that the addition of progestogens, particularly those derived from testosterone, can have additive effects on bone mineral density when used with estrogens (67). Recently, this effect also has been demonstrated with progestogens that are not derived from androgens (37). Androgens added to estrogens also have shown additive effects on bone mineral density in a 2-year study (68).

Several studies have been undertaken to determine if combinations of antiresorptive agents can be used synergistically in the prevention of bone loss. Available investigations of cyclical etidronate with or without estrogen, alendronate with or without hormone therapy or added to ongoing estrogen treatment, risedronate, and estrogen therapy combined or alone all show small additional increases in bone density (approximately 1–3% in 2 years) with the combination therapy (68–72). Recently, combination alendronate and raloxifene have demonstrated similar bone density increases as noted previously (73). Estrogen therapy with and without calcitriol therapy also produced larger increases in bone mineral density than hormone therapy alone (74).

Whether the increases in bone mineral density from any of these combined therapies results in better fracture protection is not known. The long-term safety of combination therapies has not been adequately evaluated, and the costs are universally higher.

Although calcium and vitamin D can be used as therapy by themselves, they also should be considered adjuvant therapy for all individuals. This is particularly true for adolescents and men and women older than 65 years. In women, calcium and vitamin D consumption are frequently inadequate. All calcium products work by the same mechanism regardless of the source (natural or synthetic). Doses vary by source and chemical composition (eg, carbonate, citrate, gluconate), which may affect bioavailability. The recommendations for these supplements (see box) apply to elemental calcium. Care should be made to advise patients of the differences in elemental calcium content (usually on the product label) in an attempt to make sure they ultimately receive enough calcium.

es, has led many to suggest withholding treatment until certain treatment thresholds have been reached.

The National Osteoporosis Foundation has chosen a T score of −2 for women without risk factors and −1.5 for women with additional risk factors as the threshold for therapeutic treatment (77). The Z score may help in determining an alternative strategy, particularly when the Z score is less than −1 and the patient would not have qualified for therapy based solely on the criteria discussed previously. Under these circumstances, a secondary cause for the bone loss should be sought (see box).

Monitoring a patient's response to treatment requires central bone densitometry. Although peripheral devices generally are sensitive enough to detect small differences in density, peripheral sites seldom change enough to make longitudinal measurements on individuals worthwhile. In addition, the high content of cortical bone in some peripheral areas is less likely to reflect early trabecular changes in the axial skeleton.

Follow-up densitometry measurements are another area of controversy. Although the precision of densitometric measurements in the best centers is within 2–3%, the average clinical measurement is far less precise. Repeat DXA testing in untreated postmenopausal women typically is not useful until 3–5 years have passed because 5-year postmenopausal bone mineral density reductions average only approximately 0.5 stan-

▶ Are complementary and alternative therapies beneficial for the prevention of osteoporosis?

Although some data suggest that isoflavones (a class of phytoestrogens found in rich supply in soy beans and soy products as well as in red clover) may favorably affect bone health, few randomized, controlled clinical studies with humans have been conducted, and those that have all involved small numbers of subjects in trials of short duration. Studies to date do not support the use of isoflavones to prevent or treat osteoporosis. Ipriflavone, a synthetic isoflavone available without a prescription in the United States, has not demonstrated a reliable positive effect on bone density, bone turnover markers, or fracture risk in women with osteoporosis (75).

▶ When should treatment for osteoporosis begin and how should patients be followed?

Lower bone mineral density T scores generally indicate more severe osteoporosis and higher risk of fracture. Every decrease of 1 standard deviation from age-adjusted bone density represents approximately a 10–12% change in bone mineral density and an increase in the risk of fracture by a factor of approximately 2 (76). Although few would withhold treatment from a women with osteoporosis (T score less than −2.5), whether to treat a women with higher bone density scores has become subject for debate. The controversy focuses on the extremely low risk of fracture in young women with osteopenia and all women without additional risk factors. The high costs and potential side effects of long-term therapy until "old age," when fracture risk increasdard deviations from the mean (both T scores and Z scores) in that time frame. This magnitude of change is at the usual detection limit of the assay methodology. For women receiving osteoporosis therapy, bone mineral density monitoring before 2 years of therapy are completed does not provide clinically useful information and may lead to erroneous assumptions about the effect of therapy.

Not observing an increase in bone mineral density is not evidence of treatment failure. In one study, most women who appeared to have lost more than 4% of bone mineral density during the first year of treatment (with either alendronate or raloxifene) showed substantial gains the second year while remaining on the same therapy (78). The apparent decrease in density could be caused by imprecision in the DXA measurement. A decrease in vertebral bone mineral density greater than 4–5% indicates a need to evaluate the patient's compliance with therapy and dosing instructions and to search for secondary causes of bone loss.

Summary of Recommendations

The following recommendations are based on good and consistent scientific evidence (Level A):

▶ Treatment should be initiated to reduce fracture risk in postmenopausal women who have experienced a fragility or low-impact fracture.

▶ Treatment should be instituted in those post-menopausal women with bone mineral density T scores less than −2 by central DXA in the absence of risk factors and in women with T scores less than −1.5 in the presence of 1 or more risk factors.

▶ First-line pharmacologic options determined by the FDA to be safe and effective for osteoporosis prevention (bisphosphonates [alendronate and risedronate], raloxifene, and estrogen) should be used.

▶ First-line pharmacologic options determined by the FDA to be safe and effective for osteoporosis treatment (bisphosphonates [alendronate and risedronate], raloxifene, calcitonin, and PTH) should be used.

The following recommendations are based on limited or inconsistent scientific evidence (Level B):

▶ Women should be counseled about the following preventive measures:

— Adequate calcium consumption, using dietary supplements if dietary sources are not adequate

— Adequate vitamin D consumption (400–800 IU daily) and the natural sources of this nutrient

— Regular weight-bearing and muscle-strengthening exercises to reduce falls and prevent fractures

— Smoking cessation

— Moderation of alcohol intake

— Fall prevention strategies

▶ Bone mineral density testing should be recommended to all postmenopausal women aged 65 years or older.

▶ Bone mineral density testing may be recommended for postmenopausal women younger than 65 years who have 1 or more risk factors for osteoporosis (see box "Risk Factors for Osteoporotic Fracture in Postmenopausal Women").

▶ Bone mineral density testing should be performed on all postmenopausal women with fractures to confirm the diagnosis of osteoporosis and determine disease severity.

▶ In the absence of new risk factors, screening should not be performed more frequently than every 2 years.

The following recommendations are based primarily on consensus and expert opinion (Level C):

▶ Women should be counseled on the risks of osteoporosis and related fragility fractures. Such counseling should be part of the annual gynecologic examination.

References

1. Looker AC, Wahner HW, Dunn WL, Calvo MS, Harris TB, Heyse SP, et al. Updated data on proximal femur bone mineral levels of US adults. Osteoporos Int 1998;8: 468–89. (Level III)

2. World Health Organization. Assessment of fracture risks and its application to screening for postmenopausal osteoporosis. WHO Technical Report Series 843. Geneva: WHO; 1994. (Level III)

3. Jergas M, Genant HK. Current methods and recent advances in the diagnosis of osteoporosis. Arthritis Rheum 1993;36:1649–62. (Level III)

4. Nordin BE. Guidelines for bone densitometry. Med J Aust 1994;160:517–20. (Level III)

5. Siris ES, Miller PD, Barrett-Connor E, Faulkner KG, Wehren LE, Abbott TA, et al. Identification and fracture outcomes of undiagnosed low bone mineral density in postmenopausal women: results from the National

Osteoporosis Risk Assessment. JAMA 2001;286: 2815–22. (Level II-2)

6. Boot AM, de Ridder MA, Pols HA, Krenning EP, de Muinck Keizer-Schrama SM. Bone mineral density in children and adolescents: relation to puberty, calcium intake, and physical activity. J Clin Endocrinol Metab 1997;82:57–62. (Level II-3)

7. Pocock NA, Eisman JA, Hopper JL, Yeates MG, Sambrook PN, Eberl S. Genetic determinants of bone mass in adults. A twin study. J Clin Invest 1987;80: 706–10. (Level II-3)

8. Slemenda CW, Christian JC, Williams CJ, Norton JA, Johnston CC Jr. Genetic determinants of bone mass in adult women: a reevaluation of the twin model and the potential importance of gene interaction on heritability estimates. J Bone Miner Res 1991;6:561–7. (Level II-3)

9. Seeman E, Hopper JL, Bach LA, Cooper ME, Parkinson E, McKay J, et al. Reduced bone mass in daughters of women with osteoporosis. N Engl J Med 1989;320:554–8. (Level II-2)

10. Bauer DC, Browner WS, Cauley JA, Orwoll ES, Scott JC, Black DM, et al. Factors associated with appendicular bone mass in older women. The Study of Osteoporotic Fractures Research Group. Ann Intern Med 1993;118: 657–65. (Level II-2)

11. Evans RA, Marel GM, Lancaster EK, Kos S, Evans M, Wong SY. Bone mass is low in relatives of osteoporotic patients. Ann Intern Med 1988;109:870–3. (Level II-2)

12. Looker AC, Johnston CC Jr, Wahner HW, Dunn WL, Calvo MS, Harris TB, et al. Prevalence of low femoral bone density in older U.S. women from NHANES III. J Bone Miner Res 1995;10:796–802. (Level II-3)

13. Bassey EJ, Ramsdale SJ. Increase in femoral bone density in young women following high-impact exercise. Osteoporos Int 1994;4:72–5. (Level I)

14. Taaffe DR, Robinson TL, Snow CM, Marcus R. High-impact exercise promotes bone gain in well-trained female athletes. J Bone Miner Res 1997;12:255–60. (Level II-2)

15. Welsh L, Rutherford OM. Hip bone mineral density is improved by high-impact aerobic exercise in post-menopausal women and men over 50 years. Eur J Appl Physiol Occup Physiol 1996;74:511–7. (Level III)

16. NIH Consensus Development Panel on Osteoporosis Prevention, Diagnosis, and Therapy. Osteoporosis prevention, diagnosis, and therapy. JAMA 2001;285:785–95. (Level III)

17. Prince RL, Price RI, Ho S. Forearm bone loss in hemiplegia: a model for the study of immobilization osteoporosis. J Bone Miner Res 1988;3:305–10. (Level II-3)

18. Thomas WC Jr. Exercise, age, and bones. South Med J 1994;87:S23–5. (Level III)

19. Gutin B, Kasper MJ. Can vigorous exercise play a role in osteoporosis prevention? A review. Osteoporos Int 1992;2:55–69. (Level III)

20. Marcocci C, Golia F, Bruno-Bossio G, Vignali E, Pinchera A. Carefully monitored levothyroxine suppressive therapy is not associated with bone loss in premenopausal women. J Clin Endocrinol Metab 1994;78:818–23. (Level II-2)

21. Kanis JA, Johnell O, Oden A, Jonsson B, Dawson A, Dere W. Risk of hip fracture derived from relative risks: an analysis applied to the population of Sweden. Osteoporos Int 2000;11:120–7. (Level II-2)

22. Hodgson SF, Watts NB, Bilezikian JP, Clarke BL, Gray TK, Harris DW, et al. American Association of Clinical Endocrinologists 2001 medical guidelines for clinical practice for the preventions and management of post-menopausal osteoporosis. Endocr Pract 2001;7:293–312. (Level III)

23. Osteoporosis: review of the evidence for prevention, diagnosis and treatment and cost-effectiveness analysis. Executive summary. Osteoporos Int 1998;8(suppl 4): S3–6. (Level III)

24. Bauer DC, Gluer CC, Cauley JA, Vogt TM, Ensrud KE, Genant HK, et al. Broadband ultrasound attenuation predicts fractures strongly and independently of densitometry in older women: a prospective study. Study of Osteoporotic Fractures Research Group. Arch Intern Med 1997;157:629–34. (Level II-1)

25. Hans D, Dargent-Molina P, Schott AM, Sebert JL, Cormier C, Kotzki PO, et al. Ultrasonographic heel measurements to predict hip fracture in elderly women: the EPIDOS prospective study. Lancet 1996;348:511–4. (Level II-1)

26. Cheng XG, Nicholson PH, Boonen S, Lowet G, Brys P, Aerssens J, et al. Prediction of vertebral strength in vitro by spinal bone densitometry and calcaneal ultrasound. J Bone Miner Res 1997;12:1721–8. (Level II-1)

27. Lochmuller EM, Zeller JB, Kaiser D, Eckstein F, Landgraf J, Putz R, et al. Correlation of femoral and lumbar DXA and calcaneal ultrasound, measured in situ with intact soft tissues, with the in vitro failure loads of the proximal femur. Osteoporo Int 1998;591–8. (Level II-1)

28. Lochmuller EM, Eckstein F, Kaiser D, Zeller JB, Landgraf J, Putz R, et al. Prediction of vertebral failure loads from spinal and femoral dual-energy X-ray absorptiometry, and calcaneal ultrasound: an in situ analysis with intact soft tissues. Bone 1998;23:417–24. (Level II-1)

29. Marcus R, Holloway L, Wells B, Greendale G, James MK, Wasilauskas C, et al. The relationship of biochemical markers of bone turnover to bone density changes in postmenopausal women: results from the Postmenopausal Estrogen/Progestin Interventions (PEPI) trial. J Bone Miner Res 1999;14:1583–95. (Level I)

30. Miller PD, Baran DT, Bilezikian JP, Greenspan SL, Lindsay R, Riggs BL, et al. Practical clinical application of biochemical markers of bone turnover: Consensus of an expert panel. J Clin Densitom 1999;2:323–42. (Level III)

31. Fiatarone MA, Marks EC, Ryan ND, Meredith CN, Lipsitz LA, Evans WJ. High-intensity strength training in nonagenarians: effects on skeletal muscle. JAMA 1990; 263:3029–34. (Level III)

32. Dalsky GP, Stocke KS, Ehsani AA, Slatopolsky E, Lee WC, Birge SJ Jr. Weight-bearing exercise training and lumbar bone mineral content in postmenopausal women. Ann Intern Med 1988;108:824–8. (Level II-2)

33. Felson DT, Kiel DP, Anderson JJ, Kannel WB. Alcohol consumption and hip fractures: the Framingham Study. Am J Epidemiol 1988;128:1102–10. (Level II-2)

34. Rapuri PB, Gallagher JC, Balhorn KE, Ryschon KL. Alcohol intake and bone metabolism in elderly women. Am J Clin Nutr 2000;72:1206–13. (Level II-2)

35. Felson DT, Zhang Y, Hannan MT, Kannel WB, Kiel DP. Alcohol intake and bone mineral density in elderly men and women. The Framingham Study. Am J Epidemiol 1995;142:485–92. (Level II-2)

36. Rossouw JE, Anderson GL, Prentice RL, LaCroix AZ, Kooperberg C, Stefanick ML, et al. Risks and benefits of estrogen plus progestin in healthy postmenopausal women: principal results from the Women's Health Initiative randomized controlled trial. JAMA 2002;288: 321–33. (Level I)

37. Lindsay R, Gallagher JC, Kleerekoper M, Pickar JH. Effect of lower doses of conjugated equine estrogens with and without medroxyprogesterone acetate on bone in early postmenopausal women. JAMA 2002;287:2668–76. (Level I)

38. Recker RR, Davies KM, Dowd RM, Heaney RP. The effect of low-dose continuous estrogen and progesterone therapy with calcium and vitamin D on bone in elderly women. A randomized, controlled trial. Ann Intern Med 1999;130:897–904. (Level I)

39. Genant HK, Lucas J, Weiss S, Akin M, Emkey R, McNaney-Flint H, et al. Low-dose esterified estrogen therapy: effects on bone, plasma estradiol concentrations, endometrium, and lipid levels. Estratab/Osteoporosis Study Group. Arch Intern Med 1997;157:2609–15. (Level I)

40. Weiss SR, Ellman H, Dolker M. A randomized controlled trial of four doses of transdermal estradiol for preventing postmenopausal bone loss. Transdermal Estradiol Investigator Group. Obstet Gynecol 1999;94:330–6. (Level I)

41. Schneider DL, Barrett-Connor EL, Morton DJ. Timing of postmenopausal estrogen for optimal bone mineral density. The Rancho Bernardo Study. JAMA 1997;277:543–7. (Level II-3)

42. Gallagher JC, Baylink DJ, Freeman R, McClung M. Prevention of bone loss with tibolone in postmenopausal women: results of two randomized, double-blind, placebo-controlled, dose-finding studies. J Clin Endocrinol Metab 2001;86:4717–26. (Level I)

43. Lindsay R, Tohme JF. Estrogen treatment of patients with established postmenopausal osteoporosis. Obstet Gynecol 1990;76:290–5. (Level II-2)

44. Felson DT, Zhang Y, Hannan MT, Kiel DP, Wilson PW, Anderson JJ. The effect of postmenopausal estrogen therapy on bone density in elderly women. N Engl J Med 1993;329:1141–6. (Level II-2)

45. Quigley ME, Martin PL, Burnier AM, Brooks P. Estrogen therapy arrests bone loss in elderly women. Am J Obstet Gynecol 1987;156:1516–23. (Level II-1)

46. Black DM, Thompson DE, Bauer DC, Ensrud K, Musliner T, Hochberg MC, et al. Fracture risk reduction with alendronate in women with osteoporosis: the Fracture Intervention Trial. FIT Research Group [published erratum appears in J Clin Endocrinol Metab 2001; 86:938]. J Clin Endocrinol Metab 2000;85:4118–24. (Level I)

47. McClung M, Clemmesen B, Daifotis A, Gilchrist NL, Eisman J, Weinstein RS, et al. Alendronate prevents postmenopausal bone loss in women without osteoporosis. A double-blind, randomized, controlled trial. Alendronate Osteoporosis Prevention Study Group. Ann Intern Med 1998;128:253–61. (Level I)

48. Ravn P, Bidstrup M, Wasnich RD, Davis JW, McClung MR, Balske A, et al. Alendronate and estrogen-progestin in the long-term prevention of bone loss: four-year results from the early postmenopausal intervention cohort study. A randomized, controlled trial. Ann Intern Med 1999;131: 935–42. (Level I)

49. McClung MR, Geusens P, Miller PD, Zippel H, Bensen WG, Roux C, et al. Effect of risedronate on the risk of hip fracture in elderly women. Hip Intervention Program Study Group. N Engl J Med 2001;344:333–40. (Level I)

50. Mortensen L, Charles P, Bekker PJ, Digennaro J, Johnston CC Jr. Risedronate increases bone mass in an early postmenopausal population: two years of treatment plus one year of follow-up. J Clin Endocrinol Metab 1998;83: 396–402. (Level I)

51. Tonino RP, Meunier PJ, Emkey R, Rodriguez-Portales JA, Menkes CJ, Wasnich RD, et al. Skeletal benefits of alendronate: 7-year treatment of postmenopausal osteoporotic women. Phase III Osteoporosis Treatment Study Group. J Clin Endocrinol Metab 2000;85:3109–15. (Level I)

52. Reginster J, Minne HW, Sorensen OH, Hooper M, Roux C, Brandi ML, et al. Randomized trial of the effects of risedronate on vertebral fractures in women with established postmenopausal osteoporosis. Vertebral Efficacy with Risedronate Therapy (VERT) Study Group. Osteoporos Int 2000;11:83–91. (Level I)

53. Harris ST, Watts NB, Genant HK, McKeever CD, Hangartner T, Keller M, et al. Effects of risedronate treatment on vertebral and nonvertebral fractures in women with postmenopausal osteoporosis: a randomized controlled trial. Vertebral Efficacy With Risedronate Therapy (VERT) Study Group. JAMA 1999;282:1344–52. (Level I)

54. Lufkin EG, Whitaker MD, Nickelsen T, Argueta R, Caplan RH, Knickerbocker RK, et al. Treatment of established postmenopausal osteoporosis with raloxifene: a randomized trial. J Bone Miner Res 1998;12:1747–54. (Level I)

55. Delmas PD, Bjarnason NH, Mitlak BH, Ravoux AC, Shah AS, Huster WJ, et al. Effects of raloxifene on bone mineral density, serum cholesterol concentrations, and uterine endometrium in postmenopausal women. N Engl J Med 1997;337:1641–7. (Level I)

56. Ettinger B, Black DM, Mitlak BH, Knickerbocker RK, Nickelsen T, Genant HK, et al. Reduction of vertebral fracture risk in postmenopausal women with osteoporosis treated with raloxifene: results from a 3-year randomized clinical trial. Multiple Outcomes of Raloxifene

Evaluation (MORE) Investigators [published erratum appears in JAMA 1999;282:2124]. JAMA 1999;282: 637–45. (Level I)

57. Cauley JA, Norton L, Lippman ME, Eckert S, Krueger KA, Purdie DW, et al. Continued breast cancer risk reduction in postmenopausal women treated with raloxifene: 4-year results from the MORE trial. Multiple Outcomes of Raloxifene Evaluation [published erratum appears in Breast Cancer Res Treat 2001;67:191]. Breast Cancer Res Treat 2001;65:125–34. (Level I)

58. Cummings SR, Eckert S, Krueger KA, Grady D, Powles TJ, Cauley JA, et al. The effect of raloxifene on risk of breast cancer in postmenopausal women: results from the MORE randomized trial. Multiple Outcomes of Raloxifene Evaluation [published erratum appears in JAMA 1999;282:2124]. JAMA 1999;281:2189–97. (Level I)

59. Hulley S, Grady D, Bush T, Furberg C, Herrington D, Riggs B, et al. Randomized trial of estrogen plus progestin for secondary prevention of coronary heart disease in postmenopausal women. Heart and Estrogen/progestin Replacement Study (HERS) Research Group. JAMA 1998;280:605–13. (Level I)

60. Fisher B, Costantino JP, Wickerham DL, Redmond CK, Kavanah M, Cronin WM, et al. Tamoxifen for prevention of breast cancer: report of the National Surgical Adjuvant Breast and Bowel Project P-1 Study. J Natl Cancer Inst 1998;90:1371–88. (Level I)

61. Chesnut CH 3rd, Silverman S, Andriano K, Genant H, Gimona A, Harris S, et al. A randomized trial of nasal spray salmon calcitonin in postmenopausal women with established osteoporosis: the Prevent Recurrence of Osteoporotic Fractures Study. PROOF Study Group. Am J Med 2000;109:267–76. (Level I)

62. Pun KK, Chan LW. Analgesic effect of intranasal salmon calcitonin in the treatment of osteoporotic vertebral fractures. Clin Ther 1989;11:205–9. (Level II-3)

63. Dempster DW, Cosman F, Kurland ES, Zhou H, Nieves J, Woelfert L, et al. Effects of daily treatment with parathyroid hormone on bone microarchitecture and turnover in patients with osteoporosis: a paired biopsy study. J Bone Miner Res 2001;16:1846–53. (Level II-3)

64. Lindsay R, Nieves J, Formica C, Henneman E, Woelfert L, Shen V, et al. Randomised controlled study of effect of parathyroid hormone on vertebral-bone mass and fracture incidence among postmenopausal women on oestrogen with osteoporosis. Lancet 1997;350:550–5. (Level I)

65. Neer RM, Arnaud CD, Zanchetta JR, Prince R, Gaich GA, Reginster JY, et al. Effect of parathyroid hormone (1-34) on fractures and bone mineral density in postmenopausal women with osteoporosis. N Engl J Med 2001;344: 1434–41. (Level I)

66. Black DM, Greenspan SL, Ensrud KE, Palermo L, McGowan JA, Lang TF, et al. The effects of parathyroid hormone and alendronate alone or in combination in post-menopausal osteoporosis. N Engl J Med 2003;349: 1207–15. (Level I)

67. Speroff L, Rowan J, Symons J, Genant H, Wilborn W. The comparative effect on bone density, endometrium, and lipids of continuous hormones as replacement therapy (CHART study). A randomized controlled trial. JAMA 1996;276:1397–403. (Level I)

68. Barrett-Connor E, Young R, Notelovitz M, Sullivan J, Wiita B, Yang HM, et al. A two-year, double-blind comparison of estrogen-androgen and conjugated estrogens in surgically menopausal women. Effects on bone mineral density, symptoms and lipid profiles. J Reprod Med 1999; 44:1012–20. (Level I)

69. Lindsay R, Cosman F, Lobo RA, Walsh BW, Harris ST, Reagan JE, et al. Addition of alendronate to ongoing hormone replacement therapy in the treatment of osteoporosis: a randomized, controlled clinical trial. J Clin Endocrinol Metab 1999;84:3076–81. (Level I)

70. Wimalawansa SJ. A four-year randomized controlled trial of hormone replacement and bisphosphonate, alone or in combination, in women with postmenopausal osteoporosis. Am J Med 1998;104:219–26. (Level I)

71. Harris ST, Eriksen EF, Davidson M, Ettinger MP, Moffett AH Jr, Baylink DJ et al. Effect of combined risedronate and hormone replacement therapies on bone mineral density in postmenopausal women. J Clin Endocrinol Metab 2001;86:1890–7. (Level I)

72. Bone HG, Greenspan SL, McKeever C, Bell N, Davidson M, Downs RW. Alendronate and estrogen effects in postmenopausal women with low bone mineral density. Alendronate/Estrogen Study Group. J Clin Endocrinol Metab 2000;85:720–6. (Level I)

73. Johnell O, Jonsson B, Jonsson L, Black D. Cost effectiveness of alendronate (fosamax) for the treatment of osteoporosis and prevention of fractures. Pharmacoeconomics 2003;21:305–14. (Cost-effectiveness analysis)

74. Gallagher JC, Fowler SE, Detter JR, Sherman SS. Combination treatment with estrogen and calcitriol in the prevention of age-related bone loss. J Clin Endocrinol Metab 2001;86:3618–28. (Level I)

75. Alexandersen P, Toussaint A, Christiansen C, Devogelaer JP, Roux C, Fechtenbaum J, et al. Ipriflavone in the treatment of postmenopausal osteoporosis: a randomized controlled trial. JAMA 2001;285:1482–8. (Level I)

76. Marshall D, Johnell O, Wedel H. Meta-analysis of how well measures of bone mineral density predict occurrence of osteoporotic fractures. BMJ 1996;312:1254–9. (Meta-analysis)

77. National Osteoporosis Foundation. Physician's guide to prevention and treatment of osteoporosis. Washington, DC: NOF; 2003. (Level III)

78. Cummings SR, Palermo L, Browner W, Marcus R, Wallace R, Pearson J, et al. Monitoring osteoporosis therapy with bone densitometry: misleading changes and regression to the mean. Fracture Intervention Trial Research Group. JAMA 2000;283:1318–21. (Level I)

The MEDLINE database, the Cochrane Library, and ACOG's own internal resources and documents were used to conduct a literature search to locate relevant articles published between January 1985 and October 2003. The search was restricted to articles published in the English language. Priority was given to articles reporting results of original research, although review articles and commentaries also were consulted. Abstracts of research presented at symposia and scientific conferences were not considered adequate for inclusion in this document. Guidelines published by organizations or institutions such as the National Institutes of Health and the American College of Obstetricians and Gynecologists were reviewed, and additional studies were located by reviewing bibliographies of identified articles. When reliable research was not available, expert opinions from obstetrician–gynecologists were used.

Studies were reviewed and evaluated for quality according to the method outlined by the U.S. Preventive Services Task Force:

I Evidence obtained from at least 1 properly designed randomized controlled trial.

II-1 Evidence obtained from well-designed controlled trials without randomization.

II-2 Evidence obtained from well-designed cohort or case–control analytic studies, preferably from more than 1 center or research group.

II-3 Evidence obtained from multiple time series with or without the intervention. Dramatic results in uncontrolled experiments also could be regarded as this type of evidence.

III Opinions of respected authorities, based on clinical experience, descriptive studies, or reports of expert committees.

Based on the highest level of evidence found in the data, recommendations are provided and graded according to the following categories:

Level A—Recommendations are based on good and consistent scientific evidence.

Level B—Recommendations are based on limited or inconsistent scientific evidence.

Level C—Recommendations are based primarily on consensus and expert opinion.

ISSN 1099-3630

**The American College of
Obstetricians and Gynecologists
409 12th Street, SW
PO Box 96920
Washington, DC 20090-6920**

12345/87654

Osteoporosis. ACOG Practice Bulletin No. 50. American College of Obstetricians and Gynecologists. Obstet Gynecol 2004;103:203–16.

ACOG PRACTICE BULLETIN

CLINICAL MANAGEMENT GUIDELINES FOR
OBSTETRICIAN–GYNECOLOGISTS

NUMBER 38, SEPTEMBER 2002

(Replaces Committee Opinion Number 163, November 1995)

This Practice Bulletin was developed by the ACOG Committee on Practice Bulletins—Obstetrics with the assistance of Richard Depp, MD, and James Lemons, MD. The information is designed to aid practitioners in making decisions about appropriate obstetric and gynecologic care. These guidelines should not be construed as dictating an exclusive course of treatment or procedure. Variations in practice may be warranted based on the needs of the individual patient, resources, and limitations unique to the institution or type of practice.

Perinatal Care at the Threshold of Viability

The survival rate for extremely preterm or extremely low-birth-weight (LBW) newborns born at the threshold of viability (25 or fewer completed weeks of gestation) improved in the early 1990s, largely as the result of a greater use of assisted ventilation in the delivery room and surfactant therapy. Increased use of antenatal and neonatal corticosteroids also may have influenced survival rates (1–4). However, this improvement in survival has not been associated with an equal improvement in morbidity. The incidence of chronic lung disease, sepsis, and poor growth remains high and may even have increased. There is concern that the treatment of extremely preterm and extremely LBW newborns may result in unforeseen effects into adulthood (4, 5), and that the neurodevelopmental outcome and cognitive function of extremely preterm and extremely LBW infants may be suboptimal (6–8). The purpose of this document is to describe the potential consequences of extremely preterm birth and to provide clinical management guidelines based on the best available data.

Background and Research Limitations

Early preterm birth or birth of an extremely LBW newborn (<1,000 g), especially those weighing less than 750 g, poses a variety of complex medical, social, and ethical considerations. The impact of such births on the infants, their families, the health care system, and society is profound. Although the prevalence of such births is less than 1%, they account for nearly one half of all cases of perinatal mortality (9). Until recently, discussion of clinical management and ethical and economic considerations of extremely preterm births were hampered by conflicting and insufficiently detailed outcome data (1, 3, 4).

Although early reports on birth outcomes before 26 weeks of gestation often were helpful in counseling patients, most reports had one or more relative weaknesses that limited their clinical value. For example, denominators differed from study to study, being reported variously as all births (stillbirths and liveborns), only liveborns, or only liveborns who survived long enough to be admitted to a neonatal intensive care unit. Potential survival may be overstated by as much as 100% at 23 weeks of gestation and by 56% at 24 weeks of gestation if the denominator included only infants admitted to the neonatal intensive care unit instead of using all fetal deaths and live births (10). The length of time that constituted survival also varied widely. Many studies failed to obtain complete outcome data, and children from lower socioeconomic backgrounds were more likely to be lost to follow-up.

Until the 1990s, when ultrasonography became more widely used, outcomes were largely reported only in terms of birth weight because of the uncertainty of gestational age. Studies based on birth weight were confounded by the inclusion of infants with intrauterine growth restriction (11); such newborns exhibited neurodevelopment consistent with their age and not their weight and, therefore, had an advantage when compared with newborns of the same size who were gestationally less mature (12, 13). Studies based on gestational age also could be inaccurate; use of the Ballard estimate of gestational age at birth consistently yields an age 10 days older than the age determined by the best obstetric estimate (14). In addition, the influence of sex on survival rates was rarely considered.

Data derived from many years of experience in caring for patients at a single institution often were limited by small numbers of infants, with few representatives among the lowest birth weight categories. In addition, many series included infants cared for over a relatively long time, during which many changes in management practices were likely. For these reasons, it is controversial whether individual institutions should use their own data on morbidity and survival rates for extremely preterm and extremely LBW births when counseling patients and their families. All of these concerns are important because at the threshold of viability, gestational age, weight, sex, and management are each important determinants of survival.

Information from large multicenter studies, such as those sponsored by the National Institute of Child Health and Human Development (NICHD), provides sufficiently detailed data to assist the perinatal team in developing an evidence-based approach to managing the extremely preterm and extremely LBW fetus. Data from the NICHD Neonatal Research Network are divided into subgroups based on gestational age in weeks or birth weight. Data by week of gestation are particularly im-

portant for these newborns because even a few days difference in age can be associated with a dramatic difference in expected outcome. Death and disability rates are inversely related to gestational age in newborns at 22–25 completed weeks of gestation (9, 15, 16).

Clinical Considerations and Recommendations

▶ *How should the patient and her family be counseled about the likelihood of survival of an extremely preterm or extremely LBW infant?*

An effort should be made to provide patients with information specific to the gestational age, estimated weight, and sex of their fetus. A multidisciplinary team approach to counseling may be helpful in ensuring that the information provided is consistent and represents a range of concerns and areas of clinical care. Counseling from a practitioner with additional experience and expertise in extremely preterm and extremely LBW births may be appropriate.

Data are now available from the most recent NICHD Neonatal Research Network trial, a large prospective study of 4,633 infants weighing between 400 g and 1,500 g at birth, conducted at 14 tertiary centers across the United States between 1995 and 1996 (14). In this study, gestational age was determined by the best obstetric estimate, using last menstrual period, standard obstetric parameters, and ultrasound examination. All liveborn infants were included, including those not admitted to the neonatal intensive care unit. Because mortality was defined as death occurring before patient discharge, the reported rates do not include deaths during labor or deaths after 120 days of life; conversely, survival rates refer to those infants who lived to at least 120 days. This study showed that a significant increase in survival of newborns occurs for each completed week from 21 weeks of gestation (0% survival) to 25 weeks of gestation (75% survival) (Table 1). In terms of birth weight (Table 2), survival was 11% at a birth weight of 400 g, 26% at birth weights of 500–601 g, and increased progressively to 75% at birth weights of 701–800 g (14). Infants delivered before 24 weeks of gestation (ie, up to 23 6/7 weeks) were not likely to survive, and those that did survive were not likely to be neurologically intact.

When gestational age, birth weight, and sex are combined (Fig. 1), it becomes evident that at each gestational age, a lower birth weight carries a higher mortal-

Table 1. Newborn Deaths by Gestational Age

Completed Weeks of Gestation	Number of Deaths	Percentage of Deaths
21	12	100
22	56	79
23	216	70
24	301	50
25	379	25
26	436	20
27	519	10
28	569	8
29	535	5
30	472	3
31	362	5
32	225	7
33	185	5
34–42	156	5

Data from Lemons JA, Bauer CR, Oh W, Korones SB, Papile LA, Stoll BJ, et al. Very low birth weight outcomes of the National Institute of Child Health and Human Development Neonatal Research Network, January 1995 through December 1996. NICHD Neonatal Research Network. Pediatrics 2001;107:E1.

Table 2. Newborn Deaths by Birth Weight

Birth Weight (g)	Number of Deaths	Percentage of Deaths
401–500	195	89
501–600	317	71
601–700	449	38
701–800	439	25
801–900	419	12
901–1,000	462	10
1,001–1,100	398	8
1,101–1,200	430	5
1,201–1,300	465	5
1,301–1,400	488	3
1,401–1,500	571	3

Data from Lemons JA, Bauer CR, Oh W, Korones SB, Papile LA, Stoll BJ, et al. Very low birth weight outcomes of the National Institute of Child Health and Human Development Neonatal Research Network, January 1995 through December 1996. NICHD Neonatal Research Network. Pediatrics 2001;107:E1.

ity risk. This effect is most pronounced in the lower ranges of gestational age and birth weight. In addition, when infants of similar gestational age and weight are compared, mortality rates are higher for males than for females. For example, a male born at 24 weeks of gestation weighing 700 g has a predicted mortality rate of 51%, whereas a female of the same age and weight has a predicted mortality rate of 35% (14).

These data apply to liveborn infants. Many of the smallest infants do not survive labor, do not respond to resuscitation, or are so small that resuscitation in the delivery room is not attempted. Among those who survive resuscitation in the delivery room, most deaths occur within the first 3 days of life (15, 16). It is significant that the small proportion of infants weighing less than 500 g who do survive resuscitative efforts in the delivery room usually are female, small-for-gestational-age newborns (4).

▶ *How should patients and their families be counseled about the morbidity associated with extremely preterm or extremely LBW infants?*

Two recent large, prospective studies addressing morbidity—one using gestational age and one using birth weight—provide useful data. A gestational-age-based population study of 811 extremely preterm newborns

used data collected in 1995 and found that disabilities in mental and psychomotor development, neuromotor function, or sensory and communication function were present in about one half of the large cohort of survivors at 30 months of corrected age (16). Approximately one quarter met the criteria for severe disability (16). Male newborns had lower psychomotor scores and were significantly more likely to have cerebral palsy than female newborns. A similar disadvantage for male newborns has been reported by others (2, 17).

The most recent NICHD Neonatal Research Network study, which used data based on the birth weights of infants delivered at 14 tertiary care centers, reported similar results. Of all infants weighing 501–750 g, 100% had growth failure, 50% had intraventricular hemorrhage, 25% had grades III–IV intraventricular hemorrhage, and 78% had respiratory distress syndrome (RDS) (14). The major morbidities influencing later development in these children included chronic lung disease, severe brain injury (intraventricular hemorrhage and periventricular leukomalacia), necrotizing enterocolitis, nosocomial infections, and retinopathy of prematurity.

▶ *What are the risk factors for cerebral palsy at the threshold of viability?*

A study from the NICHD Neonatal Research Network provided the first multicenter, prospective outcome data regarding the neurodevelopmental, neurosensory, and functional outcome of 1,151 extremely LBW newborns evaluated from birth to 18–22 months corrected age (Table 3) (2). Importantly, the sample size was sufficient

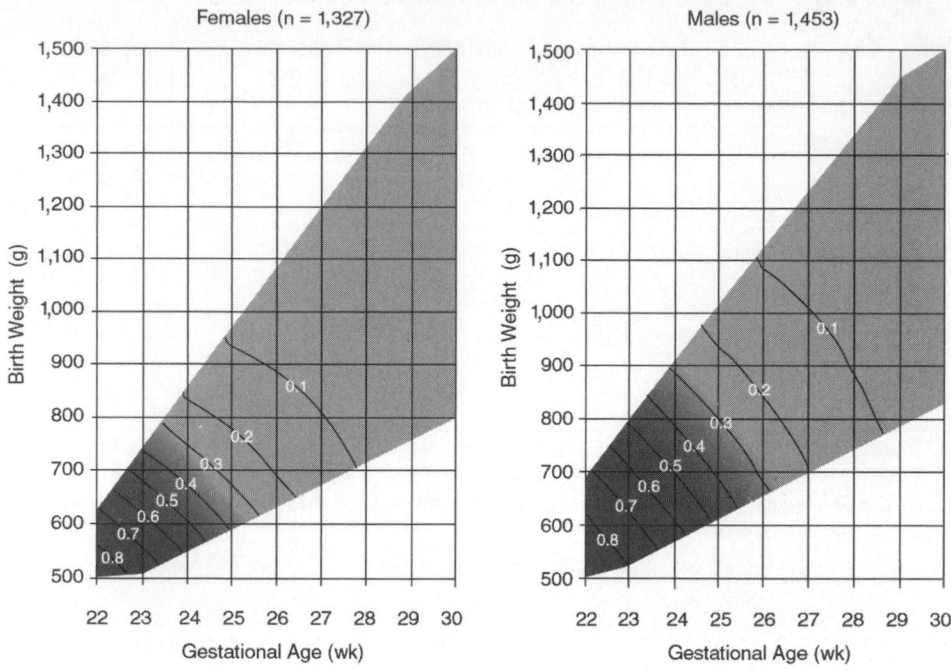

Females (n = 1,327)   Males (n = 1,453)

Figure 1. Estimated mortality risk by birth weight and gestational age based on singleton infants born in NICHD Neonatal Research Network Centers between January 1, 1995 and December 31, 1996. (Reproduced with permission from *Pediatrics*, Vol. 107, Page(s) e1, Figure 1, Copyright 2001.)

to overcome some of the limitations that hampered the clinical applicability of earlier longitudinal outcome studies. One quarter of the children had an abnormal neurologic examination, approximately one third had a Bayley II Mental Development Index score less than 70 or a Psychomotor Developmental Index score less than 70 (normal for both these indices is >80), and 10% had visual or hearing impairment. Significant risk factors associated with cerebral palsy were grades III–IV intraventricular hemorrhage, periventricular leukomalacia (odds ratio [OR], 3.05), and necrotizing enterocolitis (OR, 2.01). Risk factors for abnormal neurologic examination or Mental Development Index or Psychomotor Developmental Index scores less than 70 included grades III–IV intraventricular hemorrhage, periventricular leukomalacia, chronic lung disease, use of postnatal steroids, necrotizing enterocolitis, a mother with less than a high school education, and male sex of the fetus.

▶ *How does the assessment of gestational age affect counseling?*

Gestational age often is well established. However, if gestational age is uncertain, it is important that the clinician consider a wide range of prognoses and care options and counsel the patient about a range of possible outcomes. Even relatively small discrepancies of 1 or 2 weeks in gestational age or 100–200 g in birth weight may have major implications for survival and long-term morbidity.

In some cases—for example, in patients with little or no prenatal care—the gestational age is not established, and the clinician must consider data from fetal ultrasound measurements obtained near the time of anticipated delivery. Such measurements generally are not used to determine estimated gestational age unless they are the only data available. Although no single method has been determined to be superior, most ultrasound fetal weight formulas that include measurements of the fetal head, abdomen, and femur will yield a weight estimate within 15% of the actual weight (for weights <1,500 g) and a gestational age estimate within 2 weeks of the actual gestational age (from 20 to 30 weeks) (18). If there is a discrepancy of 2 weeks or more between the age based on menstrual dating and the age based on ultrasound measurements, or the woman is uncertain about the date of her last menstrual period, the physician may decide to make management decisions based on the ultrasound measurements, especially if measurements indicate a gestational age older than previously thought. If the measurements suggest a younger fetus, the possibility that the fetus is growth restricted should always be considered.

Table 3. Neurologic and Sensory Findings at 18 Months by Birth Weight*

Neurologic Finding	401–500 g (%) n = 14	501–600 g (%) n = 94	601–700 g (%) n = 202	701–800 g (%) n = 224
Normal examination	57	71	70	72
Cerebral palsy	29	17	21	17
Seizure disorder	0	4	5	6
Any visual impairment	21	10	12	13
Unilateral blindness	7	2	1	3
Bilateral blindness	14	1	4	2
Hearing impairment	7	11	14	9
Wears hearing aid	0	3	7	4

*Eighteen percent of the cohort were small for gestational age. Because these data are based on birth weight, it is likely the figures include intrauterine-growth-restricted infants who were gestationally more mature.

Reproduced and modified with permission from *Pediatrics*, Vol. 105, Page(s) 1216–1226, Table 3, Copyright 2000.

Ultrasonography also may provide useful information regarding the presence or absence of fetal malformations that may alter the prognosis of the fetus. However, fetal measurement and anatomic evaluation can be difficult in cases of multiple gestation or reduced amniotic fluid volume. Evaluation of multiple gestation also can be problematic because the prognosis for one infant may differ from that of the other(s).

▶ *Does the mode of delivery affect neonatal outcome?*

Few studies have evaluated the influence of obstetric management on the outcome of infants at the threshold of viability. Retrospective, nonrandomized studies have consistently failed to document a benefit of cesarean delivery for the extremely preterm fetus (19–23). It has even been difficult to document improved outcome with cesarean delivery for the extremely preterm fetus in breech position (20, 21, 24).

No prospective randomized studies of antenatal transfer of the extremely LBW infant to a tertiary care center have been reported. Retrospective data are difficult to analyze because the rapidity of labor, the severity of antepartum complications and the stability of the mother, the distance to the nearest high-risk nursery, and other factors all influence transfer decisions. However, data from retrospective studies have demonstrated a decreased mortality risk for very LBW infants delivered at hospitals with a level III neonatal intensive care unit compared with delivery at hospitals with level I or level II neonatal intensive care units (25, 26). Therefore, based on limited data, maternal transport to a tertiary care center should be considered when possible.

▶ *Is there a benefit to the use of antenatal corticosteroids for extremely preterm births?*

Although antenatal corticosteroids decrease the incidence of RDS in newborns at 29–34 weeks of gestation, randomized controlled trials have not shown a benefit in newborns treated between 24 and 28 weeks of gestation (27). In the largest randomized trial conducted on patients with intact membranes at 24–28 weeks of gestation, there was no benefit in the overall incidence or severity of RDS, but there was a significant reduction in the incidence of grades III and IV intraventricular hemorrhage ($P = 0.01$) (28). Although the precise impact of corticosteroids on RDS in pregnancies between 22 and 25 weeks of gestation has not been fully determined, the National Institutes of Health consensus conference statements on antenatal corticosteroid use recommended that all pregnant women at risk of preterm delivery between 24 and 34 weeks of gestation be considered candidates for a single course of corticosteroids (27, 29).

▶ *What are the current recommendations and ethical considerations regarding resuscitation and continued support of the extremely preterm fetus?*

Ethical decisions regarding the extent of resuscitative efforts and the subsequent support of the neonate are complex (30–32). The decision to withhold or withdraw support should not be made entirely on the basis of gestational age or birth weight, but should be individualized based on the newborn's condition at birth, survival and morbidity data, and the parents' preferences.

Each member of the health care team should make every effort to maintain a consistent theme in their discussions with family members regarding the assessment, prognosis, and recommendations for care. However, parents should understand that decisions about neonatal management made before delivery may be altered depending on the condition of the neonate at birth, the postnatal gestational age assessment, and the newborn's response to resuscitative and stabilization measures. It also is important that parents understand that the outcome depends on many factors (such as infection), some of which may not be obvious before delivery or even at the time of resuscitation. Recommendations regarding the extent of continuing support depend on frequent reevaluations of the neonate's condition, trends, and prognosis. The course of an individual newborn may change with time.

There are circumstances in which the withdrawal of life support may be appropriate, recognizing that the views of the parents are of prime importance. Compassionate care should be provided to the infant, including careful handling, maintenance of a neutral thermal environment, and gentle monitoring of vital signs.

Because it is difficult to predict how an individual extremely preterm newborn will develop, proactive programs to assess and support the infant through early school years are desirable (4). When the extremely preterm newborn does not survive, support should be provided to the family by physicians, nurses, and other staff after the infant's death. Perinatal loss support groups, intermittent contact by telephone, and a later conference with the family to review the medical events surrounding the infant's death and to evaluate the grieving response of the parents often are helpful.

Summary of Recommendations

The following recommendations are based on good and consistent scientific evidence (Level A):

▶ In general, parents of anticipated extremely preterm fetuses can be counseled that the neonatal survival rate for newborns increases from 0% at 21 weeks of gestation to 75% at 25 weeks of gestation, and from 11% at 401–500 g birth weight to 75% at 701–800 g birth weight. In addition, females generally have a better prognosis than males.

▶ In general, parents of anticipated extremely preterm fetuses can be counseled that infants delivered

before 24 weeks of gestation are less likely to survive, and those who do are not likely to survive intact. Disabilities in mental and psychomotor development, neuromotor function, or sensory and communication function are present in approximately one half of extremely preterm fetuses.

The following recommendations are based on limited or inconsistent scientific evidence (Level B):

▶ Based on data from retrospective studies, maternal transport to a tertiary care center before delivery should be considered when possible.

▶ The effects of aggressive resuscitation at birth on the outcome of the extremely preterm fetus also are unclear. Therefore, management decisions regarding the extremely preterm fetus must be individualized.

▶ The effect of antenatal steroid use in the extremely preterm fetus is unclear; however, it is recommended that all women at risk of preterm delivery between 24 and 34 weeks of gestation be considered candidates for a single course of corticosteroids.

▶ Prospectively collected outcome data for extremely preterm fetuses are available. Whenever possible, data specific to the age, weight, and sex of the individual extremely preterm fetus should be used to aid management decisions made by obstetricians and parents of fetuses at risk for preterm delivery before 26 completed weeks of gestation. This information may be developed by each institution and should indicate the population used in determining estimates of survivability.

The following recommendations are based primarily on consensus and expert opinion (Level C):

▶ When extremely preterm birth is anticipated, the estimated gestational age and weight should be carefully assessed, the prognosis for the fetus should be determined, and each member of the health care team should make every effort to maintain a consistent theme in their discussion with family members regarding the assessment, prognosis, and recommendations for care.

▶ Because it is difficult to predict how an individual extremely preterm newborn will develop, proactive programs to assess and support the infant through early school years are desirable. When the extremely preterm newborn does not survive, support should be provided to the family by physicians, nurses, and other staff after the infant's death.

References

1. Cole FS. Extremely preterm birth—defining the limits of hope. N Engl J Med 2000;343:429–30. (Level III)

2. Vohr BR, Wright LL, Dusick AM, Mele L, Verter J, Steichen JJ, et al. Neurodevelopmental and functional outcomes of extremely low birth weight infants in the National Institute of Child Health and Human Development Neonatal Research Network, 1993–1994. Pediatrics 2000;105:1216–26. (Level II-2)

3. McCormick MC. Conceptualizing child health status: observations from studies of very premature infants. Perspect Biol Med 1999;42:372–86. (Level III)

4. Hack M, Fanaroff AA. Outcomes of children of extremely low birthweight and gestational age in the 1990's. Early Hum Dev 1999;53:193–218. (Level III)

5. Hack M, Flannery DJ, Schluchter M, Carter L, Borawski E, Klein N. Outcomes in young adulthood for very-low-birth-weight infants. N Engl J Med 2002;346;149–57. (Level II-2)

6. Hack M, Taylor HG, Klein N, Eiben R, Schatschneider C, Mercuri-Minich N. School-age outcomes in children with birth weights under 750 g. N Engl J Med 1994;331:753–9. (Level II-2)

7. Hack M, Friedman H, Fanaroff AA. Outcomes of extremely low birth weight infants. Pediatrics 1996;98: 931–7. (Level II-3)

8. Peterson BS, Vohr B, Staib LH, Cannistraci CJ, Dolberg A, Schneider KC, et al. Regional brain volume abnormalities and long-term cognitive outcome in preterm infants. JAMA 2000;284:1939–47. (Level II-2)

9. Bottoms SF, Paul RH, Iams JD, Mercer BM, Thom EA, Roberts JM. Obstetric determinants of neonatal survival: influence of willingness to perform cesarean delivery on survival of extremely low-birth-weight infants. National Institute of Child Health and Human Development Network of Maternal-Fetal Medicine Units. Am J Obstet Gynecol 1997;176:960–6. (Level II-2)

10. Evans DJ, Levene MI. Evidence of selection bias in preterm survival studies: a systematic review. Arch Dis Child Fetal Neonatal Ed 2001;84:F79–84. (Level III)

11. Arnold CC, Kramer MS, Hobbs CA, McLean FH, Usher RH. Very low birth weight: a problematic cohort for epidemiologic studies of very small or immature neonates. Am J Epidemiol 1991;134:604–13. (Level II-3)

12. Pena IC, Teberg AJ, Finello KM. The premature small-for-gestational-age infant during the first year of life: comparison by birth weight and gestational age. J Pediatr 1988;113:1066–73. (Level II-2)

13. McCarton CM, Wallace IF, Divon M, Vaughan HG Jr. Cognitive and neurologic development of the premature, small for gestational age infant through age 6: comparison by birth weight and gestational age. Pediatrics 1996;98: 1167–78. (Level II-2)

14. Lemons JA, Bauer CR, Oh W, Korones SB, Papile L, Stoll BJ, et al. Very low birth weight outcomes of the National Institute of Child Health and Human Development Neonatal Research Network, January 1995 through December 1996. NICHD Neonatal Research Network. Pediatrics 2001;107:E1. (Level III)

15. Stevenson DK, Wright LL, Lemons JA, Oh W, Korones SB, Papile LA, et al. Very low birth weight outcomes of the National Institute of Child Health and Human Development Neonatal Research Network, January 1993 through December 1994. Am J Obstet Gynecol 1998;179: 1632–9. (Level II-3)

16. Wood NS, Marlow N, Costeloe K, Gibson AT, Wilkinson AR. Neurologic and developmental disability after extremely preterm birth. EPICure Study Group. N Engl J Med 2000;343:378–84. (Level II-2)

17. Tin W, Wariyar U, Hey E. Changing prognosis for babies of less than 28 weeks gestation in the north of England between 1983 and 1994. Northern Neonatal Network. BMJ 1997;314:107–11. (Level III)

18. Hadlock FP, Harrist RB, Sharman RS, Deter RL, Park SK. Estimation of fetal weight with the use of head, body, and femur measurements—a prospective study. Am J Obstet Gynecol 1985;151:333–7. (Level II-2)

19. Hack M, Fanaroff AA. Outcomes of extremely low birth weight infants between 1982 and 1988. N Engl J Med 1989;321:1642–7. (Level II-3)

20. Malloy MH, Rhoads GG, Schramm W, Land G. Increasing cesarean section rates in very low-birth weight infants. Effect on outcome. JAMA 1989;262:1475–8. (Level II-2)

21. Malloy MH, Onstad L, Wright E. The effect of cesarean delivery on birth outcome in very low birth weight infants. National Institute of Child Health and Human Development Neonatal Research Network. Obstet Gynecol 1991;77:498–503. (Level II-2)

22. Worthington D, Davis LE, Grausz JP, Sobocinski K. Factors influencing survival and morbidity with very low birth weight delivery. Obstet Gynecol 1983;62:550–5. (Level II-2)

23. Kitchen W, Ford GW, Doyle LW, Rickards AL, Lissenden JV, Pepperell RJ, et al. Cesarean section or vaginal delivery at 24 to 28 weeks' gestation: comparison of survival and neonatal and two-year morbidity. Obstet Gynecol 1985;66:149–57. (Level II-2)

24. Gravenhorst JB, Schreuder A, Veen S, Brand R, Verloove-Vanhorick SP, Verweij RA, et al. Breech delivery in very preterm and very low birthweight infants in The Netherlands. Br J Obstet Gynaecol 1993;100:411–5. (Level II-3)

25. Phibbs CS, Bronstein JM, Buxton E, Phibbs RH. The effects of patient volume and level of care at the hospital of birth on neonatal mortality. JAMA 1996;276:1054–9. (Level II-3)

26. Yeast JD, Poskin M, Stockbauer JW, Shaffer S. Changing patterns in regionalization of perinatal care and the impact on neonatal mortality. Am J Obstet Gynecol 1998;178: 131–5. (Level II-3)

27. Effect of corticosteroids for fetal maturation on perinatal outcomes. NIH Consensus Statement 1994;12:1–24. (Level III)

28. Garite TJ, Rumney PJ, Briggs GG, Harding JA, Nageotte MP, Towers CV, et al. A randomized, placebo-controlled trial of betamethasone for the prevention of respiratory distress syndrome at 24 to 28 weeks' gestation. Am J Obstet Gynecol 1992;166:646–51. (Level I)

29. Antenatal corticosteroids revisited: repeat courses. NIH Consensus Statement 2000;17:1–18. (Level III)

30. Rhoden NK. Treating Baby Doe: the ethics of uncertainty. Hastings Cent Rep 1986;16:34–42. (Level III)

31. Lantos JD, Meadow W, Miles SH, Ekwo E, Paton J, Hageman JR, et al. Providing and forgoing resuscitative therapy for babies of very low birth weight. J Clin Ethics 1992;3:283–7. (Level II-2)

32. Allen MC, Donohue PK, Dusman AE. The limit of viability—neonatal outcome of infants born at 22 to 25 weeks' gestation. N Engl J Med 1993;329:1597–1601. (Level II-3)

The MEDLINE database, the Cochrane Library, and ACOG's own internal resources and documents were used to conduct a literature search to locate relevant articles published between between January 1985 and January 2001. The search was restricted to articles published in the English language. Priority was given to articles reporting results of original research, although review articles and commentaries also were consulted. Abstracts of research presented at symposia and scientific conferences were not considered adequate for inclusion in this document. Guidelines published by organizations or institutions such as the National Institutes of Health and the American College of Obstetricians and Gynecologists were reviewed, and additional studies were located by reviewing bibliographies of identified articles. When reliable research was not available, expert opinions from obstetrician–gynecologists were used.

Studies were reviewed and evaluated for quality according to the method outlined by the U.S. Preventive Services Task Force:

I Evidence obtained from at least one properly designed randomized controlled trial.

II-1 Evidence obtained from well-designed controlled trials without randomization.

II-2 Evidence obtained from well-designed cohort or case–control analytic studies, preferably from more than one center or research group.

II-3 Evidence obtained from multiple time series with or without the intervention. Dramatic results in uncontrolled experiments could also be regarded as this type of evidence.

III Opinions of respected authorities, based on clinical experience, descriptive studies, or reports of expert committees.

Based on the highest level of evidence found in the data, recommendations are provided and graded according to the following categories:

Level A—Recommendations are based on good and consistent scientific evidence.

Level B—Recommendations are based on limited or inconsistent scientific evidence.

Level C—Recommendations are based primarily on consensus and expert opinion.

ISSN 1099-3630

**The American College of Obstetricians and Gynecologists
409 12th Street, SW
PO Box 96920
Washington, DC 20090-6920**

12345/65432

Perinatal care at the threshold of viability. ACOG Practice Bulletin No. 38. American College of Obstetricians and Gynecologists. Obstet Gynecol 2002;100:617–24.

ACOG PRACTICE BULLETIN

CLINICAL MANAGEMENT GUIDELINES FOR
OBSTETRICIAN–GYNECOLOGISTS

NUMBER 20, SEPTEMBER 2000

(Replaces Educational Bulletin Number 177, February 1993)

This Practice Bulletin was developed by the ACOG Committee on Practice Bulletins—Obstetrics with the assistance of Kim Boggess, MD. The information is designed to aid practitioners in making decisions about appropriate obstetric and gynecologic care. These guidelines should not be construed as dictating an exclusive course of treatment or procedure. Variations in practice may be warranted based on the needs of the individual patient, resources, and limitations unique to the institution or type of practice.

Perinatal Viral and Parasitic Infections

Many viral and parasitic infections are associated with significant maternal and fetal consequences if acquired during pregnancy. In the United States, some of the most commonly encountered infections with subsequent perinatal effects include cytomegalovirus (CMV), parvovirus B19, varicella zoster virus (VZV), and toxoplasmosis. The purpose of this document is to describe these infections, their modes of transmission, and their maternal and fetal effects, and to offer guidelines for counseling about and management of these infections during pregnancy.

Background

In general, perinatal infections have more severe fetal consequences when they occur early in gestation, because first-trimester infections may disrupt organogenesis. Second- and third-trimester infections can cause neurologic impairment or growth disturbances. In utero infection may be associated with certain ultrasound findings, including intrauterine growth restriction, echogenic bowel, intracranial or intrahepatic calcifications, hydrocephalus, microcephaly, isolated ascites, pericardial or pleural effusions, or nonimmune hydrops, although congenital infections also can be asymptomatic.

Cytomegalovirus

Cytomegalovirus is a double-stranded DNA herpesvirus that is transmitted by contact with infected blood, saliva, or urine, or by sexual contact. The incubation period of CMV is 28–60 days, with a mean of 40 days. Infection induces an immunoglobulin M (IgM) antibody response that disappears within 30–60 days. Viremia can be detected 2–3 weeks following primary infection. Primary CMV infection in adults generally is asymptomatic. Occasionally, patients experience a mononucleosislike syndrome, with leukocytosis, lymphocytosis, abnormal liver function tests, fever, malaise, myalgias, and chills (1). After the initial infection, CMV remains latent in host cells; recurrent infection can occur following reactivation of latent virus. In rare cases, recurrent CMV infection can occur by infection with a new strain of virus.

Prevalence of both primary and recurrent infection in pregnant women varies regionally from 0.7% to 4% for primary infection and up to 13.5% for recurrent infection (2). Vertical transmission of CMV may occur as a result of transplacental infection after primary or recurrent CMV infection, exposure to contaminated genital tract secretions at parturition, or breastfeeding. Most infants with congenital CMV are asymptomatic at birth. Clinical findings of symptomatic congenital CMV infection include jaundice, petechiae, thrombocytopenia, hepatospleno-megaly, growth restriction, and nonimmune hydrops (3, 4). The annual cost of treating the complications of CMV infections in the United States is estimated to be approximately $2 billion (2), which reflects the 50–80% seropositivity rate of pregnant women.

Cytomegalovirus is the most common congenital infection, occurring in 0.2–2.2% of all neonates (5), and is the leading cause of congenital hearing loss. Vertical transmission may occur at any stage of pregnancy, with the overall risk of infection greatest when the infection occurs during the third trimester. However, more serious fetal sequelae occur after maternal CMV infection during the first trimester. With primary maternal CMV infection, the risk of transmission to the fetus is 30–40% (6). Of those infected in utero following a primary infection, 10% will have signs and symptoms of CMV infection at birth and develop sequelae (7). Approximately 30% of severely infected infants die, and 80% of survivors have severe neurologic morbidity (5, 8). The incidence of severe fetal infection is much lower after recurrent maternal infection than after primary infection. Vertical transmission after a recurrent infection is 0.15–2% (8, 9). Infants infected after maternal CMV reactivation generally are asymptomatic at birth. Congenital hearing loss is typically the most severe sequela of secondary infection, and congenital infection following recurrent infection is unlikely to produce multiple sequelae (9). Cytomegalovirus infection acquired as a result of exposure to infected cervical secretions or breast milk is typically asymptomatic and is not associated with severe neonatal sequelae.

Parvovirus B19

Parvovirus B19 is a single-stranded DNA virus that causes the childhood exanthem erythema infectiosum, also known as fifth disease. In immunocompetent adults, the most common symptoms of parvovirus B19 infection are a reticular rash on the trunk and peripheral arthropathy,

although approximately 33% of infections are asymptomatic (10). Another manifestation of parvovirus B19 infection is transient aplastic crisis, which is more common in those with an underlying hemoglobinopathy. Most infections are mild; most individuals recover completely from parvovirus B19 infection and require only supportive care.

Transmission of parvovirus B19 most commonly occurs through respiratory secretions and hand-to-mouth contact. The infected person generally is infectious 5–10 days after exposure prior to the onset of the rash or other symptoms and is no longer infectious with the onset of the rash (11). Both IgM and IgG are produced in response to infection. The IgM response, which persists for 1 to several months, is indicative of a recent infection. IgG antibodies persist indefinitely and, in the absence of IgM, indicate prior infection and immunity. Prevalence of seropositivity to parvovirus B19 increases with age and is greater than 60% in adolescents and adults (11). The risk of maternal infection of parvovirus B19 varies with level of exposure to the infected individual. Exposure to a household member infected with parvovirus B19 is associated with an approximate 50% risk of seroconversion (12–15). The risk of transmission in a child care setting or classroom is lower, ranging from approximately 20% to 50% (15–17).

Recent maternal infection with parvovirus B19 constitutes a low risk for fetal morbidity (18), although some cases have been associated with adverse fetal effects. Transplacental transmission has been reported to be as high as 33% (19), and fetal infection with parvovirus B19 has been associated with spontaneous abortion, hydrops fetalis, and stillbirth. The rate of fetal loss among women with serologically proven parvovirus B19 infection ranges from 2% to 9% (20–22). In utero, parvovirus B19 infection is responsible for up to 18% of cases of nonimmune hydrops fetalis in some series (23, 24). Hydrops fetalis results from aplastic anemia, myocarditis, or chronic fetal hepatitis. Severe effects are seen most frequently among fetuses when maternal parvovirus B19 infection occurs at less than 20 weeks of gestation (20). Stillbirth resulting from maternal infection has occurred from 1 to 11 weeks after maternal infection. However, hydrops is unlikely to develop if it has not occurred by 8 weeks after maternal infection (23). Long-term development appears to be normal in fetuses with congenital parvovirus B19 infection that do not succumb to the disease (25, 26).

Varicella Zoster Virus

Varicella zoster virus is a DNA herpesvirus that is highly contagious and is transmitted by respiratory droplets or close contact. The attack rate among susceptible contacts is 60–90% after exposure. The incubation period after infection is 10–20 days, with a mean of 14 days (27). The period of infectivity begins 48 hours before the rash appears and lasts until the vesicles crust over. The primary infection causes chickenpox, which is characterized by fever, malaise, and a maculopapular pruritic rash that becomes vesicular. After the primary infection, VZV remains dormant in sensory ganglia and can be reactivated to cause a vesicular erythematous skin rash known as herpes zoster. The antibody to VZV develops within a few days after the onset of infection, and prior infection with VZV confers lifelong immunity.

Varicella infection is uncommon in pregnancy (occurring in 0.4–0.7 per 1,000 patients), because of the high prevalence of natural immunity (28). Pregnancy complicated by maternal varicella infection is associated with untoward maternal, fetal, and neonatal effects. The disease usually is a benign and self-limited illness in children; however, varicella national mortality data indicate that although less than 5% of varicella cases occur among adults 20 years of age or older, that group contributes to 55% of varicella-related deaths (29). Severe complications, such as encephalitis and pneumonia, are more common in adults than in children; VZV pneumonia in pregnancy is a risk factor for maternal mortality (30, 31).

In pregnancy, varicella may be transmitted across the placenta, resulting in congenital or neonatal chickenpox. The risk of congenital varicella syndrome is limited to exposure during the first 20 weeks of gestation, occurs uncommonly (up to 2%), and is characterized by skin scarring, limb hypoplasia, chorioretinitis, and microcephaly (32–34). Neonatal VZV infection is associated with a high neonatal death rate when maternal disease develops from 5 days before delivery up to 48 hours postpartum as a result of the relative immaturity of the neonatal immune system and the lack of protective maternal antibody (35, 36).

Toxoplasmosis

Toxoplasmosis is caused by the intracellular parasite *Toxoplasma gondii*. *T gondii* exists in several forms: a trophozoite, which is the invasive form, and a cyst or an oocyst, which are latent forms. Human infection is acquired by consuming cysts in undercooked meat of infected animals, by insect contamination of food, by contact with oocysts from the feces of infected cats (the only definitive hosts), or by contact with infected materials or insects in soil. Infection with *T gondii* usually is asymptomatic, although after an incubation of 5–18 days, some nonspecific symptoms may occur. Most often, toxoplasmosis presents as asymptomatic cervical lym-

phadenopathy, with symptoms occurring in only 10–20% of adult cases. Other symptoms include fever, malaise, night sweats, myalgias, and hepatosplenomegaly. Parasitemia can occur after infection, which, in pregnant women, can seed the placenta and cause subsequent fetal infection. Congenital transmission of *T gondii* from an infected woman was the first form of transmission to be recognized, and transmission depends on the time of acquisition of maternal infection. The later in gestation that the infection occurs, the more likely transmission is to occur. The rate of vertical transmission increases from 10% to 15% in the first trimester, to 25% in the second trimester, and to more than 60% in the third trimester (37, 38). The severity of infection depends on gestational age at the time of transmission. The earlier the fetus is infected, the more severe the disease. Most infected infants do not have clinical signs of infection at birth, but 55–85% will develop sequelae, including chorioretinitis (leading to severe impairment of vision), hearing loss, or mental retardation (39–41). Other clinical manifestations of congenital toxoplasmosis include rash, hepatosplenomegaly, ascites, fever, periventricular calcifications, ventriculomegaly, and seizures (42–44).

After an acute infection, IgM antibodies appear early and reach maximum levels in 1 month. IgG antibodies appear after IgM antibodies, are detectable within a few weeks after infection, and confer immunity. High titers of both IgG and IgM may persist for years. In the immunocompetent adult, the clinical course is benign and self-limited.

Clinical Considerations and Recommendations

Cytomegalovirus

▶ *How is maternal CMV infection diagnosed?*

The majority of adult CMV infections are asymptomatic, which makes diagnosis of primary infection difficult. Cytomegalovirus may be detected by culture or polymerase chain reaction (PCR) of infected blood, urine, saliva, cervical secretions, or breast milk, although diagnosis of CMV infection in adults usually is confirmed by serologic testing. Serum samples collected 3–4 weeks apart, tested in parallel for anti-CMV IgG, are essential for the diagnosis of primary infection. Seroconversion from negative to positive or a significant increase (greater than fourfold, eg, from 1:4 to 1:16) in anti-CMV IgG titers is evidence of infection. The presence of CMV-specific IgM is a useful but not completely reliable indication of a primary infection. IgM titers may not be positive during an acute infection, or they may persist for months after the primary infection (45). A small proportion of women with recurrent infection will demonstrate anti-CMV IgM (7). The reported sensitivity of CMV IgM serologic assays ranges from 50% to 90% (45).

▶ *How is fetal CMV infection diagnosed?*

Congenital CMV may be suspected prenatally after a documented maternal primary infection or, more typically, after detection of ultrasound findings suggestive of infection (46). These include abdominal and liver calcifications, calcification of the lateral border of the lateral ventricles, hydrops, echogenic bowel, ascites, hepatosplenomegaly, and ventriculomegaly (46–53). Fetuses that demonstrate abnormalities, particularly if they involve the central nervous system, generally have a much poorer prognosis (46, 54).

Cytomegalovirus has been diagnosed prenatally by detection of anti-CMV IgM in fetal blood (55–57), although this test has a high false-positive rate (58). In addition, IgM is not detectable in the first half of pregnancy, presumably because of the immaturity of the fetal immune system, limiting the usefulness of fetal serologic testing. Testing for fetal thrombocytopenia or abnormal liver function has been suggested as a method to diagnose congenital CMV. However, these tests are not specific for CMV, and normal results do not preclude severe infection.

Cytomegalovirus can be detected in the amniotic fluid of infected fetuses by either culture or PCR. The sensitivity of CMV culture ranges from 50% to 69%, compared with a sensitivity of 77–100% for PCR. Negative and positive predictive values are comparable between amniotic fluid culture and PCR (55–57, 59–64). The sensitivity of amniotic fluid testing for prenatal diagnosis of congenital CMV infection is markedly lower if performed before 21 weeks of gestation (65), and the time interval between maternal infection and testing may influence the reliability (62). Although these tests are promising, neither amniotic fluid culture nor PCR can detect all cases of congenital CMV infection. In addition, the detection of CMV in amniotic fluid does not predict the severity of congenital CMV infection. A combination of amniotic fluid culture and PCR has been suggested to have a sensitivity of 80–100% in identifying infected fetuses (56). Fetal blood sampling is less sensitive than amniotic fluid testing (64). Specific ultrasonographic findings may further assist in the accurate diagnosis of a congenitally infected infant with a poor prognosis.

▶ *How are maternal, fetal, and congenital neonatal infections with cytomegalovirus treated?*

Currently, no therapies are available for the treatment of maternal or fetal CMV infection. Antiviral treatment with ganciclovir or foscarnet is approved only for treatment of CMV retinitis in patients with acquired immunodeficiency syndrome (AIDS). However, ganciclovir has been shown in vitro to cross the placenta by simple diffusion (66), and there are reports of its postnatal use for the treatment of congenital CMV (67–69). Ganciclovir and CMV hyperimmune gamma globulin have shown promise for the treatment of neonates with congenital CMV infection (70–72). The effectiveness of treatment in the prevention of long-term neurologic sequelae has not been proven.

A live attenuated vaccine using the Towne 125 strain has been developed, and appears to be safe, somewhat protective (73–76), and economically beneficial (77). There is reluctance to embrace vaccination because of concerns about the ability of the vaccine strain to reactivate and potentially infect the host, the potential for viral shedding from the cervix or breast milk, and the possible oncogenic potential of vaccine virus (78). However, the science in this area is advancing rapidly, and new treatment options may become available.

▶ *How should women at high risk be counseled about prevention of CMV?*

Factors associated with an increased risk of CMV infection include history of abnormal cervical cytology, lower socioeconomic status, birth outside North America, first pregnancy at younger than 15 years, and infection with other sexually transmitted diseases. The greatest impact obstetrician–gynecologists can have on reducing CMV disease is by educating patients about preventive measures. Counseling should cover careful handling of potentially infected articles, such as diapers, and thorough hand-washing when around young children or immunocompromised individuals, explaining that careful attention to hygiene is effective in helping to prevent transmission (3, 12, 79). In addition, women should be counseled, when appropriate, about the avoidance of high-risk behaviors, such as intravenous drug use and sharing of needles. Condom use should be encouraged as a method of contraception.

▶ *Should women at high risk be screened before or during pregnancy?*

Currently, routine serologic testing for CMV during pregnancy is not recommended (4, 7, 80, 81). Maternal IgM antibody screening is limited for differentiating primary from recurrent infection, which makes it difficult to use such results in counseling patients about fetal risk. In addition, maternal immunity does not eliminate the possibility of fetal infection.

Although the virus is not highly contagious, some groups of women are at higher risk for the acquisition of CMV infection. Eleven percent of seronegative child care workers demonstrate seroconversion within 10 months of hire (82), and 53% of families of young children have one or more family members seroconvert within a year (83, 84). In two cross-sectional studies, increasing parity had an independent effect on increasing CMV seroprevalence, demonstrating the possibility of child-to-mother transmission (85). Therefore, women with young children or those who work with young children should be advised that the risk of infection can be reduced significantly by safe-handling techniques, such as the use of latex gloves and rigorous hand-washing after handling diapers or after exposure to respiratory secretions (3, 12, 86).

Parvovirus B19

▶ *Which methods are available to diagnose maternal parvovirus B19 infection?*

Maternal serology is the most commonly used test to diagnose acute infection with parvovirus B19. Enzyme-linked immunosorbent assay (ELISA), radioimmunoassay, and Western blot tests can measure the antibody to parvovirus B19 (20). The sensitivity of IgM and IgG assays is generally 79% (10, 87). Identification of parvovirus-specific IgM in maternal serum is diagnostic of a primary infection, although a laboratory with experience should measure titers, because false-positive results can occur. Previous exposure and infection with parvovirus B19 is indicated by the presence of antiparvovirus B19 IgG in the absence of IgM and has not been associated with adverse perinatal outcome.

Parvovirus B19 can be identified by direct visualization of viral particles in infected tissues or serum by electron microscopy or by identification of characteristic intranuclear inclusions within erythroblasts (88).

▶ *What methods are available for diagnosing fetal parvovirus B19 infection?*

Diagnosis of fetal parvovirus B19 infection can be accomplished by isolation of viral particles in abortuses or placental specimens (89, 90). Polymerase chain reaction also has been used to detect parvovirus B19 in fetal specimens, including autopsy tissue, serum, amniotic fluid, and placenta (91–95).

Sensitivity of PCR for detection of parvovirus may be as high as 100%, although data are limited by small sample sizes (94, 96). Reliable serologic tests for specific IgM antibodies in the fetus are not available. As with other intrauterine infections, IgM antibodies appear in the fetal circulation after 22 weeks of gestation, limiting the usefulness of such tests.

Ultrasonography has been the mainstay for diagnosing fetal parvovirus infection. Severely infected fetuses typically have evidence of hydrops fetalis. Serial ultrasound examinations for up to 10 weeks after maternal infection are indicated. If the fetus shows no signs of hydrops fetalis, additional tests are unnecessary.

▶ *How are maternal, fetal, and congenital neonatal infections with parvovirus B19 managed?*

After documented exposure to parvovirus B19, the woman should have serologic testing to determine if she is immune with evidence of antiparvovirus IgG. If nonimmune, the test should be repeated in 3–4 weeks and paired samples tested to document whether the woman is seropositive for parvovirus. If seroconversion does not occur, the fetus is not at risk for in utero infection. If seroconversion does occur, the fetus should be monitored for 10 weeks by serial ultrasound examination to evaluate for presence of hydrops fetalis, placentomegaly, and growth disturbances (9).

In a series of 618 pregnant women exposed to parvovirus, only 311 (50.3%) were susceptible to infection. Of those susceptible, only 52 contracted parvovirus. None of the 52 infants exposed to maternal parvovirus developed hydrops fetalis (14). However, if hydrops fetalis develops, percutaneous umbilical blood sampling should be performed to determine the fetal hematocrit, leukocyte and platelet count, and viral DNA in preparation for supportive care using transfusion (97, 98). Intrauterine transfusion should be considered if anemia is present (21, 99).

▶ *Should seronegative women with work-related exposure be taken out of work?*

When outbreaks of parvovirus B19 infection occur in situations in which prolonged, close-contact exposure occurs, as in schools, homes, or child care centers, options for prevention of transmission are limited (20). Exposure cannot be eliminated by identifying and excluding persons with acute parvovirus B19 infection; up to 20% are asymptomatic, and those with infection are infectious before they develop symptoms. Exclusion of pregnant women from the workplace during endemic periods is controversial, and a policy to routinely exclude members of high-risk groups from work during an outbreak of parvovirus B19 is not recommended (14, 20).

Varicella Zoster Virus

▶ *How is maternal VZV infection diagnosed?*

Usually, this diagnosis is based on clinical findings, and laboratory testing is not needed, especially if a rash occurs after known exposure. If laboratory diagnosis is required, the VZV antigen can be demonstrated within skin lesions or vesicular fluid by immunofluorescence. Varicella infection also can be documented by the detection of the fluorescence antibody to the membrane antigen or of the VZV antibody by ELISA (28).

▶ *How is fetal VZV infection diagnosed?*

Although two small studies estimate the rate of congenital varicella syndrome after maternal infection with VZV to be 1–2% (32, 34), these studies were subject to bias, and these rates may be overestimated. The risk of congenital varicella syndrome is small; however, the outcome for the affected infant is serious enough that a reliable method of prenatal diagnosis would be valuable.

Fetal varicella can be suspected by the presence of ultrasonographic abnormalities. Ultrasound findings suggestive of congenital varicella include hydrops, hyperechogenic foci in the liver and bowel, cardiac malformations, limb deformities, microcephaly, and intrauterine growth restriction. In one series, five fetuses with congenital VZV demonstrated some ultrasound findings that suggested infection, and all the infants died by 4 months of age (100). However, not all fetuses with congenital VZV that have ultrasound abnormalities do poorly (101). Although the sensitivity of ultrasonography is unknown, it is the preferred method of diagnosis of congenital VZV.

Invasive prenatal diagnosis in women who acquire VZV in the first half of pregnancy may serve to provide reassurance if test results are negative (102). However, if the virus is present, identifying it by culture or viral DNA by PCR in chorionic villi, amniotic fluid or fetal blood, or the viral-specific antibody does not accurately predict the severity of fetal infection (101, 103).

▶ *What therapies are available and effective for maternal, fetal, and congenital neonatal infections with varicella?*

Oral acyclovir, if instituted within 24 hours of the rash, has been shown to reduce the duration of new lesion formation and the total number of new lesions and to improve constitutional symptoms in children, adolescents, and adults (104–106). Oral acyclovir appears to be safe and can be prescribed for pregnant women if lesions develop (107). Maternal varicella complicated by pneumonia should be treated with intravenous acyclovir, because intravenous acyclovir may reduce maternal morbidity and mortality associated with varicella pneumonia (31, 108).

Maternal treatment with acyclovir has not been shown to ameliorate or prevent the fetal effects of congenital varicella syndrome (109). Varicella-zoster immune globulin (VZIG) should be given to infants born to women who develop varicella between 5 days before and 2 days after delivery, although this does not universally prevent neonatal varicella (110). Infants who develop varicella within the first 2 weeks of life should be treated with intravenous acyclovir (107, 111).

▶ *What preventive strategies are effective for varicella?*

Nonpregnant women of childbearing age should be questioned about previous infection with varicella preconceptionally and offered vaccination if no report of chickenpox is elicited. Varicella vaccine has been available since March 1995 and is approved for use in healthy susceptible persons 12 months or older (112). Conception should be delayed until 1 month after the second vaccination dose is given.

Among women who do not recall a history of varicella, 70–90% have detectable antibodies (112). Antenatal VZV screening of all pregnant women with negative or indeterminate varicella histories is not believed to be cost-effective by some (113). However, others argue that from a cost-effectiveness/cost-benefit standpoint, management based on immune testing is preferable to universal VZIG administration when caring for pregnant women exposed to VZV with a negative or indeterminate infection history (114). Patients known to be nonimmune to VZV should be counseled to avoid contact with individuals who have chickenpox. If exposure does occur, prophylactic intervention with VZIG early in the incubation period can prevent or attenuate the disease manifestations of VZV in susceptible contacts at high risk from this infection (106). Expeditious determination of the VZV membrane antigen or equivalent anti-VZV antibody status in pregnant women exposed to VZV appears to be a rapid, satisfactory method for determining who should promptly receive VZIG passive immunization (115). Although VZIG is effective in reducing the severity of maternal varicella when administered up to 72 hours after exposure, it should be given as soon as possible (116, 117). Maternal administration of VZIG does not ameliorate or prevent fetal infection.

Toxoplasmosis

▶ *How is maternal toxoplasmosis infection diagnosed?*

Isolation of *T gondii* from blood or body fluids establishes that the infection is acute; however, serologic testing for the detection of the specific antibody to *T gondii* is the primary method of diagnosis. Numerous antibody assays are available. The Sabin-Feldman dye test is the IgG test with which all others are compared, but it is performed at only a few reference laboratories. Indirect fluorescent antibody, indirect hemagglutination and agglutination tests, and ELISA also are available to detect the antitoxoplasma antibody. However, serologic assays for toxoplasmosis are not well standardized and have a high false-positive rate. IgM titers may persist at high levels (eg, ≥1:512) for years in healthy individuals (118). Both IgG and IgM testing should be used for the initial evaluation of patients suspected to have toxoplasmosis. Testing of serial specimens 3 weeks apart in parallel gives the most accurate assessment if the initial test results are equivocal. In cases in which clinical suspicion is high, specimens should be saved for repeat testing because of the wide variation between laboratories. Repeat testing in a well-recognized reference laboratory should be performed if there is evidence of a primary infection.

▶ *Which methods are available for diagnosing and monitoring fetal infection?*

Ultrasonography can demonstrate severe congenital toxoplasmosis; suggestive findings include ventriculomegaly, intracranial calcifications, microcephaly, ascites, hepatosplenomegaly, and intrauterine growth restriction. Testing fetal blood samples after 20 weeks of gestation for the presence of specific IgM is the most sensitive test in diagnosing congenital toxoplasmosis (119). Using fetal blood for antibody testing or mouse inoculation, amniotic fluid for PCR, or fetal ultrasonography to detect ventriculomegaly, 77–93% of infected infants were identified prenatally, although no single test was very sensitive (43, 120). Successful identification of *T gondii* intrauterine infection with PCR testing of amniotic fluid allows for earlier testing than fetal blood sampling, with high sensitivity (37, 121–124), although false-positive and false-negative findings do occur (125).

▶ *How are maternal, fetal, and congenital neonatal infections with toxoplasmosis treated?*

Treatment of the pregnant woman with acute toxoplasmosis reduces but does not eliminate the risk of congen-

ital infection (42, 43). Identification of acute maternal infection necessitates immediate institution of treatment until results of fetal testing are known. Spiramycin, which concentrates in the placenta, may reduce the risk of fetal transmission by 60% (126), but as a single agent, it does not treat established fetal infection. Spiramycin is available only through the U.S. Food and Drug Administration after serologic confirmation at a reference laboratory; it is recommended for pregnant women at risk unless fetal infection is documented. If fetal infection is established, pyrimethamine, sulfonamides, and folinic acid are added to the regimen because they more effectively eradicate parasites in the placenta and in the fetus than spiramycin alone (127). With treatment, even early fetal infection with toxoplasmosis can result in successful pregnancy outcomes (128).

Treatment of infants with symptomatic congenital toxoplasmosis consists of pyrimethamine and sulfadiazine, alternating monthly with spiramycin, for 1 year (127). Treatment will diminish or resolve intracranial calcifications if present, suggesting improved neurologic function (129).

▶ *Should women be screened for toxoplasmosis during pregnancy?*

A multicenter study in the United States found that approximately 38% of pregnant women have evidence of prior toxoplasmosis infection (130). Evidence of previous infection signifies that the future mother is not at risk of giving birth to a child with congenital toxoplasmosis. Serologic screening as a way to prevent congenital toxoplasmosis would have the most impact in countries with a high frequency of seropositivity, and routine prenatal screening is performed in France and Austria (39). However, in the United States, routine screening during pregnancy currently is not recommended, except in women infected with human immunodeficiency virus (HIV). Serologic screening during pregnancy may yield equivocal results, because IgM antibodies can persist for long periods (131). Exceptional circumstances may justify toxoplasmosis titer screening for pregnant women who are cat owners. One study in Belgium demonstrated a 63% reduction in the rate of maternal toxoplasmosis infection after institution of an educational program that recommended avoiding eating undercooked or raw meat, wearing gloves when working with soil, and avoiding caring for cats unless they are strictly "indoor cats" whose food is rigidly controlled (131).

Summary

The following recommendations are based on limited and inconsistent scientific data (Level B):

▶ Pregnant women who are seronegative for VZV and exposed to chickenpox should receive VZIG.

▶ Pregnant women who develop chickenpox should be treated with oral acyclovir to minimize maternal symptoms; if pneumonia develops, they should be treated with intravenous acyclovir.

▶ Pregnant women who have acute parvovirus B19 infection during pregnancy should be monitored with serial ultrasound examinations for at least 10 weeks following infection for the presence of hydrops fetalis.

▶ Fetuses with evidence of hydrops should undergo fetal blood sampling and transfusion as needed.

▶ Pregnant women who acquire toxoplasmosis should be treated with spiramycin. When diagnosed, fetal toxoplasmosis should be treated with a combination of pyrimethamine, sulfadiazine, and folinic acid, alternating with spiramycin.

The following recommendations are based primarily on consensus and expert opinion (Level C):

▶ Routine serologic screening of all pregnant women for CMV and toxoplasmosis is not recommended.

▶ Nonpregnant women of reproductive age who have no history of varicella infection should be offered varicella vaccine.

▶ The diagnosis of toxoplasmosis should be confirmed by a reliable reference laboratory.

▶ Pregnant women exposed to parvovirus B19 should have serologic screening performed to determine if they are at risk for seroconversion.

▶ Pregnant women should be counseled about methods to prevent acquisition of CMV or toxoplasmosis during pregnancy.

References

1. Klemola E, Kaariainen L. Cytomegalovirus as a possible cause of a disease resembling infectious mononucleosis. Br Med J 1965;5470:1099–1102 (Level III)

2. Fowler KB, Stagno S, Pass RF. Maternal age and congenital cytomegalovirus infection: screening of two diverse newborn populations, 1980–1990. J Infect Dis 1993;168:552–556 (Level II-3)

3. Adler SP, Finney JW, Manganello AM, Best AM. Prevention of child-to-mother transmission of cytomegalovirus by changing behaviors: a randomized controlled trial. Pediatr Infect Dis J 1996;15:240–246 (Level II-1)

4. Daniel Y, Gull I, Peyser MR, Lessing JB. Congenital cytomegalovirus infection. Eur J Obstet Gynecol Reprod Biol 1995;63:7–16 (Level III)

5. Stagno S, Pass RF, Dworsky ME, Alford CA Jr. Maternal cytomegalovirus infection and perinatal transmission. Clin Obstet Gynecol 1982;25:563–576 (Level III)

6. Stagno S, Pass RF, Cloud G, Britt WJ, Henderson RE, Walton PD, et al. Primary cytomegalovirus infection in pregnancy. Incidence, transmission to fetus, and clinical outcome. JAMA 1986;256:1904–1908 (Level II-2)

7. Hagay ZJ, Biran G, Ornoy A, Reece EA. Congenital cytomegalovirus infection: a long-standing problem still seeking a solution. Am J Obstet Gynecol 1996;174:241–245 (Level III)

8. Stagno S, Whitley RJ. Herpesvirus infections of pregnancy. Part 1: Cytomegalovirus and Epstein-Barr virus infections. N Engl J Med 1985;313:1270–1274 (Level II-3)

9. Fowler KB, Stagno S, Pass RF, Britt WJ, Boll TJ, Alford CA. The outcome of congenital cytomegalovirus infection in relation to maternal antibody status. N Engl J Med 1992;326:663–667 (Level II-2)

10. Chorba T, Coccia P, Holman RC, Tattersall P, Anderson LJ, Sudman J, et al. The role of parvovirus B19 in aplastic crisis and erythema infectiosum (fifth disease). J Infect Dis 1986;154:383–393 (Level II-2)

11. Thurn J. Human parvovirus B19: historical and clinical review. Rev Infect Dis 1988;10:1005–1011 (Level III)

12. Cytomegalovirus (CMV) infection and prevention. Atlanta, Georgia: Centers for Disease Control and Prevention, 1998 (Level III)

13. Rice PS, Cohen BJ. A school outbreak of parvovirus B19 infection investigated using salivary antibody assays. Epidemiol Infect 1996;116:331–338 (Level II-3)

14. Harger JH, Adler SP, Koch WC, Harger GF. Prospective evaluation of 618 pregnant women exposed to parvovirus B19: risks and symptoms. Obstet Gynecol 1998;91:413–420 (Level II-3)

15. Valeur-Jensen AK, Pedersen CB, Westergaard T, Jensen IP, Lebech M, Andersen PK, et al. Risk factors for parvovirus B19 infection in pregnancy. JAMA 1999;281:1099–1105 (Level II-2)

16. Gillespie SM, Cartter ML, Asch S, Rokos JB, Gary GW, Tsou CJ, et al. Occupational risk of human parvovirus B19 infection for school and day-care personnel during an outbreak of erythema infectiosum. JAMA 1990;263:2061–2065 (Level II-3)

17. Cartter ML, Farley TA, Rosengren S, Quinn DL, Gillespie SM, Gary GW, et al. Occupational risk factors for infection with parvovirus B19 among pregnant women. J Infect Dis 1991;163:282–285 (Level II-2)

18. Guidozzi F, Ballot D, Rothberg AD. Human B19 parvovirus infection in an obstetric population. A prospective study determining fetal outcome. J Reprod Med 1994;39:36–38 (Level III)

19. Public Health Laboratory Service Working Party on Fifth Disease. Prospective study of human parvovirus (B19) infection in pregnancy. BMJ 1990;300:1166–1170 (Level II-3)

20. Risks associated with human parvovirus B19 infection. MMWR Morbid Mortal Wkly Rep 1989;38:81–88, 93–97 (Level III)

21. Rodis JF, Quinn DL, Gary GW Jr, Anderson LJ, Rosengren S, Cartter ML, et al. Management and outcomes of pregnancies complicated by human B19 parvovirus infection: a prospective study. Am J Obstet Gynecol 1990;163:1168–1171 (Level III)

22. Gratacos E, Torres PJ, Vidal J, Antolin E, Costa J, Jimenez de Anta MT, et al. The incidence of human parvovirus B19 infection during pregnancy and its impact on perinatal outcome. J Infect Dis 1995;171:1360–1363 (Level II-2)

23. Yaegashi N, Okamura K, Yajima A, Murai C, Sugamura K. The frequency of human parvovirus B19 infection in nonimmune hydrops fetalis. J Perinat Med 1994;22:159–163 (Level III)

24. Jordan JA. Identification of human parvovirus B19 infection in idiopathic nonimmune hydrops fetalis. Am J Obstet Gynecol 1996;174:37–42 (Level II-3)

25. Miller E, Fairley CK, Cohen BJ, Seng C. Immediate and long term outcome of human parvovirus B19 infection in pregnancy. Br J Obstet Gynaecol 1998;105:174–178 (Level II-3)

26. Rodis JF, Rodner C, Hansen AA, Borgida AF, Deoliveira I, Shulman Rosengren S, et al. Long-term outcome of children following maternal human parvovirus B19 infection. Obstet Gynecol 1998;91:125–128 (Level II-2)

27. Preblud SR, Orenstein WA, Bart KJ. Varicella: clinical manifestations, epidemiology and health impact in children. Pediatr Infect Dis 1984;3:505–509 (Level III)

28. Enders G. Serodiagnosis of Varicella-Zoster virus infection in pregnancy and standardization of the ELISA IgG and IgM antibody tests. Dev Biol Stand 1982;52:221–236 (Level III)

29. Varicella-related deaths among adults—United States, 1997. MMWR Morb Mortal Wkly Rep 1997;46:409–412 (Level III)

30. Paryani SG, Arvin AM. Intrauterine infection with varicella-zoster virus after maternal varicella. N Engl J Med 1986;314:1542–1546 (Level II-3)

31. Smego RA Jr, Asperilla MO. Use of acyclovir for varicella pneumonia during pregnancy. Obstet Gynecol 1991;78:1112–1116 (Level III)

32. Enders G, Miller E, Cradock-Watson J, Bolley I, Ridehalgh M. Consequences of varicella and herpes zoster in pregnancy: prospective study of 1739 cases. Lancet 1994;343:1548–1551 (Level II-2)

33. Jones KL, Johnson KA, Chambers CD. Offspring of women infected with varicella during pregnancy: a prospective study. Teratology 1994;49:29–32 (Level II-2)

34. Pastuszak AL, Levy M, Schick B, Zuber C, Feldkamp M, Gladstone J, et al. Outcome after maternal varicella infection in the first 20 weeks of pregnancy. N Engl J Med 1994;330:901–905 (Level II-2)

35. Brunell PA. Placental transfer of varicella-zoster antibody. Pediatrics 1966;38:1034–1038 (Level III)

36. Brunell PA. Fetal and neonatal varicella-zoster infections. Semin Perinatol 1983;7:47–56 (Level III)

37. Hohlfeld P, Daffos F, Costa JM, Thulliez P, Forestier F, Vidaud M. Prenatal diagnosis of congenital toxoplasmosis with a polymerase-chain-reaction test on amniotic fluid. N Engl J Med 1994;331:695–699 (Level II-2)

38. Foulon W, Villena I, Stray-Pedersen B, Decoster A, Lappalainen M, Pinon JM, et al. Treatment of toxoplasmosis during pregnancy: a multicenter study of impact on fetal transmission and children's sequelae at age 1 year. Am J Obstet Gynecol 1999;180:410–415 (Level II-3)

39. Stray-Pedersen B. Toxoplasmosis in pregnancy. Baillieres Clin Obstet Gynaecol 1993;7:107–137 (Level III)

40. Wilson CB, Remington JS, Stagno S, Reynolds DW. Development of adverse sequelae in children born with subclinical congenital Toxoplasma infection. Pediatrics 1980;66:767–774 (Level II-3)

41. de Roever-Bonnet H, Koppe JG, Loewer-Seger DH. Follow-up of children with congenital toxoplasma infection and children who became serologically negative after 1 year of age, all born in 1964–1965. In: Thalhammer O, Baumgarten K, Pollak A, eds. Perinatal medicine: Sixth European Congress, Vienna. Littleton, Massachusetts: PSG Publishing Company, 1979:61–75 (Level III)

42. Desmonts G, Couvreur J. Congenital toxoplasmosis. A prospective study of 378 pregnancies. N Engl J Med 1974;290:1110–1116 (Level II-3)

43. Daffos F, Forestier F, Capella-Pavlovsky M, Thulliez P, Aufrant C, Valenti D, et al. Prenatal management of 746 pregnancies at risk for congenital toxoplasmosis. N Engl J Med 1988;318:271–275 (Level II-3)

44. Remington JS, McLeod R, Desmonts G. Toxoplasmosis. In: Remington JS, Klein JO, eds. Infectious disease of the fetus and newborn infant. 4th ed. Philadelphia: WB Saunders, 1995:140–267 (Level III)

45. Stagno S, Tinker MK, Elrod C, Fuccillo DA, Cloud G, O'Beirne AJ. Immunoglobulin M antibodies detected by enzyme-linked immunosorbent assay and radioimmunoassay in the diagnosis of cytomegalovirus infections in pregnant women and newborn infants. J Clin Microbiol 1985;21:930–935 (Level II-3)

46. Drose JA, Dennis MA, Thickman D. Infection in utero: US findings in 19 cases. Radiology 1991;178:369–374 (Level III)

47. Stein B, Bromley B, Michlewitz H, Miller WA, Benacerraf BR. Fetal liver calcifications: sonographic appearance and postnatal outcome. Radiology 1995; 197:489–492 (Level III)

48. Ghidini A, Sirtori M, Vergani P, Mariani S, Tucci E, Scola GC. Fetal intracranial calcifications. Am J Obstet Gynecol 1989;160:86–87 (Level III)

49. Yamashita Y, Iwanaga R, Goto A, Kaneko S, Yamashita F, Wasedna N, et al. Congenital cytomegalovirus infection associated with fetal ascites and intrahepatic calcifications. Acta Paediatr Scand 1989;78:965–967 (Level III)

50. Forouzan I. Fetal abdominal echogenic mass: an early sign of intrauterine cytomegalovirus infection. Obstet Gynecol 1992;80:535–537 (Level III)

51. Twickler DM, Perlman J, Maberry MC. Congenital cytomegalovirus infection presenting as cerebral ventriculomegaly on antenatal sonography. Am J Perinatol 1993;10:404–406 (Level III)

52. Weiner Z. Congenital cytomegalovirus infection with oligohydramnios and echogenic bowel at 14 weeks' gestation. J Ultrasound Med 1995;14:617–618 (Level III)

53. Yaron Y, Hassan S, Geva E, Kupferminc MJ, Yavetz H, Evans MI, et al. Evaluation of fetal echogenic bowel in the second trimester. Fetal Diagn Ther 1999;14:176–180 (Level II-3)

54. Bale JF Jr, Blackman JA, Sato Y. Outcome in children with symptomatic congenital cytomegalovirus infection. J Child Neurol 1990;5:131–136 (Level III)

55. Lynch L, Daffos F, Emanuel D, Giovangrandi Y, Meisel R, Forestier F, et al. Prenatal diagnosis of fetal cytomegalovirus infection. Am J Obstet Gynecol 1991;165: 714–718 (Level III)

56. Donner C, Liesnard C, Content J, Busine A, Aderca J, Rodesch F. Prenatal diagnosis of 52 pregnancies at risk for congenital cytomegalovirus infection. Obstet Gynecol 1993;82:481–486 (Level III)

57. Nicolini U, Kustermann A, Tassis B, Fogliani R, Galimberti A, Percivalle E, et al. Prenatal diagnosis of congenital human cytomegalovirus infection. Prenat Diagn 1994;14:903–906 (Level III)

58. Stango S. Cytomegalovirus. In: Remington JS, Klein JO, eds. Infectious disease of the fetus and newborn infant. 4th ed. Philadelphia: WB Saunders, 1995:312–353 (Level III)

59. Hohlfeld P, Vial Y, Maillard-Brignon C, Vaudaux B, Fawer CL. Cytomegalovirus fetal infection: prenatal diagnosis. Obstet Gynecol 1991;78:615–618 (Level III)

60. Lamy ME, Mulongo KN, Gadisseux JF, Lyon G, Gaudy V, Van Lierde M. Prenatal diagnosis of fetal cytomegalovirus infection. Am J Obstet Gynecol 1992;166:91–94 (Level III)

61. Hogge WA, Buffone GJ, Hogge JS. Prenatal diagnosis of cytomegalovirus (CMV) infection: a preliminary report. Prenat Diagn 1993;13:131–136 (Level III)

62. Revello MG, Baldanti F, Furione M, Sarasini A, Percivalle E, Zavattoni M, et al. Polymerase chain reaction for prenatal diagnosis of congenital human cytomegalovirus infection. J Med Virol 1995;47:462–466 (Level II-3)

63. Lipitz S, Yagel S, Shalev E, Achiron R, Mashiach S, Schiff E. Prenatal diagnosis of fetal primary cytomegalovirus infection. Obstet Gynecol 1997;89: 763–767 (Level II-3)

64. Lazzarotto T, Guerra B, Spezzacatena P, Varani S, Gabrielli L, Pradelli P, et al. Prenatal diagnosis of congenital cytomegalovirus infection. J Clin Microbiol 1998;36:3540–3544 (Level II-3)

65. Donner C, Liesnard C, Brancart F, Rodesch F. Accuracy of amniotic fluid testing before 21 weeks' gestation in prenatal diagnosis of congenital cytomegalovirus infection. Prenat Diagn 1994;14:1055–1059 (Level II-3)

66. Gilstrap LC, Bawdon RE, Roberts SW, Sobhi S. The transfer of the nucleoside analog ganciclovir across the perfused human placenta. Am J Obstet Gynecol 1994;170:967–972; discussion 972–973 (Level III)

67. Attard-Montalto SP, English MC, Stimmler L, Snodgrass GJ. Ganciclovir treatment of congenital cytomegalovirus infection: a report of two cases. Scand J Infect Dis 1993;25:385–388 (Level III)

68. Fukuda S, Miyachi M, Sugimoto S, Goshima A, Futamura M, Morishima T. A female infant successfully treated by ganciclovir for congenital cytomegalovirus infection. Acta Paediatr Jpn 1995;37:206–210 (Level III)

69. Stronati M, Revello MG, Cerbo RM, Furione M, Rondini G, Gerna G. Ganciclovir therapy of congenital human cytomegalovirus hepatitis. Acta Paediatr 1995;84: 340–341 (Level III)

70. Nigro G, Scholz H, Bartmann U. Ganciclovir therapy for symptomatic congenital cytomegalovirus infection in infants: a two-regimen experience. J Pediatr 1994;124: 318–322 (Level II-3)

71. Barbi M, Binda S, Primache V, Novelli C. Cytomegalovirus in peripheral blood leukocytes of infants with congenital or postnatal infection. Pediatr Infect Dis J 1996;15:898–903 (Level II-3)

72. Whitley RJ, Cloud G, Gruber W, Storch GA, Demmler GJ, Jacobs RF, et al. Ganciclovir treatment of symptomatic congenital cytomegalovirus infection: results of a phase II study. National Institute of Allergy and Infectious Diseases Collaborative Antiviral Study Group. J Infect Dis 1997;175:1080–1086 (Level II-3)

73. Plotkin SA, Starr SE, Friedman HM, Gonczol E, Brayman K. Vaccines for the prevention of human cytomegalovirus infection. Rev Infect Dis 1990;12 (Suppl 7):S827–S838 (Level III)

74. Plotkin SA, Starr SE, Friedman HM, Brayman K, Harris S, Jackson S, et al. Effect of Towne live virus vaccine on cytomegalovirus disease after renal transplant. A controlled trial. Ann Intern Med 1991;114:525–531 (Level I)

75. Plotkin SA, Higgins R, Kurtz JB, Morris PJ, Campbell DA Jr, Shope TC, et al. Multicenter trial of Towne strain attenuated virus vaccine in seronegative renal transplant recipients. Transplantation 1994;58:1176–1178 (Level I)

76. Adler SP, Hempfling SH, Starr SE, Plotkin SA, Riddell S. Safety and immunogenicity of the Towne strain cytomegalovirus vaccine. Pediatr Infect Dis J 1998; 17:200–206 (Level II-3)

77. Porath A, McNutt RA, Smiley LM, Weigle KA. Effectiveness and cost benefit of a proposed live cytomegalovirus vaccine in the prevention of congenital disease. Rev Infect Dis 1990;12:31–40 (Level III)

78. Scott LL, Hollier LM, Dias K. Perinatal herpesvirus infections. Herpes simplex, varicella, and cytomegalovirus. Infect Dis Clin North Am 1997;11:27–53 (Level III)

79. Raynor BD. Cytomegalovirus infection in pregnancy. Semin Perinatol 1993;17:394–402 (Level III)

80. Adler SP. Cytomegalovirus and pregnancy. Curr Opin Obstet Gynecol 1992;4:670–675 (Level III)

81. Grangeot-Keros L, Simon B, Audibert F, Vial M. Should we routinely screen for cytomegalovirus antibody during pregnancy? Intervirology 1998;41:158–162 (Level III)

82. Pass RF, August AM, Dworsky M, Reynolds DW. Cytomegalovirus infection in day-care center. N Engl J Med 1982;307:477–479 (Level II-2)

83. Olson LC, Ketusinha R, Mansuwan P, Snitbhan R. Respiratory tract excretion of cytomegalovirus in Thai children. J Pediatr 1970;77:499–504 (Level II-3)

84. Yeager AS. Transmission of cytomegalovirus to mothers by infected infants: another reason to prevent transfusion-acquired infections. Pediatr Infect Dis 1983;2: 295–297 (Level III)

85. Tookey PA, Ades AE, Peckham CS. Cytomegalovirus prevalence in pregnant women: the influence of parity. Arch Dis Child 1992;67:779–783 (Level II-3)

86. Biomedical Research Institute. CMV: diagnosis, prevention, and treatment. 2nd ed. St. Paul, Minnesota: Children's Hospital of St. Paul & Children's Biomedical Research Institute, 1989 (Level III)

87. Anderson LJ, Tsou C, Parker RA, Chorba TL, Wulff H, Tattersall P, et al. Detection of antibodies and antigens of human parvovirus B19 by enzyme-linked immunosorbent assay. J Clin Microbiol 1986;24:522–526 (Level II-2)

88. Schwarz TF, Nerlich A, Hottentrager B, Jager G, Wiest I, Kantimm S, et al. Parvovirus B19 infection of the fetus. Histology and in situ hybridization. Am J Clin Pathol 1991;96:121–126 (Level III)

89. Schwarz TF, Nerlich A, Hillemanns P. Detection of parvovirus B19 in fetal autopsies. Arch Gynecol Obstet 1993;253:207–213 (Level III)

90. Sifakis S, Ergazaki M, Sourvinos G, Koffa M, Koumantakis E, Spandidos DA. Evaluation of Parvo B19, CMV and HPV viruses in human aborted materi-al using the polymerase chain reaction technique. Eur J Obstet Gynecol Reprod Biol 1998;76:169–173 (Level II-3)

91. Clewley JP. Polymerase chain reaction assay of parvovirus B19 DNA in clinical specimens. J Clin Microbiol 1989;27:2647–2651 (Level II-3)

92. Salimans MM, van de Rijke FM, Raap AK, van Elsacker-Niele AM. Detection of parvovirus B19 DNA in fetal tissues by in situ hybridisation and polymerase chain reaction. J Clin Pathol 1989;42:525–530 (Level III)

93. Kovacs BW, Carlson DE, Shahbahrami B, Platt LD. Prenatal diagnosis of human parvovirus B19 in nonimmune hydrops fetalis by polymerase chain reaction. Am J Obstet Gynecol 1992;167:461–466 (Level III)

94. Torok TJ, Wang QY, Gary GW Jr, Yang CF, Finch TM, Anderson LJ, et al. Prenatal diagnosis of intrauterine infection with parvovirus B19 by the polymerase chain reaction technique. Clin Infect Dis 1992;14:149–155 (Level III)

95. Rogers BB, Mak SK, Dailey JV, Saller DN Jr, Buffone GJ. Detection of parvovirus B19 DNA in amniotic fluid by PCR DNA amplification. Biotechniques 1993;15: 406–408, 410 (Level III)

96. Torok TJ. Human parvovirus B19. In: Remington JS, Klein JO, eds. Infectious disease of the fetus and newborn infant. 4th ed. Philadelphia: WB Saunders, 1995:668–702 (Level III)

97. Peters MT, Nicolaides KH. Cordocentesis for the diagnosis and treatment of human fetal parvovirus infection. Obstet Gynecol 1990;75:501–504 (Level III)

98. Levy R, Weissman A, Blomberg G, Hagay ZJ. Infection by parvovirus B 19 during pregnancy: a review. Obstet Gynecol Surv 1997;52:254–259 (Level III)

99. Fairley CK, Smoleniec JS, Caul OE, Miller E. Observational study of effect of intrauterine transfusions on outcome of fetal hydrops after parvovirus B19 infection. Lancet 1995;346:1335–1337 (Level II-3)

100. Pretorius DH, Hayward I, Jones KL, Stamm E. Sonographic evaluation of pregnancies with maternal varicella infection. J Ultrasound Med 1992;11:459–463 (Level III)

101. Lecuru F, Taurelle R, Bernard JP, Parrat S, Lafay-pillet MC, Rozenberg F, et al. Varicella zoster virus infection during pregnancy: the limits of prenatal diagnosis. Eur J Obstet Gynecol Reprod Biol 1994;56:67–68 (Level III)

102. Kustermann A, Zoppini C, Tassis B, Della Morte M, Colucci G, Nicolini U. Prenatal diagnosis of congenital varicella infection. Prenat Diagn 1996;16:71–74 (Level III)

103. Isada NB, Paar DP, Johnson MP, Evans MI, Holzgreve W, Qureshi F, et al. In utero diagnosis of congenital varicella zoster virus infection by chorionic villus sampling and polymerase chain reaction. Am J Obstet Gynecol 1991;165:1727–1730 (Level III)

104. Balfour HH Jr, Rotbart HA, Feldman S, Dunkle LM, Feder HM Jr, Prober CG, et al. Acyclovir treatment of varicella in otherwise healthy adolescents. The Collaborative Acyclovir Varicella Study Group. J Pediatr 1992;120:627–633 (Level I)

105. Wallace MR, Bowler WA, Murray NB, Brodine SK, Oldfield EC 3d. Treatment of adult varicella with oral acyclovir. A randomized, placebo-controlled trial. Ann Intern Med 1992;117:358–363 (Level I)

106. Ogilvie MM. Antiviral prophylaxis and treatment in chickenpox. A review prepared for the UK Advisory Group on Chickenpox on behalf of the British Society for the Study of Infection. J Infect 1998;36(Suppl 1): 31–38 (Level III)

107. Kesson AM, Grimwood K, Burgess MA, Ferson MJ, Gilbert GL, Hogg G, et al. Acyclovir for the prevention and treatment of varicella zoster in children, adolescents and pregnancy. J Paediatr Child Health 1996;32:211–217 (Level III)

108. Cox SM, Cunningham FG, Luby J. Management of varicella pneumonia complicating pregnancy. Am J Perinatol 1990;7:300–301 (Level III)

109. American Academy of Pediatrics Committee on Infectious Diseases: the use of oral acyclovir in otherwise healthy children with varicella. Pediatrics 1993; 91:674–676 (Level III) [erratum Pediatrics 1993;91:858]

110. Miller E, Cradock-Watson JE, Ridehalgh MK. Outcome in newborn babies given anti-varicella-zoster immunoglobulin after perinatal maternal infection with varicella-zoster virus. Lancet 1989;8659:371–373 (Level II-3)

111. Williams H, Latif A, Morgan J, Ansari BM. Acyclovir in the treatment of neonatal varicella. J Infect 1987;15: 65–67 (Level III)

112. Centers for Disease Control and Prevention. Prevention of varicella: recommendations of the Advisory Committee on Immunization Practices (ACIP). MMWR Morb Mortal Wkly Rep 1996;45(RR-11):1–36 (Level III)

113. Glantz JC, Mushlin AI. Cost-effectiveness of routine antenatal varicella screening. Obstet Gynecol 1998;91: 519–528 (Level III)

114. Rouse DJ, Gardner M, Allen SJ, Goldenberg RL. Management of the presumed susceptible varicella (chickenpox)-exposed gravida: a cost-effectiveness/cost-benefit analysis. Obstet Gynecol 1996;87:932–936 (Level III)

115. McGregor JA, Mark S, Crawford GP, Levin MJ. Varicella zoster antibody testing in the care of pregnant women exposed to varicella. Am J Obstet Gynecol 1987; 157:281–284 (Level II-3)

116. Brunell PA, Ross A, Miller LH, Kuo B. Prevention of varicella by zoster immune globulin. N Engl J Med 1969;280:1191–1194 (Level II-1)

117. Varicella-zoster immune globulin for the prevention of chickenpox. Recommendations of the Immunization Practices Advisory Committee, Centers for Disease Control. Ann Intern Med 1984;100:859–865 (Level III)

118. Montoya JG, Remington JS. Toxoplasma gondii. In: Mandell GL, Bennett JE, Dolin R, eds. Principles and practices in infectious disease. 5th ed. New York: Churchill Livingstone, 2000:2858–2888 (Level III)

119. Fricker-Hidalgo H, Pelloux H, Racinet C, Grefenstette I, Bost-Bru C, Goullier-Fleuret A, et al. Detection of Toxoplasma gondii in 94 placentae from infected women by polymerase chain reaction, in vivo, and in vitro cultures. Placenta 1998;19:545–549 (Level II-3)

120. Hezard N, Marx-Chemla C, Foudrinier F, Villena I, Quereux C, Leroux B, et al. Prenatal diagnosis of congenital toxoplasmosis in 261 pregnancies. Prenat Diagn 1997;17:1047–1054 (Level II-3)

121. Grover CM, Thulliez P, Remington JS, Boothroyd JC. Rapid prenatal diagnosis of congenital Toxoplasma infection by using polymerase chain reaction and amniotic fluid. J Clin Microbiol 1990;28:2297–2301 (Level II-2)

122. van de Ven E, Melchers W, Galama J, Camps W, Meuwissen J. Identification of Toxoplasma gondii infections by BI gene amplification. J Clin Microbiol 1991;29:2120–2124 (Level III)

123. Cazenave J, Forestier F, Bessieres MH, Broussin B, Begueret J. Contribution of a new PCR assay to the prenatal diagnosis of congenital toxoplasmosis. Prenat Diagn 1992;12:119–127 (Level II-2)

124. Jenum PA, Holberg-Petersen M, Melby KK, Stray-Pedersen B. Diagnosis of congenital Toxoplasma gondii infection by polymerase chain reaction (PCR) on amniotic fluid samples. The Norwegian experience. APMIS 1998;106:680–686 (Level II-3)

125. Guy EC, Pelloux H, Lappalainen M, Aspock H, Hassl A, Melby KK, et al. Interlaboratory comparison of polymerase chain reaction for the detection of Toxoplasma gondii DNA added to samples of amniotic fluid. Eur J Clin Microbiol Infect Dis 1996;15:836–839 (Level III)

126. Mombro M, Perathoner C, Leone A, Nicocia M, Moiraghi Ruggenini A, et al. Congenital toxoplasmosis: 10-year follow up. Eur J Pediatr 1995;154:635–639 (Level II-3)

127. Stray-Pedersen B. Treatment of toxoplasmosis in the pregnant mother and newborn child. Scand J Infect Dis Suppl 1992;84:23–31 (Level III)

128. Berrebi A, Kobuch WE, Bessieres MH, Bloom MC, Rolland M, Sarramon MF, et al. Termination of pregnancy for maternal toxoplasmosis. Lancet 1994;344:36–39 (Level II-3)

129. Patel DV, Holfels EM, Vogel NP, Boyer KM, Mets MB, Swisher CN, et al. Resolution of intracranial calcifications in infants with treated congenital toxoplasmosis. Radiology 1996;199:433–440 (Level II-3)

130. Sever JL, Ellenberg JH, Ley AC, Madden DL, Fuccillo DA, Tzan NR, et al. Toxoplasmosis: maternal and pediatric findings in 23,000 pregnancies. Pediatrics 1988; 82:181–192 (Level II-3)

131. Foulon W. Congenital toxoplasmosis: is screening desirable? Scand J Infect Dis Suppl 1992;84:11–17 (Level II-3)

The MEDLINE database, the Cochrane Library, and ACOG's own internal resources and documents were used to conduct a literature search to locate relevant articles published between January 1985 and January 2000. The search was restricted to articles published in the English language. Priority was given to articles reporting results of original research, although review articles and commentaries also were consulted. Abstracts of research presented at symposia and scientific conferences were not considered adequate for inclusion in this document. Guidelines published by organizations or institutions such as the National Institutes of Health and the American College of Obstetricians and Gynecologists were reviewed, and additional studies were located by reviewing bibliographies of identified articles. When reliable research was not available, expert opinions from obstetrician–gynecologists were used.

Studies were reviewed and evaluated for quality according to the method outlined by the U.S. Preventive Services Task Force:

I   Evidence obtained from at least one properly designed randomized controlled trial.

II-1 Evidence obtained from well-designed controlled trials without randomization.

II-2 Evidence obtained from well-designed cohort or case–control analytic studies, preferably from more than one center or research group.

II-3 Evidence obtained from multiple time series with or without the intervention. Dramatic results in uncontrolled experiments also could be regarded as this type of evidence.

III   Opinions of respected authorities, based on clinical experience, descriptive studies, or reports of expert committees.

Based on the highest level of evidence found in the data, recommendations are provided and graded according to the following categories:

Level A—Recommendations are based on good and consistent scientific evidence.

Level B—Recommendations are based on limited or inconsistent scientific evidence.

Level C—Recommendations are based primarily on consensus and expert opinion.

ISSN 1099-3630

The American College of
Obstetricians and Gynecologists
409 12th Street, SW
PO Box 96920
Washington, DC 20090-6920
12345/43210

ACOG PRACTICE BULLETIN

CLINICAL MANAGEMENT GUIDELINES FOR
OBSTETRICIAN–GYNECOLOGISTS
NUMBER 41, DECEMBER 2002

This Practice Bulletin was developed by the ACOG Committee on Practice Bulletins—Gynecology with the assistance of Richard S. Legro, MD. The information is designed to aid practitioners in making decisions about appropriate obstetric and gynecologic care. These guidelines should not be construed as dictating an exclusive course of treatment or procedure. Variations in practice may be warranted based on the needs of the individual patient, resources, and limitations unique to the institution or type of practice.

Polycystic Ovary Syndrome

Polycystic ovary syndrome (PCOS) is a condition of unexplained hyperandrogenic chronic anovulation that most likely represents a heterogenous disorder. Its etiology remains unknown, and treatment is largely symptom based and empirical. Recent findings suggest PCOS has substantial metabolic sequelae, including risk of diabetes and possibly cardiovascular disease, and that primary treatment should focus on metabolic sequelae. The purpose of this document is to examine the best available evidence on the diagnosis and clinical management of PCOS.

Background

Incidence, Definition, and Diagnostic Criteria

Although there is no universally accepted definition of PCOS, diagnostic criteria established by the National Institutes of Health in 1990 define it as hyperandrogenism and chronic anovulation in cases in which secondary causes (such as adult-onset congenital adrenal hyperplasia, hyperprolactinemia, and androgen-secreting neoplasms) have been excluded (1). Insulin resistance has been noted consistently among many women with unexplained hyperandrogenic chronic anovulation, but it is not included in the diagnostic criteria (2). Ultrasonograms of women with unexplained hyperandrogenic chronic anovulation frequently show ovaries that appear polycystic (3); however, polycystic ovaries are a nonspecific finding and also are frequently noted in women with no endocrine or metabolic abnormalities. Hyperandrogenic chronic anovulation occurs in approximately 4–6% of women, with no significant differences in the prevalence of hirsutism or elevated circulating androgen levels between white and black women (4).

Hyperandrogenism can be established on the basis of clinical findings (eg, hirsutism or acne) or hormone measurement or both. However, not all women with hirsutism will have androgen excess, and not all women with androgen excess will have hirsutism (5). In the largest clinical trial to date of women with PCOS, 50–60% of the 400 women prospectively identified as having hyperandrogenic chronic anovulation had no evidence of hirsutism (6).

Etiology

No gene or specific environmental substance has been identified as causing PCOS. Selective insulin resistance may be central to the etiology of the syndrome: skeletal muscle is profoundly resistant, and other tissues (hypothalamus, adrenal, ovary) remain sensitive to the effects of insulin (7). Thus, compensatory hyperinsulinemia may result in decreased levels of sex hormone binding globulin (SHBG) and serve as a trophic stimulus to androgen production in the adrenal gland and ovary. Insulin also may have direct hypothalamic effects, such as abnormally stimulating appetite and gonadotropin secretion.

Clinical Manifestations

Women with PCOS commonly present with infertility or menstrual disorders. For this reason, much attention has been focused on the risks of ovulation induction among women with PCOS because they are at increased risk for ovarian hyperstimulation syndrome, multiple pregnancy, and first-trimester pregnancy loss. In addition, women with PCOS appear to be at increased risk for complications of pregnancy, including gestational diabetes and hypertensive disorders (8–10); the risk of these complications is further exacerbated by multiple pregnancy.

Chronic anovulation (11), obesity (12), hyperinsulinemia (13), and decreased levels of SHBG (14) are all associated with endometrial cancer. Insulin resistance and its associated conditions, such as acanthosis nigricans, centripetal fat distribution, obesity, and obesity-related sleep disorders (15), are all common with PCOS. In turn, all of these conditions are risk factors for long-term metabolic sequelae, such as type 2 diabetes and cardiovascular disease.

Differential Diagnosis

The differential diagnosis of PCOS includes other causes of androgen excess (see box "Factors to Consider in the Differential Diagnosis of Polycystic Ovary Syndrome"). Essential components of the history and physical examination are necessary to diagnose the underlying cause of oligoovulation (see box "Suggested Diagnostic Evaluation for Polycystic Ovary Syndrome"). The history should focus on the onset and duration of the various signs of androgen excess, the menstrual history, and concomitant medications, including the use of exogenous androgens. A family history of diabetes and cardiovascular disease (especially first-degree relatives with premature onset of

cardiovascular disease [male younger than 55 years and female younger than 65 years]) is important. Lifestyle factors, such as smoking, alcohol consumption, diet, and exercise, are particularly important in these women.

The physical examination should include an evaluation of balding, acne, clitoromegaly, and body hair distribution, as well as a pelvic examination to look for ovarian enlargement. The presence and severity of acne should be noted. Signs of insulin resistance, such as obesity, centripetal fat distribution, and the presence of acanthosis nigricans, should be recorded. Acanthosis nigricans is a dermatologic condition marked by velvety, mossy, verrucous, hyperpigmented skin. It has been noted on the back of the neck, in the axillae, underneath the breasts, and even on the vulva. The presence of acanthosis nigricans appears to be more a sign of insulin resistance than a distinct disease unto itself. Other pathologic conditions associated with acanthosis nigricans should be considered, such as insulinoma and malignant disease, especially adenocarcinoma of the stomach.

Because Cushing's syndrome is extremely rare (1 in 1,000,000) and screening tests are not 100% sensitive or specific (16), routine screening for Cushing's syndrome in all women with hyperandrogenic chronic anovulation is not indicated. Those who have co-existing signs of Cushing's syndrome, including a moon facies, buffalo hump, abdominal striae, centripetal fat distribution, or hypertension, should be screened. Proximal myopathies and easy bruising, not present in women with PCOS, also may help identify patients with Cushing's syndrome.

Androgen-secreting tumors of the ovary or adrenal gland are invariably accompanied by elevated circulating androgen levels. However, there is no absolute level that is pathognomonic for a tumor, just as there is no mini-

---

Factors to Consider in the Differential Diagnosis of Polycystic Ovary Syndrome

Androgen secreting tumor

Exogenous androgens

Cushing's syndrome

Nonclassical congenital adrenal hyperplasia

Acromegaly

Genetic defects in insulin action

Primary hypothalamic amenorrhea

Primary ovarian failure

Thyroid disease

Prolactin disorders

Suggested Diagnostic Evaluation
for Polycystic Ovary Syndrome

Physical

- Blood pressure
- Body mass index (weight in kg divided by height in m²) (kg/m²)
  - 25–30 = overweight, >30 = obese
- Waist–hip ratio to determine body fat distribution
  - Value >0.72 = abnormal
- Presence of stigmata of hyperandrogenism or insulin resistance
  - Acne, hirsutism, androgenic alopecia, acanthosis nigricans

Laboratory

- Documentation of biochemical hyperandrogenemia
  - Total testosterone and/or bioavailable or free testosterone
- Exclusion of other causes of hyperandrogenism
  - Thyroid-stimulating hormone levels (thyroid dysfunction)
  - Prolactin (hyperprolactinemia)
  - 17-Hydroxyprogesterone (nonclassical congenital adrenal hyperplasia caused by 21-hydroxylase deficiency): random normal level <4 ng/mL or morning fasting level <2 ng/mL
  - Consider screening for Cushing's syndrome and other rare disorders such as acromegaly
- Evaluation for metabolic abnormalities
  - 2-hour oral glucose tolerance test (fasting glucose <110 mg/dL = normal, 110–125 mg/dL = impaired, >126 mg/dL = type 2 diabetes) followed by 75-g oral glucose ingestion and then 2-hour glucose level (<140 mg/dL = normal glucose tolerance, 140–199 mg/dL = impaired glucose tolerance, >200 mg/dL = type 2 diabetes)
- Fasting lipid and lipoprotein level (total cholesterol, high-density lipoprotein, triglycerides, [low-density lipoprotein usually calculated by Friedewald equation])

Optional Tests to Consider

- Ultrasound examination of ovaries for baseline evaluation and morphology before ovulation induction or in cases of virilization or rapid conversion to an androgen excess state
- Gonadotropin determinations to determine cause of amenorrhea
- Fasting insulin levels in younger women, those with severe stigmata of insulin resistance and hyperandrogenism, or those undergoing ovulation induction
- 24-hour urine test for urinary free cortisol with late onset of polycystic ovary syndrome symptoms or stigmata of Cushing's syndrome

mum androgen level that excludes a tumor. In the past, testosterone levels greater than 2 ng/mL and dehydroepiandrosterone sulfate (DHEAS) levels greater than 700 μg/dL were regarded as suspicious for a tumor of, respectively, ovarian and adrenal etiology, but these cutoff levels have poor sensitivity and specificity (17).

The best measurement of circulating androgens to document unexplained androgen excess is uncertain. Evaluation of testosterone or bioavailable testosterone is useful for documenting ovarian hyperandrogenism. Evaluation of DHEAS levels may be useful in cases of rapid virilization (as a marker of adrenal origin), but its utility in assessing common hirsutism is questionable. Both the adrenal glands and ovaries contribute to the circulating androgen pool in women. The adrenal gland preferentially secretes weak androgens, such as dehydroepiandrosterone (DHEA) or DHEAS (up to 90% of adrenal origin). These hormones, in addition to androstenedione, may serve as prohormones for more potent androgens, such as testosterone or dihydrotestosterone. The ovary is the preferential source of testosterone, and it is estimated that 75% of circulating testosterone originates from the ovary (mainly through peripheral conversion of prohormones by liver, fat, and skin, but also through direct secretion). Androstenedione, largely of ovarian origin, is the only circulating androgen that is higher in premenopausal women than men, yet its androgenic potency is only 10% of testosterone. Dihydrotestosterone is the most potent androgen, although it circulates in negligible quantities and results primarily from the intracellular 5-α-reduction of testosterone.

Mild elevations in prolactin are common in women with PCOS (18). A prolactin level can identify prolactinomas that secrete large amounts of prolactin and that may stimulate ovarian androgen production, but this is an extremely rare cause of hyperandrogenic chronic anovulation. Evaluating serum levels of thyroid-stimulating hormone also is useful given the protean manifestations and frequency of thyroid disease in women.

Clinical Considerations and Recommendations

▶ *Who should be screened for nonclassical congenital adrenal hyperplasia, and how should screening be performed?*

Nonclassical congenital adrenal hyperplasia, often referred to as late-onset congenital adrenal hyperplasia, can present in adult women with anovulation and hirsutism and is almost exclusively caused by genetic defects in the steroidogenic enzyme, 21-hydroxylase (CYP21). In Europe and the United States, congenital adrenal hyperplasia occurs with the highest frequency among Ashkenazi Jews, followed by Hispanics, Yugoslavs, Native American Inuits in Alaska, and Italians (19).

To screen for nonclassical congenital adrenal hyperplasia caused by CYP21 mutations, a fasting level of 17-hydroxyprogesterone should be obtained in the morning. A value less than 2 ng/mL is considered normal. If the sample is obtained in the morning and during the follicular phase, some investigators have proposed cutoffs as high as 4 ng/mL (20). Specificity decreases if the sample is obtained in the luteal phase. High levels of 17-hydroxyprogesterone should prompt an adrenocorticotropic hormone stimulation test.

▶ *Does PCOS increase the risk of developing type 2 diabetes?*

Retrospective studies of women with PCOS have noted a twofold to fivefold increased risk of diabetes in women with PCOS when compared with a control population (21, 22). In a prospective, cohort study, 11.9% of women older than 30 years with PCOS had a physician's diagnosis of type 2 diabetes, compared with only 1.4% of controls (23). Recent studies have suggested as many as 40% of women with PCOS demonstrate glucose intolerance when the less stringent World Health Organization criteria are applied (2-hour glucose levels ≥140 mg/dL) (24). Undiagnosed diabetes approaches 10% in these PCOS cohorts. The risk factors associated with glucose intolerance in women with PCOS—age, high body mass index (BMI), high waist–hip ratios, and family history of diabetes—are identical to those in other populations (25).

Currently, the American Diabetes Association does not recommend screening for insulin resistance with measures of insulin or other markers of the insulin resistance syndrome (26). Although insulin sensitivity can be much more precisely quantified by direct measurement of insulin effects on glucose metabolism in target tissues, both in vivo and in vitro, dynamic tests such as the euglycemic glucose clamp or frequently sampled intravenous glucose tolerance test are too intensive and unwieldy to have widespread clinical utility. Thus, routine screening for insulin resistance is not useful in the larger population of women with PCOS. However, it may be useful to screen selected women with PCOS for hyperinsulinemia—for example, those with severe hyperandrogenism and acanthosis nigricans, younger women, or those undergoing ovulation induction. Fasting glucose levels are poor predictors of glucose intolerance risk in

women with PCOS. Women with PCOS should be screened for type 2 diabetes and impaired glucose tolerance with a fasting glucose level followed by a 2-hour glucose level after a 75-g glucose load (27). This finding has taken on new significance with the findings of the Diabetes Prevention program that both lifestyle interventions and metformin significantly reduce the risk of developing diabetes in women with impaired glucose tolerance (28).

▶ *Does PCOS have a long-term impact on the development of cardiovascular disease?*

No prospective studies have documented an increased risk of cardiovascular events in women with PCOS. However, a number of studies using surrogate endpoints for cardiovascular disease risk have suggested women with PCOS are at increased risk (29, 30). A recent cohort study found an increased prevalence of subclinical atherosclerosis in those with PCOS (7.2%) when compared with controls of similar ages (0.7%) (31). This difference was detected only in women aged 45 years or older.

Women with PCOS display a number of well-recognized risk factors for both diabetes and cardiovascular disease, such as obesity and impaired glucose tolerance (32). Dyslipidemia is a common metabolic abnormality among women with PCOS. The prevalence of borderline or high lipid levels according to National Cholesterol Education Program guidelines (33) approaches 70% in women with PCOS (34). Low-density lipoprotein (LDL) levels are disproportionately elevated in women with PCOS (34–36) when compared with other insulin-resistant states (37).

Insulin resistance has been associated with other distinct patterns of dyslipidemia, including decreased levels of high-density lipoprotein (HDL); increased levels of small, dense LDL; and elevated levels of triglycerides. A large cohort study looked at the effect of aging on the pattern of dyslipidemia in women with PCOS (35). Subjects were first evaluated in their 30s and underwent repeat lipid phenotyping over time (36). Later evaluations showed persistent lipid abnormalities in women with PCOS, but these abnormalities tended to persist and plateau, whereas in the control population, lipid abnormalities worsened (36).

All women with PCOS should be screened for cardiovascular risk by determination of BMI and waist–hip ratio and measurement of fasting lipid and lipoprotein levels (total cholesterol, HDL cholesterol, and triglycerides). Regular exercise and weight control are proven methods to reduce cardiovascular morbidity and mortality. These modalities should be considered before prescription drugs are used.

▶ *In a woman with PCOS who is not attempting to conceive, what is the best medical maintenance therapy to treat anovulation and amenorrhea?*

Combination Oral Contraceptives

Oral contraceptives have been the mainstay of long-term management of PCOS. They offer benefit through a variety of mechanisms, including suppression of pituitary luteinizing hormone secretion, suppression of ovarian androgen secretion, and increased circulating SHBG. Individual preparations may have different doses and drug combinations and thus have varying risk–benefit ratios. For instance, various progestins have been shown to have different effects on circulating SHBG levels (38), but whether that translates into a clinical benefit is uncertain. The "best" oral contraceptive for women with PCOS is not known. Oral contraceptives also are associated with a significant reduction in the risk for endometrial cancer (38), but the magnitude of the effect in women with PCOS is not known.

Progestin

Both depot and intermittent oral medroxyprogesterone acetate (10 mg for 10 days) have been shown to suppress pituitary gonadotropins and circulating androgens in women with PCOS (39). No studies have addressed the long-term use of these compounds to treat hirsutism. The regimen of cyclic oral progestin therapy that most effectively prevents endometrial cancer in women with PCOS is unknown. However use of medroxyprogesterone acetate has been associated with decreases in SHBG in women with PCOS (40). Progestin-only oral contraceptives are an alternative for endometrial protection, but they are associated with a high incidence of breakthrough bleeding (41).

Insulin-Sensitizing Agents

Drugs initially developed to treat type 2 diabetes also have been used to treat PCOS. Most studies have focused on agents that improve peripheral insulin sensitivity by decreasing circulating insulin levels. These agents include biguanides (metformin) (42, 43), thiazolidinediones (troglitazone, pioglitazone, and rosiglitazone), and an experimental insulin sensitizer drug known as D-chiro-inositol (44). They do not increase insulin secretion, as do sulfonylureas, and are, thus, rarely associated with hypoglycemia, a risk for those who are normoglycemic when fasting (as are most women with PCOS). These drugs often are referred to as insulin-sensitizing agents, but their individual effects and risk–benefit ratios

vary. There are class differences, for example, biguanides tend to decrease weight and thiazolidinediones to increase weight. Within a class there also can be significant differences in the risk–benefit ratio, for instance a known increased risk of hepatotoxicity with troglitazone (no longer available) compared with the minimal risk with rosiglitazone. These differences should discourage aggregating all of these agents into a single category when considering their use. Nonetheless, improving insulin sensitivity is associated with a decrease in circulating androgen levels, improved ovulation rate, and improved glucose tolerance. It is difficult to separate the effects of improving insulin sensitivity from those of lowering serum androgens, as any "pure" improvement in insulin sensitivity can increase SHBG and, thus, decrease bioavailable androgen. None of the agents noted are currently approved by the U.S. Food and Drug Administration (FDA) for treatment of PCOS. Despite encouraging preliminary results, troglitazone was removed from the world wide market because of hepatotoxicity.

Small studies of 3–6 months' duration with metformin in women with PCOS suggested improvement in ovulatory function in about one half of those studied (45–47). Circulating androgen levels also appear to decrease with long-term treatment. There are no studies of treatment for 1 year or more with a thiazolidinedione in women with PCOS. The effects of either metformin or thiazolidinediones on preventing endometrial hyperplasia or neoplasia in women with PCOS are unknown.

▶ *In a woman with PCOS who is not attempting to conceive, what is the best medical maintenance therapy to prevent cardiovascular disease and diabetes?*

Combination Oral Contraceptives and Progestins

In the general population, oral contraceptive use has not been associated with an increased risk of developing type 2 diabetes (48). There is no convincing evidence that the use of oral contraceptives contributes to the risk of diabetes in women with PCOS. However, suppression of androgens with oral contraceptives is associated with a significant elevation in circulating triglycerides as well as in HDL levels, as demonstrated in a large, 3-year study of women with PCOS (49). Most of these effects were achieved at 12 months, with little change in circulating lipid values between 12 months and 36 months (49). Other studies with fewer participants or of shorter duration showed similar or no effects on circulating lipids (50). There is no evidence to suggest that women with PCOS experience more cardiovascular events than the general population when they use oral contraceptives. The effect of progestins alone on metabolic risk factors varies and is not well understood.

Insulin-Sensitizing Agents

A National Institutes of Health sponsored trial demonstrated that metformin can prevent the development of diabetes in high-risk populations (eg, those with impaired glucose tolerance) (28). The use of troglitazone in this trial was terminated because of its hepatotoxicity. Among women with PCOS who use metformin, glucose tolerance improves or stays steady over time (46). Metformin also may be associated with weight loss, but results are inconsistent. Currently, data are insufficient to warrant use of insulin-sensitizing agents prophylactically to prevent diabetes in women with PCOS. However, results of ongoing prevention trials may favor more aggressive management of impaired glucose tolerance to prevent diabetes.

Multiple studies have documented improvement with the use of insulin-sensitizing agents in the cardiovascular risk profile of patients with diabetes or insulin resistance syndrome, but the role of these agents in primary or secondary prevention of cardiovascular disease is uncertain (51). However, similar improvements in lipid profiles have not been noted consistently in women with PCOS. The cardioprotective effects of insulin-sensitizing agents in women with PCOS are still unknown. Another area where there is theoretic appeal, but little data to guide therapy, is the use of statins to prevent cardiovascular disease in young women with PCOS or the metabolic syndrome of insulin resistance.

▶ *In women with PCOS who are attempting to conceive, which methods of ovulation induction are effective?*

There is no evidence-based schema to guide the initial and subsequent choices of ovulation induction methods in women with PCOS. Treatment should begin with a regimen of regular exercise and weight control and then proceed to other methods if necessary (52). The pregnancy classification of common medications used to treat PCOS are varied (see Table 1).

Clomiphene Citrate or Gonadotropins

Clomiphene citrate has traditionally been the first-line treatment agent for anovulatory women, including those with PCOS. Up to 80% of women with PCOS will ovulate in response to clomiphene treatment, and 50% of these women will conceive (53). One half of all women who are going to conceive using clomiphene will do so with the 50-mg starting dose, and another 20% will do so with the 100-mg per day dosage (54). Most pregnancies

Table 1. Pregnancy Categories of Common Medications Used in the Treatment of Polycystic Ovary Syndrome

Pregnancy Category	Drug	Class
B	Metformin	Insulin sensitizing agent
	Micronized progesterone	Progestin
C	Rosiglitazone	Insulin sensitizing agent
	Pioglitazone	Insulin sensitizing agent
	Dexamethasone	Corticosteroid
	Clomiphene citrate	Ovulation induction
	Eflornithine hydrochloride cream	Antihirsutism agent
D	Spironolactone	Antiandrogen
	Flutamide	Antiandrogen
X	Multiple formulations (atorvastatin, etc)	Statins
	Finasteride	Antiandrogen
	Leuprolide	Gonadotropin-releasing hormone agonist
	Medroxyprogesterone acetate	Progestin
	Multiple formulations	Oral contraceptives
	Multiple formulations	Gonadotropins

will occur within the first six ovulatory cycles. Increasing the duration of treatment adds little to the pregnancy rate. A recent meta-analysis showed clomiphene citrate to be effective in women with ovulatory dysfunction and estrogen production (55). There are no clear prognostic factors for response, although increased weight is associated with a larger dose requirement and a greater likelihood of failure (56).

Alternative clomiphene regimens have been developed, including prolonging the period of administration (57) and adding dexamethasone. Dexamethasone as adjunctive therapy with clomiphene citrate has been shown to increase ovulation rates in women with PCOS with higher DHEAS levels (>2000 ng/mL) (57, 58).

Gonadotropins frequently are used to induce ovulation in women with PCOS for whom clomiphene treatment has failed (59). In a large trial of gonadotropins in women with PCOS, women were randomized to either an aggressive or low-dose follicle-stimulating hormone protocol. Higher pregnancy rates (40% versus 20%, respectively) and less multifollicular ovulation (27% versus 74%) were achieved with the low-dose protocol (60). There were fewer cases of multiple pregnancy, ovarian hyperstimulation, and multifollicular ovulation (74% versus 27%) (60). Low-dose therapy with gonadotropins offers a higher rate of monofollicular development (approximately 50% or greater) with a significantly lower risk of ovarian hyperstimulation syndrome (20–25%) that results in cycle cancellation or more serious sequelae (60, 61).

Ovarian Drilling

The value of laparoscopic ovarian drilling with laser or diathermy as a primary treatment for subfertile women with anovulation and PCOS is undetermined (62). Neither drilling by laser nor diathermy has any obvious advantages, and there is insufficient evidence to suggest a difference in ovulation or pregnancy rates when drilling is compared with gonadotropin therapy as a secondary treatment for women who do not respond to clomiphene (62). A recent randomized trial found no difference in pregnancy or miscarriage rates between ovarian surgery or 3 months of ovulation induction with gonadotropins (63). Multiple pregnancy rates are reduced in those women who conceive after laparoscopic drilling. In some cases, the fertility benefits of ovarian drilling may be temporary (64), and drilling does not appear to improve metabolic abnormalities in women with PCOS (65).

Insulin-Sensitizing Agents

Metformin

Most randomized trials using metformin have shown that it improves ovulatory frequency in women with PCOS (43, 45, 46, 66, 67), although several have not shown a benefit (68–70). The dosage most frequently used has been 1,500 mg per day, and more recent studies have used 2,000 mg per day in divided doses. Metformin also has been used successfully as an adjunctive agent with both clomiphene citrate (43) and gonadotropins (67, 71). In a small study, metformin significantly improved the pregnancy rate in clomiphene-resistant women with PCOS when compared with placebo (72). Studies have been hampered by small numbers, inconsistent use of a placebo, selection bias (primarily women who are clomiphene-resistant), and lack of a dose-ranging study.

Metformin carries a small risk of lactic acidosis, most commonly among women with poorly controlled diabetes and impaired renal function. Gastrointestinal symptoms (diarrhea, nausea, vomiting, abdominal bloating, flatulence, and anorexia) are the most common adverse reactions and may be ameliorated by starting at a small dose and gradually increasing the dose or by using the sustained-release version now available in the United States.

Metformin has no known human teratogenic risk or embryonic lethality in humans and appears safe in pregnancy (73). Some clinicians advocate its use during early pregnancy to reduce the miscarriage rate, but the documentation for this claim is poor (74).

Thiazolidinediones

Thiazolidinediones are peroxisome proliferator activating receptor (PPAR-γ) agonists and are thought to improve insulin sensitivity through a postreceptor mechanism. In a large, randomized, controlled, multicenter trial, troglitazone demonstrated a dose-response effect in improving ovulation and hirsutism (6). These benefits appeared to be mediated through decreases in hyperinsulinemia and decreases in free testosterone levels (with corresponding increases in SHBG). Newer thiazolidinediones, such as rosiglitazone and pioglitazone, appear to be safer in terms of hepatotoxicity but also have been associated with embryotoxicity in animal studies, and little has been published on their effects in women with PCOS.

▶ *In obese women with PCOS, does weight loss improve ovarian function?*

Obesity contributes substantially to reproductive and metabolic abnormalities in women with PCOS. Multiple studies have shown that weight loss can improve the fundamental aspects of the endocrine syndrome of PCOS by decreasing circulating androgen levels and causing spontaneous resumption of menses (75, 76). These changes have been reported with weight loss as little as 5% of the initial weight (77). Other benefits include decreased circulating insulin levels (75, 77). The decrease in unbound testosterone levels after weight loss may be largely mediated through increases in SHBG (77). There also may be decreases in circulating luteinizing hormone levels (76), although not uniformly (78). Changes in body weight have been associated with improved ovulation and pregnancy rates. Longer-term effects from improvement in ovarian function also have been reported. In one study, hirsutism improved in approximately 50% of women who lost weight (79).

Although there is much interest in the therapeutic effects of a high protein diet for women with PCOS, few studies support the benefits. Further, there are theoretic concerns about the adverse effects of high protein on renal function in a population at high risk for diabetes, as well as the adverse effects of the increased fat composition of such diets on dyslipidemia. Only limited studies on the effects of exercise on PCOS have been performed (80). It is reasonable to assume that exercise would have the same beneficial effects in women with PCOS as women with type 2 diabetes, which exist even with no changes in body weight (81).

In the general population, weight loss can result in significant improvement in the risk for diabetes and cardiovascular disease (82). These data support the utility of lifestyle modification, ie, improved diet and increased exercise, as primary treatments for all obese women with PCOS.

▶ *How effective are the various medical agents in treating hirsutism in women with PCOS?*

Most medical methods, while improving hirsutism, do not produce the dramatic results women desire, and treatment often is palliative rather than curative. In general, combination therapies appear to produce better results than single-agent approaches (83–85); however, randomized trials have not established a primary treatment for hirsutism in PCOS.

Oral Contraceptives

No oral contraceptive has been approved by the FDA for the treatment of hirsutism. A number of observational or nonrandomized studies have noted improvement in hirsutism in women with PCOS who use oral contraceptives (86), but there are no definitive data to confirm their benefit in improving hirsutism in PCOS. Few studies have compared outcomes of different types of oral contraceptives, and no one type of pill has been shown to be superior in treating hirsutism in women with PCOS (87). A number of studies have found additive benefit when oral contraceptives are combined with other treatment modalities, such as flutamide (83). If a woman is taking an oral contraceptive that contains drospirenone, it may be necessary to reduce her dose of spironolactone and evaluate her levels of potassium.

Antiandrogens

None of the antiandrogen agents were developed to treat hyperandrogenism in women or are approved by the FDA for that indication. They have been used empirically in women with PCOS. These compounds primarily antagonize the binding of testosterone and other androgens to the androgen receptor. Androgen antagonism may result in improvements in other metabolic variables, such as circulating lipid levels (88). Randomized trials have found that spironolactone, flutamide, and finasteride all have similar efficacy in improving hirsutism (89). All appear to offer some benefit, although the best choice for hirsutism in PCOS is unknown. As a class, antiandrogens are teratogenic and pose a risk of feminization of the external genitalia in a male fetus (ambiguous genitalia) if the patient conceives. Therefore, they are frequently used in combination with oral contraceptives.

Spironolactone

Spironolactone, a diuretic and aldosterone antagonist, also binds to the androgen receptor as an antagonist (90). It has other mechanisms of action, including inhibition of ovarian and adrenal steroidogenesis, competition for androgen receptors in hair follicles, and direct inhibition of 5-α-reductase activity. The usual dosage is 25–100 mg twice per day, and the dosage is titrated to balance efficacy while avoiding side effects. A full clinical effect may take 6 months or more. Approximately 20% of women using spironolactone will experience increased menstrual frequency (91). Because it can cause and exacerbate hyperkalemia, spironolactone should be used cautiously in women with renal impairment. Rarely, exposure has resulted in ambiguous genitalia in male infants. Although spironolactone has had long and extensive use as an antiandrogen and multiple clinical trials have shown a benefit, the overall quality of the trials and small numbers enrolled have limited the ability of a meta-analysis to document its benefit in the treatment of hirsutism (92).

Flutamide

Flutamide, an androgen-receptor agonist, is another nonsteroidal antiandrogen that has been shown to be effective against hirsutism in observational trials (93, 94). The most common side effect is dry skin, but its use has been associated with hepatitis in rare cases. The common dosage is 250 mg per day. The risk of teratogenicity with this compound is significant, and contraception should be used. Administration of flutamide to a population of women with PCOS resulted in significantly decreased LDL cholesterol levels (88).

Finasteride

Finasteride inhibits both forms of the enzyme 5-α-reductase (type I, predominantly found in the skin, and type II, predominantly found in the prostate and reproductive tissues). It is available as a 5-mg tablet for the treatment of prostate cancer and a 1-mg tablet for the treatment of male alopecia. It has been found to be effective for the treatment of hirsutism (95, 96). Finasteride is better tolerated than other antiandrogens, with minimal hepatic and renal toxicity; however, it has well-documented risk for teratogenicity in male fetuses, and adequate contraception should be used.

Insulin-Sensitizing Agents

Insulin sensitizers may treat hirsutism by improving both hyperinsulinemia and hyperandrogenemia concurrently. In a 12-month study, only the highest dose of troglitazone was found to significantly—although modestly—

improve hirsutism in women with PCOS (6). In small studies with metformin, hirsutism was unchanged (50, 97) or showed only slight improvement (47, 98). Studies of longer duration are needed to detect differences between classes of insulin-sensitizing agents and their long-term benefits.

Eflornithine

An inhibitor of the enzyme ornithine decarboxylase, topical eflornithine has been approved by the FDA for treating hirsutism. It appears to be well tolerated, and may have notable benefit after 6 months of use. A variety of adverse skin conditions have been reported in a small percentage of patients. Any additional benefit or decreased efficacy in women with PCOS is unknown at present.

▶ **Is there a role for adjuvant cosmetic management of hirsutism?**

Mechanical hair removal (shaving, plucking, waxing, depilatory creams, electrolysis, and laser vaporization) often is the front line of treatment used by women (99). There is no evidence that shaving can increase hair follicle density or size of the hair shaft (100). Judicious plucking can be helpful if tolerated, but care must be taken to avoid folliculitis, pigmentation, and scarring.

In electrolysis, a direct current is passed down a needle inserted into the hair follicle, destroying the follicle. Unlike mechanical and chemical depilatory methods, electrolysis can permanently reduce hirsutism by destroying the follicle. Electrolysis satisfactorily removes hair from women and men with hypertrichosis (generalized increased hair distribution). However, electrolysis is tedious, its success is highly operator-dependent, and it may be impractical for treating large numbers of hairs. The regulation of electrology practice varies among states. Concomitant medical management directed at decreasing androgen levels usually is recommended for excess androgen states, otherwise new vellus hairs will differentiate into terminal hairs, causing recurrence of hirsutism.

Laser treatment removes hair because follicular melanin absorbs the laser wavelengths of light, which selectively thermally damage the target without damaging surrounding tissue. Women with dark hair and light skin are ideal candidates, and the approach appears to be most effective during anagen. Because of the skew of hair follicles among varying segments of the hair growth cycle, multiple treatments may be necessary. Most studies have been observational, nonrandomized studies with no specific focus on women with PCOS. Randomized studies have demonstrated a benefit over control areas

(101). The success of laser treatment is operator-dependent, and concomitant medical management generally is needed for women with hirsutism.

Summary of Recommendations

The following recommendations are based on good and consistent scientific evidence (Level A):

▶ All women with PCOS should be screened for glucose intolerance with a 2-hour glucose level after a 75-g fasting glucose challenge.

▶ All women with PCOS should be screened for dyslipidemia with a fasting lipoprotein profile, including total cholesterol, LDL, HDL, and triglyceride determinations.

▶ Interventions that improve insulin sensitivity, including weight loss, use of metformin, and use of thiazolidinediones, are useful in improving ovulatory frequency in women with PCOS.

▶ Use of clomiphene citrate is appropriate because it effectively results in pregnancy in women with PCOS.

The following recommendations are based on limited or inconsistent scientific evidence (Level B):

▶ Improvements in insulin sensitivity, by weight loss or by the use of insulin-sensitizing agents, may favorably improve many risk factors for diabetes and cardiovascular disease in women with PCOS.

▶ When using gonadotropins to induce ovulation, low-dose therapy is recommended because it offers a high rate of monofollicular development and a significantly lower risk of ovarian hyperstimulation in women with PCOS.

▶ The benefit and role of surgical therapy in ovulation induction in women with PCOS is uncertain.

The following recommendations are based primarily on consensus and expert opinion (Level C):

▶ Although eflornithine hydrochloride cream has been effective in treating facial hirsutism in women, additional benefits or risks for women with PCOS are unknown.

▶ All women with a suspected diagnosis of PCOS should be screened with a 17-hydroxyprogesterone value for nonclassical congenital adrenal hyperplasia.

▶ Combining medical interventions may be the most effective way to treat hirsutism. Combined therapy with an ovarian suppression agent and an antiandrogen appears effective in treating hirsutism in women with PCOS. The best pill or antiandrogen is unknown.

▶ The ideal choice of ablative procedures for long-term management of hirsutism in women with PCOS is unknown.

▶ The optimal progestin, duration, and frequency of treatment to prevent endometrial cancer in women with PCOS is unknown.

▶ The effects of insulin-sensitizing agents on early pregnancy are unknown; metformin appears safe, but any additional effect at reducing pregnancy loss is uncertain.

▶ The best or initial treatment for hirsutism, ovulation induction, or prevention of long-term metabolic sequelae for women with PCOS is unknown. All of these conditions may benefit from lifestyle modification as initial treatment.

References

1. Zawadri JK, Dunaif A. Diagnostic criteria for polycystic ovary syndrome: towards a rational approach. In: Dunaif A, Givens JR, Haseltine FP, Merriam GR, editors. Polycystic ovary syndrome. Current issues in endocrinology and metabolism. 1st ed. Boston (MA): Blackwell Scientific Publications; 1992. p. 377–84. (Level III)

2. Dunaif A. Insulin resistance and polycystic ovary syndrome: mechanisms and implications for pathogenesiy. Endorc Rev 1997;18:774–800. (Level III)

3. Franks S. Polycystic ovary syndrome. N Engl J Med 1995;333:853–61. (Level III)

4. Knochenhauer ES, Key TJ, Kahsar-Miller M, Waggoner W, Boots LR, Azziz R. Prevalence of the polycystic ovary syndrome in unselected black and white women of the southeastern United States: a prospective study. J Clin Endocrinol Metab 1998;83:3078–82. (Level II-3)

5. Lobo RA, Goebelsmann U, Horton R. Evidence for the importance of peripheral tissue events in the development of hirsutism in polycystic ovary syndrome. J Clin Endocrinol Metab 1983;57:393–7. (Level II-2)

6. Azziz R, Ehrmann D, Legro RS, Whitcomb RW, Hanley R, Fereshetian AG, et al. Troglitazone improves ovulation and hirsutism in the polycystic ovary syndrome: a multicenter, double blind, placebo-controlled trial. J Clin Endocrinol Metab 2001;86:1626–32. (Level I)

7. Poretsky L. On the paradox of insulin-induced hyperandrogenism in insulin-resistant states. Endocr Rev 1991; 12:3–13. (Level III)

8. Urman B, Sarac E, Dogan L, Gurgan T. Pregnancy in infertile PCOD patients. Complications and outcome. J Reprod Med 1997;42:501–5. (Level II-2)

9. Anttila L, Karjala K, Penttila RA, Ruutiainen K, Ekblad U. Polycystic ovaries in women with gestational diabetes. Obstet Gynecol 1998;92:13–6. (Level II-2)

10. Holte J, Gennarelli G, Wide L, Lithell H, Berne C. High prevalence of polycystic ovaries and associated clinical, endocrine, and metabolic features in women with previous gestational diabetes mellitus. J Clin Endocrinol Metab 1998;83:1143–50. (Level II-2)

11. Ho SP, Tan KT, Pang MW, Ho TH. Endometrial hyperplasia and the risk of endometrial carcinoma. Singapore Med J 1997;38:11–5. (Level II-2)

12. Dahlgren E, Friberg LG, Johansson S, Lindstrom B, Oden A, Samsioe G, et al. Endometrial carcinoma; ovarian dysfunction—a risk factor in young women. Eur J Obstet Gynecol Reprod Biol 1991;41:143–50. (Level II-3)

13. Troisi R, Potischman N, Hoover RN, Siiteri P, Brinton LA. Insulin and endometrial cancer. Am J Epidemiol 1997;146:476–82. (Level II-2)

14. Potischman N, Hoover RN, Brinton LA, Siiteri P, Dorgan JF, Swanson CA, et al. Case-control study of endogenous steroid hormones and endometrial cancer. J Nat Cancer Inst 1996;88:1127–35. (Level II-2)

15. Vgontzas AN, Legro RS, Bixler EO, Grayev A, Kales A, Chrousos GP. Polycystic ovary syndrome is associated with obstructive sleep apnea and daytime sleepiness: role of insulin resistance. J Clin Endocrinol Metab 2001; 86:517–20. (Level II-2)

16. Tsigos C, Chrousos GP. Differential diagnosis and management of Cushing's syndrome. Ann Rev Med 1996;47: 443–61. (Level III)

17. Waggoner W, Boots LR, Azziz R. Total testosterone and DHEAS levels as predictors of androgen-secreting neoplasms: a population study. Gynecol Endocrinol 1999;3: 394–400. (Level II-3)

18. Robinson S, Rodin DA, Deacon A, Wheeler MJ, Clayton RN. Which hormone tests for the diagnosis of polycystic ovary syndrome? Br J Obstet Gynaecol 1992;99:232–8. (Level II-2)

19. New MI, Speiser PW. Genetics of adrenal steroid 21-hydroxylase deficiency. Endocr Rev 1986;7:331–49. (Level III)

20. Azziz R, Hincapie LA, Knochenhauer ES, Dewailly D, Fox L, Boots LR. Screening for 21-hydroxylase-deficient nonclassic adrenal hyperplasia among hyperandrogenic women: a prospective study. Fertil Steril 1999;72: 915–25. (Level II-2)

21. Wild S, Pierpoint T, McKeigue P, Jacobs H. Cardiovascular disease in women with polycystic ovary syndrome at long-term follow-up: a retrospective cohort study. Clin Endocrinol (Oxf) 2000;52:595–600. (Level II-2)

22. Cibula D, Cifkova R, Fanta M, Poledne R, Zivny J, Skibova J. Increased risk of non-insulin dependent diabetes mellitus, arterial hypertension and coronary artery disease in perimenopausal women with a history of the polycystic ovary syndrome. Hum Reprod 2000;15:785–9. (Level II-2)

23. Talbott EO, Zborowski JV, Sutton-Tyrrell K, McHugh-Pemu KP, Guzick DS. Cardiovascular risk in women with polycystic ovary syndrome. Obstet Gynecol Clin North Am 2001;28:111–33, vii. (Level III)

24. Legro RS, Kunselman AR, Dodson WC, Dunaif A. Prevalence and predictors of risk for type 2 diabetes mellitus and impaired glucose tolerance in polycystic ovary syndrome: a prospective, controlled study in 254 affected women. J Clin Endocrinol Metab 1999;84:165–9. (Level II-2)

25. Haffner SM. Risk factors for non-insulin-dependent diabetes mellitus. J Hyperten Suppl 1995;13:S73–6. (Level III)

26. Consensus Development Conference on Insulin Resistance. 5-6 November 1997. American Diabetes Association. Diabetes Care 1998;21:310–4. (Level III)

27. Harris MI, Eastman RC, Cowie CC, Flegal KM, Eberhardt MS. Comparison of diabetes diagnostic categories in the U.S. population according to the 1997 American Diabetes Association and 1980-1985 World Health Organization diagnostic criteria. Diabetes Care 1997;20:1859–62. (Level III)

28. Knowler WC, Barrett-Connor E, Fowler SE, Hamman RF, Lachin JM, Walker EA, et al. Reduction in the incidence of type 2 diabetes with lifestyle intervention or metformin. N Engl J Med 2002;346:393–403. (Level I)

29. Birdsall MA, Farquhar CM, White HD. Association between polycystic ovaries and extent of coronary artery disease in women having cardiac catheterization. Ann Intern Med 1997;126:32–5. (Level II-2)

30. Guzick DS, Talbott EO, Sutton-Tyrrell K, Herzog HC, Kuller LH Jr, Wolfson SK. Carotid atherosclerosis in women with polycystic ovary syndrome: initial results from a case-control study. Am J Obstet Gynecol 1996; 174:1224–9; discussion 1229–32. (Level II-2)

31. Talbott EO, Guzick DS, Sutton-Tyrrell K, McHugh-Pemu KP, Zborowski JV, Remsberg KE, et al. Evidence for association between polycystic ovary syndrome and premature carotid atherosclerosis in middle-aged women. Arterioscler Thromb Vasc Biol 2000;20: 2414–21. (Level II-2)

32. Barzilay JI, Spiekerman CF, Wahl PW, Kuller LH, Cushman M, Furberg CD, et al. Cardiovascular disease in older adults with glucose disorders: comparison of American Diabetes Association criteria for diabetes mellitus with WHO criteria. Lancet 1999;354:622–5. (Level II-3)

33. Executive Summary of The Third Report of the National Cholesterol Education Program (NCEP) Expert Panel on Detection, Evaluation, And Treatment of High Blood Cholesterol in Adults (Adult Treatment Panel III). JAMA 2001;285:2486–97. (Level III)

34. Legro RS, Kunselman AR, Dunaif A. Prevalence and predictors of dyslipidemia in women with polycystic ovary syndrome. Am J Med 2001;111:607–13. (Level II-2)

35. Talbott E, Guzick D, Clerici A, Berga S, Detre K, Weimer K, et al. Coronary heart disease risk factors in women with polycystic ovary syndrome. Arterioscler Thromb Vasc Biol 1995;15:821–26. (Level II-2)

36. Talbott E, Clerici A, Berga SL, Kuller L, Guzick D, Detre K, et al. Adverse lipid and coronary heart disease risk profiles in young women with polycystic ovary syndrome: results of a case-control study. J Clin Epidemiol 1998;51:415–22. (Level II-2)

37. Laakso M. Dyslipidaemias, insulin resistance and atherosclerosis. Ann Med 1992;24:505–9. (Level III)

38. Vessey MP, Painter R. Endometrial and ovarian cancer and oral contraceptives—findings in a large cohort study. Br J Cancer 1995;71:1340–2. (Level II-2)

39. Anttila L, Koskinen P, Erkkola R, Irjala K, Ruutiainen K. Serum testosterone, androstenedione and luteinizing hormone levels after short-term medroxyprogesterone acetate treatment in women with polycystic ovarian disease. Acta Obstet Gynecol Scand 1994;73:634–6. (Level II-2)

40. Wortsman J, Khan MS, Rosner W. Suppression of testosterone-estradiol binding globulin by medroxyprogesterone acetate in polycystic ovary syndrome. Obstet Gynecol 1986;67:705–9. (Level II-2)

41. Kovacs G. Progestogen-only pills and bleeding disturbances. Hum Reprod 1996;11 (supp1 2):20–3. (Level III)

42. Nestler JE, Jakubowicz DJ. Lean women with polycystic ovary syndrome respond to insulin reduction with decreases in ovarian p450c17 alpha activity and serum androgens. J Clin Endocrinol Metab 1997;82:4075–9. (Level II-2)

43. Nestler JE, Jakubowicz DJ, Evans WS, Pasquali R. Effects of metformin on spontaneous and clomiphene-induced ovulation in the polycystic ovary syndrome. N Engl J Med 1998;338:1876–80. (Level II-1)

44. Nestler JE, Jakubowicz DJ, Reamer P, Gunn RD, Allan G. Ovulatory and metabolic effects of D-chiro-inositol in the polycystic ovary syndrome. N Engl J Med 1999;340: 1314–20. (Level I)

45. Pasquali R, Gambineri A, Biscotti D, Vicennati V, Gagliardi L, Colitta D, et al. Effect of long-term treatment with metformin added to hypocaloric diet on body composition, fat distribution, and androgen and insulin levels in abdominally obese women with and without the polycystic ovary syndrome. J Clin Endocrinol Metab 2000;85:2767–74. (Level I)

46. Moghetti P, Castello R, Negri C, Tosi F, Perrone F, Caputo M, et al. Metformin effects on clinical features, endocrine and metabolic profiles, and insulin sensitivity in polycystic ovary syndrome: a randomized, double-blind, placebo-controlled 6-month trial, followed by open, long-term clinical evaluation. J Clin Endocrinol Metab 2000;85:139–46. (Level I)

47. Kolodziejczyk B, Duleba AJ, Spaczynski RZ, Pawelczyk L. Metformin therapy decreases hyperandrogenism and hyperinsulinemia in women with polycystic ovary syndrome. Fertil Steril 2000;73:1149–54. (Level II-2)

48. Chasan-Taber L, Willett WC, Stampfer MJ, Hunter DJ, Colditz GA, Spielgelman D, et al. A prospective study of oral contraceptives and NIDDM among U.S. women. Diabetes Care 1997;20:330–5. (Level II-2)

49. Falsetti L, Pasinetti E. Effects of long-term administration of an oral contraceptive containing ethinylestradiol and cyproterone acetate on lipid metabolism in women with polycystic ovary syndrome. Acta Obstet Gynecol Scand 1995;74:56–60. (Level II-2)

50. Morin-Papunen LC, Vauhkonen I, Koivunen RM, Ruokonen A, Martikainen HK, Tapanainen JS. Endocrine and metabolic effects of metformin versus ethinyl estradiol-cyproterone acetate in obese women with polycystic ovary syndrome: a randomized study. J Clin Endocrinol Metab 2000;85:3161–8. (Level I)

51. Ginsberg H, Plutzky J, Sobel BE. A review of metabolic and cardiovascular effects of oral antidiabetic agents: beyond glucose-level lowering. J Cardiovasc Risk 1999; 6:337–46. (Level III)

52. Kim LH, Taylor AE, Barbieri RL. Insulin sensitizers and polycystic ovary syndrome: can a diabetes medication treat infertility? Fertil Steril 2000;73:1097–8. (Level III)

53. Adashi EY. Ovulation induction : clomiphene citrate. In: Adashi EY, Rock JA, Rosenwaks Z, editors. Reproductive endocrinology, surgery, and technology. vol. 1. Philadelphia (PA): Lippincott-Raven; 1996. p. 1181–1206. (Level III)

54. Gysler M, March CM, Mishell DR Jr, Bailey EJ. A decade's experience with an individualized clomiphene treatment regimen including its effect on the postcoital test. Fertil Steril 1982;37:161–7. (Level II-3)

55. Hughes E, Collins J, Vandekerckhove P. Clomiphene citrate for ovulation induction in women with oligo-amenorrhoea (Cochrane Review). In: The Cochrane Library, Issue 3, 2002. Oxford: Update Software. (Level III)

56. Shepard MK, Balmaceda JP, Leija CG. Relationship of weight to successful induction of ovulation with clomiphene citrate. Fertil Steril 1979;32:641–5. (Level II-2)

57. Lobo RA, Granger LR, Davajan V, Mishell DR Jr. An extended regimen of clomiphene citrate in women unresponsive to standard therapy. Fertil Steril 1982;37: 762–6. (Level II-3)

58. Daly DC, Walters CA, Soto-Albors CE, Tohan N, Riddick DH. A randomized study of dexamethasone in ovulation induction with clomiphene citrate. Fertil Steril 1984;41:844–8. (Level I)

59. Fauser BC, Donderwinkel P, Schoot DC. The step-down principle in gonadotrophin treatment and the role of GnRH analogues. Baillieres Clin Obstet Gynaecol 1993;7:309–30. (Level III)

60. Homburg R, Levy T, Ben-Rafael Z. A comparative prospective study of conventional regimen with chronic low-dose administration of follicle-stimulating hormone for anovulation associated with polycystic ovary syndrome. Fertil Steril 1995;63:729–33. (Level II-2)

61. Sagle MA, Hamilton-Fairley D, Kiddy DS, Franks S. A comparative, randomized study of low-dose human menopausal gonadotropin and follicle-stimulating hormone in women with polycystic ovarian syndrome. Fertil Steril 1991;55:56–60. (Level I)

62. Farquhar C, Vandekerckhove P, Lilford R. Laparoscopic "drilling" by diathermy or laser for ovulation induction in anovulatory polycystic ovary syndrome (Cochrane Review). In: The Cochrane Library, Issue 3, 2002. Oxford: Update Software. (Meta-analysis)

63. Farquhar CM, Williamson K, Gudex G, Johnson NP, Garland J, Sadler L. A randomized controlled trial of laparoscopic ovarian diathermy versus gonadotropin therapy for women with clomiphene citrate-resistant polycystic ovary syndrome. Fertil Steril 2002;78:404–11. (Level I)

64. Donesky BW, Adashi EY. Surgically induced ovulation in the polycystic ovary syndrome: wedge resection revisited in the age of laparoscopy. Fertil Steril 1995;63: 439–63. (Level III)

65. Lemieux S, Lewis GF, Ben-Chetrit A, Steiner G, Greenblatt EM. Correction of hyperandrogenemia by laparoscopic ovarian cautery in women with polycystic ovarian syndrome is not accompanied by improved insulin sensitivity or lipid-lipoprotein levels. J Clin Endocrinol Metab 1999;84:4278–82. (Level II-2)

66. Nestler JE, Jakubowicz DJ. Decreases in ovarian cytochrome P450c17 alpha activity and serum free testosterone after reduction of insulin secretion in polycystic ovary syndrome. N Engl J Med 1996;335:617–23. (Level I)

67. De Leo V, la Marca A, Ditto A, Morgante G, Cianci A. Effects of metformin on gonadotropin-induced ovulation in women with polycystic ovary syndrome. Fertil Steril 1999;72:282–5. (Level I)

68. Crave JC, Fimbel S, Lejeune H, Cugnardey N, Dechaud H, Pugeat M. Effects of diet and metformin administration on sex hormone-binding globulin, androgens, and insulin in hirsute and obese women. J Clin Endocrinol Metab 1995;80:2057–62. (Level I)

69. Acbay O, Gundogdu S. Can metformin reduce insulin resistance in polycystic ovary syndrome? Fertil Steril 1996;65:946–9. (Level II-2)

70. Ehrmann DA, Cavaghan MK, Imperial J, Sturis J, Rosenfield RL, Polonsky KS. Effects of metformin on insulin secretion, insulin action, and ovarian steroidogenesis in women with polycystic ovary syndrome. J Clin Endocrinol Metab 1997;82:524–30. (Level II-2)

71. Stadtmauer LA, Toma SK, Riehl RM, Talbert LM. Metformin treatment of patients with polycystic ovary syndrome undergoing in vitro fertilization improves outcomes and is associated with modulation of the insulin-like growth factors. Fertil Steril 2001;75:505–9. (Level II-2)

72. Vandermolen DT, Ratts VS, Evans WS, Stovall DW, Kauma SW, Nestler JE. Metformin increases the ovulatory rate and pregnancy rate from clomiphene citrate in patients with polycystic ovary syndrome who are resistant to clomiphene citrate alone. Fertil Steril 2001;75: 310–5. (Level I)

73. Callahan TL, Hall JE, Ettner SL, Christiansen CL, Greene MF, Crowley WF Jr. The economic impact of multiple-gestation pregnancies and the contribution of assisted-reproduction techniques to their incidence. N Engl J Med 1994;331:244–9. (Level III)

74. Glueck CJ, Phillips H, Cameron D, Sieve-Smith L, Wang P. Continuing metformin throughout pregnancy in women with polycystic ovary syndrome appears to safely reduce first-trimester spontaneous abortion: a pilot study. Fertil Steril 2001;75:46–52. (Level III)

75. Clark AM, Thornley B, Tomlinson L, Galletley C, Norman RJ. Weight loss in obese infertile women results in improvement in reproductive outcome for all forms of fertility treatment. Hum Reprod 1998;13:1502–5. (Level II-3)

76. Huber-Buchholz MM, Carey DG, Norman RJ. Restoration of reproductive potential by lifestyle modification in obese polycystic ovary syndrome: role of insulin sensitivity and luteinizing hormone. J Clin Endocrinol Metab 1999;84:1470–4. (Level II-2)

77. Kiddy DS, Hamilton-Fairley D, Bush A, Short F, Anyaoku V, Reed MJ, et al. Improvement in endocrine and ovarian function during dietary treatment of obese women with polycystic ovary syndrome. Clin Endocrinol (Oxf) 1992;36:105–11. (Level II-2)

78. Guzick DS, Wing R, Smith D, Berga SL, Winters SJ. Endocrine consequences of weight loss in obese, hyperandrogenic, anovulatory women. Fertil Steril 1994;61: 598–604. (Level I)

79. Pasquali R, Antenucci D, Casimirri F, Venturoli S, Paradisi R, Fabbri R, et al. Clinical and hormonal characteristics of obese amenorrheic hyperandrogenic women before and after weight loss. J Clin Endocrinol Metab 1989;68:173–9. (Level II-3)

80. Jaatinen TA, Anttila L, Erkkola R, Koskinen P, Laippala P, Ruutiainen K, et al. Hormonal responses to physical exercise in patients with polycystic ovarian syndrome. Fertil Steril 1993;60:262–7. (Level II-2)

81. Braun B, Zimmermann MB, Kretchmer N. Effects of exercise intensity on insulin sensitivity in women with non-insulin-dependent diabetes mellitus. J Appl Physiol 1995;78:300–6. (Level II-2)

82. Ehrmann DA, Schneider DJ, Sobel BE, Cavaghan MK, Imperial J, Rosenfield RL, et al. Troglitazone improves defects in insulin action, insulin secretion, ovarian steroidogenesis, and fibrinolysis in women with polycystic ovary syndrome. J Clin Endocrinol Metab 1997;82: 2108–16. (Level II-2)

83. Ciotta L, Cianci A, Marletta E, Pisana L, Agliano A, Palumbo G. Treatment of hirsutism with flutamide and a low-dosage oral contraceptive in polycystic ovarian disease patients. Fertil Steril 1994;62:1129–35. (Level II-2)

84. Azziz R, Ochoa TM, Bradley EL Jr, Potter HD, Boots LR. Leuprolide and estrogen versus oral contraceptive pills for the treatment of hirsutism: a prospective randomized study. J Clin Endocrinol Metab 1995;80: 3406–11. (Level I)

85. De Leo V, Fulghesu AM, la Marca A, Morgante G, Pasqui L, Talluri B, et al. Hormonal and clinical effects of GnRH agonist alone, or in combination with a combined oral contraceptive or flutamide in women with severe hirsutism. Gynecol Endrocrinol 2000;14:411–6. (Level I)

86. Falsetti L, Gambera A, Tisi G. Efficacy of the combination ethinyl oestradiol and cyproterone acetate on endocrine, clinical and ultrasonographic profile in polycystic ovarian syndrome. Hum Reprod 2001;16:36–42. (Level II-2)

87. Sobbrio GA, Granata A, D'Arrigo F, Arena D, Panacea A, Trimarchi F, et al. Treatment of hirsutism related to micropolycystic ovary syndrome (MPCO) with two low-dose oestrogen oral contraceptives: a comparative randomized evaluation. Acta Eur Fertil 1990;21:139–41. (Level I)

88. Diamanti-Kandarakis E, Mitrakou A, Raptis S, Tolis G, Duleba AJ. The effect of a pure antiandrogen receptor blocker, flutamide, on the lipid profile in the polycystic ovary syndrome. J Clin Endocrinol Metab 1998;83: 2699–705. (Level II-2)

89. Moghetti P, Tosi F, Tosti A, Negri C, Misciali C, Perrone F, et al. Comparison of spironolactone, flutamide, and finasteride efficacy in the treatment of hirsutism: a randomized, double blind, placebo-controlled trial. J Clin Endocrinol Metab 2000;85:89–94. (Level I)

90. Eil C, Edelson SK. The use of human skin fibroblasts to obtain potency estimates of drug binding to androgen receptors. J Clin Endocrinol Metab 1984;59:51–5. (Level II-3)

91. Helfer EL, Miller JL, Rose LI. Side-effects of spironolactone therapy in the hirsute woman. J Clin Endocrinol Metab 1988;66:208–11. (Level III)

92. Farquhar C, Lee O, Toomath R, Jepson R. Spironolactone versus placebo or in combination with steroids for hirsutism and/or acne (Cochrane Review). In: Cochrane Library, Issue 3, 2002. Oxford: Update Software. (Meta-analysis)

93. Pucci E, Genazzani AD, Monzani F, Lippi F, Angelini F, Gargani M, et al. Prolonged treatment of hirsutism with flutamide alone in patients affected by polycystic ovary syndrome. Gynecol Endocrinol 1995;9:221–8. (Level II-2)

94. Fruzzetti F, De Lorenzo D, Ricci C, Fioretti P. Clinical and endocrine effects of flutamide in hyperandrogenic women. Fertil Steril 1993;60:806–13. (Level II-1)

95. Moghetti P, Castello R, Magnani CM, Tosi F, Negri C, Armanini D, et al. Clinical and hormonal effects of the 5 alpha-reductase inhibitor finasteride in idiopathic hirsutism. J Clin Endocrinol Metab 1994;79:1115–21. (Level II-2)

96. Fruzzetti F, de Lorenzo D, Parrini D, Ricci C. Effects of finasteride, a 5 alpha-reductase inhibitor, on circulating androgens and gonadotropin secretion in hirsute women. J Clin Endocrinol Metab 1994;79:831–5. (Level II-2)

97. Morin-Papunen LC, Koivunen RM, Ruokonen A, Martikainen HK. Metformin therapy improves the menstrual pattern with minimal endocrine and metabolic effects in women with polycystic ovary syndrome. Fertil Steril 1998;69:691–6. (Level II-2)

98. Ibanez L, Valls C, Potau N, Marcos MV, de Zegher F. Sensitization to insulin in adolescent girls to normalize hirsutism, hyperandrogenism, oligomenorrhea, dyslipidemia, and hyperinsulinism after precocious pubarche. J Clin Endocrinol Metab 2000;85:3526–30. (Level II-2)

99. Richards RN, Uy M, Meharg G. Temporary hair removal in patients with hirsutism: a clinical study. Cutis 1990; 45:199–202. (Level III)

100. Peereboom-Wynia JD. Effect of various methods of depilation on density of hairgrowth in women with idiopathic hirsutism. Arch Dermatol Forsch 1972;243: 164–76. (Level II-2)

101. Dierickx CC. Hair removal by lasers and intense pulsed light sources. Semin Cutan Med Surg 2000;19:267–75. (Level III)

The MEDLINE database, the Cochrane Library, and ACOG's own internal resources and documents were used to conduct a literature search to locate relevant articles published between January 1985 and January 2001. The search was restricted to articles published in the English language. Priority was given to articles reporting results of original research, although review articles and commentaries also were consulted. Abstracts of research presented at symposia and scientific conferences were not considered adequate for inclusion in this document. Guidelines published by organizations or institutions such as the National Institutes of Health and the American College of Obstetricians and Gynecologists were reviewed, and additional studies were located by reviewing bibliographies of identified articles. When reliable research was not available, expert opinions from obstetrician–gynecologists were used.

Studies were reviewed and evaluated for quality according to the method outlined by the U.S. Preventive Services Task Force:

I Evidence obtained from at least one properly designed randomized controlled trial.

II-1 Evidence obtained from well-designed controlled trials without randomization.

II-2 Evidence obtained from well-designed cohort or case–control analytic studies, preferably from more than one center or research group.

II-3 Evidence obtained from multiple time series with or without the intervention. Dramatic results in uncontrolled experiments could also be regarded as this type of evidence.

III Opinions of respected authorities, based on clinical experience, descriptive studies, or reports of expert committees.

Based on the highest level of evidence found in the data, recommendations are provided and graded according to the following categories:

Level A—Recommendations are based on good and consistent scientific evidence.

Level B—Recommendations are based on limited or inconsistent scientific evidence.

Level C—Recommendations are based primarily on consensus and expert opinion.

ISSN 1099-3630

The American College of Obstetricians and Gynecologists
409 12th Street, SW, PO Box 96920
Washington, DC 20090-6920

12345/65432

Polycystic ovary syndrome. ACOG Practice Bulletin No. 41. American College of Obstetricians and Gynecologists. Obstet Gynecol 2002; 100:1389–402.

ACOG PRACTICE BULLETIN

CLINICAL MANAGEMENT GUIDELINES FOR
OBSTETRICIAN–GYNECOLOGISTS
NUMBER 60, MARCH 2005

This Practice Bulletin was developed by the ACOG Committee on Practice Bulletins—Obstetrics with the assistance of Steven G. Gabbe, MD. The information is designed to aid practitioners in making decisions about appropriate obstetric and gynecologic care. These guidelines should not be construed as dictating an exclusive course of treatment or procedure. Variations in practice may be warranted based on the needs of the individual patient, resources, and limitations unique to the institution or type of practice.

Pregestational Diabetes Mellitus

Pregestational diabetes mellitus represents one of the most challenging medical complications of pregnancy. This document provides an overview of the current understanding of pregestational diabetes mellitus and suggests management guidelines during pregnancy. Because few well-designed studies have been performed, many of the guidelines are based on expert and consensus opinion.

Background

Definition and Prevalence

More than 8 million women in the United States have pregestational diabetes mellitus, and it is observed in 1% of all pregnancies (1, 2). Type 2 pregestational diabetes mellitus is most common and is characterized by onset later in life; peripheral insulin resistance; relative insulin deficiency; obesity; and the development of vascular, renal, and neuropathic complications. The rapidly increasing incidence of type 2 pregestational diabetes mellitus is caused, in part, by increasing obesity in the United States (3). Although 90% of diabetes cases encountered during pregnancy are gestational diabetes mellitus (GDM), more than one half of these women eventually develop type 2 pregestational diabetes mellitus later in life. Type 1 diabetes mellitus tends to occur early in life. In contrast to type 2 pregestational diabetes mellitus, type 1 pregestational diabetes mellitus is characterized by an autoimmune process that destroys the pancreatic β cells, leading to the need for insulin therapy.

Management of Diabetes During Pregnancy

Pregnancy is characterized by increased insulin resistance and reduced sensitivity to insulin action. Late in the first trimester, relatively higher levels of estrogen enhance insulin sensitivity and, when associated with nausea and vomiting, increase the risk for maternal hypoglycemia. The increase in insulin resistance is largely the result of a mixture of placental hormones, including human placental lactogen, progesterone, prolactin, placental growth hormone, and cortisol. More recently, tumor necrosis factor α and leptin have been implicated as contributors to the insulin resistant state of pregnancy (4). Insulin resistance is greatest in the third trimester.

The management of diabetes in pregnancy must focus on excellent glucose control achieved using a careful combination of diet, exercise, and insulin therapy (5–8). Patients may need to be seen every 1–2 weeks during the first two trimesters and weekly after 28–30 weeks of gestation. During pregnancy, caloric requirements are increased approximately 300 kcal higher than basal needs in patients with a singleton fetus (9, 10). Carbohydrate counting increases dietary flexibility and is extremely useful as long as the total daily caloric intake is considered to avoid excessive weight gain. A registered dietitian may be of value in providing an individualized nutrition program. Women with normal body weights usually require 30–35 kcal/kg/d. Women who are less than 90% of desirable body weight may need to increase their caloric requirements to 30–40 kcal/kg, whereas those who are more than 120% of desirable body weight should decrease their caloric intake to 24 kcal/kg/d. Caloric composition includes 40–50% from complex, high-fiber carbohydrates; 20% from protein; and 30–40% from primarily unsaturated fats. The calories may be distributed as follows: 10–20% at breakfast; 20–30% at lunch; 30–40% at dinner; and up to 30% for snacks, especially a bedtime snack to reduce nocturnal hypoglycemia (9). Artificial sweeteners, including saccharin, aspartame, and acesulfame-k, may be safely used in moderate amounts. Patients should be encouraged to keep a log of food intake several days each week so that this information can be correlated with insulin dosages, exercise, and glucose values.

Most insulin used in the treatment of pregestational diabetes mellitus is biosynthetic human insulin. Insulin requirements will increase throughout pregnancy, most markedly in the period between 28–32 weeks of gestation (11). On average, insulin needs increase from a range of 0.7–0.8 U/kg/d in the first trimester, to 0.8–1 U/kg/d in the second trimester, to 0.9–1.2 U/kg/d in the third trimester (7, 12). The goal of therapy is to maintain capillary glucose levels as close to normal as possible, including a fasting glucose level of 95 mg/dL or less, premeal values of 100 mg/dL or less, 1-hour postprandial levels of 140 mg/dL or less, and 2-hour postprandial values of 120 mg/dL or less. During the night, glucose levels should not decrease to less than 60 mg/dL. Mean capillary glucose levels should be maintained at an average of 100 mg/dL with a glycosylated hemoglobin A_{1C} (Hb A_{1C}) concentration no higher than 6% (13, 14).

Short- or rapid-acting insulins (short-acting regular insulin, insulin lispro, and insulin aspart) are administered before meals to reduce glucose elevations associated with eating (15, 16) (Table 1). Although insulin lispro may be used in place of regular insulin, the two are not interchangeable. Regular insulin should be given approximately 30 minutes before eating. Insulin lispro should be given immediately before eating (17). Although its rapid onset of action improves compliance and patient satisfaction, insulin lispro can cause significant hypoglycemia in the unprepared patient.

Longer acting insulins are used to restrain hepatic glucose production between meals and in the fasting state (see Table 1). Intermediate-acting insulin (15, 16) usually is given before breakfast with a rapid- or short-acting insulin and before the evening meal or at bedtime. Bedtime dosing is preferred because an injection given with the evening meal may increase the risks of nocturnal hypoglycemia. Extended insulin zinc suspension has a prolonged duration of action that may make it difficult to determine the timing of its effect, especially if it is given twice daily. Glargine is a recently developed human insulin analog produced with recombinant DNA (18). The absorption of this insulin analog is delayed, creating a steady basal insulin state with no peak and a 24-hour duration. Glargine cannot be mixed in the same syringe with other insulins. Experience with glargine in pregnancy has been limited. In patients who are highly insulin resistant, regular U500 (concentrated) insulin may be valuable (14).

Frequent self-monitoring of blood glucose is essential to achieve euglycemia without significant hypoglycemia during pregnancy (19). Capillary glucose levels should be checked using a glucose meter and recorded in the fasting state, before and 1 or 2 hours after each meal,

Table 1. Action Profile of Commonly Used Insulins

Type	Onset of Action	Peak of Action (hours)	Duration of Action (hours)
Insulin lispro	1–15 minutes	1–2	4–5
Insulin aspart	1–15 minutes	1–2	4–5
Regular insulin	30–60 minutes	2–4	6–8
Isophane insulin suspension	1–3 hours	5–7	13–18
Insulin zinc suspension	1–3 hours	4–8	13–20
Extended insulin zinc suspension	2–4 hours	8–14	18–30
Insulin glargine	1 hour	No peak	24

Modified from Gabbe SG, Graves CR. Management of diabetes mellitus complicating pregnancy. Obstet Gynecol 2003;102:857–68.

and before bed. Results may differ depending on whether the meter tests whole blood, serum, or plasma. Fasting glucose levels reflect the action of overnight basal insulin, whereas glucose concentrations before meals indicate daytime basal insulin activity (15). Levels after meals reveal the effect of the meal and recent insulin doses. In selected patients, especially those on insulin pumps, glucose determinations at 2–3 AM may help detect nocturnal hypoglycemia caused by excessive basal insulin or an inadequate bedtime snack or nocturnal hyperglycemia caused by insufficient basal insulin or pump failure. Generally, insulin doses are changed by 20% in response to hyperglycemia or hypoglycemia. A Hb A_{1C} measurement provides an indication of glycemic control over the past 2–3 months and should be performed during each trimester. An Hb A_{1C} value of 8% reflects a mean glucose level of 180 mg/dL, with each 1% higher or lower than 8% equal to a change of 30 mg/dL (13). Patients should check urine ketones when their glucose levels exceed 200 mg/dL and immediately report positive results to their health care teams.

Even with meticulous monitoring, hypoglycemia is more frequent in pregnancy than at other times, particularly in patients with type 1 pregestational diabetes mellitus. Patients should be questioned to determine if they can recognize when their glucose levels decrease to less than 60 mg/dL. Patients and their families should be taught how to respond quickly and appropriately to hypoglycemia. A glass of milk is preferable to fruit juices containing high levels of glucose. In addition, patients should have glucagon on hand for severe hypoglycemia and loss of consciousness.

Maternal Morbidity

Pregnancy has been associated with exacerbation of many diabetes-related complications. Poorly controlled pregestational diabetes mellitus leads to serious end-organ damage that may eventually become life threatening. In turn, preexisting diabetes-related end-organ disease may have deleterious effects on obstetric outcomes.

Diabetic retinopathy, the leading cause of blindness between ages 24 and 64 years, is classified as 1) background retinopathy, characterized by retinal microaneurysms and dot-blot hemorrhages; and 2) proliferative retinopathy, marked by neovascularization (20). The rapid institution of strict glycemic control in women with diabetes during pregnancy has been associated with acute progression of retinopathy, particularly in women with hypertensive disorders, including preeclampsia (21). Proliferative retinopathy is best treated with laser therapy, ideally before conception (22). Women with diabetes who become pregnant should have a comprehensive eye examination in the first trimester and be monitored closely throughout pregnancy (23).

Diabetic nephropathy is estimated to occur in 5–10% of pregnancies (24, 25). Most studies have failed to demonstrate permanent deterioration in renal function associated with pregnancy in women with mild-to-moderate diabetic nephropathy. However, progression to end-stage renal disease has been reported in women with serum creatinine levels exceeding 1.5 mg/dL or severe proteinuria (>3 g per 24 hours) (26). Women with preexisting diabetic nephropathy are at significantly higher risk for several adverse obstetric complications, including hypertensive disorders, uteroplacental insufficiency, and iatrogenic preterm birth, because of worsening renal function (27, 28). Before conception, a baseline evaluation of renal function by serum creatinine and assessment of urinary protein excretion (urine albumin-to-creatinine ratio or 24-hour albumin excretion) is recommended with follow-up measurements at regular intervals throughout pregnancy (29).

Chronic hypertension is observed in approximately 5–10% of pregnant patients with pregestational diabetes mellitus (30). Hypertension, especially in the presence of nephropathy, increases the risk of preeclampsia, uteroplacental insufficiency, and stillbirth (31). Ideally, hypertension should be controlled before conception. In nonpregnant patients, treatment is likely to include an angiotensin-converting enzyme inhibitor or an angiotensin II receptor blocker. Because of their adverse fetal effects, these medications should be discontinued before conception and should not be used during pregnancy.

Symptomatic coronary artery disease in women with pregestational diabetes mellitus is most commonly seen in those with long-standing disease, nephropathy, and hypertension (32). Preexisting symptomatic coronary artery disease may be a potential contraindication to pregnancy because of the pregnancy-associated hemodynamic changes that may result in myocardial infarction and death (9). Diabetic neuropathy is not well-studied in pregnancy but may manifest as recalcitrant nausea and vomiting secondary to gastroparesis (33).

Diabetic Ketoacidosis

Diabetic ketoacidosis is a life-threatening emergency observed in 5–10% of all pregnancies complicated by pregestational diabetes mellitus (34, 35). Because diabetic ketoacidosis is caused by an absolute or relative insulin deficiency, it is most commonly observed in women with type 1 pregestational diabetes mellitus. Enhanced insulin resistance probably plays a role in the higher incidence of diabetic ketoacidosis observed during pregnancy, as well as the propensity for diabetic ketoacidosis to develop more rapidly and at less severe levels of hyperglycemia and even normal glucose levels. Common risk factors for diabetic ketoacidosis during pregnancy include new onset diabetes; infections, such as influenza and urinary tract infection; poor patient compliance; insulin pump failure; and treatment with β-mimetic tocolytic medications and antenatal corticosteroids (36).

Typical clinical presentation of diabetic ketoacidosis in pregnancy includes abdominal pain, nausea and vomiting, and altered sensorium. Abnormal laboratory findings commonly include a low arterial pH (<7.3), a low serum bicarbonate level (<15 mEq/L), an elevated anion gap, and positive serum ketones (36). Continuous fetal heart rate monitoring commonly demonstrates recurrent late decelerations. However, this pattern usually resolves as the maternal condition improves, and delivery is rarely indicated.

Treatment regimens are based on aggressive hydration and intravenous insulin (see box). Because hypoglycemia and hypokalemia are frequent complications of diabetic ketoacidosis therapy, glucose and potassium concentrations should be monitored closely. Although maternal mortality is rare, fetal mortality has ranged from 35% of cases to, more recently, 10% of cases (35, 37).

Perinatal Morbidity and Mortality

The perinatal mortality rate in pregnancies complicated by pregestational diabetes mellitus has decreased markedly in recent years. Overall perinatal outcome is best when glucose control is achieved before conception and in the absence of maternal vascular disease (7, 38). The relationship between maternal end-organ disease and adverse pregnancy outcome was first illustrated by Priscilla White, whose classification system attempted to predict perinatal risk according to the age at onset of diabetes; duration of diabetes; and the presence of renal (class F), proliferative retinal (class R), and cardiac (class H) complications (39).

Major congenital anomalies are the leading cause of perinatal mortality in pregnancies complicated by pregestational diabetes mellitus, occurring in 6–12% of infants of women with diabetes (40). Studies have linked the increased rate of congenital malformations, as well as spontaneous abortion, to poor preconceptional glucose control (41, 42). Hyperglycemia during organogenesis (5–8 weeks after the last menstrual period) is thought to play a critical role in abnormal development (43); however, hypoglycemia has not been associated with adverse fetal outcome (44). Glycosylated hemoglobin levels correlate directly with the frequency of anomalies. A level less than 1% higher than the upper limit of normal, or approximately 5–6%, is associated with a fetal malformation rate close to that observed in normal pregnancies

Management of Diabetic Ketoacidosis During Pregnancy

1. Laboratory assessment
   - Obtain arterial blood gases to document degree of acidosis present; measure glucose, ketones, and electrolyte levels at 1- to 2-hour intervals
2. Insulin
   - Low-dose, intravenous
   - Loading dose: 0.2–0.4 U/kg
   - Maintenance: 2–10 U/h
3. Fluids
   - Isotonic sodium chloride
   - Total replacement in first 12 hours equals 4–6 L
   - 1 L in first hour
   - 500–1,000 mL/h for 2–4 hours
   - 250 mL/h until 80% replaced
4. Glucose
   - Begin 5% dextrose in normal saline when plasma level reaches 250 mg/dL (14 mmol/L)
5. Potassium
   - If initially normal or reduced, an infusion rate up to 15–20 mEq/h may be required; if elevated, wait until levels decrease into the normal range, then add to intravenous solution in a concentration of 20–30 mEq/L
6. Bicarbonate
   - Add one ampule (44 mEq) to 1 L of 0.45 normal saline if pH is <7.1

Reprinted with permission from Elsevier. Landon MB, Catalano PM, Gabbe SG. Diabetes mellitus. In: Gabbe SG, Niebyl JR, Simpson JL, editors. Obstetrics: normal and problem pregnancies. 4th edition. New York (NY): Churchill Livingstone; 2002. p. 1102.

(2–3%), whereas an Hb A_{1C} concentration near 10% is associated with a fetal anomaly rate of 20–25% (40, 45). Complex cardiac defects; central nervous system anomalies, such as anencephaly and spina bifida; and skeletal malformations, including sacral agenesis are most common (14, 46, 47).

Adverse perinatal outcomes later in pregnancy also are increased in women with pregestational diabetes mellitus (14). Facilitated diffusion of glucose across the placenta leads to transient fetal hyperglycemia. Subsequent stimulation of the fetal pancreatic β cells results in fetal hyperinsulinemia with several fetal and neonatal consequences. Because insulin is a potent growth hormone, excessive fetal growth occurs, particularly in adipose tissue (48). The fetus of a woman with poorly controlled diabetes is at increased risk of intrauterine fetal death and is more likely to weigh more than 4,000 g with a disproportionate concentration of fat around the shoulders and chest, which more than doubles the risk of shoulder dystocia at vaginal delivery (14). Elevated postprandial values may be most closely related to the risk for macrosomia (49, 50).

The neonatal consequences of poorly controlled pregestational diabetes mellitus during pregnancy include profound hypoglycemia, a higher rate of respiratory distress syndrome, polycythemia, organomegaly, electrolyte disturbances, and hyperbilirubinemia. Long-term outcomes for type 1 diabetes mellitus include obesity and carbohydrate intolerance (51–54).

Obstetric Complications

Spontaneous preterm labor appears to be more common in women with pregestational diabetes mellitus (55). The increased incidence of hydramnios may be a cause of preterm labor in some patients with pregestational diabetes mellitus, particularly those with poor glycemic control (56).

Preeclampsia is observed in 15–20% of pregnancies complicated by type 1 diabetes mellitus without nephropathy and approximately 50% in the presence of nephropathy (55, 57). Preeclampsia also is more likely in women with hypertension and poor glucose control (24, 25, 27). In the setting of hypertension and nephropathy, the risk of fetal intrauterine growth restriction is more than doubled. The rate of primary cesarean delivery is increased in women with pregestational diabetes mellitus (56, 58).

Clinical Considerations and Recommendations

▶ *Is there a role for preconceptional counseling?*

Preconceptional counseling for women with pregestational diabetes mellitus has been reported to be beneficial and cost-effective and should be encouraged (59). Because fewer than one third of women with diabetes mellitus seek preconceptional counseling (60), any visit to a health care provider should be used as an opportunity to review the aspects of diabetes management during pregnancy. Preconceptional counseling should focus on the importance of euglycemic control before pregnancy, as well as the adverse obstetric and maternal outcomes that can result from poorly controlled diabetes. A search

for underlying vasculopathy is advisable and, in selected patients, may include a retinal examination by an ophthalmologist, a 24-hour urine collection for protein excretion and creatinine clearance, and electrocardiography. Because up to 40% of young women with type 1 diabetes mellitus also may have thyroid dysfunction, thyroid function studies also should be obtained (61). Multivitamins containing at least 400 µg of folic acid should be prescribed to all women contemplating pregnancy. This is particularly important in women with diabetes given their increased risk of neural tube defects. Higher doses of folic acid may be beneficial in some cases, especially in the presence of other risk factors for neural tube defects.

▶ *Is there a role for continuous subcutaneous insulin infusion during pregnancy?*

With continuous subcutaneous insulin infusion therapy (the insulin pump), insulin can be delivered in a pattern that closely resembles physiologic insulin secretion (62–64). A rapid-acting insulin, such as insulin lispro, is most appropriate for infusion pumps (65). Usually 50–60% of the total daily dose is administered at a continuous basal rate, with boluses before meals and snacks comprising 40–50% of the total daily dose (64). Patients who use continuous subcutaneous insulin infusion must be highly motivated and compliant. The advantages of the pump include improved patient satisfaction, a decrease in severe hypoglycemia, and better control of hyperglycemia. Major disadvantages include the increased cost of the pump and pump supplies. In addition, if the delivery of insulin is interrupted or impaired by battery failure or infection at the infusion site, diabetic ketoacidosis may develop rapidly (66).

▶ *Is there a role for oral hypoglycemic agents in pregnancy?*

Oral hypoglycemic agents, used widely in the treatment of nonpregnant patients, have not been well studied in pregnancy (67). However, glyburide, a second-generation sulfonylurea, does not cross the placenta and has been used to treat GDM. Its onset of action is approximately 4 hours and its duration of action is approximately 10 hours. In a study of 404 pregnant women with treatment initiated between 11 and 33 weeks of gestation, glyburide was found to be comparable to insulin in improving glucose control without evidence of adverse maternal and neonatal complications. Metformin has been used as a treatment for infertility in polycystic ovary syndrome (68). Metformin is a category B drug, and although there are more reports of its use during pregnancy (69), the long-term effects of in utero exposure have not been well studied. The use of all oral agents for control of type 2 diabetes mellitus during pregnancy should be limited and individualized until data regarding the safety and efficacy of these drugs become available.

▶ *What fetal assessment is appropriate in women with pregestational diabetes mellitus?*

An ultrasound examination early in gestation can be used not only to demonstrate fetal viability but to accurately date the pregnancy as well. Most major anomalies can be detected at 18–20 weeks of gestation by a specialized (or targeted) ultrasound examination that includes a carefully performed assessment of fetal cardiac structure, including the great vessels (70, 71). Echocardiography also may be indicated in cases of suspected cardiac defects or when the fetal heart and great vessels cannot be visualized by ultrasonography. Thereafter, periodic ultrasound examinations may be used to confirm appropriate fetal growth.

Antepartum fetal monitoring, including fetal movement counting, the nonstress test, the biophysical profile, and the contraction stress test when performed at appropriate intervals, is a valuable approach and can be used to monitor the pregnancies of women with pregestational diabetes mellitus (72–74). Initiation of testing is appropriate for most patients at 32–34 weeks of gestation. However, testing at earlier gestational ages may be warranted in some pregnancies complicated by additional high-risk conditions. In response to a report of an increased stillbirth rate in patients with a reactive nonstress test within 1 week of delivery, twice weekly testing has been widely adopted (75). Daily fetal movement counting is a simple technique for antepartum assessment that also should be considered. However, if maternal glucose control deteriorates, fetal condition may change, and repeat testing for fetal well-being may be indicated. Doppler velocimetry of the umbilical artery may be useful in monitoring pregnancies with vascular complications and poor fetal growth (76).

▶ *When and how should delivery occur?*

Optimal timing of delivery relies on balancing the risk of intrauterine fetal death with the risks of preterm birth. In poorly controlled patients, an amniocentesis for fetal lung maturity is advised for delivery before 39 weeks of gestation. If corticosteroids are administered to accelerate lung maturation, an increased insulin requirement over the next 5 days should be anticipated, and the patient's glucose levels should be closely monitored (77). Early delivery may be indicated in some patients with vasculopathy, nephropathy, poor glucose control, or a prior stillbirth. In contrast, patients with well-controlled diabetes may be allowed to progress to their expected date of delivery as long as antenatal testing remains reassuring (78). Expectant management beyond the estimated due date generally is not recommended. Although an ultrasound estimate of fetal weight may help to rule out macrosomia, ultrasonography has not proved to be more accurate than clinical assessment in determining the size of the large fetus (79–81). To prevent traumatic birth injury, cesarean delivery may be considered if the estimated fetal weight is greater than 4,500 g in women with diabetes (74). Induction of labor in pregnancies with a fetus with suspected macrosomia has not been found to reduce birth trauma and may increase the cesarean delivery rate (82).

▶ *How should glucose control be managed during labor?*

During induction of labor, maternal glycemia can be controlled with an intravenous infusion of regular insulin titrated to maintain hourly readings of blood glucose levels less than 110 mg/dL (6, 13, 83) (see box). Avoiding intrapartum maternal hyperglycemia may prevent fetal hyperglycemia and reduce the likelihood of subsequent neonatal hypoglycemia (54). During active labor, insulin may not be needed. Patients who are using an insulin pump may continue their basal infusion during labor.

Insulin Management During Labor and Delivery

- Usual dose of intermediate-acting insulin is given at bedtime.

- Morning dose of insulin is withheld.

- Intravenous infusion of normal saline is begun.

- Once active labor begins or glucose levels decrease to less than 70 mg/dL, the infusion is changed from saline to 5% dextrose and delivered at a rate of 100–150 cc/h (2.5 mg/kg/min) to achieve a glucose level of approximately 100 mg/dL.

- Glucose levels are checked hourly using a bedside meter allowing for adjustment in the insulin or glucose infusion rate.

- Regular (short-acting) insulin is administered by intravenous infusion at a rate of 1.25 U/h if glucose levels exceed 100 mg/dL.

Data from Coustan DR. Delivery: timing, mode, and management. In: Reece EA, Coustan DR, Gabbe SG, editors. Diabetes in women: adolescence, pregnancy, and menopause. 3rd ed. Philadelphia (PA): Lippincott Williams & Wilkins; 2004; and Jovanovic L, Peterson CM. Management of the pregnant, insulin-dependent diabetic woman. Diabetes Care 1980;3:63–8.

Insulin requirements decrease rapidly after delivery. One half of the predelivery dose may be reinstituted after starting regular food intake (13). For patients with cesarean delivery, rapid-acting insulin may be used to treat glucose values greater than 140–150 mg/dL after a regular meal pattern has been established.

▶ *Are special postpartum considerations necessary?*

Breastfeeding should be encouraged in women with pregestational diabetes mellitus. An additional 500 kcal/d more than the prepregnancy caloric intake is required. Small snacks before breastfeeding may reduce the risks of hypoglycemia (9).

Family planning options include low-dose combination oral contraceptives for women without vasculopathy who do not smoke, whereas progestin-only pills can be prescribed for women with vascular disease (84). Barrier methods, although less effective, will not affect glucose control or vasculopathy. Limited data suggest no increased complications for intrauterine device use in women with diabetes (85, 86). Sterilization should be considered for women with serious vasculopathy or for those who have completed their families.

Summary of Recommendations and Conclusions

The following recommendations are based on limited or inconsistent scientific evidence (Level B):

▶ Suspected fetal macrosomia is not an indication for induction of labor because induction does not improve maternal or fetal outcomes.

▶ Antepartum fetal monitoring, including fetal movement counting, the nonstress test, the biophysical profile, and the contraction stress test when performed at appropriate intervals, is a valuable approach and can be used to monitor the pregnancies of women with pregestational diabetes mellitus.

▶ Adequate maternal glucose control should be maintained near physiologic levels before conception and throughout pregnancy to decrease the likelihood of spontaneous abortion, fetal malformation, fetal macrosomia, intrauterine fetal death, and neonatal morbidity.

▶ Patients and their families should be taught how to respond quickly and appropriately to hypoglycemia.

▶ Preconceptional counseling for women with pregestational diabetes mellitus has been reported to be beneficial and cost-effective and should be encouraged.

▶ The use of oral agents for control of type 2 diabetes mellitus during pregnancy should be limited and individualized until data regarding the safety and efficacy of these drugs become available.

▶ To prevent traumatic birth injury, cesarean delivery may be considered if the estimated fetal weight is greater than 4,500 g in women with diabetes.

References

1. Lethbridge-Cejku M, Schiller JS, Bernadel L. Summary health statistics for U.S. adults: National Health Interview Survey, 2002. National Center for Health Statistics. Vital Health Stat 2004;10(222):1–160. (Level II-3)

2. Martin JA, Hamilton BE, Sutton PD, Ventura SJ, Menacker F, Munson ML. Births: final data for 2002. Natl Vital Stat Rep 2003;52(10):1–113. (Level II-3)

3. Narayan KM, Boyle JP, Thompson TJ, Sorensen SW, Williamson DF. Lifetime risk for diabetes mellitus in the United States. JAMA 2003;290:1884–90. (Level II-3)

4. Ryan EA. Hormones and insulin resistance during pregnancy. Lancet 2003;362:1777–8. (Level III)

5. Gabbe SG, Mestman JH, Freeman RK, Goebelsmann UT, Lowensohn RI, Nochimson D, et al. Management and outcome of pregnancy in diabetes mellitus, classes B to R. Am J Obstet Gynecol 1977;129:723–32. (Level II-2)

6. Jovanovic L, Peterson CM. Management of the pregnant, insulin-dependent diabetic woman. Diabetes Care 1980; 3:63–8. (Level II-3)

7. Jovanovic L, Druzin M, Peterson CM. Effect of euglycemia on the outcome of pregnancy in insulin-dependent diabetic women as compared with normal control subjects. Am J Med 1981;71:921–7. (Level II-2)

8. Garner P. Type I diabetes mellitus and pregnancy. Lancet 1995;346:157–61. (Level III)

9. American Diabetes Association. Prepregnancy counseling and management of women with preexisting diabetes or previous gestational diabetes. In: Medical management of pregnancy complicated by diabetes. 3rd ed. Alexandria (VA): ADA; 2000. p. 4–19. (Level III)

10. Franz MJ, Bantle JP, Beebe CA, Brunzell JD, Chiasson JL, Garg A, et al. Evidence-based nutrition principles and recommendations for the treatment and prevention of diabetes and related complications. American Diabetes Association. Diabetes Care 2003;26 (suppl):S51–61. (Level III)

11. Steel JM, Johnstone FD, Hume R, Mao JH. Insulin requirements during pregnancy in women with type I diabetes. Obstet Gynecol 1994;83:253–8. (Level II-3)

12. Langer O, Anyaegbunam A, Brustman L, Guidetti D, Levy J, Mazze R. Pregestational diabetes: insulin requirements throughout pregnancy. Am J Obstet Gynecol 1988; 159:616–21. (Level II-3)

13. Landon MB, Catalano PM, Gabbe SG. Diabetes mellitus. In: Gabbe SG, Niebyl JR, Simpson JL, editors. Obstetrics: normal and problem pregnancies. 4th edition. New York (NY): Churchill Livingstone; 2002. p. 1081–116. (Level III)

14. Gabbe SG, Graves CR. Management of diabetes mellitus complicating pregnancy. Obstet Gynecol 2003;102: 857–68. (Level III)

15. DeWitt DE, Hirsch IB. Outpatient insulin therapy in type 1 and type 2 diabetes mellitus: scientific review. JAMA 2003;289:2254–64. (Level III)

16. DeWitt DE, Dugdale DC. Using new insulin strategies in the outpatient treatment of diabetes: clinical applications. JAMA 2003;289:2265–9. (Level III)

17. Holleman F, Hoekstra JB. Insulin lispro [published erratum appears in N Engl J Med 2003;349:1487]. N Engl J Med 1997;337:176–83. (Level III)

18. Bolli GB, Owens DR. Insulin glargine. Lancet 2000;356: 443–5. (Level III)

19. Landon MB, Gabbe SG, Piana R, Mennuti MT, Main EK. Neonatal morbidity in pregnancy complicated by diabetes mellitus: predictive value of maternal glycemic profiles. Am J Obstet Gynecol 1987;156:1089–95. (Level II-3)

20. Frank RN. Diabetic retinopathy. N Engl J Med 2004;350: 48–58. (Level III)

21. Rosenn B, Miodovnik M, Kranias G, Khoury J, Combs CA, Mimouni F, et al. Progression of diabetic retinopathy in pregnancy: association with hypertension in pregnancy. Am J Obstet Gynecol 1992;166:1214–8. (Level II-3)

22. Klein BE, Moss SE, Klein R. Effect of pregnancy on progression of diabetic retinopathy. Diabetes Care 1990;13: 34–40. (Level II-2)

23. Fong DS, Aiello L, Gardner TW, King GL, Blankenship G, Cavallerano JD, et al. Retinopathy in diabetes. American Diabetes Association. Diabetes Care 2004;27 (suppl):S84–7. (Level III)

24. Gordon M, Landon MB, Samuels P, Hissrich S, Gabbe SG. Perinatal outcome and long-term follow-up associated with modern management of diabetic nephropathy. Obstet Gynecol 1996;87:401–9. (Level II-3)

25. Miodovnik M, Rosenn BM, Khoury JC, Grigsby JL, Siddiqi TA. Does pregnancy increase the risk for development and progression of diabetic nephropathy? Am J Obstet Gynecol 1996;174:1180–9; discussion 1189–91. (Level II-2)

26. Purdy LP, Hantsch CE, Molitch ME, Metzger BE, Phelps RL, Dooley SL, et al. Effect of pregnancy on renal function in patients with moderate-to-severe diabetic renal insufficiency. Diabetes Care 1996;19:1067–74. (Level III)

27. Combs CA, Rosenn B, Kitzmiller JL, Khoury JC, Wheeler BC, Miodovnik M. Early-pregnancy proteinuria in diabetes related to preeclampsia. Obstet Gynecol 1993; 82:802–7. (Level II-2)

28. Khoury JC, Miodovnik M, LeMasters G, Sibai B. Pregnancy outcome and progression of diabetic nephropathy. What's next? J Matern Fetal Neonatal Med 2002;11: 238–44. (Level II-2)

29. Preconception care of women with diabetes. American Diabetes Association. Diabetes Care 2004;27 (suppl 1): S76–8. (Level III)

30. Hinton AC, Sibai BM. Hypertensive disorders in pregnancy. In: Reece EA, Coustan DR, Gabbe SG, editors. Diabetes in women: adolescence, pregnancy, and menopause. 3rd ed. Philadelphia (PA): Lippincott Williams & Wilkins; 2004. p. 363–70. (Level III)

31. Simpson LL. Maternal medical disease: risk of antepartum fetal death. Semin Perinatol 2002;26:42–50. (Level III)

32. Gordon MC, Landon MB, Boyle J, Stewart KS, Gabbe SG. Coronary artery disease in insulin-dependent diabetes mellitus of pregnancy (class H): a review of the literature. Obstet Gynecol Surv 1996;51:437–44. (Level III)

33. Airaksinen KE, Anttila LM, Linnaluoto MK, Jouppila PI, Takkunen JT, Salmela PI. Autonomic influence on pregnancy outcome in IDDM. Diabetes Care 1990;13:756–61. (Level II-2)

34. Rodgers BD, Rodgers DE. Clinical variables associated with diabetic ketoacidosis during pregnancy. J Reprod Med 1991;36:797–800. (Level III)

35. Cullen MT, Reece EA, Homko CJ, Sivan E. The changing presentations of diabetic ketoacidosis during pregnancy. Am J Perinatol 1996;13:449–51. (Level III)

36. Montoro MN. Diabetic ketoacidosis in pregnancy. In: Reece EA, Coustan DR, Gabbe SG, editors. Diabetes in women: adolescence, pregnancy, and menopause. 3rd ed. Philadelphia (PA): Lippincott Williams & Wilkins; 2004. p. 345–50. (Level III)

37. Chauhan SP, Perry KG Jr, McLaughlin BN, Roberts WE, Sullivan CA, Morrison JC. Diabetic ketoacidosis complicating pregnancy. J Perinatol 1996;16:173–5. (Level II-3)

38. Pregnancy outcomes in the Diabetes Control and Complications Trial. Am J Obstet Gynecol 1996;174:1343–53. (Level I)

39. White P. Pregnancy complicating diabetes. Am J Med 1949;7:609–16. (Level II-3)

40. Kitzmiller JL, Buchanan TA, Kjos S, Combs CA, Ratner RE. Pre-conception care of diabetes, congenital malformations, and spontaneous abortions. Diabetes Care 1996; 19:514–41. (Level III)

41. Mills JL, Simpson JL, Driscoll SG, Jovanovic-Peterson L, Van Allen M, Aarons JH, et al. Incidence of spontaneous abortion among normal women and insulin-dependent diabetic women whose pregnancies were identified within 21 days of conception. N Engl J Med 1988;319: 1617–23. (Level II-2)

42. Rosenn B, Miodovnik M, Combs CA, Khoury J, Siddiqi TA. Glycemic thresholds for spontaneous abortion and congenital malformations in insulin-dependent diabetes mellitus. Obstet Gynecol 1994;84:515–20. (Level II-3)

43. Freinkel N. Diabetic embryopathy and fuel-mediated organ teratogenesis: lessons from animal models. Horm Metab Res 1988;20:463–75. (Level III)

44. Rosenn BM, Miodovnik M, Holcberg G, Khoury JC, Siddiqi TA. Hypoglycemia: the price of intensive insulin

therapy for pregnant women with insulin-dependent diabetes mellitus. Obstet Gynecol 1995;85:417–22. (Level II-3)

45. Greene MF, Hare JW, Cloherty JP, Benacerraf BR, Soeldner JS. First-trimester hemoglobin A1 and risk for major malformation and spontaneous abortion in diabetic pregnancy. Teratology 1989;39:225–31. (Level II-3)

46. Sheffield JS, Butler-Koster EL, Casey BM, McIntire DD, Leveno KJ. Maternal diabetes mellitus and infant malformations. Obstet Gynecol 2002;100:925–30. (Level II-3)

47. Wren C, Birrell G, Hawthorne G. Cardiovascular malformations in infants of diabetic mothers. Heart 2003;89: 1217–20. (Level II-3)

48. Modanlou HD, Komatsu G, Dorchester W, Freeman RK, Bosu SK. Large-for-gestational-age neonates: anthropometric reasons for shoulder dystocia. Obstet Gynecol 1982;60:417–23. (Level II-3)

49. Jovanovic-Peterson L, Peterson CM, Reed GF, Metzger BE, Mills JL, Knopp RH, et al. Maternal postprandial glucose levels and infant birth weight: the Diabetes in Early Pregnancy Study. The National Institute of Child Health and Human Development—Diabetes in Early Pregnancy Study. Am J Obstet Gynecol 1991;164:103–11. (Level II-2)

50. Combs CA, Gunderson E, Kitzmiller JL, Gavin LA, Main EK. Relationship of fetal macrosomia to maternal postprandial glucose control during pregnancy. Diabetes Care 1992;15:1251–7. (Level II-2)

51. Silverman BL, Rizzo T, Green OC, Cho NH, Winter RJ, Ogata ES, et al. Long-term prospective evaluation of offspring of diabetic mothers. Diabetes 1991;40 (suppl 2): 121–5. (Level II-2)

52. Silverman BL, Metzger BE, Cho NH, Loeb CA. Impaired glucose tolerance in adolescent offspring of diabetic mothers. Relationship to fetal hyperinsulinism. Diabetes Care 1995;18:611–7. (Level II-2)

53. Sobngwi E, Boudou P, Mauvais-Jarvis F, Leblanc H, Velho G, Vexiau P, et al. Effect of a diabetic environment in utero on predisposition to type 2 diabetes. Lancet 2003; 361:1861–5. (Level II-2)

54. Oh W. Neonatal outcome and care. In: Reece EA, Coustan DR, Gabbe SG, editors. Diabetes in women: adolescence, pregnancy, and menopause. 3rd ed. Philadelphia (PA): Lippincott Williams & Wilkins; 2004. p. 451–9. (Level III)

55. Reece EA, Sivan E, Francis G, Homko CJ. Pregnancy outcomes among women with and without microvascular disease (White's classes B to FR) versus non-diabetic controls. Am J Perinatol 1998;15:549–55. (Level II-2)

56. Cousins L. Obstetric complications in diabetic pregnancies. In: Reece EA, Coustan DR, Gabbe SG, editors. Diabetes in women: adolescence, pregnancy, and menopause. 3rd ed. Philadelphia (PA): Lippincott Williams & Wilkins; 2004. p. 351–62. (Level III)

57. Siddiqi T, Rosenn B, Mimouni F, Khoury J, Miodovnik M. Hypertension during pregnancy in insulin-dependent diabetic women. Obstet Gynecol 1991;77:514–9. (Level II-3)

58. Remsberg KE, McKeown RE, McFarland KF, Irwin LS. Diabetes in pregnancy and cesarean delivery. Diabetes Care 1999;22:1561–7. (Level II-3)

59. Rosenn B, Miodovnik M, Combs CA, Khoury J, Siddiqi TA. Pre-conception management of insulin-dependent diabetes: improvement of pregnancy outcome. Obstet Gynecol 1991;77:846–9. (Level II-3)

60. Janz NK, Herman WH, Becker MP, Charron-Prochownik D, Shayna VL, Lesnick TG, et al. Diabetes and pregnancy. Factors associated with seeking pre-conception care. Diabetes Care 1995;18:157–65. (Level II-2)

61. Umpierrez GE, Latif KA, Murphy MB, Lambeth HC, Stentz F, Bush A, et al. Thyroid dysfunction in patients with type 1 diabetes: a longitudinal study. Diabetes Care 2003;26:1181–5. (Level II-3)

62. Coustan DR, Reece EA, Sherwin RS, Rudolf MC, Bates SE, Sockin SM, et al. A randomized clinical trial of the insulin pump vs intensive conventional therapy in diabetic pregnancies. JAMA 1986;255:631–6. (Level II-1)

63. Carta Q, Meriggi E, Trossarelli GF, Catella G, Dal Molin V, Menato G, et al. Continuous subcutaneous insulin infusion versus intensive conventional insulin therapy in type I and type II diabetic pregnancy. Diabete Metab 1986;12: 121–9. (Level II-1)

64. Gabbe SG, Holing E, Temple P, Brown ZA. Benefits, risks, costs, and patient satisfaction associated with insulin pump therapy for the pregnancy complicated by type 1 diabetes mellitus. Am J Obstet Gynecol 2000;182: 1283–91. (Level II-3)

65. Continuous subcutaneous insulin infusion. American Diabetes Association. Diabetes Care 2004;27(suppl): S110. (Level III)

66. Lindenbaum C, Menzin A, Ludmir J. Diabetic ketoacidosis in pregnancy resulting from insulin pump failure. A case report. J Reprod Med 1993;38:306–8. (Level III)

67. Langer O, Conway DL, Berkus MD, Xenakis EM, Gonzales O. A comparison of glyburide and insulin in women with gestational diabetes mellitus. N Engl J Med 2000;343:1134–8. (Level I)

68. Heard MJ, Pierce A, Carson SA, Buster JE. Pregnancies following use of metformin for ovulation induction in patients with polycystic ovary syndrome. Fertil Steril 2002;77:669–73. (Level III)

69. Glueck CJ, Goldenberg N, Pranikoff J, Loftspring M, Sieve L, Wang P. Height, weight, and motor-social development during the first 18 months of life in 126 infants born to 109 mothers with polycystic ovary syndrome who conceived on and continued metformin through pregnancy. Hum Reprod 2004;19:1323–30. (Level II-3)

70. Greene MF, Benacerraf BR. Prenatal diagnosis in diabetic gravidas: utility of ultrasound and maternal serum alphafetoprotein screening. Obstet Gynecol 1991;77:520–4. (Level II-3)

71. Albert TJ, Landon MB, Wheller JJ, Samuels P, Cheng RF, Gabbe S. Prenatal detection of fetal anomalies in pregnancies complicated by insulin-dependent diabetes mellitus. Am J Obstet Gynecol 1996;174:1424–8. (Level II-3)

72. Kjos SL, Leung A, Henry OA, Victor MR, Paul RH, Medearis AL. Antepartum surveillance in diabetic pregnancies: predictors of fetal distress in labor. Am J Obstet Gynecol 1995;173:1532–9. (Level II-3)

73. Landon MB, Gabbe SG. Fetal surveillance and timing of delivery in pregnancy complicated by diabetes mellitus. Obstet Gynecol Clin North Am 1996;23:109–23. (Level III)

74. Rouse DJ, Owen J, Goldenberg RL, Cliver SP. The effectiveness and costs of elective cesarean delivery for fetal macrosomia diagnosed by ultrasound. JAMA 1996;276: 1480–6. (Decision analysis)

75. Barrett JM, Salyer SL, Boehm FH. The nonstress test: an evaluation of 1,000 patients. Am J Obstet Gynecol 1981; 141:153–7. (Level II-3)

76. Landon MB, Langer O, Gabbe SG, Schick C, Brustman L. Fetal surveillance in pregnancies complicated by insulin-dependent diabetes mellitus. Am J Obstet Gynecol 1992;167:617–21. (Level II-3)

77. Mathiesen ER, Christensen AB, Hellmuth E, Hornnes P, Stage E, Damm P. Insulin dose during glucocorticoid treatment for fetal lung maturation in diabetic pregnancy: test of an algorithm. Acta Obstet Gynecol Scand 2002;81: 835–9. (Level II-2)

78. Kjos SL, Henry OA, Montoro M, Buchanan TA, Mestman JH. Insulin-requiring diabetes in pregnancy: a randomized trial of active induction of labor and expectant management. Am J Obstet Gynecol 1993;169:611–5. (Level I)

79. Miller JM Jr, Brown HL, Khawli OF, Pastorek JG 2nd, Gabert HA. Ultrasonographic identification of the macro-somic fetus. Am J Obstet Gynecol 1988;159:1110–4. (Level II-3)

80. Johnstone FD, Prescott RJ, Steel JM, Mao JH, Chambers S, Muir N. Clinical and ultrasound prediction of macrosomia in diabetic pregnancy. Br J Obstet Gynaecol 1996; 103:747–54. (Level II-3)

81. Chauhan SP, Hendrix NW, Magann EF, Morrison JC, Kenney SP, Devoe LD. Limitations of clinical and sonographic estimates of birth weight: experience with 1034 parturients. Obstet Gynecol 1998;91:72–7. (Level II-2)

82. Sanchez-Ramos L, Bernstein S, Kaunitz AM. Expectant management versus labor induction for suspected fetal macrosomia: a systematic review. Obstet Gynecol 2002; 100:997–1002. (Meta-analysis)

83. Garber AJ, Moghissi ES, Bransome ED Jr, Clark NG, Clement S, Cobin RH, et al. American College of Endocrinology position statement on inpatient diabetes and metabolic control. American College of Endocrinology Task Force on Inpatient Diabetes Metabolic Control. Endocr Pract 2004;10 (suppl 2):4–9. (Level III)

84. Garg SK, Chase HP, Marshall G, Hoops SL, Holmes DL, Jackson WE. Oral contraceptives and renal and retinal complications in young women with insulin-dependent diabetes mellitus. JAMA 1994;271:1099–102. (Level II-2)

85. Kimmerle R, Weiss R, Berger M, Kurz KH. Effectiveness, safety and acceptability of a copper intrauterine device (CU Safe 300) in type 1 diabetic women. Diabetes Care 1993;16:1227–30. (Level II-2)

86. World Health Organization. Medical eligibility criteria for contraceptive use. 3rd ed. Geneva: WHO; 2004. (Level III)

The MEDLINE database, the Cochrane Library, and ACOG's own internal resources and documents were used to conduct a literature search to locate relevant articles published between January 1985 and October 2004. The search was restricted to articles published in the English language. Priority was given to articles reporting results of original research, although review articles and commentaries also were consulted. Abstracts of research presented at symposia and scientific conferences were not considered adequate for inclusion in this document. Guidelines published by organizations or institutions such as the National Institutes of Health and the American College of Obstetricians and Gynecologists were reviewed, and additional studies were located by reviewing bibliographies of identified articles. When reliable research was not available, expert opinions from obstetrician–gynecologists were used.

Studies were reviewed and evaluated for quality according to the method outlined by the U.S. Preventive Services Task Force:

I Evidence obtained from at least one properly designed randomized controlled trial.

II-1 Evidence obtained from well-designed controlled trials without randomization.

II-2 Evidence obtained from well-designed cohort or case–control analytic studies, preferably from more than one center or research group.

II-3 Evidence obtained from multiple time series with or without the intervention. Dramatic results in uncontrolled experiments also could be regarded as this type of evidence.

III Opinions of respected authorities, based on clinical experience, descriptive studies, or reports of expert committees.

Based on the highest level of evidence found in the data, recommendations are provided and graded according to the following categories:

Level A—Recommendations are based on good and consistent scientific evidence.

Level B—Recommendations are based on limited or inconsistent scientific evidence.

Level C—Recommendations are based primarily on consensus and expert opinion.

ISSN 1099-3630

**The American College of
Obstetricians and Gynecologists
409 12th Street, SW
PO Box 96920
Washington, DC 20090-6920**

12345/98765

Pregestational diabetes mellitus. ACOG Practice Bulletin No. 60. American College of Obstetricians and Gynecologists. Obstet Gynecol 2005;105:675–85.

ACOG PRACTICE BULLETIN

CLINICAL MANAGEMENT GUIDELINES FOR
OBSTETRICIAN–GYNECOLOGISTS

NUMBER 1, JUNE 1998

This Practice Bulletin was developed by the ACOG Committees on Practice Bulletins— Obstetrics and Gynecology with the assistance of Brian M. Mercer, MD. The information is designed to aid practitioners in making decisions about appropriate obstetric and gynecologic care. These guidelines should not be construed as dictating an exclusive course of treatment or procedure. Variations in practice may be warranted based on the needs of the individual patient, resources, and limitations unique to the institution or type of practice.

Premature Rupture of Membranes

Preterm delivery occurs in approximately 11% of all births in the United States and is a major factor contributing to perinatal morbidity and mortality. Despite extensive research in this area, the rate of preterm birth has increased by 17% over the past 15 years (1). Premature rupture of membranes (PROM) is a complication in one quarter to one third of preterm births. In both term and preterm births, numerous controversies exist regarding optimal methods of clinical assessment and treatment of PROM. Management hinges on evaluation of the relative risks of infection, cord accident, operative delivery, and of the gestational age in patients not in labor. The purpose of this document is to review the current understanding of this condition and to provide management guidelines that have been validated by appropriately conducted outcome-based research. Additional guidelines based on consensus and expert opinion also are presented to permit a review of most clinical aspects of PROM.

Background

The definition of PROM is rupture of membranes before the onset of labor. When membrane rupture occurs before 37 weeks of gestation, it is referred to as preterm PROM. Premature rupture of membranes can result from a wide array of pathologic mechanisms acting individually or in concert (2). The gestational age at membrane rupture has significant implications regarding the etiology and consequences of PROM. Management may be dictated by the presence of overt intrauterine infection, advanced labor, or fetal compromise. When such factors are not present, especially with preterm PROM, other interventions may have a significant impact on maternal and infant morbidity. An accurate assessment of gestational age and knowledge of the maternal, fetal, and neonatal risks are essential to appropriate evaluation, counseling, and management of patients with PROM.

Etiology

Membrane rupture may occur for a variety of reasons. At term, weakening of the membranes may result from physiologic changes combined with shearing forces created by uterine contractions (2, 3). Intrauterine infection has been shown to play an important role in preterm PROM, especially at earlier gestational ages (4). Factors associated with an increase in PROM include lower socioeconomic status, sexually transmissible infections, prior preterm delivery (especially due to PROM), vaginal bleeding, cervical conization, and cigarette smoking during pregnancy (2, 5–7). Uterine distention (hydramnios, twins), emergency cervical cerclage, prior antepartum antibiotic treatment, and preterm labor also may be associated with PROM (2, 6, 8). In many cases, however, PROM may occur in the absence of recognized risk factors.

Term Premature Rupture of Membranes

At term, PROM complicates approximately 8% of pregnancies and is generally followed by the onset of labor and delivery. In a large randomized trial, half of women with PROM who were managed expectantly delivered within 5 hours, and 95% delivered within 28 hours of membrane rupture (9). Other studies have reported similar rates (10).

The most significant maternal risk of term PROM is intrauterine infection, a risk that increases with the duration of membrane rupture (6, 9–12). Fetal risks associated with PROM include umbilical cord compression and ascending infection.

Preterm Premature Rupture of Membranes

Regardless of management or clinical presentation, birth within 1 week is the most likely outcome of any patient with PROM prior to term. A review of 13 randomized trials reported that approximately 75% of patients with preterm PROM who were managed expectantly delivered within 1 week (13). The earlier in gestation that PROM occurs, the greater the potential for pregnancy prolongation. With expectant management, 2.8–13% of women can anticipate cessation of fluid leakage (12, 14).

Of women with preterm PROM, clinically evident intraamniotic infection occurs in 13–60% and postpartum infection occurs in 2–13% (14–18). The incidence of infection increases with decreasing gestational age at membrane rupture (19, 20) and increases with digital vaginal examination (21). With appropriate management, however, serious maternal sequelae are uncommon (13, 16). Fetal malpresentation is increased with preterm PROM. Abruptio placentae affects 4–12% of pregnancies with preterm PROM (22, 23).

The most significant risks to the fetus after preterm PROM are complications of prematurity. At all gestational ages prior to term, respiratory distress has been reported to be the most common complication (15, 24). Other serious forms of morbidity, including necrotizing enterocolitis and intraventricular hemorrhage, also are associated with prematurity but are less common nearer to term. The presence of maternal infection poses the additional risk of neonatal infection. Infection, cord accident, and other factors contribute to the 1–2% risk of antenatal fetal demise after preterm PROM (13).

Midtrimester Premature Rupture of Membranes

Premature rupture of membranes occurring before and around the time of neonatal viability often is referred to as midtrimester PROM. Premature rupture of membranes at 16–26 weeks of gestation complicates almost 1% of pregnancies (7, 25). Before the 1970s, delivery in the second trimester was generally associated with neonatal death resulting from complications of prematurity. Primarily because of advances in neonatal intensive care over the past two decades, neonates are surviving at increasingly younger gestational ages. Currently, overall infant survival after delivery at 24–26 weeks of gestation is reported to be between 50% and 75% (24, 26, 27). Survival rates in pregnancies complicated by PROM are comparable (28–30) but decreased in the presence of infection or deformations.

A small number of patients with midtrimester PROM will have an extended latency period. In a review of 12 studies evaluating patients with midtrimester PROM, the mean latency period ranged from 10.6 to 21.5 days (25). Although delivery occurred within 1 week of membrane rupture in 57% of patients, in 22% of patients pregnancy continued for 1 month. Most studies of midtrimester PROM have been retrospective and include only those patients amenable to expectant management. Patients usually are excluded from analysis in the presence of labor, infection, prolapsed membranes, and fetal demise, thus potentially exaggerating the latency period to delivery and deceptively decreasing the apparent maternal and infant morbidity.

Reported maternal complications of midtrimester PROM include intraamniotic infection, endometritis, abruptio placentae, retained placentae, and postpartum hemorrhage. Maternal sepsis is a rare but serious complication reported to affect approximately 1% of cases (25, 29).

The incidence of stillbirth subsequent to PROM at 16–25 weeks of gestation ranges from 3.8% to 21.7% (7, 15, 31) compared with 0–2% with PROM at 30–36 weeks of gestation (32, 33). This increased rate of death may be explained by increased susceptibility of the umbilical cord to compression or of the fetus to hypoxia and intrauterine infection. Alternatively, this finding may reflect the lack of intervention for fetal compromise prior to neonatal viability. The fetal survival rate subsequent to PROM at less than 24 weeks of gestation has been reported to be about 30%, compared with a 57% survival rate with rupture at 24–26 weeks of gestation (25).

Several trials have described outcomes of survivors after PROM at 16–26 weeks of gestation (7, 29–31, 34, 35). Although up to 69% of these neonates were reported as having normal neurologic development, these results may be biased by a lack of follow-up. Generalized developmental delay, delayed motor development, and other less frequent complications, including cerebral palsy, chronic lung disease, blindness, hydrocephalus, and mental retardation, also were reported to occur.

A variety of conditions that are associated with fetal lung compression or oligohydramnios or both can result in pulmonary hypoplasia. Reported risks of pulmonary hypoplasia after PROM at 16–26 weeks of gestation vary from less than 1% to 27% (18, 29). Pulmonary hypoplasia rarely occurs with membrane rupture subsequent to 26 weeks of gestation, presumably because alveolar growth adequate to support postnatal development already has occurred (36, 37). Prolonged oligohydramnios also is associated with in utero deformation including abnormal facies (ie, low-set ears and epicanthal folds) and limb positioning abnormalities.

When leakage of amniotic fluid occurs after amniocentesis, the outcome is better than after spontaneous preterm PROM. In one study of 603 women who had second-trimester amniocentesis for prenatal diagnosis of genetic disorders, seven women (1.2%) experienced PROM, and leakage stopped in all with conservative management (8).

Clinical Considerations and Recommendations

▶ *How is premature rupture of membranes diagnosed?*

An accurate diagnosis is crucial to the management of suspected membrane rupture. Most cases can be diagnosed on the basis of the history and physical examination (38). Other causes of discharge include urinary leakage, excess vaginal discharge with advanced dilatation or membrane prolapse, cervicitis, bloody show, semen, and vaginal douches. Symptoms suggestive of PROM should be confirmed. Delay in evaluation may result in a missed opportunity for intervention.

Examination should be performed in a manner that minimizes the risk of introducing infection, particularly prior to term. Digital cervical examinations increase the risk of infection and add little information to that available with speculum examination (21, 39). Thus, digital examinations should be avoided unless prompt labor and delivery are anticipated. Sterile speculum examination can confirm the diagnosis of PROM as well as provide an opportunity to inspect for cervicitis or umbilical cord or fetal prolapse, assess cervical dilatation and effacement, and obtain cultures as appropriate (40).

The diagnosis of membrane rupture is confirmed by the visualization of amniotic fluid in the posterior vaginal fornix or clear fluid passing from the cervical canal. If the diagnosis remains in question, the pH of the vaginal sidewalls or fluid pool can be assessed.

The pH of the vaginal secretions is generally 4.5–6.0 whereas amniotic fluid usually has a pH of 7.1–7.3. Nitrazine paper will turn blue with a pH above 6.0–6.5. False-positive results may occur in the presence of blood or semen contamination, alkaline antiseptics, or bacterial vaginosis. Alternatively, false-negative results may occur with prolonged leakage and minimal residual fluid. More information can be obtained by swabbing the posterior fornix (avoiding cervical mucus) and allowing the vaginal fluid to dry on a microscope slide. The presence of arborization (ferning) under microscopic visualization further suggests membrane rupture.

When the clinical history or physical examination is unclear, ultrasound examination may be useful to document oligohydramnios, which in the absence of fetal urinary tract malformations or significant growth restriction is suggestive of membrane rupture. Membrane rupture can be diagnosed unequivocally with ultrasonographically guided transabdominal instillation of indigo carmine dye (1 mL in 9 mL sterile normal saline), followed by observation for passage of blue fluid from the vagina within 30 minutes of amniocentesis.

▶ *What is the optimal method of initial management for a patient with PROM at term?*

Fetal heart rate monitoring may be used to assess fetal status. Dating criteria should be reviewed to assign gestational age because virtually all aspects of subsequent care will hinge on that information. Group B streptococcal status and the need for intrapartum prophylaxis should be determined (41).

▶ *When should labor be induced in patients with term PROM?*

Fetal presentation, gestational age, and status should be established before determining whether labor should be induced. The decision to induce labor involves an assessment of the relative risks of infection or fetal compromise (which may increase with the duration of PROM) versus the risks of failed induction and operative vaginal delivery (which may increase with induced as opposed to spontaneous labor).

If the condition of the cervix is unfavorable, there is little difference in outcome when comparing induction to expectant management. Options evaluated ranged from immediate induction to observation for up to 24–72 hours prior to induction (9, 42–45). While time from admission to delivery is shortened with induction, time in labor is longer, and the need for operative vaginal delivery seems to be higher (44, 46).

Risk of cesarean delivery and risk of neonatal infectious complications do not appear to depend on the mode of management (expectant versus induction), although the risks of maternal infection may increase with expectant management (9, 43, 45). Thus, it is reasonable for consideration of the patient's wishes and hospitalization costs to influence management.

▶ What does the initial evaluation involve once PROM has been confirmed?

Fetal presentation, gestational age, and status should be determined. The gravida with evident intrauterine infection, abruptio placentae, or evidence of fetal compromise is best cared for by expeditious delivery. In the absence of an indication for immediate delivery, swabs for diagnosis of *Chlamydia trachomatis* and *Neisseria gonorrhoeae* may be obtained from the cervix if appropriate. The need for group B streptococcal intrapartum prophylaxis should be determined (41).

▶ When should one elect delivery for the fetus near term in the presence of premature rupture of membranes?

After initial assessment, relative maternal and fetal risks with expectant management, neonatal risks with early delivery, and the potential neonatal benefit from expectant management can then be determined. Because serious neonatal morbidity is uncommon with demonstrated pulmonary maturity and delivery after 32–36 weeks of gestation (33), amniotic fluid may be collected from the vaginal pool or by amniocentesis for assessment of fetal pulmonary maturity.

If pulmonary maturity has been documented after PROM at 32–36 weeks of gestation, labor induction may be considered. Available clinical trial data concerning expectant management versus immediate induction at 30–34 weeks of gestation (32) and at 32–36 weeks of gestation

(33) show increased risks of chorioamnionitis and prolonged hospitalization with expectant management but equal risks of respiratory distress syndrome, intraventricular hemorrhage, necrotizing enterocolitis, and neonatal death. It is noteworthy that in the studies cited (32, 33), which were conducted in major centers with neonatal intensive care units, antibiotics (32, 33) or antenatal corticosteroids (32) were not utilized. Although it is uncertain whether the use of prophylactic antibiotics and antenatal corticosteroids will improve the outcome of expectant management at these gestational ages, it is clear that delivery of a preterm infant should take place in a facility with experience in the management of such infants.

The gravida who experiences PROM before 30–32 weeks of gestation and whose condition is stable is generally best served by expectant management. The prophylactic use of antibiotics and antenatal corticosteroids can help reduce the risks of gestational age-dependent neonatal morbidity.

▶ What general approaches are utilized in patients with preterm PROM managed expectantly?

Expectant management of preterm PROM generally consists of modified bed rest to potentially enhance amniotic fluid reaccumulation and complete pelvic rest to avoid infection. Patients should be assessed periodically for evidence of infection or labor. In a patient with preterm PROM, a temperature exceeding 38.0°C (100.4°F) may be indicative of infection, although some investigators have suggested that fever, with additional factors such as uterine tenderness and maternal or fetal tachycardia, is a more accurate indicator of maternal infection (15, 47). Leukocyte counts are nonspecific in the absence of clinical evidence of infection, especially if antenatal corticosteroids have been administered.

If the presence of intraamniotic infection is suspected and additional diagnostic confirmation is required, amniocentesis may be considered (48). The diagnosis of intraamniotic infection may be suggested by an amniotic fluid glucose concentration of less than 20 mg/dL, by a positive Gram stain, or a positive amniotic fluid culture (49–51). The presence of amniotic fluid leukocytes alone is not diagnostic of infection. In a case-control study comparing amniotic fluid tests used to predict infection, investigators concluded interleukin-6 was the only test that had significant clinical value in predicting neonatal complications (51). Other investigators have rejected amniocentesis because of a low success rate and the need for repeat procedures (52).

▶ *Should tocolytics be considered in patients with preterm PROM in labor?*

Prophylactic tocolysis after preterm PROM has been shown to prolong latency in the short term (53–55), while therapeutic tocolysis (ie, instituting tocolysis only after contractions have ensued) has not been shown to prolong latency (56). No study to date has demonstrated that tocolytics benefit neonatal outcome, but none has utilized antibiotics or antenatal corticosteroids. As detailed below, use of both antibiotics and antenatal corticosteroids improves outcome in patients with preterm PROM who are not having contractions. The effect of tocolysis to permit antibiotic and antenatal corticosteroid administration in the patient with preterm PROM who is having contractions has yet to be investigated.

▶ *Should antenatal corticosteroids be administered to patients with preterm PROM?*

Two meta-analyses have evaluated the impact of corticosteroid use after preterm PROM on respiratory distress syndrome. These studies produced somewhat conflicting results. While both found significant reduction in respiratory distress syndrome with antenatal corticosteroid administration, one found the opposite result after deleting the study with the lowest quality score after having accepted it based on predetermined criteria (57). The other meta-analysis demonstrated a significant benefit with corticosteroids (58), including reduced rates of neonatal periventricular hemorrhage, necrotizing enterocolitis, and death.

A more recent trial of corticosteroid use after preterm PROM demonstrated a significant reduction in respiratory distress syndrome with corticosteroid administration (18% versus 44%) (59). All patients in this study also received prophylactic antibiotics. Further, multivariate analysis of prospective observational trials also has suggested a benefit of antenatal corticosteroid use regardless of membrane rupture (60).

The National Institutes of Health Consensus Development Panel recommends corticosteroid use for women with PROM prior to 30–32 weeks of gestation in the absence of intraamniotic infection (61). The available data indicate that the benefit of antenatal corticosteroids may outweigh the risk in these patients between 24 and 32 weeks of gestation. Should the pregnancy extend beyond the week that antenatal corticosteroids have known benefit, it is unclear if repeat therapy is efficacious.

Because of the possible adverse fetal effects and possible effects on maternal immune status of repeated weekly courses of antenatal corticosteroids, it would seem reasonable to adopt a rescue approach to therapy in the treatment of perterm labor rather than a routine readministration regimen. Following the initial course of antenatal corticosteroids, repeated doses should only be given on an as-needed basis (ie, if the woman is retreated for threatened preterm birth).

▶ *Should antibiotics be administered to patients with preterm PROM in an effort to prolong the latency period?*

A large number of randomized prospective clinical trials assessing the utility of adjunctive antibiotic therapy during expectant management of preterm PROM have been published over the past 10 years and are summarized in two meta-analyses. One meta-analysis demonstrated significant prolongation of pregnancy and reduced chorioamnionitis, postpartum endometritis, neonatal sepsis, pneumonia, and intraventricular hemorrhage with antibiotic treatment compared with expectant management alone (13). The other meta-analysis indicated significant reduction in neonatal sepsis and intraventricular hemorrhage (62). An additional large, multicenter trial utilizing antibiotics but no antenatal corticosteroids or tocolytics demonstrated a significant reduction in perinatal morbidity, including respiratory distress syndrome and necrotizing enterocolitis (47). In that same study, patients negative for group B streptococci also experienced longer pregnancies and less neonatal sepsis and pneumonia. A recent prospective, double-blinded trial that did utilize antenatal corticosteroids for all patients found similar perinatal benefits associated with the use of antibiotics (63).

A number of regimens appear to be effective in prolonging the latency period. Investigators in the National Institute of Child Health and Human Development trial (47) demonstrated significant perinatal benefit with a combination of ampicillin and erythromycin administered intravenously for the first 48 hours, followed by oral amoxicillin and erythromycin for an additional 5 days if delivery did not occur. The other clinical trial utilized intravenous ampicillin followed by oral amoxicillin or intravenous ampicillin/sulbactam followed by oral amoxicillin/clavulanate (63). The available clinical data provide no basis for selecting one of the prophylactic regimens over the other. The administration of antibiotics to prolong the latency period must be distinguished from well-established protocols directed at prevention of group B streptococcal infection in term and preterm patients (41). Either of the prophylactic antibiotic regimens utilized by the aforementioned clinical trials would appropriately treat group B streptococcal infections. Once labor begins, however, the need for group B streptococcal prophylaxis needs to be determined.

▶ *Can women with preterm PROM be managed at home?*

Generally, hospitalization for bed rest and pelvic rest is indicated after preterm PROM. Recognizing that latency is frequently brief, that intrauterine and fetal infection may occur suddenly, and that the fetus is at risk for umbilical cord compression, ongoing surveillance of both mother and fetus is necessary.

One clinical trial of discharge after preterm PROM suggested that gravidas can be discharged before delivery to reduce health care costs (64). Those with preterm PROM and no evidence of intrauterine infection, labor, or fetal compromise were evaluated in hospital for 72 hours. Those with negative cervical cultures and no evident labor, intrauterine infection, or fetal compromise were then randomly assigned to either continued inpatient management or discharge. Only 67 of 349 women (18%) were eligible for discharge after 72 hours. There were no identifiable differences in latency, or in the incidences of intraamniotic infection, variable decelerations, or cesarean delivery. Infant outcomes also were similar.

While the potential for a reduction in health care costs with antepartum discharge is enticing, it is important to ensure that such management will not be associated with increased risks and costs related to perinatal morbidity and mortality. Any cost savings from antenatal discharge may be rapidly lost with a small increase in neonatal intensive care unit stay. Further study regarding the risks and benefits of home care after preterm PROM is warranted.

▶ *What is the optimal form of antepartum fetal surveillance for patients with preterm PROM managed expectantly?*

Fetal testing offers the opportunity to identify occult umbilical cord compression. One study demonstrated a 32% incidence of variable decelerations after preterm PROM (38). In addition, nonreactive nonstress tests have been associated with perinatal infection. With daily fetal evaluation, one study demonstrated the last test before delivery to be nonreactive in 78% of patients who subsequently developed infection (versus 14% for those with a reactive test) (65). Biophysical profile test scores of 6 or less within 24 hours of delivery also have been demonstrated to correlate with positive amniotic fluid cultures and perinatal infection. At least eight studies have confirmed this association (66). Most of these studies have included daily fetal assessment after preterm PROM. An abnormal test should lead to reassessment of the clinical circumstances and may lead to a decision to proceed to delivery.

However, no evidence exists that any specific form or frequency of fetal surveillance directly improves perinatal outcome.

▶ *What is the optimal management for a patient with preterm PROM and a cervical cerclage?*

A retrospective comparative study demonstrated prolongation of pregnancy but increased maternal and perinatal morbidity and perinatal mortality when the cerclage was left in place following PROM (67). Two additional studies found no significant increase in maternal or perinatal morbidity in patients with cerclage removal when compared with patients with PROM and no cerclage (68, 69).

There are limited data to suggest removal of cerclage after PROM, but management with antibiotics or antenatal corticosteroids has not been addressed. The optimal management of preterm PROM in the presence of a cerclage is yet to be determined.

▶ *How does management differ in patients with second-trimester PROM?*

Initial management of gravidas with midtrimester PROM should reflect the potential for neonatal survival. Those presenting at 24–26 weeks of gestation may be considered viable (24, 70) and treated with expectant management. Given the lack of clinical trial data regarding optimal management of these patients, the recommendations reflect general clinical practice.

Women presenting with PROM before presumed viability should be counseled regarding the impact of immediate delivery and the potential risks and benefits of expectant management. Counseling should include a realistic appraisal of neonatal outcomes, including the availability of obstetric monitoring and neonatal intensive care facilities. Because of advances in perinatal care, morbidity and mortality rates continue to improve rapidly (24). An attempt should be made to provide parents with the most up-to-date information possible.

Although no evidence or consensus exists regarding the benefit of an initial period of inpatient observation in these patients, evaluation for the confirmation of PROM, evidence of infection, and the presence of associated fetal anomalies is essential if expectant management is to be considered. In addition to clinical follow-up, it may be useful to instruct patients to abstain from intercourse, limit their activities, and monitor their temperatures. Hospitalization for the duration of amniotic fluid leakage also may be appropriate.

Summary

Reports of patient care and outcome use ranges of gestational age. These ranges may be arbitrary. The recommendations that follow are based on available published data supplemented by consensus and expert opinion, with the recognition that the recommendations may not apply uniformly to patients at the extremes of gestational age.

The following recommendations are based on good and consistent scientific evidence (Level A):

▶ With term PROM, labor may be induced at the time of presentation or patients may be observed for up to 24–72 hours for the onset of spontaneous labor.

▶ Antibiotics prolong the latency period and improve perinatal outcome in patients with preterm PROM and should be administered according to one of several published protocols if expectant management is to be pursued prior to 35 weeks of gestation.

▶ Antenatal corticosteroids should be administered to gravidas with PROM before 32 weeks of gestation to reduce the risks of respiratory distress syndrome, neonatal intraventricular hemorrhage, necrotizing enterocolitis, and neonatal death.

▶ Digital cervical examinations should not be performed in patients with PROM who are not in labor and in whom immediate induction of labor is not planned.

▶ Patients with PROM prior to 30–32 weeks of gestation should be managed conservatively if no maternal or fetal contraindications exist.

The following recommendations are based primarily on consensus and expert opinion (Level C):

▶ Tocolysis may be utilized in patients with preterm PROM to permit administration of antenatal corticosteroids and antibiotics.

▶ Antenatal corticosteroids may be administered to gravidas with PROM up to 34 weeks of gestation.

References

1. Ventura SJ, Martin JA, Curtin SC, Mathews TJ. Report of final natality statistics, 1995. Monthly vital statistics report; vol 45, no. 11, supp. Hyattsville, Maryland: National Center for Health Statistics, 1997 (Level III)

2. French JI, McGregor JA. The pathobiology of premature rupture of membranes. Semin Perinatol 1996;20:344–368 (Level III)

3. Lavery JP, Miller CE, Knight RD. The effect of labor on the rheologic response of chorioamniotic membranes. Obstet Gynecol 1982;60:87–92 (Level II-3)

4. McGregor JA, French JI. Evidence-based prevention of preterm birth and rupture of membranes: infection and inflammation. J SOGC 1997;19:835–852 (Level III)

5. Harger JH, Hsing AW, Tuomala RE, Gibbs RS, Mead PB, Eschenbach DA, et al. Risk factors for preterm premature rupture of fetal membranes: a multicenter case-control study. Am J Obstet Gynecol 1990;163:130–137 (Level II-2)

6. Novak-Antolic Z, Pajntar M, Verdenik I. Rupture of the membranes and postpartum infection. Eur J Obstet Gynecol Reprod Biol 1997;71:141–146 (Level II-3)

7. Taylor J, Garite TJ. Premature rupture of the membranes before fetal viability. Obstet Gynecol 1984;64:615–620 (Level II-3)

8. Gold RB, Goyert GL, Schwartz DB, Evans MI, Seabolt LA. Conservative management of second trimester postamniocentesis fluid leakage. Obstet Gynecol 1989;74:745–747 (Level III)

9. Hannah ME, Ohlsson A, Farine D, Hewson SA, Hodnett ED, Myhr TL, et al. Induction of labor compared with expectant management for prelabor rupture of the membranes at term. N Engl J Med 1996;334:1005–1010 (Level I)

10. Wagner MV, Chin VP, Peters CJ, Drexler B, Newman LA. A comparison of early and delayed induction of labor with spontaneous rupture of membranes at term. Obstet Gynecol 1989;74:93–97 (Level II-1)

11. Guise JM, Duff P, Christian JS. Management of term patients with premature rupture of membranes and an unfavorable cervix. Am J Perinatol 1992;9:56–60 (Level II-2)

12. Johnson JWC, Egerman RS, Moorhead J. Cases with ruptured membranes that "reseal." Am J Obstet Gynecol 1990;163:1024–1032 (Level II-2)

13. Mercer BM, Arheart KL. Antimicrobial therapy in expectant management of preterm premature rupture of the membranes. Lancet 1995;346:1271–1279 (Meta-analysis)

14. Mercer BM. Management of premature rupture of membranes before 26 weeks' gestation. Obstet Gynecol Clin North Am 1992;19:339–351 (Level III)

15. Beydoun SN, Yasin SY. Premature rupture of the membranes before 28 weeks: conservative management. Am J Obstet Gynecol 1986;155:471–479 (Level II-3)

16. Garite TJ, Freeman RK. Chorioamnionitis in the preterm gestation. Obstet Gynecol 1982;59:539–545 (Level II-3)

17. Simpson GF, Harbert GM Jr. Use of β-methasone in management of preterm gestation with premature rupture of membranes. Obstet Gynecol 1985;66:168–175 (Level II-2)

18. Vergani P, Ghidini A, Locatelli A, Cavallone M, Ciarla I, Cappellini A, et al. Risk factors for pulmonary hypoplasia in second-trimester premature rupture of membranes. Am J Obstet Gynecol 1994;170:1359–1364 (Level II-3)

19. Hillier SL, Martius J, Krohn M, Kiviat N, Holmes KK, Eschenbach DA. A case-control study of chorioamnionic infection and histologic chorioamnionitis in prematurity. N Engl J Med 1988;319:972–978 (Level II-3)

20. Morales WJ. The effect of chorioamnionitis on the developmental outcome of preterm infants at one year. Obstet Gynecol 1987;70:183–186 (Level II-3)

21. Schutte MF, Treffers PE, Kloosterman GJ, Soepatmi S. Management of premature rupture of membranes: the risk of vaginal examination to the infant. Am J Obstet Gynecol 1983;146:395–400 (Level II-3)

22. Ananth CV, Savitz DA, Williams MA. Placental abruption and its association with hypertension and prolonged rupture of membranes: a methodologic review and meta-analysis. Obstet Gynecol 1996;88:309–318 (Meta-analysis)

23. Gonen R, Hannah ME, Milligan JE. Does prolonged preterm premature rupture of the membranes predispose to abruptio placentae? Obstet Gynecol 1989;74:347–350 (Level II-2)

24. Fanaroff AA, Wright LL, Stevenson DK, Shankaran S, Donovan EF, Ehrenkranz RA, et al. Very-low-birth-weight outcomes of the National Institute of Child Health and Human Development Neonatal Research Network, May 1991 through December 1992. Am J Obstet Gynecol 1995; 173:1423–1431 (Level II-3)

25. Schucker JL, Mercer BM. Midtrimester premature rupture of the membranes. Semin Perinatol 1996;20:389–400 (Level III)

26. Hack M, Taylor HG, Klein N, Eiben R, Schatschneider C, Mercuri-Minich N. School-age outcomes in children with birth weights under 750 g. N Engl J Med 1994;331:753–759 (Level II-2)

27. Kilpatrick SJ, Schlueter MA, Piecuch R, Leonard CH, Rogido M, Sola A. Outcome of infants born at 24–26 weeks' gestation: I. Survival and cost. Obstet Gynecol 1997;90:803–808 (Level II-3)

28. Bottoms SF, Paul RH, Iams JD, Mercer BM, Thom EA, Roberts JM, et al. Obstetric determinants of neonatal survival: influence of willingness to perform cesarean delivery on survival of extremely low-birth-weight infants. Am J Obstet Gynecol 1997;176:960–966 (Level II-3)

29. Moretti M, Sibai BM. Maternal and perinatal outcome of expectant management of premature rupture of the membranes in midtrimester. Am J Obstet Gynecol 1988;159: 390–396 (Level II-3)

30. Rib DM, Sherer DM, Woods JR Jr. Maternal and neonatal outcome associated with prolonged premature rupture of membranes below 26 weeks' gestation. Am J Perinatol 1993;10:369–373 (Level II-3)

31. Bengtson JM, VanMarter LJ, Barss VA, Greene MF, Tuomala RE, Epstein MF. Pregnancy outcome after premature rupture of the membranes at or before 26 weeks' gestation. Obstet Gynecol 1989;73:921–926 (Level II-3)

32. Cox SM, Leveno KJ. Intentional delivery versus expectant management with preterm ruptured membranes at 30–34 weeks' gestation. Obstet Gynecol 1995;86:875–879 (Level I)

33. Mercer BM, Crocker LG, Boe NM, Sibai BM. Induction versus expectant management in premature rupture of the membranes with mature amniotic fluid at 32 to 36 weeks: a randomized trial. Am J Obstet Gynecol 1993;169:775–782 (Level I)

34. Major CA, Kitzmiller JL. Perinatal survival with expectant management of midtrimester rupture of membranes. Am J Obstet Gynecol 1990;163:838–844 (Level II-3)

35. Morales WJ, Talley T. Premature rupture of membranes at <25 weeks: a management dilemma. Am J Obstet Gynecol 1993;168:503–507 (Level II-3)

36. Rotschild A, Ling EW, Puterman ML, Farquharson D. Neonatal outcome after prolonged preterm rupture of the membranes. Am J Obstet Gynecol 1990;162:46–52 (Level II-3)

37. van Eyck J, van der Mooren K, Wladimiroff JW. Ductus arteriosus flow velocity modulation by fetal breathing movements as a measure of fetal lung development. Am J Obstet Gynecol 1990;163:558–566 (Level II-3)

38. Smith CV, Greenspoon J, Phelan JP, Platt LD. Clinical utility of the nonstress test in the conservative management of women with preterm spontaneous premature rupture of the membranes. J Reprod Med 1987;32:1–4 (Level II-3)

39. Lenihan JP Jr. Relationship of antepartum pelvic examinations to premature rupture of the membranes. Obstet Gynecol 1984;83:33–37 (Level II-1)

40. Munson LA, Graham A, Koos BJ, Valenzuela GJ. Is there a need for digital examination in patients with spontaneous rupture of the membranes? Am J Obstet Gynecol 1985; 153:562–563 (Level II-3)

41. American College of Obstetricians and Gynecologists. Prevention of early-onset group B streptococcal disease in newborns. ACOG Committee Opinion 173. Washington, DC: ACOG, 1996 (Level III)

42. Ingemarsson I. Controversies: premature rupture of membranes at term—no advantage of delaying induction >24 hours. J Perinat Med 1996;24:573–579 (Level III)

43. Mozurkewich EL, Wolf FM. Premature rupture of membranes at term: a meta-analysis of three management schemes. Obstet Gynecol 1997;89:1035–1043 (Meta-analysis)

44. Ottervanger HP, Keirse MJ, Smit W, Holm JP. Controlled comparison of induction versus expectant care for prelabor rupture of the membranes at term. J Perinatol Med 1996;24: 237–242 (Level I-1)

45. Sanchez-Ramos L, Chen AH, Kaunitz AM, Gaudier FL, Delke I. Labor induction with intravaginal misoprostol in term premature rupture of membranes: a randomized study. Obstet Gynecol 1997;89:909–912 (Level I)

46. Alcalay M, Hourvitz A, Reichman B, Luski A, Quint J, Barkai G, et al. Prelabour rupture of membranes at term: early induction of labour versus expectant management. Eur J Obstet Gynecol Reprod Biol 1996;70:129–133 (Level I)

47. Mercer BM, Miodovnik M, Thurnau GR, Goldenberg RL, Das AF, Ramsey RD, et al. Antibiotic therapy for reduction of infant morbidity after preterm premature rupture of the membranes: a randomized controlled trial. JAMA 1997;278: 989–995 (Level I)

48. Gomez R, Romero R, Edwin SS, David C. Pathogenesis of preterm labor and preterm premature rupture of membranes associated with intraamniotic infection. Infect Dis Clin North Am 1997;11:135–176 (Level III)

49. Belady PH, Farkouh LJ, Gibbs RS. Intra-amniotic infection and premature rupture of the membranes. Clin Perinatol 1997;24:43–57 (Level III)

50. Broekhuizen FF, Gilman M, Hamilton PR. Amniocentesis for gram stain and culture in preterm premature rupture of the membranes. Obstet Gynecol 1985;66:316–321 (Level II-3)

51. Romero R, Yoon BH, Mazor M, Gomez R, Gonzalez R, Diamond MP, et al. A comparative study of the diagnostic performance of amniotic fluid glucose, white blood cell count, interleukin-6, and Gram stain in the detection of microbial invasion in patients with preterm premature rupture of membranes. Am J Obstet Gynecol 1993;169:839–851 (Level II-2)

52. Ohlsson A, Wang E. An analysis of antenatal tests to detect infection in preterm premature rupture of the membranes. Am J Obstet Gynecol 1990;162:809–818 (Level III)

53. Christensen KK, Ingemarsson I, Leideman T, Solum H, Svenningsen N. Effect of ritodrine on labor after premature rupture of the membranes. Obstet Gynecol 1980;55:187–190 (Level I)

54. Levy DL, Warsof SL. Oral ritodrine and preterm premature rupture of membranes. Obstet Gynecol 1985;66:621–623 (Level II-1)

55. Weiner CP, Renk K, Klugman M. The therapeutic efficacy and cost-effectiveness of aggressive tocolysis for premature labor associated with premature rupture of the membranes. Am J Obstet Gynecol 1988;159:216–222 (Level I)

56. Garite TJ, Keegan KA, Freeman RK, Nageotte MP. A randomized trial of ritodrine tocolysis versus expectant management in patients with premature rupture of membranes at 25 to 30 weeks of gestation. Am J Obstet Gynecol 1987;157:388–393 (Level II-1)

57. Ohlsson A. Treatments of preterm premature rupture of the membranes: a meta-analysis. Am J Obstet Gynecol 1989;160:890–906 (Meta-analysis)

58. Crowley PA. Antenatal corticosteroid therapy: a meta-analysis of the randomized trials, 1972 to 1994. Am J Obstet Gynecol 1995;173:322–335 (Meta-analysis)

59. Lewis DF, Brody K, Edwards MS, Brouillette RM, Burlison S, London SN. Preterm premature ruptured membranes: a randomized trial of steroids after treatment with antibiotics. Obstet Gynecol 1996;88:801–805 (Level I)

60. Wright LL, Verter J, Younes N, Stevenson D, Fanaroff AA, Shankaran S, et al. Antenatal corticosteroid administration and neonatal outcome in very low birth weight infants: the NICHD Neonatal Research Network. Am J Obstet Gynecol 1995;173:269–274 (Level II-3)

61. National Institutes of Health. National Institutes of Health Consensus Development Conference Statement: Effect of corticosteroids for fetal maturation on perinatal outcomes, February 28–March 2, 1994. Am J Obstet Gynecol 1995;173:246–252 (Level III)

62. Egarter C, Leitich H, Karas H, Wieser F, Husslein P, Kaider A, et al. Antibiotic treatment in preterm premature rupture of membranes and neonatal morbidity: a meta-analysis. Am J Obstet Gynecol 1996;174:589–597 (Meta-analysis)

63. Lovett SM, Weiss JD, Diogo MJ, Williams PT, Garite TJ. A prospective double-blind, randomized, controlled clinical trial of ampicillin-sulbactam for preterm premature rupture of membranes in women receiving antenatal corticosteroid therapy. Am J Obstet Gynecol 1997;176:1030–1038 (Level I)

64. Carlan SJ, O'Brien WF, Parsons MT, Lense JJ. Preterm premature rupture of membranes: a randomized study of home versus hospital management. Obstet Gynecol 1993;81:61–64 (Level I)

65. Vintzileos AM, Campbell WA, Nochimson DJ, Weinbaum PJ. The use of the nonstress test in patients with premature rupture of the membranes. Am J Obstet Gynecol 1986;155:149–153 (Level II-3)

66. Hanley ML, Vintzileos AM. Biophysical testing in premature rupture of the membranes. Semin Perinatol 1996;20:418–425 (Level III)

67. Ludmir J, Bader T, Chen L, Lindenbaum C, Wong G. Poor perinatal outcome associated with retained cerclage in patients with premature rupture of membranes. Obstet Gynecol 1994;84:823–826 (Level II-2)

68. Yeast JD, Garite TR. The role of cervical cerclage in the management of preterm premature rupture of the membranes. Am J Obstet Gynecol 1988;158:106–110 (Level II-2)

69. Blickstein I, Katz Z, Lancet M, Molgilner BM. The outcome of pregnancies complicated by preterm rupture of the membranes with and without cerclage. Int J Gynecol Obstet 1989;28:237–242 (Level II-2)

70. American College of Obstetricians and Gynecologists. Perinatal care at the threshold of viability. ACOG Committee Opinion 163. Washington, DC: ACOG, 1995 (Level III)

The MEDLINE database, the Cochrane Library, and ACOG's own internal resources and documents were used to conduct a literature search to locate relevant articles published between 1980 and August 1997. The search was restricted to articles published in the English language. Priority was given to articles reporting results of original research although review articles and commentaries also were consulted. Abstracts of research presented at symposiums and scientific conferences were not considered adequate for inclusion in this document. Guidelines published by organizations or institutions such as the National Institutes of Health and ACOG were reviewed, and additional studies were located by reviewing bibliographies of identified articles. When reliable research was not available, expert opinions from obstetrician–gynecologists were used. Studies were reviewed and evaluated for quality according to the method outlined by the U.S. Preventive Services Task Force.

I   Evidence obtained from at least one properly designed randomized controlled trial.

II-1   Evidence obtained from well-designed controlled trials without randomization.

II-2   Evidence obtained from well-designed cohort or case-control analytic studies, preferably from more than one center or research group.

II-3   Evidence obtained from multiple time series with or without the intervention. Dramatic results in uncontrolled experiments also could be regarded as this type of evidence.

III   Opinions of respected authorities, based on clinical experience, descriptive studies, or reports of expert committees.

Based on the highest level of evidence found in the data, the recommendations are graded according to the following categories:

A   The recommendation is based on good and consistent scientific evidence

B   The recommendation is based on limited or inconsistent scientific evidence

C   The recommendation is based primarily on consensus and expert opinion

ISSN 1099-3630   12345/21098

ACOG PRACTICE BULLETIN

CLINICAL MANAGEMENT GUIDELINES FOR
OBSTETRICIAN–GYNECOLOGISTS

NUMBER 15, APRIL 2000

This Practice Bulletin was developed by the ACOG Committee on Practice Bulletins—Gynecology with the assistance of Ann J. Davis, MD and Susan R. Johnson, MD, MS. The information is designed to aid practitioners in making decisions about appropriate obstetric and gynecologic care. These guidelines should not be construed as dictating an exclusive course of treatment or procedure. Variations in practice may be warranted based on the needs of the individual patient, resources, and limitations unique to the institution or type of practice.

Premenstrual Syndrome

Premenstrual syndrome (PMS) is a common problem for many women. Determining the appropriate clinical management of this condition often creates frustration for both physicians and patients. Until recently, the difficulty in managing PMS was largely attributed to imprecise diagnostic criteria, poorly designed clinical trials, and the promotion of treatment options for which there was no scientific support. In the mid-1980s, however, rigorous criteria for the diagnosis of PMS were defined. Since then, most studies of pathophysiology and treatment have met recognized standards of scientific design. This document will examine the evidence for commonly used approaches in the treatment of PMS and identify those that are effective.

Background

Premenstrual syndrome has been defined as "the cyclic occurrence of symptoms that are of sufficient severity to interfere with some aspects of life and that appear with consistent and predictable relationship to the menses" (1). Although the symptoms themselves are not unique, the restriction of the symptoms to the luteal phase of the menstrual cycle is pathognomonic of PMS (2).

Epidemiology

Premenstrual symptoms are common and are considered a normal aspect of ovulatory cycles. Most surveys have found that as many as 85% of menstruating women report one or more premenstrual symptoms. Severe symptoms that meet the criteria for PMS, however, are much less common, with only 5–10% of women reporting significant impairment in their lifestyles because of PMS (3, 4).

Risk Factors

Advancing age often is cited as a risk factor for PMS, based on surveys that find women are most likely to seek treatment after age 30 years. However, this syndrome can occur in menstruating women of any age. Genetics appears to play a role in PMS; the concordance rate of PMS is twice as high among monozygotic twins as among dizygotic twins (5, 6). Although women with PMS have a high rate of affective disorders, a causal relationship has not yet been demonstrated (7, 8).

There are no significant personality profile differences between women with PMS and asymptomatic women (9). Furthermore, PMS is not more likely to be diagnosed in women with higher levels of stress (10). However, women who have PMS may not tolerate stress as well as women who do not have PMS. Premenstrual symptoms seem to affect women irrespective of culture or socioeconomic status, although specific symptoms may vary in frequency by culture (11–13).

Etiology

The etiology of PMS is incompletely understood, but considerable progress has been made in the past decade in understanding some facets of the pathophysiology. Circulating sex steroid levels (progesterone, estrogen, and testosterone) are normal, although there may be an underlying neurobiologic vulnerability to normal fluctuations of one or more of these hormones (14, 15). Most likely, the biochemical changes involve central-nervous-system–mediated neurotransmitter interactions with sex steroids. Serotoninergic dysregulation is currently the most plausible theory. Among the several studies supporting this theory is a well-designed study in which women with severe PMS responded better to selective serotonin reuptake inhibitors (SSRIs) than to noradrenergic antidepressants such as maprotiline (16). Because not all women with PMS respond to SSRIs, other etiologic factors probably are involved.

Clinical Considerations and Recommendations

Establishing evidenced-based recommendations for PMS is difficult for many reasons. Definitions and inclusion criteria for PMS vary significantly among studies. In addition, the PMS patient populations studied in rigorous trials also may be different from the patient population of a given practitioner. For example, many recent PMS trials have properly included only women with the full-blown syndrome, including mood-related symptoms, whereas many women seek care from their practitioners for a less severe condition, with primarily somatic symptoms.

▶ *How is the diagnosis of PMS established?*

The key elements of the diagnosis are a) symptoms consistent with PMS; b) restriction of these symptoms to the luteal phase of the menstrual cycle assessed prospectively; c) impairment of some facet of the woman's life; and d) exclusion of other diagnoses that may better explain the symptoms.

The National Institute of Mental Health criteria for diagnosis are 1) a marked change of about 30% in the intensity of symptoms measured instrumentally, from cycle days 5 to 10 (as compared with those premenstrually), within the 6-day interval prior to menses and 2) documentation of these changes for at least two consecutive cycles (17). Another definition of PMS developed for research purposes by the University of California at San Diego is based on women's prospective self-reports. Their definition requires that patients have the cyclic manifestation of at least 1 of 6 behavioral symptoms and 1 of 4 somatic symptoms (see the box). Dysfunction in social or economic performance is included in this definition. Finally, the *Diagnostic and Statistical Manual of Mental Disorders*, fourth edition, includes similar criteria for the diagnosis of premenstrual dysphoric disorder, which identifies women with PMS who have more severe emotional symptoms (18).

The diagnosis of PMS should be based on prospective symptom diaries, because as many as half of the

---

Diagnostic Criteria for Premenstrual Syndrome

Premenstrual syndrome can be diagnosed if the patient reports at least one of the following affective and somatic symptoms during the 5 days before menses in each of the three prior menstrual cycles*:

Affective

    Depression

    Angry outbursts

    Irritability

    Anxiety

    Confusion

    Social withdrawal

Somatic

    Breast tenderness

    Abdominal bloating

    Headache

    Swelling of extremities

*These symptoms are relieved within 4 days of the onset of menses, without recurrence until at least cycle day 13. The symptoms are present in the absence of any pharmacologic therapy, hormone ingestion, or drug or alcohol use. The symptoms occur reproducibly during two cycles of prospective recording. The patient suffers from identifiable dysfunction in social or economic performance.

Adapted from Mortola JF, Girton L, Yen SC. Depressive episodes in premenstrual syndrome. Am J Obstet Gynecol 1989;161:1682–1687 women reporting a luteal phase pattern will be found to have some other pattern when such diaries are examined. Because some women experience cycle-to-cycle variability in symptoms, reviewing 2–3 months of prospective charting is preferable to reviewing a single cycle (19).

In the clinical setting, a simple system in which the woman records the dates of her menstrual periods and notes her symptoms on a daily basis is usually sufficient (20). However, a variety of standardized instruments and diaries developed for research purposes are also available. The most commonly used are the Calendar of Premenstrual Experiences (COPE) (21) and the Prospective Record of the Impact and Severity of Menstruation (PRISM) (22). Another type of instrument, the Visual Analogue Scales (VAS), may be especially appropriate in non-English-reading populations (23).

A careful medical and psychologic history and physical examination in conjunction with the prospective symptom diary usually will direct the clinician toward the correct diagnosis. Laboratory testing should be restricted to the identification of other disorders suggested by the evaluation, such as measuring levels of thyroid-stimulating hormone when hypothyroidism is suspected. Routine measurement of steroid hormones or gonadotropins is not useful.

▶ *How is PMS objectively differentiated from similar conditions?*

Only a small portion of women presenting for evaluation and treatment of PMS are likely to have PMS. For example, in a sample of women who responded to a newspaper recruitment for a PMS study, the most common symptoms reported were consistent with PMS: irritability, depression, mood swings, anxiety, mastalgia, abdominal bloating, weight gain, fatigue, aggression, headache, tension, muscle aches, food cravings, and breast swelling (24). However, individuals who respond to such recruitment may not be representative of the general population. In this study, after a complete evaluation, 60% of the women also were found to have psychiatric disorders.

The phenomenon of *menstrual magnification* (sometimes called premenstrual or perimenstrual exacerbation) helps explain this situation. Many medical and psychiatric conditions are exacerbated in the late luteal or menstrual phase of the cycle, leading a woman to believe that she must be experiencing PMS. The underlying mechanism of this increase in symptoms is not understood.

The differential diagnosis of PMS therefore includes any medical and psychiatric condition that either has some of the many symptoms associated with PMS or is subject to menstrual magnification. Depressive disorders, which share a similar set of symptoms, are the most com-

mon consideration (25). Depressive disorders also are subject to the magnification effect, making the distinction from PMS even more difficult. A key feature of depressive disorders, however, is that symptoms are almost always present every day of the cycle. Other psychiatric conditions that may be magnified are panic disorder and generalized anxiety disorder.

The most common medical disorders subject to menstrual magnification are migraines, seizure disorders, irritable bowel syndrome, asthma, chronic fatigue syndrome, and allergies. Endocrine abnormalities such as thyroid and adrenal disorders also should be considered. The diagnosis of these conditions usually is straightforward because the key symptoms are not part of the typical PMS symptom set, and emotional symptoms are not prominent, as they are in PMS.

Finally, women in the period of transition to menopause may have symptoms typical of PMS, especially mood disturbance, fatigue, and hot flashes. Because menstrual periods often are less predictable, these women may be less aware of the relationship of the symptoms to the menstrual cycle. The correct diagnosis usually can be made by considering the patient's age, a history of recent menstrual cycle changes, and a symptom diary showing sporadic or daily occurrence of symptoms.

▶ *Which patients require therapeutic intervention for PMS?*

Premenstrual syndrome, by definition, is associated with symptoms that interfere with some part of the patient's normal life, but there are usually no medical sequelae if the disorder is not treated. Therefore, the decision to treat the disorder should be based on the patient's desire for an improvement in her symptoms. Furthermore, because there is a wide range of symptom severity, the treatment approach should match the patient's needs.

▶ *What is the evidence supporting the effectiveness of the following common treatments for PMS?*

A wide variety of supportive, lifestyle, and dietary supplementation approaches to PMS have been recommended over the years, and a few of these have been demonstrated to have real benefit. Therefore, these strategies can be recommended to women with mild to moderate symptoms as a primary therapy and to women with severe symptoms as adjunctive therapy.

Women with severe symptoms or with symptoms resistant to nonmedical approaches should be considered for drug therapy. Although no drugs currently are specifically approved by the U.S. Food and Drug Administration for the treatment of PMS, several available drugs have been found to be effective for PMS and can be prescribed.

Supportive Therapy. Supportive therapy has been employed as a central component in PMS management, although it has not been studied rigorously. Reassurance and informational counseling may relieve many anxieties and increase the patient's sense of control. Women anecdotally report relief when they are informed that PMS is a common medical problem with a physiologic basis. Supportive therapy may contribute in part to the high response rate to placebos for virtually every form of treatment used for PMS.

The value of more formal psychologic interventions has not been conclusively demonstrated. The best evidence is for relaxation therapy. In one small comparative study, relaxation therapy had its greatest effects in women with the most severe symptoms (26). In a study of cognitive behavior therapy, the comparison group who received information about PMS, relaxation training, and lifestyle and nutrition guidelines fared nearly as well as the study group who received cognitive restructuring training (27).

Aerobic Exercise. Aerobic exercise has been found in epidemiologic studies to be associated with fewer reported PMS symptoms, and exercise has been found to reduce symptoms among people with depressive disorders. Limited evidence supports a similar role for this intervention in PMS. In a 3-month randomized trial of 23 women with prospectively diagnosed PMS, the group taking regular moderate aerobic exercise reported more improvement than the control group who did nonaerobic exercise (28). In another small prospective but not randomized study, two groups of women who exercised aerobically reported fewer PMS symptoms at the end of a 6-month trial than did a nonexercising comparison group (29). Although the evidence base is modest at this time, aerobic exercise can be recommended to all women with PMS because of its numerous other health benefits.

Dietary Supplementation. Calcium and magnesium have each been shown to be effective in the treatment of PMS. However, most of these trials have tested small numbers of patients and must be validated in larger trials before strong evidence-based recommendations can be made. One large well-designed multicenter trial of 466 women with PMS reported that 1,200 mg/d of calcium carbonate was efficacious in reducing total symptom scores (30). Two small trials have found that 200–400 mg of magnesium may be somewhat effective (31, 32).

Minimal data are available on the effectiveness of vitamin E and the treatment of premenstrual syndrome. Vitamin E has been recommended as a treatment for mastalgia. In one randomized, double-blind, controlled study comparing vitamin E 400 IU/d during the luteal phase with placebo, vitamin E was found to improve significantly affective and somatic symptoms in PMS patients (33). Although effectiveness probably is minimal, no serious side effects are reported with vitamin E 400 IU/d, and as an antioxidant it has other beneficial effects.

In one study, mood symptomatology and carbohydrate food cravings were shown to be improved by carbohydrate-rich beverages (34). This small, well-designed study should be repeated with larger numbers of subjects before evidence-based recommendations can be made. One hypothesis to explain these benefits is that diets rich in carbohydrates increase levels of tryptophan, the precursor to serotonin.

Well-designed scientific studies have not demonstrated that primrose oil is effective in the treatment of PMS. However, it may be useful in treating breast tenderness (35).

On the basis of a recent systematic review of several weak clinical studies, vitamin B_6 is considered to be of limited clinical benefit in the treatment of PMS (36). Dosages in excess of 100 mg/d may cause medical harm, including peripheral neuropathy (36).

Selective Serotonin Reuptake Inhibitors. The SSRIs are the initial drugs of choice for severe PMS. Fluoxetine is the most studied drug of this group. Its use has been studied in almost 1,000 women in rigorous trials. The largest, a 6-month, multicenter trial, evaluated 313 women with PMS who were prescribed dosages of 20–60 mg/d (37). Investigators observed 44% dropouts at dosages of 60 mg/d and 11% at dosages of 20 mg/d. This study, along with several smaller, shorter-duration placebo-controlled trials, have consistently reported the efficacy of fluoxetine. The dosage in these trials generally was 20 mg/d throughout the menstrual cycle administered as a single morning dose to avoid insomnia. One study reported efficacy in 64 women with PMS over a mean treatment time of 18 months (38). In this 18-month study, symptoms recurred in most of the women not taking fluoxetine and resolved when treatment was restarted.

Other SSRI drugs that have had a beneficial effect similar to that of fluoxetine are sertraline, paroxetine, clomipramine, fluvoxamine, and nefazodone. In the largest study of sertraline, in which there were 233 subjects, dosages ranged from 50 to 150 mg/d (39).

Intermittent therapy, with an SSRI given only during the symptomatic phase, also has been efficacious in several small, randomized, double-blind, placebo-controlled trials (40–42). This method of administration has many advantages: it is less expensive, reduces the overall rate of side effects, and is more acceptable to many women. The drug is started between 7 and 14 days before the next menstrual period, with the start day individualized to begin the medication at or just before the expected onset of symptoms.

Side effects associated with fluoxetine include headaches, nausea, and jitteriness. Insomnia often can be avoided by early-morning dosing or, if appropriate, by lowering the dosage. Decreased libido also is problematic in some patients. In cases in which improvement of libido is not seen after dosage changes, alternative therapies may be considered (4).

Other Pharmacologic Approaches. Some placebo-controlled trials have shown alprazolam, an anxiolytic medication, to be effective as a treatment for PMS (43–45), and some have not (46). There is a potential for dependency and development of tolerance with this medication, especially if dosing is not limited to the luteal phase. Sedation also can be a bothersome side effect in some patients, and withdrawals can be problematic. Alprazolam may potentially be useful for PMS patients who are not relieved by other interventions. It may be especially useful if agitation and anxiety are the primary symptoms.

Because complaints of fluid retention are common in the luteal phase, diuretic therapy has been advocated. No evidence exists that thiazide diuretics are of benefit. Spironolactone, an aldosterone antagonist with antiandrogenic properties, is the only diuretic that has been shown to be of benefit in PMS. Several randomized, double-blind, placebo-controlled trials have shown a significant reduction in somatic and affective complaints (47–51). Usual dosage in most studies is 100 mg/d in the morning during the 14-day luteal phase. However, not all reports evaluating spironolactone for PMS have shown benefit.

Historically, natural progesterone has been one of the most commonly employed therapies in women with PMS, but careful scientific scrutiny has not supported an overall benefit of this hormone when compared with placebo, whether administered as a vaginal suppository (52) or as oral micronized progesterone (45). Progesterone may be helpful for specific symptoms, such as breast tenderness and bloating, or specific psychologic symptoms, such as worrying (53).

▶ *What is the role of hormonal suppression in the treatment of PMS?*

Oral Contraceptives. Although oral contraceptives are widely prescribed for the treatment of PMS, few data support their effectiveness. In one randomized trial, a triphasic formulation reduced physical symptoms but not mood alterations (54). In another study comparing triphasic and monophasic regimens, the monophasic formulation was less likely to cause mood alterations (55). Many patients experience breast tenderness, nausea, mood alterations, and other side effects the first few months of oral contraceptive use. The evidence suggests that oral contraceptives should be considered if symptoms are primarily physical, but may not be effective if mood symptoms are more prevalent.

Gonadotropin-Releasing Hormone Agonists. Improvement in PMS symptoms with gonadotropin-releasing hormone (GnRH) agonists has been reported in the majority of well-designed studies (56–57) but not in all of them (58). The hypoestrogenic side effects and cost of GnRH agonists limit the usefulness of this method except in severe cases of PMS unresponsive to other treatment.

If this therapy is to be used for more than a few months, bone loss becomes a concern. The most commonly used approach is add-back estrogen therapy (with progestin if indicated). Add-back therapy also may result in a return of symptoms, although studies are limited and sometimes confusing. In a double-blind, placebo-controlled study of 10 women, both estrogen add-back therapy alone and progesterone therapy alone were associated with a significant recurrence of symptoms (15). Another small rigorous study evaluated eight women with PMS. Administration of the GnRH agonist resulted in an improvement of approximately 75% in luteal phase symptom scores. The addition of estrogen as well as progesterone was associated with worsening symptoms, but a similar worsening also was seen with placebo (59). If hormone therapy results in a return of symptoms, alendronate should be considered for osteoporosis prevention.

Bilateral Salpingo-Oophorectomy. Surgery for PMS is controversial because it is irreversible, it is associated with morbidity and mortality, and the resulting hypoestrogenemia must be addressed to prevent long-term complications. If employed, this approach should be reserved for those severely affected patients who meet strict diagnostic criteria and who do not respond to any potentially effective therapy other than GnRH agonists (60). These limitations are critical, because a major cause of therapeutic failure with any of the described treatments is an incorrect diagnosis of PMS. It is advisable to perform a diagnostic trial with an agonist for a minimum of 3 months to determine if oophorectomy will be effective. An additional advantage to an extended trial with an agonist is the opportunity to assess the woman's tolerance for estrogen replacement therapy.

Summary

The following recommendations are based on good and consistent scientific evidence (Level A):

▶ Women in whom PMS has been diagnosed should meet standard diagnostic criteria and should have the timing of their symptoms confirmed using a prospective symptom calendar.

▶ Risk factors such as increased imposed stress and specific personality profiles are not helpful in differentiating women with PMS from those without PMS.

▶ The SSRIs, particularly fluoxetine and sertraline, have been shown to be effective in treating PMS.

▶ The bulk of scientific evidence does not support the usefulness of natural progesterone or primrose oil in the treatment of PMS.

The following recommendations are based on limited or inconsistent scientific evidence (Level B):

▶ The use of GnRH agonists and surgical oophorectomy have been shown to be effective in PMS. However, the side effects of GnRH agonists and oophorectomy limit their usefulness in most patients.

▶ Treatment with the anxiolytic alprazolam is effective in some patients. Its side effects limit its use as a first-line approach.

▶ Carbohydrate-rich foods and beverages may improve mood symptoms and food cravings in women with PMS and are a reasonable first-line approach in many patients.

▶ Calcium supplements have been shown to be effective in the treatment of PMS.

▶ Magnesium, vitamin B_6, and vitamin E may have minimal effectiveness in the treatment of PMS.

Oral contraceptives may improve physical symptoms of PMS.

The following recommendations are based primarily on consensus and expert opinion (Level C):

▶ Supportive therapy is central to the management of all PMS patients.

▶ Aerobic exercise can be recommended to PMS patients.

▶ As an overall clinical approach, treatments should be employed in increasing orders of complexity. Using this principle, in most cases, the therapies should be used in the following order:

Step 1. Supportive therapy, complex carbohydrate diet, aerobic exercise, nutritional supplements (calcium, magnesium, vitamin E), spironolactone

Step 2. The SSRIs (fluoxetine or sertraline as the initial choice); for women who do not respond, consider an anxiolytic for specific symptoms

Step 3. Hormonal ovulation suppression (oral contraceptives or GnRH agonists)

References

1. Gise LH, Kase NG, Berkowitz RL, eds. Contemporary issues in obstetrics and gynecology. Vol 2. The premenstrual syndromes. New York: Churchill Livingstone, 1988 (Level III)

2. Mortola JF. Issues in the diagnosis and research of premenstrual syndrome. Clin Obstet Gynecol 1992;35:587–598 (Level III)

3. Stout AL, Steege JF. Psychosocial assessment of women seeking treatment for premenstrual syndrome. J Psychosom Res 1985;29:621–629 (Level III)

4. Steiner M. Premenstrual syndromes. Annu Rev Med 1997;48:447–455 (Level III)

5. Kendler KS, Silberg JL, Neale MC, Kessler RC, Heath AC, Eaves LJ. Genetic and environmental factors in the aetiology of menstrual, premenstrual and neurotic symptoms: a population-based twin study. Psychol Med 1992;22: 85–100 (Level II-3)

6. Condon JT. The premenstrual syndrome: a twin study. Br J Psychiatry 1993;162:481–486 (Level II-3)

7. Halbreich U, Endicott J. Relationship of dysphoric premenstrual changes to depressive disorders. Acta Psychiatr Scand 1985;71:331–338 (Level III)

8. DeJong R, Rubinow DR, Roy-Byrne P, Hoban MC, Grover GN, Post RM. Premenstrual mood disorder and psychiatric illness. Am J Psychiatry 1985:142:1359–1361 (Level III)

9. Trunnell EP, Turner CW, Keye WR. A comparison of the psychological and hormonal factors in women with and without premenstrual syndrome. J Abnorm Psychol 1988;97:429–436 (Level II-2)

10. Beck LE, Girvertz R, Mortola JF. The predictive role of psychosocial stress on symptom severity in premenstrual syndrome. Psychosom Med 1990;52:536–543 (Level III)

11. Adenaike OC, Abidoye RO. A study of the incidence of premenstrual syndrome in a group of Nigerian women. Public Health 1987;101:49–58 (Level III)

12. Hasin M, Dennerstein L, Gotts G. Menstrual cycle related complaints: a cross-cultural study. J Psychosom Obstet Gynaecol 1988;9:35–42 (Level II-3)

13. Stout AL, Grady TA, Steege JF, Blazer DG, George LK, Melville ML. Premenstrual symptoms in black and white community samples. Am J Psychiatry 1986;143;1436–1439 (Level III)

14. Freeman EW. Premenstrual syndrome: current perspectives on treatment and etiology. Curr Opin Obstet Gynecol 1997;9:147–153 (Level III)

15. Schmidt PJ, Nieman LK, Danaceau MA, Adams LF, Rubinow DR. Differential behavioral effects of gonadal

steroids in women with and in those without premenstrual syndrome. N Engl J Med 1998;338:209–216 (Level I)

16. Eriksson E, Hedberg MA, Andersch B, Sundblad C. The serotonin reuptake inhibitor paroxetin is superior to the noradrenaline reuptake inhibitor maprotiline in the treatment of premenstrual syndrome. Neuropsychopharmacology 1995;12:167–176 (Level II-2)

17. Hamilton JA, Parry BL, Alagna S, Blumenthal S, Herz E. Premenstrual mood changes: a guide to evaluation and treatment. Psychiatr Ann 1984;14:426-435 (Level III)

18. American Psychiatric Association. Diagnostic and statistical manual of mental disorders: DSM-IV. 4th ed. Washington, DC: APA, 1994:714–718 (Level III)

19. Hart WG, Coleman GJ, Russell JW. Assessment of premenstrual symptomatology: a re-evaluation of the predictive validity of self-report. J Psychosom Res 1987;31: 185–190 (Level III)

20. Johnson SR. Clinician's approach to the diagnosis and management of premenstrual syndrome. Clin Obstet Gynecol 1992;35:637–657 (Level III)

21. Mortola JF, Girton L, Beck L, Yen SS. Diagnosis of premenstrual syndrome by a simple, prospective, and reliable instrument: the calendar of premenstrual experiences. Obstet Gynecol 1990;76:302–307 (Level II-2)

22. Reid RL. Premenstrual syndrome. Curr Probl Obstet Gynecol Fertil 1985;8(2):1–57 (Level III)

23. McCormack HM, Horne DJ, Sheather S. Clinical applications of visual analogue scales: a critical review. Psychol Med 1988;18:1007–1019 (Level I)

24. Corney RH, Stanton R. A survey of 658 women who report symptoms of premenstrual syndrome. J Psychosom Res 1991;35:471–482 (Level III)

25. Plouffe L Jr, Stewart KS, Craft KS, Maddox MS, Rausch JL. Diagnostic and treatment results from a southeastern academic center-based premenstrual syndrome clinic: the first year. Am J Obstet Gynecol 1993;169:295–303; discussion 303–307 (Level III)

26. Goodale IL, Domar AD, Benson H. Alleviation of premenstrual syndrome symptoms with the relaxation response. Obstet Gynecol 1990;75:649–655 (Level I)

27. Christensen AP, Oei TP. The efficacy of cognitive behaviour therapy in treating premenstrual dysphoric changes. J Affect Disord 1995;33:57–63 (Level II-3)

28. Steege JF, Blumenthal JA. The effects of aerobic exercise on premenstrual symptoms in middle-aged women: a preliminary study. J Psychosom Res 1993;37:127–133 (Level II-1)

29. Prior JC, Vigna Y, Sciarretta D, Alojado N, Schulzer M. Conditioning exercise decreases premenstrual symptoms: a prospective, controlled 6-month trial. Fertil Steril 1987;47:402–408 (Level II-2)

30. Thys-Jacobs, Starkey P, Bernstein D, Tian J. Calcium carbonate and the premenstrual syndrome: effects on premenstrual and menstrual symptoms. Premenstrual Syndrome Study Group. Am J Obstet Gynecol 1998;179:444–452 (Level I)

31. Facchinetti F, Borella P, Sances G, Fioroni L, Nappi RE, Genazzani AR. Oral magnesium successfully relieves premenstrual mood changes. Obstet Gynecol 1991;78: 177–181 (Level I)

32. Walker AF, De Souza MC, Vickers MF, Abeyasekera S, Collins ML, Trinca LA. Magnesium supplementation alleviates premenstrual symptoms of fluid retention. J Womens Health 1998;7:1157–1165 (Level I)

33. London RS, Murphy L, Kitlowski KE, Reynolds MA. Efficacy of alpha-tocopherol in the treatment of the premenstrual syndrome. J Reprod Med 1987;32:400–404 (Level I)

34. Sayegh R, Schiff I, Wurtman J, Spiers P, McDermott J, Wurtman R. The effect of a carbohydrate-rich beverage on mood, appetite, and cognitive function in women with premenstrual syndrome. Obstet Gynecol 1995,86:520–528 (Level II-2)

35. Budeiri D, Li Wan Po A, Dorman JC. Is evening primrose oil of value in the treatment of premenstrual syndrome? Control Clin Trials 1996;17:60–68 (Level III)

36. Wyatt KM, Dimmock PW, Jones PW, Shaughn O'Brien PM. Efficacy of vitamin B-6 in the treatment of premenstrual syndrome: systematic review. BMJ. 1999;318: 1375–1381 (Level III)

37. Steiner M, Steinberg S, Stewart D, Carter D, Berger C, Reid R, et al. Fluoxetine in the treatment of premenstrual dysphoria. Canadian Fluoxetine/Premenstrual Dysphoria Collaborative Study Group. N Engl J Med 1995;332: 1529–1534 (Level I)

38. Pearlstein TB, Stone AB. Long-term fluoxetine treatment of late luteal phase dysphoric disorder. J Clin Psychiatry 1994;55:332–335 (Level II-2)

39. Yonkers KA, Halbreich U, Freeman E, Brown C, Endicott J, Frank E, et al. Symptomatic improvement of premenstrual dysphoric disorder with sertraline treatment. A randomized controlled trial. Sertraline Premenstrual Dysphoric Collaborative Study Group. JAMA 1997; 278:983–988 (Level I)

40. Steiner M, Korzekwa M, Lamont J, Wilkins A. Intermittent fluoxetine dosing in the treatment of women with premenstrual dysphoria. Psychopharmacol Bull 1997;33:771–774 (Level II-3)

41. Young SA, Hurt PH, Benedek DM, Howard RS. Treatment of premenstrual dysphoric disorder with sertraline during the luteal phase: a randomized, double-blind, placebo-controlled crossover trial. J Clin Psychiatry 1998;59:76–80 (Level II-1)

42. Wikander I, Sundblad C, Andersch B, Dagnell I, Zylberstein D, Bengtsson F, et al. Citalopram in premenstrual dysphoria: is intermittent treatment during luteal phases more effective than continuous medication throughout the menstrual cycle? J Clin Psychopharmacol 1998;18:390–398 (Level I)

43. Harrison WM, Endicott J, Nee J. Treatment of premenstrual dysphoria with alprazolam. A controlled study. Arch Gen Psychiatry 1990;47:270–275 (Level I)

44. Smith S, Rinehart JS, Ruddock VE, Schiff I. Treatment of premenstrual syndrome with alprazolam: results of a dou-

ble-blind, placebo-controlled, randomized crossover clinical trial. Obstet Gynecol 1987;70:37–43 (Level I)

45. Freeman EW, Rickels K, Sondheimer SJ, Polansky M. A double-blind trial of oral progesterone, alprazolam, and placebo in treatment of severe premenstrual syndrome. JAMA 1995;274:51–57 (Level I)

46. Schmidt PJ, Grover GN, Rubinow DR. Alprazolam in the treatment of premenstrual syndrome: a double-blind, placebo-controlled trial. Arch Gen Psychiatry 1993;50:467–473 (Level I)

47. O'Brien PM, Craven D, Selby C, Symonds EM. Treatment of premenstrual syndrome by spironolactone. Br J Obstet Gynaecol 1979;86:142–147 (Level I)

48. Vellacott ID, Shroff NE, Pearce MY, Stratford ME, Akbar FA. A double-blind, placebo-controlled evaluation of spironolactone in the premenstrual syndrome. Curr Med Res Opin 1987;10:450–456 (Level I)

49. Wang M, Hammarback S, Lindhe BA, Backstrom T. Treatment of premenstrual syndrome by spironolactone: a double-blind, placebo controlled study. Acta Obstet Gynecol Scand 1995;74:803–808 (Level I)

50. Burnet RB, Radden HS, Easterbrook EG, McKinnon RA. Premenstrual syndrome and spironolactone. Aust N Z J Obstet Gynaecol 1991;31:366–368 (Level I)

51. Hellberg D, Claesson B, Nilsson S. Premenstrual tension: a placebo-controlled efficacy study with spironolactone and medroxyprogesterone acetate. Int J Gynaecol Obstet 1991;34:243–248 (Level II-1)

52. Freeman E, Rickels K, Sondheimer SJ, Polansky M. Ineffectiveness of progesterone suppository treatment for premenstrual syndrome. JAMA 1990;264:349–353 (Level I)

53. Baker ER, Best RG, Manfredi RL, Demers LM, Wolf GC. Efficacy of progesterone vaginal suppositories in alleviation of nervous symptoms in patients with premenstrual syndrome. J Assist Reprod Genet 1995;12:205–209 (Level II-1)

54. Graham CA. Sherwin BB. A prospective treatment study of premenstrual symptoms using a triphasic oral contraceptive. Psychosom Res 1992;36:257–266 (Level II-2)

55. Backstrom T, Hansson-Malmstrom Y, Lindhe BA, Cavilli-Bjorkman B, Nordenstrom S. Oral contraceptives in premenstrual syndrome: a randomized comparison of triphasic and monophasic preparations. Contraception 1992;46:253–268 (Level II-1)

56. Johnson SR. Premenstrual syndrome therapy. Clin Obstet Gynecol 1998;41:405–421 (Level III)

57. Freeman EW, Sondheimer SJ, Rickels K. Gonadotropin-releasing hormone agonist in treatment of premenstrual symptoms with and without ongoing dysphoria: a controlled study. Psychopharmacol Bull 1997;33:303–309 (Level I)

58. West CP, Hillier H. Ovarian suppression with the gonadotrophin-releasing hormone agonist goserelin (Zoladex) in management of the premenstrual tension syndrome. Hum Reprod 1994;9:1058–1063 (Level I)

59. Mortola JF, Girton L, Fischer U. Successful treatment of severe premenstrual syndrome by combined use of gonadotropin-releasing hormone agonist and estrogen/progestin. J Clin Endocrinol Metab 1991;72:252A–252F (Level III)

60. Casson P, Hahn PM, Van Vugt DA, Reid RL. Lasting response to ovariectomy in severe intractable premenstrual syndrome. Am J Obstet Gynecol 1990;162:99–105 (Level II-3)

The MEDLINE database, the Cochrane Library, and ACOG's own internal resources and documents were used to conduct a literature search to locate relevant articles published between January 1985 and May 1999. The search was restricted to articles published in the English language. Priority was given to articles reporting results of original research, although review articles and commentaries also were consulted. Abstracts of research presented at symposia and scientific conferences were not considered adequate for inclusion in this document. Guidelines published by organizations or institutions such as the National Institutes of Health and the American College of Obstetricians and Gynecologists were reviewed, and additional studies were located by reviewing bibliographies of identified articles. When reliable research was not available, expert opinions from obstetrician–gynecologists were used.

Studies were reviewed and evaluated for quality according to the method outlined by the U.S. Preventive Services Task Force:

I   Evidence obtained from at least one properly designed randomized controlled trial.

II-1   Evidence obtained from well-designed controlled trials without randomization.

II-2   Evidence obtained from well-designed cohort or case–control analytic studies, preferably from more than one center or research group.

II-3   Evidence obtained from multiple time series with or without the intervention. Dramatic results in uncontrolled experiments also could be regarded as this type of evidence.

III   Opinions of respected authorities, based on clinical experience, descriptive studies, or reports of expert committees.

Based on the highest level of evidence found in the data, recommendations are provided and graded according to the following categories:

Level A—Recommendations are based on good and consistent scientific evidence.

Level B—Recommendations are based on limited or inconsistent scientific evidence.

Level C—Recommendations are based primarily on consensus and expert opinion.

ISSN 1099-3630

**The American College of
Obstetricians and Gynecologists
409 12th Street, SW
PO Box 96920
Washington, DC 20090-6920**

12345/43210

ACOG PRACTICE BULLETIN

CLINICAL MANAGEMENT GUIDELINES FOR
OBSTETRICIAN–GYNECOLOGISTS

NUMBER 27, MAY 2001

*(Replaces Educational Bulletin Number 228, September 1996,
and Committee Opinion Number 160, October 1995)*

This Practice Bulletin was developed by the ACOG Committee on Practice Bulletins— Obstetrics with the assistance of Katharine Wenstrom, MD. The information is designed to aid practitioners in making decisions about appropriate obstetric and gynecologic care. These guidelines should not be construed as dictating an exclusive course of treatment or procedure. Variations in practice may be warranted based on the needs of the individual patient, resources, and limitations unique to the institution or type of practice.

Prenatal Diagnosis of Fetal Chromosomal Abnormalities

The prevalence of chromosomal abnormalities in clinically recognized early pregnancy loss is approximately 50% (1). Aneuploid fetuses account for 6–11% of all stillbirths and neonatal deaths (2). Chromosome defects compatible with life but causing significant morbidity occur in 0.65% of newborns, and another 0.2% have structural chromosomal rearrangements that will eventually affect reproduction (3). Although it is not possible to identify all aneuploidies antenatally, screening and diagnostic programs to detect the most common autosomal trisomy in liveborn infants, Down syndrome, are well established. This document will provide clinical management guidelines for the prenatal detection of these aneuploidies.

Background

Down syndrome and other autosomal trisomies primarily occur as the result of meiotic nondisjunction, which increases with maternal age. Genetic amniocentesis has been offered to women who will be age 35 years and older at delivery because at this age the incidence of trisomy starts to increase rapidly and because the midtrimester risk of Down syndrome roughly equals the most often quoted risk of procedure-related pregnancy loss (1/200) (Table 1). However, only 12.9% of all children are born to women age 35 years and older (4). Therefore, even if all women older than 35 years requested amniocenteses, only a minority of Down syndrome pregnancies would be identified. Because younger women have the majority of pregnancies, younger women give birth to the majority of children with Down syndrome (5).

Table 1. Midtrimester and Term Risk of Down Syndrome or Any Aneuploidy

Maternal Age	Midtrimester		Term Liveborn	
	DS	All Aneuploidies	DS	All Aneuploidies
33	1/417	1/208	1/625	1/345
34	1/333	1/152	1/500	1/278
35	1/250	1/132	1/384	1/204
36	1/192	1/105	1/303	1/167
37	1/149	1/83	1/227	1/130
38	1/115	1/65	1/175	1/103
39	1/89	1/53	1/137	1/81
40	1/69	1/40	1/106	1/63
41	1/53	1/31	1/81	1/50
42	1/41	1/25	1/64	1/39
43	1/31	1/19	1/50	1/30
44	1/25	1/15	1/38	1/24
45	1/19	1/12	1/30	1/19

Abbreviation: DS, Down syndrome.

Adapted from Hook EB, Cross PK, Schreinemachers DM. Chromosomal abnormality rates at amniocentesis and in live-born infants. JAMA 1983;249:2034–2038. Copyrighted 1983, American Medical Association.

Screening and Testing for Genetic Abnormalities

Of Down syndrome pregnancies, 97% occur in families with no previous history of the syndrome (6). Screening tests are used to identify those women who are not known to be at high risk but are nevertheless carrying a fetus with Down syndrome. Screening tests have a high false-positive rate because the threshold for declaring a screening test result positive is set to capture most individuals who truly have the condition at the expense of including some who do not. Women with positive screening test results should be offered a definitive diagnostic test such as amniocentesis or chorionic villus sampling (CVS).

Second-Trimester Screening

Maternal Serum Screening

Until the mid-1980s, there was no way to identify younger women at risk of having children with Down syndrome. Down syndrome screening for younger women was initiated when researchers discovered that the mean level of maternal serum alpha fetoprotein (AFP) in pregnancies complicated by fetal Down syndrome is 0.7 multiples of the (normal) median (MoM) (7–9).

It was soon discovered that human chorionic gonadotropin (hCG) levels are higher (2.04 MoM) and unconjugated estriol levels are lower (0.79 MoM) in Down syndrome pregnancies (10–13). The relative risks derived from maternal serum levels of these three analytes are used to modify the maternal age-related risk. This protocol has been validated extensively and has become the preferred Down syndrome screening test for women younger than 35 years (13–16). At a cutoff chosen to produce a 5% or greater screen-positive rate, the multiple-marker screening test identifies approximately 60% of all Down syndrome pregnancies in women younger than 35 years. In women 35 years and older, it detects 75% or more of all Down syndrome cases and certain other aneuploidies. The screen-positive rate increases with maternal age (Table 2) (17). Some laboratories use the midtrimester Down syndrome risk of a 35-year-old woman as the screen-positive cutoff. Other laboratories select a screen-positive cutoff that will result in an acceptable balance between a high detection rate and a low screen-positive rate (usually 1:190 or 1:200). The basis of these screening protocol calculations of risk is the maternal age-related risk of Down syndrome, a risk based on previously lower rates of birth to women older than 35 years, which may now be obsolete. Screening protocols may benefit from revision using current data on maternal age.

Maternal blood sampling can be performed between 15 and 20 weeks of gestation but is most accurate when performed between 16 and 18 weeks of gestation. Accurate pregnancy dating is essential. If the estimated date of delivery is changed after the test results have returned, it is important to recalculate the results or provide the laboratory with a new blood sample if the original specimen was drawn at less than 15 weeks of gestation.

Table 2. Multiple-Marker Down Syndrome Screening Test Detection and Screen-Positive Rates, According to Maternal Age

Maternal Age	Screen-Positive Rate (%)	Detection Rate (%) (with Estriol)
20	2.4	41
25	2.9	44
30	5.0	52
35	14.0	71
40	40.0	91

Modified with permission from Haddow JE, Palomaki GE, Knight GJ, Cunningham GC, Lustig LS, Boyd PA. Reducing the need for amniocentesis in women 35 years of age or older with serum markers for screening. N Engl J Med 1994;330:1114–1118. Copyright ©1994 Massachusetts Medical Society. All rights reserved.

The multiple-marker screening test also can detect approximately 60–75% of fetuses with trisomy 18 when a separate analysis is performed that uses low levels of all three analytes with or without consideration of maternal age (18, 19). Although serum screening does not detect other aneuploidies with great frequency, the aneuploidies likely to be missed by serum screening usually are ultimately lethal (eg, trisomy 13) or are sex-chromosome abnormalities not associated with profound mental retardation or other severe physical or developmental limitations.

The contribution of estriol measurement is a subject of debate, with some centers offering AFP plus hCG alone. Some investigators consider free beta subunits of hCG (β-hCG) to be superior to the intact hCG molecule, but neither has been definitively proven to be superior. New analytes also are constantly being tested. Dimeric inhibin A is the most promising new second-trimester analyte and is now used by some commercial laboratories in combination with the three traditional analytes. With a screen-positive rate of 5% or less, this new four-analyte combination appears to detect 67–76% of Down syndrome cases in women younger than 35 years (20, 21).

Ultrasound Screening

Aneuploid fetuses may have major anatomic malformations, often discovered by chance during an ultrasound examination performed for another indication. All abnormalities involving a major organ or structure, with a few notable exceptions, or the finding of two or more minor structural abnormalities in the same fetus, indicate high risk for fetal aneuploidy (22–24) (Table 3). Structural anomalies can have many etiologies; if an aneuploidy is suspected, only a karyotype analysis of fetal cells can provide a definitive diagnosis.

Table 3. Aneuploid Risk of Major Anomalies

Structural Defect	Population Incidence	Aneuploidy Risk	Most Common Aneuploidy
Cystic hygroma	1/120 EU–1/6,000 B	60–75%	45X (80%); 21,18,13,XXY
Hydrops	1/1,500–4,000 B	30–80%*	13,21,18,45X
Hydrocephalus	3–8/10,000 LB	3–8%	13,18, triploidy
Hydranencephaly	2/1,000 IA	Minimal	
Holoprosencephaly	1/16,000 LB	40–60%	13,18,18p-
Cardiac defects	7–9/1,000 LB	5–30%	21,18,13,22,8,9
Complete atrioventricular canal		40–70%	21
Diaphragmatic hernia	1/3,500–4,000 LB	20–25%	13,18,21,45X
Omphalocele	1/5,800 LB	30–40%	13,18
Gastroschisis	1/10,000–15,000 LB	Minimal	
Duodenal atresia	1/10,000 LB	20–30%	21
Bowel obstruction	1/2,500–5,000 LB	Minimal	
Bladder outlet obstruction	1–2/1,000 LB	20–25%	13,18
Prune belly syndrome	1/35,000–50,000 LB	Low	18,13,45X
Facial cleft	1/700 LB	1%	13,18, Deletions
Limb reduction	4–6/10,000 LB	8%	18
Club foot	1.2/1,000 LB	6%	18,13,4p-,18q-
Single umbilical artery	1%	Minimal	

Abbreviations: EU, early ultrasonography; B, birth; LB, livebirth; IA, infant autopsy.

*30% if diagnosed ≥24 weeks; 80% if diagnosed ≤17 weeks

Data from Shipp TD, Benacerraf BR. The significance of prenatally identified isolated clubfoot: is amniocentesis indicated? Am J Obstet Gynecol 1998;178:600–602; and Nyberg DA, Crane JP. Chromosome abnormalities. In: Nyberg DA, Mahony BS, Pretorius DH. Diagnostic ultrasound of fetal anomalies: text and atlas. Chicago: Year Book Medical, 1990:676–724

First-Trimester Screening

Maternal Serum Analytes

Many maternal serum analytes have been evaluated for possible use for first-trimester Down syndrome screening, although preliminary data remain controversial and testing is not yet standard of care. The most discriminatory analytes at this gestational age appear to be β-hCG and pregnancy-associated plasma protein A (PAPP-A) (25, 26). The median free β-hCG in affected Down syndrome pregnancies is approximately 1.79 MoM, whereas the median PAPP-A is approximately 0.43 MoM. Because of the low correlation between these two analytes, each contributes unique biologic information to the screening test. The combination of free β-hCG, PAPP-A, and maternal age appears to yield detection and false-positive rates comparable to second-trimester serum screening (63% and 5.5%, respectively) (27). Unfortunately, free β-hCG may not be higher in Down syndrome pregnancies until 12 weeks of gestation, and PAPP-A seems to lose its discrimination value after 13 weeks of gestation, making accurate assessment of gestational age and careful timing of the screening test essential (28).

Nuchal Lucency Measurement

Nuchal lucency measurement has been suggested as another screening test for Down syndrome in the first trimester. The ultrasound finding of an increase in the size of the normal, clear area behind the fetal neck early in pregnancy is associated with an increased incidence of Down syndrome, congenital heart disease, and other congenital anomalies. Although the precise etiology and significance of the nuchal lucency are unknown, the finding may reflect accumulation of lymph fluid related to delayed development of the lymphatic ducts. An increased nuchal lucency measurement in combination with maternal age has been reported to identify 27–89% of Down syndrome pregnancies, with a screen-positive rate of 2.8–9.3% (28). Some of this wide variation may result from differences in techniques for measuring and criteria for defining an increase. Other factors include differences in study population, ultrasonographic technique, sonographer training, definition of screen positivity, and the quality of both pregnancy and pediatric follow-up. Much of the early work was derived from women at high risk (eg, prior to scheduled CVS or amniocentesis in women age 35 years or older), and results of trials in unselected low-risk women have produced conflicting results (29–31). Variability in Down syndrome detection rates is likely to be caused by the existence of significant methodologic limitations for many of the studies. Many

of the reports provide minimal information on the extent of pregnancy or pediatric follow-up; therefore, underascertainment of cases of Down syndrome is likely.

Clinical Considerations and Recommendations

▶ *Who is at high risk and should be offered prenatal diagnosis for fetal aneuploidy?*

Women with singleton pregnancies who will be age 35 years or older at delivery should be offered prenatal diagnosis. The midtrimester risk that a pregnant 35-year-old woman is carrying a fetus with Down syndrome is 1/250 (32); the risk of any aneuploidy is 1/132 (Table 1). These numbers are higher than the term risks because a large proportion of aneuploid pregnancies are spontaneously aborted before term delivery. The risks at term are 1/384 for Down syndrome and 1/204 for all aneuploidies.

In addition to women age 35 years and older, patients with a risk of fetal aneuploidy high enough to justify an invasive diagnostic procedure include the following:

- *Women who have previously had pregnancies complicated by autosomal trisomy.* The chance that such a woman could have another pregnancy with the same or a different autosomal trisomy is approximately 1% until her age-related risk exceeds 1%; then it is assumed to equal her age-related risk.

- *A fetus with a major structural defect identified by ultrasonography.* The discovery of one major or two or more minor fetal structural abnormalities increases the likelihood of aneuploidy sufficiently to warrant fetal genetic testing (22–24). However, detection of a fetal defect known not to be associated with aneuploidy (eg, fetal cleft lip discovered during an ultrasound examination ordered because the mother has a cleft lip) or an isolated malformation not usually associated with aneuploidy may not require further testing (Table 3).

- *Women who have previously had a pregnancy complicated by a sex chromosome aneuploidy.* If the previous child had an extra X chromosome, the chromosome may be maternal or paternal in origin. If it is maternal, it is age related. As with autosomal trisomies, the recurrence risk is 1% until the maternal age-related risk exceeds 1%. A woman whose previous child was karyotype 47,XYY is not at high risk of recurrence, because the extra chromosome in this situation is paternal in origin. The karyotype 45,X has a very low recurrence risk. Parents of children with 47,XYY or 45,X karyotypes may still request prenatal diagnosis in future pregnancies for reassurance.

- *Men or women with a chromosome translocation.* Women or men carrying balanced translocations, although phenotypically normal themselves, are at risk of producing unbalanced gametes, resulting in abnormal offspring. For most translocations, the observed risk of abnormal liveborn children is less than the theoretic risk, because a portion of these gametes result in nonviable conceptions. In general, carriers of chromosome translocations identified after the birth of an abnormal child have a 5–30% risk of having unbalanced offspring in the future, while those identified for other reasons (eg, during an infertility work-up) have a 0–5% risk (1). Genetic counseling may be helpful in such situations.

- *Men or women who are carriers of chromosome inversions.* An inversion occurs when two breaks occur in the same chromosome, and the intervening genetic material is inverted before the breaks are repaired. Although no genetic material is lost or duplicated, the rearrangement may alter gene function. Each carrier's risk is related to the method of ascertainment, the chromosome involved, and the size of the inversion and, thus, should be determined individually. The observed risk is approximately 5–10% if the inversion is identified after the birth of an abnormal child and 1–3% if ascertainment occurs by some other means (1). One exception is a pericentric inversion of chromosome 9, which is a population variant of no clinical consequence.

- *Parental aneuploidy.* Women with trisomy 21 or 47,XXX and men with 47,XYY usually are fertile and have a 30% risk of having trisomic offspring. In men with a normal karyotype who have oligospermia and undergo intracytoplasmic sperm injection to conceive, there is an increased incidence of abnormal karyotype in the sperm. However, this has not been reflected in an increase in karyotypically abnormal offspring in these pregnancies.

▶ *How is fetal aneuploidy diagnosed?*

Amniocentesis. Traditional genetic amniocentesis usually is offered between 15 and 20 weeks of gestation. Many large, multicenter studies have confirmed the safety of genetic amniocentesis, as well as its cytogenetic diagnostic accuracy (greater than 99%) (33). The fetal loss rate is approximately 0.5% (34), and minor complications occur infrequently. These include transient vaginal spotting or amniotic fluid leakage in approximately 1–2% of all cases and chorioamnionitis in less than one in 1,000

cases. Needle injuries to the fetus have been reported but are very rare when amniocentesis is performed under continuous ultrasound guidance. Amniotic fluid cell culture failure is uncommon.

Safe performance of genetic amniocentesis requires specialized training and ongoing experience. Several studies have confirmed that the incidence of pregnancy loss, blood-contaminated specimens, leaking of amniotic fluid, and the need for more than one needle puncture are related to the experience of the operator, the use of a small-gauge needle, and ultrasound guidance (35–37).

Early amniocentesis, performed from 11 weeks to 13 weeks of gestation, has been widely studied, and the technique is similar to traditional amniocentesis (38–40). However, early amniocentesis results in significantly higher pregnancy loss and complication rates than traditional amniocentesis. In a recent multicenter randomized trial, the spontaneous pregnancy loss rate following early amniocentesis was 2.5%, compared with 0.7% with traditional amniocentesis (41). The overall incidence of talipes was 1.4% after the early procedure, compared with 0.1% (the same as the background rate) after traditional amniocentesis, and membrane rupture was more likely after the early procedure. Finally, significantly more amniotic fluid culture failures occurred after the early procedure, necessitating an additional invasive procedure for diagnosis. For these reasons, many centers no longer offer early amniocentesis.

Chorionic Villus Sampling. Indications for CVS are similar to those for amniocentesis, except for a few rare genetic conditions that require chorionic villi for diagnosis. Chorionic villus sampling generally is performed at 10–12 weeks of gestation. The primary advantage of CVS over amniocentesis is that results are available much earlier in pregnancy, which provides reassurance for parents when results are normal and, when results are abnormal, allows earlier and safer methods of pregnancy termination.

Placental villi may be obtained through transcervical or transabdominal access to the placenta. Skill in ultrasound-guided procedures and extensive specialized training are required before attempting CVS, and maintenance of skills with regularly scheduled procedures is essential. Some active cervical infections (such as chlamydia or herpes) are a contraindication to transcervical CVS. Relative contraindications to CVS include vaginal infection, vaginal bleeding or spotting, extreme anteversion or retroversion of the uterus, and patient body habitus precluding easy access to the uterus or clear visualization of intrauterine structures with ultrasonography (42–44).

Several major collaborative trials report success rates of more than 99% with cytogenetic analysis and total pregnancy loss rates of 0.6–0.8% for CVS in excess of traditional amniocentesis (33, 45–48, 49). As with early amniocentesis, the reported excess loss rate may result from the CVS procedure itself, but it also may incorporate the expected spontaneous loss rate between 9 and 16 weeks of gestation. Patients considering CVS should be counseled that there may be a slightly higher risk of pregnancy loss associated with CVS than with traditional amniocentesis (34).

Although there have been reports of an association between CVS and limb reduction and oromandibular defects, the risk for these anomalies is unclear (50). In an analysis by the World Health Organization, an incidence of limb reduction defects of 6 per 10,000 was reported, which is not significantly different from the incidence in the general population (49). However, a workshop on CVS and limb reduction defects sponsored by the U.S. National Center for Environmental Health and the Centers for Disease Control and Prevention concluded that oromandibular–limb hypogenesis appeared to be more common after CVS. It found the risk is highest when CVS is performed before 9 menstrual weeks (51). In addition, a panel convened by the National Institute of Child Health and Development and the American College of Obstetricians and Gynecologists concluded that oro-mandibular–limb hypogenesis appeared to be more common among CVS-exposed infants and appeared to correlate, but may not be limited to, CVS performed earlier than 7 weeks (50). Women considering CVS who are concerned about the possible association of CVS with limb defects can be reassured that when the procedure is performed after 9 menstrual weeks, the risk is low and probably not higher than the general population risk.

Cordocentesis. Cordocentesis, also known as percutaneous umbilical blood sampling (PUBS), involves puncturing the umbilical vein under direct ultrasound guidance. Karyotype analysis of fetal blood usually can be accomplished within 24–48 hours. The procedure-related pregnancy loss rate, including all indications for the procedure, has been reported to be less than 2% (34, 52).

▶ *Is there a role for chromosomal analysis when a fetal ultrasound marker of aneuploidy is identified during an ultrasound examination undertaken for an unrelated indication?*

A variety of second-trimester ultrasound findings have been associated with Down syndrome. Although identification of a major anomaly indicates the need for diagnostic follow-up, ultrasound markers are less strongly associated with aneuploidy. Many of these ultrasound markers have not been well studied in unselected, low-risk women. It is, therefore, unclear how to interpret many of these findings in a given patient particularly in

conjunction with age and serum screening results. Some ultrasound markers associated with Down syndrome include nuchal fold thickness, shortened femur or humerus, pyelectasis, and hyperechogenic bowel. Although some ultrasound markers have been confirmed by multiple investigators to be associated with Down syndrome, others have been described in only one series or have been found to have contradictory associations with Down syndrome across studies (53, 54). The lack of uniformity in the definition of an abnormal finding (eg, how to define a shortened femur) and the lack of consensus on which markers are most significant make this screening approach complex.

Several series have attempted to determine which of these ultrasound markers are most predictive of fetal Down syndrome; short femur and humerus (alone or in combination) and nuchal fold thickening appear to be most promising (55, 56). Most series have found that a combination of two or more positive findings substantially increases risk and warrants further counseling regarding invasive testing. The degree to which an individual patient's risk is increased over age-related and serum analyte calculated risk is unclear. These ultrasound markers have been associated with aneuploidy only if identified in the second trimester.

▶ *Is ultrasonographic screening useful in pregnant women identified to be at high-risk for fetal aneuploidy?*

For the woman at high risk for fetal Down syndrome, usually by virtue of age or multiple-marker screening test results, an ultrasound examination may support the need for prenatal diagnosis. This is particularly true if one of the ultrasound markers for Down syndrome is present or if a gross fetal abnormality is seen. Much more commonly, the ultrasound examination is normal. It has been suggested that the absence of any ultrasound evidence for Down syndrome may decrease the risk sufficiently in high-risk women to avoid amniocentesis. Most invasive testing for Down syndrome occurs in women with a risk just above established cutoffs. Therefore, even a small decrease in the risk of Down syndrome, as determined by normal ultrasound results, may put such women in a lower risk category and avoid the need for invasive testing. This decrease in risk could have a significant impact on the overall number of invasive diagnostic tests performed.

Some studies suggest that the risk for Down syndrome may be reduced by 45–80% over the risk cited before the normal ultrasound examination with knowledgeable interpretation of these markers (57–59). These rates are based on ultrasound examinations performed by experienced operators. Several small studies have been published describing rates of Down syndrome detection between 68% and 93% using various scoring indexes combining maternal age and ultrasound markers. These studies report false-positive rates between 17% and 27% (58, 60, 61).

Risk adjustment is possible only if the ultrasound abnormalities are rigidly defined and the portion of Down syndrome fetuses with them is known. Many investigators have suggested that these measures are laboratory specific, and data may not apply in other centers (62). In addition, ultrasound markers often include anatomic abnormalities as well as biometric measures. The reproducibility of significant ultrasound findings and the magnitude of the decrease in risk for aneuploidy are not yet firmly established. The use of ultrasonographic screening for Down syndrome in high-risk women to avoid invasive testing (eg, women age 35 years and older) is, therefore, controversial and should be limited to specialized centers (55, 57, 63).

▶ *How should a finding of an isolated choroid plexus cyst be further evaluated?*

Choroid plexus cysts arise in the choroid plexus of the lateral ventricle and are typically recognized by ultrasonography in the early to middle second trimester. Choroid plexus cysts may be associated with trisomy 18 (64, 65), which has prompted consideration of the need for invasive testing of the fetus if detected. A meta-analysis reported that the risk of trisomy 18 associated with isolated choroid plexus cysts in all women (all ages combined) is 1/374 (64). Another analysis evaluated published data from more than 200,000 ultrasound examinations and determined that only in women age 32 and older, the presence of an isolated choroid plexus cyst increases the midtrimester risk of trisomy 18 enough to justify genetic testing of the fetus (65). Two recent studies found that with an isolated choroid plexus cyst, testing was justified only if serum screening results were abnormal or the patient was older than 35 years (66, 67). However, in these studies, cysts were commonly noted at the time of genetic amniocentesis; thus, the mother's age at diagnosis also may affect incidence. Therefore, with detection of an isolated choroid plexus cyst, further testing is necessary only if serum screening results are abnormal or the patient is older than 32 years at delivery.

▶ *Is there a role for serum screening in women who will be age 35 years and older at delivery?*

Because the maternal age-related risk of Down syndrome is the basis of the serum screening protocol, both the Down syndrome detection rate and the screen positive rate increase with maternal age (Table 2) (13). The screen-positive rate for all women age 35 years and older is approximately 25%; for women age 40 years, it is 40%; and by age 44, it is approximately 70% (17, 68).

Counseling should include discussion of age-specific multiple-marker screening detection rates and screen-positive rates, the detection rate of aneuploidies other than Down syndrome, the identity and prognosis of the aneuploidies likely to be missed by serum screening, and the risks and benefits of replacing a diagnostic test with a screening test. Counseling should be provided by a practitioner familiar with these components.

▶ *How does prenatal diagnosis differ in multiple gestations?*

Diagnostic options are more limited in multiple gestations (69). In women with twins, the risk of trisomy 21 should be calculated by considering the maternal age-related risk of Down syndrome and the probability that either or both fetuses could be affected. Counseling in this situation should include a discussion of options for pregnancy management if only one fetus is found to be affected. These options include terminating the entire pregnancy, selective second-trimester termination of the affected fetus, and continuing the pregnancy. It has been estimated that the midtrimester risk of fetal Down syndrome in a twin pregnancy in women age 33 years is approximately the same as the risk for that of a singleton pregnancy in women age 35 years, thus justifying counseling for amniocentesis (70, 71).

Scant data exist concerning fetal loss with twin gestation and amniocentesis or CVS. According to some small series, the fetal loss rate with amniocentesis in multiple gestations is approximately 3.5%; this was not higher than the background loss rate for twins in the second trimester in one series with a control group (52, 72, 73). Similar information for twin gestations from small, nonrandomized series exists for CVS (73–75).

A complex counseling issue arises in the presence of a monochorionic twin gestation, in which case the likelihood of discordance in the karyotype is low, and patients may opt for having a karyotype analysis performed on a single fetus. However, in order to offer this option to a patient, the diagnosis of monochorionic twin gestation must have been made with a high degree of confidence. There are no data concerning loss rates following amniocentesis in higher-order multiple gestations.

▶ *Can women who are younger than 35 years (at delivery) elect to have genetic amniocentesis?*

Because of the inherent risk of fetal aneuploidy (Table 1), women younger than 35 years may request genetic amniocentesis. Each patient should weigh the risk of amniocentesis against her desire to determine whether the fetus has an abnormal karyotype, in the context of her own values and beliefs. Consequently, some patients younger than 35 years may request genetic amniocentesis primarily rather than only after abnormal maternal serum or ultrasound screening.

▶ *Should Down syndrome screening be performed in the patient who would decline pregnancy termination?*

Prenatal diagnosis is not performed solely for the purposes of pregnancy termination; it can provide useful information for the physician and the patient. If it is determined that the fetus has an aneuploidy, management of pregnancy, labor, and delivery can be optimized (76).

Summary of Recommendations

The following recommendation is based on good and consistent scientific evidence (Level A):

▶ Early amniocentesis (<13 weeks) is not recommended because of the higher risk of pregnancy loss and complications compared with traditional amniocentesis (15–17 weeks).

The following recommendations are based primarily on consensus and expert opinion (Level C):

▶ Women with singleton pregnancies who will be age 35 years or older at delivery should be offered prenatal diagnosis for fetal aneuploidy.

▶ Patients with a risk of fetal aneuploidy high enough to justify an invasive diagnostic procedure include women with a previous pregnancy complicated by an autosomal trisomy or sex chromosome aneuploidy, a major fetal structural defect identified by ultrasonography, either parent with a chromosome translocation, and carriers of a pericentric chromosome inversion or parental aneuploidy.

▶ A combination of one major or two or more minor ultrasound markers of Down syndrome substantially increases risk and warrants further counseling regarding invasive testing.

▶ The use of ultrasonographic screening for Down syndrome in high-risk women (eg, women age 35 years and older) to avoid invasive testing should be limited to specialized centers.

▶ With an isolated choroid plexus cyst, testing is indicated only if serum screening results are abnormal or the patient will be older than 32 years at delivery.

▶ Cervical infections with chlamydia or herpes are contraindications to transcervical CVS.

▶ Counseling for amniocentesis in a twin pregnancy in women age 33 years is indicated because the midtrimester risk of fetal Down syndrome is approximately the same as for that of a singleton pregnancy at age 35 years.

▶ Nondirective counseling before genetic amniocentesis does not require a patient to commit to pregnancy termination if the result is abnormal.

References

1. Gardner RJM, Sutherland GR. Pregnancy loss and infertility. In: Chromosome abnormalities and genetic counseling. 2nd ed. New York: Oxford University Press, 1996: 311–321. Oxford Monographs on Medical Genetics No. 29 (Level III)

2. Alberman ED, Creasy MR. Frequency of chromosomal abnormalities in miscarriages and perinatal deaths. J Med Genet 1977;14:313–315 (Level III)

3. Milunsky A, Milunsky J. Genetic counseling: preconception, prenatal, and perinatal. In: Milunsky A, ed. Genetic disorders and the fetus: diagnosis, prevention, and treatment. 4th ed. Baltimore: The Johns Hopkins University Press, 1998:1–52 (Level III)

4. Ventura SJ, Martin JA, Curtin SC, Mathews TJ, Park MM. Births: final data for 1998. Natl Vital Stat Rep 2000; 48(3):1–100 (Level III)

5. Shah YG, Eckl CJ, Stinson SK, Woods JR Jr. Biparietal diameter/femur length ratio, cephalic index, and femur length measurements: not reliable screening techniques for Down syndrome. Obstet Gynecol 1990;75:186–188 (Level II-2)

6. Adams MM, Erickson JD, Layde PM, Oakley GP. Down's syndrome. Recent trends in the United States. JAMA 1981;246:758–760 (Level III)

7. Cuckle HS, Wald NJ, Lindenbaum RH. Maternal serum alpha-fetoprotein measurement: a screening test for Down syndrome. Lancet 1984;1(8383):926–929 (Level II-2)

8. Cuckle HS, Wald NJ, Thompson SG. Estimating a woman's risk of having a pregnancy associated with Down's syndrome using her age and serum alpha-fetoprotein level. Br J Obstet Gynaecol 1987;94:387–402 (Level II-2)

9. Combining maternal serum α-fetoprotein measurements and age to screen for Down syndrome in pregnant women under age 35. New England Regional Genetics Group Prenatal Collaborative Study of Down Syndrome Screening. Am J Obstet Gynecol 1989;160:575–581 (Level II-3)

10. Bogart MH, Pandian MR, Jones OW. Abnormal maternal serum chorionic gonadotropin levels in pregnancies with

fetal chromosome abnormalities. Prenat Diagn 1987;7: 623–630 (Level II-2)

11. Wald NJ, Cuckle HS, Densem JW, Nanchahal K, Canick JA, Haddow JE, et al. Maternal serum unconjugated oestriol as an antenatal screening test for Down's syndrome. Br J Obstet Gynaecol 1988;95:334–341 (Level II-2)

12. Wald NJ, Cuckle HS, Densem JW, Nanchahal K, Royston P, Chard T, et al. Maternal serum screening for Down's syndrome in early pregnancy. BMJ 1988;297:883–887 (Level II-2)

13. Haddow JE, Palomaki GE, Knight GJ, Williams J, Pulkkinen A, Canick JA, et al. Prenatal screening for Down's syndrome with use of maternal serum markers. N Engl J Med 1992;327:588–593 (Level II-3)

14. Cheng EY, Luthy DA, Zebelman AM, Williams MA, Lieppman RE, Hickok DE. A prospective evaluation of a second-trimester screening test for fetal Down syndrome using maternal serum alpha-fetoprotein, hCG, and unconjugated estriol. Obstet Gynecol 1993;81:72–77 (Level II-2)

15. Burton BK, Prins GS, Verp MS. A prospective trial of prenatal screening for Down syndrome by means of maternal serum α-fetoprotein, human chorionic gonadotropin, and unconjugated estriol. Am J Obstet Gynecol 1993;169: 526–530 (Level II-3)

16. Wenstrom KD, Williamson RA, Grant SS, Hudson JD, Getchell JP. Evaluation of multiple-marker screening for Down syndrome in a statewide population. Am J Obstet Gynecol 1993;169:793–797 (Level II-2)

17. Haddow JE, Palomaki GE, Knight GJ, Cunningham GC, Lustig LS, Boyd PA. Reducing the need for amniocentesis in women 35 years of age or older with serum markers for screening. N Engl J Med 1994;330:1114–1118 (Level II-2)

18. Canick JA, Palomaki GE, Osathanondh R. Prenatal screening for trisomy 18 in the second trimester. Prenat Diagn 1990;10:546–548 (Level III)

19. Palomaki GE, Haddow JE, Knight GJ, Wald NJ, Kennard A, Canick JA, et al. Risk-based prenatal screening for trisomy 18 using alpha-fetoprotein, unconjugated oestriol and human chorionic gonadotropin. Prenat Diagn 1995;15:713–723 (Level II-3)

20. Wald NJ, Densem JW, George L, Muttukrishna S, Knight PG. Prenatal screening for Down's syndrome using inhibin-A as a serum marker. Prenat Diagn 1996;16: 143–153 (Level II-2)

21. Wenstrom KD, Owen J, Chu DC, Boots L. Prospective evaluation of free beta-subunit of human chorionic gonadotropin and dimeric inhibin A for aneuploidy detection. Am J Obstet Gynecol 1999;181:887–892 (Level II-2)

22. Marchese CA, Carozzi F, Mosso R, Savin E, Campogrande M, Viora E, et al. Fetal karyotype in malformations detected by ultrasound [abstract]. Am J Hum Genet 1985;37:A223 (Abstract)

23. Williamson RA, Weiner CP, Patil S, Benda J, Varner MW, Abu-Yousef MM. Abnormal pregnancy sonogram: selective indication for fetal karyotype. Obstet Gynecol 1987;69:15–20 (Level III)

24. Wladimiroff JW, Sachs ES, Reuss A, Stewart PA, Pijpers L, Niermeijer MF. Prenatal diagnosis of chromosome abnormalities in the presence of fetal structural defects. Am J Med Genet 1988;29:289–291 (Level II-3)

25. Wald NJ, George L, Smith D, Densem JW, Petterson K. Serum screening for Down's syndrome between 8 and 14 weeks of pregnancy. International Prenatal Screening Research Group. Br J Obstet Gynaecol 1996;103:407–412 (Level III)

26. Haddow JE, Palomaki GE, Knight GJ, Williams J, Miller WA, Johnson A. Screening of maternal serum for fetal Down's syndrome in the first trimester. N Engl J Med 1998;338:955–961 (Level II-3)

27. Canick JA, Kellner LH, Saller DN Jr, Palomaki GE, Walker RP, Osathanondh R. Second-trimester levels of maternal urinary gonatropin peptide in Down syndrome pregnancy. Prenat Diagn 1995;15:739–744 (Level II-2)

28. Wald NJ, Kennard A, Hackshaw A, McGuire A. Antenatal screening for Down's syndrome. Health Technol Assess 1998;2:i–iv, 1–112 (Level III)

29. Pajkrt E, de Graaf IM, Mol BW, van Lith JM, Bleker OP, Bilardo CM. Weekly nuchal translucency measurements in normal fetuses. Obstet Gynecol 1998;91:208–211 (Level III)

30. Kornman LH, Morssink LP, Beekhius JR, DeWolf BT, Heringa MP, Mantingh A. Nuchal translucency cannot be used as a screening test for chromosomal abnormalities in the first trimester of pregnancy in a routine ultrasound practice. Prenat Diagn 1996;16:797–805 (Level II-3)

31. Hafner E, Schuchter K, Leibhart E, Philipp K. Results of routine fetal nuchal translucency measurement at weeks 10–13 in 4233 unselected pregnant women. Prenat Diagn 1998;18:29–34 (Level II-3)

32. Hook EB, Cross PK, Schreinmachers DM. Chromosomal abnormality rates at amniocentesis and in live born infants. JAMA 1983;249(15):2034–2038 (Level II-3)

33. Jackson LG, Zachary JM, Fowler SE, Desnick RJ, Golbus MS, Ledbetter DH, et al. A randomized comparison of transcervical and transabdominal chorionic-villus sampling. The U.S. National Institute of Child Health and Human Development Chorionic-Villus Sampling and Amniocentesis Study Group. N Engl J Med 1992;327: 594–598 (Level I)

34. Gardner RJM, Sutherland GR. Prenatal diagnostic procedures. In: Chromosome abnormalities and genetic counseling. 2nd ed. New York: Oxford University Press, 1996:336–344. Oxford Monographs on Medical Genetics No. 29 (Level III)

35. Mennuti MT, DiGaetano A, McDonnell A, Cohen AW, Liston RM. Fetal-maternal bleeding associated with genetic amniocentesis: real-time versus static ultrasound. Obstet Gynecol 1983;62:26–30 (Level II-2)

36. Romero R, Jeanty P, Reece EA, Grannum P, Bracken M, Berkowitz R, et al. Sonographically monitored amniocen-

tesis to decrease intraoperative complications. Obstet Gynecol 1985;65:426–430 (Level II-2)

37. Leschot NJ, Verjaal M, Treffers PE. Risks of midtrimester amniocentesis; assessment in 3000 pregnancies. Br J Obstet Gynaecol 1985;92:804–807 (Level II-3)

38. Nicolaides K, Brizot M de L, Patel F, Snijders R. Comparison of chorionic villus sampling and amniocentesis for fetal karyotyping at 10–13 weeks' gestation. Lancet 1994;344:435–439 (Level II-1)

39. Johnson JM, Wilson RD, Winsor EJ, Singer J, Dansereau J, Kalousek DK. The early amniocentesis study: a randomized clinical trial of early amniocentesis versus midtrimester amniocentesis. Fetal Diagn Ther 1996;11: 85–93 (Level I)

40. Sundberg K, Bang J, Smidt-Jensen S, Brocks V, Lundsteen C, Parner J, et al. Randomised study of risk of fetal loss related to early amniocentesis versus chorionic villus sampling. Lancet 1997;350:697–703 (Level I)

41. Randomised trial to assess safety and fetal outcome of early and midtrimester amniocentesis. The Canadian Early and Mid-trimester Amniocentesis Trial (CEMAT) Group. Lancet 1998;351:242–247 (Level I)

42. Infection and chorionic villus sampling [letter]. Lancet 1985;2:609–610 (Level III)

43. Brambati B, Oldrini A, Ferrazzi E, Lanzani A. Chorionic villus sampling: an analysis of the obstetric experience of 1,000 cases. Prenat Diagn 1987;7:157–169 (Level II-3)

44. Brambati B, Lanzani A, Oldrini A. Transabdominal chorionic villus sampling. Clinical experience of 1159 cases. Prenat Diagn 1988;8:609–617 (Level III)

45. Multicentre randomised clinical trial of chorion villus sampling and amniocentesis. First report. Canadian Collaborative CVS-Amniocentesis Clinical Trial Group. Lancet 1989;1(8628):1–6 (Level I)

46. Rhoads GG, Jackson LG, Schlesselman SE, de la Cruz FF, Desnick RJ, Golbus MS, et al. The safety and efficacy of chorionic villus sampling for early prenatal diagnosis of cytogenetic abnormalities. N Engl J Med 1989;320: 609–617 (Level I)

47. Ledbetter DH, Martin AO, Verlinsky Y, Pergament E, Jackson L, Yang-Feng T, et al. Cytogenetic results of chorionic villus sampling: high success rate and diagnostic accuracy in the United States collaborative study. Am J Obstet Gynecol 1990;162:495–501 (Level II-2)

48. Medical Research Council European trial of chorion villus sampling. MRC working party on the evaluation of chorion villus sampling. Lancet 1991;337:1491–1499 (Level I)

49. Kuliev A, Jackson L, Froster U, Brambati B, Simpson JL, Verlinsky Y, et al. Chorionic villus sampling safety. Report of World Health Organization/EURO meeting in association with the Seventh International Conference on Early Prenatal Diagnosis of Genetic Diseases, Tel-Aviv, Israel, May 21, 1994. Am J Obstet Gynecol 1996;174:807–811 (Level III)

50. Holmes LB. Report of National Institute of Child Health and Human Development Workshop on Chorionic Villus Sampling and Limb and Other Defects, October 20, 1992. Teratology 1993;48:7–13 (Level III)

51. Botto LD, Olney RS, Mastroiacovo P, Khoury MJ, Moore CA, Alo CJ, et al. Chorionic villus sampling and transverse digital deficiencies: evidence for anatomic and gestational-age specificity of the digital deficiencies in two studies. Am J Med Genet 1996;62:173–178 (Level II-2)

52. Ghidini A, Sepulveda W, Lockwood CJ, Romero R. Complications of fetal blood sampling. Am J Obstet Gynecol 1993;168:1339–1344 (Level III)

53. Bromley B, Lieberman E, Laboda L, Benacerraf BR. Echogenic intracardiac focus: a sonographic sign for fetal Down syndrome. Obstet Gynecol 1995;86:998–1001 (Level II-3)

54. Petrikovsky BM, Challenger M, Wyse LJ. Natural history of echogenic foci within ventricles of fetal heart. Ultrasound Obstet Gynecol 1995;5:92–94 (Level III)

55. Vintzileos AM, Egan JF. Adjusting the risk for trisomy 21 on the basis of second-trimester ultrasonography. Am J Obstet Gynecol 1995;172:837–844 (Level II-3)

56. Bahado-Sing RO, Deren O, Tan A, D'Ancona RL, Hunter D, Copel JA, et al. Ultrasonographically adjusted midtrimester risk of trisomy 21 and significant chromosomal defects in advanced maternal age. Am J Obstet Gynecol 1996;175:1563–1568 (Level II-3)

57. Nyberg DA, Luthy DA, Cheng EY, Sheley RC, Resta RG, Williams MA. Role of prenatal ultrasonography in women with positive screen for Down syndrome on the basis of maternal serum markers. Am J Obstet Gynecol 1995;173: 1030–1035 (Level II-3)

58. Sohl BD, Scioscia AL, Budorick NE, Moore TR. Utility of minor ultrasonographic markers in the prediction of abnormal fetal karyotype at a prenatal diagnostic center. Am J Obstet Gynecol 1999;181:898–903 (Level II-3)

59. Vintzileos AM, Guzman ER, Smulian JC, Day-Salvatore DL, Knuppel RA. Indication-specific accuracy of second-trimester genetic ultrasonography for the detection of trisomy 21. Am J Obstet Gynecol 1999;181(5 Pt 1): 1045–1048 (Level II-3)

60. Bromley B, Lieberman E, Benacerraf BR. The incorporation of maternal age into the sonographic scoring index for the detection at 14–20 weeks of fetuses with Down's syndrome. Ultrasound Obstet Gynecol 1997;10:321–324 (Level II-2)

61. Bromley B, Shipp T, Benacerraf BR. Genetic sonogram scoring index: accuracy and clinical utility. J Ultrasound Med 1999;18:523–528; quiz 529–530 [erratum J Ultrasound Med 1999;18:594] (Level II-3)

62. Landwehr JB Jr, Johnson MP, Hume RF, Yaron Y, Sokol RJ, Evans MI. Abnormal nuchal findings on screening ultrasonography: aneuploidy stratification on the basis of ultrasonographic anomaly and gestational age at detection. Am J Obstet Gynecol 1996;175:995–999 (Level II-3)

63. Bahado-Singh R, Oz U, Kovanci E, Cermik D, Copel J, Mahoney MJ, et al. A high-sensitivity alternative to "routine" genetic amniocentesis: multiple urinary analytes, nuchal thickness, and age. Am J Obstet Gynecol 1999; 180(1 Pt 1):169–173 (Level II-3)

64. Gross SJ, Shulman LP, Tolley EA, Emerson DS, Felker RE, Simpson JL, et al. Isolated fetal choroid plexus cysts

and trisomy 18: a review and meta-analysis. Am J Obstet Gynecol 1995;172:83–87 (Meta-analysis)

65. Gupta JK, Khan KS, Thornton JG, Lilford RJ. Management of fetal choroid plexus cysts. Br J Obstet Gynaecol 1997;104:881–886 (Level III)

66. Brown T, Kliewer MA, Hertzberg BS, Ruiz C, Stamper TH, Rosnes J, et al. A role for maternal serum screening in detecting chromosomal abnormalities in fetuses with isolated choroid plexus cysts: a prospective multicentre study. Prenat Diagn 1999;19:405–410 (Level II-2)

67. Sullivan A, Giudice T, Vavelidis F, Thiagarajah S. Choroid plexus cysts: Is biochemical testing a valuable adjunct to targeted ultrasonography? Am J Obstet Gynecol 1999;181: 260–265 (Level II-2)

68. Wenstrom KD, Desai R, Owen J, DuBard MB, Boots L. Comparison of multiple-marker screening with amniocentesis for detection of fetal aneuploidy in women equal to or greater than 35. Am J Obstet Gynecol 1995;173: 1287–1292 (Level II-2)

69. Jenkins TM, Wapner RJ. The challenge of prenatal diagnosis in twin pregnancies. Curr Opin Obstet Gynecol 2000;12:87–92 (Level III)

70. Meyers C, Adam R, Dungan J, Prenger V. Aneuploidy in twin gestations: when is maternal age advanced? Obstet Gynecol 1997;89:248–251 (Level II-3)

71. Rodis JF, Egan JF, Craffey A, Ciarleglio L, Greenstein RM, Scorza WE. Calculated risk of chromosomal abnormalities in twin gestations. Obstet Gynecol 1990;76: 1037–1041 (Level III)

72. Librach CL, Doran TA, Benzie RJ, Jones JM. Genetic amniocentesis in seventy twin pregnancies. Am J Obstet Gynecol 1984;148:585–591 (Level II-3)

73. Wapner RJ, Johnson A, Davis G, Urban A, Morgan P, Jackson L. Prenatal diagnosis in twin gestations: a comparison between second-trimester amniocentesis and first-trimester chorionic villus sampling. Obstet Gynecol 1993;82:49–56 (Level II-2)

74. De Catte L, Liebaers I, Foulon W, Bonduelle M, Van Assche E. First trimester chorionic villus sampling in twin gestations. Am J Perinatol 1996;13:413–417 (Level II-2)

75. van den Berg C, Braat AP, Van Opstal D, Halley DJ, Kleijer WJ, den Hollander NS, et al. Amniocentesis or chorionic villus sampling in multiple gestations? Experience with 500 cases. Prenat Diagn 1999;19: 234–244 (Level II-3)

76. Clark SL, DeVore GR. Prenatal diagnosis for couples who would not consider abortion. Obstet Gynecol 1989;73: 1035–1037 (Level III)

The MEDLINE database, the Cochrane Library, and ACOG's own internal resources and documents were used to conduct a literature search to locate relevant articles published between January 1985 and April 2000. The search was restricted to articles published in the English language. Priority was given to articles reporting results of original research, although review articles and commentaries also were consulted. Abstracts of research presented at symposia and scientific conferences were not considered adequate for inclusion in this document. Guidelines published by organizations or institutions such as the National Institutes of Health and the American College of Obstetricians and Gynecologists were reviewed, and additional studies were located by reviewing bibliographies of identified articles. When reliable research was not available, expert opinions from obstetrician–gynecologists were used.

Studies were reviewed and evaluated for quality according to the method outlined by the U.S. Preventive Services Task Force:

I Evidence obtained from at least one properly designed randomized controlled trial.

II-1 Evidence obtained from well-designed controlled trials without randomization.

II-2 Evidence obtained from well-designed cohort or case–control analytic studies, preferably from more than one center or research group.

II-3 Evidence obtained from multiple time series with or without the intervention. Dramatic results in uncontrolled experiments also could be regarded as this type of evidence.

III Opinions of respected authorities, based on clinical experience, descriptive studies, or reports of expert committees.

Based on the highest level of evidence found in the data, recommendations are provided and graded according to the following categories:

Level A—Recommendations are based on good and consistent scientific evidence.

Level B—Recommendations are based on limited or inconsistent scientific evidence.

Level C—Recommendations are based primarily on consensus and expert opinion.

ISSN 1099-3630

The American College of
Obstetricians and Gynecologists
409 12th Street, SW
PO Box 96920
Washington, DC 20090-6920

12345/54321

ACOG PRACTICE BULLETIN

CLINICAL MANAGEMENT GUIDELINES FOR
OBSTETRICIAN–GYNECOLOGISTS
NUMBER 21, OCTOBER 2000

This Practice Bulletin was developed by the ACOG Committee on Practice Bulletins—Gynecology with the assistance of Linda A. Barbour, MD and Kathryn L. Hassell, MD. The information is designed to aid practitioners in making decisions about appropriate obstetric and gynecologic care. These guidelines should not be construed as dictating an exclusive course of treatment or procedure. Variations in practice may be warranted based on the needs of the individual patient, resources, and limitations unique to the institution or type of practice.

Prevention of Deep Vein Thrombosis and Pulmonary Embolism

In the United States, venous thromboembolism remains a leading cause of death and morbidity among hospitalized patients. Overall, approximately 60,000 deaths per year are attributed to venous thromboembolism and the subsequent complications, including postthrombotic syndrome, venous insufficiency, pulmonary hypertension, and pulmonary dysfunction (1). Venous thromboembolism often has no symptoms, and pulmonary embolism is not suspected clinically in 70–80% of patients in whom it is detected postmortem. Most patients who die from pulmonary embolism do so within 30 minutes of the event, reinforcing the need for rapid and accurate diagnosis. Fatal pulmonary embolism is a common preventable cause of death in hospitalized patients. Venous thromboembolism also predisposes patients to long-term morbidity from postthrombotic syndrome. The purpose of this document is to review the current literature on the prevention of thromboembolism in gynecologic patients, discuss the rationale behind sometimes conflicting guidelines, and offer evidence-based recommendations to address the most clinically relevant issues in the management of these patients.

Background

Detection of Deep Vein Thrombosis

Detection of deep vein thrombosis (DVT) is difficult, especially when patients are asymptomatic. Thus, the occurrence of venous thromboembolism in surgical patients varies from one study to another. Most trials examining the efficacy of DVT prophylaxis in general surgical and gynecologic patients have used the fibrinogen I-125 uptake test to diagnose DVT. This technique is sensitive for detecting DVT only distally (calf) and is poor at detecting DVT in the upper thigh (2, 3). Because of concerns about the transmission of bloodborne diseases, the fibrinogen I-125 uptake test is no longer commercially available in the United States or in many European countries. Equally inhibiting is the limited sensitivity and predictive value of duplex compression ultrasonography and impedance plethysmography to detect asymptomatic proximal vein thrombosis (4–8). Compression ultrasound examination of the femoral and popliteal veins and calf trifurcation has been found to be a highly sensitive (>90%) and specific (>99%) method of detecting proximal vein DVT, but less reliable (50%) for detecting calf vein DVT (6, 8).

Diagnosis of pelvic vein thrombosis and internal iliac thrombosis is exceedingly difficult even with magnetic resonance imaging, which is considered the imaging modality of choice (9). Fatal pulmonary emboli have been reported at postmortem examination to be from internal iliac or pelvic veins, for which there is no highly sensitive diagnostic imaging technique. Because diagnosis is difficult, perioperative prophylaxis has become the mainstay of management.

Prophylaxis in Gynecologic Surgery

The prevalence of venous thromboembolism after surgery varies and depends on multiple risk factors. Most events occur within 7 days postoperatively in gynecologic surgical patients; however, patients continue to be at risk for the first 3 weeks after discharge, probably secondary to decreased ambulation. Patients undergoing surgery for cancer or orthopedic surgery are at the highest risk for later complications from venous thromboembolism; the risk of pulmonary embolism continues for 30 days after surgery (10). Postoperative venous thromboembolism, as diagnosed by the fibrinogen I-125 uptake test, ranges from 7% to 29% in general gynecologic surgery and up to 45% in patients with malignant disease (11–13). Pulmonary embolism occurs in 0.1–5% of cases depending on the level of risk. Unfortunately, pulmonary embolism occurs without clinical evidence of DVT in 50–80% of cases and is fatal in approximately 10–20% of cases (14).

In a univariate analysis of all characteristics identified to be statistically significantly related to venous thromboembolism, significant variables included recurrent malignant disease, a prior history of DVT, duration of anesthesia greater than 5 hours, prior pelvic radiation, venous stasis changes or venous varicosities, and age older than 45 years (11). The same analysis concluded that the type of surgery, specifically radical vulvectomy

with inguinal lymphadenopathy or pelvic exenteration (ie, surgeries that result in extensive periods of immobilization), was a significant variable in determining risk.

Hypercoagulable States

It is now estimated that nearly half of patients with thrombosis have an identifiable thrombotic disorder (15, 16) as a result of the discovery of the factor V Leiden mutation (resistance to activated protein C) and the prothrombin gene mutation G20210A. The most commonly identified hypercoagulable states are listed in Table 1. It has been observed that approximately 50–60% of patients with a hereditary form of thrombosis will not experience a thrombotic event until an environmental risk factor such as oral contraceptive use, pregnancy, orthopedic trauma, immobilization, or surgery is present (17, 18). Currently, the coexistence of multiple inherited risk factors has been acknowledged, which markedly increases the risk of thrombosis (16). Antiphospholipid antibody syndrome is an acquired hypercoagulable state that often manifests as venous or arterial thrombosis, thrombocytopenia, recurrent fetal loss, intrauterine growth restriction, or early preeclampsia (19, 20). Hyperhomocystinemia may be acquired or inherited and is associated with an increased risk of venous thromboembolism and early atherosclerotic disease with arterial thrombosis.

Preoperative patients should be classified according to levels of risk of thrombosis to determine the benefits and risks of pharmacologic and physical methods of preventing venous thromboembolism. Table 2 summarizes the classification of risk level based on published data.

Prophylaxis Alternatives

Graduated Compression Stockings

The use of graduated compression stockings, which reduce stasis, is by far the simplest of the prophylactic approaches and has the advantages of being inexpensive, easy to use, and free of side effects if properly fitted (21). Graduated compression stockings reduce the prevalence of DVT (especially calf) in medium-risk patients when compared with placebo according to a meta-analysis of all randomized controlled trials (21), including one study of gynecologic surgery (22). However, patients with malignant disease and other high-risk conditions have not been evaluated in sufficient numbers to reach conclusions about the use of graduated compression stockings in these settings (23).

Pneumatic Compression

If used at induction of anesthesia and continued until patients are fully ambulatory, pneumatic compression

Table 1. Common Hypercoagulable States

Abnormality	Prevalence in Patients with Thrombosis	Testing Methods	Can patients be tested during pregnancy?	Is the test reliable during acute thrombosis?	Is the test reliable while on anti-coagulation?
Factor V Leiden	40–70%*	APC resistance assay	No	Yes	Yes
		DNA analysis	Yes	Yes	Yes
Prothrombin gene mutation G20210A	8–30%[†]	DNA analysis	Yes	Yes	Yes
Antiphospholipid antibody	10–15%[‡]	Functional assay (eg, dilute Russell viper venom time)	Yes	Yes	Yes
		Anticardiolipin antibodies	Yes	Yes	Yes
		β_2-Glycoprotein-1 antibodies	Yes	Yes	Yes
Protein C deficiency	—	Protein C activity	Yes	No	No
Protein S deficiency	10–15%[§]	Protein S total and free antigen	Yes	No	No
AT-III deficiency	—	AT-III activity	Yes	No	No
Hyperhomocystinemia	8–25%	Fasting plasma homocystine	Yes	Unclear	Yes

* Bokarewa MI, Bremme K, Blombäck M. Arg[506]-Gln mutation in factor V and risk of thrombosis during pregnancy. Br J Haematol 1996;92:473–478; Hellgren M, Svensson PJ, Dahlbäck B. Resistance to activated protein C as a basis for venous thromboembolism associated with pregnancy and oral contraceptives. Am J Obstet Gynecol 1995;173:210–213; Faioni EM, Razzari C, Martinelli I, Panzeri D, Franchi F, Mannucci PM. Resistance to activated protein C in unselected patients with arterial and venous thrombosis. Am J Hematol 1997;55:59–64

† Grandone E, Margaglione M, Colaizzo D, D'Andrea G, Cappucci G, Brancaccio V, et al. Genetic susceptibility to pregnancy-related venous thromboembolism: roles of factor V Leiden, prothrombin G20210A, and methylenetetrahydrofolate reductase C677T mutations. Am J Obstet Gynecol 1998;179:1324–1328; Martinelli I, Taioli E, Bucciarelli P, Akhavan S, Mannucci PM. Interaction between the G20210A mutation of the prothrombin gene and oral contraceptive use in deep vein thrombosis. Arterioscler Thromb Vasc Biol 1999;19:700–703; Salomon O, Steinberg DM, Zivelin A, Gitel S, Dardik R, Rosenberg N, et al. Single and combined prothrombotic factors in patients with idiopathic venous thromboembolism: prevalence and risk assessment. Arterioscler Thromb Vasc Biol 1999;19:511–518

‡ Ginsberg JS, Wells PS, Brill-Edwards P, Donovan D, Moffat K, Johnston M, et al. Antiphospholipid antibodies and venous thromboembolism. Blood 1995;86:3685–3691

§ Aiach M, Borgel D, Gaussem P, Emmerich J, Alhenc-Gelas M, Gandrille S. Protein C and protein S deficiencies. Semin Hematol 1997;34:205–216; De Stefano V, Leone G, Mastrangelo S, Tripodi A, Rodeghiero F, Castaman G, et al. Clinical manifestations and management of inherited thrombophilia: retrospective analysis and follow-up after diagnosis of 238 patients with congenital deficiency of antithrombin III, protein C, protein S. Thromb Haemost 1994;72:352–358; Pabinger I, Schneider B. Thrombotic risk in hereditary antithrombin III, protein C, or protein S deficiency. A cooperative, retrospective study. Gesellschaft fur Thrombose- und Hamostaseforschung (GTH) Study Group on Natural Inhibitors. Arterioscler Thromb Vasc Biol 1996;16:742–748

appears to be effective in reducing DVT in medium-risk and high-risk patients (21, 23–25). Pneumatic compression may be useful in reducing leg DVT in high-risk patients with malignant disease; however, its efficacy in preventing pulmonary embolism is unknown because of limited sample sizes (26). Patient compliance is essential for the effectiveness of pneumatic compression.

Low-Dose Heparin

Low-dose unfractionated heparin has been shown to be effective as prophylaxis for DVT and pulmonary embolism in moderate-risk patients without underlying malignancy or other clinical risk factors. A review of ran-

domized trials published before 1988, which included gynecologic patients, showed that low-dose heparin decreased DVT by nearly 70% and pulmonary embolism by 40–50% (27). Unfractionated heparin, 5,000 U administered every 8 hours postoperatively, does appear to be effective prophylaxis for DVT in patients undergoing gynecologic oncologic surgery, as demonstrated in a randomized unblinded trial (28). Although the efficacy in reducing postoperative venous thrombosis was similar between low-dose heparin and intermittent pneumatic calf compression, patients receiving low-dose heparin required significantly more postoperative transfusions (25). In a randomized, multicenter, double-blinded trial

Table 2. Classification of Risk Levels for Venous Thromboembolism Among Gynecologic Surgery Patients

Classification	Definition
Low risk (<3% risk of DVT*)	Age ≤40 y and Surgery lasting <30 min
Moderate risk (10–40% risk of DVT)	Age >40 y and Surgery of any duration No other clinical risk factors
High risk (40–70% risk of DVT; 1–5% risk of pulmonary embolism)	Age >40 y plus risk factors: • Prior DVT or pulmonary embolism • Varicose veins • Infection • Malignancy • Estrogen therapy • Obesity • Prolonged surgery

*DVT indicates deep vein thrombosis.

Data from NIH Consensus Conference. Prevention of venous thrombosis and pulmonary embolism. JAMA 1986;256:744–749

of 631 patients with evaluable venograms who were undergoing abdominal or pelvic surgery for cancer, low-dose heparin, 5,000 U every 8 hours, was as good as low-molecular-weight heparin (LMWH) (enoxaparin, 40 mg once a day) in the prevention of DVT (29). A trial of patients undergoing gynecologic surgery, in which 84% of the patients had underlying malignancy, used two different preoperative regimens of unfractionated heparin and compared them with no perioperative prophylaxis. The findings of this study suggest that two to nine doses of heparin preoperatively were not statistically better in preventing DVT than only one preoperative dose of 5,000 U administered 2 hours before the surgery (28). Both regimens used heparin every 8 hours postoperatively until discharge.

Low-Molecular-Weight Heparin

Low-molecular-weight heparin has been used in numerous trials for prophylaxis in abdominal surgery with at least the same efficacy as unfractionated heparin in preventing DVT. This finding has been substantiated in a meta-analysis of 36 double-blinded randomized controlled trials, 25 of which were in the general surgery population (30, 31). Some data suggest there is a lower bleeding risk with LMWH compared with unfractionated heparin (30). Once-daily administration and a lower rate of heparin-induced thrombocytopenia are additional advantages of LMWH over unfractionated heparin (23). A randomized, double-blinded multicenter trial that used

the fibrinogen I-125 uptake test compared two different doses of dalteparin (2,500 antifactor-Xa U versus 5,000 antifactor-Xa U) in the general surgery population in which 66% of patients had malignant disease (32). It found the efficacy overall was better in the high-dose LMWH group than in the low-dose LMWH group (6.6% DVT and 12.7% DVT, respectively) in preventing DVT, but bleeding complications were higher in the high-dose group (4.7% versus 2.7%). However, in the subgroup with malignant disease, efficacy remained better in the high-dose group than the low-dose group (8.5% DVT versus 14.9% DVT) but bleeding complications were no different (4.6% versus 3.6%). In a randomized study of 80 patients undergoing pelvic or abdominal surgery for malignancy that used the fibrinogen I-125 uptake test, dalteparin (5,000 antifactor-Xa U) was equally effective as unfractionated heparin, 5,000 U administered every 8 hours. Seventy-five percent of the patients had gynecologic cancers, and there was no difference in blood loss between the groups (33).

Anesthesia Concerns

The use of major conduction anesthesia (spinal or epidural) in patients receiving heparin or LMWH thromboembolic prophylaxis is controversial (34). Intraoperative or postoperative anticoagulation after regional anesthesia is thought to be safe; however, the safety of LMWH, unfractionated heparin, or oral anticoagulants administered before the procedure is unclear. In a retrospective review of 61 reported cases of spinal hematoma associated with epidural or spinal anesthesia, 42 (61%) were associated with a hemostatic abnormality (35). At least 25 patients received heparin intravenously or subcutaneously, and in 15 of 32 patients with indwelling catheters, the spinal hematomas occurred immediately after the removal of the epidural catheter. Unfractionated low-dose heparin appeared not to pose a significant risk for spinal hematoma in over 5,000 patients who received it in combination with a single-dose spinal or epidural anesthesia, nor did antiplatelet prophylaxis (36). Low-molecular-weight heparin, however, may pose a risk if it is used preoperatively, intraoperatively, or within 3 hours postoperatively in patients receiving continuous epidural analgesia. In 1997, the U.S. Food and Drug Administration issued a public health advisory regarding reported cases of epidural or spinal hematomas with concurrent use of enoxaparin and spinal or epidural anesthesia or spinal puncture (37). Many of the epidural or spinal hematomas caused neurologic injury, including long-term or permanent paralysis, and approximately 75% of the patients were elderly women undergoing orthopedic surgery.

Clinical Considerations and Recommendations

▶ *Who are candidates for perioperative DVT thromboprophylaxis?*

Candidates for surgical prophylaxis include patients who are found to have deficiencies of protein C, protein S, or antithrombin III (AT-III), who have the factor V Leiden or prothrombin gene mutation G20210A without a personal history of thrombosis, or who experience orthopedic trauma (15, 18, 38–40), especially if they have a strong family history of thrombosis.

In addition, Table 2 outlines a risk stratification adopted from the 1986 National Institutes of Health Consensus Conference (41). Most of the evidence for determining risk status was obtained from the control arms of more than 100 trials conducted primarily among patients older than 40 years who were undergoing general surgery.

▶ *Which prophylactic methods should be considered for low-, medium-, and high-risk patients undergoing gynecologic surgery?*

Patients in the low-risk category (as defined in Table 2) who are undergoing gynecologic surgery probably do not need any thromboprophylactic agent as long as they are quickly mobilized.

Patients in the moderate-risk category would likely benefit from prophylaxis with either graduated compression stockings, pneumatic compression, low-dose unfractionated heparin (5,000 U every 8 hours) in which the first dose is given before surgery, or low-dose LMWH (dalteparin, 2,500 U once a day, or enoxaparin, 40 mg once a day). However, the need for prophylaxis should include consideration of the length and complexity of surgery, the patient's age, and the evaluation of other risk factors. In the United States, dalteparin and enoxaparin are considerably more expensive alternatives to standard heparin and have not been shown to be significantly more efficacious or associated with less bleeding risks in comparison with low-dose unfractionated heparin in moderate-risk patients. Prophylaxis with thigh-high graduated compression stockings has not been as extensively studied for moderate-risk patients compared with standard heparin.

High-risk patients should be offered standard heparin, 5,000 U every 8 hours (28). A more expensive alternative for high-risk patients is LMWH given as either dalteparin, 5,000 antifactor-Xa U once a day, or enoxa-

parin, 40 mg once a day (the first dose given the evening before surgery). However, it is not clear that the latter approach offers any advantage or is significantly more efficacious (29, 32). Pneumatic compression appears to be as effective (23) but has not been as well studied as heparin and LMWH.

Adding graduated compression stockings or pneumatic compression to anticoagulant therapy may be a good alternative for high-risk patients, especially those undergoing radical vulvectomy with inguinal lymphadenectomy or pelvic exenteration for malignancy (23, 25), although no clinical trials have confirmed this approach.

▶ *Should patients discontinue oral contraceptives or hormone replacement therapy before surgery?*

There are no studies to confirm the clinical benefit of stopping oral contraceptives preoperatively (42). The hypercoagulable changes induced by oral contraceptives do not return to normal for 4–6 weeks after discontinuation of therapy (43). The risk of postoperative thromboembolism has been reported to be 0.96% for oral contraceptive users and 0.5% for nonusers (44). However, the risk of stopping oral contraceptives 4–6 weeks before major surgery must be balanced against the risks of pregnancy (which carries a much higher risk of DVT and pulmonary embolism than does oral contraceptive use), the effects of surgery and anesthesia on pregnancy, and the possibility of subsequent termination of pregnancy with its associated physical and psychologic risks.

Discontinuation of hormone replacement therapy (HRT) before major gynecologic surgery to prevent deep vein thrombosis or pulmonary embolism has not been evaluated in randomized clinical trials. However, three retrospective case-control studies have evaluated the risk of hospital admission for deep vein thrombosis in HRT users (45–47). These studies reported that the current users of HRT had an increased risk of VTE (odds ratio 2.1 to 3.6) when compared with matched HRT nonusers, and that past use did not affect this risk. However, the absolute risk for both users and nonusers of HRT was low. One analysis of nearly 350,000 women aged 50–79 years reported that of these, 292 women were admitted to the hospital with DVT or pulmonary embolism, which represents only a modest increase in morbidity (risk of 1.3 per 10,000 per year for nonusers; risk of less than 2 additional cases per 10,000 women per year in HRT users) (47). For women with other risk factors who are undergoing gynecologic surgery, the benefit of stopping HRT has not yet been established.

▶ *Which patients should be tested for clotting abnormalities, and which tests should be ordered?*

Because of its high prevalence in the Caucasian population, all patients who are not Hispanic, Asian, or African American who have a history of DVT may be tested for the factor V Leiden mutation (16, 48–54). In non-Caucasian patients, the decision to test should be individualized. Patients with histories of extensive or recurrent thrombosis or family histories of thrombosis may have the factor V Leiden mutation in combination with another congenital or acquired disorder (55). Patients with a strong family history of thrombosis who are negative for the factor V Leiden mutation may benefit from testing for the prothrombin gene mutation G20210A and deficiencies in the natural inhibitors, including protein C, protein S, and AT-III. Patients with a history of thrombosis, recurrent fetal loss, early or severe preeclampsia, severe unexplained intrauterine growth restriction, or unexplained thrombocytopenia may be tested for antiphospholipid antibodies. Fasting plasma homocystine levels may be assessed, especially in women of childbearing age who have had venous or arterial thrombosis, because elevated levels can be treated with vitamins (folic acid, vitamin B_{12}, and vitamin B_6). The specific tests and optimal timing for testing are described in Table 1.

▶ *Should women on prolonged heparin be evaluated for heparin-induced osteoporosis or heparin-induced thrombocytopenia?*

Heparin-induced osteoporosis appears to occur predominantly in patients taking heparin for 7 weeks or longer (56, 57) and is not an issue for those taking prophylactic or short-term doses.

Heparin-induced thrombocytopenia is uncommon with the use of porcine heparin (1–3%) and is less common with LMWH (<1%), but immune-related thrombocytopenia can have severe thrombotic consequences (58). Platelet counts should be monitored at the initiation of standard heparin therapy and periodically up to 15 days after starting heparin (59). If the platelet count is unchanged at that time, further platelet counts are not needed because the vast majority of immune, heparin-induced thrombocytopenia occurs within 15 days of starting standard heparin therapy. If confirmed, heparin therapy should be stopped immediately. A low-molecular-weight heparinoid (danaparoid sodium) is available in the United States and was shown to be efficacious in

93% of 88 patients with heparin-induced thrombocytopenia and thrombosis not related to pregnancy (60). Lepirudin (recombinant hirudin), a direct thrombin inhibitor, also is available for intravenous use in patients with heparin-induced thrombocytopenia (59).

▶ *What special considerations should be given when using low-molecular-weight heparin in patients undergoing regional anesthesia?*

Low-molecular-weight heparin has a longer half-life than standard heparin, and its anticoagulant activity cannot be measured using an activated partial thromboplastin time. If used in low doses as a once-a-day regimen, at least 12 hours should lapse after administration before offering central neural blockade. No regional anesthesia should be employed within 12 hours of an injection of LMWH, and LMWH should be withheld for at least 2 hours after removal of an epidural catheter (35, 36, 61). The safety of a twice-daily dose of LMWH in patients receiving epidural anesthesia has not been studied sufficiently, and it is not known whether 24 hours is an adequate amount of time to wait after the last injection. In institutions in which an antifactor-Xa level can be obtained in a timely manner, it may be reasonable to offer spinal or epidural anesthesia as long as the antifactor-Xa levels are not above the prophylactic range. However, the safety of this practice has not been evaluated prospectively.

▶ *Which prophylactic methods are considered cost-effective?*

It is estimated that half of patients with proximal DVT and one third of patients with distal DVT develop a postthrombotic syndrome characterized by pain, swelling, and occasional ulceration of the skin and legs (62). Prophylaxis with either graduated compression stockings, pneumatic compression, low-dose standard heparin, or LMWH is less expensive than no prophylaxis in patients undergoing general abdominal surgery (63, 64). Routine surveillance is the most expensive strategy because of the lack of sensitivity of noninvasive tests to diagnose DVT (63). Although a cost analysis in Europe determined LMWH to be more cost-effective than unfractionated heparin (63), LMWH is substantially more expensive in the United States than in Europe. A cost-analysis in the United States determined that pneumatic compression was more cost-effective than either LMWH or unfractionated heparin (65).

Summary

The following recommendations are based on good and consistent scientific evidence (Level A):

▶ Alternatives for thromboprophylaxis for moderate-risk patients undergoing gynecologic surgery include the following:

1. Thigh-high graduated compression stockings placed intraoperatively and continued until the patient is fully ambulatory

2. Pneumatic compression placed intraoperatively and continued until the patient is fully ambulatory

3. Unfractionated heparin (5,000 U) administered 2 hours before surgery and continued postoperatively every 8 hours until discharge

4. Low-molecular-weight heparin (dalteparin, 2,500 antifactor-Xa U, or enoxaparin, 40 mg) administered 12 hours before surgery and once a day postoperatively until discharge

▶ Alternatives for prophylaxis for high-risk patients undergoing gynecologic surgery, especially for malignancy, include:

1. Pneumatic compression placed intraoperatively and continued until the patient is fully ambulatory

2. Unfractionated heparin (5,000 U) administered 8 hours before surgery and continued postoperatively until discharge

3. Dalteparin (5,000 antifactor-Xa U) administered 12 hours before surgery and then once a day thereafter

4. Enoxaparin (40 mg) administered 12 hours before surgery and then once a day thereafter

The following recommendations are based primarily on consensus and expert opinion (Level C):

▶ Low-risk patients who are undergoing gynecologic surgery do not require specific prophylaxis other than early ambulation.

▶ Postoperative prophylaxis should be continued for 7 days or until discharge.

References

1. Hirsh J, Hoak J. Management of deep vein thrombosis and pulmonary embolism. A statement for healthcare professionals. Council on Thrombosis (in consultation with the Council on Cardiovascular Radiology), American Heart Association. Circulation 1996;93:2212–2245 (Level III)

2. Lensing AW, Hirsh J. 125I-fibrinogen leg scanning: reassessment of its role for the diagnosis of venous thrombosis in post-operative patients. Thromb Haemost 1993;69:2–7 (Level III)

3. Weinmann EE, Salzman EW. Deep vein thrombosis. N Engl J Med 1994;331:1630–1641 (Level III)

4. Agnelli G, Cosmi B, Ranucci V, Renga C, Mosca S, Lupattelli L, et al. Impedance plethysmography in the diagnosis of asymptomatic deep vein thrombosis in hip surgery. A venography-controlled study. Arch Intern Med 1991;151:2167–2171 (Level II-2)

5. Borris LC, Christiansen HM, Lassen MR, Olsen AD, Schøtt P. Comparison of real-time B-mode ultrasonography and bilateral ascending phlebography for detection of postoperative deep vein thrombosis following elective hip surgery. The Venous Thrombosis Group. Thromb Haemost 1989;61:363–365 (Level II-2)

6. Jongbloets LM, Lensing AW, Koopman MM, Büller HR, ten Cate JW. Limitations of compression ultrasound for the detection of symptomless postoperative deep vein thrombosis. Lancet 1994;343:1142–1144 (Level II-2)

7. Lensing AW, Doris CI, McGrath FP, Cogo A, Sabine MJ, Ginsberg J, et al. A comparison of compression ultrasound with color Doppler ultrasound for the diagnosis of symptomless postoperative deep vein thrombosis. Arch Intern Med 1997;157:765–768 (Level II-2)

8. Wells PS, Lensing AW, Davidson BL, Prins MH, Hirsh J. Accuracy of ultrasound for the diagnosis of deep venous thrombosis in asymptomatic patients after orthopedic surgery. A meta-analysis. Ann Intern Med 1995;122:47–53 (Meta-analysis)

9. Spritzer CE, Evans AC, Kay HH. Magnetic resonance imaging of deep venous thrombosis in pregnant women with lower extremity edema. Obstet Gynecol 1995; 85:603–607 (Level III)

10. Bergqvist D. Prolonged prophylaxis against postoperative venous thromboembolism. Haemostasis 1996;26(suppl 4):379–387 (Level III)

11. Clarke-Pearson DL, DeLong ER, Synan IS, Coleman RE, Creasman WT. Variables associated with postoperative deep venous thrombosis: a prospective study of 411 gynecology patients and creation of a prognostic model. Obstet Gynecol 1987;69:146–150 (Level III)

12. Clarke-Pearson DL, Jelovsek FR, Creasman WT. Thromboembolism complicating surgery for cervical and uterine malignancy: incidence, risk factors, and prophylaxis. Obstet Gynecol 1983;61:87–94 (Level II-2)

13. Crandon AJ, Koutts J. Incidence of post-operative deep vein thrombosis in gynaecological oncology. Aust NZ J Obstet Gynaecol 1983;23:216–219 (Level III)

14. Farquharson DI, Orr JW Jr. Prophylaxis against thromboembolism in gynecologic patients. J Reprod Med 1984;29:845–862 (Level III)

15. Bauer KA. Management of patients with hereditary defects predisposing to thrombosis including pregnant women. Thromb Haemost 1995;74:94–100 (Level III)

16. Florell SR, Rodgers GM. Inherited thrombotic disorders: an update. Am J Hematol 1997;54:53–60 (Level III)

17. De Stefano V, Leone G, Mastrangelo S, Tripodi A, Rodeghiero F, Castaman G, et al. Clinical manifestations and management of inherited thrombophilia: retrospective analysis and follow-up after diagnosis of 238 patients with congenital deficiency of antithrombin III, protein C, protein S. Thromb Haemost 1994;72:352–358 (Level III)

18. Middledorp S, Henkens CM, Koopman MM, van Pampus EC, Hamulyák K, van der Meer J, et al. The incidence of venous thromboembolism in family members of patients with factor V Leiden mutation and venous thrombosis. Ann Intern Med 1998;128:15–20 (Level II-2)

19. Petri M. Pathogenesis and treatment of the antiphospholipid antibody syndrome. Med Clin North Am 1997;81:151–177 (Level III)

20. Shapiro GA. Antiphospholipid syndrome in obstetrics and gynecology. Semin Thromb Hemost 1994;20:64–70 (Level III)

21. Wells PS, Lensing AW, Hirsh J. Graduated compression stockings in the prevention of postoperative venous thromboembolism. A meta-analysis. Arch Intern Med 1994;154:67–72 (Meta-analysis)

22. Turner GM, Cole SE, Brooks JH. The efficacy of graduated compression stockings in the prevention of deep vein thrombosis after major gynaecological surgery. Br J Obstet Gynaecol 1984;91:588–591 (Level I)

23. Clagett GP, Anderson FA Jr, Heit J, Levine MN, Wheeler HB. Prevention of venous thromboembolism. Chest 1995;108 (suppl 4):312S–334S (Level III)

24. Clarke-Pearson DL, Synan IS, Hinshaw WM, Coleman RE, Creasman WT. Prevention of postoperative venous thromboembolism by external pneumatic calf compression in patients with gynecologic malignancy. Obstet Gynecol 1984;63:92–98 (Level I)

25. Clarke-Pearson DL, Synan IS, Dodge R, Soper JT, Berchuck A, Coleman RE. A randomized trial of low-dose heparin and intermittent pneumatic calf compression for the prevention of deep venous thrombosis after gynecologic oncology surgery. Am J Obstet Gynecol 1993;168:1146–1153; discussion 1153–1154 (Level I)

26. Clagett GP, Reisch JS. Prevention of venous thromboembolism in general surgical patients. Results of meta-analysis. Ann Surg 1988;208:227–240 (Meta-analysis)

27. Collins R, Scrimgeour A, Yusuf S, Peto R. Reduction in fatal pulmonary embolism and venous thrombosis by perioperative administration of subcutaneous heparin. Overview of results of randomized trials in general orthopedic and urologic surgery. N Engl J Med 1988;318:1162–1173 (Level III)

28. Clarke-Pearson DL, DeLong E, Synan IS, Soper JT, Creasman WT, Coleman RE. A controlled trial of two low-dose-heparin regimens for the prevention of postoperative deep vein thrombosis. Obstet Gynecol 1990;75:684–689 (Level I)

29. Enoxacan Study Group. Efficacy and safety of enoxaparin versus unfractionated heparin for prevention of deep vein thrombosis in elective cancer surgery: a double-blind randomized multicentre trial with venographic assessment. Br J Surg 1997;84:1099–1103 (Level I)

30. Kakkar VV, Boeckl O, Boneu B, Bordenave L, Brehm OA, Brücke P, et al. Efficacy and safety of a low-molecular-weight heparin and standard unfractionated heparin for prophylaxis of postoperative venous thromboembolism: European multicenter trial. World J Surg 1997;21:2–8; discussion 8–9 (Level I)

31. Koch A, Bouges S, Ziegler S, Dinkel H, Daures JP, Victor N. Low molecular weight heparin and unfractionated heparin in thrombosis prophylaxis after major surgical intervention: update of previous meta-analyses. Br J Surg 1997;84:750–759 (Meta-analysis)

32. Bergqvist D, Burmark US, Flordal PA, Frisell J, Hallböök T, Hedberg M, et al. Low molecular weight heparin started before surgery as prophylaxis against deep vein thrombosis: 2500 versus 5000 XaI units in 2070 patients. Br J Surg 1995;82:496–501 (Level I)

33. Fricker JP, Vergnes Y, Schach R, Heitz A, Eber M, Grunebaum L, et al. Low dose heparin versus low molecular weight heparin (Kabi 2165, Fragmin) in the prophylaxis of thromboembolic complications of abdominal oncological surgery. Eur J Clin Invest 1988;18:561–567 (Level I)

34. Haljamäe H. Thromboprophylaxis, coagulation disorders, and regional anesthesia. Acta Anaesthesiol Scand 1996;40:1024–1040 (Level III)

35. Vandermeulen EP, Van Aken H, Vermylen J. Anticoagulants and spinal-epidural anesthesia. Anesth Analg 1994;79:1165–1177 (Level III)

36. Horlocker TT. Regional anesthesia and analgesia in the patient receiving thromboprophylaxis. Reg Anesth 1996;21:503–507 (Level III)

37. U.S. Department of Health and Human Services. FDA Public Health Advisory. Subject: Reports of epidural or spinal hematomas with the concurrent use of low molecular weight heparin and spinal/epidural anesthesia or spinal puncture. Rockville, Maryland: Food and Drug Administration, December 1997 (Level III)

38. Friederich PW, Sanson BJ, Simioni P, Zanardi S, Huisman MV, Kindt I, et al. Frequency of pregnancy-related venous thromboembolism in anticoagulant factor-deficient

women: implications for prophylaxis. Ann Intern Med 1996;125:955–960 (Level III)

39. Pabinger I, Schneider B. Thrombotic risk in hereditary antithrombin III, protein C, or protein S deficiency. A cooperative, retrospective study. Gesellschaft fur Thrombose- und Hamostaseforschung (GTH) Study Group on Natural Inhibitors. Arterioscler Thromb Vasc Biol 1996;16:742–748 (Level III)

40. Thomas DP, Roberts HR. Hypercoagulability in venous and arterial thrombosis. Ann Intern Med 1997;126: 638–644 (Level III)

41. Prevention of venous thrombosis and pulmonary embolism. NIH Consensus Development. JAMA 1986; 256:744–749 (Level III)

42. Hutchison GL. Oral contraception and post-operative thromboembolism: an epidemiological review. Scott Med J 1989;34:547–549 (Level III)

43. Robinson GE, Burren T, Mackie IJ, Bounds W, Walshe K, Faint R, et al. Changes in hemostasis after stopping the combined contraceptive pill: implications for major surgery. BMJ 1991;302:269–271 (Level III)

44. Vessey M, Mant D, Smith A, Yeates D. Oral contraceptives and venous thromboembolism: findings in a large prospective study. Br Med J (Clin Res Ed) 1986;292:526 (Level II-2)

45. Daly E, Vessey MP, Hawkins MM, Carson JL, Gough P, Marsh S. Risk of venous thromboembolism in users of hormone replacement therapy. Lancet 1996;348:977–980 (Level II-2)

46. Jick H, Derby LE, Myers MW, Vasilakis C, Newton KM. Risk of hospital admission for idiopathic venous thromboembolism among users of postmenopausal oestrogens. Lancet 1996;348:981–983 (Level II-2)

47. Perez Gutthann S, Garcia Rodríguez LA, Castellsague J, Duque Oliart A. Hormone replacement therapy and risk of venous thromboembolism: population based case-control study. BMJ 1997;314:796–800 (Level II-2)

48. Bokarewa MI, Bremme K, Blombäck M. Arg506-Gln mutation in factor V and risk of thrombosis during pregnancy. Br J Haematol 1996;92:473–478 (Level II-3)

49. Dahlbäck B. Resistance to activated protein C as risk factor for thrombosis: molecular mechanisms, laboratory investigation, and clinical management. Semin Hematol 1997;34:217–234 (Level III)

50. Dizon-Townson DS, Nelson LM, Jang H, Varner MW, Ward K. The incidence of the factor V Leiden mutation in an obstetric population and its relationship to deep vein thrombosis. Am J Obstet Gynecol 1997;176:883–886 (Level III)

51. Faioni EM, Razzari C, Martinelli I, Panzeri D, Franchi F, Mannucci PM. Resistance to activated protein C in unselected patients with arterial and venous thrombosis. Am J Haematol 1997;55:59–64 (Level II-2)

52. Hellgren M, Svensson PJ, Dahlbäck B. Resistance to activated protein C as a basis for venous thromboembolism associated with pregnancy and oral contraceptives. Am J Obstet Gynecol 1995;173:210–213 (Level II-2)

53. Rintelen C, Mannhalter C, Ireland H, Lane DA, Knöbl P, Lechner K, et al. Oral contraceptives enhance the risk of clinical manifestation of venous thrombosis at a young age in females homozygous for factor V Leiden. Br J Haematol 1996;93:487–490 (Level III)

54. Vandenbroucke JP, Koster T, Briët E, Reitsma PH, Bertina RM, Rosendaal FR. Increased risk of venous thrombosis in oral-contraceptive users who are carriers of factor V Leiden mutation. Lancet 1994;344:1453–1457 (Level II-2)

55. Rosendaal FR. Thrombosis in the young: epidemiology and risk factors. A focus on venous thrombosis. Thromb Haemost 1997;78:1–6 (Level III)

56. Barbour LA. Current concepts of anticoagulant therapy in pregnancy. Obstet Gynecol Clin North Am 1997;24: 499–521 (Level III)

57. Dahlman TC. Osteoporotic fractures and the recurrence of thromboembolism during pregnancy and the puerperium in 184 women undergoing thromboprophylaxis with heparin. Am J Obstet Gynecol 1993;168:1265–1270 (Level III)

58. Warkentin TE, Levine MN, Hirsh J, Horsewood P, Roberts RS, Gent M, et al. Heparin-induced thrombocytopenia in patients treated with low-molecular weight heparin or unfractionated heparin. N Engl J Med 1995;332: 1330–1335 (Level II-2)

59. Hirsh J, Warkentin TE, Raschke R, Granger C, Ohman EM, Dalen JE. Heparin and low-molecular-weight heparin: mechanism of action, pharmacokinetics, dosing considerations, monitoring, efficacy and safety. Chest 1998;114 (suppl 5):489S–510S (Level III)

60. Magnani HN. Heparin-induced thrombocytopenia (HIT): an overview of 230 patients treated with Orgaran (Org 10172). Thromb Haemost 1993;70:554–561 (Level II-3)

61. Hynson JM, Katz JA, Bueff HU. Epidural hematoma associated with enoxaparin. Anesth Analg 1996;82:1072–1075 (Level III)

62. Prandoni P, Lensing AW, Cogo A, Cuppini S, Villalta S, Carta M. The long-term clinical course of acute deep venous thrombosis. Ann Intern Med 1996;125:1–7 (Level III)

63. Bergqvist D, Lindgren B, Mätzsch T. Comparison of the cost of preventing postoperative deep vein thrombosis with either unfractionated or low molecular weight heparin. Br J Surg 1996;83:1548–1152 (Level II-2)

64. Bergqvist D, Jendteg S, Johansen L, Persson U, Ödegaard K. Cost of long-term complications of deep venous thrombosis of the lower extremities: an analysis of a defined patient population in Sweden. Ann Intern Med 1997;126:454–457 (Level II-2)

65. Maxwell GL, Myers ER, Clarke-Pearson DL. Cost-effectiveness of deep venous thrombosis prophylaxis in gynecologic oncology surgery. Obstet Gynecol 2000;95:206–214 (Level III)

The MEDLINE database, the Cochrane Library, and ACOG's own internal resources and documents were used to conduct a literature search to locate relevant articles published between January 1985 and April 2000. The search was restricted to articles published in the English language. Priority was given to articles reporting results of original research, although review articles and commentaries also were consulted. Abstracts of research presented at symposia and scientific conferences were not considered adequate for inclusion in this document. Guidelines published by organizations or institutions such as the National Institutes of Health and the American College of Obstetricians and Gynecologists were reviewed, and additional studies were located by reviewing bibliographies of identified articles. When reliable research was not available, expert opinions from obstetrician–gynecologists were used.

Studies were reviewed and evaluated for quality according to the method outlined by the U.S. Preventive Services Task Force:

I   Evidence obtained from at least one properly designed randomized controlled trial.

II-1   Evidence obtained from well-designed controlled trials without randomization.

II-2   Evidence obtained from well-designed cohort or case–control analytic studies, preferably from more than one center or research group.

II-3   Evidence obtained from multiple time series with or without the intervention. Dramatic results in uncontrolled experiments also could be regarded as this type of evidence.

III   Opinions of respected authorities, based on clinical experience, descriptive studies, or reports of expert committees.

Based on the highest level of evidence found in the data, recommendations are provided and graded according to the following categories:

Level A—Recommendations are based on good and consistent scientific evidence.

Level B—Recommendations are based on limited or inconsistent scientific evidence.

Level C—Recommendations are based primarily on consensus and expert opinion.

ISSN 1099-3630

The American College of Obstetricians and Gynecologists
409 12th Street, SW
PO Box 96920
Washington, DC 20090-6920   12345/43210

ACOG PRACTICE BULLETIN

CLINICAL MANAGEMENT GUIDELINES FOR
OBSTETRICIAN–GYNECOLOGISTS

NUMBER 4, MAY 1999

(Replaces Educational Bulletin Number 147, October 1990)

This Practice Bulletin was developed by the ACOG Committee on Practice Bulletins—Obstetrics with the assistance of Michael L. Socol, MD, and T. Flint Porter, MD, MPH. The information is designed to aid practitioners in making decisions about appropriate obstetric and gynecologic care. These guidelines should not be construed as dictating an exclusive course of treatment or procedure. Variations in practice may be warranted based on the needs of the individual patient, resources, and limitations unique to the institution or type of practice.

Prevention of Rh D Alloimmunization

Before the introduction of anti-D immune globulin (formerly referred to as Rho[D] immune globulin), hemolytic disease of the fetus and newborn affected 9–10% of pregnancies and was a major cause of perinatal morbidity and mortality (1, 2). Among Rh D-alloimmunized pregnancies, mild-to-moderate hemolytic anemia and hyperbilirubinemia occur in 25–30% of fetuses/neonates, and hydrops fetalis occurs in another 25% of such cases (3). The administration of anti-D immune globulin is successful in reducing the rate of developing antibodies to the D antigen. Protocols for the antenatal and postpartum administration of anti-D immune globulin have been responsible for the dramatic decrease in alloimmunization and subsequent hemolytic disease in the past two decades. However, Rh D alloimmunization remains a clinical concern, with many cases due to failure to follow established protocols. Finally, there is concern that overuse of anti-D immune globulin may lead to a worldwide shortage. The purpose of this document is to provide direction for the appropriate and efficient management of patients at risk in order to further decrease the frequency of Rh D alloimmunization.

Background

Nomenclature

Nomenclature of blood group systems, including the Rh system, may appear confusing to the clinician. According to the *American Medical Association Manual of Style*, erythrocyte antigen and phenotype terminology should use single letters or dual letters depending on the antigen in question (eg, O, AB, Le, Rh) (4). A second designation should be used for specific subtypes (eg, Rh D, Rh C). This publication uses the designation Rh D to signify the erythrocyte antigen.

Women who carry the Rh D antigen are identified as Rh D positive, and those who do not carry the Rh D antigen are identified as Rh D negative. The use of immune globulin to counter the Rh D antigen is referred to as anti-D immune globulin.

Causes of Rh D Alloimmunization

One study indicates that 17% of Rh D-negative women who do not receive anti-D immune globulin prophylaxis during pregnancy will become alloimmunized (5). Nearly 90% of these cases result from fetomaternal hemorrhage at delivery. Approximately 10% of cases result from spontaneous antenatal fetomaternal hemorrhage, and most of these cases occur in the third trimester. The amount of Rh D-positive blood required to cause alloimmunization is small. Most women who become alloimmunized do so as a result of fetomaternal hemorrhage of less than 0.1 mL (6).

Several first- and second-trimester clinical events may cause Rh D alloimmunization. Therapeutic and spontaneous abortions are associated respectively with a 4–5% and a 1.5–2% risk of alloimmunization in susceptible (nonalloimmunized) women (6–8). Ectopic pregnancy also is associated with alloimmunization in susceptible women. Threatened abortion infrequently causes alloimmunization, although approximately 10% of women with threatened abortion have evidence of fetomaternal hemorrhage (9).

Clinical procedures, which may breach the integrity of the choriodecidual space, also may cause Rh D alloimmunization. Chorionic villus sampling is associated with a 14% risk of fetomaternal hemorrhage (10) of more than 0.6 mL (11), and amniocentesis is associated with a 7–15% risk of fetomaternal hemorrhage, even if the placenta is not traversed (5, 12). Likewise, cordocentesis and other percutaneous fetal procedures pose a risk for fetomaternal hemorrhage, although the actual risk of alloimmunization has not been quantified (13, 14). External cephalic version, whether or not it is successful, results in fetomaternal hemorrhage in 2–6% of cases (15, 16).

Anti-D Immune Globulin to Prevent Alloimmunization

The correct administration of anti-D immune globulin dramatically reduces the rate of alloimmunization. Initial studies proved that the postpartum administration of a single dose of anti-D immune globulin to susceptible Rh D-negative women within 72 hours of delivery reduced the alloimmunization rate by 90% (17). It was subsequently recognized that third-trimester antenatal alloimmunization posed a lingering and significant problem; later it was shown that the routine antenatal administration of anti-D immune globulin to Rh D-negative women at 28–29 weeks

of gestation reduced the rate of third-trimester alloimmunization from nearly 2% to 0.1% (6). With the effectiveness of anti-D immune globulin clearly demonstrated, authorities recommended its administration to Rh D-negative women who were undergoing clinical events or procedures associated with potential fetomaternal hemorrhage.

In the United States, recommendations for the administration of anti-D immune globulin were introduced in the 1970s. The current antenatal immunoprophylaxis regimen of a single dose of 300 µg at 28 weeks of gestation was based on recommendations from the 1977 McMaster Conference, and is associated with a low failure rate (18). The efficacy of the single antenatal dose of 300 µg at 28 weeks of gestation is comparable to the same dose given at both 28 weeks and 34 weeks of gestation (6). In one study of antenatal prophylaxis, three women who delivered more than 12 weeks after their antenatal dose was administered became alloimmunized. Based on these limited data, some authorities recommend that if delivery has not occurred within 12 weeks of the injection, at 28 weeks of gestation, a second 300 µg dose of anti-D immune globulin should be given (5).

In the United Kingdom, recommendations (19, 20) differ somewhat from those in the United States in that antenatal prophylaxis is given at both 28 weeks and 34 weeks of gestation, and the dose for each antenatal administration, as well as the dose given after delivery, is 100 µg. These recommendations are based on two studies (21, 22) that demonstrated the superiority of a regimen of 100 µg of anti-D immune globulin at 28 weeks and 34 weeks of gestation and postpartum compared with a regimen of only postpartum administration. The British regimen uses less anti-D immune globulin (300 µg versus 600 µg) to achieve similarly low rates of alloimmunization (7, 20), but requires a third injection at 34 weeks of gestation.

Anti-D immune globulin is extracted by cold alcohol fractionation from plasma donated by individuals with high-titer D immune globulin G antibodies. It has been shown experimentally that one prophylactic dose of 300 µg of anti-D immune globulin can prevent Rh D alloimmunization after an exposure to up to 30 mL of Rh D-positive blood or 15 mL of fetal cells (23). For exposure to larger volumes of Rh D-positive blood, more anti-D immune globulin is required. Accordingly, the American Association of Blood Banks and the National Blood Transfusion Service of the United Kingdom recommend that Rh D-negative mothers delivering Rh D-positive infants undergo a test to screen for fetomaternal hemorrhage in excess of the amount covered by the standard dose of anti-D immune globulin. This test will determine if additional anti-D immune globulin is necessary (24, 25). In the past, the American College of Obstetricians and Gynecologists recommended that only women with certain high-risk conditions, such as those experiencing abruptio placenta or manual removal of the placenta, be screened for excess fetomaternal hemorrhage. However, this policy has been shown to miss 50% of cases requiring more than the standard postpartum dose of anti-D immune globulin (26).

The risk of transmission of viral infections (human immunodeficiency virus [HIV] and hepatitis B and hepatitis C viruses) through anti-D immune globulin is minimal to absent (27). All plasma lots used for the production of anti-D immune globulin have been tested for viral infection since 1985. Moreover, the fractionation process used to prepare anti-D immune globulin effectively removes any viral particles that may be present.

Failure to Prevent Rh D Alloimmunization

In spite of recommendations for immunoprophylaxis, 0.1–0.2% of susceptible Rh D-negative women still become alloimmunized (21). There are two primary reasons for the continuing problem.

One reason women become alloimmunized is failure to implement recommended immunoprophylaxis protocols, resulting in preventable Rh D alloimmunizations. Two recent studies from the United Kingdom emphasize the scope of the problem. One study of more than 900 Rh D-negative women reported that only 59% received recommended treatment with anti-D immune globulin after potentially alloimmunizing clinical events (8). Another study showed that 16% of 63 cases of Rh D alloimmunization occurred because of failure to follow recommendations for administration of anti-D immune globulin (28). Preventable Rh D alloimmunization occurs in susceptible Rh D-negative women for the following three reasons:

1. Failure to administer an antenatal dose of anti-D immune globulin at 28–29 weeks of gestation

2. Failure to recognize clinical events that place patients at risk for alloimmunization and failure to administer anti-D immune globulin appropriately

3. Failure to administer or failure to administer timely anti-D immune globulin postnatally to women who have given birth to an Rh D-positive or untyped fetus

The second reason for the continuing problem of Rh D alloimmunization is the small rate (0.1–0.2%) of spontaneous immunization despite the recommended prophylaxis protocol. These cases most often occur in pregnancies during which there have been no prior overt sensitizing events. This problem may become the largest single cause of new Rh D alloimmunization, because alloimmunization from other causes has decreased proportionally (28).

Potential Shortage of Anti-D Immune Globulin

Anti-D immune globulin is collected by apheresis from volunteer donors who have high titers of circulating anti-Rh D antibodies. The donated plasma is pooled and fractionated by commercial manufacturers, and anti-D immune globulin is prepared in varying doses. The number of potential donors may be dwindling worldwide, raising concern about future supplies of anti-D immune globulin (29, 30). Experts in the United Kingdom estimate that supplies of anti-D immune globulin are inadequate for immunoprophylaxis of all susceptible Rh D-negative women, both primigravidas and multiparas, if standard recommendations are followed (19). In Australia, a shortage prompted importation of anti-D immune globulin. Subsequently, some physicians proposed strictly limiting the dose given for first-trimester indications and discontinuing administration of anti-D immune globulin after external cephalic version (unless fetomaternal hemorrhage is documented), ectopic pregnancy, or threatened miscarriage (31). Others disagreed, considering it unethical to withhold anti-D immune globulin in any situation. Estimates regarding future needs compared with potential supply in the United States have not been published; however, limiting doses for first-trimester indications and using lower doses of Rh D immune globulin for antenatal prophylaxis may be necessary.

Cost-Effectiveness of Rh D Prophylaxis Programs

The cost-effectiveness of preventing perinatal mortality and morbidity secondary to Rh D hemolytic disease of the newborn is an important consideration. Economic analysis of anti-D immune globulin prophylaxis is based on the cost of anti-D immune globulin and the number of alloimmunizations that would be prevented. In 1977, the McMaster Conference concluded that routine postnatal prophylaxis was cost-effective but that routine antenatal treatment should be undertaken only if supplies of anti-D immune globulin were adequate and if cases of hemolytic disease of the newborns occurred that might have been prevented by antenatal treatment (7). Some experts concluded that antenatal prophylaxis is effective only in primigravidas (32), and the debate regarding the cost-effectiveness of antenatal prophylaxis of all pregnant women remains unsettled (20, 32–37). The Scottish National Blood Transfusion Service has concluded that the administration of 100 µg of anti-D immune globulin at 28 weeks and 34 weeks of gestation is cost-effective only in primigravidas (38). Others estimate that the most cost-effective antenatal regimen is a single dose of 250 μg of anti-D immune globulin at 28 weeks of gestation (39).

The use of anti-D prophylaxis in the case of certain clinical events is even more controversial. For example, the risk of Rh D alloimmunization from threatened abortion in the first trimester is uncertain, though probably very small. The cost-effectiveness of anti-D immune globulin for threatened abortion, which has never been studied, is questionable (19).

In summary, the cost-effectiveness of antenatal Rh D immune globulin to all Rh D-negative pregnant women and in all circumstances wherein fetomaternal hemorrhage might occur has not been proved. Available data support that third-trimester antenatal prophylaxis is cost-effective in primigravidas. As long as the supply of anti-D immune globulin is adequate and data do not exist to support other recommendations, most experts believe that it is unethical to withhold anti-D immune globulin from any patient at risk of Rh D alloimmunization (19). Recommendations for the use of anti-D immune globulin in this document will be made accordingly.

Clinical Considerations and Recommendations

▶ *Should anti-D immune globulin ever be withheld from a woman undergoing sterilization?*

The use of anti-D immune globulin following postpartum and postabortal sterilization should be guided by the patient's desire for protection against any chance of alloimmunization. Proponents of its use maintain that anti-D immune globulin administration will preserve the future option of transfusing Rh D-positive blood in times of emergency (40). Opponents of this view cite the low probability of sensitization with the previous pregnancy and the improbability of receiving Rh D-incompatible blood (41).

▶ *How should one deal with the issue of paternity?*

If the father is known to be Rh D negative, antenatal prophylaxis is unnecessary. If there is doubt about the father's identity or his blood type, anti-D immune globulin prophylaxis should be given.

▶ *Is it necessary to repeat antibody screening in patients at 28 weeks of gestation prior to the administration of anti-D immune globulin?*

The American Association of Blood Banks recommends that the physician should consider a repeat antibody screen prior to the administration of antenatal anti-D immune globulin if the patient was screened for antibodies prior to 28 weeks of gestation (24). The primary rationale for repeating the antibody screen is to identify women who have become alloimmunized before 28 weeks of gestation in order to manage their pregnancies properly. However, the incidence of Rh D alloimmunization occurring prior to 28 weeks of gestation is reported to be as low as 0.18% (18), and the cost-effectiveness of routinely repeating the antibody test has not been studied. The consequences of antenatal Rh D alloimmunization can be severe, but the decision to obtain a repeat antibody screen should be dictated by individual circumstances and left to the judgment of the physician.

▶ *Is anti-D immune globulin indicated in a sensitized pregnancy?*

If Rh D antibodies are present, anti-D immune globulin is not beneficial, and management should proceed in accordance with protocols for Rh D-alloimmunized pregnancies.

▶ *How should a D^u blood type be interpreted, and what management should be undertaken?*

In the past, a woman whose blood was typed as D^u was thought to have blood cells positive for a variant of the Rh D antigen. Nomenclature and practice have changed in recent years, and currently the D^u designation has been changed to "weak D positive" (24). Patients with this designation are considered Rh D positive and should not receive anti-D immune globulin. In some centers, the D^u antigen is not assessed, and women may unnecessarily receive anti-D immune globulin. In the rare circumstance of delivery by a woman whose antenatal Rh status is negative or unknown and whose postpartum screen reveals a D^u-positive or weak D-positive result, anti-D immune globulin should be given, and the possibility of fetomaternal hemorrhage should be investigated (24).

▶ *Is threatened abortion an indication for anti-D immune globulin prophylaxis?*

Whether to administer anti-D immune globulin to a patient with threatened abortion and a live embryo or fetus at or before 12 weeks of gestation is controversial, and no evidence-based recommendation can be made. The Rh D antigen has been reported on fetal erythrocytes as early as 38 days of gestation (42), and fetomaternal hemorrhage has been documented in women with threatened abortion from 7 to 13 weeks of gestation (9). However, Rh D alloimmunization apparently attributable to threatened abortion is exceedingly rare. Experts have compared the overall benefit with the cost of the widespread use of anti-D immune globulin for a condition as common as threatened abortion (19, 43), and, thus, many physicians do not routinely administer anti-D immune globulin to women with threatened abortion and a live embryo or fetus up to 12 weeks of gestation.

▶ *How much anti-D immune globulin should be given for first-trimester events and procedures?*

Because the red cell mass of the first-trimester fetus is small, the dose of anti-D immune globulin necessary for first-trimester events is 50 µg to protect against sensitization by 2.5 mL of red blood cells (5, 44). If therapeutic or spontaneous abortion occurs after the first trimester, the standard 300 µg dose is recommended (5).

▶ *Should anti-D immune globulin be given in cases of molar pregnancy?*

Although reported (45), the risk of Rh D alloimmunization in cases of hydatidiform mole is unknown. In theory, Rh D alloimmunization would not occur in cases of classic complete molar pregnancy because organogenesis does not occur, and Rh D antigens are probably not present on trophoblast cells, although this theory has been disputed (46–48). In partial and transitional molar pregnancies, however, the embryo may not die until after erythrocyte production has begun, making maternal exposure to the Rh D antigen possible (49). Given that the diagnosis of partial versus complete molar pregnancy depends on pathologic and cytogenetic evaluations, it seems reasonable to administer anti-D immune globulin to Rh D-negative women who are suspected of molar pregnancy and who undergo uterine evacuation.

▶ *Should anti-D immune globulin be given in cases of intrauterine fetal death occurring in the second or third trimester?*

Fetal death is due to fetomaternal hemorrhage in 11–13% of cases in which no obvious other cause (eg, maternal hypertensive disease, fetal anomalies) is found (50, 51). Rh D alloimmunization has been reported in cases of fetal death from massive fetomaternal hemorrhage (52), although the influence of this cause on the overall problem of Rh D alloimmunization is unknown. The efficacy of anti-D immune globulin in this clinical situation has not been tested in properly designed trials. However, authorities agree that anti-D immune globulin should be administered to Rh D-negative women who experience fetal death in the second or third trimester. All such cases should be screened for excessive fetomaternal hemorrhage to determine if additional anti-D immune globulin is required (25, 53).

▶ *Is second- or third-trimester antenatal hemorrhage an indication for anti-D immune globulin prophylaxis?*

In patients with second- or third-trimester antenatal hemorrhage, the risk of Rh D alloimmunization is uncertain. Although the efficacy of anti-D immune globulin in this clinical situation has not been tested in properly designed trials, authorities agree that anti-D immune globulin should be administered to Rh D-negative women with second- or third-trimester hemorrhage (25, 53). Man-agement of the patient with persistent or intermittent antenatal bleeding is complex. Though unproven, one commonly used strategy is to monitor the Rh D-negative patient with continuing antenatal hemorrhage with serial indirect Coombs testing approximately every 3 weeks. If the result is positive, indicating the persistence of anti-D immune globulin, no additional treatment is necessary. If the Coombs test is negative, excessive fetomaternal hemorrhage may have occurred, and a Kleihauer-Betke test should be performed in order to determine the amount of additional anti-D immune globulin necessary.

▶ *Is anti-D immune globulin prophylaxis indicated after abdominal trauma in susceptible pregnant women?*

Although the exact risk of Rh D alloimmunization is unknown, abdominal trauma may be associated with fetomaternal hemorrhage, which may lead to alloimmunization (54–57). The efficacy of anti-D immune globulin in this clinical situation has not been tested in properly designed trials. However, authorities agree that anti-D immune globulin should be administered to Rh D-negative women who have experienced abdominal trauma (25, 53). Also, all of these patients should be screened for excessive fetomaternal hemorrhage.

▶ *What should be done if an Rh D-negative patient is discharged without receiving anti-D immune globulin after a potentially sensitizing event?*

Volunteers have been shown to receive partial protection if anti-D immune globulin was given as late as 13 days after exposure (58). The longer prophylaxis is delayed the less likely it is that the patient will be protected, but it has been recommended that a patient may still receive some benefit from anti-D immune globulin as late as 28 days postpartum (5).

▶ *How long does the effect of anti-D immune globulin last?*

The half-life of anti-D immune globulin is 24 days, although titers decrease over time. If delivery occurs within 3 weeks of the standard antenatal anti-D immune globulin administration, the postnatal dose may be withheld in the absence of excessive fetomaternal hemorrhage (53). The same is true when anti-D immune globulin is given for antenatal procedures, such as external cephalic version or amniocentesis, or for third-trimester bleeding. An excessive amount of fetal erythrocytes not covered by anti-D immune globulin administration can be assumed to have entered maternal blood if either the results of the Kleihauer-Betke test are positive or the results of the indirect Coombs test are negative.

▶ *Should administration of anti-D immune globulin be repeated in patients with a postdate pregnancy?*

One study found that three patients became alloimmunized to the Rh D antigen when delivery occurred more than 12 weeks after the standard prophylaxis at 28 weeks of gestation (5). Based on these limited data, some experts have recommended that if delivery has not occurred within 12 weeks after injection at 28 weeks of gestation, a second antenatal dose should be given (5). Because this recommendation is based on so few cases, the final decision whether to administer a second dose should be left to the physician's judgment.

▶ *Should all Rh D-negative women be screened for excessive fetomaternal hemorrhage after delivery of an Rh D-positive infant?*

The risk of excessive fetomaternal hemorrhage exceeding 30 mL (the amount covered by the standard 300 µg dose of anti-D immune globulin) at the time of delivery is approximately 1 in 1,250 (5). Previous American College of Obstetricians and Gynecologists documents have recommended that only pregnancies designated as high risk be screened for excessive fetomaternal hemorrhage, including cases of abdominal trauma, abruptio placentae, placenta previa, intrauterine manipulation, multiple gestation, or manual removal of the placenta. However, such a screening program has been reported to detect only 50% of patients who required additional anti-D immune globulin (26). Based on this finding, the American Association of Blood Banks has recommended that all Rh D-negative women who deliver Rh D-positive infants be screened using the Kleihauer-Betke or rosette test (24).

Summary

The reduction in the incidence of Rh D alloimmunization is a prototype for the effectiveness of preventive medicine. Some controversies remain, however, such as the use of anti-D immune globulin in patients with either threatened abortion or antenatal hemorrhage. Similarly, it may not be cost-effective either to screen all Rh D-negative patients with an indirect Coombs test at 24–28 weeks of gestation or to screen all postpartum patients for excessive fetomaternal hemorrhage.

The following recommendations are based on good and consistent scientific evidence (Level A):

The Rh D-negative woman who is not Rh D-alloimmunized should receive anti-D immune globulin:

▶ At approximately 28 weeks of gestation, unless the father of the baby is also known to be Rh D negative

▶ Within 72 hours after the delivery of an Rh D-positive infant

▶ After a first-trimester pregnancy loss

▶ After invasive procedures, such as chorionic villus sampling, amniocentesis, or fetal blood sampling

The following recommendations are based primarily on consensus and expert opinion (Level C):

Anti-D immune globulin prophylaxis should be considered if the patient has experienced:

▶ Threatened abortion

▶ Second- or third-trimester antenatal bleeding

▶ External cephalic version

▶ Abdominal trauma

References

1. Mollison PL, Engelfreit CP, Contreras M. Haemolytic disease of the newborn in blood. In: Transfusion in clinical medicine. 8th ed. Oxford: Blackwell Scientific Publications, 1987:637–687 (Level III)

2. Huchcroft S, Gunton P, Bowen T. Compliance with postpartum Rh isoimmunization prophylaxis in Alberta. Can Med Assoc J 1985;133:871–875 (Level II-3)

3. Tannirandorn Y, Rodeck CH. New approaches in the treatment of haemolytic disease of the fetus. Baillieres Clin Haematol 1990;3:289–320 (Level III)

4. Iverson C, Flanagin A, Fontanarosa PB, Glass RM, Glitman P, Lantz JC, et al. American Medical Association manual of style. 9th ed. Baltimore: Williams and Wilkins, 1998 (Level III)

5. Bowman JM. Controversies in Rh prophylaxis. Who needs Rh immune globulin and when should it be given? Am J Obstet Gynecol 1985;151:289–294 (Level III)

6. Bowman JM. The prevention of Rh immunization. Transfus Med Rev 1988;2:129–150 (Level III)

7. McMaster conference on prevention of Rh immunization. 28–30 September, 1977. Vox Sang 1979;36:50–64 (Level III)

8. Howard HL, Martlew VJ, McFadyen IR, Clarke CA. Preventing Rhesus D haemolytic disease of the newborn by giving anti-D immunoglobulin: are the guidelines being adequately followed? Br J Obstet Gynaecol 1997;104: 37–41 (Level II-3)

9. Von Stein GA, Munsick RA, Stiver K, Ryder K. Fetomaternal hemorrhage in threatened abortion. Obstet Gynecol 1992;79:383–386 (Level II-2)

10. Brambati B, Guercilena S, Bonnachi I, Oldrini A, Lanzani A, Piceni L. Feto-maternal transfusion after chorionic villus sampling: clinical implications. Hum Reprod 1986;1:37–40 (Level II-3)

11. Blakemore KJ, Baumgarten A, Schoenfeld-Dimaio M, Hobbins JC, Mason EA, Mahoney MJ. Rise in maternal

serum alpha-fetoprotein concentration after chorionic villus sampling and the possibility of isoimmunization. Am J Obstet Gynecol 1986;155:988–993 (Level III)

12. Blajchman MA, Maudsley RF, Uchida I, Zipursky A. Letter: Diagnostic amniocentesis and fetal-maternal bleeding. Lancet 1974;1:993–994 (Level III)

13. Daffos F, Capella-Pavlovsky M, Forestier F. Fetal blood sampling during pregnancy with use of a needle guided by ultrasound: a study of 606 consecutive cases. Am J Obstet Gynecol 1985;153:655–660 (Level II-3)

14. Pielet BW, Socol ML, MacGregor SN, Ney JA, Dooley SL. Cordocentesis: an appraisal of risks. Am J Obstet Gynecol 1988;159:1497–1500 (Level III)

15. Lau TK, Stock A, Rogers M. Fetomaternal hemorrhage after external cephalic version at term. Aust N Z J Obstet Gynaecol 1995;35:173–174 (Level II-3)

16. Marcus RG, Crewe-Brown H, Krawitz S, Katz J. Fetomaternal haemorrhage following successful and unsuccessful attempts at external cephalic version. Br J Obstet Gynaecol 1975;82:578–580 (Level III)

17. Freda VJ, Gorman JG, Pollack W, Bowe E. Prevention of Rh hemolytic disease—ten years' clinical experience with Rh immune globulin. N Engl J Med 1975;292:1014–1016 (Level III)

18. Bowman JM, Chown B, Lewis M, Pollock JM. Rh isoimmunization during pregnancy: antenatal prophylaxis. Can Med Assoc J 1978;118:623–627 (Level III)

19. Robson SC, Lee D, Urbaniak S. Anti-D immunoglobulin in RhD prophylaxis. Br J Obstet Gynaecol 1998;105:129–134 (Level III)

20. Statement from the consensus conference on anti-D prophylaxis. 7 and 8 April 1997. The Royal College of Physicians of Edinburgh. The Royal College of Obstetricians and Gynaecologists, UK. Vox Sang 1998;74:127–128 (Level III)

21. Tovey LA, Townley A, Stevenson BJ, Taverner J. The Yorkshire antenatal anti-D immunoglobulin trial in primigravidae. Lancet 1983;2:244–246 (Level II-2)

22. Huchet J, Dallemagne S, Huchet C, Brossard Y, Larsen M, Parnet-Mathieu F. Antepartum administration of preventive treatment of Rh-D immunization in rhesus-negative women. Parallel evaluation of transplacental passage of fetal blood cells. Results of a multicenter study carried out in the Paris region. J Gynecol Obstet Biol Reprod (Paris) 1987;16:101–111 (Level II-2)

23. Pollack W, Ascari WQ, Kochesky RJ, O'Connor RR, Ho TY, Tripodi D. Studies on Rh prophylaxis. 1. Relationship between doses of anti-Rh and size of antigenic stimulus. Transfusion 1971;11:333–339 (Level II-1)

24. Snyder EL. Prevention of hemolytic disease of the newborn due to anti-D. Prenatal/perinatal testing and Rh immune globulin administration. American Association of Blood Banks Association Bulletin 1998;98(2):1–6 (Level III)

25. National Blood Transfusion Service Immunoglobulin Working Party. Recommendations for the use of anti-D immunoglobulin. 1991;137–145 (Level III)

26. Ness PM, Baldwin ML, Niebyl JR. Clinical high-risk designation does not predict excess fetal-maternal hemorrhage. Am J Obstet Gynecol 1987;156:154–158 (Level II-3)

27. Centers for Disease Control and Prevention. Lack of transmission of human immunodeficiency virus through Rho (D) immune globulin (human). MMWR 1987;36:728–729 (Level II-3)

28. Hughes RG, Craig JI, Murphy WG, Greer IA. Causes and clinical consequences of Rhesus (D) haemolytic disease of the newborn: a study of a Scottish population, 1985–1990. Br J Obstet Gynaecol 1994;101:297–300 (Level III)

29. Beveridge HE. Dwindling supplies of anti-D. Med J Aust 1997;167:509–510 (Level III)

30. Nelson M, Popp HJ, Kronenberg H. Dwindling supplies of anti-D. Med J Aust 1998;168:311 (Level III)

31. de Crespigny L, Davison G. Anti-D administration in early pregnancy—time for a new protocol. Aust N Z J Obstet Gynaecol 1995;35:385–387 (Level III)

32. Tovey LA, Taverner JM. A case for the antenatal administration of anti-D immunoglobulin to primigravidae. Lancet 1981;1:878–881 (Level III)

33. Clarke C, Whitfield AG. Rhesus immunization during pregnancy: the cause for antenatal anti-D. BMJ 1980;280:903–904 (Level III)

34. Tovey GH. Should anti-D immunoglobulin be given antenatally? Lancet 1980;2:466–468 (Level II-3)

35. Bowman JM, Friesen AD, Pollack JM, Taylor WE. WinRho: Rh immune globulin prepared by ion exchange for intravenous use. Can Med Assoc J 1980;123:1121–1127 (Level II-3)

36. Bowman JM, Pollock JM. Failures of intravenous Rh immune globulin prophylaxis: an analysis of the reasons for such failures. Transfus Med Rev 1987;1:101–112 (Level III)

37. Torrance GW, Zipursky A. Cost-effectiveness of antepartum prevention of Rh immunization. Clin Perinatol 1984;11:267–281 (Level III)

38. Cairns JA. Economics of antenatal prophylaxis. Br J Obstet Gynaecol 1998;105(suppl 18):19–22 (Level III)

39. Vick S, Cairns J, Urbaniak S, Whitfield C, Raafat A. Cost-effectiveness of antenatal anti-D prophylaxis. Health Econ 1996;5:319–328 (Cost-effectiveness analysis)

40. Gorman JG, Freda VJ. Rh immune globulin is indicated for Rh-negative mothers undergoing sterilization. Am J Obstet Gynecol 1972;112:868–869 (Level III)

41. Scott JR, Guy LR. Is Rh immunoglobulin indicated in patients having puerperal sterilization? Obstet Gynecol 1975;46:178–180 (Level II-3)

42. Bergstrom H, Nillson L, Ryttinger L. Demonstration of Rh antigens in a 38-day old fetus. Am J Obstet Gynecol 1967;1:130–133 (Level III)

43. Haines P. An overview from a panel member. Br J Obstet Gynaecol 1998;105(suppl 18):5–6 (Level III)

44. Stewart FH, Burnhill MS, Bozorgi N. Reduced dose of Rh immunoglobulin following first trimester pregnancy termination. Obstet Gynecol 1978;51:318–322 (Level II-1)

45. Price JR. RH sensitization by hydatiform mole. N Engl J Med 1968;278:1021 (Level III)

46. Fischer HE, Lichtiger B, Cox I. Expression of Rh0(D) antigen in choriocarcinoma of the uterus in an Rh0(D)-negative patient: report of a case. Hum Pathol 1985;16:1165–1167 (Level III)

47. van't Veer MB, Overbeeke MA, Geertzen HG, van der Lans SM. The expression of Rh-D factor in human trophoblast. Am J Obstet Gynecol 1984;150:1008–1010 (Level III)

48. Goto S, Nishi H, Tomoda Y. Blood group Rh-D factor in human trophoblast determined by immunofluorescent method. Am J Obstet Gynecol 1980;137:707–712 (Level III)

49. Morrow CP, Curtin JP. Tumors of the placental trophoblast. In: Synopsis of gynecologic oncology. 5th ed. New York: Churchill Livingstone, 1998:315–351 (Level III)

50. Laube DW, Schauberger CW. Fetomaternal bleeding as a cause for "unexplained" fetal death. Obstet Gynecol 1982;60:649–651 (Level III)

51. Owen J, Stedman CM, Tucker TL. Comparison of predelivery versus postdelivery Kleihauer-Betke stains in cases of fetal death. Am J Obstet Gynecol 1989;161:663–666 (Level III)

52. Stedman CM, Quinlan RW, Huddleston JF, Cruz AC, Kellner KR. Rh sensitization after third-trimester fetal death. Obstet Gynecol 1988;71:461–463 (Level III)

53. American Association of Blood Banks. Technical Manual. 12th ed. Bethesda, Maryland: American Association of Blood Banks, 1996 (Level III)

54. Rose PG, Strohm PL, Zuspan FP. Fetomaternal hemorrhage following trauma. Am J Obstet Gynecol 1985;153:844–847 (Level II-2)

55. Chhibber G, Zacher M, Cohen AW, Kline AJ. Rh isoimmunization following abdominal trauma: a case report. Am J Obstet Gynecol 1984;149:692 (Level III)

56. Kettel LM, Branch DW, Scott JR. Occult placental abruption after maternal trauma. Obstet Gynecol 1988;71:449–453 (Level III)

57. Dahmus MA, Sibai BM. Blunt abdominal trauma: are there any predictive factors for abruptio placentae or maternal-fetal distress? Am J Obstet Gynecol 1993;169:1054–1059 (Level III)

58. Samson D, Mollison PL. Effect on primary Rh immunization of delayed administration of anti-Rh. Immunology 1975;28:349–357 (Level II-1)

The MEDLINE database, the Cochrane Library, and ACOG's own internal resources and documents were used to conduct a literature search to locate relevant articles published between January 1980 and December 1998. The search was restricted to articles published in the English language. Priority was given to articles reporting results of original research, although review articles and commentaries also were consulted. Abstracts of research presented at symposia and scientific conferences were not considered adequate for inclusion in this document. Guidelines published by organizations or institutions such as the National Institutes of Health and the American College of Obstetricians and Gynecologists were reviewed, and additional studies were located by reviewing bibliographies of identified articles. When reliable research was not available, expert opinions from obstetrician–gynecologists were used.

Studies were reviewed and evaluated for quality according to the method outlined by the U.S. Preventive Services Task Force:

I   Evidence obtained from at least one properly designed randomized controlled trial.

II-1 Evidence obtained from well-designed controlled trials without randomization.

II-2 Evidence obtained from well-designed cohort or case–control analytic studies, preferably from more than one center or research group.

II-3 Evidence obtained from multiple time series with or without the intervention. Dramatic results in uncontrolled experiments could also be regarded as this type of evidence.

III Opinions of respected authorities, based on clinical experience, descriptive studies, or reports of expert committees.

Based on the highest level of evidence found in the data, recommendations are provided and graded according to the following categories:

Level A—Recommendations are based on good and consistent scientific evidence.

Level B—Recommendations are based on limited or inconsistent scientific evidence.

Level C—Recommendations are based primarily on consensus and expert opinion.

ISSN 1099-3630   12345/32109

The American College of
Obstetricians and Gynecologists
409 12th Street, SW
PO Box 96920
Washington, DC 20090-6920

ACOG PRACTICE BULLETIN

CLINICAL MANAGEMENT GUIDELINES FOR
OBSTETRICIAN–GYNECOLOGISTS

NUMBER 47, OCTOBER 2003

This Practice Bulletin was developed by the ACOG Committee on Practice Bulletins— Obstetrics with the assistance of Mara Dinsmoor, MD. The information is designed to aid practitioners in making decisions about appropriate obstetric and gynecologic care. These guidelines should not be construed as dictating an exclusive course of treatment or procedure. Variations in practice may be warranted based on the needs of the individual patient, resources, and limitations unique to the institution or type of practice.

Prophylactic Antibiotics in Labor and Delivery

The use of antibiotics to prevent infections during pregnancy and the puerperium is clearly different from the use of antibiotics to treat established infections. Prophylactic antibiotics are frequently prescribed on an "empiric" basis, which for many years was thought to have few adverse consequences. Concerns about the emergence of resistant strains of common bacteria, in addition to the emergence of strains with increased virulence, have resulted in increased scrutiny of the use of antibiotics, particularly in the hospital setting. Cost considerations also affect the use and choice of prophylactic agents. The purpose of this Practice Bulletin is to present a review of clinical situations in which prophylactic antibiotics are frequently prescribed and to weigh the evidence supporting the use of antibiotics in these scenarios.

Background

Appropriate and effective prophylactic agents are active against most but not necessarily all potential pathogens, which usually are the endogenous flora. The goal of prophylaxis is to attain therapeutic levels of antibiotic agents in tissues at the time of microbial contamination; optimally, the agent of choice also should be long-acting, inexpensive, and have a low incidence of side effects.

Antibiotic prophylaxis is distinguished from antibiotic treatment by the following 2 characteristics (1): 1) short courses are used (within 24 hours), frequently in single doses, and 2) to be effective, antibiotic prophylaxis is administered shortly before or at the time of bacterial inoculation. Delaying administration by even a few hours eliminates the benefit of prophylaxis.

Risks of Widespread Use of Antibiotics

Development of Resistant Organisms

Although it may be difficult for the individual practitioner to recognize or acknowledge the risks of inappropriate antibiotic use for his or her individual patient, the impact of increasing use of antibiotics can be felt clearly, even in the hospital setting. Antimicrobial prophylaxis has been shown to result in marked changes in an individual's skin flora, with an increase in the resistant flora postoperatively (2). In several studies, postoperative colonization rates with resistant staphylococci were 66–91%, although none of the patients had been colonized preoperatively (2). This appears to be a result of selection of resistant endogenous flora, as well as nosocomial acquisition of resistant microorganisms.

Awareness of the potential adverse effects on neonates of resistant bacterial infections has been increasing. A comparison of very-low-birthweight neonates (ie, <1,500 g) born between 1998 and 2000 with those born between 1991 and 1993 found a reduction in early-onset neonatal sepsis from group B streptococci (GBS) and an increase in sepsis caused by *Escherichia coli* (3). Sepsis in very-low-birthweight neonates with ampicillin-resistant *E coli* is more likely to be fatal than infection with susceptible strains (4). Some authors have noted similar increases in the rates of neonatal infections with gram-negative organisms, but others have not (5–7). Some authors have reported changes in the resistance patterns of the isolated strains of *E coli*, particularly after maternal antibiotic administration (4–5, 8–11). The increases in *E coli* sepsis and the increasing resistance to ampicillin appear to be confined almost entirely to the preterm and low-birthweight population (12). In addition to resistant *E coli*, GBS isolates resistant to erythromycin and clindamycin have been reported (13, 14).

In the past, resistance has been combated by the development of new classes or modifications of older drugs; however, it seems increasingly unlikely that the pharmaceutical industry will be able to keep pace with the rapid emergence of resistant organisms (15). In the past 2 decades, increasing difficulties have been encountered in treating multidrug-resistant tuberculosis as well as increasingly resistant strains of *Staphylococcus aureus*, enterococci, and *Streptococcus pneumoniae* (16).

Other Risks

The incidence of allergic reactions or anaphylaxis after antibiotic administration is unclear. Anaphylaxis to penicillin is estimated to occur in 1 in 2,500–25,000 recipients; less severe reactions occur in approximately 10% of recipients (12). It has been estimated that approximately 5% of patients receiving an antibiotic in the hospital will have a significant adverse reaction (17). Skin reactions (urticaria, rash, pruritus) to cephalosporins occur in 1–3% of patients; however, the risk of anaphylaxis is thought to be much lower (0.001–0.1%) (18). A case of anaphylaxis to penicillin after administration for GBS prophylaxis has been reported, and there are reports of exfoliative dermatitis and severe immune hemolytic anemia associated with cephalosporin therapy (18–20).

Pharmacokinetics of Antibiotics

It has long been assumed that the pharmacokinetics of antibiotics in pregnancy are different from those in the nonpregnant patient. As a result of the increase in the glomerular filtration rate during pregnancy that begins early in the first trimester, those medications that are excreted by renal filtration may be expected to have shorter half-lives and may be expected to reach lower peak serum levels in pregnant women. Because of the increased plasma volume in pregnancy, the volume of distribution is greater and the concentration of plasma proteins is lower than in the nonpregnant state, potentially leading to lower plasma and serum levels of antibiotics. Hormone-mediated increases in binding proteins also may result in changes in the distribution of drugs, whereas decreases in gastric emptying time and changes in gastric acidity may change the oral absorption of drugs. In addition, much of the drug may be sequestered in the fetal compartment such that it is not available to the woman. Overall, these considerations are believed to result in a reduction in the amount of the drug available to the woman and, potentially, a need for increased antibiotic dosage.

Most of these pharmacokinetic effects have not been well studied, and most of the studies that do exist on the pharmacokinetics of antibiotics during pregnancy have concentrated primarily on the rapidity and extent of transplacental transfer. Antibiotics that are known or suspected to achieve decreased levels in pregnancy include the penicillins (including expanded-spectrum penicillins), cephalosporins, aminoglycosides, nitrofurantoin, and erythromycin (21). Levels of clindamycin and trimethoprim–sulfamethoxazole probably are unchanged (21).

When therapeutic levels of antibiotics in the fetal compartment are desired, agents known to have efficient transplacental transfer should be used. Examples of such clinical situations include prophylaxis for preterm premature rupture of membranes (PROM) to prolong the latency period and maternal intrapartum prophylaxis for GBS. Antibiotics that are known to reach concentrations of 30–90% of maternal serum in the second trimester and beyond include ampicillin, cephalothin, clindamycin, imipenem, and the aminoglycosides (21, 22).

Clinical experience suggests that ampicillin and penicillin reach therapeutic levels in fetal blood within 4 hours of maternal administration (12). After intravenous administration of cefazolin, therapeutic levels are reached in fetal plasma within 1 hour and in amniotic fluid within 1–2 hours (23). Antibiotics that do not appear to cross the placenta well include erythromycin, azithromycin, and dicloxacillin (21, 24, 25). The risk of neonatal GBS colonization decreases significantly 4 hours after administration of maternal prophylaxis (26). Therefore, neonates are considered at risk for disease when their mothers received antibiotics for less than 4 hours before delivery, and some institutions may require a sepsis workup for such neonates.

Clinical Considerations and Recommendations

▶ *Is antibiotic prophylaxis appropriate for patients undergoing cervical cerclage?*

Few studies have evaluated the use of antibiotics during the performance of a prophylactic cervical cerclage. Because the rate of complications (including infectious complications) after prophylactic cerclage (when performed before any evidence of cervical dilation or shortening) is low (1–5%), a study with a sufficiently large sample size to determine whether prophylactic antibiotic therapy is of benefit would be extremely difficult to implement (27).

Emergency cerclage, performed later in pregnancy and when cervical dilatation and effacement are present, has a higher rate of complications, including chorioamnionitis and rupture of membranes (27, 28). In addition, the risk of preexistent, often subclinical, chorioamnionitis as a cause of the cervical insufficiency is significant, averaging approximately 33% (27, 29). However, evidence is insufficient to recommend antibiotic prophylaxis for either prophylactic or emergency cerclage.

▶ *Is antibiotic prophylaxis appropriate for patients undergoing cesarean delivery?*

High-Risk Patients

A number of well-designed studies have documented the efficacy of prophylactic antibiotics in reducing the rates of postpartum endometritis and wound infection in patients who have undergone cesarean delivery and are at high risk for such infections (30). High-risk patients include those who have cesarean deliveries after rupture of membranes or after labor, or both, and patients who undergo emergency procedures for which preoperative cleansing may have been inadequate. Other patients who may be at increased risk for postoperative infection include those whose surgeries last for more than 1 hour and those who experience high blood loss. Compared with placebo, the use of antibiotic prophylaxis generally will reduce the rate of febrile morbidity and postpartum endometritis from an average of 35–40% to 15% or less (30–32). The risks of febrile morbidity, urinary tract infection, and wound infection also are reduced by antibiotic prophylaxis, particularly in those patient populations in whom the baseline risk is high (30). Therefore, prophylactic antibiotic use in high-risk patients is beneficial.

Low-Risk Patients

Whether patients at lower risk for infection benefit from antibiotic therapy is less clear. No differences in rates of wound infection, endometritis, urinary tract infection, pneumonia, or febrile morbidity were noted in a study that randomized 480 women to receive either cefoxitin or placebo at the time of elective cesarean delivery (before labor or rupture of membranes) (33). In a prospective study of 82 women undergoing elective cesarean delivery, the incidence of febrile morbidity in general and endometritis in particular was reduced by antibiotic prophylaxis (34). The Cochrane review concluded that prophylactic antibiotics significantly reduced the risk of endometritis after elective cesarean delivery (relative risk [RR], 0.24; 95% confidence interval [CI], 0.25–0.35), although the elective group included nonlaboring patients with ruptured membranes of up to 6 hours of duration (30). A meta-analysis of 4 studies of women undergoing cesarean delivery before labor who had intact membranes concluded that antibiotic prophylaxis resulted in a significant decrease in postoperative fever (RR, 0.25; 95% CI, 0.14–0.44) and a significant decrease in endometritis (RR, 0.05; 95% CI, 0.01–0.38) (35).

A number of antibiotics have been shown to be efficacious for prophylaxis, including cefazolin, cefotetan, cefuroxime, ampicillin, piperacillin, cefoxitin, and ampicillin–sulbactam. One retrospective study of 2,280 non-elective cesarean deliveries reported that cefazolin and cefoxitin were equally efficacious in preventing endometritis, with cefazolin costing 80% less than cefoxitin (36). A randomized double-blind study of 377 women undergoing cesarean delivery also revealed no significant differences in outcome between those given cefazolin and those given cefotetan (37). A randomized study of 10 different prophylaxis regimens in 1,580 patients showed that 4 agents were significantly more effective in preventing postpartum endometritis: single doses of ampicillin (2 g), cefazolin (2 g), piperacillin (4 g), and cefotetan (1 g) (38). A meta-analysis of 51 antibiotic trials confirmed that ampicillin and first-generation cephalosporins had similar efficacy when compared with second- and third-generation cephalosporins (39) for cesarean delivery prophylaxis. Ampicillin may no longer be an appropriate choice, given the increasing prevalence of ampicillin-resistant *E coli*. Because those antibiotics with a narrower spectrum have been shown to be as efficacious as the newer, broad-spectrum agents, the practitioner should choose from among those with a narrower spectrum.

Single-dose therapy, usually given when the umbilical cord is clamped, has been shown to be as efficacious as multidose therapy in most studies (38, 40–42). Single-dose therapy also reduces costs, potential toxicity, and the risk of colonization with resistant organisms. Irrigation of the uterine and skin incisions with antibiotic solutions is no more efficacious or safe than intravenous administration in preventing postpartum infection (39).

▶ Is antibiotic prophylaxis appropriate for patients with preterm PROM?

Numerous trials have evaluated the prophylactic use of intravenous antibiotics to prolong latency and improve maternal and neonatal outcomes following preterm PROM (43–48). Regardless of the antibiotic prescribed or the duration of treatment, most trials described a statistically significant—but not always clinically significant—prolongation of the latency period. However, these same studies generally did not show an improvement in neonatal outcome.

The Maternal-Fetal Medicine Units Network multicenter trial revealed a reduction in neonatal morbidity and mortality with antibiotic prophylaxis, including reductions in respiratory distress syndrome, necrotizing enterocolitis, intraventricular hemorrhage, and early-onset sepsis (49). In this study, neonates of GBS-positive women did not receive the same benefit, and none of the patients received antenatal corticosteroids.

Several meta-analyses have concluded that antibiotic prophylaxis after preterm PROM is effective in prolonging pregnancy, reducing maternal infectious complications, and reducing neonatal infectious morbidity (45, 50, 51). However, a large multicenter trial from the United Kingdom reported that pregnancy was prolonged by the use of erythromycin, amoxicillin–clavulanic acid, or

both, but only the use of erythromycin resulted in reduced neonatal morbidity. The use of amoxicillin–clavulanic acid alone or in combination with erythromycin resulted in no reduction in morbidity and a 2.5-fold increase in necrotizing enterocolitis (0.7–1.8%, *P* = .0005) (52). Two other studies have found increases in necrotizing enterocolitis after antibiotic prophylaxis for preterm PROM; one used ampicillin prophylaxis and the other used ampicillin plus gentamicin and clindamycin, followed by amoxicillin–clavulanic acid (43, 48).

Certain broad-spectrum antibiotics lead to improved latency and may be particularly useful in cases of extreme prematurity. However, this prolongation does not necessarily result in better neonatal outcomes. Therefore, emerging data concerning resistant organisms make it necessary to assess the risks and benefits for each patient. For example, at 26 weeks of gestation, it may be more beneficial to use antibiotics in an effort to prolong pregnancy, whereas at 33 weeks of gestation, the risk of neonatal sepsis may outweigh the benefit of antibiotic use.

▶ Is antibiotic prophylaxis appropriate for prevention of bacterial endocarditis?

Although obstetric delivery sometimes can be associated with brief bacteremia, it appears to be rare, occurring in only 1–5% of patients (53, 54). The current recommendations of the American College of Cardiology and the American Heart Association suggest that prophylaxis for bacterial endocarditis be administered intrapartum to patients at risk only in the presence of suspected bacteremia or active infection (55, 56) (Table 1). Antibiotic prophylaxis is considered optional for patients experiencing uncomplicated delivery who are at high risk for endocarditis (those with prosthetic valves, prior endocarditis, complex congenital heart disease, or surgical systemic pulmonary shunts or conduits). Patients who require antibiotic prophylaxis for dental procedures do not necessarily require prophylaxis for obstetric delivery, because the risk of significant bacteremia with pathogenic organisms after some dental procedures is higher (60–90%) than for obstetric procedures. If antibiotic prophylaxis is used, the recommended regimen is 2 g of ampicillin (intramuscularly [IM] or intravenously [IV]) plus 1.5 mg/kg of IV gentamicin (to a maximum of 120 mg), followed by 1 g of ampicillin (IM or IV) or 1 g of oral amoxicillin 6 hours later. In patients who are allergic to penicillin, vancomycin (1 g IV over 1–2 hours) should be substituted for ampicillin. Ideally, prophylaxis should be administered shortly before delivery (within 30 minutes) and should not be given for more than 6–8 hours total. In those patients who are at moderate risk (see

Table 1) for endocarditis, the regimen is the same, except that the gentamicin and the second dose of ampicillin may be eliminated.

▶ *Is antibiotic prophylaxis appropriate for patients undergoing manual removal of the placenta?*

Several studies document the increased risk of postpartum endometritis after manual removal of the placenta during cesarean delivery, even in the presence of antibiotic prophylaxis (57–59). Although it is common practice to administer prophylactic antibiotics to patients who give birth vaginally and in whom a manual removal of the placenta has been performed, no data exist to either support or refute this practice.

Summary of Recommendations

The following recommendations are based on good and consistent scientific evidence (Level A):

▶ All high-risk patients undergoing cesarean delivery should be given antibiotic prophylaxis.

▶ For prophylaxis with cesarean delivery, narrow-spectrum antibiotics, such as a first-generation cephalosporin, should be used.

▶ Antibiotic prophylaxis may be considered for patients with PROM, particularly in cases of extreme prematurity, to prolong the latency period between membrane rupture and delivery.

Table 1. American College of Cardiology/American Heart Association Recommendations for Antibiotic Prophylaxis to Prevent Bacterial Endocarditis

Cardiac Lesion	Prophylaxis for Uncomplicated Delivery	Prophylaxis for Suspected Bacteremia*
High-Risk Category		
Prosthetic cardiac valves (both homograft and bioprosthetic)	Optional	Recommended
Prior bacterial endocarditis	Optional	Recommended
Complex cyanotic congenital cardiac malformations	Optional	Recommended
Surgically constructed systemic pulmonary shunts or conduits	Optional	Recommended
Moderate-Risk Category		
Congenital cardiac malformations (except repaired atrial septal defect, ventricular septal defect, or patent ductus arteriosus, or isolated secundum atrial septal defect)	Not recommended	Recommended
Acquired valvular dysfunction (most commonly rheumatic heart disease)	Not recommended	Recommended
Hypertrophic cardiomyopathy	Not recommended	Recommended
Mitral valve prolapse with valvar regurgitation or thickened leaflets or both	Not recommended	Recommended
Negligible-Risk Category†		
Mitral valve prolapse without valvar regurgitation	Not recommended	Not recommended
Physiologic, functional, or innocent heart murmurs	Not recommended	Not recommended
Previous Kawasaki disease without valvar dysfunction	Not recommended	Not recommended
Previous rheumatic fever without valvar dysfunction	Not recommended	Not recommended
Cardiac pacemakers and implanted defibrillators	Not recommended	Not recommended
Prior coronary bypass graft surgery	Not recommended	Not recommended

*Eg, intraamniotic infection.

†Risk for developing endocarditis is not higher than the general population.

Data from Bonow RO, Carabello B, de Leon AC Jr, Edmunds LH Jr, Fedderly BJ, Freed MD, et al. Guidelines for the management of patients with valvular heart disease: executive summary. A report of the American College of Cardiology/American Heart Association Task Force on Practice Guidelines (Committee on Management of Patients with Valvular Heart Disease). Circulation 1998;98:1949–84. Dajani AS, Taubert KA, Wilson W, Bolger AF, Bayer A, Ferrieri P, et al. Prevention of bacterial endocarditis: recommendations by the American Heart Association. JAMA 1997;277:1794–801.

The following recommendations are based primarily on consensus and expert opinion (Level C):

▶ Evidence is insufficient to recommend perioperative antibiotic prophylaxis at the time of prophylactic or emergency cervical cerclage.

▶ Prophylaxis for bacterial endocarditis is optional in patients with the following cardiac conditions who are undergoing uncomplicated obstetric delivery: prosthetic cardiac valves, prior bacterial endocarditis, complex cyanotic congenital cardiac malformations, and surgically constructed systemic pulmonary shunts or conduits.

▶ Patients with the above cardiac conditions who are undergoing obstetric delivery complicated by intraamniotic infection should receive prophylaxis.

▶ Although the evidence is inconclusive, for low-risk patients undergoing cesarean delivery, use of prophylactic antibiotics is recommended.

References

1. Kaiser AB. Antimicrobial prophylaxis in surgery. N Engl J Med 1986;315:1129–38. (Level III)

2. Archer GL. Alteration of cutaneous staphylococcal flora as a consequence of antimicrobial prophylaxis. Rev Infect Dis 1991;13:S805–9. (Level III)

3. Stoll BJ, Hansen N, Fanaroff AA, Wright LL, Carlo WA, Ehrenkranz RA, et al. Changes in pathogens causing early-onset sepsis in very-low-birth-weight infants. N Engl J Med 2002;347:240–7. (Level II-2)

4. Schuchat A, Zywicki SS, Dinsmoor MJ, Mercer B, Romaguera J, O'Sullivan MJ, et al. Risk factors and opportunities for prevention of early-onset neonatal sepsis: a multicenter case-control study. Pediatrics 2000;105: 21–6. (Level II-2)

5. Towers CV, Carr MH, Padilla G, Asrat T. Potential consequences of widespread antepartal use of ampicillin. Am J Obstet Gynecol 1998;179:879–83. (Level III)

6. Levine EM, Ghai V, Barton JJ, Strom CM. Intrapartum antibiotic prophylaxis increases the incidence of gram-negative neonatal sepsis. Infect Dis Obstet Gynecol 1999;7:210–3. (Level II-2)

7. Baltimore RS, Huie SM, Meek JI, Schuchat A, O'Brien KL. Early-onset neonatal sepsis in the era of group B streptococcal prevention. Pediatrics 2001;108:1094–8. (Level III)

8. Stiver HG, Forward KR, Tyrrell DL, Krip G, Livingstone RA, Fugere P, et al. Comparative cervical microflora shifts after cefoxitin or cefazolin prophylaxis against infection following cesarean section. Am J Obstet Gynecol 1984; 149:718–21. (Level I)

9. Terrone DA, Rinehart BK, Einstein MH, Britt LB, Martin JN Jr, Perry KG. Neonatal sepsis and death caused by resistant Escherichia coli: possible consequences of extended maternal ampicillin administration. Am J Obstet Gynecol 1999;180:1345–8. (Level III)

10. Towers CV, Briggs GG. Antepartum use of antibiotics and early-onset neonatal sepsis: the next 4 years. Am J Obstet Gynecol 2002;187:495–500. (Level II-2)

11. Friedman S, Shah V, Ohlsson A, Matlow AG. Neonatal escherichia coli infections: concerns regarding resistance to current therapy. Acta Paediat 2000;89:686–9. (Level III)

12. Schrag S, Gorwitz R, Fultz-Butts K, Schuchat A. Prevention of perinatal group B streptococcal disease. Revised guidelines from CDC. MMWR Recomm Rep 2002;51(RR-11):1–22. (Level III)

13. Bland ML, Vermillion ST, Soper DE, Austin M. Antibiotic resistance patterns of group B streptococci in late third-trimester rectovaginal cultures. Am J Obstet Gynecol 2001;184:1125–6. (Level II-3)

14. Pearlman MD, Pierson CL, Faix RG. Frequent resistance of clinical group B streptococci isolates to clindamycin and erythromycin. Obstet Gynecol 1998;92:258–61. (Level II-3)

15. Gold HS, Moellering RC Jr. Antimicrobial-drug resistance. N Engl J Med 1996;335:1445–53. (Level III)

16. Report of the ASM task force of antibiotic resistance. Antimicrob Agents Chemother 1995; (suppl):1–23. (Level III)

17. Moellering RC Jr. Principles of anti-infective therapy. In: Mandell GL, Bennett JE, Dolin R, editors. Mandell, Douglas, and Bennett's principles and practice of infectious diseases. Vol 1. 5th ed. Philadelphia (PA): Churchill Livingstone; 2000. p. 223–35. (Level III)

18. Kelkar PS, Li JT. Cephalosporin allergy. N Engl J Med 2001;345:804–9. (Level III)

19. Garratty G, Leger RM, Arndt PA. Severe immune hemolytic anemia associated with prophylactic use of cefotetan in obstetric and gynecologic procedures. Am J Obstet Gynecol 1999;181:103–4. (Level II-3)

20. Dunn AB, Blomquist J, Khouzami V. Anaphylaxis in labor secondary to prophylaxis against group B Streptococcus. A case report. J Reprod Med 1999;44:381–4. (Level III)

21. Sweet RL, Gibbs RS. Antimicrobial agents. In: Infectious diseases of the female genital tract. 4th ed. Philadelphia (PA): Lippincott Williams & Wilkins; 2002. p. 609–60. (Level III)

22. Heikkila A, Renkonen OV, Erkkola R. Pharmacokinetics and transplacental passage of imipenem during pregnancy. Antimicrob Agents Chemother 1992;36:2652–5. (Level III)

23. Fiore Mitchell T, Pearlman MD, Chapman RL, Bhatt-Mehta V, Faix RG. Maternal and transplacental pharmacokinetics of cefazolin. Obstet Gynecol 2001;98:1075–9. (Level II-3)

24. Heikkinen T, Laine K, Neuvonen PJ, Ekblad U. The transplacental transfer of the macrolide antibiotics erythromycin, roxithromycin and azithromycin. BJOG 2000; 107:770–5. (Level III)

25. Philipson A, Sabath LD, Charles D. Transplacental passage of erythromycin and clindamycin. N Engl J Med 1973;288:1219–21. (Level II-1)

26. de Cueto M, Sanchez MJ, Sampedro A, Miranda JA, Herruzo AJ, Rosa-Fraile M. Timing of intrapartum ampicillin and prevention of vertical transmission of group B streptococcus. Obstet Gynecol 1998;91:112–4. (Level III)

27. Harger JH. Cerclage and cervical insufficiency: an evidence-based analysis [published erratum appears in Obstet Gynecol 2003;101:205]. Obstet Gynecol 2002;100: 1313–27. (Level III)

28. Charles D, Edwards WR. Infectious complications of cervical cerclage. Am J Obstet Gynecol 1981;141:1065–71. (Level II-3)

29. Romero R, Gonzalez R, Sepulveda W, Brandt F, Ramirez M, Sorokin Y, et al. Infection and labor. VIII. Microbial invasion of the amniotic cavity in patients with suspected cervical incompetence: prevalence and clinical significance. Am J Obstet Gynecol 1992;167:1086–91. (Level II-3)

30. Smaill F, Hofmeyr GJ. Antibiotic prophylaxis for cesarean section (Cochrane Review). In: The Cochrane Library, Issue 2, 2003. Oxford: Update Software. (Level I)

31. Watts DH, Krohn MA, Hillier SL, Eschenbach DA. Bacterial vaginosis as a risk factor for post-cesarean endometritis. Obstet Gynecol 1990;75:52–8. (Level II-2)

32. Gibbs RS, St Clair PJ, Castillo MS, Castaneda YS. Bacteriologic effects of antibiotic prophylaxis in high-risk cesarean section. Obstet Gynecol 1981;57:277–82. (Level I)

33. Bagratee JS, Moodley J, Kleinschmidt I, Zawilski W. A randomised controlled trial of antibiotic prophylaxis in elective caesarean delivery. BJOG 2001;108:143–8. (Level I)

34. Duff P, Smith PN, Keiser JF. Antibiotic prophylaxis in low-risk cesarean section. J Reprod Med 1982;27:133–8. (Level II-2)

35. Chelmow D, Ruehli MS, Huang E. Prophylactic use of antibiotics for nonlaboring patients undergoing cesarean delivery with intact membranes: a meta-analysis. Am J Obstet Gynecol 2001:184:656–61. (Level III)

36. Currier JS, Tosteson TD, Platt R. Cefazolin compared with cefoxitin for cesarean section prophylaxis: the use of a two-stage study design. J Clin Epidemiol 1993;46:625–30. (Level II-2)

37. Carlson C, Duff P. Antibiotic prophylaxis for cesarean delivery: is an extended-spectrum agent necessary? Obstet Gynecol 1990;76:343–6. (Level I)

38. Faro S, Martens MG, Hammill HA, Riddle G, Tortolero G. Antibiotic prophylaxis: is there a difference? Am J Obstet Gynecol 1990;162:900–7; discussion 907–9. (Level I)

39. Hopkins L, Smaill F. Antibiotic prophylaxis regimens and drugs for cesarean section (Cochrane Review). In: The Cochrane Library, Issue 2, 2003. Oxford: Update Software. (Level I)

40. Gonik B. Single- versus three-dose cefotaxime prophylaxis for cesarean section. Obstet Gynecol 1985;65:189–93. (Level I)

41. Roex AJ, Puyenbroek JI, van Loenen AC, Arts NF. Single-versus three-dose cefoxitin prophylaxis in caesarean section: a randomized clinical trial. Eur J Obstet Gynecol Reprod Biol 1987;25:293–8. (Level I)

42. Saltzman DH, Eron LJ, Tuomala RE, Protomastro LJ, Sites JG. Single-dose antibiotic prophylaxis in high-risk patients undergoing cesarean section. A comparative trial. J Reprod Med 1986;31:709–12. (Level I)

43. Christmas JT, Cox SM, Andrews W, Dax J, Leveno KJ, Gilstrap LC. Expectant management of preterm ruptured membranes: effects of antimicrobial therapy. Obstet Gynecol 1992;80:759–62. (Level I)

44. Ernest JM, Givner LB. A prospective, randomized, placebo-controlled trial of penicillin in preterm premature rupture of membranes. Am J Obstet Gynecol 1994;170: 516–21. (Level I)

45. Kenyon S, Boulvain M, Nelson J. Antibiotics for preterm rupture of membranes (Cochrane Review). In: The Cochrane Library, Issue 2, 2003. Oxford: Update Software. (Level I)

46. Mercer BM, Miodovnik M, Thurnau GR, Goldenberg RL, Das AF, Ramsey RD, et al. Antibiotic therapy for reduction of infant morbidity after preterm premature rupture of the membranes. A randomized controlled trial. National Institute of Child Health and Human Development Maternal-Fetal Medicine Units Network. JAMA 1997; 278:989–95. (Level I)

47. Mercer BM, Moretti ML, Prevost RR, Sibai BM. Erythromycin therapy in preterm premature rupture of the membranes: a prospective, randomized trial of 220 patients. Am J Obstet Gynecol 1992;166:794–802. (Level I)

48. Owen J, Groome LJ, Hauth JC. Randomized trial of prophylactic antibiotic therapy after preterm amnion rupture. Am J Obstet Gynecol 1993;169:976–81. (Level I)

49. Mercer BM, Miodovnik M, Thurnau GR, Goldenberg RL, Das AF, Ramsey RD, et al. Antibiotic therapy for reduction of infant morbidity after preterm premature rupture of the membranes: a randomized controlled trial. National Institute of Child Health and Human Development Maternal-Fetal Medicine Units Network. JAMA 1997; 278:989–95. (Level I)

50. Mercer BM, Arheart KL. Antimicrobial therapy in expectant management of preterm premature rupture of the membranes [published erratum appears in: Lancet 1996;347:410]. Lancet 1995;346:1271–9. (Meta-analysis)

51. Egarter C, Leitich H, Karas H, Wieser F, Husslein P, Kaider A, et al. Antibiotic treatment in preterm premature rupture of membranes and neonatal morbidity: a meta-analysis. Am J Obstet Gynecol 1996;174:589–97. (Meta-analysis)

52. Kenyon SL, Taylor DJ, Tarnow-Mordi W; ORACLE Collaborative Group. Broad-spectrum antibiotics for preterm, prelabour rupture of the fetal membranes: the ORACLE I randomised trial. ORACLE Collaborative Group [published erratum appears in: Lancet 2001;358: 156]. Lancet 2000;357:979–88. (Level I)

53. Durack DT. Prevention of infective endocarditis. N Engl J Med 1995;332:38–44. (Level III)

54. Sugrue D, Blake S, Troy P, MacDonald D. Antibiotic prophylaxis against infective endocarditis after normal delivery—is it necessary? Br Heart J 1980;44:499–502. (Level III)

55. Bonow RO, Carabello B, de Leon AC Jr, Edmunds LH Jr, Fedderly BJ, Freed MD, et al. Guidelines for the management of patients with valvular heart disease: executive summary. A report of the American College of Cardiology/American Heart Association Task Force on Practice Guidelines (Committee on Management of Patients with Valvular Heart Disease. Circulation 1998;98:1949–84. (Level III)

56. Dajani AS, Taubert KA, Wilson W, Bolger AF, Bayer A, Ferrieri P, et al. Prevention of bacterial endocarditis: recommendations by the American Heart Association. JAMA 1997;277:1794–801. (Level III)

57. Atkinson MW, Owen J, Wren A, Hauth JC. The effect of manual removal of the placenta on post-cesarean endometritis. Obstet Gynecol 1996;87:99–102. (Level I)

58. Lasley DS, Eblen A, Yancey MK, Duff P. The effect of placental removal method on the incidence of postcesarean infections. Am J Obstet Gynecol 1997;176:1250–4. (Level I)

59. Magann EF, Washburne JF, Harris RL, Bass JD, Duff WP, Morrison JC. Infectious morbidity, operative blood loss, and length of the operative procedure after cesarean delivery by method of placental removal and site of uterine repair. J Am Coll Surg 1995;181:517–20. (Level I)

The MEDLINE database, the Cochrane Library, and ACOG's own internal resources and documents were used to conduct a literature search to locate relevant articles published between January 1985 and January 2003. The search was restricted to articles published in the English language. Priority was given to articles reporting results of original research, although review articles and commentaries also were consulted. Abstracts of research presented at symposia and scientific conferences were not considered adequate for inclusion in this document. Guidelines published by organizations or institutions such as the National Institutes of Health and the American College of Obstetricians and Gynecologists were reviewed, and additional studies were located by reviewing bibliographies of identified articles. When reliable research was not available, expert opinions from obstetrician–gynecologists were used.

Studies were reviewed and evaluated for quality according to the method outlined by the U.S. Preventive Services Task Force:

I   Evidence obtained from at least one properly designed randomized controlled trial.

II-1   Evidence obtained from well-designed controlled trials without randomization.

II-2   Evidence obtained from well-designed cohort or case–control analytic studies, preferably from more than 1 center or research group.

II-3   Evidence obtained from multiple time series with or without the intervention. Dramatic results in uncontrolled experiments also could be regarded as this type of evidence.

III   Opinions of respected authorities, based on clinical experience, descriptive studies, or reports of expert committees.

Based on the highest level of evidence found in the data, recommendations are provided and graded according to the following categories:

Level A—Recommendations are based on good and consistent scientific evidence.

Level B—Recommendations are based on limited or inconsistent scientific evidence.

Level C—Recommendations are based primarily on consensus and expert opinion.

ISSN 1099-3630

The American College of Obstetricians and Gynecologists
409 12th Street, SW, PO Box 96920, Washington, DC 20090-6920

12345/76543

Prophylactic antibiotics in labor and delivery. ACOG Practice Bulletin No. 47. American College of Obstetricians and Gynecologists. Obstet Gynecol 2003;102:875–82.

ACOG PRACTICE BULLETIN

CLINICAL MANAGEMENT GUIDELINES FOR
OBSTETRICIAN–GYNECOLOGISTS
NUMBER 7, SEPTEMBER 1999

(Replaces Technical Bulletin Number 111, December 1987)

This Practice Bulletin was developed by the ACOG Committee on Practice Bulletins— Gynecology with the assistance of Douglas W. Laube, MD. The information is designed to aid practitioners in making decisions about appropriate obstetric and gynecologic care. These guidelines should not be construed as an exclusive course of treatment or procedure. Variations in practice may be warranted based on the needs of the individual patient, resources, and limitations unique to the institution or type of practice.

Prophylactic Oophorectomy

In the United States, approximately 600,000 hysterectomies are performed each year, one half of which involve oophorectomy (1). Historically, the putative benefits of prophylactic oophorectomy have included the alleviation of symptoms related to retained ovaries and the prevention of cancer. These benefits are countered by arguments favoring the retention of ovaries, which allows continued hormone production in both premenopausal and postmenopausal women. This document will weigh the risks and benefits of prophylactic oophorectomy and provide a framework for the evaluation and counseling of patients who would be candidates for this procedure.

Background

Prophylactic oophorectomy is the removal of the ovaries for the potential benefit of preventing long-term morbidity and mortality. The term *prophylactic* implies that the ovaries are normal at the time of removal. Oophorectomy can be performed either alone as a planned surgical procedure or in conjunction with other planned surgical procedures such as hysterectomy or colectomy. *Incidental oophorectomy* is a term commonly used when the ovaries are removed at the time of another indicated surgery, and this term should not be used interchangeably with *prophylactic oophorectomy*. The term *incidental* implies that the surgery occurs by chance or without consequence. There are obvious consequences associated with oophorectomy; therefore, when oophorectomy is performed for future benefit, the surgery should be termed *prophylactic*.

Ovarian Physiology

The ovary is a complex metabolic organ consisting of follicular and stromal compartments. Follicles produce both androgens and estrogen, and stromal tissue synthesizes androgens. With the loss of all follicles around menopause, both androgen and estrogen levels decrease, but the ovary remains a source of androgens that are peripherally converted to estrogen. The role of endogenous androgens and the consequences of their removal may be significant but have not yet been clarified.

The positive effects of estrogen production on lipid metabolism and bone remodeling remain the primary argument for retention of the ovaries in premenopausal women. The benefits of estrogen are well documented (2–4), but any benefits of ovarian androgen production remain to be documented.

Cancer Prevention

In the United States, one in 70 women will develop ovarian cancer in her lifetime. Between 4% and 14% of these women will have had antecedent hysterectomies in which the ovaries were retained (5). Current screening techniques for ovarian cancer, including the use of ultrasonography and tumor markers, are neither sensitive nor specific enough to detect early cancer as part of a screening program for the general population. A high proportion of ovarian cancer is detected when it is in advanced stages. Prevention of ovarian cancer is the primary reason for prophylactic oophorectomy. Although oophorectomy does not eliminate the risk of cancer (patients still can develop peritoneal carcinoma, which acts like ovarian cancer), reported cases are rare (6).

The literature has recorded elective oophorectomy rates of between 50% and 66% in women 40–64 years of age undergoing hysterectomy (7, 8). Data from the Centers for Disease Control and Prevention collected between 1988 and 1993 concur that ovarian retention occurs in approximately 40–50% of patients undergoing hysterectomy at 40 years of age or older (1). It has been suggested that, in the United States, approximately 1,000 cases of ovarian cancer can be prevented if prophylactic oophorectomy is practiced in all women older than 40 years of age who undergo hysterectomy. This assumes an annual incidence of 24,000 new ovarian cancer cases and does not take into account the incidence of peritoneal carcinoma. The dilemma for the patient and the clinician is whether the estimated number of cancer cases prevented (1,000) is worth the number of oophorectomies performed (approximately 300,000) (9). The benefit of prophylactic oophorectomy may be offset by the consequence of estrogen loss early in life.

Factors to Consider for Prophylactic Oophorectomy

The potential risks and benefits of this procedure need to be considered within the context of the potential risks and benefits of extended hormone production or prescribed hormone replacement. The potential for alleviation of symptoms related to ovarian function should be considered, especially in patients with documented premenstrual syndrome. New developments in genetic testing, early diagnosis, refinements in diagnostic imaging, knowledge of hormone interactions with the cardiovascular and central nervous systems, and refined surgical techniques must all be considered with the individual patient.

Risk Factors for Ovarian Cancer

There is no consensus regarding the benefits of oophorectomy performed at the time of hysterectomy. Patients at greater risk for developing ovarian cancer are those with low parity, decreased fertility, and delayed childbearing if they did not use oral contraceptives (6, 10–12).

Women who have used oral contraceptives have a lower risk for invasive epithelial ovarian cancer than nonusers do. Both hospital and population studies revealed that, among those who have used oral contraceptives, the risk continues to decrease as years of use increase, although there is little additional protection conferred by oral contraceptives beyond 6 years of use. The protective benefits of higher parity, as well as longer duration of breastfeeding, also have been reported. Use of fertility drugs may be associated with a higher risk of ovarian cancer, as is a history of longer premenopausal sexual activity without contraception. There are no consistent data linking age at menarche, age at menopause, or duration of estrogen replacement therapy with development of epithelial ovarian cancer (10).

Operative Risk at the Time of Hysterectomy

There are no studies evaluating increased operative risk or morbidity at the time of abdominal hysterectomy when prophylactic oophorectomy is included. Retrospective studies looking at prophylactic oophorectomy at the time of vaginal hysterectomy have shown that the ovaries can be removed successfully in 65–97% of patients (13, 14). One study found no significant increase in operating time, estimated blood loss, length of hospital stay, or postoperative morbidity between patients who had their ovaries removed and those who did not (13). Another study found that oophorectomy added 23.4 minutes to the total operating time compared with vaginal hysterectomy alone (14).

Genetic Factors

The emergence of data suggesting the close link of ovarian cancer with familial breast–ovarian cancer syndromes has contributed to arguments favoring oophorectomy in subsets of patients identified with genetic risk factors.

The role of *BRCA1* mutations in ovarian cancer indicates that these tumors have unique biologic clinical and pathologic features (15). Recent evidence identifies the significant contribution of *BRCA1* mutations to the development of ovarian cancer, revealing that this mutation occurs in approximately 5% of women in whom cancer is diagnosed before 70 years of age (16). Although screening for *BRCA1* mutations has been suggested, it is difficult to define those women at risk based only on the number of family members affected. Because of the relatively small number (5%) of all ovarian cancers related to inherited mutations in the *BRCA1* gene, the optimal strategy for decreasing cancer mortality in these patients has yet to be determined.

BRCA2 mutations increase the risk of ovarian cancer but to a lesser degree than *BRCA1* mutations (17). The risk of ovarian cancer in families with Lynch syndrome II is reported to be 3.5 times higher than expected, with the estimated cumulative risk by 70 years of age still less than 10% (18). The mean age at diagnosis for ovarian cancer in women with Lynch syndrome II is approximately 45 years of age, roughly 20 years earlier than in the general population (19).

Clinical Considerations and Recommendations

▶ *Who are candidates for prophylactic oophorectomy?*

In determining candidates who would benefit from prophylactic oophorectomy, the advantages and disadvantages of prophylactic oophorectomy need to be evaluated (11, 20). The decision to perform prophylactic oophorectomy should be based not only on the patient's age but also on other factors that weigh individual risk for developing ovarian cancer against loss of ovarian function (see the box).

▶ *With ovary retention, what is the risk of needing a future oophorectomy for benign disease?*

The retention of ovaries following prior hysterectomy has been reported to contribute to reoperation in up to 5% of patients (21, 22), with pain in the retained ovary or ovaries the most commonly cited reason. In a retrospective study of more than 1,200 women who had at least one ovary retained after undergoing hysterectomy for benign indications, there was an approximate 4% reoperation rate (23). The author noted that the risk of having pathology in retained ovaries after hysterectomy was sig-

Patient Factors to Consider in Prophylactic Oophorectomy

Age
Parity
Previous abdominal surgery
Risk of ovarian cancer
Menopausal status
Family and personal history
Desire and willingness to use hormone replacement therapy
Risk for osteoporosis
Risk for coronary heart disease
Effect on self-image

nificantly higher in women who had only one ovary retained, compared with those who had both ovaries retained. In addition, the mean age at the time of hysterectomy was significantly lower in women who developed ovarian disorders following hysterectomy than in those who did not develop subsequent ovarian disorders. These findings suggest that the removal of one ovary at the time of hysterectomy in premenopausal women indicates the suspicion of clinical disease. The likelihood of future pathology in the retained ovary is therefore greater. Also, the younger the woman is at the time of hysterectomy, the more years there are for her to develop nonmalignant ovarian disorders that will require oophorectomy. In another study that followed a group of 84 premenopausal women undergoing radical hysterectomy, 27% experienced early loss of hormonal function or required subsequent oophorectomy (24).

▶ *Is prophylactic oophorectomy associated with increased morbidity?*

The morbidity associated with prophylactic oophorectomy is primarily related to the loss of estrogen. It is unclear whether exogenous estrogen fully compensates for the lost function of the ovaries, but it appears that estrogen replacement therapy is adequate compensation. However, there may be underlying advantages of ovarian function that have not yet been identified, particularly postmenopausal androgen production. Also, patients who do not take hormone replacement therapy will experience symptoms of early menopause, such as vasomotor hot flashes and vaginal atrophy (25), and are at a higher risk for osteoporosis (3, 26).

▶ *Should hormone replacement therapy be recommended for women undergoing prophylactic oophorectomy?*

Hormone replacement therapy should be recommended for women undergoing prophylactic oophorectomy just as it is for women undergoing natural menopause. The benefit of estrogen replacement therapy appears to be the same in natural or surgical menopause (3, 27), and the same risks and benefits should be discussed with the patient. If the patient is premenopausal, her need for estrogen replacement may be even greater because of her age and potential life span.

The favorable effects of estrogen replacement on bone metabolism have been well documented since the first reports of randomized trials. Additionally, in an evaluation of 27 premenopausal women undergoing oophorectomy, levels of lipoprotein A and cholesterol, along with other hemostatic factors, were found to be lower or not statistically different from preoperative levels, when estrogen replacement therapy was given (28). These observations are consistent with the beneficial effects of estrogen on cardiovascular hemodynamics and cardiovascular disease.

Despite the potentially favorable effects of estrogen replacement and the development of a number of promising synthetic hormone replacement medications, current estrogen replacement usage rates in postmenopausal women are low, and compliance with hormone replacement therapy is poor (29). Therefore, an unwillingness to accept hormone replacement therapy represents a potentially serious health problem, making the decision for elective oophorectomy more difficult.

▶ *What is the risk–benefit relationship associated with oophorectomy?*

The risk–benefit relationship for an individual woman is difficult to calculate. Compliance with estrogen replacement therapy and the risks of coronary artery disease and osteoporosis versus the risk of reoperation or ovarian cancer must be considered. Speroff and colleagues used Markov cohort modeling to evaluate prophylactic oophorectomy considering the influence of estrogen on coronary heart disease, breast cancer, and osteoporotic fractures (30). When compliance with estrogen replacement therapy was perfect, oophorectomy yielded longer life expectancy. When actual drug-taking behavior is considered, retaining the ovaries resulted in longer survival. While only a theoretical model, this analysis emphasizes the need to consider patient compliance with estrogen replacement therapy in decision making.

▶ *When is prophylactic oophorectomy indicated as adjunctive treatment for premenopausal women with breast cancer?*

Prophylactic oophorectomy as adjunctive treatment in the management of premenopausal breast cancer has been practiced for more than 40 years. The efficacy of this procedure has been assumed as part of an accepted endocrine management strategy for breast cancer. Today, with the use of multiagent chemotherapy, tamoxifen, and GnRH agonists, the role for oophorectomy is unclear. Large, prospective trials are currently underway to evaluate the efficacy of oophorectomy for node-positive, estrogen-sensitive breast tumors in premenopausal women.

▶ *Are there genetic risks that should be considered in the decision to perform prophylactic oophorectomy?*

Women with *BRCA1* have a 45% lifetime risk of ovarian cancer, and *BRCA2* conveys a 25% risk (12). Although large-scale prospective data are lacking, most clinicians agree that prophylactic oophorectomy in select women at high risk of inherited ovarian cancer (*BRCA1 and BRCA2*) should be considered (11, 31, 32). Multicenter studies are currently ongoing to assess the assumed benefit of prophylactic oophorectomy in this subset of patients. Because the average age of ovarian cancer in women with these genetic mutations is mid 40s, prophylactic oophorectomy should be performed at completion of childbearing or at 35 years of age.

Contemporary recommendations for women with Lynch syndrome II include at least an annual physical examination with bimanual rectovaginal examination, determinations of CA 125 levels, and transvaginal ultrasonography, with consideration of laparoscopic prophylactic bilateral oophorectomy upon completion of childbirth or by 35 years of age (11). The role of oophorectomy at the time of surgery for primary nonhereditary (sporadic) colorectal cancer is not clear. Some contemporary literature suggests that removing ovaries in this group of women decreases the likelihood of metastatic disease to the ovary (18). Prior to surgical intervention, a familial syndrome should be established by a full pedigree analysis, and the patient should be counseled as to the ethical and medical implications of this testing.

▶ *Are there other considerations in assessing the risks and benefits of prophylactic oophorectomy?*

The decision to perform prophylactic oophorectomy should be individual to the patient. Ovarian retention or removal in some patients may have a distinct bearing on their self-image. In addition to the ovarian contribution to the hormonal milieu, questions regarding the patient's self-image, reproductive function, and sexuality should be considered. Intact reproductive organs may be linked to self-perception of sexuality. Body image also may be related to the occurrence of posthysterectomy depression, although other factors, including preoperative depression, prior psychiatric disturbances, age younger than 35 years, nulliparity, and fewer than 12 years of formal education, also may serve as risk factors (33).

Summary

The following recommendations are based primarily on consensus and expert opinion (Level C):

▶ The decision to perform prophylactic oophorectomy should not be based only on age; it should be a highly individualized decision that takes into account several patient factors and choices.

▶ Removal of one ovary at the time of hysterectomy in premenopausal women may indicate the suspicion of clinical disease. The likelihood of future pathology in the retained ovary is therefore greater. The patient should be counseled before surgery that if ovarian pathology is found, bilateral oophorectomy may be indicated.

▶ Hormone replacement therapy should be considered for women undergoing prophylactic oophorectomy, and patients should be counseled about the risks and benefits of hormone replacement therapy prior to undergoing surgery.

▶ Compliance with hormone replacement therapy is important in women undergoing prophylactic oophorectomy to reduce the risk of future morbidity.

▶ Prophylactic oophorectomy should be considered for select women at high risk of inherited ovarian cancer.

▶ In addition to health risks and benefits, patient counseling should include consideration of how oophorectomy may relate to the individual patient's body image, perceptions concerning sexuality, and personal feelings.

References

1. Lepine LA, Hillis SD, Marchbanks PA, Koonin LM, Morrow B, Kieke BA, et al. Hysterectomy surveillance—United States 1980–1993. MMWR Morb Mortal Wkly Rep 1997;46:1–15 (Level II-3)

2. Bush TL, Barrett-Connor E, Cowan LD, Criqui MH, Wallace RB, Suchindran CM, et al. Cardiovascular mortality and noncontraceptive use of estrogen in women: results from the Lipid Research Clinics Program Follow-up Study. Circulation 1987;75;1102–1109 (Level II-2)

3. Ettinger B, Genant HK, Cann CE. Postmenopausal bone loss is prevented by treatment with low-dosage estrogen with calcium. Ann Intern Med 1987;106:40–45 (Level II-1)

4. Effects of estrogen or estrogen/progestin regimens on heart disease risk factors in postmenopausal women: The Postmenopausal Estrogen/Progestin Interventions (PEPI) Trial. The Writing Group of the PEPI Trial. JAMA 1995;273:199–208 (Level I)

5. Sightler SE, Boike GM, Estape RE, Averette HE. Ovarian cancer in women with prior hysterectomy: a 14-year experience at the University of Miami. Obstet Gynecol 1991;78:681–684 (Level II-3)

6. Piver MS, Jishi MF, Tsukada Y, Nava G. Primary peritoneal carcinoma after prophylactic oophorectomy in women with a family history of ovarian cancer. Cancer 1993;71:2751–2755 (Level III)

7. Dicker RC, Scally MJ, Greenspan JR, Layde PM, Ory HW, Maze JM, et al. Hysterectomy among women of reproductive age. JAMA 1982;248:323–327 (Level II-3)

8. Pokras R, Hufnagel VG. Hysterectomy in the United States, 1965–84. Am J Public Health 1988;78:852–853 (Level II-3)

9. Averette HE, Nguyen HN. The role of prophylactic oophorectomy in cancer prevention. Gynecol Oncol 1994;55:S38–S41 (Level III)

10. Whittemore AS, Harris R, Itnyre J. Characteristics relating to ovarian cancer risk: collaborative analysis of 12 US case-control studies. II. Invasive epithelial ovarian cancers in white women. Collaborative Ovarian Cancer Group. Am J Epidemiol 1992;136:1184–1203 (Level II-2)

11. NIH consensus conference. Ovarian cancer: screening, treatment, and follow-up. NIH Consensus Development Panel on Ovarian Cancer. JAMA 1995;273:491–497 (Level III)

12. Narod SA, Risch H, Moslehi R, Dorum A, Neuhausen S, Olsson H, et al. Oral contraceptives and the risk of hereditary ovarian cancer. Hereditary Ovarian Cancer Clinical Study Group. N Engl J Med 1998;339:424–428 (Level II-2)

13. Ballard LA, Walters MD. Transvaginal mobilization and removal of ovaries and fallopian tubes after vaginal hysterectomy. Obstet Gynecol 1996;87:35–39 (Level II-2)

14. Davies A, O'Connor H, Magos AL. A prospective study to evaluate oophorectomy at the time of vaginal hysterectomy. Br J Obstet Gynaecol 1996;103:915–920 (Level II-2)

15. Rubin SC, Benjamin I, Behbakht K, Takahashi H, Morgan MA, LiVolsi VA, et al. Clinical and pathological features of ovarian cancer in women with germ-line mutations of *BRCA1*. N Engl J Med 1996;335:1413–1416 (Level II-2)

16. Stratton JF, Gayther SA, Russell P, Dearden J, Gore M, Blake P, et al. Contribution of *BRCA1* mutations to ovarian cancer. N Engl J Med 1997;336:1125–1130 (Level II-3)

17. Ford D, Easton DF. The genetics of breast and ovarian cancer. Br J Cancer 1995;72:805–812 (Level III)

18. Burke W, Petersen G, Lynch P, Botkin J, Daly M, Garber J, et al. Recommendations for follow-up care of individuals with an inherited predisposition to cancer. I. Hereditary nonpolyposis colon cancer. JAMA 1997;277:915–919 (Level III)

19. Watson P, Lynch HT. Extracolonic cancer in hereditary nonpolyposis colorectal cancer. Cancer 1993;71:677–685 (Level II-3)

20. Irwin KL, Weiss NS, Lee NC, Peterson HB. Tubal sterilization, hysterectomy, and the subsequent occurrence of epithelial ovarian cancer. Am J Epidemiol 1991;134:362–369 (Level II-2)

21. Christ JE, Lotze EC. The residual ovary syndrome. Obstet Gynecol 1975;46:551–556 (Level II-3)

22. Grogan RH, Duncan CJ. Ovarian salvage in routine abdominal hysterectomy. Am J Obstet Gynecol 1955;70:1277–1283 (Level III)

23. Plockinger B, Kolbl H. Development of ovarian pathology after hysterectomy without oophorectomy. J Am Coll Surg 1994;178:581–585 (Level II-2)

24. Parker M, Bosscher J, Barnhill D, Park R. Ovarian management during radical hysterectomy in the premenopausal patient. Obstet Gynecol 1993;82:187–190 (Level II-3)

25. American College of Obstetricians and Gynecologists. Hormone replacement therapy. ACOG Educational Bulletin 247. Washington, DC: ACOG, 1998 (Level III)

26. Lindsay R, Tohme JF. Estrogen treatment of patients with established postmenopausal osteoporosis. Obstet Gynecol 1990;76:290–295 (Level II-1)

27. Lindsay R. Estrogen/progestogen therapy: prevention and treatment of postmenopausal osteoporosis. Proc Soc Exp Biol Med 1989;191:275–277 (Level III)

28. Lip GY, Blann AD, Jones AF, Beevers DG. Effects of hormone-replacement therapy on hemostatic factors, lipid factors, and endothelial function in women undergoing surgical menopause: implications for prevention of atherosclerosis. Am Heart J 1997;134:764–771 (Level II-3)

29. Ravnikar VA. Compliance with hormone therapy. Am J Obstet Gynecol 1987;156:1332–1334 (Level III)

30. Speroff T, Dawson NV, Speroff L, Haber RJ. A risk-benefit-analysis of elective bilateral oophorectomy: effect of changes in compliance with estrogen therapy on outcome. Am J Obstet Gynecol 1991;164:165–174 (Level III)

31. Struewing JP, Watson P, Easton DF, Ponder BA, Lynch HT, Tucker MA. Prophylactic oophorectomy in inherited breast/ovarian cancer families. J Natl Cancer Inst Monogr 1995;17:33–35 (Level II-2)

32. Burke W, Daly M, Garber J, Botkin J, Kahn MJ, Lynch P, et al. Recommendations for follow-up care of individuals with an inherited predisposition to cancer. II. BRCA1 and BRCA2. JAMA 1997;277:997–1003 (Level III)

33. Moore JT, Tolley DH: Depression following hysterectomy. Psychosomatics 1976;17:86–89 (Level II-3)

The MEDLINE database, the Cochrane Library, and ACOG's own internal resources were used to conduct a literature search to locate relevant articles published between January 1985 and January 1999. The search was restricted to articles published in the English language. Priority was given to articles reporting results of original research, although review articles and commentaries also were consulted. Abstracts of research presented at symposiums and scientific conferences were not considered adequate for inclusion in this document. Guidelines published by organizations or institutions such as the National Institutes of Health and ACOG were reviewed, and additional studies were located by reviewing bibliographies of identified articles. When reliable research was not available, expert opinions from obstetrician–gynecologists were used.

Studies were reviewed and evaluated for quality according to the method outlined by the U.S. Preventive Services Task Force:

I   Evidence obtained from at least one properly designed randomized controlled trial.

II-1   Evidence obtained from well-designed controlled trials without randomization.

II-2   Evidence obtained from well-designed cohort or case–control analytic studies, preferably from more than one center or research group.

II-3   Evidence obtained from multiple time series with or without the intervention. Dramatic results in uncontrolled experiments also could be regarded as this type of evidence.

III   Opinions of respected authorities, based on clinical experience, descriptive studies, or reports of expert committees.

Based on the highest level of evidence found in the data, recommendations are provided and graded according to the following categories:

Level A—Recommendations are based on good and consistent scientific evidence.

Level B—Recommendations are based on limited or inconsistent scientific evidence.

Level C—Recommendations are based primarily on consensus and expert opinion.

ISSN 1099-3630

**The American College of Obstetricians and Gynecologists
409 12th Street, SW
PO Box 96920
Washington, DC 20090-6920**

12345/32109

ACOG PRACTICE BULLETIN

CLINICAL MANAGEMENT GUIDELINES FOR
OBSTETRICIAN–GYNECOLOGISTS

NUMBER 39, OCTOBER 2002

(Replaces Committee Opinion Number 224, October 1999)

Selective Estrogen Receptor Modulators

Selective estrogen receptor modulators (SERMs) are synthetic compounds that bind estrogen receptors and produce agonistic activity in some tissues while acting as estrogen antagonists in other tissues. Although referred to collectively, their effects in different organs (eg, endometrium, urinary tract) are far from uniform. Much confusion exists about the indications for their use and the effects of these compounds. The purpose of this document is to review the use of SERMs for breast cancer risk reduction and skeletal protection as approved by the U.S. Food and Drug Administration (FDA).

This Practice Bulletin was developed by the ACOG Committee on Practice Bulletins—Gynecology with the assistance of Steven R. Goldstein, MD. The information is designed to aid practitioners in making decisions about appropriate obstetric and gynecologic care. These guidelines should not be construed as dictating an exclusive course of treatment or procedure. Variations in practice may be warranted based on the needs of the individual patient, resources, and limitations unique to the institution or type of practice.

Background

A number of compounds that exhibit the properties of SERMs are either in clinical use or are in development. Four SERMs are approved for use in the United States: 1) clomiphene, 2) tamoxifen, 3) toremifene, and 4) raloxifene. Clomiphene, tamoxifen, and toremifene belong to the triphenylethylene family of SERMs, whereas raloxifene is a benzothiophene.

Clomiphene is among the most widely prescribed drugs for the management of infertility in women (1). Tamoxifen, originally developed as a medical therapy for the treatment of breast cancer, was found to have estrogenic activity on bone remodeling and in cholesterol metabolism. It also was found to have estrogenic activity in the endometrium, resulting in an increase in the relative risk of benign and malignant neoplasms. Tamoxifen has been approved by the FDA for the treatment of breast cancer and to reduce the incidence of breast cancer in healthy women at high risk of breast cancer. More studies comparing tamoxifen with raloxifene for breast cancer prevention currently are underway. Toremifene also is indicated for the treatment of estrogen-receptor-positive breast cancer in postmenopausal women.

Raloxifene is approved for the prevention and treatment of osteoporosis in postmenopausal women. In clinical trials for the treatment of osteoporosis, raloxifene was associated with a significant reduction in new-onset cases of breast cancer when measured as a secondary endpoint in low-risk women. Based on pre-clinical studies, raloxifene appears to be a pure estrogen antagonist in the uterus. Short-term clinical studies in small series of patients have not shown a stimulatory effect on the uterus.

Tibolone has not yet received FDA approval. However, it has been used in Europe for approximately 20 years for the treatment of menopausal symptoms and the prevention of osteoporosis (2).

Other SERMs (idoxifene, droloxifene, and lev-ormeloxifene) have shown adverse gynecologic, gas-trointestinal, and genitourinary effects that resulted in the suspension of phase three trials. Specifically, these effects included uterine changes detected by ultrasonog-raphy that gave the impression of "thickening" of the endometrium as well as an increased incidence of utero-vaginal prolapse, urinary incontinence, and leukorrhea (3, 4).

Bisphosphonates act as specific inhibitors of osteo-clast mediated bone resorption. These agents reduce bone turnover by reducing the number of sights at which bones are remodeled. Thus, bone formation exceeds bone resorption at these remodeling sights leading to progres-sive gains in bone mass.

Physiologic Effects

Bone Metabolism

Bone remodeling is a continuous process that involves both resorption and formation. During menopause, bone loss accelerates in women, leading to an increased risk for osteoporosis. As antiresorptive agents, SERMs decrease bone tissue resorption by osteoclasts and there-by inhibit bone loss. Rigorous clinical trial data on the effects of SERMs on bone metabolism are limited pri-marily to raloxifene, although there also have been some studies published about other SERMs. Clomiphene has been shown to have some estrogen-agonist effects on bone in ovariectomized rat models, but there is only lim-ited clinical evidence for skeletal antiresorptive effects of clomiphene (1). Studies of tamoxifen use in premeno-pausal women indicate that after initiation of therapy there may be loss in bone mineral density for 3 years, which stabilizes after this period (5). Studies in post-menopausal women taking tamoxifen for breast cancer prevention demonstrated increases in bone mineral den-sity of 1–2% per year (5). Similar results have been observed in postmenopausal women taking tamoxifen to treat breast cancer (6).

Breast Cancer Risk Reduction

One of the mechanisms of action of SERMs for breast cancer risk reduction is mediated by competitive inhibi-tion of estrogen binding to estrogen receptors. The ratio-nale for the use of SERMs for breast cancer risk reduc-tion comes from clinical trials in breast cancer patients that indicated tamoxifen reduced the incidence of con-tralateral breast cancer in women with invasive disease (7). These results provided the rationale for testing the efficacy of tamoxifen in preventing breast cancer in women at high risk for the disease.

Cardiovascular Effects

A number of intermediate markers of cardiovascular dis-ease are altered favorably by raloxifene and tamoxifen, while others show little change. Both agents have been shown to reduce serum levels of total cholesterol and low-density lipoproteins while having no effects on high-density lipoproteins or triglycerides in postmenopausal women (8–11). Raloxifene and tamoxifen significantly decrease lipoprotein(a) levels (12, 13). Fibrinogen levels are reduced with both tamoxifen and raloxifene therapy (9, 10). Both raloxifene and tamoxifen also significantly decrease serum concentrations of homocysteine (14–17). Raloxifene therapy is not associated with an increase in C-reactive protein, whereas this marker was reduced sig-nificantly with tamoxifen (16, 18). The effect of ralox-ifene on plasminogen-activator inhibitor is neutral, whereas tamoxifen therapy has been associated with decreases in this marker (13, 16).

Although the effect on most surrogate markers for cardiovascular disease usually is favorable or neutral with the use of either raloxifene or tamoxifen, it is unclear whether either compound will have an effect on clinical outcomes of cardiovascular disease. In the Multiple Outcomes of Raloxifene Evaluation (MORE) trial, raloxifene therapy for 4 years was not associated with a reduced risk for cardiovascular events in the overall population (19). However, in a subpopulation of 1,035 women at increased risk for cardiovascular events, raloxifene was associated with a statistically significant 40% reduction in the risk for cardiovascular events (19). Neither raloxifene nor tamoxifen appears to be associat-ed with an early increased risk for cardiovascular events in randomized clinical trials of postmenopausal women who have osteoporosis or are at increased risk for breast cancer, respectively (19, 20).

Little data are available on the cardiovascular effects of other SERMs. In comparative studies, the effects of toremifene on lipid profiles have been comparable with tamoxifen (21, 22). Likewise, droloxifene appears to have a profile similar to tamoxifen (23–25).

Endometrial and Uterine Effects

In clinical trials of up to 3 years' duration, raloxifene did not cause increases in endometrial thickness or increase the incidence of vaginal bleeding, endometrial hyperplasia, or uterine cancer (26–28). In the MORE trial, fluid in the endometrial cavity (observed by transvaginal ultrasonography) was present in more women assigned to raloxifene than those assigned to placebo. The clinical significance of this finding is unknown. In contrast, tamoxifen has been associated with endometrial thickening, endometrial polyps (29), endometrial cystic atrophy (30–32), endometrial hyperplasia (29, 33), a twofold to fourfold increased risk for endometrial cancer in randomized, controlled clinical trials, and a small but increased risk of uterine sarcoma (4, 34, 35). The uterine effects of toremifene are not as well studied as those of tamoxifen. The rates of vaginal bleeding and vaginal discharge are similar in randomized trials directly comparing tamoxifen and toremifene (36, 37). However, benign uterine effects were less common with toremifene, and to date it has not been associated with endometrial hyperplasia or cancer. Levormeloxifene, idoxifene, and droloxifene also have been associated with increased endometrial thickness (3, 4).

Thromboembolic Events

Both raloxifene and tamoxifen are associated with an increased risk for venous thromboembolism. In one study, the relative risk of deep vein thrombosis or pulmonary embolism was 3.1 (95% confidence interval [CI], 1.5–6.2) for women taking raloxifene, as compared with placebo (38). The magnitude of this increased risk is similar to that observed with tamoxifen (20). The risk for venous thromboembolism with other SERMs is unknown because of the small size of the clinical trials and the rare nature of this event.

Genital Tract

Several studies suggest tamoxifen has estrogenic effects on the vagina. In a study comparing postmenopausal women who had breast cancer with fit, age-matched controls, the vaginal pH in the tamoxifen-treated group was significantly lower and was comparable with the pH levels in fertile women. Two thirds of tamoxifen-treated women had well-estrogenized vaginal smears, compared with none in the control group (39). In the National Surgical Adjuvant Breast and Bowel Project (NSABP) that studied cancer prevention, tamoxifen was associated with an increase in vaginal discharge (20), as was droloxifene (40). Although the effects of raloxifene on the vaginal mucosa have not been studied directly, raloxifene has not been associated with events related to vaginal atrophy, including vaginitis, leukorrhea, or dyspareunia (26).

Pelvic Floor Relaxation

Neither tamoxifen nor raloxifene has been associated with pelvic floor relaxation. In a posthoc analysis based on approximately 7,000 postmenopausal women who had an intact uterus when they entered the study, 3 years of raloxifene therapy was associated with a significant reduction in the risk for pelvic floor surgery (50%) (41). The mechanism by which SERMs might affect pelvic floor relaxation is not clear. The presence of estrogen receptors in pelvic floor tissues indicates this region is a target for estrogen and may respond to SERMs. Similar to their known effects on collagen metabolism in bone tissue, SERMs also may affect tissue remodeling in the pelvic floor.

Vasomotor Symptoms

In an integrated analysis of five randomized, placebo-controlled trials, younger, healthy postmenopausal women receiving raloxifene had a significantly higher incidence of hot flashes (25%) than those receiving placebo (18%), but the trial excluded women with severe vasomotor symptoms (26). However, there was no therapy difference for the severity of hot flashes or for the discontinuation of therapy because of hot flashes. The increased incidence of hot flashes in the raloxifene-treated group was observed only during the first 6 months of therapy. In older, postmenopausal women with osteoporosis, the overall incidence of hot flashes was lower but still significantly different between raloxifene (9.7%) and placebo (6.4%) (38). A higher incidence of hot flashes also has been associated with tamoxifen. Of postmenopausal women taking tamoxifen, 16% sought treatment for vasomotor symptoms (42). Extremely bothersome hot flashes also were more common in the tamoxifen-treated group of the NSABP Breast Cancer Prevention Trial (NSABP P-1 trial) (20). Hot flashes also have been associated with toremifene, idoxifene, and droloxifene therapy (43–45).

Clinical Considerations and Recommendations

▶ **Are SERMs effective in reducing the risk of breast cancer?**

Tamoxifen is approved by the FDA for breast cancer risk reduction on the basis of the results of the NSABP P-1 trial, in which it reduced the risk of both invasive and noninvasive breast cancer by approximately 50% (20, 46). The effects were primarily caused by a reduction in the risk for estrogen-receptor-positive breast cancer. Two other European trials failed to show similar efficacy (47, 48). These studies had smaller sample sizes, shorter follow-up, and allowed concomitant treatment with estrogen replacement therapy or hormone replacement therapy.

Raloxifene also acts as an estrogen antagonist in breast tissue. In the MORE trial, 4 years of raloxifene therapy was associated with a 72% reduction in the risk of invasive breast cancer (49). Similar to tamoxifen, the risk reduction was attributable to a 90% reduction in the risk of estrogen-receptor-positive breast cancer, with no apparent decrease in the risk of estrogen-receptor-negative breast cancer.

▶ *Who are appropriate candidates for SERMs?*

Because of the increase in thromboembolic events and uterine malignancy seen in women older than 50 years using tamoxifen, a delicate risk–benefit balance exists. This issue appears to be of less concern for women younger than 50 years because the NSABP P-1 trial did not show any increase in uterine malignancy or thromboembolic events in this group. To warrant tamoxifen therapy, women should be at high risk of developing breast cancer (50). Those at high risk include women with ductal carcinoma in situ and lobular carcinoma in situ who do not choose surgical therapy, women with ductal hyperplasia with atypia, and women with a high risk on the basis of personal and family history. Chemoprophylaxis has been suggested for women at high risk of developing breast cancer (46, 50).

Raloxifene is approved by the FDA for the prevention and treatment of osteoporosis. The National Osteoporosis Foundation recommends treatment for all women in whom dual-energy X-ray absorptiometry elicits a "T score" of –2 or, for those who have other risk factors, a T score less than –1.5 (51). Significant risk factors are summarized in Table 1. Other appropriate candidates to consider for preventive therapy include postmenopausal women who are currently taking hormone replacement therapy for osteoporosis prevention but would like to discontinue using it because of symptoms or fears associated with the use of hormone replacement therapy, including breast tenderness, vaginal bleeding, and fear of breast or uterine cancer. Raloxifene also is appropriate for the prevention and treatment of osteoporosis in women who have a family history of breast or endometrial cancer. Raloxifene is contraindicated in pregnant women or those who may become pregnant and in women with a current or past history of venous thromboembolic events, including deep vein thrombosis, pulmonary embolism, and retinal vein thrombosis.

Table 1. Risk Factors for Osteoporosis

Nonmodifiable	Potentially Modifiable
Personal history of fracture as an adult	Current cigarette smoking
History of fracture in first-degree relative	Low body weight (<127 lb)
Caucasian race	Estrogen deficiency:
	Early menopause (age <45 years) or bilateral ovariectomy
	Prolonged premenopausal amenorrhea (>1 year)
Advanced age	Low calcium intake
Female sex	Alcoholism
Dementia	Impaired eyesight despite adequate correction
Poor health or frailty	Recurrent falls
	Inadequate physical activity
	Poor health or frailty

Reprinted with permission from Physicians guide to prevention and treatment of osteoporosis. 1999, National Osteoporosis Foundation, Washington, DC 20037

▶ *Is raloxifene appropriate for breast cancer patients who have completed a 5-year course of tamoxifen?*

No studies have investigated the use of raloxifene after a 5-year course of tamoxifen. Women previously treated with tamoxifen may begin to lose bone mineral density when they complete their course of therapy. Their status and relative risk for osteoporosis should be evaluated and choices for prevention or therapy made accordingly.

▶ *Are SERMs effective in reducing bone loss?*

In premenopausal women, tamoxifen may cause decreases in bone mineral density for 3 years after initiation of therapy, which stabilizes after this period (5). Several large, randomized clinical trials of raloxifene for the prevention and treatment of osteoporosis in postmenopausal women have been published (8, 38, 52–54). Increases in bone mineral density of approximately 2–3% more than placebo have been demonstrated for the spine and total hip. Histomorphometry and bone turnover assessments have been performed for women taking tamoxifen and raloxifene, and both confirm the estrogenic actions of these agents on bone tissue. Both raloxifene and tamoxifen reduce biochemical indices of bone turnover by 20–50% (6, 8, 38, 55, 56). Histomorphometry studies indicate bone morphology is normal in women receiving raloxifene (57, 58).

The MORE trial examined the effect of raloxifene on fracture risk reduction in 7,705 postmenopausal women with osteoporosis. This study demonstrated a significant risk reduction of 30–50% for vertebral fracture among women treated for 3 years (38). In the NSABP P-1 trial, tamoxifen was associated with a nonsignificant decrease in the incidence of hip, vertebral, and Colles' fractures (20). However, tamoxifen has not been evaluated prospectively in women with osteoporosis, and its effects in the bone remain to be established.

▶ *In patients using SERMs, are there beneficial effects on vaginal dryness and hot flashes with the addition of estrogen?*

With tamoxifen, many patients experience vaginal dryness. However, in the NSABP P-1 trial, 29% of patients had leukorrhea described as moderately bothersome or worse (20). No clinical trials adding vaginal estrogen to systemic tamoxifen have been performed; therefore, efficacy and toxicity of this approach has not been evaluated.

Raloxifene does not differ from placebo with respect to its association with vaginal dryness (26). Still, the lack of a positive effect of raloxifene on urogenital atrophy will cause many sexually active women to experience vaginal discomfort. The addition of local estrogen therapy may improve such symptoms.

Twenty-five percent of younger postmenopausal women taking raloxifene experienced hot flashes at some point during the original clinical trials although only 1.7% discontinued therapy as a result (26). In the MORE trial, a group of older women with osteoporosis experienced a 10.6% incidence of hot flashes (38). In the NSABP P-1 trial, 68% of the women taking tamoxifen reported hot flashes that were moderately bothersome or worse, compared with 49% in the placebo group (20).

No published trials have studied the combination of systemic estrogen and SERMs to reduce vasomotor symptoms. Because the two compounds compete for the same receptors, the effect of such co-administration on other organ systems is unknown.

▶ *In patients using SERMs, are there benefits with the addition of bisphosphonates?*

Although the average increase in bone mineral density with raloxifene in the first 24 months is 2–3%, some individuals actually lose bone mineral density. This also is true of other antiresorptive agents. The addition of alendronate to raloxifene therapy significantly enhances the antiresorptive efficacy beyond that of either agent independently (59, 60). The effect on actual fracture rates and the long-term safety of such combinations of antiresorptive agents remain unknown.

▶ *How should women taking raloxifene be evaluated?*

In terms of osteoporosis treatment, efficacy often is monitored with surrogate markers of clinical outcomes. Because baseline bone mineral density is clearly predictive of future fracture risk, changes in bone mineral density in response to antiresorptive therapy traditionally have been used as a surrogate marker of efficacy in terms of osteoporosis. However, most antiresorptive agents are associated with similar fracture risk reduction despite wide variations in the magnitude of their bone mineral density response (38, 61–63). Effective treatments for osteoporosis should not be discontinued or changed because of early, treatment-associated decreases in bone mineral density, especially because frequent bone mineral density monitoring may be misleading (64). Therefore, although bone mineral density has been used in most clinical studies to monitor the efficacy of treatment, the frequency of bone mineral density testing for the screening and monitoring of therapy has not been standardized.

Based on limited studies, raloxifene does not appear to induce proliferation, hyperplasia, or malignancy of the endometrium (8, 28) nor does it cause polyps, as does tamoxifen (65). Routine gynecologic care according to established clinical principles seems to be appropriate for patients taking raloxifene or tamoxifen. Specific or heightened uterine surveillance is not routinely required for patients taking SERMS. Vaginal bleeding should be investigated. Nongynecologic surveillance (eg, lipid profiles, dual-energy X-ray absorptiometry, mammography) should be based on individual patient history as well as the established guidelines for those procedures.

▶ *Does tamoxifen increase the risk of uterine cancer?*

Before the NSABP P-1 trial, only women who had breast cancer were treated with tamoxifen. The NSABP P-1 trial showed a 50% reduction in preinvasive and invasive breast cancer in women with a high risk of breast cancer (20). An increase in endometrial cancer also was reported in these women. The overall relative risk of endometrial cancer with tamoxifen was 2.53 (95% CI, 1.35–4.97). In women older than 50 years, the relative risk increased to 4.01 (95% CI, 1.70–10.90), while in women younger than 50 years, there was no statistically significant difference (20). An increased risk of uterine sarcoma has been observed in women taking tamoxifen (35). This effect is small and similar to that of estrogen.

New data suggest it may be possible to identify breast cancer patients at high and low risk for developing atypical hyperplasia with tamoxifen therapy on the basis of the presence or absence of benign endometrial polyps before beginning tamoxifen therapy (65). Among women taking tamoxifen for up to 5 years, those who had polyps that were removed before initiation of tamoxifen therapy had an incidence of atypical hyperplasia 18 times greater than those who had uterine cavities that were without lesion (11.7% versus 0.7%).

The risk of endometrial cancer does not appear to increase with raloxifene use. In a group of women with osteoporosis receiving raloxifene, the relative risk of endometrial carcinoma was 0.8 over a 3-year period of follow-up (95% CI, 0.21–2.67) (25).

▶ *How should the risk of breast cancer be assessed?*

A woman's decisions relating to her breast health— whether a program of intensive surveillance with mammography and ultrasonography, chemopreventive agents, or possibly even prophylactic mastectomy—depend on her awareness of the medical options, her own personal preferences, and, importantly, an individualized estimate of the probability of her developing breast cancer over a defined period. Such an estimate also is useful for designing prevention trials in high-risk subsets of the population. Such prevention trials differ from therapeutic clinical trials because they expose asymptomatic, healthy women to potentially toxic interventions for prolonged periods to reduce their risk of developing breast cancer. Risk estimates for various individual risk factors are available (Table 2), but risk estimates for combinations of risk factors (eg, the Gail model) (66) are clearly preferable. The usefulness of the Gail model is limited in patients with second-degree relatives with breast cancer (eg, paternal transmission) and is falsely increased in patients with multiple breast biopsies.

▶ *How long should patients take SERMs?*

For chemoprevention of breast cancer, the duration of use of tamoxifen has not been established. Based on the NSABP P-1 trial, tamoxifen use for 5 years is currently recommended (20). There is no known additional benefit in its use for more than 5 years (67). The use of raloxifene for osteoporosis prevention is not time-limited (38).

Summary of Recommendations

The following recommendations are based on good and consistent scientific evidence (Level A):

▶ Consideration should be given to tamoxifen therapy for women at high risk for developing breast cancer.

Table 2. Factors That Increase the Relative Risk for Breast Cancer in Women

Relative Risk	Factor
Relative risk >4	Certain inherited genetic mutations for breast cancer
	Two or more first-degree relatives with breast cancer diagnosed at an early age
	Personal history of breast cancer
	Age (≥65 years vs <65 years, although risk increases across all ages until age 80 years)
Relative risk 2.1–4	One first-degree relative with breast cancer
	Nodular densities on mammogram (>75% of breast volume)
	Atypical hyperplasia
	High-dose ionizing radiation to the chest
	Ovaries not surgically removed (age <40 years)
Relative risk 1.1–2	High socioeconomic status
	Urban residence
	Northern U.S. residence
Reproductive factors	Early menarche (age <12 years)
	Late menopause (age ≥55 years)
	No term pregnancies (for breast cancer diagnosed at age ≥40 years)
	Late age at first term pregnancy (≥30 years)
	Never breastfed a child
Other factors that affect circulating hormones or genetic susceptibility	Postmenopausal obesity
	Alcohol consumption
	Recent hormone replacement therapy
	Recent oral contraceptive use
	Tall stature
	Personal history of cancer of endometrium, ovary, or colon
	Jewish heritage

Reprinted and adapted with permission from Elsevier Science. Hulka BS, Stark AT. Breast cancer: cause and prevention. Lancet 1995;346:883–7.

▶ Raloxifene is appropriate therapy for women who are candidates for chemoprevention of osteoporosis.

▶ Raloxifene is appropriate therapy for women with established osteoporosis to prevent osteoporotic fractures.

▶ Neither raloxifene nor tamoxifen should be used in women with a history of venous thromboembolic events, including pulmonary emboli, deep vein thrombosis, or retinal vein thrombosis.

▶ Any abnormal uterine bleeding should be investigated in women taking tamoxifen or raloxifene.

The following recommendations are based primarily on consensus and expert opinion (Level C):

▶ Because there are no data on the use of raloxifene in women who have completed a 5-year course of tamoxifen therapy, such women should have an individual assessment of their risk of osteoporosis, and decisions about prevention or treatment should be made accordingly.

▶ The use of tamoxifen for chemoprevention should be limited to 5 years.

▶ Co-administration of local vaginal estrogen therapy may be used for the relief of vaginal dryness in patients receiving raloxifene or tamoxifen therapy.

▶ Individualized risk assessment should be performed to determine whether a patient is a candidate for breast cancer risk reduction by chemoprevention, unless she has ductal carcinoma in situ or lobular carcinoma in situ in which case, the benefit of chemoprevention already has been documented.

References

1. Young RL, Goldzieher JW, Elkind-Hirsch K, Hickox PG, Chakraborty PK. A short-term comparison of the effects of clomiphene citrate and conjugated equine estrogen in menopausal/castrate women. Int J Fertil 1991;36:167–71. (Level I)

2. Modelska K, Cummings S. Tibolone for postmenopausal women: systematic review of randomized trials. J Clin Endocrinol Metab 2002;87:16–23. (Level III)

3. Hendrix SL, McNeeley SG. Effect of selective estrogen receptor modulators on reproductive tissues other than endometrium. Ann N Y Acad Sci 2001;949:243–50. (Level III)

4. Fleischer AC, Wheeler JE, Yeh IT, Kravitz B, Jensen C, MacDonald B. Sonographic assessment of the endometrium in osteopenic postmenopausal women treated with idoxifene. J Ultrasound Med 1999;18:503–12. (Level I)

5. Powles TJ, Hickish T, Kanis JA, Tidy A, Ashley S. Effect of tamoxifen on bone mineral density measured by dual-energy x-ray absorptiometry in healthy premenopausal and postmenopausal women. J Clin Oncol 1996;14:78–84. (Level I)

6. Love RR, Mazess RB, Barden HS, Epstein S, Newcomb PA, Jordan VC, et al. Effects of tamoxifen on bone mineral density in postmenopausal women with breast cancer. N Engl J Med 1992;326:852–56. (Level I)

7. Rutqvist LE, Cedermark B, Glas U, Mattsson A, Skoog L, Somell A, et al. Contralateral primary tumors in breast cancer patients in a randomized trial of adjuvant tamoxifen therapy. J Natl Cancer Inst 1991;83:1299–306. (Level I)

8. Delmas PD, Bjarnason NH, Mitlak BH, Ravoux AC, Shah AS, Huster WJ, et al. Effects of raloxifene on bone mineral density, serum cholesterol concentrations, and uterine endometrium in postmenopausal women. N Engl J Med 1997;337:1641–47. (Level I)

9. Walsh BW, Kuller LH, Wild RA, Paul S, Farmer M, Lawrence JB, et al. Effects of raloxifene on serum lipids and coagulation factors in healthy postmenopausal women. JAMA 1998;279:1445–51. (Level I)

10. Grey AB, Stapleton JP, Evans MC, Reid IR. The effect of the anti-estrogen tamoxifen on cardiovascular risk factors in normal postmenopausal women. J Clin Endocrinol Metab 1995;80:3191–5. (Level I)

11. Guetta V, Lush RM, Figg WD, Waclawiw MA, Cannon RO 3rd. Effects of the antiestrogen tamoxifen on low-density lipoprotein concentrations and oxidation in postmenopausal women. Am J Cardiol 1995;76:1072–73. (Level I)

12. Mijatovic V, van der Mooren MJ, Kenemans P, de Valk-de Roo GW, Netelenbos C. Raloxifene lowers serum lipoprotein(A) in healthy postmenopausal women: a randomized, double-blind, placebo-controlled comparison with conjugated equine estrogens. Menopause 1999;6:134–7. (Level I)

13. Shewmon DA, Stock JL, Rosen CJ, Heinilouma KM, Hogue MM, Morrison A, et al. Tamoxifen and estrogen lower circulating lipoprotein(a) concentrations in healthy postmenopausal women. Arterioscler Thromb 1994;14:1586–93. (Level I)

14. Cattaneo M, Baglietto L, Zighetti ML, Bettega D, Robertson C, Costa A, et al. Tamoxifen reduces plasma homocysteine levels in healthy women. Br J Cancer 1998;77:2264–66. (Level I)

15. Anker G, Lonning PE, Ueland PM, Refsum H, Lien EA. Plasma levels of the atherogenic amino acid homocysteine in post-menopausal women with breast cancer treated with tamoxifen. Int J Cancer 1995;60:365–68. (Level II-2)

16. Walsh BW, Paul S, Wild RA, Dean RA, Tracy RP, Cox DA, et al. The effects of hormone replacement therapy and raloxifene on C-reactive protein and homocysteine in healthy postmenopausal women: a randomized, controlled trial. J Clin Endocrinol Metab 2000;85:214–8. (Level I)

17. De Leo V, la Marca A, Morgante G, Lanzetta D, Setacci C, Petraglia F. Randomized control study of the effects of raloxifene on serum lipids and homocysteine in older women. Am J Obstet Gynecol 2001;184:350–53. (Level I)

18. Cushman M, Costantino JP, Tracy RP, Song K, Buckley L, Roberts JD, et al. Tamoxifen and cardiac risk factors in healthy women: Suggestion of an anti-inflammatory effect. Arterioscler Thromb Vasc Biol 2001;21:255–61. (Level I)

19. Barrett-Connor E, Grady D, Sashegyi A, Anderson PW, Cox DA, Hoszowski K, et al. Raloxifene and cardiovascular events in osteoporotic postmenopausal women: four-year results from the MORE (Multiple Outcomes of Raloxifene Evaluation) randomized trial. JAMA 2002;287:847–57. (Level I)

20. Fisher B, Costantino JP, Wickerham DL, Redmond CK, Kavanah M, Cronin WM, et al. Tamoxifen for prevention of breast cancer: report of the National Surgical Adjuvant Breast and Bowel Project P-1 Study. J Natl Cancer Inst 1998;90:1371–88. (Level I)

21. Saarto T, Blomqvist C, Ehnholm C, Taskinen MR, Elomaa I. Antiatherogenic effects of adjuvant anti-estrogens: a randomized trial comparing the effects of tamoxifen and toremifene on plasma lipid levels in post-menopausal women with node-positive breast cancer. J Clin Oncol 1996;14:429–33. (Level I)

22. Gylling H, Pyrhonen S, Mantyla E, Maenpaa H, Kangas L, Miettinen TA. Tamoxifen and toremifene lower serum cholesterol by inhibition of delta 8-cholesterol conversion to lathosterol in women with breast cancer. J Clin Oncol 1995;13:2900–5. (Level I)

23. Herrington DM, Pusser BE, Riley WA, Thuren TY, Brosnihan KB, Brinton EA, et al. Cardiovascular effects of droloxifene, a new selective estrogen receptor modula-tor, in healthy postmenopausal women. Arterioscler Thromb Vasc Biol 2000;20:1606–12. (Level I)

24. Herrington DM, Brosnihan KB, Pusser BE, Seely EW, Ridker PM, Rifai N, et al. Differential effects of E and droloxifene on C-reactive protein and other markers of inflammation in healthy postmenopausal women. J Clin Endocrinol Metab 2001;86:4216–22. (Level I)

25. Cummings SR, Eckert S, Krueger KA, Grady D, Powles TJ, Cauley JA, et al. The effect of raloxifene on risk of breast cancer in postmenopausal women: results from the MORE randomized trial. Multiple Outcomes of Raloxifene Evaluation. JAMA 1999;281:2189–97. (Level I)

26. Davies GC, Huster WJ, Lu Y, Plouffe L Jr, Lakshmanan M. Adverse events reported by postmenopausal women in controlled trials with raloxifene. Obstet Gynecol 1999;93: 558–65. (Level III)

27. Goldstein SR, Scheele WH, Rajagopalan SK, Wilkie JL, Walsh BW, Parsons AK. A 12-month comparative study of raloxifene, estrogen, and placebo on the post-menopausal endometrium. Obstet Gynecol 2000;95: 95–103. (Level I)

28. Fugere P, Scheele WH, Shah A, Strack TR, Glant MD, Jolly E. Uterine effects of raloxifene in comparison with continuous-combined hormone replacement therapy in postmenopausal women. Am J Obstet Gynecol 2000;182: 568–74. (Level I)

29. Goldstein SR. Unusual ultrasonographic appearance of the uterus in patients receiving tamoxifen. Am J Obstet Gynecol 1994;170:447–51. (Level III)

30. McGonigle KF, Shaw SL, Vasilev SA, Odom-Maryon T, Roy S, Simpson JF. Abnormalities detected on trans-vaginal ultrasonography in tamoxifen-treated postmeno-pausal breast cancer patients may represent endometrial cystic atrophy. Am J Obstet Gynecol 1998;178:1145–50. (Level II-3)

31. Tomas E, Kauppila A, Blanco G, Apaja-Sarkkinen M, Laatikainen T. Comparison between the effects of tamox-ifen and toremifene on the uterus in postmenopausal breast cancer patients. Gynecol Oncol 1995;59:261–6. (Level I)

32. Kennedy MM, Baigrie CF, Manek S. Tamoxifen and the endometrium: review of 102 cases and comparison with HRT-related and non-HRT-related endometrial pathology. Int J Gynecol Pathol 1999;18:130–7. (Level II-2)

33. Fisher B, Costantino JP, Redmond CK, Fisher ER, Wickerham DL, Cronin WM. Endometrial cancer in tamoxifen-treated breast cancer patients: findings from the National Surgical Adjuvant Breast and Bowel Project (NSABP) B-14. J Natl Cancer Inst 1994;86:527–37. (Level I)

34. Tamoxifen for early breast cancer: an overview of the randomised trials. Early Breast Cancer Trialists' Collaborative Group. Lancet 1998;351:1451–67. (Meta-analysis)

35. Wickerham DL, Fisher B, Wolmark N, Bryant J, Costantino J, Bernstein L, et al. Association of tamoxifen and uterine sarcoma. Clin Oncol 2002;20:2758–60. (Level III)

36. Pyrhonen S, Ellmen J, Vuorinen J, Gershanovich M, Tominaga T, Kaufmann M, et al. Meta-analysis of trials comparing toremifene with tamoxifen and factors predict-ing outcome of antiestrogen therapy in postmenopausal women with breast cancer. Breast Cancer Res Treat 1999; 56:133–43. (Meta-analysis)

37. Marttunen MB, Cacciatore B, Hietanen P, Pyrhonen S, Tiitinen A, Wahlstrom T, et al. Prospective study on gynaecological effects of two antioestrogens tamoxifen and toremifene in postmenopausal women. Br J Cancer 2001;84:897–902. (Level I)

38. Ettinger B, Black DM, Mitlak BH, Knickerbocker RK, Nickelsen T, Genant HK, et al. Reduction of vertebral frac-ture risk in postmenopausal women with osteoporosis treated with raloxifene: results from a 3-year randomized clinical trial. Multiple Outcomes of Raloxifene Evaluation (MORE) Investigators. JAMA 1999;282:637–45. (Level I)

39. Miodrag A, Ekelund P, Burton R, Castleden CM. Tamoxifen and partial oestrogen agonism in post-menopausal women. Age Ageing 1991;20:52–4. (Level II-2)

40. Bruning PF. Droloxifene, a new anti-oestrogen in post-menopausal advanced breast cancer: preliminary results of a double-blind dose-finding phase II trial. Eur J Cancer 1992;28A:1404–7. (Level I)

41. Goldstein SR, Neven P, Zhou L, Taylor YL, Ciaccia AV, Plouffe L. Raloxifene effect on frequency of surgery for pelvic floor relaxation. Obstet Gynecol 2001;98:91–6. (Level III)

42. Loprinzi CL, Zahasky KM, Sloan JA, Novotny PJ, Quella SK. Tamoxifen induced hot flashes. Clin Breast Cancer 2000;1:52–6. (Level III)

43. Dowsett M, Dixon JM, Horgan K, Salter J, Hills M, Harvey E. Antiproliferative effects of idoxifene in a place-bo-controlled trial in primary human breast cancer. Clin Cancer Res 2000;6:2260–67. (Level I)

44. Haarstad H, Lonning PE, Gundersen S, Wist E, Raabe N, Kvinnsland S. Influence of droloxifene on metastatic breast cancer as first-line endocrine treatment. Acta Oncol 1998;37:365–68. (Level III)

45. Gershanovich M, Garin A, Baltina D, Kurvet A, Kangas L, Ellmen J. A phase III comparison of two toremifene doses to tamoxifen in postmenopausal women with advanced breast cancer. Eastern European Study Group. Breast Cancer Res Treat 1997;45:251–62. (Level I)

46. Chlebowski RT, Collyar DE, Somerfield MR. Pfister DG. American Society of Clinical Oncology technology assessment on breast cancer risk reduction strategies: tamoxifen and raloxifene. J Clin Oncol 1999;17:1939–55. (Level III)

47. Powles T, Eeles R, Ashley S, Easton D, Chang J, Downsett M, et al. Interim analysis of the incidence of breast cancer in the Royal Marsden Hospital tamoxifen randomised chemoprevention trial. Lancet 1998;352: 98–101. (Level I)

48. Veronesi U, Maisonneuve P, Costa A, Sacchini V, Maltoni C, Robertson C, et al. Prevention of breast cancer with tamoxifen: preliminary findings from the Italian randomised trial among hysterectomised women. Italian Tamoxifen Prevention Study. Lancet 1998;352:93–7. (Level I)

49. Cauley JA, Norton L, Lippman ME, Eckert S, Krueger KA, Purdie DW, et al. Continued breast cancer risk reduction in postmenopausal women treated with raloxifene: 4-year results from the MORE trial. Breast Cancer Res Treat 2001;65:125–34. (Level I)

50. Ruffin MT 4th, August DA, Kelloff GJ, Boone CW, Weber BL, Brenner DE. Selection criteria for breast cancer chemoprevention subjects. J Cell Biochem suppl 1993;17G:234–41. (Level III)

51. National Osteoporosis Foundation. Physician's guide to prevention and treatment of osteoporosis. Washington, DC: NOF; 1999. (Level III)

52. Johnston CC Jr, Bjarnason NH, Cohen FJ, Shah A, Lindsay R, Mitlak BH, et al. Long-term effects of raloxifene on bone mineral density, bone turnover, and serum lipid levels in early postmenopausal women: three-year data from 2 double-blind, randomized, placebo-controlled trials. Arch Intern Med 2000;160:3444–50. (Level I)

53. Meunier PJ, Vignot E, Garnero P, Confavreux E, Paris E, Liu-Leage S, et al. Treatment of postmenopausal women with osteoporosis or low bone density with raloxifene. Raloxifene Study Group Osteoporos Int 1999;10:330–6. (Level I)

54. Lufkin EG, Whitaker MD, Nickelsen T, Argueta R, Caplan RH, Knickerbocker RK, et al. Treatment of established postmenopausal osteoporosis with raloxifene: a randomized trial. J Bone Miner Res 1998;13:1747–54. (Level I)

55. Draper MW, Flowers DE, Huster WJ, Neild JA, Harper KD, Arnaud C. A controlled trial of raloxifene (LY139481) HCl: impact on bone turnover and serum lipid profile in healthy postmenopausal women. J Bone Miner Res 1996;11:835–42. (Level I)

56. Grey AB, Stapleton JP, Evans MC, Tatnell MA, Ames RW, Reid IR. The effect of the antiestrogen tamoxifen on bone mineral density in normal late postmenopausal women. Am J Med 1995;99:636–41. (Level I)

57. Prestwood KM, Gunness M, Muchmore DB, Lu Y, Wong M, Raisz LG. A comparison of the effects of raloxifene and estrogen on bone in postmenopausal women. J Clin Endocrinol Metab 2000;85:2197–202. (Level I)

58. Ott SM, Oleksik A, Lu Y, Harper K, Lips P. Bone histomorphometric and biochemical marker results of a 2-year placebo-controlled trial of raloxifene in postmenopausal women. J Bone Miner Res 2002;17:341–8. (Level I)

59. Black DM, Cummings SR, Karpf DB, Cauley JA, Thompson DE, Nevitt MC, et al. Randomised trial of effect of alendronate on risk of fracture in women with existing vertebral fractures. Fracture Intervention Trial Research Group. Lancet 1996;348:1535–41. (Level I)

60. Johnell O, Scheele WH, Lu Y, Reginster JY, Need AG, Seeman E. Additive effects of raloxifene and alendronate on bone density and biochemical markers of bone remodeling in postmenopausal women with osteoporosis. J Clin Endocrinol Metab 2002;87:985–92. (Level I)

61. Harris ST, Watts NB, Genant HK, McKeever CD, Hangartner T, Keller M, et al. Effects of risedronate treatment on vertebral and nonvertebral fractures in women with postmenopausal osteoporosis: a randomized controlled trial. Vertebral Efficacy With Risedronate Therapy (VERT) Study Group. JAMA 1999;282:1344–52. (Level I)

62. Chesnut CH 3rd, Silverman S, Andriano K, Genant H, Gimona A, Harris S, et al. A randomized trial of nasal spray salmon calcitonin in postmenopausal women with established osteoporosis: the prevent recurrence of osteoporotic fractures study. PROOF Study Group. Am J Med 2000;109:267–76. (Level I)

63. Sarkar S, Mitlak BH, Wong M, Stock JL, Black DM, Harper KD. Relationships between bone mineral density and incident vertebral fracture risk with raloxifene therapy. J Bone Miner Res 2002;17:1–10. (Level I)

64. Cummings SR, Palermo L, Browner W, Marcus R, Wallace R, Pearson J, et al. Monitoring osteoporosis therapy with bone densitometry: misleading changes and regression to the mean. Fracture Intervention Trial Research Group. JAMA 2000;283:1318–21. (Level I)

65. Berliere M, Charles A, Galant C, Donnez J. Uterine side effects of tamoxifen: a need for systematic pretreatment screening. Obstet Gynecol 1998;91:40–4. (Level II-2)

66. Gail MH, Brinton LA, Byar DP, Corle DK, Green SB, Schairer C, et al. Projecting individualized probabilities of developing breast cancer for white females who are being examined annually. J Natl Cancer Inst 1989;81:1879–86. (Level III)

67. Bryant J, Fisher B, Dignam J. Duration of adjuvant tamoxifen therapy. J Natl Cancer Inst Monogr 2001;30: 56–61. (Level III)

The MEDLINE database, the Cochrane Library, and ACOG's own internal resources and documents were used to conduct a literature search to locate relevant articles published between January 1985 and November 2001. The search was restricted to articles published in the English language. Priority was given to articles reporting results of original research, although review articles and commentaries also were consulted. Abstracts of research presented at symposia and scientific conferences were not considered adequate for inclusion in this document. Guidelines published by organizations or institutions such as the National Institutes of Health and the American College of Obstetricians and Gynecologists were reviewed, and additional studies were located by reviewing bibliographies of identified articles. When reliable research was not available, expert opinions from obstetrician–gynecologists were used.

Studies were reviewed and evaluated for quality according to the method outlined by the U.S. Preventive Services Task Force:

I   Evidence obtained from at least one properly designed randomized controlled trial.
II-1   Evidence obtained from well-designed controlled trials without randomization.
II-2   Evidence obtained from well-designed cohort or case–control analytic studies, preferably from more than one center or research group.
II-3   Evidence obtained from multiple time series with or without the intervention. Dramatic results in uncontrolled experiments could also be regarded as this type of evidence.
III   Opinions of respected authorities, based on clinical experience, descriptive studies, or reports of expert committees.

Based on the highest level of evidence found in the data, recommendations are provided and graded according to the following categories:

Level A—Recommendations are based on good and consistent scientific evidence.

Level B—Recommendations are based on limited or inconsistent scientific evidence.

Level C—Recommendations are based primarily on consensus and expert opinion.

ISSN 1099-3630

The American College of Obstetricians and Gynecologists
409 12th Street, SW
PO Box 96920
Washington, DC 20090-6920

12345/65432

Selective estrogen receptor modulators. ACOG Practice Bulletin No. 39. The American College of Obstetricians and Gynecologists. Obstet Gynecol 2002;100:835–44.

ACOG PRACTICE BULLETIN

CLINICAL MANAGEMENT GUIDELINES FOR
OBSTETRICIAN–GYNECOLOGISTS

NUMBER 40, NOVEMBER 2002

(Replaces Practice Pattern Number 7, October 1997)

This Practice Bulletin was developed by the ACOG Committee on Practice Bulletins—Obstetrics with the assistance of Robert J. Sokol, MD, and Sean C. Blackwell, MD. The information is designed to aid practitioners in making decisions about appropriate obstetric and gynecologic care. These guidelines should not be construed as dictating an exclusive course of treatment or procedure. Variations in practice may be warranted based on the needs of the individual patient, resources, and limitations unique to the institution or type of practice.

Shoulder Dystocia

Shoulder dystocia is most often an unpredictable and unpreventable obstetric emergency. Failure of the shoulders to deliver spontaneously places both the pregnant woman and fetus at risk for injury. Several maneuvers to release impacted shoulders have been developed, but the urgency of this event makes prospective studies impractical for comparing their effectiveness. The purpose of this document is to provide clinicians with information based on published studies regarding management of deliveries at risk for or complicated by shoulder dystocia.

Background

Shoulder dystocia is most often defined as a delivery that requires additional obstetric maneuvers following failure of gentle downward traction on the fetal head to effect delivery of the shoulders (1). Retraction of the delivered fetal head against the maternal perineum (turtle sign) may be present and may assist in the diagnosis. Shoulder dystocia is caused by the impaction of the anterior fetal shoulder behind the maternal pubis symphysis. It also can occur from impaction of the posterior fetal shoulder on the sacral promontory. Because the delivering attendant must determine whether ancillary maneuvers are actually necessary, the diagnosis of shoulder dystocia has a subjective component. Although severe cases are readily apparent, milder forms may be overdiagnosed or underdiagnosed. The reported incidence ranges from 0.6% to 1.4% among vaginal deliveries of fetuses in the vertex presentation (2–7). Differences in reported rates are partly because of clinical variation in describing shoulder dystocia and the patient population being studied.

Maternal Complications

A study of 236 shoulder dystocia cases reported an 11% rate of postpartum hemorrhage and a 3.8% rate of fourth-degree lacerations (8). These complications were not more common with rotational maneuvers or other fetal manipulation when compared with the McRoberts maneuver alone (8). It should be noted that the performance of certain "heroic" maneuvers in cases of catastrophic shoulder dystocia, such as the Zavanelli maneuver and symphysiotomy, may be associated with significant maternal morbidity (9, 10).

Neonatal Complications

Brachial plexus injuries and fractures of the clavicle and humerus are associated with shoulder dystocia. The reported incidence of brachial plexus injuries following a delivery complicated by shoulder dystocia varies widely from 4% to 40% (2, 3, 5, 6, 11–18). Fortunately, most cases resolve without permanent disability; that is, fewer than 10% of all cases of shoulder dystocia result in a persistent brachial plexus injury (3, 14–16). Data suggest that a significant proportion (34–47%) of brachial plexus injuries are not associated with shoulder dystocia; in fact, 4% occur after cesarean delivery (11, 19–21).

Some severe cases of shoulder dystocia may result in hypoxic-ischemic encephalopathy and even death (22, 23). A study of outcomes from 6,238 cases of shoulder dystocia found that asphyxia was more common among births complicated by shoulder dystocia regardless of maternal diabetic status (22).

Clinical Considerations and Recommendations

▶ *Can shoulder dystocia be predicted accurately?*

Shoulder dystocia is most often unpredictable and unpreventable. Although fetal macrosomia and maternal diabetes increase the risk of shoulder dystocia (3, 5, 6, 22, 24–28), a substantial proportion of cases occur among women who do not have diabetes and among infants with birth weights less than 4,000 g. In one study, the presence of both diabetes and macrosomia accurately predicted only 55% of cases of shoulder dystocia (5). Additional studies failed to find any combination of risk factors that could accurately predict which pregnancies would be complicated by shoulder dystocia (3, 4, 6, 25, 26). Maternal obesity is associated with macrosomia, and, thus, obese women are at risk for shoulder dystocia. Other antepartum conditions associated with shoulder dystocia include multiparity, postterm gestation, previous history of a macrosomic birth, and a previous history of shoulder dystocia (5, 29). Associated intrapartum factors include labor induction, epidural anesthesia, and operative vaginal delivery (forceps and vacuum-assisted delivery) (3, 4). In each case, risk factors can be identified, but their predictive value is not high enough to be useful in a clinical setting.

▶ *Do labor abnormalities predict shoulder dystocia?*

Three studies have specifically evaluated labor patterns in patients who develop shoulder dystocia (30–32). The largest study, comparing 276 consecutive cases of shoulder dystocia with 600 matched controls, did not identify labor patterns as predictive among any of the cohort, even those with diabetes or macrosomia (30). Another found a significant association between active-phase abnormality and shoulder dystocia, but it included only 36 patients (31). A retrospective analysis of 52 cases of shoulder dystocia reported no difference in protracted dilatation and mean duration of second stage of labor (32). Therefore, data are inadequate to suggest that the labor curve is a useful predictor of shoulder dystocia.

▶ *Does labor induction for suspected fetal macrosomia affect the risk of shoulder dystocia or brachial plexus injury?*

A small, randomized trial of 273 patients with an ultrasound-estimated fetal weight of 4,000–4,500 g comparing labor induction with expectant management reported no significant difference in the rate of shoulder dystocia (3.7% versus 4.3%) or brachial plexus palsy (0% versus 1.4%) (33). Another retrospective study found labor induction with an antenatal diagnosis of macrosomia significantly increased the cesarean delivery rate (36% versus 17%) (34). Labor induction in a woman who does not have diabetes for the sole indication of suspected macrosomia has not been shown to be effective in decreasing the occurrence of shoulder dystocia or decreasing the rate of cesarean delivery (35).

▶ *Is there any benefit to planned cesarean delivery for the prevention of shoulder dystocia in cases of suspected fetal macrosomia?*

A policy of planned cesarean delivery for suspected macrosomic fetuses (>4,000 g) in women who do not have diabetes is not recommended. Ultrasonography is not an accurate predictor of macrosomia (36–38). Furthermore, most macrosomic infants do not experience this complication. Consequently, if all fetuses suspected of being macrosomic underwent cesarean delivery, the cesarean delivery rate would increase disproportionately when compared with the reduction in the rate of shoulder dystocia (6, 24). For example, one study projected a 27% increase in the total cesarean delivery rate (increasing from 15.1% to 19.1%) if cesarean deliveries were performed for all patients with fetuses that weighed 4,000 g or more; unfortunately, the number of shoulder dystocia cases would be reduced by only 42% (6). Another study reported similar results among fetuses with estimated birth weights of 4,000 g or more; in that study, an additional 76 cesarean deliveries would have prevented only five cases of shoulder dystocia, none of which resulted in permanent injury (39). A study using a decision analysis model estimated an additional 2,345 cesarean deliveries would be required—at a cost of $4.9 million annually—to prevent one permanent injury resulting from shoulder dystocia if all fetuses suspected of weighing 4,000 g or more underwent cesarean delivery (11). Although the diagnosis of fetal macrosomia is imprecise, prophylactic cesarean delivery may be considered for suspected fetal macrosomia with estimated fetal weights greater than 5,000 g in women without diabetes and greater than 4,500 g in women with diabetes (40).

▶ *What should the obstetrician do in cases of shoulder dystocia?*

The performance of the McRoberts maneuver is a reasonable initial maneuver (41). One study described this maneuver as involving hyperflexion and abduction of the hips causing cephalad rotation of the symphysis pubis and flattening of the lumbar lordosis that frees the impacted shoulder (42). Suprapubic pressure may be used at the same time to assist in dislodging the impacted shoulder (1). In contrast, fundal pressure may further worsen impaction of the shoulder and also may result in uterine rupture (12, 17). Controversy exists as to whether episiotomy is necessary, because shoulder dystocia typically is not caused by obstructing soft tissue. Direct fetal manipulation with either rotational maneuvers or delivery of the posterior arm also may be used (43). In these circumstances, performance of a proctoepisiotomy may be helpful to create more room within the posterior vagina.

In cases of severe shoulder dystocia that are not responsive to commonly used maneuvers, more aggressive approaches may be warranted. Cephalic replacement (Zavanelli maneuver) has been described for relieving catastrophic cases (9, 10, 44–46); however, it is associated with a significantly increased risk of fetal morbidity and mortality and maternal morbidity. Intentional fracture of the fetal clavicle may help decrease the bisacromial diameter; however it may be difficult to perform in emergent situations. It is clear that brachial plexus injury can occur regardless of the procedure or procedures used to disimpact the shoulders (3, 4, 47, 48).

▶ *How should a woman with a history of delivery complicated by shoulder dystocia be counseled regarding subsequent deliveries?*

A history of shoulder dystocia is associated with a recurrence rate ranging from 1% to 16.7% (3, 26, 49–51).

However, the true incidence may remain unknown because physicians and patients often choose not to attempt a trial of labor when there is a history of a complicated delivery or an injured infant.

Because most subsequent deliveries will not be complicated by shoulder dystocia, the benefit of universal elective cesarean delivery is questionable in patients who have such a history of shoulder dystocia. Other factors that may aid in the decision-making process for mode of delivery include the present estimate of fetal weight compared with the prior pregnancy birth weight, gestational age, the presence of maternal glucose intolerance, and the severity of the prior neonatal injury. A discussion and review of the prior delivery events should be undertaken with the patient, preferably before the intrapartum period. After discussion with the patient, either method of delivery is appropriate.

Summary of Recommendations

The following recommendations are based on limited or inconsistent scientific evidence (Level B):

▶ Shoulder dystocia cannot be predicted or prevented because accurate methods for identifying which fetuses will experience this complication do not exist.

▶ Elective induction of labor or elective cesarean delivery for all women suspected of carrying a fetus with macrosomia is not appropriate.

The following recommendations are based primarily on consensus and expert opinion (Level C):

▶ In patients with a history of shoulder dystocia, estimated fetal weight, gestational age, maternal glucose intolerance, and the severity of the prior neonatal injury should be evaluated and the risks and benefits of cesarean delivery discussed with the patient.

▶ Planned cesarean delivery to prevent shoulder dystocia may be considered for suspected fetal macrosomia with estimated fetal weights exceeding 5,000 g in women without diabetes and 4,500 g in women with diabetes.

▶ There is no evidence that any one maneuver is superior to another in releasing an impacted shoulder or reducing the chance of injury. However, performance of the McRoberts maneuver is a reasonable initial approach.

References

1. Resnik R. Management of shoulder girdle dystocia. Clin Obstet Gynecol 1980;23:559–64. (Level III)

2. Hopwood HG. Shoulder dystocia: fifteen years' experience in a community hospital. Am J Obstet Gynecol 1982; 144:162–6. (Level III)

3. Baskett TF, Allen AC. Perinatal implications of shoulder dystocia. Obstet Gynecol 1995;86:14–7. (Level II-3)

4. Nocon JJ, McKenzie DK, Thomas LJ, Hansell RS. Shoulder dystocia: an analysis of risks and obstetric maneuvers. Am J Obstet Gynecol 1993;168:1732–7; discussion 1737–9. (Level II-2)

5. Acker DB, Sachs BP, Friedman EA. Risk factors for shoulder dystocia. Obstet Gynecol 1985;66:762–8. (Level II-2)

6. Gross SJ, Shime J, Farine D. Shoulder dystocia: predictors and outcome. A five-year review. Am J Obstet Gynecol 1987;156:334–6. (Level II-3)

7. Gherman RB, Ouzounian JG, Miller DA, Kwok L, Goodwin TM. Spontaneous vaginal delivery: a risk factor for Erb's palsy? Am J Obstet Gynecol 1998;178:423–7. (Level II-2)

8. Gherman RB, Goodwin TM, Souter I, Neumann K, Ouzounian JG, Paul RH. The McRoberts' maneuver for the alleviation of shoulder dystocia: how successful is it? Am J Obstet Gynecol 1997;176:656–61. (Level II-3)

9. O'Leary JA. Cephalic replacement for shoulder dystocia: present status and future role of the Zavanelli maneuver. Obstet Gynecol 1993;82:847–50. (Level III)

10. Goodwin TM, Banks E, Millar LK, Phelan JP. Catastrophic shoulder dystocia and emergency symphysiotomy. Am Obstet Gynecol 1997;177:463–4. (Level III)

11. Rouse DJ, Owen J, Goldenberg RL, Cliver SP. The effectiveness and costs of elective cesarean delivery for fetal macrosomia diagnosed by ultrasound. JAMA 1996;276: 1480–6. (Level III)

12. el Madany AA, Jallad KB, Radi FA, el Hamdan H, O'deh HM. Shoulder dystocia: anticipation and outcome. Int J Gynaecol Obstet 1990;34:7–12. (Level II-2)

13. Hassan AA. Shoulder dystocia: risk factors and prevention. Aust N Z J Obstet Gynaecol 1988;28:107–9. (Level III)

14. Morrison JC, Sanders JR, Magann EF, Wiser WL. The diagnosis and management of dystocia of the shoulder. Surg Gynecol Obstet 1992;175:515–22. (Level III)

15. al-Najashi S, al-Suleiman SA, el-Yahia A, Rahman MS, Rahman J. Shoulder dystocia—a clinical study of 56 cases. Aust & N Z J of Obstet Gynaecol 1989;29:129–32. (Level II-3)

16. Keller JD, Lopez-Zeno JA, Dooley SL, Socol ML. Shoulder dystocia and birth trauma in gestational diabetes: a five-year experience. Am J Obstet Gynecol 1991;165: 928–30. (Level II-2)

17. Gross TL, Sokol RJ, Williams T, Thompson K. Shoulder dystocia: a fetal-physician risk. Am J Obstet Gynecol 1987; 156:1408–18. (Level II-2)

18. Gonik B, Hollyer VL, Allen R. Shoulder dystocia recognition: differences in neonatal risks for injury. Am J Perinatol 1991;8:31–4. (Level II-3)

19. Gilbert WM, Nesbitt TS, Danielsen B. Associated factors in 1611 cases of brachial plexus injury. Obstet Gynecol 1999;93:536–40. (Level II-3)

20. Gherman RB, Ouzounian JG, Goodwin TM. Brachial plexus palsy: an in utero injury? Am J Obstet Gynecol 1999;180:1303–7. (Level III)

21. Graham EM, Forouzan I, Morgan MA. A retrospective analysis of Erb's palsy cases and their relation to birth weight and trauma at delivery. J Matern Fetal Med 1997; 6:1–5. (Level II-3)

22. Nesbitt TS, Gilbert WM, Herrchen B. Shoulder dystocia and associated risk factors with macrosomic infants born in California. Am J Obstet Gynecol 1998;179:476–80. (Level II-3)

23. Hope P, Breslin S, Lamont L, Lucas A, Martin D, Moore I, et al. Fatal shoulder dystocia: a review of 56 cases reported to the Confidential Enquiry into Stillbirths and Deaths in Infancy. Br J Obstet Gynaecol 1998;105: 1256–61. (Level III)

24. Langer O, Berkus MD, Huff RW, Samueloff A. Shoulder dystocia: should the fetus weighing greater than or equal to 4000 grams be delivered by cesarean section? Am J Obstet Gynecol 1991;165:831–7. (Level II-2)

25. Sandmire HF, O'Halloin TJ. Shoulder dystocia: its incidence and associated risk factors. Int J Gynaecol Obstet 1988;26:65–73. (Level II-2)

26. Bahar AM. Risk factors and fetal outcome in cases of shoulder dystocia compared with normal deliveries of a similar birthweight. Br J Obstet Gynaecol 1996;103: 868–72. (Level II-2)

27. Gonen R, Spiegel D, Abend M. Is macrosomia predictable, and are shoulder dystocia and birth trauma preventable? Obstet Gynecol 1996;88:526–9. (Level II-2)

28. Benedetti TJ, Gabbe SG. Shoulder dystocia. A complication of fetal macrosomia and prolonged second stage of labor with midpelvic delivery. Obstet Gynecol 1978; 52:526–9. (Level II-3)

29. Acker DB, Sachs BP, Friedman EA. Risk factors for shoulder dystocia in the average-weight infant. Obstet Gynecol 1986;67:614–8. (Level II-2)

30. McFarland M, Hod M, Piper JM, Xenakis EM, Langer O. Are labor abnormalities more common in shoulder dystocia? Am J Obstet Gynecol 1995;173:1211–4. (Level II-2)

31. Gemer O, Bergman M, Segal S. Labor abnormalities as a risk factor for shoulder dystocia. Acta Obstet Gynecol Scand 1999;78:735–6. (Level II-2)

32. Lurie S, Levy R, Ben-Arie A, Hagay Z. Shoulder dystocia: could it be deduced from the labor partogram? Am J Perinatol 1995;12:61–2. (Level II-2)

33. Gonen O, Rosen DJ, Dolfin Z, Tepper R, Markov S, Fejgin MD. Induction of labor versus expectant management in macrosomia: a randomized study. Obstet Gynecol 1997; 89:913–7. (Level I)

34. Leaphart WL, Meyer MC, Capeless EL. Labor induction with a prenatal diagnosis of fetal macrosomia. J Matern Fetal Med 1997;6:99–102. (Level II-2)

35. Kjos SL, Henry OA, Montoro M, Buchanan TA, Mestman JH. Insulin-requiring diabetes in pregnancy: a randomized trial of active induction of labor and expectant management. Am J Obstet Gynecol 1993;169:611–5. (Level I)

36. Smith GC, Smith MF, McNay MB, Fleming JE. The relation between fetal abdominal circumference and birthweight: findings in 3512 pregnancies. Br J Obstet Gynaecol 1997;104:186–90. (Level II-3)

37. O'Reilly-Green CP, Divon MY. Receiver operating characteristic curves of sonographic estimated fetal weight for prediction of macrosomia in prolonged pregnancies. Ultrasound Obstet Gynecol 1997;9:403–8. (Level II-3)

38. Benacerraf BR, Gelman R, Frigoletto FD Jr. Sonographically estimated fetal weights: accuracy and limitation. Am J Obstet Gynecol 1988;159:1118–21. (Level II-2)

39. Delpapa EH, Mueller-Heubach E. Pregnancy outcome following ultrasound diagnosis of macrosomia. Obstet Gynecol 1991;78:340–3. (Level II-3)

40. Rouse DJ, Owen J, Goldenberg RL, Cliver SP. The effectiveness and costs of elective cesarean delivery for fetal macrosomia diagnosed by ultrasound. JAMA 1996;276:1480–6. (Level III)

41. Gherman RB, Tramont J, Muffley P, Goodwin TM. Analysis of McRoberts' maneuver by X-ray analysis. Obstet Gynecol 2000;95:43–7. (Level III)

42. Gonik B, Stringer CA, Held B. An alternate maneuver for management of shoulder dystocia. Am J Obstet Gynecol 1983;145:882–4. (Level II)

43. O'Leary JA, Leonetti HB. Shoulder dystocia: prevention and treatment. Am J Obstet Gynecol 1990;162:5–9. (Level III)

44. Gherman R. Catastrophic shoulder dystocia—what is the etiology? Am J Obstet Gynecol 1998;178:417. (Level III)

45. Sandberg EC. The Zavanelli maneuver: a potentially revolutionary method for the resolution of shoulder dystocia. Am J Obstet Gynecol 1985;152:479–84. (Level III)

46. Sandberg EC. The Zavanelli maneuver: 12 years of recorded experience. Obstet Gynecol 1999;93:312–7. (Level III)

47. Gherman RB, Ouzounian JG, Goodwin TM. Obstetric maneuvers for shoulder dystocia and associated fetal morbidity. Am J Obstet Gynecol 1998;178:1126–30. (Level II-2)

48. McFarland MB, Langer O, Piper JM, Berkus MD. Perinatal outcome and the type and number of maneuvers in shoulder dystocia. Int J Gynaecol Obstet 1996;55:219–24. (Level II-3)

49. Smith RB, Lane C, Pearson JF. Shoulder dystocia: what happens at the next delivery? Br J Obstet Gynaecol 1994;101:713–5. (Level II-3)

50. Ginsberg NA, Moisidis C. How to predict recurrent shoulder dystocia. Am J Obstet Gynecol 2001;184:1427–9; discussion 1429–30. (Level II-2)

51. Lewis DF, Raymond RC, Perkins MB, Brooks GG, Heymann AR. Recurrence rate of shoulder dystocia. Am J Obstet Gynecol 1995;172:1369–71. (Level II-2)

The MEDLINE database, the Cochrane Library, and ACOG's own internal resources and documents were used to conduct a literature search to locate relevant articles published between January 1985 and November 2000. The search was restricted to articles published in the English language. Priority was given to articles reporting results of original research, although review articles and commentaries also were consulted. Abstracts of research presented at symposia and scientific conferences were not considered adequate for inclusion in this document. Guidelines published by organizations or institutions such as the National Institutes of Health and the American College of Obstetricians and Gynecologists were reviewed, and additional studies were located by reviewing bibliographies of identified articles. When reliable research was not available, expert opinions from obstetrician–gynecologists were used.

Studies were reviewed and evaluated for quality according to the method outlined by the U.S. Preventive Services Task Force:

I   Evidence obtained from at least one properly designed randomized controlled trial.

II-1   Evidence obtained from well-designed controlled trials without randomization.

II-2   Evidence obtained from well-designed cohort or case–control analytic studies, preferably from more than one center or research group.

II-3   Evidence obtained from multiple time series with or without the intervention. Dramatic results in uncontrolled experiments could also be regarded as this type of evidence.

III   Opinions of respected authorities, based on clinical experience, descriptive studies, or reports of expert committees.

Based on the highest level of evidence found in the data, recommendations are provided and graded according to the following categories:

Level A—Recommendations are based on good and consistent scientific evidence.

Level B—Recommendations are based on limited or inconsistent scientific evidence.

Level C—Recommendations are based primarily on consensus and expert opinion.

ISSN 1099-3630

The American College of Obstetricians and Gynecologists
409 12th Street, SW
PO Box 96920
Washington, DC 20090-6920

12345/65432

Shoulder dystocia. ACOG Practice Bulletin No. 40. American College of Obstetricians and Gynecologists. Obstet Gynecol 2002;100:1045–50.

ACOG PRACTICE BULLETIN

CLINICAL MANAGEMENT GUIDELINES FOR
OBSTETRICIAN–GYNECOLOGISTS

NUMBER 16, MAY 2000

(Replaces Educational Bulletin Number 192, May 1994)

This Practice Bulletin was developed by the ACOG Committee on Practice Bulletins—Gynecology with the assistance of Elizabeth A. Stewart, MD. The information is designed to aid practitioners in making decisions about appropriate obstetric and gynecologic care. These guidelines should not be construed as dictating an exclusive course of treatment or procedure. Variations in practice may be warranted based on the needs of the individual patient, resources, and limitations unique to the institution or type of practice.

Surgical Alternatives to Hysterectomy in the Management of Leiomyomas

Uterine leiomyomas (also called fibroids) are the most common solid pelvic tumors in women and the leading indication for hysterectomy. Although most women with uterine leiomyomas are asymptomatic and can be followed without treatment, some will require more active measures. Hysterectomy remains the most common treatment for leiomyomas because it is the only treatment that provides a cure and eliminates the possibility of recurrence. Many women seek an alternative to hysterectomy because they desire future childbearing or wish to retain their uteri even if they have completed childbearing. As alternatives to hysterectomy become increasingly available, the efficacies of these treatments and the risk of potential problems are important to delineate. The purpose of this bulletin is to review the literature about surgical alternatives to hysterectomy and to offer treatment recommendations.

Background

As benign neoplasms, uterine leiomyomas usually require treatment only when they cause symptoms. The two most common symptoms for which women seek treatment are abnormal uterine bleeding and pelvic pressure or pain. However, not all bleeding is caused by leiomyomas; therefore, other causes of abnormal bleeding should be ruled out. The most common kind of abnormal uterine bleeding associated with leiomyomas is menorrhagia. Often, menses last 7 days or more, frequently resulting in iron deficiency anemia. This heavy flow also may require frequent changes of sanitary protection, causing significant interruptions in a woman's work or social schedule.

Uterine leiomyomas are clinically apparent in 25–50% of women (1), although studies in which careful pathologic examination of the uterus is carried out suggest the prevalence may be as high as 80% (2). The lack of a simple, inexpensive, and safe long-term medical treatment means that most symptomatic leiomyomas are still managed surgically.

Leiomyomas range greatly in size. Both size and location can play a role in symptoms and potential treatments. Leiomyomas may be subserosal, submucosal, or intramural; however, some types may be combined, for example, largely intramural with a submucosal extension.

The pelvic and abdominal discomfort that women experience with leiomyomas often is referred to as pressure and often is analogous to the discomforts women experience during pregnancy due to the enlarging of the uterus. In addition to pelvic pressure, the leiomyomas may press on adjacent structures, leading to difficulty with urination or defecation or dyspareunia.

Surgical Alternatives to Hysterectomy

In choosing a surgical alternative to hysterectomy, both safety and efficacy need to be established for each procedure. It must be recognized that all surgical alternatives to hysterectomy allow the possibility for new leiomyomas to form, and preexisting leiomyomas that were too small to be detected or were intentionally not removed may exhibit significant growth, necessitating another procedure. Complications of other surgical procedures may lead to an unanticipated hysterectomy.

Myomectomy

For women who desire future childbearing or who prefer to retain their uteri, myomectomy may be an option. Myomectomy removes only the visible and accessible leiomyomas, and the uterus is reconstructed. Most myomectomies traditionally have been performed by laparotomy.

Laparoscopic Myomectomy

Endoscopic myomectomy is now a treatment option for many women. Laparoscopic myomectomy minimizes the size of the abdominal incision, although it usually requires a minimum of three small incisions. Because the laparoscope usually is inserted at the umbilicus, the uterus must be small enough to be well-visualized with this approach; thus, this technique would not be appropriate for large uteri.

Hysteroscopic Procedures

Hysteroscopic procedures are primarily efficacious for the control of leiomyoma-related bleeding and do not significantly reduce uterine size. Only if a leiomyoma is submucosal or has a submucosal component can it be removed through the vagina (ie, hysteroscopic myomectomy).

For women with primarily intramural leiomyomas or women who have simultaneous hysteroscopic myomectomies, destruction of the endometrium by endometrial ablation can decrease bleeding. Endometrial ablation can be performed for a variety of indications, and it also can be useful in the control of leiomyoma-related menorrhagia. Endometrial ablation can utilize a variety of techniques, including laser ablation, thermal ablation, physical resection, or chemical destruction. Theoretically, even if leiomyomas remain, menstrual bleeding cannot occur because there is no endometrium. These procedures require hysteroscopic expertise.

Procedures Under Development

Several innovative options are being studied as possible alternative treatments for leiomyomas. Although all of these procedures may prove to be effective treatments for leiomyomas compared with current options, the number of patients treated have been small, the follow-up periods have been relatively short, and the safety of the procedures in women desiring pregnancy has not been demonstrated.

Uterine artery embolization is a radiologic alternative to surgery that involves partial blockage of the uterine arteries and, thus, decreased blood flow to the leiomyomatous uterus. Several case series of embolizations have been reported, with 8–53 patients monitored for intervals of 3–20 months (3–5). These reports suggest that most patients have a significant decrease in bleeding symptoms, as well as a reduction in uterine size. However, uterine artery embolization may have serious consequences including infection, massive uterine bleeding, and uterine necrosis, requiring emergency surgery (6). Patients can experience significant uterine pain, ischemia, and hypoxic changes following embolization of the myoma. Therefore, uterine artery embolization is regarded as investigational. Myolysis involves delivering electric current with needles or the use of lasers to coagulate myomas at the time of laparoscopy. A large series of cases have been reported from a single center (7).

As the biology of leiomyomas is better understood, new medical treatment options may become available. Both the progesterone antagonist mifepristone (RU 486) and gonadotropin-releasing hormone (GnRH) antagonists have been shown in small studies to produce equivalent levels of uterine shrinkage and rates of amenorrhea to GnRH agonists (8–10), with the attendant advantages of normal follicular levels of estradiol (mifepristone) and rapidity of action (antagonists). Understanding the derangements of growth factors and genes that lead to leiomyoma formation and growth also may lead to new medical therapies aimed at these underlying mechanisms (11).

Clinical Considerations and Recommendations

▶ *In symptomatic women with leiomyomas and an indication for surgery, does hysterectomy produce a better outcome than myomectomy in relation to long-term morbidity (eg, pain, bleeding, recurrence, operative complications, and patient satisfaction)?*

Randomized studies are difficult to perform on this subject for which patient preference often is strong. However, reports of retrospective series have provided some information on this topic.

Abdominal Myomectomy. Although early studies suggested the morbidity associated with myomectomy was increased compared with hysterectomy, more recent studies suggest that the risks of the two procedures are similar (12–14). However, women choosing myomectomy face the additional risks of recurrence of leiomyomas and the possibility of having to proceed with hysterectomy because of intraoperative complications.

There is less outcomes research available for myomectomy than there is for hysterectomy (15). However, clinical experience and pooled results of numerous small studies suggest that there is excellent resolution of menorrhagia symptoms (overall 81% resolution; range, 40–93%) with similar results for resolution of pelvic pressure with abdominal myomectomy (1).

In the long term, however, the risk of formation of new leiomyomas limits the efficacy of myomectomy. There are a number of studies that have examined the use of ultrasonography to assess the recurrence risk of leiomyomas after abdominal myomectomy (16–19). Clearly, an estimate depends on the detection power of the measuring instrument. Thus, later studies using transvaginal ultrasonography tend to give higher estimates of recurrence (51% at 5 years) compared with earlier transabdominal ultrasound studies (27% at 10 years) but, presumably, are more accurate (16, 17). Studies have indicated that women who experience childbirth after a myomectomy appear to have a decreased recurrence risk

(16, 17). There have been conflicting reports over whether the preoperative use of GnRH agonists affects recurrence risk (18, 19).

The clinically relevant endpoint is whether a second surgical procedure is needed after conservative surgery. A summary of a small case series conducted since the 1920s suggests the risk of follow-up treatment (in this instance, defined as hysterectomy, second myomectomy, or radiation therapy) varied from 3% to 32%, with a mean risk of 15%, although no information on the length of follow-up was given (1). In a relatively large series (125 patients followed at least 5 years and up to 23 years), there was evidence that recurrence depended on the number of leiomyomas present, with a recurrence risk of 11% for a single myoma and a recurrence risk of 26% with multiple myomas (20). A more recent study of 80 patients found a similar reoperation rate of 18% after 10 years (21).

The risk of undergoing an unexpected hysterectomy at the time of myomectomy appears to be low with skilled surgical technique (<1%), even when uterine size is substantial (14, 22–24). There may, however, be higher rates of hysterectomy for surgeons inexperienced in the procedure. Blood loss and the risk of transfusion may be increased in women with larger uteri (14, 25).

Laparoscopic Myomectomy. There are a number of case series of laparoscopic myomectomies, the largest of them reporting on more than 200 patients covering a period in excess of 5 years (26–28). The two major concerns with laparoscopic myomectomy versus hysterectomy are the removal of large myomas through small abdominal incisions and the repair of the uterus. The introduction of more efficient morcellators has made the removal easier, although skilled operative technique is necessary because injury to other organs is possible. Although there are multiple techniques available for laparoscopic suturing, there is controversy as to whether the closure techniques available are equal to those achieved at laparotomy. This is most relevant to women contemplating a future pregnancy.

Recommendations differ regarding cases amenable to a laparoscopic approach; most recommend a laparotomy or a laparoscopically assisted approach with leiomyomas in excess of 5–8 cm, multiple leiomyomas, or the presence of deep intramural leiomyomas (26–28). In addition to routine surgical complications, reported complications include a 2–8% conversion rate to a more open procedure, the formation of uteroperitoneal fistulas, and the possibility of uterine rupture during a subsequent pregnancy (26–28). It appears that the risk of recurrent leiomyomas may be higher after a laparoscopic myomectomy than after a traditional myomectomy, with a 33% recurrence risk at 27 months (29).

Hysteroscopic Myomectomy. Several series of between 100 and 200 patients undergoing hysteroscopic myomectomies with good results have been published. In a series in which almost all patients were treated for menorrhagia, 16% of the submucosal resection group ultimately underwent a second surgery after a mean follow-up of 9 years (30). In the same series, women undergoing ablation with or without submucosal myomectomy had an 8% chance of undergoing a second surgery after a mean of 6 years of follow-up (30). In a series of 167 patients who were followed for 3 years after hysteroscopic myomectomy plus myolysis, approximately 5% underwent a second surgery (31). For women desiring pregnancy, fertility rates appear good: 59% of patients with submucosal leiomyomas conceived after hysteroscopic myomectomy (32).

Endometrial Ablation. Endometrial ablation appears to be an effective therapy for the control of menstrual bleeding in women with abnormal bleeding only. For leiomyomas, one study suggested endometrial ablation had a failure rate of 40%, compared with a failure rate of 5% in women with a normal uterus (33). Thus, ablation for women with clinically significant leiomyomas may prove to be a less desirable course of action than for women with idiopathic menorrhagia. Currently, there is no evidence to support the use of this procedure for women with leiomyomas; however, new techniques are being explored.

Complications with all techniques involving operative hysteroscopy include the risk of injury to intraabdominal structures either by uterine perforation or secondary to electrical or thermal injury (34). In addition, there can be significant complications as a consequence of the distending medium used. The uterine vasculature can rapidly absorb the substance distending the uterus. Fatal events have been reported with air embolism using an Nd-YAG laser with saline as the distending medium, as well as with hyponatremic encephalopathy with sorbitol as the distending medium (35, 36). Many newer technologies have been designed to minimize this risk, including systems that accurately measure inflow and outflow of hysteroscopic fluids and devices that use physiologic saline as the uterine distending medium.

▶ *In women with leiomyomas who are candidates for surgery, does the use of adjunctive medical treatment result in better outcomes?*

Preoperative Adjuvants. Gonadotropin-releasing hormone agonists have been used widely for preoperative treatment of uterine leiomyomas, both for myomectomy and hysterectomy. These medications are very effective in inducing amenorrhea and causing uterine shrinkage in a large proportion of women who take them. However, they are expensive and have significant side effects for most women in the short term and significant effects on bone density if taken over longer periods.

Currently, GnRH agonists are the only drugs available that result in clinically significant uterine shrinkage and amenorrhea. When a significant reduction in uterine volume is necessary to achieve surgical goals (eg, when the patient prefers a low-transverse incision instead of a vertical incision or an endoscopic procedure), GnRH agonists may be useful.

By inducing amenorrhea, GnRH agonists have been shown to improve hematologic parameters, shorten hospital stay, and decrease blood loss, operating time, and postoperative pain when given for 2–3 months preoperatively (37–39). However, because no study has shown a significant decrease in transfusion risk or improvement in quality of life, and the cost of these medications is substantial, the decision to use GnRH agonists preoperatively remains complex. It also is worth noting that in a study that achieved hematologic improvement with GnRH agonist treatment in 74% of women, there was a 46% improvement rate in the placebo group with iron supplementation alone (38). One surgical disadvantage to preoperative GnRH agonist therapy is that it may make the leiomyomas softer and the surgical planes less distinct. Although many studies find the operative time equivalent for laparotomies, one study of laparoscopic myomectomies found that overall operating time decreased after GnRH agonist treatment. However, in the subgroup in which the largest leiomyoma was hypoechoic, operative time was longer because of the difficulty in dissection (39).

Intraoperative Adjuvants. Several studies suggest that the infiltration of vasopressin into the myometrium decreases blood loss at the time of myomectomy. A study of 20 patients demonstrated that vasopressin significantly decreased blood loss compared with saline injection in a randomized myomectomy study (40). Two studies compared the use of physical vascular compression, primarily a tourniquet around the lower uterine segment, with pharmacologic vasoconstriction (vasopressin administration). In one study using a Penrose drain tourniquet and vascular clamps, there was no significant difference between the two techniques (25). A more recent study using a Foley catheter as a tourniquet found blood loss to be significantly greater in the tourniquet group (41). There are no studies comparing tourniquet with placebo. Additionally, one study demonstrated that injection of vasopressin into the cervix at the time of operative hysteroscopy decreased blood loss, fluid intravasation, and operative time (42).

▶ *In pregnant women who have undergone a myomectomy, does a planned cesarean delivery versus a trial of labor help prevent uterine rupture?*

No study directly addresses the issue of cesarean delivery versus a trial of labor after myomectomy. The widely quoted clinical dictum is that if the endometrial cavity is entered at the time of myomectomy, then cesarean delivery is recommended. This appears to arise from a 3-year collaborative trial of data reporting a rate of uterine rupture of approximately 0.1% (43). Most of these ruptures had cesarean deliveries as antecedents, and because myomectomy also can produce a transmural incision in the uterus, it appears to have been treated in an analogous way. However, in the original study, the incidence of uterine rupture after myomectomy was only 0.002% (43). There are rare case reports of rupture remote from term after traditional abdominal myomectomy (44, 45). Uterine rupture can carry significant consequences for both mother and fetus.

However, several case reports have demonstrated uterine rupture at 33–34 weeks of gestation following laparoscopic myomectomy (46–48) and myolysis (49, 50). Although most of the case reports detail ruptures with intramural leiomyomas, one describes a case in which the 5-cm leiomyoma was subserosal; however, in this case no suturing was performed (48). Clearly long-term follow-up is necessary to determine the safety of innovative approaches to leiomyomas in women attempting pregnancy, and patients should be counseled preoperatively regarding these issues.

▶ *In women with leiomyomas who desire to become pregnant, does removal of leiomyomas versus expectant management increase the pregnancy rate?*

It is difficult to assess the contributions of leiomyomas to infertility for several reasons. First, there is a high prevalence of leiomyomas in the population, and the incidence of leiomyomas increases with age, as does infertility. Because not all leiomyomas are symptomatic, many women may conceive without even knowing that they have them. Finally, studies to date have been case series; randomized trials have not been conducted.

It appears that distortion of the uterine cavity may cause infertility and lead to pregnancy complications (51, 52). One study examining women attempting in vitro fertilization showed a decreased implantation rate in women with distortion of the cavity (53). When myomectomies have been performed on infertile patients with no other infertility factor, pregnancy rates have been reported in the range of 40–60% after 1–2 years (54–56). However, the use of additional fertility treatments in these studies was not excluded and may have contributed to the increase as well.

Two recent studies have examined the effect of leiomyomas on the outcome of assisted reproduction when there is no distortion of the uterine cavity. Using age-matched patients with similar embryo characteristics, the first study found significant decreases in both clinical pregnancies (53% versus 37%) and delivery rates (48% versus 33%) in patients with leiomyomas (57). The second study showed both significantly decreased pregnancy rates and implantation rates with both intramural and submucosal leiomyomas but not with subserosal leiomyomas (58). Although a general problem with the myomatous uterus or other associated factors may play a role in this process, indications for myomectomy in women undergoing assisted reproductive techniques remain to be clarified.

Some surgeons feel that a prophylactic myomectomy for women with large fibroids who want to preserve future fertility may be appropriate in some circumstances. The evidence that the complication rate is low in skilled surgical hands, even with substantial uterine size, suggests myomectomy may be indicated (14, 22–24); however, the risk of recurrent myomas is high, which may make myomectomy a less effective treatment (16, 17). Consideration of multiple factors is important, including size and location of myomas, previous fertility, and the woman's age.

▶ *In menopausal women with leiomyomas, what is the effect of hormone replacement therapy on leiomyoma growth, bleeding, and pain?*

For many years, health care providers have counseled patients that leiomyomas are a self-limiting problem that will resolve when a woman completes the transition to menopause. Because leiomyomas are responsive to estrogen, the hypoestrogenism of menopause most women experience results in uterine shrinkage, and all women have cessation of physiologic menses. However, as more women elect hormone replacement therapy, there is the possibility that problems with leiomyomas may persist into menopause.

There is some evidence that women with leiomyomas who take hormone replacement therapy are more likely to have abnormal bleeding. In a study using hysteroscopy to evaluate women with abnormal bleeding who were taking hormone replacement therapy (using women with no abnormal bleeding as controls), women with structural abnormalities of the cavity, including endometrial polyps and submucosal leiomyomas, had an increased likelihood of abnormal bleeding (59).

A small pilot study examined whether hormone replacement therapy during menopause caused an increase in size of asymptomatic leiomyomas (60). This study showed a significant increase in leiomyoma dimension after 1 year of transdermal hormone replacement therapy but no increase with oral conjugated estrogens. Because the clinical magnitude of the increase associated with the transdermal route is small (14.3–19.7 mm) and the follow-up time short, it is not clear whether this will result in clinically significant changes.

▶ *In asymptomatic women with leiomyomas, does expectant management produce a better outcome than surgical treatment in relation to long-term morbidity?*

Expectant management in an asymptomatic patient should be the norm; however, in some instances an asymptomatic leiomyomatous uterus might require treatment. If there is concern that the mass is not a leiomyoma but instead a sarcoma, further evaluation is warranted. Traditionally, the major clinical sign used to make this distinction was rapid growth in uterine size. However, in a study of 1,332 hysterectomy specimens for which the preoperative diagnosis was uterine leiomyomas, sarcomas were not only rare (2–3 per 1,000) but no more common in the subgroup of women who had experienced rapidly enlarging uterine size (61). If a comparison is made between the prevalence of leiomyosarcomas discovered incidentally (1:2,000) and the mortality rate for hysterectomy for benign disease (1.0–1.6 per 1,000 for premenopausal women), the decision to proceed to hysterectomy to find potential sarcomas should be made cautiously (62). Other risk factors for sarcomas, including increasing age or a history of prior pelvic radiation, may influence this decision. Alternatively, both endometrial biopsy and magnetic resonance imaging appear to be useful in diagnosing sarcomas and differentiating them from other intrauterine lesions (63, 64).

In rare circumstances, the uterus will cause significant compression of the ureters that can lead to the compromise of renal function, which requires further evaluation. Finally, in a woman contemplating pregnancy or experiencing recurrent miscarriage, significant distortion of the uterine cavity may require intervention in an asymptomatic patient (51, 52). Proximity of the leiomyoma to the placental implantation site and large size of the leiomyoma appear to increase obstetric risk, including placental abruption and premature labor. However, no consensus exists for when myomectomy should be rec-

ommended in women desiring pregnancy but with no history of infertility (52).

Historically, it has been argued that uterine size alone should be an indication for hysterectomy. The argument has usually been twofold. The first issue was that a large leiomyomatous uterus made assessment of the ovaries and early surveillance for ovarian cancer impossible. However, the National Institutes of Health and National Cancer Institute Consensus Conference acknowledge the futility of routine pelvic examinations in the identification of early ovarian cancer. Second, the argument is made that because of increased morbidity during surgery for a large uterus, surgery is a safer option when the uterus is smaller. Although some studies have shown increased morbidity, others show no differences in perioperative complications (13, 14, 62). This currently does not appear to be a cogent argument for intervention.

▶ *In women with leiomyomas planning future pregnancies who are candidates for surgery, what is the impact on future fertility (pregnancy rate) of surgery versus expectant management?*

As with any woman with leiomyomas, asymptomatic women with leiomyomas who desire future fertility should be managed expectantly because they have no indication for surgery. For mildly symptomatic women, given the risk of recurrence, intervening as close to the desired pregnancy as practical is desirable. The consequences of postoperative adhesions after myomectomy are unclear and should be avoided, despite the availability of assisted reproductive technology. Finally, although the risk of hysterectomy appears low for most surgical alternatives to hysterectomy, it is never eliminated. This risk should be considered in determining the appropriate treatment for women planning future pregnancies.

Summary

The following recommendations are based on good and consistent scientific evidence (Level A):

▶ In women with symptomatic leiomyomas, hysterectomy provides a definitive cure.

▶ In women with symptomatic leiomyomas, abdominal myomectomy is a safe and effective option for women who wish to retain their uterus. If this option is selected, women should be counseled preoperatively about the relatively high risk of reoperation.

▶ Use of GnRH agonists preoperatively is beneficial, especially when improvement of hematologic status and uterine shrinkage are important goals. Benefits of the use of GnRH agonists should be weighed against their cost and side effects for individual patients.

▶ The use of vasopressin at the time of myomectomy appears to limit blood loss.

The following recommendation is based on limited or inconsistent scientific evidence (Level B):

▶ The clinical diagnosis of rapidly growing leiomyomas has not been shown to predict uterine sarcoma and thus should not be used as the sole indication for myomectomy or hysterectomy.

The following recommendations are based primarily on consensus and expert opinion (Level C):

▶ Laparoscopic myomectomy appears to be a safe and effective option for women with a small number of moderately sized uterine leiomyomas who do not desire future fertility. Further studies are necessary to evaluate the safety of this procedure for women planning pregnancy.

▶ Hysteroscopic myomectomy is an effective option for controlling menorrhagia in women with submucosal leiomyomas.

▶ Although endometrial ablation appears to be an effective option in controlling menorrhagia in women without leiomyomas, further studies are needed in women who have clinically significant leiomyomas.

▶ Because leiomyomas may be a factor in infertility for some patients, the issues are complex, and myomectomy should not be performed without first completing a comprehensive fertility evaluation.

▶ Although postmenopausal women with leiomyomas may have more bleeding problems and some increase in leiomyoma size while taking hormone replacement therapy, there appears to be no reason to withhold this treatment option from women who desire or need such therapy.

References

1. Buttram VC Jr, Reiter RC. Uterine leiomyomata: etiology, symptomatology, and management. Fertil Steril 1981;36:433–445 (Level III)

2. Cramer SF, Patel A. The frequency of uterine leiomyomas. Am J Clin Pathol 1990;94:435–438 (Level II-3)

3. Bradley EA, Reidy JF, Forman RG, Jarosz J, Braude PR. Transcatheter uterine artery embolisation to treat large uterine fibroids. Br J Obstet Gynaecol 1998;105:235–240 (Level III)

4. Goodwin SC, Vedantham S, McLucas B, Forno AE, Perrella R. Preliminary experience with uterine artery embolization for uterine fibroids. J Vasc Interv Radiol 1997;8:517–526 (Level III)

5. Ravina JH, Herbreteau D, Ciraru-Vigneron N, Bouret JM, Houdart E, Aymard A, et al. Arterial embolisation to treat uterine myomata. Lancet 1995;346:671–672 (Level III)

6. Barbieri RL. Ambulatory management of uterine leiomyomata. Clin Obstet Gynecol 1999;42:196–205 (Level III)

7. Goldfarb HA. Bipolar laparoscopic needles for myoma coagulation. J Am Assoc Gynecol Laparosc 1995;2:175–179 (Level II-2)

8. Kettel LM, Murphy AA, Morales AJ, Rivier J, Vale W, Yen SS. Rapid regression of uterine leiomyomas in response to daily administration of gonadotropin-releasing hormone antagonist. Fertil Steril 1993;60:642–646 (Level III)

9. Murphy AA, Kettel LM, Morales AJ, Roberts VJ, Yen SS. Regression of uterine leiomyomata in response to the antiprogesterone RU 486. J Clin Endocrinol Metab 1993;76:513–517 (Level III)

10. Murphy AA, Morales AJ, Kettel LM, Yen SS. Regression of uterine leiomyomata to the antiprogesterone RU486: dose-response effect. Fertil Steril 1995;64:187–190 (Level III)

11. Stewart EA, Nowak RA. Leiomyoma-related bleeding: a classic hypothesis updated for the molecular era. Hum Reprod Update 1996;2:295–306 (Level III)

12. Hillis SD, Marchbanks PA, Peterson HB. Uterine size and risk of complications among women undergoing abdominal hysterectomy for leiomyomas. Obstet Gynecol 1996;87:539–543 (Level II-2)

13. Iverson RE Jr, Chelmow D, Strohbehn K, Waldman L, Evantash EG. Relative morbidity of abdominal hysterectomy and myomectomy for management of uterine leiomyomas. Obstet Gynecol 1996;88:415–419 (Level II-2)

14. Ecker JL, Foster JT, Friedman AJ. Abdominal hysterectomy or abdominal myomectomy for symptomatic leiomyoma: a comparison of preoperative demography and postoperative morbidity. J Gynecol Surg 1995;11:11–18 (Level II-2)

15. Carlson KJ, Miller BA, Fowler FJ Jr. The Maine Women's Health Study: I. Outcomes of hysterectomy. Obstet Gynecol 1994;83:556–565 (Level II-3)

16. Candiani GB, Fedele L, Parazzini F, Villa L. Risk of recurrence after myomectomy. Br J Obstet Gynaecol 1991;98:385–389 (Level II-3)

17. Fedele L, Parazzini F, Luchini L, Mezzopane R, Tozzi L, Villa L. Recurrence of fibroids after myomectomy: a transvaginal ultrasonographic study. Hum Reprod 1995;10:1795–1796 (Level II-3)

18. Fedele L, Vercellini P, Bianchi S, Brioschi D, Dorta M. Treatment with GnRH agonists before myomectomy and

the risk of short-term myoma recurrence. Br J Obstet Gynaecol 1990;97:393–396 (Level I)

19. Friedman AJ, Daly M, Juneau-Norcross M, Fine C, Rein MS. Recurrence of myomas after myomectomy in women pretreated with leuprolide acetate depot or placebo. Fertil Steril 1992;58:205–208 (Level I)

20. Malone LJ. Myomectomy: recurrence after removal of solitary and multiple myomas. Obstet Gynecol 1969;34:200–203 (Level II-3)

21. Acien P, Quereda F. Abdominal myomectomy: results of a simple operative technique. Fertil Steril 1996;65:41–51 (Level II-3)

22. Smith DC, Uhlir JK. Myomectomy as a reproductive procedure. Am J Obstet Gynecol 1990;162:1476–1479; discussion 1479–1482 (Level III)

23. Chong RK, Thong PH, Tan SL, Thong PW, Salmon YM. Myomectomy: indications, results of surgery and relation to fertility. Singapore Med J 1988;29:35–37 (Level III)

24. LaMorte AI, Lalwani S, Diamond MP. Morbidity associated with abdominal myomectomy. Obstet Gynecol 1993; 82:897–900 (Level III)

25. Ginsburg ES, Benson CB, Garfield JM, Gleason RE, Friedman AJ. The effect of operative technique and uterine size on blood loss during myomectomy: a prospective randomized study. Fertil Steril 1993;60:956–962 (Level I)

26. Dubuisson JB, Chapron C, Levy L. Difficulties and complications of laparoscopic myomectomy. J Gynecol Surg 1996;12:159–165 (Level II-3)

27. Nezhat C, Nezhat F, Silfen SL, Schaffer N, Evans D. Laparoscopic myomectomy. Int J Fertil 1991;36:275–280 (Level II-3)

28. Seinera P, Arisio R, Decko A, Farina C, Crana F. Laparoscopic myomectomy: indications, surgical technique and complications. Hum Reprod 1997;12:1927–1930 (Level II-3)

29. Nezhat FR, Roemisch M, Nezhat CH, Seidman DS, Nezhat CR. Recurrence rate after laparoscopic myomectomy. J Am Assoc Gynecol Laparosc 1998;5:237–240 (Level III)

30. Derman SG, Rehnstrom J, Neuwirth RS. The long-term effectiveness of hysteroscopic treatment of menorrhagia and leiomyomas. Obstet Gynecol 1991;77:591–594 (Level II-3)

31. Phillips DR, Milim SJ, Nathanson HG, Haselkorn JS. Experience with laparoscopic leiomyoma coagulation and concomitant operative hysteroscopy. J Am Assoc Gynecol Laparosc 1997;4:425–433 (Level II-3)

32. Ubaldi F, Tournaye H, Camus M, Van der Pas H, Gepts E, Devroey P. Fertility after hysteroscopic myomectomy. Hum Reprod Update 1995;1:81–90 (Level III)

33. Yin CS, Wei RY, Chao TC, Chan CC. Hysteroscopic endometrial ablation without endometrial preparation. Int J Gynaecol Obstet 1998;62:167–172 (Level II-3)

34. Kivnick S, Kanter MH. Bowel injury from rollerball ablation of the endometrium. Obstet Gynecol 1992;79:833–835 (Level III)

35. Arieff AI, Ayus JC. Endometrial ablation complicated by fatal hyponatremic encephalopathy. JAMA 1993;270:1230–1232 (Level III)

36. Challener RC, Kaufman B. Fatal venous air embolism following sequential unsheathed (bare) and sheathed quartz fiber Nd:YAG laser endometrial ablation. Anesthesiology 1990;73:548–551 (Level III)

37. Gerris J, Degueldre M, Peters AA, Romao F, Stjernquist M, al-Taher H. The place of Zoladex in deferred surgery for uterine fibroids. Zoladex Myoma Study Group. Horm Res 1996;45:279–284 (Level I)

38. Stovall TG, Muneyyirci-Delale O, Summitt RL Jr, Scialli AR. GnRH agonist and iron versus placebo and iron in the anemic patient before surgery for leiomyomas: a randomized controlled trial. Leuprolide Acetate Study Group. Obstet Gynecol 1995;86:65–71 (Level I)

39. Zullo F, Pellicano M, De Stefano R, Zupi E, Mastrantonio P. A prospective randomized study to evaluate leuprolide acetate treatment before laparoscopic myomectomy: efficacy and ultrasonographic predictors. Am J Obstet Gynecol 1998;178:108–112 (Level I)

40. Frederick J, Fletcher H, Simeon D, Mullings A, Hardie M. Intramyometrial vasopressin as a haemostatic agent during myomectomy. Br J Obstet Gynaecol 1994;101:435–437 (Level I)

41. Fletcher H, Frederick J, Hardie M, Simeon D. A randomized comparison of vasopressin and tourniquet as hemostatic agents during myomectomy. Obstet Gynecol 1996;87:1014–1018 (Level I)

42. Phillips DR, Nathanson HG, Milim SJ, Haselkorn JS, Khapra A, Ross PL. The effect of dilute vasopressin solution on blood loss during operative hysteroscopy: a randomized controlled trial. Obstet Gynecol 1996;88:761–766 (Level I)

43. Garnet JD. Uterine rupture during pregnancy: an analysis of 133 patients. Obstet Gynecol 1964;23:898–905 (Level II-3)

44. Golan D, Aharoni A, Gonen R, Boss Y, Sharf M. Early spontaneous rupture of the post myomectomy gravid uterus. Int J Gynaecol Obstet 1990;31:167–170 (Level III)

45. Ozeren M, Ulusoy M, Uyanik E. First-trimester spontaneous uterine rupture after traditional myomectomy: case report. Isr J Med Sci 1997;33:752–753 (Level III)

46. Dubuisson JB, Chavet X, Chapron C, Gregorakis SS, Morice P. Uterine rupture during pregnancy after laparoscopic myomectomy. Hum Reprod 1995;10:1475–1477 (Level III)

47. Harris WJ. Uterine dehiscence following laparoscopic myomectomy. Obstet Gynecol 1992;80:545–546 (Level III)

48. Pelosi MA 3rd, Pelosi MA. Spontaneous uterine rupture at thirty-three weeks subsequent to previous superficial laparoscopic myomectomy. Am J Obstet Gynecol 1997;177:1547–1549 (Level III)

49. Arcangeli S, Pasquarette MM. Gravid uterine rupture after myolysis. Obstet Gynecol 1997;89:857 (Level III)

50. Vilos GA, Pispidikis JT, Botz CK. Economic evaluation of hysteroscopic endometrial ablation versus vaginal hys-

terectomy for menorrhagia. Obstet Gynecol 1996;88: 241–245 (Level II-2)

51. Garcia CR, Tureck RW. Submucosal leiomyomas and infertility. Fertil Steril 1984;42:16–19 (Level III)

52. Rice JP, Kay HH, Mahony BS. The clinical significance of uterine leiomyomas in pregnancy. Am J Obstet Gynecol 1989;160:1212–1216 (Level II-2)

53. Farhi J, Ashkenazi J, Feldberg D, Dicker D, Orvieto R, Ben Rafael Z. Effect of uterine leiomyomata on the results of in-vitro fertilization treatment. Hum Reprod 1995;10: 2576–2578 (Level II-2)

54. Babaknia A, Rock JA, Jones HW Jr. Pregnancy success following abdominal myomectomy for infertility. Fertil Steril 1978;30:644–647 (Level III)

55. Gehlbach DL, Sousa RC, Carpenter SE, Rock JA. Abdominal myomectomy in the treatment of infertility. Int J Gynaecol Obstet 1993;40:45–50 (Level III)

56. Sudik R, Husch K, Steller J, Daume E. Fertility and pregnancy outcome after myomectomy in sterility patients. Eur J Obstet Gynecol Reprod Biol 1996;65:209–214 (Level II-2)

57. Stovall DW, Parrish SB, Van Voorhis BJ, Hahn SJ, Sparks AE, Syrop CH. Uterine leiomyomas reduce the efficacy of assisted reproduction cycles: results of a matched follow-up study. Hum Reprod 1998;13:192–197 (Level II-2)

58. Eldar-Geva T, Meagher S, Healy DL, MacLachlan V, Breheny S, Wood C. Effect of intramural, subserosal, and submucosal uterine fibroids on the outcome of assisted reproductive technology treatment. Fertil Steril 1998;70: 687–691 (Level II-2)

59. Akkad AA, Habiba MA, Ismail N, Abrams K, al-Azzawi F. Abnormal uterine bleeding on hormone replacement: the importance of intrauterine structural abnormalities. Obstet Gynecol 1995;86:330–334 (Level II-2)

60. Sener AB, Seckin NC, Ozmen S, Gokmen O, Dogu N, Ekici E. The effects of hormone replacement therapy on uterine fibroids in postmenopausal women. Fertil Steril 1996;65:354–357 (Level II-1)

61. Parker WH, Fu YS, Berek JS. Uterine sarcoma in patients operated on for presumed leiomyoma and rapidly growing leiomyoma. Obstet Gynecol 1994;83:414–418 (Level II-3)

62. Reiter RC, Wagner PL, Gambone JC. Routine hysterectomy for large asymptomatic uterine leiomyomata: a reappraisal. Obstet Gynecol 1992;79:481–484 (Level II-3)

63. Schwartz LB, Diamond MP, Schwartz PE. Leiomyosarcomas: clinical presentation. Am J Obstet Gynecol 1993;168:180–183 (Level II-3)

64. Schwartz LB, Zawin M, Carcangiu ML, Lange R, McCarthy S. Does pelvic magnetic resonance imaging differentiate among the histologic subtypes of uterine leiomyomata? Fertil Steril 1998;70:580–587 (Level II-3)

The MEDLINE database, the Cochrane Library, and ACOG's own internal resources and documents were used to conduct a literature search to locate relevant articles published between January 1985 and May 1999. The search was restricted to articles published in the English language. Priority was given to articles reporting results of original research, although review articles and commentaries also were consulted. Abstracts of research presented at symposia and scientific conferences were not considered adequate for inclusion in this document. Guidelines published by organizations or institutions such as the National Institutes of Health and the American College of Obstetricians and Gynecologists were reviewed, and additional studies were located by reviewing bibliographies of identified articles. When reliable research was not available, expert opinions from obstetrician–gynecologists were used.

Studies were reviewed and evaluated for quality according to the method outlined by the U.S. Preventive Services Task Force:

I   Evidence obtained from at least one properly designed randomized controlled trial.

II-1   Evidence obtained from well-designed controlled trials without randomization.

II-2   Evidence obtained from well-designed cohort or case–control analytic studies, preferably from more than one center or research group.

II-3   Evidence obtained from multiple time series with or without the intervention. Dramatic results in uncontrolled experiments also could be regarded as this type of evidence.

III   Opinions of respected authorities, based on clinical experience, descriptive studies, or reports of expert committees.

Based on the highest level of evidence found in the data, recommendations are provided and graded according to the following categories:

Level A—Recommendations are based on good and consistent scientific evidence.

Level B—Recommendations are based on limited or inconsistent scientific evidence.

Level C—Recommendations are based primarily on consensus and expert opinion.

ISSN 1099-3630

**The American College of
Obstetricians and Gynecologists
409 12th Street, SW
PO Box 96920
Washington, DC 20090-6920**

12345/43210

ACOG *PRACTICE BULLETIN*

CLINICAL MANAGEMENT GUIDELINES FOR
OBSTETRICIAN–GYNECOLOGISTS

NUMBER 18, JULY 2000

This Practice Bulletin was developed by the ACOG Committee on Practice Bulletins— Gynecology with the assistance of Andrew M. Kaunitz, MD. The information is designed to aid practitioners in making decisions about appropriate obstetric and gynecologic care. These guidelines should not be construed as dictating an exclusive course of treatment or procedure. Variations in practice may be warranted based on the needs of the individual patient, resources, and limitations unique to the institution or type of practice.

The Use of Hormonal Contraception in Women with Coexisting Medical Conditions

Although numerous studies have addressed the safety and effectiveness of hormonal contraceptive use in healthy women, data are far less complete for women with underlying medical problems or other special circumstances. Because recommendations vary widely, substantial confusion exists with respect to contraceptive guidelines for women with coexisting medical conditions or other concerns. Using available scientific evidence, this Practice Bulletin will provide information to facilitate contraceptive counseling and selection for women with coexisting medical conditions.

Background

Decisions regarding contraception for women with coexisting medical problems may be complicated. In some cases, medications taken for certain chronic conditions may alter the effectiveness of hormonal contraception, and pregnancy in these cases may pose substantial risks to the mother as well as her fetus. Package labeling approved by the U.S. Food and Drug Administration for progestin-only oral contraceptives (OCs) is occasionally the same as that for combined estrogen-progestin preparations. For instance, current labeling for norethindrone progestin-only OCs no longer lists a history of thromboembolism as a contraindication (1). Such a history, however, remains listed as a contraindication in package labeling for norgestrel progestin-only pills and for depot medroxyprogesterone acetate (DMPA) injections.

Sometimes, simultaneous use of two contraceptive methods is appropriate. For instance, although hormonal contraception provides effective birth control for women at risk for human immunodeficiency virus or other sexually transmitted diseases (or those currently infected), such patients also should be encouraged to use male or female condoms correctly and consistently to prevent disease. For women concomitantly using major teratogens, such as isotretinoin or thalidomide, simultaneous use of two methods of contraception (eg, OCs and condoms) also may be appropriate.

This Practice Bulletin will focus on selection of hormonal contraceptives for women with coexisting medical problems. However, practitioners should recognize that the use of other nonhormonal forms of contraception, such as intrauterine devices, represent a safe, effective choice for many women.

Clinical Considerations and Recommendations

This document will address the use of combination OCs in women who have the following conditions and risk factors:

- Older than 35 years
- Smoke tobacco products
- Hypertension
- Diabetes
- Migraine headaches
- Fibrocystic breast changes, fibroadenoma, or family history of breast cancer
- Uterine fibroids
- Lipid disorders
- Breastfeeding/postpartum
- Take concomitant medication
- Anticipate surgery
- Venous thromboembolism (VTE)
- Systemic lupus erythematosus (SLE)
- Sickle cell disease

In addition, the document will review clinical settings in which the use of progestin-only contraceptives represent safe alternatives for women with contraindications to combination OCs (see the box). The effect of DMPA use on bone mineral density (BMD) will be reviewed, particularly with respect to adolescent candidates. Practitioners should be aware that patients who have any of the previously mentioned conditions or risk factors and use OCs require close monitoring and follow-up evaluation.

Indications for Contraception Methods Other Than Oral Contraceptives

In women with the following conditions, use of progestin-only oral contraceptives, depot medroxyprogesterone acetate,* or implants may be safer than combination oral contraceptives. An intrauterine device also represents an appropriate contraceptive choice for women with these conditions.

Migraine headaches

Older than 35 years and smoke cigarettes

History of thromboembolic disease

Coronary artery disease

Congestive heart failure

Cerebrovascular disease

Less than 2 weeks postpartum[†]

Hypertension with vascular disease or older than 35 years

Diabetes with vascular disease or older than 35 years

Systemic lupus erythematosus with vascular disease, nephritis, or antiphospholipid antibodies

Hypertriglyceridemia

* Because of its long duration of action and potential for hypoestrogenic effects, depot medroxyprogesterone acetate may be less appropriate than other progestin-only contraceptives for some women with these listed conditions.

[†]Use of an intrauterine device may not be an appropriate contraceptive choice.

▶ *Is combination OC use safe for women older than 35 years?*

Use of combination OCs is safe in healthy, nonsmoking women older than 35 years. Recent large U.S. population-based case–control studies found no increased risk of myocardial infarction (2) or stroke (3) among healthy, nonsmoking women older than 35 years who use OCs formulated with less than 50 μg of estrogen.

Perimenopausal women benefit from the more regular menses and positive effect on BMD (4, 5) offered by combination OCs. In addition, use of combination OCs may reduce vasomotor symptoms in perimenopausal women (6). Furthermore, the reduced risk of endometrial and ovarian cancers associated with OC use is of particular importance to older women of reproductive age.

As increasing numbers of women in their late 40s and early 50s use combination OCs, the question of when women no longer need contraception and can consider transitioning to hormone replacement therapy will arise more frequently. Assessment of follicle-stimulating hormone levels to determine when older OC users have become menopausal and thus no longer need contraception is expensive and may be misleading (7–10). Until a well-validated tool to confirm menopause is available, an alternative approach is for healthy, nonsmoking women doing well on combination OCs to discontinue OCs routinely between the ages of 50 and 55 years. By age 55, the likelihood that a woman has reached menopausal status is at least 85% (11, 12).

▶ *Is combination OC use safe for women who smoke cigarettes?*

Smoking represents the single most important preventable cause of death and disability in U.S. women (13). At every opportunity, women should be encouraged to quit smoking, regardless of hormonal contraception use.

Numerous epidemiologic studies conducted from the 1960s through the 1980s observed high relative risks of myocardial infarction among women who used OCs formulated with 50 µg or more of estrogen and smoked cigarettes, compared with women who neither smoked nor used OCs (14). The absolute rates of myocardial infarction in this study increased substantially among OC users who smoked and were in their mid-30s or older. Accordingly, package labeling for combination OCs was modified to warn clinicians and OC users of the risks associated with smoking among OC users in general and particularly among those aged 35 years and older.

Data are sparse on U.S. women older than 35 years who smoke and use OCs. Recently, epidemiologic studies assessing the risk of arterial events among U.S. women using contemporary OCs formulated with less than 50 µg of estrogen have been published. These large case–control studies found no evidence that use of these lower-dose contemporary formulations increased risks of myocardial infarction (2) or stroke (3) in nonsmokers or in women who smoked, regardless of their age. Reflecting current U.S. clinical practice, these studies included few OC users who were older than 35 years or who smoked. Therefore, unless other studies confirm the safety of contemporary combination OCs in older women who smoke, practitioners should prescribe combination OCs to such women with caution, if at all. Nonetheless, the recent U.S. studies provide evidence that combination OCs should not be denied to women younger than 30 years who smoke cigarettes (15). When considering OCs for women who are between the ages of 30 and 35 years and are smokers, the number of cigarettes smoked and the competing risk of pregnancy should be taken into account. In women who are older than 35 years and are smokers, the risk of using OCs is likely to exceed the risk of pregnancy.

▶ *Is combination OC use safe for women with chronic hypertension?*

Hypertension is a common condition associated with increased maternal and fetal risks should pregnancy occur, which emphasizes the importance of effective contraception for women with chronic hypertension.

Use of OCs appears to increase blood pressure, even with contemporary OC preparations. A small clinical trial found that an OC containing 30 µg of ethinyl estradiol and 150 µg of progestin increased the ambulatory blood pressure of normotensive women (approximately 8 mm Hg systolic and 6 mm Hg diastolic) (16). A small cross-sectional study of Italian women with mild hypertension found that those using combination OCs (most with 30 µg of estrogen) had ambulatory systolic blood pressures approximately 7 mm Hg higher than those not using OCs (17).

It is unclear if the use of contemporary OCs in women with hypertension increases the risk of vascular events. A large Danish case–control study of women with cerebral thromboembolism found that the risk of stroke was increased threefold in hypertensive women whether or not they used OCs (18). A large World Health Organization study conducted in developing and European countries observed that combination OC users with a history of hypertension had an increased risk of myocardial infarction and stroke (19). A pooled analysis of two U.S. population-based, case–control studies on OC use and myocardial infarction (2) and stroke (3) suggests that current OC use may not substantially increase the risk of stroke or myocardial infarction in women with hypertension. However, the studies included too few women who were hypertensive or older than 35 years to draw firm conclusions.

In healthy women of reproductive age, the incidence of myocardial infarction or stroke with use of low-dose OCs is extremely low. Although the relative risk of these conditions is increased in women with hypertension, the absolute risk remains low. In view of the increased risk of myocardial infarction and stroke associated with hypertension and uncertainty regarding additional risks of OCs, the decision to use OCs in these patients should be weighed against the risk of pregnancy associated with hypertension, and the noncontraceptive benefits of OCs should be taken into account. Women with well-controlled and monitored hypertension who are aged 35 years or younger are appropriate candidates for a trial of combination OCs formulated with 35 µg or less of estrogen, provided they are otherwise healthy, show no evidence of end-organ vascular disease, and do not smoke cigarettes. If blood pressure remains well-controlled with careful monitoring several months after initiating OCs, use can be continued.

Although coronary artery disease, congestive heart failure, and cerebrovascular disease are uncommon in women of reproductive age, the risk of pregnancy and delivery in these women can be substantial, making effective contraception important. Inadequate data are available to address the use of OCs in women with these conditions; therefore, given the increased risk of venous thromboembolism with combined OCs, their use is contraindicated. However, progestin-only contraceptives such as DMPA, progestin-only OCs, or levonorgestrel implants may be appropriate.

▶ *Is combination OC use safe for women with diabetes?*

Pregnancy in women with diabetes is associated with an array of serious maternal and perinatal complications, which emphasizes the importance of effective contraception in this patient population. In theory, the steroids in combination OCs might impair carbohydrate metabolism and accelerate the occurrence of vascular disease in diabetic women. Fortunately, current combination OCs do not appear to have this effect. In a cross-sectional U.S. study, 43 women with type 1 (formerly insulin-dependent) diabetes who used combination OCs for 1–7 years (mean duration, 3.4 years) were compared with a similar number of women with type 1 diabetes who were not using OCs. The overall mean age and duration of diabetes was 23 and 14 years, respectively, in this study group. Hemoglobin A_{1c} values were similar in the OC users and nonusers, which suggests that OC use did not affect control of diabetes. Likewise, the degree of nephropathy and retinopathy was similar in both groups, which suggests that OC use did not accelerate the development of diabetic vascular disease (20).

Although studies of OC use in women with type 2 (formerly non–insulin-dependent) diabetes have not been reported, two recent papers offer reassurance that combination OC use does not precipitate this disease. A prospective cohort study, which followed more than 98,000 U.S. women nurses, found that use of combination OCs did not significantly increase the risk of developing type 2 diabetes over a 4-year follow-up period; likewise, past use did not appear to increase risk (21). In a California population of Hispanic women with gestational diabetes followed for up to 7 years postpartum, use of combination OCs did not accelerate the development of type 2 diabetes. The use of progestin-only pills by the relatively small subgroup of women who nursed their infants was associated with a significantly increased risk of developing type 2 diabetes (22), an unexpected finding that is difficult to interpret.

Although the above data support the use of combination OCs in women with diabetes, based on theoretical concerns, such use should be limited to nonsmoking, otherwise healthy women with diabetes who are younger than 35 years and show no evidence of hypertension, nephropathy, retinopathy, or other vascular disease. Practitioners who provide contraception to women with diabetes should coordinate care with the physician treating the diabetes and follow such patients closely. Appropriate follow-up includes monitoring blood pressure, weight, and lipid status. Regardless of hormonal contraception use, women with the following risk factors should undergo blood glucose screening every 3 years: history of gestational diabetes, family history of diabetes in parents or siblings, obesity (body weight greater than 120% of ideal) or hypertension, and member of high-risk ethnic groups (African American, Hispanic, Native American).

▶ *Is combination OC use safe for women with migraine headaches?*

Headaches are a frequent occurrence in women of reproductive age. Most of these headaches are tension headaches, not migraines (23). Some women with migraines experience improvement in their symptoms with the use of OCs, while some women's symptoms worsen. However, in women using OCs, most migraines occur during the hormone-free interval. Because the presence of true migraine headaches affects the decision to use OCs, careful consideration of the diagnosis is important.

A large hospital-based case–control study performed at five European centers found that women with classic migraines (with aura) had a statistically significant fourfold increased risk of ischemic stroke; women with simple migraine (without aura) had a threefold increased risk that was not statistically significant (24). Women with a history of migraines using OCs (<50 μg of estrogen) had a greater than sixfold increased risk of ischemic stroke (not statistically significant [OR 6.6; 95% CI, 0.8–55]) when compared with women who were not using OCs and who had no migraine headaches. Compared with women who did not smoke, did not use OCs, and had no history of migraines, women who smoked, were using OCs, and had a history of migraines had a 34-fold increased risk of ischemic stroke (OR 34.4; 95% CI, 3.3–361).

A pooled analysis of two large, U.S. population-based case–control studies also observed a statistically significant twofold elevated risk of ischemic stroke, as well as hemorrhagic stroke (not statistically significant) among current users of OCs who reported migraine headaches compared with women with migraines who did not use OCs (3). A large Danish population-based case–control study found that among women with a history of migraine headaches, the risk of stroke was elevated approximately threefold (*P*< 0.01) (18). Neither study categorized migraines by type. The additional risk of thrombotic stroke attributable to women with migraines using OCs has been estimated as 8 per 100,000 women at age 20 years, and 80 per 100,000 women at age 40 years (25).

Although cerebrovascular events rarely occur among women with migraines who use combination OCs, the impact of a stroke on a woman of reproductive age is so devastating that clinicians should consider the use of progestin-only, intrauterine, or barrier contraceptives in this setting. Concerns remain that all women with migraines are at increased risk of stroke. However, because absolute risk remains low, the use of combination OCs may be considered for women with migraine headaches if they do not have focal neurologic signs, do not smoke, are otherwise healthy, and are younger than 35 years.

▶ *Does the use of combination OCs increase the risk of breast cancer in women with fibro-cystic breast changes, fibroadenoma, or a family history of breast cancer?*

Women with fibroadenoma, benign breast disease with epithelial hyperplasia with or without atypia, or a family history of breast cancer have an increased risk of breast cancer (26). A recently published massive reanalysis of 54 studies assessing the association of OC use and breast cancer risk, however, provides reassurance to these women and to their clinicians regarding OC use. Overall, this reanalysis found that 10 years or more after discontinuing OC use, the risk of breast cancer was identical among these former OC users and those who never used OCs. Small but significantly increased relative risks (RR) were observed in current OC users (RR, 1.24) and those who had used OCs in the previous 1–4 years (RR, 1.16) or 5–9 years earlier (RR, 1.07). The increase in risk was restricted to women with localized disease; there was an associated reduced risk of metastatic disease, which suggests that much if not all of the risk can be attributed to early diagnosis of existing disease (27).

A positive family history of breast cancer in a mother or sister, or both, or a history of benign breast disease should not be regarded as contraindications to OC use. Use of OCs has an identical effect on the risk of breast cancer for women with and without each of these two risk categories (27).

▶ *What are the effects of combination OC use in women with uterine leiomyomata?*

Use of combination OCs reduces menstrual blood loss in women with normal menses as well as in those with men-

orrhagia (28). A Swedish study conducted in the 1960s using high-dose oral contraceptives, which are not currently used, noted OC use significantly reduced bleeding in women with menorrhagia associated with uterine fibroids (29). Oral contraceptive use also reduces dysmenorrhea (28). Some practitioners routinely employ the use of combination OCs as first-line medical management in women with menorrhagia or dysmenorrhea associated with uterine leiomyomata. Several large epidemiologic studies have observed that OC use does not induce the growth of uterine fibroids and may decrease bleeding disorders in these women (30–32).

▶ *Is combination OC use safe for women with lipid disorders?*

The term "dyslipidemia" includes disorders of lipoprotein metabolism that lead to atherosclerosis. These abnormalities arise from genetic and secondary factors and are caused by excessive entry of lipoproteins into the bloodstream, an impairment in their removal, or both.

The estrogen component of combination OCs enhances removal of low-density lipoprotein (LDL) and increases levels of high-density lipoprotein (HDL) cholesterol. Both of these actions can have a favorable effect on a woman's risk of coronary artery disease. Oral estrogen also increases triglyceride levels; however, in the setting of concomitantly increased HDL and decreased LDL levels, the moderate triglyceride elevations caused by oral estrogen use do not appear to increase the risk of atherogenesis. Numerous epidemiologic studies of past use of OCs find no increased risk of cardiovascular disease, arguing against any adverse long-term effect of OCs on the risk of atherogenesis (33). The progestin component of combination OCs antagonizes these estrogen-induced lipid changes, which increases LDL levels and decreases HDL and triglyceride levels. Accordingly, among women taking combination OCs with an identical dose of estrogen, the choice (and dose) of the progestin component affects net lipid changes. It is not known whether the differential lipid effects of distinct OC formulations have any clinical significance in women with normal baseline lipid levels or those with lipid disorders.

Using guidelines from the National Cholesterol Education Program (34), experts have recommended that most women with controlled dyslipidemia can use combination OCs formulated with 35 µg or less of estrogen. In contrast, in women with uncontrolled LDL cholesterol greater than 160 mg/dL or multiple additional risk factors for coronary artery disease (including smoking, diabetes, obesity, hypertension, family history of premature coronary artery disease, HDL level <35 mg/dL, or triglyceride level >250 mg/dL), use of alternative contraceptives should be considered (35). Fasting serum lipid levels should be monitored as frequently as each month after initiating combination OC use in dyslipidemic women; less frequent monitoring is appropriate once stabilization of lipid parameters has been observed.

Ongoing communication with the patient's primary care physician (or internist) is appropriate, and the importance of a low-fat diet, daily exercise, and the achievement of ideal body weight should be emphasized (22). Concomitant hormonal contraception and lipid-lowering therapy may be appropriate in some women.

▶ *What hormonal contraceptive options are available for postpartum and lactating women?*

Postpartum women remain in a hypercoagulable state for weeks after childbirth. Product labeling for combination OCs advises deferring use until 4 weeks postpartum in nonbreastfeeding women. Because first ovulation after delivery can occur in as little as 25 days (36), some practitioners initiate the use of combination OCs in nonbreastfeeding women as early as 2 weeks after childbirth, although no data support or refute the safety of this approach. Because progestin-only OCs, DMPA, and implants do not contain estrogen, these methods may be safely initiated immediately postpartum (37).

Combination OCs are not recommended as the first choice for breastfeeding mothers because of the negative effect of contraceptive doses of estrogen on lactation. The estrogenic component of combination OCs can reduce the volume of milk production and the caloric and mineral content of breast milk in lactating women (38). However, use of combination OCs by well-nourished breastfeeding women does not appear to result in infant development problems (38). Their use can be considered once milk flow is well established.

Progestin-only contraceptives do not impair lactation and, in fact, may increase the quality and duration of lactation (39). In nursing women using progestin-only OCs, very small amounts of progestin are passed into the breast milk, and no adverse effects on infant growth have been observed (40). Product labeling for progestin-only pills may suggest that fully breastfeeding women begin tablets 6 weeks postpartum and advise partially breastfeeding women to begin at 3 weeks.

Like other progestin-only methods, DMPA use does not adversely affect breastfeeding (38). Product labeling for DMPA advises initiation of use within the first 5 days postpartum if not breastfeeding and, if exclusively breastfeeding, at 6 weeks postpartum. When initiated immediately postpartum, however, use of DMPA does not adversely affect lactation (38) or infant development (41).

Product labeling for progestin subdermal implants indicates that insertion should be deferred until 6 weeks postpartum in lactating women. Studies of the effects of implant use on lactation and infant development investigated outcomes of insertion at least 30 days postpartum (42, 43). Although the results of these studies have been reassuring, data assessing immediate postpartum implant insertion in breastfeeding women are needed. Given the lack of procoagulation effect and the apparent safety in nursing mothers with DMPA and implants, their immediate postpartum use in both lactating and nonlactating women appears reasonable.

▶ *What hormonal contraceptive options are available for women taking concomitant medications?*

For women with seizure disorders, the frequency of seizures may increase during pregnancy (44). In addition, the risk of birth defects is intrinsically increased in these women (44). Finally, many anticonvulsants are teratogens (44). Each of these observations emphasizes the importance of providing effective contraception for women with seizure disorders.

Anticonvulsants that induce hepatic enzymes can decrease serum concentrations of the estrogen or progestin component of OCs, or both (45) (see the box, "Interaction of Anticonvulsants and Combination Oral Contraceptives"). This effect has been observed with phenobarbital (46), phenytoin, carbamazepine (47), felbamate (48), and topiramate (49). Therapeutic doses of vigabatrin do not induce hepatic enzymes. Nonetheless, a small clinical trial found ethinyl estradiol levels lower than during placebo use in two of 13 volunteers taking this anticonvulsant (50). Although each of these studies demonstrated reduced serum levels of OC steroids during anticonvulsant use, and many of them demonstrated associated breakthrough bleeding, investigators did not observe ovulation or accidental pregnancy during anticonvulsant use. Although some clinicians prescribe OCs containing 50 μg of ethinyl estradiol to women taking these anticonvulsants, no published data support the enhanced contraceptive efficacy of this practice. Use of condoms in conjunction with OCs or use of DMPA or an intrauterine device may be considered for such women (see the box).

In contrast to the above anticonvulsants, use of valproic acid (51), gabapentin (52), and tiagabine (53) does not appear to decrease serum levels of contraceptive steroids in women using combination OCs. Practitioners should be aware, however, that studies of the latter agents were performed using anticonvulsant doses lower than those used in clinical practice (54).

Interaction of Anticonvulsants and Combination Oral Contraceptives

Anticonvulsants that decrease steroid levels in women taking combination oral contraceptives

    Barbiturates (including phenobarbital and primidone)

    Phenytoin

    Carbamazepine

    Felbamate

    Topiramate

    Vigabatrin

Anticonvulsants that do not decrease steroid levels in women taking combination oral contraceptives

    Valproic acid

    Gabapentin*

    Lamotrigine*

    Tiagabine*

*Pharmacokinetic study used anticonvulsant dose lower than that used in clinical practice.

Although there have been many anecdotal reports of OC failure in women taking concomitant antibiotics, pharmacokinetic evidence of lower serum steroid levels exists only for rifampin (55) and griseofulvin (56) (see the box, "Interaction of Antiinfective Agents and Combination Oral Contraceptives"). Because OC steroids are strikingly reduced in women concomitantly taking rifampin, such women should not rely on combination OCs, progestin-only OCs, or implants for contraceptive protection. Pharmacokinetic studies have not demonstrated lowered

---

Interaction of Antiinfective Agents and Combination Oral Contraceptives

Antiinfective agents that decrease steroid levels in women taking combination oral contraceptives

    Rifampin

    Griseofulvin

Antiinfective agents that do not decrease steroid levels in women taking combination oral contraceptives

    Tetracycline

    Doxycycline

    Ampicillin

    Metronidazole

    Quinolone antibiotics

OC steroid levels with concomitant use of tetracycline (57), doxycycline (58), ampicillin or metronidazole (59), or quinolone antibiotics (60–62).

Serum progestin levels during use of progestin-only OCs and implants are lower than during combined OC use. Accordingly, these low-dose progestin-only contraceptives are not appropriate choices for women using concomitant liver enzyme inducers (40, 63). The contraceptive efficacy of DMPA in women taking hepatic enzyme inducers has not been explicitly studied. A potential advantage of using DMPA in women with seizure disorders is DMPA's intrinsic anticonvulsant effect (23).

▶ *Is hormonal contraceptive use safe for women with a history of thromboembolism?*

The estrogenic component of combination OCs, which increases hepatic production of serum globulins involved in coagulation (including factor VII, factor X, and fibrinogen), increases the risk of VTE in users. Beginning in 1995, European studies clarified that, compared with nonusers, current users of OCs formulated with 35 µg or less of estrogen experience a threefold to fourfold increased risk of VTE. This risk, in absolute terms, remains lower than the increased risk of VTE during pregnancy.

The goal of screening OC candidates with respect to VTE risk is to identify those women for whom the VTE risk associated with OC use outweighs OC benefits. In addition to current use of exogenous estrogens, risk factors for VTE include pregnancy and the puerperium, personal or family history of VTE, obesity, surgery, and certain familial coagulation disorders. Although cigarette smoking, hypertension, and diabetes represent risk factors for arterial disease, including myocardial infarction and stroke, they do not increase VTE risk (64). Likewise, the presence of superficial varicose veins does not increase VTE risk (64). Health risks (including VTE) associated with pregnancy, noncontraceptive OC benefits, and the potential for effective use of contraceptives that do not increase VTE risk (eg, progestin-only OCs and intrauterine and barrier methods) should all be factored into risk–benefit considerations. Practitioners should be aware that package labeling for DMPA and for certain brands of progestin-only OCs inappropriately indicates that a history of VTE contraindicates the use of these progestin-only methods.

Women with a documented history of unexplained VTE or VTE associated with pregnancy or exogenous estrogen use should not use combination OCs unless they are currently taking anticoagulants. An OC candidate who had experienced a single episode of VTE years earlier associated with a nonrecurring risk factor (eg, VTE occurring after immobilization following a motor vehicle accident) may not currently be at increased risk for VTE. Accordingly, the decision to initiate combination OCs in such a candidate can be individualized.

▶ *Should women awaiting surgery discontinue combination OC use?*

Venous thromboembolism with pulmonary embolism remains a major cause of fatalities associated with surgical (including gynecologic) procedures. Findings of a large British prospective cohort study suggested that the risk of postoperative VTE was approximately twice as high ($P>0.05$) in OC users as in nonusers (65). A prospective study found that, among women taking OCs formulated with 30 µg of estrogen, OC-induced procoagulant changes did not substantially resolve until 6 or more weeks after OC discontinuation (66). Accordingly, the risks associated with stopping OCs 1 month or more before major surgery should be balanced against the risks of an unintended pregnancy (67). In current OC users having major surgical procedures, heparin prophylaxis should be considered (67). Because of the low perioperative risk of VTE, it currently is not considered necessary to discontinue combination OCs before laparoscopic tubal sterilization or other brief surgical procedures.

▶ *Is OC use safe in women with hypercoagulable states?*

Women with factor V Leiden mutation who use OCs experience a risk of VTE 30 times higher than non-OC users who are not carriers of the mutation (68). A clotting assay can determine activated protein C resistance, and a polymerase chain reaction test can identify the presence of factor V Leiden mutation. Such screening would identify approximately 5% of U.S. OC candidates as having factor V Leiden mutation; however, the great majority of these women will never experience VTE, even if they use combination OCs (69). Given the rarity of fatal VTE, one group of investigators concluded that screening more than 1 million combination OC candidates for thrombophilic markers would, at best, prevent two OC-associated deaths (70). Some practitioners may choose to test for factor V Leiden mutation in women with a positive family history of VTE who are considering OC use or pregnancy. In this setting, the clinician should weigh factors including age of onset of thrombosis in affected family members, the clinical setting, and severity of thrombotic episodes. The risks, benefits, and financial implications of such selective testing, however, are unknown.

Women using warfarin for chronic anticoagulation may experience menorrhagia and, rarely, hemoperitoneum following rupture of ovarian cysts. In addition, warfarin is a teratogen. Because use of combination OCs can reduce menstrual blood loss (28) and does not increase the risk of recurrent thrombosis in well-anticoagulated women (69, 71), some authorities recommend their use in such patients. Because intramuscular injection of DMPA consistently suppresses ovulation (72), DMPA represents another potential contraceptive choice in anticoagulated women.

▶ *Does the use of emergency contraception increase the risk of VTE?*

Use of postcoital (emergency) contraception may increase in the United States with the recent availability of a dedicated product. A recent retrospective cohort analysis from Britain found no cases of thromboembolism in more than 100,000 episodes of postcoital contraception use with the Yuzpe regimen (73).

▶ *Are hormonal contraceptives safe for women with SLE?*

Because the risks of maternal and perinatal morbidity as well as mortality can be high in pregnancies complicated by SLE, effective contraception is an important component of the care of such women. Particular concerns about hormonal contraception use in women with SLE relate to the increased risk of venous and arterial thrombosis in women with this disease. A small retrospective cohort study noted that while combination OC use was associated with flareups in SLE patients with renal disease, progestin-only OC use was not associated with increased disease activity (74). One retrospective cohort study of 85 women with SLE noted that among 31 patients using combination OCs, increased disease activity was not precipitated by OC use. However, deep vein thrombosis was diagnosed in two OC users; both of these women had antiphospholipid antibodies (75). A small prospective cohort study found that use of progestin-only OCs or contraceptive injections was not associated with increased SLE activity (76).

Existing data from observational studies suggest that combination OC use should be avoided in SLE patients with a history of vascular disease, nephritis, or antiphospholipid antibodies, although progestin-only methods are safe alternatives. Data are insufficient to address the use of combination OCs among women with stable or inactive disease who have no history of thrombosis, nephropathy, or antiphospholipid antibodies (77). If such women do not wish to use progestin-only methods, use of combination OCs with close monitoring can be considered in selected cases.

► *Is hormonal contraceptive use safe for women with sickle cell disease?*

In persons with sickle cell disease, abnormal hemoglobin precipitates and becomes rigid when subjected to oxygen deprivation. Vasoocclusive episodes in those with sickle cell disease, however, differ from intravascular thrombosis (78). Pregnancy in women with sickle cell disease carries increased risks of maternal complications and is associated with elevated rates of spontaneous abortion, intrauterine growth restriction, and neonatal mortality.

No well-controlled study has assessed whether VTE risk in OC users with sickle cell disease is higher than in other combination OC users. Accordingly, recommendations regarding use of combination OCs in this patient population vary widely. On the basis of studies of pregnant women with sickle cell disease, small observational studies of women with sickle cell disease who use combination OCs, and theoretical considerations, the consensus is that pregnancy carries a greater risk than combination OC use.

Two controlled studies have assessed the use of DMPA in women with sickle cell disease (79, 80). Both of these found that use of DMPA reduced the incidence of painful crises. Accordingly, DMPA may be a particularly appropriate contraceptive for women with sickle cell disease.

► *What are the effects of DMPA on bone density?*

Use of DMPA in contraceptive doses suppresses ovarian production of estradiol. Thus, there has been concern that women using DMPA for contraception might develop osteopenia. A New Zealand study of women who used DMPA for at least 5 years found significantly reduced bone density in the lumbar spine and femoral neck compared with premenopausal controls (81). A subsequent study performed by the same investigator noted that among women who had used DMPA for at least 3 years, deficits in BMD of the lumbar spine were reversible following DMPA discontinuation (82). Five recent cross-sectional studies suggest that DMPA use decreases BMD of the spine (83–87). In the largest of these studies, the median duration of DMPA use was 12 years. In this study, initiation of DMPA use before age 21 years and use for more than 15 years were identified as risk factors for osteopenia (84). None of these cross-sectional studies found evidence of osteoporosis or fractures in DMPA users.

Information on the effects of DMPA use on BMD during adolescence is limited. However, a small study compared BMD of the lumbar spine in females aged 12–21 years. In this prospective cohort study, BMD in those using no hormones was compared with those using DMPA, OCs, or implants. After 1 year of use, bone density in DMPA users decreased 1.5%, whereas it increased 1.5% in OC users, 2.5% in levonorgestrel implant users, and 2.9% in those using no hormones. None of those who initially selected an OC continued after 2 years. However, follow-up BMD measurements at 2 years showed a total decrease of 3.1% in DMPA users and total increases of 9.5% in non-hormone users and 9.3% in implant users (88).

The rate-of-loss trends in BMD seen with DMPA seem to be similar to those noted during lactation (89, 90) in that no long-term decrease occurs. Two recent cross-sectional studies of menopausal women found no long-term BMD declines in former DMPA users. In these reports, BMD in former DMPA users was not significantly different from never-users (91, 92). Estrogen supplementation (eg, conjugated estrogen, 1.25 mg daily, or equivalent doses of other estrogens) can be considered for long-term users of DMPA, including adolescents. However, no data address the effect of such an add-back regimen on BMD in women using DMPA. Caution should be exercised in prescribing DMPA for adolescents, women known to be at high risk for low BMD, and perimenopausal women.

Summary

The following recommendations are based on good and consistent scientific evidence (Level A):

► Women with fibroadenoma, benign breast disease with epithelial hyperplasia with or without atypia, or a family history of breast cancer are at little or no additional risk of breast cancer because of OC use. Therefore, OCs can be prescribed for such women if they are otherwise appropriate candidates.

► Progestin-only preparations are safe and preferable forms of hormonal contraception for lactating women. Combination OCs are not recommended as the first choice for breastfeeding mothers because of the negative impact of contraceptive doses of estrogen on lactation. However, use of combination OCs by well-nourished breastfeeding women does not appear to result in infant development problems; therefore, their use can be considered once milk flow is well established.

► Hormonal contraceptive effectiveness is compromised by the use of the antibiotics rifampin and griseofulvin; thus, women taking these antibiotics should use nonhormonal contraceptives.

► Progestin-only preparations are appropriate for women at increased risk for VTE. Combination OCs

► are not recommended for women with a documented history of unexplained VTE or VTE associated with pregnancy or exogenous estrogen use, unless they are taking anticoagulants.

► Combination OCs should be prescribed with caution, if ever, to women who are older than 35 years and are smokers. Women younger than 30 years who smoke and are otherwise healthy generally can be prescribed combination OCs.

► If desired, healthy, nonsmoking women doing well on combination OCs may continue their use until menopause.

The following recommendations are based on limited or inconsistent scientific evidence (Level B):

► Women with well-controlled and monitored hypertension aged 35 years and younger are appropriate candidates for a trial of combination OCs formulated with 35 μg or less of estrogen, provided they are otherwise healthy with no evidence of end-organ vascular disease and do not smoke cigarettes. If blood pressure remains well-controlled several months after initiating OCs, use can be continued.

► The use of combination OCs by women with diabetes should be limited to such women who do not smoke, are younger than 35 years, and are otherwise healthy with no evidence of hypertension, nephropathy, retinopathy, or other vascular disease.

► Women with migraine headaches who have focal neurologic signs are not appropriate candidates for OC use. Combination OCs can be used by women with simple migraine headaches (ie, no focal neurologic signs) if they do not smoke, are younger than 35 years, and are otherwise healthy. If such women experience increased frequency or severity of headaches or develop headaches with focal neurologic signs or symptoms, they should discontinue OC use.

► Combination OCs may be beneficial in treating dysmenorrhea and menorrhagia in women with uterine fibroids.

► The risks associated with stopping OCs 1 month or more before major surgery should be balanced against the risks of an unintended pregnancy. In current OC users undergoing major surgical procedures, heparin prophylaxis should be considered. Because of the low perioperative risk of VTE, it generally is considered unnecessary to discontinue combination OCs before laparoscopic tubal sterilization or other brief surgical procedures.

► Progestin-only OCs and contraceptive injections appear to be the hormonal contraception methods of choice for women with SLE. Use of combination OCs in women with SLE can be considered if the women have stable or inactive disease and no history of thrombosis, nephropathy, or antiphospholipid antibodies.

The following recommendations are based primarily on consensus and expert opinion (Level C):

► Most women with controlled dyslipidemia can use combination OCs formulated with 35 μg or less of estrogen. In women with uncontrolled LDL cholesterol greater than 160 mg/dL, a triglyceride level greater than 250 mg/dL, or multiple additional risk factors for coronary artery disease, alternative contraceptives should be considered.

► DMPA has noncontraceptive benefits and is the contraceptive method of choice for many women with sickle cell disease.

► Progestin-only contraceptives may be appropriate for women with coronary artery disease, congestive heart failure, or cerebrovascular disease. However, combination oral contraceptives are contraindicated in these women.

References

1. Corfman P. Labeling guidance text for progestin-only oral contraceptives. Contraception 1995;52:71–76 (Level III)

2. Sidney S, Siscovick DS, Petitti DB, Schwartz SM, Quesenberry CP, Psaty BM, et al. Myocardial infarction and use of low-dose oral contraceptives: a pooled analysis of 2 US studies. Circulation 1998;98:1058–1063 (Level II-2)

3. Schwartz SM, Petitti DB, Siscovick DS, Longstreth WT Jr, Sidney S, Raghunathan TE, et al. Stroke and use of low-dose oral contraceptives in young women: a pooled analysis of two US studies. Stroke 1998;29:2277–2284 (Level II-2)

4. Gambacciani M, Spinetti A, Taponeco F, Cappagli B, Piaggesi L, Fioretti P. Longitudinal evaluation of perimenopausal vertebral bone loss: effects of a low-dose oral contraceptive preparation on bone mineral density and metabolism. Obstet Gynecol 1994;83:392–396 (Level I)

5. Sulak PJ. Oral contraceptives: therapeutic uses and quality-of-life benefits—case presentations. Contraception 1999;59(suppl):35S–38S (Level III)

6. Casper RF, Dodin S, Reid RL. The effect of 20 μg ethinyl estradiol/1 mg norethindrone acetate (Minestrin), a low-dose oral contraceptive, on vaginal bleeding patterns, hot flashes, and quality of life in symptomatic perimenopausal women. Menopause 1997;4:139–147 (Level I)

7. Gebbie AE, Glasier A, Sweeting V. Incidence of ovulation in perimenopausal women before and during hormone replacement therapy. Contraception 1995;52:221–222 (Level II-3)

8. Burger HG. Diagnostic role of follicle-stimulating hormone (FSH) measurements during the menopausal transition—an analysis of FSH, oestradiol and inhibin. Eur J Endocrinol 1994;130:38–42 (Level III)

9. Castracane VD, Gimpel T, Goldzieher JW. When is it safe to switch from oral contraceptives to hormonal replacement therapy? Contraception 1995;52:371–376 (Level II-2)

10. Creinin MD. Laboratory criteria for menopause in women using oral contraceptives. Fertil Steril 1996;66:101–104 (Level II-3)

11. Stanford JL, Hartge P, Brinton LA, Hoover RN, Brookmeyer R. Factors influencing the age at natural menopause. J Chronic Dis 1987;40:995–1002 (Level II-3)

12. McKinlay SM, Bifano NL, McKinlay JB. Smoking and age at menopause in women. Ann Intern Med 1985;103:350–356 (Level II)

13. American College of Obstetricians and Gynecologists. Smoking and women's health. ACOG Educational Bulletin 240. Washington, DC: ACOG, 1997 (Level III)

14. Croft P, Hannaford PC. Risk factors for acute myocardial infarction in women: evidence from the Royal College of General Practitioners' oral contraception study. BMJ 1989;298:165–168 (Level II-2)

15. Schwingl PJ, Ory HW, Visness CM. Estimates of the risk of cardiovascular death attributable to low-dose oral contraceptives in the United States. Am J Obstet Gynecol 1999;180:241–249 (Level III)

16. Cardoso F, Polonia J, Santos A, Silva-Carvalho J, Ferreira-de-Almeida J. Low-dose oral contraceptives and 24-hour ambulatory blood pressure. Int J Gynaecol Obstet 1997;59:237–243 (Level II-3)

17. Narkiewicz K, Graniero GR, D'Este D, Mattarei M, Zonzin P, Palatini P. Ambulatory blood pressure in mild hypertensive women taking oral contraceptives. A case-control study. Am J Hyperten 1995;8:249–253 (Level II-2)

18. Lidegaard O. Oral contraceptives, pregnancy and the risk of cerebral thromboembolism: the influence of diabetes, hypertension, migraine and previous thrombotic disease. Br J Obstet Gynaecol 1996;102:153–159 (Level II-2)

19. WHO Collaborative Study of Cardiovascular Disease and Steroid Hormone Contraception. Ischemic stroke and combined oral contraceptives: results of an international, multicentre, case-control study. Lancet 1996;348:498–505 (Level II-2)

20. Garg SK, Chase HP, Marshall G, Hoops SL, Holmes DL, Jackson WE. Oral contraceptives and renal and retinal complications in young women with insulin-dependent diabetes mellitus. JAMA 1994;271:1099–1102 (Level II-2)

21. Chasan-Taber L, Willett WC, Stampfer MJ, Hunter DJ, Colditz GA, Spiegelman D, et al. A prospective study of oral contraceptives and NIDDM among U.S. women. Diabetes Care 1997;20:330–335 (Level II-2)

22. Kjos SL, Peters RK, Xiang A, Thomas D, Schaefer U, Buchanan T. Contraception and the risk of type 2 diabetes mellitus in Latina women with prior gestational diabetes mellitus. JAMA 1998;28:533–538 (Level II-3)

23. Mattson RH, Rebar RW. Contraceptive methods for women with neurologic disorders. Am J Obstet Gynecol 1993;168(6 Pt 2):2027–2032 (Level II-3)

24. Chang CL, Donaghy M, Poulter N. Migraine and stroke in young women: case control study. The World Health Organisation Collaborative Study of Cardiovascular Disease and Steroid Hormone Contraception. BMJ 1999;318:13–18 (Level II-2)

25. MacGregor EA, Guillebaud J. Combined oral contraceptives, migraine and ischaemic stroke. Clinical and Scientific Committee of the Faculty of Family Planning and Reproductive Health Care and the Family Planning Association. Br J Fam Plann 1998;24:53–60 (Level III)

26. Dupont WD, Page DL. Risk factors for breast cancer in women with proliferative breast disease. N Engl J Med 1985;312:146–151 (Level II-2)

27. Collaborative Group on Hormonal Factors in Breast Cancer. Breast cancer and hormonal contraceptives: collaborative reanalysis of individual data on 53,297 women with breast cancer and 100,239 women without breast cancer from 54 epidimiological studies. Lancet 1996;347:1713–1727 (Level III)

28. Larsson G, Milsom I, Lindstedt G, Rybo G. The influence of a low-dose combined oral contraceptive on menstrual blood loss and iron status. Contraception 1992;46:327–334 (Level III)

29. Nilsson L, Rybo G. Treatment of menorrhagia. Am J Obstet Gynecol 1971;110:713–720 (Level II-2)

30. Ross RK, Pike MC, Vessey MP, Bull D, Yeates D, Casagrande JT. Risk factors for uterine fibroids: reduced risk associated with oral contraceptives. BMJ (Clin Res Ed) 1986;293:359–362 (Level II-2)

31. Marshall LM, Spiegelman D, Goldman MB, Manson JE, Colditz GA, Barbieri RL, et al. A prospective study of reproductive factors and oral contraceptive use in relation to the risk of uterine leiomyomata. Fertil Steril 1998;70:432–439 (Level II-2)

32. Parazzini F, Negri E, LaVecchia C, Fedele L, Rabaiotti M, Luchini L. Oral contraceptive use and risk of uterine fibroids. Obstet Gynecol 1992;79:430–433 (Level II-2)

33. Chasen-Taber L, Stampfer MJ. Epidemiology of oral contraceptives and cardiovascular disease. Ann Intern Med 1998;128:467–477 (Level III)

34. National Cholesterol Education Program Expert Panel on Detection, Evaluation, and Treatment of High Blood Cholesterol in Adults. Report of the National Cholesterol Education Program Expert Panel on Detection, Evaluation, and Treatment of High Blood Cholesterol in Adults. Arch Intern Med 1988;148:36–69 (Level III)

35. Knopp RH, LaRosa JC, Burkman RT Jr. Contraception and dyslipidemia. Am J Obstet Gynecol 1993;168:1994–2005 (Level III)

36. Campbell OM, Gray RH. Characteristics and determinants of postpartum ovarian function in women in the United States. Am J Obstet Gynecol 1993;169:55–60 (Level II-2)

37. American College of Obstetricians and Gynecologists. Hormonal contraception. ACOG Technical Bulletin 198. Washington, DC: ACOG, 1994 (Level III)

38. World Health Organization (WHO) Task Force on Oral Contraceptives. Effects of hormonal contraceptives on breast milk composition and infant growth. Stud Fam Plann 1988;19(6 Pt 1):361–369 (Level II-2)

39. Koetsawang S. The effects of contraceptive methods on the quality and quantity of breast milk. Int J Gynaecol Obstet 1987;25(suppl):115–127 (Level III)

40. McCann MF, Potter LS. Progestin-only oral contraception: a comprehensive review. Contraception 1994;50(suppl 1): S1–S195 (Level III)

41. Karim M, Ammar R, el-Mahgoub S, el-Ganzoury B, Fikri F, Abdou I. Injected progestogen and lactation. BMJ 1971;1:200–203 (Level II-2)

42. Shaaban MM, Salem HT, Abdullah KA. Influence of levonorgestrel contraceptive implants, Norplant, initiated early postpartum upon lactation and infant growth. Contraception 1985;32:623–635 (Level II-2)

43. Abdulla KA, Elwan SI, Salem HS, Shaaban MM. Effect of early postpartum use of the contraceptive implants, NORPLANT, on the serum levels of immunoglobulins of the mothers and their breastfed infants. Contraception 1985;32:261–266 (Level II-2)

44. O'Brien MD, Gilmour-White S. Epilepsy and pregnancy. BMJ 1993;307:492–495 (Level III)

45. Back DJ, Orme ML. Pharmacokinetic drug interactions with oral contraceptives. Clin Pharmacokinet 1990;18: 472–484 (Level III)

46. Back DJ, Bates M, Bowden A, Breckenridge AM, Hall MJ, Jones H, et al. The interaction of phenobarbital and other anticonvulsants with oral contraceptive steroid therapy. Contraception 1980;22:495–503 (Level II-3)

47. Crawford P, Chadwick DJ, Martin C, Tjia J, Back DJ, Orme M. The interaction of phenytoin and carbamazepine with combined oral contraceptive steroids. Br J Clin Pharmacol 1990;30:892–896 (Level II-3)

48. Saano V, Glue P, Banfield CR, Reidenberg P, Colucci RD, Meehan JW, et al. Effects of felbamate on the pharmacokinetics of a low-dose combination oral contraceptive. Clin Pharmacol Ther 1995;58:523–531 (Level I)

49. Rosenfeld WE, Doose DR, Walker SA, Nayak RK. Effect of topiramate on the pharmacokinetics of an oral contraceptive containing norethindrone and ethinyl estradiol in patients with epilepsy. Epilepsia 1997;38:317–323 (Level II-3)

50. Bartoli A, Gatti G, Cipolla G, Barzaghi N, Veliz G, Fattore C, et al. A double-blind, placebo-controlled study on the effect of vigabatrin on in vivo parameters of hepatic microsomal enzyme induction and on the kinetics of steroid oral contraceptives in healthy female volunteers. Epilepsia 1997;38:702–707 (Level I)

51. Crawford P, Chadwick D, Cleland P, Tjia J, Cowie A, Back DJ, et al. The lack of effect of sodium valproate on the pharmacokinetics of oral contraceptive steroids. Contraception 1986;33:23–29 (Level II-3)

52. Eldon MA, Underwood BA, Randinitis EJ, Sedman AJ. Gabapentin does not interact with a contraceptive regimen of norethindrone acetate and ethinyl estradiol. Neurology 1998;50:1146–1148 (Level II-3)

53. Mengel HB, Houston A, Back DJ. An evaluation of the interaction between tiagabine and oral contraceptives in female volunteers. J Pharm Med 1994;4:141–150 (Level II-3)

54. Natsch S, Hekster YA, Keyser A, Deckers CL, Meinardi H, Renier WO. Newer anticonvulsant drugs: role of pharmacology, drug interactions and adverse reactions in drug choice. Drug Saf 1997;17:228–240 (Level III)

55. Back DJ, Breckenridge AM, Crawford F, MacIver M, Orme ML, Park BK, et al. The effect of rifampicin on norethisterone pharmacokinetics. Euro J Clin Pharmacol 1979;15:193–197 (Level III)

56. Geurts TB, Goorissen EM, Sitsen JM. Summary of drug interactions with oral contraceptives. Pearl River, New York: Parthenon Publishing, 1993:27–124 (Level III)

57. Murphy AA, Zacur HA, Charache P, Burkman RT. The effect of tetracycline on levels of oral contraceptives. Am J Obstet Gynecol 1991;164(1 Pt 1):28–33 (Level II-3)

58. Neely JL, Abate M, Swinker M, D'Angio R. The effect of doxycycline on serum levels of ethinyl estradiol, norethindrone, and endogenous progesterone. Obstet Gynecol 1991;77:416–420 (Level II-2)

59. Joshi JV, Joshi UM, Sankholi GM, Krishna U, Mandlekar A, Chowdhury V, et al. A study of interaction of low-dose combination oral contraceptive with ampicillin and metronidazole. Contraception 1980;22:643–652 (Level II-2)

60. Maggiolo F, Puricelli G, Dottorini M, Caprioli S, Bianchi W, Suter F. The effect of ciprofloxacin on oral contraceptive steroid treatments. Drugs Exp Clin Res 1991;17: 451–454 (Level II-1)

61. Back DJ, Tjia J, Martin C, Millar E, Mant T, Morrison P, et al. The lack of interaction between temafloxacin and combined oral contraceptive steroids. Contraception 1991;43:317–323 (Level II-2)

62. Csemiczky G, Alvendal C, Landgren BM. Risk for ovulation in women taking a low-dose oral contraceptive (Microgynon) when receiving antibacterial treatment with a fluoroquinolone (ofloxacin). Adv Contracep 1996;12: 101–109 (Level II-1)

63. Haukkamaa M. Contraception by Norplant subdermal capsules is not reliable in epileptic patients on anticonvulsant treatment. Contraception 1986;33:559–565 (Level II-3)

64. World Health Organization. Cardiovascular disease and steroid hormone contraception. Report of a WHO Scientific Group. World Health Organ Tech Rep Ser 1998;877:i-vii,1–89 (Level III)

65. Vessey M, Mant D, Smith A, Yeates D. Oral contraceptives and venous thromboembolism: findings in a large prospective study. BMJ (Clin Res Ed) 1986;292:526 (Level II-2)

66. Robinson GE, Burren T, Mackie IJ, Bounds W, Walshe K, Faint R, et al. Changes in haemostasis after stopping the combined contraceptive pill: implications for major surgery. BMJ 1991;302:269–271 (Level II-3)

67. Bonnar J. Can more be done in obstetric and gynecologic practice to reduce morbidity and mortality associated with venous thromboembolism? Am J Obstet Gynecol 1999; 180:784–791(Level III)

68. Vandenbroucke JP, Koster T, Briet E, Reitsma PH, Bertina RM, Rosendaal FR. Increased risk of venous thrombosis in oral-contraceptive users who are carriers of factor V Leiden mutation. Lancet 1994;344:1453–1457 (Level II-2)

69. Comp PC. Thrombophilic mechanisms of OCs. Int J Fertil Womens Med 1997;42 (suppl 1):170–176 (Level III)

70. Price DT, Ridker PM. Factor V Leiden mutation and the risks for thromboembolic disease: a clinical perspective. Ann Intern Med 1997;127:895–903 (Level III)

71. Comp PC, Zacur HA. Contraceptive choices in women with coagulation disorders. Am J Obtset Gynecol 1993;168:1990–1993 (Level III)

72. Mishell DR Jr. Pharmacokinetics of depot medroxyprogesterone acetate contraception. J Reprod Med 1996; 41(suppl):381–390 (Level III)

73. Vasilakis C, Jick SS, Jick H. The risk of venous thromboembolism in users of postcoital contraceptive pills. Contraception 1999;59:79–83 (Level II-2)

74. Jungers P, Dougados M, Pelissier C, Kuttenn F, Tron F, Lesavre P, et al. Influence of oral contraceptive therapy on the activity of systemic lupus erythematosus. Arthritis Rheum 1982;25:618–623 (Level III)

75. Julkunen HA. Oral contraceptives in systemic lupus erythematosus: side-effects and influence on the activity of SLE. Scand J Rheumatol 1991;20:427–433 (Level III)

76. Mintz G, Gutierrez G, Deleze M, Rodriguez E. Contraception with progestagens in systemic lupus erythematosus. Contraception 1984;30:29–58 (Level II-2)

77. Petri M, Robinson C. Oral contraceptives and systemic lupus erythematosus. Arthritis Rheum 1997;40:797–803 (Level III)

78. Charache S, Niebyl JR. Pregnancy in sickle cell disease. Clin Haematol 1985;14:729–746 (Level III)

79. De Ceulaer K, Gruber C, Hayes R, Serjeant GR. Medroxyprogesterone acetate and homozygous sickle-cell disease. Lancet 1982;2:229–231 (Level II-2)

80. de Abood M, de Castillo Z, Guerrero F, Espino M, Austin KL. Effect of Depo-Provera or Microgynon on the painful crises of sickle cell anemia patients. Contraception 1997;56:313–316 (Level I)

81. Cundy T, Evans M, Roberts H, Wattie D, Ames R, Reid IR. Bone density in women receiving depot medroxyprogesterone acetate for contraception. BMJ 1991;303:13–16 (Level II-2)

82. Cundy T, Cornish J, Evans M, Roberts H, Reid IR. Recovery of bone density in women who stop using medroxyprogesterone acetate. BMJ 1994;308:247–248 (Level II-2)

83. Gbolade B, Ellis S, Murby B, Randall S, Kirkman R. Bone density in the long term users of depot medroxyprogesterone acetate. Br J Obstet Gynaecol 1998;105:790–794 (Level II-3)

84. Cundy T, Cornish J, Roberts H, Elder H, Reid IR. Spinal bone density in women using depot medroxyprogesterone contraception. Obstet Gynecol 1998;92:569–573 (Level II-2)

85. Paiva LC, Pinto-Neto AM, Faundes A. Bone density among long-term users of medroxyprogesterone acetate as a contraceptive. Contraception 1998;58:351–355 (Level II-2)

86. Scholes D, Lacroix AZ, Ott SM, Ichikawa LE, Barlow WE. Bone mineral density in women using depot medroxyprogesterone acetate for contraception. Obstet Gynecol 1999;93:233–238 (Level II-2)

87. Tang OS, Tang G, Yip P, Li B, Fan S. Long-term depot-medroxyprogesterone acetate and bone mineral density. Contraception 1999;59:25–29 (Level II-2)

88. Cromer BA, Blair JM, Mahan JD, Zibners L, Naumovski Z. A prospective comparison of bone density in adolescent girls receiving depot medroxyprogesterone acetate (Depo-Provera), levonorgestrel (Norplant), or oral contraceptives. J Pediatr 1996;129:671–676 (Level II-2)

89. Kolthoff N, Eiken P, Kristensen B, Nielsen SP. Bone mineral changes during pregnancy and lactation: a longitudinal cohort study. Clin Sci (Colch) 1998;94:405–412 (Level II-3)

90. Kalkwarf HJ, Specker BL, Bianchi DC, Ranz J, Ho M. The effect of calcium supplementation on bone density during lactation and after weaning. N Engl J Med 1997;337:523–528 (Level I)

91. Orr-Walker BJ, Evans MC, Ames RW, Clearwater JM, Cundy TR, Reid IR. The effect of past use of the injectable contraceptive depot medroxyprogesterone acetate on bone mineral density in normal post-menopausal women. Clin Endocrinol (Oxf) 1998;49:615–618 (Level II-3)

92. Petitti DB, Piaggio G, Mehta S, Cravioto MC, Meirik O. Steroid hormone contraception and bone mineral density: a cross sectional study in an international population. Obstet Gynecol 2000;95:736–744 (Level II-3)

The MEDLINE database, the Cochrane Library, and ACOG's own internal resources and documents were used to conduct a literature search to locate relevant articles published between January 1985 and March 1998. The search was restricted to articles published in the English language. Priority was given to articles reporting results of original research, although review articles and commentaries also were consulted. Abstracts of research presented at symposia and scientific conferences were not considered adequate for inclusion in this document. Guidelines published by organizations or institutions such as the National Institutes of Health and the American College of Obstetricians and Gynecologists were reviewed, and additional studies were located by reviewing bibliographies of identified articles. When reliable research was not available, expert opinions from obstetrician–gynecologists were used.

Studies were reviewed and evaluated for quality according to the method outlined by the U.S. Preventive Services Task Force:

I   Evidence obtained from at least one properly designed randomized controlled trial.

II-1 Evidence obtained from well-designed controlled trials without randomization.

II-2 Evidence obtained from well-designed cohort or case–control analytic studies, preferably from more than one center or research group.

II-3 Evidence obtained from multiple time series with or without the intervention. Dramatic results in uncontrolled experiments also could be regarded as this type of evidence.

III Opinions of respected authorities, based on clinical experience, descriptive studies, or reports of expert committees.

Based on the highest level of evidence found in the data, recommendations are provided and graded according to the following categories:

Level A—Recommendations are based on good and consistent scientific evidence.

Level B—Recommendations are based on limited or inconsistent scientific evidence.

Level C—Recommendations are based primarily on consensus and expert opinion.

ISSN 1099-3630

**The American College of
Obstetricians and Gynecologists
409 12th Street, SW
PO Box 96920
Washington, DC 20090-6920**

12345/32109

ACOG PRACTICE BULLETIN

CLINICAL MANAGEMENT GUIDELINES FOR
OBSTETRICIAN–GYNECOLOGISTS

NUMBER 6, SEPTEMBER 1999

This Practice Bulletin was developed by the ACOG Committee on Practice Bulletins—Obstetrics with the assistance of Robert M. Silver, MD, Richard L. Berkowitz, MD, and James Bussel, MD. The information is designed to aid practitioners in making decisions about appropriate obstetric and gynecologic care. These guidelines should not be construed as dictating an exclusive course of treatment or procedure. Variations in practice may be warranted based on the needs of the individual patient, resources, and limitations unique to the institution or type of practice.

Thrombocytopenia in Pregnancy

Thrombocytopenia in pregnant women is diagnosed frequently by obstetricians because platelet counts are now included with automated complete blood cell counts (CBCs) obtained during routine prenatal screening (1). The condition is common, occurring in 7–8% of pregnancies (2). Thrombocytopenia can result from a variety of physiologic or pathologic conditions, several of which are unique to pregnancy. Some causes of thrombocytopenia are serious medical disorders that have the potential for profound maternal and fetal morbidity. In contrast, other conditions, such as gestational thrombocytopenia, are benign and pose no maternal or fetal risks. Because of the increased recognition of maternal and fetal thrombocytopenia, there are numerous controversies regarding obstetric management. Clinicians must weigh the risks of maternal and fetal bleeding complications against the costs and morbidity of diagnostic tests and invasive interventions.

Background

Platelet Function

Unlike other bleeding disorders in which bruising often is the initial clinical manifestation, platelet disorders, such as thrombocytopenia, usually result in bleeding into mucous membranes. Although bruising can occur, the most common manifestations of thrombocytopenia are petechiae, ecchymoses, epistaxis, gingival bleeding, and menometrorrhagia. In contrast to hemophilia, bleeding into joints usually does not occur; life-threatening bleeding is less common but can occur, resulting in hematuria, gastrointestinal bleeding, and, although rare, intracranial hemorrhage.

Definition of Thrombocytopenia

The normal range of the platelet count in nonpregnant individuals is 150,000–400,000/μL. In this population, thrombocytopenia is defined as any platelet value less than 150,000/μL, with counts of 100,000–150,000/μL indicative of mild thrombocytopenia, 50,000–100,000/μL indicative of moderate thrombocytopenia, and less than 50,000/μL indicative of severe thrombocytopenia. The definition of thrombocytopenia is somewhat arbitrary and not necessarily clinically relevant. Clinically significant bleeding usually is limited to patients with platelet counts less than 10,000/μL. Serious bleeding complications are rare, even in those with severe thrombocytopenia (3). Excessive bleeding associated with trauma or surgery is uncommon unless the patient's platelet count is less than 50,000/μL. The mean platelet count in pregnant women is lower than in nonpregnant individuals (4, 5).

Differential Diagnosis of Thrombocytopenia

Thrombocytopenia is due to either increased platelet destruction or decreased platelet production. In pregnancy, the former is responsible for most cases (2). Increased platelet destruction can be caused by an immunologic destruction, abnormal platelet activation, or platelet consumption resulting from excessive bleeding or exposure to abnormal vessels. Decreased platelet production is less common, and usually is associated with either leukemia, aplastic anemia, or folate deficiency (6, 7).

The most common cause of thrombocytopenia during pregnancy is gestational thrombocytopenia, which accounts for about two thirds of cases (2) (see the box).

Gestational Thrombocytopenia

Gestational thrombocytopenia, also termed essential thrombocytopenia or benign or incidental thrombocytopenia of pregnancy, is by far the most common cause of mild thrombocytopenia during pregnancy, affecting up to 8% of gestations (2). There are several characteristics of this condition (2). First, the thrombocytopenia is relatively mild with platelet counts usually remaining greater than 70,000/μL. However, a lower threshold for gestational thrombocytopenia has never been established. Second, women are asymptomatic with no history of bleeding. The thrombocytopenia usually is detected as part of routine prenatal screening. Third, women have no history of thrombocytopenia prior to pregnancy (except in previous pregnancies). Although gestational thrombocytopenia may recur in subsequent pregnancies (8), the recurrence risk is unknown. Fourth, platelet counts usually return to normal within 2–12 weeks following delivery.

Causes of Thrombocytopenia in Pregnancy

Gestational thrombocytopenia
Pregnancy-induced hypertension
HELLP syndrome
Pseudothrombocytopenia (laboratory artifact)
Human immunodeficiency virus (HIV) infection
Immune thrombocytopenic purpura
Systemic lupus erythematosus
Antiphospholipid syndrome
Hypersplenism
Disseminated intravascular coagulation
Thrombotic thrombocytopenic purpura
Hemolytic uremic syndrome
Congenital thrombocytopenias
Medications (heparin, quinine, quinidine, zidovudine, sulfonamides)

Finally, there is an extremely low risk of fetal or neonatal thrombocytopenia. In a large, prospectively evaluated cohort study of 756 women with gestational thrombocytopenia, only one woman's infant had a platelet count of less than 50,000/μL (9). However, this infant had thrombocytopenia due to congenital bone marrow dysfunction. Another study confirmed the extremely low risk of fetal thrombocytopenia in women with gestational thrombocytopenia (10). Thus, women with gestational thrombocytopenia are not at risk for maternal or fetal hemorrhage or bleeding complications.

Although its cause is uncertain, gestational thrombocytopenia may be due to accelerated platelet consumption (4). Antiplatelet antibodies often are detectable in women with gestational thrombocytopenia, but neither their presence nor their absence can be used to diagnose the disorder or differentiate it from immune thrombocytopenic purpura (ITP) (11). Indeed, there are no specific diagnostic tests to definitively distinguish gestational thrombocytopenia from mild ITP (1). The primary means of differentiation is to monitor platelet counts closely, to look for levels that decrease below the 50,000–70,000/μL range, and to document a normal neonatal platelet count and a restoration of normal maternal platelet values after delivery.

Thrombocytopenia with an Immunologic Basis

Thrombocytopenia with an immunologic basis during pregnancy can be broadly classified as two disorders: neonatal alloimmune thrombocytopenia and ITP, an autoimmune condition. Neonatal alloimmune thrombocytopenia has no effect on the mother but probably is responsible for more intracranial hemorrhage due to thrombocytopenia than all the other primary thrombocytopenic conditions combined. In contrast, ITP may affect both mothers and fetuses, but with appropriate management the outcome for both is excellent.

Neonatal Alloimmune Thrombocytopenia

Neonatal alloimmune thrombocytopenia is the platelet equivalent of hemolytic (Rh) disease of the newborn, developing as a result of maternal alloimmunization to fetal platelet antigens. It affects one in 1,000–2,000 live births and can be a serious and potentially life-threatening condition (12, 13). Unlike Rh disease, neonatal alloimmune thrombocytopenia can occur during a first pregnancy. Almost half of the clinically evident cases of neonatal alloimmune thrombocytopenia are discovered in the first live-born infant (14).

In typical cases of unanticipated neonatal alloimmune thrombocytopenia, the mother is healthy and has a normal platelet count, and her pregnancy, labor, and delivery are indistinguishable from those of other low-risk obstetric patients. The neonates, however, are either born with evidence of profound thrombocytopenia or develop symptomatic thrombocytopenia within hours after birth. Affected infants often manifest generalized petechiae or ecchymoses over the presenting fetal part. Hemorrhage into viscera and bleeding following circumcision or venipuncture also may ensue. The most serious complication of neonatal alloimmune thrombocytopenia is intracranial hemorrhage, which occurs in 10–20% of infants (14, 15). Fetal intracranial hemorrhage due to neonatal alloimmune thrombocytopenia can occur in utero, and 25–50% of fetal intracranial hemorrhage in untreated mothers may be detected by ultrasonography before the onset of labor (16). Ultrasonographic findings may include intracranial hemorrhage, porencephalic cysts, and obstructive hydrocephalus. These observations are in contrast to neonatal intracranial hemorrhage due to ITP, which is exceedingly rare and usually occurs during the neonatal period.

Several polymorphic, diallelic antigen systems residing on platelet membrane glycoproteins are responsible for neonatal alloimmune thrombocytopenia. Many of these antigen systems have several names because they were identified in different parts of the world concurrently. Recently, a uniform nomenclature has been adopted that describes these antigens as human platelet antigens (HPA-1 and HPA-2), with alleles designated as "a" or "b" (17). Although there are at least 10 officially recognized platelet-specific antigens at this time, more than 50% of

the reported cases in Caucasians and most of the severe cases have occurred as a result of sensitization against HPA-1a, also known as PlA1 and Zwa.

Fetal thrombocytopenia due to HPA-1a sensitization tends to be severe and can occur early in gestation. In a cohort study of 107 fetuses with neonatal alloimmune thrombocytopenia (97 with HPA-1a incompatibility) studied in utero before receiving any therapy, 50% had initial platelet counts of less than 20,000/μL (13). This percentage included 21 of 46 fetuses tested before 24 weeks of gestation. Furthermore, this series documented that the fetal platelet count decreases at a rate of more than 15,000/μL per week in the absence of therapy.

The recurrence risk of neonatal alloimmune thrombocytopenia is extremely high and approaches 100% in cases involving HPA-1a if the subsequent sibling carries the pertinent antigen (13). Thus, the recurrence risk is related to the zygosity of the father. As with red cell alloimmunization, the disease tends to be equally severe or progressively worse in subsequent pregnancies.

Immune Thrombocytopenic Purpura

Acute ITP is a self-limited disorder that usually occurs in childhood. It may follow a viral infection and rarely persists. Chronic ITP typically occurs in the second or third decade of life and has a female to male ratio of 3:1 (18). Estimates of the frequency of ITP during pregnancy vary widely, affecting one in 1,000–10,000 pregnancies (19).

Immune thrombocytopenic purpura is characterized by immunologically mediated platelet destruction. The patient produces IgG antiplatelet antibodies that recognize platelet membrane glycoproteins. This process leads to increased platelet destruction by cells of the reticuloendothelial system (18). The rate of destruction exceeds the compensatory ability of the bone marrow to produce new platelets, which leads to thrombocytopenia. Most of the platelet destruction occurs in the spleen, although other sites also are involved.

There are no pathognomonic signs, symptoms, or diagnostic tests for ITP; it is a diagnosis of exclusion. However, four findings have been traditionally associated with the condition: 1) persistent thrombocytopenia (platelet count <100,000/μL with or without accompanying megathrombocytes on the peripheral smear), 2) normal or increased numbers of megakaryocytes determined from bone marrow, 3) exclusion of other systemic disorders or drugs that are known to be associated with thrombocytopenia, and 4) absence of splenomegaly.

Most women with ITP have a history of bruising easily and petechiae, or of possible epistaxis and gingival bleeding, which precedes their pregnancy, but some women are completely asymptomatic. Important hemorrhagic symptoms rarely occur unless the platelet count is less than 20,000/μL. It is believed that the course of ITP usually is not affected by pregnancy, although there have been anecdotal reports of patients' conditions worsening during pregnancy and improving postpartum (20, 21). Pregnancy may be adversely affected by severe thrombocytopenia, and the primary risk to the mother is hemorrhage during the peripartum period.

Maternal IgG antiplatelet antibodies can cross the placenta, placing the fetus and neonate at risk for the development of thrombocytopenia. Retrospective case series of ITP in pregnancy indicate that 12–15% of infants born to mothers with ITP will develop platelet counts less than 50,000/μL (22, 23). Sometimes, this results in minor clinical bleeding such as purpura, ecchymoses, or melena. On rare occasions, fetal thrombocytopenia associated with ITP leads to intracranial hemorrhage unrelated to the mode of delivery. When it occurs, intracranial hemorrhage can result in severe neurologic impairment and even death. Serious bleeding complications are estimated to occur in 3% of infants born to women with ITP, and the rate of intracranial hemorrhage is less than 1% (22, 23). These data may overestimate the risk, as a result of publication bias. In a prospective, population-based study of almost 16,000 pregnancies delivered at a single center, no infant born to a mother with ITP suffered intracranial hemorrhage (9). The only three infants with intracranial hemorrhage had neonatal alloimmune thrombocytopenia, not ITP. The platelet count of the affected newborn usually will decrease after delivery, and the nadir may not be reached for several days (20).

Pregnancy-Induced Hypertension

Pregnancy-induced hypertension (PIH) is reported to be the cause of 21% of cases of maternal thrombocytopenia (9). The thrombocytopenia usually is moderate, and platelet counts rarely decrease below 20,000/μL. Clinical hemorrhage is uncommon unless the patient develops disseminated intravascular coagulopathy, but a decreasing maternal platelet count generally is considered a sign of worsening disease and is an indication for delivery.

In some cases, microangiopathic hemolytic anemia and elevated liver function tests are associated with thrombocytopenia in individuals with PIH. Such individuals are considered to have HELLP syndrome.

The cause of thrombocytopenia in women with severe PIH is unknown. The disease is associated with a state of accelerated platelet destruction, platelet activation, increased platelet volume, and increased megakaryocyte activity (21). Increased levels of platelet-associated IgG have been detected in patients with PIH (24). However, this finding is nonspecific and does not necessarily imply an immunologic basis for the thrombocytopenia. Platelet function also may be impaired in women with PIH, even if their platelet count is normal. It is noteworthy that the platelet count may decrease before the other clinical manifestations of PIH are apparent (25).

The neonates of mothers with PIH are at increased risk of neonatal thrombocytopenia (2). However, this is true only for infants born prematurely, and especially those with growth restriction. Term infants of mothers with PIH are no more likely to have thrombocytopenia than are controls. In a study of 1,414 mothers with hypertension, neonatal thrombocytopenia associated with PIH rarely decreased below 20,000/μL and caused no fetal bleeding complications (9).

Clinical Considerations and Recommendations

▶ *What is the appropriate workup for maternal thrombocytopenia?*

When thrombocytopenia is diagnosed in a pregnant woman, it is important that the diagnosis be as precise as possible. The differential diagnosis of thrombocytopenia in pregnancy includes gestational thrombocytopenia, pseudothrombocytopenia, HIV infection, drug-induced thrombocytopenia, PIH, HELLP syndrome, thrombotic thrombocytopenic purpura, hemolytic uremic syndrome, disseminated intravascular coagulation, systemic lupus erythematosus, antiphospholipid syndrome, and congenital thrombocytopenias. These disorders usually can be determined on the basis of a detailed medical and family history and a physical examination, with attention to blood pressure, splenomegaly, HIV serology, and adjunctive laboratory studies as appropriate.

A CBC and examination of the peripheral blood smear generally are indicated in the evaluation of maternal thrombocytopenia. A CBC is helpful to exclude pancytopenia. Evaluation of the peripheral smear serves to rule out platelet clumping that may be associated with pseudothrombocytopenia. Bone marrow biopsy rarely is needed to distinguish between inadequate platelet production and increased platelet turnover. Numerous assays have been developed for both platelet-associated (direct) antibodies and circulating (indirect) antiplatelet antibodies. Although many individuals with ITP will have elevated levels of platelet-associated antibodies and sometimes circulating antiplatelet antibodies, these assays are not recommended for the routine evaluation of maternal thrombocytopenia (26). Tests for antiplatelet antibodies are nonspecific, poorly standardized, and subject to a large degree of interlaboratory variation (1). Also, gestational thrombocytopenia and ITP cannot be differentiated on the basis of antiplatelet antibody testing (11).

If drugs and other medical disorders are excluded, the primary differential diagnosis in the first and second trimesters will be either gestational thrombocytopenia or ITP. It should be noted that although gestational thrombocytopenia can occur in the first trimester, it typically becomes manifest later in pregnancy. In general, in a woman with no history of thrombocytopenia or the milder the thrombocytopenia, the more likely she is to have gestational thrombocytopenia. If the platelet count is less than 70,000/μL, ITP is more likely to be present, and if the platelet count is less than 50,000/μL, ITP is almost certainly present. During the third trimester or postpartum period, the sudden onset of significant maternal thrombocytopenia should lead to consideration of PIH, thrombotic thrombocytopenic purpura, hemolytic uremic syndrome, acute fatty liver, or disseminated intravascular coagulation, although ITP can present this way as well.

▶ When should women with ITP receive medical therapy?

The goal of medical therapy during pregnancy in women with ITP is to minimize the risk of bleeding complications associated with severe thrombocytopenia. Because the platelet function of these patients usually is normal, it is not necessary to maintain their counts in the normal range. There is general agreement that asymptomatic pregnant women with platelet counts greater than 50,000/μL do not require treatment. Also, most authorities recommend treatment in the presence of a platelet count significantly less than 50,000/μL or in the presence of bleeding. However, the degree of thrombocytopenia in asymptomatic pregnant women that requires treatment is somewhat controversial, and consultation from a physician experienced in these matters should be considered. Higher counts (eg, >50,000/μL) are desirable for invasive procedures and delivery, which may be associated with hemorrhage, the need for surgery, or the desire to use regional anesthesia. Bleeding times are not useful in assessing platelet function in patients with ITP.

▶ What therapy should be used to treat ITP during pregnancy?

The first line of treatment for ITP is prednisone, usually initiated in a dosage of 1–2 mg/kg/d. A response to antenatal corticosteroids usually occurs within 3–7 days and reaches a maximum within 2–3 weeks. Once platelet counts reach acceptable levels, the dosage can be tapered by 10–20% per week until the lowest dosage required to maintain a platelet count greater than 50,000/μL is reached. An increase in the platelet count occurs in about 70% of patients, and up to 25% will achieve complete remission (27).

Intravenous immune globulin (IVIG) is appropriate therapy for cases refractory to steroids as well as in circumstances such as platelet counts less than 10,000/μL in the third trimester, or platelet counts less than 30,000/μL associated with bleeding or with preoperative or predelivery status. A response to therapy can be expected in as few as 6 hours or in as many as 72 hours. In 70% of cases, the platelet count will return to pretreatment levels within 30 days after treatment (26, 28). Intravenous immune globulin is costly and of limited availability. When considering use of IVIG, it is prudent to seek consultation from a physician experienced in such cases.

Splenectomy is associated with complete remission in approximately 66% of patients with ITP (18); however, it often is not successful in patients who do not respond to intravenous immunoglobulin (29). The procedure usually is avoided during pregnancy because of fetal risks and technical difficulties late in gestation. However, splenectomy can be accomplished safely during pregnancy, ideally in the second trimester. It is appropriate for severe cases (platelet counts of less than 10,000/μL) that have failed treatment with antenatal corticosteroids and IVIG (26).

Platelet transfusions should be used only as a temporary measure to control life-threatening hemorrhage or to prepare a patient for surgery. The usual increase in platelets of approximately 10,000/μL per unit of platelets transfused is not achieved in patients with ITP because of the decreased survival of donor platelets. Thus, 6–10 U of platelet concentrate should be transfused. Other drugs used to treat ITP such as colchicine, azathioprine, vinca alkaloids, cyclophosphamide, and danazol have potential adverse fetal effects.

▶ What additional specialized care should women with ITP receive?

Other than serial assessment of the maternal platelet count (every trimester in asymptomatic women in remission and more frequently in thrombocytopenic individuals), little specialized care is required. Pregnant women with ITP should be instructed to avoid nonsteroidal antiinflammatory agents, salicylates, and trauma. Individuals with splenectomies should be immunized against pneumococcus, *Hemophilus influenzae,* and meningococcus. If the diagnosis of ITP is made, consultation and ongoing evaluation with a physician experienced in such matters is appropriate.

▶ *Can fetal or neonatal intracranial hemorrhage be prevented in pregnancies complicated by ITP?*

It is logical to assume that therapies known to increase the maternal platelet count in patients with ITP also would improve the fetal platelet count. However, medical therapies such as IVIG (30) and steroids (22, 30–32) do not reliably prevent fetal thrombocytopenia or improve fetal outcome. Because some of these therapies (eg, IVIG) have not been adequately tested in appropriate trials, there are insufficient data to recommend maternal medical therapy for fetal indications.

Some investigators have recommended cesarean delivery to decrease the risk of intracranial hemorrhage by avoiding the potential trauma associated with vaginal birth (33). This strategy was based on anecdotal reports of intracranial hemorrhage associated with vaginal delivery (34) as well as the biologic plausibility of the hypothesis. Others have proposed that cesarean delivery be reserved for fetuses with platelet counts less than 50,000/μL (35, 36). This tactic was prompted by the observation that the risk of fetal bleeding is inversely proportional to the platelet count, and bleeding problems are extremely rare in fetuses with platelet counts more than 50,000/μL (31, 37).

Cesarean delivery has never been proven to prevent intracranial hemorrhage reliably. Several reports indicate that hemorrhagic complications in infants with thrombocytopenia are unrelated to the mode of delivery (22, 31, 37, 38). In a review of 474 neonates born to mothers with ITP, 29% of infants born vaginally with thrombocytopenia had a bleeding complication, compared with 30% delivered by cesarean birth (31). In this study, the rate of intracranial hemorrhage also was similar for both modes of delivery: 4% after vaginal delivery and 3% after cesarean delivery. In addition, it is unclear that intracranial hemorrhage is an intrapartum phenomenon. The neonatal platelet count often dramatically decreases after delivery. Thus, intracranial hemorrhage during the neonatal period could be mistakenly attributed to intrapartum events. No case of intracranial hemorrhage has been proven definitively to have occurred during labor (22, 23). Because cesarean delivery does not clearly prevent intraventricular hemorrhage, many obstetricians choose the mode of delivery in ITP based on obstetric considerations alone.

▶ *What tests or characteristics can be used to predict fetal thrombocytopenia in pregnancies complicated by ITP?*

No maternal test or characteristic can reliably predict the severity of thrombocytopenia in all cases of infants born to mothers with ITP. Maternal characteristics and serology, including prior splenectomy, platelet count, and the presence of platelet-associated antibodies, all correlate poorly with neonatal thrombocytopenia (39, 40). Fetal thrombocytopenia is rare in the absence of circulating antiplatelet antibodies (10), but exceptional cases have been reported (41). Also, these assays are difficult to perform and have a low positive predictive value (10).

▶ *Is there any role for fetal platelet count determination in ITP?*

At this time, most obstetricians do not obtain fetal platelet counts (42). Scalp sampling is fraught with inaccuracies and technical difficulties, and cordocentesis carries a 1–2% risk of necessitating an emergent cesarean delivery for fetal indications (43). The low incidence of intracranial hemorrhage and the lack of demonstrated difference in neonatal outcome between vaginal and cesarean deliveries also supports the opinion that the determination of fetal platelet count is unwarranted for ITP (22, 23, 31, 37, 44). A substantial minority of perinatologists (42) feel that the 5% risk of fetal thrombocytopenia of less than 20,000/μL and the attendant theoretically increased risk of an intracranial hemorrhage warrant informing patients of the availability of cordocentesis or scalp sampling during labor when choosing mode of delivery (45–47).

▶ *What is the appropriate neonatal care for infants born of pregnancies complicated by ITP?*

Regardless of the mode, delivery should be accomplished in a setting where an available clinician familiar with the disorder can treat any neonatal complications and have access to the medications needed for treatment.

▶ *Can a patient with thrombocytopenia be given regional anesthesia?*

The literature offers only limited and retrospective data to address this issue. However, two studies (48, 49) reported on a total of 184 patients with platelet counts less than 150,000/μL. Of these, 113 patients received epidural anesthesia without neurologic complication or sequelae. In all of these patients, the diagnosis was gestational thrombocytopenia. Another study of patients with platelet counts less than 100,000/μL due to preeclampsia, ITP, or infection also received epidural anesthesia without complication (50). Although the complication of greatest concern is that of epidural hematoma, there are only two cases in the literature of parturients who developed an epidural hematoma after regional anesthesia. One patient had preeclampsia and a lupus anticoagulant (51) and the other had an ependymoma (52). Cases reported in nonparturients have almost always been associated with anticoagulant therapy.

Although limited, data support the safety of epidural anesthesia in patients with platelet counts greater than 100,000/µL. In women with gestational thrombocytopenia with platelet counts less than 99,000/µL but greater than 50,000/µL, epidural anesthesia also may be safe, but its use in such patients will require a consensus among the obstetrician, anesthesiologist, and patient. When platelet counts are less than 50,000/µL, epidural anesthesia should not be given.

▶ *When should an evaluation for possible neonatal alloimmune thrombocytopenia be initiated, and what tests are useful in making the diagnosis?*

The most appropriate screening program incorporates evaluation of patients with a history of infants with otherwise unexplained bleeding or thrombocytopenia. Neonatal alloimmune thrombocytopenia should be suspected in cases of otherwise unexplained fetal or neonatal thrombocytopenia, porencephaly, or intracranial hemorrhage (either in utero or after birth). The laboratory diagnosis includes determination of platelet type and zygosity of both parents and the confirmation of maternal antiplatelet antibodies with specificity for paternal (or fetal–neonatal) platelets and the incompatible antigen. Platelet typing may be determined serologically or by genotyping because the genes and polymorphisms responsible for most cases of neonatal alloimmune thrombocytopenia have been identified. This is helpful when the father is heterozygous for the pertinent antigen because fetal platelet antigen typing can be performed using amniocytes (53). Chorionic villus sampling should not be performed because of its potential increased sensitization to antiplatelet antibodies. The laboratory evaluation of neonatal alloimmune thrombocytopenia can be complex, results may be ambiguous, and an antigen incompatibility cannot always be identified. Accordingly, testing for this disorder should be performed in an experienced regional laboratory that has special interest and expertise in neonatal alloimmune thrombocytopenia.

There is a theoretical benefit from population-based screening for platelet antigen incompatibility. However, such a program has not been shown to be clinically useful or cost-effective and is not currently recommended. Another area of controversy is the patient whose sister has had a pregnancy complicated by neonatal alloimmune thrombocytopenia. It may be worthwhile to evaluate these patients for platelet antigen incompatibility or

human leukocyte antigen phenotype. However, the theoretical advantages of testing these women must be weighed against the potential for anxiety, cost, and morbidity without proven benefit.

▶ *How can one determine the fetal platelet count in pregnancies complicated by neonatal alloimmune thrombocytopenia?*

Unfortunately, as with ITP, there are no good indirect methods to determine the fetal platelet count. Maternal antiplatelet antibody titers correlate poorly with the severity of the disease. Also, characteristics such as the outcome of previously affected siblings (eg, birth platelet count or intracranial hemorrhage recognized after delivery) do not reliably predict the severity of fetal thrombocytopenia (13). Currently, the only accurate means of estimating the fetal platelet count is to sample the fetal blood directly, although this may increase the risk of fetal exsanguination.

▶ *What is the appropriate obstetric management of neonatal alloimmune thrombocytopenia?*

The primary goal of the obstetric management of pregnancies complicated by neonatal alloimmune thrombocytopenia is to prevent intracranial hemorrhage and its associated complications. In contrast to ITP, however, the higher frequency of intracranial hemorrhage associated with neonatal alloimmune thrombocytopenia justifies more aggressive interventions. Also, strategies intended to avoid intracranial hemorrhage must be initiated antenatally because of the risk of in utero intracranial hemorrhage.

The optimal management of fetuses at risk for neonatal alloimmune thrombocytopenia (those testing positive for the incompatible antigen or those whose fathers are homozygous for the antigen) remains controversial. The management decisions for these cases should be individualized and are best made after consultation with obstetric and pediatric specialists familiar with the disorder as soon as the diagnosis is made. Several therapies have been used in an attempt to increase the fetal platelet count and to avoid intracranial hemorrhage, including maternal treatment with IVIG, with or without steroids (15, 54–60), and fetal platelet transfusions (59, 61, 62). Intravenous immune globulin administered to the mother appears to be the most consistently effective antepartum therapy for neonatal alloimmune thrombocytopenia (15). However, none of these therapies is effective in all cases. Direct fetal administration of IVIG does not reliably improve the fetal platelet count, although only a few cases have been reported. Platelet transfusions with maternal platelets are consistently effective in raising the fetal platelet count. However, the short half-life of transfused platelets requires weekly procedures and may worsen the alloimmunization.

It is unknown whether it is necessary to determine the fetal platelet count before initiating therapy. The risks of cordocentesis in the setting of neonatal alloimmune thrombocytopenia must be weighed against the ability to determine the need for and the effectiveness of therapy. Although unproven, the benefit of transfusing maternal platelets at the time of cordocentesis may reduce the risk of bleeding complications from the procedure (63). The optimal time during gestation to first assess the fetal platelet count also is controversial. When fetal blood sampling is indicated, performance at 22–24 weeks of gestation may optimize medical therapy.

Most investigators recommend determination of the fetal platelet count once fetal pulmonary maturity is achieved, but before the onset of labor (eg, 37 weeks of gestation). A trial of labor is permitted for fetuses with platelet counts greater than 50,000/μL, while those with severe thrombocytopenia are delivered by cesarean birth. Although this strategy is of unproven efficacy, the high rate of intracranial hemorrhage in neonatal alloimmune thrombocytopenia is considered to warrant these interventions. Delivery should be accomplished in a setting equipped to handle a neonate with severe thrombocytopenia.

▶ *What is appropriate obstetric management for gestational thrombocytopenia?*

Pregnancies with gestational thrombocytopenia are not at risk for maternal bleeding complications or fetal thrombocytopenia (4, 9). Thus, such interventions as the determination of the fetal platelet count or cesarean delivery are not indicated in patients with this condition. Women with gestational thrombocytopenia do not require any additional testing or specialized care, except follow-up platelet counts.

▶ *Is it necessary to treat thrombocytopenia associated with PIH?*

The primary treatment of maternal thrombocytopenia in the setting of PIH or HELLP syndrome is delivery. Although antepartum reversal of thrombocytopenia has been reported with medical therapy (64), this course of treatment is not usual (65, 66). More importantly, the underlying pathophysiology of PIH will only resolve following birth. Thus, other than to allow for medical stabilization, the effect of betamethasone on fetal pulmonary maturity, or in special cases at preterm gestations, severe thrombocytopenia due to PIH is an indication for delivery (66).

Major hemorrhage is infrequent in patients with PIH but minor bleeding such as operative site oozing during cesarean delivery is common. Platelet transfusions occasionally are needed to improve hemostasis in patients with severe thrombocytopenia or DIC. However, transfusions are less effective in these women because of accelerated platelet destruction. Therefore, platelet transfusions are best reserved for patients with severe thrombocytopenia and active bleeding. An exception is the patient undergoing cesarean delivery. Although of uncertain benefit, many authorities recommend platelet transfusions to increase the platelet count to more than 50,000/μL before cesarean delivery (66).

Platelet counts often decrease for 24–48 hours after birth, followed by a rapid recovery (67–69). Most patients will achieve normal platelet counts within a few days to a week postpartum (67, 69). However, although rare, thrombocytopenia may continue for a prolonged period, which often is associated with persistent multisystem dysfunction (68). Plasma exchange has been reported to improve the platelet count in women with HELLP syndrome (70), but the efficacy remains unproven. Although thrombocytopenia associated with PIH or HELLP syndrome may improve after treatment with steroids or uterine curettage (71, 72), the clinical benefit of these therapies also is uncertain.

Summary

The following recommendation is based on good and consistent scientific evidence (Level A):

▶ Neonatal alloimmune thrombocytopenia should be treated with IVIG as the initial approach when fetal thrombocytopenia is documented.

The following recommendations are based on limited or inconsistent scientific evidence (Level B):

▶ The mode of delivery in pregnancies complicated by ITP should be chosen based on obstetric considerations alone. Prophylactic cesarean delivery does not appear to reduce the risk of fetal or neonatal hemorrhage.

▶ Epidural anesthesia is safe in patients with platelet counts greater than 100,000/μL.

▶ Mild maternal thrombocytopenia (≥ 70,000/μL) in asymptomatic pregnant women with no history of bleeding problems is usually benign gestational thrombocytopenia. These women should receive routine prenatal care with periodic repeat platelet counts (monthly to bimonthly).

The following recommendations are based primarily on consensus and expert opinion (Level C):

▶ Platelet counts of at least 50,000/μL rarely require treatment.

▶ Neonatal alloimmune thrombocytopenia should be suspected in cases of otherwise unexplained fetal or neonatal thrombocytopenia, hemorrhage, or porencephaly.

▶ Prior to initiating any plan of treatment for a woman based on thrombocytopenia in her fetus, consultation should be sought from a physician with experience dealing with that problem.

▶ Laboratory testing for neonatal alloimmune thrombocytopenia should be performed in a regional laboratory with special interest and expertise in dealing with the problem.

References

1. Rouse DJ, Owen J, Goldenberg RL. Routine maternal platelet count: an assessment of technologically driven practice. Am J Obstet Gynecol 1998;179:573–576 (Level III)

2. Burrows RF, Kelton JG. Thrombocytopenia at delivery: a prospective survey of 6,715 deliveries. Am J Obstet Gynecol 1990;162:731–734 (Level II-3)

3. Lacey JV, Penner JA. Management of idiopathic thrombocytopenic purpura in the adult. Semin Thromb Hemost 1977;3:160–174 (Level III)

4. Burrows RF, Kelton JG. Incidentally detected thrombocytopenia in healthy mothers and their infants. N Engl J Med 1988;319:142–145 (Level II-3)

5. Nagey DA, Alger LS, Edelman BB, Heyman MR, Pupkin MJ, Crenshaw C Jr. Reacting appropriately to thrombocytopenia in pregnancy. South Med J 1986;79:1385–1388 (Level III)

6. Jih DM, Werth VP. Thrombocytopenia after a single dose of methotrexate. J Am Acad Dermatol 1998;39:349–351 (Level III)

7. Mant MJ, Connolly T, Gordon PA, King EG. Severe thrombocytopenia probably due to acute folic acid deficiency. Crit Care Med 1979;7:297–300 (Level III)

8. Ruggeri M, Schiavotto C, Castaman G, Tosetto A, Rodeghiero F. Gestational thrombocytopenia: a prospective study. Haematologica 1997;82:341–342 (Level II-3)

9. Burrows RF, Kelton JG. Fetal thrombocytopenia and its relation to maternal thrombocytopenia. N Engl J Med 1993;329:1463–1466 (Level II-3)

10. Samuels P, Bussel JB, Braitman LE, Tomaski A, Druzin ML, Mennuti MT, et al. Estimation of the risk of thrombocytopenia in the offspring of pregnant women with presumed immune thrombocytopenic purpura. N Engl J Med 1990;323:229–235 (Level II-3)

11. Lescale KB, Eddleman KA, Cines DB, Samuels P, Lesser ML, McFarland JG, et al. Antiplatelet antibody testing in thrombocytopenic pregnant women. Am J Obstet Gynecol 1996;174:1014–1018 (Level II-2)

12. Blanchette VS, Chen L, de Friedberg ZS, Hogan VA, Trudel E, Decary F. Alloimmunization to the PlA1 platelet antigen: results of a prospective study. Br J Haematol 1990;74:209–215 (Level II-3)

13. Bussel JB, Zabusky MR, Berkowitz RL, McFarland JG. Fetal alloimmune thrombocytopenia. N Engl J Med 1997; 337:22–26 (Level II-2)

14. Mueller-Eckhardt C, Kiefel V, Grubert A, Kroll H, Weisheit M, Schmidt S, et al. 348 cases of suspected neonatal alloimmune thrombocytopenia. Lancet 1989; 1:363–366 (Level II-3)

15. Bussel JB, Berkowitz RL, Lynch L, Lesser ML, Paidas MJ, Huang CL, et al. Antenatal management of alloimmune thrombocytopenia with intravenous gamma-globulin: a randomized trial of the addition of low-dose steroid to intravenous gamma-globulin. Am J Obstet Gynecol 1996;174:1414–1423 (Level I)

16. Herman JH, Jumbelic MI, Ancona RJ, Kickler TS. In utero cerebral hemorrhage in alloimmune thrombocytopenia. Am J Pediatr Hematol Oncol 1986;8:312–317 (Level III)

17. von dem Borne AE, Decary F. Nomenclature of platelet-specific antigens. Transfusion 1990;30:477 (Level III)

18. George JN, el-Harake MA, Raskob GE. Chronic idiopathic thrombocytopenic purpura. N Engl J Med 1994;331: 1207–1211 (Level III)

19. Sainio S, Joutsi L, Jarvenpaa AL, Kekomaki R, Koistinen E, Riikonen S, et al. Idiopathic thrombocytopenic purpura in pregnancy. Acta Obstet Gynecol Scand 1998; 77: 272–277 (Level III)

20. Kelton JG, Inwood MJ, Barr RM, Effer SB, Hunter D, Wilson WE, et al. The prenatal prediction of thrombocytopenia in infants of mothers with clinically diagnosed immune thrombocytopenia. Am J Obstet Gynecol 1982;144:449–454 (Level II-3)

21. McCrae KR, Samuels P, Schreiber AD. Pregnancy-associated thrombocytopenia: pathogenesis and management. Blood 1992;80:2697–2714 (Level III)

22. Payne SD, Resnik R, Moore TR, Hedriana HL, Kelly TF. Maternal characteristics and risk of severe neonatal thrombocytopenia and intracranial hemorrhage in pregnancies complicated by autoimmune thrombocytopenia. Am J Obstet Gynecol 1997;177:149–155 (Level II-3)

23. Silver RM, Branch DW, Scott JR. Maternal thrombocytopenia in pregnancy: time for a reassessment. Am J Obstet Gynecol 1995;173:479–482 (Level III)

24. Burrows RF, Hunter DJ, Andrew M, Kelton JG. A prospective study investigating the mechanism of thrombocytopenia in preeclampsia. Obstet Gynecol 1987;70:334–338 (Level II-2)

25. Redman CW, Bonnar J, Beilin L. Early platelet consumption in pre-eclampsia. BMJ 1978;1:467–469 (Level II-2)

26. George JN, Woolf SH, Raskob GE, Wasser JS, Aledort LM, Ballem PJ, et al. Idiopathic thrombocytopenic purpura: a practice guideline developed by explicit methods for the American Society of Hematology. Blood 1996;88: 3–40 (Level III)

27. Karpatkin S. Autoimmune thrombocytopenic purpura. Am J Med Sci 1971;261:127–138 (Level III)

28. Bussel JB, Pham LC. Intravenous treatment with gamma globulin in adults with immune thrombocytopenic purpu-

ra: review of the literature. Vox Sang 1987;52:206–211 (Level III)

29. Law C, Marcaccio M, Tam P, Heddle N, Kelton JG. High-dose intravenous immune globulin and the response to splenectomy in patients with idiopathic thrombocytopenic purpura. N Engl J Med 1997;336:1494–1498 (Level III)

30. Kaplan C, Daffos F, Forestier F, Tertian G, Catherine N, Pous JC, et al. Fetal platelet counts in thrombocytopenic pregnancy. Lancet 1990;336:979–982 (Level II-3)

31. Cook RL, Miller RC, Katz VL, Cefalo RC. Immune thrombocytopenic purpura in pregnancy: a reappraisal of management. Obstet Gynecol 1991;78:578–583 (Level II-3)

32. Christiaens GC, Nieuwenhuis HK, von dem Borne AE, Ouwehand WH, Helmerhorst FM, Van Dalen CM, et al. Idiopathic thrombocytopenic purpura in pregnancy: a randomized trial on the effect of antenatal low dose corticosteroids on neonatal platelet count. Br J Obstet Gynaecol 1990;97:893–898 (Level I)

33. Carloss HW, McMillan R, Crosby WH. Management of pregnancy in women with immune thrombocytopenic purpura. JAMA 1980;224:2756–2758 (Level III)

34. Jones RW, Asher MI, Rutherford CJ, Munro HM. Autoimmune (idiopathic) thrombocytopenic purpura in pregnancy and the newborn. Br J Obstet Gynaecol 1977;84:679–683 (Level III)

35. Ayromlooi J. A new approach to the management of immunologic thrombocytopenic purpura in pregnancy. Am J Obstet Gynecol 1978;130:235–236 (Level III)

36. Scott JR, Cruikshank DP, Kochenour NK, Pitkin RM, Warenski JC. Fetal platelet counts in the obstetric management of immunologic thrombocytopenic purpura. Am J Obstet Gynecol 1980;136:495–499 (Level III)

37. Burrows RF, Kelton JG. Pregnancy in patients with idiopathic thrombocytopenic purpura: assessing the risks for the infant at delivery. Obstet Gynecol Surv 1993;48:781–788 (Level III)

38. Laros RK Jr, Kagan R. Route of delivery for patients with immune thrombocytopenic purpura. Am J Obstet Gynecol 1984;148:901–908 (Level III)

39. Scott JR, Rote NS, Cruikshank DP. Antiplatelet antibodies and platelet counts in pregnancies complicated by autoimmune thrombocytopenic purpura. Am J Obstet Gynecol 1983;145:932–939 (Level II-3)

40. Burrows RF, Kelton JG. Low fetal risks in pregnancies associated with idiopathic thrombocytopenic purpura. Am J Obstet Gynecol 1990;163:1147–1150 (Level II-3)

41. Risk of thrombocytopenia in offspring of mothers with presumed immune thrombocytopenic purpura. N Engl J Med 1990;323:1841–1843 (Level III)

42. Peleg D, Hunter SK. Perinatal management of women with immune thrombocytopenic purpura: survey of United States perinatologists. Am J Obstet Gynecol 1999;180:645–649 (Level II-3)

43. Ghidini A, Sepulveda W, Lockwood CJ, Romero R. Complications of fetal blood sampling. Am J Obstet Gynecol 1993;168:1339–1344 (Level III)

44. Berry SM, Leonardi MR, Wolfe HM, Dombrowski MP, Lanouette JM, Cotton DB. Maternal thrombocytopenia.

Predicting neonatal thrombocytopenia with cordocentesis. J Reprod Med 1997;42:276–280 (Level III)

45. Garmel SH, Craigo SD, Morin LM, Crowley JM, D'Alton ME. The role of percutaneous umbilical blood sampling in the management of immune thrombocytopenic purpura. Prenat Diagn 1995;15:439–445 (Level III)

46. De Carolis S, Noia G, DeSantis M, Trivellini C, Mastromarino C, De Carolis MP, et al. Immune thrombocytopenic purpura and percutaneous umbilical blood sampling: an open question. Fetal Diagn Ther 1993;8:154–160 (Level II-2)

47. Scioscia AL, Grannum PA, Copel JA, Hobbins JC. The use of percutaneous umbilical blood sampling in immune thrombocytopenic purpura. Am J Obstet Gynecol 1988;159:1066–1068 (Level II-3)

48. Beilin Y, Zahn J, Comerford M. Safe epidural analgesia in thirty parturients with platelet counts between 69,000 and 98,000 mm-3. Anesth Analg 1997;85:385–388 (Level III)

49. Rolbin SH, Abbott D, Musclow E, Papsin F, Lie LM, Freedman J. Epidural anesthesia in pregnant patients with low platelet counts. Obstet Gynecol 1988;71:918–920 (Level III)

50. Rasmus KT, Rottman RL, Kotelko DM, Wright WC, Stone JJ, Rosenblatt RM. Unrecognized thrombocytopenia and regional anesthesia in parturients: a retrospective review. Obstet Gynecol 1989;73:943–946 (Level III)

51. Lao TT, Halpern SH, MacDonald D, Huh C. Spinal subdural haematoma in a parturient after attempted epidural anaesthesia. Can J Anaesth 1993;40:340–345 (Level III)

52. Roscoe MWA, Barrington TW. Acute spinal subdural hematoma. A case report and review of literature. Spine 1984;9:672–675 (Level III)

53. McFarland JG, Aster RH, Bussel JB, Gianopoulos JG, Derbes RS, Newman PJ. Prenatal diagnosis of neonatal alloimmune thrombocytopenia using allele-specific oligonucleotide probes. Blood 1991;78:2276–2282 (Level III)

54. Bussel JB, Berkowitz RL, McFarland JG, Lynch L, Chitkara U. Antenatal treatment of neonatal alloimmune thrombocytopenia. N Engl J Med 1988;319:1374–1378 (Level II-2)

55. Lynch L, Bussel JB, McFarland JG, Chitkara U, Berkowitz RL. Antenatal treatment of alloimmune thrombocytopenia. Obstet Gynecol 1992;80:67–71 (Level II-2)

56. Marzusch K, Schnaidt M, Dietl J, Weist E, Hofstaetter C, Golz R. High-dose immunoglobulin in the antenatal treatment of neonatal alloimmune thrombocytopenia: case report and review. Br J Obstet Gynaecol 1992;99:260–262 (Level III)

57. Mir N, Samson D, House MJ, Kovar IZ. Failure of antenatal high-dose immunoglobulin to improve fetal platelet count in neonatal alloimmune thrombocytopenia. Vox Sang 1988;55:188–189 (Level III)

58. Bowman J, Harman C, Mentigolou S, Pollack J. Intravenous fetal transfusion of immunoglobulin for alloimmune thrombocytopenia. Lancet 1992;340:1034–1035 (Level III)

59. Nicolini U, Tannirandorn Y, Gonzalez P, Fisk NM, Beacham J, Letsky EA, et al. Continuing controversy in

alloimmune thrombocytopenia: fetal hyperimmunoglobulinemia fails to prevent thrombocytopenia. Am J Obstet Gynecol 1990;163:1144–1146 (Level III)

60. Zimmermann R, Huch A. In-utero fetal therapy with immunoglobulin for alloimmune thrombocytopenia. Lancet 1992;340:606 (Level III)

61. Kaplan C, Daffos F, Forestier F, Cox WL, Lyon-Caen D, Dupuy-Montbrun MC, et al. Management of alloimmune thrombocytopenia: antenatal diagnosis and in utero transfusion of maternal platelets. Blood 1988;72:340–343 (Level III)

62. Murphy MF, Pullon HW, Metcalfe P, Chapman JF, Jenkins E, Waters AH, et al. Management of fetal alloimmune thrombocytopenia by weekly in utero platelet transfusions. Vox Sang 1990;58:45–49 (Level III)

63. Paidas MJ, Berkowitz RL, Lynch L, Lockwood CJ, Lapinski R, McFarland JG, et al. Alloimmune thrombocytopenia: fetal and neonatal losses related to cordocentesis. Am J Obstet Gynecol 1995;172:475–479 (Level II-2)

64. Clark SL, Phelan JR, Allen SH, Golde SR. Antepartum reversal of hematologic abnormalities associated with the HELLP syndrome. A report of three cases. J Reprod Med 1986;31:70–72 (Level III)

65. Weinstein L. Syndrome of hemolysis, elevated liver enzymes, and low platelet count: a severe consequence of hypertension in pregnancy. Am J Obstet Gynecol 1982;142:159–167 (Level III)

66. Sibai BM. The HELLP syndrome (hemolysis, elevated liver enzymes, and low platelets): much ado about nothing? Am J Obstet Gynecol 1990;162:311–316 (Level III)

67. Katz VL, Thorp JM Jr, Rozas L, Bowes WA Jr. The natural history of thrombocytopenia associated with preeclampsia. Am J Obstet Gynecol 1990;163:1142–1143 (Level II-3)

68. Martin JN Jr, Blake PG, Lowry SL, Perry KG Jr, Files JC, Morrison JC. Pregnancy complicated by preeclampsia-eclampsia with the syndrome of hemolysis, elevated liver enzymes, and low platelet count: how rapid is postpartum recovery? Obstet Gynecol 1990;76:737–741 (Level II-3)

69. Neiger R, Contag SA, Coustan DR. The resolution of preeclampsia-related thrombocytopenia. Obstet Gynecol 1991;77:692–695 (Level II-3)

70. Martin JN Jr, Files JC, Blake PG, Norman PH, Martin RW, Hess LW, et al. Plasma exchange for preeclampsia. I. Postpartum use for persistently severe preeclampsia-eclampsia with HELLP syndrome. Am J Obstet Gynecol 1990;162:126–137 (Level III)

71. Magann EF, Martin JN Jr, Isaacs JD, Perry KG Jr, Martin RW, Meydrech EF. Immediate postpartum curettage: accelerated recovery from severe preeclampsia. Obstet Gynecol 1993;81:502–506 (Level I)

72. Magann EF, Bass D, Chauhan SP, Sullivan DL, Martin RW, Martin JN Jr. Antepartum corticosteroids: disease stabilization in patients with the syndrome of hemolysis, elevated liver enzymes, and low platelets (HELLP). Am J Obstet Gynecol 1994;171:1148–1153 (Level I)

The MEDLINE database, the Cochrane Library, and ACOG's own internal resources were used to conduct a literature search to locate relevant articles published between January 1985 and January 1999. The search was restricted to articles published in the English language. Priority was given to articles reporting results of original research, although review articles and commentaries also were consulted. Abstracts of research presented at symposiums and scientific conferences were not considered adequate for inclusion in this document. Guidelines published by organizations or institutions such as the National Institutes of Health and ACOG were reviewed, and additional studies were located by reviewing bibliographies of identified articles. When reliable research was not available, expert opinions from obstetrician–gynecologists were used.

Studies were reviewed and evaluated for quality according to the method outlined by the U.S. Preventive Services Task Force:

I   Evidence obtained from at least one properly designed randomized controlled trial.

II-1   Evidence obtained from well-designed controlled trials without randomization.

II-2   Evidence obtained from well-designed cohort or case–control analytic studies, preferably from more than one center or research group.

II-3   Evidence obtained from multiple time series with or without the intervention. Dramatic results in uncontrolled experiments also could be regarded as this type of evidence.

III   Opinions of respected authorities, based on clinical experience, descriptive studies, or reports of expert committees.

Based on the highest level of evidence found in the data, recommendations are provided and graded according to the following categories:

Level A—Recommendations are based on good and consistent scientific evidence.

Level B—Recommendations are based on limited or inconsistent scientific evidence.

Level C—Recommendations are based primarily on consensus and expert opinion.

ISSN 1099-3630

**The American College of Obstetricians and Gynecologists
409 12th Street, SW
PO Box 96920
Washington, DC 20090-6920**   12345/32109

ACOG PRACTICE BULLETIN

CLINICAL MANAGEMENT GUIDELINES FOR
OBSTETRICIAN–GYNECOLOGISTS

NUMBER 19, AUGUST 2000

(Replaces Educational Bulletin Number 234, March 1997)

This Practice Bulletin was developed by the ACOG Committee on Practice Bulletins— Obstetrics with the assistance of Linda A. Barbour, MD, MSPH. The information is designed to aid practitioners in making decisions about appropriate obstetric and gynecologic care. These guidelines should not be construed as dictating an exclusive course of treatment or procedure. Variations in practice may be warranted based on the needs of the individual patient, resources, and limitations unique to the institution or type of practice.

Thromboembolism in Pregnancy

During pregnancy, women have a fivefold increased risk of venous thromboembolism (VTE), compared with nonpregnant women. The absolute risk of symptomatic venous thrombosis during pregnancy is between 0.5 and 3.0 per 1,000 women based on studies using radiographic documentation (1–3). Pulmonary embolism (PE) is a leading cause of maternal death in the United States (4). The prevalence and severity of this condition warrant consideration of anticoagulant therapy in pregnancy for women at risk for VTE. Such therapy includes the treatment of acute thrombotic events, prophylaxis for patients with a history of thrombotic events or identified acquired or congenital thrombophilias, and prevention and treatment of systemic embolization in women with valvular heart disease. The purpose of this document is to review the current literature on the prevention and management of thromboembolism in obstetric patients, discuss the data behind sometimes conflicting guidelines from expert panels, and offer evidence-based recommendations to address the most clinically relevant issues in the management of these patients.

Background

Numerous changes in the coagulation system account for the hypercoagulable state associated with pregnancy (see the box). Recently, it has been recognized that up to half of women who have thrombotic events during pregnancy possess an underlying congenital or acquired thrombophilia (5). The most common thrombophilias in the Caucasian population are the factor V Leiden mutation, which has a prevalence of 5% in this population, and the prothrombin gene mutation G20210A, which has a prevalence of 2% in this population (5, 6). In approximately 50% of patients with a hereditary thrombophilia, the initial thrombotic event occurs in the presence of an additional risk factor such as pregnancy, oral contraceptive use, orthopedic trauma, immobilization, or surgery (7, 8).

Pregnancy-Associated Changes in Coagulation

Increases in clotting factors (I, VII, VIII, IX, X)

Decreases in protein S

Decreases in fibrinolytic activity

Increased venous stasis

Vascular injury associated with delivery

Increased activation of platelets

Resistance to activated protein C

Risk of Thromboembolism During Pregnancy

Traditionally, it was believed that the risk of venous thrombosis was greatest in the third trimester and immediately postpartum. More recent studies using objective criteria for diagnosis have found that antepartum deep vein thrombosis (DVT) is at least as common as postpartum thrombosis and occurs with equal frequency in all three trimesters (1). However, PE is more common postpartum.

Women with a history of thromboembolism have an increased risk of recurrence when they become pregnant; however, the estimates of recurrence are based primarily on two retrospective studies and range from 7.5% to 12% (9, 10). No studies differentiated the risk of recurrence based on underlying factors such as acquired or congenital thrombophilias, use of oral contraceptives, pregnancy, orthopedic trauma, recent surgery, or the occurrence of the event in the antepartum versus postpartum period. Most of the estimates of recurrence are based on women who had their initial event during oral contraceptive use or pregnancy. Risk factors for thromboembolic disorders are noted in the box.

Anticoagulation Medications in Pregnancy

Although many terms have been used to classify anticoagulant regimens, the following terminology will be used in this document:

- Low-dose prophylaxis—a fixed dose of anticoagulant given 1–2 times per day without use of routine monitoring to verify a therapeutic prolongation of the activated partial thromboplastin time (APTT).

- Adjusted-dose prophylaxis—anticoagulant administered for prophylaxis to achieve traditional therapeutic effects, given 2–3 times per day with frequent laboratory testing to verify adequate APTT prolongation of at least 1.5 to 2.5.

Heparin

There is considerable clinical experience with heparin use in pregnancy (11). Heparin requirements appear to increase during pregnancy because of increases in heparin-binding proteins, plasma volume, renal clearance, and heparin degradation by the placenta, which reduces the bioavailability of heparin (12). There are no prospective trials that have determined adequate prophylactic doses in pregnancy. The major concerns with heparin use during pregnancy are not fetal but maternal and include heparin-induced osteoporosis and heparin-induced thrombocytopenia (HIT).

Two prospective trials of pregnant women exposed to heparin confirmed a mean bone loss of 5% (13, 14), with approximately one third sustaining a 10% or greater decrease in bone density (13). The complete reversibility of this process has not been clearly established, nor does there appear to be a clear dose-response relationship (15). In selected patients, such as those who have a strong family history of osteoporosis or are smokers, postpartum evaluation of bone density may have prognostic and therapeutic implications (13, 14).

There are two types of heparin-induced thrombocytopenia. The more common type is the benign, reversible nonimmune form, which occurs in patients within the first few days of therapy and typically resolves by 5 days. This

---

Risk Factors for Deep Vein Thrombosis and Thromboembolic Disorders

Hereditary Thrombophilia (prevalence in general population)

    Factor V Leiden mutation (5–9%)*

    AT-III deficiency (0.02–0.2%)

    Protein C deficiency (0.2–0.5%)

    Protein S deficiency (0.08%)

    Hyperhomocystinemia (1–11%)

    Prothrombin gene mutation (2–4%)

Prior history of deep vein thrombosis

Mechanical heart valve

Atrial fibrillation

Trauma/prolonged immobilization/major surgery

Other familial hypercoagulable states

Antiphospholipid syndrome

*For African Americans, about 1%; for Caucasians, 6–11%.

Data from Lockwood CJ. Heritable coagulopathies in pregnancy. Obstet Gynecol Surv 1999;54:754–765 condition does not require cessation of heparin therapy. The less common but more severe type is the immune form of HIT, which occurs within 5–14 days of full-dose heparin therapy in as many as 3% of patients (16) and may result in widespread thrombosis (17, 18). The occurrence of autoimmune thrombocytopenia from prophylactic doses of heparin has been reported, but is rare. Deep vein thrombosis and PE are the most frequent clinical presentations of the immune form of HIT. It has been recommended, therefore, that platelet counts be checked on day 5 and then periodically for the first 2 weeks of heparin therapy. If the HIT is severe, heparin therapy must be stopped and alternative anticoagulation therapy initiated; low-molecular-weight heparin (LMWH) may not be a safe alternative because it has a low cross reactivity with heparin. In such situations, consultation with someone with expertise in the field may be needed (17, 18).

Low-Molecular-Weight Heparin

Low-molecular-weight heparin may reduce three of the complications caused by standard heparin: bleeding, osteoporosis, and thrombocytopenia (16, 18, 19). However, virtually all data on LMWH come from nonpregnant patients. It has been conclusively demonstrated that LMWH does not cross the placenta into the fetal circulation (20, 21). Although the bioavailability of LMWH should be improved over standard heparin because of the reduction of heparin binding, the increases in renal clearance and volume of distribution of the drug may necessitate dosage increases in pregnancy (22, 23). Another advantage of LMWH is that dosing can be limited to once or twice daily (22, 24). If laboratory monitoring is used, monitoring peak antifactor Xa levels every 4–6 weeks should be utilized particularly when twice daily dosing is given. The APTT does not correlate well with the anticoagulant effect of LMWH.

Warfarin

Warfarin derivatives cross the placenta and in most cases are relatively contraindicated in pregnancy; therefore, they primarily are used postpartum or in patients with certain types of mechanical heart valves (25–29). Warfarin use should be restricted to the second or early third trimester in selected patients in whom prolonged high-dose heparin therapy is relatively contraindicated. A skeletal embryopathy resulting in stippled epiphyses and nasal and limb hypoplasia can occur when warfarin is given between 6 and 12 weeks of gestation (30). Midtrimester exposure may result in optic atrophy, microcephaly, and developmental delay. Bleeding can occur in the fetus at any time, resulting in a high fetal loss rate (30).

Clinical Considerations and Recommendations

▶ *Who are candidates for thromboprophylaxis in pregnancy?*

Thromboprophylaxis is defined as administration of anticoagulants because of an increased risk of VTE during pregnancy rather than treatment for an acute event. Often this can be accomplished using relatively low doses, which have a minimal effect on laboratory measures of coagulation. Such low-dose prophylaxis carries fewer risks than full therapeutic anticoagulation. There are certain high-risk conditions that require dosage adjustments to achieve higher therapeutic levels of anticoagulation (adjusted-dose heparin prophylaxis). Each patient's regimen should be individualized once the risks of heparin therapy are weighed against the benefits (31).

Patients with the following conditions are at highest risk and should have adjusted-dose heparin prophylaxis (12):

- Artificial heart valves (some investigators recommend warfarin therapy after the first trimester in certain circumstances) (26–29)

- Antithrombin-III (AT-III) deficiency (with or without a history of thrombosis; also referred to as "antithrombin deficiency") (32, 33)

- Antiphospholipid syndrome (some investigators recommend low-dose prophylaxis for this condition if there is no history of DVT) (34, 35)

- History of rheumatic heart disease with current atrial fibrillation (36)

- Homozygous factor V Leiden mutation, homozygous prothrombin G20210A mutation

- Patients receiving chronic anticoagulation for recurrent thromboembolism

Patients who are identified carriers of other inherited thrombophilias who do not have a history of thrombosis but have a strong family history of thrombosis (36) and noncarriers with a history of thromboembolic events before the current pregnancy (34) appear to be at lower risk and may be candidates for low-dose prophylaxis. However, no data exist to support or refute this approach.

It is not clear whether patients with a history of thrombosis identified with a protein C or protein S deficiency should receive low-dose or adjusted-dose heparin prophylaxis during pregnancy. It is also not known whether asymptomatic women who have been identified as carriers of inherited thrombophilia (except AT-III or homozygosity to the factor V Leiden or prothrombin G20210A mutation) and who are without a personal or family history of thromboembolism should receive heparin prophylaxis because there is marked variation in the penetrance of the thrombotic trait.

Patients with a history of idiopathic thrombosis, extensive or life-threatening thrombosis, recurrent thrombosis, thrombosis related to a high estrogen state, or who have an underlying thrombophilia or postthrombotic syndrome are likely to be at a higher risk of recurrence in pregnancy than patients with a definite transient provocation (orthopedic trauma or surgery) without any of these risk factors. The former group should consider antepartum thromboprophylaxis beginning in the first trimester and continuing until 6 weeks postpartum. It is unclear whether patients who have sustained VTE from a transient and highly thrombogenic provocation (eg, orthopedic trauma) and who have no other risk factors may benefit from antepartum prophylaxis. Their risk of recurrence is likely higher than the baseline population, and an increasing number of thrombophilic states are being identified in patients who sustain thromboses in the setting of recognized transient provocations (37). Although data are limited, some experts recommend that, at minimum, such patients be given postpartum prophylaxis with warfarin.

▶ *How should a prophylactic heparin regimen be administered during pregnancy?*

Because of the absence of adequate prospective trials, a number of different prophylactic regimens have been offered by varying consensus panels, often based on nonpregnant patient studies (34, 38, 39) (see the box).

One study determined that during pregnancy, a doubling of the dose of heparin was required to achieve the same anticoagulant response of a nonpregnant patient taking 5,000 U of heparin twice daily for low-dose prophylaxis (12). Some patients who are AT-III deficient will not respond to heparin and may require AT-III factor therapy (40).

Pregnant patients who require adjusted-dose heparin for anticoagulation for long-term prophylaxis may theoretically benefit from the higher bioavailability and more consistent therapeutic anticoagulation with LMWH (41, 42).

▶ *Who should be tested for inherited or acquired thrombophilias?*

Women who have a history of thrombosis should be offered testing, especially if such testing would affect management. It is controversial whether to test women who do not have a history of thrombosis but have a fami-

---

Prophylactic Heparin Regimens in Pregnancy

Unfractionated Heparin

Low–dose prophylaxis:

1. 5,000–7,500 U every 12 hours during the first trimester
7,500–10,000 U every 12 hours during the second trimester
10,000 U every 12 hours during the third trimester unless the APTT* is elevated. The APTT may be checked near term and the heparin dose reduced if prolonged

OR

2. 5,000–10,000 U every 12 hours throughout pregnancy

Adjusted-dose prophylaxis:

≥10,000 U twice a day to three times a day to achieve APTT of 1.5–2.5

Low-Molecular-Weight Heparin

Low-dose prophylaxis:

Dalteparin, 5,000 U once or twice daily, or enoxaparin, 40 mg once or twice daily

Adjusted-dose prophylaxis:

Dalteparin, 5,000–10,000 U every 12 hours, or enoxaparin, 30–80 mg every 12 hours

*APTT indicates activated partial thromboplastin time.

Data from Colvin BT, Barrowcliffe TW. The British Society for Haematology guidelines on the use and monitoring of heparin 1992: second revision. J Clin Pathol 1993;46:97–103. Ginsberg JS, Hirsh J. Use of antithrombotic agents during pregnancy. Chest 1998;114: 524S–530S. Maternal and Neonatal Haemostasis Working Party of the Haemostasis and Thrombosis Task. Guidelines on the presentation, investigation and management of thrombosis associated with pregnancy. J Clin Pathol 1993;46:489–496

---

ly history of thrombosis. Women who have a first-degree relative with an AT-III deficiency or homozygous factor V Leiden or prothrombin G20210A mutation may benefit from testing. Individuals with a strong family history of thrombophilias may be more likely to have multiple inherited risk factors with an increased risk of thrombosis (4–40%) during pregnancy (32, 43, 44). The coexistence of multiple inherited risk factors has been demonstrated. In one study, 15% of patients with protein C deficiency and 39% with protein S deficiency also were positive for factor V Leiden mutations, which markedly increased the risk of thrombosis for the patient (45).

Patients with a history of thrombosis, recurrent fetal loss, early or severe preeclampsia, or severe unexplained intrauterine growth restriction may be tested for antiphospholipid antibodies. Prophylactic anticoagulation for patients with antiphospholipid syndrome has been shown to improve pregnancy outcome (35, 46).

Deficiencies in protein C, protein S, and AT-III and mutations, including factor V Leiden, prothrombin G20210A, and C677T in the methylenetetrahydrofolate reductase (MTHFR) gene associated with hyperhomocystinemia, also have been associated with severe early preeclampsia, unexplained fetal loss or stillbirth, and placental abruption (47–49). However, there are no randomized clinical trials supporting the efficacy of anticoagulation therapy in preventing these conditions. It is important to discuss with the patient the implications of a positive test result for one of these thrombophilias and to determine whether patient management would be altered during the pregnancy or in the future if the test results are positive.

▶ Which tests should be ordered?

The following tests may be ordered to evaluate the risk for thromboembolic events in women with a history of thrombosis, a family history of thrombosis, or a first-degree relative with a specific mutation:

- Lupus anticoagulant (for women with a personal history of VTE)
- Anticardiolipin antibodies (for women with a personal history of VTE)
- Factor V Leiden mutation
- Prothrombin G20210A mutation
- AT-III antigen activity levels
- Fasting homocysteine levels or the MTHFR mutation
- Protein C antigen activity levels
- Protein S antigen activity levels (free and total)

Given the low prevalence of AT-III and the variable pathogenicity of protein C and protein S, consideration should be given to testing only when all other studies have yielded negative results. It is important to note that physiologic changes in normal pregnancy result in marked alterations in protein S and activated protein C resistance, which is associated with the factor V Leiden mutation; therefore, deferral of testing until after pregnancy may be warranted. For example, protein S levels decline by 40% in pregnancy (50, 51). Also, testing for AT-III, protein C, and protein S in the setting of extensive clotting, warfarin use, or heparin administration may result in falsely low values (33, 52, 53). DNA testing for the factor V Leiden,

prothrombin G20210A mutation, and the MTHFR mutation are reliable in pregnancy.

▶ How is deep vein thrombosis detected in pregnancy?

A high index of suspicion is required for the diagnosis of DVT in pregnancy because some of the symptoms of DVT are similar to the common symptoms of pregnancy. Noninvasive testing for DVT includes compression ultrasound (CUS), which uses firm compression with the ultrasound transducer probe to detect an intraluminal filling defect and impedance plethysmography (IPG), which measures impedance flow with pneumatic cuff inflation around the thigh. In the symptomatic nonpregnant patient, IPG has a sensitivity of 83% and specificity of 92% of detecting proximal DVT. Compression ultrasound has a sensitivity of 95% for proximal DVT (73% for distal DVT) and specificity of 96% for detecting all DVT (54), with a negative predictive value of 98% and a positive predictive value of 97% in the nonpregnant symptomatic patient. It has been shown that if serial (3 or more follow-up tests over 7–14 days) IPGs have normal results in a symptomatic pregnant patient with a suspected DVT, it appears safe to withhold anticoagulation (55).

If the clinical suspicion is high and noninvasive test results are negative, limited venography with abdominal shielding that results in fetal exposure less than 0.05 rads should be considered (56). If iliac or pelvic thrombosis is suspected, full venography can be performed (bilateral venography without shielding results in fetal exposure <1.0 rads) (56). Diagnosis of pelvic vein thrombosis and internal iliac thrombosis is difficult. Although the use of venography is widespread, MRI may become the imaging modality of choice in these circumstances, but its role still is not well defined in the pregnant patient (57).

▶ How is the diagnosis of pulmonary embolism made if suspected clinically?

The diagnosis of PE has traditionally been evaluated initially with ventilation–perfusion scanning (V/Q). A V/Q scan results in minimal radiation exposure to the fetus (<0.1 rads). However, any outcome other than high probability or normal requires further testing because of insufficient accuracy to rule out PE in patients for which there is a high clinical suspicion (58). Unfortunately, about 40–60% of V/Q scans are nondiagnostic in the nonpregnant population (neither high probability nor normal), and further evaluation becomes necessary. If noninvasive testing (IPG, CUS) reveals a proximal DVT, then anticoagulation therapy can be initiated. If the results of these tests are negative, but clinical suspicion is high, then pulmonary angiography should be considered (54).

Spiral computed tomography (CT) may be useful for diagnosing PE; however, there is still difficulty reliably identifying emboli below the segmental level (59). Both sensitivity and specificity of spiral CT in nonpregnant patients for central pulmonary artery embolus are approximately 94%. It also may detect abnormalities other than PE responsible for symptoms (pleural effusions, consolidation, emphysema, pulmonary masses) and may be more specific in patients with underlying cardiopulmonary disease (60–62). Magnetic resonance angiography also may be promising, but current technology limits adequate visualization of subsegmental defects (63, 64). Both techniques are unstudied in pregnancy.

► *How should heparin be administered to women with acute thrombosis or embolism during pregnancy?*

Acute thromboembolism associated with pregnancy requires an intravenous heparin bolus of 5,000 U (80 IU/kg) followed by continuous infusion of at least 30,000 IU for 24 hours titrated to achieve full anticoagulation (3, 65). Intravenous anticoagulation should be maintained for at least 5–7 days. The patient can then be changed to subcutaneous adjusted-dose heparin therapy. Subcutaneous injections should be given to pregnant patients every 8 hours to prolong the APTT at least 1.5–2.5 times control throughout the dosing interval, similar to patients who are not pregnant (58, 66). The APTT cannot gauge the adequacy of anticoagulation with therapeutic heparin in patients with antiphospholipid syndrome for which small amounts of heparin may markedly increase the APTT. Levels of antifactor Xa may be used instead.

Therapeutic heparinization with subcutaneous dosing every 8–12 hours should be continued for at least 3 months after the acute event. After 3 months of therapeutic heparinization, experts differ as to what should be done for the remainder of the pregnancy. Some recommend using a lower dose of subcutaneous heparin. Others recommend continuing therapeutic anticoagulation for the remainder of the pregnancy (34).

Low-molecular-weight heparin may be an alternative treatment for acute thromboembolism. Although the actual dosing is unclear in pregnancy, dosage should be adjusted based on maternal weight. Although laboratory testing appears not to be essential in the nonpregnant patient, the role of monitoring antifactor Xa levels is not clear in the pregnant patient. The effectiveness of LMWH is less affected by changes in maternal physiology than is heparin, but there are still changes as pregnancy progresses. Therefore, it may be warranted to periodically reevaluate antifactor Xa levels during pregnancy in a woman on adjusted-dose or full anticoagulation. Ideally, dosing should be enough to achieve a peak antifactor Xa level of 0.5–1.2 U/mL (22, 34). Some experts also check trough levels to ensure that they remain in the lower limits of the anticoagulation range. Pending further informative data, the clinician may either use peak or trough levels, or both, to assess anticoagulation.

► *How is anticoagulation managed in the intrapartum and postpartum period?*

Intrapartum care is complicated, and treatment approaches vary. In such situations, it may be helpful to consult with personnel who have expertise in the intrapartum management of such patients. Patients requiring therapeutic adjusted-dose heparin during pregnancy, including those with recent thromboembolism, and patients with mechanical heart valves may be switched to intravenous heparin at the time of labor and delivery to take advantage of its short half-life (1½ hours). Patients can then be switched to warfarin postpartum. Heparin and warfarin therapy should be overlapped for the first 5–7 days postpartum until an international normalized ratio (INR) of approximately 2.0–3.0 has been achieved (67).

Patients receiving prophylactic anticoagulation with heparin should be instructed to withhold their injections at the onset of labor. Patients requiring adjusted-dose, prophylactic anticoagulation for high-risk conditions can resume their heparin injections 4–8 hours after an uncomplicated delivery, and warfarin can be administered the following morning. Postpartum dosing for women on low-dose prophylactic heparin varies widely, although all concur that the postpartum period is one of high risk. There are no definitive studies to guide one's approach in such situations.

► *Can regional anesthesia be administered to patients receiving anticoagulants?*

The use of major conduction anesthesia (spinal or epidural) in patients receiving thromboembolic prophylaxis is controversial (68, 69). Intraoperative or postoperative anticoagulation after regional anesthesia is thought to be safe; however, the safety of LMWH, unfractionated heparin, or oral anticoagulants administered before the procedure is unclear. Because there are no studies addressing anticoagulation in pregnancy relative to the use of conduction anesthesia, data from nonpregnant patients must be used.

Unfractionated low-dose heparin (≤5,000 IU twice daily) appeared not to pose a significant risk for spinal hematoma in over 5,000 nonpregnant patients who received it in combination with spinal or epidural anesthesia (70).

Although extensive clinical testing in Europe during the past decade suggested that there was no increased risk in patients receiving perioperative LMWH thromboprophylaxis, the U.S. Food and Drug Administration reported cases of epidural or spinal hematomas in nonpregnant patients with concurrent use of enoxaparin (a low-molecular-weight heparin) and spinal or epidural anesthesia or spinal puncture (71). Many of the epidural or spinal hematomas caused neurologic injury, including long-term or permanent paralysis. The discrepancy in the incidence of epidural or spinal hematomas in the European versus the United States literature may be related to higher dosing and preference in the United States of continuous epidurals rather than single shot spinals (70, 72). In one British study of pregnant women, there were no spinal hematomas in the 43 women receiving LMWH thromboprophylaxis who also received epidural analgesia (22). However, the doses given were lower than are currently employed and usually administered once a day.

The American Society of Regional Anesthesia has recommended that patients receiving higher doses of LMWH (specifically enoxaparin, 1 mg/kg twice daily) should not receive neuraxial blocks for 24 hours from the last dose (73). Also, obtaining an antifactor Xa level before placing the block was not recommended because it was believed not to be adequately predictive of the risk of bleeding. Needle placement in patients receiving low-dose, once daily LMWH should occur at least 10–12 hours after the LMWH dose. No specific recommendations were made for patients using an intermediate dose of 30–40 mg of enoxaparin twice daily. However, given that twice daily dosing may maintain antifactor Xa levels between 0.1 and 0.2 IU/mL 12 hours after injection, it would seem prudent to delay epidural anesthesia for 24 hours after the last injection. Alternatively, patients could be switched to standard heparin at term because a normal APTT usually is sufficient to ensure the safety of epidural anesthesia in a heparin anticoagulated patient as long as the platelet count also is normal.

Summary

The following recommendations are based primarily on consensus and expert opinion (Level C):

▶ Pregnant patients with a history of isolated venous thrombosis directly related to a transient, highly thrombogenic event (orthopedic trauma, complicated surgery) in whom an underlying thrombophilia has been excluded may be offered heparin prophylaxis or no prophylaxis during the antepartum period. However, they should be counseled that their risk of thromboembolism is likely to be higher than the normal population. Prophylactic warfarin should be offered for 6 weeks postpartum.

▶ Pregnant patients with a history of idiopathic thrombosis, thrombosis related to pregnancy or oral contraceptive use, or a history of thrombosis accompanied by an underlying thrombophilia other than homozygous for the factor V Leiden mutation, heterozygous for both the factor V Leiden and the prothrombin G20210A mutation, or AT-III deficiency should be offered antepartum and postpartum low-dose heparin prophylaxis.

▶ Patients without a history of thrombosis but who have an underlying thrombophilia and have a strong family history of thrombosis also are candidates for antepartum and postpartum prophylaxis. At the minimum, postpartum prophylaxis should be offered.

▶ Pregnant patients with a history of life-threatening thrombosis, with recent thrombosis, with recurrent thrombosis, receiving chronic anticoagulation, or patients with thrombosis found to be AT-III deficient, homozygous for the factor V Leiden mutation or prothrombin G20210A mutation, heterozygous for both the factor V Leiden and the prothrombin G20210A mutation should be given adjusted-dose heparin every 8 hours to maintain the APTT at least 1.5 times control throughout the dosing interval. Low-molecular-weight heparin administered twice daily also is an alternative.

▶ Patients at risk for thrombosis should receive warfarin postpartum for 6 weeks to achieve an INR of approximately 2.0–3.0. Heparin should be given immediately postpartum with warfarin for at least 5 days until the INR is therapeutic.

▶ Patients with antiphospholipid syndrome and a history of thrombosis require adjusted-dose prophylactic anticoagulation.

▶ Patients who are candidates for either prophylactic or therapeutic heparin may be given enoxaparin or dalteparin during pregnancy. However, because of the lack of data regarding adequate dosing during pregnancy, antifactor Xa levels may be monitored.

▶ The safety of epidural anesthesia with twice-daily dosing of LMWH is of concern and should be withheld until 24 hours after the last injection.

▶ Epidural anesthesia appears to be safe in women taking unfractionated low-dose heparin if the APTT is normal.

References

1. Gherman RB, Goodwin TM, Leung B, Byrne JD, Hethumumi R, Montoro M. Incidence, clinical characteristics, and timing of objectively diagnosed venous thromboembolism during pregnancy. Obstet Gynecol 1999;94:730–734 (Level II-3)

2. Lindqvist P, Dahlback B, Marsal K. Thrombotic risk during pregnancy: a population study. Obstet Gynecol 1999;94:595–599 (Level II-2)

3. Toglia MR, Weg JG. Venous thromboembolism during pregnancy. N Engl J Med 1996;335:108–114 (Level III)

4. Berg CJ, Atrash HK, Koonin LM, Tucker M. Pregnancy-related mortality in the United States, 1987–1990. Obstet Gynecol 1996;88:161–167 (Level II-3)

5. Grandone E, Margaglione M, Colaizzo D, D'Andrea G, Cappucci G, Brancaccio V, et al. Genetic susceptibility to pregnancy-related venous thromboembolism: roles of factor V Leiden, prothrombin G20210A, and methylenetetrahydrofolate reductase C677T mutations. Am J Obstet Gynecol 1998;179:1324–1328 (Level II-2)

6. Dizon-Townson DS, Nelson LM, Jang H, Varner MW, Ward K. The incidence of the factor V Leiden mutation in an obstetric population and its relationship to deep vein thrombosis. Am J Obstet Gynecol 1997;176:883–886 (Level III)

7. De Stefano V, Leone G, Mastrangelo S, Tripodi A, Rodeghiero F, Castaman G, et al. Clinical manifestations and management of inherited thrombophilia: retrospective analysis and follow-up after diagnosis of 238 patients with congenital deficiency of antithrombin III, protein C, protein S. Thromb Haemost 1994;72:352–358 (Level III)

8. Middledorp S, Henkens CM, Koopman MM, van Pampus EC, Hamulyák K, van der Meer J, et al. The incidence of venous thromboembolism in family members of patients with factor V Leiden mutation and venous thrombosis. Ann Intern Med 1998;128:15–20 (Level II-2)

9. Badaracco MA, Vessey MP. Recurrence of venous thromboembolic disease and use of oral contraceptives. Br Med J 1974;1:215–217 (Level II-2)

10. Tengborn L, Bergqvist D, Mätzsch T, Bergqvist A, Hedner U. Recurrent thromboembolism in pregnancy and puerperium. Is there a need for thromboprophylaxis? Am J Obstet Gynecol 1989;160(1);90–94 (Level II-2)

11. Ginsberg JS, Kowalchuk G, Hirsh J, Brill-Edwards P, Burrows R. Heparin therapy during pregnancy. Risks to the fetus and mother. Arch Intern Med 1989;149:2233–2236 (Level II-3)

12. Barbour LA, Smith JM, Marlar RA. Heparin levels to guide thromboembolism prophylaxis during pregnancy. Am J Obstet Gynecol 1995;173:1869–1873 (Level III)

13. Barbour LA, Kick SD, Steiner JF, LoVerde ME, Heddleston LN, Lear JL, et al. A prospective study of heparin-induced osteoporosis in pregnancy using bone densitometry. Am J Obstet Gynecol 1994;170:862–869 (Level II-2)

14. Dahlman TC, Sjöberg HE, Ringertz H. Bone mineral density during long-term prophylaxis with heparin in pregnancy. Am J Obstet Gynecol 1994;170:1315–1320 (Level II-2)

15. Dahlman TC. Osteoporotic fractures and the recurrence of thromboembolism during pregnancy and the puerperium in 184 women undergoing thromboprophylaxis with heparin. Am J Obstet Gynecol 1993;168:1265–1270 (Level III)

16. Warkentin TE, Levine MN, Hirsh J, Horsewood P, Roberts RS, Gent M, et al. Heparin-induced thrombocytopenia in patients treated with low-molecular-weight heparin or unfractionated heparin. N Engl J Med 1995;332:1330–1335 (Level II-2)

17. Kelton JG. The clinical management of heparin-induced thrombocytopenia. Semin Hematol 1999;36(suppl 1):17–21 (Level III)

18. Hirsh J, Warkentin TE, Raschke R, Granger C, Ohman EM, Dalen JE. Heparin and low-molecular-weight heparin: mechanisms of action, pharmacokinetics, dosing considerations, monitoring, efficacy, and safety. Chest 1998;114:489S–510S (Level III)

19. Bergqvist D. Low molecular weight heparins. J Intern Med 1996:240;63–72 (Level III)

20. Forestier F, Solé Y, Aiach M, Alhenc Gelás M, Daffos F. Absence of transplacental fragmin (Kabi) during second and third trimesters of pregnancy. Thromb Haemost 1992;67:180–181 (Level III)

21. Omri A, Delaloye JF, Andersen H, Bachmann F. Low molecular weight heparin Novo (LHN-1) does not cross the placenta during the second trimester of pregnancy. Thromb Haemost 1989;61:55–56 (Level II-2)

22. Nelson-Piercy C, Letsky EA, de Swiet M. Low-molecular-weight heparin for obstetric thromboprophylaxis: experience of sixty-nine pregnancies in sixty-one women at risk. Am J Obstet Gynecol 1997;176:1062–1068 (Level III)

23. Dulitzki M, Pauzner R, Langevitz P, Pras M, Many A, Schiff E. Low-molecular-weight heparin during pregnancy and delivery: preliminary experience with 41 pregnancies. Obstet Gynecol 1996;87:380–383 (Level III)

24. Rasmussen C, Wadt B, Jacobsen B. Thromboembolic prophylaxis with low molecular weight heparin during pregnancy. Int J Gynaecol Obstet 1994;47:121–125 (Level III)

25. Orme ML, Lewis PJ, de Swiet M, Serlin MJ, Sibeon R, Baty JD, et al. May mothers given warfarin breast-feed their infants? BMJ 1977;1(6076):1564–1565 (Level III)

26. Chan WS, Anand S, Ginsberg JS. Anticoagulation of pregnant women with mechanical heart valves. Arch Intern Med 2000;160:191–196 (Level III)

27. Iturbe-Alessio I, Fonseca M, Mutchinik O, Santos MA, Zajarías A, Salazar E. Risks of anticoagulant therapy in pregnant women with artificial heart valves. N Engl J Med 1986;315:1390–1393 (Level II-2)

28. Born D, Martinez EE, Almeida PAM, Santos DV, Carvalho AC, Moron AF, et al. Pregnancy in patients with prosthetic heart valves: the effects of anticoagulation on mother, fetus, and neonate. Am Heart J 1992;124:413–417 (Level II-2)

29. Salazar E, Izaguirre R, Verdejo J, Mutchinick O. Failure of adjusted doses of subcutaneous heparin to prevent thromboembolic phenomena in pregnant patients with mechanical cardiac valve prostheses. J Am Coll Cardiol 1996;27: 1698–1703 (Level III)

30. Hall JG, Pauli RM, Wilson KM. Maternal and fetal sequelae of anticoagulation during pregnancy. Am J Med 1980;68:122–140 (Level III)

31. McColl MD, Ramsay JE, Tait RC, Walker ID, McCall F, Conkie JA, et al. Risk factors for pregnancy associated venous thromboembolism. Thromb Haemost 1997;78: 1183–1188 (Level III)

32. Conard J, Horellou MH, Van Dredan P, Lecompte T, Samama M. Thrombosis and pregnancy in congenital deficiencies in AT III, protein C or protein S: study of 78 women. Thromb Haemost 1990;63:319–320 (Level III)

33. Van Boven HH, Lane DA. Antithrombin and its inherited deficiency states. Semin Hematol 1997;34:188–204 (Level III)

34. Ginsberg JS, Hirsh J. Use of antithrombotic agents during pregnancy. Chest 1998;114:524S–530S (Level III)

35. Branch DW, Silver RM, Blackwell JL, Reading JC, Scott JR. Outcome of treated pregnancies in women with antiphospholipid syndrome: an update of the Utah experience. Obstet Gynecol 1992;80:614–620 (Level II-2)

36. Barbour LA, Pickard J. Controversies in thromboembolic disease during pregnancy: a critical review. Obstet Gynecol 1995;86:621–633 (Level III)

37. Gerhardt A, Scharf RE, Beckmann MW, Struve S, Bender HG, Pillny M, et al. Prothrombin and factor V mutations in women with a history of thrombosis during pregnancy and the puerperium. N Engl J Med 2000;342:374–380 (Level II-2)

38. Colvin BT, Barrowcliffe TW. The British Society for Haematology Guidelines on the use and monitoring of heparin 1992: second revision. BCSH Haemostasis and Thrombosis Task Force. J Clin Pathol 1993;46:97–103 (Level III)

39. Maternal and Neonatal Haemostasis Working Party of the Haemostasis and Thrombosis Task. Guidelines on the prevention, investigation and management of thrombosis associated with pregnancy. J Clin Pathol 1993;46:489–496 (Level III)

40. Lechner K, Kyrle PA. Antithrombin III concentrates—are they clinically useful? Thromb Haemost 1995;73:340–348 (Level III)

41. Barbour LA. Current concepts of anticoagulant therapy in pregnancy. Obstet Gynecol Clin North Am 1997;24: 499–521 (Level III)

42. Weitz JI. Drug therapy: low molecular weight heparin. N Engl J Med 1997;337:688–698 (Level III)

43. Miletich JP. Thrombophilia as a multigenic disorder. Semin Thromb Hemost 1998;24(suppl 1):13–20 (Level III)

44. Friederich PW, Sanson BJ, Simioni P, Zanardi S, Huisman MV, Kindt I, et al. Frequency of pregnancy-related venous thromboembolism in anticoagulant factor-deficient women: implications for prophylaxis. Ann Intern Med 1996;125:955–960 (Level III)

45. Florell SR, Rodgers GM. Inherited thrombotic disorders: an update. Am J Hematol 1997;54:53–60 (Level III)

46. Rai R, Cohen H, Dave M, Regan L. Randomised controlled trial of aspirin and aspirin plus heparin in pregnant women with recurrent miscarriage associated with phospholipid antibodies (or antiphospholipid antibodies). BMJ 1997;314:253–257 (Level I)

47. Brenner B, Mandel H, Lanir N, Younis J, Rothbart H, Ohel G, et al. Activated protein C resistance can be associated with recurrent fetal loss. Br J Haematol 1997;97:551–554 (Level II-2)

48. Dizon-Townson D, Meline L, Nelson LM, Varner M, Ward K. Fetal carriers of the factor V Leiden mutation are prone to miscarriage or placental infarction. Am J Obstet Gynecol 1997;177:402–405 (Level II-2)

49. Kupferminc MJ, Eldor A, Steinman N, Many A, Bar-Am A, Jaffa A, et al. Increased frequency of genetic thrombophilia in women with complications of pregnancy. N Engl J Med 1999;340:9–13 (Level II-2)

50. Faught W, Garner P, Jones C, Ivey B. Changes in protein C and protein S levels in normal pregnancy. Am J Obstet Gynecol 1995;172:147–150 (Level II-3)

51. Lefkowitz JB, Clarke SH, Barbour LA. Comparison of protein S functional and antigenic assays in normal pregnancy. Am J Obstet Gynecol 1996;175:657–650 (Level II-3)

52. Rao AK, Kaplan R, Sheth S. Inherited thrombophilic states. Semin Thromb Hemost 1998;24(suppl 1):3–12 (Level III)

53. Reiter W, Ehrensberger H, Steinbrückner B, Keller F. Parameters of haemostasis during acute venous thrombosis. Thromb Haemost 1995;74:596–601 (Level III)

54. Douketis JD, Ginsberg JS. Diagnostic problems with venous thromboembolic disease in pregnancy. Haemostasis 1995;25:58–71 (Level III)

55. Hull RD, Raskob GE, Carter CJ. Serial impedance plethysmography in pregnant patients with clinically suspected deep-vein thrombosis. Clinical validity of negative findings. Ann Intern Med 1990;112:663–667 (Level II-3)

56. Ginsberg JS, Hirsh J, Rainbow AJ, Coates G. Risks to the fetus of radiologic procedures used in the diagnosis of maternal venous thromboembolic disease. Thromb Haemost 1989;61:189–196 (Level III)

57. Spritzer CE, Evans AC, Kay HH. Magnetic resonance imaging of deep venous thrombosis in pregnant women with lower extremity edema. Obstet Gynecol 1995;85: 603–607 (Level III)

58. Ginsberg JS. Management of venous thromboembolism. N Engl J Med 1996;335(24):1816–1828 (Level III)

59. Hansell DM. Spiral computed tomography and pulmonary embolism: current state. Clin Radiol 1997;52:575–581 (Level III)

60. Cross JJ, Kemp PM, Walsh CG, Flower CD, Dixon AK. A randomized trial of spiral CT and ventilation perfusion

scintigraphy for the diagnosis of pulmonary embolism. Clin Radiol 1998;53:177–182 (Level I)

61. Lipchik RJ, Goodman LR. Spiral computed tomography in the evaluation of pulmonary embolism. Clin Chest Med 1999;20:731–738 (Level III)

62. Kim KI, Muller NL, Mayo JR. Clinically suspected pulmonary embolism: utility of spiral CT. Radiology 1999;210:693–697 (Level III)

63. Meaney JF, Weg JG, Chenevert TL, Stafford-Johnson D, Hamilton BH, Prince MR. Diagnosis of pulmonary embolism with magnetic resonance angiography. N Engl J Med 1997;336:1422–1427 (Level II-2)

64. Woodard PK, Yusen RD. Diagnosis of pulmonary embolism with spiral computed tomography and magnetic resonance angiography. Curr Opin Cardiol 1999;14: 442–447 (Level III)

65. Bates SM, Ginsberg JS. Thrombosis in pregnancy. Curr Opin Hematol 1997;4:335–343 (Level III)

66. Ramin SM, Ramin KD, Gilstrap LC. Anticoagulants and thrombolytics during pregnancy. Semin Perinatol 1997;21: 149–153 (Level III)

67. Hyers TM, Agnelli G, Hull RD, Weg JG, Morris TA, Samama M, et al. Antithrombotic therapy for venous thromboembolic disease. Chest 1998;114:561S–578S (Level III)

68. Haljamäe H. Thromboprophylaxis, coagulation disorders, and regional anesthesia. Acta Anaesthesiol Scand 1996;40:1024–1040 (Level III)

69. Hynson JM, Katz JA, Bueff HU. Epidural hematoma associated with enoxaparin. Anesth Analg 1996;82:1072–1075 (Level III)

70. Horlocker TT, Wedel DJ. Neuraxial block and low-molecular-weight heparin: balancing perioperative analgesia and thromboprophylaxis. Reg Anesth Pain Med 1998;23(6 Suppl 2);164–177 (Level III)

71. U.S. Department of Health and Human Services. FDA Public Health Advisory, Subject: reports of epidural or spinal hematomas with the concurrent use of low molecular weight heparin and spinal/epidural anesthesia or spinal puuncture. Rockville, Maryland: Food and Drug Administration, December 1997 (Level III)

72. Tryba M. European practice guidelines: thromboembolism prophylaxis and regional anesthesia. Reg Anesth Pain Med 1998;23(6 Suppl 2):178–182 (Level III)

73. American Society of Regional Anesthesia (ASRA). Recommendations for neuraxial anesthesia and anticoagulation. Richmond, VA: ASRA, 1998 (Level III

The MEDLINE database, the Cochrane Library, and ACOG's own internal resources and documents were used to conduct a literature search to locate relevant articles published between January 1985 and March 1998. The search was restricted to articles published in the English language. Priority was given to articles reporting results of original research, although review articles and commentaries also were consulted. Abstracts of research presented at symposia and scientific conferences were not considered adequate for inclusion in this document. Guidelines published by organizations or institutions such as the National Institutes of Health and the American College of Obstetricians and Gynecologists were reviewed, and additional studies were located by reviewing bibliographies of identified articles. When reliable research was not available, expert opinions from obstetrician–gynecologists were used.

Studies were reviewed and evaluated for quality according to the method outlined by the U.S. Preventive Services Task Force:

I Evidence obtained from at least one properly designed randomized controlled trial.

II-1 Evidence obtained from well-designed controlled trials without randomization.

II-2 Evidence obtained from well-designed cohort or case–control analytic studies, preferably from more than one center or research group.

II-3 Evidence obtained from multiple time series with or without the intervention. Dramatic results in uncontrolled experiments could also be regarded as this type of evidence.

III Opinions of respected authorities, based on clinical experience, descriptive studies, or reports of expert committees.

Based on the highest level of evidence found in the data, recommendations are provided and graded according to the following categories:

Level A—Recommendations are based on good and consistent scientific evidence.

Level B—Recommendations are based on limited or inconsistent scientific evidence.

Level C—Recommendations are based primarily on consensus and expert opinion.

ISSN 1099-3630

The American College of Obstetricians and Gynecologists
409 12th Street, SW
PO Box 96920
Washington, DC 20090-6920   12345/43210

ACOG PRACTICE BULLETIN

CLINICAL MANAGEMENT GUIDELINES FOR
OBSTETRICIAN–GYNECOLOGISTS

NUMBER 37, AUGUST 2002

(Replaces Practice Bulletin Number 32, November 2001)

This Practice Bulletin was developed by the ACOG Committee on Practice Bulletins— Obstetrics with the assistance of Sarah Kilpatrick, MD, PhD. The information is designed to aid practitioners in making decisions about appropriate obstetric and gynecologic care. These guidelines should not be construed as dictating an exclusive course of treatment or procedure. Variations in practice may be warranted based on the needs of the individual patient, resources, and limitations unique to the institution or type of practice.

Thyroid Disease in Pregnancy

Because thyroid disease is the second most common endocrine disease affecting women of reproductive age, obstetricians often care for patients who have been previously diagnosed with alterations in thyroid gland function. In addition, both hyperthyroidism and hypothyroidism may initially manifest during pregnancy. Obstetric conditions, such as gestational trophoblastic disease or hyperemesis gravidarum, may themselves affect thyroid gland function. This document will review the thyroid-related pathophysiologic changes created by pregnancy and the maternal–fetal impact of thyroid disease.

Background

Definitions

Thyrotoxicosis is the clinical and biochemical state that results from an excess production of and exposure to thyroid hormone from any etiology. In contrast, hyperthyroidism is thyrotoxicosis caused by hyperfunctioning of the thyroid gland (1). Graves' disease is an autoimmune disease characterized by production of thyroid-stimulating immunoglobulin (TSI) and thyroid-stimulating hormone-binding inhibitory immunoglobulin (TBII) that act on the thyroid-stimulating hormone (TSH) receptor to mediate thyroid stimulation or inhibition, respectively. Thyroid storm is characterized by a severe, acute exacerbation of the signs and symptoms of hyperthyroidism.

Hypothyroidism is caused by inadequate thyroid hormone production. Postpartum thyroiditis is an autoimmune inflammation of the thyroid gland that presents as new-onset, painless hypothyroidism, transient thyrotoxicosis, or thyrotoxicosis followed by hypothyroidism within 1 year postpartum.

Physiologic Changes in Thyroid Function During Pregnancy

Table 1 depicts how thyroid function test (TFT) results change in normal pregnancy and in hyperthyroid and hypothyroid states. The concentration of thyroid binding globulin (TBG) increases in pregnancy because of reduced hepatic clearance and estrogenic stimulation of TBG synthesis (2). The test results that change significantly in pregnancy are those that are influenced by serum TBG concentration. These tests include total thyroxine (TT_4), total triiodothyronine (TT_3), and resin triiodothyronine uptake (RT_3U). Although there may be a transient increase in free thyroxine (FT_4) and free thyroxine index (FTI) in the first trimester (possibly related to human chorionic gonadotropin [hCG] stimulation), this increase does not result in elevations beyond the normal nonpregnant range (3).

Plasma iodide levels decrease during pregnancy because of fetal use of iodide and increased maternal renal clearance of iodide (2). This alteration is associated with a noticeable increase in thyroid gland size in approximately 15% of women (2, 4). In two longitudinal studies of more than 600 women without thyroid disease, thyroid volume, measured by ultrasonography, significantly increased in pregnancy (with a mean increase in size of 18% that was noticeable in most women) and returned to normal in the postpartum period (4, 5). None of these women had abnormal TFT results despite their enlarged thyroid glands.

Thyroid Function and the Fetus

The fetal thyroid begins concentrating iodine at 10–12 weeks of gestation and is controlled by pituitary TSH by approximately 20 weeks of gestation. Fetal serum levels of TSH, TBG, FT_4, and free triiodothyronine (FT_3) increase throughout gestation, reaching mean adult levels at approximately 36 weeks of gestation (6). Thyroid-stimulating hormone does not cross the placenta, and only small amounts of thyroxine (T_4) and triiodothyronine (T_3) cross the placenta. In neonates with congenital hypothyroidism, enough maternal thyroid hormone crosses the placenta to prevent the overt stigmata of hypothyroidism at birth and maintain cord blood thyroid hormone levels at 25–50% of normal (7). However, thyrotropin-releasing hormone (TRH), iodine, and TSH receptor immunoglobulins do cross the placenta, as do the thioamides propylthiouracil (PTU) and methimazole.

Hyperthyroidism

Signs and Symptoms

Hyperthyroidism occurs in 0.2% of pregnancies; Graves' disease accounts for 95% of these cases (8). The signs and symptoms of hyperthyroidism include nervousness, tremors, tachycardia, frequent stools, excessive sweating, heat intolerance, weight loss, goiter, insomnia, palpitations, and hypertension. Distinctive symptoms of Graves' disease are ophthalmopathy (signs including lid lag and lid retraction) and dermopathy (signs include localized or pretibial myxedema). Although some symptoms of hyperthyroidism are similar to symptoms of pregnancy or nonthyroid disease, serum TFTs differentiate thyroid disease from nonthyroid disease.

Inadequately treated maternal thyrotoxicosis is associated with a greater risk of preterm delivery, severe preeclampsia, and heart failure than treated, controlled maternal thyrotoxicosis (9, 10). Although untreated hyperthyroidism has been associated with miscarriage (8, 11), it is difficult to find concrete data to support this claim.

Fetal and Neonatal Effects

Inadequately treated hyperthyroidism also is associated with an increase in medically indicated preterm deliveries, low birth weight (LBW), and possibly fetal loss (9, 10). In one study, all of seven fetal losses occurred in women with persistent hyperthyroidism (9).

Fetal and neonatal risks associated with Graves' disease are related either to the disease itself or to thioamide treatment of the disease. The possibility of fetal thyrotoxicosis should be considered in all women with a

Table 1. Changes in Thyroid Function Test Results in Normal Pregnancy and in Thyroid Disease

Maternal Status	TSH	FT_4	FTI	TT_4	TT_3	RT_3U
Pregnancy	No change	No change	No change	Increase	Increase	Decrease
Hyperthyroidism	Decrease	Increase	Increase	Increase	Increase or no change	Increase
Hypothyroidism	Increase	Decrease	Decrease	Decrease	Decrease or no change	Decrease

Abbreviations: TSH, thyroid-stimulating hormone; FT_4, free thyroxine; FTI, free thyroxine index; TT_4, total thyroxine; TT_3, total triiodothyronine; RT_3U, resin T3 uptake.

history of Graves' disease (8). If fetal thyrotoxicosis is diagnosed, consultation with a clinician with expertise in such conditions is warranted.

Because a large proportion of thyroid dysfunction in women is mediated by antibodies that cross the placenta (Graves' disease and chronic autoimmune thyroiditis), there is a legitimate concern for risk of immune-mediated hypothyroidism and hyperthyroidism to develop in the neonate. Women with Graves' disease have TSI and TBII that can stimulate or inhibit the fetal thyroid. The latter (TBII) may cause transient hypothyroidism in neonates of women with Graves' disease (12, 13). One to five percent of these neonates have hyperthyroidism or neonatal Graves' disease caused by the transplacental passage of maternal TSI (11). The incidence is low because of the balance of stimulatory and inhibitory antibodies with thioamide treatment (14). Maternal antibodies are cleared less rapidly than thioamides in the neonate, resulting in a sometimes delayed presentation of neonatal Graves' disease (14). The incidence of neonatal Graves' disease is unrelated to maternal thyroid function. The neonates of women who have been treated surgically or with radioactive iodine 131 (I-131) prior to pregnancy and require no thioamide treatment are at higher risk for neonatal Graves' disease because they lack suppressive thioamide (14).

Etiology and Differential Diagnosis

The most common cause of hyperthyroidism is Graves' disease. The other clinical characteristics of Graves' disease also are immune-mediated but they are less understood. The diagnosis of Graves' disease is generally made by documenting elevated levels of FT_4 or an elevated FTI, with suppressed TSH in the absence of a nodular goiter or thyroid mass. Although most patients with Graves' disease have TSH receptor, antimicrosomal, or antithyroid peroxidase antibodies, measurement of these is neither required nor recommended to establish the diagnosis (11). Other etiologies of thyrotoxicosis are excess production of TSH, gestational trophoblastic neoplasia, hyperfunctioning thyroid adenoma, toxic multinodular goiter, subacute thyroiditis, and extrathyroid source of thyroid hormone.

Hypothyroidism

It is well accepted that having one autoimmune disease increases the likelihood of developing another; autoimmune thyroid dysfunction is no exception. For example, there is a 5–8% incidence of hypothyroid disease in patients with type 1 (insulin-dependent) diabetes (15). Women with type 1 diabetes also have a 25% risk of developing postpartum thyroid dysfunction (15).

Signs and Symptoms

The classic signs and symptoms of hypothyroidism are fatigue, constipation, intolerance to cold, muscle cramps, hair loss, dry skin, prolonged relaxation phase of deep tendon reflexes, and carpal tunnel syndrome. These are initially indolent and nonspecific but may progress to weight gain, intellectual slowness, voice changes, and insomnia. If left untreated, hypothyroidism will progress to myxedema and myxedema coma. It is unusual for advanced hypothyroidism to present in pregnancy. Subclinical hypothyroidism is defined as elevated TSH with normal FTI in an asymptomatic patient. Untreated hypothyroidism is associated with an increased risk of preeclampsia, but it is not clear from the available data whether subclinical hypothyroidism carries a similar risk (16, 17).

Fetal and Neonatal Effects

In retrospective studies, a high incidence of LBW in neonates was associated with inadequately treated hypothyroidism (16, 17). The etiology of LBW in these studies was preterm delivery (medically indicated), preeclampsia, or placental abruption. One study reported two stillbirths, both of which were associated with placental abruption and preeclampsia (17). It is not clear whether hypothyroidism is associated with intrauterine growth restriction independent of other complications. Women with iodine-deficient hypothyroidism are at significant risk of having babies with congenital cretinism (growth failure, mental retardation, and other neuropsychologic deficits). In an iodine-deficient population, treatment with iodine in the first and second trimesters of pregnancy significantly reduces the incidence of the neurologic abnormalities of cretinism (18).

Untreated congenital hypothyroidism also results in cretinism. The incidence of congenital hypothyroidism is 1 per 4,000 newborns, and only 5% of neonates are identified by clinical symptoms at birth, likely because of the ameliorative effects of maternal thyroid hormone (2). All 50 states and the District of Columbia offer screening of newborns for congenital hypothyroidism. If identified and treated within the first few weeks of life, near-normal growth and intelligence can be expected (19).

Etiology and Differential Diagnosis

Most cases of hypothyroidism are the result of a primary thyroid abnormality; a small number of cases are caused by hypothalamic dysfunction. The most common etiologies of hypothyroidism in pregnant or postpartum women are Hashimoto's disease (chronic thyroiditis or chronic autoimmune thyroiditis) (1), subacute thyroiditis, thyroidectomy, radioactive iodine treatment, and iodine deficiency. In developed countries, Hashimoto's disease is the most common etiology (20) and is characterized by the production of antithyroid antibodies, including thyroid antimicrosomal and antithyroglobulin antibodies. Both Hashimoto's disease and iodine deficiency are associated with goiter (a sign of compensatory TSH production), while subacute thyroiditis is not associated with goiter.

Worldwide, the most common cause of hypothyroidism is iodine deficiency (8). Although iodine deficiency is rare in the United States, some populations may benefit from consideration of this etiology of hypothyroidism, including certain immigrant populations and those with poor nutrition.

Clinical Considerations and Recommendations

▶ *What laboratory tests are used to diagnose and manage thyroid disease during pregnancy?*

The mainstay of thyroid function evaluation is TSH testing; such testing is now performed using monoclonal antibodies, making it more sensitive than the original radioimmunoassay. The American Association of Clinical Endocrinologists (21) and the American Thyroid Association (22) recommend TSH testing as the initial test for the screening and evaluation of symptomatic disease for all men and women. The free component is the biologically active portion and is not subject to change in conditions that alter TBG, such as pregnancy. In a pregnant patient suspected of being hyperthyroid or hypothyroid, TSH and FT_4 or FTI should be measured. Free thyroxine assessment by either direct immunoradiometric or chemiluminescent methods generally is available and preferred over the equilibrium dialysis method. However, FTI can be calculated as the product of TT_4 and RT_3U if FT_4 is not available. Measurement of FT_3 usually is only pursued in patients with thyrotoxicosis with suppressed TSH but normal FT_4 measurements. Elevated FT_3 indicates T_3 toxicosis, which may occur before excessive FT_4 production develops (11, 23).

Another test of thyroid function is the TRH stimulation test, which evaluates the secretory ability of the pituitary. The various antibody tests include TSH receptor antibodies, which can be either stimulatory (TSI) or inhibitory (TBII), and antimicrosomal antibodies. The usefulness of these various antibodies in pregnancy is complex and will be discussed as follows.

Although the incidence of neonatal Graves' disease is associated with extremely high levels of maternal TSI, the clinical usefulness of evaluating these levels is not clear. In general, perinatal experts suggest there is no practical use for measuring TSI routinely (8), while endocrinologists suggest that measuring TSI in the third trimester is useful (11, 14, 24, 25). Routine evaluation of maternal TSI levels is not recommended, but such evaluation may be helpful in some circumstances.

▶ *What medications can be used to treat hyperthyroidism and hypothyroidism in pregnancy, and how should they be administered and adjusted during pregnancy?*

Hyperthyroidism in pregnancy is treated with thioamides, specifically PTU and methimazole, which decrease thyroid hormone synthesis by blocking the organification of iodide. Propylthiouracil also reduces the peripheral conversion of T_4 to T_3 and, thus, may have a quicker suppressant effect than methimazole. Traditionally, PTU has been preferred in pregnant patients because it was believed that PTU crossed the placenta less well than methimazole and because methimazole was associated with fetal aplasia cutis, a congenital skin defect of the scalp (26). However, recent data have refuted both of these arguments. One study comparing FT_4 and TSH in newborn umbilical cord blood samples of women treated with PTU with those of women treated with methimazole found no significant difference in mean FT_4 or TSH levels. Furthermore, there was no relationship between maternal dosage of thioamide and umbilical cord blood levels of TSH or FT_4 (27). A retrospective study that compared 99 women treated with PTU with 36 women treated with methimazole reported no cases of aplasia cutis and similar rates of fetal anomalies (3%) (28). Finally, there was no significant difference in the incidence of aplasia cutis between control women without thyroid disease and women with hyperthyroidism who were treated with methimazole (26).

Thioamide treatment of Graves' disease can suppress fetal and neonatal thyroid function. However, it usually is transient and rarely requires therapy. Fetal goiter also has been associated with thioamide treatment for Graves' disease, presumably caused by drug-induced fetal hypothyroidism (29). Fetal thyrotoxicosis secondary to maternal antibodies is rare, but all fetuses of women with Graves' disease should be monitored for appropriate growth and normal heart rate. However, in the absence of these findings, routine screening for fetal goiter by ultrasonography is unnecessary. All neonates of women with thyroid disease are at risk for neonatal thyroid dysfunction, and the neonate's pediatrician should be aware of the maternal diagnosis.

Women taking PTU may breastfeed because only small amounts of the medication cross into breast milk. Studies have demonstrated that TFT results were normal in neonates after 1–8 months of breastfeeding from women taking PTU (30, 31). Methimazole also is considered safe for breastfeeding; however, it is present in a higher ratio in breast milk (30).

The goal of management of hyperthyroidism in pregnancy is to maintain the FT_4 or FTI in the high normal range using the lowest possible dosage of thioamides to minimize fetal exposure to thioamides. Thus, once treatment has started, it may be helpful to measure FT_4 or FTI every 2–4 weeks and titrate the thioamide until FT_4 or FTI are consistently in the high normal range (8). In more than 90% of patients, improvement will be seen within 2–4 weeks after thioamide treatment begins (11).

One side effect of thioamides is agranulocytosis. The incidence of agranulocytosis is 0.1–0.4%; it usually presents with a fever and sore throat. If a patient on thioamides develops these symptoms, a complete blood cell count should be drawn and the medication should be discontinued. Treatment with the other thioamide carries a significant risk of cross reaction. Other major side effects of thioamides, including thrombocytopenia, hepatitis, and vasculitis, occur in less than 1% of patients; minor side effects, including rash, nausea, arthritis, anorexia, fever, and loss of taste or smell, occur in 5% of patients (11).

Beta-blockers may be used during pregnancy to ameliorate the symptoms of thyrotoxicosis until thioamides decrease thyroid hormone levels. Propranolol is the most common β-blocker used for this indication. Thyroidectomy should be reserved for women in whom thioamide treatment is unsuccessful.

Iodine 131 is contraindicated in pregnant women because of the risk of fetal thyroid ablation; therefore, women should avoid pregnancy for 4 months after I-131 treatment (23). Unfortunately, our understanding of fetal thyroid ablation and the consequent risk of fetal hypothyroidism from exposure to maternal I-131 comes from the inadvertent treatment of pregnant women (32, 33). Counseling of women exposed to I-131 in pregnancy should focus on the gestational age at exposure. If the woman was at less than 10 weeks of gestation when exposed to I-131, it is unlikely the fetal thyroid was ablated. If exposure occurred at 10 weeks of gestation or later, the woman must consider the risks of induced congenital hypothyroidism and consider whether to continue the pregnancy. Breastfeeding should be avoided for at least 120 days after treatment with I-131 (34).

Treatment of hypothyroidism in pregnant women is the same as for nonpregnant women and involves administering levothyroxine at sufficient dosages to normalize TSH levels. It takes approximately 4 weeks for the thyroxine therapy to alter the TSH level. Therefore, levothyroxine therapy should be adjusted at 4-week intervals until TSH levels are stable. Data indicate pregnancy increases maternal thyroid hormone requirements in women with hypothyroidism diagnosed before pregnancy (2, 35). In these studies, TSH levels increased while FTI decreased during pregnancy in these women, necessitating an increase in mean thyroxine dosage from 0.1 mg/day before pregnancy to 0.148 mg/day during pregnancy (35). In stable patients, it is prudent to check TSH levels every trimester in pregnant women with hypothyroidism (21).

▶ *What changes in thyroid function occur with hyperemesis gravidarum, and should TFTs be performed routinely in women with hyperemesis?*

Nausea and vomiting of pregnancy have been attributed to the high hCG levels in the first trimester, and women with hyperemesis gravidarum have been assumed to have particularly high hCG levels and to be at risk for hyperthyroidism. In a prospective study of 67 women with singleton pregnancies and hyperemesis, 66% were found to have biochemical hyperthyroidism with an undetectable level of TSH or elevated FTI or both (36). The biochemical hyperthyroidism resolved in all of the women without treatment by 18 weeks of gestation (36). Further, the women with the most severe hyperemesis had significantly higher FTIs than those with mild or moderate disease.

Complete resolution of biochemical and clinical hyperthyroidism also has been reported in other studies (37, 38). These studies have reported that some women with hyperemesis gravidarum required a short course of thioamides; however, most of these women had resolution of their signs and symptoms without treatment (38, 39). Women who required treatment throughout the remainder of their pregnancies had other symptoms of thyroid disease, including thyroid enlargement, persistent tachycardia despite fluid replacement, and abnormal response to TRH stimulation (39). In a study comparing pregnant women with hyperemesis and those without hyperemesis, there was no difference in mean TSH or FT_3 levels (40). Levels of FT_4 and hCG were significantly higher in the women with hyperemesis, but hCG levels correlated significantly and positively with FT_4 levels and negatively with TSH levels only in the hyperemesis group. Other studies have replicated these results and shown suppression of TSH when compared with controls (37). Hyperemesis gravidarum is associated with biochemical hyperthyroidism but rarely with clinical hyperthyroidism and is largely transitory, requiring no treatment. Routine measurements of thyroid function are not recommended in patients with hyperemesis gravidarum unless other overt signs of hyperthyroidism are evident.

▶ *How is thyroid storm diagnosed and treated in pregnancy?*

Thyroid storm is a medical emergency characterized by an extreme hypermetabolic state. It is rare—occurring in 1% of pregnant patients with hyperthyroidism—but has a high risk of maternal heart failure (9). Older literature described a maternal mortality of up to 25% but this has not been substantiated by more recent data (9, 41). Thyroid storm is diagnosed by a combination of the following signs and symptoms: fever; tachycardia out of proportion to the fever; changed mental status, including restlessness, nervousness, confusion, and seizures; vomiting; diarrhea; and cardiac arrhythmia (42). Often there is an identified inciting event such as infection, surgery, labor, or delivery. However, the diagnosis can be difficult to make and requires expedient treatment to avoid the severe consequences of untreated thyroid storm, which include shock, stupor, and coma. If thyroid storm is suspected, serum FT_4, FT_3, and TSH levels should be evaluated to help confirm the diagnosis, but therapy should not be withheld pending the results.

Therapy for thyroid storm consists of a standard series of drugs (see box) (8, 42). Each drug has a specific role in the suppression of thyroid function. Propylthiouracil or methimazole blocks additional synthesis of thyroid hormone, and PTU also inhibits peripheral conversion of T_4 to T_3. Saturated solution of potassium iodide and sodium iodide block the release of thyroid hormone from the gland. Dexamethasone decreases thyroid hormone release and peripheral conversion of T_4 to T_3, and propranolol inhibits the adrenergic effects of excessive thyroid hormone. Finally, phenobarbital can be used to reduce extreme agitation or restlessness and may increase the catabolism of thyroid hormone (42). In addition to pharmacologic management, general supportive measures should be undertaken, including administration of oxygen, maintenance of intravascular volume and electrolytes, use of antipyretics, use of a cooling blanket, and appropriate maternal and fetal monitoring; invasive central monitoring and continuous maternal cardiac monitoring in an intensive care setting may be indicated. Coincident with treating the thyroid storm, the perceived underlying cause of the storm should be treated. As with other acute maternal illnesses, fetal well-being should be appropriately evaluated with

---

Treatment of Thyroid Storm in Pregnant Women

1. Propylthiouracil (PTU), 600–800 mg orally, stat, then 150–200 mg orally every 4–6 hours. If oral administration is not possible, use methimazole rectal suppositories.

2. Starting 1–2 hours after PTU administration, saturated solution of potassium iodide (SSKI), 2–5 drops orally every 8 hours, *or*

   sodium iodide, 0.5–1.0 g intravenously every 8 hours, *or*

   Lugol's solution, 8 drops every 6 hours, *or*

   lithium carbonate, 300 mg orally every 6 hours.

3. Dexamethasone, 2 mg intravenously or intramuscularly every 6 hours for four doses.

4. Propranolol, 20–80 mg orally every 4–6 hours, *or* propranolol, 1–2 mg intravenously every 5 minutes for a total of 6 mg, then 1–10 mg intravenously every 4 hours.

   If the patient has a history of severe bronchospasm:

   Reserpine, 1–5 mg intramuscularly every 4–6 hours

   Guanethidine, 1mg/kg orally every 12 hours

   Diltiazem, 60 mg orally every 6–8 hours

5. Phenobarbital, 30–60 mg orally every 6–8 hours as needed for extreme restlessness.

Data from Ecker JL, Musci TJ. Thyroid function and disease in pregnancy. Curr Probl Obstet Gynecol Fertil 2000;23:109–122; and Molitch ME. Endocrine emergencies in pregnancy. Bailliere's Clin Endocrinol Metab 1992;6:167–191

---

ultrasonography, biophysical profile, or nonstress test depending on the gestational age of the fetus. In general, it is prudent to avoid delivery in the presence of thyroid storm unless fetal indications for delivery outweigh the risks to the woman.

▶ *How should a thyroid nodule or thyroid cancer during pregnancy be assessed?*

The incidence of thyroid cancer in pregnancy is 1 per 1,000 (43). Any thyroid nodule discovered during pregnancy should be diagnostically evaluated, because malignancy will be found in up to 40% of these nodules (34, 44). Pregnancy itself does not appear to alter the course of thyroid cancer (43, 45). Whether pregnancy increases the risk of recurrence of thyroid cancer or the risk that a thyroid nodule becomes cancerous is less clear

(34). In a cohort study comparing thyroid cancer in pregnant or postpartum women with nonpregnant women, there were no differences in the presenting physical findings, tumor type, tumor size, presence of metastases, time between diagnosis and treatment, recurrence rates, or death rates (43). Women in this study were monitored for a median of 20 years. These data strongly suggest that pregnancy does not affect the outcome of thyroid cancer. In addition, except for the time between diagnosis and surgery, there was no difference in outcome between those women who had thyroidectomy during pregnancy and those who had the procedure after pregnancy. Significantly more pregnant women had no symptoms, emphasizing the importance of the physical examination during pregnancy.

Another study compared pregnancy outcomes among women with thyroid cancer who fell into 1 of 3 categories: 1) before treatment, 2) after thyroidectomy but before I-131 treatment, and 3) after treatment with both thyroidectomy and I-131 (46). The study found no differences in stillbirths, LBW, or malformations among the three groups. The incidence of spontaneous abortion was significantly higher in women who had any treatment for thyroid cancer but was not different between those women who had surgery only and those who had surgery and I-131 treatment.

If a diagnosis of cancer is made, a multidisciplinary treatment plan should be determined. The options are pregnancy termination, treatment during pregnancy, and preterm or term delivery with treatment after pregnancy. This decision will be affected by the gestational age at diagnosis and the tumor characteristics. Definitive treatment for thyroid cancer is thyroidectomy and radiation. Thyroidectomy can be performed during pregnancy, preferably in the second trimester, but radiation should be deferred until after pregnancy. Breastfeeding should be avoided for at least 120 days after I-131 treatment (34).

▶ How is postpartum thyroiditis diagnosed and treated?

Postpartum thyroiditis occurs in 5% of women who do not have a history of thyroid disease (47). Studies have found that approximately 44% of women with postpartum thyroiditis have hypothyroidism, while the remaining women are evenly split between thyrotoxicosis and thyrotoxicosis followed by hypothyroidism (47, 48). In one study, goiter was present in 51% of women with postpartum thyroiditis (48). Postpartum thyroiditis also may occur after pregnancy loss and has a 70% risk of recurrence (49, 50).

The diagnosis of postpartum thyroiditis is made by documenting new-onset abnormal levels of TSH or FT_4 or both. If the diagnosis is in doubt, measuring anti-microsomal or thyroperoxidase antithyroid peroxidase antibodies may be useful to confirm the diagnosis.

The need for treatment in women with postpartum thyroiditis is less clear. In a prospective study of 605 asymptomatic pregnant and postpartum women, only five women, or 11% of the women diagnosed with postpartum thyroiditis, developed permanent hypothyroidism (48). Furthermore, none of the women with thyrotoxicosis required treatment, and only 40% of those with hypothyroidism required treatment (48). Those who were treated received T_4 for extremely high levels of TSH with suppressed T_4 or increasing goiter size. Because of the low incidence of postpartum thyroiditis and the low likelihood of requiring treatment, screening with TFTs and antimicrosomal antibodies in asymptomatic women is not warranted (47, 51).

Women who develop a goiter in pregnancy or postpartum or who develop postpartum hypothyroid or hyperthyroid symptoms (including excessive fatigue, weight gain, dry skin, dry hair, cold intolerance, persistent amenorrhea, difficulty concentrating, depression, nervousness, or palpitations) should have their TSH and FT_4 levels evaluated (47, 48, 51). As noted previously, thyroid antimicrosomal or antithyroid peroxidase antibodies also may be useful. Because some of these symptoms are common in the postpartum state, clinicians must use their judgment to determine whether the symptoms warrant evaluation. If the patient has hypothyroidism, the decision to treat depends on the severity of abnormality and symptoms. Women with the highest levels of TSH and antithyroid peroxidase antibodies have the highest risk for developing permanent hypothyroidism (48).

▶ Which pregnant patients should be screened for thyroid dysfunction?

It is appropriate to perform indicated testing of thyroid function in women with a personal history of thyroid disease or symptoms of thyroid disease. The performance of TFTs in asymptomatic pregnant women who have a mildly enlarged thyroid is not warranted. Development of a significant goiter or distinct nodules should be evaluated as in any patient.

An observational study has drawn considerable attention to the subject of maternal subclinical hypothyroidism and resulted in calls from some professional organizations for universal screening for maternal hypothyroidism (20). Investigators screened maternal serum samples—obtained in the second trimester for purposes of maternal serum alphafetoprotein screening for neural tube defects—for elevated TSH levels (20). Out of 25,216 samples, only 75 women had TSH levels above the 99.7th percentile. The investigators then compared the results of neuropsychologic testing for 62 children of hypothyroid women with those of 124 children of matched women with normal thyroid glands when the children were approximately 8 years of age. They found no significant difference in mean IQ scores between the children of hypothyroid women and controls ($P = 0.06$). There was a significant difference in mean IQ scores when the children of untreated hypothyroid women were compared with controls but not between children of untreated and treated hypothyroid women. Among the children of the untreated women, 19% had full-scale IQ scores of 85 or lower, compared with only 5% of the children of women with normal thyroid glands.

It is important to acknowledge the limitations of the current understanding of this issue. The data available are observational. There have been no intervention trials to demonstrate the efficacy of screening and treatment to improve neuropsychologic performance in the offspring of hypothyroid women. The available data are consistent with the possibility that maternal hypothyroidism is associated with a decrement in some neuropsychologic testing. However, the association needs further testing to document its validity and, if confirmed, evidence that treatment ameliorates the effect. For all of these reasons, it would be premature to recommend universal screening for hypothyroidism during pregnancy.

Summary of Recommendations

The following recommendation is based on good and consistent scientific evidence (Level A):

▶ Levels of TSH or FT_4/FTI should be monitored to manage thyroid disease in pregnancy.

The following recommendations are based on limited or inconsistent scientific evidence (Level B):

▶ Either PTU or methimazole can be used to treat pregnant women with hyperthyroidism.

▶ Thyroid function tests are not indicated in asymptomatic pregnant women with slightly enlarged thyroid glands.

The following recommendations are based primarily on consensus and expert opinion (Level C):

▶ There is no need to measure TFTs routinely in women with hyperemesis.

▶ There are insufficient data to warrant routine screening of asymptomatic pregnant women for hypothyroidism.

▶ Indicated testing of thyroid function may be performed in women with a personal history of thyroid disease or symptoms of thyroid disease.

▶ The presence of maternal thyroid disease is important information for the pediatrician to have at the time of delivery.

▶ Thyroid nodules should be investigated to rule out malignancy.

References

1. Jameson JL, Weetman AP. Disorders of the thyroid gland. In: Braunwald E, Fauci AS, Hauser SL, Kasper DL, Longo DL, Jameson JL, eds. Harrison's principles of internal medicine. 15th ed. New York: McGraw-Hill, 2001: 2060–2084 (Level III)

2. Burrow GN, Fisher DA, Larsen PR. Maternal and fetal thyroid function. N Engl J Med 1994;331:1072–1078 (Level III)

3. Ecker JL, Musci TJ. Treatment of thyroid disease in pregnancy. Obstet Gynecol Clin North Am 1997;24:575–589 (Level III)

4. Glinoer D, de Nayer P, Bourdoux P, Lemone M, Robyn C, van Steirteghem A, et al. Regulation of maternal thyroid during pregnancy. J Clin Endocrinol Metab 1990;71: 276–287 (Level II-2)

5. Rasmussen NG, Hornnes PJ, Hegedus L. Ultrasonographically determined thyroid size in pregnancy and post partum: the goitrogenic effect of pregnancy. Am J Obstet Gynecol 1989;160:1216–1220 (Level II-2)

6. Thorpe-Beeston JG, Nicolaides KH, Felton CV, Butler J, McGregor AM. Maturation of the secretion of thyroid hormone and thyroid-stimulating hormone in the fetus. N Eng J Med 1991;324:532–536 (Level II-3)

7. Utiger RD. Maternal hypothyroidism and fetal development [letter]. N Engl J Med 1999;341:601–602 (Level III)

8. Ecker JL, Musci TJ. Thyroid function and disease in pregnancy. Curr Probl Obstet Gynecol Fertil 2000;23:109–122 (Level III)

9. Davis LE, Lucas MJ, Hankins GD, Roark ML, Cunningham FG. Thyrotoxicosis complicating pregnancy. Am J Obstet Gynecol 1989;160:63–70 (Level II-2)

10. Millar LK, Wing DA, Leung AS, Koonings PP, Montoro MN, Mestman JH. Low birth weight and preeclampsia in pregnancies complicated by hyperthyroidism. Obstet Gynecol 1994;84:946–949 (Level II-2)

11. Weetman AP. Graves' disease. N Engl J Med 2000;343: 1236–1248 (Level III)

12. Matsuura N, Harada S, Ohyama Y, Shibayama K, Fukushi M, Ishikawa N, et al. The mechanisms of transient hypothyroxinemia in infants born to mothers with Graves' disease. Pediatr Res 1997;42:214–218 (Level II-2)

13. McKenzie JM, Zakarija M. Fetal and neonatal hyperthyroidism and hypothyroidism due to maternal TSH receptor antibodies. Thyroid 1992;2:155–163 (Level III)

14. Laurberg P, Nygaard B, Glinoer D, Grusssendorf M, Orgiazzi J. Guidelines for TSH-receptor antibody measurements in pregnancy: results of an evidence-based symposium organized by the European Thyroid Association. Eur J Endocrinol 1998;139:584–586 (Level III)

15. Alvarez-Marfany M, Roman SH, Drexler AJ, Robertson C, Stagnaro-Green A. Long-term prospective study of postpartum thyroid dysfunction in women with insulin dependent diabetes mellitus. J Clin Endocrinol Metab 1994;79:10–16 (Level II-2)

16. Leung AS, Millar LK, Koonings PP, Montoro M, Mestman JH. Perinatal outcome in hypothyroid pregnancies. Obstet Gynecol 1993;81:349–353 (Level II-2)

17. Davis LE, Leveno KJ, Cunningham FG. Hypothyroidism complicating pregnancy. Obstet Gynecol 1988;72:108–112 (Level II-2)

18. Cao XY, Jiang XM, Dou ZH, Rakeman MA, Zhang ML, O'Donnell K, et al. Timing of vulnerability of the brain to iodine deficiency in endemic cretinism. N Engl J Med 1994;331:1739–1744 (Level II-1)

19. Screening for congenital hypothyroidism. In: U.S. Preventive Services Task Force. Guide to clinical preventive services. 2nd ed. Baltimore: Williams & Wilkins, 1996:503–507 (Level III)

20. Haddow JE, Palomaki GE, Allan WC, Williams JR, Knight GJ, Gagnon J, et al. Maternal thyroid deficiency during pregnancy and subsequent neuropsychological development of the child. N Engl J Med 1999;341:549–555 (Level II-2)

21. American Association of Clinical Endocrinologists. AACE clinical practice guidelines for evaluation and treatment of hyperthyroidism and hypothyroidism. Jacksonville, Florida: AACE, 1996 (Level III)

22. Ladenson PW, Singer PA, Ain KB, Bagchi N, Bigos ST, Levy EG, et al. American Thyroid Association guidelines for detection of thyroid dysfunction. Arch Intern Med 2000;160:1573–1575 [erratum Arch Intern Med 2001;161: 284] (Level III)

23. Gittoes NJ, Franklyn JA. Hyperthyroidism. Current treatment guidelines. Drugs 1998;55:543–553 (Level III)

24. Davies TF, Roti E, Braverman LE, Degroot LJ. Thyroid controversy—stimulating antibodies. J Clin Endocrinol Metab 1998;83:3777–3785 (Level III)

25. Wallace C, Couch R, Ginsberg J. Fetal thyrotoxicosis: a case report and recommendations for prediction, diagnosis, and treatment. Thyroid 1995;5:125–128 (Level III)

26. Van Dijke CP, Heydendael RJ, De Kleine MJ. Methimazole, carbimazole and congenital skin defects. Ann Intern Med 1987;106:60–61 (Level II-3)

27. Momotani N, Noh JY, Ishikawa N, Ito K. Effects of propl-thiouracil and methimazole on fetal thyroid status in mothers with Graves' hyperthyroidism. J Clin Endocrinol Metab 1997;82:3633–3636 (Level II-1)

28. Wing DA, Millar LK, Koonings PP, Montoro MN, Mestman JH. A comparison of propylthiouracil versus methimazole in the treatment of hyperthyroidism in pregnancy. Am J Obstet Gyencol 1994;170:90–95 (Level II-1)

29. Davidson KM, Richards DS, Schatz DA, Fisher DA. Successful in utero treatment of fetal goiter and hypothyroidism. N Engl J Med 1991;324:543–546 (Level III)

30. Briggs GG, Freeman RK, Yaffe SJ. Drugs in pregnancy and lactation: a reference guide to fetal and neonatal risk. Baltimore: Williams & Wilkins, 1998 (Level II-2)

31. Momotani N, Yamashita R, Yoshimoto M, Noh J, Ishikawa N, Ito K. Recovery from foetal hypothyroidism: evidence for the safety of breast-feeding while taking propyl-thiouracil. Clin Endocrinol (Oxf) 1989;31:591–595 (Level II-3)

32. Berg GE, Nystrom EH, Jacobsson L, Lindberg S, Lindstedt RG, Mattsson S, et al. Radioiodine treatment of hyperthyroidism in a pregnant women. J Nucl Med 1998;39(2):357–361 (Level III)

33. Evans PM, Webster J, Evans WD, Bevan JS, Scanlon MF. Radioiodine treatment in unsuspected pregnancy. Clin Endocrinol (Oxf) 1998;48:281–283 (Level III)

34. McClellan DR, Francis GL. Thyroid cancer in children, pregnant women, and patients with Graves' disease. Endocrinol Metab Clin North Am 1996;25:27–48 (Level III)

35. Mandel SJ, Larsen PR, Seely EW, Brent GA. Increased need for thyroxine during pregnancy in women with primary hypothyroidism. N Engl J Med 1990;323:91–96 (Level II-3)

36. Goodwin TM, Montoro M, Mestman JH. Transient hyperthyroidism and hyperemesis gravidarum: clinical aspects. Am J Obstet Gynecol 1992;167:648–652 (Level II-2)

37. Kimura M, Amino N, Tamaki H, Ito E, Mitsuda N, Miyai K, et al. Gestational thyrotoxicosis and hyperemesis gravidarum: possible role of hCG with higher stimulating activity. Clin Endocrinol (Oxf) 1993;38:345–350 (Level II-2)

38. Lao TT, Chin RK, Chang AM. The outcome of hyperemetic pregnancies complicated by transient hyperthyroidism. Aust N Z J Obstet Gynaecol 1987;27:99–101 (Level II-3)

39. Shulman A, Shapiro MS, Bahary C, Shenkman L. Abnormal thyroid function in hyperemesis gravidarum. Acta Obstet Gynecol Scand 1989;68:533–536 (Level II-2)

40. Leylek OA, Cetin A, Toyaksi M, Erselcan T. Hyperthyroidism in hyperemesis gravidarum. Int J Gynaecol Obstet 1996;55:33–37 (Level II-2)

41. Burrow GN. The management of thyrotoxicosis in pregnancy. N Engl J Med 1985;313:562–565 (Level II-3)

42. Molitch ME. Endocrine emergencies in pregnancy. Baillieres Clin Endocrinol Metab 1992;6:167–191 (Level III)

43. Moosa M, Mazzaferri EL. Outcome of differentiated thyroid cancer diagnosed in pregnant women. J Clin Endocrinol Metab 1997;82:2862–2866 (Level II-2)

44. Mazzaferri EL. Management of a solitary thyroid nodule. N Engl J Med 1993;328:553–559 (Level III)

45. Vini L, Hyer S, Pratt B, Harmer C. Management of differentiated thyroid cancer diagnosed during pregnancy. Eur J Endocrinol 1999;140:404–406 (Level III)

46. Schlumberger M, De Vathaire F, Ceccarelli C, Delisle MJ, Francese C, Couette JE, et al. Exposure to radioactive

iodine-131 for scintigraphy or therapy does not preclude pregnancy in thyroid cancer patients. J Nucl Med 1996;37:606–612 (Level II-2)

47. Gerstein HC. How common is postpartum thyroiditis? A methodology overview of the literature. Arch Intern Med 1990;150:1397–1400 (Level II-2)

48. Lucas A, Pizarro E, Granada ML, Salinas I, Foz M, Sanmarti A. Postpartum thyroiditis: epidemiology and clinical evolution in a nonselected population. Thyroid 2000;10:71–77 (Level II-2)

49. Lazarus JH, Ammari F, Oretti R, Parkes AB, Richards CJ, Harris B. Clinical aspects of recurrent postpartum thyroiditis. Br J Gen Pract 1997;47:305–308 (Level II-3)

50. Marqusee E, Hill JA, Mandel SJ. Thyroiditis after pregnancy loss. J Clin Endocrinol Metab 1997;82:2455–2457 (Level II-3)

51. Screening for thyroid disease. In: U.S. Preventive Services Task Force. Guide to clinical preventive services. 2nd ed. Baltimore: Williams & Wilkins, 1996:209–218 (Level III)

The MEDLINE database, the Cochrane Library, and ACOG's own internal resources and documents were used to conduct a literature search to locate relevant articles published between January 1985 and August 2000. The search was restricted to articles published in the English language. Priority was given to articles reporting results of original research, although review articles and commentaries also were consulted. Abstracts of research presented at symposia and scientific conferences were not considered adequate for inclusion in this document. Guidelines published by organizations or institutions such as the National Institutes of Health and the American College of Obstetricians and Gynecologists were reviewed, and additional studies were located by reviewing bibliographies of identified articles. When reliable research was not available, expert opinions from obstetrician–gynecologists were used.

Studies were reviewed and evaluated for quality according to the method outlined by the U.S. Preventive Services Task Force:

I   Evidence obtained from at least one properly designed randomized controlled trial.

II-1   Evidence obtained from well-designed controlled trials without randomization.

II-2   Evidence obtained from well-designed cohort or case–control analytic studies, preferably from more than one center or research group.

II-3   Evidence obtained from multiple time series with or without the intervention. Dramatic results in uncontrolled experiments could also be regarded as this type of evidence.

III   Opinions of respected authorities, based on clinical experience, descriptive studies, or reports of expert committees.

Based on the highest level of evidence found in the data, recommendations are provided and graded according to the following categories:

Level A—Recommendations are based on good and consistent scientific evidence.

Level B—Recommendations are based on limited or inconsistent scientific evidence.

Level C—Recommendations are based primarily on consensus and expert opinion.

ISSN 1099-3630

The American College of Obstetricians and Gynecologists
409 12th Street, SW, PO Box 96920
Washington, DC 20090-6920

12345/65432

Thyroid disease in pregnancy. ACOG Practice Bulletin No. 37. American College of Obstetricians and Gynecologists. Obstet Gynecol 2002;100:387–396

ACOG PRACTICE BULLETIN

CLINICAL MANAGEMENT GUIDELINES FOR
OBSTETRICIAN–GYNECOLOGISTS

NUMBER 58, DECEMBER 2004

*(Replaces Committee Opinion Number 180, November 1996, and
Practice Pattern Number 5, August 1997)*

This Practice Bulletin was developed by the ACOG Committee on Practice Bulletins—Obstetrics with the assistance of John Seeds, MD, and Lyndon M. Hill, MD. The information is designed to aid practitioners in making decisions about appropriate obstetric and gynecologic care. These guidelines should not be construed as dictating an exclusive course of treatment or procedure. Variations in practice may be warranted based on the needs of the individual patient, resources, and limitations unique to the institution or type of practice.

Ultrasonography in Pregnancy

In the United States, approximately 65% of pregnant women have at least 1 ultrasound examination (1). The purpose of this document is to present evidence regarding methodology, indications, benefits, and risks of obstetric ultrasonography in specific clinical situations. Portions of this document were developed collaboratively by the American College of Radiology, the American Institute of Ultrasound in Medicine, and the American College of Obstetricians and Gynecologists (ACOG). Sections of the document addressing physician qualifications and responsibilities, documentation, quality control, infection control, and patient education are recommendations of ACOG.

Background

Instrumentation

For most ultrasound examinations, an instrument with real-time, 2-dimensional imaging and sector or convex array abdominal transducers, typically with frequencies ranging from 3 MHz to 7 MHz, or vaginal transducers, with frequencies ranging from 5 MHz to 9 MHz, are used. Higher frequency transducers provide better resolution but with less penetration. Selection of transducer frequency for a particular case should take into consideration this trade-off between resolution and penetration. The equipment should allow the user to perform on-screen linear and circumference measurements. A method for storing the images also is required. The equipment should be serviced at regular intervals according to the manufacturer's recommendations.

Two measurements of acoustic output are displayed on-screen with contemporary ultrasound equipment. The thermal index is an estimate of possible tissue temperature increase that may be caused by ultrasound absorption. The mechanical index is a measure of the interaction of ultrasonography with microscopic gas bubbles that are present in all tissues. The mechanical index incorporates cavitation with other possible nonthermal effects of ultrasonography. When the thermal index and mechanical index are adjusted by the user to values of less than unity (1), the likelihood of tissue effect is very low (2). Most machines allow adjustment of output and will instantly recalculate and display the new thermal index and mechanical index.

Most manufacturers now offer machines capable of 3-dimensional surface rendering of fetal anatomy, and some offer near real-time 3-dimensional imaging. Proof of a clear advantage of 3-dimensional ultrasonography in prenatal diagnosis is not present when compared with 2-dimensional imaging by an experienced clinician. Therefore, 3-dimensional imaging is not considered a required modality at this time.

Types of Examinations

The American College of Obstetricians and Gynecologists uses the terms "standard," "limited," and "specialized" to describe various types of ultrasound examinations performed during the second or third trimesters. Although the standard and limited examinations are defined by their components, the specialized examination is defined by the indications for the examination, that is, the circumstances that suggest a more thorough ultrasound examination is needed. First-trimester obstetric ultrasonography is distinct from these and is discussed separately.

Standard Examination

A standard examination is performed during the second or third trimester of pregnancy. It includes an evaluation of fetal presentation, amniotic fluid volume, cardiac activity, placental position, fetal biometry, and an anatomic survey. If technically feasible, the uterus and adnexa also are examined.

Fetal anatomy, as described in this document, may be assessed adequately by ultrasonography after approximately 16–20 weeks of gestation. It may be possible to document normal structures before this time, although some structures can be difficult to visualize because of fetal size, position, movement, abdominal scars, and increased maternal wall thickness. A second- or third-trimester ultrasound examination may pose technical limitations for an anatomic evaluation because of imaging artifacts from acoustic shadowing. When this occurs, the report of the ultrasound examination should document the nature of this technical limitation.

The essential elements of a standard examination of fetal anatomy are listed in the box. A more detailed fetal anatomic examination may be necessary if an abnormality or suspected abnormality is found on the standard examination.

Essential Elements of Fetal Anatomic Ultrasound Survey

Head and Neck
- Cerebellum
- Choroid plexus
- Cisterna magna
- Lateral cerebral ventricles
- Midline falx
- Cavum septi pellucidi

Chest
- The basic cardiac examination includes a 4-chamber view of the fetal heart. If technically feasible, an extended basic cardiac examination also can be attempted to evaluate both outflow tracts.

Abdomen
- Stomach (presence, size, and situs)
- Kidneys
- Bladder
- Umbilical cord insertion site into the fetal abdomen
- Umbilical cord vessel number

Spine
- Cervical, thoracic, lumbar, and sacral spine

Extremities
- Legs and arms (presence or absence)

Sex
- For evaluation of multiple gestations

American College of Radiology. ACR practice guideline for the performance of antepartum obstetrical ultrasound. In: ACR practice guidelines and technical standards, 2003. Philadelphia (PA): ACR; 2003. p. 625–31.

Limited Examination

A limited examination is performed when a specific question requires investigation. In an emergency, for example, a limited examination can be performed to evaluate heart activity in a bleeding patient. This evaluation also would be appropriate for verifying fetal presentation in a laboring patient; however, in most cases, a limited examination is appropriate only when the patient has had a prior complete examination.

Specialized Examination

A detailed or targeted anatomic examination is performed when an anomaly is suspected on the basis of history, biochemical abnormalities or clinical evaluation, or suspicious results from either the limited or standard ultrasound examination. Other specialized examinations might include fetal Doppler, biophysical profile, fetal echocardiography, or additional biometric studies. Specialized examinations are performed by an operator with experience and expertise in such ultrasonography who determines the components of the examination on a case-by-case basis.

First-Trimester Ultrasonography

Indications. An ultrasound examination may be of benefit in many circumstances in the first trimester of pregnancy, including, but not limited to, the following indications:

- To confirm the presence of an intrauterine pregnancy
- To evaluate a suspected ectopic pregnancy
- To define the cause of vaginal bleeding
- To evaluate pelvic pain
- To estimate gestational age
- To diagnose or evaluate multiple gestations
- To confirm cardiac activity
- As an adjunct to chorionic villus sampling, embryo transfer, or localization and removal of an intrauterine device
- To evaluate maternal pelvic masses or uterine abnormalities
- To evaluate suspected hydatidiform mole

Imaging Parameters. Ultrasonography in the first trimester may be performed either transabdominally or transvaginally. If a transabdominal examination is not definitive, a transvaginal or transperineal examination should be performed whenever possible. The following factors should be considered during the examination:

- The uterus and adnexa should be evaluated for the presence of a gestational sac. If a gestational sac is seen, its location should be documented. The gestational sac should be evaluated for the presence or absence of a yolk sac or embryo, and the crown–rump length should be recorded, when possible. The crown–rump length is a more accurate indicator of gestational age than is the mean gestational sac diameter. However, the mean gestational sac diame-

ter should be recorded when an embryo is not identified. Caution should be used in making the presumptive diagnosis of a gestational sac in the absence of a definite embryo or yolk sac. Without these findings, an intrauterine fluid collection could represent a pseudogestational sac associated with an ectopic pregnancy.

- Presence or absence of cardiac activity should be reported. With transvaginal ultrasound examinations, cardiac motion usually is observed when the embryo is 5 mm or greater in length. If an embryo less than 5 mm in length is seen without cardiac activity, an additional ultrasound examination at a later time may be needed to document cardiac activity.
- Fetal number should be reported. Amnionicity and chorionicity should be documented for all multiple pregnancies when possible.
- Evaluation of the uterus, adnexal structures, and cul-de-sac should be performed. The presence, location, and size of leiomyomata and adnexal masses should be recorded. The cul-de-sac should be evaluated by ultrasonography for the presence or absence of fluid.

Second- and Third-Trimester Ultrasonography

Indications. In 1984, the U.S. Department of Health and Human Services published a list of 27 indications for an obstetric ultrasound examination. Since then, advances in ultrasonographic technology have increased the list of indications (see box).

Imaging Parameters. The components of a standard fetal examination are as follows:

- Fetal cardiac activity, number, and presentation should be reported. Abnormal heart rate or rhythm should be reported. For multiple pregnancies, additional information should be documented: chorionicity, amnionicity, comparison of fetal sizes, estimation of amniotic fluid volume (increased, decreased, or normal) on each side of the membrane, and fetal genitalia (when visualized).
- A qualitative or semiquantitative estimate of amniotic fluid volume should be reported. Although it is acceptable for experienced examiners to estimate the amniotic fluid volume qualitatively, semiquantitative methods also have been described for this purpose (eg, amniotic fluid index, single deepest pocket, 2-diameter pocket).

• The placenta's location, appearance, and relationship to the internal cervical os should be recorded. The umbilical cord should be imaged, and the number of

---

Indications for Ultrasonography During Pregnancy

• Estimation of gestational age for patients with uncertain clinical dates, or verification of dates for patients who are to undergo scheduled elective repeat cesarean delivery, indicated induction of labor, or other elective termination of pregnancy

• Evaluation of fetal growth

• Vaginal bleeding of undetermined etiology in pregnancy

• Evaluation of incompetent cervix

• Abdominal and pelvic pain

• Determination of fetal presentation

• Suspected multiple gestation

• Adjunct to amniocentesis

• Significant uterine size and clinical dates discrepancy

• Pelvic mass

• Suspected hydatidiform mole

• Adjunct to cervical cerclage placement

• Suspected ectopic pregnancy

• Suspected fetal death

• Suspected uterine abnormality

• Biophysical evaluation for fetal well-being

• Suspected polyhydramnios or oligohydramnios

• Suspected abruptio placentae

• Adjunct to external version from breech to vertex presentation

• Estimation of fetal weight or presentation in premature rupture of membranes or premature labor

• Evaluation of abnormal serum screening value

• Follow-up observation of identified fetal anomaly

• Follow-up evaluation of placental location for identified "placenta previa"

• History of previous congenital anomaly

• Evaluation of fetal condition in late registrants for prenatal care

American College of Radiology. ACR practice guideline for the performance of antepartum obstetrical ultrasound. In: ACR practice guidelines and technical standards, 2003. Philadelphia (PA): ACR; 2003. p. 625–31.

---

vessels in the cord should be evaluated when possible. The apparent placental position early in pregnancy may not correlate well with its location at the time of delivery. Therefore, if low-lying placenta or placenta previa are suspected early in gestation, verification in the third trimester by repeat ultrasonography is indicated. Transabdominal, transperineal, or transvaginal views may be helpful in visualizing the internal cervical os and its relationship to the placenta.

• Gestational age should be assessed. First-trimester crown–rump measurement is the most accurate means of ultrasound dating of pregnancy. Beyond this period, a variety of ultrasonographic parameters, such as biparietal diameter, abdominal circumference, and femoral diaphysis length, can be used to estimate gestational age. The variability of gestational age estimations, however, increases with advancing pregnancy. Significant discrepancies between the estimated gestational age and fetal measurements from later ultrasound examinations may suggest the possibility of a fetal growth abnormality, intrauterine growth restriction (IUGR), or macrosomia.

— Biparietal diameter usually is measured at the level of the thalami and cavum septi pellucidi. The cerebellar hemispheres should not be visible in this scanning plane. The measurement is taken from the outer edge of the proximal skull to the inner edge of the distal skull. The head shape may be flattened (dolichocephaly) or rounded (brachycephaly) as a normal variant. These variants of normal fetal head development may make measurement of the head circumference more reliable than biparietal diameter for estimating gestational age.

— Head circumference is measured at the same level as the biparietal diameter, around the outer perimeter of the calvarium. This measurement is not affected by head shape.

— Femoral diaphysis length can be reliably used after 14 weeks of gestational age. The long axis of the femur shaft is most accurately measured with the beam of insonation being perpendicular to the shaft, excluding the distal femoral epiphysis.

— Abdominal circumference should be determined at the skin line on a true transverse view at the level of the junction of the umbilical vein, portal sinus, and fetal stomach when visible. Abdominal circumference measurement is used with other biometric parameters to estimate fetal weight and may allow detection of IUGR or macrosomia.

- Fetal weight can be estimated by obtaining measurements such as the biparietal diameter, head circumference, abdominal circumference, and femoral diaphysis length. Results from various prediction models can be compared with fetal weight percentiles from published nomograms. If previous studies have been performed, interval measurement changes also should be evaluated for growth. Ultrasound examinations for growth evaluation can typically be performed no less than 2 weeks apart. A shorter interval between ultrasound examinations may result in confusion as to whether anatomic changes are truly caused by growth as opposed to variations in the measurement technique itself.

- Evaluation of the maternal uterus and adnexal structures should be performed. Such evaluation will allow recognition of incidental findings of potential clinical significance. The presence, location, and size of leiomyomata and adnexal masses should be recorded. Frequently, it is not possible to image the normal maternal ovaries during the second and third trimesters.

Ultrasound Facility Accreditation

Recently, the American Institute of Ultrasound in Medicine and the American College of Radiology have offered ultrasound facility accreditation. This process involves review of equipment use and maintenance, report generation, storage of images, and ultrasonographer and physician qualifications. Practices, not individuals, may be accredited in ultrasonography for obstetrics, gynecology, or both.

Physicians who perform, evaluate, and interpret diagnostic obstetric ultrasound examinations should be licensed medical practitioners with an understanding of the indications for such imaging studies, the expected content of a complete obstetric ultrasound examination, and a familiarity with the limitations of ultrasound imaging. They should be familiar with the anatomy, physiology, and pathophysiology of the pelvis, the pregnant uterus, and the fetus. These physicians should have undergone specific training in obstetric ultrasonography either during or since their residency training and should be able to document this training. Physicians active in obstetric ultrasonography should regularly review and update their expertise in this area through postgraduate medical education. Completion of an approved residency in obstetrics and gynecology with documentation of obstetric ultrasound experience and training with certification by the American Board of Obstetrics and Gynecology is evidence of the necessary and appropriate training.

Physicians are responsible for the quality and accuracy of ultrasound examinations performed in their names regardless of whether they personally produced the images. Physicians are responsible for the quality of the documentation of examinations and the quality control and safety of the environments and the procedures.

Documentation

Appropriate documentation of an obstetric or gynecologic ultrasound examination is essential to both direct clinical care and quality assurance. Complete documentation of the biometric data produced and the maternal and fetal anatomy examined are necessary both to support clinical assessment and decision making as well as to support a conclusion that recommended guidelines were satisfied by the study. An adequate written report of findings may be provided either through the completion of a carefully designed preprinted template that includes the biometry and specific anatomic areas examined as recommended by these guidelines or through the creation of a unique narrative report that includes all findings. It should be the goal of practitioners to document in the medical record their efforts during ultrasound examinations to methodically examine all fetal anatomy and measure all relevant dimensions. The report should be complete but easy to interpret.

Quality review is facilitated by storing the appropriate images in the medical record or in another easily accessed but secure location. The images stored should include images of fetal biometry as well as anatomy. The images may be in the form of thermal paper prints or other media with appropriate storage durability. Videotape provides more extensive visual documentation for review. Absence of visual image documentation eliminates the possibility of future review or clinical reinterpretation and weakens the defense against an allegation that an incomplete or inadequate study was performed.

Quality Control, Performance Improvement, Safety, and Patient Education

Ideally, quality control is accomplished through careful recordkeeping of obstetric ultrasound examination results, reliable archival of reports and images, and clinical correlation with clinical outcomes. The ultimate quality standard of any imaging study is to correlate the study findings with clinical outcomes. Any practice active in obstetric ultrasonography should maintain such records and make every effort to correlate imaging results with ultimate clinical outcome data.

Ultrasound transducers, like any instrument used on a patient, present the possibility of microbial transmission if not properly cleaned between patients. Transabdominal ultrasonography is not completely free of this risk, although the risk is substantially lower than it is for endovaginal ultrasonography. Transabdominal transducers may be adequately cleansed between patients simply by wiping with a disposable antiseptic paper towelette. Endovaginal transducers should always be covered with a single-use disposable latex or nonlatex cover. However, disposable protective covers are not without risk of rupture or defect, and it is recommended that endovaginal transducers undergo appropriate antimicrobial cleansing, if not chemical sterilization, between uses.

Practitioners are encouraged to regularly update and review their ultrasound skills through accredited postgraduate medical education. Before an ultrasound examination is performed, patients should be counseled about the limitations of ultrasonography for diagnosis.

Clinical Considerations and Recommendations

▶ How safe is ultrasonography for the fetus?

Ultrasonography should be performed only when there is a valid medical indication, and the lowest possible ultrasonic exposure setting should be used to gain the necessary diagnostic information under the as low as reasonably achievable (ALARA) principle. From a medical standpoint, fetal ultrasonography is considered safe when properly used and when medical information about a pregnancy is needed; however, ultrasound energy delivered to the fetus cannot be assumed to be completely innocuous. Diagnostic levels of ultrasonography can produce physical effects, such as mechanical vibrations (referred to as cavitation), or an increase in tissue temperature under laboratory conditions.

Although there is no reliable evidence of physical harm to human fetuses from diagnostic ultrasound imaging, public health experts, clinicians, and industry representatives agree that casual use of ultrasonography, especially during pregnancy, should be avoided. Viewed in this light, exposing the fetus to ultrasonography with no anticipation of medical benefit is not justified (3–5). The U.S. Food and Drug Administration views the promotion, sale, or lease of ultrasound equipment for making "keepsake" fetal videos as an unapproved use of a medical device; use of ultrasonography without a physician's order may be a violation of state or local laws or regulations regarding the use of a prescription medical device (6). Specific indications are the best basis for ultrasonography in pregnancy.

▶ Should all patients be offered ultrasonography?

It has been suggested that all patients be offered routine ultrasound screening. It has been shown, for example, that 90% of infants with congenital anomalies are born to women with no risk factors (7). However, several studies conducted between 1985 and 1994 found routine ultrasound screening yielded no consistent impact on perinatal morbidity or mortality (8–11). In the screened populations, the detection rate for congenital anomalies ranged from 16% to 85%. A subsequent secondary analysis of these studies concluded that routine screening was cost-effective (12). Using a mathematical model to evaluate further the published study results, other researchers concluded that routine screening at tertiary centers would be cost-effective, but screening in nontertiary centers resulted in a net loss (13).

Given the limitations of the evidence, a physician is not obligated to perform ultrasonography in a patient who is at low risk and has no indications. However, if a patient requests ultrasonography, it is reasonable to honor the request. The decision ultimately rests with the physician and patient jointly.

▶ What gestational age represents the optimal time for an obstetric ultrasound examination?

The optimal time for obstetric ultrasound examination is the first trimester in the case of a pregnancy resulting from ovulation induction or other assisted reproductive technologies, bleeding in the first trimester, hyperemesis gravidarum, previous ectopic pregnancy, significant abdominal pain, or possibly increased risk of fetal aneuploidy. If none of these indications apply, 16–20 weeks of gestation is an appropriate time to obtain an accurate estimate of gestational age and a reasonable survey of fetal anatomy. Although gestational age derived from crown–rump length in the first trimester is statistically more precise than the average estimated gestational age found in the second trimester, the difference in precision is not clinically important, and a complete anatomic assessment is not possible in the first trimester. Therefore, the optimal timing for a single ultrasound examination in the absence of specific indications for a first-trimester examination is 16–20 weeks of gestation.

▶ How may ultrasonography be used to detect chromosomally abnormal fetuses in the second trimester in women at high risk?

A second-trimester specialized ultrasound examination may be targeted to detect fetal aneuploidy. This type of examination has been offered in some centers for the past several years and is aimed at the detection of a range of minor anatomic features associated with an increased risk of fetal aneuploidy. Advanced maternal age or an abnormal first- or second-trimester multiple marker screen indicating an increased risk for Down syndrome are among the indications for a specialized ultrasound examination. The standard ultrasound examination is less likely to detect the minor anatomic features associated with aneuploidy. There are to date no uniformly agreed-on criteria for such a specialized ultrasonogram. Furthermore, such minor anatomic markers for aneuploidy have been studied mainly in high-prevalence referral populations in which the predictive value is much higher than it would be in a low-prevalence population.

To date, no randomized controlled trials have evaluated the efficacy of a specialized ultrasound examination in the detection of karyotypically abnormal fetuses. The studies that have been performed indicate a range rather than a single estimate of sensitivity. Hence, evidence is insufficient to support or refute the general use of a specialized ultrasound examination to evaluate the entire at-risk obstetric population. The use of the ultrasound markers developed in high-prevalence patient populations in screening for Down syndrome in a low-risk population in the second trimester currently is premature.

▶ *How is ultrasonography used to detect disturbances in fetal growth?*

Intrauterine Growth Restriction

Intrauterine growth restriction is an outcome associated with a multitude of etiologies. The effect on the fetus varies depending on the etiology, time of onset, and severity of the growth restricting process. Individual prognosis, therefore, varies widely.

Generally, a birth weight below the 10th percentile for gestational age using a representative reference nomogram has been the most common definition of IUGR. By definition, 10% of infants in any population will have birth weights at or below the 10th percentile. However, IUGR could be manifest at a weight above the population determined at the 10th percentile (eg, an undernourished infant born at the 15th percentile whose genetic makeup would have resulted in greater growth). Distinctions between normal and pathologic growth often cannot be made reliably in clinical practice, especially before birth. A substantial proportion of infants with birth weights below the 10th percentile are not pathologically growth restricted but instead simply reflect familial or ethnic growth patterns.

Although defining a pathologic condition using a 10th percentile cutoff makes statistical sense, it may not be clinically relevant. One study suggests that adverse perinatal outcome generally is confined to those infants with birth weights below the 5th percentile and, in most cases, below the 3rd percentile (14).

Four standard fetal measurements generally are obtained as part of any complete obstetric ultrasound examination after the first trimester: 1) fetal abdominal circumference, 2) head circumference, 3) biparietal diameter, and 4) femur length (15). Fetal morphologic parameters can be converted to fetal weight estimates using published formulas and tables (16). All such methods carry an inherent variance or error. Contemporary ultrasound equipment calculates and displays an estimate of fetal weight on the basis of these formulas. An abdominal circumference within the normal range reliably excludes growth restriction with a false-negative rate of less than 10% (17). A small abdominal circumference or fetal weight estimate below the 10th percentile suggests the possibility of growth restriction, with the likelihood increasing as the percentile rank decreases (17). When IUGR is suspected, serial measurements of fetal biometric parameters provide an estimated growth rate. Such serial measurements are of considerable clinical value in confirming or excluding the diagnosis and assessing the progression and severity of growth restriction. Given the high incidence of genetic and structural defects associated with IUGR, a detailed ultrasound survey for the presence of fetal structural and functional defects may be indicated. The sensitivity of fetal biometry for the detection of IUGR varies between 25% and 94% (Table 1). None of the randomized controlled trials in low-risk patients support a recommendation for screening for IUGR.

Amniotic fluid volume is an important diagnostic and prognostic parameter in fetuses with IUGR (18, 19). Oligohydramnios is highly suggestive of growth failure and indicates an increased risk of fetal death. Oligohydramnios is diagnosed by ultrasonography in approximately 77–83% of pregnancies with growth-restricted fetuses (18–20). In contrast, amniotic fluid volume often is normal even in a fetus with significant growth restriction; thus, the absence of oligohydramnios should not diminish the importance of the diagnosis of IUGR.

Although Doppler velocimetry of the umbilical arteries is not useful as a screening technique for IUGR (21, 22), it has been demonstrated to be useful once IUGR has been diagnosed. Not only can Doppler velocimetry findings be normal in growth-restricted fetuses with chromosomal or other structural etiologies (23), but Doppler velocimetry has been shown to both reduce interventions and improve fetal outcome in pregnancies at risk for IUGR (24). Thus, once IUGR is sus-

Table 1. Randomized Controlled Trials Evaluating the Antenatal Diagnosis of Intrauterine Growth Restriction

Author	Year	Population	No. Screened	Intrauterine Growth Restriction	
				N	% Detected
Bakketeig*	1984	Low risk	510	41	25
Neilson†	1984	Low risk	433	33	94
Secher‡	1987	Low risk	2,771	267	31.1
Larsen§	1992	High risk	484	64	67
Duff‖	1993	Low risk	760	32	60
Ewigman¶	1993	Low risk	7,812	176	—

*Bakketeig LS, Eik-Nes SH, Jacobsen G, Ulstein MK, Brodtkorb CJ, Balstad P, et al. Randomized controlled trial of ultrasonographic screening in pregnancy. Lancet 1984;2:207–11.

†Neilson J, Munjanja SP, Whitfield CR. Screening for small for dates fetuses: a controlled trial. Br Med J (Clin Res Ed) 1984; 289:1179–82.

‡Secher NJ, Kern Hansen P, Lenstrup C, Sindberg Eriksen P, Morsing G. A randomized study of fetal abdominal diameter and fetal weight estimation for detection of light-for-gestation infants in low-risk pregnancies. Br J Obstet Gynaecol 1987;94:105–9.

§Larsen T, Larsen JF, Petersen S, Greisen G. Detection of small-for-gestational-age fetuses by ultrasound screening in a high risk population: a randomized controlled trial. Br J Obstet Gynaecol 1992;99:469–74.

‖Duff GB. A randomized controlled trail in a hospital population of ultrasound measurement screening for the small for dates baby. Aust N Z J Obstet Gynaecol 1993;33:374–8.

¶Ewigman BG, Crane JP, Frigoletto FD, LeFevre ML, Bain RP, McNellis D. Effect of prenatal ultrasound screening on perinatal outcome. RADIUS Study Group. N Engl J Med 1993;329:821–7.

pected or diagnosed, Doppler velocimetry may be useful as a part of fetal evaluation. Fetuses with normal flow patterns seem less likely to benefit from consideration of early delivery than do their counterparts with abnormal studies.

Identification of IUGR is improved by recording growth velocity or through 2 sets of examinations generally 2–4 weeks apart. Serial ultrasonograms to determine the rate of growth should be obtained approximately every 2–4 weeks. Measurements at shorter intervals (<2 weeks) may overlap and cause measurement errors.

Macrosomia

Macrosomia implies growth beyond a specific weight, usually 4,000 g or 4,500 g, regardless of gestational age (25–27). Numerous fetal body dimensions have been evaluated in an attempt to estimate fetal weight more reliably. Although all of the published formulas for estimating fetal weight show a good correlation with birth weight, the variability of the estimate generally is plus or minus 16–20% (2 standard deviations) (28). In addition, most of the formulas currently in use have a greater error when the fetus has macrosomia. For example, one study reported a mean absolute percent error for a fetal weight estimate of 12.6% for fetuses greater than 4,500 g and 8.4% for fetuses less than 4,500 g (P <.001) (29).

The initial studies of macrosomia established the accuracy of the ultrasound estimation of fetal weight (28). Among women without diabetes, ultrasound biometry used to detect macrosomia has a sensitivity of 22–44%, a specificity of 99%, a positive predictive value of 30–44%, and a negative predictive value of 97–99% (30, 31). It was only later that the clinical and ultrasonographic estimates of fetal weight were compared. These investigations reported no difference between ultrasound and clinical measurements in the prediction of macrosomia (32, 33).

The true value of ultrasonography in the management of expected fetal macrosomia may be its ability to rule out the diagnosis. The standard deviation of ultrasound estimates of fetal weight is too large to allow the weight estimate to be used independently in clinical decision making (34).

Conclusions

▶ Ultrasound examination is an accurate method of determining gestational age, fetal number, viability, and placental location. Gestational age is most accurately determined in the first half of pregnancy.

▶ The ability of ultrasonography to diagnose major fetal anomalies is well established.

▶ The diagnosis of fetal growth abnormalities with ultrasonography is not precise.

▶ Ultrasonography is safe for the fetus when used appropriately.

▶ Specific indications are the best basis for the use of ultrasonography in pregnancy.

▶ The optimal timing for a single ultrasound examination in the absence of specific indications for a first-trimester examination is at 16–20 weeks of gestation.

Summary of Recommendations

The following recommendation is based on limited or inconsistent scientific evidence (Level B):

▶ Serial ultrasonograms to determine the rate of growth should be obtained approximately every 2–4 weeks.

The following recommendations are based primarily on consensus and expert opinion (Level C):

▶ Casual use of ultrasonography, especially during pregnancy, should be avoided.

▶ Before an ultrasound examination is performed, patients should be counseled about the limitations of ultrasonography for diagnosis.

References

1. Martin JA, Hamilton BE, Sutton PD, Ventura SJ, Menacker F, Munson ML. Births: final data for 2002. Natl Vital Stat Rep 2003;52(10):1–113. (Level II-3)

2. American Institute of Ultrasound in Medicine. Acoustic output measurement standards for diagnostic ultrasound equipment. Laurel (MD): AIUM; 1998. (Level III)

3. Stark CR, Orleans M, Haverkamp AD, Murphy J. Short- and long-term risks after exposure to diagnostic ultrasound in utero. Obstet Gynecol 1984;63:194–200. (Level II-2)

4. Lyons EA, Dyke C, Toms M, Cheang M. In utero exposure to diagnostic ultrasound: a 6-year follow-up. Radiology 1988;166:687–90. (Level II-2)

5. American Institute of Ultrasound in Medicine. Bioeffects of diagnostic ultrasound with gas body contrast agents. Laurel (MD): AIUM; 2002. (Level III)

6. Rados C. FDA cautions against ultrasound "keepsake" images. FDA Consum 2004;38(1):12–6. (Level III)

7. Long G, Sprigg A. A comparative study of routine versus selective fetal anomaly ultrasound scanning. J Med Screen 1998;5:6–10. (Level III)

8. Ewigman BG, Crane JP, Frigoletto FD, LeFevre ML, Bain RP, McNellis D. Effect of prenatal ultrasound screening on perinatal outcome. RADIUS Study Group. N Engl J Med 1993;329:821–7. (Level I)

9. Saari-Kemppainen A, Karjalainen O, Ylostalo P, Heinonen OP. Fetal anomalies in a controlled one-stage ultrasound screening trial. A report from the Helsinki Ultrasound Trial. J Perinatal Med 1994;22:279–89. (Level I)

10. Bucher H, Schmidt JG. Does routine ultrasound scanning improve outcome of pregnancy? Meta-analysis of various outcome measures. BMJ 1993;307:13–7. (Meta-analysis)

11. Crane JP, LeFevre ML, Windborn RC, Evans JK, Ewigman BG, Bain RP, et al. A randomized trial of prenatal ultrasonographic screening: impact on the detection, management and outcome of anomalous fetuses. The RADIUS Study Group. Am J Obstet Gynecol 1994;171:392–9. (Level I)

12. Leivo T, Tuominen R, Saari-Kemppainen A, Ylostalo P, Karjalainen O, Heinonen OP. Cost-effectiveness of one-stage ultrasound screening in pregnancy: a report from the Helsinki ultrasound trial. Ultrasound Obstet Gynecol 1996;7:309–14. (Level III)

13. Vintzileos AM, Ananth CV, Smulian JC, Beazoglou T, Knuppel RA. Routine second-trimester ultrasonography in the United States: a cost-benefit analysis. Am J Obstet Gynecol 2000;182:655–60. (Level III)

14. McIntire DD, Bloom SL, Casey BM, Leveno KJ. Birth weight in relation to morbidity and mortality among newborn infants. N Engl J Med 1999;340:1234–8. (Level II-2)

15. Hadlock FP, Deter RL, Harrist RB, Park SK. Estimating fetal age: computer-assisted analysis of multiple fetal growth parameters. Radiology 1984;152:497–501. (Level II-3)

16. Shepard MJ, Richards VA, Berkowitz RL, Warsof SL, Hobbins JC. An evaluation of two equations for predicting fetal weight by ultrasound. Am J Obstet Gynecol 1982;142:47–54. (Level III)

17. Warsof SL, Cooper DJ, Little D, Campbell R. Routine ultrasound screen for antenatal detection of intrauterine growth retardation. Obstet Gynecol 1986;67:33–9. (Level II-2)

18. Chamberlain PF, Manning FA, Morrison I, Harman CR, Lange IR. Ultrasound evaluation of amniotic fluid volume. I. The relationship of marginal and decreased amniotic fluid volumes to perinatal outcome. Am J Obstet Gynecol 1984:150:245–9. (Level II-3)

19. Varma TR, Bateman S, Patel RH, Chamberlain GV, Pillai U. Ultrasound evaluation of amniotic fluid: outcome of pregnancies with severe oligohydramnios. Int J Gynaecol Obstet 1988;27:185–92. (Level II-2)

20. Philipson EH, Sokol RJ, Williams T. Oligohydraminios: clinical associations and predictive value for intrauterine growth retardation. Am J Obstet Gynecol 1983;146:271–8. (Level II-2)

21. Davies JA, Gallivan S, Spencer JA. Randomised controlled trial of Doppler ultrasound screening of placental perfusion during pregnancy. Lancet 1992;340:1299–303. (Level I)

22. Low JA. The current status of maternal and fetal blood flow velocimetry. Am J Obstet Gynecol 1991;164:1049–63. (Level III)

23. Wladimiroff JW, vd.Wijngaard JA, Degani S, Noordam MJ, van Eyck J, Tonge HM. Cerebral and umbilical arterial blood flow velocity waveforms in normal and growth-retarded pregnancies. Obstet Gynecol 1987;69:705–9. (Level II-2)

24. Alfirevic Z, Neilson JP. Doppler ultrasonography in high-risk pregnancies: systematic review with meta-analysis. Am J Obstet Gynecol 1995;172:1379–87. (Meta-analysis)

25. Menticoglou SM, Manning FA, Morrison I, Harman CR. Must macrosomic fetuses be delivered by a cesarean section? A review of outcome for 780 babies greater than or equal to 4500 g. Aust N Z J Obstet Gynaecol 1992;32:100–3. (Level II-2)

26. Lipscomb KR, Gregory K, Shaw K. The outcome of macrosomic infants weighing at least 4500 grams: Los Angeles county + University of Southern California experience. Obstet Gynecol 1995;85:558–64. (Level II-3)

27. Nesbitt TS, Gilbert WM, Hernchen B. Shoulder dystocia and associated risk factors with macrosomic infants born in California. Am J Obstet Gynecol 1998;179:476–80. (Level II-3)

28. Hadlock FP, Harrist RB, Carpenter RJ, Deter RL, Park SK. Sonographic estimation of fetal weight. The value of femur length in addition to head and abdomen measurements. Radiology 1984;150:535–40. (Level II-3)

29. Alsulyman OM, Ouzounian JG, Kjos SL. The accuracy of intrapartum ultrasonographic fetal weight estimation in diabetic pregnancies. Am J Obstet Gynecol 1997;177:503–6. (Level II-2)

30. Smith GC, Smith MF, McNay MG, Fleming JE. The relation between fetal abdominal circumference and birth-weight: findings in 3512 pregnancies. Br J Obstet Gynaecol 1997;104:186–90. (Level II-3)

31. O'Reilly-Green CP, Divon MY. Receiver operating characteristic curves of sonographic estimated fetal weight for prediction of macrosomia in prolonged pregnancies. Ultrasound Obstet Gynecol 1997;9:403–8. (Level II-3)

32. Chauhan SP, Lutton PM, Bailey KJ, Guerrieri JP, Morrison JC. Intrapartum clinical, sonographic, and parous patients estimates of newborn birthweight. Obstet Gynecol 1992;79:956–8. (Level II-3)

33. Raman S, Urquhart R, Yusof M. Clinical versus ultrasound estimation of fetal weight. Aust N Z J Obstet Gynaecol 1992;32:196–9. (Level II-3)

34. American College of Obstetricians and Gynecologists. Fetal macrosomia. ACOG Practice Bulletin 22. Washington, DC: ACOG; 2000. (Level III)

The MEDLINE database, the Cochrane Library, and ACOG's own internal resources and documents were used to conduct a literature search to locate relevant articles published between January 1985 and September 2004. The search was restricted to articles published in the English language. Priority was given to articles reporting results of original research, although review articles and commentaries also were consulted. Abstracts of research presented at symposia and scientific conferences were not considered adequate for inclusion in this document. Guidelines published by organizations or institutions such as the National Institutes of Health and the American College of Obstetricians and Gynecologists were reviewed, and additional studies were located by reviewing bibliographies of identified articles. When reliable research was not available, expert opinions from obstetrician–gynecologists were used.

Studies were reviewed and evaluated for quality according to the method outlined by the U.S. Preventive Services Task Force:

I   Evidence obtained from at least 1 properly designed randomized controlled trial.

II-1   Evidence obtained from well-designed controlled trials without randomization.

II-2   Evidence obtained from well-designed cohort or case–control analytic studies, preferably from more than 1 center or research group.

II-3   Evidence obtained from multiple time series with or without the intervention. Dramatic results in uncontrolled experiments also could be regarded as this type of evidence.

III   Opinions of respected authorities, based on clinical experience, descriptive studies, or reports of expert committees.

Based on the highest level of evidence found in the data, recommendations are provided and graded according to the following categories:

Level A—Recommendations are based on good and consistent scientific evidence.

Level B—Recommendations are based on limited or inconsistent scientific evidence.

Level C—Recommendations are based primarily on consensus and expert opinion.

ISSN 1099-3630

The American College of Obstetricians and Gynecologists
409 12th Street, SW, PO Box 96920, Washington, DC 20090-6920

12345/87654

Ultrasonography in pregnancy. ACOG Practice Bulletin No. 58. American College of Obstetricians and Gynecologists. Obstet Gynecol 2004;104:1449–58.

ACOG PRACTICE BULLETIN

CLINICAL MANAGEMENT GUIDELINES FOR
OBSTETRICIAN–GYNECOLOGISTS

NUMBER 63, JUNE 2005

This Practice Bulletin was developed by the ACOG Committee on Practice Bulletins—Gynecology with the assistance of Mark D. Walters, MD. The information is designed to aid practitioners in making decisions about appropriate obstetric and gynecologic care. These guidelines should not be construed as dictating an exclusive course of treatment or procedure. Variations in practice may be warranted based on the needs of the individual patient, resources, and limitations unique to the institution or type of practice.

Urinary Incontinence in Women

Numerous techniques have been developed to evaluate the types and extent of urinary incontinence. A number of treatment options exist, including behavioral, medical, and surgical approaches. The purpose of this document is to consider the best available evidence for evaluating and treating urinary incontinence in women.

Background

Etiology

Urinary incontinence affects 10–70% of women living in a community setting and up to 50% of nursing home residents (1). Prevalence of incontinence appears to increase gradually during young adult life, has a broad peak around middle age, and then steadily increases in the elderly (2). Most women with incontinence do not seek medical help (3). The estimated annual direct cost of urinary incontinence in women in the United States is $12.43 billion (4).

Among women experiencing urinary incontinence, the differential diagnosis includes genitourinary and nongenitourinary conditions (see box, "Differential Diagnosis of Urinary Incontinence in Women"). Some conditions that cause or contribute to urinary incontinence are potentially reversible (see box, "Common Causes of Transient Urinary Incontinence").

The relative likelihood of each condition causing incontinence varies with the age and health of the individual. Among ambulatory women with incontinence, the most common condition is urodynamic stress incontinence, which represents 29–75% of cases. Detrusor overactivity accounts for 7–33% of incontinence cases, with the remainder being mixed forms (3). Among older, noninstitutionalized women with incontinence evaluated in referral centers, stress incontinence is found less often, and detrusor abnormalities and mixed disorders are more common than in younger ambulatory women. More severe and troublesome incontinence probably occurs with increasing age, especially age older than 70 years (3).

Differential Diagnosis of Urinary Incontinence in Women

Genitourinary etiology

- Filling and storage disorders
  - Urodynamic stress incontinence
  - Detrusor overactivity (idiopathic)
  - Detrusor overactivity (neurogenic)
  - Mixed types
- Fistula
  - Vesical
  - Ureteral
  - Urethral
- Congenital
  - Ectopic ureter
  - Epispadias

Nongenitourinary etiology

- Functional
  - Neurologic
  - Cognitive
  - Psychologic
  - Physical impairment
- Environmental
- Pharmacologic
- Metabolic

Common Causes of Transient Urinary Incontinence

- Urinary tract infection or urethritis
- Atrophic urethritis or vaginitis
- Drug side effects
- Pregnancy
- Increased urine production
  - Metabolic (hyperglycemia, hypercalcemia)
  - Excess fluid intake
  - Volume overload
- Delirium
- Restricted mobility
- Stool impaction
- Psychologic

Diagnosis

The history and physical examination are the first and most important steps in evaluation. A preliminary diagnosis can be made with simple office and laboratory tests, with initial therapy based on these findings. If complex conditions are present, the patient does not improve after initial therapy, or surgery is being considered, definitive, specialized studies may be necessary.

History and Voiding Diary

In addition to patient history, daily urinary diaries are considered a practical and reliable method of obtaining information on voiding behavior because patient recall by history taking may be unreliable (5). Urinary diaries of diurnal voiding frequency, nocturnal voiding frequency, and number of incontinence episodes have been shown to be highly reproducible and correlated well with urodynamic diagnosis (6). Most authors recommend documentation of symptoms for a 3- to 7-day period (6–8). Consistent results have been shown between the first 3-day period and the last 4-day period, suggesting that a 3-day chart may be adequate to document symptoms, thus improving compliance (8).

After the urologic history, thorough medical, surgical, gynecologic, neurologic, and obstetric histories should be obtained. Certain medical and neurologic conditions, such as diabetes, stroke, and lumbar disk disease, may cause urinary incontinence. Furthermore, strong coughing associated with smoking or chronic pulmonary disease can markedly worsen symptoms of stress incontinence. A bowel history is important because anal incontinence and constipation are relatively more common in women with urinary incontinence and pelvic organ prolapse. A history of hysterectomy, vaginal repair, pelvic radiotherapy, or retropubic surgery should alert the physician to possible effects of prior surgery on the lower urinary tract.

A complete list of the patient's medications (including nonprescription medications) should be obtained. This is important to determine whether individual drugs may be influencing the function of the bladder or urethra, leading to urinary incontinence or voiding difficulties (Table 1).

Physical Examination

General, gynecologic, and lower neurologic examinations are needed on every woman with incontinence. Palpation of the anterior vaginal wall and urethra may elicit urethral discharge or tenderness that suggests a urethral diverticulum or other inflammatory or neoplastic conditions of the urethra. Vaginal discharge can mimic incontinence. The pelvic examination is of primary importance to assess vulvar and vaginal atrophy in menopausal women.

Table 1. Medications That Can Affect Lower Urinary Tract Function

Type of Medication	Lower Urinary Tract Effects
Diuretics	Polyuria, frequency, urgency
Caffeine	Frequency, urgency
Alcohol	Sedation, impaired mobility, diuresis
Narcotic analgesics	Urinary retention, fecal impaction, sedation, delirium
Anticholinergic agents	Urinary retention, voiding difficulty
Antihistamines	Anticholinergic actions, sedation
Psychotropic agents	
Antidepressants	Anticholinergic actions, sedation
Antipsychotics	Anticholinergic actions, sedation
Sedatives and hypnotics	Sedation, muscle relaxation, confusion
Alpha-adrenergic blockers	Stress incontinence
Alpha-adrenergic agonists	Urinary retention, voiding difficulty
Calcium-channel blockers	Urinary retention, voiding difficulty

Modified from Parsons M, Cardozo L. Female urinary incontinence in practice. London: The Royal Society of Medicine Press; 2004. p. 36. http://www.rsmpress.co.uk/bkparsons.htm.

The presence and severity of anterior vaginal relaxation, including cystocele and proximal urethral detachment and mobility, or anterior vaginal scarring, are important to estimate. Associated pelvic support abnormalities, such as posterior vaginal prolapse (rectocele or enterocele) and uterovaginal or apical prolapse, also should be noted. The amount or severity of prolapse in each vaginal segment may be measured and recorded using a method such as the Pelvic Organ Prolapse Quantification System (9). A bimanual examination is useful to rule out coexistent gynecologic pathology, and the anal sphincter should be examined for evidence of prior lacerations or weakness. A rectal examination is useful to further evaluate pelvic and anorectal pathology and fecal impaction, the latter of which may be associated with voiding difficulties and incontinence in older women. Urinary incontinence has been shown to improve or resolve after the removal of fecal impactions in institutionalized geriatric patients (10).

Urinary incontinence may be the presenting symptom of neurologic disease. The screening neurologic examination should include mental status as well as sensory and motor function of the perineum and both lower extremities. Sacral segments 2 through 4 contain the important neurons controlling micturition. The strength and tone of the bulbocavernosus muscle, levators, and external anal sphincter can be estimated digitally. Lower extremity motor function and sensory function along the sacral dermatomes are important to evaluate. The anal reflex and the bulbocavernosus reflex can be used to assess sacral reflex activity. However, these reflexes can be difficult to evaluate clinically (11).

Measuring Urethral Mobility

Predicting the amount of urethral mobility by examination of the anterior vaginal wall is inaccurate. It is difficult to differentiate between cystocele and rotational descent of the urethra with physical examination, and the two often coexist. Placement of a cotton swab in the urethra to the level of the vesical neck and measurement of the axis change with straining (ie, Q-tip test) may be used to demonstrate urethral mobility. Measuring urethral mobility aids in the diagnosis of stress incontinence and in planning treatment for this condition (eg, bladder neck suspension versus periurethral injection of bulking agents).

Because most women with primary urodynamic stress incontinence have urethral hypermobility, a nonmobile urethra should prompt consideration of urodynamic testing. The measurement of urethral mobility is not useful in differentiating urodynamic stress incontinence from abnormalities of voiding or detrusor function because these diagnoses require the measurement of detrusor pressure during filling and emptying. Other tests, such as perineal ultrasonography and magnetic resonance imaging, can be used for assessment of bladder neck mobility, but these are not commonly used in clinical practice.

Laboratory Tests

Few laboratory tests are necessary for the evaluation of incontinence. A clean midstream or catheterized urine sample should be obtained for dipstick urinalysis. If significant bacteriuria is found, antibiotics are appropriate, and the patient can be reevaluated in several weeks.

Blood testing (blood urea nitrogen, creatinine, glucose, and calcium) is recommended if compromised renal function is suspected or if polyuria (in the absence of diuretics) is present. Urine cytology is not recommended in the routine evaluation of the patient with incontinence (12, 13). However, patients with microscopic hematuria (two to five red blood cells per high-power field), those older than 50 years with persistent hematuria (14), or those with acute onset of irritative voiding symptoms in the absence of urinary tract infection may require cystoscopy and cytology to exclude bladder neoplasm.

Office Evaluation of Bladder Filling and Voiding

During office assessment, the specific circumstances leading to the involuntary loss of urine should be determined. If possible, such circumstances should be reproduced and directly observed during clinical evaluation. The amount of urine and the time required can be evaluated by normal voiding in the office setting, and the volume of residual urine can then be noted by transurethral catheterization or ultrasound examination of the bladder. A sterile urine sample can be obtained at this time if necessary. A syringe without its piston or bulb can be used to fill the bladder with sterile water to assess bladder capacity. Once the catheter is removed, a cough stress test can be performed to evaluate stress incontinence.

Urodynamic Tests

Cystometry is a test of detrusor function and can be used to assess bladder sensation, capacity, and compliance and to determine the presence and magnitude of both voluntary and involuntary detrusor contractions. Cystometry can be simple and office based or it can be multichannel, including measurement of intraabdominal, bladder, and detrusor (bladder minus intraabdominal) pressures.

Urodynamic tests also are valuable for the assessment of voiding function. Uroflowmetry is an electronic measure of urine flow rate and pattern. Combined with assessment of postvoid residual urine volume, it is a screening test for voiding dysfunction. If the uroflowmetry and postvoid residual urine volume are normal, voiding function is probably normal; however, if the uroflowmetry or postvoid residual urine volume or both are abnormal, further testing is necessary to determine the cause. More sophisticated measures of voiding function include a pressure-flow voiding study with or without videofluoroscopy. Electromyography of the striated urethral sphincter may be useful to assess neurogenic voiding dysfunction.

Normal values for postvoid residual urine volume measurements have not been established. Volumes less than 50 mL indicate adequate bladder emptying, and volumes greater than 200 mL can be considered inadequate emptying. Clinical judgment must be exercised in interpreting the significance of postvoid residual urine volumes, especially in the intermediate range of 50–200 mL. Because isolated instances of elevated residual urine volume may not be significant, the test should be repeated when abnormally high values are obtained.

Cystourethroscopy

Cystourethroscopy may help to identify bladder lesions and foreign bodies, as well as urethral diverticula, fistulas, urethral strictures, and intrinsic sphincter deficiency. It frequently is used as part of the surgical procedures to treat incontinence and is an important component of the evaluation of postoperative incontinence and other intraoperative and postoperative lower urinary tract complications.

Management Options

Absorbent products are the most common method used to actively manage urinary incontinence among community residents (3). Many individuals with mild symptoms or with incontinence that cannot be cured depend on barrier management.

Behavioral Approaches

For women who desire treatment, several behavior modifications can be incorporated, including lifestyle interventions, scheduled or prompted voiding, bladder training, and pelvic muscle rehabilitation. Lifestyle interventions that may help modify incontinence include weight loss, caffeine reduction and fluid management, reduction of physical forces (eg, work, exercise), cessation of smoking, and relief of constipation (1). Other lifestyle alterations are not well supported by published literature.

Bladder training is widely used with no reported side effects and does not limit future treatment options. Also known as bladder drills or timed voiding, it generally is used for the treatment of urge incontinence, but it also may improve symptoms of mixed and stress incontinence. This method aims to increase the time interval between voiding, by either a mandatory or self-adjusted schedule. It is most effective for patients who are physically and cognitively able and who are motivated. Bladder training generally is improved with patient education, the use of scheduled voiding, and positive reinforcement by trained health care professionals (15).

Pelvic muscle exercises, also called Kegel and pelvic floor exercises, are performed to strengthen the voluntary periurethral and perivaginal muscles (voluntary urethral sphincter and levator ani). Pelvic muscle exercises may be used alone or augmented with bladder training, biofeedback, or electrical stimulation. Health care providers can teach patients the correct method of distinguishing and contracting the pelvic muscles.

Medical Management

The urethra and bladder contain a rich supply of estrogen receptors; therefore, it is biologically feasible that estrogen therapy affects postmenopausal urogenital symptoms. However, trials have demonstrated an increase in urinary incontinence with estrogen therapy.

A number of other pharmacologic agents appear to be effective for frequency, urgency, and urge incontinence. However, the response to treatment often is unpredictable, and side effects are common with effective doses. Generally, drugs improve detrusor overactivity by inhibiting the contractile activity of the bladder. These agents can be broadly classified into anticholinergic agents, tricyclic antidepressants, musculotropic drugs, and a variety of less commonly used drugs.

Surgical Treatments

Many surgical treatments have been developed for stress urinary incontinence, but only a few—retropubic colposuspension and sling procedures—have survived and evolved with enough supporting evidence to make recommendations. Contemporary, less invasive modifications of these operations are being performed, and studies assessing their efficacy are ongoing.

Procedures. The basic goal of retropubic colposuspension is to suspend and stabilize the anterior vaginal wall, and, thus, the bladder neck and proximal urethra, in a retropubic position. This prevents their descent and allows for urethral compression against a stable suburethral layer.

Most recent studies are performed with colposuspension techniques using two or three nonabsorbable sutures on each side of the mid urethra and bladder neck. One randomized trial of patients undergoing laparoscopic Burch procedures for stress incontinence showed that two sutures on each side of the urethra resulted in a significantly higher cure rate than one suture (16).

The tension-free vaginal tape procedure is based on a theory that the pathophysiology of stress urinary incontinence is the impairment of the pubourethral ligaments (17). A narrow strip of polypropylene mesh is placed at the mid urethra to compensate for this inefficiency. The success of tension-free vaginal tape has led to the introduction of similar products with modified methods of mid-urethral sling placement (retropubic "top-down" and transobturator). The use of these other materials and modified methods compared with tension-free vaginal tape has yet to be fully evaluated.

A number of bulking agents have been used for the treatment of urodynamic stress incontinence with intrinsic sphincter deficiency in women. The bulking agents (collagen, carbon-coated beads, and fat) are injected transurethrally or periurethrally in the periurethral tissue around the bladder neck and proximal urethra. They provide a "washer" effect around the proximal urethra and the bladder neck. These agents usually are used as second-line therapy after surgery has failed, when stress incontinence persists with a nonmobile bladder neck, or among older, debilitated women for whom any form of operative treatment may be especially hazardous.

Complications. Intraoperative or immediate postoperative complications of surgery for stress incontinence include direct surgical injury to the lower urinary tract, hemorrhage, bowel injury, wound complications, retention, and urinary tract infection. Gynecologic surgeons may perform cystoscopy during or after retropubic and sling procedures to verify ureteral patency and the absence of sutures or sling material in the bladder. Most of the chronic complications after Burch colposuspension and sling procedures relate to voiding dysfunction and urge symptoms (Table 2).

Incontinence With Pelvic Organ Prolapse. Urinary incontinence frequently coexists with uterine prolapse and descent of the anterior vaginal wall. Symptoms of stress incontinence can be overt, or the patient can be asymptomatic but will develop stress incontinence if the vaginal prolapse is reduced or repaired (potential stress incontinence).

Table 2. Complication Rates Following Surgical Treatment for Stress Urinary Incontinence

Complication	Rate	Procedure
Bladder perforation	3–9%	Tension-free tape[1,2]
	2%	Colposuspension[1]
Detrusor overactivity/urge incontinence	5–27%	Burch colposuspension[3]
	0–30%	Sling[4,5]
	6%	Tension-free tape[6]
Erosion of surgical materials	≤5%	Sling[5]
Sling revision or removal	5–35%	Sling[7]
Voiding disorders	2–37%	Sling[8]
	4–11%	Tension-free tape[1,2,9]

[1]Ward K, Hilton P. Prospective multicentre randomised trial of tension-free vaginal tape and colposuspension as primary treatment for stress incontinence. United Kingdom and Ireland Tension-free Vaginal Tape Trial Group. BMJ 2002;325:67–70.

[2]Tamussino KF, Hanzal E, Kolle D, Ralph G, Riss PA. Tension-free vaginal tape operation: results of the Austrian registry. Austrian Urogynecology Working Group. Obstet Gynecol 2001;98:732–6.

[3]Dainer M, Hall CD, Choe J, Bhatia NN. The Burch procedure: a comprehensive review. Obstet Gynecol Surv 1999;54:49–60.

[4]Bezerra CA, Bruschini H, Cody DJ. Suburethral sling operations for urinary incontinence in women. The Cochrane Database of Systematic Reviews 2001, Issue 3. Art. No.: CD001754. DOI: 10.1002/14651858.CD001754.

[5]Bidmead J, Cardozo L. Sling techniques in the treatment of genuine stress incontinence. BJOG 2000;107:147–56.

[6]Nilsson CG, Falconer C, Rezapour M. Seven-year follow-up of the tension-free vaginal tape procedure for treatment of urinary incontinence. Obstet Gynecol 2004;104:1259–62.

[7]Persson J, Iosif C, Wolner-Hanssen P. Risk factors for rejection of synthetic suburethral slings for stress urinary incontinence: a case-control study. Obstet Gynecol 2002;99:629–34.

[8]Jarvis GJ. Surgery for genuine stress incontinence. Br J Obstet Gynaecol 1994; 101:371–4.

[9]Klutke C, Siegel S, Carlin B, Paszkiewicz E, Kirkemo A, Klutke J. Urinary retention after tension-free vaginal tape procedure: incidence and treatment. Urology 2001;58:697–701.

Clinical Considerations and Recommendations

▶ *When is office evaluation of bladder filling, voiding, or cystometry useful for evaluation of incontinence?*

The findings of a careful history and physical examination predict the actual incontinence diagnosis with reasonable accuracy. Whenever objective clinical findings do not correlate with or reproduce the patient's symptoms, simple bladder filling and cough stress tests are useful. When trials of therapy are used, patients must be monitored periodically to evaluate response. If the patient fails to improve to her satisfaction, appropriate further testing is indicated. Of women who have the symptom of stress incontinence as their only symptom, 10–30% are found to have bladder overactivity (alone or coexistent with urodynamic stress incontinence) or other rare conditions.

Retrograde bladder filling provides an assessment of bladder sensation and an estimate of bladder capacity. Patients without urgency and frequency who note a sensation of bladder fullness and have an estimated bladder capacity that is within normal range probably have normal bladder filling function. The definition of normal bladder capacity lacks consensus, with values that range from 300 mL to 750 mL. In addition, large bladder capacities are not always pathologic. Researchers showed that 33% of women with bladder capacities greater than 800 mL were urodynamically normal, and only 13% had true bladder atony (18).

Loss of small amounts of urine in spurts, simultaneous with coughing and in the absence of urge, strongly suggests a diagnosis of urodynamic stress incontinence (19, 20). Prolonged loss of urine, leaking 5–10 seconds after coughing, or no urine loss with provocation indicates that other causes of incontinence, especially detrusor overactivity, may be present. The inability to demonstrate the sign of stress incontinence during simple bladder filling and cough stress test correlates highly with the absence of urodynamic stress incontinence (20, 21). Interpretation of these office tests can be difficult because of artifact introduced by increases in intraabdominal pressure caused by straining or patient movement. Borderline or negative test results should be repeated to maximize their diagnostic accuracy.

Limited data support the need for cystometric testing in the routine or basic evaluation of urinary incontinence. It is indicated as part of the evaluation of more complex disorders of bladder filling and voiding, such as the presence of neurologic disease and other comorbid conditions.

Multichannel or subtracted cystometry allows more precise measurements of detrusor pressures with filling and voiding, although both false-positive and false-negative test results generally are found with cystometry. No studies have determined whether the addition of multichannel cystometry or video assessment over simple filling cystometry improves diagnostic accuracy or outcomes after treatment. Other complex urodynamic tests, such as a pressure-flow voiding study, uroflowmetry, and electromyography of the urethral sphincter, are available for the assessment of complex and neurogenic causes of urinary incontinence and voiding disorders.

Even under the most typical clinical situations, the diagnosis of incontinence based only on clinical evaluation may be uncertain. This diagnostic uncertainty may be acceptable if medical or behavioral treatment (as opposed to surgery) is planned because of the low morbidity and cost of these treatments and because the ramifications of continued incontinence are not severe. When surgical treatment of stress incontinence is planned, urodynamic testing often is recommended to confirm the diagnosis, unless the patient has an uncomplicated history and compatible physical findings of stress incontinence and has not had previous surgery for incontinence.

▶ *When are urethral pressure profilometry and leak point pressure measurements useful for evaluation of incontinence?*

Based on extensive review of the evidence, researchers found that urethral pressure profilometry is not standardized, reproducible, or able to contribute to the differential diagnosis in women with stress incontinence symptoms (22). Therefore, it does not meet the criteria for a useful diagnostic test (22). Leak point pressure measures the amount of increase in intraabdominal pressure that causes stress incontinence, although its usefulness also has not been proved (23).

▶ *When is cystoscopy useful for evaluation of incontinence?*

Cystoscopy is indicated for the evaluation of patients with incontinence who have sterile hematuria or pyuria; irritative voiding symptoms, such as frequency, urgency, and urge incontinence, in the absence of any reversible causes; bladder pain; recurrent cystitis; suburethral mass; and when urodynamic testing fails to duplicate symptoms of urinary incontinence (24). Bladder lesions are found in less than 2% of patients with incontinence (25, 26); therefore, cystoscopy should not be performed routinely in patients with incontinence to exclude neoplasm.

▶ *Are pessaries and medical devices effective for the treatment of urinary incontinence?*

Pessaries and other mechanical devices modified to selectively support the bladder neck may be effective for treating some cases of urinary incontinence, but objective evidence regarding their effectiveness has not been reported (1). Replacement of the prolapsed anterior vaginal wall with a pessary may unmask incontinence by straightening out the urethrovesical kinking that may have been responsible for either continence or some degree of urinary retention.

▶ *Are behavior modifications (eg, bladder retraining, biofeedback, weight loss) effective for the treatment of urinary incontinence?*

In one study, behavioral therapy that included group and individual instruction, individualized scheduled voiding, diary keeping, and instructions on pelvic muscle exercises resulted in a 50% reduction in the mean number of incontinence episodes (compared with a 15% reduction in controls; $P = .001$), and this was maintained for 6 months (27). Thirty-one percent of women were 100% improved (dry), 41% were at least 75% improved, and 52% were at least 50% improved. There were no differences in treatment efficacy by type of incontinence (stress, urge, mixed) (27). Data show that behavioral training with biofeedback resulted in a 63% mean reduction in incontinence episodes, compared with a 69% mean reduction following verbal feedback and a 59% mean reduction after receiving a self-help booklet (differences not significant) (28). Patient satisfaction was highest in the verbal feedback group and lowest in the self-help booklet group. For stress incontinence, behavioral training reduced the mean number of incontinence episodes by 69%; the addition of pelvic floor electrical stimulation did not result in significantly greater improvement than behavioral training alone (29). Therefore, behavioral therapy improves symptoms of urge and mixed incontinence and can be recommended as a noninvasive treatment in many women.

Researchers showed that combining drug and behavioral therapy in a stepped program can produce added benefit for patients with urge incontinence (30). However, there is not enough evidence to show whether drug therapy is better than bladder training or useful as a supplement (31).

Obesity appears to be an independent risk factor for the development of incontinence, with obese women having a 4.2-fold greater risk of stress urinary incontinence than those with a normal body mass index (32–35). Few published intervention studies have investigated incontinence after weight loss, and these addressed only the effects of massive weight loss in morbidly obese women (36, 37).

▶ *Are pelvic muscle exercises effective for the treatment of urinary incontinence?*

Pelvic floor training appears to be an effective treatment for adult women with stress and mixed incontinence (38), and pelvic muscle exercises appear better than no treatment or placebo. Pelvic muscle exercise reduces incontinence and increases vaginal pressure measurements, but direct correlations between these alterations are weak (39). Pelvic muscle exercise appears to be superior to electrical stimulation and vaginal cones in the treatment of stress incontinence (40). Bladder training, pelvic muscle exercise, or their combination appeared equal in symptom improvement and urodynamic parameters in one randomized trial (41). Generally, the effect of adding pelvic muscle training to other treatments for stress urinary incontinence and the effects of pelvic muscle exercise on urge incontinence alone remain unclear (38).

▶ *Is pharmacotherapy (eg, estrogen, tolterodine, oxybutynin, imipramine) effective for the treatment of urinary incontinence?*

The effect of postmenopausal hormone therapy (HT) on urinary incontinence has been evaluated in several randomized controlled trials. One trial studied postmenopausal women with at least one episode of incontinence weekly at baseline, randomized to receive either HT or placebo (42). Exacerbation of incontinence occurred in 39% of the HT group and 27% of the placebo group ($P = .001$). In a subset analysis of the Women's Health Initiative study, postmenopausal women both with and without symptoms of incontinence were randomized to receive a) combined HT or placebo or b) unopposed estrogen therapy or placebo (43). Both combined therapy and unopposed estrogen were found to increase the incidence of urinary incontinence among women without symptoms at baseline. For those women with symptoms at baseline, frequency increased in both the combined therapy and unopposed estrogen groups.

Other smaller studies have examined the use of oral estrogen preparations in the treatment of stress or urge incontinence and found that the use of estrogen did not reduce incontinence (44–47). Therefore, oral estrogen regimens cannot be recommended as treatment or prevention for any type of urinary incontinence.

Several meta-analyses addressing drug therapy for bladder overactivity have been published (48, 49). The anticholinergic drugs oxybutynin chloride and tolterodine have five or more randomized controlled trials each; these trials report a small beneficial effect of anticholinergic drug treatment as therapy for urge incontinence (48). However, for many of the outcomes studied, the observed differences between treatment with anticholinergic medications and placebo may be of questionable clinical significance (49). No significant difference among these agents was reported. The most typical side effect of anticholinergic therapy is dry mouth; other side effects most frequently reported were blurred vision, constipation, nausea, dizziness, and headache (48). Alternative drugs, new drugs, and new formulations of existing drugs are all available, but limited data exist on which to base recommendations.

▶ Is there a role for bulking agents in the treatment of urinary incontinence?

Most of the reported studies have used glutaraldehyde cross-linked collagen as the bulking agent. Reviewers summarized the literature on cross-linked bovine collagen for the treatment of stress incontinence and intrinsic sphincter deficiency (50). Most patients in the studies had failed incontinence surgeries and had a supported nonmobile bladder neck. Seventeen studies were cited with cure rates ranging from 7% to 83% over a 10-year period. The cure rate, defined in 15 articles as completely dry, averaged 48%. An overall average of 76% of subjects (range, 68–90%) were listed as "dry" or "improved" (50). The limitations of existing bulking agents are their durability and long-term results.

For women with extensive comorbidity precluding surgery or anesthesia or both, injection of bulking agents may provide a useful option for relief of symptoms for a 12-month period. Two or three injections are likely to be required to achieve a satisfactory result (51).

▶ When is surgery indicated for urinary incontinence?

Surgery is indicated for the treatment of stress urinary incontinence when conservative treatments have failed to satisfactorily relieve the symptoms and the patient wishes further treatment in an effort to achieve continence. It is desirable if the patient does not wish to have more children, although retaining fertility potential is not a contraindication of surgery. However, there is no evidence on the effect of subsequent pregnancy.

Not all patients with urinary incontinence need urodynamic testing before surgery. These patients include women who lose urine only with physical exertion; have normal voiding habits (<8 voiding episodes per day, <2 per night); have no associated findings on neurologic or physical examination; have no history of antiincontinence or radical pelvic surgery; possess a hypermobile urethra, pliable vaginal wall, and adequate vaginal capacity on physical examination; have a normal postvoid residual volume; and are not pregnant.

Patients who are thought to have detrusor overactivity on clinical evaluation can be given appropriate behavioral or medical therapy, and a substantial percentage of patients can be expected to respond (52). Even patients with mixed disorders (coexistent stress and urge incontinence) respond to various forms of conservative therapy (53, 54).

▶ Which type of surgery is indicated in the treatment of urinary incontinence?

Retropubic colposuspension procedures are indicated for women with the diagnosis of urodynamic stress incontinence and a hypermobile proximal urethra and bladder neck. Selection of a retropubic approach (versus a sling) depends on many factors, such as the need for laparotomy for other pelvic disease, the amount of pelvic organ prolapse and whether a vaginal or abdominal procedure will be used to suspend the vagina, the age and health status of the patient, and the preferences of the patient and surgeon. Although retropubic procedures can be used for intrinsic sphincter deficiency with urethral hypermobility, sling operations may yield better long-term results. Hysterectomy adds little to the efficacy of Burch colposuspension in curing stress incontinence (55), and it should be performed only for specific uterine pathology or for the treatment of uterine prolapse.

One consensus panel review indicated that after 48 months, retropubic suspensions and sling procedures seem to be more efficacious than transvaginal needle suspension procedures or anterior colporrhaphy (56). The authors also noted that retropubic suspensions and sling procedures are associated with slightly higher complication rates, including longer convalescence and postoperative voiding dysfunction. Clinical outcomes of the tension-free vaginal tape procedure and other mid-urethral slings were not available at the time of the consensus panel review.

Several review articles have been published summarizing the cure rates of retropubic procedures compared with other procedures for the treatment of urodynamic stress incontinence. Open abdominal retropubic suspension appears to be better than anterior vaginal repair, even in women with prolapse, judged on subjective cure rates in six trials (57).

A multicenter randomized trial found no difference between Burch colposuspension and tension-free vaginal tape procedures, with objective cure rates for urodynamic stress incontinence of 57% and 66%, respectively (58). Bladder injury was more common during the tension-free vaginal tape procedure ($P = .013$); delayed voiding, operation time ($P < .001$), and return to normal activity ($P < .001$) were all longer after colposuspension (58).

In a cohort of women who underwent Burch colposuspension, the cure rate of stress incontinence gradually decreased over 10–12 years, reaching a plateau at 69% (59). Cure rates were significantly lower in women who had previous bladder neck surgery ($P = .02$). Approximately 10% of patients required at least one additional surgery to cure their stress incontinence (59).

Only a few studies have assessed the paravaginal defect repair for stress incontinence. A prospective randomized trial found that only 61% of women were continent 3 years after a paravaginal defect repair, compared with 100% of women who were continent 3 years after a Burch colposuspension ($P = .004$) (60). The paravaginal defect repair should not be used as primary treatment of urodynamic stress incontinence.

Laparoscopic access can be used to perform a Burch colposuspension, and this technique has become popular with some physicians and patients. However, it remains to be proved whether laparoscopic colposuspension yields cure rates equal to open Burch colposuspension for stress incontinence in women. One recent randomized trial comparing open Burch colposuspension with laparoscopic colposuspension showed significantly higher objective and subjective stress incontinence cure rates in the open Burch group ($P < .001$) (61); however, the results of most other studies comparing the two techniques are inconclusive (62, 63).

Long-term objective results of the tension-free vaginal tape procedure for primary stress incontinence were shown in a multicenter trial; at a median follow-up of 56 months, 85% of patients were objectively and subjectively cured, 10.6% were improved, and 4.7% were regarded as failures (64). There were no cases of mesh erosion or permanent retention. Two randomized trials comparing the results of tension-free vaginal tape with Burch colposuspension showed similar objective and subjective cure rates from both procedures (58, 65). However, a recent randomized trial of laparoscopic Burch colposuspension and tension-free tape procedures showed higher objective cure rates for urodynamic stress incontinence for tension-free tape procedures, although quality of life and satisfaction scores were similar between procedures (66).

Two large cohort studies have assessed the results of pubovaginal fascial bladder neck sling for stress incontinence. At a mean follow-up of 51 months (range 22–68), continence rates were 88% overall (67). Preoperative urge incontinence resolved in 81 of 109 women (74%),

whereas de novo urgency developed in 7% of women. In patient questionnaires, 92% reported a high degree of satisfaction with low symptom distress scores. In another study of 251 women, permanent urinary retention developed in 2% of patients (68).

The intermediate and long-term results for suburethral slings suggest that the 10-year continence rate is similar to the 1-year continence rate (69). In fact, it appears that sling procedures that are effective after 6 months are likely to remain effective for many years (69).

▶ *For patients with both prolapse and urinary incontinence, what surgical procedures are appropriate?*

Patients with vaginal prolapse with coexistent symptomatic stress incontinence have a number of treatment options. Treatment choice often depends on patient characteristics and the surgeon's experience. If the prolapse is to be repaired abdominally, as with a sacral colpopexy, a retropubic colposuspension may be appropriate. Transvaginal prolapse repair may include a sling placed at the time of repair to treat stress incontinence.

Women who have severe pelvic organ prolapse but potential stress incontinence present a unique challenge. Data supporting specific recommendations in these patients are scarce and several opposing opinions are common. In fact, even the correct method for making the diagnosis of potential stress incontinence is controversial. For women who have significant anterior vaginal wall prolapse after their vaginal apex is suspended, appropriate repair generally is indicated. Suburethral plication of the bladder neck to stabilize a hypermobile urethra is probably appropriate in many cases. One recent randomized controlled trial of women with prolapse and potential stress incontinence showed that a tension-free vaginal tape procedure resulted in less incontinence postoperatively than a suburethral plication ($P = .01$) with similar rates of urinary retention and urge incontinence (70).

Summary of Conclusions and Recommendations

The following recommendations are based on good and consistent scientific evidence (Level A):

▶ Behavioral therapy, including bladder training and prompted voiding, improves symptoms of urge and mixed incontinence and can be recommended as a noninvasive treatment in many women.

▶ Pelvic floor training appears to be an effective treatment for adult women with stress and mixed incontinence and can be recommended as a noninvasive treatment for many women.

▶ Pharmacologic agents, especially oxybutynin and tolterodine, may have a small beneficial effect on improving symptoms of detrusor overactivity in women.

The following recommendations are based on limited or inconsistent scientific evidence (Level B):

▶ Cystometric testing is not required in the routine or basic evaluation of urinary incontinence.

▶ Bulking agents are a relatively noninvasive method of treatment for stress incontinence and can be used in women for whom any form of operative treatment is contraindicated.

▶ Long-term data suggest that Burch colposuspension and sling procedures have similar objective cure rates; therefore, selection of treatment should be based on patient characteristics and the surgeon's experience.

▶ The combination of a hysterectomy and a Burch colposuspension does not result in higher continence rates than a Burch procedure alone.

▶ Tension-free vaginal tape and open Burch colposuspension have similar success rates.

▶ Anterior colporrhaphy, needle urethropexy, and paravaginal defect repair have lower cure rates for stress incontinence than Burch colposuspension.

The following recommendations are based primarily on consensus and expert opinion (Level C):

▶ After the basic evaluation of urinary incontinence, simple cystometry is appropriate for detecting abnormalities of detrusor compliance and contractibility, measuring postvoid residual volume, and determining capacity.

▶ Patients with urinary incontinence should undergo a basic evaluation that includes a history, physical examination, measurement of postvoid residual volume, and urinalysis.

References

1. Abrams P, Cardozo L, Khoury S, Wein A, editors. Incontinence. 2nd ed. Plymouth, UK: Health Publication Ltd; 2002. (Level III)

2. Hannestad YS, Rortveit G, Sandvik H, Hunskaar S. A community-based epidemiological survey of female urinary incontinence: the Norwegian EPINCONT study. Epidemiology of Incontinence in the County of Nord-Trondelag. J Clin Epidemiol 2000;53:1150–7. (Level II-3)

3. Hunskaar S, Arnold EP, Burgio K, Diokno AC, Herzog AR, Mallett VT. Epidemiology and natural history of urinary incontinence. Int Urogynecol J Pelvic Floor Dysfunct 2000;11:301–19. (Level III)

4. Wilson L, Brown JS, Shin GP, Luc KO, Subak LL. Annual direct cost of urinary incontinence. Obstet Gynecol 2001; 98:398–406. (Level III)

5. Assessment and treatment of urinary incontinence. Scientific Committee of the First International Consultation on Incontinence. Lancet 2000;355:2153–8. (Level III)

6. Wyman JF, Choi SC, Harkins SW, Wilson MS, Fantl JA. The urinary diary in evaluation of incontinent women: a test-retest analysis. Obstet Gynecol 1988;71:812–7. (Level III)

7. Abrams P, Klevmark B. Frequency volume charts: an indispensable part of lower urinary tract assessment. Scand J Urol Nephrol Suppl 1996;179:47–53. (Level III)

8. Nygaard I, Holcomb R. Reproducibility of the seven-day voiding diary in women with stress urinary incontinence. Int Urogynecol J Pelvic Floor Dysfunct 2000;11:15–7. (Level III)

9. Bump RC, Mattiasson A, Bo K, Brubaker LP, DeLancey JO, Klarskov P, et al. The standardization of terminology of female pelvic organ prolapse and pelvic floor dysfunction. Am J Obstet Gynecol 1996;175:10–7. (Level III)

10. Ouslander JG, Schnelle JF. Incontinence in the nursing home. Ann Intern Med 1995;122:438–49. (Level III)

11. Blaivas JG, Zayed AA, Labib KB. The bulbocavernosus reflex in urology: a prospective study of 299 patients. J Urol 1981;126:197–9. (Level III)

12. Mohr DN, Offord KP, Owen RA, Melton LJ 3rd. Asymptomatic microhematuria and urologic disease. A population-based study. JAMA 1986;256:224–9. (Level III)

13. Chahal R, Gogoi NK, Sundaram SK. Is it necessary to perform urine cytology in screening patients with haematuria? Eur Urol 2001;39:283–6. (Level III)

14. Cohen RA, Brown RS. Clinical practice. Microscopic hematuria. N Engl J Med 2003;348:2330–8. (Level III)

15. Wilson D, Hay-Smith J, Bo K. Outcomes of conservative treatment. In: Cardozo L, Staskin D, editors. Textbook of female urology and urogynaecology. London: Isis Medical Media; 2001. p. 325–42. (Level III)

16. Persson J, Wolner-Hanssen P. Laparoscopic Burch colposuspension for stress urinary incontinence: a randomized comparison of one or two sutures on each side of the urethra. Obstet Gynecol 2000;95:151–5. (Level I)

17. Petros PE, Ulmsten UI. An integral theory of female urinary incontinence, experimental and clinical considerations. Acta Obstet Gynecol Scand Suppl 1990;153:7–31. (Level III)

18. Weir J, Jaques PF. Large-capacity bladder. A urodynamic survey. Urology 1974;4:544–8. (Level III)

19. Diokno AC, Wells TJ, Brink CA. Urinary incontinence in elderly women: urodynamic evaluation. J Am Geriatr Soc 1987;35:940–6. (Level III)

20. Wall LL, Wiskind AK, Taylor PA. Simple bladder filling with a cough stress test compared with subtracted cystometry for the diagnosis of urinary incontinence. Am J Obstet Gynecol 1994;171:1472–7; discussion 1477–9. (Level II-3)

21. Swift SE, Ostergard DR. Evaluation of current urodynamic testing methods in the diagnosis of genuine stress incontinence. Obstet Gynecol 1995;86:85–91. (Level II-3)

22. Weber AM. Is urethral pressure profilometry a useful diagnostic test for stress urinary incontinence? Obstet Gynecol Surv 2001;56:720–35. (Level III)

23. Weber AM. Leak point pressure measurement and stress urinary incontinence. Curr Womens Health Rep 2001; 1:45–52. (Level III)

24. Association of Professors of Gynecology and Obstetrics. Clinical management of urinary incontinence. Crofton (MD): APGO; 2004. (Level III)

25. Awad SA, Gajewski JB, Katz NO, Acker-Roy K. Final diagnosis and therapeutic implications of mixed symptoms of urinary incontinence in women. Urology 1992; 39:352–7. (Level II-2)

26. Ouslander J, Leach G, Staskin D, Abelson S, Blaustein J, Morishita L, et al. Prospective evaluation of an assessment strategy for geriatric urinary incontinence. J Am Geriatr Soc 1989;37:715–24. (Level III)

27. Subak LL, Quesenberry CP, Posner SF, Cattolica E, Soghikian K. The effect of behavioral therapy on urinary incontinence: a randomized controlled trial. Obstet Gynecol 2002;100:72–8. (Level I)

28. Burgio KL, Goode PS, Locher JL, Umlauf MG, Roth DL, Richter HE, et al. Behavioral training with and without biofeedback in the treatment of urge incontinence in older women: a randomized controlled trial. JAMA 2003;288: 2293–9. (Level I)

29. Goode PS, Burgio KL, Locher JL, Roth DL, Umlauf MG, Richter HE, et al. Effect of behavioral training with or without pelvic floor electrical stimulation on stress incontinence in women: a randomized controlled trial. JAMA 2003;290:345–52. (Level I)

30. Burgio KL, Locher JL, Goode PS. Combined behavioral and drug therapy for urge incontinence in older women. J Am Geriatr Soc 2000;48:370–4. (Level II-3)

31. Wallace SA, Roe B, Williams K, Palmer M. Bladder training for urinary incontinence in adults. The Cochrane Database of Systematic Reviews 2004, Issue 1. Art. No.: CD001308. DOI: 10.1002/14651858.CD001308.pub2. (Meta-analysis)

32. Alling Moller L, Lose G, Jorgensen T. Risk factors for lower urinary tract symptoms in women 40 to 60 years of age. Obstet Gynecol 2000;96:446–51. (Level II-3)

33. Brown JS, Seeley DG, Fong J, Black DM, Ensrud KE, Grady D. Urinary incontinence in older women: who is at risk? Study of Osteoporotic Fractures Research Group. Obstet Gynecol 1996;87:715–21. (Level II-3)

34. Parazzini F, Chiaffarino F, Lavezzari M, Giambanco V. Risk factors for stress, urge or mixed urinary incontinence in Italy. VIVA Study Group. BJOG 2003;110:927–33. (Level II-2)

35. Contreras Ortiz O. Stress urinary incontinence in the gynecological practice. Int J Gynaecol Obstet 2004;86 (suppl):S6–16. (Level III)

36. Bump RC, Sugerman HJ, Fantl JA, McClish DK. Obesity and lower urinary tract function in women: effect of surgically induced weight loss. Am J Obstet Gynecol 1992; 167:392–7; discussion 397–9. (Level II-3)

37. Deitel M, Stone E, Kassam HA, Wilk EJ, Sutherland DJ. Gynecologic-obstetric changes after loss of massive excess weight following bariatric surgery. J Am Coll Nutr 1988;7:147–52. (Level II-2)

38. Hay-Smith EJ, Bo K, Berghmans LC, Hendriks HJ, de Bie RA, van Waalwijk Doorn ES. Pelvic floor muscle training for urinary incontinence in women. The Cochrane Database of Systematic Reviews 2001, Issue 1. Art. No.: CD001407. DOI: 10.1002/14651858.CD001407. (Meta-analysis)

39. Theofrastous JP, Wyman JF, Bump RC, McClish DK, Elser DM, Bland DR, et al. Effects of pelvic floor muscle training on strength and predictions of response in the treatment of urinary incontinence. Neurourol Urodyn 2002;21:486–90. (Level I)

40. Bo K, Talseth T, Holme I. Single blind, randomised controlled trial of pelvic floor exercises, electrical stimulation, vaginal cones, and no treatment in management of genuine stress incontinence in women. BMJ 1999;318: 487–93. (Level I)

41. Elser DM, Wyman JF, McClish DK, Robinson D, Fantl JA, Bump RC. The effect of bladder training, pelvic floor muscle training, or combination training on urodynamic parameters in women with urinary incontinence. Continence Program for Women Research Group. Neurourol Urodyn 1999;18:427–36. (Level I)

42. Grady D, Brown JS, Vittinghoff E, Applegate W, Varner E, Snyder T. Postmenopausal hormones and incontinence: the Heart and Estrogen/Progestin Replacement Study. HERS Research Group. Obstet Gynecol 2001;97:116–20. (Level I)

43. Hendrix SL, Cochrane BB, Nygaard IE, Handa VL, Barnabei VM, Iglesia C, et al. Effects of estrogen with and without progestin on urinary incontinence. JAMA 2005;293:935–48. (Level I)

44. Jackson S, Shepherd A, Brookes S, Abrams P. The effect of oestrogen supplementation on post-menopausal urinary stress incontinence: a double-blind placebo-controlled trial. Br J Obstet Gynaecol 1999;106:711–8. (Level I)

45. Fantl JA, Bump RC, Robinson D, McClish DK, Wyman JF. Efficacy of estrogen supplementation in the treatment of urinary incontinence. The Continence Program for Women Research Group. Obstet Gynecol 1996;88:745–9. (Level I)

46. Wilson PD, Faragher B, Butler B, Bu'Lock D, Robinson EL, Brown AD. Treatment with oral piperazine oestrone

sulphate for genuine stress incontinence in postmenopausal women. Br J Obstet Gynaecol 1987;94:568–74. (Level I)

47. Cardozo L, Bachmann G, McClish D, Fonda D, Birgerson L. Meta-analysis of estrogen therapy in the management of urogenital atrophy in postmenopausal women: second report of the Hormones and Urogenital Therapy Committee. Obstet Gynecol 1998;92:722–7. (Meta-analysis)

48. Haeusler G, Leitich H, van Trotsenburg M, Kaider A, Tempfer CB. Drug therapy of urinary urge incontinence: a systematic review. Obstet Gynecol 2002;100:1003–16. (Level III)

49. Herbison P, Hay-Smith J, Ellis G, Moore K. Effectiveness of anticholinergic drugs compared with placebo in the treatment of overactive bladder: systematic review. BMJ 2003;326:841–4. (Meta-analysis)

50. Dmochowski RR, Appell RA. Injectable agents in the treatment of stress urinary incontinence in women: where are we now? Urology 2000;56(suppl):32–40. (Level III)

51. Pickard R, Reaper J, Wyness L, Cody DJ, McClinton S, N'Dow J. Periurethral injection therapy for urinary incontinence in women. The Cochrane Database of Systematic Reviews 2003, Issue 2. Art. No.: CD003881. DOI: 10.1002/14651858.CD003881. (Meta-analysis)

52. Davila GW, Guerette N. Current treatment options for female urinary incontinence—a review. Int J Fertil Womens Med 2004;49:102–12. (Level III)

53. Davila GW, Bernier F. Multimodality pelvic physiotherapy treatment of urinary incontinence in adult women. Int Urogynecol J 1995;6:187–94. (Level II-3)

54. Wyman JF, Fantl JA, McClish DK, Bump RC. Comparative efficacy of behavioral interventions in the management of female urinary incontinence. Continence Program for Women Research Group. Am J Obstet Gynecol 1998;179:999–1007. (Level I)

55. Langer R, Ron-El R, Neuman N, Herman A, Bukovsky I, Caspi E. The value of simultaneous hysterectomy during Burch colposuspension for urinary stress incontinence. Obstet Gynecol 1988;72:866–9. (Level I)

56. Leach GE, Dmochowski RR, Appell RA, Blaivas JG, Hadley HR, Luber KM, et al. Female Stress Urinary Incontinence Clinical Guidelines Panel summary report on surgical management of female stress urinary incontinence. The American Urological Association. J Urol 1997;158:875–80. (Level III)

57. Glazener CM, Cooper K. Anterior vaginal repair for urinary incontinence in women. The Cochrane Database of Systematic Reviews 2001, Issue 1. Art. No.: CD001755. DOI: 10.1002/14651858.CD001755. (Meta-analysis)

58. Ward K, Hilton P. Prospective multicentre randomised trial of tension-free vaginal tape and colposuspension as primary treatment for stress incontinence. United Kingdom and Ireland Tension-free Vaginal Tape Trial Group. BMJ 2002;325:67–70. (Level I)

59. Alcalay M, Monga A, Stanton SL. Burch colposuspension: a 10-20 year follow up [published erratum appears in Br J Obstet Gynaecol 1996;103:290]. Br J Obstet Gynaecol 1995;102:740–5. (Level II-3)

60. Colombo M, Milani R, Vitobello D, Maggioni A. A randomized comparison of Burch colposuspension and abdominal paravaginal defect repair for female stress urinary incontinence. Am J Obstet Gynecol 1996;175:78–84. (Level I)

61. Ankardal M, Ekerydh A, Crafoord K, Milsom I, Stjerndahl JH, Engh ME. A randomised trial comparing open burch colposuspension using sutures with laparoscopic colposuspension using mesh and staples in women with stress urinary incontinence. BJOG 2004;111: 974–81. (Level I)

62. Lapitan MC, Cody DJ, Grant AM. Open retropubic colposuspension for urinary incontinence in women. The Cochrane Database of Systematic Reviews 2003, Issue 1. Art. No.: CD002912. DOI: 10.1002/14651858. CD002912. (Meta-analysis)

63. Moehrer B, Carey M, Wilson D. Laparoscopic colposuspension: a systematic review. BJOG 2003;110:230–5. (Level III)

64. Nilsson CG, Kuuva N, Falconer C, Rezapour M, Ulmsten U. Long-term results of the tension-free vaginal tape (TVT) procedure for surgical treatment of female stress urinary incontinence. Int Urogynecol J Pelvic Floor Dysfunct 2001;12(suppl 2):S5–8. (Level II-2)

65. Liapis A, Bakas P, Creatsas G. Burch colposuspension and tension-free vaginal tape in the management of stress urinary incontinence in women. Eur Urol 2002;41: 469–73. (Level I)

66. Paraiso MF, Walters MD, Karram MM, Barber MD. Laparoscopic Burch colposuspension versus tension-free vaginal tape: a randomized trial. Obstet Gynecol 2004; 104:1249–58. (Level I)

67. Morgan TO Jr, Westney OL, McGuire EJ. Pubovaginal sling: 4-year outcome analysis and quality of life assessment. J Urol 2000;163:1845–8. (Level II-3)

68. Chaikin DC, Rosenthal J, Blaivas JG. Pubovaginal fascial sling for all types of stress urinary incontinence: long-term analysis. J Urol 1998;160:1312–6. (Level III)

69. Bidmead J, Cardozo L. Sling techniques in the treatment of genuine stress incontinence. BJOG 2000;107:147–56. (Level III)

70. Meschia M, Pifarotti P, Spennacchio M, Buonaguidi A, Gattei U, Somigliana E. A randomized comparison of tension-free vaginal tape and endopelvic fascia plication in women with genital prolapse and occult stress urinary incontinence. Am J Obstet Gynecol 2004;190:609–13. (Level I)

The MEDLINE database, the Cochrane Library, and ACOG's own internal resources and documents were used to conduct a literature search to locate relevant articles published between January 1985 and February 2005. The search was restricted to articles published in the English language. Priority was given to articles reporting results of original research, although review articles and commentaries also were consulted. Abstracts of research presented at symposia and scientific conferences were not considered adequate for inclusion in this document. Guidelines published by organizations or institutions such as the National Institutes of Health and the American College of Obstetricians and Gynecologists were reviewed, and additional studies were located by reviewing bibliographies of identified articles. When reliable research was not available, expert opinions from obstetrician–gynecologists were used.

Studies were reviewed and evaluated for quality according to the method outlined by the U.S. Preventive Services Task Force:

I   Evidence obtained from at least one properly designed randomized controlled trial.

II-1   Evidence obtained from well-designed controlled trials without randomization.

II-2   Evidence obtained from well-designed cohort or case–control analytic studies, preferably from more than one center or research group.

II-3   Evidence obtained from multiple time series with or without the intervention. Dramatic results in uncontrolled experiments also could be regarded as this type of evidence.

III   Opinions of respected authorities, based on clinical experience, descriptive studies, or reports of expert committees.

Based on the highest level of evidence found in the data, recommendations are provided and graded according to the following categories:

Level A—Recommendations are based on good and consistent scientific evidence.

Level B—Recommendations are based on limited or inconsistent scientific evidence.

Level C—Recommendations are based primarily on consensus and expert opinion.

ISSN 1099-3630

**The American College of
Obstetricians and Gynecologists
409 12th Street, SW
PO Box 96920
Washington, DC 20090-6920**

12345/98765

Urinary incontinence in women. ACOG Practice Bulletin No. 63. American College of Obstetricians and Gynecologists. Obstet Gynecol 2005;105:1533–45.

ACOG PRACTICE BULLETIN

CLINICAL MANAGEMENT GUIDELINES FOR
OBSTETRICIAN–GYNECOLOGISTS

NUMBER 28, JUNE 2001

This Practice Bulletin was developed by the ACOG Committee on Practice Bulletins— Gynecology with the assistance of Maida Taylor, MD. The information is designed to aid practitioners in making decisions about appropriate obstetric and gynecologic care. These guidelines should not be construed as dictating an exclusive course of treatment or procedure. Variations in practice may be warranted based on the needs of the individual patient, resources, and limitations unique to the institution or type of practice.

Use of Botanicals for Management of Menopausal Symptoms

Lack of confidence in the espoused benefits of hormone replacement therapy (HRT) coupled with a significant array of side effects of HRT, results in fewer than 1 in 3 women choosing to take HRT. The use of alternatives to conventional HRT has become more accessible and acceptable to many women. As more women choose these alternatives, physicians are confronted with the challenges of how to advise patients about alternative medicine and how to determine which therapies may be safe and effective. This document will examine available scientific information on alternative therapies for treatment of menopausal symptoms and provide recommendations on efficacy and potential adverse consequences.

Background

Discontent with Current Pharmaceutical Regimens

Hormone replacement therapy is associated with various side effects and complications; 30–40% of patients experience some degree of abnormal bleeding in the first year of hormone use, which often results in discontinuation of use (1). Initiating HRT also is viewed by some women as treating menopause as a medical disorder, which is seen by a large segment of the population as a natural, normal part of the aging process. In addition, many women believe that estrogen therapy may increase the risk of breast cancer, and the fear of breast cancer is most often cited as the reason for lack of initiation (2).

Complementary and Alternative Medicine

Complementary medicine can be defined as those systems, practices, interventions, modalities, professions, therapies, applications, theories, or claims that are currently not an integral part of the conventional medical system (3). Alternatively, conventional medicine refers to medicine as it is generally practiced and widely taught by medical doctors, doctors of osteopathy, and their allied health professionals (4). Alternative medicine encompasses a number of systematic medical practices based on physical assessments that differ from physiology as it is taught in Western medical institutions. The most recognizable and widely employed alternatives are biologic-based therapies such as botanical medicines, dietary supplements, vitamins, minerals, and orthomolecular medicine. In a 1998 survey, alternative medicine visits exceeded visits to conventional primary care providers, and 70% of such encounters were never discussed with the patient's regular personal physician (5). In addition, a national survey reported the highest rates of use in the groups aged 35–49 years (42%) and 50–64 years (44%) (6). Three theories were proposed by the investigator as tentative predictors of use of alternatives therapies: 1) dissatisfaction with conventional medicine; 2) viewing alternatives as more empowering because of their over-the-counter status; and 3) perceiving alternatives as more compatible with personal values or ethical or religious belief systems. Predictors of alternative care use were reported to include higher educational level, poorer health status, holistic orientation to health, having had a transformational experience changing one's world view, and several chronic health conditions such as anxiety, back problems, chronic pain, and urinary tract problems. Only 4.4% of respondents relied primarily on alternative therapies.

In 1997, out-of-pocket expenditures for alternative therapies were estimated at $27 billion, which was more than the out-of-pocket expenditures for all physician services that year (7). Recently, third-party carriers have started providing coverage for alternative therapies, sometimes assessing an extra premium for such expanded benefits.

Complementary and Alternative Medicines Used in Menopause

The symptoms associated with perimenopause and menopause stimulate a healthy concern about wellness and motivate women to undertake appropriate interventions to lower health risks associated with menopause. Interest in alternative medicine can be viewed simply as a natural extension of interest in nutrition, exercise, and other behavioral, nonpharmacologic interventions directed at maintaining well-being. Unfortunately, many of the alternatives promoted and touted as substitutes for HRT do not offer any substantiated health benefits.

According to the North American Menopause Society, nonhormonal interventions commonly used for menopause include a healthy diet, exercise, vitamins, and calcium supplements. The North American Menopause Society also indicates that more than 30% of women use acupuncture, natural estrogen, herbal supplements, or so-called plant estrogens (8). Alternative therapies to conventional HRT include botanical products, vitamins and minerals, unconventional hormones and steroids sold over-the-counter as nutritional supplements or as cosmetics, and nonproprietary single and combination estrogen and progestin preparations custom blended by compounding pharmacies.

Most studies of menopausal interventions, including phase-III clinical trials of estrogenic drugs, show a 20–30% response rate in placebo groups. Unconventional interventions need to be studied in well-controlled trials before their use can be supported. Documentation of efficacy is essential because these products should yield effective results of a magnitude large enough to warrant their costs, which are substantial.

Botanical Medicine

Up to one half of drugs commonly used today are either plant products or phytochemicals that were initially isolated from botanical material but are now synthesized by chemical processing techniques. Outside of pharmaceutical preparations, plants are used therapeutically in the form of herbs, oils, pills, teas, or tinctures (see box). In

---

Therapeutic Forms of Botanical Preparations

Bulk herbs are raw or dried plants used in toto, as pulvers or powders, or to make teas and tinctures. The powders also can be put into capsules or compounded into tablet form.

Oils are concentrates of fat-soluble chemicals from herbs, often highly concentrated, and usually used externally. Many are highly toxic if ingested.

Tablets or capsules can be compounded for ease of use and often with the intent of providing a fixed metered dose.

Teas may be used to extract solubles in herbs by adding hot water, and the "potency" is determined by the steeping time. Teas are traditionally brewed 1–2 minutes, infusions for 20–30 minutes, while preparation of a decoction requires boiling the plant material in water for 10–20 minutes.

Tinctures are alcohol-extracted concentrates usually added to water or placed directly into the mouth or under the tongue.

addition, currently used products include highly concentrated extracts of phytochemicals, synthetic derivatives, and even steroids like dehydroepiandrosterone (DHEA) and androstenedione, which are classified as food supplements because they are produced from plant precursor sterols.

Dietary Plant Estrogen/Phytoestrogens

Plants do not make estrogens in the classic sense of the term. Plants make sterol molecules, many of which exert weak estrogenic activity in animals although their effects increase when large quantities are ingested. These compounds, phytoestrogens, often possess structural similarities to more active human and animal estrogens. Plant sterols are used as the precursors for the biosynthetic production of mass-manufactured therapeutic pharmaceutical-grade steroids. A number of plants used to treat symptoms of menopause have been identified in botanical medicine texts as having estrogenic activity, but research has contradicted these traditional assumptions (9).

Phytoestrogens are classified into three groups (10):

1. Isoflavones, particularly, genistein and daidzein, are plant sterol molecules found in soy and garbanzo beans and other legumes, which are most often consumed in products like tempeh, soy, miso, and tofu. Generally, 1 g of soy protein yields 1.2–1.7 mg of isoflavones, depending on the type of soybean used as the source of the protein.

2. Lignins are a constituent of the cell wall of plants and are bioavailable as a result of the effect of intestinal bacteria on grains. The highest amounts are found in the husk of seeds used to produce oils, especially flaxseed. The whole seed added to salad or cereal, or flaxseed meal or flour can be used as a food additive.

3. Coumestans have steroidlike activity but are not a significant source of phytoestrogens for most individuals. High concentrations are found in red clover, sunflower seeds, and bean sprouts and are known to have estrogenic effects when ingested by animals.

Asian diets are typically high in soy foods and contain an average of 40–80 mg of active forms of isoflavones per day, while American diets average less than 3 mg per day. American and European diets tend to elevate plasma levels of sex hormones and decrease sex-hormone-binding-globulin concentrations, thus increasing the exposure of peripheral tissues to the effects of circulating estrogens. High-soy diets act through several mechanisms to lower effective circulating and tissue levels of steroids. High isoflavone intake may depress luteinizing hormone (LH) levels and secondarily depresses estrogen production (11, 12).

The plant lignan and isoflavonoid glycosides become hormonelike compounds with weak estrogenic and antioxidative activity through the action of intestinal flora. Red clover is a rich source of isoflavones, as well as coumestans, and is used commercially to make isoflavone supplements. These compounds exert detectable effects on circulating gonadotropins and sex steroids, suggesting that they have biological activity (12). They also can act on intracellular enzymes, protein synthesis, growth factors, cellular proliferation, differentiation, and angiogenesis. Limited observational studies on isolated populations in cross-cultural comparison suggest that the incidence of cancer and atherosclerotic disease decreases with increasing intake of bioflavonoids and that diphenolic isoflavonoids and lignans are cancer-protective compounds (13). These protective effects have accrued in populations over a lifetime. It is unclear that changing one's intake of isoflavones or soy protein at age 50 years will significantly lower the lifetime risk of these diseases. A directive advising lifelong adherence to a diet rich in a variety of fruits and vegetables while limiting the intake of animal protein and fat should apply to men and women of all ages, not just those experiencing their menopausal transition. Moreover, no single synthetic or chemical derived from soy is thought to match the benefits derived from ingesting soy foods. The effects—either beneficial or detrimental—of prolonged intake of supra-dietary levels of soy or isoflavone are unknown.

Bean products are rich sources of diphenols, which are thought to lower cancer risk by modifying hormone metabolism and production and limiting cancer cell growth. Bean foods also provide large amounts of fiber, and fiber modifies the level of sex hormones by increasing gastrointestinal motility. Fiber alters bile acid metabolism and partially interrupts the enterohepatic circulation causing increased estrogen excretion by decreasing the rate of estrogen reuptake in the enterohepatic system (14).

Manufacturing and Regulating Botanicals

The federal Dietary Supplement Health and Education Act of 1994 (DSHEA) defined dietary supplements and limited the claims that can be made on supplement labels and in supporting literature. Manufacturers are responsible for ensuring the safety of their supplement products. Supplements are neither foods nor drugs, so manufacturers do not have to provide any evidence to support purported benefits before marketing their products. The Food and Drug Administration (FDA) oversees the industry, but the Federal Trade Commission is responsible for identifying inappropriate or unsubstantiated claims and enforcing DSHEA regulations.

In 1997, the FDA proposed a new dietary supplement rule allowing supplements to make structural or functional claims, but not disease claims. Such language as "supports well-being" or "helps promote heart health" would be allowed, while statements like "lowers cholesterol" would not be permitted. Supplements that "...expressly or implicitly claim to diagnose, treat, prevent, or cure a disease...[would be] ...regarded as drugs and have to meet the safety and effectiveness standards for drugs..." (15). The American Botanical Council objects to the FDA attempting to redefine the DSHEA, while the American Medical Association supports the refined definitions.

Botanicals are subject to a high degree of variation in production. Plants grown in the field may have different amounts of active constituents due to growing conditions. Products coming out of production facilities may vary greatly in the amount of active ingredients.

The botanical industry has set up voluntary guidelines, and some manufacturers have signed agreements in kind affirming that they will produce products set to an industry-defined standard. However, without mandatory oversight, problems of adulteration, contamination, and dose standardization will continue. Consequently, buyers and their physicians need to beware.

Uses for Botanicals in Menopausal Women

A brief description of several commonly used botanicals follows. Also included are their suggested and advertised uses.

Vasomotor Symptoms

Soy Products. The effects of soy protein found in whole foods, soy protein isolates, and those of isoflavone isolates made into powders or pills may not all be the same. Even soy foods are not necessarily reliable sources of biologically active isoflavones. The alcohol processing often used in the manufacture of tofu and soy milk removes the biologically active forms, the aglyconic isoflavones. Producers of soy foods recognize that the public is interested in isoflavone supplements, and many indicate in their product labeling the amounts and forms of isoflavones found in the foodstuff. Although the mechanisms of action of soy and dietary isoflavones are not fully understood, they appear to involve binding to the estrogen receptor. For this reason, one should not assume these dietary supplements are safe for women with estrogen-dependent cancers, most importantly breast cancer.

Black Cohosh. Black cohosh was the principle ingredient in Lydia Pinkham's Vegetable Compound, an ethanolic extract sold over-the-counter in the United States and in Europe. A black cohosh extract is one of the leading botanicals sold in Germany and is the country's top selling menopausal herbal remedy. The German Commission E Monographs state that black cohosh has estrogen-like action, suppresses LH, binds to estrogen receptors, has no contraindications to its use, and that the only side effect is occasional gastric discomfort (16).

Black cohosh has been found to reduce LH levels in rats that had ovariectomies and to reduce LH levels in postmenopausal women after 8 weeks of use (17). Despite these LH effects, other studies in humans and animals indicate that black cohosh has no estrogenic effects on sex-steroid-dependent tissues. In one unpublished double-blind, randomized study, black cohosh did not affect follicle-stimulating hormone, LH, estradiol, estrone, prolactin, sex-hormone-binding globulin, endometrial thickness, or vaginal maturation index (18). No claims are made regarding cardiac or bone effects, and black cohosh is suggested only for treatment of menopausal symptoms such as hot flashes, sleep disorders, anxiety, and depression and for nonmenopausal conditions like dysmenorrhea and premenstrual syndrome.

Evening Primrose. The evening primrose plant (also called evening star) produces seeds rich in gamma linolenic acid (GLA) and also contains several anticoagulant substances. Commercial preparations made from fixed oil sources are generally 72% linolenic acid (LA) and 14% GLA. Thus, each 500-mg capsule will contain 45 mg of GLA and 365 mg of LA plus lesser amounts of oleic, palmitic, and stearic acid. Because GLA is elaborated by the placenta, and because high concentrations are found in breast milk, it is suggested that GLA is the nutritionally perfect fatty acid for humans. With respect to the gynecologic uses of GLA, evening primrose is commonly recommended for mastalgia and mastodynia, premenstrual syndrome, menopausal symptoms, and bladder symptoms.

Dong Quai. Dong Quai (also seen as Dang Gui and Tang Kuei), a type of angelica, is the most commonly prescribed Chinese herbal medicine for "female problems" (19). Dong Quai supposedly regulates and balances the menstrual cycle and is said to strengthen the uterus. Dong Quai is used in traditional Chinese medicine to nourish and "tonify" blood. It also is said to exert estrogenic activity. Most herbal practitioners seem to agree it is contraindicated during pregnancy and lactation.

Mood Disturbances

St. John's Wort. Extracts of the flower *hypericum perforatum,* known as St. John's wort, have been used for centuries to treat mild to moderate depression. The constituents include hypericin, pseudohypericin, and flavonoids. Several unconfirmed mechanisms of action for the psychotropic effects of St. John's wort have been proposed, including monamine oxidase inhibition, suppression of corticotropin-releasing hormone, and serotonin receptor blockade. Hypericin does not appear to be a monamine oxidase inhibitor (20).

Commercial preparations often contain generally recommended doses; one capsule three times a day provides a cumulative dose equivalent to the upper limit of doses found in the literature to date. Side effects are similar to, but far less than, those of standard antidepressant medications, including dry mouth, dizziness, and constipation.

Valerian Root. Valerian root, the common valerian or garden heliotrope, has been used traditionally as a tranquilizer and soporific. The active constituent has never been identified but is thought to be a gamma aminobutyric acid (GABA) derivative. Note that a similar GABA-like compound has been found in chamomile, which is also proffered as an herbal sleep aid. Before the advent of benzodiazepines and barbiturates, many psychiatric disorders were treated with valerian. Although it has no demonstrable toxicity and degrades rapidly, there have been reports of dystonic reactions and visual disturbances, perhaps mediated by other drugs used concomitantly. Little is known about the actions, effects, or potential interactions of valerian with other drugs. After L-tryptophan was taken off the market, valerian use became popular again. Most botanical texts advise against its use during pregnancy and lactation.

Loss of Libido/Vaginal Dryness/Dyspareunia

Chasteberry. Chasteberry or vitex also is known as Chaste tree, Monk's pepper, agnus castus, Indian spice, sage tree hemp, and tree wild pepper. It has been recommended by some for vaginal dryness at menopause and also for depression. Vitex contains hormonelike substances, which competitively bind receptors and produce antiandrogenic effects; it is often recommended to reduce libido in males because of its proposed value as an anti-aphrodisiac. Antithetically, vitex also is recommended by some to enhance libido in menopausal women.

In vitro and animal studies have suggested that vitex inhibits prolactin, and perhaps explains the purported benefit of recommending vitex for mastalgia and pre-menstrual syndrome. A placebo-controlled, double-blind clinical trial of 20 male subjects used 120-, 240-, and 480-mg extracts of vitex, which did not demonstrate any effect on prolactin (21). Another single-armed study in 56 women with mastodynia showed a reduction in prolactin in the treatment group compared with controls (22). Studies, the quality of which cannot be assessed, claim that vitex corrects inadequate luteal phase, and that it restores LH activity.

Ginseng. There are many types of ginseng (*Panax ginseng*)—Siberian, Korean, American, White, and Red. All are promoted as "adaptogens," which help one cope with stress and supposedly boost immunity. Ginseng also is reputed to be an aphrodisiac, a claim that is unsubstantiated by medical evidence. It also is promoted as a means of improving athletic performance and inducing weight loss without the need for diet or exercise. There is evidence that ginseng does not improve athletic performance, despite claims made (23). Reports of antioxidant effects and reduced rates of disease, particularly cancer rates, are suspect because the products in general use have been found to contain little or no active ingredients (24).

Menstrual Disorders/Menorrhagia

Wild Yam. Yam extracts, tablets, and creams claim to be progesterone substitutes and also are touted as a natural source of DHEA. Sterol structures from the plant are used as precursors in the biosynthesis of progesterone, DHEA, and other steroids, but do not have inherent biological activity. Claims are made that the plant sterol dioscorea is converted into progesterone in the body and alleviates "estrogen dominance." There is no human biochemical pathway for bioconversion of dioscorea to progesterone or DHEA in vivo. Mexican yam extract more accurately is estrogenic, containing considerable diosgenin, an estrogenlike substance found in plants. Some estrogenic effects might be expected from eating these species of yams, but only if large quantities of raw yams are consumed (25). Yams from the grocery store generally are not the varieties known to contain significant amounts of dioscorea or diosgenin. Yam extracts also are purported to be effective for uterine cramps.

Clinical Considerations and Recommendations

A limited body of scientific information about botanicals is available in English. A few publications from Europe and Asia are available in full text. Most of the literature includes in vitro effects, animal models, and open, often single-armed or nonrandomized studies. The amount and sophistication of studies of most alternative therapies do not meet the current standards for evidence-based recommendations.

▶ *Are there useful nonpharmaceutical supplements or botanicals for treatment of vasomotor symptoms, including hot flashes, flushes, and night sweats?*

Soy/Isoflavone Isolates. In one study, women given a soy protein supplement with 40 mg of protein and 76 mg of isoflavones had a 45% reduction in vasomotor symptoms compared with a 30% reduction in controls who received a placebo (26). Other research demonstrated a 40% reduction in vasomotor symptoms when diet was supplemented with soy flour, but the vaginal maturation index did not improve (27). Based on these limited studies, the use of soy may have benefits.

Black Cohosh. Although a dozen studies of women taking black cohosh extracts show an apparent reduction in symptomatology, the studies are largely unblinded, use unvalidated tools to measure outcomes, and contain small numbers of patients. Based on this limited evidence, there appears to be a positive effect on sleep disorders, mood disturbance, and hot flashes (28). There have been no reports of black cohosh toxicity. No clinical studies have reported efficacy or safety of black cohosh beyond 6 months of use. Black cohosh should not be confused with blue cohosh, *Caulophyllum thalictroides,* which has weak nicotine activity and toxic potential.

Evening Primrose. A meta-analysis of clinical trials of evening primrose oil used to treat premenstrual syndrome concluded that of the seven controlled trials, only five were properly randomized (29). In the only one of the five trials that was blinded, evening primrose was ineffective in treating premenstrual syndrome. To date, there is only one randomized, double-blind, placebo-controlled study of the use of GLA in the treatment of vasomotor symptoms during menopause (30). Although the women taking GLA had "significant improvement... in the maximum number of night time flushes," GLA provided no benefits beyond those seen with placebo.

Dong Quai. Kaiser Permanente conducted a double-blind controlled clinical trial using a daily dose of 4.5 g of dong quai (9). Dong quai and placebo both reported a 25% reduction in hot flashes. Critics of the study have noted that the dose of dong quai was lower than that often used in traditional Chinese medicine, and that dong quai is never employed as an isolated intervention. The argument is made that the botanicals must be taken together in a balanced formula and that the therapeutic outcome requires that proper synergy take place between the components. However, its benefit cannot be substantiated based on available evidence.

Dong quai is potentially toxic. It contains numerous coumarinlike derivatives and may cause excessive bleeding or interactions with other anticoagulants (31). Dong quai also contains psoralens and is potentially photosensitizing, which has led to concern about an increased risk of sun-exposure-related skin cancers (32).

Ginseng. Ginsana, the largest manufacturer of ginseng, funded a study of 384 women to investigate the effects of ginseng in menopausal women. No differences were found between treatment subjects and placebo controls in vasomotor symptoms, but significant improvements were reported in quality of life measures, particularly depression, general health, and well-being scores (33).

▶ *Are there alternative, nonpharmaceutical supplements or botanicals that have demonstrated usefulness in the treatment of sleep, mood and affective, cognitive, and other behavioral disorders associated with menopause syndrome?*

St. John's Wort. A meta-analysis of 15 controlled trials encompassing 1,757 cases found that St. John's wort hypericin in doses less than 1.2 mg per day produced a 61% improvement in mild to moderate depression, while doses up to 2.7 mg per day produced a 75% improvement (34). Its efficacy in the treatment of severe depression is not documented. Some have suggested that St. John's wort is helpful in treating seasonal affective disorder. No clinical studies have reported results or safety parameters beyond 2 years of use.

St. John's wort is also potentially photosensitizing (24), and concern has been raised about an increased rate of cataracts. The issue of possible interactions between St. John's wort and selective serotonin reuptake inhibitors or monamine oxidase inhibitors has been raised. Some consultants advise against using St. John's wort for weeks to months after stopping these drugs. Interaction with anesthetic agents has also been reported (35).

Valerian Root. In 1998, the U.S. Pharmacopeia (USP) stated in its monograph on valerian: "Studies supporting this use are not good enough to prove that it is effective. Therefore, USP advisory panels do not support its use" (36). There is a case report of high-output congestive heart failure, tachycardia, and delirium attributed to acute withdrawal from valerian (37). Based on available data, valerian appears not to be useful, and may be harmful.

▶ *Are there alternative, nonpharmaceutical supplements or botanicals that have been shown to be useful for treatment of decreased libido, vaginal dryness, or dyspareunia?*

Soy/Isoflavones. Findings regarding the effects of soy supplements on vaginal maturation index are inconsistent with some showing improvements (11) and others showing no change (12). Different isoflavones may have a differential impact on estrogen-sensitive tissues, so that various types of dietary soy may affect the lower genital tract with a significant degree of variability (12, 27). Therefore, some soy products may be useful in the treatment of vaginal dryness and dyspareunia, although sources of isoflavones and beneficial amounts have yet to be clarified.

Chasteberry or Vitex. Although vitex's supposed anti-hormonal activity serves as the basis for advising its use in treating mastalgia, all claims of efficacy in women are poorly documented. Although studies of vitex use in menopause are limited, a recent randomized trial assessed the effects of vitex in women with premenstrual syndrome, which may apply to women with similar complaints in menopause. After three cycles of vitex, significant improvements in mood alteration, anger, headache, and breast fullness were reported on a self assessment screening tool. However, other menstrual symptoms, like bloating, remained unchanged. Physician ratings of patients' conditions also indicated better effects than with placebo (38).

Ginseng. No published studies have documented that ginseng has an effect on libido in menopausal women. Moreover, 54 ginseng products examined by the American Botanical Council proved to have little ginseng (60%) or no ginseng (25%), and many were heavily adulterated with caffeine (24). Other analyses have found significant variation in the active ingredient, ginsenosides, as well as high levels of pesticides or lead. Ginseng may hold some promise in the treatment of fatigue, depression, immunosuppression, and other health problems, but it cannot be recommended as a treatment for menopause. For its other indications, caution is advised given the poor production standards and lack of quality evidence for the claims made.

▶ *Are there alternative, nonpharmaceutical supplements or botanicals that are useful for the treatment of menstrual disorders during perimenopause and menopause?*

Wild and Mexican Yam. Based on the lack of bioavailability, the hormones in wild and Mexican yam would not be expected to have any efficacy. Wild yam extracts are neither estrogenic nor progestational, and although many yam extract products contain no yam, some are laced with progesterone. Perhaps some may even contain medroxyprogesterone. Oral ingestion does not produce serum levels. There are no published reports demonstrating the efficacy of wild yam cream. A 1-month supply costs more than $25, while a month of commercially produced vaginal estrogen cream costs less than $20 (39).

▶ *Are there useful alternative, nonpharmaceutical supplements or botanicals for the prevention of coronary heart disease and osteoporosis?*

Soy/Isoflavone Isolates. There is some evidence to indicate that high isoflavone intake may favorably affect lipid profile and is, by extension, thought to reduce cardiac disease risk. However, study results are conflicting. A study in Finland found an inverse relationship between isoflavone intake and coronary heart disease in both women and men (40), but similar benefits have not been demonstrated in the United States (41). A meta-analysis showed higher soy intake is associated with significant improvement in lipid profiles (42). Soy protein intake of approximately 47 g per day correlated with a statistically significant 9.3% reduction in serum cholesterol, a 12.9% reduction in serum low-density lipoprotein cholesterol, a 10.5% reduction in serum triglycerides, and an insignificant 2.4% increase in high-density lipoproteins. Isoflavone isolates containing 40 mg of isoflavone isolates have been shown to induce a 23% increase in arterial compliance after 1 year of use, an increase equal to that seen in women receiving conjugated equine estrogens (43).

Dietary soy or isolated isoflavone supplements may have a salutary effect on bone mass. Ipriflavone, a synthetic version of genistein, slows bone reabsorption and stimulates collagen synthesis in bone. Pharmaceutical quality ipriflavone is approved in Europe and Japan for treatment of osteoporosis using 600 mg per day. Ipriflavone with supplemental calcium has been found to decrease bone loss in natural menopause in some studies (44, 45), but not others (46), to decrease bone loss after surgically induced menopause (47), and in women with gonadotropin-agonist-induced bone loss (48).

▶ *Does the use of alternative therapies require any special medical monitoring?*

No published studies have investigated the role of clinical monitoring in patients using alternative medicine therapies. However, alternative steroid products may pose a risk for consequences of excessive steroid ingestion. Androgens are associated with abnormal liver functions as well as potential hyperandrogenicity. Estrogens compounded by an alternative therapy pharmacy may produce varying serum estradiol levels in women or increased estrogen bioactivity without detectable changes in circulating estradiol. Risks of excessive levels include hepatic effects and increased risk of deep vein thrombosis.

Although most botanicals appear to be harmless, products may be adulterated or contaminated. In addi-

Counseling Patients About Complementary and Alternative Medicine

- All patients should be asked about their use of herbal therapies and dietary supplements. Use of these products should be documented in the patient's chart.

- "Natural" is not an assurance of safety or efficacy.

- Potentially dangerous drug–herb interactions occur.*

- Lack of standardization of botanicals may result in variability of content and efficacy from batch to batch, from a single manufacturer, or between manufacturers.

- Lack of quality control and regulation may result in contamination, adulteration, or potential misidentification of plant products.

- Errors in compounding may result in toxic or lethal outcomes in custom-blended herbal preparations.

- Botanicals should not be used by women planning to become pregnant in the near future or during pregnancy or lactation without professional advice.

- Botanicals should not be taken in larger than recommended doses or for longer than recommended duration.

- Several botanicals have known adverse effects and toxicities.

- Infants, children, and the elderly should not use botanicals without professional advice.

- Patients should be counseled in a rational, judicious, and balanced manner about the relative risks and benefits of conventional therapies and alternative interventions.

- Adverse events and outcomes should be documented in the chart, therapy discontinued, and reported to the U.S. Food and Drug Administration.

- Because the expected placebo response for menopausal treatment ranges from 10% to 30%, a small positive response to any treatment, conventional or alternative, may not necessarily represent a pharmacologic effect. Anecdotal experience is not a substitute for well-constructed clinical trials. Nonetheless, the effect of support, counseling, and empathetic care should not be discounted or dismissed.

*For a complete listing of potentially dangerous drug–herb interactions see Newall CA, Anderson LA, Phillipson JD. Herbal medicines: a guide for health-care professionals. London: Pharmaceutical Press, 1996.

Modified from Cirigliano M, Sun A. Advising patients about herbal therapies [letter]. JAMA 1998;280:1565–1566. Copyright 1998, American Medical Association.

tion, all menopausal women taking any pharmaceutical or alternative preparation should have blood pressure readings, mammograms, and Pap tests at recommended intervals. Women using estrogen supplements who are relying on unconventional estrogenic or progestational therapies such as transdermal progesterone cosmetic creams should be monitored according to standard guidelines for women taking unopposed estrogen—that is, endometrial surveillance should be considered. In counseling patients, the risk of adverse effects from these therapies must be weighed against the costs associated with any routine testing. Further guidelines for counseling patients regarding the use of complementary and alternative medicine are shown in the box. Also, it is important for clinicians to be aware of issues surrounding referral to alternative care providers (3).

Summary of Recommendations

Given the general lack of standardization of products, the relatively short duration of therapy and follow-up in the available data, and the difficulty of interpreting the available clinical data, few recommendations can be made with confidence. The following conclusions can be drawn in reference to short-term (≤ 2 years) use of botanical and alternative medicine for the management of menopause.

The following recommendations are based primarily on consensus and expert opinion (Level C):

▶ Soy and isoflavones may be helpful in the short-term (≤ 2 years) treatment of vasomotor symptoms. Given the possibility that these compounds may interact with estrogen, these agents should not be considered free of potential harm in women with estrogen-dependent cancers.

▶ St. John's wort may be helpful in the short-term (≤ 2 years) treatment of mild to moderate depression in women.

▶ Black cohosh may be helpful in the short-term (≤ 6 months) treatment of women with vasomotor symptoms.

▶ Soy and isoflavone intake over prolonged periods may improve lipoprotein profiles and protect against osteoporosis. Soy in foodstuffs may differ in biological activity from soy and isoflavones in supplements.

References

1. Ettinger B, Pressman A, Bradley C. Comparison of continuation of postmenopausal hormone replacement therapy: transdermal versus oral estrogen. Menopause 1998;5: 152–156 (Level II-3)

2. Creasman WT. Is there an association between hormone replacement therapy and breast cancer? J Womens Health 1998;7:1231–1246 (Level III)

3. American College of Obstetricians and Gynecologists. Complementary and alternative medicine. ACOG Committee Opinion 227. Washington, DC: ACOG, 1999 (Level III)

4. National Center for Complementary and Alternative Medicine. Expanding horizons of healthcare. Bethesda, Maryland: NCCAM, 2000, NCCAM Clearinghouse publication no. X-38 (Level III)

5. Eisenberg DM, Davis RB, Ettner SL, Appel S, Wilkey S, Van Rompay M, et al. Trends in alternative medicine use in the United Sates, 1990–1997: results of a follow-up national survey. JAMA 1998;280:1569–1575 (Level III)

6. Astin JA. Why patients use alternative medicine: results of a national study. JAMA 1998;279:1548–1553 (Level III)

7. Eisenberg DM. Advising patients who seek alternative medical therapies. Ann Intern Med 1997;127:61–69 (Level III)

8. Kaufert P, Boggs PP, Ettinger B, Woods NF, Utian WH. Women and menopause: beliefs, attitudes, and behaviors. The North American Menopause Society 1997 Menopause Survey. Menopause 1998;5:197–202 (Level III)

9. Hirata JD, Swiersz LM, Zell B, Small R, Ettinger B. Does dong quai have estrogenic effects in postmenopausal women? A double-blind, placebo-controlled trial. Fertil Steril 1997;68:981–986 (Level I)

10. Kurzer MS, Xu X. Dietary phytoestrogens. Annu Rev Nutr 1997;17:353–381 (Level III)

11. Wilcox G, Wahlqvist ML, Burger HG, Medley G. Oestrogenic effects of plant foods in postmenopausal women. BMJ 1990;301:905–906 (Level II-3)

12. Baird DD, Umbach DM, Lansdell L, Hughes CL, Setchell KD, Weinberg CR, et al. Dietary intervention study to assess estrogenicity of dietary soy among postmenopausal women. J Clin Endocrinol Metab 1995;80:1685–1690 (Level I)

13. Tham DM, Gardner CD, Haskell WL. Clinical review 97: Potential health benefits of dietary phytoestrogens: a review of the clinical, epidemiological, and mechanistic evidence. J Clin Endocrinol Metab 1998;83:2223–2235 (Level III)

14. Rose DP, Lubin M, Connolly JM. Effects of diet supplementation with wheat bran on serum estrogen levels in the follicular and luteal phases of the menstrual cycle. Nutrition 1997;13:535–539 (Level II-3)

15. Mitka M. FDA never promised an herb garden—but sellers and buyers eager to see one grow [news]. JAMA 1998;280:1554–1556 (Level III)

16. Blumenthal M, ed. The complete German Commission E monographs: therapeutic guide to herbal medicines. Austin, Texas: American Botanical Council, 1998 (Level III)

17. Duker EM, Kopanski L, Jarry H, Wuttke W. Effects of extracts from Cimicifuga racemosa on gonadotropin release in menopausal women and ovariectomized rats. Planta Med 1991;57:420–424 (Level II-3)

18. Liske E, Wustenberg P. Therapy of climacteric complaints with cimicifuga racemosa: herbal medicine with clinically proven evidence [abstract]. Menopause 1998;5:250 (Level III)

19. Beinfield H, Korngold E. Between heaven and earth: a guide to Chinese medicine. New York: Ballantine Books, 1991 (Level III)

20. Bennett DA Jr, Phun L, Polk JF, Voglino SA, Zlotnik V, Raffa RB. Neuropharmacology of St. John's Wort (Hypericum). Ann Pharmacother 1998;32:1201–1208 (Level III)

21. Merz PG, Schrodter A, Rietbrock S, Gorkow Ch, Loew D. Prolktinsekretion und Vertraglichkeit unter der Behandlung mit einem Agnus-castus-Spezialextrakt (B1095E1). Erste Ergebnisse zum Einflub auf die Prolaktinsekretion. In: Loew D, Rietbrock N, eds. Phytopharmaka in Forschung und klinischer Anwendung. Darmstadt: Steinkopff, 1995:93–97 (German)

22. Wuttke W, Gorkow Ch, Jarry J. Dompainergic compounds in Vitex agtnus castus. In: Loew D, Rietbrock N, eds. Phytopharmaka in Forschung und kinischer Anwendug. Darmstadt: Steinkopff, 1995:81–91 (German)

23. Allen JD, McLung J, Nelson AG, Welsch M. Ginseng supplementation does not enhance healthy young adults' peak aerobic exercise performance. J Am Coll Nutr 1998; 17:462–466 (Level II-1)

24. O'Hara M, Kiefer D, Farrell K, Kemper K. A review of 12 commonly used medicinal herbs. Arch Fam Med 1998; 7:523–536 (Level III)

25. Mirkin G. Estrogen in yams. JAMA 1991;265:912 (Level III)

26. Albertazzi P, Pansini F, Bonaccorsi G, Zanotti L, Forini E, De Aloysio D. The effect of dietary soy supplementation on hot flushes. Obstet Gynecol 1998;91:6–11 (Level II-1)

27. Murkies AL, Lombard C, Strauss BJ, Wilcox G, Burger HG, Morton MS. Dietary flour supplementation decreases post-menopausal hot flushes: effect of soy and wheat. Maturitas 1995;21:189–195 (Level I)

28. Warnecke G. Influence of a phytopharmaceutical on climacteric complaints. Die Medizinische Welt 1985; 36:871–874 (German)

29. Budeiri D, Li Wan Po A, Dornan JC. Is evening primrose oil of value in the treatment of premenstrual syndrome? Control Clin Trials 1996;17:60–68 (Level III)

30. Chenoy R, Hussain S, Tayob Y, O'Brien PM, Moss MY, Morse PF. Effect of oral gamolenic acid from evening primrose oil on menopausal flushing. BMJ 1994; 308:501–503 (Level I)

31. Fugh-Berman A. Herb-drug interactions. Lancet 2000; 355:134–138 [erratum Lancet 2000;355:1020] (Level III)

32. Tyler VE. The honest herbal: a sensible guide to the use of herbs and related remedies. 3rd ed. Binghamton, New York: Pharmaceutical Products Press, 1993 (Level III)

33. Wiklund IK, Mattsson LA, Lindgren R, Limoni C. Effects of a standardized ginseng extract on quality of life and physiological parameters in symptomatic postmenopausal women: a double-blind, placebo-controlled trial. Swedish Alternative Medicine Group. Int J Clin Pharmacol Res 1999;19:89–99 (Level I)

34. Linde K, Ramirez G, Mulrow CD, Pauls A, Weidenhammer W, Melchart D. St. John's wort for depression—an overview and meta-analysis of randomised clinical trials. BMJ 1996;313:253–258 (Meta-analysis)

35. Koupparis LS. Harmless herbs: a cause for concern [letter]? Anaesthesia 2000;55:101–102 (Level III)

36. U.S. Pharmacopeia Botanical monograph series: information for the health care professional and consumer. Rockville, Maryland: US Pharmacopeial Convention, Inc., 1998 (Level III)

37. Garges HP, Varia I, Doraiswany PM. Cardiac complications and delirium associated with valerian root withdrawal [letter]. JAMA 1998;280:1566–1567 (Level III)

38. Schellenberg R. Treatment for the premenstrual syndrome with agnus castus fruit extract: prospective, randomised, placebo controlled study. BMJ 2001;322:134–137 (Level I)

39. Gorski T. Wild yam cream threatens women's health. Nutr Forum 1997;14:23–24 (Level III)

40. Knekt P, Jarvinen R, Reunanen A, Maatela J. Flavonoid intake and coronary mortality in Finland: a cohort study. BMJ 1996;312:478–481 (Level II-3)

41. Rimm EB, Katan MB, Ascherio A, Stampfer MJ, Willett WC. Relation between intake of flavonoids and risk for coronary heart disease in male health professionals. Ann Intern Med 1996;125:384–389 (Level II-3)

42. Anderson JW, Johnstone BM, Cook-Newell ME. Meta-analysis of the effects of soy protein intake on serum lipids. N Engl J Med 1995;333:276–282 (Meta-analysis)

43. Nestel PJ, Pomeroy S, Kay S, Komesaroff, Behrsing J, Cameron JD, et al. Isoflavones from red clover improve systemic arterial compliance but not plasma lipids in menopausal women. J Clin Endocrinol Metab 1999;84:895–898 [erratum J Clin Endocrinol Metab 1999;84:3647] (Level II-3)

44. Valente M, Bufalino L, Castiglione GN, D'Angelo R, Mancuso A, Galoppi P, et al. Effects of 1-year treatment with ipriflavone on bone in postmenopausal women with low bone mass. Calcif Tissue Int 1994;54:377–380 (Level I)

45. Gambacciani M, Ciaponi M, Cappagli B, Piaggesi L, Genazzani AR. Effects of combined low dose of the isoflavone derivative ipriflavone and estrogen replacement on bone mineral density and metabolism in postmenopausal women. Maturitas 1997;28:75–81 (Level I)

46. Alexandersen P, Toussaint A, Christiansen C, Devogelaer JP, Roux C, Fechtenbaum J, et al. Ipriflavone in the treatment of postmenopausal osteoporosis: a randomized controlled trial. JAMA 2001;285:1482–1488 (Level I)

47. Gambacciani M, Spinetti A, Cappagli B, Taponeco F, Felipetto R, Parrini D, et al. Effects of ipriflavone administration on bone mass and metabolism in ovariectomized women. J Endocrinol Invest 1993;16:333–337 (Level I)

48. Gambacciani M, Spinetti A, Piaggesi L, Cappagli B, Taponeco F, Manetti P, et al. Ipriflavone prevents the bone mass reduction in premenopausal women treated with gonadotropin hormone-releasing hormone agonists. Bone Miner 1994;26:19–26 (Level I)

Web Resources

The National Library of Medicine (http://www.nlm.nih.gov/)

The National Center for Complementary and Alternative Medicine (http://nccam.nih.gov)

The NIH Office of Dietary Supplements (http://dietary-supplements.info.nih.gov)

The Richard and Hinda Rosenthal Center for Complementary & Alternative Medicine (http://cpmcnet.columbia.edu/dept/rosenthal/)

The American Botanical Council (http://www.herbalgram.org)

Health World Online (http://www.healthy.net)

Quackwatch (http://www.quackwatch.com)

ConsumerLab (http://www.consumerlab.com)

The MEDLINE database, the Cochrane Library, and ACOG's own internal resources and documents were used to conduct a literature search to locate relevant articles published between January 1985 and January 2001. Priority was given to articles reporting results of original research, although review articles and commentaries also were consulted. Abstracts of research presented at symposia and scientific conferences were not considered adequate for inclusion in this document. Guidelines published by organizations or institutions such as the National Institutes of Health and the American College of Obstetricians and Gynecologists were reviewed, and additional studies were located by reviewing bibliographies of identified articles. When reliable research was not available, expert opinions from obstetrician–gynecologists were used.

Studies were reviewed and evaluated for quality according to the method outlined by the U.S. Preventive Services Task Force:

I   Evidence obtained from at least one properly designed randomized controlled trial.

II-1   Evidence obtained from well-designed controlled trials without randomization.

II-2   Evidence obtained from well-designed cohort or case–control analytic studies, preferably from more than one center or research group.

II-3   Evidence obtained from multiple time series with or without the intervention. Dramatic results in uncontrolled experiments could also be regarded as this type of evidence.

III   Opinions of respected authorities, based on clinical experience, descriptive studies, or reports of expert committees.

Based on the highest level of evidence found in the data, recommendations are provided and graded according to the following categories:

Level A—Recommendations are based on good and consistent scientific evidence.

Level B—Recommendations are based on limited or inconsistent scientific evidence.

Level C—Recommendations are based primarily on consensus and expert opinion.

ISSN 1099-3630

**The American College of
Obstetricians and Gynecologists
409 12th Street, SW
PO Box 96920
Washington, DC 20090-6920**

12345/54321

ACOG PRACTICE BULLETIN

CLINICAL MANAGEMENT GUIDELINES FOR
OBSTETRICIAN–GYNECOLOGISTS

NUMBER 54, JULY 2004

(Replaces Practice Bulletin Number 5, July 1999)

This Practice Bulletin was developed by the ACOG Committee on Practice Bulletins— Obstetrics with the assistance of T. Flint Porter, MD and Carolyn M. Zelop, MD. The information is designed to aid practitioners in making decisions about appropriate obstetric and gynecologic care. These guidelines should not be construed as dictating an exclusive course of treatment or procedure. Variations in practice may be warranted based on the needs of the individual patient, resources, and limitations unique to the institution or type of practice.

Vaginal Birth After Previous Cesarean Delivery

A trial of labor after previous cesarean delivery has been accepted as a way to reduce the overall cesarean delivery rate (1). Although vaginal birth after cesarean delivery (VBAC) is appropriate for most women with a history of a low-transverse cesarean delivery, several factors increase the likelihood of a failed trial of labor, which in turn leads to increased maternal and perinatal morbidity. The purpose of this document is to review the current risks and benefits of VBAC in various situations and provide practical management guidelines.

Background

Between 1970 and 1988, the cesarean delivery rate in the United States increased dramatically from 5% to nearly 25% (1–3). The rapid growth was likely a result of increased pressure that discouraged physicians from performing vaginal breech deliveries and midpelvic forceps deliveries. At the same time, increasing reliance on continuous electronic monitoring of fetal heart rate and uterine contraction patterns led to an increase in the number of cesarean deliveries performed for presumed fetal compromise and dystocia, respectively. With few exceptions, major improvements in newborn outcomes as a result of the increased cesarean delivery rate are yet to be proved (4).

Changing Concepts

The dictum "once a cesarean, always a cesarean," which dominated obstetric practice in the United States for nearly 70 years (5), began changing gradually approximately 30 years ago as improvements in obstetric care made a trial of labor after a previous cesarean delivery safer for both the woman and the fetus. Based on the findings of several large series that documented the relative safety of a trial of labor after a previous cesarean delivery (6–9), organizations such as the National Institutes of Health and the American College of Obstetricians and

Gynecologists enthusiastically embraced VBAC as a way to decrease the cesarean delivery rate in the United States.

The national enthusiasm for VBAC led to a decrease in the cesarean delivery rate, which reached 20.7% in 1996 (10). During the same period (1989–1996), the VBAC rate increased from less than 18.9% to 28.3%. Some third-party payers and managed care organizations even mandated that all women who had previous cesarean deliveries undergo trials of labor (11, 12). Many physicians were pressured into offering VBAC to unsuitable candidates or to women who wanted to have a repeat cesarean delivery. As the VBAC rate increased, so did the number of well-publicized reports of uterine rupture and other complications during trials of labor after previous cesarean deliveries (11, 13, 14). As a result, many physicians and hospitals have discontinued the practice altogether. This abrupt change in practice has contributed to the cesarean delivery rate in the United States increasing again, reaching an all-time high of 26.1% in 2002, while the VBAC rate has decreased by 55% to 12.6% (15).

Supportive Evidence

Despite thousands of citations in the world's literature, there are currently no randomized trials comparing maternal or neonatal outcomes for both repeat cesarean delivery and VBAC. Instead, VBAC recommendations have been based on data from large clinical series suggesting that the benefits of VBAC outweigh the risks in most women with a previous low-transverse cesarean delivery (6–9, 16–18). Most have been conducted in university or tertiary-level centers with full-time in-house obstetric and anesthesia coverage (19). Only a few studies have documented the relative safety of VBAC in smaller community hospitals or facilities where resources may be more limited (17, 20–22). Furthermore, the early series of women attempting a trial of labor after a previous cesarean delivery focused on successful VBAC and maternal mortality. It has become apparent that women who fail a trial of labor are at risk for several maternal complications, including uterine rupture, hysterectomy, the need for transfusion, and endometritis (16, 19, 23), as well as perinatal morbidity and mortality (24, 25).

Clinical Considerations and Recommendations

▶ *Who are candidates for a trial of labor?*

The preponderance of evidence suggests that most patients who have had a low-transverse uterine incision from a previous cesarean delivery and who have no con-

traindications for vaginal birth are candidates for a trial of labor. Following are selection criteria useful in identifying candidates for VBAC:

- One previous low-transverse cesarean delivery
- Clinically adequate pelvis
- No other uterine scars or previous rupture
- Physician immediately available throughout active labor capable of monitoring labor and performing an emergency cesarean delivery
- Availability of anesthesia and personnel for emergency cesarean delivery

Based on the findings from several retrospective studies, it may be reasonable to offer a trial of labor to women in the following other specific obstetric circumstances.

More Than One Previous Cesarean Delivery

Women who have had 2 previous low-transverse cesarean deliveries have traditionally been considered candidates for a trial of labor. However, the few studies that address this issue report a risk of uterine rupture ranging between 1% and 3.7% (9, 26, 27). In the only study that controlled for other potential confounding variables, the risk of uterine rupture during labor was nearly 5 times greater for women with 2 previous cesarean deliveries when compared with women who had 1 previous cesarean delivery (27). Women with a previous vaginal delivery followed by a cesarean delivery were only approximately one fourth as likely to sustain uterine rupture during a trial of labor (27). Therefore, for women with 2 prior cesarean deliveries, only those with a prior vaginal delivery should be considered candidates for a spontaneous trial of labor.

Macrosomia

Although macrosomia (usually birth weight greater than 4,000 g or 4,500 g, regardless of gestational age) is associated with a lower likelihood of successful VBAC (28–31), 60–90% of women attempting a trial of labor who give birth to infants with macrosomia are successful (30, 31). The rate of uterine rupture appears to be increased only in those women without a previous vaginal delivery (31).

Gestation Beyond 40 Weeks

Awaiting spontaneous labor beyond 40 weeks of gestation decreases the likelihood of successful VBAC, but the risk of uterine rupture does not increase (32, 33). In one study of more than 1,200 women attempting a trial of labor after 40 weeks of gestation, only labor induction was associated with an increased risk of uterine rupture (33).

Previous Low-Vertical Incision

In 1 case series and 4 retrospective studies, women with a previous low-vertical uterine incision were just as likely to have successful VBAC as women with a previous low-transverse uterine incision (34–37). In addition, there was no increase in maternal or perinatal morbidity.

Unknown Uterine Scar Type

The type of uterine incision performed at the time of a prior cesarean delivery cannot be confirmed in some patients. Many authorities question the safety of offering VBAC under these circumstances; others suggest that the uterine scar type usually can be inferred based on the indication for the prior cesarean delivery. Two case series, both carried out at large tertiary care facilities, reported rates of VBAC success and uterine rupture similar to those from other contemporaneous studies of women with documented previous low-transverse uterine incisions (38, 39). In one small, randomized controlled trial (n = 197) comparing labor augmentation with no intervention in women with a previous cesarean delivery and unknown scar, 5 uterine scar disruptions occurred in the group that received labor augmentation while no scar disruptions occurred in the group without augmentation (40).

Twin Gestation

The safety of VBAC in women with twin gestations has been examined in small case series and 2 small, retrospective studies (41–44). In the 2 trials, which included a total of only 45 women with twin gestations, the rates of successful VBAC and uterine rupture did not differ significantly between study subjects and women with singleton gestations who also were attempting VBAC.

▶ *What is the success rate for trials of labor?*

Most published series of women attempting a trial of labor after a previous cesarean delivery indicate that 60–80% have successful vaginal births (17, 23, 45–48). The earliest studies usually included only those subjects who met strict inclusion criteria, excluding those who were not felt to be appropriate VBAC candidates. However, in a population-based study of nearly 40,000 women from hospitals throughout California, 61.4% of women who attempted VBAC were successful (17).

There is no completely reliable way to predict whether a trial of labor will be successful in an individual patient (49–52). Generally, success rates for women whose first cesarean delivery was performed for a nonrecurring indication are similar to those of patients who have not undergone a previous cesarean delivery (46, 53, 54). Most women who have undergone a cesarean delivery because of dystocia also can have a successful VBAC, but the percentage may be lower (50–80%) than for those with nonrecurring indications (75–86%) (46, 55–58). If the prior cesarean delivery for dystocia was performed before complete cervical dilation (5–9 cm), 67–73% of VBAC attempts are successful compared with only 13% if the prior cesarean delivery was performed after complete cervical dilation (56). Other aspects of obstetric history also influence the likelihood of a successful VBAC. Women who have given birth vaginally at least once are 9–28 times more likely to have a successful trial of labor than women who have not undergone vaginal delivery (14, 59). If the most recent delivery was a successful VBAC, the likelihood of failure is reduced by 30–90% (52, 60). Factors that negatively influence the likelihood of successful VBAC include labor augmentation and induction (52, 61, 62), maternal obesity (63, 64), gestational age beyond 40 weeks (33), birth weight greater than 4,000 g (30), and interdelivery interval of less than 19 months (65).

▶ *What are the risks and benefits associated with VBAC?*

Neither elective repeat cesarean delivery nor VBAC is without risk. Generally, successful VBAC is associated with shorter maternal hospitalizations, less blood loss and fewer transfusions, fewer infections, and fewer thromboembolic events than cesarean delivery (8, 16, 23, 25). However, a failed trial of labor may be associated with major maternal complications, such as uterine rupture, hysterectomy, and operative injury (16, 18, 23, 25, 48), as well as increased maternal infection and the need for transfusion (23). Neonatal morbidity also is increased with a failed trial of labor, as evidenced by the increased incidence of arterial umbilical cord blood gas pH levels below 7, 5-minute Apgar scores below 7, and infection (25, 47, 66). However, multiple cesarean deliveries also carry maternal risks, including an increased risk of placenta previa and accreta (67, 68). Based on these risks, one decision model analysis found it is reasonable to consider a trial of labor if the chance of success is 50% or greater, and the desire for future pregnancy after cesarean delivery is at least 10–20% (67).

The incidence of maternal death with VBAC is extremely low. In a recent meta-analysis, only 3 maternal deaths were reported among the more than 27,000 women who attempted a trial of labor after a prior cesarean delivery (25). Although the incidence of perinatal death is low (generally less than 1%), it is more likely to occur during a trial of labor than an elective repeat cesarean delivery (18, 25, 47, 69). Uterine rupture has been associated with fetal death, as well as severe neonatal neurologic injury (24, 70–72).

Uterine rupture during a trial of labor after a previous cesarean delivery is a life-threatening complication that has been directly attributed to attempted VBAC. In most cases, the cause of uterine rupture is unknown, but poor obstetric outcomes can result even in women who are appropriate candidates for VBAC. The exact incidence of uterine rupture is difficult to determine because reports in the literature have sometimes grouped true, catastrophic uterine ruptures together with asymptomatic scar dehiscences. Additionally, early case series included ruptures in the absence of labor as well as ruptures during labor in women with previous classical incisions (24). The rate of uterine rupture is largely dependent on the type and location of the previous incision. Uterine rupture rates in women with previous classical incisions and T-shaped incisions range between 4% and 9% (73). Although uterine rupture occurs more often in women undergoing a trial of labor than women who elect repeat cesarean delivery, rupture rates during attempted VBAC generally are less than 1% (17, 18, 25).

The risk of uterine rupture also is influenced by obstetric history. A previous vaginal birth significantly reduces the risk of uterine rupture (74). The risk of uterine rupture appears to be inversely related to the length of time between deliveries, ie, the longer the interval between deliveries, the lower the risk of rupture (75–77). Women who attempt VBAC who have interdelivery intervals of less than 24 months have a 2–3-fold increased risk of uterine rupture when compared with women who attempt VBAC more than 24 months after their last delivery (76). Finally, the findings of one nonrandomized trial suggest that compared with a double layer closure, a single layer closure of the hysterotomy incision in the primary cesarean delivery may increase the risk of uterine rupture 4-fold during a subsequent trial of labor (78).

Common signs of uterine rupture are a nonreassuring fetal heart rate pattern with decelerations or bradycardia (18). Other findings are more variable and include uterine or abdominal pain, loss of station of the presenting part, vaginal bleeding, and hypovolemia.

▶ *What factors should be taken into consideration when evaluating the cost-effectiveness of a trial of labor after a previous cesarean delivery and an elective repeat cesarean delivery?*

A true analysis of the cost-effectiveness of VBAC should include hospital and physician costs, the method of reimbursement, potential professional liability expenses, and the probability that a woman will continue with child-

bearing after her first attempt at VBAC (79). Higher costs may be incurred by a hospital if a woman has a prolonged labor or has significant complications or if the newborn is admitted to a neonatal intensive care unit. Additionally, evidence suggests that cost savings are not achieved unless at least 70% of women who attempt a trial of labor are successful (80–82).

▶ *Should women with a previous cesarean delivery undergo induction or augmentation of labor?*

Spontaneous labor is more likely to result in a successful VBAC rather than labor induction or augmentation (52, 61, 62). A meta-analysis of studies published before 1989 found no relationship between the use of oxytocin and rupture of the uterine scar (83). In contrast, several more recent large studies have shown an increased risk (37, 61, 62, 84). In one large retrospective study of more than 20,000 women, uterine rupture was nearly 5 times more common among women undergoing labor induction with oxytocin compared with those who had an elective repeat cesarean delivery (37). However, uterine rupture occurred in less than 1% of women in both groups. Furthermore, among the women attempting VBAC, the rate of uterine rupture was not different between those who received oxytocin and those who labored spontaneously.

There is considerable evidence that cervical ripening with prostaglandin preparations increases the likelihood of uterine rupture (37, 61, 85–87). In a review of Washington State birth records, the rate of uterine rupture during labor induced with prostaglandin was 24.5 in 1,000, which was 15-fold higher than that of women electing to have a repeat cesarean delivery (37). Likewise, misoprostol has been associated with an unacceptably high rate of uterine rupture in women with a previous cesarean delivery (88–91). Therefore, the use of prostaglandins for induction of labor in most women with a previous cesarean delivery should be discouraged.

▶ *How should midtrimester delivery be accomplished in women with a previous cesarean delivery?*

Some women with a history of a cesarean delivery will require delivery during the midtrimester in a subsequent pregnancy, usually because of fetal demise or the presence of anomalies. The published data on midtrimester VBAC are limited to single cases and small case series that report both successful and failed VBAC, as well as uterine rupture during a trial of labor (92–94). The induction agents in these reports are typically prostaglandin preparations, including misoprostol. A second-trimester hysterotomy is associated with its own risks, and the decision to attempt a trial of labor in the midtrimester should probably be based on individual circumstances, including but not limited to the number of previous cesarean deliveries, gestational age, placentation, and the woman's desire to preserve reproductive function.

▶ *What are contraindications for VBAC?*

A trial of labor is not recommended in patients at high risk for uterine rupture. Circumstances under which a trial of labor should not be attempted are as follows:

- Previous classical or T-shaped incision or extensive transfundal uterine surgery
- Previous uterine rupture
- Medical or obstetric complication that precludes vaginal delivery
- Inability to perform emergency cesarean delivery because of unavailable surgeon, anesthesia, sufficient staff, or facility
- Two prior uterine scars and no vaginal deliveries

In addition, a combination of factors that would not ordinarily constitute a compelling case to proceed with a primary cesarean delivery might be considered sufficient to choose repeat cesarean delivery instead of VBAC in some situations.

▶ *How should patients be counseled?*

The enthusiasm for VBAC varies greatly among patients and physicians. It is reasonable for women to undergo a trial of labor in a safe setting, but the potential complications should be discussed thoroughly and documented. If the type of previous incision is in doubt, attempts should be made to obtain the patient's medical records. After thorough counseling that weighs the individual benefits and risks of VBAC, the ultimate decision to attempt this procedure or undergo a repeat cesarean delivery should be made by the patient and her physician. Global mandates for a trial of labor after a previous cesarean delivery are inappropriate because individual risk factors are not considered. It should be recognized that there are repeat elective cesarean deliveries that are clinically indicated (95). The informed consent process and the plan of management should be documented in the medical record.

▶ *How does management of labor differ for patients undergoing VBAC?*

Despite extensive data on VBAC, there is relatively little information on how labor should be conducted. Management of labor varies in different situations.

External Cephalic Version

There are limited data about external cephalic version for breech presentation and VBAC. The data suggest that it may be as successful in VBAC candidates as in women who have not undergone a previous cesarean delivery (96).

Analgesia

Vaginal birth after cesarean delivery is not a contraindication to epidural anesthesia, and adequate pain relief may encourage more women to choose a trial of labor (97, 98). Success rates for VBAC are similar in women who do and do not receive epidural analgesia, as well as in those women who receive other types of pain relief (99, 100). Epidural analgesia rarely masks the signs and symptoms of uterine rupture.

Intrapartum Management

Once labor has begun, a patient attempting VBAC should be evaluated promptly. Most authorities recommend continuous electronic monitoring. However, no data suggest monitoring with intrauterine pressure catheters is superior to external monitoring. Personnel who are familiar with the potential complications of VBAC should be present to watch for nonreassuring fetal heart rate patterns and inadequate progress in labor.

Augmentation

The safety of oxytocin for augmentation of contractions during a trial of labor after a previous low-transverse cesarean delivery has been examined in several studies. Reported uterine rupture rates vary widely in the early studies (0.4–8%), which may reflect the inadvertent inclusion of asymptomatic scar dehiscence among cases of catastrophic uterine rupture (83, 101, 102). Nevertheless, in a recent study of 1,072 patients receiving oxytocin augmentation, the rate of symptomatic uterine rupture was 1% compared with 0.4% in those who labored spontaneously (84). In a nested case–control study, there was no association between uterine rupture and oxytocin dosing intervals, total oxytocin received, and mean duration of oxytocin administration (103).

Delivery

There is nothing unique about the delivery of the fetus during a trial of labor. The need to explore the uterus after a successful vaginal delivery is controversial. Most asymptomatic scar dehiscences heal well, and there are no data to suggest that future pregnancy outcome is better if the dehiscence is surgically repaired. Excessive vaginal bleeding or signs of hypovolemia at delivery require prompt and complete assessment of the previous scar and the entire genital tract.

▶ *How should future pregnancies be managed after uterine rupture?*

If the site of the ruptured scar is confined to the lower segment of the uterus, the rate of repeat rupture or dehiscence in labor is 6% (104). If the scar includes the upper segment of the uterus, the repeat rupture rate is 32% (104, 105). Therefore, women who have had a previous uterine rupture should give birth by repeat cesarean delivery before the onset of labor.

Summary of Recommendations

The following recommendations are based on good and consistent scientific evidence (Level A):

▶ Most women with one previous cesarean delivery with a low-transverse incision are candidates for VBAC and should be counseled about VBAC and offered a trial of labor.

▶ Epidural anesthesia may be used for VBAC.

The following recommendations are based on limited or inconsistent scientific evidence (Level B):

▶ Women with a vertical incision within the lower uterine segment that does not extend into the fundus are candidates for VBAC.

▶ The use of prostaglandins for cervical ripening or induction of labor in most women with a previous cesarean delivery should be discouraged.

The following recommendations are based primarily on consensus and expert opinion (Level C):

▶ Because uterine rupture may be catastrophic, VBAC should be attempted in institutions equipped to respond to emergencies with physicians immediately available to provide emergency care.

▶ After thorough counseling that weighs the individual benefits and risks of VBAC, the ultimate decision to attempt this procedure or undergo a repeat cesarean delivery should be made by the patient and her physician. This discussion should be documented in the medical record.

▶ Vaginal birth after a previous cesarean delivery is contraindicated in women with a previous classical uterine incision or extensive transfundal uterine surgery.

References

1. Curtin SC. Rates of cesarean birth and vaginal birth after previous cesarean, 1991–95. Monthly vital statistics report; vol. 45, no. 11, suppl 3. Hyattsville (MD): National Center for Health Statistics; 1997. (Level II-3)

2. Rates of cesarean delivery—United States, 1991. MMWR Morb Mortal Wkly Rep 1993;42:285–9. (Level II-3)

3. Stafford RS. Alternative strategies for controlling rising cesarean section rates. JAMA 1990;263:683–7. (Level III)

4. Scheller JM, Nelson KB. Does cesarean delivery prevent cerebral palsy or other neurologic problems of childhood? Obstet Gynecol 1994;83:624–30. (Level III)

5. Cragin EB. Conservatism in obstetrics. N Y Med J 1916; 104:1–3. (Level III)

6. Cowan RK, Kinch RA, Ellis B, Anderson R. Trial of labor following cesarean delivery. Obstet Gynecol 1994;83: 933–6. (Level II-3)

7. Flamm BL, Newman LA, Thomas SJ, Fallon D, Yoshida MM. Vaginal birth after cesarean delivery: results of a 5-year multicenter collaborative study. Obstet Gynecol 1990;76:750–4. (Level II-3)

8. Flamm BL, Goings JR, Liu Y, Wolde-Tsadik G. Elective repeat cesarean delivery versus trial of labor: a prospective multicenter study. Obstet Gynecol 1994;83:927–32. (Level II-2)

9. Miller DA, Diaz FG, Paul RH. Vaginal birth after cesarean: a 10-year experience. Obstet Gynecol 1994;84:255–8. (Level III)

10. Vaginal birth after cesarean birth–California, 1996–2000. MMWR Morb Mortal Wkly Rep 2002;51:996–8. (Level II-3)

11. Sachs BP, Kobelin C, Castro MA, Frigoletto F. The risks of lowering the cesarean-delivery rate. N Engl J Med 1999;340:54–7. (Level III)

12. Studnicki J, Remmel R, Campbell R, Werner DC. The impact of legislatively imposed practice guidelines on cesarean section rates: the Florida experience. Am J Med Qual 1997;12:62–8. (Level III)

13. Phelan JP. VBAC: time to reconsider? OBG Manage 1996;8(11):62, 64–8. (Level III)

14. Flamm BL. Once a cesarean, always a controversy. Obstet Gynecol 1997;90:312–5. (Level III)

15. Martin JA, Hamilton BE, Sutton PD, Ventura SJ, Menacker F, Munson ML. Births: final data for 2002. Natl Vital Stat Rep 2003;52(10):1–113. (Level II-3)

16. McMahon MJ, Luther ER, Bowes WA Jr, Olshan AF. Comparison of a trial of labor with an elective second cesarean section. N Engl J Med 1996;335:689–95. (Level II-2)

17. Gregory KD, Korst LM, Cane P, Platt LD, Kahn K. Vaginal birth after cesarean and uterine rupture rates in California. Obstet Gynecol 1999;94:985–9. (Level II-3)

18. Kieser KE, Baskett TF. A 10-year population-based study of uterine rupture. Obstet Gynecol 2002;100:749–53. (Level II-3)

19. Yap OW, Kim ES, Laros RK Jr. Maternal and neonatal outcomes after uterine rupture in labor. Am J Obstet Gynecol 2001;184:1576–81. (Level II-3)

20. Raynor BD. The experience with vaginal birth after cesarean delivery in a small rural community practice. Am J Obstet Gynecol 1993;168:60–2. (Level III)

21. Blanchette H, Blanchette M, McCabe J, Vincent S. Is vaginal birth after cesarean safe? Experience at a community hospital. Am J Obstet Gynecol 2001;184:1478–84; discussion 1484–7. (Level II-2)

22. Poma PA. Rupture of a cesarean-scarred uterus: a community hospital experience. J Natl Med Assoc 2000;92: 295–300. (Level II-2)

23. Hibbard JU, Ismail MA, Wang Y, Te C, Karrison T, Ismail MA. Failed vaginal birth after a cesarean section: how risky is it? I. Maternal morbidity. Am J Obstet Gynecol 2001;184:1365–71; discussion 1371–3. (Level II-2)

24. Leung AS, Farmer RM, Leung EK, Medearis AL, Paul RH. Risk factors associated with uterine rupture during trial of labor after cesarean delivery: a case-control study. Am J Obstet Gynecol 1993;168:1358–63. (Level II-2)

25. Mozurkewich EL, Hutton EK. Elective repeat cesarean delivery versus trial of labor: a meta-analysis of the literature from 1989 to 1999. Am J Obstet Gynecol 2000;183:1187–97. (Meta-analysis)

26. Asakura H, Myers SA. More than one previous cesarean delivery: a 5-year experience with 435 patients. Obstet Gynecol 1995;85:924–9. (Level III)

27. Caughey AB, Shipp TD, Repke JT, Zelop CM, Cohen A, Lieberman E. Rate of uterine rupture in women with one or two prior cesarean deliveries. Am J Obstet Gynecol 1999;181:872–6. (Level II-2)

28. Flamm BL, Goings JR. Vaginal birth after cesarean section: is suspected fetal macrosomia a contraindication? Obstet Gynecol 1989;74:694–7. (Level II-2)

29. Phelan JP, Eglinton GS, Horenstein JM, Clark SL, Yeh S. Previous cesarean birth. Trial of labor in women with macrosomic infants. J Reprod Med 1984;29:36–40. (Level II-2)

30. Zelop CM, Shipp TD, Repke JT, Cohen A, Lieberman E. Outcomes of a trial of labor following previous cesarean delivery among women with fetuses weighing >4000 g. Am J Obstet Gynecol 2001;185:903–5. (Level II-2)

31. Elkousy MA, Sammel M, Stevens E, Peipert JF, Macones G. The effect of birth weight on vaginal birth after cesarean delivery success rates. Am J Obstet Gynecol 2003;188:824–30. (Level II-2)

32. Yeh S, Huang X, Phelan JP. Postterm pregnancy after previous cesarean section. J Reprod Med 1984;29:41–4. (Level II-2)

33. Zelop CM, Shipp TD, Cohen A, Repke JT, Lieberman E. Trial of labor after 40 weeks' gestation in women with prior cesarean. Obstet Gynecol 2001;97:391–3. (Level II-2)

34. Martin JN Jr, Perry KG Jr, Roberts WE, Meydrech EF. The case for trial of labor in the patient with a prior low-segment vertical cesarean incision. Am J Obstet Gynecol 1997;177:144–8. (Level III)

35. Naef RW 3rd, Ray MA, Chauhan SP, Roach H, Blake PG, Martin JN Jr. Trial of labor after cesarean delivery with a lower-segment, vertical uterine incision: is it safe? Am J Obstet Gynecol 1995;172:1666–73; discussion 1673–4. (Level II-2)

36. Shipp TD, Zelop CM, Repke JT, Cohen A, Caughey AB, Lieberman E. Intrapartum uterine rupture and dehiscence in patients with prior lower uterine segment vertical and transverse incisions. Obstet Gynecol 1999;94:735–40. (Level II-2)

37. Lydon-Rochelle M, Holt VL, Easterling TR, Martin DP. Risk of uterine rupture during labor among women with a prior cesarean delivery. N Engl J Med 2001;345:3–8. (Level II-2)

38. Pruett KM, Kirshon B, Cotton DB, Poindexter AN 3rd. Is vaginal birth after two or more cesarean sections safe? Obstet Gynecol 1988;72:163–5. (Level III)

39. Beall M, Eglinton GS, Clark SL, Phelan JP. Vaginal delivery after cesarean section in women with unknown types of uterine scar. J Reprod Med 1984;29:31–5. (Level II-2)

40. Grubb DK, Kjos SL, Paul RH. Latent labor with an unknown uterine scar. Obstet Gynecol 1996;88:351–5. (Level I)

41. Miller DA, Mullin P, Hou D, Paul RH. Vaginal birth after cesarean section in twin gestation. Am J Obstet Gynecol 1996;175:194–8. (Level II-2)

42. Strong TH Jr, Phelan JP, Ahn MO, Sarno AP Jr. Vaginal birth after cesarean delivery in the twin gestation. Am J Obstet Gynecol 1989;161:29–32. (Level III)

43. Sansregret A, Bujold E, Gauthier RJ. Twin delivery after a previous caesarean: a twelve-year experience. J Obstet Gynaecol Can 2003;25:294–8. (Level II-2)

44. Myles T. Vaginal birth of twins after a previous cesarean section. J Matern Fetal Med 2001;10:171–4. (Level II-2)

45. Flamm BL. Vaginal birth after cesarean section. In: Flamm BL, Quilligan EJ, editors. Cesarean section: guidelines for appropriate utilization. New York (NY): Springer-Verlag; 1995. p. 51–64. (Level III)

46. Bujold E, Gauthier RJ. Should we allow a trial of labor after a previous cesarean for dystocia in the second stage of labor? Obstet Gynecol 2001;98:652–5. (Level III)

47. Rageth JC, Juzi C, Grossenbacher H. Delivery after previous cesarean: a risk evaluation. Swiss Working Group of Obstetric and Gynecologic Institutions. Obstet Gynecol 1999;93:332–7. (Level III)

48. Chauhan SP, Martin JN Jr, Henrichs CE, Morrison JC, Magann EF. Maternal and perinatal complications with uterine rupture in 142,075 patients who attempted vaginal birth after cesarean delivery: a review of the literature. Am J Obstet Gynecol 2003;189:408–17. (Level III)

49. Pickhardt MG, Martin JN Jr, Meydrech EF, Blake PG, Martin RW, Perry KG Jr, et al. Vaginal birth after cesarean delivery: are there useful and valid predictors of success or failure? Am J Obstet Gynecol 1992;166:1811–5; discussion 1815–9. (Level II-3)

50. Thurnau GR, Scates DH, Morgan MA. The fetal-pelvic index: a method of identifying fetal-pelvic disproportion in women attempting vaginal birth after previous cesarean delivery. Am J Obstet Gynecol 1991;165:353–8. (Level II-2)

51. Troyer LR, Parisi VM. Obstetric parameters affecting success in a trial of labor: designation of a scoring system. Am J Obstet Gynecol 1992;167:1099–104. (Level II-3)

52. Macones GA, Hausman N, Edelstein R, Stamilio DM, Marder SJ. Predicting outcomes of trials of labor in women attempting vaginal birth after cesarean delivery: a comparison of multivariate methods with neural networks. Am J Obstet Gynecol 2001;184:409–13. (Level II-2)

53. Bedoya C, Bartha JL, Rodriguez I, Fontan I, Bedoya JM, Sanchez-Ramos J. A trial of labor after cesarean section in patients with or without a prior vaginal delivery. Int J Gynaecol Obstet 1992;39:285–9. (Level II-2)

54. Shipp TD, Zelop CM, Repke JT, Cohen A, Caughey AB, Lieberman E. Labor after previous cesarean: influence of prior indication and parity. Obstet Gynecol 2000;95:913–6. (Level II-2)

55. Demianczuk NN, Hunter DJ, Taylor DW. Trial of labor after previous cesarean section: prognostic indicators of outcome. Am J Obstet Gynecol 1982;142:640–2. (Level II-3)

56. Hoskins IA, Gomez JL. Correlation between maximum cervical dilatation at cesarean delivery and subsequent vaginal birth after cesarean delivery. Obstet Gynecol 1997;89:591–3. (Level II-2)

57. Impey L, O'Herlihy C. First delivery after cesarean delivery for strictly defined cephalopelvic disproportion. Obstet Gynecol 1998;92:799–803. (Level II-2)

58. Jongen VH, Halfwerk MG, Brouwer WK. Vaginal delivery after previous caesarean section for failure of second stage of labour. Br J Obstet Gynaecol 1998;105:1079–81. (Level II-2)

59. McNally OM, Turner MJ. Induction of labour after 1 previous Caesarean section. Aust N Z J Obstet Gynaecol 1999;39:425–9. (Level II-2)

60. Caughey AB, Shipp TD, Repke JT, Zelop C, Cohen A, Lieherman E. Trial of labor after cesarean delivery: the effect of previous vaginal delivery. Am J Obstet Gynecol 1998;179:938–41. (Level II-2)

61. Ravasia DJ, Wood SL, Pollard JK. Uterine rupture during induced trial of labor among women with previous cesarean delivery. Am J Obstet Gynecol 2000;183:1176–9. (Level II-3)

62. Sims EJ, Newman RB, Hulsey TC. Vaginal birth after cesarean: to induce or not to induce. Am J Obstet Gynecol 2001;184:1122–4. (Level II-2)

63. Chauhan SP, Magann EF, Carroll CS, Barrilleaux PS, Scardo JA, Martin JN Jr. Mode of delivery for the morbidly obese with prior cesarean delivery: vaginal versus repeat cesarean section. Am J Obstet Gynecol 2001;185:349–54. (Level II-2)

64. Carroll CS Sr, Magann EF, Chauhan SP, Klauser CK, Morrison JC. Vaginal birth after cesarean section versus elective repeat cesarean delivery: weight-based outcomes. Am J Obstet Gynecol 2003;188:1516–20; discussion 1520–2. (Level II-2)

65. Huang WH, Nakashima DK, Rumney PJ, Keegan KA Jr, Chan K. Interdelivery interval and the success of vaginal birth after cesarean delivery. Obstet Gynecol 2002;99:41–4. (Level II-2)

66. Hook B, Kiwi R, Amini SB, Fanaroff A, Hack M. Neonatal morbidity after elective repeat cesarean section and trial of labor. Pediatrics 1997;100:348–53. (Level II-2)

67. Mankuta DD, Leshno MM, Menasche MM, Brezis MM. Vaginal birth after cesarean section: trial of labor or repeat cesarean section? A decision analysis. Am J Obstet Gynecol 2003;189:714–9. (Decision analysis)

68. Ananth CV, Smulian JC, Vintzileos AM. The association of placenta previa with history of cesarean delivery and abortion: a metaanalysis. Am J Obstet Gynecol 1997;177:1071–8. (Meta-analysis)

69. Smith GC, Pell JP, Cameron AD, Dobbie R. Risk of perinatal death associated with labor after previous cesarean delivery in uncomplicated term pregnancies. JAMA 2002;287:2684–90. (Level II-2)

70. Farmer RM, Kirschbaum T, Potter D, Strong TH, Medearis AL. Uterine rupture during trial of labor after previous cesarean section. Am J Obstet Gynecol 1991;165:996–1001. (Level II-2)

71. Jones RO, Nagashima AW, Hartnett-Goodman MM, Goodlin RC. Rupture of low transverse cesarean scars during trial of labor. Obstet Gynecol 1991;77:815–7. (Level III)

72. Scott JR. Mandatory trial of labor after cesarean delivery: an alternative viewpoint. Obstet Gynecol 1991;77:811–4. (Level III)

73. Scott JR. Avoiding labor problems during vaginal birth after cesarean delivery. Clin Obstet Gynecol 1997;40:533–41. (Level III)

74. Zelop CM, Shipp TD, Repke JT, Cohen A, Lieberman E. Effect of previous vaginal delivery on the risk of uterine rupture during a subsequent trial of labor. Am J Obstet Gynecol 2000;183:1184–6. (Level II-2)

75. Shipp TD, Zelop CM, Repke JT, Cohen A, Lieberman E. Interdelivery interval and risk of symptomatic uterine rupture. Obstet Gynecol 2001;97:175–7. (Level II-2)

76. Bujold E, Mehta SH, Bujold C, Gauthier RJ. Interdelivery interval and uterine rupture. Am J Obstet Gynecol 2002;187:1199–202. (Level II-2)

77. Esposito MA, Menihan CA, Malee MP. Association of interpregnancy interval with uterine scar failure in labor: a case-control study. Am J Obstet Gynecol 2000;183:1180–3. (Level II-2)

78. Bujold E, Bujold C, Hamilton EF, Harel F, Gauthier RJ. The impact of a single-layer or double-layer closure on uterine rupture. Am J Obstet Gynecol 2002;186:1326–30. (Level II-2)

79. Grobman WA, Peaceman AM, Socol ML. Cost-effectiveness of elective cesarean delivery after one prior low transverse cesarean. Obstet Gynecol 2000;95:745–51. (Cost-benefit analysis)

80. Clark SL, Scott JR, Porter TF, Schlappy DA, McClellan V, Burton DA. Is vaginal birth after cesarean less expensive than repeat cesarean delivery? Am J Obstet Gynecol 2000;182:599–602. (Cost-benefit analysis)

81. Chung A, Macario A, El-Sayed YY, Riley ET, Duncan B, Druzin ML. Cost-effectiveness of a trial of labor after previous cesarean. Obstet Gynecol 2001;97:932–41. (Level II-2)

82. DiMaio H, Edwards RK, Euliano TY, Treloar RW, Cruz AC. Vaginal birth after cesarean delivery: an historic cohort cost analysis. Am J Obstet Gynecol 2002;186:890–2. (Cost-benefit analysis)

83. Rosen MG, Dickinson JC, Westhoff CL. Vaginal birth after cesarean: a meta-analysis of morbidity and mortality. Obstet Gynecol 1991;77:465–70. (Meta-analysis)

84. Zelop CM, Shipp TD, Repke JT, Cohen A, Caughey AB, Lieberman E. Uterine rupture during induced or augmented labor in gravid women with one prior cesarean delivery. Am J Obstet Gynecol 1999;181:882–6. (Level II-2)

85. Stone JL, Lockwood CJ, Berkowitz G, Alvarez M, Lapinski R, Valcamonico A, et al. Use of cervical prostaglandin E2 gel in patients with previous cesarean section. Am J Perinatol 1994;11:309–12. (Level II-2)

86. Blanco JD, Collins M, Willis D, Prien S. Prostaglandin E2 gel induction of patients with a prior low transverse cesarean section. Am J Perinatol 1992;9:80–3. (Level II-2)

87. Norman M, Ekman G. Preinductive cervical ripening with prostaglandin E2 in women with one previous cesarean section. Acta Obstet Gynecol Scand 1992;71:351–5. (Level II-2)

88. Bennett BB. Uterine rupture during induction of labor at term with intravaginal misoprostol. Obstet Gynecol 1997;89:832–3. (Level III)

89. Wing DA, Lovett K, Paul RH. Disruption of prior uterine incision following misoprostol for labor induction in women with previous cesarean delivery. Obstet Gynecol 1998;91:828–30. (Level III)

90. Choy-Hee L, Raynor BD. Misoprostol induction of labor among women with a history of cesarean delivery. Am J Obstet Gynecol 2001;184:1115–7. (Level II-2)

91. Plaut MM, Schwartz ML, Lubarsky SL. Uterine rupture associated with the use of misoprostol in the gravid patient with a previous cesarean section. Am J Obstet Gynecol 1999;180:1535–42. (Level III)

92. Oteri O, Hopkins R. Second trimester therapeutic abortion using mifepristone and oral misoprostol in a woman with two previous caesarean sections and a cone biopsy. J Matern Fetal Med 1999;8:300–1. (Level III)

93. Berghahn L, Christensen D, Droste S. Uterine rupture during second-trimester abortion associated with misoprostol. Obstet Gynecol 2001;98:976–7. (Level III)

94. Rouzi AA. Second-trimester pregnancy termination with misoprostol in women with previous cesarean sections. Int J Gynaecol Obstet 2003;80:317–8. (Level III)

95. Gregory KD, Henry OA, Gellens AJ, Hobel CJ, Platt LD. Repeat cesareans: how many are elective? Obstet Gynecol 1994;84:574–8. (Level II-3)

96. Flamm BL, Fried MW, Lonky NM, Giles WS. External cephalic version after previous cesarean section. Am J Obstet Gynecol 1991;165:370–2. (Level II-2)

97. Johnson C, Oriol N. The role of epidural anesthesia in trial of labor. Reg Anesth 1990;15:304–8. (Level III)

98. Sakala EP, Kaye S, Murray RD, Munson LJ. Epidural analgesia. Effect on the likelihood of a successful trial of labor after cesarean section. J Reprod Med 1990;35:886–90. (Level II-2)

99. Flamm BL, Lim OW, Jones C, Fallon D, Newman LA, Mantis JK. Vaginal birth after cesarean section: results of a multicenter study. Am J Obstet Gynecol 1988;158:1079–84. (Level II-2)

100. Stovall TG, Shaver DC, Solomon SK, Anderson GD. Trial of labor in previous cesarean section patients, excluding classical cesarean sections. Obstet Gynecol 1987;70:713–7. (Level II-3)

101. Horenstein JM, Phelan JP. Previous cesarean section: the risks and benefits of oxytocin usage in a trial of labor. Am J Obstet Gynecol 1985;151:564–9. (Level II-2)

102. Flamm BL, Goings JR, Fuelberth NJ, Fischermann E, Jones C, Hersh E. Oxytocin during labor after previous cesarean section: results of a multicenter study. Obstet Gynecol 1987;70:709–12. (Level II-3)

103. Goetzl L, Shipp TD, Cohen A, Zelop CM, Repke JT, Lieberman E. Oxytocin dose and the risk of uterine rupture in trial of labor after cesarean. Obstet Gynecol 2001;97:381–4. (Level II-2)

104. Ritchie EH. Pregnancy after rupture of the pregnant uterus. A report of 36 pregnancies and a study of cases reported since 1932. J Obstet Gynaecol Br Commonw 1971;78:642–8. (Level III)

105. Reyes-Ceja L, Cabrera R, Insfran E, Herrera-Lasso F. Pregnancy following previous uterine rupture: study of 19 patients. Obstet Gynecol 1969;34:387–9. (Level III)

The MEDLINE database, the Cochrane Library, and ACOG's own internal resources and documents were used to conduct a literature search to locate relevant articles published between January 1985 and March 2004. The search was restricted to articles published in the English language. Priority was given to articles reporting results of original research, although review articles and commentaries also were consulted. Abstracts of research presented at symposia and scientific conferences were not considered adequate for inclusion in this document. Guidelines published by organizations or institutions such as the National Institutes of Health and the American College of Obstetricians and Gynecologists were reviewed, and additional studies were located by reviewing bibliographies of identified articles. When reliable research was not available, expert opinions from obstetrician–gynecologists were used.

Studies were reviewed and evaluated for quality according to the method outlined by the U.S. Preventive Services Task Force:

I   Evidence obtained from at least 1 properly designed randomized controlled trial.

II-1   Evidence obtained from well-designed controlled trials without randomization.

II-2   Evidence obtained from well-designed cohort or case–control analytic studies, preferably from more than 1 center or research group.

II-3   Evidence obtained from multiple time series with or without the intervention. Dramatic results in uncontrolled experiments also could be regarded as this type of evidence.

III   Opinions of respected authorities, based on clinical experience, descriptive studies, or reports of expert committees.

Based on the highest level of evidence found in the data, recommendations are provided and graded according to the following categories:

Level A—Recommendations are based on good and consistent scientific evidence.

Level B—Recommendations are based on limited or inconsistent scientific evidence.

Level C—Recommendations are based primarily on consensus and expert opinion.

ISSN 1099-3630

**The American College of
Obstetricians and Gynecologists
409 12th Street, SW
PO Box 96920
Washington, DC 20090-6920**

12345/87654

Vaginal birth after previous cesarean delivery. ACOG Practice Bulletin No. 54. American College of Obstetricians and Gynecologists. Obstet Gynecol 2004;104:203–12.

Technology Assessments

Genetics and Molecular Diagnostic Testing (No. 1)   1027
Hysteroscopy (No. 4)   1046
Saline Infusion Sonohysterography (No. 3)   1050

Technology Assessments

ACOG

TECHNOLOGY ASSESSMENT

IN OBSTETRICS AND GYNECOLOGY

NUMBER 1, JULY 2002

This Technology Assessment was developed by the ACOG Committee on Genetics with the assistance of Deborah A. Driscoll, MD, FACOG; Katherine D. Wenstrom, MD, FACOG, and John Williams III, MD, FACOG. This document reflects emerging clinical and scientific advances as of the date issued and is subject to change. The information should not be construed as dictating an exclusive course of treatment or procedure to be followed. Variations in practice may be warranted based on the needs of the individual patient, resources, and limitations unique to the institution or type of practice.

THE AMERICAN COLLEGE
OF OBSTETRICIANS
AND GYNECOLOGISTS
WOMEN'S HEALTH CARE PHYSICIANS

Genetics and Molecular Diagnostic Testing

Knowledge of human genetics has increased dramatically in the past few decades. The genetic basis of disease and the response to therapy is rapidly being elucidated and may soon become a part of routine medical practice. A draft of the human genome was published in 2001 (1). This project produced a detailed map of the genes, markers, and other landmarks along each chromosome. It is hoped that these maps will facilitate the development of genetic screening and diagnostic tests, as well as novel therapies, technologies, and strategies for prevention. Obstetricians and gynecologists, who deal with inheritance and the genetic transmission of traits and disease on a daily basis, will be called on to incorporate genetics and recent developments in genetic testing into their medical practice. This document reviews the basics of genetic transmission and genetic technologies in current use. (See the "Glossary" for definitions of terms for genetics and molecular diagnostic testing.)

ORGANIZATION OF THE GENOME

There are 2 meters of DNA, including approximately 30,000 genes, in each human nucleus. The DNA is wrapped very compactly around basic proteins called histones to form nucleosomes, which are then organized into solenoid structures and looped around a nonhistone protein scaffold to form chromatin. As the cell enters prophase, the chromatin begins to condense until it assumes the familiar structure of metaphase chromosomes. Each chromosome is composed of densely packed nontranscribed DNA near the centromeres, called heterochromatin, and less densely packed transcribed DNA called euchromatin.

Seventy-five percent of the genome is unique, single copy DNA, and the remainder consists of various classes of repetitive DNA. Surprisingly, virtually all of the repetitive DNA and a large portion of the single copy DNA have no apparent or recognized function. Less than 10% of the genome encodes genes. The single copy DNA contains all of the genes necessary to make and sustain the organism, while the repetitive DNA contains unique markers that identify each individual and can be used to study genetic variation between individuals.

Genes

A gene is a unique series of four purine and pyrimidine bases that ultimately specifies an amino acid sequence for a polypeptide chain of a protein. The basic gene contains one or more exons, which are DNA sequences that will be transcribed into messenger RNA (mRNA), and introns (or intervening sequences), which are noncoding or nontranscribed regions that separate exons (Fig. 1). The regions upstream and downstream to the exons are called the 5′ untranslated region and the 3′ untranslated region, respectively. These regions are transcribed, but not translated (as the name implies), and they are important in gene regulation.

The processes of transcription and translation are more complex than previously recognized. The transcription of DNA to mRNA requires transcription factors. Enhancers and silencer DNA sequences located upstream or downstream of a gene can increase and decrease transcriptional activity of the gene, respectively. Transcription is initiated when the enzyme RNA polymerase II binds to the pro-

moter, a DNA sequence upstream of a gene. RNA polymerase moves along a single strand of DNA and forms a complementary strand of mRNA. Once the mRNA is formed, a cap or chemically modified guanine nucleotide is added to the 5′ end to prevent the mRNA from being degraded, and a chain of 100–200 adenine bases (poly-A tail) is added to the 3′ end. Before the mRNA leaves the nucleus, the introns are excised by a process called gene splicing. The mature mRNA then moves to the ribosomes for translation. The protein product usually is created in a precursor form, and undergoes cleavage into a smaller active protein or combines with other polypeptides to form a larger functional protein. The protein may be further modified in the Golgi apparatus of the cell by glycosylation. Some genes contain more than one promoter in different parts of the gene or have alternative splice sites, which allows the same gene to encode different protein products.

Gene expression also is controlled by methylation of the regulatory region, which prevents gene transcription and effectively turns the gene off.

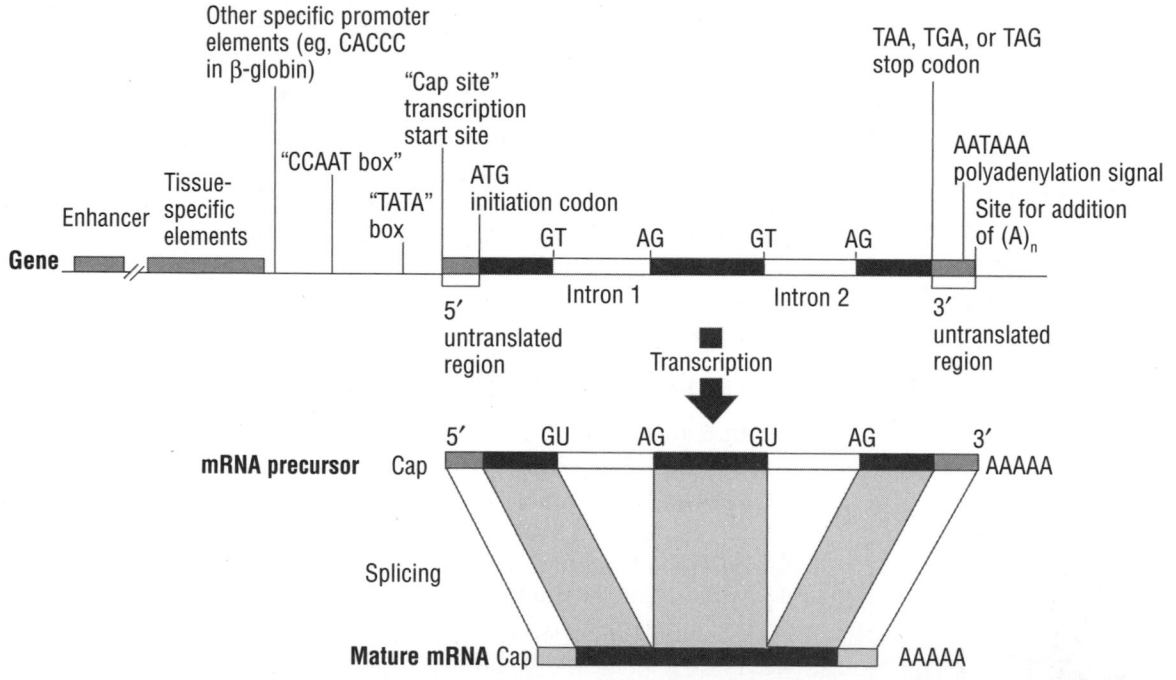

Fig. 1. Structure of a typical gene. In this example, the gene has three exons (solid dark regions) and two introns (white regions), a 5′ untranslated region and 3′ untranslated region. The intron splice donor site (GT) and the splice acceptor site (AG) identify where introns are removed in mRNA production. The upstream region (5′) contains an enhancer, tissue specific elements, and promoter elements, such as the CCAAT box and TATA box, which regulate expression. Typical locations for the translation initiation site (ATG), translation stop codons (TAA, TAG, TGA), and the polyadenylation signal (AATAAA) are shown. (Gelehrter TD, Ginsburg D, Collins FS. Principles of medical genetics. 2nd ed. Baltimore: Williams and Wilkins, 1997)

Methylation serves the important function of controlling tissue-specific gene activation. The expression of genes that are not essential for each specific tissue type is prevented by methylation, while necessary genes remain active. For example, the globin genes are methylated in all nonerythroid tissues but are not methylated in reticulocytes, ensuring that only red blood cells produce hemoglobin. Methylation also allows the temporal control of gene expression. Parental alleles may demonstrate different patterns of methylation that are not tissue specific (see section on "Imprinting").

Many genes exist in several alternate forms called alleles. These are normal variants within the population. For example, there are several normal alleles for the genes that determine blood type and Rh status. In contrast, a mutation is an alteration in the DNA sequence that results in a change in protein structure or function, which may have adverse effects. Mutations can occur in the germline (eg, gametes) and can be transmitted from one generation to the next, or can occur only in the somatic cells and can be associated with cancer. There are many types of mutations, such as single purine or pyrimidine base substitutions (missense, nonsense), deletions and insertions of one or more bases, and visible chromosome deletions and duplications. Mutations occur infrequently in the population. The distinction between an allele and a mutation can be blurred; many normal alleles probably result from ancient mutations that either did not affect survival or conferred some selective advantage.

The vast majority (99.8%) of DNA is identical in all humans. However, minor differences that distinguish one person from another do exist. These differences, called polymorphisms, generally consist of a single nucleotide change and occur every 200 to 500 base pairs. Polymorphisms, in general, do not produce deleterious effects. Some polymorphisms may modify gene function (eg, splice variant or thymidine tract in intron 8 of the cystic fibrosis [CF] gene can influence the amount of mRNA produced). In most cases, polymorphisms are normal variants, which often are used to track the transmission of disease genes (see sections on "Restriction Fragment Length Polymorphism Analysis" and "Linkage Analysis").

When newly discovered genes are analyzed, it can be difficult to distinguish a normal allele from a polymorphism or a mutation. For example, more than 100 variations of the *BRCA1* gene, one of the major genes associated with familial breast and ovarian cancers, have been identified. It is not currently known whether all of these variations are actually mutations associated with disease, or if some could be polymorphisms or allelic variants. The ability to distinguish alleles from mutations is essential for molecular diagnosis and screening programs.

SINGLE GENE (MENDELIAN) DISORDERS

A mendelian trait or disease is determined by a single gene. Diseases caused solely by abnormalities in a single gene are relatively rare. The phenotype of many single gene disorders is influenced by modifying genes, or by the independent actions of a combination of additional genes, often with environmental influences.

Autosomal Dominant

All genes come in pairs; one copy of the gene is present on each of a pair of chromosomes. The influence of each gene in determining the phenotype is described as either dominant or recessive. If one of the genes in a pair specifies the phenotype in preference to the other gene, that gene and the trait or disease it specifies are considered to be dominant. The carrier of a gene causing an autosomal dominant disease has a 50% chance of passing on the affected gene with each conception.

The phenotype of an individual carrying a dominant gene is determined by several factors. One factor is penetrance. Penetrance indicates whether or not the mutant gene is expressed. If a dominant gene produces some kind of recognizable phenotypic expression in all individuals who carry it, it is said to have complete penetrance. A gene that is not expressed in all individuals who carry it has incomplete penetrance. For individuals, penetrance is an all-or-nothing phenomenon, but penetrance in a population can be quantitated. For example, a phenotype that is expressed in 80% of individuals who carry the gene has 80% penetrance.

Incomplete penetrance may account for some autosomal dominant diseases that appear to "skip" generations. Alternatively, the individual carrying the dominant gene may have very mild phenotypic abnormalities that have been overlooked, the disease may have a late onset, the gene carrier is either too young or died before the gene's effects were manifest, or phenotypic expression of the dominant gene could require the presence of a second mutated gene or certain epigenetic phenomena. An example of such a disease is retinoblastoma.

The degree to which a penetrant gene is expressed (the range of phenotypic features) is called expressivity. If all individuals carrying the affected gene do not have identical phenotypes, the gene has variable expressivity. Such a gene can produce a range of phenotypic features from mild to severe. An example of a disease with variable expressivity is neurofibromatosis.

Autosomal Recessive

Autosomal recessive traits or diseases occur only when both copies of the gene in question are the same. Individuals who have only one abnormal gene (heterozygotes or carriers) may have some phenotypic alteration recognized at the biochemical or cellular level, but only individuals who have two copies of the affected gene (homozygotes) have the disease. Many enzyme deficiency diseases are autosomal recessive. The enzyme level in the carrier of an abnormal recessive gene will be approximately 50% of normal, but because enzymes are made in great excess, this reduction usually is not enough to cause disease. However, the reduced enzyme level can be used for genetic screening purposes. For example, to identify carriers of Tay–Sachs disease, hexosaminidase A levels are measured. Carriers of recessive conditions that do not produce any physical or quantitative biochemical change in the heterozygote can be identified only by molecular methods (eg, Canavan disease).

The carrier of a gene causing an autosomal recessive disease usually is recognized after the birth of an affected child, after the diagnosis of an affected family member, or as the result of a genetic screening program. A couple whose child has an autosomal recessive disease has a 25% recurrence risk with each conception. The likelihood that a normal sibling of an affected child is a carrier of the gene is 2 out of 3 (one fourth of all offspring will be homozygous normal, two fourths will be heterozygote carriers, and one fourth will be homozygous abnormal; thus, 3 of 4 children will be phenotypically normal and 2 of these 3 will be carriers). Carrier children will not have affected children unless their partners are gene carriers or are affected. Because genes leading to rare autosomal recessive conditions have a low prevalence in the general population, the chance that the partner will be a gene carrier is low unless the couple is related (consanguineous). When individuals inherit two different mutated alleles that result in abnormal phenotypes, they are called compound heterozygotes. For example, an individual who inherits a ΔF508 and W1282X mutation in the CF gene has CF without expressing two identical alleles.

Co-Dominant

If the genes in a gene pair are different from each other, but both are expressed in the phenotype, they are considered to be co-dominant. For example, the genes responsible for the hemoglobinopathies are co-dominant. The individual with one hemoglobin gene directing the production of sickle hemoglobin, and the other directing the production of hemoglobin C, will produce both S and C hemoglobins. Likewise, the genes that determine blood type are co-dominant, because an individual is capable of expressing both A and B red cell antigens simultaneously.

X-Linked

X-linked diseases usually are recessive, and primarily affect men because men have only one copy of the X chromosome. Examples of X-linked recessive disorders are color blindness, hemophilia A (classical hemophilia or factor VIII deficiency), and Duchenne muscular dystrophy. Women carrying an X-linked recessive gene generally are unaffected unless unfavorable lyonization (the inactivation of one X chromosome in every cell) results in the X chromosome carrying the abnormal gene being active in the majority of cells.

When a woman carries a gene causing an X-linked recessive condition, there is a 50% chance of passing on the gene with each conception; each of her sons has a 50% chance of being affected and each of her daughters has a 50% chance of being a carrier. When a man has an X-linked disease, all of his sons will be unaffected (because they receive the Y chromosome from their father) and all of his daughters will be carriers (because they receive the affected X chromosome from their father). X-linked dominant disorders have been described, and affect females predominantly because they tend to be lethal in male offspring. An example of this is X-linked hypophosphatemia.

DUPLICATION AND DELETION SYNDROMES

A deletion refers to a region of a chromosome that is missing, while a duplication is the presence of an extra copy of a region of a chromosome. The carrier of a deletion is effectively monosomic for the genes in the missing segment, while the carrier of a duplication is trisomic for the duplicated genes. Deletions and duplications usually are described by their location (eg, duplication 4p) or by the two chromosomal break points defining the missing or extra segment (4p15.2→16.1). If the deletion is a common one, it may be defined by an eponym (eg, del 1q32-q41 also is called Van der Woude's syndrome). Terminal deletions and duplications are caused simply by chromosome breakage with loss or gain of the terminal chromosome segment. Interstitial deletions and duplications occur during prophase of meiosis when homologous chromosomes align and crossovers occur. If the chromosomes are misaligned during this process, the unaligned loop containing the mismatched segment could be deleted. Alternatively, misalignment could lead to unequal crossing over, so that one chromosome has a deletion and the other a duplication. A similar problem with meiosis can produce deletions and duplications in the offspring of individuals who are carriers of chromosome inversions. Deletions and duplications also occur as a result of malsegregation during meiosis in carriers of balanced translocations.

When a deletion or duplication is identified in a fetus or child, the parents should be tested to see if it arose de novo in their offspring or if either parent is a carrier or has a translocation. Deletions and duplications may be identified by routine or high resolution cytogenetic analysis. Microdeletions and duplications, which are too small to be detected by traditional cytogenetic techniques, can now be recognized with molecular techniques, such as fluorescence in situ hybridization (FISH) (see section on "Fluorescence In Situ Hybridization").

Chromosome deletions and duplications can result in a constellation of phenotypic abnormalities with widely varying pathophysiology or pathogenesis because the genes that are in close proximity to one another on a chromosome may have completely unrelated functions and control independent traits. Deletion syndromes usually cause more serious phenotypic and functional abnormalities than duplication syndromes. Monosomy generally has more severe consequences than trisomy.

Syndromes caused by a microdeletion involving genes physically located together in a chromosome segment are called contiguous gene deletion syndromes, and their study has yielded a great deal of information about gene location and function. Although deletions can occur in any area of any chromosome, some deletions occur more frequently than would be expected by chance alone. Several common chromosome deletion syndromes have been recognized, such as DiGeorge syndrome, which most often results from a microdeletion of the

long arm of chromosome 22 (del 22q11.2). Affected individuals typically have conotruncal cardiac defects; thymus and parathyroid gland hypoplasia or aplasia; atypical facies, including short palpebral fissures, micrognathia with a short philtrum, and ear anomalies; and learning and speech difficulties. Deletions of the terminal portions of the short arms of chromosomes 4 (4 p- or Wolf-Hirschhorn syndrome) and 5 (5 p- or cri du chat syndrome) also occur more frequently than would be expected by chance alone.

NONMENDELIAN PATTERNS OF INHERITANCE

Hereditary Unstable DNA

Mendel's first law states that genes are passed unchanged from parent to progeny. Barring the occurrence of new mutations, this law still applies to many genes or traits. However, it is now known that certain genes are inherently unstable, and their size and, consequently, their function may be altered as they are transmitted from parent to child. These genes generally contain a region of triplet repeats, such as $(CGG)_n$. The number of triplet repeats in gametes can increase as meiosis is completed prior to fertilization. If the number of triplet repeats reaches a critical level, the gene containing the triplets becomes methylated and is turned off, resulting in phenotypic abnormalities. Some triplet regions expand only during female meiosis, while others can expand when transmitted by either parent. Some triplet regions have been passed from parent to child for many generations without expansion, for unknown reasons.

An example of a genetic disease caused by such triplet repeats is fragile X syndrome. Fragile X syndrome is the most common form of all familial mental retardation, accounting for 4–8% of all individuals with mental retardation in all ethnic and racial groups. Affected individuals have mild to severe mental retardation, autistic behavior, attention deficit hyperactivity disorder, speech and language problems, a narrow face with a large jaw, long prominent ears, and macro-orchidism (in postpubertal males). Some children also have seizures. The incidence of the full fragile X syndrome generally is quoted as 1 per 1,500 males and 1 per 2,500 females.

Until recently, fragile X syndrome was diagnosed using a cytogenetic technique. Cells were cultured in a folate deficient medium, which resulted in fragile sites identified cytogenetically as nonstaining gaps or constrictions on the long arm of the X chromosome (Xq27-28). This technique was unreliable for carrier testing, and less than half the cells from affected males manifested the fragile site. Fortunately, the fragile X gene can now be directly examined using molecular techniques (see section on "Trinucleotide Repeat Analysis").

The fragile X mutation is now known to be a region of unstable DNA in the X chromosome. The region is best described as a series of CGG (cytosine–guanine–guanine) repeats at Xq27. The number of repeats and the degree of methylation determines whether or not an individual is affected. Individuals carrying 2–49 repeats are phenotypically normal. Individuals carrying 50–199 repeats are phenotypically normal but have a premutation, which can expand as it is passed on to their offspring, who would then be affected. Those with more than 200 repeats have the full mutation and, if methylation occurs, usually are affected. However, not all individuals carrying the full mutation are mentally retarded. Phenotypic variability results from lyonization (in females) and mosaicism for the size of the expansion, the degree of methylation, or both during mitosis in the zygote. Therefore, the phenotype cannot be predicted by analysis of either the parental gene or fetal cells.

The number of repeats usually remains stable when the gene is transmitted by a male. However, when the gene passes through female meiosis, it can expand. The risk of expansion generally correlates with the number of repeats in the premutation. Premutations with 100 or more repeats expand on transmission 100% of the time. The risk of expansion of mutations with 50–99 repeats increases proportionally with expansion size. If a female carries a premutation, which then increases in size as she transmits it to her offspring, it is possible for her to have a child with fragile X syndrome even though she is unaffected and has no family history of mental retardation.

The number of CGG repeats and the methylation status of the gene can be determined using restriction endonuclease digestion and Southern blot analysis (see section on "Trinucleotide Repeat Analysis"). It is now apparent that triplet repeat expansion is responsible for a number of primarily neurologic diseases, such as myotonic dystrophy, Huntington's chorea, and Friedreich's ataxia. The expansion of triplet repeats is an important mechanism of genetic disease, and is likely to play an important part in diseases for which preconceptional counseling and prenatal diagnosis may be considered.

Imprinting

Another tenet of mendelian genetics is that gene function is not influenced by the sex of the parent transmitting the gene. In contrast to this rule, it is now apparent that the function of certain genes is altered by the sex of the parent from whom they were inherited, by a process known as "imprinting." Imprinting is a mechanism for epigenetic control of gene expression; that is, it changes the phenotype without permanently altering the genotype. An imprinted gene is inherited in an inactivated (transcriptionally silent) state, as the result of methylation of the promoter region. The extent of the imprinting, and thus the degree of inactivation, is determined by the sex of the transmitting parent.

When a gene is inherited in an imprinted or inactivated state, gene function is necessarily directed entirely by the active co-gene inherited from the other parent. It appears that imprinting exerts an effect in part by controlling the dosage of specific genes. Certain important genes appear to be monoallelic; that is, under normal circumstances only one member of the gene pair is functional (as opposed to most of the genes in the genome, which are biallelic). Only a fraction of human genes are imprinted. With imprinted genes, however, normal development occurs only when both a paternally derived and a maternally derived copy of the gene is present.

Imprinting was first recognized in association with genetic disease. Two very distinct genetic diseases with dissimilar phenotypes were discovered to be associated with the same chromosomal deletion, at 15q11-13. One of the diseases is Prader-Willi syndrome, which is characterized by obesity; hyperphagia; short stature; small hands, feet, and external genitalia; and mild mental retardation. The other disorder is Angelman's syndrome, which includes normal stature and weight, severe mental retardation, absent speech, seizure disorder, ataxia and jerky arm movements, and paroxysms of inappropriate laughter. Cytogenetic analysis has confirmed that both diseases are associated with the same deletion. If the maternally derived chromosome 15 is deleted, the result is Angelman's syndrome; if the paternally derived chromosome 15 is deleted, the result is Prader-Willi syndrome. Furthermore, a deletion is not required to produce the phenotype. If an individual has two normal intact copies of chromosome 15, but both came from the man (see section on "Uniparental Disomy"), the phenotype is consistent with Angelman's syndrome, because the maternal contribution is missing. Likewise, two complete copies of chromosome 15 of maternal origin produces Prader-Willi syndrome. Studies of the methylation patterns in individuals with the 15q11-13 deletion have shown that differential methylation (imprinting) is responsible for these observed phenotypic differences.

Several clinical examples from obstetrics illustrate the developmental importance of imprinting. Complete hydatidiform mole, which has an exclusively paternally derived diploid chromosome complement, is characterized by the abundant growth of placental tissue, but no fetal structures. Conversely, ovarian teratoma, which has a maternally derived diploid chromosome complement, is characterized by the growth of various fetal tissues, but no placental structures. Triploidy, characterized by a conceptus with three complete haploid chromosome complements (69 chromosomes), has two distinct phenotypes. If the extra haploid chromosome complement comes from the man, the embryo will be lost early in gestation and the placenta will be large and cystic, and severe early onset preeclampsia is likely to develop; if the extra chromosome complement comes from the woman, the fetus will be anomalous and the placenta will be extremely small. These observations confirm that both the paternally derived and maternally derived imprinted genes must be present for normal fetal development to occur.

Uniparental Disomy

Uniparental disomy is a situation in which both members of one pair of chromosomes are inherited from one parent. Every gene on each of the chromosomes in question will have come from one parent. This usually occurs as the result of "correction" of a trisomic zygote by loss of a chromosome. When a conceptus with three copies of a chromosome loses one chromosome and retains the two chromosomes transmitted by the other parent, this results in heterodisomy (inheritance of two different homologous chromosomes from one parent). Less frequently, "rescue" of a monosomic conceptus with only one chromosome from one parent may occur by duplication of the chromosome during mitosis producing a cell with two copies of the same chromosome or uniparental isodisomy. For some chromosomes, uniparental disomy can result in functional or developmental fetal abnormalities, particularly if imprinting of the genes on that chromosome exists. Recent studies have demonstrated clinically significant uniparental disomy for chromosomes 6, 7, 11, 14, and 15. Uniparental disomy has no effect on the majority of chromosomes.

Mitochondrial Inheritance

Every human cell contains hundreds of mitochondria. Because each mitochondrian contains its own genome and associated replication systems, each behaves as a virtually autonomous organism. The human oocyte contains approximately 100,000 mitochondria in the cytoplasm and mitochondrial DNAs. In contrast, a sperm contains only 100 mitochondria, which are selectively eliminated during fertilization. Therefore, mitochondria are inherited exclusively from the woman. Because mitochondria contain genetic information, mitochondrial inheritance allows the transmission of genes directly from the woman to her offspring without the possibility of recombination.

If a mutation occurs in the mitochondrial DNA, it may segregate into a daughter cell during cell division and thus be propagated. Over time, the percentage of mutant mitochondrial DNAs in different cell lines can drift towards either normal or pure mutant. If an oocyte containing largely mutant mitochondrial DNAs is fertilized, the offspring might have a mitochondrial disease. Several mitochondrial genetic diseases have been described. These include myoclonic epilepsy with ragged red fibers (MERRF), Leber's hereditary optic neuropathy, Kearns–Sayre syndrome, Leigh syndrome (ataxia, hypotonia, spasticity, and optic abnormalities), and pigmentary retinopathy.

Germline Mosaicism

Some cytogenetically normal individuals have mosaicism (the presence of two or more populations of cells with different characteristics within one tissue or organ) confined to their gonads. Gonadal or germline mosaicism can arise as the result of a mitotic error occurring in the zygote; if the error occurs in cells destined to become the gonad, a portion of the germ cells may be abnormal. Because spermatogonia and oogonia continue to divide throughout fetal development, gonadal mosaicism also could occur as the result of a meiotic error in the dividing germ cells of the embryo. Germline mosaicism may explain the occurrence of a "new" (not previously occurring in a family) autosomal dominant mutation causing a disease, such as achondroplasia or osteogenesis imperfecta, or a new X-linked disease, such as Duchenne muscular dystrophy. It also explains the recurrence of such diseases in more than one offspring in a previously unaffected family. Because of the potential for germline mosaicism, the recurrence risk after the birth of a child with a disease caused by a new mutation is approximately 6%.

Multifactorial and Polygenic Inheritance

Polygenic traits are determined by the combined effects of many genes; multifactorial traits are determined by multiple genes and environmental factors. It is now believed that the majority of inherited traits are multifactorial or polygenic. Traits determined by single genes and transmitted by strict mendelian inheritance, without the contribution of modifier genes, are probably relatively rare. Birth defects caused by multifactorial or polygenic inheritance are recognized by their tendency to recur in families, but not according to a mendelian inheritance pattern. Other characteristics that distinguish multifactorial traits from those with other inheritance patterns are listed in the box. When counseling couples regarding their offspring's risk of a familial multifactorial trait, it is important to consider the affected relative's degree of relatedness to the fetus, not the parents. The empiric recurrence risk for first-degree relatives (the fetus's parents or siblings) usually is quoted as 2–3%, but the risk declines exponentially with successively more distant relationships. Multifactorial traits generally fall into one of the three following categories: 1) continuously variable, 2) threshold, or 3) complex disorders.

Continuously variable traits have a normal distribution in the general population. By convention, abnormality is defined as a trait or measurement greater than two standard deviations above or below the population mean. These are typically measurable or quantitative traits like height or head size, and are believed to result from the individually small effects of many genes combined with environmental factors. Such traits tend to be less extreme in the offspring of affected individuals, because of the statistical principle of regression to the mean.

Multifactorial Inheritance

1. The disorder is familial, but there is no apparent pattern of inheritance.
2. The risk to first-degree relatives is the square root of the population risk.
3. The risk is sharply lower for second-degree relatives.
4. The recurrence risk is higher if more than one family member is affected.
5. The risk is higher if the defect is more severe (ie, the recurrence risk for bilateral cleft lip is higher than for unilateral cleft lip).
6. If the defect is more common in one sex, the recurrence risk is higher if the affected individual is of the less commonly affected sex.

Threshold traits do not appear until a certain threshold of liability is exceeded. Factors creating liability to the malformation are assumed to be continuously distributed in the population; only individuals who are at the extreme of this distribution exceed the threshold and have the trait or defect. The phenotypic abnormality is thus an all or none phenomenon. Individuals in high-risk families have enough abnormal genes or environmental influences that their liability is close to the threshold; for unknown reasons, some factor or factors increases the liability for certain family members still further and the threshold is crossed, resulting in the defect. Cleft lip and palate and pyloric stenosis are examples of threshold traits.

Certain threshold traits have a predilection for one gender, indicating that males and females have a different liability threshold. When a family includes an affected member who is the less frequently affected sex, this indicates that even more abnormal genes or environmental influences are present, and the affected individual (and possibly the family) has a more extreme position in the normal distribution of predisposing factors. The affected person's first-degree relatives (eg, their siblings) have a higher liability for that particular trait. For example, pyloric stenosis is more common in males. If a girl is born with pyloric stenosis, this indicates that she or her parents have even more abnormal genes or predisposing factors than usually are necessary to produce pyloric stenosis. After the birth of a girl with pyloric stenosis, the recurrence risk for her siblings or for her future children will be higher than expected; male siblings or offspring will have the highest liability because they are the most susceptible sex and they will inherit more than the usual number of predisposing genes.

The recurrence risk for threshold traits also is higher if the defect is severe, again indicating the presence of more abnormal genes or influences. For example, the recurrence risk after the birth of a child with bilateral cleft lip and palate is 8%, compared with only 4% after unilateral cleft lip without cleft palate.

Complex disorders of adult life are traits in which many genes determine an individual's susceptibility to environmental factors, with disease resulting from the most unfavorable combination of both. This category includes common diseases, such as heart disease and hypertension. These disorders usually are familial and behave as threshold traits but with a very strong environmental influence. The genetic mechanisms of many common adult diseases have not yet been elucidated, although several associated genes have been identified. In some cases, the identity of the associated gene provides a clue to the pathogenesis of the disease; in others, the related gene may simply be used as a disease marker. Premature cardiovascular diseases, for example, are associated with the gene for apolipoprotein E, a gene that likely influences the pathology of the disease. In contrast, the association of type 1 diabetes with HLA-DR3/4 is less clear.

MOLECULAR DIAGNOSTIC TESTING

Advances in our understanding of the molecular basis of inherited disorders have led to the development of DNA-based tests, which may be used for the confirmation of a diagnosis, prenatal diagnosis, and carrier testing. Molecular diagnostic testing is now widely available for a number of single gene disorders, such as Tay–Sachs disease, Canavan disease, sickle cell disease, CF, muscular dystrophies, and fragile X syndrome. Molecular-cytogenetic testing has been developed for the detection of chromosomal abnormalities, including aneuploidy and submicroscopic deletions and duplications.

DNA can be obtained from many sources, including blood lymphocytes, skin, hair, cheek cells, and paraffin tissue blocks. Most diagnostic laboratories prefer either blood samples or buccal swabs for DNA testing. Cultured amniocytes, chorionic villi, and fetal blood are used for prenatal DNA testing of the fetus.

MUTATION DETECTION

Once a gene has been cloned and mutations have been identified, direct testing for the mutation is possible. This is the most accurate diagnostic method. Direct mutation tests usually are performed by commercial and hospital-based laboratories for common mutations, which are well characterized and account for the majority of cases. In some cases, the mutations are unique to a specific ethnicity. For example, two specific mutations in the aspartoacylase gene account for 97% of the mutations that cause Canavan disease in the Ashkenazi Jewish population. For some genetic disorders, the mutations are unique or specific to an individual family; therefore, mutation testing may not be routinely provided by a commercial laboratory. In these cases, there may be only one or two academic or hospital laboratories in the country that offer the testing. (This information is provided by GeneTests, a genetic testing resource web site at www.genetests.org.) In general, initial screening of a gene for mutations usually takes place in research laboratories under approved protocols and is not practical for diagnostic testing. Once a mutation has been identified, it may be possible to offer diagnostic or carrier testing to individuals at risk.

There are a variety of methods available for detecting mutations. The methodology usually is determined by the nature of the specific mutation. Allele specific oligonucleotide hybridization and restriction fragment length polymorphisms analysis frequently are used to detect point mutations. Southern blot analysis and polymerase chain reaction (PCR) often are used to detect gene deletions associated with disorders such as Duchenne muscular dystrophy and spinal muscular atrophy. A combination of PCR and Southern blot analysis are used to determine the number of trinucleotide repeats for disorders such as fragile X syndrome and myotonic dystrophy.

Southern Blot Analysis

Southern blot analysis provides a basis for studying genetic disorders at the DNA level. This procedure, named after its inventor E. M. Southern, separates DNA fragments according to size and allows the identification of specific DNA fragments using radiolabeled DNA probes.

The steps to prepare a Southern blot are shown in Figure 2. First, DNA is extracted from nucleated cells (leukocytes, trophoblasts, or amniocytes) or tissue, and digested into small pieces with a restriction enzyme. Then, the DNA is loaded into an agarose gel, an electric current is applied, and DNA fragments migrate down the gel according to size (smaller fragments move faster). The DNA contained within the agarose gel is still double stranded and must be denatured by alkali treatment into single-stranded pieces and then transferred to a nitrocellulose or nylon membrane. The membrane contains many thousands of fixed DNA fragments. Specific DNA fragments can be detected using a DNA probe labeled with a radionuclide, such as ^{32}P, although nonradioactive substances such as biotin–avidin may be used. The probes may be complementary DNA (cDNA), genomic DNA (exons, introns, or regulatory regions), or short pieces of single-stranded DNA called oligonucleotides, which usually range in size from 20 to 50 base pairs. The DNA probe will hybridize only with DNA fragments on the blot that are complementary. To visualize the DNA fragment, the blot is exposed to X-ray film at

Fig. 2. Southern blot analysis. (Jameson JL. Principles of molecular medicine. Totowa, NJ: Humana Press, 1998:16)

-70°C, a process called autoradiography. The film is developed, and the presence or absence of DNA bands or fragments can be determined.

Polymerase Chain Reaction

The development of the PCR has greatly simplified DNA analysis and shortened laboratory time. Polymerase chain reaction allows the exponential amplification of the targeted gene or DNA sequence. Only minute quantities of DNA, typically 0.1–1 µg, are necessary for PCR. DNA can be amplified from a single cell. One important prerequisite of PCR, which is not required for Southern blot analysis, is that the sequence of the gene, or at least the borders of the region of DNA to be amplified, must be known.

The PCR procedure has three steps (Fig. 3). First, DNA is denatured by heating to render it single stranded. Second, the PCR primers (primer A and B), which are short pieces of DNA (oligonucleotides) 20–30 base pairs in length exactly com-

plementary to the ends of each piece of the double-stranded DNA to be amplified, anneal to their complementary regions of the DNA. Third, synthesis of the complementary strand of DNA occurs in the presence of the enzyme Taq polymerase and nucleotides triphosphates (dATP, dCTP, dGTP, and dTTP). The reaction cycle of denaturation, annealing, and extension is repeated 25–30 times to produce millions of copies of DNA.

Typically, fragments several kilobases (kb) in size can be amplified, but sequences up to 10 kb have been successfully amplified. The exact cycling parameters and conditions for PCR must be determined empirically for each set of primers. Polymerase chain reaction is very sensitive; therefore, extreme care must be taken to avoid amplification of contaminant DNA from aerosolized secretions or sloughed skin cells. These precautions are particularly important when DNA from a single cell is being amplified.

Restriction Fragment Length Polymorphism Analysis

Restriction fragment length polymorphism analysis can be used when a mutation either creates or destroys a restriction endonuclease site. To detect the mutation, DNA around the site of the mutation is amplified by the PCR, incubated with the appropriate restriction enzyme, and analyzed by agarose gel electrophoresis. When a mutation creates a new restriction site, two DNA fragments will be detected if the mutation is present (Fig. 4A). An individual without the mutation will demonstrate a single fragment. This method frequently is used for the prenatal genetic diagnosis of sickle cell disease. Sickle cell disease is caused by a single base pair substitution (adenine to thymidine) in codon 6 of the β-subunit of hemoglobin, which results in the loss of the MstII restriction site. Individuals with sickle cell disease are homozygous for this mutation.

Allele Specific Oligonucleotide Hybridization (Dot Blot)

Allele specific oligonucleotide hybridization (dot blot) frequently is used to detect point mutations. A segment of DNA surrounding the mutation is amplified by PCR and then an aliquot is spotted onto a filter membrane. The membrane is hybridized with an oligonucleotide probe specific for the normal sequence and one specific for the mutation. A positive hybridization signal is detected only when the sequence of the PCR product on the membrane is

Fig. 3. Polymerase chain reaction. (Jameson JL. Principles of molecular medicine. Totowa, NJ: Humana Press, 1998:15)

complementary to the sequence of the oligonucleotide. For example, testing an individual who is heterozygous for the mutant allele will reveal a positive hybridization signal with both the normal sequence and the mutant oligonucleotide probe. DNA from individuals homozygous for the mutation will only hybridize to the mutant oligonucleotide (Fig. 4B). This technique is used for the detection of point mutations for many single gene disorders, including CF, Tay–Sachs disease, Gaucher's disease, Canavan disease, and sickle cell disease.

Deletion Analysis

Intragenic deletions can be detected by PCR or Southern blot analysis or both. Polymerase chain reaction can be used to determine the absence or presence of exons within a gene. A sample of DNA is amplified by PCR and then the PCR products are

Fig. 4. Mutation detection. **(A)** Restriction fragment length polymorphism (RFLP) analysis. The region of DNA surrounding the mutation is amplified by specific PCR primers, digested with a restriction enzyme, and analyzed by agarose-gel electrophoresis. In this example, the mutation creates a new restriction site. Individuals homozygous for the mutation have two DNA fragments (Lane 2) while an individual with two normal copies has one single fragment (Lane 1). A heterozygous individual has one normal uncut fragment and two cut fragments (Lane 3). **(B)** Allele specific oligonucleotide (ASO) hybridization. The amplified DNA from an individual homozygous for the mutation only hybridizes to the mutant oligonucleotide (MUT) whereas a heterozygous individual (HET) hybridizes to both the normal (wild-type) and the mutant. A normal individual will only hybridize to the normal oligonucleotide (WT). (Korf B. Molecular diagnosis. N Engl J Med 1995;332: 1500. Copyright © 1995 Massachusetts Medical Society. All rights reserved.)

analyzed by gel electrophoresis, stained with ethidium bromide to detect the absence or presence of DNA fragments (Fig. 5). The absence of a DNA fragment indicates the presence of a deletion. This method is used routinely for diagnostic and prenatal testing for Duchenne muscular dystrophy, an X-linked disorder. Approximately 60% of patients with Duchenne muscular dystrophy have intragenic deletions in the dystrophin gene and the majority of these can be detected by PCR. Most laboratories use a multiplex strategy to examine multiple exons in one PCR. However, PCR is not useful to determine carrier status in the mothers of affected males. This requires Southern blot analysis with cDNA probes from the dystrophin gene and scanning densitometry to assess gene dosage. Testing of females at risk to be carriers based on their family history is less reliable when an affected relative is not available for DNA testing. Dosage analysis also can be used to test male patients with Duchenne muscular dystrophy with a negative result by multiplex PCR to detect duplications within the dystrophin gene, which occur in approximately 6% of patients with Duchenne muscular dystrophy.

Linkage Analysis

When the location of a gene is known but the gene has not yet been characterized, or when the mutations have not been identified, linkage analysis may be performed to predict the likelihood that a relative or fetus has inherited a disease-causing gene within an at-risk family. Linkage analysis requires that 1) at least two generations of family members, including affected individuals, are available and willing to be tested, and 2) highly polymorphic markers such as restriction fragment length polymorphisms, or short tandem repeat polymorphisms close to or within the gene are available. These polymorphic markers result from normal genetic variation and are not disease causing but may be used to track the inheritance of genetic diseases within families. The closer a marker is to a gene, the higher the likelihood that the marker and gene are transmitted or inherited together (linkage). The accuracy of linkage analysis depends on the correct diagnosis, the informativeness of the markers within the family, and the distance between the marker and the disease-causing gene. Markers closest to or within a gene are less likely to undergo recombination and will provide the

Fig. 5. Multiplex gene deletion analysis. Exons A–D are simultaneously amplified with 4 sets of PCR primers. When an exon is deleted, the DNA fragment is absent. In lane 2 exon A is absent, in lane 3 exons B and C, and in lane 4 exon C. Lane 1 shows no evidence of a deletion; all 4 DNA products are present. (Korf B. Molecular diagnosis. N Engl J Med 1995; 332:1219. Copyright © 1995 Massachusetts Medical Society. All rights reserved.)

most accurate prediction. Although linkage analysis is less accurate than direct mutation detection, under the specified circumstances it may provide families with helpful information.

TRINUCLEOTIDE REPEAT ANALYSIS

The detection of trinucleotide repeat expansions, associated with diseases such as fragile X syndrome, myotonic dystrophy, and Huntington's disease, often requires a combination of PCR and Southern blot analysis (Fig. 6). The size of normal alleles, premutation alleles, and, in some cases, full mutations can be determined by using PCR. However, full mutations associated with a large expansion (eg, >200 repeats in fragile X syndrome) may need to be detected using Southern blot analysis. It also is used to assess the methylation status in fragile X patients and pregnancies with the full mutation. The repeat region not only expands to more than 200 repeats but also becomes hypermethylated in affected individu-

als. DNA is digested with restriction enzymes including a methylation-sensitive enzyme such as BsshII, gel electrophoresed, and hybridized with a DNA probe from the repeat region of the fragile X gene (FMR-1).

FLUORESCENCE IN SITU HYBRIDIZATION

Fluorescence in situ hybridization (FISH) is performed on either metaphase chromosome preparations from cultured lymphocytes, amniocytes, or villi, or interphase nuclei from blood, tissue, chorionic villi, or amniotic fluid. After the chromosomes or nuclei are fixed on a microscope slide, they are hybridized with a fluorochrome-labeled DNA probe specific for a particular region of a chromosome. The probe will hybridize to complementary DNA sequences that can be visualized using a fluorescence microscope. Fluorescence in situ hybridization is used as an adjunct to routine cytogenetic analysis for the detection of submicroscopic chromosome

Fig. 6. Trinucleotide repeat analysis by PCR and Southern blot. A region of DNA containing the CGG repeat is amplified and the product is analyzed on an agarose gel. The DNA fragment from a carrier with a premutation is larger because of the expanded number of repeats. Sometimes the expansion is so large that the DNA fails to amplify and the number of repeats cannot be detected using PCR. In this case, a Southern blot is performed (left panel) and the DNA from an individual with a full mutation appears as a much larger band. (Korf B. Molecular diagnosis. N Engl J Med 1995;332: 1501. Copyright © 1995 Massachusetts Medical Society. All rights reserved.)

deletions and duplications. These deletions and duplications often are several 1,000 base pairs but are too small to be detected by conventional cytogenetics. DNA probes have been developed for the common deletion and duplication syndromes (Table 1). It also may be used to identify or confirm the presence of a subtle chromosomal rearrangement (eg, translocation) or characterize a marker chromosome. Fluorescence in situ hybridization of interphase nuclei is used prenatally for the rapid detection of common aneuploidies, such as trisomy 21. However, this is generally reserved for cases where confirmation of a chromosomal abnormality may influence a couple's reproductive options or obstetric management.

COMPARATIVE GENOMIC HYBRIDIZATION

Comparative genomic hybridization is a relatively new DNA-based cytogenetic technique to identify subtle chromosome deletions and duplications that have not been detected using traditional cytogenetic methods. To accomplish this, DNA from a patient is labeled with a green fluorochrome and normal control DNA is labeled with a red fluorochrome, which can be visualized with a fluorescence microscope. The DNA is hybridized to normal metaphase chromosomes. Wherever a chromosome region is duplicated, the metaphase chromosome will hybridize with the excess green-labeled DNA and appear green. Conversely, deletions will appear red. Clinically, comparative genomic hybridization is primarily used to detect cytogenetic changes in tumors but, it also has been used to identify subtle unbalanced translocations, the origin of marker or supernumerary chromosomes, and intrachromosomal duplications.

MICROARRAY TECHNOLOGY

DNA chip technology is a high throughput method used primarily to study gene expression. Miniature arrays of cDNA clones are spotted onto a glass slide and hybridized with labeled cDNA prepared from the tissue of interest. If a gene is strongly expressed in the tissue, the hybridization signal will be intense. This technique can analyze the gene expression of thousands of genes at one time. In the future, oligonucleotide arrays also may be used to search for gene mutations and polymorphisms. Chips containing gene specific oligonucleotides matching normal and single nucleotides substitution sequences

Table 1. Microdeletion Syndromes

Syndrome	Chromosome Deletion
Aniridia/Wilm's tumor	11p13
Angelman's	15q11-13
DiGeorge/velocardiofacial	22q11.2
Langer-Giedion	8q24
Miller-Dieker	17p13.3
Prader-Willi	15q11-13
Smith-Magenis	17p11.2
Williams	7q11.23

are hybridized with fluorescent-labeled DNA. Improvements in chip technology will enable whole genome expression screening as well as improved mutation detection in the future.

INDICATIONS FOR MOLECULAR TESTING

A variety of molecular diagnostic tests are available to determine whether an individual or fetus has inherited a disease-causing gene mutation. In general, testing is offered to individuals or couples identified as being at risk for a genetic disorder based on their family history, medical history, or ethnicity. Determination of an individual's carrier status for a genetic disorder provides a more accurate estimate of their risk of having an affected offspring and allows an individual or couple to consider prenatal testing options. This information also may assist couples with their reproductive decisions. Furthermore, it can identify other family members or relatives at risk for the disorder or at risk for being a carrier.

Molecular testing also may be used in clinical and prenatal situations to confirm a diagnosis. For example, screening for CF mutations may determine whether an infertile male with congenital bilateral absence of the vas deferens is a CF carrier. Prenatal molecular testing for some genetic disorders may be offered when a congenital anomaly is identified antenatally. For example, FISH for the 22q11.2 deletion may establish a cause when a conotruncal cardiac defect is detected by ultrasonography. Establishing an etiology enables clinicians to provide couples with accurate genetic risk assessments, prognostic information, and recommendations for obstetric and neonatal management.

Prior to diagnostic and carrier testing for genetic disorders, patients should be informed of the natural history of the disorder and current therapy, the inheritance and their risk of inheriting or transmitting the gene, benefits and limitations of testing, and the implications of negative and positive results. Preconceptional and prenatal testing also should include a discussion of reproductive options including prenatal testing, adoption, donor programs, and termination of pregnancy. Written informed consent should be obtained from all individuals undergoing genetic screening. Patients should understand that molecular testing is voluntary and that every effort will be made to ensure confidentiality of their medical records and test results.

ACCURACY AND LIMITATIONS OF MOLECULAR TESTING

Direct detection of a point mutation, deletion, or duplication is the most accurate test. However, the accuracy of molecular diagnosis also is dependent on an accurate diagnosis. If an affected relative is not available to identify the presence of a mutation or if medical records are not available to confirm the diagnosis, this may decrease the accuracy of testing for a specific mutation and for the suspected genetic disorder.

One of the limitations of molecular diagnostic testing is test sensitivity. There are a number of factors that determine the ability to detect mutations. Many genetic disorders result from a variety of genetic alterations. For example, more than 800 mutations have been reported in patients with CF. The mutation detection rates for many genetic disorders, including neurofibromatosis, CF, and hemophilia, are less than 100%. Therefore, the absence of a mutation does not exclude the possibility that an individual may be a carrier. Furthermore, there may be ethnic differences in the detection rates; 97% of CF mutations have been identified in the Ashkenazi Jewish population while only 30% in Asian Americans. The incidence and carrier risk for some genetic disorders also is dependent on ethnicity and has led to the current recommendations for carrier screening for specific genetic disorders. Differences in test sensitivity and the prevalence of mutations must be considered for each individual genetic disorder and discussed with the patient prior to testing. Disease prevalence and test sensitivity should be taken into account in future recommendations for molecular-based carrier testing.

Another limitation to molecular testing is genetic heterogeneity. In some cases, there may be more than one gene or chromosomal locus responsible for a genetic disorder. For example, at least two genes have been identified that cause tuberous sclerosis, an autosomal dominant disorder. Conversely, mutations in a single gene can cause different phenotypes. For example, mutations in fibroblast growth factor receptor 3 (FGFR3) are associated with several types of skeletal disorders, including achondroplasia, hypochondroplasia, thanatophoric dysplasia, and with craniosynostosis (eg, Crouzon's disease, coronal synostosis).

In some diseases, the identification of a genetic mutation cannot precisely predict the phenotype because of reduced penetrance or phenotypic variability or both. For example, 85% of women with a *BRCA1* mutation develop breast cancer during their lifetime; therefore, the finding of a *BRCA1* mutation indicates a strong predisposition to breast cancer but it does not indicate which women with the mutation will develop a malignancy. Some genetic disorders are highly variable even within families with the same mutation. Therefore, it may only be possible to provide patients with a description of the natural history of the disorder and an estimate of the frequency of specific features in patients with similar mutations. The lack of genotype phenotype correlation for some genetic disorders, such as CF, also can limit the ability to accurately predict the course of the disease. Therefore, when molecular testing indicates that a patient or fetus has inherited a mutation, it is helpful to consult a geneticist or someone with expertise in the specific disorder to provide current information regarding the prognosis, as well as, the limitations and accuracy of testing.

APPLICATIONS IN OBSTETRICS AND GYNECOLOGY

Genetics is taking an increasingly prominent role in the practice of obstetrics and gynecology. Gene identification, characterization of disease-causing mutations, and advances in genetic technology have led to an increased number of available genetic tests, which may be used for the diagnosis of genetic disorders, carrier detection, and prenatal or preimplantation genetic diagnosis. Testing for a specific genetic disorder most often occurs in an obstetric setting based on either the family history or the couple's ethnicity. Genetic counseling should be offered to couples at risk so they can review the nature of the disorder, the inheritance pattern, their specific risk for being a carrier and for having a child with the disorder, the current availability of prenatal and postnatal testing as well the accuracy and limitations of testing, and their reproductive options. Most molecular genetic testing for disorders, such as Duchenne muscular dystrophy, fragile X syndrome, neurofibromatosis, and hemophilia, is performed when a couple is at high risk based on their family history. Initially, testing is performed to determine whether the parent is a carrier. If the parent is a carrier, prenatal testing by amniocentesis or chorionic villus sampling is possible. Some couples may consider preimplantation genetic diagnosis. Single gene disorders and chromosomal abnormalities, such as deletions and translocations, may be identified in an embryo conceived through in vitro fertilization by testing a single blastomere. Genetic testing for disorders prevalent in specific ethnic populations such as CF for Caucasians and Tay–Sachs and Canavan disease for individuals of Eastern European Jewish ancestry, is used to determine if an individual is a carrier. Prenatal molecular diagnostic testing is available for couples who are both carriers of sickle cell disease and thalassemia determined by hemoglobin electrophoresis. The genetic testing options in pregnancy are rapidly growing with the completion of the human genome project; however, a thorough family history is essential to identify a couple at risk.

Genetic testing during pregnancy may establish a diagnosis that may influence obstetric management. For example, PCR of amniotic fluid is used to determine the Rh status of the fetus to determine if the fetus is at risk for hemolytic disease of the newborn when the woman is Rh sensitized and the man is a heterozygous carrier of antigen D. The fetus at risk will need close surveillance during the pregnancy. A specific molecular diagnostic test may be considered when the finding of a fetal malformation by ultrasonography raises the suspicion of a genetic disorder. For example, mutation testing for CF in a fetus with echogenic bowel, fibroblast growth factor receptor 2 (FGFR2) for suspected Apert's syndrome (craniosynostosis), and 22q11.2 deletion testing when a conotruncal cardiac defect is detected. Identification of an etiology provides the physician and couple with a better understanding of the prognosis that influences not only the obstetric and neonatal care of the infant but also a couple's reproductive decisions. Furthermore, it establishes an accurate assessment of the recurrence risk for this family and their relatives.

Some of the genes responsible for the inherited forms of some types of cancer (such as breast, ovarian, and colon) have been identified. Risk assess-

ment for relatives in these families may include genetic testing in addition to evaluating other risk factors, such as family history. In some families, breast and ovarian cancer is attributed to an inherited genetic mutation, BRCA1 or BRCA2. The genes responsible for hereditary nonpolyposis colorectal cancer, juvenile polyposis, and familial adenomatosis polyposis, have been identified. It is likely that other genes that contribute to cancer will be identified in the future, which may be useful for cancer risk assessment and management.

Genetic screening and testing should be considered a component of an infertility evaluation. Preconceptional genetic screening and counseling can identify couples at risk for having offspring with a genetic disorder and provide them with information that enables them to make informed decisions regarding their reproductive options. Genetic causes of severe oligospermia and azoospermia include balanced translocations, Klinefelter's syndrome (47,XXY), and Y chromosome abnormalities and microdeletions. Cytogenetic studies and PCR-based Y chromosome deletion testing should be considered. Approximately two thirds of males with congenital bilateral absence of the vas deferens have at least one CF mutation. Men with congenital bilateral absence of the vas deferens should be offered CF carrier testing. Partners of carriers and individuals with CF should be tested to assess their risk for having a child with CF. This information may be useful for an infertile couple considering their reproductive options, such as testicular aspiration and biopsy with intracytoplasmic sperm injection, preimplantation genetic diagnosis with in vitro fertilization, donor gamete, adoption, and prenatal testing.

SUMMARY

Human genetics and molecular testing is playing an increasingly important role in obstetric and gynecologic practice. It is essential that obstetricians and gynecologists are aware of the advances in our understanding of genetic disease and the fundamental principles of molecular testing and genetic screening as genetics is integrated into routine medical practice. In the future, elucidation of the genetic basis for reproductive disorders, common diseases, and cancer with improved high throughput technology for genetic testing will expand testing opportunities and influence treatment options and prevention strategies.

REFERENCE

1. The human genome. Science 2001;291:1145–1434

RESOURCES

Bell J. The new genetics in clinical practice. BMJ 1998;316: 618–620

Blackwood MA, Weber BL. BRCA1 and BRCA2: from molecular genetics to clinical medicine. J Clin Oncol 1998;16: 1969–1977

Brown PO, Botstein D. Exploring the new world of the genome with DNA microassays. Nat Genet 1999;21(suppl):33–37

Caskey CT. Medical genetics. JAMA 1997;277:1869–1870

Collins FS. Genetics: an explosion of knowledge is transforming clinical practice. Geriatrics 1999;54:41–47;quiz 48

Cooper DN, Schmidtke J. Diagnosis of human genetic disease using recombinant DNA. 4th ed. Hum Genet 1993;92:211–236

Davis JG. Predictive genetic tests: problems and pitfalls. Ann N Y Acad Sci 1997;833:42–46

Jameson JL. Principles of molecular medicine. Totowa, New Jersey: Humana Press, 1998

Korf B. Molecular diagnosis (1). N Engl J Med 1995;332: 1218–1220

Korf B. Molecular diagnosis (2). N Engl J Med 1995;332: 1499–1502

Makowski DR. The Human Genome Project and the clinician. J Fla Med Assoc 1996;83:307–314

Mark HF, Jenkins R, Miller WA. Current applications of molecular cytogenetic technologies. Ann Clin Lab Sci 1997;27: 47–56

Pyeritz RE. Family history and genetic risk factors: forward to the future. JAMA 1997;278:1284–1285

SOURCES OF ONLINE INFORMATION

Tutorial in Genetics (HHMI)
www.hhmi.org/GeneticTrail/
Online Mendelian Inheritance in Man
www3.ncbi.nlm.nih.gov/Omim/
MEDLINE
www.ncbi.nlm.nih.gov/PubMed/
GeneTests
www.genetests.org
Genome Database
www.gob.org
Biochemical testing information
biochemgen.ucsd.edu/wbgtests/dz.tst.htm
Alliance of Genetic Support Groups
medhlp.netusa.net/www/agsg.htm
National Human Genome Research
www.nhgri.nih.gov

Centers for Disease Control and Prevention
www.cdc.gov/genetics
Gene Clinics
www.geneclinics.org

GLOSSARY

Allele: One of two or more alternate forms of a gene.

Allele specific oligonucleotides: Synthetic oligonucleotide designed to hybridize to a specific sequence, and under the right conditions, to fail to hybridize to a related sequence. Allele specific oligonucleotides also are used as PCR primers in several methods similarly designed to distinguish between closely related alleles.

Autosomal Dominant: An allele located on an autosome (nonsex chromosome) that expresses itself phenotypically in the presence of the same or a different allele (ie, in a homozygous or heterozygous condition).

Autosomal Recessive: An allele located on an autosome that does not express itself phenotypically in the presence of a dominant allele (ie, in a heterozygous condition). It is only phenotypically expressed in a homozygous condition.

Chimera: An organism with tissues composed of two or more genetically distinct cell types.

Chromatin: An intranuclear and intrachromosomal complex made up of DNA, and histone and nonhistone proteins.

Co-Dominant: Alleles that are different from each other, but both are expressed in the phenotype.

Codon: A section of DNA (three nucleotide pairs in length) that codes for a single amino acid.

Comparative Genomic Hybridization: A cytogenetic method based on a combination of fluorescence microscopy and digital image analysis. Differentially labeled test DNA and normal reference DNA are hybridized simultaneously to normal chromosome spreads. Hybridization is detected with two different fluorochromes. Deletions, duplications, or amplifications are seen as changes in the ratio of the intensities of the two fluorochromes along the target chromosomes.

Complementary DNA (cDNA) Probe: A DNA sequence that is exactly complementary to mRNA, lacking introns and regulatory regions.

Contiguous Gene Deletion Syndrome: A syndrome caused by a deletion involving genes that are physically located together in a chromosome segment.

Constitutive Heterochromatin: Condensed genetically inactive chromatin located in the same regions of both homologous chromosomes.

DNA: A double-helical structure composed of two coils of nucleotide chains connected by nitrogen bases.

DNA Hybridization: A process whereby labeled nucleic acid molecules (oligonucleotide probe) bind to a DNA sequence on a target (Southern blot, metaphase chromosomes, or interphase nuclei) that is complementary to its own.

DNA Methylation: A process for control of tissue specific gene expression. Methylation "turns off" the regulatory region of a gene, thereby preventing DNA transcription.

Epigenetic: Non–DNA/RNA related process that affects genotype and phenotype (ie, methalization).

Exon: A region of a gene made up of DNA sequences that will be transcribed into mRNA.

Expressivity: The degree to which a genotype is expressed in the phenotype (range of phenotypic features).

Fluorescence in situ Hybridization (FISH): A procedure for detecting specific nucleic acid sequences in morphologically preserved chromosomes, cells, and tissue sections using fluorescent labeled oligonucleotide probes.

Gene: A unit of heredity responsible for the inheritance of a specific trait that occupies a fixed chromosomal site and corresponds to a sequence of nucleotides along a DNA molecule.

Genome: The entire complement of genetic material in a chromosome set.

Genomic Imprinting: The existence of parent-of-origin differences in the expression of certain genes.

Germline Mosaicism: Mosaicism that is confined to the gonad.

Hereditary Unstable DNA (Triplet Repeat Expansion): Gene containing a region of triplet codon repeats such as $(CGC)_n$. The number of triplet repeats can increase during meiosis. If the expansion of repeats reaches a critical number, the gene becomes methylated and is turned off, resulting in phenotypic abnormalities.

Heterochromatin: Chromatin that remains condensed throughout interphase. It contains DNA that is genetically inactive and replicates late in the S phase of the cell cycle. There are two types of heterochromatin: constitutive and facultative.

Hybridization (Dot Blot): A semiquantitative technique for evaluating the relative abundance of nucleic acid sequences in a mixture or the extent of similarity between homologous sequences.

Imprinting: The imposition of a stable behavior pattern in a young animal by exposure, during a particular period in its development, to one of a restricted set of stimuli.

Intron: A region of a gene, made up of noncoding DNA sequences that lies between exons.

Karyotype: The chromosome constitution of an individual.

Linkage: The association of genes on the same chromosome.

Methylation: (see DNA Methylation)

Mitochondrial Inheritance: Mitochondria are inherited exclusively from women. Because they contain DNA, mitochondrial inheritance allows transmission of genes directly from the woman to her offspring.

Mosaicism: The presence of two or more populations of cells with different characteristics within one tissue or organ.

Multifactorial Inheritance: Inheritance of traits that are determined by a combination of genetic and environmental factors.

Mutation: An alteration of DNA sequencing in a gene that results in a heritable change in protein structure or function that frequently has adverse effects.

   Deletion: A mutation that is generated by removal of a sequence of DNA, with the regions on either side being joined together.

   Expansion (see Hereditary Unstable DNA)

   Frame-shift: A mutation caused by deletions or insertions that are not a multiple of three base pairs. Results in a change in the reading frame in which triplet codons are translated into protein.

   Insertion: A mutation caused by the presence of an additional sequence of nucleotide pairs in DNA.

   Inversion: A mutation involving the removal of a DNA sequence, its rotation through 180 degrees, and its reinsertion in the same location.

   Missense: A mutation that alters a codon so that it encodes a different amino acid.

Northern Blot: A technique for transferring RNA from an electrophoresis gel to a nitrocellulose filter on which it can be hybridized to a complementary DNA (cDNA) probe.

Nucleotide: A component of a DNA or RNA molecule composed of a nitrogenous base, one deoxyribose or ribose sugar, and one phosphate group. In DNA, adenine specifically joins to thymine and guanine joins to cytosine. In RNA, uracil replaces thymine.

Oligonucleotide Primer: A short sequence of nucleotides that is necessary to hybridize to a DNA or RNA strand using the enzymes DNA polymerase or reverse transcriptase.

Penetrance: The ability of a mutant gene to be expressed in an individual who carries the gene.

Phenotype: Observable physical characteristics of an organism resulting from the expression of the genotype and its interaction with the environment.

Polygenic Inheritance: Inheritance of traits that are determined by the combined effects of many genes.

Polymerase Chain Reaction (PCR): A method for enzymatically amplifying a short sequence of DNA through repeated cycles of denaturation, binding with an oligonucleotide primer and extension of the primers by a DNA polymerase.

Polymorphisms: Minor differences that distinguish one individual from another.

Recombinant DNA: A new DNA sequence formed by the combination of two nonhomologous DNA molecules.

Restriction Endonuclease: An enzyme that recognizes and cleaves a specific DNA sequence (usually 4–10 nucleotide bases long).

Restriction Fragment Length Polymorphism: A polymorphic difference in DNA sequence between individuals that can be recognized by restriction endonucleases.

Southern Blot: A technique used to detect specific DNA sequences by separating restriction enzyme digested DNA fragments on an electrophoresis gel, transferring (blotting) these fragments from the gel onto a membrane or nitrocellulose filter, followed by hybridization with a labeled probe to a specific DNA sequence.

Spectral Karyotype: A molecular cytogenetic method in which all of the chromosomes in a metaphase spread are visualized in different colors (multicolor FISH).

Uniparental Disomy: Inheritance of two copies of part or all of a chromosome from one parent and no copy from the other parent.

Uniparental Heterodisomy: Inheritance of two homologous chromosomes from one parent.

Uniparental Isodisomy: Inheritance of two identical chromosomes from one parent.

Threshold Traits: Traits that are not manifested until a certain threshold of liability is exceeded.

Transcription: The process of RNA synthesis from a DNA template that is directed by RNA polymerase.

Triplet Repeat Expansion (see Hereditary Unstable DNA)

Trinucleotide Repeat Analysis (Repeats): Unstable DNA sequences found in several human genes. Normally the triplets are repeated in tandem 5–50 times. When the number rises above the normal range, mutant disease syndromes appear.

X-inactivation: A process by which one of the X chromosomes in each somatic cell of females is rendered inactive. This results in a balance in gene expression between the X chromosomal and autosomal genes, which is necessary because males have only one X chromosome.

X-linked: An allele for a trait or disorder that is located on the X chromosome, and may be either dominant or recessive.

Western Blot: A technique, conceptually related to the Southern and Northern blot that is used to detect specific proteins.

The American College of
Obstetricians and Gynecologists
409 12th Street, SW
PO Box 96920
Washington, DC 20090-6920

12345/65432

Genetics and molecular diagnostic testing. ACOG Technology Assessment in Obstetrics and Gynecology No. 1. American College of Obstetricians and Gynecologists. Obstet Gynecol 2002;100:193–211

ACOG
TECHNOLOGY ASSESSMENT
IN OBSTETRICS AND GYNECOLOGY

NUMBER 4, AUGUST 2005

This Technology Assessment was developed by the ACOG Committee on Gynecologic Practice. This document reflects emerging clinical and scientific advances as of the date issued and is subject to change. The information should not be construed as dictating an exclusive course of treatment or procedure to be followed. Variations in practice may be warranted based on the needs of the individual patient, resources, and limitations unique to the institution or type of practice.

THE AMERICAN COLLEGE
OF OBSTETRICIANS
AND GYNECOLOGISTS
WOMEN'S HEALTH CARE PHYSICIANS

Hysteroscopy

ABSTRACT: *Hysteroscopy is an effective, minimally invasive procedure for the diagnosis and treatment of intrauterine pathology. Selection of a distending medium requires consideration of the advantages, disadvantages, and risks associated with various media as well as their compatibility with electrosurgical or laser energy. Preoperative discussions with patients should address risks and benefits of the procedure, comorbidities, analgesia or anesthesia, and possible preoperative cervical dilation. Pregnancy, genital tract infection, and uterine carcinoma are contraindications to hysteroscopy. Possible complications include hemorrhage, fluid overload, perforation, visceral injury, infection, and embolization.*

Hysteroscopy is performed to view and treat pathology within the uterine cavity. Diagnostic hysteroscopy allows visualization of the endocervical canal, endometrial cavity, and fallopian tube ostia. Common abnormal findings include polyps, leiomyomata, intrauterine adhesions, and müllerian anomalies. Operative hysteroscopy incorporates the use of mechanical, electrosurgical, or laser instruments to treat intracavitary disease.

INSTRUMENTATION

Hysteroscopes are available in both flexible and rigid models, all of which contain a telescope consisting of light bundles. Flexible hysteroscopes range in diameter from 2.7 mm to 5 mm and have a bendable tip that can be deflected in two directions ranging from 120 degrees to 160 degrees. Most also contain an operating channel for tubal catheterization or endometrial biopsy. Rigid hysteroscopes may consist of two or three pieces and range from 1 mm to 5 mm in diameter. Their tips have varying viewing angles (0, 12, 15, 30, and 70 degrees). An outer sheath fits over the telescope to allow inflow of a distending medium into the intrauterine cavity. This system allows fluid to return on the outside of the outer sheath passively from the intrauterine cavity through the cervix.

Continuous flow hysteroscopes consist of two channels to allow fluid to flow into the intrauterine cavity while debris and cloudy intrauterine fluid exit through perforations in the outer sheath to the outflow port. Fluid exiting the outflow port can be collected through tubing and returned to a device for the accurate measurement of fluid volume.

Operative hysteroscopes typically range from 8 mm to 10 mm in diameter and contain a working element. These hysteroscopes contain a retractable hand piece wherein electrosurgical tips (eg, rollerballs, loops, and vaporizing tips), lasers, or mechanical instruments (eg, scissors) can be attached.

DISTENDING MEDIA

The uterine cavity requires distension for adequate visualization. Several distending media are available, and each has inherent advantages and disadvantages. It is critically important to understand which media are compatible with electrosurgical and laser energy. Furthermore, the risks associated with various media should be understood.

Carbon Dioxide Gas

Carbon dioxide (CO_2), a colorless gas, is used in outpatient settings for diagnostic purposes. The advantages include the ease of cleaning and maintaining equipment and a clear view of the cavity in the absence of active bleeding or bubbles. To minimize the risk of gas embolization, the flow of CO_2 should be limited to 100 mL/min with intrauterine pressures less than 100 mm Hg. Insufflators designed for use in laparoscopy must not be used for hysteroscopy.

Fluid Media

Fluid media have historically been divided into electrolyte and nonelectrolyte media, based on compatibility with electrosurgical procedures. However, it is now possible to use electrolyte media with bipolar electrosurgical systems. It also is important to understand which media are hypoosmolar. Media also are categorized by viscosity.

Low-Viscosity, Electrolyte-Poor Fluid. Low-viscosity, electrolyte-poor fluids include glycine, 1.5%, sorbitol, 3%, and mannitol, 5%. These fluids have been widely used for operative hysteroscopy. They are compatible with radiofrequency energy, which cuts, desiccates, and fulgurates intrauterine tissue. Monopolar devices require electrolyte-poor fluids. If electrolyte-containing fluid is used, the electrical current will dissipate away from the electrode, rendering it ineffective. Glycine, 1.5%, and sorbitol, 3%, are hypoosmolar. The use of these fluids can cause hyponatremia and decreased serum osmolality, with the potential for cerebral edema and death. Some clinicians have recommended mannitol, 5%, which is isoosmolar and acts as its own diuretic. It

may cause hyponatremia but not decreased serum osmolality (1).

Low-Viscosity Electrolyte Fluid. Normal saline and lactated Ringer's solution are electrolyte fluids. The use of these fluids is advantageous because they are readily available and are isotonic. These solutions are the distending media of choice during diagnostic hysteroscopy and in operative cases where mechanical, laser, or bipolar energy is used. Although the risk of hyponatremia and decreased serum osmolality can be reduced by using these media, pulmonary edema can still occur, and careful attention should be paid to fluid input and output.

High-Viscosity Fluid. Dextran 70 is a colorless, viscous, polysaccharide liquid. The advantage of using this liquid is that it is immiscible with blood and, therefore, provides excellent visibility, especially in the presence of blood in the endometrial cavity. The major disadvantage of using dextran 70 is that it is sticky and, when dry, tends to harden and crystallize onto the equipment. It also can be a powerful plasma expander, and the volume usually is limited to 300 mL and must not exceed 500 mL. For every 100 mL absorbed, the plasma volume may expand by an additional 860 mL (2). Other concerns include anaphylaxis and disseminated intravascular coagulation. Beet sugar allergy is an absolute contraindication.

PREOPERATIVE CONSIDERATIONS

A preoperative consultation allows the patient and physician to discuss the hysteroscopic procedure, weigh its inherent risks and benefits, and review the patient's medical history for any comorbid conditions. Appropriate analgesia or anesthesia should also be considered depending on the venue (ie, office versus operating room). Preoperative placement of laminar or osmotic dilators or pretreatment with misoprostol for cervical ripening may facilitate cervical dilation and decrease operative time (3).

CONTRAINDICATIONS

Known viable pregnancy, known genital tract infections, and known uterine carcinomas are contraindications to hysteroscopy. Theoretically, hysteroscopy may cause reflux of neoplastic cells into the peritoneal cavity, although it is unclear if this adversely affects the prognosis (4, 5). However, hysteroscopy is acceptable as part of the evaluation of abnormal uterine bleeding.

PREVENTION AND MANAGEMENT OF COMPLICATIONS

The most common perioperative complications associated with operative hysteroscopy are hemorrhage (2.4%), fluid overload (1.5%) (6), and cervical laceration (1–11%) (7). Other complications include uterine perforation, visceral injury, infection, CO_2 and air embolism, and, rarely, death. Late complications may include intrauterine adhesions and infertility.

Hemorrhage

Hemorrhage may occur during hysteroscopic resection of the endometrium, myomata, uterine septa, or synechia. For cases in which there is continued bleeding, electrosurgical coagulation can be used (8). Alternative strategies such as injection of vasopressin at the bleeding site, Foley catheter balloon tamponade (9), or irrigation of the uterine cavity with epsilon aminocaproic acid can be attempted. In extreme cases, uterine artery embolization or hysterectomy may be necessary.

Fluid Overload

Complications from fluid overload may best be avoided by limiting excess fluid absorption, recognizing and treating fluid overload promptly, and selecting a distending medium that minimizes risk.

The best way to limit excess fluid intravasation is to monitor the fluid deficit closely and frequently throughout the procedure. Newer methods of fluid monitoring based on measurement of fluid weight have made this more accurate; however, some of these systems can be expensive and may not be available in all settings. One difficulty in estimating fluid input and output is that commercially purchased 3-liter bags may be overfilled by up to 150–300 mL (10). Dilutional hyponatremia can be rapidly evaluated by serum sodium analysis.

Guidelines for fluid monitoring and the limits of fluid excess have been published (1) and adapted by the American College of Obstetricians and Gynecologists' Committee on Gynecologic Practice as follows:

- Hydration of patients undergoing hysteroscopy should be closely monitored preoperatively and intraoperatively.

- With low-viscosity, electrolyte-poor fluids, a deficit of 750 mL implies excessive intravasation, and the fluid deficit should be monitored at an extremely close interval. In elderly patients, patients with comorbid conditions, and patients with cardiovascular compromise, consideration should be given to terminating the procedure immediately.

- Depending on patient size and other factors, if fluid deficit reaches 1,000–1,500 mL of a non-electrolyte solution or 2,500 mL of an electrolyte solution, further infusion should be stopped and the procedure should be promptly concluded. Electrolytes should be assessed, administration of diuretics considered, and further diagnostic and therapeutic intervention begun as indicated.

- In an outpatient setting with limited acute care and laboratory services, consideration should be given to discontinuing procedures at a lower fluid deficit threshold.

- An automated fluid monitoring system facilitates early recognition of excessive deficit in real-time totals.

- In the absence of automated monitoring, an individual should be designated to frequently measure intake and outflow and report the deficit to the operative team.

The treatment of fluid overload from hypotonic agents may require consultation and possibly transfer to an acute care facility. Whereas most women recover, seizures, permanent brain damage, and death have been reported with serum sodium levels of 116 ± 2 mmol/L (11). Although the rate at which severe hyponatremia should be corrected is controversial, most authors agree that if acute hyponatremia has existed for less than 24 hours, there are few long-term complications from rapid correction. Therapy is most often provided in the form of hypertonic saline in conjunction with loop-acting diuretics. Serum sodium levels should be increased by 1–2 mEq/L/h but by no more than 12 mEq/L in the first 24 hours (12). When patients present with hyponatremia of greater than 48 hours postoperatively, rapid correction should not be undertaken because it can lead to neurologic compromise, seizures, and death. Consultation is strongly encouraged in these situations and often requires slower correction in an intensive care setting.

Perforation

Prior to performing hysteroscopy, a pelvic examination should be performed to determine uterine position. If resistance is encountered during insertion of the hysteroscope, the cervix may need further dilation. Midline uterine perforation rarely leads to significant morbidity unless a laser or electrosurgical device is used. Lateral uterine or cervical perforations can result in significant bleeding. Laparoscopy may be useful to determine the extent of damage, including the existence of bowel or bladder injury.

Embolization

Air and CO_2 emboli are rare complications of hysteroscopy and may result in circulatory collapse. For such emboli to occur, there must be both vascular access and a pressure gradient between the site of access and the right side of the heart. In the conscious patient, chest pain and dyspnea may be noted. Other findings can include decreased oxygen saturation, the presence of a "mill wheel" heart murmur, hypotension, bradycardia, or tachycardia. In the anesthetized patient, cardiopulmonary status shows signs of collapse with sudden hypotension, decrease in oxygenation and/or in end-tidal CO_2, or cardiac dysrhythmias (13).

Management of this emergency consists of placing the patient in a left lateral decubitus position with the head tilted downward 5 degrees. This maneuver favors the movement of air in the right ventricle and right ventricular outflow tract toward the apex of the right ventricle (14). The air may be aspirated by passing a catheter down the jugular vein into the right ventricle, or possibly by performing cardiocentesis.

SUMMARY

Hysteroscopy is an effective procedure for the diagnosis and treatment of intrauterine pathology. It is minimally invasive and can be used with a high degree of safety. Knowledge of potential dangers relating to distending media and intraoperative complications will enhance its safety.

REFERENCES

1. Loffer FD, Bradley LD, Brill AI, Brooks PG, Cooper JM. Hysteroscopic fluid monitoring guidelines. The ad hoc committee on hysteroscopic training guidelines of the American Association of Gynecologic Laparoscopists. J Am Assoc Gyn Laparosc 2000;7:167–8.
2. Lukacsko P. Noncardiogenic pulmonary edema secondary to intrauterine instillation of 32% dextran 70. Fertil Steril 1985;44:560–1.
3. Thomas JA, Leyland N, Durand N, Windrim RC. The use of oral misoprostol as a cervical ripening agent in operative hysteroscopy: a double-blind, placebo-controlled trial. Am J Obstet Gynecol 2002;186:876–9.
4. Obermair A, Geramou M, Gucer F, Denison U, Graf AH, Kapshammer E, et al. Does hysteroscopy facilitate tumor cell dissemination? Incidence of peritoneal cytology from patients with early stage endometrial carcinoma following dilatation and curettage (D&C) versus hysteroscopy and D&C. Cancer 2000;88:139–43.
5. Arikan G, Reich O, Weiss U, Hahn T, Reinisch S, Tamussino K, et al. Are endometrial carcinoma cells disseminated at hysteroscopy functionally viable? Gynecol Oncol 2001;83:221–6.
6. Overton C, Hargreaves J, Maresh M. A national survey of the complications of endometrial destruction for menstrual disorders: the MISTLETOE study. Minimally Invasive Surgical Techniques—Laser, EndoThermal or Endoresection. Br J Obstet Gynaecol 1997;104:1351–9.
7. Preutthipan S, Herabutya Y. Vaginal misoprostol for cervical priming before operative hysteroscopy: a randomized control trial. Obstet Gynecol 2000;96:890–4.
8. Loffer FD. Complications of hysteroscopy—their cause, prevention, and correction. J Am Assoc Gynecol Laparosc 1995;3:11–26.
9. Goldrath MH. Uterine tamponade for the control of acute uterine bleeding. Am J Obstet Gynecol 1983;147:869–72.
10. Vulgaropulos SP, Haley LC, Hulka JF. Intrauterine pressure and fluid absorption during continuous flow hysteroscopy. Am J Obstet Gynecol 1992;167:386–390; discussion 390–1.
11. Arieff AI. Management of hyponatraemia. BMJ 1993; 307:305–8.
12. Witz CA, Silverberg CM, Burns WN, Schenken RS, Olive DL. Complications associated with the absorption of hysteroscopic fluid media. Fertil Steril 1993;60:745–56.
13. Stoloff DR, Isenberg RA, Brill AI. Venous air and gas emboli in operative hysteroscopy. J Am Assoc Gynecol Laparosc 2001;8:181–92.
14. deWet C, Harrison L, Jacobsohn E. Air embolism. In: Atlee JL, editor. Complications in anesthesia. Philadelphia (PA):WB Saunders;1999. p. 323–5.

The American College of Obstetricians and Gynecologists
409 12th Street, SW
PO Box 96920
Washington, DC 20090-6920

12345/98765

Hysteroscopy. ACOG Technology Assessment in Obstetrics and Gynecology No. 4. American College of Obstetricians and Gynecologists. Obstet Gynecol 2005;106:439–42.

ACOG
TECHNOLOGY ASSESSMENT
IN OBSTETRICS AND GYNECOLOGY

NUMBER 3, SEPTEMBER 2003

This Technology Assessment was developed by the ACOG Committee on Gynecologic Practice with the assistance of Daniel Breitkopf, MD, Steven R. Goldstein, MD, and John W. Seeds, MD. This document reflects emerging clinical and scientific advances as of the date issued and is subject to change. The information should not be construed as dictating an exclusive course of treatment or procedure to be followed. Variations in practice may be warranted based on the needs of the individual patient, resources, and limitations unique to the institution or type of practice.

THE AMERICAN COLLEGE
OF OBSTETRICIANS
AND GYNECOLOGISTS
WOMEN'S HEALTH CARE PHYSICIANS

Saline Infusion Sonohysterography

ABSTRACT: Saline infusion sonohysterography consists of ultrasonographic imaging of the uterus and uterocervical cavity, using real-time ultrasonography during injection of sterile saline into the uterus. When properly performed, saline infusion sonohysterography can provide information about the uterus and endometrium. The most common indication for sonohysterography is abnormal uterine bleeding. Sonohysterography should not be performed in a woman who is pregnant or who could be pregnant or in a woman with a pelvic infection or unexplained pelvic tenderness. Physicians who perform or supervise diagnostic saline infusion sonohysterography should have training, experience, and demonstrated competence in gynecologic ultrasonography and saline infusion sonohysterography. Portions of this document were developed jointly with the American College of Radiology and the American Institute of Ultrasound in Medicine.

This document has been developed to provide assistance to qualified physicians performing saline infusion sonohysterography. Properly performed sonohysterography can provide information about the uterus and endometrium. Additional studies may be necessary for a complete diagnosis. However, adherence to the following recommendations will maximize the diagnostic benefit of sonohysterography.

The clinical aspects of this document include sections addressing indications and contraindications, specifications of the examination, and equipment specifications that were developed collaboratively by the American College of Radiology, the American Institute of Ultrasound in Medicine, and the American College of Obstetricians and Gynecologists (ACOG). Sections of the document addressing physician qualifications and responsibilities, documentation, quality control, performance improvement, safety, infection control, and patient education are recommendations of the ACOG Committee on Gynecologic Practice.

Saline infusion sonohysterography consists of ultrasonographic imaging of the uterus and uterocervical cavity, using real-time ultrasonography during injection of sterile saline into the uterine cavity. The goal of sonohysterography is to detect abnormalities of the uterus and endometrium using real-time ultrasonography and static images with sufficient anatomic detail for diagnosis of normal and abnormal findings.

INDICATIONS AND CONTRAINDICATIONS

The indications for sonohysterography include, but are not limited to, the following factors:

- Abnormal bleeding in premenopausal and post-menopausal women
- Infertility and habitual abortion
- Congenital abnormalities or anatomic variants of the uterine cavity or both
- Preoperative and postoperative evaluation of the uterine cavity, especially with regard to uterine myomata, polyps, and cysts
- Suspected uterine cavity synechiae
- Further evaluation of suspected abnormalities seen on endovaginal ultrasonography, including focal or diffuse endometrial thickening or debris
- Inadequate imaging of the endometrium by endovaginal ultrasonography

The most common indication for sonohysterography is abnormal uterine bleeding in both premenopausal and postmenopausal women.

Sonohysterography should not be performed in a woman who is pregnant or who could be pregnant. This usually is avoided by scheduling the examination in the follicular phase of the menstrual cycle, after the menstrual flow has essentially ceased, but before the patient has ovulated. In a patient with regular menstrual cycles, saline infusion sonohysterography should not, in most cases, be performed later than the 10th day of the menstrual cycle. Sonohysterography should not be performed in patients with a pelvic infection or unexplained pelvic tenderness, which may be caused by chronic pelvic inflammatory disease. Pelvic organ tenderness should be assessed during a preliminary endovaginal ultrasound examination. Active vaginal bleeding is not a contraindication to the procedure but may make the interpretation more challenging.

PHYSICIAN QUALIFICATIONS AND RESPONSIBILITIES

Physicians who perform or supervise diagnostic saline infusion sonohysterography should be skilled in vaginal ultrasonography and transcervical placement of catheters. They should understand the indications, limitations, and possible complications of the procedure. Physicians should have training, experience, and demonstrated competence in gynecologic ultrasonography and saline infusion sonohysterography. Physicians are responsible for the documentation of the examination, quality control, and patient safety.

SPECIFICATIONS OF THE EXAMINATION

Patient Preparation

Referring physicians may elect to prescribe prophylactic antibiotics if patients routinely take them for other invasive procedures. If painful, dilated, or obstructed fallopian tubes (or a combination of these conditions) are found before saline infusion, and the patient is not taking prophylactic antibiotics, the examination should be delayed until treatment can be administered. In the presence of nontender hydrosalpinges, consideration may be given to administering antibiotics at the time of the examination. A pregnancy test is advised when clinically indicated. Patients should be asked if they have a latex allergy before latex sheaths are used.

Procedure

Preliminary unenhanced endovaginal ultrasonography with measurements of the endometrium and evaluation of the uterus and ovaries should be performed before saline infusion sonohysterography. After the external os is cleansed, the cervical canal and/or uterine cavity should be catheterized using aseptic technique, and sterile saline should be administered under real-time ultrasonographic imaging. Imaging should include real-time scanning of the endometrium and cervical canal.

Images

Appropriate images, in at least 2 planes, using a high-frequency endovaginal ultrasound probe should be produced and recorded to demonstrate normal and abnormal findings. Precatheterization images should be obtained, including the thickest bilayer endometrial measurement on a sagittal image.

The uterine cavity is filled with sterile saline, and representative images with a complete survey of the uterine cavity are obtained as necessary for diagnostic evaluation. If a balloon catheter is used for the examination, images should be obtained at the end of the procedure with the balloon deflated to fully evaluate the endometrial cavity, particularly the cervical canal and lower uterine segment.

Documentation

Appropriate documentation of a saline infusion sonohysterography examination is essential for clinical care and quality assessment and improvement. Documentation of biometry and anatomy is necessary to support clinical assessment and decision making as well as to establish that recommended guidelines were followed. An adequate written report should include patient identification, procedural technique, measurements, morphologic descriptions, and interpretation. Images of key findings and written reports from ultrasound examinations are considered part of the medical record and should be documented and stored appropriately. (In the *Current Procedural Terminology* [CPT], saline infusion sonohysterography is referred to as hysterosonography.)

Equipment Specifications

Saline infusion sonohysterography must be conducted with an endovaginal transducer. If a patient has an enlarged uterus, additional transabdominal images may be required to fully evaluate the endometrium. The transducer should be adjusted to operate at the highest clinically appropriate frequency under the "as low as reasonably achievable" ALARA principle.

Quality Control, Infection Control, and Patient Education

Quality control is accomplished through careful record keeping, reliable archiving of reports and images, and clinical correlation with outcomes. Endovaginal transducers should always be covered with a single-use disposable latex or nonlatex cover. However, because no such disposable protective cover is without risk of rupture or defect, it is recommended that endovaginal transducers undergo appropriate antimicrobial and antiviral cleansing between patients.

The saline infusion sonohysterography procedure should be fully explained to the patient in advance. Because of the sensitive nature of the transvaginal examination, it may be advisable to have a chaperon present.

Bibliography

Bree RL, Bowerman RA, Bohm-Velez M, Benson CB, Doubilet PM, DeDreu S, et al. US evaluation of the uterus in patients with postmenopausal bleeding: A positive effect on diagnostic decision making. Radiology 2000;216:260–4.

Cohen JR, Luxman D, Sagi J, Yovel I, Wolman I, David MP. Sonohysterography for the diagnosis of endometrial thickening in postmenopausal bleeding—a preliminary report. J Am Assoc Gynecol Laparosc 1994;1:S7–8.

Doubilet PM. Society of Radiologists in Ultrasound Consensus Conference statement on postmenopausal bleeding. J Ultrasound Med 2001;20:1037–42.

Dubinsky TJ, Parvey HR, Gormaz G, Makland N. Transvaginal hysterosonography in the evaluation of small endoluminal masses. J Ultrasound Med 1995;14:1–6.

Dubinsky TJ, Stroehlein K, Abu-Ghazzeh Y, Parvey HR, Makland N. Prediction of benign and malignant endometrial disease: hysterosonographic-pathologic correlation. Radiology 1999;210:393–7.

Goldstein RB, Bree RL, Benson CB, Benacerraf BR, Bloss JD, Carlos R, et al. Evaluation of the woman with postmenopausal bleeding: Society of Radiologists in Ultrasound-Sponsored Consensus Conference statement. J Ultrasound Med 2001; 20:1025–36.

Goldstein SR. Use of ultrasonohysterography for triage of perimenopausal patients with unexplained uterine bleeding. Am J Obstet Gynecol 1994;170:565–70.

Hann LE, Gretz EM, Bach AM, Francis SM. Sonohysterography for evaluation of the endometrium in women treated with tamoxifen. AJR Am J Roentgenol 2001;177:337–42.

Laifer-Narin S, Ragavendra N, Parmenter EK, Grant EG. False-normal appearance of the endometrium on conventional transvaginal sonography: comparison with saline hysterosonography. AJR Am J Roentgenol 2002;178:129–33.

Laifer-Narin SL, Ragavendra N, Lu DS, Sayre J, Perrella RR, Grant EG. Transvaginal saline hysterosonography: characteristics distinguishing malignant and various benign conditions. AJR Am J Roentgenol 1999;172:1513–20.

Lev-Toaff AS, Toaff ME, Liu JB, Merton DA, Goldberg BB. Value of sonohysterography in the diagnosis and management of abnormal uterine bleeding. Radiology 1996;201:179–84.

Merrill JA. Management of postmenopausal bleeding. Clin Obstet Gynecol 1981;24:285–99.

Parsons AK, Lense JJ. Sonohysterography for endometrial abnormalities: preliminary results. J Clin Ultrasound 1993; 21:87–95.

Schwartz LB, Snyder J, Horan C, Porges RF, Nachtigall LE, Goldstein SR. The use of transvaginal ultrasound and saline infusion sonohysterography for the evaluation of asymptomatic postmenopausal breast cancer patients on tamoxifen. Ultrasound Obstet Gynecol 1998;11:48–53.

Sheth S, Hamper UM, Kurman RJ. Thickened endometrium in the postmenopausal woman: sonographic-pathologic correlation. Radiology 1993;187:135–9.

Syrop CH, Sahakian V. Transvaginal sonographic detection of endometrial polyps with fluid contrast augmentation. Obstet Gynecol 1992;79:1041–3.

**The American College of
Obstetricians and Gynecologists
409 12th Street, SW
PO Box 96920
Washington, DC 20090-6920**

12345/76543

Saline infusion sonohysterography. ACOG Technology Assessment in Obstetrics and Gynecology No. 3. American College of Obstetricians and Gynecologists. Obstet Gynecol 2003;102:659–62.

Policy Statements

AAFP/ACOG Joint Statement on Cooperative Practice
and Hospital Privileges *(July 1980, Revised March 1998)*   1057

Abortion Policy *(January and July 1997, Reaffirmed July 2004)*   1059

Access to Women's Health Care *(July 1988, Amended September 1999,
Amended and Reaffirmed July 2003)*   1062

Cervical Cancer Prevention in Low-Resource Settings *(March 2004)*   1063

Joint Statement of ACOG/AAP on Human Immunodeficiency
Virus Screening *(May 1999)*   1066

Joint Statement of Practice Relationships Between Obstetrician–Gynecologists
and Certified Nurse-Midwives/Certified Midwives *(October 2002)*   1068

Tobacco Advertising Aimed at Women and Adolescents *(July 1990, Reaffirmed July 2000,
Revised July 2004)*   1069

Policy Statements

ACOG *Statement of Policy*

As issued by the ACOG Executive Board

This document was developed by a joint task force of the American Academy of Family Physicians and the American College of Obstetricians and Gynecologists.

AAFP--ACOG JOINT STATEMENT ON COOPERATIVE PRACTICE AND HOSPITAL PRIVILEGES

Access to maternity care is an important public health concern in the United States. Providing comprehensive perinatal services to a diverse population requires a cooperative relationship among a variety of health professionals, including social workers, health educators, nurses and physicians. Prenatal care, labor and delivery, and postpartum care have historically been provided by midwives, family physicians and obstetricians. All three remain the major caregivers today. A cooperative and collaborative relationship among obstetricians, family physicians and nurse midwives is essential for provision of consistent, high-quality care to pregnant women.

Regardless of specialty, there should be shared common standards of perinatal care. This requires a cooperative working environment and shared decision making. Clear guidelines for consultation and referral for complications should be developed jointly. When appropriate, early and ongoing consultation regarding a woman's care is necessary for the best possible outcome and is an important part of risk management and prevention of professional liability problems. All family physicians and obstetricians on the medical staff of the obstetric unit should agree to such guidelines and be willing to work together for the best care of patients. This includes a willingness on the part of obstetricians to provide consultation and back-up for family physicians who provide maternity care. The family physician should have knowledge, skills and judgment to determine when timely consultation and/or referral may be appropriate.

The most important objective of the physician must be the provision of the highest standards of care, regardless of specialty. Quality patient care requires that all providers should practice within their degree of ability as determined by training, experience and current competence. A joint practice committee with obstetricians and family physicians should be established in health care organizations to determine and monitor standards of care and to determine proctoring guidelines. A collegial working relationship between family physicians and obstetricians is essential if we are to provide access to quality care for pregnant women in this country.

The American College of Obstetricians and Gynecologists
409 12th Street, SW, PO Box 96920 • Washington, DC 20090-6920 Telephone 202-638-5577

A.   Practice privileges

The assignment of hospital privileges is a local responsibility and privileges should be granted on the basis of training, experience and demonstrated current competence. All physicians should be held to thesame standards for granting of privileges, regardless of specialty, in order to assure the provision of high-quality patient care. Prearranged, collaborative relationships should be established to ensure ongoing consultations, as well as consultations needed for emergencies.

The standard of training should allow any physician who receives training in a cognitive or surgical skill to meet the criteria for privileges in that area of practice. Provisional privileges in primary care, obstetric care and cesarean delivery should be granted regardless of specialty as long as training criteria and experience are documented. All physicians should be subject to a proctorship period to allow demonstration of ability and current competence. These principles should apply to all health care systems.

B. Interdepartmental relationships

Privileges recommended by the department of family practice shall be the responsibility of the department of family practice. Similarly, privileges recommended by the department of obstetrics-gynecology shall be the responsibility of the department of obstetrics-gynecology. When privileges are recommended jointly by the departments of family practice and obstetrics-gynecology, they shall be the joint responsibility of the two departments.

Published July 1980
Reformatted July 1988
Revised and Retitled March 1998

ACOG *Statement of Policy*

As issued by the ACOG Executive Board

ABORTION POLICY

The following statement is the American College of Obstetricians and Gynecologists' (ACOG) general policy related to abortion, with specific reference to the procedure referred to as "intact dilatation and extraction" (intact D & X).

1. The abortion debate in this country is marked by serious moral pluralism. Different positions in the debate represent different but important values. The diversity of beliefs should be respected.

2. ACOG recognizes that the issue of support of or opposition to abortion is a matter of profound moral conviction to its members. ACOG, therefore, respects the need and responsibility of its members to determine their individual positions based on personal values or beliefs.

3. Termination of pregnancy before viability is a medical matter between the patient and physician, subject to the physician's clinical judgment, the patient's informed consent and the availability of appropriate facilities.

4. The need for abortions, other than those indicated by serious fetal anomalies or conditions which threaten maternal welfare, represents failures in the social environment and the educational system.

The most effective way to reduce the number of abortions is to prevent unwanted and unintended pregnancies. This can be accomplished by open and honest education, beginning in the home, religious institutions and the primary schools. This education should stress the biology of reproduction and the responsibilities involved by boys, girls, men and women in creating life and the desirability of delaying pregnancies until circumstances are appropriate and pregnancies are planned.

In addition, everyone should be made aware of the dangers of sexually transmitted diseases and the means of protecting each other from their transmission. To accomplish these aims, support of the community and the school system is essential.

The medical curriculum should be expanded to include a focus on the components of reproductive biology which pertain to conception control. Physicians should be encouraged to apply these principles in their own practices and to support them at the community level.

Society also has a responsibility to support research leading to improved methods of contraception for men and women.

5. Informed consent is an expression of respect for the patient as a person; it particularly respects a patient's moral right to bodily integrity, to self-determination regarding sexuality and reproductive capacities, and to

The American College of Obstetricians and Gynecologists
409 12th Street, SW, PO Box 96920 • Washington, DC 20090-6920 Telephone 202-638-5577

the support of the patient's freedom within caring relationships.

A pregnant woman should be fully informed in a balanced manner about all options, including raising the child herself, placing the child for adoption, and abortion. The information conveyed should be appropriate to the duration of the pregnancy. The professional should make every effort to avoid introducing personal bias.

6. ACOG supports access to care for all individuals, irrespective of financial status, and supports the availability of all reproductive options. ACOG opposes unnecessary regulations that limit or delay access to care.

7. If abortion is to be performed, it should be performed safely and as early as possible.

8. ACOG opposes the harassment of abortion providers and patients.

9. ACOG strongly supports those activities which prevent unintended pregnancy.

The College continues to affirm the legal right of a woman to obtain an abortion prior to fetal viability. ACOG is opposed to abortion of the healthy fetus that has attained viability in a healthy woman. Viability is the capacity of the fetus to survive outside the mother's uterus. Whether or not this capacity exists is a medical determination, may vary with each pregnancy and is a matter for the judgment of the responsible attending physician.

Intact Dilatation and Extraction

The debate regarding legislation to prohibit a method of abortion, such as the legislation banning "partial birth abortion," and "brain sucking abortions," has prompted questions regarding these procedures. It is difficult to respond to these questions because the descriptions are vague and do not delineate a specific procedure recognized in the medical literature. Moreover, the definitions could be interpreted to include elements of many recognized abortion and operative obstetric techniques.

ACOG believes the intent of such legislative proposals is to prohibit a procedure referred to as "intact dilatation and extraction" (Intact D & X). This procedure has been described as containing all of the following four elements:

1. deliberate dilatation of the cervix, usually over a sequence of days;
2. instrumental conversion of the fetus to a footling breech;
3. breech extraction of the body excepting the head; **and**
4. partial evacuation of the intracranial contents of a living fetus to effect vaginal delivery of a dead but otherwise intact fetus.

Because these elements are part of established obstetric techniques, it must be emphasized that unless all four elements are present in sequence, the procedure is not an intact D & X. Abortion intends to terminate a pregnancy while preserving the life and health of the mother. When abortion is performed after 16 weeks, intact D & X is one method of terminating a pregnancy.

The physician, in consultation with the patient, must choose the most appropriate method based upon the patient's individual circumstances.

According to the Centers for Disease Control and Prevention (CDC), only 5.3% of abortions performed in the United States in 1993, the most recent data available, were performed after the 16th week of pregnancy. A preliminary figure published by the CDC for 1994 is 5.6%. The CDC does not collect data on the specific method of abortion, so it is unknown how many of these were performed using intact D & X. Other data show that second trimester transvaginal instrumental abortion is a safe procedure.

Terminating a pregnancy is performed in some circumstances to save the life or preserve the health of the mother.

Intact D & X is one of the methods available in some of these situations. A select panel convened by ACOG could identify no circumstances under which this procedure, as defined above, would be the only option to save the life or preserve the health of the woman. An intact D & X, however, may be the best or most appropriate procedure in a particular circumstance to save the life or preserve the health of a woman, and only the doctor, in consultation with the patient, based upon the woman's particular circumstances can make this decision. The potential exists that legislation prohibiting specific medical practices, such as intact D & X, may outlaw techniques that are critical to the lives and health of American women. **The intervention of legislative bodies into medical decision making is inappropriate, ill advised, and dangerous.**

Approval by the Executive Board
General policy: January 1993
Reaffirmed and revised: July 1997
Intact D & X statement: January 1997
Combined and reaffirmed: September 2000
Reaffirmed: July 2004

ACOG *Statement of Policy*

As issued by the ACOG Executive Board

ACCESS TO WOMEN'S HEALTH CARE

Excellence in women's health care is an essential element of the long-term physical, intellectual, social and economic well-being of any society. It is a basic determinant of the health of future generations.

The American College of Obstetricians and Gynecologists is the representative organization of physicians who are qualified specialists in providing health services unique to women. ACOG calls for quality health care appropriate to every woman's needs throughout her life and for assuring that a full array of clinical services be available to women without costly delays or the imposition of geographic, financial, attitudinal or legal barriers.

The College and its membership are committed to facilitating both access to and quality of women's health care. Fellows should exercise their responsibility to improve the health status of women and their offspring both in the traditional patient-physician relationships and by working within their community and at the state and national levels to assure access to high-quality programs meeting the health needs of all women.

In addition, it is critical that all Americans be provided with adequate and affordable health coverage. There remains a considerable and increasing portion of the American population that does not have health insurance coverage. As a result, those individuals often defer obtaining preventive and medical services, jeopardizing the health and well-being of themselves and their families. The College supports universal coverage that is designed to improve the individual and collective health of society. Expanding health coverage to all Americans must become a high priority.

Approved by the Executive Board July 1988
Amended September 1999
Amended and Reaffirmed July 2003

The American College of Obstetricians and Gynecologists
409 12th Street, SW, PO Box 96920 • Washington, DC 20090-6920 Telephone 202-638-5577

ACOG *Statement of Policy*

As issued by the ACOG Executive Board

A joint policy statement from the American College of Obstetricians and Gynecologists, the Society of Obstetricians and Gynaecologists of Canada, the Central American Federation of Associations and Societies of Obstetrics and Gynecology, the Gynaecologic Oncologists of Canada, the Society of Canadian Colposcopists, the Society of Gynecologic Oncologists, and the Royal College of Obstetricians and Gynaecologists.

CERVICAL CANCER PREVENTION IN LOW-RESOURCE SETTINGS

Cervical cancer is the third most common cancer in the world and the leading cause of cancer death among women in developing countries (1). Worldwide, an estimated 470,000 new cases occur and 233,000 women die annually from cervical cancer (2, 3). Eighty percent of these deaths occur where resources are the most limited (4).

Where organized comprehensive detection, treatment, and referral programs have been implemented, the incidence and mortality of this cancer have decreased dramatically (5). However, implementing programs characteristic of industrialized countries—including testing, treatment, quality assurance, follow-up, and information system components on a widespread basis—requires considerable resources and a high level of program coordination. These programs are impractical and unaffordable in low-resource settings. Yet, women deserve access to services that can safely, effectively, and affordably prevent cervical cancer.

Given the recognized obstacles to implementing cytology-based screening and the limited range of treatment methods available in low-resource settings, other program options are needed. Such options must be feasible and sustainable, and the optimal strategy for a particular setting will necessarily vary given local resource constraints; disease prevalence; and capacity for training, supervision, and infrastructure.

One evidence-based approach designed to prevent cervical cancer in low-resource settings is the "single-visit approach." This approach links a detection method with an immediate management option, such as an offer of treatment or referral, provided by appropriately trained and supervised personnel. There is growing evidence that a single-visit approach, incorporating visual inspection of the cervix with acetic acid wash (VIA), followed by an immediate offer of treatment with cryotherapy for eligible lesions, is a safe, acceptable, and cost-effective approach to cervical cancer prevention (6–9).

The American College of Obstetricians and Gynecologists

409 12th Street, SW, PO Box 96920 • Washington, DC 20090-6920 Telephone 202 638 5577

The American College of Obstetricians and Gynecologists, the Society of Obstetricians and Gynaecologists of Canada, the Central American Federation of Associations and Societies of Obstetrics and Gynecology, the Gynaecologic Oncologists of Canada, the Society of Canadian Colposcopists, the Society of Gynecologic Oncologists, and the Royal College of Obstetricians and Gynaecologists recognize the value of VIA linked to immediate cryotherapy (or referral). It is a viable option for reducing over time the incidence of cervical cancer in settings where services are limited and where other approaches are considered impractical or too expensive.

The obstetric–gynecologic organizations supporting this statement have an important role to play in increasing the capacity of obstetric–gynecologic associations worldwide to include feasible and sustainable cervical cancer prevention programs as part of their national women's health strategies. In turn, national societies of obstetrics and gynecology have an important responsibility to educate both policy makers and the public about the importance of programs aimed at preventing cervical cancer in their countries.

Recognizing both the worldwide burden of this disease and the increasingly important role that women play in socioeconomic development, funding agencies should be aware of the public health importance of cervical cancer. They should be prepared to help underwrite cost-effective, resource-appropriate interventions to prevent unnecessary deaths caused by this disease.

References
1. World Health Organization. State of the art new vaccines: research and development. Initiative for Vaccine Research. Geneva: WHO; 2003. Available at: http://www.who.int/vaccine_research/documents/en/stateofart_excler.pdf. Retrieved November 21, 2003.
2. Program for Appropriate Technology in Health. Cervical cancer prevention. Reproductive Health Outlook. Seattle (WA): PATH; 2003. Available at: http://www.rho.org/assets/RHO_cxca_10-9-03.pdf. Retrieved November 21, 2003.
3. International Agency for Research on Cancer. GLOBOCAN 2000 database: cancer incidence, mortality, and prevalence worldwide. Lyons (FR): IARC; 2001.
4. Parkin DM, Pisani P, Ferlay J. Estimates of the worldwide incidence of eighteen major cancers in 1985. Int J Cancer 1993;54:594–606.
5. Sankaranarayanan R, Budukh AM, Rajkumar R. Effective screening programmes for cervical cancer in low- and middle-income developing countries. Bull World Health Organ 2001;79:954–62.
6. Gaffikin L, Blumenthal PD, Emerson M, Limpaphayom K; Royal Thai College of Obstetricians and Gynaecologists (RTCOG)/JHPIEGO Corporation Cervical Cancer Prevention Group [corrected]. Safety, acceptability, and feasibility of a single visit approach to cervical cancer prevention in rural Thailand: a demonstration project. Lancet 2003;361:814-20.

7. Mandelblatt J, Lawrence W, Gaffikin L, Limpaphayom KK, Lumbiganon P, Warakamin S, et al. Costs and benefits of different strategies to screen for cervical cancer in less-developed countries. J Natl Cancer Inst 2002;94:1469–83.
8. Goldie SJ, Kuhn L, Denny L, Pollack A, Wright TC. Policy analysis of cervical cancer screening strategies in low-resource settings: clinical benefits and cost effectiveness [published erratum appears in JAMA 2001;286:1026]. JAMA 2001;285:3107–15.
9. Martin-Hirsch PL, Paraskevaidis E, Kitchener H. Surgery for cervical intraepithelial neoplasia (Cochrane Review). In: The Cochrane Library, Issue 4, 2003. Chichester, UK: John Wiley & Sons, Ltd.

ACOG *Statement of Policy*

As issued by the ACOG Executive Board

This document was developed jointly by the
American Academy of Pediatrics and the
American College of Obstetricians and Gynecologists.

JOINT STATEMENT ON HUMAN IMMUNODEFICIENCY VIRUS SCREENING

The problem of perinatal transmission of HIV infection was first appreciated in 1982. In 1991, the Institute of Medicine (IOM) recommended a policy of routine counseling and offering testing (with specific informed consent) for HIV infection to all pregnant women. Since 1991, there have been major advances in the treatment of HIV infection, including demonstration in 1994 of the efficacy of zidovudine to reduce perinatal transmission. The U.S. Public Health Service subsequently issued guidelines for use of zidovudine to reduce perinatal transmission and for counseling and voluntary testing for pregnant women. Dramatic declines in reported pediatric AIDS cases have been observed as a consequence of implementation of these guidelines. However, for a variety of reasons, screening pregnant women in the United States has been far from universal and infected babies continue to be born to undiagnosed infected women. Further reduction in the rate of perinatal HIV infection will require wider application of both screening to identify infected women, and treatments, which have demonstrated efficacy in reducing vertical transmission.

The IOM recently completed a study of interventions that would be helpful to further HIV infection in the United States (Reducing the Odds). They have recommended that "the United States should adopt a national policy of universal HIV testing, with patient notification, as a routine component of prenatal care". Early diagnosis of HIV infection in pregnant women allows them to institute effective antiretroviral therapy for their own health and to reduce the risk of HIV transmission to their infants. The use of "patient notification" provides women the opportunity to decline to be tested but eliminates the obligation to provide extensive pretest counseling, which has been a barrier to testing in many settings. Care providers would be charged with responsibility for the details of how the notification would take place. The IOM has recommended universal testing for two reasons. First, attempts to identify those "at risk" for infection inevitably fail to identify some infected individuals. Second, universal testing of all pregnant women avoids stereotyping and stigmatizing any social or ethnic group. The IOM recognizes in its report that many states now have laws requiring a formal, and in many cases written informed consent process prior to testing. They recommend that the Federal government adopt policies that will encourage these states to change their laws.

The American College of Obstetricians and Gynecologists

409 12th Street, SW, PO Box 96920 • Washington, DC 20090-6920 Telephone 202-638-5577

The AAP and the ACOG strongly support efforts to further reduce the rate of perinatal transmission of HIV in the United States. We therefore support the recommendation of the IOM for universal HIV testing with patient notification as a routine component of prenatal care. If a patient declines testing, this should be noted in the medical record. We recognize that current laws in some states may prevent implementation of this recommendation at this time. We encourage our members and Fellows to include counseling as a routine part of care, but not as a prerequisite for, and barrier to, prenatal HIV testing.

Approved by the ACOG Executive Board
Approved by the AAP Executive Board
May 1999

ACOG *Statement of Policy*

As issued by the ACOG Executive Board

JOINT STATEMENT OF PRACTICE RELATIONSHIPS BETWEEN OBSTETRICIAN-GYNECOLOGISTS AND CERTIFIED NURSE-MIDWIVES/CERTIFIED MIDWIVES*

The American College of Obstetricians and Gynecologists (ACOG) and the American College of Nurse-Midwives (ACNM) recognize that in those circumstances in which obstetrician-gynecologists and certified nurse-midwives/certified midwives collaborate in the care of women, the quality of those practices is enhanced by a working relationship characterized by mutual respect and trust as well as professional responsibility and accountability. When obstetrician-gynecologists and certified nurse-midwives/certified midwives collaborate, they should concur on a clear mechanism for consultation, collaboration and referral based on the individual needs of each patient.

Recognizing the high level of responsibility that obstetrician-gynecologists and certified nurse-midwives/certified midwives assume when providing care to women, ACOG and ACNM affirm their commitment to promote appropriate standards for education and certification of their respective members, to support appropriate practice guidelines, and to facilitate communication and collegial relationships between obstetrician-gynecologists and certified nurse-midwives/certified midwives.

*Certified nurse-midwives are registered nurses who have graduated from a midwifery education program accredited by the ACNM Division of Accreditation and have passed a national certification examination administered by the ACNM Certification Council, Inc. Certified midwives are graduates of a Division of Accreditation accredited, university-affiliated midwifery education program, have successfully completed the same science requirements and ACNM Certification Council, Inc., national certification examination as certified nurse-midwives and adhere to the same professional standards as certified nurse-midwives.

American College of Nurse-Midwives
American College of Obstetricians and Gynecologists
October 1, 2002

The American College of Obstetricians and Gynecologists
409 12th Street, SW, PO Box 96920 • Washington, DC 20090-6920 Telephone 202 638 5577

ACOG *Statement of Policy*

As issued by the ACOG Executive Board

TOBACCO ADVERTISING AIMED AT WOMEN AND ADOLESCENTS

The American College of Obstetricians and Gynecologists opposes the unconscionable targeting of women of all ages by the tobacco industry.

The health risks of tobacco use to women are well documented. It also is well known that smoking by a pregnant woman may be harmful to her fetus. It is unnecessary to catalogue all of these risks here. Because of these well-known dangers, it is irresponsible for tobacco companies to single out women, especially those who are young, educationally or otherwise disadvantaged women, and encourage them to smoke.

Specifically, tobacco companies must stop targeting their advertising to encourage adolescent women to smoke cigarettes. The health of all women and future generations demands that consideration.

Approved by the Executive Board July 1990
Reaffirmed July 2000
Revised and approved July 2004

The American College of Obstetricians and Gynecologists
409 12th Street, SW, PO Box 96920 • Washington, DC 20090-6920 Telephone 202 638 5577

Title Index

Title Index

Title Index

AAFP/ACOG Joint Statement on Cooperative Practice and Hospital Privileges (PS) **1057**

Abortion Policy (PS) **1059**

Access to Women's Health Care (PS) **1062**

Advanced Paternal Age: Risks to the Fetus (CO189) **5**

Air Travel During Pregnancy (CO264) **7**

Analgesia and Cesarean Delivery Rates (CO269) **9**

Antenatal Corticosteroid Therapy for Fetal Maturation (CO273) **11**

Antepartum Fetal Surveillance (PB9) **337**

Antibiotic Prophylaxis for Gynecologic Procedures (PB23) **348**

Antiphospholipid Syndrome (PB68) **357**

Appropriate Use of Laparoscopically Assisted Vaginal Hysterectomy (CO311) **13**

Assessment of Fetal Lung Maturity (EB230) **267**

Assessment of Risk Factors for Preterm Birth (PB31) **366**

At-Risk Drinking and Illicit Drug Use: Ethical Issues in Obstetric and Gynecologic Practice (CO294) **15**

Avoiding Inappropriate Clinical Decisions Based on False-Positive Human Chorionic Gonadotropin Test Results (CO278) **26**

Benefits and Risks of Sterilization (PB46) **374**

Breast Cancer Screening (PB42) **386**

Breastfeeding: Maternal and Infant Aspects (EB258) **274**

Cervical Cancer Prevention in Low-Resource Settings (PS) **1063**

Cervical Cancer Screening in Adolescents (CO300) **29**

Cervical Cytology Screening (PB45) **398**

Cervical Insufficiency (PB48) **409**

Chronic Hypertension in Pregnancy (PB29) **418**

Chronic Pelvic Pain (PB51) **427**

Circumcision (CO260) **34**

Coding Responsibility (CO249) **36**

Complementary and Alternative Medicine (CO227) **37**

Compounded Bioidentical Hormones (CO322) **40**

Coping with the Stress of Medical Professional Liability Litigation (CO309) **42**

Diagnosis and Management of Preeclampsia and Eclampsia (PB33) **444**

Diagnosis and Treatment of Cervical Carcinomas (PB35) **453**

Diagnosis and Treatment of Gestational Trophoblastic Disease (PB53) **466**

Dystocia and the Augmentation of Labor (PB49) **479**

Elective Coincidental Appendectomy (CO323) **44**

Emergency Oral Contraception (PB69) **489**

Endometriosis in Adolescents (CO310) **46**

Exercise During Pregnancy and the Postpartum Period (CO267) **53**

External Cephalic Version (PB13) **500**

Fetal Macrosomia (PB22) **507**

Fetal Pulse Oximetry (CO258) **56**

First-Trimester Screening for Fetal Aneuploidy (CO296) **58**

Follow-up of Abnormal Screening Mammography (CO272) **61**

Fragile X Syndrome (CO161) **62**

Genetic Evaluation of Stillbirths and Neonatal Deaths (CO257) **64**

Genetics and Molecular Diagnostic Testing (TA1) **1027**

Gestational Diabetes (PB30) **518**

Guidelines for Adolescent Health Research (CO302) **67**

Guidelines for Diagnostic Imaging During Pregnancy (CO299) **71**

Gynecologic Herpes Simplex Virus Infections (PB57) **532**

Health Care for Homeless Women (CO312) **76**

Hemoglobinopathies in Pregnancy (PB64) **539**

Hepatitis Virus Infections in Obstetrician-Gynecologists (CO203) **82**

Human Papillomavirus (PB61) **548**

Hysteroscopy (TA4) **1046**

Immunization During Pregnancy (CO282) **84**

Inappropriate Reimbursement Practices by Third Party Payers (CO250) **90**

Inappropriate Use of the Terms Fetal Distress and Birth Asphyxia (CO326) **94**

Induced Abortion and Breast Cancer Risk (CO285) **96**

Induction of Labor (PB10) **562**

Induction of Labor for Vaginal Birth After Cesarean Delivery (CO271) **99**

Induction of Labor with Misoprostol (CO228) **101**

Influenza Vaccination and Treatment During Pregnancy (CO305) **103**

Informed Refusal (CO306) **105**

Intrapartum Fetal Heart Rate Monitoring (PB70) **572**

Intrauterine Device (PB59) **581**

Intrauterine Growth Restriction (PB12) **591**

Joint Statement of ACOG/AAP on Human Immunodeficiency Virus Screening (May 1999) (PS) **1066**

Joint Statement of Practice Relationships Between Obstetrician-Gynecologists and Certified Nurse-Midwives/Certified Midwives (October 2002) (PS) **1068**

Length of Hospital Stay for Gynecologic Procedures (CO191) **107**

Management of Abnormal Cervical Cytology and Histology (PB66) **603**

Management of Anovulatory Bleeding (PB14) **623**

Management of Asymptomatic Pregnant or Lactating Women Exposed to Anthrax (CO268) **108**

Management of Endometrial Cancer (PB65) **631**

Management of Herpes in Pregnancy (PB8) **644**

Management of Infertility Caused by Ovulatory Dysfunction (PB34) **653**

Management of Isoimmunization in Pregnancy (EB227) **290**

Management of Postterm Pregnancy (PB55) **665**

Management of Preterm Labor (PB43) **673**

Management of Recurrent Early Pregnancy Loss (PB24) **682**
Maternal Decision Making, Ethics, and the Law (CO321) **111**
Maternal Phenylketonuria (CO230) **122**
Medical Management of Abortion (PB67) **694**
Medical Management of Endometriosis (PB11) **706**
Medical Management of Tubal Pregnancy (PB3) **719**
Meningococcal Vaccination for Adolescents (CO314) **124**
Mode of Term Singleton Breech Delivery (CO265) **127**
Multiple Gestation: Complicated Twin, Triplet, and
    High-Order Multifetal Pregnancy (PB56) **726**
Nausea and Vomiting of Pregnancy (PB52) **741**
Neural Tube Defects (PB44) **754**
New U.S. Food and Drug Administration Labeling on
    Cytotec (Misoprostol) Use and Pregnancy (CO283) **129**
Newborn Screening (CO287) **131**
Nongynecologic Procedures (CO253) **134**
Nonmedical Use of Obstetric Ultrasonography (CO297) **135**
Nonobstetric Surgery in Pregnancy (CO284) **137**
Nonsurgical Diagnosis and Management of
    Vaginal Agenesis (CO274) **138**
Obesity in Pregnancy (CO315) **142**
Obstetric Analgesia and Anesthesia (PB36) **765**
Obstetric Aspects of Trauma Management (EB251) **297**
Obstetric Management of Patients
    with Spinal Cord Injuries (CO275) **147**
Operative Vaginal Delivery (PB17) **780**
Optimal Goals for Anesthesia Care in Obstetrics (CO256) **150**
Osteoporosis (PB50) **788**
Pain Relief During Labor (CO295) **153**
Partner Consent for Participation in Women's Reproductive
    Health Research (CO307) **154**
Partnering with Patients to Improve Safety (CO320) **157**
Patient Safety in Obstetrics and Gynecology (CO286) **160**
Performance and Interpretation of Imaging Studies by
    Obstetrician-Gynecologists (CO243) **163**
Perinatal Care at the Threshold of Viability (PB38) **802**
Perinatal Risks Associated with Assisted Reproductive
    Technology (CO324) **165**
Perinatal Viral and Parasitic Infections (PB20) **810**
Placenta Accreta (CO266) **169**
Placental Pathology (CO125) **171**
Polycystic Ovary Syndrome (PB41) **823**
Pregestational Diabetes Mellitus (PB60) **837**
Premature Rupture of Membranes (PB1) **848**
Premenstrual Syndrome (PB15) **858**
Prenatal and Perinatal Human Immunodeficiency Virus
    Testing: Expanded Recommendations (CO304) **172**
Prenatal and Preconceptional Carrier Screening for
    Genetic Diseases in Individuals of Eastern European
    Jewish Descent (CO298) **178**
Prenatal Diagnosis of Fetal Chromosomal
    Abnormalities (PB27) **867**
Prevention of Deep Vein Thrombosis
    and Pulmonary Embolism (PB21) **879**
Prevention of Early-Onset Group B Streptococcal
    Disease in Newborns (CO279) **182**
Prevention of Rh D Alloimmunization (PB4) **889**
Primary and Preventive Care: Periodic
    Assessments (CO292) **190**

Professional Liability and Gynecology-Only
    Practice (CO288) **198**
Prophylactic Antibiotics in Labor and Delivery (PB47) **897**
Prophylactic Oophorectomy (PB7) **905**
Psychosocial Risk Factors: Perinatal Screening
    and Intervention (EB255) **304**
Racial and Ethnic Disparities in Women's Health (CO317) **199**
Reading the Medical Literature: Applying Evidence
    to Practice **329**
Response to Searle's Drug Warning
    on Misoprostol (CO248) **203**
Role of the Obstetrician-Gynecologist in the Diagnosis and
    Treatment of Breast Disease (CO186) **205**
Routine Storage of Umbilical Cord Blood for Potential Future
    Transplantation (CO183) **207**
Rubella Vaccination (CO281) **210**
Safety of Lovenox in Pregnancy (CO276) **211**
Saline Infusion Sonohysterography (TA3) **1050**
Scheduled Cesarean Delivery and the Prevention of Vertical
    Transmission of HIV Infection (CO234) **213**
Screening for Canavan Disease (CO212) **216**
Screening for Tay-Sachs Disease (CO318) **218**
Selective Estrogen Receptor Modulators (PB39) **911**
Sexually Transmitted Diseases in Adolescents (CO301) **220**
Shoulder Dystocia (PB40) 921
Smoking Cessation During Pregnancy (CO316) **228**
Statement on Surgical Assistants (CO240) **234**
Surgical Alternatives to Hysterectomy in the Management
    of Leiomyomas (PB16) **927**
Tamoxifen and Endometrial Cancer (CO232) **235**
Teratology (EB236) **311**
The Importance of Preconception Care in the Continuum of
    Women's Health Care (CO313) **238**
The Role of the Generalist Obstetrician-Gynecologist in the
    Early Detection of Ovarian Cancer (CO280) **240**
The Role of the Obstetrician-Gynecologist
    in the Assessment and Management of Obesity (CO319) **243**
The Uninsured (CO308) **248**
The Use of Hormonal Contraception in Women
    with Coexisting Medical Conditions (PB18) **936**
Thrombocytopenia in Pregnancy (PB6) **950**
Thromboembolism in Pregnancy (PB19) **961**
Thyroid Disease in Pregnancy (PB37) **971**
Tobacco Advertising Aimed at Women
    and Adolescents (PS) **1069**
Tubal Ligation with Cesarean Delivery (CO205) **252**
Ultrasonography in Pregnancy (PB58) **981**
Update on Carrier Screening for Cystic Fibrosis (CO325) **253**
Urinary Incontinence in Women (PB63) **991**
Use and Abuse of the Apgar Score (CO174) **257**
Use of Botanicals for Management of
    Menopausal Symptoms (PB28) **1004**
Use of Progesterone to Reduce Preterm Birth (CO291) **260**
Uterine Artery Embolization (CO293) **262**
Vaginal Birth After Previous Cesarean Delivery (PB54) **1015**
Viral Hepatitis in Pregnancy (EB248) **318**

CO: Committee Opinion; EB: Educational Bulletin; PB: Practice Bulletin; PS: Policy Statement; TA: Technology Assessment

Subject Index

Subject Index

Subject Index

Note: Page numbers followed by *b*, *f*, or *t* indicate boxes, figures, or tables, respectively.

A

AAP. *See* American Academy of Pediatrics
Abbe-McIndoe operation, 140
Abdominal bloating, in ovarian cancer, 241
Abdominal circumference, fetal, 595, 984, 987
Abdominal film, fetal radiation exposure from, 73*b*
Abdominal hysterectomy, antibiotic prophylaxis in, 349*t*, 350. *See also* Hysterectomy
Abdominal myomectomy, 929
Abdominal pain
  cyclic, in müllerian aplasia, 139
  versus nausea and vomiting of pregnancy, 742–743
  in ovarian cancer, 241
Abdominal palpation, for fetal weight estimate, 510–511
Abdominal size, in ovarian cancer, 241
Abdominal trauma, in pregnancy
  blunt, 298–299
  penetrating, 299
  and Rh D alloimmunization, 301, 893
ABO incompatibility, 290
Abortion
  induced, and breast cancer risk, 96–97. *See also specific types*
  medical, 694–702
    background of, 694–699
    candidates for, 699
    clinical considerations and recommendations in, 699–702
    confirmation of, 700
    contraindications to, 699
    counseling in, 697, 701
    emergency contraception versus, 490
    failed
      definition of, 698
      management of, 698–699
    follow-up dilation and curettage in, 698–699
    and future fertility, 701
    gestational age and, 699
    incomplete, 698–699
    infection risk in, 699

Abortion *(continued)*
  medical *(continued)*
    medications currently used in, 694–695
    methotrexate for, 695
    methotrexate–misoprostol for, 695–696, 696*t*
    mifepristone for, 694–695
    mifepristone–misoprostol for, 695, 696*t*, 697
    misoprostol for, 203–204, 695–697
    nonsteroidal antiinflammatory drugs and, 700–701
    pretreatment laboratory testing for, 699
    pretreatment ultrasonography for, 699–700
    side effects of, 697, 698*t*
    versus surgical, 697, 697*t*
    symptom management in, 697
    teratogenic effects of, 701
  policy statement on, 1059–1061
  septic, intrauterine devices and, 585–586
  spontaneous
    air travel and, 7
    herpes simplex virus infection and, 646
    intrauterine devices and, 585–586
    obesity and, 142
    and Rh D alloimmunization, 890, 893
  surgical, antibiotic prophylaxis in, 349*t*, 351
  threatened, and Rh D alloimmunization, 890, 892
  tubal sterilization after, 374–375, 377
Abruptio placentae
  chronic hypertension and, 419
  external cephalic version and, 501
  maternal smoking and, 228
  trauma and, 298–301
Abscess, during breastfeeding, 284–285
Abstinence, encouragement of, among adolescents, 223
Abuse (domestic, physical, or sexual)
  as barrier to care, 306
  chronic pelvic pain in, 430, 436
  in postpartum period, 307
  in pregnancy, 298, 307
Acanthosis nigricans
  differential diagnosis in, 824
  in polycystic ovary syndrome, 824

Acardiac twin, 734
Acceleration, in fetal heart rate, 573*t*, 574
Access to health care, policy statement on, 1062
Accreditation, for ultrasonography, 985
Accuracy, definition of, 334
Acephalus twin, 734
Acetaminophen, for mastitis, 284
Achondroplasia, paternal age and, 5
Acidemia, 257
  lactic, 257, 660
  metabolic, and fetal heart rate, 337–338
ACIP. *See* Advisory Committee on Immunization Practices
ACMG. *See* American College of Medical Geneticists
Acne, in polycystic ovary syndrome, 823–824
Acoustic stimulation, in nonstress test, 339
Acquired immunodeficiency syndrome (AIDS). *See* Human immunodeficiency virus (HIV) infection
Actinomyces israelii infection, intrauterine devices and, 585
Active Bacterial Core Surveillance/Emerging Infections Program, 183
Active management, of labor, 483
Acupuncture, for chronic pelvic pain, 436
Acute chest syndrome, 540
Acute fatty liver, in multiple gestation, 729
Acyclovir
  for herpes simplex virus infection, 534–535, 535*t*, 647–648, 648*t*
  use during pregnancy, 648
  for varicella zoster virus infection, 815
Add-back therapy, with gonadotropin-releasing hormone agonists, 50, 711, 862
Addison's disease, and ovulatory dysfunction, 657
Adenocarcinoma(s)
  cervical
    in situ (AIS), 603, 608–611
    treatment of, 459, 608–611
  endometrial, 632–633
ADHD. *See* Attention deficit hyperactivity disorder
Adhesiolysis, 435

Adolescent(s)
  age at first sexual intercourse, 30, 221
  age for first visit to obstetrician–gyne-
      cologist, 32
  alcohol abuse among
      special issues in, 21–22
      and sexually transmitted disease risk,
          221
  anovulatory bleeding in, 625–626
  cervical cancer screening in, 29–32,
      222, 401, 606
      abnormal results in, management of,
          30–31
      initiation of, 30
      need for additional research on,
          32
      patient and parent education on,
          32
  condom use among, 221
  confidentiality for, 21–22, 31*b*,
      221–222
  consent by, 68, 221–222
  drug abuse among, 21–22, 221
  endometrial cancer in, 626
  endometriosis in, 46–51
      complementary and alternative medi-
          cine for, 51
      diagnosis of, 47–49, 48*f*
      empiric therapy for, 47–48
      history in, 47
      imaging studies of, 47
      incidence of, 46–47
      müllerian anomalies and, 46, 49
      physical examination in, 47
      presentation and characteristics of,
          47
      serum markers in, 47
      surgical diagnosis of, 48–49
      surgical management of, 50–51
      treatment of, 48*f*, 49–51
      typical lesions in, 49
  high-risk, follow-up difficulties for, 30
  homeless, 76
  human papillomavirus infection in,
      220
      risk factors for, 30, 32*b*
      screening for, 29–32
  meningococcal vaccine for, 124–126
      Advisory Committee on
          Immunization Practices Centers
          for Disease Control and
          Prevention recommendations
          on, 125
      American College of Obstetricians
          and Gynecologists recommen-
          dations on, 125–126
  morbidity in, leading causes of, 191
  mortality in, leading causes of, 191
  periodic assessments in, 191
  pregnancy in, unintended, 307
  sexual history of, 30, 31*b*

Adolescent(s) (*continued*)
  sexually transmitted diseases in,
      220–224
      barriers to care in, 221–222
      costs of, 221–222
      epidemiology of, 220–221
      in nonpregnant patients, 222–223
      partner notification of, 224
      in pregnancy, 223–224
      prevention guidelines for, 222–224
      publications on, 226
      reporting of, 224
      risk factors for, 221
      screening guidelines for, 222–224
      treatment of, guidelines for, 224
      victims of sexual assault, 224
      web site resources on, 226–227
  tobacco advertising aimed at, policy
      statement on, 1069
Adolescent health research
  background of, 67–68
  guidelines for, 67–70
  legal issues in, 68
  parental consent for, waiving of
      requirement for, 68–70
  permission and assent in, 68
  regulations on, 68–69
Adrenocorticotropic hormone, for nausea
      and vomiting of pregnancy,
      747*t*
Advisory Committee on Immunization
      Practices (ACIP), meningococ-
      cal vaccine recommendations
      of, 125
Advocates for Youth, 226
Aerobic capacity, in pregnancy, air travel
      and, 8
Aerobic exercise
  during pregnancy, 53–55
      absolute contraindications to, 54*b*
      relative contraindications to, 54*b*
  for premenstrual syndrome, 861
AFI. *See* Amniotic fluid index
AFP. *See* Alpha-fetoprotein
African American(s)
  cystic fibrosis in, 254*t*
  endometrial cancer in, 631–632
  group B streptococcal disease in, 183
  health care insurance among, 201
  health disparities for, 199–202
  macrosomia in, 509
  obesity in, 243
  osteoporosis in, 790
  sickle cell disease in, 540
AGC. *See* Atypical glandular cells
Age
  and anovulatory bleeding, 625
  at first sexual intercourse, 30, 221
  for first visit to obstetrician–gynecolo-
      gist, 32
  gestational. *See* Gestational age

Age (*continued*)
  maternal
      and Down syndrome, 867–868, 868*t*,
          873
      and multiple gestation, 728
      and serum screening, 873
  and ovulatory dysfunction, 655
  paternal, advanced, 5
  periodic assessments based on,
      190–194
  and premenstrual syndrome, 858
  and urinary incontinence, 991
Agranulocytosis, thioamides and, 975
AIDS. *See* Human immunodeficiency
      virus (HIV) infection
Air travel, during pregnancy, 7–8
AIUM. *See* American Institute of
      Ultrasound in Medicine
Alan Guttmacher Institute, 226
Alanine aminotransferase
  in hepatitis, 320
  in preeclampsia, 446
ALARA principle, 986
Alcohol use, 15–23
  adolescent
      special issues in, 21–22
      and sexually transmitted disease risk,
          221
  breastfeeding contraindicated in, 276
  brief intervention in, 16, 19
  costs of, 15
  epidemiology of, 15–16
  ethical basis for care in, 16–19
      beneficence, 16–17, 19
      justice, 17–18, 20
      nonmaleficence, 17, 19
      respect for autonomy, 18–20
  ethical responsibilities in
      to neonates, 20–21
      to pregnant patients, 19–20
  fetal effects of, 15, 20–21, 311, 315*t*
  guidance for physicians in, 22–23
  and intrauterine growth restriction,
      592–593
  legal sanctions in, 19–20, 114
  maternal decision making versus fetal
      protection in, 111–119
  and osteoporosis, 793
  physician's knowledge gaps about, 16,
      19
  and recurrent pregnancy loss, 684
  screening for
      tools for, 17, 18*b*
      universal, 16, 19
  treatment referral in, 16, 19–20
Alendronate, for osteoporosis prevention,
      794–795
Alesse, 491*t*
Allele(s), 1029, 1043
Allele-specific oligonucleotide(s),
      1043

Allele-specific oligonucleotide hybridization, 1036–1037, 1037*f*

Allis clamp scalp stimulation, 577

Alloimmune disorders, and recurrent pregnancy loss, 685, 688

Alpha-fetoprotein (AFP)
in Down syndrome, 868–869
in neural tube defects, 758–759
and risk of poor pregnancy outcome, 759, 759*t*

Alprazolam, for premenstrual syndrome, 862

Alternative systems of medical practice, 37

Alveolar period, of lung development, 268

ALTS. *See* Atypical Squamous Cells of Undetermined Significance/Low Grade Squamous Intraepithelial Lesion Triage Study

Amantadine, during pregnancy, 104

Amaurosis fugax, antiphospholipid syndrome and, 359

Ambulation, and course of labor, 482

Amenorrhea
hypothalamic, 654–655
intrauterine devices and, 586
ovulatory dysfunction and, 653
in polycystic ovary syndrome, therapy for, 827
primary, in müllerian aplasia, 139
in women of reproductive age, 625

Amenorrhea method, lactational, 282–283, 283*f*

American Academy of Family Physicians, 226

American Academy of Pediatrics (AAP), 226
on breastfeeding, 275, 275*b*, 286
on group B streptococcal disease prophylaxis, 183
on newborn screening, 132–133

American College of Medical Geneticists (ACMG), cystic fibrosis carrier screening guidelines of, 253–254

American Institute of Ultrasound in Medicine (AIUM), on nonmedical use of obstetric ultrasonography, 135–136

American Social Health Association, 226

American Society for Colposcopy and Cervical Pathology (ASCCP), 551

American Society for Reproductive Medicine (ASRM), endometriosis classifications of, 708*f*, 709

Aminoglycosides, pharmacokinetics of, 899

Aminopterin, teratogenicity of, 315*t*, 756

Amitriptyline, for chronic pelvic pain, 432

Amniocentesis, 871, 1042
for Canavan disease, 217
versus chorionic villus sampling, 871
complications of, 871
for Down syndrome, 867
early, 871
elective, in women younger than 35 years, 873–874
for fetal lung maturity assessment, 268
in isoimmunization, 292
in multiple gestation, 728, 873
for neural tube defects, 758–759
pregnancy loss rate with, 871
and premature rupture of membranes, 850
in preterm labor and delivery, 677–678
traditional, 871
training for, 871
for twin–twin transfusion syndrome, 733–734

Amnioinfusion, for nonreassuring fetal heart rate, 578

Amniotic fluid analysis
for fetal lung maturity assessment, 269–271, 270*t*
in stillbirths and neonatal deaths, 65–66

Amniotic fluid embolism, oxytocin and, 567

Amniotic fluid index (AFI), 340, 343

Amniotic fluid volume, 339–340, 343
in intrauterine growth restriction, 595, 987
in postterm pregnancy, 667
ultrasound assessment of, 343, 983, 987

Amniotomy
complications of, 566–567
for labor induction, 484–485, 562–564, 566–567

Amoxicillin, prophylactic
for anthrax, 109–110
for bacterial endocarditis, 353*t*
for preterm premature rupture of membranes, 852

Amoxicillin–clavulanic acid, prophylactic, 900

Ampicillin
oral contraception use with, 942
pharmacokinetics of, 899
prophylactic
for bacterial endocarditis, 353*t*, 900–901
for cesarean delivery, 899–900
for group B streptococcal disease, 186*t*
for preterm premature rupture of membranes, 852, 900

Ampicillin–sulbactam, prophylactic, for cesarean delivery, 899

Anal–genital contact, among adolescents
as "abstinent behavior," 223
and sexually transmitted disease risk, 222–223

Analgesia
for chronic pelvic pain, 433
for intrauterine device insertion, 583
for medical abortion, 697
obstetric, 153, 765–775
anticoagulation and, 966–967
background of, 765–769
and breastfeeding, 773–774
chronic hypertension and, 423
clinical considerations and recommendations, 770–774
epidural, 153, 766–767
administration of, 766–767
and cesarean delivery rates, 9–10, 771–772
and chronic back pain, 770
enoxaparin contraindicated before, 212
in external cephalic version, 502
and fetal heart rate, 575
and fever, 768*t*, 771
and hematoma, 767, 772, 882, 955–956, 966–967
indications for, 766
and operative delivery rates, 771
patient-controlled, 770, 774
in preeclampsia, 448
and progress of labor, 482
side effects of, 767, 768*t*
spinal analgesia combined with, 767
thrombocytopenia and, 955–956
for vaginal birth after cesarean delivery, 1019
maternal aspiration risk in, 773
and maternal mortality, 769
maternal request for, 153
methods of, 765–769
nurses' role in, 153
parenteral, 765–766, 766*t*
selection of agent for, factors in, 770
transplacental passage of, 770
in preeclampsia, 448, 773
regional, 766–767
contraindications to, 769, 769*b*
side effects of, 767, 768*t*
spinal, 767
and hematoma, 767, 772, 882, 966–967
side effects of, 767, 768*t*
spinal epidural, 767
third-party payment for, 153, 766
thrombocytopenia and, 955–956
for vaginal birth after cesarean delivery, 150–152, 1019
postoperative, optimal agents for, 774

Anaphylaxis, antibiotics and, 350, 898

Androgen(s)
  and anovulatory bleeding, 625
  measurement of, 825
  for osteoporosis, in combination therapy, 795
  in polycystic ovary syndrome, 654, 823–825
  teratogenicity of, 315t
Androgen insensitivity, versus vaginal agenesis, 139
Androgen-secreting tumors, 824–825
Androstenedione, in polycystic ovary syndrome, 654, 825
Anencephaly, 755t
Anesthesia. See also Analgesia
  deep vein thrombosis prophylaxis and, 882, 884
  obstetric, 765–775
    anticoagulation and, 966–967
    availability of personnel and facilities for, 150–151
    available methods of, 765–769
    background of, 765–769
    and breastfeeding, 773–774
    chronic hypertension and, 423
    clinical considerations and recommendations, 770–774
    and fetal heart rate, 575
    general, 769
    local, 769
    maternal aspiration risk in, 773
    and maternal mortality, 769
    for obese patients, 143
    optimal goals for, 150–152
    in preeclampsia, 448, 773
    third-party payment for, 153, 766
    thrombocytopenia and, 955–956
  in pregnancy, for nonobstetric surgery, 137
Anesthesiologists
  availability and qualifications of, 150–152
  consultation with, 774, 775b
  relationship with obstetricians, 152
Aneuploidy
  midtrimester risk of, 867, 868t
  parental, 871
  prenatal diagnosis of, 867–874
    background of, 867–870
    clinical considerations and recommendations in, 870–874
    methods of, 871–872
    in multiple gestation, 873
  recurrent preembryonic or embryonic, 683
  screening for
    first-trimester, 58–60, 870
    indications for, 870–871
    maternal serum, 868–870
    second-trimester, 868–869
    ultrasonography, 869, 872–873, 986–987

Aneuploidy (continued)
  structural anomalies in, 869, 869t
  term risk of, 867, 868t
Angelman's syndrome
  assisted reproductive technology and, 167
  genetics of, 1032–1033, 1040t
Angiotensin-converting enzyme (ACE) inhibitors, teratogenicity of, 315t, 422
Animal studies, of teratogens, 312
Aniridia, 1041t
Annexin V, antibody against, 359
Anovulation, 624, 654
  causes of, 624, 624b
  hyperandrogenic, 625, 823–824
  in polycystic ovary syndrome, 823, 827
Anovulatory bleeding
  acute, treatment of, 628
  in adolescents (13–18 years), 625–626
  age considerations in, 625
  background of, 623–625
  clinical considerations and recommendations in, 626
  definition of, 623
  diagnosis of, 624
  endometrial evaluation in, indications for, by age, 626
  estrogen therapy for, 626–628
  management of, 623–628
  medical therapies for, by age, 626–627
  pathophysiology of, 624
  physical examination in, 624
  surgical treatment of, 627–628
  in women of later reproductive age (40 years to menopause), 625–627
  in women of reproductive age (19–39 years), 625–627
Anthrax
  active infections of, 109
  cutaneous, 108
  exposure to, management of, 108–110
    in asymptomatic pregnant or lactating women, 109–110
    in bioterrorism, 109
    prophylaxis in, 109–110
  gastrointestinal, 109
  inhalational, 109
Anthrax vaccine, during pregnancy, 87t
Antiandrogens, for hirsutism, 830
Antibiotic(s)
  adverse reactions to, 350, 898
  for mastitis, 284–285
  oral contraception use with, 942, 942b
  pharmacokinetics of, 898–899
  for preterm labor, 675–677
  prophylaxis, 348–354, 897–902
    background of, 348–350, 897
    for bacterial endocarditis, 352, 352b–353b, 353t, 585, 900–901, 901t

Antibiotic(s) (continued)
  prophylaxis (continued)
    for cervical cerclage, 414, 899
    for cesarean delivery, 187–188, 350, 899–900
    clinical considerations and recommendations in, 350–354, 899–902
    cost-effectiveness of, 354
    for gynecologic procedures, 348–354, 349t
    for hysterectomy, 349t, 350
    intrapartum, for group B streptococcal disease, 183–188, 898–899
      benefit versus risk analysis of, 186
      culture-based approach in, 183–188, 184f, 185b
      hospital compliance with, 184
      in premature rupture of membranes, 183–188, 187f, 852, 900
      recommended regimens for, 186, 186t
      resistance to, 186
      risk-based approach in, 183–184
    in intrauterine device insertion, 349t, 351, 584–585
    in labor and delivery, 897–902
    for manual removal of placenta, 901
    pharmacology of, 349–350
    for preterm premature rupture of membranes, 183–188, 187f, 852, 898–900
    spectrum of activity, 349–350
    theory of, 349
    versus treatment regimens, 897
  resistance to, 350, 898
  widespread use of, risks of, 898
Antibody titers, 291–292
Anticardiolipin antibodies, 357–361, 361t, 685, 688
Anticholinergic drugs
  for nausea and vomiting of pregnancy, 745, 747t
  for urinary incontinence, 997–998
Anticoagulation
  adjusted-dose prophylaxis, 962
  for antiphospholipid syndrome, 361–362
  for deep vein thrombosis prophylaxis, 881–883
  and epidural hematoma, 772, 882, 966–967
  in intrapartum and postpartum period, 966
  low-dose prophylaxis, 962
  in multiple gestation, 729–730
  in pregnancy, 211–212, 962–968
    indications for, 963–964
    and regional anesthesia, 966–967
  and spinal hematoma, 772, 882, 966–967

Anticonvulsants
  and intrauterine growth restriction, 593
  oral contraception use with, 941, 942b
Anti-D alloimmunization. *See* Anti-D
    immune globulin prophylaxis;
    Rh D alloimmunization
Antidepressants
  for chronic pelvic pain, 432–433
  for smoking cessation, 230
Anti-D immune globulin prophylaxis,
    890–894
  antenatal administration of, 890
  in antenatal hemorrhage, 893
  antibody screening before, 892
  cost-effectiveness of, 891–892
  discharge without, follow-up in, 893
  duration of effects, 893
  in external cephalic version, 503
  failure of, 891
  in fetal death, 893
  for first-trimester events and proce-
      dures, 893
  in hydatidiform mole, 469, 893
  infection transmission via, 891
  in medical abortion, 699
  paternity and, 892
  postpartum administration of, 890
  potential shortage of, 891
  recommendations for, 890
  repeat, in postterm pregnancy, 894
  in sensitized pregnancy, 892
  for sterilization procedures, 892
  in threatened abortion, 892
  in trauma, 301, 893
Antiemetics
  with emergency contraception, 493
  for nausea and vomiting of pregnancy,
      745–748, 746f, 747t
Antihistamines, for nausea and vomiting
    of pregnancy, 745, 746f, 747t
Antihypertensive agents
  for chronic hypertension, in pregnancy,
      422
  for preeclampsia, 448, 448b
Antinuclear antibodies, and recurrent
    pregnancy loss, 685
Antioxidants, for preeclampsia prevention,
    449
Antiphospholipid syndrome, 357–363,
    880, 881t
  antepartum surveillance in, 362
  antibodies in, 358–359
  background of, 357–359
  catastrophic, 359
  clinical considerations and recommen-
      dations in, 360–363
  conditions associated with, 360
  diagnosis of, laboratory criteria for, 361,
      361t, 688
  and fetal death, 357, 360
  indications for testing, 360–361, 361t

Antiphospholipid syndrome *(continued)*
  and intrauterine growth restriction, 357,
      360, 592
  management of, 688
    long-term, 362
    during pregnancy and postpartum
        period, 361–362
  medical complications of, 359
  obstetric complications of, 357, 360
  and placental insufficiency, 357, 360
  and preeclampsia, 357, 360
  and preterm delivery, 357, 360
  primary, 357
  and recurrent pregnancy loss, 360,
      684–685, 688
  secondary, 357
  testing for, 688
  and thrombocytopenia, 357, 359
  thromboprophylaxis in, 963
  and thrombosis, 357, 359, 880, 881t
Antithrombin III deficiency, 881t
  and deep vein thrombosis, 884
  and recurrent pregnancy loss, 684, 688
  and thromboembolism, in pregnancy,
      963–965
Antiviral influenza drugs, during preg-
    nancy, 104
Apert syndrome, 5, 1042
Apgar, Virginia, 257
Apgar score
  components of, 257, 258t
  factors affecting, 257
  macrosomia and, 510
  1-minute, 258
  5-minute, 258
  postterm pregnancy and, 666
  and subsequent disability, 258
  use and abuse of, 257–258
Appendectomy, elective coincidental, 44–45
  definition of, 44
  risk–benefit analysis of, 44–45
Arcuate uterus, and recurrent pregnancy
    loss, 684
Arnold-Chiari malformation, 755, 760
Arrest, of labor, 480
  cesarean delivery for, 481
  diagnosis of, 2-hour rule for, 480–481
  requiring delivery, criteria for, 480–481
  risk factors for, 481
  support from allied personnel in, 481
5A's (Ask, Advise, Assess, Assist, and
    Arrange), in smoking interven-
    tion, 229–230, 230b
ASC. *See* Atypical squamous cells
ASCCP. *See* American Society for
    Colposcopy and Cervical
    Pathology
ASC-H. *See* Atypical squamous cells—
    cannot exclude HSIL
ASC-US. *See* Atypical squamous cells of
    undetermined significance

Asherman's syndrome, and recurrent
    pregnancy loss, 684
Ashkenazi Jews
  Canavan disease in, 178–181, 179t,
      180b, 216–217
  carrier status screening for, 178–181,
      179t, 216–219, 1042
  clinical features of diseases common
      among, 180b
  cystic fibrosis in, 178–181, 179t,
      253–255, 254t
  Tay-Sachs disease in, 178–181, 179t,
      180b, 218–219
Asians and Asian Americans
  cystic fibrosis in, 254t
  diet of, 1006
  macrosomia in, 509
  osteoporosis in, 790
Aspartate aminotransferase
  in hepatitis, 320
  in preeclampsia, 446
Asphyxia, birth, inappropriate use of
    term, 94–95, 257–258
Aspiration
  fine-needle, 206, 454
  maternal, anesthesia and, 773
Aspirin
  for antiphospholipid syndrome,
      361–362, 688
  for intrauterine growth restriction, 596
ASRM. *See* American Society for
    Reproductive Medicine
Assistants, surgical, statement on, 234
Assisted reproductive technology
  counseling in, 166
  definition of, 165
  in müllerian aplasia, 139–140
  multiple pregnancy risk of, 166–167,
      728
  perinatal risks associated with,
      165–167
  in polycystic ovary syndrome, 654
Asthma, maternal smoking and, 229
Asynclitism, and operative vaginal birth,
    782b
Atad Ripener Device, 563
Atherosclerosis, polycystic ovary syn-
    drome and, 826
Athletes, pregnant, exercise by, 55
Atrioventricular canal, complete, in aneu-
    ploidy, 869t
At-risk drinking, 15–23. *See also* Alcohol
    use
Attention deficit hyperactivity disorder
    (ADHD), maternal smoking
    and, 307
Atypical glandular cells (AGC), 400, 603,
    604b
  favor neoplasia, 608
  management of, 608–609
  not otherwise specified (AGC-NOS), 608

Atypical squamous cells (ASC), 400, 603, 604*b*
cannot exclude HSIL (ASC-H), 400, 603, 604*b*, 607–608
management of, 606–607
Atypical squamous cells of undetermined significance (ASC-US), 400, 551, 603, 604*b*
Atypical Squamous Cells of Undetermined Significance/Low Grade Squamous Intraepithelial Lesion Triage Study (ALTS), 551, 604–605
Augmentation of labor. *See* Labor augmentation
Auscultation, intermittent, versus electronic fetal heart rate monitoring, 574–575
Autoimmune disorders, and recurrent pregnancy loss, 684–685
Autoimmune hepatitis, 321*t*
Autonomic dysreflexia, spinal cord injury and, 148
Autonomy, respect for, vii
in alcohol abuse, 18–20
in drug abuse, 18–20
in informed refusal, 106
in maternal decision making, 111–119
Autopsy, in stillbirths and neonatal deaths, 64–66
Autosomal dominant diseases, 1029–1030
in Ashkenazi Jews
carrier screening for, 178–181, 179*t*
clinical features of, 180*b*
paternal age and, 5
Autosomal dominant trait, 1030, 1043
Autosomal recessive diseases, 1030
Autosomal recessive trait, 1030, 1043
Aventis Pharmaceuticals, warnings on enoxaparin, 211–212
Aviane, 491*t*
AWARE Foundation, 226
Azithromycin
pharmacokinetics of, 899
prophylactic, for intrauterine device insertion, 584–585
Azoospermia
genetic causes of, 1042
perinatal risks associated with, 166–167

B

Bacillus anthracis, 109. *See also* Anthrax
Back pain, chronic, epidural analgesia and, 770
Bacterial endocarditis, 349
antibiotic prophylaxis for, 352, 352*b*–353*b*, 353*t*, 585, 900–901, 901*t*
cardiac conditions associated with, 352, 352*b*

Bacterial vaginosis
intrauterine devices and, 584
and postoperative infection, 348–349
and preterm delivery, 367–369
and recurrent pregnancy loss, 687–688
Bacteriuria testing, indications for, 195*t*
Bacteroides, and preterm labor, 366–367
Bariatric surgery, 143–144, 245*t*, 246
counseling in, 144
pregnancy complications after, 143
procedures for, 143–144
Barium enema, fetal radiation exposure from, 73*b*
Barrier contraception, during breastfeeding, 281
Barriers to care, 305–306
for adolescents, 221–222
for homeless women, 78–79
Basal body temperature charts, 653, 657
Bean foods, 1006
Beckwith-Wiedemann syndrome, assisted reproductive technology and, 167
Bed rest
for intrauterine growth restriction, 596
for preterm labor prevention, 673
Behavioral state alteration, fetal, 337–338
Behavior therapy, for obesity, 245, 245*t*
The Belmont Report, 155
Beneficence, vii
in alcohol abuse, 16–17, 19
in drug abuse, 16–17, 19
Benzamides, for nausea and vomiting of pregnancy, 747*t*
Benzodiazepines, for nausea and vomiting of pregnancy, 747*t*
Beta agonists, and fetal heart rate, 577–578
Beta blockers
for chronic hypertension, in pregnancy, 422
for hyperthyroidism, in pregnancy, 975
Beta$_2$-glycoprotein I, antibodies against, 359
Betamethasone
antenatal
for fetal maturation, 11–12, 676
for preterm labor and delivery, 676
and fetal heart rate, 575–576
Beta-mimetic agonists, for preterm labor, 675, 675*t*, 676
Bethesda System, of cervical cytology reporting, 399–400, 603–604, 604*b*
BFP STS. *See* Biologic false-positive serologic test for syphilis
Bias
confounding, 334
definition of, 334
information, 334
selection, 334
Bicarbonate, for diabetic ketoacidosis, in pregnancy, 840*b*

Bichloracetic acid, for human papillomavirus infection, 554
Bicornuate uterus, and recurrent pregnancy loss, 684, 686–687
Biest (biestrogen), 40
Biguanides, for polycystic ovary syndrome, 826, 828
Bilateral salpingo-oophorectomy
for endometriosis, 713–714
for premenstrual syndrome, 862
Biliopancreatic diversion, 143–144
Billing denials, inappropriate, 90–93
Bioelectromagnetic applications, 38
Bioidentical hormones, compounded, 40–41
definition of, 40
Food and Drug Administration regulations for, 41
safety, efficacy, and quality of, 41
salivary level testing of, 41
Biologic false-positive serologic test for syphilis (BFP STS), antibody in, 359
Biologic therapy, alternative, 38
Biophysical profile (BPP), 339–340
components of, 339
follow-up of, 342, 344
in intrauterine growth restriction, 596
modified, 340
in postterm pregnancy, 667
scoring in, 339–340
Bioterrorism, anthrax exposure in, 109
Biotinidase deficiency, newborn screening for, 132–133
Biparietal diameter, 595, 984, 987
Birth asphyxia, inappropriate use of term, 94–95, 257–258
Birth control pill. *See* Oral contraception
Birth weight. *See also* Low birth weight; Macrosomia
assisted reproductive technology and, 165–166
homelessness and, 78
maternal smoking and, 228–229
in multiple gestation, 727*t*
nausea and vomiting of pregnancy and, 744
newborn deaths by, 803–804, 804*f*–805*f*
percentiles, for gestational age, 507, 508*t*
thyroid disease and, 972–973
Bishop pelvic scoring system, 562–563, 563*t*
Bisphosphonates, 912
for add-back therapy, with gonadotropin-releasing hormone agonists, 711
for osteoporosis, 794, 795, 912
with selective estrogen receptor modulators therapy, 915

Black cohosh, for menopausal symptoms, 1007, 1009
Bladder catheterization, antibiotic prophylaxis in, 352–353
Bladder filling and voiding, office evaluation of, 993–994, 996
Bladder outlet obstruction, in aneuploidy, 869t
Bladder training, 994
Bleeding
  anovulatory, management of, 623–628
  uterine
    with leiomyoma, 927
    in medical abortion, 697
    noncyclic, differential diagnosis of, 624, 625b
Blocking factors, and recurrent pregnancy loss, 685, 688
Blood, in amniotic fluid, and fetal lung maturity tests, 269–271
Blood dyscrasias
  anovulatory bleeding in, 625–626
  and epidural hematoma, 772
Blood transfusion
  hepatitis B transmission via, 319
  intrauterine fetal, in isoimmunization, 294
  in sickle cell disease, in pregnancy, 544
Bloom syndrome
  carrier screening for, 178–181, 179t
  clinical features of, 180b
Blunt abdominal trauma, in pregnancy, 298–299
BMD. See Bone mineral density
BMI. See Body mass index
Bodily integrity, and maternal decision making, 116
Body mass index (BMI), 142–144
  and obesity management, 243–246, 244t
  in ovulatory dysfunction, 654, 657–658
Bone
  cortical, 789
  trabecular, 789
Bone mass
  age at peak, 789
  ethnicity and, 790
  factors affecting, 790, 790b
  genetics and, 790
  loss of, 789–790. See also Osteoporosis
  secondary cause of loss, workup for, 796b, 797
  race and, 790
Bone mineral density (BMD)
  breastfeeding and, 275
  depot medroxyprogesterone acetate and, 944
  gonadotropin-releasing hormone agonists and, 50

Bone mineral density (BMD) (continued)
  in osteoporosis, 788–797. See also Osteoporosis
  testing of, 788–789
    alternatives to dual-energy X-ray absorptiometry in, 792–793
    cost-effectiveness of, 789
    indications for, 195t, 791–792
    methods of, 790–791
    peripheral quantitative computed tomography for, 792
    quantitative ultrasonography for, 792
    for treatment indication and monitoring, 796–797
Bone remodeling, 789
Bone resorption, 789
Bone turnover, biochemical markers of, 792–793, 793b
Botanicals
  background of, 1004–1008
  clinical considerations and recommendations for, 1008–1011
  for dyspareunia, 1008–1010
  for heart disease prevention, 1010
  for loss of libido, 1008–1010
  manufacture and regulation of, 1006–1007
  for menopausal symptoms, 1004–1011
  monitoring use of, 1010–1011
  for mood disturbances, 1007–1008
  for osteoporosis prevention, 1010
  preparations of, therapeutic forms of, 1005–1006, 1005b
  for vaginal dryness, 1008–1010
  for vasomotor symptoms, 1007–1009
Bottle supplements, and breastfeeding, 283
Bowel obstruction, in aneuploidy, 869t
Bowel preparation, preoperative, antibiotic prophylaxis in, 351–352
BPP. See Biophysical profile
Brachial plexus injury
  incidence of, 510
  macrosomia and, 510–511, 513
  shoulder dystocia and, 922
Bradycardia, fetal, 573t, 574–575
BRCA1 and BRCA2 genes, 1042
  and breast cancer, 392–393, 1042
  and ovarian cancer, 242, 907–908, 1042
  variations of, 1029
Breast abscess, during breastfeeding, 284–285
Breast cancer
  breastfeeding and
    detection concerns in, 286–287
    preventive effects of, 275
  diagnosis of, early, guidelines for, 205–206
  ethnic disparities in, 200
  genetic counseling in, 393
  genetics of, 392, 1042
  incidence of, 386

Breast cancer (continued)
  induced abortion and, 96–97
  inflammatory, versus mastitis, 284
  mathematical model of, 387
  mortality from, 386
  oral contraception and, 940
  prevention of, tamoxifen for, 236
  prophylactic oophorectomy in, 908
  racial disparities in, 200
  raloxifene for, 914
  risk of
    age-specific, 386, 387t
    assessment of, 916
    lifetime, 386
    relative, factors in, 391, 391t, 916, 916t
  role of obstetrician–gynecologist in, 205–206
  screening for, 386–393. See also Mammography
  selective estrogen receptor modulators for
    preventive use of, 912–917
    therapeutic use of, 911
  tamoxifen for, 911–914
  in uninsured women, 249
Breast Cancer Detection Demonstration Project, 388
Breast engorgement, 284
Breastfeeding, 274–287
  American Academy of Pediatrics statement on, 275, 275b, 286
  abscess during, 284–285
  after delivery, 279
  analgesia and, 773–774
  anesthesia and, 773–774
  benefits of, 274–275
    for families and society, 275
    for infants, 274–275, 275b
    for women, 275
  bottle supplements and, 283
  and breast cancer
    detection concerns in, 286–287
    preventive effects of, 275
  capability for, 276
  complications of, 284–285
  as contraception (lactational amenorrhea method), 282–283, 283f
  contraception during, 280–283
    hormonal, 281–282, 282b, 941
    nonhormonal, 281, 281b
  contraindications to, 276–277
  diabetes mellitus and, 843
  dietary requirements for, 280
  duration of, 286
  education on, 277–280
    during antenatal period, 278
    during first obstetric visit, 278
    during hospital stay, 279–280
    during periodic gynecologic examinations, 278
  resources for, 279b

Breastfeeding *(continued)*
  expectations in daily life, 285
  Healthy People 2010 goal for, 288
  hepatitis infection and, 277, 319
  herpes simplex virus infection and,
      277, 649–650
  at home, after hospital discharge,
      280
  interruption of, 284
  latch-on for, 280, 284, 284*b*
  and mastitis, 284–285
  medications and, 277, 277*t*
  milk supply for, maintenance of,
      283–284
  obstacles to, 275–276
  and ovarian cancer, 275
  pacifiers and, 283
  phone-in resource for, 280
  positioning for, 284, 284*b*
  of premature infants, 276
  rates of, 274, 288
  rooming-in and, 279
  rubella vaccine during, 210
  and sexuality, 280
  sore nipples with, 284
  spousal or partner support for, 280
  supporting, 287, 288*b*
  thyroid disease treatment and, 975
  weaning from, 286
  by working mothers, 275–276, 285
Breast mass. *See also* Breast cancer
  nonpalpable, management of, 393
  palpable, evaluation of, 392
Breast milk. *See also* Breastfeeding
  expressing of, 285
  storage of, 285
Breast self-examination, 389–390
Breech presentation
  delivery of
    cesarean, 127–128, 500
    mode, in singleton birth, 127–128
  external cephalic version for, 127–128,
      500–504, 1019
  incidence of, 500
  in neural tube defects, 760
Bromocriptine
  adverse effects of, 660
  contraindicated during breastfeeding,
      277*t*
  for ovulation induction, 656–657,
      659–660
Bronchopulmonary dysplasia, 268
Buclizine, for nausea and vomiting of
      pregnancy, 747*t*
Bulk herbs, 1005*b*
Bulking agents, for urinary incontinence,
      995, 998
Bupivacaine, epidural, 767
Bupropion, for smoking cessation,
      230
Burch colposuspension, 995, 998–999

Butorphanol
  adverse effects of, 770
  contraindications to, 770
  and fetal heart rate, 576, 576*t*
  parenteral, obstetric, 765–766, 766*t*, 770
Butyrophenones, for nausea and vomiting
      of pregnancy, 747*t*

C
CA 125
  in endometrial cancer, 634
  in endometriosis, 47, 707–708
  in ovarian cancer, 240–242
Cabergoline, for ovulation induction,
      656–657
Caffeine, and recurrent pregnancy loss,
      684
CAH. *See* Congenital adrenal hyperplasia
Cajun descent, Tay-Sachs disease in indi-
      viduals of, 178, 218–219
Calcitonin
  for add-back therapy, with
      gonadotropin-releasing hor-
      mone agonists, 711
  salmon, for osteoporosis, 795
Calcium channel blockers
  for chronic hypertension, in pregnancy,
      422
  for preterm labor, 675, 675*t*, 676
Calcium requirements
  for breastfeeding, 280
  recommended daily, 795, 796*b*
Calcium supplementation
  for intrauterine growth restriction, 596
  for osteoporosis prevention, 795
  for preeclampsia prevention, 449
  for premenstrual syndrome, 861
Caloric intake
  in gestational diabetes, 523
  in pregestational diabetes, in pregnancy,
      838
  in suspected macrosomia, 511
Canadian National Breast Cancer Study,
      389
Canalicular period, of lung development,
      268
Canavan disease
  carrier screening for, 178–181, 179*t*,
      216–217, 1042
  clinical features of, 180*b*, 216
  etiology of, 216
  prenatal diagnosis of, 217
Cancer. *See* specific types
Captopril, teratogenicity of, 315*t*, 422
Carbamazepine
  oral contraception use with, 941
  teratogenicity of, 315*t*, 756
Carbohydrates, for premenstrual syndrome,
      861
Carbon dioxide gas, for hysteroscopy,
      1047

Carboplatin, for endometrial cancer, 637
Carcinosarcoma, endometrial, 632
Cardiac defects, in aneuploidy, 869*t*
Cardiovascular disease, in polycystic
      ovary syndrome, 826–828
Cardiovascular risk factors, periodic
      assessments of
  ages 13–18 years, 191
  ages 19–39 years, 192
  ages 40–64 years, 193
  ages 65 and older, 194
Cardiovascular system, during pregnancy,
      53–54
Carrier(s), 1030
Carrier screening, 1030, 1041–1042
  of Ashkenazi Jews, 178–181, 179*t*,
      216–219, 1042
  for Canavan disease, 178–181, 179*t*,
      216–217, 1042
  for cystic fibrosis, 178–181, 179*t*,
      253–255, 1040, 1042
  informed consent for, 181, 1041
  for Tay-Sachs disease, 178–181, 179*t*,
      218–219, 1030, 1042
Case–control study, 331
Case study, 332
Category A substances, 312
Category B substances, 312
Category C substances, 312
Category D substances, 312
Category E substances, 312–313
Catheterization, antibiotic prophylaxis in,
      352–353
Caucasians, osteoporosis in, 790
CCI. *See* Correct Coding Initiative
CDC. *See* Centers for Disease Control
      and Prevention
CDE system, 291
Cefazolin, prophylactic
  for cesarean delivery, 899–900
  for group B streptococcal disease, 186*t*
  for gynecologic procedures, 349, 349*t*
Cefotetan, prophylactic, for cesarean
      delivery, 899–900
Cefoxitin, prophylactic, for cesarean
      delivery, 899–900
Cell death, ionizing radiation and, 72
Centers for Disease Control and
      Prevention (CDC)
  Mother-Infant Rapid Intervention at
      Delivery (MIRIAD) Study
      Group of, 174, 176
  recommendations of
    on group B streptococcal disease
        prophylaxis, 183
    on hepatitis B vaccine, 323
    on human immunodeficiency virus
        testing, 173, 176
    for human papillomavirus treatment,
        553–554
    on meningococcal vaccine, 125

Centers for Disease Control and
    Prevention (CDC) (continued)
  recommendations of (continued)
    on rubella vaccine, 210
    on sexually transmitted disease
      screening, for adolescents, 223
  resources of, 227
Central adiposity, 244
Cephalohematoma, with vacuum extrac-
    tion, 784–785
Cephalopelvic disproportion, 480
Cephalosporin(s)
  as alternative to penicillin, 353–354,
    898
  hypersensitivity reactions to, 353–354
  prophylactic, for cesarean delivery, 900
Cephalothin, pharmacokinetics of, 899
Cerebral palsy
  Apgar score and, 258
  hypoxic event sufficient to cause, crite-
    ria for, 95, 95b
  multiple gestation and, 727, 727t
  nonreassuring fetal heart rate and, 574
  threshold of viability and, 804–805,
    806t
Cervical atresia, and endometriosis, 707
Cervical biopsy, and cervical cerclage,
    414
Cervical cancer, 453–462
  adenocarcinoma, treatment of, 459,
    608–611
  adjuvant therapy for, 458
  background of, 453–454
  chemotherapy for, 457–459
  clinical considerations and recommen-
    dations in, 454–462
  diagnosis of, 454
  early-stage (stage Ib-IIa), treatment of,
    457–458
  fertility preservation in, 457, 611
  follow-up in, 460
  histology of, 454
  human papillomavirus infection and,
    29, 400–401, 453–454,
    550–551, 604–605
  hysterectomy for, 456–457, 461
  imaging studies in, 454–455
  incidence of, 398
  International Federation of Gynecology
    and Obstetrics nomenclature
    for, 454, 455b
  late-stage (stage IIb or later), treatment
    of, 458–459
  long-term monitoring in, 459–460
  management of, 454
  microinvasive
    definition of, 456–457
    diagnosis and treatment of, 456–457
    volumetric measurements of,
      456–457
  mortality from, 398

Cervical cancer (continued)
  in pregnancy
    continuation versus termination of
      pregnancy in, 460
    episiotomy site and, 461
    mode of delivery in, 461
    treatment of, 460–462
  prevalence of, 453
  prevention, in low-resource settings,
    policy statement on,
    1063–1065
  racial and ethnic disparities in, 200
  radiation therapy for, 456–459,
    461–462
  recurrence of, 459–460
  risk factors for, 453–454
  screening for, 398–405, 550–551,
    603–613. See also Cervical
    cytology screening
    in adolescents, 29–32, 222, 401,
      606
    in pregnancy, 460, 461f, 612
  squamous cell, treatment of, 459
  stage 0, 455b
  stage I, 455b
  stage Ib1 versus stage Ib2, 456
  stage II, 455b
  stage III, 455b
  stage IV, 455b
  staging of, 454–456, 455b
  surgical evaluation of, 456
  surgical management of, 456–457,
    461
  in uninsured women, 249
Cervical cerclage, 411
  antibiotic prophylaxis for, 414, 899
  cervical biopsy and, 414
  complications of, 413–414, 413t
  diethylstilbestrol exposure and, 414
  early or first-trimester, 413
  elective, 411–412
  emergency, 412–414
  indications for, 411–412
  McDonald technique of, 411
  morbidity in, 413–414
  in multiple gestation, 731
  postoperative displacement of, 413
  and premature rupture of membranes,
    413–414, 413t
  preterm premature rupture of mem-
    branes with, 853
  prevalence of, 409–410
  removal of, 414
  Shirodkar technique of, 411
  success rate of, 410
  therapeutic, 412
  tocolytic therapy with, 414
Cervical cytology screening, 398–405,
    550–552
  abnormal results of, management of,
    30–31, 603–613

Cervical cytology screening (continued)
  in adolescents, 29–32, 222, 401, 606
    abnormal results in, management of,
      30–31
    need for additional research on, 32
    patient and parent education on,
      30–31
  background of, 398–401, 603–606
  Bethesda System in, 399–400,
    603–604, 604b
  clinical considerations and recommen-
    dations in, 401–405, 606–612
  conventional method of, 399
  cytologic findings in, 603–604
  discontinuation of, 402–403
  effectiveness of methods in, 403
  errors in, 399
  follow-up in, 605–606
  frequency of
    method of screening and, 403
    optimal, 401–402
  histologic findings in, 603–604
  human papillomavirus testing with,
    403–404, 549–552, 605–606,
    611–612
  initiation of, 401
  interpretation of, 603–604
  liquid-based methods of, 399, 403,
    550–552
  in low-resource settings, policy state-
    ment on, 1063–1065
  new devices for, 399
  in pregnancy, 460, 461f, 612
  reporting results of, 399–400, 603–604
  sensitivity of, 605
  techniques of, 399
  value of, 398–399
Cervical dilatation, and epidural analgesia,
    9–10
Cervical incompetence. See Cervical
    insufficiency
Cervical Incompetence Prevention
    Randomized Cerclage Trial
    (CIPRACT), 412
Cervical insufficiency, 409–415
  background of, 409–411
  causes of, 410
  clinical considerations and recommen-
    dations in, 411–414
  definition of, 409
  diagnostic criteria for, 410–411
  emerging theories of, 410
  historic features of, 411, 412b
  incidence of, 409–410
  prevalence of, 409–410
  recommendations on, 415
  treatment of, 411
Cervical intraepithelial neoplasia (CIN),
    400, 550–552, 603–604
  CIN 1, management of, 609–610
  CIN 2, management of, 610

Cervical intraepithelial neoplasia (CIN),
    (continued)
  CIN 3, management of, 610
  excision versus ablation in, 610
  human immunodeficiency virus infec-
      tion and, 610
  hysterectomy for, 612
  management of, 603–613
  monitoring after treatment for, 611–612
  natural history of, 400–401, 604–605
  in pregnancy, 612
  tests for, sensitivity and specificity of,
      605t
Cervical ripening, 562–563
  criteria for, 564–565
  inpatient versus outpatient, 566
  methods of, 563
    complications of, 565–566
    effectiveness of, comparison of, 565
  misoprostol for, 101–102, 563
    Food and Drug Administration label-
        ing on, 129–130
    recommendations on, 130, 130b
    Searle's drug warning on, response
        to, 203–204
  for vaginal birth after cesarean delivery,
      99–100
Cervix
  functional versus nonfunctional, 409
  incompetent. *See* Cervical insufficiency
  length of, 368–369, 369t, 412–413
    measurement by digital examination,
        730–731
    measurement by ultrasonography,
        730
    in multiple gestation, 730–731
  in postterm pregnancy, favorable or
      unfavorable, 667–668
  short, management of
    in second trimester, 412–413
    in third trimester, 413
  status of, Bishop scoring system for,
      562–563, 563t
  ultrasound screening of, 368–369, 369t,
      410–411, 730
Cesarean delivery
  after myomectomy, 931
  analgesia and, 9–10, 771–772
  anesthesia for, availability of, 150–152
  antibiotic prophylaxis in, 187–188,
      350, 899–900
  for breech presentation, 127–128, 500
  chronic hypertension and, 419
  in diabetes mellitus, 842
  for dystocia, 481
  external cephalic version, 502
  fetal heart rate monitoring and, 56–57
  gestational diabetes and, 518–519,
      525–526
  group B streptococcal prophylaxis in,
      187–188

Cesarean delivery *(continued)*
  in herpes simplex virus infection, 649
  for intracranial hemorrhage prevention,
      955
  for macrosomia, 509–513, 922–923
  maternal decision making versus fetal
      protection in, 112, 116
  maternal obesity and, 143–144
  for multiple gestation, 734
  for neural tube defects, 760
  perimortem, 301
  postoperative analgesia for, 774
  in postterm pregnancy, 666
  in preeclampsia, 448
  previous
    and placenta accreta, 169
    vaginal birth after. *See* Vaginal birth
        after cesarean delivery
  scheduled, and prevention of vertical
      human immunodeficiency virus
      transmission, 213–215
  for threshold of viability, 806
  trauma and, 300
  tubal sterilization with, 252, 377
Cetirizine, for nausea and vomiting of
    pregnancy, 747t
CGG repeats, 1032
Chagas disease, and intrauterine growth
    restriction, 593
Chasteberry, for menopausal symptoms,
    1008, 1010
Chemical methods, for tubal sterilization,
    376
Chemotherapy
  for cervical cancer, 457–459
  for endometrial cancer, 637
Chest X-ray, fetal radiation exposure
    from, 73b
Chickenpox. *See* Varicella zoster virus
    infection
Child abuse, behavior during pregnancy
    as, 112
Child-centered approach, to maternal and
    child health, 113
Chimera, 1043
Chinese medicine, traditional, 37
Chlamydial infection
  in adolescents, 220, 222–223
    during pregnancy, 223–224
    screening guidelines for, 222–224
  and ectopic pregnancy, 719
  and recurrent pregnancy loss, 687–688
  screening for, before intrauterine device
      insertion, 584
Chlorambucil, for gestational trophoblastic
    disease, 474
Chloroprocaine, obstetric use of, 769
Chlorpromazine, for nausea and vomiting
    of pregnancy, 747t
Cholestasis of pregnancy, jaundice in,
    321t

Chorioamnionitis
  cervical cerclage and, 413–414, 413t
  dystocia and, 481
  premature rupture of membranes and,
      851
Choriocarcinoma, gestational, 468–469
  diagnosis of, 469
  histology of, 468
  incidence of, 466–467
Chorionic villus sampling (CVS),
      871–872, 1042
  versus amniocentesis, 871
  for Canavan disease, 217
  complications of, 872
  contraindications to, 871
  indications for, 871
  in multiple gestation, 728, 873
  pregnancy loss rate with, 871–872
  and Rh D alloimmunization, 890
  in stillbirths and neonatal deaths, 65–66
  success rates of, 871–872
Choroid plexus cyst, evaluation of, 873
Chromatin, 1027, 1043
Chromatography, in fetal lung maturity
    assessment, 269
Chromosomal abnormalities
  deletion, 1030–1031, 1037–1038,
      1038f, 1044
  duplication, 1030–1031
  fetal
    assisted reproductive technology
        and, 166–167
    first-trimester screening for, 58–60,
        870
    and intrauterine growth restriction,
        593, 596–597
    prenatal diagnosis of, 58–60, 867–874
      background of, 867–870
      clinical considerations and recom-
          mendations in, 870–874
      ultrasonography for, 869, 872–873,
          986–987
  insertion, 1044
  inversion, 1044
  molecular diagnostic testing for,
      1035–1043
  parental
    as indication for prenatal screening,
        871
    and recurrent pregnancy loss, 683, 686
CIPRACT. *See* Cervical Incompetence
      Prevention Randomized
      Cerclage Trial
Ciprofloxacin, for anthrax prophylaxis,
      109–110
Cirrhosis, hepatitis and, 320
Cisplatin
  for cervical cancer, 458–459
  for endometrial cancer, 637
  for gestational trophoblastic disease,
      473–474

Clavicular fracture, macrosomia and, 510

Cleft lip or palate, and breastfeeding, 276

Clindamycin
  pharmacokinetics of, 899
  prophylactic
    for group B streptococcal disease, 185b, 186, 186t
    for gynecologic procedures, 354
    for preterm premature rupture of membranes, 900

Clinical breast examination, 389–390
  effectiveness of, 390–391
  frequency of, 390–391

Clinical classification system, for gestational trophoblastic disease, 472–473, 473t

Clinical Laboratory Improvement Amendments (CLIA), 399

Clinical trials, 154–155, 330–331

Clomiphene citrate, 911–917
  indications for, 911
  for ovulation induction, 627, 655–656
    administration of, 658
    complications with, 658
    dosage of, 658
    glucocorticoids with, 659, 828
    monitoring with, 658
    and ovarian cancer, 661
    in polycystic ovary syndrome, 654, 828–829
    postcoital test in, 661
    in premature ovarian failure, 655
  physiologic effects of, 912–913
  pregnancy category of, 828t

Clomipramine, for premenstrual syndrome, 861–862

Clostridium sordellii infection, in medical abortion, 699

Club foot
  amniocentesis and, 871
  in aneuploidy, 869t

Coagulopathy, 880, 881t
  and deep vein thrombosis, 880, 884
  and oral contraception use, 943
  in pregnancy, 961–962, 962b
  and recurrent pregnancy loss, 684, 688
  and thromboembolism, in pregnancy, 961, 963–965

Cocaine
  contraindicated during breastfeeding, 277t
  and fetal heart rate, 576, 576t
  and intrauterine growth restriction, 593
  teratogenicity of, 315t

Code of conduct, viii–x

Code of Federal Regulations: Title 45-Public Welfare; Part 46: Protection of Human Subjects (45 CFR Part 46), 67–70

Code of professional ethics, vii–x

Coding and reimbursement, 90–93
  for smoking cessation program, 232
  for tubal ligation, 252

Coding responsibility, 36

Co-dominant genes, 1030, 1043

Codon, 1043

Cohort study, 331

Cold-knife conization, 457, 609–611

Colic, maternal smoking and, 229

Collaborative Review of Sterilization, 377–378

College students, meningococcal vaccine for, 125

Colon cancer, endometrial cancer with, 632

Color, in Apgar score, 257, 258t

Colostrum, 274–275

Colposcopy, 456, 551, 605–613
  for adenocarcinoma in situ, 608
  for atypical glandular cells, 608
  for atypical squamous cells, 606–607
  for atypical squamous cells, cannot exclude high-grade squamous intraepithelial lesions, 607–608
  with biopsy, 605–606, 609
  endocervical curettage with, 609
  for high-grade squamous intraepithelial lesions, 607–608
  inconclusive results of, management of, 611
  for low-grade squamous intraepithelial lesions, 607–608
  sensitivity and specificity of, 605–606, 605t
  without biopsy, 605–606

Colposuspension, 995, 998–999

Communication, physician–patient, 157–159
  ethical guidelines on, 161
  improvement of, 161

Comparative genomic hybridization, 1040, 1043

Complementary and alternative medicine (CAM), 37–39
  for chronic pelvic pain, 436
  classification of, 37–38
  counseling about, 1011, 1011b
  definition of, 37, 1005
  for endometriosis, in adolescents, 51
  ethical responsibility in, 37
  for menopausal symptoms, 1004–1011
  monitoring use of, 1010–1011
  for osteoporosis prevention, 796
  predictors for use of, 1005
  referral for, 38
  regulation of, 38
  reimbursement for, 39, 1005
  resources on, 39
  safety of, 38

Complementary DNA (cDNA) probe, 1043

Complex disorders of adult life, 1034–1035

Compounded bioidentical hormones, 40–41
  definition of, 40
  Food and Drug Administration regulations for, 41
  safety, efficacy, and quality of, 41
  salivary level testing of, 41

Compression stockings, graduated, 880, 883

Computed tomography
  in cervical cancer, 454–455
  contrast agents in, use during pregnancy, 74
  in endometriosis, 708
  peripheral quantitative, in osteoporosis, 792
  in pulmonary embolism, 966
  radiation exposure from, 72, 73b
  in trauma, during pregnancy, 300

Condoms
  effectiveness of, versus tubal sterilization, 377
  for genital herpes prevention, 536
  for human papillomavirus prevention, 552–553, 555
  latex versus polyurethane, 223
  use of
    by adolescents, 221, 223
    during breastfeeding, 281

Condylomata acuminata, 548

Confidence interval, 334

Confidentiality
  for adolescents, 221–222
    in alcohol and drug abuse, 21–22
    in sexual history taking, 31b
  in liability litigation, 43

Conflicts of interest, viii–ix

Confounder, 334

Confounding bias, 334

Confounding variable, 334

Congenital adrenal hyperplasia (CAH)
  newborn screening for, 132–133
  nonclassical, screening for, 825–826

Congenital anomalies
  assisted reproductive technology and, 166
  enoxaparin sodium and, 211
  pregestational diabetes and, 840

Conization, cold-knife, 457, 609–611

Consent
  informed
    for carrier screening, 181
    in maternal decision making, 114–116
    physician–patient communication and, 158
    for research, 67–68
    from minors, legal issues of, 68, 221–222

Consent *(continued)*
  parental
    for adolescent health research, waiving of requirement for, 68–70
    for evaluation of stillbirths and neonatal deaths, 64
  partner
    methods of obtaining, 156*b*
    potential adverse effects of, 155
    reasons for, 155
    recommendations on, 156
    for reproductive health research, 154–155
    requirement for, inconsistencies in, 155
Constitutive heterochromatin, 1043
Consultations, precertification for reimbursement for, 92
Contiguous gene deletion syndrome, 1043
Continuously variable traits, 1034
Contraception. *See also specific methods*
  during breastfeeding, 280–283
    hormonal, 281–282, 282*b*
    nonhormonal, 281, 281*b*
  breastfeeding as (lactational amenorrhea method), 282–283, 283*f*
  in diabetes mellitus, 843
  emergency, 489–495
    access to, 492, 494
    antiemetics as adjunct to, 493
    awareness of, 492
    background of, 490–492
    candidates for, 492
    clinical considerations and recommendations in, 492–495
    clinical follow-up in, 494
    drug interactions of, 492
    effectiveness of, 493
    effects on pregnancy, 491–492
    initiation of, timing of, 493
    intrauterine device for, 494, 587
    mechanism of action, 490
    versus medical abortion, 490
    regimens for, 490, 491*t*
    regular contraceptive use after, 494
    repeated use of, safety of, 494
    resources on, 495
    screening procedures for, 492–493
    side effects of, 490
    and thromboembolism, 943
  hormonal, and coexisting medical conditions, 936–945
  sterilization as, 374
  two methods of, indications for, 936–937
  for uninsured women, 249
Contraction stress test, 338–339
  contraindications to, 339, 342–343
  equivocal–hyperstimulatory, 339
  equivocal–suspicious, 339
  follow-up of, 342

Contraction stress test *(continued)*
  interpretation of, 338–339
  negative, 338
  positive, 339
  technique of, 338
  unsatisfactory, 339
Contrast agents, use during pregnancy, 74
Controlled trials
  with randomization, 330–331
  without randomization, 331
Conversion disorder, nausea and vomiting of pregnancy as, 743
Cooperative practice, policy statement on, 1057–1058
Copper intrauterine device, 582, 582*t*
Cordocentesis, 872, 890
Correct Coding Initiative (CCI), 91
Cortical bone, 789
Corticosteroids
  antenatal
    for fetal maturation, 11–12, 271–272, 676
    for preterm labor and delivery, 676, 732
    for preterm premature rupture of membranes, 852
    rescue therapy with, 11
  for antiphospholipid syndrome, 362
  and fetal heart rate, 575–576, 576*t*
  for intrauterine growth restriction, 594
  for nausea and vomiting of pregnancy, 745–748, 746*f*, 747*t*
  and osteoporosis, 790, 791*b*
  in ovulation induction, 659, 828
Cost-benefit analysis, 332–334
Cost-effectiveness analysis, 332–334
Coumestans, 1006
Counseling, in periodic assessments
  ages 13–18 years, 191
  ages 19–39 years, 192
  ages 40–64 years, 193
  ages 65 and older, 194
CPT. *See Current Procedural Terminology*
Craniorachischisis, 755*t*
Cretinism, 973
Cross product ratio, 335
Cross-sectional studies, 332
Crown–rump measurements, for gestational age estimation, 267–268, 984
Cryosurgery, for human papillomavirus infection, 554
Cryotherapy, for cervical intraepithelial neoplasia, 610
Cryselle, 491*t*
Cuff cellulitis, postoperative, 348–349
Culture-based approach, in group B streptococcal prophylaxis, 183–188, 184*f*, 185*b*

Cunnilingus, sexually transmitted disease transmission via, 222
Current Procedural Terminology (CPT), 90
Cushing's syndrome
  ovulatory dysfunction in, 657, 824
  versus polycystic ovary syndrome, 824
  in pregnancy, 420
CVS. *See* Chorionic villus sampling
Cyclophosphamide
  contraindicated during breastfeeding, 277*t*
  for gestational trophoblastic disease, 474
Cyclosporine, contraindicated during breastfeeding, 277*t*
Cystic fibrosis
  carrier screening for, 178–181, 179*t*, 253–255, 1040, 1042
  clinical features of, 255
  ethnicity and, 253–254, 254*t*
  newborn screening for, 132
  patient information on, 255
Cystic fibrosis transmembrane regulator (CFTR) gene, 254–255
Cystic hygroma, in aneuploidy, 869*t*
Cystometry, in urinary incontinence, 994, 996
Cystoscopy, in urinary incontinence, 996
Cystourethroscopy, 994
Cytokines, in recurrent pregnancy loss, 685
Cytomegalovirus infection
  clinical considerations and recommendations in, 812–814
  clinical features of, 810–811
  congenital, 811
  fetal, diagnosis of, 813
  hepatitis or jaundice with, 321*t*, 811
  intrauterine growth restriction with, 593
  maternal, diagnosis of, 812–813
  mother-to-child transmission of, 811
  perinatal, 810–814
  prevalence of, 811
  prevention of, 813
  primary, 810
  recurrent, 811
  risk factors for, 813
  screening for women at high risk for, 813–814
  teratogenicity of, 316*t*, 811
  treatment of, 813
  vaccine against, development of, 813
Cytotec. *See* Misoprostol

D

Dactinomycin, for gestational trophoblastic disease, 473–474
Daidzein, 1006
Dalkon Shield, 581, 586

Dalteparin, safety in pregnancy, 212
Danazol
  for endometriosis, 50, 709–710
  teratogenicity of, 315*t*
Dang Gui, 1007, 1009
D antigen, 290–292, 889–894, 1042. *See
    also* Rh D alloimmunization
Davydov procedure, 141
Day care problems, as barrier to care, 306
D&C. *See* Dilation and curettage
Deaths, fetal. *See* Fetal death (loss)
Deaths, neonatal
  counseling in, 66
  genetic evaluation of, 64–66
  laboratory studies of, 65–66
  management of, 65, 65*b*
  obstetric history in, 65
  parental consent for evaluation of, 64
  physical examination in, 65
  placental examination in, 65
  sample procurement for study of, 65,
    66*b*
Deceleration, in fetal heart rate, 574
  early, 573*t*
  late, 573*t*
  in preterm fetus, 575
  prolonged, 573*t*
  recurrent, 574
  variable, 573*t*
Decision analysis, 332, 333*f*
Decision making, maternal, 111–119
  bodily integrity in, 116
  coercive or punitive actions against,
    116–119
    American College of Obstetricians
      and Gynecologists opposition
      to, 119
    counterproductive effects of, 118
    criminalization of behavior by, 119
    "moral failings" viewpoint of,
      117–118
    vulnerable women affected by,
      118–119
  ethical considerations in, 113–118
  informed consent in, 114–116
  informed refusal in, 116–117
  limitations of obstetrics and, 116–117
  recent cases on, 112
  recommendations on, 118–119
Decubital ulcers, spinal cord injury and,
    148
Deep vein thrombosis, 879–885
  background of, 879–882
  clinical considerations and recommen-
    dations in, 883–885
  detection of, 879–880, 965
  hypercoagulable states and, 880, 884
  in pregnancy, diagnosis of, 965
  prophylaxis
    anesthesia concerns in, 882, 884
    approaches in, 880–883

Deep vein thrombosis *(continued)*
  prophylaxis *(continued)*
    coagulopathy testing in, 884
    graduated compression stockings for,
      880, 883
    in gynecologic surgery, 880
    hormone therapy discontinuation for,
      883
    for low-, medium-, and high-risk
      patients, 883
    low-dose heparin for, 881–884
    low-molecular-weight heparin for,
      882–884
    oral contraceptive discontinuation
      for, 883
    perioperative, indications for, 883
    pneumatic compression for,
      880–881, 883
    side effect evaluation in, 884
    risk levels for, 880, 882*t*, 883
Deferoxamine, for thalassemia, 545
Dehydroepiandrosterone (DHEA), 825
Dehydroepiandrosterone sulfate (DHEAS)
  measurement of, 825
  in polycystic ovary syndrome, 654, 825
  as tumor marker, 825
Deletion, chromosomal, 1030–1031,
    1037–1038, 1038*f*, 1044
Dental dams, for genital herpes preven-
    tion, 536
Depot medroxyprogesterone, for
    endometriosis, in adolescents,
    49–50
Depot medroxyprogesterone acetate
    (DMPA)
  anticonvulsant effect of, 942
  and bone density, 944
  during breastfeeding, 281–282, 941
  with concomitant medications,
    942–943
Descriptive studies, 332
Desensitization, for nausea and vomiting
    of pregnancy, 749
Desflurane, 769
Desipramine, for chronic pelvic pain, 432
Detrusor overactivity, 991, 994
Dexamethasone
  antenatal, for fetal maturation, 11–12,
    676
  and fetal heart rate, 576
  in ovulation induction, 828
  pregnancy category of, 828*t*
  for thyroid storm, in pregnancy, 976,
    976*t*
DHEA. *See* Dehydroepiandrosterone
DHEAS. *See* Dehydroepiandrosterone
    sulfate
Diabetes mellitus
  and air travel during pregnancy, 7
  and breastfeeding, 843
  contraception in, 843, 939

Diabetes mellitus *(continued)*
  and fetal lung maturity, 271–272
  gestational, 518–527
    background of, 518–520
    and cesarean delivery, 518–519,
      525–526
    clinical considerations and recom-
      mendations in, 520–527
    definition of, 518
    delivery in, timing and mode of,
      525–526
    diagnosis of, 521–522
    diagnostic criteria for, 522, 522*t*
    diet therapy for, 523
    exercise and, 53, 524
    fetal assessment in, 524–525
    fetal complications of, 518–519
    glucose monitoring in, 522
    history of, and postpartum screening,
      526–527
    maternal complications of, 518–519
    maternal obesity and, 142–143
    in multiple gestation, 728
    oral antidiabetic agents for, 524
    and perinatal mortality, 519
    and preeclampsia, 518–519
    prevalence of, 518
    risk factors for, 520
    screening for
      approach in, 520
      controversy over, 519–520
      gestational age and, 520–521
      method for, 521
      threshold value in, 521
      venous versus capillary blood in,
        521
    treatment of
      controversy over, 519–520
      goals of, 519–520
      insulin in, 523–524
  and macrosomia, 507–509, 511, 519,
    525–526
  and neural tube defects, 841
  in nonpregnant state, criteria for, 526*t*
  oral contraception and, 939
  in polycystic ovary syndrome, 824,
    826, 827–828
  preconceptional care of, 238
  preconceptional counseling in, 841
  pregestational, 837–843
    background of, 837–841
    clinical considerations and recom-
      mendations in, 841–843
    definition of, 837
    delivery timing and mode in, 842
    fetal surveillance in, 842
    glucose control in, during labor,
      842–843, 842*b*
    incidence of, 837
    insulin therapy for, 838–839, 838*t*,
      841–843

Diabetes mellitus (continued)
  pregestational (continued)
    management during pregnancy,
      837–839
    maternal morbidity in, 839
    obstetric complications of, 841
    perinatal mortality and morbidity in,
      840–841
    postpartum considerations in, 843
    treatment of, before ovulation induc-
      tion, 657
  prevention of, 827–828
  and recurrent pregnancy loss, 683–684
  type 1, 518, 837
  type 2, 518, 837
Diabetic ketoacidosis, during pregnancy,
    839–840
  clinical presentation of, 840
  risk factors for, 840
  treatment of, 840, 840b
Diabetic nephropathy, during pregnancy,
    839
Diabetic retinopathy, during pregnancy,
    839
Diagnostic imaging, 71–74. See also
    specific modalities
Diaphragm, effectiveness of, versus tubal
    sterilization, 377
Diaphragmatic hernia, in aneuploidy,
    869t
Diarrhea
  antibiotics and, 350
  medical abortion and, 697, 698t
Diazepam, for nausea and vomiting of
    pregnancy, 747t
Dicloxacillin
  for mastitis, 284–285
  pharmacokinetics of, 899
Didelphic uterus, and recurrent pregnancy
    loss, 684
Diego antibodies, 291t
Diet
  for breastfeeding, 280
  in complementary and alternative
    medicine, 38
  for diabetes mellitus, 519–520
  for gestational diabetes, 523
  and nausea and vomiting of pregnancy,
    744–745
  for obesity, 245–246, 245t
  for ovulatory dysfunction, 654–655
  for premenstrual syndrome, 861
  for suspected macrosomia, 511
Dietary plant estrogen, 1006
Dietary Supplement and Health Education
    Act (1994), 38, 1006
Diethylstilbestrol
  and cervical cerclage, 414
  and ectopic pregnancy, 719
  teratogenicity of, 315t
DiGeorge syndrome, 1031, 1040t

Digital examination, for cervical length
    measurement, 730–731
Digital scalp stimulation, 577
Dihydrotestosterone, 825
Dilation and curettage (D&C)
  antibiotic prophylaxis in, 349t, 351
  follow-up, in medical abortion,
    698–699
  for hydatidiform mole, 469–470
Dilation and extraction, intact (intact D &
    X), policy statement on,
    1059–1061
Dilators
  for cervical ripening, 563, 566, 568
  for vaginal agenesis, 140
Dimenhydrinate, for nausea and vomiting
    of pregnancy, 746f, 747t
Dinoprostone (prostaglandin E₂)
  administration of, 565
  adverse effects of, 565
  cost-effectiveness of, 568
  for labor induction, 563–568
Diphenhydramine, for nausea and vomit-
    ing of pregnancy, 747t
Diphenols, 1006
Diphtheria–tetanus vaccine, during preg-
    nancy, 88t
Discordant growth, in multiple gestation,
    732
Disseminated intravascular coagulopathy,
    maternal, in multiple gestation,
    733
Distending media, for hysteroscopy, 1047
Diuretics
  for chronic hypertension, in pregnancy,
    422
  for premenstrual syndrome, 862
Dizziness, medical abortion and, 697, 698t
DMPA. See Depot medroxyprogesterone
    acetate
DNA, 1027, 1043
  hereditary unstable, 1031–1032, 1044
  recombinant, 1044
  repetitive, 1027
  sampling of, 1035
  single copy, 1027
  testing of, 1035–1043
DNA chip technology, 1040
DNA hybridization, 1043
DNA methylation, 1028–1029, 1044
DNA sequences, 1028
Domestic violence
  as barrier to care, 306
  in postpartum period, 307
  in pregnancy, 298, 307
Dong Quai, for menopausal symptoms,
    1007, 1009
Dopamine agonists, for ovulation induc-
    tion, 656–657, 659–660
Dopamine antagonists, for nausea and
    vomiting of pregnancy, 747t

Doppler studies
  in breast cancer evaluation, 390
  of fetal heart rate, 572
  middle cerebral artery, 343–344
  in placenta accreta, 169
  umbilical artery, 340, 343–344, 595,
    987–988
Dormitory residents, meningococcal vac-
    cine for, 125
Dot blot, 1036–1037, 1044
Double balloon device, for cervical ripen-
    ing, 563
Double uterus, and recurrent pregnancy
    loss, 684
Down syndrome
  maternal age and, 867–868, 868t,
    873
  midtrimester or term risk of, 867,
    868t
  nuchal lucency measurement in, 870,
    872
  prenatal screening for, 867–874
    background of, 867–870
    clinical considerations and recom-
      mendations in, 870–874
    first-trimester, 58–60, 870
    indications for, 870–871
    maternal serum, 868–869, 868t,
      873
    in multiple gestation, 873
    multiple-marker test in, 868–869,
      868t
    second-trimester, 868–869
    ultrasonography, 869–870, 872–873
    in women who would decline preg-
      nancy termination, 874
Doxepin, for chronic pelvic pain,
    432
Doxorubicin
  contraindicated during breastfeeding,
    277t
  for endometrial cancer, 637
Doxycycline
  oral contraception use with, 942
  prophylactic, 349t, 584–585
    for anthrax, 109–110
    for gynecologic procedures, 349t,
      350, 354
Doxylamine, for nausea and vomiting of
    pregnancy, 745, 746f, 747t
Drinking, 15–23. See also Alcohol use
Droloxifene, 912–913
Droperidol, for nausea and vomiting of
    pregnancy, 747t
Drug abuse. See Substance abuse
Dual energy X-ray absorptiometry
    (DXA), 788, 790–791,
    796–797
Dᵘ blood type, 892
Duchenne muscular dystrophy, grandfa-
    ther effect and, 5

Duffy antibodies, 291, 291t
Duodenal atresia, in aneuploidy, 869t
Duplication, chromosomal, 1030–1031
D&X, intact. *See* Dilation and extraction, intact
DXA. *See* Dual-energy X-ray absorptiometry
Dyslipidemia
oral contraception and, 940–941
polycystic ovary syndrome and, 826
Dysmaturity syndrome, 666
Dysmenorrhea
chronic pelvic pain in, 429–430, 433
complementary and alternative medicine for, 436
in endometriosis, 47, 707
Dyspareunia
botanicals for, 1008–1010
chronic pelvic pain in, 429–430, 433
in endometriosis, 707
Dystocia, 479–485
adverse outcomes associated with, 481
ambulation and, 482
background of, 479–481
caregiver support in, 481, 483
cesarean delivery for, 481
clinical considerations and recommendations in, 481–485
definition of, 480
diagnosis of, intrauterine pressure catheters in, 482
epidural analgesia and, 482
hydration and, 483
and labor augmentation, 479–485
pelvimetry in, 482–483
postterm pregnancy and, 666
prediction of, 481–482
risk factors for, 481
shoulder, 921–923
background of, 921–922
causes of, 921
clinical considerations and recommendations in, 922–923
definition of, 921
history of, counseling in, 923
incidence of, 921
labor abnormalities and, 922
in macrosomia, 508, 508f, 510, 513, 782, 922–923
cesarean delivery in, 922–923
labor induction in, 922
management of, 923
maternal complications of, 921–922
McRoberts maneuver for, 921–923
neonatal complications of, 922
prediction of, 922
risk factors for, 922
Zavanelli maneuver for, 922–923

E

Early Reproductive Events and Breast Cancer Workshop, 97
Eastern European Jewish descent, individuals of
Canavan disease in, 178–181, 179t, 180b, 216–217
carrier screening for, 178–181, 179t, 216–219, 1042
clinical features of diseases common among, 180b
cystic fibrosis in, 178–181, 179t, 253–255, 254t
Tay-Sachs disease in, 178–181, 179t, 180b, 218–219
Eating disturbances, in ovarian cancer, 241
Echocardiography, fetal, in pregestational diabetes, 842
Eclampsia, 444–449
analgesia use in, 448, 773
anesthesia use in, 448
background of, 444–446
definition of, 445
management of, 448
neurologic or cerebral manifestations of, 446
prevention of, 449
Ectopic pregnancy, 719–724
background of, 719–721
clinical considerations and recommendations in, 721–724
diagnosis of, 720–721
etiology of, 719–720
expectant management of, 723
human chorionic gonadotropin concentration in, 720–724
incidence of, 719
intrauterine devices and, 585
maternal smoking and, 228
medical management of
contraindications to, 721b
cost-effectiveness of, 723
counseling in, 723, 723b
effects of, 720
indications for, 721–722, 721b
potential problems with, 722–723
side effects of, 722–723, 722b
methotrexate for, 720–723
pain in resolution, versus rupture, 722–723
and Rh D alloimmunization, 890
serum progesterone levels in, 721
success rates in, 721
tubal sterilization and, 378
ultrasonography in, 720–721
EDD. *See* Estimated date of delivery
Education
for imaging studies, 163
patient
on breastfeeding, 277–280
on cervical cytology screening, 30–31

Education *(continued)*
patient *(continued)*
on sonohysterography, 1052
on ultrasonography, during pregnancy, 985–986
Eflornithine
for hirsutism, 831
pregnancy category of, 828t
Elderly
morbidity in, leading causes of, 194
mortality in, leading causes of, 194
periodic assessments in, 194
Electrocautery, for human papillomavirus infection, 554–555
Electrocoagulation, for tubal sterilization, 375–376
Electrolysis, for hirsutism, 831
Embolization
in hysteroscopy, 1049
uterine artery, 262–263, 928
Emergency contraception, 489–495
access to, 492, 494
antiemetics as adjunct to, 493
awareness of, 492
background of, 490–492
candidates for, 492
clinical considerations and recommendations in, 492–495
clinical follow-up in, 494
drug interactions of, 492
effectiveness of, 493
effects on pregnancy, 491–492
initiation of, timing of, 493
intrauterine device for, 494, 587
mechanism of action, 490
versus medical abortion, 490
regimens for, 490, 491t
regular contraceptive use after, 494
repeated use of, safety of, 494
resources on, 495
screening procedures for, 492–493
side effects of, 490
and thromboembolism, 943
Enalapril, teratogenicity of, 315t, 422
Encephalocele, 755t
Endocarditis, bacterial, 349
antibiotic prophylaxis for, 352, 352b–353b, 353t, 585, 900–901, 901t
cardiac conditions associated with, 352, 352b
Endocervical curettage, with colposcopy, 609
Endometrial ablation, 434
for anovulatory bleeding, 627–628
hysteroscopic-assisted, 627–628
for leiomyoma, 928, 930
thermal balloon, 627
Endometrial biopsy, antibiotic prophylaxis in, 349t, 351

Endometrial cancer, 631–639
    in adolescents, 626
    anovulatory bleeding in, evaluation of, 626
    background of, 631–633
    cervical involvement in, treatment of, 637
    chemotherapy for, 637
    clear cell, 633
    clinical considerations and recommendations in, 633–639
    with colon cancer, 632
    comorbid conditions with, 633, 638
    diagnosis of, stage at, 631
    epidemiology of, 631–632
    ethnic disparities in, 631–632
    etiology of, 632
    follow-up in, 638
    histologic considerations in, 632–633
    incidence of, 631
    intraperitoneal disease in, treatment of, 637
    lifetime risk of, 631
    mortality in, 631
    nodal metastases in
        assessment for, 635
        therapy for, 636–637
    in obese patient, 638
    obesity and, 243
    papillary, 633
    physical examination in, 633–634
    posthysterectomy findings of, 636
    postoperative treatment of, 635–636
    precursor of, 632–633
    preoperative evaluation of, 633–634
    progestin for, 637–638
    prognosis of, 633, 635f
    racial disparities in, 631–632
    radiation therapy for, 635–637
    referral to gynecologic oncologist in, 637–638
    retroperitoneal node assessment in, 635
    risk factors for, 632, 632t
    staging of
        appropriate, 634–635
        International Federation of Gynecology and Obstetrics system of, 633, 634t
        surgical, 633–635
        survival by mode of, 633, 635f
        tumor–node–metastases system of, 633, 634t
    tamoxifen and, 235–236, 913, 915–916
    type I, 632
    type II, 632
    in women of later reproductive age, 626
    in women of reproductive age, 626
    5-year survival rate in, 631

Endometrial hyperplasia, 632–633
    atypical, 632–633, 637–638
    selective estrogen receptor modulators and, 913
    World Health Organization classification of, 632, 632b
Endometriomas, ovarian, 708, 713
Endometriosis, 706–714
    in adolescents, 46–51
        lesions in, 49
        treatment of, 48f, 49–51
    asymptomatic, incidental findings of, 712
    background of, 706–709
    classification of, 708f, 709
    clinical considerations and recommendations in, 709–714
    clinical presentation of, 47, 707
    complementary and alternative medicine for, 51, 436
    diagnosis of, 47–49, 48f, 707–708
    empiric therapy for, 47–48, 712
    etiology of, 706–707
    familial association of, 706
    gonadotropin-releasing hormone agonists for, 47–50, 433–434, 709–714
    histologic features of, 707
    history in, 47
    imaging studies of, 47, 708, 713
    incidence of, 46–47, 706
    and infertility, 707, 709–710, 712
    laparoscopy in, 48–49, 432, 710
    medical management of, 709–714
        in extrapelvic disease, 713
        versus no therapy
            in asymptomatic women, 711
            in fertility preservation, 709, 712
            in pain management, 709, 712–713
            in women who have completed childbearing, 712
        postoperative, 710–711
        presence of endometrioma and, 713
        versus surgical treatment, 709–710
        with surgical treatment, 710–711
    müllerian anomalies and, 46, 49
    oral contraceptives for, 49–51, 433, 709–714
    pain in, 430, 432–434, 707, 709–714
    physical examination in, 47
    in premenarcheal girls, 46
    presacral neurectomy for, 435
    recurrence of, estrogen therapy and, 713–714
    serum markers in, 47, 707–708
    suppressive therapy in, postoperative, 713–714
    surgical diagnosis of, 48–49
    surgical management of, 50–51, 434–435, 713–714
    visual inspection for, 707

Endometritis, medical abortion and, 699
Endothelin(s), in preeclampsia, 446
Engerix-B, 322
Enoxaparin sodium (Lovenox)
    anesthesia concerns with, 882
    for deep vein thrombosis prophylaxis, 882
    safety in pregnancy, 211–212
Enpresse, 491t
Enteral nutrition, for nausea and vomiting of pregnancy, 748
Enzymatic assays, for fetal lung maturity, 271
Enzyme immunoassay (EIA), for human immunodeficiency virus, 174
Enzyme-linked immunosorbent assay (ELISA)
    for herpes simplex virus, 533–534
    for human immunodeficiency virus, 173
    for toxoplasmosis, 816
    for varicella zoster virus, 815
Ephedrine
    for nonreassuring fetal heart rate, 578
    use with regional analgesia, 767
Epidural analgesia, 153, 766–767
    administration of, 766–767
    and cesarean delivery rates, 9–10, 771–772
    and chronic back pain, 770
    enoxaparin contraindicated before, 212
    in external cephalic version, 502
    and fetal heart rate, 575
    and fever, 768t, 771
    and hematoma, 767, 772, 882, 955–956, 966–967
    indications for, 766
    maternal request for, 153
    and operative delivery rates, 771
    patient-controlled, 770, 774
    in preeclampsia, 448
    and progress of labor, 482
    side effects of, 767, 768t
    spinal analgesia combined with, 767
    thrombocytopenia and, 955–956
    for vaginal birth after cesarean delivery, 1019
Epigenetic control of gene expression, 1032, 1044
Episiotomy
    and cervical cancer, 461
    local anesthesia for, 769
    in shoulder dystocia, 923
Erb-Duchenne paralysis, macrosomia and, 510
Ergotamine, contraindicated during breastfeeding, 277t
Errors, 160–162
    in cervical cytology screening, 399
    medication, 158, 161
    surgical, reduction of, 161

Errors *(continued)*
system problems and, 161–162
type I, 335
type II, 335
Erythroblastosis fetalis, 291–295
Erythromycin
for mastitis, 285
pharmacokinetics of, 899
prophylactic
for group B streptococcal disease, 185*b*, 186, 186*t*
for preterm premature rupture of membranes, 852, 900
Escherichia coli, antibiotic-resistant, 898
Essure device, 375
Estimated date of delivery (EDD)
days beyond, 666. *See also* Postterm pregnancy
determination of, 666
Estriol
salivary, and preterm delivery, 367–368
serum, in Down syndrome, 868–869, 868*t*
Estrogen
in anovulatory bleeding, 624–625
compounded bioidentical preparations of, 40–41
declining levels in women older than 40 years, 627
dietary plant, 1006
in endometrial cancer, 632
and nausea and vomiting of pregnancy, 743
Estrogen–progestin oral contraception
during breastfeeding, 282
emergency use of, 490
for polycystic ovary syndrome, 827–828
Estrogen therapy
add-back, with gonadotropin-releasing hormone agonists, 711, 862
for anovulatory bleeding, 626–628
contraindications to, 627
and endometriosis recurrence, 713–714
for osteoporosis, 793–794
after prophylactic oophorectomy, 908
and urinary incontinence, 994, 997
for vasomotor symptoms, with selective estrogen receptor modulators, 915
Ethic(s)
in adolescent health research, 67–70
in alcohol and drug abuse, 15–23
American College of Obstetricians and Gynecologists code of, vii–x
in complementary and alternative medicine, 37
framing, in perinatal medicine, 113–114
in maternal decision making, 111–119

Ethic(s) *(continued)*
in maternal–fetal relationship, 114–116
in nonmedical use of obstetric ultrasonography, 135–136
in physician–patient relationship, 161–162
in storage of newborn screening blood spots, 133
in umbilical cord blood storage, 207–208
Ethical foundations, vii–viii
Ethics in Obstetrics and Gynecology, vii
Ethnic disparities
in bone mass, 790
in endometrial cancer, 631–632
in health care financing, 200–201
in infant, fetal, and perinatal mortality, 200, 200*t*
in intrauterine growth restriction, 592
in macrosomia, 509
in preterm delivery, 200, 367
in women's health, 199–202
American College of Obstetricians and Gynecologists recommendations on, 201–202
examples of, 200
understanding causes of, 200–201
Etidronate, for osteoporosis prevention, 795
Etoposide, for gestational trophoblastic disease, 473–474
Etretinate, teratogenicity of, 316*t*
Evaluation of Cesarean Delivery, 9–10
Evening primrose, for menopausal symptoms, 1007, 1009
Evidence
level I, 330–331
level II-1, 331
level II-2, 331–332
level II-3, 332
level III, 332
Evidence-based medicine, 329–335
Evidence-based recommendations, development of, 334
Exanthem erythema infectiosum, 811
Exchange transfusion, prophylactic, in sickle cell disease, 544
Exencephaly, 755*t*
Exercise
for chronic pelvic pain, 434
for gestational diabetes, 53, 524
for obesity, 245, 245*t*
for polycystic ovary syndrome, 829–830
during postpartum period, 55
during pregnancy, 53–55
absolute contraindications to, 54*b*
by competitive athlete, 55
and prevention of gestational diabetes, 53
relative contraindications to, 54*b*

Exercise *(continued)*
during pregnancy *(continued)*
safety of activities for, 54
supine position contraindicated in, 53–54
warning signs for termination of, 54*b*
for premenstrual syndrome, 861
weight-bearing, and bone loss, 790, 793
Exons, 1028, 1028*f*, 1044
Expectant management
of diabetes mellitus, during pregnancy, 842
of ectopic pregnancy, 723
of leiomyoma, 931–932
of postterm pregnancy, 667–668
of premature rupture of membranes, 851, 853
Expert opinion, 332
Expressivity, genetic, 1044
External cephalic version, 127–128, 500–504
adverse effects of, 501
anesthesia and, 502
background of, 500
benefits and risks of, 501
candidates for, 500–501
and cesarean delivery rates, 502
clinical considerations and recommendations in, 500–504
contraindications to, 501
cost implications of, 504
goal of, 500
protocol for, 502–503, 503*f*
success rates for, 501–502
success versus failure of, predictive factors in, 501–502
tocolysis use in, 502
for vaginal birth after cesarean delivery, 1019
Extremely low birth weight
antenatal corticosteroids in, 806
and cerebral palsy, 804–805, 806*t*
clinical considerations and recommendations in, 803–807
mode of delivery in, 806
morbidity associated with, counseling about, 804
mortality in, counseling on, 803–804, 804*f*–805*f*
perinatal care in, 802–807
resuscitation and support in, 806–807

F

Facial cleft, in aneuploidy, 869*t*
Factor V Leiden mutation, 880, 881*t*
and deep vein thrombosis, 880, 884
and oral contraception use, 943
and recurrent pregnancy loss, 684, 688
and thromboembolism, in pregnancy, 961, 963–965

Failure to progress, in labor, 480

Falls, in osteoporosis, 793

Falope ring, 376

False-positive results, in human chorionic gonadotropin testing, 26–27

Falun (Sweden) Meeting Committee, 389

Famciclovir, for herpes simplex virus infection, 534, 535t, 648, 648t

Familial dysautonomia
  carrier screening for, 178–181, 179t
  clinical features of, 180b

Fanconi anemia group C
  carrier screening for, 178–181, 179t
  clinical features of, 180b

Fasting, before anesthesia use, 773

Fasting glucose testing, 195t, 521, 526–527, 526t

Felbamate, oral contraception use with, 941

Fellatio, sexually transmitted disease transmission via, 222

Femur length, fetal, 595, 872, 984, 987

Fentanyl
  adverse effects of, 770
  and fetal heart rate, 770
  parenteral, obstetric, 766, 766t, 770
  spinal epidural, 767
  transplacental passage of, 770

Ferguson v. City of Charleston, 20, 119

Fetal alcohol syndrome, 15, 20–21, 311, 893

Fetal behavioral state alteration, 337–338

Fetal breathing, in biophysical profile, 339–340

Fetal death (loss)
  amniocentesis and, 871
  antiphospholipid syndrome and, 357, 360
  chorionic villus sampling and, 871–872
  chronic hypertension and, 419
  enoxaparin sodium and, 212
  ethnic disparities in, 200, 200t
  gestational diabetes and, 519
  hyperthyroidism and, 972
  intrauterine growth restriction and, 593–594, 594t
  labor induction in, 568
  maternal smoking and, 228
  in multiple gestation, 732–733
  in postterm pregnancy, 666–667, 667f
  pregestational diabetes and, 840–841
  premature rupture of membranes and, 849–850
  racial and ethnic disparities in, 200, 200t
  trauma and, 298–299

Fetal distress, inappropriate use of term, 94–95

Fetal heart rate (FHR)
  acceleration in, 573t, 574
  analgesia and, 575, 767–770
  anesthesia and, 575, 767–770
  baseline, 573t
  baseline variability in, 573t
  in contraction stress test, 338–339
  deceleration in, 574
    early, 573t
    late, 573t
    prolonged, 573t
    recurrent, 574
    variable, 573t
  external cephalic version and, 501
  medications affecting, 575–576, 576t
  monitoring of, 572–578
    background of, 572–574
    and cesarean delivery rates, 56–57
    clinical considerations and recommendations in, 574–578
    diagnostic value of, 56
    efficacy of, 574–575
    electronic, 572–578
    external, 572
    false-positive rate of, 577
    fetal pulse oximetry with, 56–57, 577
    frequency of use, 572
    versus intermittent auscultation, 574–575
    internal, 572
    interobserver and intraobserver variability in, 575
    interpretation of, guidelines for, 573–574
    in isoimmunization, 294
    in oxytocin augmentation, 485
    in preterm fetus, 575
    with prostaglandin use, 566
    purpose of, 572
    review of, guidelines for, 574
    in trauma, 300–301
  nonreassuring pattern of, 577–578
    ancillary tests in, 577
    and cerebral palsy, 574
    fetal stimulation in, 577
    initial assessment of, 577
    persistent, intrauterine resuscitation for, 577–578
  in nonstress test, 339
  patterns of, definitions of, 573–574, 573t
  reassuring pattern of, 576

Fetal heart response, physiology of, 337–338

Fetal lung development, 268

Fetal lung maturity
  assessment of, 267–272
  associated conditions and, 271
  corticosteroids and, 271–272, 676
  gestational age and, 267–268, 271

Fetal lung maturity *(continued)*
  intrauterine growth restriction and, 594
  in multiple gestation, 734
  physiology and pathophysiology of, 268
  in premature rupture of membranes, 851–852
  in preterm labor and delivery, 676
  tests of, 267–272
    amniocentesis for, 268
    biochemical, 268
    biophysical, 268
    cascade or sequential, 272
    classification of, 268
    comparison of, 270t, 272
    direct, 268, 270t
    fluorescence polarization, 270t, 271
    foam stability index, 269, 270t
    indirect tests, 268
    lamellar body counts, 270t, 271
    lecithin–sphingomyelin ratio, 269, 270t
    optical density, 270t, 271
    phosphatidylglycerol, 269, 270t, 272
    in premature rupture of membranes, 272
    "shake," 269, 270t
    strategies for, 272
    ultrasonography, 267–268, 271

Fetal–maternal hemorrhage
  and Rh D alloimmunization, 890–891, 894
  screening for, 890–891, 894
  trauma and, 301

Fetal maturation, antenatal corticosteroids for, 11–12. *See also* Fetal lung maturity

Fetal movement
  assessment of, 338, 344
  in biophysical profile, 339–340
  in nonstress test, 339

Fetal protection, versus maternal decision making, 111–119

Fetal pulse oximetry, 56–57

Fetal rights, 114

Fetal surgery
  fetal risks in, 760
  maternal risks in, 113, 760
  for neural tube defects, 760

Fetal surveillance, antepartum, 337–345
  abnormal result in, response to, 342
  in antiphospholipid syndrome, 362
  background of, 337–340
  in chronic hypertension, 422
  clinical considerations and recommendations in, 340–345
  comparison of tests for, 342–343
  effectiveness of, 340
  false-negative rate of, 341
  false-positive rate of, 342

Fetal surveillance, antepartum
(*continued*)
follow-up in, 342
frequency of, 341
in gestational diabetes, 524–525
indications for, 341
in intrauterine growth restriction, 596
in multiple gestation, 733
normal result in, reassurance from, 341–342
in postterm pregnancy, 666–667
predictive value of, 341
in preeclampsia, 447
in pregestational diabetes, 842
in preterm premature rupture of membranes, 853
with prostaglandin use, 566
in sickle cell disease, 544
techniques of, 338–340
timing of initiation, 341
Fetal tone, in biophysical profile, 339–340
Fetal weight, estimation of
accuracy of, 510–511
in gestational diabetes, 525–526
Hadlock's formula for, 511
Leopold's maneuvers for, 510–511
maternal, 510–511
symphysis–fundal height in, 510
ultrasonography for, 510–511, 525–526, 985, 987, 989
Fever, analgesia and, 767, 768t, 771
FHR. *See* Fetal heart rate
Fibrinogen I-125 uptake test, for deep vein thrombosis, 879–880
Fibroadenoma, breast, oral contraception and, 940
Fibrocystic breast changes, oral contraception and, 940
Fibroids. *See* Leiomyoma(s)
Fibronectin, fetal, and preterm delivery, 367–369, 369t, 676, 731
Fifth disease, 811
FIGO. *See* International Federation of Gynecology and Obstetrics
Filshie clip, 376
Fimbriectomy, 375
Finasteride
for hirsutism, 830
pregnancy category of, 828t
Fine-needle aspiration
of breast mass, 206
of cervical lesion, 454
First-trimester screening
criteria for, 59–60
for Down syndrome, 870
for fetal aneuploidy, 58–60, 870
First-trimester ultrasonography, 983
imaging parameters in, 983
indications for, 983

FISH. *See* Fluorescence in situ hybridization
Fitness, periodic assessments of
ages 13–18 years, 191
ages 19–39 years, 192
ages 40–64 years, 193
ages 65 and older, 194
Fluid media, for hysteroscopy, 1047
high-viscosity, 1047
low-viscosity, electrolyte-poor, 1047
low-viscosity electrolyte, 1047
Fluid overload, in hysteroscopy, 1048
Fluid therapy, for diabetic ketoacidosis, in pregnancy, 840b
Fluorescence in situ hybridization (FISH), 1039–1040, 1044
Fluorescence polarization, 270t, 271
Fluoride supplementation
contraindicated for osteoporosis prevention, 795
indications for, 195t
Fluoroquinolone(s), for anthrax prophylaxis, 109–110
5-Fluorouracil
for cervical cancer, 459
for gestational trophoblastic disease, 473
Fluoxetine
for premenstrual syndrome, 861–862
side effects of, 862
Flushes, menopausal, botanicals for, 1008–1009
Flutamide
for hirsutism, 830
pregnancy category of, 828t
Fluvoxamine, for premenstrual syndrome, 861–862
FMR-1 gene, 62–63, 63t
Foam stability index, 269, 270t
Folic acid
and neural tube defects, 756–758
requirements in pregnancy, 757–758
Folic acid antagonists
and intrauterine growth restriction, 593
teratogenicity of, 315t, 756
Folic acid supplementation
preconceptional, 238
in sickle cell disease, 543–544
Folinic acid
for postmolar gestational trophoblastic disease prophylaxis, 470
for toxoplasmosis, 816
Follicle-stimulating hormone (FSH)
in anovulatory bleeding, 625
in ovulation induction, 655–656, 660
in ovulatory dysfunction, 654–655, 657
Follow-up, physician–patient relationship and, 158

Food and Drug Administration
on dietary supplements, 1006–1007
on hormonal contraception during breastfeeding, 281–282
on mifepristone use, for medical abortion, 695
on misoprostol use during pregnancy, 129–130
pregnancy risk categories of, 312–313
on vacuum extraction, 783
Forceps delivery, 780–786
clinical considerations and recommendations in, 784–786
complications of, 781–782, 783t
contraindications to, 784
criteria for, 781, 781b
epidural analgesia and, 771
incidence of, 780–781
long-term infant consequences of, 783
for macrosomia, 513, 782
rotational midforceps, role in current practice, 785
station classification in, 781
types of, 781, 781b
Foscarnet, for cytomegalovirus infection, 813
Fractures, in osteoporosis
prevention of, 793–794
risk factors for, 790, 790b
Fragile X syndrome, 62–63
genetics of, 62–63, 63t, 1031–1032
testing for, recommendations on, 63
Frame-shift mutation, 1044
French-Canadian descent, Tay-Sachs disease in individuals of, 178, 218–219
Frequent moves, as barrier to care, 306
FSH. *See* Follicle-stimulating hormone

G

G. D. Searle & Co., drug warning on misoprostol, response to, 101–102
Gabapentin, oral contraception use with, 941
Galactorrhea, 624, 654
Galactosemia
breastfeeding contraindicated in, 276
newborn screening for, 132–133
Ganciclovir, for cytomegalovirus infection, 813
Gardnerella vaginalis, and preterm labor, 366–367
Gastric banding, 143–144
Gastric ulcers, prevention of, 129–130, 203–204
Gastroplasty, vertical banded, 143–144
Gastroschisis, in aneuploidy, 869t
Gaucher's disease
carrier screening for, 178–181, 179t
clinical features of, 180b

GDM. *See* Gestational diabetes mellitus
Gene(s), 1028–1029
  co-dominant, 1030, 1043
  definition of, 1028, 1044
  hereditary unstable, 1031–1032
  mutation of, 1029
  polymorphisms of, 1029
  structure of, 1028, 1028*f*
  variants (alleles) of, 1029
Gene expression, 1028–1029, 1032, 1044
General anesthesia, obstetric, 769
Genetic(s), 1027–1043
  glossary of terms in, 1043–1045
  knowledge of, increase in, 1027
Genetic counseling, 1041–1042
  in breast cancer, 393
  indications for, 195*t*
  on paternal age, 5
Genetic disorders, 58–60, 867–874
  prenatal diagnosis of
    background of, 867–870
    clinical considerations and recommendations in, 870–874
  single gene (mendelian), 1029–1030
Genetic evaluation, of stillbirths and neonatal deaths, 64–66
Genetic testing, 1035–1043
  accuracy of, 1041
  applications in obstetrics and gynecology, 1041–1042
  in Ashkenazi Jews, 178–181, 179*t*, 216–219, 1042
  indications for, 195*t*, 1040–1041
  limitations of, 1041
Genistein, 1006
Genital herpes. *See* Herpes simplex virus infection, genital
Genital warts. *See* Human papillomavirus infection
Genome
  definition of, 1044
  mapping of, 1027
  organization of, 1027–1029
Genomic imprinting, 167, 1032–1033, 1044
Gentamicin, prophylactic
  for bacterial endocarditis, 353*t*, 900–901
  for preterm premature rupture of membranes, 900
Germline mosaicism, 1033
Gestational age
  assessment of
    for labor induction, 564, 564*b*
    in postterm pregnancy, 666
    at threshold of viability, 805–806
    ultrasonography in, 267–268, 984–985
  birth weight percentiles for, 507, 508*t*
  and fetal lung maturity, 267–268, 271
  and macrosomia, 509

Gestational age *(continued)*
  and medical abortion, 699
  newborn deaths by, 803–804, 804*f*–805*f*
  optimal, for ultrasonography, 986
  at premature rupture of membranes, 848
  and preterm labor and delivery, 674*f*, 676
  and screening for gestational diabetes, 520–521
Gestational diabetes mellitus (GDM), 518–527
  background of, 518–520
  and cesarean delivery, 518–519, 525–526
  clinical considerations and recommendations in, 520–527
  definition of, 518
  delivery in, timing and mode of, 525–526
  diagnosis of, 521–522
  diagnostic criteria for, 522, 522*t*
  diet therapy for, 523
  exercise and, 53, 524
  fetal assessment in, 524–525
  fetal complications of, 518–519
  glucose monitoring in, 522
  history of, and postpartum screening, 526–527
  insulin therapy for, 523–524
  and macrosomia, 508–509, 511, 519, 525–526
  maternal complications of, 518–519
  maternal obesity and, 142–143
  in multiple gestation, 728
  oral antidiabetic agents for, 524
  and perinatal mortality, 519
  and preeclampsia, 518–519
  prevalence of, 518
  risk factors for, 520
  screening for
    approach in, 520
    controversy over, 519–520
    gestational age and, 520–521
    method for, 521
    threshold value in, 521
    venous versus capillary blood in, 521
  treatment of
    controversy over, 519–520
    goals of, 519–520
Gestational sac, ultrasonography of, 983
Gestational thrombocytopenia, 951
Gestational trophoblastic disease, 466–475
  background of, 466–469
  clinical considerations and recommendations in, 469–475
  incidence of, 466–467

Gestational trophoblastic disease *(continued)*
  malignant (metastatic), 468–469
    cerebral metastases from, 474
    classification of, 472–473
    Clinical Classification system for, 472–473, 473*t*
    clinical diagnosis of, 469
    clinical presentation of, 468
    evaluation of, 473
    good-prognosis, 472, 473*t*
    high-risk, treatment of, 474
    histologic considerations in, 468
    International Federation of Gynecology and Obstetrics scoring system for, 472, 472*t*
    low-risk, treatment of, 474
    oral contraception after, 475
    poor-prognosis, 472, 473*t*
    staging, 472–473
    surveillance after therapy, 474–475
    treatment of, 473
    World Health Organization prognostic index score of, 472
  nonmetastatic
    classification of, 472, 473*t*
    treatment of, 473–474
    postmolar, 467–469, 470
    recommendations in, 469–475
Gestrinone, 434
Ginger, for nausea and vomiting of pregnancy, 745
Ginseng, for menopausal symptoms, 1008–1010
Glucocorticoids, in ovulation induction, 659, 828
Glucose control, during labor, 842–843
Glucose intolerance, and recurrent pregnancy loss, 684, 687
Glucose monitoring
  in gestational diabetes, 522–523
  in pregestational diabetes, 838–839
Glucose testing, 195*t*, 520–523, 526–527, 526*t*
Glucose tolerance test (GTT), 520–523, 526–527, 526*t*
Glyburide
  for gestational diabetes, 524
  for pregestational diabetes, during pregnancy, 841–842
GnRH. *See* Gonadotropin-releasing hormone
Goiter, 977
Gonadotropin(s)
  and ovarian cancer, 661
  for ovulation induction, 656, 657*f*, 660–661, 828–829
Gonadotropin-releasing hormone (GnRH), in ovulatory dysfunction, 654–655

Gonadotropin-releasing hormone (GnRH) agonists
  add-back therapy with, 50, 711, 862
  bone mineral density loss with, 50
  for chronic pelvic pain, 433–434
  for endometrioma, 713
  for endometriosis, 47–50, 433–434, 709–714
  for leiomyoma, 928–930
  long-term therapy with, 711
  for ovulatory dysfunction, 655
  for premenstrual syndrome, 862
Gonorrhea
  in adolescents, 220, 222
  during pregnancy, 223–224
  reporting and partner notification of, 224
  screening for, before intrauterine device insertion, 584
Goserelin, 433
Gothenburg Breast Cancer Screening Trial, 388
Graduated compression stockings, 880, 883
Graft-versus-host disease, umbilical cord blood and risk of, 207
Grandfather effect, 5
Graves' disease
  definition of, 971
  in pregnancy, 972–973
    differential diagnosis of, 973
    etiology of, 973
    fetal and neonatal effects of, 972–973
    laboratory tests in, 974
    signs and symptoms of, 972
    treatment of, 974–975
Griseofulvin, interaction with oral contraception, 942
Group B streptococcal disease
  antibiotic susceptibility testing in, 185b
  culture collection and processing in, 184–186, 185b
  early-onset, in newborns
    factors associated with, 183
    incidence of, 182–183
    prevention of, 182–188
  intrapartum antibiotic prophylaxis against, 183–188, 898–899
    benefit versus risk analysis of, 186
    in cesarean delivery, 187–188
    culture-based approach in, 183–188, 184f, 185b
    hospital compliance with, 184
    in premature rupture of membranes, 183–188, 187f, 852, 900
    recommended regimens for, 186, 186t
    resistance to, 186
    risk-based approach in, 183–184
  invasive, 182–183
  late-onset, in newborns, 182

GTT. See Glucose tolerance tesst
Guidelines for Adolescent Health Research, 69
Guidelines for Women's Health Care, 190
Gunshot wounds, 299
Guthrie, Robert, 131
Guthrie test, 131–132
Gynecologic infections, 348–349
Gynecologic Oncology Group, 633
Gynecologic procedures, antibiotic prophylaxis for, 348–354
Gynecology-only practice, professional liability in, 198

H
Hadlock's formula, for fetal weight estimate, 511
Halogenated anesthesia, 769
Haloperidol, for nausea and vomiting of pregnancy, 747t
Hashimoto's thyroiditis, and hypothyroidism, 973–974
HBcAg. See Hepatitis B core antigen
HBeAg. See Hepatitis B e antigen
HBsAg. See Hepatitis B surface antigen
Headache
  medical abortion and, 697, 698t
  migraine, and oral contraception use, 939–940
  postdural puncture, 767
Head circumference, fetal, 595, 984, 987
Health behaviors, periodic assessments of
  ages 13–18 years, 191
  ages 19–39 years, 192
  ages 40–64 years, 193
  ages 65 and older, 194
Health care financing, racial and ethnic disparities in, 200–201
Health Care for the Homeless, 80b
Health disparities
  definition of, 199
  racial and ethnic, 199–202
    American College of Obstetricians and Gynecologists recommendations on, 201–202
    examples of, 200
    understanding causes of, 200–201
Health insurance
  individuals lacking, 248–250
    capacity of health care system to serve, 249
    reproductive health and health care of, 249
  racial and ethnic disparities in, 201
Health Insurance Plan of Greater New York, breast cancer screening study of, 387–389
Health literacy, 158
Healthy People 2010, 17, 287
Healthy Start Prenatal Risk Screening Instrument, 304–305, 305b, 310f

Hearing loss
  cytomegalovirus infection and, 811
  newborn screening for, 132–133
Heart disease
  ethnic disparities in, 200
  obesity and, 243
  prevention of, botanicals for, 1010
  racial and ethnic disparities in, 200
  risk factors for, periodic assessments of, 191–194
Heart rate
  in Apgar score, 257, 258t
  fetal. See Fetal heart rate
Heart valves, prosthetic
  enoxaparin contraindicated in pregnant women with, 211–212
  thromboprophylaxis with, 963
HELLP syndrome, 419, 423, 445–447, 729, 957
Hematocrit, before medical abortion, 699
Hematologic values, normal fetal, 292, 293t
Hematoma
  maternal
    epidural and spinal analgesia and, 767, 772, 882, 955–956, 966–967
    operative vaginal delivery and, 782
    subgaleal, fetal, vacuum extraction and, 783
Hematopoietic stem cells, from umbilical cord blood, 207–208
Hemoconcentration, in preeclampsia, 446
Hemodynamic monitoring, in preeclampsia and eclampsia, 448
Hemoglobin
  adult, 539
  fetal, 539
  normal fetal values of, 293t
  structure of, 539
  testing of
    indications for, 195t
    before medical abortion, 699
Hemoglobin Bart's disease, 540
Hemoglobin H disease, 540
Hemoglobinopathies
  background of, 539–541
  clinical considerations and recommendations in, 541–545
  hematologic features of, 543t
  newborn screening for, 132
  in pregnancy, 539–545
  prenatal testing for, 542–543
  screening for, 541–542, 542f
Hemoglobin S, 539–540
Hemophilia A, grandfather effect and, 5
Hemorrhage
  antenatal, anti-D immune globulin in, 893
  enoxaparin sodium and, 212

Hemorrhage *(continued)*
  fetal–maternal
    and Rh D alloimmunization,
      890–891, 894
    screening for, 890–891, 894
    trauma and, 301
  in hysteroscopy, 1048
  intracranial fetal and neonatal
    in idiopathic thrombocytopenic pur-
      pura, 953, 955
    in neonatal alloimmune thrombocy-
      topenia, 952
    prevention of, 955
    with vacuum extraction, 782–783,
      783*t*
  in placenta accreta, 169–170
  retinal fetal and neonatal, with vacuum
    extraction, 782–783
Heparin
  adverse effects of, 884
  anesthesia concerns with, 882, 884,
    966–967
  for antiphospholipid syndrome,
    361–362, 688
  for deep vein thrombosis prophylaxis,
    882–884
  and epidural and spinal hematoma,
    772, 882, 966–967
  in intrapartum and postpartum period,
    966
  for intrauterine growth restriction, 596
  low-molecular-weight. *See* Low-molec-
    ular-weight heparin
  and osteoporosis, 790, 791*b*, 884, 962
  postpartum prophylactic, for obese
    patients, 143
  during pregnancy, 962–968
    for acute thromboembolism, 966
    indications for, 963–964
    regimens for, 964, 964*b*
  and thrombocytopenia, 884, 962–963
Hepatitis. *See also specific types*
  autoimmune, 321*t*
  clinical manifestations of, 320
  diagnosis of, 320–322
  epidemiology of, 318–320
  etiology of, 318–320
  general supportive measures in, 322
  general tests in, 320–321
  in health care workers, precautions
    against, 323
  immunotherapy for, 322–323
  jaundice in, 320, 321*t*
  management of, 322–323
  natural history of, 318–320
  and nausea and vomiting of pregnancy,
    748
  in obstetrician–gynecologists, 82
  in pregnancy, 318–324
  specific tests in, 321–322
Hepatitis A immune globulin, 89*t*, 318, 322

Hepatitis A vaccine, 318, 322
  indications for, 195*t*
  during pregnancy, 86*t*
Hepatitis A virus infection, 318
  and breastfeeding, 277
  clinical manifestations of, 320
  diagnosis of, 321
  epidemiology of, 318
  etiology of, 318
  management of, 322
  natural history of, 318
  in pregnancy, 318
  transmission of, 318
Hepatitis B core antigen (HBcAg), 319,
    321
Hepatitis B e antigen (HBeAg), 319
Hepatitis B immune globulin, 321–323
  during breastfeeding, 277
  for neonates, 319
  during pregnancy, 88*t*
Hepatitis B surface antigen (HBsAg),
    319, 321
Hepatitis B vaccine, 220, 319, 322–323
  indications for, 195*t*
  for neonates, 319
  for obstetrician–gynecologists, 82
  during pregnancy, 86*t*
Hepatitis B virus infection, 319
  acute, 319, 321
  in adolescents, 220, 223
  and breastfeeding, 277
  chronic, 319, 321
  clinical manifestations of, 320
  diagnosis of, 321
  epidemiology of, 319
  etiology of, 319
  in health care workers, precautions
    against, 323
  management of, 322–323
  mother-to-child transmission of, 319
  natural history of, 319
  in obstetrician–gynecologists, 82
  perinatal management of, 323
  in pregnancy, 319
  reporting and partner notification of, 224
  screening for, 323
  transmission of, 319
Hepatitis C virus infection, 319
  and breastfeeding, 277, 319
  diagnosis of, 321–322
  hepatitis D co-infection with, 319–320
  management of, 323
  mother-to-child transmission of, 319
  in obstetrician–gynecologists, 82
  testing for, indications for, 195*t*
Hepatitis D virus infection, 319–320
  chronic, 320
  clinical manifestations of, 320
  diagnosis of, 322
  management of, 323
  mother-to-child transmission of, 320

Hepatitis E virus infection, 320
  clinical manifestations of, 320
  diagnosis of, 322
  epidemiology of, 320
  mother-to-child transmission of, 320
  natural history of, 320
Hepatitis G virus infection, 320
  clinical manifestations of, 320
  diagnosis of, 322
  mother-to-child transmission of, 320
Hepatocellular carcinoma, hepatitis and,
    320
Herbal medicine, 38
  for chronic pelvic pain, 436
  interactions of, with emergency contra-
    ception, 492
  for menopausal symptoms, 1004–1011
Hereditary unstable DNA, 1031–1032,
    1044
Heroin, and intrauterine growth restric-
    tion, 593
Herpes simplex virus infection
  and breastfeeding, 277, 649–650
  genital, 532–536
    antiviral therapy for, 534–535, 535*t*,
      647–648, 648*t*
    asymptomatic patient in
      postexposure prophylaxis for, 534
      postexposure testing for, 534
    background of, 532–533, 644–645
    cesarean delivery in, 649
    clinical considerations and recom-
      mendations in, 533–536,
      647–650
    clinical presentation of, 645–646,
      645*b*
    diagnosis of, 533–534, 647
    etiology of, 644–645
    first clinical episodes of, treatment
      of, 534, 535*t*
    incidence of, 645
    intermittent reactivation of, 533
    invasive procedures in, 649
    living with, counseling about,
      535–536
    nonprimary first episode, 645–646,
      645*b*
    in pregnancy, management of,
      644–650
    premature rupture of membranes in,
      649
    prevalence of, 532–533
    primary, 645, 645*b*
    recurrent, 532–533, 645*b*, 646
      prevention of, 534–535
      treatment of, 534, 535*t*, 647
    screening for, in pregnancy or at
      delivery, 648
    severe episodes of, treatment of, 535,
      535*t*
    spectrum of disease in, 533

Herpes simplex virus infection (continued)
  genital (continued)
    suppressive therapy for, 535, 535t,
      648, 648t
    transmission of, 646–647
      maternal–fetal, 646
      during pregnancy, 646–647
      prevention of, 536
      via sexual and direct contact, 646
    vaccine against, development of, 536
    vaginal delivery in, 649
    viral shedding in, 533, 645–646
  neonatal, 645–646, 649–650
  type 1, 532–533, 644
  type 2, 532–533, 644
Herpes zoster infection, breastfeeding
    precautions in, 276–277
Heterochromatin, 1027, 1043, 1044
Heterophilic antibodies, and false-positive
    human chorionic gonadotropin
    test results, 26–27, 468,
    471–472
Heterozygotes, 1030
Hexoprenaline, and fetal heart rate,
    577–578
Hexosaminidase A
  pseudodeficiency of, 219
  in Tay-Sachs disease, 178, 218–219,
    1030
Hexosaminidase B, in Sandhoff disease,
    218
High-altitude exercise, contraindicated
    during pregnancy, 54
High forceps delivery, 781b
High-grade squamous intraepithelial
    lesions (HSILs), 400, 603, 604b
  in adolescents, 30, 32
  atypical squamous cells suggestive of, 400
  management of, 607–608
High-risk factors, periodic assessments
    based on, 190, 195t–196t
Hip film, fetal radiation exposure from, 73b
Hirsutism
  adjuvant cosmetic management of, 831
  in ovulatory dysfunction, 624–625, 654
  in polycystic ovary syndrome,
    823–824, 830–831
  treatment of, 830–831
Hispanic(s)
  cystic fibrosis in, 254t
  group B streptococcal disease in, 183
  health care insurance among, 201
  health disparities for, 199–202
  macrosomia in, 509
  obesity in, 243
  osteoporosis in, 790
History, patient, in periodic assessments
  ages 13–18 years, 191
  ages 19–39 years, 192
  ages 40–64 years, 193
  ages 65 and older, 194

HIV. See Human immunodeficiency virus
Holoprosencephaly, in aneuploidy, 869t
Holorachischisis, 755t
Homelessness, 76–80
  common characteristics of, 77b
  definition of, 77b
  impact on women, 77–78
  prevention of, 80
  risk factors for, 76–77
Homeless women
  gynecologic health of, 77
  health care for, 76–80
    barriers to, 78–79
    federal program for, 80b
    J. C. Lewis Health Center for, 79b
    preventive, 78
    recommendations for improving, 79
    use patterns of, 78
  obstetric health of, 77–78
  population of, 76–77
  violence against, 77
Home uterine activity monitoring
    (HUAM), 367–368, 731
Homocystinuria, newborn screening for,
    133
Homozygotes, 1030
Hormonal contraception. See also Oral
    contraception
  during breastfeeding, 281–282, 282b,
    941
  and coexisting medical conditions,
    936–945
    background of, 936–937
    clinical considerations and recom-
      mendations in, 937–945
  concomitant medications with,
    941–942
Hormonal disorders, and recurrent preg-
    nancy loss, 683–684
Hormone(s), compounded bioidentical,
    40–41
Hormone therapy
  after prophylactic oophorectomy, 908
  discontent with, 1004
  discontinuation, for deep vein thrombo-
    sis prophylaxis, 883
  and endometriosis recurrence, 713–714
  and leiomyomas, 931–932
  and urinary incontinence, 997
Hospital practices, for supporting breast-
    feeding, 279–280, 279b
Hospital privileges, policy statement on,
    1057–1058
Hospital stay, length of, for gynecologic
    procedures, 107
Hot flashes
  botanicals for, 1008–1009
  selective estrogen receptor modulators
    and, 913, 915
Housing problems, as barrier to care, 306
HPV. See Human papillomavirus infection

HUAM. See Home uterine activity moni-
    toring
Hulka-Clemens clip, 376
Human chorionic gonadotropin (hCG)
  beta subunit of, 720
  in confirmation of complete abortion,
    700
  in Down syndrome, 868–870
  in ectopic pregnancy, 720–724
  free beta, in first-trimester screening,
    59
  in hydatidiform mole, 467–472
  in malignant gestational trophoblastic
    disease, 469, 474–475
  microheterogeneity of, 27
  and nausea and vomiting of pregnancy,
    743
  in nonmetastatic gestational trophoblas-
    tic disease, 473–474
  for ovulation induction, 659
  in recurrent pregnancy loss, 687
  tests for, false-positive results of, 468,
    471–472
    avoiding inappropriate clinical deci-
      sions based on, 26–27
    causes of, 26–27
    methods for identifying, 27, 471–472
Human immunodeficiency virus (HIV)
    infection
  in adolescents, 220–224
  breastfeeding contraindicated in, 276
  care provider risk of, 213
  and cervical intraepithelial neoplasia,
    610
  during pregnancy, 223–224
  prevention of mother-to-child transmis-
    sion, 172, 174
    scheduled cesarean delivery and,
      213–215
    zidovudine for, 172, 213–214
  racial and ethnic disparities in, 200
  reporting and partner notification of,
    224
  screening for
    indications for, 195t
    perinatal, 172–176
    policy statement on, 1066–1067
    prenatal, 172–176
      conventional algorithm for, 173
      opt-in versus opt-out approach in,
        173, 176
      repeat, in third trimester, 173–174
      rapid, in obstetric setting, 174–175
        false-positive rates in, 174
        oral, fluid-based, 175
        positive predictive value of, by
          HIV prevalence rates, 174, 175t
        positive results in, management of,
          175
    recommendations on, 175–176
    routine newborn, 132

Human leukocyte antigens, and recurrent pregnancy loss, 685, 688
Human papillomavirus (HPV) infection, 548–556
  in adolescents, 220
    need for additional research on, 32
    risk factors for, 30, 32b
    screening for, 29–32
  background of, 548–551
  and cervical cancer, 29, 400–401, 453–454, 550–551, 604–605
  clinical considerations and recommendations in, 556
  counseling about, 555–556
  cytologic effects of, 549
  epidemiology of, 548–549
  immunocompromised states and, 30, 32b
  incidence of, 548–549
  natural history of, 550
  neonatal, 550, 555–556
  nomenclature and taxonomy for, 550
  patient-applied therapies for, 553–554
  patient questions about, 555–556
  ping-pong effect of, 555
  and pregnancy, 555–556
  prevalence of, 548–549, 604
  prevention of, 552–553
  provider-applied medication for, 554–555
  reinfection with, 555
  risk factors for, 549–550
  subclinical, 549
  testing for, 403–404, 549–552, 605, 611–612
    follow-up in, 606–607
    recommendations on, 551
    for women older than 30 years, 551–552, 605
  transmission of, 549–550
  types of, 550
  typical lesions of, 548
  vaccine against, development of, 553
Humeral length, fetal, in Down syndrome, 872
Hybrid Capture II, 403–404, 552
Hybridization, 1044. *See also specific types*
Hydatidiform moles, 467–468
  classification of, 467, 467t
  clinical features of, 467t
  co-existent fetus with, 470–471
  complete, 467, 467t, 1033
  diagnosis of, 467–469
  evacuation of
    management after, 468–470
    methods for, 469
    monitoring after, 470
    prophylactic chemotherapy after, 470
  future pregnancies after, 470
  genetics of, 1033

Hydatidiform moles *(continued)*
  human chorionic gonadotropin values in, 467–471
  incidence of, 466–467
  malignant sequelae of, 467–468. *See also* Gestational trophoblastic disease, malignant
  management of, 469–470
  medical complications of, 467, 469–470
  oral contraception after, 470
  partial, 467, 467t
  pathology of, 467t
  pulmonary complications of, 469
  Rh D alloimmunization in, 469, 893
Hydralazine, for preeclampsia, 448, 448b
Hydranencephaly, in aneuploidy, 869t
Hydration
  and course of labor, 483
  for preterm labor prevention, 673
  for regional analgesia, 767
Hydrocephalus, in aneuploidy, 869t
Hydromorphone, postoperative use of, 774
Hydrops, in aneuploidy, 869t
Hydrops fetalis, parvovirus B19 infection and, 811, 814
17 α-Hydroxyprogesterone caproate (17P), for preterm birth prevention, 260–261
5-Hydroxytryptamine 3 agonists, for nausea and vomiting of pregnancy, 745, 747t
Hydroxyurea, for cervical cancer, 459
Hydroxyzine, for nausea and vomiting of pregnancy, 747t
Hygroscopic dilators, for cervical ripening, 563, 566, 568
Hymen, imperforate, versus vaginal agenesis, 139
Hyperandrogenism
  differential diagnosis of, 824–825
  in polycystic ovary syndrome, 823–824
Hypercarbia, 257
Hypercoagulable states, 880, 881t
  and deep vein thrombosis, 880, 884
  and oral contraception use, 943
  in pregnancy, 961–962, 962b
  and recurrent pregnancy loss, 684, 688
  and thromboembolism, in pregnancy, 961, 963–965
Hyperemesis gravidarum, 741–749. *See also* Nausea, of pregnancy
Hyperglycemia
  and congenital anomalies, 840
  in pregestational diabetes, 839–840
Hypergonadotropic hypoestrogenic anovulation, 654–655
Hyperhomocystinemia, 880, 881t
Hypericum perforatum (St. John's wort), 1007–1008

Hyperinsulinemia, in polycystic ovary syndrome, 824
Hyperprolactinemia
  ovulation induction in, 656–657, 659–660
  in ovulatory dysfunction, 624, 654–655
  in polycystic ovary syndrome, 825
Hypersplenism, anovulatory bleeding in, 625
Hypertension
  chronic
    oral contraception and, 938
    in pregnancy, 418–424
      adjunctive tests in, 420
      agents contraindicated in, 422
      background of, 418–420
      clinical considerations and recommendations in, 420–424
      clinical tests in, 420
      definition of, 418–419
      diabetes mellitus and, 839
      diagnostic criteria for, 418, 419b
      documentation of, 418–419
      effects of, 419–420
      fetal surveillance in, 422
      intrapartum concerns in, 423
      physiologic changes of pregnancy and, 420
      versus preeclampsia, 419, 423
      timing of delivery in, 422–423
      treatment of, 421–422
  essential, in pregnancy, evaluation of, 420–421
  pregnancy-induced
    air travel contraindicated with, 7
    definition of, 444
    in hydatidiform mole, 468–469
    in multiple gestation, 729
    obesity and, 142–143
    thrombocytopenia in, 953, 957
Hyperthermia, exercise-induced, teratogenicity of, 54
Hyperthyroidism
  definition of, 971
  in hydatidiform mole, 469
  and nausea and vomiting of pregnancy, 748, 975–976
  and osteoporosis, 790
  and ovulatory dysfunction, 654
  in pregnancy, 972–973
    differential diagnosis of, 973
    etiology of, 973
    fetal and neonatal effects of, 972–973
    laboratory tests in, 974
    medications for, 974–975
    signs and symptoms of, 972
Hypnosis, for nausea and vomiting of pregnancy, 749
Hypoglycemia, in pregestational diabetes, 839

Hypoglycemic agents, oral
   for gestational diabetes, 524
   for pregestational diabetes, during
      pregnancy, 841–842
Hypogonadotropic hypogonadism,
      654–655, 657*f*
Hypotension
   oxytocin and, 567
   regional analgesia and, 767, 768*t*
Hypothalamic amenorrhea, 654–655
Hypothyroidism
   congenital
      and cretinism, 973
      incidence of, 973
      newborn screening for, 132–133,
         973
   definition of, 971
   and ovulatory dysfunction, 654
   in pregnancy, 973–974
      differential diagnosis of, 973–974
      etiology of, 973–974
      fetal and neonatal effects of, 973
      laboratory tests in, 974
      medications for, 974–975
      signs and symptoms of, 973
   and recurrent pregnancy loss, 687
Hypoxemia, and fetal heart rate,
      337–338
Hypoxia
   air travel and, 8
   Apgar score and, 257–258
   in respiratory distress syndrome, 268
Hypoxic event, sufficient to cause cerebral
      palsy, 95, 95*b*
Hysterectomy
   for anovulatory bleeding, 627–628
   antibiotic prophylaxis in, 348–349,
      349*t*, 350
   for cervical cancer, 456–457, 461
   for cervical intraepithelial neoplasia,
      612
   for chronic pelvic pain, 434–435
   for endometrial cancer, 637
   endometrial cancer findings in, 636
   for endometriosis, 713–714
   for hydatidiform mole, 470
   infections associated with, 348–349
   for leiomyoma, versus myomectomy,
      929–930
   for nonmetastatic gestational tro-
      phoblastic disease, 473–474
   prophylactic oophorectomy with, 906
   tubal sterilization and, 379
   vaginal
      antibiotic prophylaxis in, 349*t*, 350
      for endometrial cancer, 637
      laparoscopically assisted, 13–14
Hysterosalpingography
   antibiotic prophylaxis in, 349*t*, 350
   in cervical insufficiency, 410
   of uterine anatomic anomalies, 686

Hysteroscope(s), 1046–1047
   continuous flow, 1046
   flexible, 1046
   operative, 1047
   rigid, 1046
Hysteroscopic-assisted endometrial abla-
      tion, 627–628
Hysteroscopy, 1046–1049
   antibiotic prophylaxis in, 349*t*,
      350–351
   carbon dioxide gas for, 1047
   complications of, 1048
   contraindications to, 1047
   diagnostic, 1046
   distending media for, 1047
   embolization in, 1049
   fluid media for, 1047
      high-viscosity, 1047
      low-viscosity, electrolyte-poor, 1047
      low-viscosity electrolyte, 1047
   fluid overload in, 1048
   hemorrhage in, 1048
   instrumentation for, 1046–1047
   for leiomyoma, 928, 930
   operative, 1046
   perforation in, 1048–1049
   preoperative considerations in, 1047
   of uterine anatomic anomalies, 686–687

I

Ibuprofen, for intrauterine device insertion,
      583
ICD-9-CM Coding Clinic, 90
ICSI. *See* Intracytoplasmic sperm injec-
      tion
Idiopathic thrombocytopenic purpura
   anovulatory bleeding in, 625
   in pregnancy, 951–953
      diagnosis of, 952
      epidemiology of, 952
      fetal and neonatal intracranial hem-
         orrhage in, 953
      fetal platelet count in, 955
      fetal thrombocytopenia in, 953, 955
      neonatal care in, 955
      pathophysiology of, 952
      prevention of hemorrhage in, 955
      specialized care for, 954
Idoxifene, 912–913
Illicit drug use, 15–23. *See also*
      Substance abuse
Imaging studies. *See also specific types*
   compensation for, 164
   education for, 163
   in fetal lung maturity assessment,
      267–268, 271
   performance and interpretation of,
      163–164
   in pregnancy, 71–74, 981–989
   timeliness of, 163–164
Imipenem, pharmacokinetics of, 899

Imipramine, for chronic pelvic pain, 432
Imiquimod, for human papillomavirus
      infection, 554
Immune globulins, during pregnancy,
      88*t*–89*t*
Immune thrombocytopenic purpura. *See*
      Idiopathic thrombocytopenic
      purpura
Immunization. *See also specific types*
   periodic assessments of
      ages 13–18 years, 191
      ages 19–39 years, 192
      ages 40–64 years, 193
      ages 65 and older, 194
   during postpartum period, 84
   preconceptional, 84
   during pregnancy, 84, 85*t*–89*t*, 103–104
Immunocompromised states. *See also*
      Human immunodeficiency virus
      infection
   causes of, 30, 32*b*
   and human papillomavirus infection, 30
Immunofluorescence assay, for human
      immunodeficiency virus, 173
Immunoglobulin A, in colostrum,
      274–275
Impedance plethysmography, in deep vein
      thrombosis, 880, 965
Imperforate hymen, versus vaginal agene-
      sis, 139
The Importance of Newborn Screening
      (March of Dimes), 133
Imprinting, 167, 1032–1033, 1044
Inactivated bacterial vaccines, during
      pregnancy, 87*t*
Incidence, definition of, 335
Incontinence, urinary, 991–1000
Indigestion, in ovarian cancer, 241
Indirect Coombs' test, 290–291, 893–894
Indomethacin, for preterm labor, 675*t*
Induction of labor. *See* Labor induction
Induction of ovulation. *See* Ovulation
      induction
Infant mortality
   by birth weight, 803–804, 804*f*–805*f*
   ethnic disparities in, 200, 200*t*
   by gestational age, 803–804, 804*f*–805*f*
   racial and ethnic disparities in, 200,
      200*t*
   at threshold of viability, 803–804
Infection control
   in sonohysterography, 1052
   in ultrasonography, 985–986
Infertility. *See also* Assisted reproductive
      technology
   female
      endometriosis and, 707, 709–710,
         712
      ovulatory dysfunction and, 653–662
      uterine artery embolization and,
         262–263

Infertility *(continued)*
genetic screening and testing in, 1042
male
perinatal risks associated with, 166–167
testing for, 657
Influenza treatment, during pregnancy, 103–104
Influenza vaccine
indications for, 196*t*
during pregnancy, 86*t*, 103–104
Information bias, 334
Information sharing, physician–patient, 157
Informed consent
for carrier screening, 181, 1041
in maternal decision making, 114–116
physician–patient communication and, 158
from partner, 154–155
for research, 67–68
Informed refusal, 105–106, 116–117
Inhalational anesthesia, 769
Inheritance
mendelian, 1029–1030
mitochondrial, 1033, 1044
multifactorial, 1034–1035, 1034*b*, 1044
nonmendelian, 1031–1035
polygenic, 1034–1035, 1044
Inhibin B, in ovulatory dysfunction, 655
Iniencephaly, 755*t*
Insertion, chromosomal, 1044
Institute of Medicine (IOM), prenatal weight gain guidelines of, 143
Institutional Review Boards (IRBs), 67–70, 155
Insulin, in anovulatory bleeding, 625
Insulin resistance
in polycystic ovary syndrome, 824, 826
in pregnancy, 837–838
Insulin-sensitizing agents
for hirsutism, 830–831
for ovulation induction, 829
for polycystic ovary syndrome, 827–831
Insulin therapy
commonly used agents in, 838, 838*t*
continuous subcutaneous, in pregnancy, 841
for diabetic ketoacidosis, in pregnancy, 840*b*
for gestational diabetes, 523–524
during labor, 842–843, 842*b*
longer acting, 838
for pregestational diabetes, 838–839, 838*t*, 841–843
short- or rapid-acting, 838
Intact dilation and extraction (intact D & X), policy statement on, 1059–1061

Interdepartmental relationships, policy statement on, 1057–1058
Interference from others, as barrier to care, 306
Interferon alfa, for hepatitis, 322–323
Intermittent auscultation, versus electronic fetal heart rate monitoring, 574–575
Internal iliac thrombosis, diagnosis of, 880
International Federation of Gynecology and Obstetrics (FIGO)
cervical cancer staging system of, 454–456, 455*b*
endometrial cancer staging system of, 633, 634*t*
gestational trophoblastic disease criteria of, 468
gestational trophoblastic disease scoring system of, 472, 472*t*
Interstitial cystitis
chronic pelvic pain in, 430, 432
diagnostic criteria for, 432
evaluation of, 432
Interstitial cystitis symptom index, 432
Intervention studies, 330–331
Intimate partner violence, 298, 307
Intracranial hemorrhage, fetal and neonatal
in idiopathic thrombocytopenic purpura, 953, 955
in neonatal alloimmune thrombocytopenia, 952
prevention of, 955
with vacuum extraction, 782–783, 783*t*
Intracranial pressure, in neural tube defects, 755
Intracytoplasmic sperm injection (ICSI), 165–7
Intrauterine device (IUD), 581–587
and actinomycosis, 585
background of, 581–583
and bacterial vaginosis, 584
candidate selection for, 582, 583*b*
clinical considerations and recommendations, 583–587
contraindications to, 582, 583*b*
copper versus levonorgestrel system, 582, 582*t*
currently available, 582
and ectopic pregnancy, 585
effectiveness of, versus tubal sterilization, 377–378
for emergency contraception, 494, 587
historical perspective on, 581–582
insertion of, 583
antibiotic prophylaxis in, 349*t*, 351, 584–585
difficulties in, 584
sexually transmitted disease screening before, 584

Intrauterine device (IUD) *(continued)*
mechanism of action, 582
and menstrual flow, 586
in nulliparous women, 584
and pelvic inflammatory disease, 583–584
removal of
difficulties in, 584
in menopausal women, 586
and pregnancy outcome, 585–586
safety of, versus tubal sterilization, 378
use during breastfeeding, 281
Intrauterine fetal transfusion, in isoimmunization, 294
Intrauterine growth restriction (IUGR), 591–597
amniotic fluid volume in, 595, 987
antenatal diagnosis of, 594–595
antiphospholipid syndrome and, 357, 360, 592
background of, 591–595
chronic hypertension and, 419, 422
clinical considerations and recommendations in, 595–597
clinical evaluation for, 594–595
definitions of, 591–592, 987
delivery indications in, 595, 597
diabetes mellitus and, 841
ethnic disparities in, 592
etiology of, 592–593, 596–597
fetal morbidity and mortality in, 593–594, 594*t*
fetal surveillance in, 596
genetic disorders and, 593, 596–597
geographic disparities in, 592
infections and, 593
interventions for, 596
malnutrition and, 593
maternal exercise and, 54
maternal medical conditions and, 592
maternal smoking and, 228, 592–593, 596
monitoring of, 595–596
multiple gestation and, 593, 727, 727*t*, 730, 732
neonatal mortality in, 594
placental disease and, 592–593
preeclampsia and, 592
racial disparities in, 592
risk factors for, 592, 592*b*, 594
screening for, 595
substance abuse and, 592–593
teratogen exposure and, 593
ultrasonography in, 595–596, 987–988, 988*t*
umbilical artery Doppler velocimetry in, 343–345, 595, 987–988
Intravenous immunoglobulin (IVIG)
for antiphospholipid syndrome, 362
for neonatal alloimmune thrombocytopenia, 956

Intravenous immunoglobulin (IVIG)
    (continued)
    for recurrent pregnancy loss, 689
    for thrombocytopenia, in pregnancy, 954
Intravenous pyelography, fetal radiation
    exposure from, 73*b*
Intravesical potassium sensitivity test, 432
Intron, 1044
Invasive mole, 468
Inversion, chromosomal, 1044
Investigational studies, uncontrolled, 332
In vitro fertilization, 165–167
Iodine, and thyroid function, 972–974
IOM. *See* Institute of Medicine
Ionizing radiation
    and carcinogenesis, 72–73
    and cell death, 72
    from computed tomography, 72
    fetal exposure to, from common proce-
        dures, 72, 73*b*
    measures of, 72, 72*t*
    teratogenicity of, 72, 317*t*
    from X-rays, during pregnancy, 71–74
Ipriflavone, for osteoporosis, 796
IRBs. *See* Institutional Review Boards
Iron chelation therapy, for thalassemia,
    545
Iron supplementation, for breastfed
    infants, 286
Irregular bleeding, emergency contracep-
    tion and, 491
Irritable bowel syndrome
    chronic pelvic pain in, 430–431
    diagnostic criteria for, 430–431, 431*b*
Irving method, for tubal sterilization, 376
Isoflavones, 1006
    for heart disease prevention, 1010
    for menopausal symptoms, 1007–1009
    for osteoporosis, 796
    for osteoporosis prevention, 1010
Isoflurane, 769
Isoimmunization, in pregnancy, 290–295
    amniocentesis in, 292
    ancillary testing in, 294
    antibody titers in, 291–292
    clinically significant antibodies in, 291,
        291*t*
    clinical management of, 291–294
    intrauterine fetal transfusion in, 294
    Liley graph in, 292, 293*f*
    versus normal hematologic values, 292,
        293*t*
    percutaneous umbilical cord blood
        sampling in, 292
    perinatal outcome in, 294
    Rh D, 290–292, 889–894. *See also* Rh
        D alloimmunization
Isotretinoin, teratogenicity of, 316*t*
IUD. *See* Intrauterine device
IUGR. *See* Intrauterine growth restriction
IVIG. *See* Intravenous immunoglobulin

J

J. C. Lewis Health Center, 79*b*
Jaundice
    in cytomegalovirus infection, 321*t*, 811
    in hepatitis, 320, 321*t*
    in pregnancy, differential diagnosis of,
        320, 321*t*
Jejunoileal bypass, 143–144
Jews, Ashkenazi
    Canavan disease in, 178–181, 179*t*,
        180*b*, 216–217
    carrier screening for, 178–181, 179*t*,
        216–219, 1042
    clinical features of diseases common
        among, 180*b*
    cystic fibrosis in, 178–181, 179*t*,
        253–255, 254*t*
    Tay-Sachs disease in, 178–181, 179*t*,
        180*b*, 218–219
Johns Hopkins AIDS Service, 227
Justice, vii
    in alcohol abuse, 17–18, 20
    in drug abuse, 17–18, 20
    in maternal decision making, 116

K

Kanamycin, teratogenicity of, 316*t*
Karyotype
    in aneuploidy, 869, 873
    definition of, 1044
    in intrauterine growth restriction,
        596–597
    in monochorionic twin gestation, 873
    in recurrent pregnancy loss, 683, 686
    spectral, 1045
Keepsakes, obstetric ultrasonography for,
    135–136, 986
Kegel exercises, for urinary incontinence,
    994, 997
Kell antibodies, 291, 291*t*
Kelley, Florence, 113
Ketamine, chronic hypertension and, 423
Ketorolac, for preterm labor, 675*t*
Kick counts, 338, 344
Kidd antibodies, 291*t*
Kielland's forceps rotation, 785
Kleihauer-Betke test, 301, 893–894
Knife wounds, 299
Kyphosis, chronic pelvic pain in, 431

L

Labetalol
    for hypertension, in pregnancy, 422–423
    for preeclampsia, 448, 448*b*
Labor
    active management of, 483
    active phase of, 479
    ambulation and course of, 482
    amniotomy and, 484–485
    antibiotic prophylaxis in, 897–902

Labor *(continued)*
    arrest of, 480
        cesarean delivery for, 481
        diagnosis of, 2-hour rule for,
            480–481
        requiring delivery, criteria for,
            480–481
        risk factors for, 481
        second-stage, 480
        support from allied personnel in, 481
    caregiver support in, 481, 483
    definition of, 479
    failure to progress in, 480
    hydration and, 483
    latent phase of, 479
    pain in, 765
    pain relief during, 153, 765–774. *See*
        also Analgesia, obstetric;
        Anesthesia, obstetric
    protraction of, 480
    spinal cord injuries and, 148
    trial of. *See also* Vaginal birth after
        cesarean delivery
        after myomectomy, 931
        candidates for, 1016–1017
        cost-effectiveness of, 1018
        risks and benefits of, 1017–1018
        success rate for, 1017
Laboratory testing, in periodic assess-
    ments
    ages 13–18 years, 191
    ages 19–39 years, 192
    ages 40–64 years, 193
    ages 65 and older, 194
Labor augmentation
    amniotomy for, 484–485
    contraindications to, 480
    definition of, 480
    dystocia and, 479–485
    indications for, 480
    oxytocin for, 480–481, 484
        epidural analgesia and, 771
        fetal monitoring with, 485
        low-dose versus high-dose regimens,
            483, 483*t*
    in twin gestation, 484
    in vaginal birth after cesarean delivery,
        1018–1019
Labor induction, 562–568
    amniotomy for, 484–485, 562–564,
        566–567
    background of, 562–564
    clinical considerations and recommen-
        dations in, 564–568
    contraindications to, 564
    criteria for, 564–565
    gestational age assessment for, 564,
        564*b*
    indications for, 564
    intact versus ruptured membranes in,
        567–568

Labor induction *(continued)*
  in intrauterine demise, 568
  for macrosomia, 512–513, 922
  membrane stripping for, 562–563, 567
  methods of, 563–564
    complications of, 566–567
    cost-effectiveness of, 568
  misoprostol for, 101–102, 129–130, 203–204, 563–568
    complications with, 565–566
    cost-effectiveness of, 568
    Food and Drug Administration labeling on, 129–130
    in fetal demise, 568
    in postterm pregnancy, 668
    recommendations on, 130, 130b
    Searle's warning on, response to, 203–204
  oxytocin for, 562–568
    administration of, 567
    complications with, 566–567
    dosage of, 567, 567t
    in fetal demise, 568
  prostaglandin E₂ for, 563–568
    administration of, 565
    adverse effects of, 565
    cost-effectiveness of, 568
    in fetal demise, 568
    fetal surveillance with, 566
    in postterm pregnancy, 668
    in postterm pregnancy, 667–668
  in premature rupture of membranes, 567–568, 850–851
  and shoulder dystocia, 922
  situations necessitating precaution in, 564
  for vaginal birth after cesarean delivery, 99–100, 1018
Lactational amenorrhea method, 282–283, 283f
Lactic acidemia, 257, 660
Lamellar body(ies), 268
Lamellar body counts, 270t, 271
Laminaria, for cervical ripening, 563, 566, 568
Langer-Giedion syndrome, 1040t
Language barriers, 306
Laparoscopically assisted vaginal hysterectomy, 13–14, 350
Laparoscopic myomectomy, 928–929
Laparoscopy
  antibiotic prophylaxis in, 349t, 350
  in cervical cancer, 454
  in chronic pelvic pain, 432
  in endometrial cancer, 637
  in endometriosis, 48–49, 432, 710
  in müllerian aplasia, 139, 141
  for tubal sterilization, 375
Laparotomy, antibiotic prophylaxis in, 349t, 350

Large for gestational age. *See also* Macrosomia
  definition of, 507
  maternal obesity and, 144
Laryngeal papillomatosis, 556
Laser therapy
  for cervical intraepithelial neoplasia, 610
  for endometriosis, in adolescents, 50
  for hirsutism, 831
  for human papillomavirus infection, 554–555
Latch-on, for breastfeeding, 280, 284, 284b
Latex allergy, neural tube defects and, 759
Lathrop, Julia, 113
Lead, teratogenicity of, 315t
Leak point pressure measurement, 996
Lecithin, 268
Lecithin–sphingomyelin ratio, 269, 270t
  blood in amniotic fluid and, 269
  determination of, 269
  meconium in amniotic fluid and, 269
  storage conditions and, 269
LEEP. *See* Loop electrosurgical excision procedure
Leiomyoma(s), 927–933
  adjunctive medical treatment for, 928, 930
    intraoperative, 930
    preoperative, 930
  background of, 927–928
  clinical considerations and recommendations for, 929–933
  endometrial ablation for, 928, 930
  expectant management of, versus surgical removal, 931–932
  hormone therapy and, 931–932
  hysteroscopic procedures for, 928, 930
  and lipid disorders, 940–941
  long-term morbidity in, 932
  in menopausal women, 931–932
  myolysis for, 928
  myomectomy for, 928
    abdominal, 929
    versus hysterectomy, 929–930
    hysteroscopic, 930
    laparoscopic, 928–929
    trial of labor versus cesarean delivery after, 931
  oral contraception and, 940
  pregnancy after, 931–932
  procedures under development for, 928–929
  and recurrent pregnancy loss, 684
  size of, 928
  surgical alternatives for, 927–933
  symptoms of, 927–928
  uterine artery embolization for, 262–263, 928

Length of hospital stay, for gynecologic procedures, 107
Leopold maneuvers, for fetal weight estimate, 510–511
Lesbians, sexually transmitted disease transmission among, 222
Lessina, 491t
Leukemia, anovulatory bleeding in, 625–626
Leukocyte immunization, paternal, for recurrent pregnancy loss, 688
Leuprolide, 433, 828t
Levlen, 491t
Levlite, 491t
Levobupivacaine, epidural, 767
Levonorgestrel
  during breastfeeding, 281–282
  emergency use of, 490
Levonorgestrel intrauterine system, 582, 582t
  for menorrhagia, 586
  and menstrual flow, 586
Levora, 491t
Levormeloxifene, 912–913
Levothyroxine, for hypothyroidism, 975
Lewis antibodies, 291
Liability
  in gynecologic-only practice, 198
  in tubal ligation, 252
Liability litigation
  confidentiality in, 43
  coping with stress of, 42–43
  emotional responses to, 42
  family communication about, 43
Libido, loss of, botanicals for, 1008–1010
Lidocaine
  for herpes simplex virus infections, 534
  obstetric use of, 769
Ligation, for tubal sterilization, 376
Lignins, 1006
Lignocaine, for intrauterine device insertion, 583
Liley graph, 292, 293f
Limb reduction
  in aneuploidy, 869t
  chorionic villus sampling and, 872
Linkage, definition of, 1044
Linkage analysis, 1038–1039
Lipid disorder(s)
  oral contraception and, 940–941
  polycystic ovary syndrome and, 826
Lipid profile assessment, indications for, 196t
Lisinopril, teratogenicity of, 422
Listeria monocytogenes, and recurrent pregnancy loss, 684
Literacy, health, 158

Lithium
contraindicated during breastfeeding, 277t
teratogenicity of, 315t
Liver, in preeclampsia, 446
Liver enzyme inducers, interaction with oral contraception, 942
Live virus vaccines, during pregnancy, 85t–86t
Local anesthesia, obstetric, 769
Loop electrosurgical excision procedure (LEEP), 457, 606, 608, 610–612
Lo/Ovral, 491t
Lordosis, exaggerated, chronic pelvic pain in, 431
Lovenox. See Enoxaparin sodium
Low birth weight
extremely
antenatal corticosteroids in, 806
and cerebral palsy, 804–805, 806t
clinical considerations and recommendations in, 803–807
mode of delivery in, 806
morbidity associated with, counseling about, 804
mortality in, counseling on, 803–804, 804f–805f
perinatal care in, 802–807
resuscitation and support in, 806–807
homelessness and, 78
hyperthyroidism and, 972
hypothyroidism and, 973
nausea and vomiting of pregnancy and, 744
Low forceps delivery, 781b
Low-grade squamous intraepithelial lesion (LSIL), 400, 551, 603, 604b, 607–608
Low-molecular-weight heparin
anesthesia concerns with, 882, 884, 966–967
for deep vein thrombosis prophylaxis, 882–884
and epidural or spinal hematoma, 772, 882, 966–967
during pregnancy, 211–212, 962–968
Low-Ogestrel, 491t
LSIL. See Low-grade squamous intraepithelial lesion
Lung development, fetal, 268
Lung maturity, fetal. See Fetal lung maturity
Lung profile, 272
Lupus anticoagulant antibodies, 357–361, 361t, 685, 688
Luteal phase deficiency, 655
evaluation for, 687
and premenstrual syndrome, 862
and recurrent pregnancy loss, 683, 687

Luteinizing hormone
in anovulatory bleeding, 625
in ovulation induction, 655–656
in ovulation testing, 653
in ovulatory dysfunction, 654
Lutera, 491t
Lutheran antibodies, 291t
Lydia Pinkham's Vegetable Compound, 1007
Lymphangiography, in cervical cancer, 454–455
Lynch syndrome II, ovarian cancer in, 907–908
Lynestrenol, 434

M
Macrosomia, 507–514
background of, 507–508
cesarean delivery for, 509–513, 922–923
clinical considerations and recommendations in, 510–514
definition of, 507–508
diagnosis of, 509
ethnic disparities in, 509
fetal morbidity and mortality in, 510
fetal weight estimates in, accuracy of, 510–511
frequency of occurrence, 508
gender differences in, 509
gestational age and, 509
interventions for, 511
labor induction for, 512–513, 922
management of labor and delivery in, 513
maternal diabetes mellitus and, 507–509, 511, 519, 525–526
maternal morbidity in, 509–510
maternal obesity and, 142–144, 508–509, 511
operative vaginal delivery for, 508, 508f, 513, 782
postterm pregnancy and, 666
racial disparities in, 509
risk factors for, 508–509
risks associated with, 509–510
and shoulder dystocia, 508, 508f, 510, 513, 782, 922–923
ultrasonography in, 510–511, 989
vaginal birth after cesarean section in, 1016
Magnesium
for chronic pelvic pain, 436
for premenstrual syndrome, 861
Magnesium sulfate
and fetal heart rate, 576, 576t
for preeclampsia and eclampsia, 423, 447–448
for preterm labor, 675, 675t, 676
Magnetic field therapy, for chronic pelvic pain, 436

Magnetic resonance angiography, in pulmonary embolism, 966
Magnetic resonance imaging
in breast cancer evaluation, 390
in cervical cancer, 454–455
in deep vein thrombosis, 965
in endometriosis, 708
during pregnancy, 73
Magnet therapy, 38
Maine Women's Health Study, 434
Malabsorptive procedures, in obesity surgery, 143–144
Malaria, and intrauterine growth restriction, 596
Male factor infertility, perinatal risks associated with, 166–167
Malmstrom cup, for vacuum extraction, 784–785
Malnutrition, and intrauterine growth restriction, 593
Mammography
fetal radiation exposure from, 73b
indications for, 196t
magnified, 205–206
screening, 386–393
abnormal, follow-up of, 61
adverse consequences of, 389
before age 40, 392
background of, 386–390
current guidelines for, 386–387
false-positive, 389
frequency and timing of, 388–389, 391
meta-analyses of, 388
psychosocial effects of, 389
radiation risk in, 389
rationale for, 387–388
recommendations on, 205
upper age range for, 392, 392f
value of, studies documenting, 387–388
Manual healing methods, 38
Maple syrup urine disease, newborn screening for, 132–133
March of Dimes, on newborn screening, 133
Marfan syndrome, paternal age and, 5
Maryland Women's Health Study, 434–435
Massachusetts Teratogen Information Service, 313
Mastitis, 284–285
abscess with, 284–285
causative agents of, 284
clinical features of, 284
differential diagnosis of, 284
treatment of, 284–285
Materiality of patient viewpoint, 105–106
Maternal and Child Health Bureau, 113

Maternal decision making, 111–119
  bodily integrity in, 116
  coercive and punitive actions against, 116–119
    American College of Obstetricians and Gynecologists opposition to, 119
    counterproductive effects of, 118
    criminalization of behavior by, 119
    "moral failings" viewpoint of, 117–118
    vulnerable women affected by, 118–119
  ethical considerations in, 113–118
  informed consent in, 114–116
  informed refusal in, 116–117
  limitations of obstetrics and, 116–117
  recent cases on, 112
  recommendations on, 118–119
Maternal–fetal surgery, 113
  fetal risks in, 760
  maternal risks in, 113, 760
  for neural tube defects, 760
Maternal mortality
  anesthesia-related, 769
  ethnic disparities in, 200
  nausea and vomiting of pregnancy and, 744
  racial disparities in, 200
  trauma and, 297–298
Maternal serum analytes, 870
Maternal serum screening. *See also specific types*
  for chromosome abnormalities, 58–60, 868–870, 873
  combined with nuchal translucency screening, 59–60
  for Down syndrome, 868–870, 873
  maternal age and, 873
Maturation, fetal, antenatal corticosteroids for, 11–12. *See also* Fetal lung maturity
Mayer–Rokitansky–Küster–Hauser syndrome, 138–141
McDonald procedure, of cervical cerclage, 411
McRoberts maneuver, 921–923
M-cup, for vacuum extraction, 784–785
Mean corpuscular volume
  normal fetal values of, 293*t*
  in thalassemia, 542
Measles–mumps–rubella (MMR) vaccine
  during breastfeeding, 210
  indications for, 196*t*
  interval from receiving until pregnancy, 210
  during postpartum period, 84, 210
  during pregnancy, 85*t*, 210
  shortage of, 210

Mechanical index, in ultrasonography, 981–982
Meclizine, for nausea and vomiting of pregnancy, 747*t*
Meconium, and fetal lung maturity tests, 269–271
Medical liability litigation
  confidentiality in, 43
  coping with stress of, 42–43
  emotional responses to, 42
  family communication about, 43
Medical literature, in development of American College of Obstetricians and Gynecologists guidelines, 329–335
Medical Research Council Vitamin Study Research Group, 756
Medication
  physician–patient communication about, 158
  safe practices for, 161
Mediterranean ancestry, and hemoglobinopathies, 540–541, 542*f*
Medium chain acyl-CoA dehydrogenase deficiency, newborn screening for, 132–133
Medroxyprogesterone acetate
  for add-back therapy, with gonadotropin-releasing hormone agonists, 50
  for chronic pelvic pain, 434
  for endometrioma, 713
  for endometriosis, 49–50, 434, 709–710
  for osteoporosis, 793
  for polycystic ovary syndrome, 827
  pregnancy category of, 828*t*
Membrane stripping
  complications of, 567
  for labor induction, 562–563, 567
Menarche, early, and endometriosis, 707
Mendelian disorders, 1029–1030
Meningitis, group B streptococcal disease and, 182–183
Meningocele, 755*t*
Meningococcal vaccine
  for adolescents, 124–126
    Advisory Committee on Immunization Practices, Centers for Disease Control and prevention recommendations on, 125
    American College of Obstetricians and Gynecologists recommendations on, 125–126
  conjugate (MCV4), 124–125
  polysaccharide (MPSV4), 124–125
  during pregnancy, 87*t*
Meningomyelocele, 755, 755*t*
Menometrorrhagia, definition of, 623–624

Menopause
  bone mass loss in, 789
  leiomyomas in, 931–932
  symptom management in
    botanicals for, 1004–1011
    complementary and alternative medicine for, 1005
    discontent with current pharmaceutical regimens for, 1004
Menorrhagia
  definition of, 623–624
  with leiomyoma, 927
  levonorgestrel intrauterine system for, 586
  surgical treatment of, 627–628
  in women of reproductive age, 625
Menstrual cycle, tubal sterilization and, 375, 379
Menstrual flow
  and endometriosis, 707
  intrauterine devices and, 586
  with leiomyoma, 927
Menstrual magnification, 860
Meperidine
  adverse effects of, 770
  and breastfeeding, 774
  and fetal heart rate, 576, 576*t*, 770
  parenteral, obstetric, 765–766, 766*t*, 770
  patient-controlled, avoidance of, 774
  transplacental passage of, 770
Mercury, organic, teratogenicity of, 316*t*
Messenger RNA, 1028
Meta-analysis, 332, 333*f*
Metabolic acidemia, 257, 337–338
Metabolic disorders, and recurrent pregnancy loss, 683–684
Metformin
  adverse effects of, 660
  for diabetes mellitus, during pregnancy, 841–842
  for hirsutism, 831
  for ovulation induction, 654, 656, 660–661, 829
  for polycystic ovary syndrome, 654, 656, 660–661, 826, 828–829, 831
  pregnancy category of, 828*t*
Methadone, and intrauterine growth restriction, 593
Methimazole
  contraindicated during breastfeeding, 975
  for hyperthyroidism, 974–975
Methionine, 756–757
Methotrexate
  adverse effects of, 720, 722–723, 722*b*
  contraindicated during breastfeeding, 277*t*

Methotrexate *(continued)*
  for ectopic pregnancy, 720–723
    contraindications to, 721*b*
    cost-effectiveness of, 723
    counseling on, 723, 723*b*
    indications for, 721–722, 721*b*
    potential problems with, 722–723
    protocols for, 722
  for gestational trophoblastic disease
    in high-risk metastatic disease, 474
    in low-risk metastatic disease, 474
    in nonmetastatic disease, 473
    prophylactic use of, 470
    therapeutic use of, 473
  and intrauterine growth restriction, 593
  mechanism of action, 695, 720
  for medical abortion, 695–696, 696*t*
  teratogenicity of, 315*t*, 701
Methylation, DNA, 1028–1029, 1044
Methyldopa, for chronic hypertension, in
    pregnancy, 422
Methylenetetrahydrofolate reductase,
    757
Methylprednisolone, for nausea and vom-
    iting of pregnancy, 745–748,
    746*f*, 747*t*
Metoclopramide, for nausea and vomiting
    of pregnancy, 745, 746*f*, 747*t*
Metronidazole
  oral contraception use with, 942
  prophylactic use of, 349*t*, 354
Metrorrhagia
  definition of, 623–624
  in women of reproductive age, 625
Mexican yam, for menopausal symptoms,
    1008, 1010
Microarray technology, 1040
Microdeletion, chromosomal, 1031,
    1039–1040, 1040*t*
Micronized progesterone, 828*t*
Middle cerebral artery Doppler velocime-
    try, 343–345
Midforceps delivery, 781*b*, 785
Midwives, certified, practice relationships
    with, policy statement on, 1068
Mifepristone, 694–695
  for labor induction, in fetal demise,
    568
  for leiomyoma, 928–929
  mechanism of action, 694
  for medical abortion, 694–695
    alternative regimens for, 695
    confirmation of complete result, 700
    contraindications to, 699
    failure of, management of, 698–699
    Food and Drug Administration-
      approved protocol for, 695
    gestational age and, 699
    infection risk with, 699
    misoprostol use with, 695, 696*t*, 697
  medical applications of, 694–695

Migraine headaches, and oral contracep-
    tion use, 939–940
Milk ducts, clogged, 284
Miller-Dieker syndrome, 1040*t*
Mind–body interventions, 37
Minilaparotomy, for tubal sterilization,
    375
Misoprostol, 695
  adverse effects of, 565–566
  fetal surveillance with, 566
  for geriatric ulcer prevention, 129–130,
    203–204
  for labor induction, 101–102, 129–130,
    130*b*, 203–204, 563
    complications with, 565–566
    cost-effectiveness of, 568
    in fetal demise, 568
    in postterm pregnancy, 668
  for medical abortion, 203–204,
    695–697, 696*t*
    confirmation of complete result, 700
    contraindications to, 699
    failure of, management of, 698–699
    gestational age and, 699
    infection risk with, 699
    methotrexate use with, 695–696,
      696*t*
    mifepristone use with, 695, 696*t*,
      697
    tamoxifen use with, 695
  oral, 695
  pharmacokinetics of, 695
  during pregnancy, Food and Drug
    Administration labeling on,
    129–130
  Searle's drug warning on, response to,
    203–204
  teratogenicity of, 701
  vaginal administration of, 695
Missense mutation, 1029, 1044
Mitochondrial inheritance, 1033, 1044
MNS antibodies, 291*t*
Molar pregnancy. *See* Hydatidiform moles
Molecular diagnostic testing, 1035–1043
  accuracy of, 1041
  applications in obstetrics and gyne-
    cology, 1041–1042
  in Ashkenazi Jews, 178–181, 179*t*,
    216–219, 1042
  indications for, 1040–1041
  limitations of, 1041
Monochorionic twin pregnancy, 728, 730,
    733–734, 873
Mononucleosis, jaundice in, 321*t*
Monosomy, 1031
Mood disturbances, botanicals for,
    1007–1009
Morbidity, leading causes of, 191–194,
    197*b*
Morning-after pill. *See* Emergency con-
    traception

Morning sickness. *See* Nausea, of preg-
    nancy
Morphine
  and breastfeeding, 774
  and fetal heart rate, 576, 576*t*
  parenteral, obstetric, 766*t*
  patient-controlled, 774
  postoperative use of, 774
Mortality. *See also* Fetal death (loss);
    Stillbirths
  infant
    by birth weight, 803–804, 804*f*–805*f*
    ethnic disparities in, 200, 200*t*
    by gestational age, 803–804,
      804*f*–805*f*
    racial disparities in, 200, 200*t*
    at threshold of viability, 803–804
  leading causes of, 191–194, 197*b*
  maternal
    anesthesia-related, 769
    ethnic disparities in, 200
    nausea and vomiting of pregnancy
      and, 744
    racial disparities in, 200
    trauma and, 297–298
Mosaicism
  definition of, 1044
  germline, 1033
  placental, and intrauterine growth
    restriction, 592–593
Mother-Infant Rapid Intervention at
    Delivery Study Group, 174,
    176
Mother-to-child transmission
  of cytomegalovirus infection, 811
  of genital herpes, 645–646, 649–650
  of group B streptococcal disease, pre-
    vention of, 182–188
  of hepatitis B, 319
  of hepatitis C, 319
  of hepatitis D, 320
  of hepatitis E, 320
  of hepatitis G, 320
  of human immunodeficiency virus, pre-
    vention of, 172, 174
    scheduled cesarean delivery and,
      213–215
    zidovudine for, 172, 213–214
  of human papillomavirus, 550,
    555–556
  of parvovirus B19 infection, 811
  of toxoplasmosis, 812
  of varicella zoster virus infection,
    812
Motor vehicle crashes, in pregnancy,
    297–298, 301
Movement, fetal
  assessment of, 338, 344
  in biophysical profile, 339–340
  in nonstress test, 339
Moves, frequent, as barrier to care, 306

Mucolipidosis IV
  carrier screening for, 178–181, 179t
  clinical features of, 180b
Müllerian anomalies, and endometriosis, 46, 49
Müllerian aplasia (agenesis), 138–141
  counseling in, 139–140
  diagnosis of, 138–141
  differential diagnosis of, 139
  evaluation of patient with, 139–140
  incidence of, 138
  management of, 138–141
  neovagina creation in
    nonsurgical, 140
    surgical, 140–141
  reproductive potential in, 139–140
  support of "buddies" in, 140
Multifactorial inheritance, 1034–1035, 1034b, 1044
Multiple gestation, 726–735
  acute fatty liver in, 729
  antepartum fetal surveillance in, 733
  assisted reproductive technology and, 166–167, 728
  background of, 727–728
  and cerebral palsy, 727, 727t
  cervical length in, 730–731
  clinical considerations and recommendations in, 730–735
  complications of, 728–730
  death of one fetus in, management of, 732–733
  delivery mode in, 734
  delivery timing in, 734
  discordant growth in, 732
  gestational diabetes in, 728
  home uterine activity monitoring in, 731
  hypertension and preeclampsia in, 729
  intrauterine growth restriction in, 593, 727, 727t, 730, 732
  maternal age and, 728
  morbidity and mortality in, 727, 727t
  and neonatal intensive care stays, 727, 727t
  ovulation induction and, 661
  prenatal diagnosis of, 728
  prenatal screening and diagnosis in, 873
  preterm labor and delivery in, 677, 727
    antenatal corticosteroids for, 732
    management of, 731–732
    prediction of, 730–731
    tocolytic therapy for, 731–732
  prolonging, interventions for, 731
  prophylactic cerclage for, 731
  rare complications of, 734
  reduction of, 730
  rest at home in, 731
  restriction of activities in, 731
  routine hospitalization for, 731

Multiple gestation (continued)
  second-twin delivery in, 733
  selective fetal termination in, 730
  thromboembolism in, 729–730
  vaginal birth after cesarean delivery in, 1017
Multiple Outcomes of Raloxifene Evaluation, 912, 915
Multiplex gene detection analysis, 1037–1038, 1038f
Multivitamins, and prevention of nausea and vomiting of pregnancy, 744
Mumps vaccine
  during postpartum period, 84
  during pregnancy, 85t
Muscular dystrophy, Duchenne, grandfather effect and, 5
Mutation, genetic, 1029
  definition of, 1044
  detection of, 1035–1039
  types of, 1044
Mycoplasma infection
  and preterm labor, 366–367
  and recurrent pregnancy loss, 687–688
Myeloschisis, 755t
Myocardial infarction, oral contraception and, 937–945
Myolysis, for leiomyoma, 928
Myomectomy, for leiomyoma, 928–930
  abdominal, 929
  adjunctive medical treatment with, 931
  versus hysterectomy, 929–930
  hysteroscopic, 930
  laparoscopic, 928–929
  trial of labor versus cesarean delivery after, 931

N

N-acetylaspartic acid, in Canavan disease, 216–217
Nafarelin, 433
Nalbuphine
  adverse effects of, 770
  and fetal heart rate, 576, 576t, 770
  parenteral, obstetric, 765–766, 766t, 770
  for pruritus, 774
  transplacental passage of, 770
Naloxone, for parenteral analgesia toxicity, 770
Naltrexone, for pruritus, 774
National Breast Cancer and Cervical Cancer Early Detection Program, 549
National Commission for the Protection of Human Subjects of Biomedical and Behavioral Research, 68
National Health and Nutrition Examination Survey, 142

National High Blood Pressure Education Program Working Group, 418–419, 421, 444
National Institute of Child Health and Human Development Research Planning Workshop, 573–574
National Institute on Alcohol Abuse and Alcoholism (NIAAA), 16–17, 18b
National Sexually Transmitted Disease Hotline, 227
National Surgical Adjuvant Breast and Bowel Project (NSABP), 913–916
National Women's Health Information Center, 227
Natural killer cells, in recurrent pregnancy loss, 685, 688
Nausea
  emergency contraception and, 491, 493
  medical abortion and, 697, 698t
  of pregnancy, 741–749
    clinical considerations and recommendations in, 744–749
    definition of, 741–742
    diagnosis of, 748
    differential diagnosis of, 742–743, 742b
    enteral or parenteral nutrition for, 748
    etiology of, 743–744
    as evolutionary adaptation, 743
    fetal effects of, 744
    hormones and, 743
    hospitalization for, indications for, 742, 748
    incidence of, 741–742
    laboratory assessment of, 748
    maternal effects of, 744
    nonpharmacologic therapies for, 744–745
    pharmacologic therapies for, 745–748, 746f, 747t
    psychologic theories of, 743
    psychotherapy for, 749
    radiologic assessment of, 748
    risk factors for, 743–744
    thyroid disease and, 748, 975–976
    timing of, 742
Needle biopsy
  of breast mass, 206
  of cervical lesion, 454
Nefazodone, for premenstrual syndrome, 861–862
Negative predictive value, 335
Neisseria meningitidis, 124
  serogroup B, 125
  vaccine against
    for adolescents, 124–126
    during pregnancy, 87t

Nellcor N-400 Fetal Oxygen Saturation Monitoring System, 56–57
Neonatal alloimmune thrombocytopenia, 951–952
  antigen systems in, 952
  evaluation for, 956
  fetal platelet count in, 956
  incidence of, 952
  intracranial hemorrhage in, 952
  obstetric management of, 956–957
  recurrent risk of, 952
Neonatal deaths
  counseling in, 66
  genetic evaluation of, 64–66
  laboratory studies of, 65–66
  management of, 65, 65b
  obstetric history in, 65
  parental consent for evaluation of, 64
  physical examination in, 65
  placental examination in, 65
  sample procurement for study of, 65, 66b
Neonatal intensive care unit stays, multiple gestation and, 727, 727t
Neovagina creation
  nonsurgical, 140
  surgical, 140–141
Nerve stimulation, for chronic pelvic pain, 435
Neural tube defects, 754–761
  alpha-fetoprotein screening for, 758–759
  amniocentesis for, 758–759
  background of, 754–757
  clinical consequences of, 755
  cranial, 754, 755t
  diabetes mellitus and, 841
  diagnosis of, 758–759
  embryology of, 754
  environmental factors in, 756
  ethnicity and, 756
  etiology of, 755–756
  fetal surgery for, 760
  folic acid and, 756–757
  genetics of, 755–756, 756t
  maternal obesity and, 144
  obstetric management of, 759–760
  pathophysiology of, 754–755
  prevention of, 757–758
  race and, 756
  spinal, 754–755, 755t
  two-hit hypothesis of, 760
  ultrasound screening for, 759
Neuraxial analgesia, 153. See also Epidural analgesia
Neurofibromatosis, paternal age and, 5
Newborn screening, 131–133
  American Academy of Pediatrics recommendation for, 132–133
  core panel for, 133

Newborn screening (continued)
  costs of, 132
  emerging technology in, 133
  Guthrie test for, 131–132
  inequities in, state-to-state, 132
  legal mandates for, 132–133
  March of Dimes advocacy of, 133
  for phenylketonuria, 122, 131–133
  sensitivity and specificity of, 132
  storage of blood spots obtained for, 133
Nicotine replacement therapy, 230–232
Niemann-Pick disease type A
  carrier screening for, 178–181, 179t
  clinical features of, 180b
Night sweats, botanicals for, 1008–1009
Nipple(s)
  inverted, and breastfeeding, 276
  sore, breastfeeding and, 284
Nipple stimulation, for contraction stress test, 338
Nitric oxide, in preeclampsia, 446
Nonmaleficence, vii
  in alcohol abuse, 17, 19
  in drug abuse, 17, 19
Nonobstetric surgery, in pregnancy, 137
Nonreassuring fetal heart rate, 577–578
  ancillary tests in, 577
  and cerebral palsy, 574
  fetal stimulation in, 577
  initial assessment of, 577
  persistent, intrauterine resuscitation for, 577–578
Nonreassuring fetal status, as preferred terminology, 94–95
Nonsense mutation, 1029
Nonsteroidal antiinflammatory drugs (NSAIDs)
  for endometriosis, 49–50, 709
  for intrauterine device insertion, 583
  and medical abortion, 700–701
  postoperative use of, 774
  for preterm labor, 675–676
Nonstress test, 339
  acoustic stimulation for, 339
  in biophysical profile, 339–340
  follow-up of, 342, 344
  in intrauterine growth restriction, 596
  nonreactive, 339
  reactive, 339
Nordette, 491t
Norethindrone acetate
  for add-back therapy, with gonadotropin-releasing hormone agonists, 50
  for endometriosis, 434
Norgestrel, emergency use of, 490
Northern blot, 1044
Nortriptyline, for chronic pelvic pain, 432
Notification, partner, of sexually transmitted diseases, 224

NSAIDs. See Nonsteroidal antiinflammatory drugs
Nuchal fold thickness, in Down syndrome, 872
Nuchal translucency screening, 58–60, 870, 872
Nuclear medicine studies, during pregnancy, 73–74
Nucleotide, definition of, 1044
Null hypothesis, 335
Nurse-midwives, certified, practice relationships with, policy statement on, 1068
Nurses, role in pain management, 153
Nutrition
  in complementary and alternative medicine, 38
  enteral, for nausea and vomiting of pregnancy, 748
  and intrauterine growth restriction, 593, 596
  parenteral, for nausea and vomiting of pregnancy, 748
  periodic assessments of
    ages 13–18 years, 191
    ages 19–39 years, 192
    ages 40–64 years, 193
    ages 65 and older, 194
  psychosocial evaluation of, 306–307
Nutritional therapy, for chronic pelvic pain, 436

O
Obesity
  with anovulation, 624–625
  assessment of, 244–245
  bariatric surgery for, 143–144, 245t, 246
    counseling in, 144
    pregnancy complications after, 143
    procedures for, 143–144
  body mass calculations in, 244, 244t
  childhood, maternal smoking and, 229
  conditions associated with, 243
  definition of, 142, 243
  and endometrial cancer, 638
  epidemiology of, 243
  management of, 245–246
  maternal, breastfeeding and, 275
  and ovulatory dysfunction, 657–658
  patient resources on, 247
  pharmacotherapy for, 245–246, 245t
  physician resources on, 247
  in polycystic ovary syndrome, 824, 829–830
  in pregnancy, 142–144
    and cesarean delivery, 143–144
    and fetal risks, 144
    and gestational diabetes, 142–143
    and gestational hypertension, 142–143

Obesity *(continued)*
  in pregnancy *(continued)*
    and intrapartum complications, 143
    and macrosomia, 142–144, 508–509, 511
    and preterm delivery, 144
    recommendations for care in, 144
    and spontaneous abortion, 142
    and surgical complications, 143
  prevalence of, 142
  role of obstetrician–gynecologist in, 243–246
  and shoulder dystocia, 922
  treatment of, guide to selecting, 245t
  and urinary incontinence, 997
  weight loss for, assessing readiness for, 245, 246t
Observational studies, 331–332
Obstetrician–gynecologists
  cooperative practices and hospital privileges of, policy statement on, 1057–1058
  generalist, role in early detection of ovarian cancer, 240–242
  hepatitis virus infections in, 82
  imaging study performance and interpretation by, 163–164
  relationship with anesthesiologists, 152
  relationship with nurse-midwives/midwives, policy statement on, 1068
  relationship with patients
    ethics in, 161–162
    and follow-up, 158
    and health literacy, 158
    information sharing in, 157
    and informed consent, 158
    and medication information, 158
    partnership in, 157–159, 162
    and patient safety, 160–162
  role in breast cancer, 205–206
  role in obesity, 243–246
Occlusion methods, for tubal sterilization, 375–376
Occupational exposures, and recurrent pregnancy loss, 684
Odds ratio, 335, 335t
Ogestrel, 491t
Oils, botanical, 1005, 1005b
Oligohydramnios
  assessment for, 340, 343
  as indication for delivery, 343, 345
  in intrauterine growth restriction, 595, 987
  in postterm pregnancy, 667
  in premature rupture of membranes, 850
Oligomenorrhea
  intrauterine devices and, 586
  ovulatory dysfunction and, 653
  in women older than 40 years, 627

Oligonucleotide primer, 1044
Oligo-ovulation, 654
Oligospermia
  genetic causes of, 1042
  perinatal risks associated with, 166–167
Oliguria, in preeclampsia, 446
Omphalocele, in aneuploidy, 869t
Oncologist, gynecologist, referral to, 241, 637–638
Ondansetron
  for nausea and vomiting of pregnancy, 745, 746f, 747t
  for pruritus, 774
Oophorectomy
  for endometriosis, 713–714
  future, ovary retention and risk of, 907
  incidental, 905
  for premenstrual syndrome, 862
  prophylactic, 905–909
    background of, 905–907
    for breast cancer, 908
    for cancer prevention, 905–909
    candidates for, 907, 907b
    clinical considerations and recommendations in, 907–909
    factors to consider for, 906–907
    genetic factors and, 906–908
    hormone replacement therapy after, 908
    with hysterectomy, operative risk of, 906
    morbidity in, 907
    for ovarian cancer, 906
    risks versus benefits of, 908–909
Open peritoneal lavage, in pregnancy, 300
Operative vaginal delivery, 780–786
  alternative instruments for, after failed attempt, 784
  analgesia and, 771
  background of, 780–781
  clinical considerations and recommendations in, 784–786
  clinical issues in, 781–783
  complications of, 781–783, 783t
  contraindications to, 784
  incidence of, 780–781
  indications for, 780
  long-term infant consequences of, 783
  for macrosomia, 508, 508f, 513, 782
  methods of, 780
  predelivery considerations in, 782b
  trial of, 784
Optical density, and fetal lung maturity test, 270t, 271
Opt-in versus opt-out approach, in human immunodeficiency virus testing, 173, 176

Oral contraception
  after hydatidiform mole, 470
  after malignant gestational trophoblastic disease, 475
  for anovulatory bleeding, 626–627
  antibiotic use with, 942, 942b
  anticonvulsant use with, 941, 942b
  and breast cancer, 940
  during breastfeeding, 281–282, 941
  cerebrovascular risks of, 937–945
  and chronic hypertension, 938–939
  for chronic pelvic pain, 433
  and coexisting medical conditions, 936–945
    background of, 936–937
    clinical considerations and recommendations in, 937–945
  concomitant medications with, 941–942
  contraindications to, 362, 936, 937b
  and diabetes mellitus, 939
  discontinuation, for deep vein thrombosis prophylaxis, 883
  effectiveness of, versus tubal sterilization, 377
  emergency, 489–495, 491t
  for endometrioma, 713
  for endometriosis, 49–51, 433, 709–714
  and fibrocystic breast changes, 940
  for hirsutism, 830
  and hypercoagulable states, 943
  and leiomyoma, 940
  and migraine headache, 939–940
  and ovarian cancer, 906
  for polycystic ovary syndrome, 827–828, 830
  postpartum use of, 941
  for premenstrual syndrome, 862
  preoperative discontinuation of, 943
  and sickle cell disease, 944
  simultaneous use of other method with, 936–937
  smoking and, 938
  and systemic lupus erythematosus, 943
  for women older than 35 years, 937–938
Oral–genital contact, among adolescents
  as "abstinent behavior," 223
  and sexually transmitted disease risk, 222–223
OraQuick Rapid HIV-1 Antibody Test, 174–175
Organic mercury, teratogenicity of, 316t
Organization of Teratogen Information Services, 313
Orlistat, 245–246
Oseltamivir, during pregnancy, 104
Osteoblasts, 789
Osteoclasts, 789
Osteopenia, 788–789, 789t

Osteoporosis, 788–797
  background of, 788–789
  biochemical markers of bone turnover in, 792–793, 793b
  clinical considerations and recommendations in, 791–797
  combination of antiresorptive therapies for, 795
  complementary and alternative medicine for, 796
  definitions of, 788–789, 789t
  drugs associated with, 790, 791b
  estrogen for, 793–794
  ethnicity and, 790
  exercise for, 790, 793
  fractures in
    prevention of, 793–794
    risk factors for, 790, 790b
  heparin-induced, 790, 791b, 884, 962
  lifestyle changes for, 793
  medical conditions associated with, 790, 791b
  pathophysiology of, 789
  prevention of, 793–797, 1010
  progestin for, 793–794
  race and, 790
  risk factors for, 914, 914b
  screening for, 788–789
    alternatives to dual-energy X-ray absorptiometry in, 792–793
    cost-effectiveness of, 789
    indications for, 195t, 791–792
    methods of, 790–791
    peripheral quantitative computed tomography for, 792
    quantitative ultrasonography in, 792
    selective estrogen receptor modulators for, 794–795, 911–912, 914–915
  treatment of, 793–797
    indications for, 796–797
    monitoring of, 796–797
Outlet forceps delivery, 781b
Ovarian cancer
  breastfeeding and, 275
  CA 125 levels in, 240–242
  early detection of, role of generalist obstetrician–gynecologist in, 240–242
  epidemiology of, 240
  genetics of, 242, 906–908, 1042
  hereditary, 242
  misconception as "silent" cancer, 240–241
  oncologist referral for, criteria for, 241
  ovulation induction and, 661, 906
  physical examination in, 241
  poor prognosis in, 240
  in postmenopausal women, 241
  prevention of, oophorectomy for, 905–909

Ovarian cancer (continued)
  risk factors for, 906
  staging of, 241–242
  surgical evaluation for, 241–242
  symptoms of, 240–241
  tubal sterilization and, 379
  ultrasonography in, 242
Ovarian diathermy, for ovulation induction, 659, 829
Ovarian drilling, 829
Ovarian endometrioma, 708, 713
Ovarian failure, premature, 654–655
Ovarian function, uterine artery embolization and, 262–263
Ovarian hyperstimulation, controlled, 656
Ovarian teratoma, 1033
Ovary(ies)
  physiology of, 905–906
  removal of
    for endometriosis, 713–714
    for premenstrual syndrome, 862
    prophylactic, 905–909. See also Oophorectomy, prophylactic
Overweight, definition of, 142, 243, 244t
Ovral, 491t
Ovrette, 491t
Ovulation
  cycle of, 624
  detection of, 653, 657
Ovulation induction, 655–657
  clomiphene citrate for, 627, 655–656, 658–659, 661, 828–829
  dopamine agonists for, 656–657, 659–660
  glucocorticoids for, 659
  gonadotropins for, 656, 660, 828–829
  human chorionic gonadotropin for, 659
  in hyperprolactinemia, 656–657, 659–660
  metformin for, 654, 656, 829
  and multiple gestation, 661
  and ovarian cancer, 661, 906
  ovarian drilling and diathermy for, 659, 829
  in polycystic ovary syndrome, 654, 654b, 656–661, 828–829
  postcoital test in, 661
  in premature ovarian failure, 655
  weight loss and, 657–658
Ovulatory dysfunction
  age-related, 655
  background of, 653–657
  clinical considerations and recommendations in, 657–662
  diagnosis of, 657
  etiology of, 653–654
  in hyperprolactinemia, 624, 654–655
  in hypothalamic amenorrhea, 654–655
  infertility caused by, management of, 653–662
  in luteal phase deficiency, 655
  obesity and, 657–658

Ovulatory dysfunction (continued)
  in polycystic ovary syndrome, 654, 654b
  in premature ovarian failure, 654–655
  treatment of, 655–657
Oxybutynin chloride, for urinary incontinence, 997–998
Oxygen therapy, maternal, for intrauterine growth restriction, 596
Oxytocin
  for active management of labor, 483
  adverse effects of, 566, 567
  breastfeeding and, 275
  for cervical ripening, 563
  for labor augmentation, 480–481
    epidural analgesia and, 771
    fetal monitoring with, 485
    low-dose versus high-dose regimens, 483, 483t
    in twin gestation, 484
    in vaginal birth after cesarean delivery, 1019
  for labor induction, 562–568
    administration of, 567
    complications with, 566–567
    dosage of, 567, 567t
    in fetal demise, 568
Oxytocin antagonists, for preterm labor, 675

P
Pacifiers, and breastfeeding, 283
Paclitaxel, for endometrial cancer, 637
Pain
  abdominal
    cyclic, in müllerian aplasia, 139
    versus nausea and vomiting of pregnancy, 742–743
    in ovarian cancer, 241
  chronic pelvic, 427–437
  definition of, 427
Pain management. See also Analgesia; Anesthesia
  in labor, 153, 765–774
  in medical abortion, 697
  postoperative, optimal agents for, 774
Pancreatitis, and nausea and vomiting of pregnancy, 748
P antibodies, 291t
Pap test. See also Cervical cytology screening
  in adolescents, 29–32, 222
    abnormal results in, management of, 30–31
    need for additional research on, 32
    patient and parent education on, 32
  ethnic disparities in obtaining, 201
  lack of health insurance for, 249
  racial disparities in obtaining, 201
Paraaortic node metastases, in endometrial cancer, 636–637

Paracervical block, 769
Paramethadione, teratogenicity of, 316t
Parasitic infections, perinatal, 810–817
Parathyroid hormone
  for add-back therapy, with gonado-
    tropin-releasing hormone
    agonists, 711
  human recombinant, for osteoporosis,
    795
Parental consent
  for adolescent health research, waiving
    of requirement for, 68–70
  for evaluation of stillbirths and neo-
    natal deaths, 64
Parenteral analgesia, obstetric, 765–766,
    766t
  selection of agent for, 770
  transplacental passage of, 770
Parenteral nutrition, for nausea and vom-
    iting of pregnancy, 748
Parkland method, for tubal sterilization,
    376
Paroxetine, for premenstrual syndrome,
    861–862
Partner consent
  methods of obtaining, 156b
  potential adverse effects of, 155
  reasons for, 155
  recommendations on, 156
  for reproductive health research,
    154–155
  requirement for, inconsistencies in, 155
Partner interference, as barrier to care, 306
Partner notification, of sexually transmitted
    diseases, 224
Partnership with patients, 157–159, 162
Partner violence, 298, 306–307
Parvovirus B19 infection
  clinical considerations and recommen-
    dations in, 814–815
  fetal, diagnosis of, 814
  management of, 814
  maternal, diagnosis of, 814
  mother-to-child transmission of, 811
  perinatal, 811, 814
  transmission of, 811
  work-related exposure of seronegative
    women, 814–815
Paternal age, advanced, 5
Paternal leukocyte immunization, for
    recurrent pregnancy loss, 688
Paternity, and Rh D alloimmunization, 892
Patient choice, in maternal decision
    making, 114–115
Patient-controlled epidural analgesia, 770,
    774
Patient history, in periodic assessments
  ages 13–18 years, 191
  ages 19–39 years, 192
  ages 40–64 years, 193
  ages 65 and older, 194

Patient–physician relationship. See
    Physician–patient relationship
Patient safety, 160–162
  culture of, encouragement of, 160
  objectives for, 160–162
  physician–patient partnership and, 162
  as priority, 162
  system problems in, identification and
    correction of, 161–162
PCOS. See Polycystic ovary syndrome
PCR. See Polymerase chain reaction
Pelvic examination
  in ovarian cancer, 241–242
  in urinary incontinence, 992–993
Pelvic floor exercises, for urinary inconti-
    nence, 994, 997
Pelvic floor injury, operative vaginal
    delivery and, 782
Pelvic floor relaxation, selective estrogen
    receptor modulators and, 913
Pelvic fractures, in pregnancy, 299
Pelvic inflammatory disease (PID)
  antibiotic prophylaxis against,
    350–351, 354
  chronic pelvic pain in, 430
  and ectopic pregnancy, 719
  in homeless women, 77
  intrauterine devices and, 583–584
  tubal sterilization and, 380
Pelvic muscle exercises, for urinary
    incontinence, 994, 997
Pelvic node metastases, in endometrial
    cancer, 635–637
Pelvic organ prolapse, and urinary incon-
    tinence, 993, 995, 999
Pelvic Organ Prolapse Quantification
    System, 993
Pelvic pain
  chronic, 427–437
    acupuncture for, 436
    adhesiolysis for, 435
    analgesics for, 433
    antidepressants for, 432–433
    background of, 427–432
    clinical considerations and recom-
      mendations in, 432–437
    complementary and alternative medi-
      cine for, 436
    counseling for, 435–436
    definition of, 427–428
    diagnostic imaging in, 432
    diagnostic studies of, 431–432
    endometrial ablation for, 434
    in endometriosis, 430, 432–434, 707,
      709–714
    etiology of, 428–430
    exercise for, 434
    gonadotropin-releasing hormone
      agonists for, 433–434
    gynecologic conditions causing or
      exacerbating, 428b

Pelvic pain (continued)
  chronic (continued)
    herbal and nutritional therapy for, 436
    hormonal therapy for, 433–434
    hysterectomy for, 434–435
    in interstitial cystitis, 430, 432
    in irritable bowel syndrome,
      430–431
    laparoscopy in, 432
    magnetic field therapy for, 436
    management of, 432–436
    in musculoskeletal disorders, 431
    nongynecologic conditions causing
      or exacerbating, 429t
    nonmedical treatments of, efficacy
      of, 434
    obstetric history and, 431
    past surgery and, 431
    in pelvic inflammatory disease, 430
    in physical and sexual abuse, 430, 436
    physical therapy for, 434
    populations at increased risk for,
      430–431
    presacral neurectomy for, 435
    prevalence of, 428
    progestins for, 434
    psychotherapy for, 435–436
    sacral nerve stimulation for, 435
    surgical treatment of, 434–435
    trigger points in, local anesthetic
      injection of, 433
    uterine nerve ablation for, 435
  in endometriosis, in adolescents, 46–47
  in ovarian cancer, 241
Pelvic vein thrombosis, diagnosis of, 880
Pelvimetry
  in dystocia management, 482–483
  before operative vaginal delivery, 782b
Penetrance, genetic, 1029–1030, 1044
Penetrating trauma, in pregnancy, 299
Penicillin(s)
  hypersensitivity reactions to, 350, 898
    alternative treatments in, 353–354,
      898
    types of, 353
  for mastitis, 284–285
  pharmacokinetics of, 899
  prophylactic
    for anthrax, 109–110
    for group B streptococcal disease,
      186, 186t
Peptostreptococcus, and preterm labor,
    366–367
Percutaneous umbilical cord blood sam-
    pling
  in isoimmunization, 292, 294
  loss rate with, 292, 294
  in parvovirus B19 infection, 814
Perforation, in hysteroscopy, 1048–1049
Performance improvement, in ultrasono-
    graphy, 985–986

Pergolide, for ovulation induction, 656–657, 660

Perimenopausal women, anovulatory bleeding in, 625–627

Perimenstrual exacerbation, 860

Perimortem cesarean delivery, 301

Perinatal infections, 810–817
  background of, 810–811
  clinical considerations and recommendations in, 812–817

Perinatal mortality
  ethnic disparities in, 200, 200t
  gestational diabetes and, 519
  intrauterine growth restriction and, 593–594, 594t
  maternal smoking and, 228
  in postterm pregnancy, 666–667, 667f
  pregestational diabetes and, 840–841
  racial disparities in, 200, 200t

Periodic assessments, 190–197
  based on age, 190–194
    ages 13–18 years, 191
    ages 19–39 years, 192
    ages 40–64 years, 193
    ages 65 and older, 194
  based on risk factors, 190, 195t–196t

Peripheral bone densitometry, 792

Peritoneal lavage, in pregnancy, 300

Perphenazine, for nausea and vomiting of pregnancy, 747t

Pessaries, for urinary incontinence, 997

PET. See Positron emission tomography

PGE₂. See Prostaglandin E₂

Prostaglandin E₂ (PGE₂)
  administration of, 565
  adverse effects of, 565
  cost-effectiveness of, 568
  in fetal demise, 568
  fetal surveillance with, 566
  for labor induction, 563–568, 668

Pharmacologic therapy, 38. See also specific drugs and disorders

Phencyclidine, contraindicated during breastfeeding, 277t

Phenindione, contraindicated during breastfeeding, 277t

Phenobarbital, for thyroid storm, in pregnancy, 976, 976t

Phenothiazines, for nausea and vomiting of pregnancy, 745, 747t

Phenotype, 1029–1030, 1044

Phenylketonuria
  cause of, 122
  genetics of, 122
  maternal, 122–123
  neonatal screening for, 122, 131–133

Phenytoin
  and intrauterine growth restriction, 593
  oral contraception use with, 941
  teratogenicity of, 316t, 756

Pheochromocytoma, in pregnancy, 420

Phosphatidylcholine (lecithin), 268–269, 270t

Phosphatidylglycerol, 268–269, 270t, 272

Physical abuse, chronic pelvic pain in, 430, 436

Physical examination, in periodic assessments
  ages 13–18 years, 191
  ages 19–39 years, 192
  ages 40–64 years, 193
  ages 65 and older, 194

Physical therapy, for chronic pelvic pain, 434

Physician conduct and practice, ethical code on, vii–ix

Physician–patient relationship
  ethics in, 161–162, vii–viii
  and follow-up, 158
  and health literacy, 158
  information sharing in, 157
  and informed consent, 158
  and medication information, 158
  partnership in, 157–159, 162
  and patient safety, 160–162

Phytoestrogens, 1006

PID. See Pelvic inflammatory disease

Piercings, and sexually transmitted disease risk, 221

Pilot Breast Cancer Prevention Trial, 236

Pioglitazone
  for ovulation induction, 829
  for polycystic ovary syndrome, 826, 829
  pregnancy category of, 828t

Piperacillin, prophylactic, for cesarean delivery, 899–900

Pituitary gland tumor, prolactin-secreting, 655

Placenta
  examination of, 171
  manual removal of, antibiotic prophylaxis for, 901
  pathology of, 171. See also specific types
  storage of, 171
  in stillbirths and neonatal deaths, examination of, 65

Placenta accreta, 169–170
  etiology of, 169
  imaging studies in, 169
  incidence of, 169
  management of, 170
  morbidity and mortality in, 169
  risk factors for, 169

Placental abnormalities
  air travel and, 8
  and intrauterine growth restriction, 592–593

Placental insufficiency, antiphospholipid syndrome and, 357, 360

Placental mosaicism, and intrauterine growth restriction, 592–593

Placental site trophoblastic tumors, 468–469
  histology of, 468
  incidence of, 467

Placenta previa
  and intrauterine growth restriction, 593
  maternal smoking and, 228

Plan B, 490, 491t

Planned Parenthood Federation of America, Inc., 227

Plant-derived hormones, compounded bioidentical, 40–41

Platelet function, 950–951

Platelet transfusion, for thrombocytopenia, in pregnancy, 954, 956–957

PMS. See Premenstrual syndrome

Pneumatic compression, 880–881, 883

Pneumococcal vaccine
  indications for, 196t
  during pregnancy, 87t

Podofilox, for human papillomavirus infection, 554

Poliomyelitis vaccine, during pregnancy, 85t

Polycystic ovary syndrome (PCOS), 823–832
  anovulatory bleeding in, 625
  background of, 823–824
  cardiovascular disease in, 826
  clinical manifestations of, 824
  combination oral contraceptives for, 827–828
  comorbidities, prevention of, 827–828
  definition of, 654, 823–824
  diabetes mellitus in, 824, 826
  diagnostic criteria for, 823–824
  diagnostic evaluation for, 825b
  differential diagnosis of, 824–825, 824b
  etiology of, 824
  hirsutism in, 823–824
    adjuvant cosmetic management of, 831
    treatment of, 830–831
  incidence of, 654, 823–824
  insulin resistance in, 824, 826
  insulin-sensitizing agents for, 827–828
  maintenance therapy for, 827–828
  metformin for, 654, 656, 660–661, 826, 828–829, 831
  morphologic features of, 654
  obesity in, 824, 829–830
  ovulation induction in, 654, 654b, 656–661, 828–829
    clomiphene citrate for, 828–829
    clomiphene–glucocorticoids for, 659, 828
    gonadotropins in, 660, 828–829

Polycystic ovary syndrome *(continued)*
ovulation induction in *(continued)*
human chorionic gonadotropin for, 659
metformin for, 654, 656, 660–661, 829
ovarian drilling and diathermy for, 659, 829
thiazolidinediones for, 829
weight loss for, 657–658
ovulatory dysfunction in, 654
physical examination in, 824
pregnancy categories of drugs used in, 828*t*
pregnancy complications in, 824
progestin for, 827–828
and recurrent pregnancy loss, 683
treatment of, 654
weight loss for, 829–830
Polygenic inheritance, 1034–1035, 1044
Polymenorrhea
definition of, 623–624
ovulatory dysfunction and, 653
Polymerase chain reaction (PCR), 1036, 1037*f*, 1044
in cytomegalovirus infection, 812–813
for deletion analysis, 1037–1038, 1038*f*
in herpes simplex virus infection, 533
in parvovirus B19 infection, 814
in toxoplasmosis, 816
for trinucleotide repeat analysis, 1039, 1039*f*
in varicella zoster virus infection, 815
Polymorphisms, 1029, 1044
Pomeroy tubal sterilization method, 375–376
PORTEC. *See* Postoperative Radiation Therapy in Endometrial Carcinoma
Portia, 491*t*
Positive predictive value, 335
Positron emission tomography (PET), in cervical cancer, 455
Postcoital contraception. *See* Emergency contraception
Postoperative Radiation Therapy in Endometrial Carcinoma (PORTEC), 633, 635–637
Postpartum period
exercise during, 55
immunization during, 84
Postterm pregnancy, 665–669
antenatal fetal surveillance in, 666–667
frequency of, 667
initiation of, 666–667
methods of, 667
background of, 665–666
cervix in, favorable or unfavorable, 667–668
clinical considerations and recommendations in, 666–669

Postterm pregnancy *(continued)*
etiologic factors in, 665
fetal risks in, 666
gestational age assessment in, 666
labor induction versus expectant management in, 667–668
maternal risks in, 666
perinatal mortality in, 667, 667*f*
prevention of, interventions for, 666
prostaglandins in, 668
Rh D alloimmunization prophylaxis in, 894
vaginal birth after cesarean delivery in, 668–669, 1016–1017
Posture, and chronic pelvic pain, 431
Postvoid residual urine volume, 994
Potassium, for diabetic ketoacidosis, in pregnancy, 840*b*
Potassium iodide, for thyroid storm, in pregnancy, 976, 976*t*
Potassium sensitivity test, intravesical, 432
Power (statistical), 335
Practice Bulletins. *See* Practice guidelines
Practice guidelines, 329–335
evidence-based recommendations in, development of, 334
implications for practice, 334
literature analysis for, 330
literature searches for, 330
selection of topics for, 330
study designs for, types of, 330–334
Practice Patterns. *See* Practice guidelines
Practice privileges, policy statement on, 1057–1058
Practice relationships with nurse-midwives/midwives, policy statement on, 1068
Prader-Willi syndrome, 1032–1033, 1040*t*
Preconceptional screening, for Ashkenazi Jews, 178–181, 179*t*, 216–219
Preconception and Prenatal Carrier Screening for Cystic Fibrosis: Clinical and Laboratory Guidelines, 253
Preconception care
core considerations in, 239
importance of, 238–239
Predictive value, 335
Prednisone
for antiphospholipid syndrome, 361–362
for nausea and vomiting of pregnancy, 745
and osteoporosis, 790, 791*b*
for thrombocytopenia, in pregnancy, 954
Preeclampsia, 444–449
analgesia use in, 448, 773
anesthesia use in, 448, 773

Preeclampsia *(continued)*
antiphospholipid syndrome and, 357, 360
background of, 444–446
blood pressure measurement in, 447
versus chronic hypertension, 419, 423
chronic hypertension and, 419–420, 423
clinical considerations and recommendations in, 446–449
definition of, 444–445
delivery mode in, 448
diagnostic criteria for, 445, 445*b*
epidemiology of, 445
fetal changes in, 446
fetal surveillance in, 447
gestational diabetes and, 518–519
and HELLP syndrome, 446
hematologic changes in, 446
hepatic changes in, 446
and intrauterine growth restriction, 592
invasive hemodynamic monitoring in, 448
management of
during labor and delivery, 447–448
optimal, 447
outpatient, 447
maternal obesity and, 142–143
in multiple gestation, 729
neurologic and cerebral manifestations of, 446
pathophysiology of, 445
pregestational diabetes and, 841
prevention of, 449
renal changes in, 446
risk factors for, 445
30-15 rule for, 445
screening for, 446–447
severe
diagnosis of, 445*b*
jaundice in, 321*t*
superimposed, 445
vascular changes in, 446
Pregnancy
air travel during, 7–8
alcohol and drug abuse during
epidemiology of, 15–16
ethical basis for care in, 16–19
ethical responsibilities in, 19–21
fetal effects of, 15
legal sanctions in, 19–20
screening for, 16–17, 18*b*
anticoagulation in, 211–212, 962–963
cervical cancer in, 460–462
cervical cytology screening in, 460, 461*f*, 612
coagulation changes in, 961–962, 962*b*
diagnostic imaging during, 71–74, 981–989
ectopic. *See* Ectopic pregnancy

Pregnancy *(continued)*
exercise during, 53–55
absolute contraindications to, 54*b*
by competitive athlete, 55
and prevention of gestational
diabetes, 53
relative contraindications to, 54*b*
safety of activities for, 54
supine position contraindicated in,
53–54
warning signs for termination of, 54*b*
genital herpes in, management of,
644–650
hemoglobinopathies in, 539–545
in homeless women, 77–78
human papillomavirus infection and,
555–556
hypertension in
chronic, 418–424
essential, evaluation of, 420–421
pregnancy-induced, 7, 142–143, 444,
468–469, 729, 953, 957
immunization during, 84, 85*t*–89*t*,
103–104
isoimmunization in, management of,
290–295
jaundice in, differential diagnosis of,
320, 321*t*
loss of. *See* Pregnancy loss
maternal decision making in, versus
fetal protection, 111–119
molar. *See* Hydatidiform moles
nausea and vomiting of, 741–749
nonobstetric surgery in, 137
obesity in, 142–144
postterm, management of, 665–669
psychosocial risk factors in, screening
and intervention for, 304–308
smoking cessation during, 228–232
thrombocytopenia in, 950–958
thromboembolism in, 961–968
thyroid disease in, 971–978
thyroid function changes in, 972, 972*t*
trauma in, management of, 297–302
unintended, 307–308
definition of, 307
risk factors in, 307–308
Pregnancy-associated plasma protein-A,
in first-trimester screening, 59,
870
Pregnancy-induced hypertension, air travel
contraindicated with, 7
Pregnancy loss
definition of, 682
early, recurrent, 682–689
alloimmune disorders and, 685, 688
antiphospholipid syndrome and, 360,
684–685, 688
autoimmune disorders and, 684–685
background of, 682–683
causes of, 683–686

Pregnancy loss *(continued)*
early, recurrent *(continued)*
chromosomal analysis in, 686
clinical considerations and recommendations in, 686
definition of, 683, 686
diagnosis of, 686
environmental factors in, 684
genetic abnormalities and, 683, 686
hormonal disorders and, 683–684
immunotherapy for, 688–689
infectious causes of, 684, 687–688
intravenous immunoglobulin for, 689
luteal phase deficiency and, 683, 687
metabolic disorders and, 683–684
occupational factors in, 684
paternal lymphocyte immunization
for, 688
personal habits and, 684
thrombophilia and, 684, 688
unexplained, 685–686
uterine anatomic anomalies and, 684,
686–687
uterine evaluation in, 686–687
sporadic, 682–683
Pregnancy Riskline, 313
Premature ovarian failure, 654–655
Premature rupture of membranes (PROM),
848–854
amniocentesis and, 850
background of, 848–850
cervical cerclage and, 413–414, 413*t*
clinical considerations and recommendations in, 850–854
definition of, 848
delivery indications in, 851
diagnosis of, 850
etiology of, 849
fetal lung maturity assessment in, 272
gestational age at, 848
group B streptococcal prophylaxis in,
183–188, 187*f*, 852, 900
in herpes simplex virus infection, 649
initial evaluation of, 851
labor induction in, 567–568, 850–851
latency period in, 849, 852
maternal smoking and, 228
midtrimester, 849–850
fetal complications of, 849–850
maternal complications of, 849
preterm, 849
antenatal corticosteroids for, 852
antepartum fetal surveillance in, 853
antibiotics for, 852, 898–900
with cervical cerclage, management
of, 853
definition of, 848
expectant management of, 851, 853
home management of, 853
tocolytic therapy for, 852
and preterm birth, 673, 674*f*

Premature rupture of membranes (PROM)
(continued)
second-trimester, management of, 853
term, 849, 850
Prematurity, threshold of viability in, perinatal care at, 802–807
Premenstrual exacerbation, 860
Premenstrual syndrome (PMS), 858–863
aerobic exercise for, 861
background of, 858–859
bilateral salpingo-oophorectomy for,
862
clinical considerations and recommendations in, 859–863
definition of, 858
diagnosis of, 859–860
diagnostic criteria for, 859, 859*b*
dietary supplementation for, 861
differential diagnosis of, 860
epidemiology of, 858
etiology of, 859
gonadotropin-releasing hormone agonists for, 862
hormonal suppression for, 862
oral contraceptives for, 862
risk factors for, 858–859
selective serotonin reuptake inhibitors
for, 859, 861–862
symptom diaries in, 859–860
therapy for, 860–863
effectiveness of, 860–862
indications for, 860
supportive, 861
Prenatal care
ethnic disparities in, 201
racial disparities in, 201
for uninsured women, 249
Prenatal diagnosis, 58–60, 867–874. *See
also specific disorders and tests*
Presacral neurectomy, for chronic pelvic
pain, 435
Preterm labor and delivery
air travel and, 7–8
amniocentesis in, 677–678
antenatal corticosteroids for, 676, 732
antibiotics for, 675–677
antiphospholipid syndrome and, 357,
360
assisted reproductive technology and,
165
background of, 673–676
bacterial infections and, 366–367
bacterial vaginosis and, 367–369
biologic markers for, 367–368
clinical considerations and recommendations in, 676–678
contractions without cervical changes
in, 677
definition of, 366, 673
demographic characteristics and, 367
ethnic disparities in, 200, 367

Preterm labor and delivery *(continued)*
external cephalic version and, 501
fetal fibronectin levels and, 367–369, 369t, 676, 731
fetal lung maturation in, 267–272
gestational age and, 674f, 676
incidence of, 673, 674f
interventions in, candidates for, 676
management of, 673–678, 731–732
maternal obesity and, 144
maternal smoking and, 367
in multiple gestation, 677, 727, 730–731
pathophysiology of, 366–367
predicting risk of, 367, 730–731
pregestational diabetes and, 841
premature rupture of membranes and, 673, 674f
prevention of
cervical ultrasonography and, 368–369, 369t
efficacy of treatments for, 677
home uterine activity monitoring and, 367–368, 731
nonpharmacologic methods of, 673
progesterone for, 260–261, 261t
progression of, identifying patients at risk for, 676
racial disparities in, 200, 367
risk factors for, 260, 367
assessment of, 366–370
background of, 366–368
clinical considerations and recommendations in, 368–369
recommendations on, 369–370
salivary estriol and, 367–368
tocolytic therapy for, 675, 675t, 731–732
combination of agents in, 676–677
first-line agent for, 676–677
maintenance, 677
and neonatal outcome, 676
for recurrent symptoms, 677
Prevalence, definition of, 335
Preventive care, periodic assessments in, 190–197
Primary care, periodic assessments in, 190–197
Primrose oil, for premenstrual syndrome, 861
Private antigens, 291t
Prochlorperazine, for nausea and vomiting of pregnancy, 747t
Professional relations, viii–ix
Progenitor cells, from umbilical cord blood, 207
Progesterone
for anovulatory bleeding, 627
compounded bioidentical preparations of, 40–41
in ectopic pregnancy, 721

Progesterone *(continued)*
for luteal phase deficiency, 687
in ovulation testing, 653
for premenstrual syndrome, 862
for preterm birth prevention, 260–261, 261t
Progestin
for add-back therapy, with gonadotropin-releasing hormone agonists, 711
for chronic pelvic pain, 434
for endometrial hyperplasia and cancer, 637–638
for endometriosis, 49–50, 434, 709
for osteoporosis, 793–794, 795
for polycystic ovary syndrome, 827–828
with tamoxifen therapy, 236
Progestin-only oral contraception
during breastfeeding, 281–282, 941
emergency use of, 490
for polycystic ovary syndrome, 827
PROM. *See* Premature rupture of membranes
Prolactin, elevated levels of
ovulation induction with, 656–657, 659–660
in ovulatory dysfunction, 624, 654–657, 659–660
in polycystic ovary syndrome, 825
Promethazine, for nausea and vomiting of pregnancy, 745, 746f, 747t
Propranolol, for thyroid storm, in pregnancy, 976, 976t
Propylthiouracil (PTU)
contraindicated during breastfeeding, 975
for hyperthyroidism, in pregnancy, 974–975
for thyroid storm, in pregnancy, 976, 976t
Prospective cohort study, 331
Prostaglandin(s). *See also* Misoprostol; Prostaglandin E₂
administration of, 565
adverse effects of, 565–566
in anovulatory bleeding, 624
cost-effectiveness of, 568
fetal surveillance with, 566
for labor induction, 101–102, 563–568
in postterm pregnancy, 668
for vaginal birth after cesarean delivery, 99–100, 1018
in preeclampsia, 446
Prosthetic heart valves, enoxaparin contraindicated in pregnant women with, 211–212
Protein C deficiency, 880, 881t
and deep vein thrombosis, 880, 884
and recurrent pregnancy loss, 684, 688
and thromboembolism, in pregnancy, 964–965

Protein S deficiency, 880, 881t
and deep vein thrombosis, 880, 884
and recurrent pregnancy loss, 684, 688
and thromboembolism, in pregnancy, 964–965
Proteinuria
definition of, 445
in preeclampsia, 444–445, 445b
Prothrombin, antibody against, 359
Prothrombin G20210A mutation, 880, 881t
and deep vein thrombosis, 880, 884
and recurrent pregnancy loss, 684, 688
and thromboembolism, in pregnancy, 961, 964–965
Protraction disorders, of labor, 480
Prudent use, of obstetric ultrasonography, 135
Prune belly syndrome, in aneuploidy, 869t
Pruritic urticarial papules and pustules of pregnancy, in multiple gestation, 730
Pruritus
analgesia and, 767, 768t, 774
antibiotics and, 898
Pseudomembranous colitis, antibiotic-induced, 350
Pseudopregnancy, in endometriosis treatment, 49
Psychosocial risk factors
periodic assessments of
ages 13–18 years, 191
ages 19–39 years, 192
ages 40–64 years, 193
ages 65 and older, 194
in pregnancy
barriers to care in, 305–306
in discharge planning, 305
frequent moves, 306
intimate partner violence, 307
nutrition, 306–307
safety, 306
screening and intervention for, 304–308
screening tools for, 304–305, 305b, 310f
stress, 307
substance use, 307
tobacco use, 307
unintended pregnancy, 307–308
Psychotherapy, for chronic pelvic pain, 435–436
PTU. *See* Propylthiouracil
Public antigens, 291t
Pudendal block, 769
Pulmonary embolism, 879–885
in multiple gestation, 729
in pregnancy, diagnosis of, 965–966
prevention of, 880–882
Pulmonary hypoplasia, in premature rupture of membranes, 850

Pulmonary profile, 272
Pulmonary tree development, 268
Pulsatility index (S-D/A), 340
Pulse oximetry, fetal, 56–57, 577
"Pump" twin, 734
P-value, 335
Pyridoxine
    for nausea and vomiting of pregnancy,
        745, 746*f*
    for premenstrual syndrome, 861
Pyrimethamine, for toxoplasmosis, 816

Q

Quadruplet pregnancy, 727, 727*t*. *See also*
    Multiple gestation
Quality control
    in sonohysterography, 1052
    in ultrasonography, 985–986
Quitlines, smoking, 229

R

Rabies immune globulin, during preg-
    nancy, 88*t*
Rabies vaccine, during pregnancy, 86*t*
Racial disparities
    in endometrial cancer, 631–632
    in health care financing, 200–201
    in infant, fetal, and perinatal mortality,
        200, 200*t*
    in intrauterine growth restriction, 592
    in macrosomia, 509
    in osteoporosis, 790
    in preterm delivery, 200, 367
    in women's health, 199–202
        American College of Obstetricians
            and Gynecologists recommen-
            dations on, 201–202
        examples of, 200
        understanding causes of, 200–201
Rad, 72, 72*t*
Radiation exposure
    and carcinogenesis, 72–73
    and cell death, 72
    from computed tomography, 72
    fetal, from common procedures, 72,
        73*b*
    measures of, 72, 72*t*
    teratogenicity of, 72, 317*t*
    from X-rays, during pregnancy, 71–74
Radiation therapy
    for cervical cancer, 456–459, 461–462
    for endometrial cancer, 635–637
Radioactive iodine, contraindicated
    during breastfeeding, 277*t*
    during pregnancy, 73–74, 975
Raloxifene, 911–917
    and bone metabolism, 912
    for breast cancer prevention, 914
    for breast cancer treatment, 914
    cardiovascular effects of, 912
    duration of therapy, 916

Raloxifene *(continued)*
    endometrial and uterine effects of, 913
    genital tract effects of, 913
    indications for, 911–912
    monitoring with, 915
    for osteoporosis prevention, 794–795,
        911–912, 914–916
    physiologic effects of, 912–913
    and thromboembolism, 913
    and vasomotor symptoms, 913, 915
Randomized controlled trials, 330–331
Rape, of homeless women, 77
Rapid human immunodeficiency virus
    testing, 174–175
RBRVS. *See* Resource Based Relative
    Value Scale
Reassuring fetal heart rate, 576
Recombinant DNA, 1044
Recombivax HB, 322
Red blood cells, normal fetal values of,
    293*t*
Red clover, 1006
Reduction, of multiple gestation, 730
Reflex irritability, in Apgar score, 257,
    258*t*
Refusal, informed, 105–106, 116–117
Regional analgesia, obstetric, 766–767
    anticoagulation and, 966–967
    contraindications to, 769, 769*b*
    and maternal mortality, 769
    in preeclampsia, 773
    side effects of, 767, 768*t*
    thrombocytopenia and, 955–956
Reimbursement, third-party
    for analgesia, 153, 766
    for anesthesia, 153, 766
    appealing denial of, steps for, 91*b*
    billing staff's knowledge about, 93
    for complementary and alternative
        medicine, 39, 1005
    for consultations, precertification of, 92
    for diagnostic tests performed at time
        of evaluation and management
        services, 92
    inappropriate practices in, 90–93
    qualifying circumstances for, failure to
        recognize, 91
    for same-day diagnostic and therapeu-
        tic procedures, denial of, 91–92
    for smoking cessation program, 232
Relative odds, 335
Relative risk, 335
Relaxation therapy, for nausea and vomit-
    ing of pregnancy, 749
Relaxin, recombinant human and porcine,
    for cervical ripening, 563
Renal artery stenosis, 420
Reporting, of sexually transmitted diseases,
    224
Reproductive health research, partner con-
    sent for, 154–155

Rescue therapy, with antenatal cortico-
    steroids, 11
Research
    adolescent health
        background of, 67–68
        guidelines for, 67–70
        legal issues in, 68
        parental consent for, waiving of
            requirement for, 68–70
        permission and assent in, 68
        regulations on, 68–69
    reproductive health, partner consent for,
        154–155
Research subject, definition of, 155
Resistance index (S-D/S), 340
Resource Based Relative Value Scale
    (RBRVS), 90
Respect for autonomy, vii
    in alcohol abuse, 18–20
    in drug abuse, 18–20
    in informed refusal, 106
    in maternal decision making, 111–119
Respiration, in Apgar score, 257, 258*t*
Respiratory acidemia, 257
Respiratory distress syndrome, 268
    complications of, 268
    etiology of, 268
    hydatidiform mole evacuation and, 469
    maternal diabetes mellitus and, 271
Rest, in multiple gestation, 731
Restriction endonuclease, 1044
Restriction fragment length polymorphism
    analysis, 1036, 1037*f*, 1044
Restriction of activities, in multiple gesta-
    tion, 731
Restrictive procedures, in obesity surgery,
    143–144
Resuscitation
    intrauterine, for persistent nonreassuring
        fetal heart pattern, 577–578
    for newborns at threshold of viability,
        806–807
Retinal hemorrhage, with vacuum extrac-
    tion, 782–783
Retinoids, teratogenicity of, 316*t*
Retroperitoneal node assessment, in
    endometrial cancer, 635
Retropubic colposuspension, 995, 998
Retrospective cohort study, 331
Reveal test, for human immunodeficiency
    virus, 174
Rh D alloimmunization, 290–292,
    889–894
    antibody titers in, 291–292, 892
    background of, 889–892
    causes of, 890
    clinical considerations and recommen-
        dations in, 892–894
    fetal–maternal hemorrhage screening
        in, 894
    nomenclature in, 889–890

Rh D alloimmunization *(continued)*
  prophylaxis, 890–894
    antenatal administration of, 890
    in antenatal hemorrhage, 893
    antibody screening before, 892
    cost-effectiveness of, 891–892
    discharge without, follow-up in, 893
    duration of effects, 893
    in external cephalic version, 503
    failure of, 891
    in fetal death, 893
    in first-trimester events and procedures, 893
    in hydatidiform mole, 469, 893
    infection transmission via, 891
    in medical abortion, 699
    paternity issues in, 892
    postpartum administration of, 890
    potential shortage of agent for, 891
    recommendations for, 890
    repeat, in postterm pregnancy, 894
    in sensitized pregnancy, 892
    in sterilization procedures, 892
    in threatened abortion, 892
    in trauma, 301, 893
  testing for, 1042
Rifampin, interaction with oral contraception, 942
Rimantadine, during pregnancy, 104
Risedronate, for osteoporosis prevention, 794–795
Risk-based approach, in group B streptococcal prophylaxis, 183–184
Risk factors. *See also specific disorders*
  periodic assessments of, 190, 195t–196t
    ages 13–18 years, 191
    ages 19–39 years, 192
    ages 40–64 years, 193
    ages 65 and older, 194
  psychosocial
    periodic assessment of, 191–194
    in pregnancy, 304–308
Ritodrine, for preterm labor, 675t
RNA, messenger, 1028
RNA polymerase, 1028
Roentgen, 72, 72t
Rooming-in, 279
Ropivacaine, epidural, 767
Rosiglitazone
  for ovulation induction, 829
  for polycystic ovary syndrome, 826, 829
  pregnancy category of, 828t
Rotational midforceps delivery, 785
Rubella titer assessment, indications for, 196t
Rubella vaccine, 210
  during breastfeeding, 210
  interval from receiving until pregnancy, 210
  during postpartum period, 84, 210

Rubella vaccine *(continued)*
  during pregnancy, 85t, 210
  shortage of, 210
Rubella virus infection
  and intrauterine growth restriction, 593
  teratogenicity of, 311, 316t

S
Sabin-Feldman dye test, for toxoplasmosis, 816
Sacral nerve stimulation, for chronic pelvic pain, 435
Safety, patient, 160–162
  culture of, encouragement of, 160
  objectives for, 160–162
  physician–patient partnership and, 162
  as priority, 162
  problems, as barrier to care, 306
  system problems in, identification and correction of, 161–162
Safety restraint use, during pregnancy, 297, 301
St. John's wort, for menopausal symptoms, 1007–1009
Saline infusion, for cervical ripening, 563
Saline infusion sonohysterography, 1050–1052
Salivary estriol, and preterm delivery, 367–368
Salivary testing, of compounded bioidentical hormone levels, 41
Salmon calcitonin, for osteoporosis, 795
Same-day procedures, reimbursement denied for, 91–92
Sandhoff disease, 218
Scalp blood sampling, fetal, 577
Scalp electrode, for fetal heart rate monitoring, 572
Scalp injury, in vacuum extraction, 782
Scalp stimulation, fetal, 577
Scope of practice, vi
Scopolamine, for nausea and vomiting of pregnancy, 747t
Screening. *See also specific disorders*
  maternal serum and nuchal translucency, 59–60
  newborn, 131–133
    American Academy of Pediatrics recommendation for, 132–133
    core panel for, 133
    costs of, 132
    emerging technology in, 133
    Guthrie test for, 131–132
    inequities in, state-to-state, 132
    legal mandates for, 132–133
    March of Dimes advocacy of, 133
    for phenylketonuria, 122, 131–133
    sensitivity and specificity of, 132
    storage of blood spots obtained for, 133

Screening *(continued)*
  nuchal translucency and maternal serum, 59–60
  in periodic assessments
    ages 13–18 years, 191
    ages 19–39 years, 192
    ages 40–64 years, 193
    ages 65 and older, 194
Scuba diving, contraindicated during pregnancy, 54
Searle & Co. drug warning on misoprostol, response to, 101–102
Seasonale, 491t
Seatbelts, in pregnancy, 297, 301
Second-trimester screening, for Down syndrome, 868–869
Second-trimester ultrasonography, 983–985
  imaging parameters for, 983–985
  indications for, 983
SEER. *See* Surveillance, Epidemiology, and End Result
Selection bias, 334
Selective estrogen receptor modulators (SERMs), 911–917
  approved agents, 911
  background of, 911–912
  bisphosphonates with, 915
  and bone metabolism, 912, 914–915
  for breast cancer prevention, 912–917
  for breast cancer treatment, 911
  candidates for, 914
  cardiovascular effects of, 912
  clinical considerations and recommendations for, 913–917
  duration of therapy, 916
  endometrial and uterine effects of, 913, 915–916
  and endometrial cancer, 235–236
  estrogen therapy with, 915
  genital tract effects of, 913
  indications for, 911–912
  for osteoporosis prevention, 794–795, 911–912, 914–915
  and pelvic floor relaxation, 913
  physiologic effects of, 912–913
  thromboembolic effects of, 913
  vasomotor symptoms with, 913, 915
Selective fetal termination, 730
Selective serotonin reuptake inhibitors (SSRIs)
  for chronic pelvic pain, 432–433
  for premenstrual syndrome, 859, 861–862
  side effects of, 862
Semen analysis, 657
Sensitivity
  calculation of, 335t
  definition of, 335

Sepsis, group B streptococcal disease and, 182–183

Septate uterus, and recurrent pregnancy loss, 684, 686–687

Septic abortion, intrauterine devices and, 585–586

SERMs. *See* Selective estrogen receptor modulators

Serotonin, in premenstrual syndrome, 859

Serotonin agonists, for nausea and vomiting of pregnancy, 745, 747*t*

Serotonin reuptake inhibitors
  for chronic pelvic pain, 432–433
  for premenstrual syndrome, 859, 861–862
  side effects of, 862

Sertraline
  for chronic pelvic pain, 432
  for premenstrual syndrome, 861–862

Serum screening, maternal. *See also specific types*
  for chromosome abnormalities, 58–60, 868–870, 873
  combined with nuchal translucency screening, 59–60
  for Down syndrome, 868–870, 873
  maternal age and, 873

Serum Urine and Ultrasound Screening Study, 59

Serving the Family from Birth to the Medical Home (AAP), 132–133

17P therapy, for preterm birth prevention, 260–261

Sevoflurane, 769

Sex chromosome abnormalities, assisted reproductive technology and, 166–167

Sex hormone binding globulin (SHBG), in polycystic ovary syndrome, 824, 827

Sexual abuse, chronic pelvic pain in, 430, 436

Sexual assault victims
  adolescent, sexually transmitted disease risk of, 224
  homeless women, 77

Sexuality
  periodic assessments of
    ages 13–18 years, 191
    ages 19–39 years, 192
    ages 40–64 years, 193
    ages 65 and older, 194
  prophylactic oophorectomy and, 909

Sexuality Information and Education Council of the United States, 227

Sexually transmitted diseases (STDs)
  in adolescents, 220–224
    barriers to care in, 221–222
    costs of, 221–222
    epidemiology of, 220–221
    nonpregnant, 222–223

Sexually transmitted diseases (STDs) *(continued)*
  in adolescents *(continued)*
    pregnant, 223–224
    prevention guidelines for, 222–224
    publications on, 226
    reporting and partner notification of, 224
    risk factors for, 221
    screening guidelines for, 222–224
    treatment of, guidelines for, 224
    victims of sexual assault, 224
    web site resources on, 226–227
  in homeless women, 77
  screening for
    indications for, 196*t*
    before intrauterine device insertion, 584

"Shake" test, of fetal lung maturity, 269, 270*t*

SHBG. *See* Sex hormone binding globulin

Shirodkar procedure, of cervical cerclage, 411

Shoulder dystocia, 921–923
  background of, 921–922
  causes of, 921
  clinical considerations and recommendations in, 922–923
  definition of, 921
  history of, counseling in, 923
  incidence of, 921
  labor abnormalities and, 922
  in macrosomia, 508, 508*f*, 510, 513, 782, 922–923
    cesarean delivery in, 922–923
    labor induction in, 922
  management of, 923
  maternal complications of, 921–922
  McRoberts maneuver for, 921–923
  neonatal complications of, 922
  prediction of, 922
  risk factors for, 922
  Zavanelli maneuver for, 922–923

Sibutramine hydrochloride, 245–246

Sickle cell disease, 539–540
  acute chest syndrome in, 540
  clinical features of, 540
  diagnosis of, 540
  ethnicity and, 540
  genetics of, 1030
  hematologic features of, 543*t*
  newborn screening for, 132–133
  oral contraception in, 944
  painful crises in, 544
  in pregnancy
    air travel contraindicated in, 7
    fetal surveillance in, 544
    management of, 543–544
    transfusion therapy in, 544
  prenatal testing for, 542–543
  screening for, 541–542, 542*f*

Sickle cell trait, 539–540

Single blood spot, for newborn screening, 133

Single-energy X-ray absorptiometry, 792

Single gene disorders, 1029–1030

Single umbilical artery, in aneuploidy, 869*t*

Single-visit approach, in cervical cancer prevention, 1063–1065

Skin examination, indications for, 196*t*

Sleep disorders, menopausal, botanicals for, 1009

Sling procedures, for urinary incontinence, 995, 998–999

Small bowel series, fetal radiation exposure from, 73*b*

Small for gestational age, 592. *See also* Intrauterine growth restriction
  assisted reproductive technology and, 165
  definition of, 592

Smith-Magenis syndrome, 1041*t*

Smoking
  advertisements for, policy statement on, 1069
  and ectopic pregnancy, 719
  and oral contraception use, 938
  and osteoporosis, 793
  during pregnancy
    cessation of, 228–232
      5A's (Ask, Advise, Assess, Assist, and Arrange) in, 229–230, 230*b*
      coding and reimbursement in, 232
      intervention for, 229–230
      pharmacotherapy for, 230–232
      resources for, 231*b*
      support systems for, 232
    consequences of, 228–229, 307
    epidemiology of, 228
    and intrauterine growth restriction, 228, 592–593, 596
    and preterm delivery, 367
    and recurrent pregnancy loss, 684

Societal responsibilities, viii, x

Society of Adolescent Medicine, research guidelines of, 68–69

The Society of Obstetricians and Gynecologists of Canada, 227

Sodium pentothal, 769

Sonohysterography
  antibiotic prophylaxis in, 350–351
  contraindications to, 1051
  documentation of, 1052
  equipment specifications in, 1052
  images in, 1051
  indications for, 1051
  infection control in, 1052
  patient education on, 1052
  patient preparation for, 1051
  physician qualifications and responsibilities in, 1051
  procedure of, 1051

Sonohysterography (continued)
   quality control in, 1052
   saline infusion, 1050–1052
   specifications of examination in, 1051–1052
   of uterine anatomic anomalies, 686
Sore nipples, breastfeeding and, 284
Southern blot analysis, 1035–1036, 1036f, 1044–1045
   for deletion analysis, 1037–1038
   for trinucleotide repeat analysis, 1039, 1039f
Soy
   for heart disease prevention, 1010
   isoflavones from, 1006
   for menopausal symptoms, 1007–1009
   for osteoporosis prevention, 1010
Specificity
   calculation of, 335t
   definition of, 335
Spectral karyotype, 1045
Sperm abnormalities, perinatal risks associated with, 166–167
Sphingomyelin, 269, 270t
Spina bifida, 754–755, 755t. See also Neural tube defects
   clinical consequences of, 755
   obstetric management of, 759–760
Spinal analgesia, 767
   and hematoma, 767, 772, 882, 966–967
   side effects of, 767, 768t
Spinal cord injuries
   ascertainment of labor in, 148
   and autonomic dysreflexia, 148
   complications of, 147–148
   and decubital ulcers, 148
   general support in, 148–149
   obstetric management of, 147–149
   and pulmonary function, 148
   and urinary tract infections, 147–148
Spinal epidural analgesia, 575, 767
Spiral computed tomography
   in pulmonary embolism, 966
   radiation exposure from, 72–73
Spiramycin, for toxoplasmosis, 816
Spironolactone
   for hirsutism, 830
   pregnancy category of, 828t
   for premenstrual syndrome, 862
Splenectomy, for thrombocytopenia, in pregnancy, 954
Sporadic pregnancy loss, 682–683
Squamous cell carcinoma, cervical, treatment of, 459
SSRIs. See Selective serotonin reuptake inhibitors
Stab wounds, 299
Staphylococcus aureus
   antibiotic-resistant, 898
   and mastitis, 284
   and postoperative infection, 349

Staphylococcus epidermidis, and postoperative infection, 349
State child health insurance program (sCHIP), maternal versus fetal care in, 113–114
Statins, pregnancy category of, 828t
Statistical power, 335
STDs. See Sexually transmitted diseases
Stem cells, from umbilical cord blood, 207–208
Stereotactic needle biopsy, of breast mass, 206
Sterilization, 374–381. See also Tubal sterilization; Vasectomy
   background of, 374–376
   clinical considerations and recommendations in, 377–381
Stillbirths
   counseling in, 66
   genetic evaluation of, 64–66
   laboratory studies of, 65–66
   management of, 65, 65b
   maternal obesity and, 144
   obstetric history in, 65
   parental consent for evaluation of, 64
   physical examination of, 65
   placental examination in, 65
   in postterm pregnancy, 666
   premature rupture of membranes and, 849–850
   sample procurement for study of, 65, 66b
Stimulation, fetal, for nonreassuring heart rate, 577
Streptococcal disease, group B
   antibiotic susceptibility testing in, 185b
   culture collection and processing in, 184–186, 185b
   early-onset, in newborns
      factors associated with, 183
      incidence of, 182–183
      prevention of, 182–188
   intrapartum antibiotic prophylaxis against, 183–188, 898–899
      benefit versus risk analysis of, 186
      in cesarean delivery, 187–188
      culture-based approach in, 183–188, 184f, 185b
      hospital compliance with, 184
      in premature rupture of membranes, 183–188, 187f, 852, 900
      recommended regimens for, 186, 186t
      resistance to, 186
      risk-based approach in, 183–184
   invasive, 182–183
   late-onset, in newborns, 182
Streptococcus agalactiae. See Streptococcal disease, group B
Streptococcus pneumoniae, antibiotic-resistant, 898

Streptomycin, teratogenicity of, 316t
Stress
   of medical liability litigation, 42–43
   physical, and preterm delivery, 367
   in pregnancy, 307
   and premenstrual syndrome, 859
Stress incontinence, 991
Stress test, contraction, 338–339
   contraindications to, 339, 342–343
   equivocal–hyperstimulatory, 339
   equivocal–suspicious, 339
   follow-up of, 342
   interpretation of, 338–339
   negative, 338
   positive, 339
   technique of, 338
   unsatisfactory, 339
Stroke, oral contraception and, 937–942
Study designs, 330–334
Subgaleal hematoma, fetal, vacuum extraction and, 783
Substance abuse, 15–23, 307
   adolescent
      special issues in, 21–22
      and sexually transmitted disease risk, 221
   breastfeeding contraindicated in, 276
   brief intervention in, 16, 19
   costs of, 15–16
   epidemiology of, 15–16
   ethical basis for care in, 16–19
      beneficence, 16–17
      justice, 17–18, 20
      nonmaleficence, 17
      respect for autonomy, 18–20
   ethical responsibilities in
      to neonates, 20–21
      to pregnant patients, 19–20
   guidance for physicians in, 22–23
   and intrauterine growth restriction, 592–593
   legal sanctions in, 19–20, 114
   maternal decision making versus fetal protection in, 111–119
   physicians' knowledge gaps about, 16, 19
   screening for
      tools for, 17, 18b
      universal, 16, 19
   treatment referral in, 16, 19–20
Sudden infant death syndrome (SIDS), smoking during pregnancy and, 229
Sulfadiazine, for toxoplasmosis, 816
Sulfonamides, for toxoplasmosis, 816
Sulfonylureas, contraindicated in gestational diabetes, 524
Sulindac, for preterm labor, 675t
Supine position, during exercise, contraindicated during pregnancy, 53–54

Surfactant, 268
  deficiency of, 268
  in fetal lung maturity tests, 269–271,
    270t
Surfactant therapy, 268
Surgery, nonobstetric, in pregnancy, 137.
    See also specific procedures
Surgical assistants, statement on, 234
Surgical errors, reduction of, 161
Surveillance, Epidemiology, and End
    Results (SEER) program, 633
Survival sex, by homeless women, 77
Swedish Two-County breast cancer
    screening trial, 388–389
Symphysis–fundal height, for fetal weight
    estimate, 510
Syphilis
  in adolescents
    during pregnancy, 223–224
    screening for, 222
  biologic false-positive serologic test
    for, antibody in, 359
  and intrauterine growth restriction, 593
  reporting and partner notification of, 224
  teratogenicity of, 316t
Systemic lupus erythematosus, oral con-
    traception in, 943
Systolic to diastolic ratio, 340, 343

T

T-ACE, 17, 18b
Tachycardia, fetal, 573t, 574–575
Tachysystole, uterine
  definition of, 565
  misoprostol and, 101–102, 203–204,
    565–566
Tamoxifen, 911–917
  and bone metabolism, 912, 914–915
  for breast cancer, 235–236, 911, 916
  cardiovascular effects of, 912
  duration of therapy, 916
  endometrial or uterine effects of,
    235–236, 913, 915–916
  genital tract effects of, 913
  indications for, 911
  with misoprostol, for medical abortion,
    695
  for osteoporosis prevention, 794–795
  physiologic effects of, 912–913
  thromboembolic effects of, 913
  and vasomotor symptoms, 913, 915
Tandem mass spectrometry, for newborn
    screening, 133
Tang Kuei, 1007, 1009
Tattoos, and sexually transmitted disease
    risk, 221
Tay-Sachs disease
  carrier screening for, 178–181,
    218–219, 1030, 1042
  clinical features of, 180b
  pathophysiology of, 218

TBG. See Thyroid binding globulin
Tea, botanical, 1005, 1005b
Technetium Tc 99m scan, during preg-
    nancy, 73
Tension-free vaginal tape procedure, 995,
    998–999
Teratogen(s), 311–313, 315t–317t
  agents not documented as, 313, 313b
  counseling regarding, 312–313
  current information on, sources for,
    313, 314b
  factors influencing effect of, 311
  Food and Drug Administration risk
    categories of, 312–313
  and intrauterine growth restriction, 593
  study of, 312
  susceptibility to, individual variation in,
    311
  threshold phenomena of, 311
Teratology, 311–313. See also Teratogen(s)
Teratoma, ovarian, 1033
Terbutaline
  and fetal heart rate, 576t, 577–578
  for preterm labor, 675t
Term gestation, confirmation of, 564,
    564b
Test hypothesis, 335
Testosterone
  in anovulatory bleeding, 625
  teratogenicity of, 315t
Tetanus–diphtheria vaccine, during preg-
    nancy, 88t
Tetanus immune globulin, during preg-
    nancy, 88t
Tetanus prophylaxis, in pregnancy, 300
Tetracycline
  oral contraception use with, 942
  teratogenicity of, 316t
Thalassemia(s), 540–541
  alpha, 540–541, 541t
  beta, 541
  hematologic features of, 543t
  in pregnancy, management of,
    544–545
  prenatal testing for, 542–543
  screening for, 541–542, 542f
Thalidomide, teratogenicity of, 316t
Theca lutein cysts, with hydatidiform
    mole, 469–470
Thermal balloon ablation, 627
Thermal index, in ultrasonography,
    981–982
Thermoregulatory symptoms, in medical
    abortion, 697, 698t
Thiazolidinediones
  for hirsutism, 830–831
  for ovulation induction, 829
  for polycystic ovary syndrome, 826,
    828–831
Thioamides, for hyperthyroidism,
    974–975

Third-party payment
  for analgesia, 153, 766
  for anesthesia, 153, 766
  appealing denial of, steps for, 91b
  billing staff's knowledge about, 93
  for complementary and alternative
    medicine, 39, 1005
  for consultations, precertification of,
    92
  for diagnostic tests performed at time
    of evaluation and management
    services, 92
  inappropriate reimbursement practices
    in, 90–93
  qualifying circumstances for, failure to
    recognize, 91
  for same-day procedures, denial of,
    91–92
  for smoking cessation program, 232
Third-trimester testing, for human
    immunodeficiency virus,
    173–174
Three-dimensional ultrasonography, 982
Threshold of viability
  antenatal corticosteroids at, 806
  cerebral palsy risk factors at, 804–805,
    806t
  gestational age assessment at, 805–806
  mode of delivery and, 806
  morbidity associated with, counseling
    on, 804
  mortality in, counseling on, 803–804,
    804f–805f
  perinatal care at, 802–807
    background of, 802–803
    clinical considerations and recom-
      mendations in, 803–807
    research limitations and, 802–803
    resuscitation and support in, 806–807
Threshold phenomena, of teratogens, 311
Threshold traits, 1034–1035, 1045
Thrombocytopenia
  in antiphospholipid syndrome, 357, 359
  definition of, 951
  and epidural or spinal hematoma, 772,
    955–956
  fetal and neonatal, 951
  gestational, 951, 957
  heparin-induced, 884, 962–963
  in preeclampsia, 446
  in pregnancy, 950–958
    background of, 950–953
    causes of, 951, 951b
    clinical considerations and recom-
      mendations in, 953–958
    differential diagnosis of, 951
    fetal and neonatal intracranial hem-
      orrhage in, 952–953, 955
    idiopathic thrombocytopenic pur-
      pura, 951–955
    with immunologic basis, 951–953

Thrombocytopenia (continued)
in pregnancy (continued)
maternal workup for, 953–954
neonatal alloimmune, 951–952, 956–957
obstetric management of, 956–957
in pregnancy-induced hypertension, 953, 957
and regional anesthesia, 955–956
specialized care in, 954
treatment of, 954
Thromboembolism
emergency contraception and, 943
in multiple gestation, 729–730
oral contraception and, 942–943
postpartum, maternal obesity and, 143
in pregnancy, 961–968
acute, treatment of, 966
air travel and, 8
background of, 961–963
clinical considerations and recommendations in, 963–968
prophylaxis
anticoagulants for, 962–963
candidates for, 963–964
enoxaparin sodium for, 211
heparin for, 962–964, 964b
and regional anesthesia, 966–967
risk of, 962
testing in, 965
thrombophilia and, 964–965
risk levels for, preoperative, 880, 882t
selective estrogen receptor modulators and, 913
Thrombophilia
and recurrent pregnancy loss, 684, 688
and thromboembolism, in pregnancy, 964–965
Thrombosis
antiphospholipid syndrome and, 357, 359, 880, 881t
deep vein. See Deep vein thrombosis
Thromboxane A_2, in preeclampsia, 446
Thyroid antibodies, and recurrent pregnancy loss, 685, 687
Thyroid binding globulin (TBG)
fetal levels of, 972
in pregnancy, 972
Thyroid cancer, in pregnancy, assessment of, 976–977
Thyroid disease
definition in, 971
and nausea and vomiting of pregnancy, 748, 975–976
and osteoporosis, 790
and ovulatory dysfunction, 624–625, 654
in pregnancy, 971–978
background of, 971–974
clinical considerations and recommendations in, 974–978

Thyroid disease (continued)
in pregnancy (continued)
laboratory tests in, 974
medications for, 974–975
screening for, 977–978
and recurrent pregnancy loss, 684–685, 687
Thyroid function
changes in pregnancy, 972, 972t
and fetus, 972
Thyroiditis
and hypothyroidism, 973–974
postpartum
definition of, 971
diagnosis of, 977
treatment of, 977
Thyroid nodule, in pregnancy, assessment of, 976–977
Thyroid-releasing hormone stimulation test, 974
Thyroid-stimulating hormone
in anovulatory bleeding, 625
changes in pregnancy, 972, 972t
fetal levels of, 972
measurement of
indications for, 196t
in pregnancy, 974
in nausea and vomiting of pregnancy, 748, 975–976
in recurrent pregnancy loss, 687
Thyroid storm, in pregnancy, 971
diagnosis of, 976
treatment of, 976, 976b
Thyrotoxicosis, 971. See also Hyperthyroidism
Thyroxine
changes in pregnancy, 972, 972t
fetal levels of, 972
measurement of, 974
in nausea and vomiting of pregnancy, 748, 975–976
Tiagabine, oral contraception use with, 941
Tibolone, for osteoporosis prevention, 794–795, 912
Tinctures, botanical, 1005, 1005b
TNM. See Tumor–node–metastases
Tobacco advertising, policy statement on, 1069
Tobacco use, 307. See also Smoking
Tocolytic therapy
in cervical cerclage, 414
contraindications to, 675t
in external cephalic version, 502
fetal and neonatal side effects of, 675t
maternal side effects of, 675t
in nonreassuring fetal heart rate pattern, 577
for preterm labor, 675, 675t
combination of agents in, 676–677
first-line agent for, 676–677

Tocolytic therapy (continued)
for preterm labor (continued)
maintenance, 677
in multiple gestation, 731–732
and neonatal outcome, 676
for recurrent symptoms, 677
for preterm premature rupture of membranes, 852
To Err is Human: Building a Safer Health System, 160
Tolterodine, for urinary incontinence, 997–998
Tone, in Apgar score, 257, 258t
Topiramate, oral contraception use with, 941
Toremifene, 911–917
endometrial and uterine effects of, 913
indications for, 911
physiologic effects of, 912–913
and vasomotor symptoms, 913
Toxoid vaccines, during pregnancy, 88t
Toxoplasma gondii, 812. See also Toxoplasmosis
Toxoplasmosis
clinical considerations and recommendations in, 816
congenital, 812
fetal, diagnosis of, 816
and intrauterine growth restriction, 593
management of, 816
maternal, diagnosis of, 816
mother-to-child transmission of, 812
newborn screening for, 132
perinatal, 812, 816
and recurrent pregnancy loss, 684
screening for, during pregnancy, 816
teratogenicity of, 317t
Trabecular bone, 789
Traditional Chinese medicine, 37
Training, for imaging studies, 163
Transabdominal cervicoisthmic cerclage, 411, 414
Transcervical approach, in tubal sterilization, 375
Transcription, genetic, 1028, 1045
Transfusion
blood
hepatitis B transmission via, 319
intrauterine fetal, in isoimmunization, 294
in sickle cell disease, in pregnancy, 544
platelet, for thrombocytopenia, in pregnancy, 954, 956–957
Transient ischemic attacks, antiphospholipid syndrome and, 359
Translation, genetic, 1028
Transplantation, umbilical cord blood storage for, 207–208
Transportation, as barrier to care, 306

Transvaginal approach, in tubal sterilization, 375
Transverse vaginal septum, versus vaginal
agenesis, 139
Trauma, in pregnancy, 297–302
blunt abdominal, 298–299
causes of, 298
epidemiology of, 297
fetal assessment in, 300–301
fetal–maternal hemorrhage in, 301
fetal mortality in, 298
incidence of, 297–298
management of, 299–301
maternal mortality in, 298
penetrating, 299
perimortem cesarean delivery in, 301
Rh D alloimmunization in, 301, 893
types of, 298–299
Travel, air, during pregnancy, 7–8
Trichloroacetic acid, for human papillomavirus infection, 554
Tricyclic antidepressants, for chronic
pelvic pain, 432–433
Triest (triestrogen), 40
Triiodothyronine
fetal levels of, 972
in pregnancy, 972, 972t
Tri-Levlen, 491t
Trimethadione
and intrauterine growth restriction,
593
teratogenicity of, 316t
Trimethobenzamide, for nausea and vomiting of pregnancy, 745, 746f,
747t
Trinucleotide repeat analysis, 1039,
1039f, 1045
Triphasil, 491t
Triplet pregnancy. *See also* Multiple gestation
assisted reproductive technology and,
728
morbidity and mortality in, 727, 727t
Triplet repeat expansion, 1031–1032,
1044
Triploidy, 1033
Trisomy, 1031
Trisomy 18
choroid plexus cyst in, 873
first-trimester screening for, 58–60
prenatal diagnosis of, 869
Trisomy 21. *See* Down syndrome
Trivora, 491t
Troglitazone
hepatotoxicity of, 828
for hirsutism, 830–831
for ovulation induction, 829
for polycystic ovary syndrome, 826,
828–831
Trypanosomiasis, and intrauterine growth
restriction, 593

T score, in bone mineral density testing,
788–789, 789t, 792, 796–797,
914
Tubal ligation, 376
Tubal pregnancy. *See* Ectopic pregnancy
Tubal sterilization, 374–376
with cesarean delivery, 252, 377
clinical considerations and recommendations in, 377–381
coding for, 252
complications of, 377
counseling in, 380, 380b
and ectopic pregnancy, 378
effectiveness of
versus intrauterine device, 377–378
versus other contraceptive methods,
377–378
versus vasectomy, 378–379
and hysterectomy, 379
liability in, 252
and menstrual cycle, 375, 379
methods of, 375–376
chemical, 376
mechanical, 376
occlusion, 375–376
noncontraceptive benefits of, 379–380
postabortion, 374–375, 377
postpartum, 374–375
prevalence of, 374
regret over, 380
safety of, 377
versus intrauterine device, 378
versus vasectomy, 378–379
timing of, 374–375
transcervical approaches in, 375
transvaginal approach in, 375
Tuberculosis
breastfeeding contraindicated in, 276
skin test for, indications for, 196t
Tumor–node–metastases (TNM) staging,
of endometrial cancer, 633, 634t
TWEAK, 17, 18b
Twin pregnancy. *See also* Multiple gestation
acardiac or acephalus twin in, 734
assisted reproductive technology and,
728
hydatidiform mole–fetus, 470–471
labor augmentation in, 484
monochorionic, 728, 730, 733–734, 873
monozygotic, 728
morbidity and mortality in, 727, 727t
second-twin delivery in, 733
vaginal birth after cesarean delivery in,
1017
Twin–twin transfusion syndrome,
733–734
Two-hour rule, for diagnosing labor
arrest, 480–481
Two-hit hypothesis, of neural tube defects,
760

Two-patient model, of maternal–fetal
dyad, 114
Typhoid vaccine, during pregnancy, 87t

U

U.S. MaternaCare, 250
Uchida method, for tubal sterilization,
376
Ulcers
decubital, spinal cord injury and, 148
gastric, prevention of, misoprostol for,
129–130, 203–204
Ultrasonography
in amniotic fluid assessment, 343, 983,
987
in aneuploidy screening, 869, 869t,
872–873, 986–987
for breast cancer evaluation, 205–206,
390, 392
cervical, 368–369, 369t, 410–411, 730
in cervical insufficiency, 410–411
in chronic pelvic pain, 432
in cytomegalovirus infection, perinatal,
813
in deep vein thrombosis, 880, 965
in ectopic pregnancy, 720–721
in endometriosis, 47, 708
in gestational age assessment, 267–268,
984–985
in gestational diabetes, 524–526
in hydatidiform mole, 467–468, 471
in hysteroscopy (sonohysterography),
1050–1052
in intrauterine growth restriction,
595–596, 987–988, 988t
in macrosomia, 510–511, 989
in medical abortion
for confirmation of complete abortion, 700
pretreatment, 699–700
in neural tube defects, 759
nuchal translucency in, 58–60, 870, 872
in ovarian cancer evaluation, 242
in ovulation testing, 653
in parvovirus B19 infection, perinatal,
814
in placenta accreta, 169
in pregestational diabetes, 842
in pregnancy, 73, 981–989. *See also*
specific applications
background of, 981–986
clinical considerations and recommendations for, 986–989
documentation in, 985
facility accreditation for, 985
for fetal anatomic survey, 982, 982b
fetal effects of, 986
for fetal lung maturity assessment,
267–268, 271
for fetal weight estimate, 510–511,
525–526, 985, 987, 989

Ultrasonography *(continued)*
  in pregnancy *(continued)*
    first-trimester, 983
      imaging parameters in, 983
      indications for, 983
    indications for, 983, 984*b*
    instrumentation for, 981–982
    limited examination, 982
    in nausea and vomiting evaluation, 748
    nonmedical use of, 135–136, 986
    offering of, 986
    optimal gestational age for, 986
    patient education on, 985–986
    performance improvement in, 985–986
    for postterm prevention, 666
    prudent use of, 135
    quality control in, 985–986
    requests for, 986
    safety of, 985–986
    second- and third-trimester, 983–985
      imaging parameters for, 983–985
      indications for, 983
    specialized examination, 983, 986–987
    standard examination, 982, 982*b*
    three-dimensional, 982
    in trauma evaluation, 300–301
    types of examination, 982–985
  in premature rupture of membranes, 850
  in preterm labor and delivery, 676
  quantitative, in osteoporosis, 792
  in toxoplasmosis, perinatal, 816
  in uterine anatomic anomalies, 686
  in varicella zoster virus infection, perinatal, 815
Umbilical artery, single, in aneuploidy, 869*t*
Umbilical artery Doppler velocimetry, 340
  effectiveness of, 343–344
  in intrauterine growth restriction, 343–345, 595, 987–988
Umbilical blood gas parameters, 338
Umbilical cord
  prolapse of
    amniotomy and, 566–567
    premature rupture of membranes and, 849–850
  in stillbirths and neonatal deaths, examination of, 65
Umbilical cord blood
  percutaneous sampling of
    in isoimmunization, 292, 294
    loss rate with, 292, 294
    in parvovirus B19 infection, 814
  storage of
    for-profit companies for, 208
    for potential future transplantation, 207–208
    scientific, legal, and ethical issues in, 207–208

Unborn Victims of Violence Act (2004), 114
Uncontrolled investigational studies, 332
Uni-Gold test, for human immunodeficiency virus, 174
Uninsured, 248–250
  capacity of health care system to serve, 249
  reproductive health and health care of, 249
Unintended pregnancy, 307–308
  definition of, 307
  risk factors in, 307–308
Uniparental disomy, 1033, 1045
Uniparental heterodisomy, 1045
Uniparental isodisomy, 1045
Ureaplasma urealyticum
  and preterm labor, 366–367
  and recurrent pregnancy loss, 687–688
Urethral mobility, measurement of, 993
Urethral pressure profile, 996
Uric acid test, for preeclampsia, 446
Urinary frequency, in ovarian cancer, 241
Urinary incontinence, 991–1000
  age and, 991
  background of, 991–995
  behavioral therapy for, 994, 997
  bulking agents for, 995, 998
  clinical considerations and recommendations in, 996–1000
  cost of, 991
  cystometry in, 994, 996
  cystoscopy in, 996
  cystourethroscopy in, 994
  diagnosis of, 992–994
  differential diagnosis of, 991, 992*b*
  etiology of, 991
  history and voiding diary in, 992
  laboratory tests in, 993
  leak point pressure measurement in, 996
  management of, 994–995
  medical therapy for, 994, 997–998
  medications and, 992, 993*t*
  obesity and, 997
  office evaluation of, 993–994, 996
  pelvic muscle (Kegel) exercises for, 994, 997
  pelvic organ prolapse and, 993, 995, 999
  pessaries and mechanical devices for, 997
  physical examination in, 992–993
  prevalence of, 991
  surgery for, 995
    complications of, 995, 995*t*
    indications for, 998
    procedures in, 995, 998–999
  transient, causes of, 991, 992*b*
  urethral mobility in, 993
  urethral pressure profile in, 996
  urodynamic stress, 991
  urodynamic tests in, 994

Urinary tract infections
  chronic pelvic pain in, 430, 432
  evaluation of, 432
  spinal cord injury and, 147–148
Urine test, for human chorionic gonadotropin, 27
Urodynamic stress incontinence, 991
Urodynamic studies
  antibiotic prophylaxis in, 349*t*, 352–353
  in urinary incontinence, 994
Uroflowmetry, 994
Uterine activity
  and fetal heart rate, 338–339
  minimally effective, definition of, 480
  monitoring of, home, 367–368, 731
Uterine artery embolization, 262–263
  complications of, 262–263
  for leiomyoma, 262–263, 928
  pregnancy outcomes after, 263
Uterine bleeding
  anovulatory. *See* Anovulatory bleeding
  with leiomyoma, 927
  in medical abortion, 697
  noncyclic, differential diagnosis of, 624, 625*b*
Uterine fibroids. *See* Leiomyoma(s)
Uterine fundal height measurement
  in fetal weight estimation, 510
  in intrauterine growth restriction, 594–595
Uterine hyperstimulation
  misoprostol and, 101–102, 203–204, 565–566
  with nonreassuring fetal heart rate pattern, 577–578
  oxytocin and, 566–567
  prostaglandin E$_2$ and, 565
Uterine nerve ablation, 435
Uterine synechiae, 684, 687
Uterus
  anatomic anomalies of, and recurrent pregnancy loss, 684, 686–687
  hypertonic, with nonreassuring fetal heart rate pattern, 577–578
  rupture of
    management of future pregnancies after, 1020
    misoprostol use and, 129–130, 203–204, 566
    myomectomy and, 931
    trauma and, 299
    in vaginal birth after cesarean delivery, 99–100, 1017–1020

V

Vaccine(s). *See also specific types*
  periodic assessments of
    ages 13–18 years, 191
    ages 19–39 years, 192
    ages 40–64 years, 193
    ages 65 and older, 194

Vaccine(s) *(continued)*
during postpartum period, 84
preconceptional, 84
during pregnancy, 84, 85*t*–89*t*,
103–104
Vacuum extraction, 780–786
clinical considerations and recommendations in, 784–786
complications of, 781–783, 783*t*
contraindications to, 784
equipment, 784–785
Food and Drug Administration advisory
and recommendations on, 783
incidence of, 780–781
long-term infant consequences of, 783
for macrosomia, 782
techniques for, 784–785
Vaginal agenesis, 138–141
counseling in, 139–140
diagnosis of, 138–141
etiology of, 138
incidence of, 138
management of, 138–141
neovagina creation in
nonsurgical, 140
surgical, 140–141
reproductive potential in, 139–140
support of "buddies" in, 140
Vaginal atresia, and endometriosis, 707
Vaginal birth after cesarean delivery
(VBAC), 1015–1020
analgesia in, 150–152, 1019
anesthesia in, 150–152, 1019
augmentation of labor for, 1018–1019
background of, 1015–1016
candidates for, 1016–1017
changing concepts in, 1015–1016
clinical considerations and recommendations for, 1016–1020
contraindications to, 1019
cost-effectiveness of, 1018
counseling on, 1019
delivery of fetus in, 1019–1020
external cephalic version for, 1019
induction of labor for, 99–100, 1018
intrapartum management in, 1019
in macrosomia, 1016
management of labor in, 1019–1020
midtrimester, 1018–1019
more than one previous cesarean
delivery and, 1016
in obese patients, 143
in postterm pregnancy, 668–669,
1016–1017
previous low-vertical incision and, 1017
risks and benefits of, 1017–1018
success rate for, 1017
supportive evidence for, 1016
in twin gestation, 1017
unknown uterine scar type and, 1017
uterine rupture in, 99–100, 1017–1020

Vaginal delivery
in breech presentation, 127–128
in cervical cancer, 461
in herpes simplex virus infection, 649
indications for, 780–781, 781*b*
macrosomia and, 508, 508*f*, 513
for neural tube defects, 760
operative, 780–786
alternative instruments for, after
failed attempt, 784
analgesia and, 771
background of, 780–781
clinical considerations and recommendations in, 784–786
clinical issues in, 781–783
complications of, 781–783, 783*t*
contraindications to, 784
incidence of, 780–781
indications for, 780
long-term infant consequences of,
783
for macrosomia, 508, 508*f*, 513, 782
methods of, 780
predelivery considerations in, 782*b*
trial of, 784
pelvic fracture and, 299
in preeclampsia, 448
spinal cord injury and, 148
Vaginal discharge, selective estrogen
receptor modulators and, 913
Vaginal dryness, botanicals for,
1008–1010
Vaginal hysterectomy
antibiotic prophylaxis in, 349*t*, 350
for endometrial cancer, 637
laparoscopically assisted, 13–14
Vaginal pH
in premature rupture of membranes,
850
selective estrogen receptor modulators
and, 913
Vaginal prolapse, and urinary incontinence,
993, 995, 999
Vaginal tape procedure, for urinary incontinence, 995, 998–999
Vaginosis, bacterial
intrauterine devices and, 584
and postoperative infection, 348–349
and preterm delivery, 367–369
and recurrent pregnancy loss, 687–688
Valacyclovir, for herpes simplex virus
infection, 534, 535*t*, 648, 648*t*
Valerian root, for menopausal symptoms,
1008–1009
Valproic acid
oral contraception use with, 941
teratogenicity of, 316*t*
Vancomycin, prophylactic
for bacterial endocarditis, 353*t*
for group B streptococcal disease,
186*t*

Varicella zoster immune globulin
neonatal use of, 815
during pregnancy, 89*t*, 815
Varicella zoster vaccine, 815
indications for, 196*t*
during pregnancy, 86*t*
Varicella zoster virus infection
breastfeeding precautions in, 276–277
clinical considerations and recommendations in, 815
congenital or neonatal, 812
fetal, diagnosis of, 815
and intrauterine growth restriction, 593
management of, 815
maternal, diagnosis of, 815
perinatal, 811–812, 815
prevention of, 815
screening for, 815
teratogenicity of, 317*t*
Vasectomy, 376
complications of, 376
effectiveness of, versus tubal sterilization, 378–379
failure rates of, 376
late sequelae of, 376
prevalence of, 374, 376
recommendations on, 381
safety of, versus tubal sterilization,
378–379
Vasomotor symptoms
botanicals for, 1007–1009
estrogen therapy for, 915
selective estrogen receptor modulators
and, 913, 915
Vasopressin, in leiomyoma surgery, 930
Vasospasm, in preeclampsia, 446
VBAC. *See* Vaginal birth after cesarean
delivery
Vecchietti procedure, 141
Velocardiofacial syndrome, 1031, 1041*t*
Ventilation–perfusion scanning, 965
Veracity, vii
Vertical banded gastroplasty, 143–144
Vertical transmission
of cytomegalovirus infection, 811
of genital herpes, 645–646, 649–650
of group B streptococcal disease, prevention of, 182–188
of hepatitis B, 319
of hepatitis C, 319
of hepatitis D, 320
of hepatitis E, 320
of hepatitis G, 320
of human immunodeficiency virus, prevention of, 172, 174
scheduled cesarean delivery and,
213–215
zidovudine for, 172, 213–214
of human papillomavirus, 550,
555–556
of parvovirus B19 infection, 811

Vertical transmission (*continued*)
of toxoplasmosis, 812
of varicella zoster virus infection, 812
Vibroacoustic stimulation, fetal, 577
Vigabatrin, oral contraception use with, 941
Violence, against homeless women, 77
Viral infections, perinatal, 810–817
Vitamin A, teratogenicity of, 316t
Vitamin B₁, for chronic pelvic pain, 436
Vitamin B₆ (pyridoxine)
for nausea and vomiting of pregnancy, 745, 746f
for premenstrual syndrome, 861
Vitamin D supplementation
for breastfed infants, 286
for osteoporosis prevention, 795
Vitamin E
for preeclampsia prevention, 449
for premenstrual syndrome, 861
Vitex, for menopausal symptoms, 1008, 1010
Voiding diary, 992
Vomiting
emergency contraception and, 491, 493
medical abortion and, 697, 698t
of pregnancy, 741–749
clinical considerations and recommendations in, 744–749
definition of, 741–742
diagnosis of, 748
differential diagnosis of, 742–743, 742b
enteral nutrition for, 748
etiology of, 743–744
as evolutionary adaptation, 743
fetal effects of, 744
hormones and, 743
hospitalization for, indications for, 742, 748
incidence of, 741–742
laboratory assessment of, 748
maternal effects of, 744
nonpharmacologic therapies for, 744–745
parenteral nutrition for, 748
pharmacologic therapies for, 745–748, 746f, 747t
psychologic theories of, 743
psychotherapy for, 749
radiologic assessment of, 748
risk factors for, 743–744
thyroid disease and, 748, 975–976
timing of, 742

von Willebrand's disease, anovulatory bleeding in, 625
Vulva-to-vulva sex, sexually transmitted disease transmission via, 222

W

Waist circumference, 244
Walking, and course of labor, 482
Warfarin
in intrapartum and postpartum period, 966
intrauterine growth restriction with, 593
oral contraception use with, 943
during pregnancy, 963
Warts, genital. *See* Human papillomavirus infection
Weaning, 286
Weight. *See also* Birth weight; Macrosomia; Obesity
fetal, estimation of
accuracy of, 510–511
in gestational diabetes, 525–526
Hadlock's formula for, 511
Leopold's maneuvers for, 510–511
maternal, 510–511
symphysis–fundal height in, 510
ultrasonography for, 510–511, 525–526, 985, 987, 989
normal, definition of, 142
Weight-bearing exercise, and bone loss, 790, 793
Weight gain, prenatal
recommendations on, 143
spinal cord injury and, 148–149
Weight loss
for obesity, 245–246, 246t
in ovarian cancer, 241
for ovulatory dysfunction, 657–658
for polycystic ovary syndrome, 829–830
Wernicke's encephalopathy, nausea and vomiting of pregnancy and, 744
Western blot assay, 1045
for herpes simplex virus, 534
for human immunodeficiency virus, 173
WHO. *See* World Health Organization
Wild yam, for menopausal symptoms, 1008, 1010
Williams syndrome, 1041t
Wilm's tumor, 1040t
Women's Health Initiative, 793–794, 997

Working mothers, breastfeeding by, 285
World Health Organization (WHO)
endometrial hyperplasia classification of, 632, 632b
gestational trophoblastic disease prognostic index score of, 472
osteopenia and osteoporosis definitions of, 788–789, 789t
Wound complications, postcesarean delivery, in obese patients, 143
Wrist pressure or stimulation, for nausea and vomiting of pregnancy, 745

X

Xg antibodies, 291t
X-inactivation, 1045
X-linked diseases, 5, 1030, 1045
X-ray(s)
during pregnancy
and carcinogenesis, 72–73
and cell death, 72
contrast agent use in, 74
fetal exposure from common procedures, 72, 73b
guidelines for, 71–74
teratogenicity of, 72
radiation exposure in, measures of, 72, 72t

Y

Yam, for menopausal symptoms, 1008, 1010
Y chromosome abnormalities
assisted reproductive technology and, 166–167
testing for, 1042
Yellow fever vaccine, during pregnancy, 85t
Yuzpe regimen, and thromboembolism, 943

Z

Zanamivir, during pregnancy, 104
Zavanelli maneuver, 922–923
Zidovudine
and fetal heart rate, 576t
for prevention of mother-to-child human immunodeficiency virus transmission, 172, 213–214
Zinc supplementation, for intrauterine growth restriction, 596
Z score, in bone mineral density testing, 788–789